MW01628665

A COMPENDIUM OF NEUROPSYCHOLOGICAL TESTS

A COMPENDIUM OF NEUROPSYCHOLOGICAL TESTS

Fundamentals of Neuropsychological Assessment and Test Reviews for Clinical Practice

FOURTH EDITION

Elisabeth M. S. Sherman, Jing Ee Tan, and Marianne Hrabok

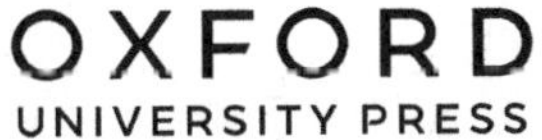

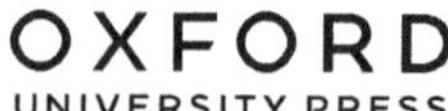

Oxford University Press is a department of the University of Oxford. It furthers the University's objective of excellence in research, scholarship, and education by publishing worldwide. Oxford is a registered trade mark of Oxford University Press in the UK and certain other countries.

Published in the United States of America by Oxford University Press
198 Madison Avenue, New York, NY 10016, United States of America.

© Oxford University Press 2022

All rights reserved. No part of this publication may be reproduced, stored in a retrieval system, or transmitted, in any form or by any means, without the prior permission in writing of Oxford University Press, or as expressly permitted by law, by license, or under terms agreed with the appropriate reproduction rights organization. Inquiries concerning reproduction outside the scope of the above should be sent to the Rights Department, Oxford University Press, at the address above.

You must not circulate this work in any other form
and you must impose this same condition on any acquirer.

CIP data is on file at the Library of Congress
ISBN 978–0–19–985618–3

This material is not intended to be, and should not be considered, a substitute for medical or other professional advice. Treatment for the conditions described in this material is highly dependent on the individual circumstances. And, while this material is designed to offer accurate information with respect to the subject matter covered and to be current as of the time it was written, research and knowledge about medical and health issues is constantly evolving and dose schedules for medications are being revised continually, with new side effects recognized and accounted for regularly. Readers must therefore always check the product information and clinical procedures with the most up-to-date published product information and data sheets provided by the manufacturers and the most recent codes of conduct and safety regulation. The publisher and the authors make no representations or warranties to readers, express or implied, as to the accuracy or completeness of this material. Without limiting the foregoing, the publisher and the authors make no representations or warranties as to the accuracy or efficacy of the drug dosages mentioned in the material. The authors and the publisher do not accept, and expressly disclaim, any responsibility for any liability, loss, or risk that may be claimed or incurred as a consequence of the use and/or application of any of the contents of this material.

Printed by Integrated Books International, United States of America

This book is dedicated to the memory of Dr. Esther Strauss, mentor, role model, and friend. Esther was one of the first female neuropsychologists whom we saw gracefully mix science, scholarship, and family. She was humble and hard-working; she taught us that the most daunting tasks of scholarship don't require innate stores of superlative brilliance or rarified knowledge; they simply require putting one's head down and getting to work. Over the years, we saw her navigate life with warmth, humor, and intelligence, and witnessed her dedication to and love of neuropsychology. She died too soon, in 2009, three years after the last edition of this book was published; her imprint is still there in the words of this book. She is deeply missed.

We also want to acknowledge and remember Dr. Otfried Spreen. Otfried was a pioneer in neuropsychology who helped shape neuropsychology as we know it today through successive generations of students, academics, and clinicians who relied on his writings and scholarly work as roadmaps on how to understand and best practice neuropsychology. The very first edition of this book was a compilation of tests used at the University of Victoria Neuropsychology Laboratory at a time where few commercial tests existed and neuropsychologists relied on researchers for normative data. We hope that the current edition lives up to Otfried's initial vision of a useful compilation of tests for practicing clinicians.

CONTENTS

PREFACE

KNOW YOUR TOOLS

How well do you know your tools? Although most of us have a fairly good grasp of the main advantages and limitations of the tests we use, if we dig below the surface, we see that this knowledge can at times be quite shallow. For example, how many neuropsychologists know the test-retest reliability coefficients for all the tests in their battery or can describe the sensitivity and specificity of their tests? This is not because the information is lacking (although this is also at times a problem), and it isn't because the information is difficult to find. Indeed, most of the information one could ever want on neuropsychological tests can be found on the office shelves of practicing neuropsychologists, in the test manuals of the tests we most frequently use. The rest can be easily obtained via literature searches or online. A working knowledge of neuropsychological tests is hampered by the most common of modern-day afflictions: lack of time, too many priorities, and, for want of a better term, information overload.

Understanding the tests we use requires enough time to read test manuals and to regularly survey the research literature for pertinent information as it arises. However, there are simply too many manuals and too many studies for the average neuropsychologist to stay up to date on the strengths and weaknesses of every test used. The reality is that many tests have lengthy manuals several hundred pages long, and some tests are associated with literally hundreds, even thousands, of research studies. The longer the neuropsychological battery, the higher the stack of manuals and the more voluminous the research. A thorough understanding of every test's psychometric properties and research base, in addition to expert competency in administration, scoring, and interpretation, requires hours and hours of time, which for most practicing neuropsychologists is simply not feasible.

Our own experience bears this out. As is always the case prior to launching a revision of the *Compendium*, there was a large number of tests to review since the previous edition, and this was compounded by the release of several major test batteries and complex scales such as the Wechsler Adult Intelligence Scale, Fourth Edition (WAIS-IV), Wechsler Memory Scale, Fourth Edition (WMS-IV), Advanced Clinical Solutions (ACS), and Minnesota Multiphasic Personality Test-2 Restructured Form (MMPI-2-RF) since the previous edition. As an example, the ACS has an online manual that is almost 400 pages long, in addition to an administration and scoring manual of more than 150 pages; the MMPI-2-RF has multiple test manuals and entire books dedicated to its use. In parallel, since the previous edition of this book, there was an exponential increase in the number of research studies involving neuropsychological tests. As authors and practicing clinicians, we were elated at the amount of new scholarship on neuropsychological assessment, yet dismayed as our offices became stacked with paperwork and our virtual libraries and online cloud storage repeatedly reached maximum storage capacity. The sheer volume of literature that we reviewed for this book was staggering, and completing this book was the most challenging professional task we have encountered. Our wish for this book is that our efforts will have been worth it. At the very least, we hope that the time we spent on this book will save the readers some time of their own.

The essential goal for this book was to create a clinical reference that would provide, in a relatively easy-to-read, searchable format, major highlights of the most commonly used neuropsychological tests in the form of comprehensive, empirically based critical reviews. To do this, we balanced between acting as clinicians and acting as researchers: we were researchers when we reviewed the details of the scientific literature for each test, and we were clinicians when providing commentary on tests, focusing as much on the practicalities of the test as on the scientific literature. As every neuropsychologist knows, there are some exquisitely researched tests that are terrible to use in clinical practice because they are too long, too cumbersome, or too complicated, and this was essential to convey to the readership so that the book could be of practical utility to everyday clinicians like ourselves.

In addition to the core focus on test reviews, the book was also designed to provide an overview of foundational psychometric concepts relevant to neuropsychological practice including overviews of models of test validity and basics of reliability which have been updated since the previous edition. As well, woven throughout the text is a greater emphasis on performance validity and symptom validity in each review, as well as updated criteria for malingered neurocognitive dysfunction. The current edition of this book presents a needed updating based on the past several years of research on malingering and performance validity in neuropsychology.

"Know Your Tools" continues to be the guiding principle behind this edition of the *Compendium of Neuropsychological Tests*. We hope that after reading this book, users will gain a greater understanding of critical issues relevant to the broader practice of neuropsychological assessment, a strong working knowledge of the specific strengths and weaknesses of the tests they use, and, most importantly, an enhanced understanding of clinical neuropsychological assessment grounded in clinical practice and research evidence.

CHANGES COMPARED TO PRIOR EDITIONS

Users will notice several changes from the previous edition. Arguably the biggest change is the exclusive focus on adult tests and norms. Not including pediatric tests and norms had to be done to prevent the book from ballooning into absurd proportions. As some of us have combined adult and pediatric practices, this was a painful albeit necessary decision. Fortunately, pediatric neuropsychological tests are already well covered elsewhere (e.g., Baron, 2018).

Since its first publication in 1991, the *Compendium of Neuropsychological Tests* has been an essential reference text to guide the reader through the maze of literature on tests and to inform clinicians and researchers of the psychometric properties of their instruments so that they can make informed choices and sound interpretations. The goals of the fourth edition of the *Compendium* remain the same, although admittedly, given the continued expansion of the field, our coverage is necessarily selective; in the end, we had to make very hard decisions about which tests to include and which tests to omit. Ultimately, the choice of which tests to include rested on practice surveys indicating the tests most commonly used in the field; we selectively chose those with at least a 10% utilization rate based on surveys. Several surveys were key in making these decisions (Dandachi-FitzGerald, Ponds, & Merten, 2013; LaDuke, Barr, Brodale, & Rabin, 2017; Martin, Schroeder, & Odland, 2015; Rabin, Paolillo, & Barr, 2016; Young, Roper, & Arentsen, 2016). As well, a small number of personal or sentimental favorites made it to the final edition, including some dear to Esther and Otfried. All the reviews were extensively revised and updated, and many new tests were added, in particular a number of new cognitive screening tests for dementia, as well as additional performance and symptom validity tests not covered in the prior edition. We can therefore say fairly confidently that the book does indeed include most of the neuropsychological tests used by most neuropsychologists.

Nevertheless, we acknowledge that some readers may find their favorite test missing from the book. For example, we did not cover computerized concussion assessment batteries or some specialized computerized batteries such as the Cambridge Neuropsychological Test Automated Battery (CANTAB). To our great regret, this was impossible for both practical and logistical reasons. These reasons included but were not limited to a lower rate of usage in the field according to survey data, but also the need to avoid more weekday evenings, early mornings, weekends, and holidays with research papers to review for this book, a regular albeit inconvenient habit in our lives for the last several years. Hopefully the reviews of computerized assessment batteries already in the literature will compensate for this necessary omission; a few did manage to slip into the book as well, such as the review of the CNS Vital Signs (CNS VS).

Because of the massive expansion of research studies on tests, most reviews also had to be expanded. To make room for these longer reviews, some of the general introductory chapters were not carried over from the prior edition, as most of the information is available in other books and resources (e.g., Lezak, Howieson, Bigler, & Tranel, 2012). We retained the chapter on psychometrics and gave validity and reliability their own chapter to better cover changing models in the field. We also retained the chapter on performance validity, symptom validity, and malingering given their critical importance in assessment.

In this edition, we also elected not to include any scales covering the assessment of psychopathology, unless they also functioned as symptom validity scales. Psychopathology scales are not specific to neuropsychological assessment and are reviewed in multiple other sources, including several books. We retained some scales and questionnaires measuring neuropsychological constructs such as executive function, however. Last, for this edition, we included a look-up box at the beginning of each review outlining the main features of each test. We hope that this change will make it easier for readers to locate critical information and to compare characteristics across measures.

ORGANIZATION OF THE BOOK

The first chapter in this volume presents basic psychometric concepts in neuropsychological assessment and provides an overview of critical issues to consider in evaluating tests for clinical use. The second chapter presents new ways of looking at validity and reliability as well as psychometric and practical principles involved in evaluating validity and reliability evidence. (Note the important table in this chapter entitled, "Top 10 Reasons for Not Using Tests," a personal favorite courtesy of Susan Urbina [2014].) Chapter 3 presents an overview of malingering, including updated malingering criteria.

Chapters 4 to 16 address the specific domains of dementia screening, premorbid estimation, intelligence, neuropsychological batteries and related scales, attention, executive functioning, memory, language, visual-spatial skills, sensory function, motor function, performance validity, and symptom validity. Tests are assigned in a rational manner to each of the separate domains—with the implicit understanding that there exists considerable commonality and overlap across tests measuring purportedly discrete domains. This is especially true of tests measuring attention and of those measuring executive functioning.

To promote clarity, each test review follows a fixed format and includes Domain, Age Range, Administration Time, Scoring Format, Reference, Description, Administration, Scoring, Demographic Effects, Normative Data, Evidence for Reliability, Evidence for Validity, Performance/Symptom Validity, and Comment. In each review, we take the bird's-eye view while grounding our impressions in the nitty-gritty of the scientific research; we have also tried to highlight clinical issues relevant to a wide variety of examinees and settings, with emphasis on diversity.

CAUTIONS AND CAVEATS

First, a book of this scope and complexity will unfortunately—and necessarily—contain errors. As well, it is possible that in shining a spotlight on a test's limitations, we have inadvertently omitted or distorted some information supportive of its strengths and assets. For that, we apologize in advance. We encourage readers to inform us of omissions, misinterpretations, typographical errors, and inadvertent scientific or clinical blunders so that we can correct them in the next edition.

Second, while this book presents relevant research on tests, it is not intended as an exhaustive survey of neuropsychological test research, and as such, will not include every relevant or most up-to-date research study for each test profiled. Our aim is to provide a general overview of research studies while retaining mention of some older studies as historical background, particularly for some of the older measures included in the book. The reader is encouraged to use the book as a jumping-off point for more detailed reading and exploration of research relevant to neuropsychological tests.

Third, neuropsychology as a field still has a considerable way to go in terms of addressing inclusivity and diversity, particularly with regard to ethnicity and gender. Many older tests and references have ignored diversity altogether or have used outdated terms or ways of classifying and describing people. As much as possible we have attempted to address this, but our well-meaning efforts will necessarily fall short.

We also want to make it explicit that norms based on ethnicity/race including the ones in this book are not to be interpreted as reflecting physical/biological/genetic differences and that the selection of which norms to use should be a decision based on what is best for the particular patient's clinical situation. We acknowledge the Position Statement on Use of Race as a Factor in Neuropsychological Test Norming and Performance Prediction by the American Academy of Clinical Neuropsychology (AACN), as follows:

> *The field of neuropsychology recognizes that environmental influences play the predominant role in creating racial disparities in test performance. Rather than attributing racial differences in neuropsychological test scores to genetic or biological predispositions, neuropsychology highlights environmental factors to explain group differences including underlying socioeconomic influences; access to nutritional, preventative healthcare, and educational resources; the psychological and medical impact of racism and discrimination; the likelihood of exposure to environmental toxins and pollutants; as well as measurement error due to biased expectations about the performance of historically marginalized groups and enculturation into the groups on which tests were validated. The above is only a partial list of factors leading to differences in performance among so-called racial groups, but none of these factors, including those not enumerated here, is thought to reflect any biological predisposition that is inherent to the group in question. Race, therefore, is often a proxy for factors that are attributable to inequity, injustice, bias, and discrimination. (https://theaacn.org/wp-content/uploads/2021/11/AACN-Position-Statement-on-Race-Norms.pdf)*

ACKNOWLEDGMENTS

We first acknowledge the immense contribution to the field of neuropsychology by Otfried Spreen and Esther Strauss, who first had the idea that neuropsychology needed a compendium for its tests and norms. They created the first *Compendium* in 1991 and were authors for the subsequent editions in 1998, with Elisabeth Sherman joining them as an additional author in the 2006 edition. Both Otfried and Esther sadly passed away after the 2006 edition was published, leaving a large void in the field. We hope that this book does justice to their aim in creating the *Compendium* and that the fourth edition continues their legacy of providing the field of neuropsychology with the essential reference text on neuropsychological tests and testing.

We express our gratitude to the numerous authors whose published work has provided the basis for our reviews and who provided additional information, clarification, and helpful comments. Thank you to Travis White at Psychological Assessment Resources, David Shafer at Pearson, Jamie Whitaker at Houghton Mifflin Harcourt, and Paul Green for graciously providing us with test materials for review, and to all the other test authors and publishers who kindly provided us with materials. We are indebted to them for their generous support.

We also wish to thank those who served as ad hoc reviewers for some test reviews. Special thanks to Glenn Larrabee, Jim Holdnack, and Brian Brooks who provided practical and scholarly feedback on some of the reviews and to Kevin Bianchini and Grant Iverson for some spirited discussions and resultant soul-searching on malingering. Thanks also to Amy Kovacs at Psychological Assessment Resources and Joseph Sandford at BrainTrain for checking some of the reviews for factual errors. An immense debt of gratitude is owed to Shauna Thompson, M.Ed., for her invaluable help at almost every stage of this book and especially for the heavy lifting at the very end that got this book to print.

Finally, we thank our families for their love and understanding during the many hours, days, months, and years it took to write this book. Elisabeth wishes to thank Michael Brenner, who held up the fort while the book went on, and on, and on; she also dedicates this book to her three reasons: Madeleine, Tessa, and Lucas. Special thanks to Tessa in particular for her flawless editing and reference work.

Jing wishes to thank Sheldon Tay, who showered her with love and encouragement through the evenings and weekends she spent writing, and for rearranging his life around her writing schedule.

Marianne extends gratitude to Jagjit, for support, love, dedication, humor, and his "can do" attitude that sustained her during this book; to their children Avani, Saheli, and Jorah, for continuous light and inspiration; to her Mom, who spent many hours of loving, quality time with her grandkids so Marianne could focus on writing; and to her family for support and believing in her always.

REFERENCES

Baron, I. S. (2018). *Neuropsychological evaluation of the child: Domains, methods, and case studies* (2nd ed.). New York: Oxford University Press.

Dandachi-FitzGerald, B., Ponds, R. W. H. M., & Merten, T. (2013). Symptom validity and neuropsychological assessment: A survey of practices and beliefs of neuropsychologists in six European countries. *Archives of Clinical Neuropsychology, 28*(8), 771–783. https://doi.org/10.1093/arclin/act073

LaDuke, C., Barr, W., Brodale, D. L., & Rabin, L. A. (2017). Toward generally accepted forensic assessment practices among clinical neuropsychologists: A survey of professional practice and common test use. *Clinical Neuropsychologist*, 1–20. https://doi.org/10.1080/13854046.2017.1346711

Lezak, M. D., Howieson, D. B., Bigler, E. D., & Tranel, D. (2012). *Neuropsychological assessment* (5th ed.). New York: Oxford University Press.

Martin, P. K., Schroeder, R. W., & Odland, A. P. (2015). Neuropsychologists' validity testing beliefs and practices: A survey of North American professionals. *Clinical Neuropsychologist, 29*(6), 741–776. https://doi.org/10.1080/13854046.2015.1087597

Rabin, L. A., Paolillo, E., & Barr, W. B. (2016). Stability in test-usage practices of clinical neuropsychologists in the United States and Canada over a 10-year period: A follow-up survey of INS and NAN members. *Archives of Clinical Neuropsychology, 31*(3), 206–230. https://doi.org/10.1093/arclin/acw007

Rabin, L., Spadaccini, A., Brodale, D., Charcape, M., & Barr, W. (2014). Utilization rates of computerized tests and test batteries among clinical neuropsychologists in the US and Canada. *Professional Psychology: Research and Practice, 45*, 368–377.

Young, J. C., Roper, B. L., & Arentsen, T. J. (2016). Validity testing and neuropsychology practice in the VA healthcare system: Results from recent practitioner survey. *Clinical Neuropsychologist, 30*(4), 497–514. https://doi.org/10.1080/13854046.2016.1159730

1 | PSYCHOMETRICS IN NEUROPSYCHOLOGICAL ASSESSMENT

DANIEL J. SLICK AND ELISABETH M.S. SHERMAN

OVERVIEW

The process of neuropsychological assessment depends to a large extent on the reliability and validity of neuropsychological tests. Unfortunately, not all neuropsychological tests are created equal, and, like any other product, published tests vary in terms of their "quality," as defined in psychometric terms such as reliability, measurement error, temporal stability, sensitivity, specificity, and predictive validity and with respect to the care with which test items are derived and normative data are obtained. In addition to commercially available tests, numerous tests developed primarily for research purposes have found their way into clinical usage; these vary considerably with regard to psychometric properties. With few exceptions, when tests originate from clinical research contexts, there is often validity data but little else, which makes estimating measurement precision and stability of test scores a challenge.

Regardless of the origins of neuropsychological tests, their competent use in clinical practice demands a good working knowledge of test standards and of the specific psychometric characteristics of each test used. This includes familiarity with the Standards for Educational and Psychological Testing (American Educational Research Association [AERA] et al., 2014) and a working knowledge of basic psychometrics. Texts such as those by Nunnally and Bernstein (1994) and Urbina (2014) outline some of the fundamental psychometric prerequisites for competent selection of tests and interpretation of obtained scores. Other neuropsychologically focused texts such as Mitrushina et al. (2005), Lezak et al. (2012), Baron (2018), and Morgan and Ricker (2018) also provide guidance. This chapter is intended to provide a broad overview of some important psychometric concepts and properties of neuropsychological tests that should be considered when critically evaluating tests for clinical usage.

THE NORMAL CURVE

Within general populations, the frequency distributions of a large number of physical, biological, and psychological attributes approximate a bell-shaped curve, as shown in Figure 1–1. This *normal curve* or *normal distribution*, so named by Karl Pearson, is also known as the *Gaussian* or *Laplace-Gauss distribution*, after the 18th-century mathematicians who first defined it. It should be noted that Pearson later stated that he regretted his choice of "normal" as a descriptor for the normal curve because it had "the disadvantage of leading people to believe that all other distributions of frequency are in one sense or another 'abnormal.' That belief is, of course, not justifiable" (Pearson, 1920, p. 25).

The normal distribution is central to many commonly used statistical and psychometric models and analytic methods (e.g., classical test theory) and is very often the implicitly or explicitly assumed population distribution for psychological constructs and test scores, though this assumption is not always correct.

DEFINITION AND CHARACTERISTICS

The normal distribution has a number of specific properties. It is unimodal, perfectly symmetrical, and asymptotic at the tails. With respect to scores from measures that are normally distributed, the *ordinate*, or height of the curve at any point along the *x* (test score) axis, is the proportion of persons within the sample who obtained a given score. The ordinates for a range of scores (i.e., between two points on the *x* axis) may also be summed to give the proportion of persons who obtained a score within the specified range. If a specified normal curve accurately reflects a population distribution, then ordinate values are also equivalent to the probability of observing a given score or range of scores when randomly sampling from the population. Thus, the normal curve may also be referred to as a *probability distribution*.

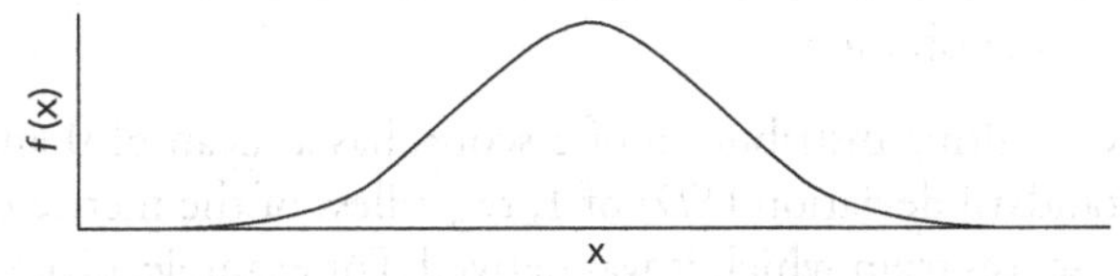

Figure 1–1 The normal curve.

The normal curve is mathematically defined as follows:

$$f(x) = \frac{1}{\sqrt{2\pi\sigma^2}} e - (x - \mu)^2 \quad [1]$$

Where:

x = measurement values (test scores)
μ = the mean of the test score distribution
σ = the standard deviation of the test score distribution
π = the constant *pi* (3.14 ...)
e = the base of natural logarithms (2.71 ...)
$f(x)$ = the height (ordinate) of the curve for any given test score

RELEVANCE FOR ASSESSMENT

As noted previously, because it is a frequency distribution, the area under any given segment of the normal curve indicates the frequency of observations or cases within that interval. From a practical standpoint, this provides psychologists with an estimate of the "normality" or "abnormality" of any given test score or range of scores (i.e., whether it falls in the center of the bell shape, where the majority of scores lie, or instead at either of the tail ends, where few scores can be found).

STANDARDIZED SCORES

An individual examinee's raw score on a test has little value on its own and only takes on clinical meaning by comparing it to the raw scores obtained by other examinees in appropriate normative or *reference samples*. When reference sample data are normally distributed, then raw scores may be *standardized* or converted to a metric that denotes rank relative to the participants comprising the reference sample. To convert raw scores to standardized scores, scores may be linearly transformed or "standardized" in several ways. The simplest standard score is the *z score*, which is obtained by subtracting the sample mean score from an obtained score and dividing the result by the sample standard deviation, as show below:

$$z = (x - X) / SD \quad [2]$$

Where:

x = measurement value (test score)
X = the mean of the test score distribution
SD = the standard deviation of the test score distribution

The resulting distribution of z scores has a mean of 0 and a standard deviation (SD) of 1, regardless of the metric of raw scores from which it was derived. For example, given a mean of 25 and an SD of 5, a raw score of 20 translates into a z score of -1.00. In addition to the z score, linear transformation can be used to produce other standardized scores that have the same properties. The most common of these are T scores (mean [M] = 50, SD = 10) and standardized scores used in most IQ tests ($M = 10$, $SD = 3$, and $M = 100$, $SD = 15$). It must be remembered that z scores, T scores, and all other standardized scores are derived from *samples*; although these are often treated as population values, any limitations of generalizability due to reference sample composition or testing circumstances must be taken into consideration when standardized scores are interpreted.

THE MEANING OF STANDARDIZED TEST SCORES

As well as facilitating translation of raw scores to estimated population ranks, standardization of test scores, by virtue of conversion to a common metric, facilitates comparison of scores across measures—as long as critical assumptions are met, including that raw score distributions of tests being compared are approximately normal. In addition, if standardized scores are to be compared, they should be derived from similar samples or, more ideally, from the same sample. A T score of 50 on a test normed on a population of university students does not have the same meaning as an "equivalent" T score on a test normed on a population of older adults. When comparing standardized scores, one must also take into consideration both the reliability of the two measures and their intercorrelation before determining if a significant difference exists (see Crawford & Garthwaite, 2002). In some cases (e.g., tests with low precision), relatively large disparities between standardized scores may not actually reflect reliable differences and therefore may not be clinically meaningful. Furthermore, statistically significant or reliable differences between test scores may be common in a reference sample; therefore, the base rate of score differences in reference samples must also be considered. One should also keep in mind that when raw test scores are not normally distributed, standardized scores will not accurately reflect actual population rank, and differences between standardized scores will be misleading.

Note also that comparability across tests does not imply equality in meaning and relative importance of scores. For example, one may compare standardized scores on measures of pitch discrimination and intelligence, but it will rarely be the case that these scores are of equal clinical or practical significance.

STANDARDIZED PERCENTILES

The standardized scores just described are useful but also somewhat abstract. In comparison, a more easily understandable and clinically useful metric is the *percentile*, which denotes the percentage of scores that fall at or below a given test score. It is critically important to distinguish between percentile scores that are derived directly from raw untransformed test score distributions and percentile scores that are derived from linear transformations of raw test scores because the two types of percentile scores will only be equivalent when reference sample distributions are normally distributed, and they may diverge quite markedly when reference sample distributions are non-normal. Unfortunately, there is no widely used nomenclature to distinguish between the two types of percentiles, and so it may not always be clear which type is being referred to in test documentation and research publications. To ensure clarity within this chapter, percentile scores derived from linear transformations of raw test scores are always referred to as *standardized percentiles*.

When raw scores have been transformed into standardized scores, the corresponding standardized percentile rank can be easily looked up in tables available in most statistical texts or quickly obtained via online calculators. *Z* score conversions to percentiles are shown in Table 1–1. Note that this method for deriving percentiles should only be used when raw score distributions are normally distributed. When raw score distributions are substantially non-normal, percentiles derived via linear transformation will not accurately correspond to actual percentile ranks within the reference samples from which they were derived.

INTERPRETATION OF STANDARDIZED PERCENTILES

An important property of the normal curve is that the relationship between raw or *z* scores (which for purposes of this discussion are equivalent since they are linear transformations of each other) and percentiles is not linear. That is, a constant difference between raw or *z* scores will be associated with a variable difference in percentile scores as a function of the distance of the two scores from the mean. This is due to the fact that there are proportionally more observations (scores) near the mean than there are farther from the mean; otherwise, the distribution would be rectangular, or non-normal. This can readily be seen in Figure 1–2, which shows the normal distribution with demarcation of *z* scores and corresponding percentile ranges. Because percentiles have a nonlinear relationship with raw scores, they cannot be used for some arithmetic procedures such as calculation of average scores; standardized scores must be used instead.

The nonlinear relation between *z* scores and percentiles has important interpretive implications. For example, a one-point difference between two *z* scores may be interpreted differently depending on where the two scores fall on the normal curve. As can be seen, the difference between a *z* score of 0 and a *z* score of +1.00 is 34 percentile points, because 34% of scores fall between these two *z* scores (i.e., the scores being compared are at the 50th and 84th percentiles). However, the difference between a *z* score of +2.00 and a *z* score of +3.00 is less than three percentile points because only 2.5% of the distribution falls between these two points (i.e., the scores being compared are at the 98th and 99.9th percentiles). On the other hand, interpretation of percentile score differences is also not straightforward in that an equivalent "difference" between two percentile rankings may entail different clinical implications depending on whether the scores occur at the tail end of the curve or if they occur near the middle of the distribution. For example, the 30 percentile point difference between scores at the 1st and 31st percentiles will be more clinically meaningful than the same 30 percentile point difference between scores at the 35th and 65th percentiles.

INTERPRETING EXTREME STANDARDIZED SCORES

A final critical issue with respect to the meaning of standardized scores has to do with extreme observations. In clinical practice, one may encounter standardized scores that are either extremely low or extremely high. The meaning and comparability of such scores will depend critically on the characteristics of the normative samples from which they are derived.

For example, consider a hypothetical case in which an examinee obtains a raw score that is below the range of scores found in a normative sample. Suppose further that the examinee's raw score translates to a *z* score of −5.00, nominally indicating that the probability of encountering this score in the normative sample would be 3 in 10 million (i.e., a percentile ranking of .00003). This represents a considerable extrapolation from the actual normative data, as (1) the normative sample did not include 10 million individuals, and (2) not a single individual in the normative sample obtained a score anywhere close to the examinee's score. The percentile value is therefore an extrapolation and confers a false sense of precision. While one may be confident that it indicates impairment, there may be no basis to assume that it represents a meaningfully "worse" performance than a *z* score of −3.00, or of −4.00.

The *estimated prevalence value* of an obtained standard score can be calculated to determine whether interpretation of extreme scores may be appropriate. This is simply accomplished by inverting the percentile score corresponding to the *z* score (i.e., dividing 1 by the percentile score). For example, a *z* score of −4 is associated with an estimated frequency of occurrence or prevalence of approximately 0.00003. Dividing 1 by this value gives a rounded result of 33,333. Thus, the estimated prevalence value of this score in the population is 1 in 33,333. If the normative sample from which a *z* score is derived is considerably smaller than the denominator of the estimated prevalence value (i.e., 33,333

TABLE 1–1 Score Conversion Table

STANDARD SCORES[a]	T SCORES	SCALED SCORES[b]	PERCENTILES	−Z / +Z	PERCENTILES	SCALED SCORES[b]	T SCORES	STANDARD SCORES[a]
≤55	≤20	≤1	≤0.1	≤3.00≥	≥99.9	≥19	≥80	≥145
56–60	21–23	2	<1	2.67–2.99	>99	18	77–99	140–144
61–67	24–27	3	1	2.20–2.66	99	17	73–76	133–139
68–70	28–30	4	2	1.96–2.19	98	16	70–72	130–132
71–72	31		3	1.82–1.95	97		69	128–129
73–74	32–33		4	1.70–1.81	96		67–68	126–127
75–76	34	5	5	1.60–1.69	95	15	66	124–125
77			6	1.52–1.59	94			123
78	35		7	1.44–1.51	93		65	122
79	36		8	1.38–1.43	92		64	121
80		6	9	1.32–1.37	91	14		120
81	37		10	1.26–1.31	90		63	119
			11	1.21–1.25	89			
82	38		12	1.16–1.20	88		62	118
83			13	1.11–1.15	87			117
84	39		14	1.06–1.10	86		61	116
			15	1.02–1.05	85			
85	40	7	16	.98–1.01	84	13	60	115
			17	.94–.97	83			
86	41		18	.90–.93	82		59	114
87			19	.86–.89	81			113
			20	.83–.85	80			
88	42		21	.79–.82	79		58	112
			22	.76–.78	78			
89			23	.73–.75	77			111
	43		24	.70–.72	76		57	
90		8	25	.66–.69	75	12		110
			26	.63–.65	74			
91	44		27	.60–.62	73		56	109
			28	.57–.59	72			
			29	.54–.56	71			
92			30	.52–.53	70			108
	45		31	.49–.51	69		55	
93			32	.46–.48	68			107
			33	.43–.45	67			
94	46		34	.40–.42	66		54	106
			35	.38–.39	65			
			36	.35–.37	64			
95		9	37	.32–.34	63	11		105
	47		38	.30–.31	62		53	
96			39	.27–.29	61			104
			40	.25–.26	60			
			41	.22–.24	59			
97	48		42	.19–.21	58		52	103
			43	.17–.18	57			
			44	.14–.16	56			
98			45	.12–.13	55			102
	49		46	.09–.11	54		51	
99			47	.07–.08	53			101
			48	.04–.06	52			
			49	.02–.03	51			
100	50	10	50	.00–.01	50	10	50	100

[a] $M = 100$, $SD = 15$.

[b] $M = 10$, $SD = 3$.

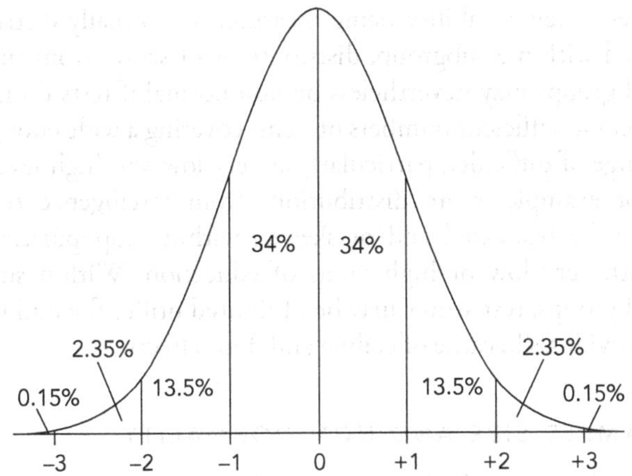

Figure 1–2 The normal curve demarcated by *z* scores.

in the example), then some caution may be warranted in interpreting the percentile. In addition, whenever such extreme scores are being interpreted, examiners should also verify that the examinee's raw score falls within the range of raw scores in the normative sample. If the normative sample size is substantially smaller than the estimated prevalence sample size *and* the examinee's score falls outside the sample range, then standardized scores and associated percentiles should be interpreted with considerable caution. Regardless of the *z* score value, it must also be kept in mind that interpretation of the associated percentile value may not be justifiable if the normative sample has a significantly non-normal distribution. In sum, the clinical interpretation of extreme scores depends to a large extent on how extreme the score is and on the properties of the reference samples involved. One can have more confidence that a percentile is reasonably accurate if (1) the score falls within the range of scores in the reference sample, (2) the reference sample is large and accurately reflects relevant population parameters, and (3) the shape of the reference sample distribution is approximately normal, particularly in tail regions where extreme scores are found.

NON-NORMALITY

Although ideal from a psychometric standpoint, normal distributions appear to be the exception rather than the rule when it comes to normative data for psychological measures, even for very large samples. In a landmark study, Micceri (1989) analyzed 400 reference samples for psychological and education tests, including 30 national tests and 131 regional tests. He found that extremes of asymmetry and multimodality were the norm rather than the exception and so concluded that the "widespread belief in the naïve assumption of normality" of score distributions for psychological tests is not supported by the actual data (p. 156).

The primary factors that lead to non-normal test score distributions have to do with test design, reference sample characteristics, and the constructs being measured. More concretely, these factors include (1) test item sets that do not cover a full range of difficulty resulting in floor/ceiling effects, (2) the existence of distinct unseparated subpopulations within reference samples, and (3) the abilities being measured are not normally distributed in the population.

SKEW

As with the normal curve, some varieties of non-normality may be characterized mathematically. *Skew* is a formal measure of asymmetry in a frequency distribution that can be calculated using a specific formula (see Nunnally & Bernstein, 1994). It is also known as the *third moment of a distribution* (the mean and variance are the first and second moments, respectively). A true normal distribution is perfectly symmetrical about the mean and has a skew of zero. A non-normal but symmetric distribution will also have a skew value that is at or near zero. Negative skew values indicate that the left tail of the distribution is heavier (and often more elongated) than the right tail, which may be truncated, while positive skew values indicate that the opposite pattern is present (see Figure 1–3). When distributions are skewed, the mean and median are not identical; the mean will not be at the midpoint in rank, and *z* scores will not accurately translate into sample percentile rank values. The error in mapping of *z* scores to sample percentile ranks increases as skew increases.

TRUNCATED DISTRIBUTIONS

Significant skew often indicates the presence of a truncated distribution, characterized by restriction in the range of scores on one side of a distribution but not the other, as is the case, for example, with reaction time measures, which cannot be lower than several hundred milliseconds, but can reach very high positive values in some individuals. In fact, distributions of scores from reaction time measures, whether aggregated across trials on an individual level or across individuals, are often characterized by positive skew and positive outliers. Mean values may therefore be positively biased with respect to the "central tendency" of the distribution as defined by other indices, such as the median. Truncated distributions are also commonly seen for error scores. A good example of this is failure to maintain set (FMS) scores on the Wisconsin Card Sorting Test (see

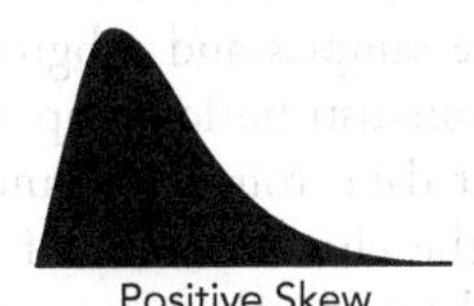
Positive Skew

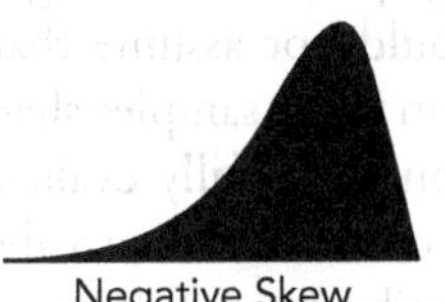
Negative Skew

Figure 1–3 Skewed distributions.

review in this volume). In a normative sample of 30- to 39-year-old persons, observed raw scores range from 0 to 21, but the majority of persons (84%) obtain scores of 0 or 1, and less than 1% obtain scores greater than 3.

FLOOR AND CEILING EFFECTS

Floor and ceiling effects may be defined as the presence of truncated tails in the context of limitations in range of item difficulty. For example, a test may be said to have a *high floor* when a large proportion of the examinees obtain raw scores at or near the lowest possible score. This may indicate that the test lacks a sufficient number and range of easier items. Conversely, a test may be said to have a *low ceiling* when the opposite pattern is present (i.e., when a high number of examinees obtain raw scores at or near the highest possible score). Floor and ceiling effects may significantly limit the usefulness of a measure. For example, a measure with a high floor may not be suitable for use with low functioning examinees, particularly if one wishes to delineate level of impairment.

MULTIMODALITY AND OTHER TYPES OF NON-NORMALITY

Multimodality is the presence of more than one "peak" in a frequency distribution (see the histogram in Figure 1–4 for an example). Pronounced multimodality strongly suggests the presence of two or more distinct subpopulations within a reference sample, and test developers who are confronted with such data should strongly consider evaluating grouping variables (e.g., level of education) that might separate examinees into subgroups that have better shaped score distributions. Another form of non-normality is the *uniform* or *near-uniform distribution* (a distribution with no or minimal peak and relatively equal frequency across all scores), though this type of distribution is rarely seen in psychological data.

SUBGROUPS VERSUS LARGER REFERENCE SAMPLES

Score distributions for a general population and subpopulations may not share the same shape. Scores may be normally distributed within an entire population but not normally distributed within specific subgroups, and the converse may also be true. Scores from general populations and subgroups may even be non-normal in different ways (e.g., positively vs. negatively skewed). Therefore, test users should not assume that reference samples and subgroups from those samples share a common distribution shape but should carefully evaluate relevant data from test manuals or other sources to determine the characteristics of the distributions of any samples or subsamples they may utilize to obtain standardized scores. It should also be noted that even when an ability being measured is normally distributed within a subgroup, distributions of scores from such subgroups may nevertheless be non-normal if tests do not include sufficient numbers of items covering a wide enough range of difficulty, particularly at very low and high levels. For example, score distributions from intelligence tests may be truncated and/or skewed within subpopulations with very low or high levels of education. Within such subgroups, test scores may be of limited utility for ranking individuals because of ceiling and floor effects.

SAMPLE SIZE AND NON-NORMALITY

The degree to which a given distribution approximates the underlying population distribution increases as the number of observations (N) increases and becomes less accurate as N decreases. This has important implications for norms derived from small samples. A larger sample will produce a more normal distribution, but only if the underlying population distribution from which the sample is obtained is normal. In other words, a large N does not "correct" for non-normality of an underlying population distribution. However, small samples may yield non-normal test score distributions due to random sampling errors, even when the construct being measured is normally distributed within the population from which the sample is drawn. That is, one may not automatically assume, given a non-normal distribution in a small sample, that the population distribution is in fact non-normal (note that the converse may also be true).

NON-NORMALITY AS A FUNDAMENTAL CHARACTERISTIC OF CONSTRUCTS BEING MEASURED

Depending on the characteristics of the construct being measured and the purpose for which a test is being designed, a normal distribution of reference sample scores may not be expected or even desirable. In some cases, the population distribution of the construct being measured may not be normally distributed (e.g., reaction time). Alternatively, test developers may want to identify and/or discriminate between persons at only one end of a continuum of abilities. For example, the executive functioning scales reviewed in this volume are designed to detect deficits and not executive functioning strengths; aphasia scales work the same way. These tests focus on the characteristics of only one side of the distribution of the general population (i.e., the lower end), while the characteristics of the other side of the distribution are less of a concern. In such cases, measures may even be deliberately designed to have floor or ceiling effects when administered to a general population. For example, if one is not interested in one tail (or even one-half) of the distribution, items that would provide discrimination in that region may be omitted to save administration time. In this case, a test with a high floor or low ceiling in the general population (and with positive or negative skew) may be more desirable than a test with a normal distribution. Nevertheless, all things being equal, a more normal-looking distribution of scores within the targeted subpopulation is usually desirable, particularly if tests are to be used across the range of abilities (e.g., intelligence tests).

IMPLICATIONS OF NON-NORMALITY

When reference sample distributions are substantially non-normal, any standardized scores derived by linear transformation, such as T scores and standardized percentiles, will not accurately correspond to actual percentile ranks within the reference sample (and, by inference, the reference population). Depending on the degree of non-normality, the degree of divergence between standardized scores and percentiles derived directly from reference sample raw scores can be quite large. For a concrete example of this problem, consider the histogram in Figure 1–4, which shows a hypothetical distribution (n = 1,000) of raw scores from a normative sample for a psychological test. To simplify the example, the raw scores have a mean of 50 and a standard deviation of 10, and therefore no linear transformation is required to obtain T scores. From a glance, it is readily apparent that the distribution of raw scores is grossly non-normal; it is bimodal with a truncated lower tail and significant positive skew, consistent with a significant floor effect and the likely existence of two distinct subpopulations within the normative sample.

A normal curve derived from the sample mean and standard deviation is overlaid on the histogram in Figure 1–4 for purposes of comparing the assumed distribution of raw scores corresponding to T scores with the actual distribution of raw scores. As can be seen, the shapes of the assumed and actual distributions differ quite considerably. Percentile scores derived directly from the raw test scores are also shown for given T scores to further illustrate the degree of error that can be associated with standardized scores derived via linear transformation when reference sample distributions are non-normal. For example, a T score of 40 nominally corresponds to the 16th percentile, but, with respect to the hypothetical test being considered here, a T score of 40 actually corresponds to a level of performance that falls below the 1st percentile within the reference sample. Clearly, the difference between percentiles derived directly from the sample distribution as opposed to standardized percentiles is not trivial and has significant implications for clinical interpretation. Therefore, whenever reference sample distributions diverge substantially from normality, percentile scores derived directly from untransformed raw test scores must be used rather than scaled scores and percentiles derived from linear transformations, and tables with such data should be provided by test publishers as appropriate. Ultimately, regardless of what information test publishers provide, it is always incumbent on clinicians to evaluate the degree to which reference sample distributions depart from normality in order to determine which types of scores should be used.

CORRECTIONS FOR NON-NORMALITY

Although the normal curve is from many standpoints an ideal or even expected distribution for psychological data, reference sample scores do not always conform to a normal distribution. When a new test is constructed, non-normality can be "corrected" by examining the distribution of scores on the prototype test, adjusting test properties, and resampling until a normal distribution is reached. For example, when a test is first administered during a try-out phase and a positively skewed distribution is obtained (i.e.,

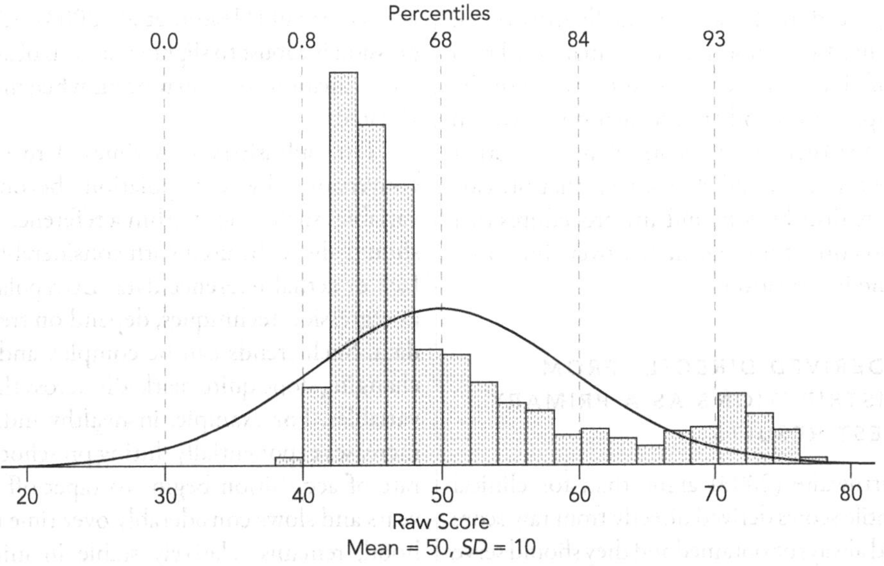

Figure 1–4 A non-normal test score distribution.

with most scores clustering at the tail end of the distribution), the test likely has too high a floor. Easy items can then be added so that the majority of scores fall in the middle of the distribution rather than at the lower end (Urbina, 2014). When this is successful, the greatest numbers of individuals obtain about 50% of items correct. This level of difficulty usually provides the best differentiation between individuals at all ability levels (Urbina, 2014).

When confronted with reference samples that are not normally distributed, some test developers resort to a variety of "normalizing" procedures, such as log transformations on the raw data, before deriving standardized scores. A discussion of these procedures is beyond the scope of this chapter, and interested readers are referred to Urbina (2014). Although they can be useful in some circumstances, normalization procedures are by no means a panacea because they often introduce problems of their own with respect to interpretation. Urbina (2014) states that scores should only be normalized if (1) they come from a large and representative sample, or (2) any deviation from normality arises from defects in the test rather than characteristics of the sample. Furthermore, it is preferable to modify test content and procedures during development (e.g., by adding or modifying items) to obtain a more normal distribution of scores rather than attempting to transform non-normal scores into a normal distribution. Whenever normalization procedures are used, test publishers should describe in detail the nature of any sample non-normality that is being corrected, the correction procedures used, and the degree of success of such procedures (i.e., the distribution of scores after application of normalizing procedures should be thoroughly described). The reasons for correction should also be justified, and percentile conversions derived directly from un-normalized raw scores should also be provided as an option for users. Despite the limitations inherent in methods for correcting for non-normality, Urbina (2014) notes that most test developers will probably continue to use such procedures because normally distributed test scores are required for some statistical analyses. From a practical point of view, test users should be aware of the mathematical computations and transformations involved in deriving scores for their instruments. When all other things are equal, test users should choose tests that provide information on score distributions and any procedures that were undertaken to correct non-normality over those that provide partial or no information.

PERCENTILES DERIVED DIRECTLY FROM RAW SCORE DISTRIBUTIONS AS A PRIMARY METRIC FOR TEST RESULTS

Crawford and Garthwaite (2009) argue that, for clinical assessments, percentile scores derived directly from raw score distributions should always be obtained and they should serve as the primary metric for interpretation and presentation of test results in reports. These researchers state that "percentile ranks express scores in a form that is of greater relevance to the neuropsychologist than any alternative metric because they tell us directly how common or uncommon such scores are in the normative population" (p. 194). They note that when reference sample distributions are normally distributed, standardized scores are also useful, particularly for certain arithmetical and psychometric procedures for which percentiles cannot be used, such as averaging scores. However, raw score percentiles must always be used instead of standardized scores whenever reference samples are non-normal as the latter have minimal meaning in such cases. Crawford, Garthwaite, and Slick (2009) also advance the preceding argument and, in addition, provide a proposed set of reporting standards for percentiles as well as detailed methods for calculating accurate confidence intervals for raw score percentiles—including a link to free software for performing the calculations on Dr. John Crawford's website (https://homepages.abdn.ac.uk/j.crawford/pages/dept/psychom.htm). It is good practice to include confidence intervals when percentiles are presented in reports, particularly in high-stakes assessments where major decisions rely on finite score differences (e.g., determination of intellectual disability for criminal-forensic or disability purposes).

EXTRAPOLATION AND INTERPOLATION

Despite the best efforts of test publishers to obtain optimum reference samples, there are times when such samples fall short with respect to score ranges or cell sizes for subgroups such as age categories. In these cases, test developers may turn to extrapolation and/or interpolation for purposes of obtaining a full range of scaled scores, using techniques such as multiple regression. For example, Heaton and colleagues have published sets of norms that use multiple regression to derive scaled scores that are adjusted for demographic characteristics, including some for which reference sample sizes are very small (Heaton et al., 2003). Although multiple regression is robust to slight violations of assumptions, substantial estimation errors may occur when model assumptions are violated.

Test publishers sometimes derive standardized score conversions by extrapolation beyond the bounds of variables such as age within a reference sample. Such norms should always be used with considerable caution due to the lack of actual reference data. Extrapolation methods, such as regression techniques, depend on trends in the reference data. Such trends can be complex and difficult to model, changing slope quite markedly across the range of predictor variables. For example, in healthy individuals, vocabulary increases exponentially during preschool years, but then the rate of acquisition begins to taper off during early school years and slows considerably over time through early adulthood, remains relatively stable in middle age, and then shows a minor decrease with advancing age. Modeling such complex curves in a way that allows for accurate extrapolation is certainly a challenge, and even a well-fitting model that is extended beyond actual data points provides only an educated guess that may not be accurate.

Interpolation, utilizing the same types of methods as are employed for extrapolation, is sometimes used for deriving standardized scores when there are gaps in reference samples with respect to variables such as age or years of education. When this is done, the same limitations and interpretive cautions apply. Whenever test publishers use extrapolation or interpretation to derive scaled scores, the methods employed should be adequately described, any violations of underlying assumptions of statistical models utilized should be noted, and estimation error metrics should be reported.

MEASUREMENT ERROR

A good working understanding of conceptual issues and methods of quantifying measurement error is essential for competent clinical practice. We start our discussion of this topic with concepts arising from classical test theory.

TRUE SCORES

A central element of classical test theory is the concept of a *true score*, or the score an examinee would obtain on a measure in the absence of any measurement error (Lord & Novick, 1968). True scores can never be known. Instead, they are estimated and are conceptually defined as the mean score an examinee would obtain across an infinite number of equivalent randomly sampled parallel forms of a test, assuming that the examinee's scores were not systematically affected by test exposure, practice, or other time-related factors such as maturation (Lord & Novick, 1968). In contrast to true scores, *obtained scores* are the actual scores yielded by tests. Obtained scores include any measurement error associated with a given test. That is, they are the sum of true scores and error. Note that measurement error in the classical model arises only from test characteristics; measurement error arising from particular characteristics of individual examinees or testing circumstances is not explicitly addressed or accounted for.

In the classical model, the relation between obtained and true scores is expressed in the following formula, where error (e) is random and all variables are assumed to be normally distributed:

$$x = t + e \qquad [3]$$

Where:

x = obtained score
t = true score
e = error

When test reliability is less than perfect, as is always the case, the net effect of measurement error across examinees is to bias obtained scores outward from the population mean. That is, scores that are above the mean are most likely higher than true scores, while those that are below the mean are most likely lower than true scores (Lord & Novick, 1968). *Estimated true scores* correct this bias by regressing obtained scores toward the normative mean, with the amount of regression depending on test reliability and deviation of the obtained score from the mean. The formula for estimated true scores (t') is:

$$t' = X + [r_{xx}(x - X)] \qquad [4]$$

Where:

X = mean test score
r_{xx} = test reliability (internal consistency reliability)
x = obtained score

If working with z scores, the formula is simpler:

$$t' = r_{xx} \times z \qquad [5]$$

Formula 4 shows that an examinee's estimated true score is the sum of the mean score of the group they belong to (i.e., the normative sample) and the deviation of their obtained score from the normative mean weighted by test reliability (as derived from the same normative sample). Furthermore, as test reliability approaches unity (i.e., r = 1.0), estimated true scores approach obtained scores (i.e., there is little measurement error, so estimated true scores and obtained scores are nearly equivalent). Conversely, as test reliability approaches zero (i.e., when a test is extremely unreliable), estimated true scores approach the mean test score. That is, when a test is highly reliable, greater weight is given to obtained scores than to the normative mean score; but, when a test is very unreliable, greater weight is given to the normative mean score than to obtained scores. Practically speaking, estimated true scores will always be closer to the mean than obtained scores (except, of course, where the obtained score is at the mean).

THE USE OF TRUE SCORES IN CLINICAL PRACTICE

Although the true score model is abstract, it has practical utility and important implications for test score interpretation. For example, what may not be immediately obvious from Formulas 4 and 5 is readily apparent in Table 1–2: estimated true scores translate test reliability (or lack thereof) into the same metric as actual test scores.

As can be seen in Table 1–2, the degree of regression to the mean of true scores is inversely related to test reliability and directly related to degree of deviation from the

TABLE 1–2 Estimated True Score Values for Three Observed Scores at Three Levels of Reliability

	RELIABILITY	OBSERVED SCORES (M = 100, SD = 15) 110	120	130
Test 1	.95	110	119	129
Test 2	.80	108	116	124
Test 3	.65	107	113	120

NOTE: Estimated true scores rounded to whole values.

reference mean. This means that the more reliable a test is, the closer obtained scores are to true scores and that the further away the obtained score is from the sample mean, the greater the discrepancy between true and obtained scores. For a highly reliable measure such as Test 1 (r = .95), true score regression is minimal even when an obtained score lies a considerable distance from the sample mean; in this example, a standard score of 130, or two *SD*s above the mean, is associated with an estimated true score of 129. In contrast, for a test with low reliability, such as Test 3 (r = .65), true score regression is quite substantial. For this test, an obtained score of 130 is associated with an estimated true score of 120; in this case, fully one-third of the observed deviation from the mean is "lost" to regression when the estimated true score is calculated.

Such information has important implications with respect to interpretation of test results. For example, as shown in Table 1–2, as a result of differences in reliability, obtained scores of 120 on Test 1 and 130 on Test 3 are associated with essentially equivalent estimated true scores (i.e., 119 and 120, respectively). If only obtained scores are considered, one might interpret scores from Test 1 and Test 3 as significantly different even though these "differences" actually disappear when measurement precision is taken into account. It should also be noted that this issue is not limited to comparisons of scores from the same individual across different tests but also applies to comparisons between scores from different individuals from the same test when the individuals come from different groups and the test in question has different reliability levels across those groups.

Regression to the mean may also manifest as pronounced asymmetry of confidence intervals centered on true scores, relative to obtained scores, as discussed in more detail later. Although calculation of true scores is encouraged as a means of translating reliability coefficients into more concrete and useful values, it is important to consider that any significant difference between characteristics of an examinee and the sample from which a mean sample score and reliability estimate were derived may invalidate the process. For example, it makes little sense to estimate true scores for severely brain-injured individuals on measures of cognition using test parameters from healthy normative samples because mean scores within brain-injured populations are likely to be substantially different from those seen in healthy normative samples; reliabilities may differ substantially as well. Instead, one may be justified in deriving estimated true scores using data from a comparable clinical sample if this is available. These issues underscore the complexities inherent in comparing scores from different tests in different populations.

THE STANDARD ERROR OF MEASUREMENT

Examiners may wish to quantify the margin of error associated with using obtained scores as estimates of true scores. When the reference sample score *SD* and the internal consistency reliability of a test are known, an estimate of the *SD* of obtained scores about true scores may be calculated. This value is known as the *standard error of measurement*, or *SEM* (Lord & Novick, 1968). More simply, the *SEM* provides an estimate of the amount of error in a person's observed score. It is a function of the reliability of the test and of the variability of scores within the sample. The *SEM* is inversely related to the reliability of the test. Thus, the greater the reliability of the test, the smaller the *SEM* is, and the more confidence the examiner can have in the precision of the score.

The *SEM* is defined by the following formula:

$$SEM = SD\sqrt{1-r_{xx}} \qquad [6]$$

Where:

SD = the standard deviation of the test, as derived from an appropriate normative sample

r_{xx} = the reliability coefficient of the test (usually internal reliability)

CONFIDENCE INTERVALS

While the *SEM* can be considered on its own as an index of test precision, it is not necessarily intuitively interpretable, and there is often a tendency to focus excessively on test scores as point estimates at the expense of consideration of associated estimation error ranges. Such a tendency to disregard imprecision is particularly inappropriate when interpreting scores from tests with lower reliability. Clinically, it is therefore very important to report, in a concrete and easily understandable manner, the degree of precision associated with specific test scores. One method of doing this is to use *confidence intervals*.

The *SEM* is used to form a confidence interval (or range of scores) around estimated true scores within which obtained scores are most likely to fall. The distribution of obtained scores about the true score (the error distribution) is assumed to be normal, with a mean of zero and an *SD* equal to the *SEM*; therefore, the bounds of confidence intervals can be set to include any desired range of probabilities by multiplying by the appropriate z value. Thus, if an individual were to take a large number of randomly parallel versions of a test, the resulting obtained scores would fall within an interval of ±1 *SEM* of the estimated true scores 68% of the time and within 1.96 *SEM* 95% of the time (see Table 1–1).

Obviously, confidence intervals for unreliable tests (i.e., with a large *SEM*) will be larger than those for highly reliable tests. For example, we may again use data from Table 1–2. For a highly reliable test such as Test 1, a 95% confidence interval for an obtained score of 110 ranges from 103 to 116. In contrast, the confidence interval for Test 3, a less reliable test, is considerably larger, ranging from 89 to 124.

It is important to bear in mind that confidence intervals for obtained scores that are based on the *SEM* are centered on *estimated true scores* and are based on a model that deals with performance across a large number of randomly parallel forms. Such confidence intervals will be symmetric around obtained scores only when obtained scores are at the test mean or when reliability is perfect. Confidence intervals will be asymmetric about obtained scores to the same degree that true scores diverge from obtained scores. Therefore, when a test is highly reliable, the degree of asymmetry will often be trivial, particularly for obtained scores within one *SD* of the mean. For tests of lesser reliability, the asymmetry may be marked. For example, in Table 1–2, consider the obtained score of 130 on Test 2. The estimated true score in this case is 124 (see Equations 4 and 5). Using Equation 5 and a *z*-multiplier of 1.96, we find that a 95% confidence interval for the obtained scores spans ±13 points, or from 111 to 137. This confidence interval is substantially asymmetric about the obtained score.

It is also important to note that *SEM*-based confidence intervals should not be used for estimating the likelihood of obtaining a given score at retesting with the same measure as effects of prior exposure are not accounted for. In addition, Nunnally and Bernstein (1994) point out that use of *SEM*-based confidence intervals assumes that error distributions are normally distributed and homoscedastic (i.e., equal in spread) across the range of scores obtainable for a given test. However, this assumption may often be violated. A number of alternate error models do not require these assumptions and may thus be more appropriate in some circumstances (see Nunnally & Bernstein, 1994, for a detailed discussion). In addition, there are quite a number of alternate methods for estimating error intervals and adjusting obtained scores for regression to the mean and other sources of measurement error (Glutting et al., 1987). There is no universally agreed upon method for estimating measurement errors, and the most appropriate methods may vary across different types of tests and interpretive uses, though the majority of methods will produce roughly similar results in many cases. In any case, a review of alternate methods for estimating and correcting for measurement error is beyond the scope of this book; the methods presented were chosen because they continue to be widely used and accepted, and they are relatively easy to grasp conceptually and mathematically. Ultimately, the choice of which specific method is used for estimating and correcting for measurement error is far less important than the issue of whether *any* such estimates and corrections are calculated and incorporated into test score interpretation. That is, test scores should never be interpreted in the absence of consideration of measurement error.

THE STANDARD ERROR OF ESTIMATION

In addition to estimating confidence intervals for obtained scores, one may also be interested in estimating confidence intervals for estimated true scores (i.e., the likely range of true scores about the estimated true score). For this purpose, one may construct confidence intervals using the *standard error of estimation* (SE_E; Lord & Novick, 1968). The formula for this is:

$$SE_E = SD\sqrt{r_{xx}(1-r_{xx})} \quad [7]$$

Where:

SD = the standard deviation of the variable being estimated

r_{xx} = the test reliability coefficient

The SE_E, like the *SEM*, is an indication of test precision. As with the *SEM*, confidence intervals are formed around estimated true scores by multiplying the SE_E by a desired z value. That is, one would expect that, over a large number of randomly parallel versions of a test, an individual's true score would fall within an interval of ±1 SE_E of the estimated true scores 68% of the time, and fall within 1.96 SE_E 95% of the time. As with confidence intervals based on the *SEM*, those based on the SE_E will usually not be symmetric around obtained scores. All of the other caveats detailed previously regarding *SEM*-based confidence intervals also apply.

The choice of constructing confidence intervals based on the *SEM* versus the SE_E will depend on whether one is more interested in true scores or obtained scores. That is, while the *SEM* is a gauge of test accuracy in that it is used to determine the expected range of *obtained* scores about true scores over parallel assessments (the range of error in *measurement* of the true score), the SE_E is a gauge of estimation accuracy in that it is used to determine the likely range within which *true* scores fall (the range of error of *estimation* of the true score). Regardless, both *SEM*-based and SE_E-based confidence intervals are symmetric with respect to estimated true scores rather than the obtained scores, and the boundaries of both will be similar for any given level of confidence interval when a test is highly reliable.

THE STANDARD ERROR OF PREDICTION

When the standard deviation of obtained scores for an alternate form is known, one may calculate the likely range of obtained scores expected on retesting with a parallel form. For this purpose, the *standard error of prediction* (SE_P; Lord & Novick, 1968) may be used to construct confidence intervals. The formula for this is:

$$SE_p = SD_y\sqrt{1-r_{xx}^2} \quad [8]$$

Where:

SD_y = the standard deviation of the parallel form administered at retest
r_{xx} = the reliability of the form used at initial testing

In this case, confidence intervals are formed around estimated true scores (derived from initial obtained scores) by multiplying the SE_P by a desired *z* value. That is, one would expect that, when retested over a large number of randomly sampled parallel versions of a test, an individual's obtained score would fall within an interval of ±1 SE_P of the estimated true scores 68% of the time and fall within 1.96 SE_E 95% of the time. As with confidence intervals based on the *SEM*, those based on the SE_P will generally not be symmetric around obtained scores. All of the other caveats detailed previously regarding the *SEM*-based confidence intervals also apply. In addition, while it may be tempting to use SE_P-based confidence intervals for evaluating significance of change at retesting with the same measure, this practice violates the assumptions that a parallel form is used at retest and, particularly, that no prior exposure effects apply.

STANDARD ERRORS AND TRUE SCORES: PRACTICAL ISSUES

Nunnally and Bernstein (1994) note that most test manuals do "an exceptionally poor job of reporting estimated true scores and confidence intervals for expected obtained scores on alternative forms. For example, intervals are often erroneously centered about obtained scores rather than estimated true scores. Often the topic is not even discussed" (p. 260). As well, in general, confidence intervals based on age-specific *SEM*s are preferable to those based on the overall *SEM* (particularly at the extremes of the age distribution, where there is the most variability) and can be constructed using age-based *SEM*s found in most manuals.

As outlined earlier, estimated true scores and their associated confidence intervals can contribute substantially to the process of interpreting test results, and an argument can certainly be made that these should be preferred to obtained scores for clinical purposes and also for research. Nevertheless, there are compelling practical reasons to primarily focus on obtained scores, the most important of which is that virtually all data in test manuals and independent research concerning psychometric properties of tests are presented in the metric of obtained scores. In addition, a particular problem with the use of the SE_P for test-retest comparisons is that it is based on a psychometric model that typically does not apply: in most cases, retesting is carried out using the same test that was originally administered rather than a parallel form. Usually, obtained test-retest scores are interpreted rather than the estimated true scores, and test-retest reliability coefficients for obtained scores are usually lower—and sometimes much lower—than internal consistency reliability coefficients. In addition, the SE_P does not account for practice/exposure effects, which can be quite substantial when the same test is administered a second time. As a result, SE_P-based confidence intervals will often be miscentered and too small, resulting in high false-positive rates when used to identify significant changes in performance over time. For more discussion regarding the calculation and uses of the *SEM*, SE_E, SE_P, and alternative error models, see Dudek (1979), Lord and Novick (1968), and Nunnally and Bernstein (1994).

SCREENING, DIAGNOSIS, AND OUTCOME PREDICTION OF TESTS

In some cases, clinicians use tests to measure *how much* of an attribute (e.g., intelligence) an examinee has, while in other cases tests are used to help determine whether or not an examinee has a specific attribute, condition, or illness that may be either *present or absent* (e.g., Alzheimer's disease). In the latter case, a special distinction in test use may be made. *Screening tests* are those which are broadly or routinely used to detect a specific attribute or illness, often referred to as a *condition of interest* (COI) among persons who are not "symptomatic" but who may nonetheless have the COI (Streiner, 2003). *Diagnostic tests* are used to assist in ruling in or out a specific condition in persons who present with "symptoms" that suggest the diagnosis in question. Another related use of tests is for purposes of prediction of outcome. As with screening and diagnostic tests, the outcome of interest may be defined in binary terms—it will either occur or not occur (e.g., the examinee will be able to handle independent living or not). Thus, in all three cases, clinicians will be interested in the relation between a measure's distribution of scores and an attribute or outcome that is defined in binary terms. It should be noted that tests used for screening, diagnosis, and prediction may be used when the COI or outcome to be predicted consists of more than two categories (e.g., mild, moderate, and severe). However, only the binary case will be considered in this chapter.

Typically, data concerning screening or diagnostic accuracy are obtained by administering a test to a sample of persons who are also classified, with respect to the COI, by a so-called gold standard. Those who have the condition according to the gold standard are labeled COI^+, while those who do not have the condition are labeled COI^-. In medicine, the gold standard may be a highly accurate diagnostic test that is more expensive and/or has a higher level of associated risk of morbidity than some new diagnostic method that is being evaluated for use as a screening measure or as a possible replacement for the existing gold standard. In neuropsychology, the situation is often more complex as the COI may be a psychological construct or behavior (e.g., cognitive impairment, malingering) for which consensus with respect to fundamental definitions is lacking or diagnostic gold standards may not exist.

The simplest way to relate test results to binary diagnoses or outcomes is to utilize a *cutoff score*. This is a single point along the continuum of possible scores for a given test. Scores at or above the cutoff classify examinees as belonging to one of two groups; scores below the cutoff classify examinees as belonging to the other group. Those who have the COI according to the test are labeled as *test positive* (Test$^+$), while those who do not have the COI are labeled *test negative* (Test$^-$).

Table 1–3 shows the relation between examinee classifications based on test results versus classifications based on a gold standard measure. By convention, test classification is denoted by row membership and gold standard classification is denoted by column membership. Cell values represent the total number of persons from the sample falling into each of four possible outcomes with respect to agreement between a test and a respective gold standard. Agreements between gold standard and test classifications are referred to as *true-positive* and *true-negative* cases, while disagreements are referred to as *false-positive* and *false-negative* cases, with *positive* and *negative* referring to the presence or absence of a COI per classification by the gold standard. When considering outcome data, observed outcome is substituted for the gold standard. It is important to keep in mind while reading the following section that while gold standard measures are often implicitly treated as 100% accurate, this may not always be the case. Any limitations in accuracy or applicability of a gold standard or outcome measure need to be accounted for when interpreting classification accuracy statistics. See Mossman et al. (2012) and Mossman et al. (2015) for thorough discussions of this problem and methods to account for it when validating diagnostic measures.

TABLE 1–3 Classification/Prediction Accuracy of a Test in Relation to a "Gold Standard" or Actual Outcome

	GOLD STANDARD		
TEST RESULT	COI$^+$	COI$^-$	ROW TOTAL
Test Positive	A (True Positive)	B (False Positive)	A + B
Test Negative	C (False Negative)	D (True Negative)	C + D
Column total	A + C	B + D	N = A + B + C + D

NOTE: COI = condition of interest.

SENSITIVITY, SPECIFICITY, AND LIKELIHOOD RATIOS

The general accuracy of a test with respect to a specific COI is reflected by data in the *columns* of a classification accuracy table (Streiner, 2003). The column-based indices include *sensitivity*, *specificity*, and the *positive* and *negative likelihood ratios* (LR$^+$ and LR$^-$). The formulas for calculation of the column-based classification accuracy statistics from data in Table 1–4 are given below:

$$\text{Sensitivity} = A/(A + C) \quad [9]$$

$$\text{Specificity} = D/(D + B) \quad [10]$$

$$LR^+ = \text{Sensitivity}/(1 - \text{Specificity}) \quad [11]$$

$$LR^- = \text{Specificity}/(1 - \text{Sensitivity}) \quad [12]$$

Sensitivity is defined as the proportion of COI$^+$ examinees who are correctly classified as such by a test. Specificity is defined as the proportion of COI$^-$ examinees who are correctly classified as such by a test. The *positive likelihood ratio* (LR$^+$) combines sensitivity and specificity into a single index of overall test accuracy indicating the odds (likelihood) that a positive test result has come from a COI$^+$ examinee. For example, a likelihood ratio of 3.0 may be interpreted as indicating that a positive test result is three times as likely to have come from a COI$^+$ examinee as from a COI$^-$ one. The LR$^-$ is interpreted conversely to the LR$^+$. As the LR approaches 1, test classification approximates random assignment of examinees. That is, a person who is Test$^+$ is equally likely to be COI$^+$ or COI$^-$. For purposes of working examples, Table 1–4 presents hypothetical test and gold standard data.

Using Equations 9 to 12, the hypothetical test demonstrates moderate sensitivity (.75) and high specificity (.95), with an LR$^+$ of 15 and an LR$^-$ of 3.8. Thus, for the hypothetical measure, a positive result is 15 times more likely to be obtained by an examinee who has the COI than by one who does not, while a negative result is 3.8 times more likely to be obtained by an examinee who does not have the COI than by one who does.

TABLE 1–4 Classification/Prediction Accuracy of a Test in Relation to a "Gold Standard" or Actual Outcome (Hypothetical Data)

	GOLD STANDARD		
TEST RESULT	COI$^+$	COI$^-$	ROW TOTAL
Test Positive	30	2	32
Test Negative	10	38	48
Column total	40	40	N = 80

NOTE: COI = condition of interest.

Note that sensitivity, specificity, and $LR^{+/-}$ are parameter estimates that have associated errors of estimation that can be quantified. The magnitude of estimation error is inversely related to sample size and can be quite large when sample size is small. The formulas for calculating standard errors for sensitivity, specificity, and the LR are complex and will not be presented here (see McKenzie et al., 1997). Fortunately, these values may also be easily calculated using a number of readily available computer programs. Using one of these (Mackinnon, 2000) with data from Table 1–4, the 95% confidence interval for sensitivity was found to be .59 to .87, while that for specificity was .83 to .99. LR^+ was 3.8 to 58.6, and LR^- was 2.2 to 6.5. Clearly, the range of measurement error is not trivial for this hypothetical study. In addition to appreciating issues relating to estimation error, it is also important to understand that while column-based indices provide useful information about test validity and utility, a test may nevertheless have high sensitivity and specificity but still be of limited clinical value in some situations, as will be detailed later.

POSITIVE AND NEGATIVE PREDICTIVE VALUE

As opposed to being concerned with test accuracy at the *group* level, clinicians are typically more concerned with test accuracy in the context of diagnosis and other decision making at the level of *individual* examinees. That is, clinicians wish to determine whether or not an individual examinee does or does not have a given COI. In this scenario, clinicians must consider indices derived from the data in the *rows* of a classification accuracy table (Streiner, 2003). These row-based indices are positive predictive value (PPV) and negative predictive value (NPV). The formulas for calculation of these from data in Table 1–3 are given here:

$$PPV = A/(A + B) \qquad [13]$$

$$NPV = D/(C + D) \qquad [14]$$

PPV is defined as the probability that an individual with a positive test result has the COI. Conversely, NPV is defined as the probability that an individual with a negative test result does *not* have the COI. For example, predictive power estimates derived from the data presented in Table 1–4 indicate that PPV = .94 and NPV = .79. Thus, in the hypothetical dataset, 94% of persons who obtain a positive test result actually have the COI, while 79% of people who obtain a negative test result do not in fact have the COI. When predictive power is close to .50, examinees are approximately equally likely to be COI^+ as COI^-, regardless of whether they are $Test^+$ or $Test^-$. When predictive power is less than .50, test-based classifications or diagnoses will be incorrect more often than not. However, predictive power values at or below .50 may still be informative. For example, if the population prevalence of a COI is .05 and the PPV based on test results is .45, a clinician can rightly conclude that an examinee is much more likely to have the COI than members of the general population, which may be clinically relevant.

As with sensitivity and specificity, PPV and NPV are parameter estimates that should always be considered in the context of estimation error. Unfortunately, standard errors or confidence intervals for estimates of predictive power are rarely listed when these values are reported; clinicians are thus left to their own devices to calculate them. Fortunately, these values may be easily calculated using a number of freely available computer programs (see Crawford, Garthwaite, & Betkowska, 2009; Mackinnon, 2000). Using one of these (Mackinnon, 2000) with data from Table 1–4, the 95% confidence intervals for PPV and NPV given the base rate in the study were found to be .94 to .99 and .65 to .90, respectively. Clearly, the confidence interval range is not trivial for this small dataset.

BASE RATES

Of critical importance to clinical interpretation of test scores, PPV and NPV vary with the base rate or prevalence of a COI.

The prevalence of a COI is defined with respect to Table 1–3 as:

$$(A + C)/N \qquad [15]$$

As should be readily apparent from inspection of Table 1–4, the prevalence of the COI in the sample is 50%. Formulas for deriving predictive power for any level of sensitivity and specificity and a specified prevalence are given here:

$$PPV = \frac{\text{Prevalence} \times \text{Sensitivity}}{(\text{Prevalence} \times \text{Sensitivity}) + [(1 - \text{Prevalence}) \times (1 - \text{Specificity})]} \qquad [16]$$

$$NPV = \frac{1 - \text{Prevalence} \times \text{Specificity}}{[(1 - \text{Prevalence}) \times \text{Specificity}] + [\text{Prevalence} \times (1 - \text{Sensitivity})]} \qquad [17]$$

From inspection of these formulas, it should be apparent that, regardless of sensitivity and specificity, predictive power will vary between 0 and 1 as a function of prevalence. Application of Formulas 16 and 17 to the data presented in Table 1–4 across the range of possible base rates provides the range of possible PPV and NPV values depicted in Figure 1–5 (note that Figure 1–5 was produced by a spreadsheet developed for analyzing the predictive power of tests and is freely available from Daniel Slick at dslick@gmail.com).

As can be seen in Figure 1–5, the relation between predictive power and prevalence is curvilinear and asymptotic,

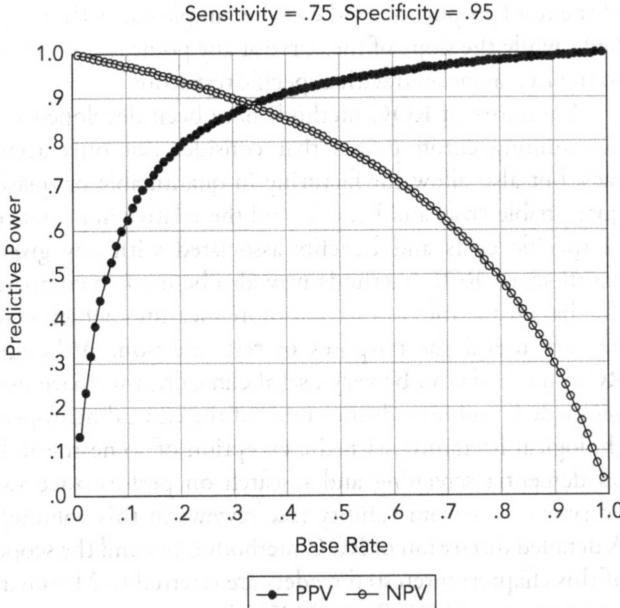

Figure 1–5 Relation of predictive power to prevalence—hypothetical data.

with endpoints at 0 and 1. For any given test cutoff score, PPV will always increase with base rate, while NPV will simultaneously decrease. For the hypothetical test being considered, one can see that both PPV and NPV are moderately high (at or above .80) when the COI base rate ranges from 20% to 50%. The tradeoff between PPV and NPV at high and low base rate levels is also readily apparent; as the base rate increases above 50%, PPV exceeds .95 while NPV declines, falling below .50 as the base rate exceeds 80%. Conversely, as the base rate falls below 30%, NPV exceeds .95 while PPV rapidly drops off, falling below 50% as the base rate falls below 7%.

From the foregoing, it is apparent that the predictive power values derived from data presented in Table 1–4 would not be applicable in settings where base rates vary from the 50% value in the hypothetical dataset. This is important because, in practice, clinicians may often be presented with PPV values based on data where "prevalence" values are near 50%. This is due to the fact that, regardless of the prevalence of a COI in the population, some diagnostic validity studies employ equal-sized samples of COI^{+} and COI^{-} individuals to facilitate statistical analyses. In contrast, the actual prevalence of COIs may differ substantially from 50% in various clinical settings and circumstances (e.g., screening vs. diagnostic use). For examples of differing PPV and NPV across different base rates, see Chapter 16, on the Minnesota Multiphasic Personality Inventory, 2 (MMPI-2) and Minnesota Multiphasic Personality Inventory, 2 Restructured Form (MMPI-2-RF).

For example, suppose that the data from Table 1–4 were from a validity trial of a neuropsychological measure designed for administration to young adults for purposes of predicting development of schizophrenia. The question then arises: Should the measure be used for broad screening given a lifetime schizophrenia prevalence of .008? Using Formula 16, one can determine that for this purpose the measure's PPV is only .11 and thus the "positive" test results would be incorrect 89% of the time.

Conversely, the prevalence of a COI may in some settings be substantially higher than 50%. As an example of the other extreme, the base rate of head injuries among persons admitted to an acute hospital head injury rehabilitation service is essentially 100%, in which case the use of neuropsychological tests to determine whether or not examinees had sustained a head injury would not only be redundant, but very likely lead to false-negative errors (such tests could, of course, be legitimately used for other purposes, such as grading injury severity). Clearly, clinicians need to carefully consider published data concerning sensitivity, specificity, and predictive power in light of intended test use and, if necessary, calculate PPV and NPV values and COI base rate estimates applicable to specific groups of examinees seen in their own practices. In addition, it must be kept in mind that PPV and NPV values calculated for individual examinees are estimates that have associated measurement errors that allow for construction of confidence intervals. Crawford, Garthwaite, and Betkowska (2009) provide details on the calculation of such confidence intervals and also a free computer program that performs the calculations.

DIFFICULTIES WITH ESTIMATING AND APPLYING BASE RATES

Prevalence or base rate estimates may be based on large-scale epidemiological studies that provide good data on the rate of occurrence of COIs in the general population or within specific subpopulations and settings (e.g., prevalence rates of various psychiatric disorders in inpatient psychiatric settings). However, in some cases, no prevalence data may be available, or reported prevalence data may not be applicable to specific settings or subpopulations. In these cases, clinicians who wish to determine predictive power must develop their own base rate estimates. Ideally, these can be derived from data collected within the same setting in which the test will be employed, though this is typically time-consuming and many methodological challenges may be faced, including limitations associated with small sample sizes. Methods for estimating base rates in such contexts are beyond the scope of this chapter; interested readers are directed to Mossman (2003), Pepe (2003), and Rorer and Dawes (1982).

DETERMINING THE OPTIMUM CUTOFF SCORE: ROC ANALYSES AND OTHER METHODS

The foregoing discussion has focused on the diagnostic accuracy of tests using specific cutoff points, presumably ones that are optimal for given tasks such as diagnosing dementia or detecting noncredible performance. A number of methods for determining an optimum cutoff point are available, and, although they may lead to similar results, the differences between them are not trivial. Many of these methods are mathematically complex and/or computationally demanding, thus requiring computer applications.

The determination of an optimum cutoff score for detection or diagnosis of a COI is often based on simultaneous evaluation of sensitivity and specificity or predictive power across a range of scores. In some cases, this information, in tabular or graphical form, is simply inspected and a score is chosen based on a researcher's or clinician's comfort with a particular error rate. For example, in malingering research, cutoffs that minimize false-positive errors or hold them below a low threshold are often explicitly chosen (i.e., by convention, a specificity of .90 or higher), even though such cutoffs are associated with relatively large false-negative error rates (i.e., lower detection of examinees with the COI, malingering).

A more formal, rigorous, and often very useful set of tools for choosing cutoff points and for evaluating and comparing test utility for diagnosis and decision making falls under the rubric of *receiver operating characteristics* (ROC) analyses. Clinicians who use tests for diagnostic or other decision-making purposes should be familiar with ROC procedures. The statistical procedures utilized in ROC analyses are closely related to and substantially overlap those of Bayesian analyses. The central graphic element of ROC analyses is the ROC graph, which is a plot of the true-positive proportion (*y* axis) against the false-positive proportion (*x* axis) associated with each specific score in a range of test scores. Figure 1–6 shows an example a ROC graph. The area under the curve is equivalent to the overall accuracy of the test (proportion of the entire sample correctly classified), while the slope of the curve at any point is equivalent to the LR^+ associated with a specific test score.

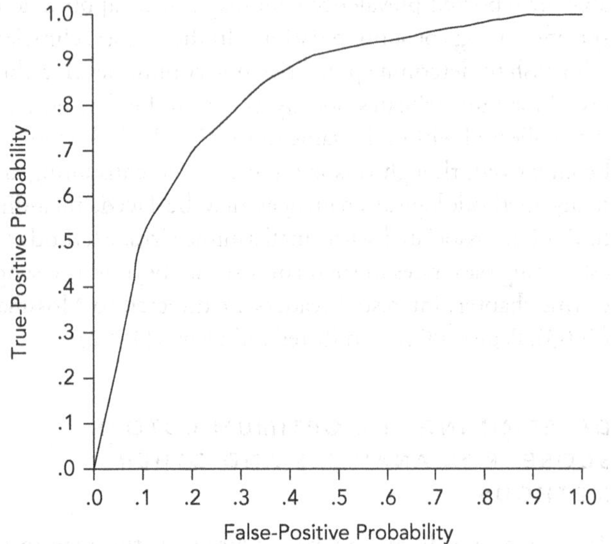

Figure 1–6 *An ROC graph.*

A number of ROC methods have been developed for determining cutoff points that consider not only accuracy, but also allow for factoring in quantifiable or quasi-quantifiable costs and benefits and the relative importance of specific costs and benefits associated with any given cutoff score. ROC methods may also be used to compare the diagnostic utility of two or more measures, which may be very useful for purposes of test selection. Although ROC methods can be very useful clinically, they have not yet made broad inroads into most of the clinical neuropsychological literature, with the exception of some research on dementia screening and research on performance validity and symptom validity (see reviews in this volume). A detailed discussion of ROC methods is beyond the scope of this chapter; interested readers are referred to Mossman and Somoza (1992), Pepe (2003), Somoza and Mossman (1992), and Swets, Dawes, and Monahan (2000).

EVALUATION OF PREDICTIVE POWER ACROSS A RANGE OF CUTOFF SCORES AND BASE RATES

As noted earlier, it is important to recognize that positive and negative predictive power are *not* properties of tests but rather are properties of specific test scores in specific contexts. The foregoing sections describing the calculation and interpretation of predictive power have focused on methods for evaluating the value of a single cutoff point for a given test for purposes of classifying examinees as COI^+ or COI^-. However, by focusing exclusively on single cutoff points, clinicians are essentially transforming continuous test scores into binary scores, thus discarding much potentially useful information, particularly when scores are considerably above or below a cutoff. Lindeboom (1989) proposed an alternative approach in which predictive power across a range of test scores and base rates can be displayed in a single Bayesian probability table. In this approach, test scores define the rows and base rates define the columns of a table; individual table cells contain the associated PPV and NPV for a specific score and specific base rate. Such tables have rarely been constructed for standardized measures, but examples can be found in some test manuals (e.g., the Victoria Symptom Validity Test; Slick et al., 1997). The advantage of this approach is that it allows clinicians to consider the diagnostic confidence associated with an examinee's specific score, leading to more accurate assessments. A limiting factor for use of Bayesian probability tables is that they can only be constructed when sensitivity and specificity values for an entire range of scores are available, which is rarely the case for most tests. In addition, predictive power values in such tables are subject to any validity limitations of underlying data and should include associated standard errors or confidence intervals.

COMBINING RESULTS OF MULTIPLE SCREENING/DIAGNOSTIC TESTS

Often, more than one test that provides data relevant to a specific diagnosis is administered. In these cases, clinicians may wish to integrate predictive power estimates *across* measures. There may be a temptation to use the PPV associated with a score on one measure as the "base rate" when the PPV for a score from a second measure is calculated. For example, suppose that the base rate of a COI is 15%. When a test designed to detect the COI is administered, an examinee's score translates to a PPV of 65%. The examiner then administers a second test designed to detect the COI, but when PPV for the examinee's score on the second test is calculated, a "base rate" of 65% is used rather than 15% because the former is now the assumed prior probability that the examinee has the COI given their score on the first test administered. The resulting PPV for the examinee's score on the second measure is now 99%, and the examiner concludes that the examinee has the COI. While this procedure may seem logical, it will produce an inflated PPV estimate for the second test score whenever the two measures are correlated, which will almost always be the case when both measures are designed to screen for or diagnose the same COI.

A more defensible method for combining results of multiple diagnostic tests is to derive empirically derived classification rules based on the number of positive findings from a set of screening/diagnostic tests. While this approach to combining test results can produce more accurate classifications, its use of binary data (positive or negative findings) as inputs does not capitalize on the full range of data available from each test, and so accuracy may not be optimized. To date, this approach to combining test results has primarily been used with performance/symptom validity tests, and there have been some interesting debates in the literature concerning the accuracy and clinical utility of the derived classification rules; see Larrabee (2014a, 2014b), Bilder et al. (2014), and Davis and Millis (2014).

A preferred psychometric method for integrating scores from multiple screening/diagnostic measures, one that utilizes the full range of data from each test, is to construct group membership (i.e., COI^+ vs. COI^-) prediction equations using methods such as logistic regression or multiway frequency analyses. These methods can be used clinically to generate binary classifications or classification probabilities, with the latter being preferred because it is a better gauge of accuracy. Ideally, the derived classification formulas should be well validated before being utilized clinically. More details on methods for combining classification data across measures may be found in Franklin and Krueger (2003) and Pepe (2003).

WHY ARE CLASSIFICATION ACCURACY STATISTICS NOT UBIQUITOUS IN NEUROPSYCHOLOGICAL RESEARCH AND CLINICAL PRACTICE?

Of note, the mathematical relations between sensitivity, specificity, base rates, and predictive power were first elucidated by Thomas Bayes and published in 1763; methods for deriving predictive power and other related indices of confidence in decision making are thus often referred to as *Bayesian* statistics. Note that in Bayesian terminology, the prevalence or base rate of a COI is known as the *prior probability*, while PPV and NPV are known as *posterior probabilities*. Conceptually, the difference between the prior and posterior probabilities associated with information added by a test score is an index of the diagnostic utility of a test. There is an entire literature concerning Bayesian methods for statistical analysis of test utility. These will not be covered here, and interested readers are referred to Pepe (2003).

Needless to say, Bayes's work predated the first diagnostic applications of psychological tests as we know them today. However, although neuropsychological tests are routinely used for diagnostic decision making, information on the predictive power of most tests is often absent from both test manuals and applicable research literature. This is so despite the fact that the importance and relevance of Bayesian approaches to the practice of clinical psychology was well described 60 years ago by Meehl and Rosen (1955). Bayesian statistics are finally making major inroads into the mainstream of neuropsychology, particularly in the research literature concerning symptom/performance validity measures, in which estimates of predictive power have become de rigueur, although these are still typically presented without associated standard errors, thus greatly reducing the utility of the data.

ASSESSING CHANGE OVER TIME

Neuropsychologists are often interested in tracking changes in function over time. In these contexts, three interrelated questions arise:

- To what degree do changes in examinee test scores reflect "real" changes in function as opposed to measurement error?
- To what degree do real changes in examinee test scores reflect clinically significant changes in function as opposed to clinically trivial changes?
- To what degree do changes in examinee test scores conform to expectations, given the application of treatments or the occurrence of other events or processes occurring between test and retest, such as head injury, dementia, or brain surgery?

A number of statistical/psychometric methods have been developed for assessing changes observed over repeated administrations of neuropsychological tests; these differ considerably with respect to mathematical models and assumptions regarding the nature of test data. As with most areas of psychometrics, the problems and processes involved in decomposing observed scores (i.e., change scores) into measurement error and "true" scores are often complex. Clinicians are certainly not aided by the lack of agreement about which methods to use for analyzing test-retest data, limited retest data for many tests, and limited coverage and direction concerning retest procedures in most test manuals. Only a relatively brief discussion of this important area of psychometrics is presented here. Interested readers are referred to other sources (e.g., Duff, 2012; Heilbronner et al., 2010; Hinton-Bayre & Kwapil, 2017; Holdnack et al., 2013) for a more in-depth review.

REFERENCE SAMPLE CHANGE SCORE DISTRIBUTIONS

If a reference or normative sample is administered a test twice, a distribution of observed change scores ("change score" = retest score minus baseline score) can be obtained. When such information is available, individual examinee change scores can be transformed into standardized scores or percentiles derived directly from raw change scores, with the latter being preferable when the distribution of change scores is non-normal. These change scores provide information on the degree of unusualness of any observed changes in performance over time. Unfortunately, use of this method of evaluating change is usually complicated by a number of factors. First, retest samples tend to be relatively small for many tests, thus limiting generalizability. This is particularly important when change scores vary with demographic variables (e.g., age and level of education) and/or initial test score level (e.g., normal vs. abnormal) because retest samples typically are restricted with respect to both. Second, retest samples are often obtained within a short period of time after initial testing, typically less than 2 months, whereas in clinical practice typical test-retest intervals are often much longer. Thus any effects of extended test-retest intervals on change score distributions are not reflected in most change score data presented in test manuals or otherwise available. Last, change score information is often presented in the form of summary statistics (e.g., mean and *SD*), which only allow for the creation of linear scaled scores that have limited utility if change scores are not normally distributed.

THE RELIABLE CHANGE INDEX

Jacobson and Truax (1991; see also Jacobson et al., 1999) proposed a psychometric method for determining if changes in test scores over time are reliable (i.e., not an artifact of imperfect test reliability). This method involves calculation of a *reliable change index* (RCI). The RCI is an indicator of the probability that an observed difference between test-retest scores from the same examinee on the same test can be attributed to measurement error (i.e., to imperfect reliability). When there is a low probability that the observed change is due to measurement error, one may infer that it reflects other factors, such as progression of illness, treatment effects, and/or prior exposure to the test.

The RCI is calculated using the *standard error of the difference* (SE_D), an index of measurement error derived from classical test theory. It is the standard deviation of expected test-retest difference scores about a mean of 0 given an assumption that no actual change has occurred. The formula for the SE_D is:

$$SE_D = \sqrt{2 \cdot (SEM)^2} \qquad [18]$$

where *SEM* is the standard error of measurement, as previously defined in Formula 6. Inspection of Formula 18 reveals that tests with a large *SEM* will have a large SE_D. The RCI for a specific score is calculated by dividing the observed amount of change by the SE_D, transforming observed change scores into SE_D units. The formula is given below:

$$(S_2 - S_1)/SE_D \qquad [19]$$

Where:

S_1 = an examinee's initial test score
S_2 = an examinee's score at retest on the same measure

The resulting RCI scores can be either negative or positive and can be thought of as a type of *z* score that can be interpreted with reference to upper or lower tails of a normal probability distribution. Therefore, RCI scores falling outside a range of −1.96 to 1.96 would be expected to occur less than 5% of the time as a result of measurement error alone, assuming that an examinee's true retest score had not changed since the first test. The assumption that an examinee's true score has not changed can therefore be rejected at $p < .05$ (two-tailed) when their RCI score is above 1.96 or below −1.96.

The RCI is often calculated using *SD* (to calculate *SEM*) and reliability estimates obtained from test normative samples. However, as these values may not be applicable to the clinical group to which an examinee belongs, care must be taken in interpretation of the RCI in such circumstances. It may be preferable to use *SD* and reliability estimates from samples similar to an examinee, if these are available. Because the SE_D value is constant for any given combination of test and reference sample, it can be used to construct RCI confidence intervals applicable to any initial test score obtained from a person similar to the reference sample, using the formula below:

$$RCI - CI = S_1 - (z \cdot SE_D) \qquad [20]$$

Where:

S_1 = Initial test score
z = z score associated with a given confidence range (e.g., 1.64 for a 90% C.I.)

Retest scores falling outside the desired confidence interval about initial scores can be considered evidence of a significant change. Note that while a "significant" RCI value may be considered as a prerequisite, it is *not* by itself sufficient evidence that clinically significant change has occurred. Consider RCIs in the context of highly reliable tests: relatively small score changes at retest can produce significant RCIs, but both the initial test score and retest score may remain within the same classification range (e.g., normal) so that the clinical implications of observed change may be minimal. In addition, use of the RCI implicitly assumes that no practice effects pertain. When practice effects are present, significant RCI values may partially or wholly reflect effects of prior test exposure rather than a change in underlying functional level.

To allow RCIs to be used with tests that have practice effects, Chelune et al. (1993, as cited in Strauss et al., 2006; see also Chelune, 2003) suggest a modification to the calculation of the RCI in which the mean change score for a reference group is subtracted from the observed change score of an individual examinee and the result is used as an *adjusted change score* for purposes of calculating an adjusted RCI. Alternatively, an RCI confidence interval calculated using Formula 21 could have its endpoints adjusted by addition of the mean change score.

$$\text{Adj. RCI} - \text{CI} = (S_1 + M_C) \pm (z \cdot SE_D) \qquad [21]$$

Where:

S_1 = Initial test score
M_C = Mean change score (Retest − Test)
z = z score associated with a given confidence range (e.g., 1.64 for a 90% C.I.)

This approach appears to offer some advantages over the traditional RCI, particularly for tests where large practice effects are expected. However, adjusting for practice in this way is problematic in a number of ways, first and foremost of which is the use of a constant term for the practice effect, which will not reflect any systematic variability in practice effects across individuals. Second, neither standard nor adjusted RCIs account for regression toward the mean because the associated estimated measurement error is not adjusted proportionally for the extremity of observed change.

Two final issues with the use of RCIs arise from their foundation in classical test theory, a model that assumes that an equivalent parallel form is administered at retest rather than the same measure that was used initially, which is rarely the case in actual clinical practice. RCIs use internal consistency reliability (Cronbach's α) to estimate measurement error because the measurement model is only concerned with test-intrinsic measurement error and not with any other sources of error, such as those arising from examinees and testing environments. In contrast, test-retest reliability coefficients are a more accurate reflection of variability in change over time based on actual test-retest data rather than a theoretical model, and they often differ considerably from internal reliability coefficients, in many cases being substantially smaller. In addition, the RCI model assumes that change scores are normally distributed, when in reality large departures from normality are not uncommon. Therefore, clinicians should very carefully consider whether or not to use RCIs, especially when internal consistency and test-retest reliability coefficients differ markedly and/or test-retest score distributions are non-normal.

Last, RCIs should be interpreted with regard to base rates because healthy people show some changes over serial assessments detected by RCIs; to be clinically meaningful, the number of RCI scores exceeding the RCI must be greater than the base rate of low scores for the population in question. For more information on this, see Brooks et al. (2016; see also Nelson, 2015).

STANDARDIZED REGRESSION-BASED CHANGE SCORES

The RCI may provide useful information regarding the likelihood of a meaningful change in the function being measured by a test, but, as noted earlier, it may have limited validity in some circumstances. Many quantifiable factors not accounted for by RCI may influence or predict retest scores, including test-retest interval, baseline ability level (Time 1 score), scores from other tests, and examinee characteristics such as gender, education, age, acculturation, and neurological or medical conditions. In addition, while RCI scores factor in measurement error, it is operationalized as a constant and so does not account for regression to the mean (i.e., the increase in measurement error associated with more extreme scores). One method for evaluating change that does allow clinicians to account for additional predictors and also controls for regression to the mean is the use of *linear regression models* (Crawford & Howell, 1998; Hermann et al., 1991).

With linear regression models, predicted retest scores are derived and then compared with observed retest scores for purposes of determining if deviations from predicted values are significant. In the preferred method, this is accomplished by dividing the difference between obtained retest scores and regression-predicted retest scores by the *standard error for individual predicted scores* ($SE_{\hat{Y}}$). Because score differences are divided by a standard error, the resulting value is standardized. The resulting standardized score is in fact a t statistic that can be translated into a probability value using an appropriate program or table. Small probability values indicate that the observed retest score differs significantly from the predicted value. The $SE_{\hat{Y}}$ is used because, unlike the standard error of the regression, it is not constant across cases but increases as individual values of independent variables deviate from the mean, thus accounting for regression to the mean on a case-by-case basis (Crawford & Howell, 1998). Thus, persons who are outliers with respect to their scores on predictor variables will have larger margins of error associated with their predicted scores, and thus larger score changes will be required to reach significance for these individuals.

As with other standardized scores (e.g., *z* scores), standardized regression-based change scores (SRB scores) from different measures can be directly compared regardless of the original test score metric. However, a number of inferential limitations of such comparisons, described in the section on standardized scores earlier in this chapter, still apply. Regression models can also be used when one wishes to consider change scores from multiple tests simultaneously; these are more complex and will not be covered here. Examples of regression equations for measuring change developed for specific neuropsychological tests are presented throughout this volume.

LIMITATIONS OF STANDARDIZED REGRESSION-BASED CHANGE SCORES

It is important to understand the limitations of regression methods. Whenever SRB scores are derived, it is imperative to assess model fit and check for violations of assumptions of the linear model (linear relationship, multivariate normality, minimal multicollinearity, minimal auto-correlation, and homoscedasticity; see Pedhazur, 1997, pp. 33–34). SRB models that do not fit the data well or that violate assumptions should not be used, and other types of prediction models such as nonlinear regression should be considered instead. Regression equations based on smaller sample sizes will lead to large error terms so that meaningful predicted-obtained differences may be missed. Equations from large-scale studies or from cross-validation efforts are therefore preferred. In order to maximize validity, sample characteristics should match populations seen clinically, and predictor variables should be carefully chosen to match data that will likely be available to clinicians. Test users should generally avoid interpolation; that is, they should avoid applying a regression equation to an examinee's data (predictor variables and test-retest scores) when the data values fall outside the ranges for corresponding variables comprising the regression equation. For example, if a regression equation is developed for predicting IQ at retest from a sample with initial IQ scores ranging from 85 to 125, it should not be applied to an examinee whose initial IQ is 65.

It is critical to understand that SRB scores do not necessarily indicate whether a clinically significant change from baseline level has occurred—for which use of RCIs may be more appropriate. Instead, SRB scores are an index of the degree to which observed change conforms to established trends in a reference population. These trends may consist of increases or decreases in performance over time in association with combinations of influential predictor variables, such as type and severity of illness, treatment type, baseline cognitive level, gender, age, and test-retest interval. For example, healthy individuals may obtain high scores at retesting, while individuals with progressive neurological disease may obtain decreased scores. The following two examples will illustrate this point.

In the first example, consider a hypothetical scenario of a treatment for depression that is associated with improved post-treatment scores on a depression inventory, such that in a clinical reference sample, the test-retest correlation is high and the average improvement in scores at retest exceeds the threshold for clinical significance as established by RCI. In the simplest case (i.e., using only scores from Time 1), regression-predicted retest scores would be equivalent to the mean score change observed in the clinical reference sample. In this case, an examinee who at retest obtained a depression score at or near the post-treatment mean would obtain a *nonsignificant* SRB score but a *significant* RCI score, indicating that they demonstrated the typically seen clinically significant improvement in response to treatment. Conversely, an examinee who obtained an unchanged depression score following treatment would obtain a *significant* SRB score but a *nonsignificant* RCI score, indicating that they did not show the typically seen significant improvement in response to treatment.

In the second example, consider a hypothetical scenario of a memory test that has significant prior exposure (i.e., learning) effects such that, in the normative sample, the test-retest correlation is high and the average improvement in scores at retest exceeds the threshold for clinical significance as established by RCI. As with the depression score example, in the simplest case (i.e., using only scores from Time 1), regression-predicted retest scores would be equivalent to the mean score change observed in the reference sample. In this case, an examinee who at retest obtained a memory score at or near the retest mean would obtain a *nonsignificant* SRB score but a *significant* RCI score, indicating that they demonstrated the typically seen prior exposure/learning effect (note the difference in interpretation from the previous example—the improvement in score is assumed to reflect treatment effects in the first case and to be artifactual in the second case). Conversely, an examinee who obtained an unchanged memory score following treatment would obtain a *significant* SRB score but a *nonsignificant* RCI score, indicating that they did not show the typically seen prior exposure/learning effect. Conceivably, in the context of a clinical referral, the latter finding might be interpreted as reflective of memory problems.

CLINICALLY SIGNIFICANT CHANGE

Once a clinician has determined that an observed test score change is reliable, they will need to determine whether the change is clinically meaningful. This is because a reliable change is not necessarily evidence in and of itself of clinical significance. A trivial change can be reliable using precise and exact psychometric tools with little error variance but matter nothing clinically.

Jacobson and Truax (1991) proposed that clinically significant change occurs, in the context of treatment, when an examinee's score (e.g., on the Beck Depression Inventory) moves from within the clinically depressed range into the normal population range. A reliable change from the impaired to the average range could similarly be interpreted as significant change, but a change of one *SD*, or half an *SD* could also be evidence of clinically significant change, depending on the condition and the tests used. However, there are at present no widely accepted criteria for defining clinically significant change within the context of neuropsychological assessment. Rather, the determination of clinical significance of any observed change that is reliable will depend greatly on the specific context of the assessment and the judgment of the clinician, based on psychometric methods for determining whether change should be interpreted as significant in the first place. For more information, see Heilbronner, Sweet, Attix, and colleagues (2010).

NORMAL VARIABILITY AND BASE RATES OF LOW SCORES

Normal variation or *normal variability* refers to the fact that many healthy individuals demonstrate considerable variability in performance across a battery of neuropsychological tests. Research on normal variation indicates that it is not uncommon for healthy adults to obtain a wide range of scores on a battery of neuropsychological tests or a single test with multiple subtests, including a non-insignificant number of scores in the impaired range (e.g., Binder et al., 2009). Additionally, the number of low scores obtained by healthy adults varies with factors such as IQ and level of education. These studies show that the development and routine application of comprehensive norms for normal variability and base rates of low scores will be greatly beneficial to the field of clinical neuropsychology.

Taking a more basic psychometric approach, Ingraham and Aiken (1996) have shown that the likelihood that a profile of tests scores will exceed criteria for "abnormality" increases as (1) the number of tests in a battery *increases*, (2) the *z* score cutoff used to classify a test score as abnormal *decreases*, and (3) the number of abnormal test scores required to reach criteria *decreases*. Ingraham and Aiken (1996) developed a mathematical model that may be used for determining the likelihood of obtaining an abnormal test result from a given number of tests. Implicit in this model is an assumption that some "abnormal" test scores are spurious. As Ingraham and Aiken note, the problem of determining whether a profile of test scores meets criteria for abnormality is considerably complicated by the fact that most neuropsychological measures are intercorrelated, and therefore the probabilities of obtaining abnormal results from each test are not independent. However, they provide some suggested guidelines for adapting their model or using other methods to provide useful approximations. Expanding further on Ingraham and Aiken's work, Crawford et al. (2007) provide a model for estimating the percentage of the population with abnormally low scores or abnormally large score differences from a given set of intercorrelated neuropsychological tests. Of great benefit to clinicians, they also provide free computer software to perform the calculations.

The accumulated research and normative data indicate that clinicians should always consider available data on base rates of low scores when interpreting results. When these data are not available, mathematical models can be used to estimate the prevalence of low scores in healthy populations. In either case, the data show that a conservative approach is warranted when interpreting a small number of large score discrepancies or abnormal scores from a battery of tests (see also Brooks, Holdnack, & Iverson, 2011; Brooks, Iverson, & Holdnack, 2013; Heyanka, Holster, & Golden, 2013; Holdnack, Tulsky, Brooks, Slotkin, Gershon, Heinemann, & Iverson, 2017; Zakzanis & Jeffay, 2011).

A FINAL WORD ON THE VALUE OF NEUROPSYCHOLOGICAL TESTS

Though progress has been made, much work remains to be done in developing more psychometrically sound and clinically efficient and useful neuropsychological measures. At times, the technical limitations of many tests that are currently available with regard to measurement error, reliability, validity, diagnostic accuracy, and other important psychometric characteristics may lead to questions regarding their worth in clinical practice. Indeed, informed consideration may, quite appropriately, lead neuropsychologists to limit or completely curtail their use of some measures. The extreme argument would be to completely exclude any tests that entail measurement error, effectively eliminating all forms of objective measurement of human characteristics. However, it is important to keep in mind the limited and unreliable nature of human judgment—even expert judgment—when left to its own devices. Indeed, "this fallibility in the judgments made by humans about fellow humans is one of the primary reasons that psychological tests have been developed and applied in ever-increasing numbers over the past century" (p. 393; Dahlstom, 1993). In this context, neuropsychological tests need not be perfect, or even psychometrically exceptional; they need only meaningfully improve clinical decision making and significantly reduce errors of judgment—those errors stemming from prejudice, personal bias, halo effects, ignorance, and stereotyping—made by people when judging other people (Dahlstom, 1993; see also Meehl, 1973). The judicious selection, appropriate administration, and well-informed interpretation of standardized tests will usually achieve this result.

REFERENCES

American Educational Research Association, American Psychological Association, & National Council on Measurement in Education. (2014). *Standards for educational and psychological testing.* Washington, DC: American Psychological Association.

Baron, I. S. (2018). *Neuropsychological evaluation of the child: Domains, methods, and case studies* (2nd ed.). New York: Oxford University Press.

Bilder, R. M., Sugar, C. A., & Hellemann, G. S. (2014). Cumulative false positive rates given multiple performance validity tests: Commentary on Davis and Millis (2014) and Larrabee (2014). *The Clinical Neuropsychologist, 28*(8), 1212–1223.

Binder, L. M., Iverson, G. L., & Brooks, B. L. (2009). To err is human: "Abnormal" neuropsychological scores and variability are common in healthy adults. *Archives of Clinical Neuropsychology, 24*(1), 31–46.

Brooks, B. L., Holdnack, J. A., & Iverson, G. L. (2011). Advanced clinical interpretation of the WAIS-IV and WMS-IV: prevalence of low scores varies by level of intelligence and years of education. *Assessment, 18*, 156–167.

Brooks, B. L., Iverson, G. L., & Holdnack, J. A. (2013). Understanding and using multivariate base rates with the WAIS-IV/WMS-IV. In J. A. Holdnack, L. W. Drozdick, L. G. Weiss, & G. L. Iverson (Eds.), *WAIS-IV/WMS-IV/ACS: Advanced clinical interpretation* (pp. 75–102). San Diego, CA: Elsevier Science.

Brooks, B. L., Holdnack, J. A., & Iverson, G. L. (2016). To change is human: "Abnormal" reliable change memory scores are common in healthy adults and older adults. *Archives of Clinical Neuropsychology, 31*(8), 1026–1036.

Chelune, G. J. (2003). Assessing reliable neuropsychological change. In R. D. Franklin (Ed.), *Prediction in forensic and neuropsychology: Sound statistical practices* (pp. 65–88). Mahwah, NJ: Lawrence Erlbaum Associates.

Crawford, J. R., & Garthwaite, P. H. (2002). Investigation of the single case in neuropsychology: Confidence limits on the abnormality of test scores and test score differences. *Neuropsychologia, 40*, 1196–1208.

Crawford, J. R., & Garthwaite, P. H. (2009). Percentiles please: The case for expressing neuropsychological test scores and accompanying confidence limits as percentile ranks. *The Clinical Neuropsychologist, 23*(2), 193–204.

Crawford, J. R., Garthwaite, P. H., & Betkowska, K. (2009). Bayes' theorem and diagnostic tests in neuropsychology: Interval estimates for post-test probabilities. *The Clinical Neuropsychologist, 23*(4), 624–644.

Crawford, J. R., Garthwaite, P. H., & Gault, C. B. (2007). Estimating the percentage of the population with abnormally low scores (or abnormally large score differences) on standardized neuropsychological test batteries: A generic method with applications. *Neuropsychology, 21*(4), 419–430.

Crawford, J. R., Garthwaite, P. H., & Slick, D. J. (2009). On percentile norms in neuropsychology: Proposed reporting standards and methods for quantifying the uncertainty over the percentile ranks of test scores. *The Clinical Neuropsychologist, 23*(7), 1173–1195.

Crawford, J. R., & Howell, D. C. (1998). Regression equations in clinical neuropsychology: An evaluation of statistical methods for comparing predicted and obtained scores. *Journal of Clinical and Experimental Neuropsychology, 20*(5), 755–762.

Dahlstom, W. G. (1993). Small samples, large consequences. *American Psychologist, 48*(4), 393–399.

Davis, J. J., & Millis, S. R. (2014). Reply to commentary by Bilder, Sugar, & Helleman (2014 this issue) on minimizing false positive error with multiple performance validity tests. *The Clinical Neuropsychologist, 28*(8), 1224–1229.

Dudek, F. J. (1979). The continuing misinterpretation of the standard error of measurement. *Psychological Bulletin, 86*(2), 335–337.

Duff, K. (2012). Evidence-based indicators of neuropsychological change in the individual patient: Relevant concepts and methods. *Archives of Clinical Neuropsychology, 27*(3), 248–261.

Franklin, R. D., & Krueger, J. (2003). Bayesian inference and belief networks. In R. D. Franklin (Ed.), *Prediction in forensic and neuropsychology: Sound statistical practices* (pp. 65–88). Mahwah, NJ: Lawrence Erlbaum Associates.

Glutting, J. J., McDermott, P. A., & Stanley, J. C. (1987). Resolving differences among methods of establishing confidence limits for test scores. *Educational and Psychological Measurement, 47*(3), 607–614.

Heaton, R. K., Taylor, M. J., & Manly, J. (2003). Demographic effects and use of demographically corrected norms with the WAIS-III and WMS-III. In D. S. Tulsky, D. H. Saklofske, G. J. Chelune, R. K. Heaton, R. Ivnik, R. Bornstein, A. Prifitera, & M. F. Ledbetter (Eds.), *Clinical interpretation of the WAIS-III and WMS-III* (pp. 181–210). New York: Academic Press.

Heilbronner, R. L., Sweet, J. J., Attix, D. K., Krull, K. R., Henry, G. K., & Hart, R. P. (2010). Official position of the American Academy of Clinical Neuropsychology on serial neuropsychological assessments: The utility and challenges of repeat test administrations in clinical and forensic contexts. *The Clinical Neuropsychologist, 24*(8), 1267–1278. doi: 10.1080/13854046.2010.526785.

Hermann, B. P., Wyler, A. R., VanderZwagg, R., LeBailly, R. K., Whitman, S., Somes, G., & Ward, J. (1991). Predictors of neuropsychological change following anterior temporal lobectomy: Role of regression toward the mean. *Journal of Epilepsy, 4*, 139–148.

Heyanka, D. J., Holster, J. L., & Golden, C. J. (2013). Intraindividual neuropsychological test variability in healthy individuals with high average intelligence and educational attainment. *The International Journal of Neuroscience, 123*(8), 526–531.

Hinton-Bayre, A. D., & Kwapil, K. J. (2017). Best practice approaches for evaluating significant change for individuals. In S. C. Bowden (Ed.), *Neuropsychological assessment in the age of evidence-based practice* (pp. 121–154). New York: Oxford University Press.

Holdnack, J. A., Dorzdick, L. W., Iverson, G. L., & Chelune, G. J. (2013). Serial assessments with the WAIS-IV and WMS-IV. In J. A. Holdnack, L. W. Drozdick, L. G. Weiss, & G. L. Iverson (Eds.), *WAIS-IV, WMS-IV, and ACS: Advanced clinical interpretation.* New York: Elsevier.

Holdnack, J. A., Tulsky, D, S., Brooks, B. L., Slotkin, J., Gershon, R., Heinemann, A. W., & Iverson, G. L. (2017). Interpreting patterns of low scores on the NIH toolbox cognition battery. *Archives of Clinical Neuropsychology, 32*(5), 574–584.

Ingraham, L. J., & Aiken, C. B. (1996). An empirical approach to determining criteria for abnormality in test batteries with multiple measures. *Neuropsychology, 10*(1), 120–124.

Jacobson, N. S., Roberts, L. J., Berns, S. B., & McGlinchey, J. B. (1999). Methods for defining and determining the clinical significance of treatment effects description, application, and alternatives. *Journal of Consulting and Clinical Psychology, 67*(3), 300–307.

Jacobson, N. S., & Truax, P. (1991). Clinical significance: A statistical approach to defining meaningful change in psychotherapy research. *Journal of Consulting and Clinical Psychology, 59*, 12–19.

Larrabee, G. J. (2014a). False-positive rates associated with the use of multiple performance and symptom validity tests. *Archives of Clinical Neuropsychology, 29*(4), 364–373.

Larrabee, G. J. (2014b). Minimizing false positive error with multiple performance validity tests: Response to Bilder, Sugar, & Hellemann (2014 this issue). *The Clinical Neuropsychologist, 28*(8), 1230–1242.

Lezak, M. D., Howieson, D. B., Bigler, E. D., & Tranel, D. (2012). *Neuropsychological assessment* (5th ed.). New York: Oxford University Press.

Lindeboom, J. (1989). Who needs cutting points? *Journal of Clinical Psychology, 45*(4), 679–683.

Lord, F. M., & Novick, M. R. (1968). *Statistical theories of mental test scores.* Reading, MA: Addison-Wesley.

Mackinnon, A. (2000). A spreadsheet for the calculation of comprehensive statistics for the assessment of diagnostic tests and inter-rater agreement. *Computers in Biology and Medicine, 30,* 127–134.

McKenzie, D., Vida, S., Mackinnon, A. J., Onghena, P., & Clarke, D. (1997). Accurate confidence intervals for measures of test performance. *Psychiatry Research, 69,* 207–209.

Meehl, P. E. (1973). Why I do not attend case conferences. In P. E. Meehl (Ed.), *Psychodiagnosis: Selected papers* (pp. 225–302). Minneapolis: University of Minnesota Press.

Meehl, P. E., & Rosen, A. (1955). Antecedent probability and the efficiency of psychometric signs, patterns, or cutting scores. *Psychological Bulletin, 52,* 194–216.

Micceri, T. (1989). The unicorn, the normal curve, and other improbable creatures. *Psychological Bulletin, 105*(1), 156–166.

Mitrushina, M. N., Boone, K. B., Razani, J., & D'Elia, L. F. (2005). *Handbook of normative data for neuropsychological assessment* (2nd ed.). New York: Oxford University Press.

Morgan, J. E., & Ricker, J. H. (2018). *Textbook of clinical neuropsychology* (2nd ed.). New York: Oxford University Press.

Mossman, D. (2003). Daubert, cognitive malingering, and test accuracy. *Law and Human Behavior, 27*(3), 229–249.

Mossman, D., Miller, W. G., Lee, E. R., Gervais, R. O., Hart, K. J., & Wygant, D. B. (2015). A Bayesian approach to mixed group validation of performance validity tests. *Psychological Assessment, 27*(3), 763–776.

Mossman, D., & Somoza, E. (1992). Balancing risks and benefits: Another approach to optimizing diagnostic tests. *Journal of Neuropsychiatry and Clinical Neurosciences, 4*(3), 331–335.

Mossman, D., Wygant, D. B., & Gervais, R. O. (2012). Estimating the accuracy of neurocognitive effort measures in the absence of a "gold standard." *Psychological Assessment, 24*(4), 815–822.

Nelson, L. D. (2015). False-positive rates of reliable change indices for concussion test batteries: A Monte Carlo simulation. *Journal of Athletic Training, 50*(12), 1319–1322. doi: 10.4085/1062-6050-51.1.09. Epub 2015 Dec 17.

Nunnally, J. C., & Bernstein, I. H. (1994). *Psychometric theory* (3rd ed.). New York: McGraw-Hill.

Pearson, K. (1920). Notes on the history of correlation. *Biometrika, 13,* 25–45.

Pedhazur, E. (1997). *Multiple regression in behavioral research.* New York: Harcourt Brace.

Pepe, M. S. (2003). *The statistical evaluation of medical tests for classification and prediction.* New York: Oxford University Press.

Rorer, L. G., & Dawes, R. M. (1982). A base-rate bootstrap. *Journal of Consulting and Clinical Psychology, 50*(3), 419–425.

Slick, D. J., Hopp, G., Strauss, E., & Thompson, G. (1997). *The Victoria Symptom Validity Test.* Odessa, FL: Psychological Assessment Resources.

Strauss, E., Sherman, E. M. S., & Spreen, O. (2006). *A compendium of neuropsychological tests: Administration, norms, and commentary* (3rd ed.). New York: Oxford University Press.

Somoza, E., & Mossman, D. (1992). Comparing diagnostic tests using information theory: The INFO-ROC technique. *Journal of Neuropsychiatry and Clinical Neurosciences, 4*(2), 214–219.

Streiner, D. L. (2003). Diagnosing tests: Using and misusing diagnostic and screening tests. *Journal of Personality Assessment, 81*(3), 209–219.

Swets, J. A., Dawes, R. M., & Monahan, J. (2000). Psychological science can improve diagnostic decisions. *Psychological Science in the Public Interest, 1*(1), 1–26.

Urbina, S. (2014). *Essentials of psychological testing* (2nd ed.). Hoboken, NJ: Wiley.

Zakzanis, K. K., & Jeffay, E. (2011). Neurocognitive variability in high-functioning individuals: implications for the practice of clinical neuropsychology. *Psychological Reports, 108*(1), 290–300.

2 | VALIDITY AND RELIABILITY IN NEUROPSYCHOLOGICAL ASSESSMENT: NEW PERSPECTIVES

ELISABETH M. S. SHERMAN

THE CASE FOR UPGRADING OUR TOOLS AND OUR KNOWLEDGE

> We have made a methodical comparison between the admission certificates filled out for the same children within only a few days' interval by the doctors. . . . We have compared several hundreds of these certificates, and we think we may say without exaggeration that they looked as if they had been drawn by chance out of a sack.
>
> (Binet & Simon, 1907, p. 76)

Thankfully, this passage describes events that occurred long ago and not modern hospital admission records. It describes the conclusions reached by psychologists Binet and Simon (1907), who, in the early 1900s, while in the midst of their groundbreaking work on human intelligence and prior to the common use of standardized tests to measure intellectual ability, had reviewed the diagnoses that had been assigned to children with intellectual deficits by staff psychiatrists in four Paris hospitals: Sainte-Anne, Bicêtre, la Salpêtrière, and Vaucluse (Dahlstrom, 1993). The specific categories they reviewed were the three intellectual disability categories of "*l'idiotie*," "*l'imbécilité*," and "*la débilité mentale*." In so doing, Binet and Simon documented one of the earliest contemporary examples of weak—if not random—diagnoses assigned by clinicians unaided by validated methodological tools. It was a defining event that spurred innovators such as Binet and Simon to substantially improve assessment methods in ways that we still benefit from today and of which were born many of the fundamental notions that we now take for granted, including test validity, interrater reliability, and test-retest reliability.

The field of assessment has progressed greatly since these early days. In the not too distant past, assessing an examinee for a specific problem used to be hampered by a lack of appropriate standardized tests. Some senior neuropsychologists may even recall constructing their own testing materials to capture a specific clinical problem not adequately covered by existing instruments. The problem is now not of scarcity, but of abundance: today, there are literally thousands of cognitive tests and rating scales designed for evaluating specific cognitive and behavioral problems. Faced with this vast library of instruments, how do we choose the right test? Although the goal is easy—choose the best test for assessing a particular problem in a particular examinee for a particular purpose—in practice, there is so much information to analyze before choosing a suitable test that the clinician can easily become overwhelmed, leading users to employ tools they actually know little about. The problem is now not one of access to good tests, but access to good information that tells the user which test might be more useful than another for assessing a specific problem. This book is an attempt to provide that information for test users in a readable, easily accessible way and, most importantly, to update the knowledge base on tests so that users can make the best decisions about test selection and test interpretation.

Having up-to-date information on tests is an obvious prerequisite for good test usage and the premise of this book. But does our understanding of the fundamentals—that is, of the twin concepts of test validity and reliability—also need updating? Common mistakes still appear in our thinking, such as asking questions such as "Is this test reliable?" or "Has this test been validated?" Both these questions are unanswerable. They can only be answered once rephrased in terms of specifics, such as, "Is this test reliable enough to use in dementia screening?" or "Is there enough validation evidence to use this test to predict return to work after head injury?" Validity and reliability appear to be simple concepts, but they require updating, just as our tests and test interpretations require updating as the field moves forward. In the past few years, many established notions about validity and reliability have been increasingly questioned—and in some cases completely turned on their heads. These include sacrosanct notions including, surprisingly, whether classical test theory is still relevant in clinical assessment, whether the alpha coefficient as a measure of internal consistency has any real utility, and whether internal reliability even matters if a test is good at predicting outcomes.

From a practical perspective, a working knowledge of validity makes it easier for clinicians to choose which tests and scores to use in different circumstances and for different purposes. For instance, some tests fail to reach standards for clinical diagnostic purposes but would be perfectly appropriate for large-scale screening. Conversely, a test that clearly taps a specific psychological construct may not have any utility as a diagnostic measure of that construct but may show great utility in predicting a specific outcome of considerable practical utility. For example, an executive functioning test like the Trail Making Test is of no practical utility for making a diagnosis of adult attention deficit hyperactivity disorder (ADHD), even though ADHD is defined by the presence of executive dysfunction, but it is useful for predicting driving capacity in older adults, likely because it taps executive functioning as well as speed and scanning. The value of a test score is always interpreted in relation to a specific group, for a specific purpose.

VALIDITY IN NEUROPSYCHOLOGICAL ASSESSMENT

CHANGING DEFINITIONS OF TEST VALIDITY

As one begins to review the literature on validity, one has to agree with Newton and Shaw, who provide one of the more readable, comprehensive bird's-eye views of the field of test validity (2014). That is, it is very difficult to fully grasp the concept of test validity due to the sheer size and heterogeneity of the literature, but, most surprising, there exists at present no generally accepted, comprehensive, consensus theory of test validity. They describe the field of test validity as one of piecemeal insights, concepts, and arguments searching for the missing holy grail; even the more well-known theories have been described as "viscous" and "confused" (Newton & Shaw, 2014). Instead, the field has relied on testing standards for defining validity; that is, starting with the first standards in the 1950s, the periodically updated *Standards for Educational and Psychological Testing* (American Educational Research Association, American Psychological Association, & National Council on Measurement in Education Joint Committee [AERA, APA, & NCME], 2014). However, standards are not the same as a consensus theory of validity, and, although extremely useful, the *Standards* have been described as shorthand, oversimplified, sometimes ambiguous, and occasionally contradictory summaries of validity theories—more like a collection of heuristic principles than a definitive theory of validity—while validity continues to be heavily debated within the field despite more than 100 years of work on the question (Newton & Shaw, 2014).

One major problem is that the field of test validity uses terms that overlap with that of other disciplines—most notably, with validity in research (Newton & Shaw, 2014). Validity in research describes the evidence upon which research conclusions are based; validity for testing describes the evidence upon which testing conclusions (i.e., test interpretations) are based. The conceptual overlap between validity as a concept for research and validity as a concept for test measurement has caused all manner of confusion, in part because some of the developers of research validity theories also developed measurement validity theories (e.g., Campbell). According to Newton and Shaw, the field of research validity borrowed ideas from measurement validity, and because test validation requires research, which itself requires validation, test measurement validity then incorporated concepts borrowed from research validity (Newton & Shaw, 2014). One such concept is the idea of internal and external validity, which was first applied in research, and the concept of ecological validity, also first applied in research, which originally meant the generalization of research findings across research conditions. Ecological validity then became attached to the concept of test validity, particularly in the field of neuropsychology. To further complicate things, even the term "construct validity" is used in research, outside of the field of test validity, to describe research findings that inform on the underlying construct (Newton & Shaw, 2014).

Furthermore, the meaning of test validity has changed over time, sometimes in the same theoretical models, and some of the key theoretical accounts are simply hard to read and downright confusing (Newton & Shaw, 2014). This confusion is not helped by an exponential expansion of terms for validity subtypes—in their recent count, Newton and Shaw found more than 150 types of validity, with almost 30 being synonyms of each other. Examples include ecological, essential, external, external test, extra-test, cross-cultural, incremental, known-groups, predictive, response, structural, and theoretic validity, to name just a few.

THE HISTORY OF TEST VALIDITY

There were four waves in the history of test validity: namely, the genesis of validity from the 1800s to 1951, the fragmentation of validity from 1952 to 1974, the (re)unification of validity from 1974 to 1999, and, finally, the deconstruction of validity from 2000 to the present, fueled by a desire to simplify overcomplicated validation practices originating in earlier theories (Newton & Shaw, 2014)

Initially, the concept of test validity was spurred by the invention of the correlation coefficient by Pearson in 1896; correlations were then applied to test scores, leading to the use of the correlation coefficient as an index of test validity in the 1920s and to the notion of the validity coefficient, which tied validity to classical test theory (Markus & Borsboom, 2013). This paired well with the view of validity as being based on logical analysis of test content, with those in educational measurement typically focusing on content validity, usually in terms of item match to educational curricula, and those in aptitude measurement focusing on empirical correlation with criterion measures, using the newly minted validity coefficient (Newton & Shaw, 2014).

Cronbach and Meehl (1955) were some of the first theorists to embed the idea of construct validity into a scientific framework, emphasizing that validation was neither entirely logical (content-based) nor entirely empirical (criterion-based), but instead required generation and testing of predictions to determine the construct that accounted for test performance, particularly for tests that tapped neither achievement (content) or aptitude (predicting an outcome), but which were designed to measure a psychological attribute (personality tests; Newton & Shaw, 2014).

Nevertheless, validity stayed anchored to the concept of test-centered validity into the 1970s. Most neuropsychologists are familiar with the tripartite model of validity, which proposes three separate types of validity: content validity, construct validity, and criterion validity. The tripartite model of validity can be traced back to its historical roots and understood in a historical context originating more than 40 years ago (Urbina, 2014). It was incorporated into the 1985 *Standards* (Markus & Borsboom, 2013) and remained the main model for test validity for many years. Nevertheless, theorists were also beginning to unify the three separate validity components under the broader term of "construct validity" as the field moved toward validity models centered on test interpretations and external utility of tests rather than on test-test correlations. Some of the limitations of criterion-based validity in particular were that it did not contribute to theory development, as tests became validated only against specific criterion measures, and that there was no way to validate the specific criterion measures themselves (Strauss & Smith, 2009). Most validity theoreticians now agree that the tripartite model is an outdated model of test validity (Borsboom et al., 2004; Lissitz, 2009; Markus & Borsboom, 2013; Strauss & Smith, 2009). Consequently, traditional terms associated with or stemming from the tripartite model of validity are no longer part of the *Standards* (AERA, APA, & NCME, 2014), including the notions of concurrent, predictive, convergent, and divergent validity which were earlier components of criterion validity.

The tripartite model remained strongly ingrained in the field until the publication of the construct validity model by Messick (1989). Messick's model did not include different types of validity, as did its predecessors; instead, it proposed a unitary theory of construct validity defined as an overall judgment of the extent to which empirical evidence and theoretical rationales supported the adequacy and effectiveness of interpretations and actions resulting from test scores. In so doing, Messick's model moved validity further away from tests and toward test score interpretations, eliminating the notion of different kinds of validity in favor of different kinds of *evidence* for validation. In the model, construct validity depended on six different types of evidence, including content-related, substantive, structural, generalizability, external, and consequential evidence, forming the "evidential basis for score interpretation" (Messick, 1995, p. 743). The *Standards* (AERA, APA, & NCME, 1999) then followed suit with a model very much like Messick's, where evidence based on test content, response processes, internal structure, relations to other variables, and consequences of testing were included. Notably, the most controversial aspect of Messick's model was to include the consequences of test use as a component of validity; this concept remains embedded in the general understanding of validity, including the most current *Standards*, which also include the consequences of testing as a component of validity, although the *Standards* are somewhat vague on how this specifically applies. Some have argued that including the consequences of testing in a model for test validation conflates professional ethics, morality, and politics with test validity (see Urbina, 2014, for a more in-depth discussion of this issue). Newton and Shaw hail Messick's model as undeniably comprehensive and acknowledge that it came to dominate the world of educational and psychological measurement. It solidified the notion that all validity is construct validity and "recast all validation as laborious scientific enquiry into score meaning, encouraging evaluators to accumulate as much evidence and analysis as they could lay their hands on" (p. 22). Unfortunately, they also concluded that Messick's validity model was "very confusing, if not confused" and that it caused a legacy of rift in the field. Different approaches to investigate validity became different kinds of validity, even though the field had more or less agreed that construct validity was, in fact, simply validity.

Markus and Borsboom (2013) aptly note that unified models of test validity like Messick's require multiple kinds of validity evidence and therefore place a large burden on test developers. Note Table 2–1, which lists standard methods through which the various kind of evidence can be appraised by test users, now considered de rigueur in most large-scale test manuals. Markus and Borsboom conclude that "not every cook needs to perform the tasks of a chef, and not every builder needs to perform the tasks of an architect" (p. 12), echoing the general sentiment toward reducing the amount of evidence needed to bolster the validity of test score interpretations. This thinking is already evident in the newest *Standards*, which clearly state that not all evidence is needed for all possible usages of test scores, only the ones applicable to the particular testing situation.

Specifically, test validation is the process through which evidence is accumulated to provide the scientific basis for score interpretation. It is the process of constructing and evaluating arguments for and against the intended interpretation of test scores and their relevance to the proposed use (ADRA, APA, & MCME, 2014). A key concept in test validity is that there must be evidence for each proposition that underlies a proposed test score interpretation for a specific use. For instance, in the *Standards*, a score that predicts a given criterion

TABLE 2–1 Examples of Types of Information to Consider in Evaluating the Validity of Test Scores

Does the score tap the right content domain?	Is there evidence of. . . . Definition of construct Formulation of hypotheses to measure construct Explanation of theoretical model on which test is based Review of literature with supporting evidence Clear definition of proposed test usage Systematic review of test domain from which items are to be sampled Collection of sample of items large enough to be representative of domain and with sufficient range of difficulty for target population Selection of panel of judges for expert review, based on specific selection criteria (e.g., academic and practical backgrounds or expertise within specific subdomains) Evaluation of items by expert panel based on specific criteria such as accuracy, relevance, and bias Structural equation modeling
Are the scores reliable?	Is there evidence of. . . . Internal, test-retest, alternate form, and interrater reliability Determination of practice effects and effects of prior exposure
Does the test score relate in expected ways to other test scores?	Is there evidence of. . . . Factor analysis Intra-test correlations Correlations with other tests tapping similar domains Correlations with other tests tapping different domains
Does the test predict useful outcomes?	Is there evidence of. . . . Sensitivity to developmental and age-related changes Differential diagnostic sensitivity Clinical group differences Effect sizes Classification accuracy statistics (e.g., sensitivity, specificity, positive predictive power, negative predictive power) for accurate classification of individuals based on test scores Meta-analysis Treatment sensitivity and responsiveness Prediction studies to relate scores to specific outcomes

does not require evidence that it samples a specific content domain, and a score that samples a given content domain does not require evidence of criterion prediction. However, a score that samples a given domain and predicts a criterion must have evidence supporting both propositions. Therefore, the older view that tests had to fulfill criteria for all the different kinds of validity evidence, including content, construct, criterion, and predictive, no longer applies according to the *Standards*. No type of evidence is deemed inherently preferable to another, according to the *Standards*. Last, once the basis for a given test score interpretation has been confirmed, whether to use a specific test score rests on additional considerations, such as cost-benefit analysis and consideration of any negative consequences of use (ADRA, APA, & MCME, 2014), relating the *Standards* to the responsible use and ethics of test use. That is, does using the test outweigh any negative consequences?

CURRENT DEFINITIONS OF TEST VALIDITY

Given this history, where are we now with regards to a theory of test validity? As always, we turn to the *Standards* to provide the best gauge of current thinking on validity. Specifically, the 2014 *Standards for Educational and Psychological Testing* (ADRA, APA, & NCME, 2014) state that "Validity is the degree to which evidence and theory support the interpretation of test scores for the proposed use of the test" (p. 11).

In the previous edition of this book, we defined validity as the degree to which a test actually measures what it is intended to measure, a definition that has its roots in the validity coefficient (Newton & Shaw, 2014). Note the current definition's important shift away from tests and scores to interpretation. That is, a *test* or a *score* cannot be said to have validity or to lack validity. Rather, it is the *interpretation* of the test score that is either supported or not supported by validity evidence. That is, validity is not a property of a test or of a score, but instead is a property of the meaning attached to a test score in the specific context of test usage.

In their review, Newton and Shaw (2014) provide some of the most useful insights on the relationships among validity, measurement accuracy, and decision-making. They note that validity is concerned with accuracy of measurement but is equally concerned with the potential to make correct decisions based on those measurements. The two are inseparable, and, therefore, test validity is best understood as being tantamount to validity for decision making—although this view continues to be contested. Essentially, validity is therefore less like truth and more like plausibility (Newton & Shaw, 2014), which fits with the idea of making an informed judgment on the utility of a test based on the available evidence. Borsboom proposes to do away with the whole notion of construct validity as we now know it and to simply define validity as a property of measurement instruments that codes whether these instruments are sensitive to variation in a targeted attribute, consistent with the older notion that a test is valid if it measures what it should measure, and to anchor validity to causality (Borsboom et al., 2009; Borsboom et al., 2004).

The *Standards* introduce the notion of propositions—that is, specific claims that support the proposed interpretation for the particular purpose of testing that determine what type of evidence is important for the validation of the test (ADRA, APA, & MCME, 2014; Table 2–2).

Following a similar example in the *Standards*, when IQ scores are interpreted as a way to determine school placement for giftedness, evidence for the following propositions would be important: (1) that IQ tests are able to determine giftedness; (2) that the content of the particular IQ test is relevant to the assessment of giftedness; (3) that the test scores produce a range of scores, including those signifying giftedness; (4) that IQ test scores are not unduly influenced by extraneous variables, such as gender or ethnicity, or time of test administration; (5) that people who score highly on the IQ test will do better in a giftedness program than those who do not; and so on. Each of these propositions would then be evaluated in terms of the evidence available. Other interpretations would require different propositions that would require evidence as proof of validity. For instance, using the same IQ test as a predictor of intellectual disability rather than giftedness would require different propositions (e.g., that IQ scores correlate with scales measuring activities of daily living and predict degree of assistance needed in everyday life and so on).

TABLE 2–2 Important Concepts in Test Validity

	DEFINITION
Test validity	The degree to which all the accumulated evidence supports the intended interpretation of test scores for the proposed use A property of the meaning attached to a test score in the specific context of test usage, determined by evaluating the evidence for that interpretation
Construct	A concept, attribute or characteristic that a test score is designed to measure
Test validation	The process through which evidence is accumulated to provide the scientific basis for score interpretation
Propositions	Claims that support the proposed interpretation for the particular purpose of testing
Construct underrepresentation	The degree to which a test score fails to capture important aspects of the construct; also known as construct deficiency
Construct-irrelevant variance	The degree to which test scores are affected by processes that are extraneous to the test's intended purpose; also known as construct contamination

SOURCE: Adapted from the Standards for Educational and Psychological Testing (ADRA, APA, & NCME, 2014).

The *Standards* specify that because interpretation of a test score for a given use typically involves more than one proposition, strong evidence for one proposition does not invalidate the need for strong evidence for other propositions. However, realistically, it may be the case that a small number of compelling pieces of evidence for few propositions are preferable in most cases to weak evidence for several propositions.

Realistically, many tests in neuropsychological practice are used in multiple ways that require evidence to support a number of different test score interpretations and propositions. For example, take the Rey Auditory-Verbal Learning Test (RAVLT). The same RAVLT scores can generate a number of different interpretations and usages. Based on the review of the RAVLT in this volume, the reader can see that RAVLT scores can be used to quantify memory functioning in healthy people, detect memory decline over time, diagnose mild cognitive impairment (MCI), differentiate Alzheimer's disease (AD) from frontotemporal dementia, predict risk of all-cause dementia over a decade, predict risk of memory deficits related to epilepsy surgery, evaluate executive dysfunction in psychiatric conditions, predict reduced hippocampal volume in schizophrenia, and serve as a performance validity indicator useful in detect feigning and exaggeration of memory deficits. All of these different usages require different kinds of evidence, but some interpretations of scores (i.e., that a low score on the RAVLT indicates poor memory relative to the general population) have more evidentiary basis than others (i.e., that a low score on the RAVLT means that your hippocampus is small). Technically speaking, if the RAVLT were only used to predict hippocampal volume and had been only validated for that purpose, then it would not need studies showing that the scores are predictive of other things such as risk of dementia or that it correlates well with other memory tests. Most users will require that a test like the RAVLT have evidence supporting several levels of test score interpretation—a useful test is one that serves several purposes, particularly in neuropsychological batteries where real estate is at a premium (i.e., the best tests will serve multiple purposes while keeping the test battery as brief as possible).

As will be amply evident as the reader proceeds through this book, most well-known neuropsychological tests have multiple sources of evidence for validity in the form of factor-analytic studies, correlational studies, and clinical studies using test scores to predict specific outcomes to support various test score interpretations. It is the rare test that will have only one kind of evidence to support its use in a particular clinical scenario, but this may change as the field moves from multifactorial tests to those measuring very narrow and specific abilities. Notably, the *Standards* do not require that evidence include specific techniques, such as

TABLE 2–3 Types of Evidence for Establishing the Validity of Test Interpretations

TYPE OF EVIDENCE
Content-oriented evidence
Evidence regarding cognitive processes
Evidence regarding internal structure
Evidence regarding relationships with conceptually related constructs
Evidence regarding relationships with criteria
Evidence based on consequences of testing

SOURCE: Adapted from the Standards for Educational and Psychological Testing (ADRA, APA, & NCME, 2014), and Urbina (2014).

factor analysis, item analysis, or correlational matrices, only that the evidence support the interpretation of the test score in a specific context. Types of evidence for establishing the validity of test score interpretations are shown in Table 2–3, similar to those in Messick's model.

CONSTRUCT UNDERREPRESENTATION, CONSTRUCT OVERREPRESENTATION, AND CONSTRUCT-IRRELEVANT VARIANCE

Construct underrepresentation is the degree to which a test fails to capture important aspects of the construct; this is also known as *construct deficiency*. Conversely, *construct overrepresentation* is the degree to which test scores are affected by processes that are extraneous to the test's intended purpose; this is also known as *construct contamination*. Construct underrepresentation occurs when a test fails to capture all the aspects of the construct (ADRA, APA, & MCME, 2014). An example would be a visual memory test that includes only subtests that tap visual working memory and none that tap long-term visual memory, or using the Boston Naming Test as a reflection of an examinee's language ability when it provides only a narrow view of the broad concept of language. *Construct-irrelevant variance* occurs when test scores are unduly influenced by factors other than the construct of interest (ADRA, APA, & MCME, 2014; Table 2–2). An example is an attention test that requires high arithmetic ability, linguistic ability, and response speed and can therefore be failed for multiple reasons other than attention problems.

WHO DECIDES IF A TEST SCORE INTERPRETATION IS VALID?

Knowing the different kinds of evidence relevant to validity is a central requirement for responsible and competent test use. The shift from test to interpretation also highlights another shift: the shift from test developer to test user. As was stated in the previous *Standards*, validation is the joint responsibility of the test developer and of the test user. That is, the test user is ultimately the final judge of whether a particular test interpretation is appropriate. This parallels a similar situation inherent to medico-legal settings in which neuropsychologists are asked to provide an opinion based on the preponderance of the evidence (i.e., based on the degree of probable accuracy of the available evidence, rather than simply on the amount of available evidence). In the same way, the test user must make a determination of test validity based on the preponderance of the validation evidence (ADRA, APA, & MCME, 2014). The test user is therefore ultimately responsible for evaluating the evidence for and against the interpretation in the specific circumstances in which the test is given. Importantly, the decision may vary depending on the stakes involved (ADRA, APA, & MCME, 2014). More extensive and higher level evidence will be required for high-stakes testing interpretations, such as those involving the determination of disability, medico-legal opinion, and criminal responsibility.

Because specific intrinsic and extrinsic factors can affect validity, including deviations from standard administration, unusual testing environments, and variables relating to examinees themselves, when a test score interpretation differs from that specified by the test developer, it is the test user who must furnish the evidence that the particular interpretation remains valid for the particular "off-label" use of the test score (ADRA, APA, & NCME, 2014).

THE VALIDATION THAT NEVER ENDS

In the previous edition of this book, we stated that determining test validity was never actually finalized because evidence for or against a specific test score interpretation must be continually updated as populations, testing contexts, and the scientific literature change over time. This concept was the basis for Messick's view that validation is a "never-ending process" (Messick, 1989) that can, by its very nature, never provide a final, conclusive opinion on whether a test measures a specific construct. This view has been seriously challenged. Specifically, Borsboom has argued that the conceptualization of validity as beyond our understanding makes construct validity into "a black hole from which nothing can escape" because it can never yield a definitive answer as to whether a test score actually measures a specific construct or not. He argues that construct validity should be addressed *before* or *during* test construction, not afterward (Borsboom, 2006). Therefore, instruments with weak construct validity would simply never see the light of day, and tests where the user has to continually ask, "What does this test measure?" or "How does this test work?" would simply not be sent out for use in the real world (Borsboom, 2006). To be fair to test developers, although the argument is compelling, few large-scale, modern, commercially available neuropsychological instruments are created without first undergoing extensive piloting and trial versions, therefore ensuring that tests arrive to market with considerable evidence of their validity already established, as we have witnessed over successive editions of this book. While the first edition contained several tests with limited norms and validity evidence, most neuropsychological tests in current usage tend toward comprehensive, well-validated tests rather than the small-sample, "homemade," bedside tests that characterized the field in the early days. As to whether test validation is ever "finished" for a specific test score, a better way to frame the question would be to ask whether the evidence is sufficient for using the test in a specific examinee, for a specific goal, at the specific point in time when the test is being used.

WHAT IS AN ADEQUATE VALIDITY COEFFICIENT?

While the validity coefficient is but one aspect of validity, one classic method for presenting validity evidence is through intercorrelations among tests that are believed to measure similar and dissimilar constructs. Realistically, many tests do not yield clear-cut correlation matrices with high correlations to similar tests and low correlations to dissimilar tests; in fact, some tests manuals include very few dissimilar measures in their validation sections. Whenever large numbers of correlations among measures are presented, there tends to be expected and unexpected relationships between variables, and dissociable relations between tests may not occur in a clear-cut manner. Some of the common variance may be due to global factors, such as underlying innate intelligence, or to the fact that most neuropsychological tests require multiple basic abilities.

Validity coefficients involving psychological test scores are thought to rarely exceed .30 or .40, given the complexities involved in measuring and predicting human behavior (Nunnally & Bernstein, 1994). The tests reviewed in this volume indicate that, generally speaking, two tests that tap the same cognitive domain and use similar testing formats tend to have much higher correlations than .40, typically in the .70 to .80 range. Similarly, correlations between two versions of the same test (i.e., two consecutive IQ test versions) may have correlations as high as .90 or more. Typically, tests that tap similar domains but have very different testing formats, such as an objective attention test and a subjective rating scale of attention skills in everyday life, may attain only modest correlations, in the .30 range and, in some cases, even lower than that. Importantly, tests with even quite modest correlations with specific outcome variables (say, a correlation of .30 between an executive functioning test and risk of substance abuse) may be of considerable utility depending on the circumstances in which they will be used, particularly if they serve to significantly increase the test's "hit rate" over chance or in combination with other variables (Urbina, 2014). Urbina (2014) also emphasizes that coefficients in the .20s and .30s are not uncommon in predictive validity studies and must be considered in the light of the multifactorial nature of test scores and evaluated against the predictive ability of other alternative predictors which are often lacking.

RELIABILITY IN NEUROPSYCHOLOGY

Reliability refers to measurement precision (accuracy) and consistency (Newton & Shaw, 2014; Urbina, 2014). It is a property of test scores, not of tests (Urbina, 2014). A reliable test score will be minimally affected by measurement error, whereas an unreliable score will be greatly affected by measurement error. *Measurement error* can be conceptualized as all the factors that distort the test score and which do not reflect the actual construct being measured. Measurement error as a whole includes different kinds of error, including errors introduced by interscorer differences, time sampling, content sampling, and inter-item inconsistency (Urbina, 2014).

Whether a test score is reliable is determined through evaluation of different kinds of reliability evidence that tell us the degree to which the score is free from measurement error. These include the consistency across test items (*internal reliability* or internal consistency), consistency over time (*test-retest reliability* or test stability), consistency across alternate forms (*alternate form reliability*), and consistency across raters (*interrater reliability*). Reliability coefficients can be conceptualized as falling along a continuum where scores are perfectly unreliable (r = .00) or perfectly reliable (r = 1.00).

HOW DOES RELIABILITY FIT IN WITH VALIDITY?

In the field of measurement, one often hears that it is possible to have a reliable score that is not valid, but it is impossible to have a valid score that is not reliable. High reliability does not necessarily translate into high validity; some constructs that can be measured with a high degree of precision are of little value clinically. Similarly, current thinking now indicates that it is perhaps acceptable to use a test score that is slightly unreliable yet valid for a specific purpose. Interestingly, the notion that reliability defines the upper limit of validity—that is, that a reliable test may have good validity, but an unreliable test will always have poor validity—is now seen by some as incorrect and best viewed as a maxim rather than as a fact (Markus & Borsboom, 2013). The notion can be traced back to early classical test theory models where validity was defined by the size of the correlation coefficient between a test and a criterion measure; this could be adjusted upward or downward based on the reliability coefficient of the tests (i.e., using the attenuation formula). The notion that reliability is the essential quality that limits validity is based on a validity theory to which few now subscribe because it focuses exclusively on test scores, not on test score interpretations (Markus & Borsboom, 2013). If validity equals measurement quality, then reliability can be seen as a technical component of validity, one that taps measurement consistency but which is only one component of validity (Newton & Shaw, 2014).

Nevertheless, some general principles continue to be reasonable. This includes, when faced with deciding between test scores with varying reliability, choosing the score with slightly lower but adequate evidence of reliability if that score has evidence of superior validity (Nunnally & Bernstein, 1994).

CAN ALL CONSTRUCTS BE MEASURED RELIABLY?

There are some neuropsychological domains that are difficult to measure in a highly reliable manner. Thus, even though there is the assumption that questionable reliability is always a function of measurement error, reliability may depend on the nature of the cognitive process measured and on the nature of the population evaluated. For example, many executive functioning test scores have relatively modest reliabilities, suggesting that this ability is difficult to assess reliably. Other tests may yield low coefficients in groups with atypical score distributions, such as the very old, the very young, or individuals with brain disorders. In the end, a score with high reliability will always be preferred to that with low reliability, but only if it has sufficient validity evidence for the purpose for which it was designed.

INTERNAL RELIABILITY

Internal reliability, a core concept in classical test theory, reflects the *extent to which the individual items within a test measure the same cognitive domain or construct*. Low internal reliability generally means that a test is made up of items that do not measure the same construct or are more heterogeneous than those of tests with high internal reliability. IQ tests are a class of tests that typically are designed to have scores with very high internal reliability, whereas instruments designed to sample a variety of content domains over few items will have lower internal reliabilities (e.g., cognitive screeners such as the Repeatable Battery for the Assessment of Neuropsychological Status [RBANS]). Generally speaking, a score based on a test with more items will typically have higher internal consistency than a scale with few items.

Internal reliability is usually assessed with an estimate of the average correlation among items within the test. The most well-known method is to use Cronbach's alpha coefficient as an estimate of internal reliability. Cronbach's alpha is the average of all the correlations between items. However, the method has been criticized for being an inadequate measure of internal reliability, first, because it provides a lower bound of the true reliability and, second, because it does not adequately measure whether a test is in fact unidimensional, and this is best assessed via other methods such as confirmatory factor analysis (Bowden & Finch, 2017). High internal reliability cannot be equated with a single-factor solution of unidimensionality, which is incorrect; a one-factor test can have any alpha value (Sijtsma, 2009). Instead, internal reliability informs only on the average degree of interrelatedness of items but says very little about internal consistency per se; for these reasons, the alpha coefficient is now viewed by some as obsolete, with other coefficients such as the greatest lower bound (glb) or omega (ω) coefficient recommended instead (Sijtsma, 2009). One recommendation is to use ω when all items are normally distributed, followed by alpha, and to use glb when the proportion of asymmetrical items is high (Trizano-Hermosilla & Alvarado, 2016; see also Revelle & Zinbarg, 2009).

TABLE 2–4 Methods for Evaluating Internal Reliability

METHOD	DESCRIPTION
Cronbach's alpha	Provides a general estimate of reliability based on all the possible ways of splitting test items Based on the average intercorrelation between test items and any other set of items
Split-half or Spearman-Brown	Obtained by correlating two halves of items from the same test
Kuder-Richardson	Used for items with dichotomous answers (i.e., yes/no, true/false), or heterogeneous tests where split-half methods must be used (i.e., the mean of all the different split-half coefficients if the test were split into all possible ways)

Internal reliability can also be evaluated by calculating the *split-half* or *Spearman-Brown reliability coefficient*, or the *Kuder-Richardson reliability coefficient* (also known as KR20). Descriptions of these different methods are presented in Table 2–4.

One major limitation of internal reliability as a measure of test validation is that it, by definition, provides information on only a single administration of a test, contrary to classical test theory which is based on infinite parallel forms of a test, and thus provides little information about accuracy (Sijtsma, 2009). In addition, there is no such thing as a single internal consistency estimate for a given test score. Like other kinds of reliability, internal reliability varies with sample characteristics. That is, internal consistency can vary across different age groups and different clinical groups for the same test score.

TEST-RETEST RELIABILITY AND PRACTICE EFFECTS

One of the biggest mistakes test users can make is to confound real change with expected variability attributable to measurement error and practice effects. Two scores will almost always be different to some degree from test to retest in the absence of real change, but these apparent score differences are readily explainable once the psychometric properties of the test are understood (Bowden & Finch, 2017). This requires a basic understanding of test-retest coefficients and practice effects.

Test-retest reliability provides an estimate of the correlation between scores on a test administered twice over a given time interval. A test score with high test-retest reliability will show little change over time. IQ tests are an example of tests designed a priori to capture stable estimates of an individual's ability levels; these typically have high test-retest correlations. Tests measuring dynamic (i.e., changeable) abilities such as attention or mood may have lower test-retest reliabilities than tests measuring domains that are more trait-like and stable. In most neuropsychological contexts, the evaluation will tap different domains that are expected to vary along a continuum of stable to changeable, but a minimum degree of test-retest stability is expected for all test scores, typically at least .60 or higher depending on the domain assessed.

The size of the test-retest coefficient is influenced by subject characteristics as well as by the interval between test and retest. Across tests, there is no standard time interval for test-retest reliability, which complicates comparisons across tests. Most stability coefficients and practice effects provided in test manuals are based on a single sample of healthy adults retested over a relatively brief interval, typically over intervals of 2–6 weeks. This contrasts sharply with the typical clinical scenario, where a patient would be reassessed after 6 months to a year, for example, to assess for recovery from brain injury or to track ongoing decline from a progressive neurological condition such as dementia. Only some tests provide test-retest reliability coefficients and expected practice effects for longer intervals that mirror more closely what happens clinically. Rarely, some tests provide reliability estimates over longer intervals of a year or more, but these are exceptions in the field.

As a general rule, the shorter the time interval between test and retest, the higher the retest reliability coefficient. However, the extent to which the time interval affects the test-retest coefficient will depend on the type of ability evaluated (i.e., stable vs. more variable) and the type of individual being assessed because some groups are intrinsically more variable than others. Score fluctuations over time may depend on examinee characteristics, including age (e.g., younger adults tending to produce more stable scores than older adults) and neurological status (e.g., healthy people tending to produce more stable scores than brain-injured people). Because this may not necessarily occur in expected patterns across age or demographics, test-retest reliability estimates should ideally be provided for both a range of healthy individuals and a range of clinical populations.

One of the most significant influences on tests readministered after a period of time is the *practice effect.* Readministering a test would be expected to yield better performance at retest, and this is the case in most instances. However, not all persons necessarily show a positive practice effect on retest, especially in some clinical populations. An examinee may approach tests that they had difficulty with previously with heightened anxiety that leads to decreased performance, or with increased boredom and disengagement once familiar with the test leading to more random responses and lower scores. Conversely, practice effects and other effects of prior exposure may also plateau after several exposures, leading to a more accurate measurement of the construct being assessed; tests whose practice effects plateau are typically those involving attention or speed. Notably, readministering questionnaires measuring subjective psychological or cognitive symptoms may yield slight improvements in test scores over time due to prior exposure to test items without necessarily signifying a change in clinical status.

The actual nature of the test may also change with reexposure. For instance, tests that rely on a one-time novelty effect—for example, requiring the examinee to solve a problem or deduce a strategy—may not be performed in the same way once the examinee has prior familiarity with the testing paradigm. Examples include the Wisconsin Card Sorting Test and the Category test, both reviewed in this volume. Thus, some tests may simply not be amenable to being administered multiple times in the same examinee.

The size of a retest reliability coefficient does not indicate the magnitude of practice effects, and reliability coefficients do not provide information on which individuals retain their relative place in the distribution from baseline to retest and which individuals encounter score increases or decreases on retesting. A test score can have a high test-retest coefficient yet have a retest mean that is several points higher than its baseline score. Overall, two main questions must be answered to properly interpret scores in a retest situation: (a) What is the magnitude of the typical expected practice effect? and (b) Is the practice effect expected to be consistent across individuals in the group from which the examinee originates? The practical problem for clinicians is that while most test manuals provide some information on mean practice effects across groups, there are no good methods in test manuals for determining the probability of a known practice effect occurring for an individual examinee. This is because the majority of practice effects are estimated in healthy subjects, not clinical subjects, and are averaged for the group, with little information provided regarding the distribution of practice effects across individuals. The average practice effect may only apply for a subset of the sample itself. Certain subgroups may benefit more from prior exposure than others (e.g., individuals with above average intelligence), just as some subgroups may demonstrate more stable scores. Nevertheless, practice effects, as long as they are relatively systematic and accurately assessed, do not make tests unusable for clinical practice. The key is knowing the expected practice effect, adjusting retest scores accordingly, and comparing change scores against a cumulative frequency distribution to determine how frequently a particular test-retest difference occurs in the normative sample (see Chapter 1).

Last, it must be kept in mind that factors other than prior exposure may affect test-retest reliability. Variability in scores on the same measure over time can be related to situational variables such as examinee state, examiner state, examiner identity (same vs. different at retest), and environmental conditions (same vs. different at retest). With all the different sources of error that can potentially confound measurement at retest, it is quite remarkable that so many tests reviewed in this volume have strong test-retest reliability coefficients.

ALTERNATE FORM RELIABILITY

Alternate forms are designed to eliminate the confounding effects of practice when a test is administered more than once. However, alternate forms can introduce another type of error variance, called *content sampling error*, in addition to the time sampling error that accumulates when a test is repeatedly administered over time (Lineweaver & Chelune, 2003). Thus, tests with alternate forms must employ rigorous psychometric standards to avoid introducing new sources of error. Practically speaking, it can be very challenging to create alternate forms with the exact same difficulty level, leading to score differences on retest that are not due to real change. Nevertheless, even though psychometrically equivalent alternate forms are possible, prior exposure to similar stimuli and procedures can improve retest scores because of format familiarity and procedural learning effects despite the use of different test items. Thus, it is possible for mean scores to be higher when retesting with an alternate form even though the examinee may not have been previously exposed to the actual content of the test items. Ideally, practice effects for alternate forms also need to be known or ruled out. Practically speaking, this information is usually lacking for tests.

INTERRATER RELIABILITY

Interrater reliability refers to the degree of consensus between different raters in scoring items. Test manuals provide specific and detailed instructions on how to administer and score tests according to standard procedures in order to reduce the chances of introducing additional error due to different examiners and scorers. However, some degree of examiner variance remains in individually administered tests, particularly when scores involve a degree of judgment in the scoring procedure. Although many tests are administered and scored in a straightforward manner, such that a wrong answer is unequivocally wrong, there are other tests that have a subjective component that requires detailed scoring instructions because of the potential for examiner variance. When this is the case, an estimate of the consistency of scores across examiners is needed as additional evidence for the reliability of the test. See Table 2–5 for examples of statistical methods for evaluating interrater reliability.

ALTERNATIVES TO CLASSICAL TEST THEORY

GENERALIZABILITY THEORY

Classical test theory considers all error to be attributable to random variation among theoretically parallel test forms and is thus unable to handle error that arises out of specific sources, such as the use of different raters or different testing situations (Markus & Borsboom, 2013). *Generalizability theory*, also known as *G theory*, is a method to directly address sources of error other than random error, to identify each type of error, and to evaluate the single and combined effect of different sources of error, including, unlike other approaches, the impact of interaction effects between different kinds of error (Brennan, 2001; Cronbach et al., 1972; Shavelson & Webb, 1991; Urbina, 2014).

TABLE 2–5 Statistical Methods for Evaluating Interrater Reliability

METHOD	EXPLANATION
Percent agreement	This technique is used for nominal data such as classifications or ratings. The number of times each rating is assigned by each rater is divided by the total number of ratings. This method assumes that the data are nominal, and it does not adjust for chance agreement between raters.
Kappa	Cohen's kappa is used for comparing two raters; Fleiss's kappa for more than two raters. This technique takes into account the amount of agreement that would be expected to occur by chance. However, the data are treated as nominal.
Pearson's product-moment correlation Spearman's rank correlation	Pearson's coefficient is used for continuous data, Spearman's for ordinal data. Both involve pairwise correlations between the scores of raters. However, because this technique does not take into account the magnitude of the score differences between raters, the scores of two raters could yield a perfect correlation, yet not agree (e.g., Rater 1 = 1, 2, 3, 4; Rater 2 = 7, 8, 9, 10).
Intraclass correlation coefficient (ICC)	The ICC reflects the proportion of variance of an observation due to between-subject variability in the true scores. The ICC will be high when there is little variation between the scores assigned to each item by the raters.
Mean differences and confidence intervals (Bland-Altman plot)	This technique provides information on agreement between raters, and identifies any biases among raters through the derivation of two indices: (a) the mean of the differences between the two raters, and (b) confidence intervals reflecting agreement. If the raters tend to agree, the mean will be near zero. If one rater is usually higher than the other by a consistent amount, the mean will be greater than zero, but the confidence interval will be narrow. If the raters tend to disagree, but without a consistent pattern of one rating higher than the other, the mean will be near zero but the confidence interval will be wide. This information can be graphed using a Bland-Altman plot.

In generalizability theory, the estimate of reliability is the generalizability coefficient. Like classical test theory, this estimate depends on the amount of variance in the population studied. The generalizability coefficient is therefore not a property of the test itself, but of the interaction of the test and the population in which it was administered (Markus & Borsboom, 2013). Generalizability theory uses the general linear model; *between-groups variance* is considered an estimate of true score variance, and *within-group variance* is considered an estimate of error variance. The generalizability coefficient is the ratio of estimated true variance to the sum of the estimated true variance and estimated error variance.

Although it requires a considerable amount of data on all sources of error for the same sample (i.e., test-retest variance, alternate form variance, inter-scorer variance), it provides a more accurate estimation of the reliability of scores by differentiating between sources of variance and by parsing variance effects. Generalizability theory identifies the sources of systematic and unsystematic error variance among the overall undifferentiated error variance in test scores and provides an estimate of magnitude for each error type (Webb & Shavelson, 2005). It therefore has the potential to provide test developers with critical information on how to decrease error if major sources of error can be identified and corrected.

ITEM RESPONSE THEORY

Item response theory (IRT) refers to a variety of complex mathematical procedures and mathematical models used to develop and evaluate tests that consider the test taker and the test items as two separate but equally critical dimensions. Unlike classical test theory, where the focus is on the overall test, in IRT, the focus is on the examinee's performance on test items, with each item carefully selected and calibrated to provide information on a specific construct via mathematical models of the relationship between the abilities or latent traits the test is measuring. Unlike classical test theory that considers a test score to be a sampling from a theoretically infinite populations of observations, IRT considers the test score to be a manifestation of an underlying latent variable (Markus & Borsboom, 2013). As well, unlike classical test theory and generalizability theory, which both provide reliability estimates based on the use of a specific test in a specific population (i.e., test-by-population interaction), in modern test theory, latent variable models evaluate measurement precision conditionally on the latent variable (Markus & Borsboom, 2013). In IRT, reliability is determined based on individual test items with regard to difficulty level and discriminability (Urbina, 2014). As explained by Urbina (2014), IRT item selection is optimally suited to test taker levels and inappropriate items are removed, resulting in a shorter, more reliable test with more informative test items. The *Rasch model* is one type of IRT model, although some consider it separate from IRT. A detailed review of IRT and Rasch models is beyond the scope of this book.

WHAT KIND OF RELIABILITY EVIDENCE MATTERS MOST?

As we have discussed, tests cannot be described simply as "reliable" or "unreliable." Rather, the relative importance of one kind of reliability evidence over another will depend on how the test score will be used, with whom, and for what purpose. For instance, a demanding attention test may be highly reliable in healthy young adults but yield unreliable scores in older individuals due to the test introducing too much measurement error stemming from normal age-related decreases in visual and motor functioning.

Given the different kinds of reliability evidence, which one matters most when choosing a test for clinical use? Some have argued that evidence for internal reliability is most important—thus, if alpha is low (regardless of other levels of reliability evidence), a test score should not be considered reliable. However, some tests yield scores with relatively low alpha values yet possess high test-retest reliability. Examples are tests that are made up of heterogeneous items that yield stable scores at retest, such as certain dementia screening instruments. Internal consistency is therefore not necessarily the primary index of reliability, but should be evaluated within the broader context of test-retest and interrater reliability (Cicchetti, 1994).

What about test-retest reliability? Does it need to be considered if the test will only be used once and is not likely to be administered again in future? Test-retest coefficients are essential for evaluating a test's utility because they provide a measure of the degree to which test scores are replicable and stable. For example, a clinician must be reasonably certain that the IQ or memory score obtained now is a good estimate of that person's functioning in future if that score is to be used for educational planning or for making a diagnosis regarding a permanent condition such as cognitive disability or dementia. Test scores will have limited clinical utility if they cannot be trusted to give a reasonable estimate of a person's functioning in the future. In most clinical applications, it is the evidence for test-retest reliability that is the most important aspect of reliability to scrutinize.

Overall, selecting tests—and equally important, selecting test scores—requires that a clinician use an informed and pragmatic rather than a dogmatic approach to evaluating the utility of test scores for clinical decision making. If the goal is to measure a specific, narrowly defined construct or content area, then high internal reliability might be the most important consideration. High test-retest reliability is usually a requirement of most clinical situations, but it may be considered less important if the test is specifically designed to measure state variables that fluctuate. For example, if a depression symptom scale is composed entirely of extremely stable items that are completely resistant to change, it will not be sensitive to treatment-related effects and would be a poor choice for determining whether a patient has benefited from an antidepressant drug regimen. One way around the problem of low test-retest reliability may be to use multiple measures of the specific construct and seek converging evidence to support clinical inferences. Test-retest correlations will necessarily be lower than those for internal reliability because they are subject to more sources of variation, as are, for the same reasons, long-term test-retest correlations versus those measured over shorter intervals (Urbina, 2014).

HOW TO SELECT A GOOD TEST

The selection of neuropsychological measures requires a careful and thoughtful process that involves sifting through multiple sources of psychometric evidence. This depends heavily on test publishers' ability to include comprehensive information in test manuals that clinicians need for selecting and administering tests, but it is equally incumbent on clinicians to review this information carefully before proceeding to use a particular test. Just because a test has a particular construct in its name is no guarantee that the test actually measures that construct.

Pragmatically speaking, all the theoretical validity models in the world will be of no utility to the practicing clinician unless they can be translated into specific, step-by-step procedures for evaluating the potential utility of tests, to say nothing of the validity of specific test score interpretations stemming from the use of the test. Table 2–6 presents a comprehensive but not exhaustive list of specific features that users can look for when evaluating a test for possible use and what to look for in test manuals. Few tests will satisfy each condition, but a good test should have sufficient evidence satisfying a number of points in the table. This evidence might include factor analysis, subtest intercorrelations, correlations with other tests, and responsivity to treatment effects. Obviously, not all tests will have sufficient evidence to be useful for all examinees and usages, but test users should have a sufficiently broad knowledge of neuropsychological tools to be able to select one test over another for a specific examinee or usage based on the quality of the validation evidence available. In essence, we have used this model to critically evaluate all the tests reviewed in this volume.

WHEN NOT TO TEST

Last, and most importantly, and even though this book is all about testing, sometimes it is simply not appropriate to test. Urbina (2014) provides a useful reminder of the very real circumstances in which tests should not be used; these speak for themselves and are reproduced in Table 2–7.

TABLE 2–6 Questions to Ask When Choosing Tests for Clinical Use

Does it have the right content?

- Has the operationalization of the construct (i.e., the translation of theory into test items) been done carefully (e.g., systematic review of the domain from which items are to be sampled)?
- Does the test have a large enough sample of items to be representative of the domain measured?
- Do the items have sufficient range of difficulty for the target population?
- Were items generated with care, using experts in the field or items from previously validated scales?
- Was the final item pool evaluated by experts in the field for accuracy and relevance?
- Has bias been adequately evaluated?

Is it a good measure of the construct you need to assess?

- Is there a theoretical model?
- Is there a literature review with supporting evidence?
- Has the construct being measured been well defined?
- Were hypotheses generated to measure the construct?
- Does the test score correlate highly with other test scores measuring the same construct?
- Does it have low correlations with test scores measuring different constructs?
- Do factor-analytic studies support the construct measured by the test score as it is operationalized in the test?
- Are factor-analytic and correlational findings consistent with the theoretical background for the construct measured?

Will the test be able to predict the right outcomes?

- Is the test score sensitive to expected developmental, demographic, or other differences in the sample?
- Do group difference studies support the test score?
- Do classification accuracy statistics (e.g., positive and negative predictive power) support the use of the test score?
- Are there meta-analytic studies on the test score's usage in the population of interest?
- Is the test score sensitive to treatment effects (e.g., responsiveness)?

TABLE 2–7 Top 10 Reasons for Not Using Tests

1. The purpose of the testing is unknown or unclear to the user.
2. The test user is not completely familiar with all of the necessary test documentation or trained on the procedures related to the test.
3. The test user does not know where the test results will go or how they will be used, or cannot safeguard their use.
4. The information that is sought from testing is already available or can be gathered more efficiently through other sources.
5. The test taker is not willing or able to cooperate with the testing.
6. The test taker is likely to incur some harm due to the testing process itself.
7. The environmental setting and conditions for the testing are inadequate.
8. The test format or materials are inappropriate in light of the test taker's age, sex, cultural/linguistic background, disability status, or any other condition that might invalidate the test data.
9. The test norms are outdated, inadequate, or inapplicable for the test taker.
10. The documentation on the reliability and validity of test scores is inadequate.

SOURCE: From Urbina (2014).

REFERENCES

American Educational Research Association, American Psychological Association, & National Council on Measurement in Education. (1999). *Standards for educational and psychological testing*. Washington, DC: American Psychological Association.

American Educational Research Association, American Psychological Association, & National Council on Measurement in Education, Joint Committee on Standards for Educational and Psychological Testing (US). (2014). *Standards for educational and psychological testing*. Washington, DC: AERA.

Binet, A., & Simon, T. (1907). *Les enfants anormaux*. Paris: Armond Colin.

Borsboom, D. (2006). The attack of the psychometricians. *Psychometrika, 71*(3), 425–440.

Borsboom, D., Cramer, A. O. J., Kievit, R. A., Scholten, A. Z., & Franić, S. (2009). The end of construct validity. In R. W. Lissitz (Ed.), *The concept of validity: Revisions, new directions, and applications* (pp. 135–170). Charlotte, NC: IAP Information Age Publishing.

Borsboom, D., Mellenbergh, G. J., & van Heerden, J. (2004). The concept of validity. *Psychological Review, 111*(4), 1061–1071.

Bowden, S., & Finch, S. (2017). When is a test reliable enough and why does it matter? In S. Bowden (Ed.), *Neuropsychological assessment in the age of evidence-based practice: Diagnostic and treatment recommendations* (pp. 95–119). New York: Oxford University Press.

Brennan, R. L. (2001). *Generalizability theory*. New York: Springer-Verlag.

Cicchetti, D. V. (1994). Guidelines, criteria, and rules of thumb for evaluating normed and standardized assessment instruments in psychology. *Psychological Assessment, 6*(4), 284–290.

Cronbach, L. J., & Meehl, P. E. (1955). Construct validity in psychological tests. *Psychological Bulletin, 52*(4), 281–302.

Cronbach, L. J., Gleser, G. C., Nanda, H., & Rajaratnam, N. (1972). *The dependability of behavioral measurements: Theory of generalizability for scores and profiles*. New York: Wiley.

Dahlstrom, W. G. (1993). Small samples, large consequences. *American Psychologist, 48*(4), 393–399.

Lineweaver, T. T., & Chelune, G. J. (2003). Use of the WAIS III and WMS III in the context of serial assessments: Interpreting reliable and meaningful change. In D. S. Tulsky, D. H. Saklofske, G. J. Chelune, R. K. Heaton, R. Ivnik, R. Bornstein, A. Prifitera, & M. F. Ledbetter (Eds.), *Clinical interpretation of the WAIS III and WMS III* (pp. 303–337). New York: Academic Press.

Lissitz, R. W. (Ed.). (2009). *The concept of validity: Revisions, new directions and applications* (1st ed.). Charlotte, NC: Information Age Publishing.

Markus, K. A., & Borsboom, D. (2013). *Frontiers of test validity theory: Measurement, causation, and meaning*. New York: Routledge.

Messick, S. (1989). Validity. In R. L. Linn (Ed.), *Educational measurement* (3rd ed., pp. 13–103). New York: American Council on Education/Macmillan.

Messick, S. (1995). Validity of psychological assessment: Validation of inferences from persons' responses and performances as scientific inquiry into score meaning. *American Psychologist, 50*(9), 741–749.

Newton, P., & Shaw, S. (2014). *Validity in educational and psychological assessment*. Washington, DC: SAGE.

Nunnally, J. C., & Bernstein, I. H. (1994). *Psychometric theory* (3rd ed.). New York: McGraw Hill.

Revelle, W., & Zinbarg, R. E. (2009). Coefficients alpha, beta, omega, and the glb: Comments on Sijtsma. *Psychometrika, 74*(1), 145. https://doi.org/10.1007/s11336-008-9102-z

Shavelson, R. J., & Webb, N. M. (1991). *Generalizability theory: A primer*. Newbury Park, CA: SAGE.

Sijtsma, K. (2009). On the use, the misuse, and the very limited usefulness of Cronbach's alpha. *Psychometrika, 74*(1), 107. https://doi.org/10.1007/s11336-008-9101-0

Strauss, M. E., & Smith, G. T. (2009). Construct validity: advances in theory and methodology. *Annual Review of Clinical Psychology, 5*, 1–25. https://doi.org/10.1146/annurev.clinpsy.032408.153639

Trizano-Hermosilla, I., & Alvarado, J. M. (2016). Best alternatives to Cronbach's alpha reliability in realistic conditions: Congeneric and asymmetrical measurements. *Frontiers in Psychology, 7*. https://doi.org/10.3389/fpsyg.2016.00769

Urbina, S. (2014). *Essentials of psychological testing* (2nd ed.). Hoboken, NJ: Wiley.

Webb, N. M., & Shavelson, R. J. (2005). Generalizability theory: Overview. In B. S. Everitt & D. C. Howell (Eds.), *Encyclopedia of statistics in behavioral science, Vol. 2* (pp. 717–719). Chichester, UK: John Wiley & Sons.

3 | PERFORMANCE VALIDITY, SYMPTOM VALIDITY, AND MALINGERING CRITERIA

ELISABETH M. S. SHERMAN

WHY VALIDITY TESTING MATTERS

Neuropsychological opinion is critical in determining whether cognitive deficits are legitimate. This is because neuropsychologists are one of the few assessment professionals—if not the only assessment professionals—who have sophisticated, evidence-based tools to make this determination. Neuropsychological opinion is therefore virtually irreplaceable in settings where there are external incentives for successfully feigning, exaggerating, or fabricating cognitive deficits.

External incentives are intrinsic to certain kinds of referrals sent to neuropsychologists. External incentives may be financial, such as financial settlements in personal injury litigation and wage replacement in disability and workers' compensation claims, but may also include avoidance of duties, such as discharge from military duty and avoidance of criminal prosecution or, in some countries, avoidance of the death penalty in criminal sentencing. Certain diagnoses bring with them financial support and access to services (intellectual disability), accommodations in academic and work settings (Attention Deficit/Hyperactivity Disorder [ADHD], learning disability), and access to controlled substances (ADHD, chronic pain). As highlighted elsewhere in this book, the percentage of examinees who feign, exaggerate, or fabricate cognitive deficits during neuropsychological evaluation ranges from 5% in general medical evaluations to 20–40% in personal injury and disability evaluations and up to 50% or higher in criminal justice, penal, and military settings.

However, there is increased awareness among practitioners that examinees seen in traditional clinical settings such as clinics, hospitals, schools, and nonforensic private practices may also not perform to the best of their ability for a variety of reasons and that tools are required to identify invalid performance so that test results can be interpreted correctly. Apart from the issue of external incentives, examinees may simply choose to or not be able to fully engage in the assessment process due to situational factors such as illness, oppositional behavior, disengagement, discomfort, fatigue, or other factors. Regardless of the reason, neuropsychologists need to be able to detect which scores accurately reflect the examinee's actual cognitive level and symptom picture and which do not. This is a prerequisite of accurate clinical assessment.

WHAT IS A VALIDITY TEST?

Regardless of the setting or the reason for the assessment, examiners need to have confidence that the scores they have obtained are valid. An examinee's performance is deemed to be valid when it provides an accurate estimate of that examinee's actual skill level, as measured for a specific purpose and circumstance. Validity tests are designed specifically to check the accuracy of test scores to help the examiner identify scores that are not reflective of the examinee's actual skill level or symptom picture. This is different from the term *validity* as usually defined in psychometrics, which involves gathering evidence about whether a test measures what it is intended to measure (i.e., test validity). In contrast, a *validity test* tells the user whether a test score adequately captured a reasonably good estimate of the examinee's ability or symptoms. Validity testing is the direct assessment of cognition and of self-reported symptoms using standardized measures designed for that purpose. Validity testing allows practitioners to make decisions about examinee behavior (i.e., Is the examinee likely feigning or exaggerating symptoms?) and about the utility of scores (i.e., Is the score interpretable?).

Measures designed to assess the validity of cognitive test scores, including the validity of domains like memory or attention, are known as *performance validity tests* (PVTs; Larrabee, 2012). PVTs flag results indicative of invalid performance. Measures designed to assess the validity of self- or informant-reported symptoms or behaviors, such as those measured by most standardized questionnaires, are known as *symptom validity tests* (SVTs; Larrabee, 2012). SVTs flag self-reported symptoms indicative of distortion (i.e., overreporting, implausible reporting, or inconsistent reporting). PVTs and SVTs are not tests of malingering. The determination of malingering depends on meeting accepted, multidimensional malingering criteria that encompass not only PVTs and SVTs, but also the totality of the assessment findings including psychometric, observational, and documentary sources of evidence.

Most PVTs are standalone tests added to the neuropsychological battery. However, *embedded PVTs*—that is, PVTs included within existing cognitive tests—are increasingly used in the field; many cognitive tests reviewed in this volume serve the dual purpose of providing information on cognitive function while also serving as embedded PVTs. Conversely, most of the commonly used SVTs in neuropsychology are embedded SVTs; that is, they are part of a more comprehensive questionnaire that assesses a number of different facets of psychopathology. Although a few standalone SVTs do exist, to date, almost none have been developed specifically for neuropsychological evaluations. Reviews for the most commonly used PVTs and SVTs in neuropsychology are included in this book.

The methods by which PVTs and SVTs detect invalid performance and noncredible symptom report vary across tests. Most are designed to identify scores that are not credible by virtue of being too low (e.g., cognitive test scores) or too negative or implausible (self-reported symptoms) to be believable; that is, they identify scores that are indicative of exaggeration of cognitive problems or enhancement of symptoms to an extent that cannot be attributable to a bona fide cognitive, medical, or psychiatric condition.

WHEN SHOULD CLINICIANS USE VALIDITY TESTS?

The answer to this question is simple: with every assessment. Some clinicians are reluctant to employ PVTs and SVTs routinely. This may relate to inaccurate information about these tests. Although perception is slowly changing, many clinicians still believe that PVTs and SVTs (1) are applicable only to forensic referrals and are not needed as part of day-to-day clinical assessments, (2) are necessary only when a clinician already suspects malingering, (3) yield results equivalent to a diagnosis of malingering when failed, and (4) cannot be used reliably with some groups, such as older examinees or people with cognitive deficits. None of these perceptions are accurate, as will be seen throughout this book.

More importantly, however, validity tests increase a clinician's confidence that the data obtained are an adequate representation of a person's true functioning and provide objective evidence that the test results can be confidently combined with clinical judgment, background history, additional assessment data, knowledge of disease or disorder, and all other collateral information to yield an accurate picture of that examinee's functioning. Validity tests are therefore not simply malingering rule-in tools but are instead essential aspects of test interpretation. In the same vein, examiners have an ethical obligation to ensure that their opinions, diagnoses, and recommendations are accurate, which comes from having valid data deemed to be representative of true abilities (Bush, 2013). Fulfilling this obligation is supported and facilitated by using PVTs and SVTs. Consistent with this view, position papers put forth by the National Academy of Neuropsychology (Bush et al., 2005) and the American Academy of Clinical Neuropsychology (Heilbronner et al., 2009) recommend the routine clinical use of validity tests.

For these reasons, it is strongly recommended that PVTs and SVTs be used regularly in all assessments, including those conducted within academic, medical, and nonforensic private practice settings, regardless of whether known external incentives, a high base rate of noncredible performance, or suspicion of underperforming are present. In this book, we specifically provide cutoffs for PVTs and SVTs that minimize false positives (i.e., that provide specificities of .90 and higher for detection of invalid scores). This protects credible patients, albeit at the expense of not identifying all malingerers; as Boone has noted, this is akin to a built-in safeguard against false-positive identification of malingering (2013).

TERMINOLOGY

The terms *feigning, exaggeration,* and *fabrication* are sometimes used interchangeably in the literature to describe examinee behaviors related to invalid performance or invalid symptom report. However, although there is some overlap between terms, they designate different kinds of behavior. *Feigning* and *fabrication* involve creating symptoms de novo for a problem or condition that is not present (e.g., pretending to forget test items when they were recalled, reporting pain symptoms when none exist, claiming long-term cognitive effects from an injury that never happened, falsifying health history). *Exaggeration* consists of embellishing or amplifying existing symptoms stemming from a condition that is present (e.g., a brain-injured examinee exaggerating cognitive symptoms, an examinee with minor whiplash reporting incapacitating headache, an examinee using a cane for a minor leg injury). Last, the term *induction*, seen more in the medical than neuropsychological literature, refers to deliberately creating a condition or symptom in oneself or someone else to cause impairment or disease (e.g., injecting oneself with a toxic or psychoactive substance).

In neuropsychology, examinees are sometimes said to have shown "poor effort" when test scores are invalid. Although it has appealing face validity, the term *effort* is problematic because high effort can be expended toward producing feigned yet believable impairment. In the medical domain, purely descriptive terms such as *abnormal illness behavior* and *medically unexplained symptoms* have replaced older terms such as *psychogenic symptoms* to avoid the problem of inferring intent.

Although the field has not yet reached consensus on precise terms when referring to examinee behaviors indicative of feigning or exaggeration of deficits or of self-reported symptoms, it is recommended that terms that imply knowledge of the examinee's internal states and motivations, such as *poor effort* or *psychogenic symptoms*, be replaced by those that refer to more behavioral or observational descriptions (e.g., *invalid performance, invalid symptom report*). Other terms such as *suboptimal performance* may appear useful but imply different meanings depending on the context (i.e., Does suboptimal mean below maximum potential, or faked?). Instead, phrases such as "invalid performance due to exaggeration of cognitive deficits" or "invalid symptom report due to overreporting of symptoms" can be used to summarize test results. When appropriate, these findings may then be attributed to a specific cause depending on the case and referral question (e.g., attributed to malingering, somatic symptom disorder, factitious disorder, or other factors).

THE SLICK, SHERMAN, AND IVERSON MALINGERED NEUROCOGNITIVE DYSFUNCTION CRITERIA

Unlike other branches of psychology or psychiatry, neuropsychology has developed a comprehensive set of criteria for determining the presence of malingering of cognitive deficits: the Slick et al. (1999) criteria for malingered neurocognitive dysfunction. The Slick et al. criteria have been used extensively for over 20 years and continue to stand the test of time as the malingering criteria with the most empirical research. They have assumed a prominent role in the literature as a gold-standard validation criterion for a number of PVTs and SVTs. The American Academy of Clinical Neuropsychology (Heilbronner et al., 2009) deemed them more representative of the current state of neuropsychological knowledge on malingering than other malingering criteria, including those of the *Diagnostic and Statistical Manual of Mental Disorders* (DSM). The Slick et al. criteria are considered a major milestone in the field's operationalization of cognitive malingering; as such, in the years since publication, they have strongly influenced the development of malingering detection methods (Bender & Frederick, 2018; Chafetz et al., 2015) and influenced the development of other malingering criteria such as the Malingered Pain-Related Disability (MPRD) criteria (Bianchini et al., 2005). The Slick et al. criteria have been referenced numerous times since their publication in 1999 (Garcia-Willingham et al., 2018), with almost 800 citations to date (www.researchgate.net).

In the original malingering framework, the term *malingered neurocognitive dysfunction* (MND) was defined as "the volitional exaggeration or fabrication of cognitive dysfunction for the purpose of obtaining substantial material gain or avoiding or escaping formal duty or responsibility" (Slick et al., 1999, p. 552). "Substantial material gain" was defined as anything of nontrivial value, such as financial compensation for personal injury. "Formal duties" were defined as actions people are legally obligated to perform, such as military service, and "formal responsibilities" were those that involved accountability in legal proceedings, such as competency to stand trial. "Malingering" was defined according to three different "diagnostic categories": (1) *Definite MND*, defined by clear and compelling evidence of volitional exaggeration or fabrication of cognitive dysfunction; (2) *Probable MND*, defined by evidence strongly suggestive of volitional exaggeration or fabrication of cognitive dysfunction; and (3) *Possible MND*, defined by the presence of evidence suggestive of volitional exaggeration or fabrication of cognitive dysfunction or by meeting criteria for definite or probable MND except that other primary etiologies (i.e., psychiatric, neurological, or developmental factors) could not be ruled out. Determining the specific criteria for the subtypes required reference to Criterion B (evidence from neuropsychological testing) and Criterion C (evidence from self-report), yielding a total of 13 possible criteria to support or rule out the three MND subtypes. Thus, the Slick et al. model included evidence from self-report and SVTs in addition to PVTs. However, Criterion C (i.e., evidence based on self-report including SVTs) was deemed insufficient for a diagnosis of MND, but instead provided additional evidence in support of the diagnosis.

LIMITATIONS OF THE MND CRITERIA

The Slick et al. criteria were long overdue for a revision. Updates were needed to address advances in the field of malingering research since publication of the criteria including updates to the methods for determining malingering and related terminology. At the time of publication in 1999, the terms "PVT" and "SVT" were not yet well-known in the field, and the Slick et al. criteria referred to "forced-choice measures" or "psychometric measures" to refer to these kinds of tests. The authors noted that psychometric methods and instruments for detecting malingering were "in a relatively early stage of development," with most being experimental and lacking adequate normative data (p. 555). This is clearly no longer the case, as illustrated by the multitude of books, book chapters, and peer-reviewed scientific papers on PVTs and SVTs, many of which have cutoffs that were derived based on their ability to detect MND as defined by the Slick et al. model.

The MND criteria also needed simplification and streamlining of redundant content, as some have noted (Boone, 2011; Larrabee, 2005). Most importantly, the specific recommendations made by Boone (2011) and Larrabee (2005), and the points made by Rogers and colleagues (Rogers et al., 2011a, 2011b) needed to be addressed, along with revisions published in book chapters by the authors that addressed some but not all criticisms (Sherman, 2015; Slick & Sherman, 2012). Specifically, questions were raised about the number of PVT failures needed to reach criteria, the specificity and false-positive rate for PVT cutoffs, the role of SVTs, the definition of exclusionary criteria, and the clarification of discrepancies indicative of feigning or fabrication. Last, and practically speaking, the MND criteria were lengthy and cumbersome, and this limited their ease of use and uptake in general clinical settings.

OTHER KINDS OF MALINGERING

Of course, neuropsychologists do not only assess cognition; most also assess for mental health conditions and measure the subjective impact of medical and psychiatric conditions. This is primarily done by empirically measuring self-reported symptoms using standardized questionnaires; less often, according to surveys, this is done using structured clinical interviews. Thus, the current standard of practice for most neuropsychological evaluations is to include rating scales that measure the nature and severity of a variety of self-reported symptoms, including cognitive symptoms, somatic symptoms, and psychiatric symptoms, with the choice of scales depending on the type of referral and clinical presentation. A typical battery may therefore include assessment of mental health conditions such as depression, anxiety, and posttraumatic stress disorder (PTSD) or assess subjective symptomatology arising from neurological conditions (e.g., concussion, multiple sclerosis, stroke, dementia) or from general medical conditions (e.g., pain disorders). Items or entire scales may be devoted to tapping self-reported memory problems, executive dysfunction, headache severity, dizziness, musculoskeletal pain, sleep disturbance, or fatigue, to name but a few examples.

One of the distinct benefits of using well-designed standardized tools to measure self-reported symptoms is that scales that include validity indexes allow a determination of whether self-reported symptoms are bona fide or indicative of feigning or exaggeration. The use of standardized tools to empirically assess self-reported cognitive, somatic, and psychiatric symptoms is one of the strengths of the field compared to disciplines that depend solely on clinical interview and observation.

The increased use of standardized self-report scales in neuropsychological settings has revealed that malingering tends to occur according to three main symptom clusters—malingering of cognitive disturbance (performance-based or self-reported), malingering of physical symptoms, and malingering of psychiatric symptoms—and that the type of symptom exaggeration will depend on the nature of the setting and of the external incentive. For example, a malingering examinee aiming to appear brain-injured may feign memory problems and headache to fit with assumptions about brain injury; another may feign chronic pain and psychological distress to obtain a disability pension after a workplace accident not involving brain injury. Another examinee may feign cognitive problems but not psychiatric symptoms when seeking income replacement for intellectual disability. Conversely, in criminal settings, a malingering examinee may feign severe cognitive deficits and severe psychiatric symptoms including dramatic psychotic symptoms to avoid criminal prosecution, a presentation virtually unseen in other settings associated with cognitive malingering such as ADHD clinics, where exaggeration may be more selective (e.g., involving attention and memory, but not extreme psychiatric disturbance).

The original MND criteria were aimed at detection of cognitive malingering, yet SVTs designed to detect psychiatric malingering were included in the criteria as evidence supportive of MND. At the time the MND criteria were created, there were a limited number of SVTs, and the research on cognitive malingering prediction using SVTs was sparse. Since then, although the two kinds of malingering can certainly co-occur, particularly in criminal settings, it is now clear that psychiatric SVTs are much less predictive of MND than are other kinds of SVTs, most notably those tapping cognitive or somatic symptoms (see Minnesota Multiphasic Personality Inventory-2 [MMPI-2] and Minnesota Multiphasic Personality Inventory-2 Restructured Form [MMPI-2-RF] reviews, for example, in this volume). Although the presence of one kind of malingering may increase the odds of another kind of malingering, using psychiatric malingering to bolster a diagnosis of cognitive malingering conflates the three types of malingering and leads to lack of clarity in the field because each kind of malingering can occur on its own and represents a distinct type of symptom exaggeration. Generally speaking, malingering examinees presenting for neuropsychological assessment may do so with one type of malingering or with a mixed picture of exaggerated cognitive, somatic, and psychiatric symptoms and with varying degrees of each symptom cluster depending on the case. The MND model did not clearly differentiate between cognitive, somatic, and psychiatric malingering as measured by SVTs in its criteria.

OTHER DEFINITIONS AND CONCEPTUAL FRAMEWORKS OF MALINGERING

THE DSM-5 DEFINITION OF MALINGERING

In the fifth edition of the *Diagnostic and Statistical Manual of Mental Disorders* (DSM-5; American Psychiatric Association, 2013), malingering is conceptualized as a condition that may be the focus of clinical attention but that

TABLE 3–1 DSM-5 Malingering Definition

Motivation	External incentive
Deception	Intentional
One or more of	1. Medico-legal context 2. Marked discrepancy between claimed stress or disability and objective findings and observations 3. Lack of cooperation during diagnosis or treatment 4. Presence of antisocial personality disorder

SOURCE: Adapted from American Psychiatric Association (2013).

TABLE 3–2 Clinical Decision Model for Establishing Malingered PTSD

A. Known motivation for malingering
B. Two or more of the following:
Irregular employment
Prior insurance claims
Capacity for recreation, but not for work
Lack of nightmares or nightmares that are inconsistent with presentation
Antisocial personality traits
Evasiveness and contradictions
Unwillingness to cooperate or hostile behaviour in the evaluation
C. Confirmatory evidence of malingering (one or more of the following criteria):
Admission of malingering
Incontrovertible proof of malingering
Unambiguous psychometric evidence of malingering
Strong corroborative evidence of malingering

SOURCE: Adapted from Resnick et al. (2018).

is not a mental health diagnosis. Malingering is classified in DSM-5 under "Non-Adherence to Medical Treatment." Conceptualizing malingering in neuropsychological assessment as "non-adherence to neuropsychological assessment" may be a useful way to help maintain a behavioral, nonjudgmental approach to malingering detection as one of several factors that can affect test validity. However, in DSM-5, malingering is defined as the intentional production of false or exaggerated *physical* or *psychological* symptoms (Table 3–1). Thus, technically speaking, cognitive malingering cannot be defined as malingering in DSM-5 because DSM-5 covers only somatic and psychiatric malingering. The DSM-5 definition depends heavily on characteristics of the setting or of the examinee in addition to other elements that are not well-defined, including marked discrepancies between claims and objective findings or observations, or lack of cooperation during diagnosis or treatment.

Given the significant advances in the field of malingering, the DSM-5 criteria are poorly defined and vague, and they give equal value to criteria that may have quite different sensitivity to malingering detection (e.g., marked discrepancies vs. lack of cooperation in assessment and treatment). In particular, the criteria regarding antisocial personality disorder may have minimal useful predictive utility regarding the likelihood of malingering (e.g., Gillard, 2018). Some have concluded that the DSM-5 criteria have ignored more than 30 years of empirical and theoretical work on malingering and were derived mainly for traditional psychiatric settings, rendering them both conceptually and practically flawed (Berry & Nelson, 2010). The DSM-5 model is thus considered inadequate for identifying malingering in the context of neuropsychological assessment.

THE RESNICK ET AL. MODEL FOR MALINGERED PTSD

There are few models of malingering of psychiatric symptoms other than DSM-5. One potentially useful model for identifying psychiatric malingering is the clinical decision model proposed by Resnick and colleagues for identifying malingering of PTSD (e.g., Resnick et al., 2018). This is defined by a combination of external incentives, examinee characteristics (e.g., irregular employment, prior insurance claims, antisocial personality traits), and evidence of malingering defined according to degree of proof. Although it has potential as a first step in better defining this aspect of psychiatric malingering, the model has significant limitations. This includes a majority of criteria depending heavily on the personal characteristics and background of the examinee, fairly vague and circular criteria such as "evidence for malingering" as part of the malingering criteria themselves, and inclusion of criteria that may be quite common in the general population (e.g., job dissatisfaction, lack of nightmares). The only SVT criterion in the model is poorly defined (e.g., "psychometric evidence of malingering"), and the model relies heavily on evidence outside the evaluation itself that is also vaguely defined and circular (e.g., "strong corroborative evidence of malingering"). Although the model has potential in helping better define criteria for malingered PTSD, it needs more research and refinement before applying it in high-stakes clinical assessments; it is nevertheless shown here for information purposes (Table 3–2).

THE BIANCHINI ET AL. CRITERIA FOR MALINGERED PAIN-RELATED DISABILITY

Bianchini and colleagues developed criteria specifically aimed at the detection of malingered pain-related disability (MPRD) for use in neuropsychological assessment (Bianchini et al., 2005). These were derived based on the MND model and are an advancement in the field of somatic malingering. Exaggeration of pain is one of the most common presentations of malingering in neuropsychological assessment settings relating to personal injury, disability evaluations, and unexplained medical conditions (see Boone, 2017, for a comprehensive review, as well as Greve et al., 2012, among others). Although a detailed review of MPRD is beyond the scope of this chapter, the MPRD criteria are referenced in several PVT and SVT reviews in this volume as they have been used to calibrate and validate PVT and SVT cutoffs for use in examinees presenting with pain. PVT and SVT cutoffs with high probability of detecting MPRD are often found to be different from those for other conditions such as traumatic brain injury (see, e.g., tables in reviews for the MMPI-2-RF and the Word Memory Test [WMT]). The Bianchini et al. criteria are shown in Table 3–3.

Like the MND criteria, the Bianchini criteria have been criticized, most notably for using evidence of cognitive malingering (i.e., PVT test failure) as criteria for pain malingering (Bender, 2018). Like the MND criteria, the Bianchini et al. criteria use failure on SVTs that measure psychiatric overreporting to support the diagnosis of MPRD even though somatic malingering and psychiatric malingering may represent different dimensions of malingering. Thus, like the MND, the MPRD model may conflate cognitive, somatic, and psychiatric malingering; some examinees may indeed exaggerate pain but not cognitive problems or psychological symptoms. Of note, these criteria also require evidence from the physical evaluation (e.g., Waddell's signs) provided by other practitioners such as physicians, physiotherapists, or

TABLE 3–3 Diagnostic Categories for the Diagnosis of Malingered Pain-Related Disability

I. Definite MPRD
1. Presence of substantial external incentive [Criterion A]
2. "Definitive" evidence of intent [Criterion C1 or D1]
3. Behaviors meeting the criteria for "definitive" intent [C1 or D1] are not fully accounted for by psychiatric, neurologic, or developmental factors [Criterion E]

II. Probable MPRD
1. Evidence of significant external incentive [Criterion A]
2. Two or more types of "probable" evidence of intent from Criterion B [B1–B5], Criterion C [C2–C5], and/or Criterion D [D2–D6]. This evidence must be well-validated and have a known error rate.
3. Behavior meeting necessary criteria from groups B, C, and D are not fully accounted for by psychiatric, neurologic, or developmental factors [Criterion E]

III. Possible MPRD
1. Evidence of significant external incentive [Criterion A]
2. Evidence does not rise to the level sufficient for a diagnosis of Probable MPRD.
Only one type of quantitative "probable" evidence of intent from Criterion B [B1–B5], Criterion C [C2–C5] and/or Criterion D [D2–D6].
OR
One or more forms of qualitative evidence of intent from Criterion B [B1–B5], Criterion C [C2–C5] and/or Criterion D [D2–D6].
OR
Evidence sufficient for a diagnosis of MPRD is present BUT Criterion E is not met.

Criterion A: Evidence of significant external incentive. At least one clearly identified and substantial external incentive for exaggeration or fabrication of symptoms is present at the time of examination (e.g., personal injury settlement, disability pension, evasion of criminal prosecution, release from military service, obtaining drugs).

Criterion B: Evidence from physical evaluation. Evidence that the patient's physical abilities, capacities, and/or limitations as demonstrated in formal physical evaluation (e.g., medical physical examination, physical therapy/occupational therapy examination, Functional Capacity Evaluation) are consistent with exaggeration or feigning of physical disability.
1. Probable effort bias. Performance on one or more well-validated measures of physical capacity (e.g., Jamar Grip Test) is consistent with exaggeration of diminished physical capacity.
2. Discrepancy between subjective report of pain and physiological reactivity (e.g., no heart-rate increase with significant change in subjective pain report).
3. Nonorganic findings. The presence on physical examination or functional capacity evaluation of signs or symptoms not consistent with known physiological mechanisms (e.g., Waddell's signs). Reported symptoms/complaints are substantially different than would be expected given the medical findings (clear nonorganic findings).
4. Discrepancy between the patient's physical presentation during formal evaluation and their physical capacities documented when they are not aware of being observed. Such observation may occur in the context of formal evaluation, be documented via surveillance videography, or derive from the report of reliable collateral informants (e.g., friends or relatives).

Criterion C: Evidence from cognitive/perceptual (neuropsychological) testing. Evidence that patient's cognitive capacities as indicated by formal cognitive testing (e.g., in the context of psychological or neuropsychological evaluation) are consistent with exaggeration or feigning of cognitive disability.
1. Definite negative response bias. Below chance performance ($p < .05$) on one or more forced-choice measures of cognitive or perceptual function.
2. Probable response bias. Performance on one or more well-validated tests designed to measure exaggeration or fabrication of cognitive or perceptual symptoms is consistent with exaggeration of diminished cognitive capacity.
3. Discrepancy between cognitive/neuropsychological test data and known patterns of brain functioning. A pattern of neuropsychological test performance is present that is discrepant from currently accepted models of normal and abnormal central nervous system function and the documented history of the patient (e.g., no head injury associated with the injury in question; exceptions may include cervical injury patients with concussions or use of narcotic analgesics or other sedating medications). The discrepancy is consistent with an attempt to feign or exaggerate cognitive deficit.

(continued)

TABLE 3–3 Continued

4. Discrepancy between test data and observed behavior. Performance on two or more neuropsychological tests is discrepant with observed levels of cognitive function in a way that suggests exaggeration of cognitive dysfunction (e.g., well-educated patient with no apparent expressive language deficit who scores in moderate or severely impaired range on measures of verbal fluency; patient who presents as globally impaired but drove self to the evaluation). Such observations may occur in the context of formal evaluation, be documented via surveillance videography, or derive from the report of reliable collateral informants (e.g., patient's friends or relatives).

Criterion D: Evidence from self-report. Evidence that the patient's self-reported symptoms, complaints, or limitations are consistent with exaggeration or feigning of physical, cognitive, or emotional/psychological disability.

1. Compelling inconsistency. Compelling inconsistencies occur when the difference in the way a patient presents when being evaluated compared with when they are not aware of being evaluated is such that it is not reasonable to believe the patient is not purposely controlling the difference. (Note that it may be possible to document compelling inconsistencies related to physical examination or cognitive test data; such circumstances would meet this criterion. However, conservative application of these criteria suggests that many, if not most, of these inconsistencies would be best used to meet other criteria).
2. Self-reported history is discrepant with documented history. For example, minimization or denial of concurrent or prior illness/injury (broadly defined) in a manner that emphasizes the injury for which compensation is sought. Also included would be overstatement of academic, vocational, or other achievement in a way that exaggerates the magnitude of loss due to the injury in question.
3. Self-reported symptoms are discrepant with known patterns of physiological or neurological functioning (e.g., whole body pain in a patient with small right-sided cervical disc bulge with no evidence of nerve root irritation; complaints of remote memory loss).
4. Self-reported symptoms are discrepant with observations of behavior. Reported symptoms in a given behavioral domain. (i.e., physical, cognitive, emotional) are markedly inconsistent with behavioral observations (e.g., patient complains that he is unable to move extremity and is observed to do so when distracted). Such observation may occur in the context of formal evaluation, be documented via surveillance videography, or derive from the report of reliable collateral informants (e.g., patient's friends or relatives).
5. Evidence from formal psychological evaluation that the person has significantly misrepresented their current status (e.g., exaggerated physical symptoms or exaggerated or minimized psychological symptoms/distress) in a manner that emphasizes the injury for which compensation is sought. For example, responses during interview or on self-report measures of psychological or physical function suggest impairment in the context of elevations on well-validated validity scales or indices consistent with exaggeration of physical (e.g., MMPI-2 FBS) or emotional symptoms (e.g., MMPI-2 F, Fb, or Fp) or evidence of vehement denial of psychological problems in a manner consistent with extreme defensiveness regarding psychological symptoms in order to further emphasize physical complaints (e.g., MMPI-2 L or K).

Criterion E: Behavior meeting necessary criteria from groups B, C, and D are not fully accounted for by psychiatric, neurologic, or developmental factors. The behaviors meeting the above criteria represent a likely volitional act aimed at achieving some secondary gain and cannot be fully accounted for by other disorders that result in significantly diminished capacity to appreciate laws or mores against malingering or inability to conform behavior to such standards. The simple presence of objectively documented pathology, illness, or injury (including psychiatric illness) expressly does not preclude a diagnosis of MPRD.

NOTE: MMPI-2 FBS = Minnesota Multiphasic Personality Inventory-2 Fake Bad Scale; MPRD = Malingered Pain-Related Disability.

SOURCE: From Bianchini et al. (2005).

occupational therapists. Although physical evidence of malingering may be available to neuropsychologists who work in multidisciplinary settings such as pain clinics, this type of evidence is more difficult to obtain in medicolegal or independent practice settings where information on physical findings may be nonstandardized or based on prior records that may be outdated at the time of the neuropsychological evaluation.

RECONCEPTUALIZING MALINGERING IN NEUROPSYCHOLOGICAL ASSESSMENT

There is a need in the field for a new method to identify cognitive, somatic, and psychiatric malingering designed for use in neuropsychological assessment. Table 3–4 presents revised and expanded malingering criteria that include all three domains relevant to malingering assessment: cognitive, somatic, and psychiatric. The malingering model is based on the original MND criteria model but expands and better defines criteria to include all three malingering presentations. The intent of these revised criteria is to replace the 1999 MND criteria and to create additional criteria for the identification of somatic malingering and psychiatric malingering for use in neuropsychological assessment.

The proposed *Multidimensional Criteria for Cognitive, Somatic, and Psychiatric Malingering* therefore yield four main types of malingering: (1) *malingering of cognitive dysfunction* based on revised and updated MND criteria, (2) *malingering of somatic symptoms*, (3) *malingering of psychiatric symptoms*, and (4) *malingering with mixed presentation.*

The multidimensional malingering criteria take into account the recommendations and criticisms of the 1999 MND criteria and of those of other malingering models. Specifically, they were created in order to (1) simplify diagnostic categories for clinical use, (2) expand and clarify external incentives, (3) more clearly include the role of compelling inconsistencies as prima facie evidence of malingering, (4) update and redefine the number of PVT and SVT failures needed to reach criteria, (5) address the issue of false positives on tests to determine malingering, (6) address

TABLE 3–4 Multidimensional Malingering Criteria for Neuropsychological Assessment

Malingering is the volitional feigning or exaggeration of neurocognitive, somatic, or psychiatric symptoms for the purpose of obtaining material gain and services or avoiding formal duty, responsibility, or undesirable outcome. It is indicated by clear and compelling evidence based on the four criteria listed as follows (Criteria A–D).

A. PRESENCE OF AN EXTERNAL INCENTIVE

A clearly identifiable and substantial external incentive for feigning or exaggeration of deficits or symptoms is present at the time of examination.

External incentives for malingering include access to a desirable outcome such as financial settlement, disability payment, wage replacement, social assistance, access to services or accommodations in community, academic, or work settings, or access to prescription medication.

External incentives may also include avoidance of an undesirable outcome such as those related to criminal proceedings (e.g., avoiding being deemed competent to stand trial or avoiding criminal sentencing), military service (e.g., avoiding deployment), or work or school settings (e.g., avoiding probation, suspension, expulsion, or termination). Avoidance of an undesirable outcome in the context of malingering may also be adaptive (e.g., feigning illness to avoid being returned to an abusive situation). External incentives for malingering may also include avoiding having to fulfill more basic duties and responsibilities such as avoiding work, school, examinations, or home responsibilities.

The kinds of evaluations associated with external incentives for malingering include those related to personal injury litigation, determination of disability benefits and workers' compensation, social services eligibility, criminal proceedings, military evaluations, and evaluations for specific clinical diagnoses that are associated with external incentives, such as those for brain injury, intellectual disability, chronic pain and related conditions, unexplained medical or neurological symptoms, ADHD, and learning disability, among others.

B. INVALID PRESENTATION ON EXAMINATION INDICATIVE OF FEIGNING OR EXAGGERATION

On examination of the examinee, there is either (a) compelling inconsistencies indicative of deliberate exaggeration or feigning of deficits or symptoms or (b) psychometric evidence of exaggeration or feigning of deficits or symptoms on performance validity tests (PVTs) or symptom validity tests (SVTs).

Compelling inconsistencies are observations during the examination that indicate definitive evidence of feigning or exaggeration. They are defined as clear and compelling evidence indicative of feigning or exaggeration of neurocognitive, somatic, or psychiatric deficits or symptoms observed or documented during the evaluation (e.g., unequivocal demonstration of disputed capacity when the examinee thinks they are unobserved; clear discrepancies between skills observed during the interview or while in the evaluation setting that are highly implausible and that indicate feigning, dissimulation, or distortion of symptoms). Note that compelling inconsistencies that are documented in written, audio, video, or electronic form such as social media would be included under Criterion C (Marked Discrepancies) because they form part of the records or documentation for the case rather than part of the direct examination of the patient.

Performance validity tests (PVTs) are objective tests designed to detect invalid cognitive performance.

Symptom validity tests (SVTs) are self-report scales or structured interviews that measure *overreporting* of self-reported cognitive, somatic, or psychiatric symptoms.

To meet criteria for *Invalid Presentation on Examination Indicative of Feigning or Exaggeration*, the examinee must present with one or more of the following criteria.

1. ***Invalid Neurocognitive Presentation.*** **One or more of a, b, or c must be present.**
   a. *One or more compelling inconsistencies pertaining to cognitive deficits or symptoms are observed or documented during the evaluation.*
   b. *Invalid scores on PVTs.*
   Psychometric evidence of invalid cognitive test performance based on (a) using at minimum two or more PVTs that alone or in combination have a low false-positive rate (i.e., .10), while (b) taking into account the ratio of failed PVT scores to total number of PVTs administered, (c) minimizing PVT redundancy, and (d) using PVT cutoffs that have been validated in clinical studies. Obtaining one PVT in the significantly below-chance range also would meet this criterion (i.e., significantly below-chance performance on forced-choice tests based on binomial probability theory).
   c. *Psychometric evidence of exaggerated cognitive symptoms on SVTs.*
   Psychometric evidence of exaggerated symptom reporting using SVTs that alone or in combination have a low false-positive rate (i.e., .10). For example, one or more SVT scores measuring primarily feigned or exaggerated cognitive symptoms in the invalid range using (a) SVTs with an acceptable false-positive rate, (b) SVTs that provide non-redundant information, and (c) SVTs that have cutoffs that have been validated in clinical studies would meet this criterion.
2. ***Invalid Somatic Symptom Presentation.*** **One or both of a or b must be present.**
   a. *One or more compelling inconsistencies pertaining to somatic symptoms are observed or documented during the evaluation.*
   b. *Psychometric evidence of exaggerated somatic symptoms on SVTs.*
   Psychometric evidence of exaggerated symptom reporting using SVTs that alone or in combination have a low false-positive rate (i.e., .10). For example, one or more SVT scores measuring primarily feigned or exaggerated somatic symptoms in the invalid range using (a) SVTs with an acceptable false-positive rate, (b) SVTs that provide non-redundant information, and (c) SVTs that have cutoffs that have been validated in clinical studies would meet this criterion.
3. ***Invalid Psychiatric Presentation.*** **One or both of a or b must be present.**
   a. *One or more compelling inconsistencies pertaining to psychiatric symptoms are observed or documented during the evaluation.*
   b. *Psychometric evidence of exaggerated psychiatric symptoms on SVTs.*
   Psychometric evidence of exaggerated symptom reporting using SVTs that alone or in combination have a low false-positive rate (i.e., .10). For example, one or more SVT scores measuring primarily feigned or exaggerated psychiatric symptoms in the invalid range using (a) SVTs with an acceptable false-positive rate, (b) SVTs that provide non-redundant information, and (c) SVTs that have cutoffs that have been validated in clinical studies would meet this criterion.
4. ***Invalid Mixed Symptom Presentation.***
   Evidence of compelling inconsistency and/or psychometric evidence of invalid or exaggerated PVT or SVT results across two or more of cognitive, somatic, or psychiatric domains.

   For example, the following would each satisfy this criterion:

   - Two or more compelling inconsistencies across domains (i.e., two or more of B1a, B2a, or B3a).
   - Psychometric evidence in more than one domain (i.e., two or more among B1b, B1c, B2b, or B3b).
   - One or more compelling inconsistencies combined with psychometric evidence of invalid or exaggerated deficits or symptoms in one or more domains (i.e., one or more compelling inconsistencies with one or more of either of B1b, B1c, B2b, or B3b).

(continued)

TABLE 3–4 Continued

C. MARKED DISCREPANCIES

One or more *marked* discrepancies between *obtained test data/symptom report* and the types of evidence below are present, as follows.

1. ***Natural history and pathogenesis of the condition in question.***
   Information obtained by self-report or through tests or scales is markedly discrepant from currently accepted models of normal and abnormal neurological, medical, or psychiatric functioning in a way that suggests feigning or exaggeration of deficits or symptoms.
2. ***Records and other media.***
   Information obtained by self-report or through tests or scales is markedly inconsistent with records or other documented history (e.g., audio, video, social media) in a way that suggests feigning or exaggeration of deficits or symptoms.
3. ***Reliable collateral informant report.***
   Information obtained by self-report or through tests or scales is markedly discrepant from day-to-day level of function described by at least one reliable collateral informant with minimal stakes in the outcome of the evaluation, in a way that suggests feigning or exaggeration of dysfunction.

D. BEHAVIORS MEETING CRITERION B ARE NOT FULLY ACCOUNTED FOR BY ANOTHER DEVELOPMENTAL, MEDICAL, OR PSYCHIATRIC CONDITION

Behaviors meeting Criterion B are assumed to reflect an informed, rational, and volitional attempt toward acquiring or achieving outcomes as defined in Criterion A and cannot be fully accounted for by significant developmental, medical, or psychiatric conditions that result in significantly diminished capacity to appreciate laws or mores against malingering, or inability to conform behavior to such standards. Examples of significant developmental, medical, and psychiatric conditions are listed as follows:

- Moderate to severe dementia
- Moderate to severe intellectual disability (e.g., IQ < 60)
- Severe psychiatric, neurological, or other medical disorders associated with cognitive impairment sufficient to preclude independence in basic activities of daily living

Malingering can co-occur in conditions associated with cognitive deficits including mild intellectual disability, mild dementia, or mild cognitive impairment. Similarly, malingering can co-occur in psychiatric or neurological conditions defined by somatoform symptoms (e.g., somatic symptom disorder, conversion disorder/functional neurological symptom disorder, factitious disorder, unexplained medical symptoms) and in the presence of other psychiatric conditions (e.g., depression).

SPECIFIERS

The four specifiers for the clinical presentation of malingering are described as follows.

Malingering of Neurocognitive Dysfunction
In addition to meeting Criteria A, C, and D, the individual meets Criterion B1a, B1b, or B1c for feigned or exaggerated cognitive dysfunction, that is, *one or more* of the following:

- A compelling inconsistency pertaining to cognitive deficits or symptoms
- Invalid cognitive performance as demonstrated by performance validity tests
- Invalid cognitive symptom report demonstrated by symptom validity tests

Malingering of Somatic Symptoms
In addition to meeting Criteria A, C, and D, the individual meets Criterion B2a or B2b for feigned or exaggerated somatic symptoms, that is, either of the following:

- A compelling inconsistency pertaining to somatic symptoms
- Invalid somatic symptom report as demonstrated by symptom validity tests

Malingering of Psychiatric Symptoms
In addition to meeting Criteria A, C, and D, the individual meets Criterion B3a or B3b for feigned or exaggerated psychiatric symptoms, that is, either of the following:

- A compelling inconsistency pertaining to psychiatric symptoms
- Invalid psychiatric symptom report on symptom validity tests

Malingering with Mixed Presentation
In addition to meeting Criteria A, C, and D, the individual meets Criterion B4 for feigned or exaggerated symptoms in more than one domain (i.e., cognitive, somatic, and/or psychiatric).

SOURCE: Sherman, Slick, and Iverson (2020).

the issue of increased false positives with increased number of PVTs and SVTs administered, (7) better define the role of SVTs in malingering determination, (8) add specifiers related to malingering presentation, and, most importantly, (9) clearly define the exclusionary criteria based on the past decade of research on malingering in neuropsychology. The details underlying these changes and their methodology are described in detail elsewhere (Sherman, Slick, & Iverson, 2020). Further research and validation of the criteria will help advance and refine methods and standards for malingering detection and allow a broader determination of malingering for use in neuropsychological assessment.

DIFFERENTIAL DIAGNOSIS OF CONDITIONS ASSOCIATED WITH FEIGNED, EXAGGERATED, OR UNEXPLAINED SYMPTOMS

Importantly, a number of different conditions should be considered before attributing invalid performance or overreporting to malingering. To do so, neuropsychologists need to have a working knowledge of disorders seen in neuropsychological practice that present with feigned, exaggerated, or unexplained symptoms, with or without the presence of deception or external incentives. For example,

TABLE 3–5 Overview of Conditions Associated with Feigned, Exaggerated, or Unexplained Symptoms

	DEFINING FEATURES	INVOLVES DELIBERATE DECEPTION	EXTERNAL INCENTIVE REQUIRED
Malingering of neurocognitive dysfunction Malingering of somatic symptoms Malingering of psychiatric symptoms	The volitional feigning or exaggeration of cognitive, somatic, or psychiatric symptoms for the purpose of obtaining material gain or avoiding formal duty or responsibility	Yes	Yes
Factitious disorder	The feigning, exaggeration, or induction of physical or psychological symptoms in order to deceive; the intent is to assume the sick role	Yes	No[a, b]
Somatic symptom disorder	Technically restricted only to the overreporting or exaggeration of physical symptoms such as pain; the intent is to assume the sick role	No	No[b]
Conversion disorder (functional neurological symptom disorder)	Involves voluntary motor or sensory symptoms that are incompatible with known medical conditions (e.g., nonepileptic seizures, unexplained paralysis); technically, conversion does not include cognitive symptoms	No	No[b]
Illness anxiety disorder (hypochondriasis)	Intense fear and preoccupation about having a medical condition, or fear and preoccupation in excess of actual symptoms; thought to be a form of anxiety disorder; may manifest in neuropsychology settings as irrational fear of severe sequelae after a minor medical event (e.g., fear of progressive memory loss after a single concussion)	No	No[b]
Dissociative amnesia	Inability to recall basic autobiographical information most often in the form of memory loss for specific events or generalized amnesia for personal history, not compatible with known patterns of brain injury or disease; often occurs along with other psychiatric disorders, but is thought to be a type of dissociative disorder; if seen in criminal settings (i.e., amnesia for a crime one has committed) it may reflect malingering, not dissociation	No	No[b]

[a] In the Diagnostic and Statistical Manual of Mental Disorders (DSM-IV), the co-occurrence of an external incentive was an exclusionary criterion; this is no longer the case in DSM-5, and so factitious disorder can occur in the presence of external incentives and malingering.

[b] Condition may nevertheless co-occur with external incentives and malingering.

the DSM-5 makes distinctions between disorders involving intentional deception (i.e., malingering, factitious disorder) and those that do not (i.e., somatic symptom disorder, conversion disorder/functional neurological symptom disorder). However, it specifies that the presence of external incentives is not necessarily specific to malingering: external incentives can be present in disorders other than malingering and are no longer part of exclusionary criteria for some conditions such as factitious disorder (American Psychiatric Association, 2013). Table 3–5 contrasts various conditions associated with exaggerated or unexplained symptoms, including malingering, factitious disorder, somatic symptom disorder, conversion disorder/functional neurological symptom disorder, illness anxiety disorder (previously known as hypochondriasis), and dissociative amnesia. All of these conditions may present with noncredible or implausible symptoms and should be considered in the differential diagnosis. As well, none of these conditions exclude malingering and all can co-occur with malingering. For more information on differential diagnosis of malingering in neuropsychological assessment, see Sherman et al. (2020) as well as the many excellent comprehensive sources on these topics, such as Boone (2013, 2017), Larrabee (2012), Carone and Bush (2013), Morgan and Ricker (2018), Morgan and Sweet (2009), and Rogers and Bender (2018), among others.

Clinicians are often reluctant to diagnose malingering but are also especially reluctant to diagnose clinical conditions such as factitious disorder, somatic symptom disorder, and conversion disorder, all of which tend to be chronic and associated with high personal and healthcare costs. Factitious disorder in particular is a severe and incapacitating condition associated with poor outcome. It is certainly true that correctly identifying disorders involving deception and unexplained symptoms is a diagnostic challenge made more complicated by the fact that these can co-occur in the presence of bona fide medical conditions and, in some cases, may be more likely to occur in those with a previous medical condition (e.g., somatic symptom disorder). However, unlike most disciplines, neuropsychology has tools uniquely suited to this diagnostic challenge. Most important, because early detection can help avert escalation and poor outcome in some of these disorders, a clear understanding of the distinguishing features of these disorders paired with a nonjudgmental, proactive attitude to assessment is recommended.

REFERENCES

American Psychiatric Association. (2013). *Diagnostic and Statistical Manual of Mental Disorders* (5th ed.). Washington, DC: Author.

Berry, D. T. R., & Nelson, N. W. (2010). DSM-5 and malingering: A modest proposal. *Psychological Injury and Law, 3*(4), 295–303.

Bender, S. D. (2018). Malingered traumatic brain injury. In R. Rogers & S. D. Bender (Eds.), *Clinical assessment of malingering and deception* (4th ed., pp. 122–150). New York: Guilford Press.

Bender, S. D., & Frederick, R. (2018). Neuropsychological models of feigned cognitive deficits. In R. Rogers & S. D. Bender (Eds.), *Clinical assessment of malingering and deception* (4th ed., pp. 42–60). New York: Guilford Press.

Bianchini, K. J., Greve, K. W., & Glynn, G. (2005). On the diagnosis of malingered pain-related disability: Lessons from cognitive malingering research. *The Spine Journal, 5*(4), 404–417. https://doi.org/10.1016/j.spinee.2004.11.016

Boone, K. B. (2011). Clarification or confusion? A review of Rogers, Bender, and Johnson's "A Critical Analysis of the MND Criteria for Feigned Cognitive Impairment: Implications for Forensic Practice and Research." *Psychological Injury and Law, 4*(2), 157–162. https://doi.org/10.1007/s12207-011-9106-3

Boone, K. B. (2013). *Clinical practice of forensic neuropsychology: An evidence-based approach*. New York: Guilford Press.

Boone, K. B. (2017). *Neuropsychological evaluation of somatoform and other functional somatic conditions*. New York: Routledge.

Bush, S. S. (2013). Ethical considerations in mild traumatic brain injury cases and symptom validity assessment. In D. A. Carone & S. S. Bush (Eds.), *Mild traumatic brain injury: Symptom assessment validity and malingering* (pp. 45–56). New York: Springer.

Bush, S. S., Ruff, R. M., Tröster, A. I., Barth, J. T., Koffler, S. P., Pliskin, N. H., . . . Silver, C. H. (2005). Symptom validity assessment: Practice issues and medical necessity NAN policy & planning committee. *Archives of Clinical Neuropsychology, 20*(4), 419–426. https://doi.org/10.1016/j.acn.2005.02.002

Carone, D. A., & Bush, S. S. (2013). *Mild traumatic brain injury: Symptom assessment validity and malingering.* New York: Springer.

Chafetz, M. D., Williams, M. A., Ben-Porath, Y. S., Bianchini, K. J., Boone, K. B., Kirkwood, M. W., . . . Ord, J. S. (2015). Official position of the American Academy of Clinical Neuropsychology Social Security Administration Policy on validity testing: Guidance and recommendations for change. *The Clinical Neuropsychologist, 29*(6), 723–740. https://doi.org/10.1080/13854046.2015.1099738

Garcia-Willingham, N. E., Bosch, C. M., Walls, B. D., & Berry, D. T. (2018). Assessment of feigned cognitive impairment using standard neuropsychological tests. In R. Rogers & S. D. Bender (Eds.), *Clinical assessment of malingering and deception* (4th ed., pp. 329–358). New York: Guilford Press.

Gillard, N. D. (2018). Psychopathy and deception. In R. Rogers & S. D. Bender (Eds.), *Clinical assessment of malingering and deception* (4th ed., pp. 174–187). New York: Guilford Press.

Greve, K. W., Bianchini, K. J., & Ord, J. (2012). The psychological assessment of persons with chronic pain. In G. J. Larrabee (Ed.), *Forensic neuropsychology: A scientific approach* (2nd ed., pp. 302–335). New York: Oxford University Press.

Heilbronner, R. L., Sweet, J. J., Morgan, J. E., Larrabee, G. J., Millis, S. R., & Conference Participants. (2009). American Academy of Clinical Neuropsychology Consensus Conference Statement on the neuropsychological assessment of effort, response bias, and malingering. *The Clinical Neuropsychologist, 23*(7), 1093–1129. https://doi.org/10.1080/13854040903155063

Larrabee, G. J. (2005). Assessment of malingering. In G. J. Larrabee (Ed.), *Forensic neuropsychology: A scientific approach*. New York: Oxford University Press.

Larrabee, G. J. (2012). Performance validity and symptom validity in neuropsychological assessment. *Journal of the International Neuropsychological Society, 18*(4), 625–630.

Morgan, J. E., & Ricker, J. H. (2018). *Textbook of clinical neuropsychology* (2nd ed.). New York: Oxford University Press.

Morgan, J. E., & Sweet, J. J. (2009). *Neuropsychology of malingering casebook*. New York: Psychology Press.

Resnick, P. J., West, S. G., & Wooley, C. N. (2018). The malingering of posttraumatic disorders. In R. Rogers & S. D. Bender (Eds.), *Clinical assessment of malingering and deception* (4th ed., pp. 188–211). New York: Guilford Press.

Rogers, R., & Bender, S. D. (2018). *Clinical assessment of malingering and deception* (4th ed.). New York: The Guilford Press.

Rogers, R., Bender, S. D., & Johnson, S. F. (2011a). A commentary on the MND model and the Boone critique: "Saying it doesn't make it so." *Psychological Injury and Law, 4*(2), 163–167. https://doi.org/10.1007/s12207-011-9108-1

Rogers, R., Bender, S. D., & Johnson, S. F. (2011b). A critical analysis of the MND criteria for feigned cognitive impairment: Implications for forensic practice and research. *Psychological Injury and Law, 4*(2), 147–156. https://doi.org/10.1007/s12207-011-9107-2

Sherman, E. M. S. (2015). Terminology and diagnostic concepts. In M. K. Kirkwood (Ed.), *Validity testing in child and adolescent assessment* (pp. 23–41). New York: Guilford Press.

Sherman, E.M.S., Slick, D.J., & Iverson, G.I. (2020). Multidimensional malingering criteria for neuropsychological assessment: A twenty-year update of the Malingered Neurocognitive Dysfunction criteria. *Archives of Clinical Neuropsychology*. https://academic.oup.com/acn/article/doi/10.1093/arclin/acaa019/5830790

Slick, D. J., & Sherman, E. M. S. (2013). Differential diagnosis of malingering. In D. A. Carone & S. S. Bush (Eds.), *Mild traumatic brain injury: Symptom assessment validity and malingering* (pp. 57–72). New York: Springer.

Slick, D. J., Sherman, E. M., & Iverson, G. L. (1999). Diagnostic criteria for malingered neurocognitive dysfunction: Proposed standards for clinical practice and research. *The Clinical Neuropsychologist, 13*(4), 545–561. https://doi.org/10.1076/1385-4046(199911)13:04;1-Y;FT545

4 | PREMORBID ESTIMATION

NATIONAL ADULT READING TEST (NART)

TEST NAME	**National Adult Reading Test (NART)**
DOMAIN	Premorbid intellectual functioning
AGE RANGE	18+ years
ADMINISTRATION TIME	10 minutes
SCORING FORMAT	Hand scored
REFERENCES	Blair, J. R., & Spreen, O. (1989). Predicting premorbid IQ: A revision of the National Adult Reading Test. *The Clinical Neuropsychologist, 3,* 129–136. Del Ser, T., González-Montalvo, J., Martínez-Espinosa, S., Delgado-Villapalos, C., & Bermejo, F. (1997). Estimation of premorbid intelligence in Spanish people with the Word Accentuation Test and its application to the diagnosis of dementia. *Brain and Cognition, 33*(3), 343–356. Grober, E., & Sliwinski, M. (1991). Development and validation of a model for estimating premorbid verbal intelligence in the elderly. *Journal of Clinical and Experimental Neuropsychology, 13,* 933–949. Nelson, H. E., & Willison, J. (1991). *National Adult Reading Test (NART): Test manual* (2nd ed.). Windsor, UK: NFER Nelson. Ryan, J. J., & Paolo, A. M. (1992). A screening procedure for estimating premorbid intelligence in the elderly. *The Clinical Neuropsychologist, 6,* 53–62.

DESCRIPTION

The National Adult Reading Test or NART-2 (Nelson, 1982; Nelson & O'Connell, 1978; Nelson & Willison, 1991) is a reading test of 50 irregularly spelled words (e.g., ache, naive, thyme) for the determination of premorbid intellectual function. Because the words are short, examinees do not have to analyze a complex visual stimulus, and because they are irregular, phonological decoding or intelligent guesswork will not provide the correct pronunciation. Therefore, it has been argued that performance depends more on previous knowledge than on current cognitive capacity (Nelson & O'Connell, 1978). The value of the test lies in (a) the high correlation between reading ability and intelligence in the general population (Crawford, Stewart, Cochrane et al., 1989), (b) the fact that word reading tends to produce a fairly accurate estimate of preinjury IQ (Crawford et al., 2001; Moss & Dowd, 1991), and (c) the fact that the ability to pronounce irregular words is generally retained in conditions with cognitive decline (Crawford, Parker, & Besson, 1988; Fromm et al., 1991; Sharpe & O'Carroll, 1991; Stebbins, Gilley, Wilson, Bernard, & Fox, 1990).

The test was initially developed by Nelson (1982) in England for use with the Wechsler Adult Intelligence Scale (WAIS). Nelson and Willison (1991) and Ryan and Paolo (1992) restandardized the NART (NART-2) for the WAIS-R on a British sample and an American sample of people 75 years and older, respectively. Bright et al. (2016)

and Watt et al. (2017) updated the NART and/or NART-2 on a British and an Australian sample, respectively. Blair and Spreen (1989) modified the test for use with North American populations (NAART) and validated it against the WAIS-R. Grober and Sliwinski (1991) also developed their own North American version, the AMNART.

In addition to these three main versions, other modifications have also appeared in the literature. A short version, the NAART35, was developed by Uttl (2002) and appears to provide a reliable and valid measure of verbal intelligence. An abbreviated NART (Short NART) is based on the first half of the test (Beardsall & Brayne, 1990). Various local versions of the NART have been developed, including New Zealand English (NZART; Starkey & Halliday, 2011), Australian English (Lucas et al., 2003), Italian (Colombo et al., 2002), Swedish (NART-SWE; Rolstad et al., 2008), and Japanese (JART; Matsuoka et al., 2006). A Spanish adaptation, the Word Accentuation Test (or Test de Acentuación de Palabras [TAP]; Del Ser et al., 1997), has also been developed for European Spanish speakers and modified for use in Spanish speakers in South America as the Word Accentuation Test (WAT-BA; Burin et al., 2000) and North America (WAT-C; Krueger et al., 2006). The various versions, tests predicted, and the populations the prediction models are derived from are presented in Table 4–1.

Another useful modification is to place the words into sentences (e.g., the Cambridge Contextual Reading Test or CCRT: Beardsall & Huppert, 1994; C-AUSNART: Lucas et al., 2003). The provision of semantic and syntactic cues (context) results in a larger number of words being read correctly and, hence, in a higher estimate of IQ, particularly among people with dementia and poor-to-average readers (Beardsall & Huppert, 1994; Conway & O'Carroll, 1997; Watt & O'Carroll, 1999).

As seen in Table 4–1, many versions of the NART are used to predict older WAIS editions. We do not recommend using NART versions that reference older editions of the WAIS because they are likely to underestimate IQ due to the Flynn effect. As such, only NART versions related to WAIS-III and later are presented in this chapter.

TABLE 4–1 National Adult Reading Test (NART) Versions

TEST	TEST PREDICTED	POPULATION
NART (original)	WAIS	British (Nelson, 1982)
	WAIS-IV	British (Bright, Hale, Gooch, Myhill, & van der Linde, 2016)
	WAIS-IV	Australian (Watt, Ong, & Crowe, 2017)
NART-2	WAIS-R FAS PASAT Raven's SPM	British (Nelson & Willison, 1991) American, age 75 and older (Ryan & Paolo, 1992)
NAART	WAIS-R Vocabulary	North American (Blair & Spreen, 1989)
NAART-35	WAIS-R Vocabulary	North American (Uttl, 2002)
AMNART	WAIS-R	North American (Grober & Sliwinski, 1991)
C-AUSNART	WAIS-R	Australian (Lucas et al., 2003)
JART	WAIS-R	Japanese (Matsuoka et al., 2006)
NZART	WASI	New Zealander (Starkey & Halliday, 2011)
NART-SWE	WAIS-III	Swedish (Rolstad et al., 2008)
WAT (or TAP in Spanish)	WAIS	European Spanish (Del Ser et al., 1997)
WAT-BA	WAIS-III	Argentinean Spanish, age 65–85 (Burin et al., 2000)
WAT-C	WAIS-III	American Spanish (Krueger et al., 2006)

ADMINISTRATION

NART-2

The examinee is presented with the word card (Figure 4–1) and is instructed to read each word. "I want you to read slowly down this list of words starting here. After each word please wait until I say 'next' before reading the next word. I must warn you that there are many words that you probably won't recognize; in fact most people don't know them, so just have a guess at these, OK? Go ahead." The examinee should be encouraged to attempt every word.

NZART

Starkey and Halliday (2011) developed a local New Zealand version of the NART (NZART). The NZART word list is presented in Figure 4–2. The administration procedure is identical to the NART.

Ache	Procreate	Leviathan
Debt	Quadruped	Aeon
Psalm	Catacomb	Detente
Depot	Superfluous	Gauche
Chord	Radix	Drachm
Bouquet	Assignate	Idyll
Deny	Gist	Beatify
Capon	Hiatus	Banal
Heir	Simile	Sidereal
Aisle	Rarefy	Puerperal
Subtle	Cellist	Topiary
Nausea	Zealot	Demense
Equivocal	Abstemious	Campanile
Naive	Gouge	Labile
Thyme	Placebo	Syncope
Courteous	Facade	Prelate
Gaoled	Aver	

Figure 4–1 The National Adult Reading Test (NART).

SOURCE: From the New Adult Reading Test. Nelson and O'Connell (1978).

Debt	Hiatus	Facetious
Choir	Meringue	Ochre
Aisle	Debris	Impugn
Chaos	Inertia	Zealot
Māori	Placebo	Façade
Nausea	Chameleon	Tourniquet
Grotesque	Equivocal	Hippocrates
Fatigue	Crochet	Quadruped
Cologne	Tacit	Indict
Subtle	Colonel	Caveat
Naïve	Reify	Corps
Psalm	Cognac	Abstemious
Torque	Amygdaloid	Topiary
Sieve	Risqué	Idyll
Whenua	Epitome	Vivace
Thyme	Indices	Labile
Lingerie	Chassis	Détente
Kaitiaki	Superfluous	Caecum
Insatiable	Leviathan	Talipes
Courteous	Subpoena	Syncope

Figure 4–2 *New Zealand Adult Reading Test (NZART).*
SOURCE: Starkey and Halliday (2011).

WORD ACCENTUATION TEST (WAT)

Del Ser et al. (1997) developed a Spanish reading task (WAT) with an ambiguous graphic clue for the Spanish reader consisting of 30 infrequent words written in capital letters without the usual accent marks to facilitate pronunciation (Figure 4–3). The test was developed in Spain, and since Spanish has marked geographical differences, different versions have been developed for use in Argentina (WAT-BA; Burin et al., 2000) as well as in the United States (WAT-C; Krueger et al., 2006). The Word Accentuation Test-Buenos Aires (WAT-BA) comprises 44 items. The Word Accentuation Test-Chicago (WAT-C; Krueger et al., 2006) comprises 40 items. Unfortunately, only the original WAT includes a table to convert WAT scores to estimated IQ. Interested readers may refer to the respective published papers for the other word lists.

ACULLA	CUPULA
ALELI	ANOMALO
ALEGORIA	APATRIDA
CONCAVO	DIAMETRO
ACME	PUGIL
CANON	GRISU
DESCORTES	TACTIL
ACOLITO	BULGARO
ABOGACIA	CELIBE
RABI	HUSSAR
MANCHU	MOARE
AMBAR	POLIGAMO
SILICE	ALBEDRIO
PIFANO	VOLATILE
DISCOLOR	BALADI

Figure 4–3 *Word Accentuation Test (WAT).*
SOURCE: Del Ser et al. (1997).

SCORING

The use of a pronunciation guide and a recording device is recommended to facilitate scoring. Each incorrectly pronounced word counts as one error. Slight variations in pronunciation are acceptable when they are due to regional accents. The total number of errors is tabulated. The error score is then entered into the appropriate prediction equation (Table 4–2) to estimate premorbid IQ scores.

WAT total scores (not errors) are converted to WAIS-III Full-Scale IQ (FSIQ) using the data presented in Table 4–3 (Gomar et al., 2011). This table should be used to estimate WAIS-III FSIQ based on five subtests (i.e., Vocabulary, Similarities, Matrix Reasoning, Block Design, Digit Span) for European Spanish-speaking individuals between ages 18 and 65.

PREDICTION OF OTHER COGNITIVE TESTS

The NART can also be used to estimate premorbid performance on other cognitive tasks, including the FAS verbal fluency task (Crawford et al., 1992), the Paced Auditory Serial Addition Test (PASAT; Crawford et al., 1998), and the Raven's Standard Progressive Matrices (Freeman & Godfrey, 2000; Van den Broek & Bradshaw, 1994). The equations are provided in Table 4–4.

VALIDATION OF NART SCORES

Crawford, Allan, Cochrane, and Parker (1990) developed a regression equation to predict NART scores from demographic variables (years of education, social class, age, and gender) using a healthy UK sample. The equation is as follows:

$$\text{Predicted NART error score} = 37.9 - 1.77\,(\text{education}) + 2.7\,(\text{class}) - .07\,(\text{age}) - 0.03\,(\text{gender})$$
$$\text{SEE} = 6.93$$

Note. Social class coding: 1 = professional (e.g., architect, church minister); 2 = intermediate (e.g., computer programmer, teacher); 3 = skilled (e.g., carpenter, salesperson); 4 = semiskilled (e.g., assembly line worker, waiter); 5 = unskilled (e.g., cleaner, laborer). Gender coding: male = 1, female = 2.

TABLE 4–2 National Adult Reading Test (NART) Equations to Predict Wechsler Adult Intelligence Scale Tests (WAIS-IV, WAIS-III, and WASI)

Australian data, aged 18–65 using NART/NART-2 and demographics to predict WAIS-IV (Watt et al., 2017)

Predicted WAIS-IV FSIQ = 133.62 – 1.282 × (NART/NART-2 error)
Predicted VCI = 127.78 – 1.189 * (NART/NART-2 errors)
Predicted PRI = 128.32 – 1.027 * (NART/NART-2 errors)
Predicted WMI = 130.56 – 1.199 * (NART/NART-2 errors)
Predicted PSI = 120.63 – 0.604 * (NART/NART-2 errors)
Predicted WAIS-IV FSIQ = 123.20 – (1.172 × (NART/NART-2 error)) – (0.118 × age) – (1.524 × sex) + (0.944 × education)
Predicted VCI = 126.78 – 1.180 * (NART/NART-2 errors) – 0.142 * (age) – 0.383 * (sex) + 0.394 * (education)
Predicted PRI = 124.35 – 0.916 * (NART/NART-2 errors) – 0.091 * (age) – 3.711 * (sex) + 0.685 * (education)
Predicted WMI = 124.08 – 1.013 * (NART/NART-2 errors) – 0.054 * (age) – 6.059 * (sex) + 0.910 * (education)
Predicted PSI = 89.81 – 0.519 * (NART/NART-2 errors) – 0.091 * (age) + 6.575 * (sex) + 1.428 * (education)
Where male = 0, female = 1; education = number of years of formal education. FSIQ, Full Scale IQ; VCI, Verbal Comprehension Index; PRI, Perceptual Reasoning Index; WMI, Working Memory Index; PSI, Processing Speed Index

British data, age 18–70 using NART to predict WAIS-IV (Bright et al., 2016)

Predicted WAIS-IV FSIQ = –0.9775 × NART error + 126.41, SE_E = 9.25
Predicted WAIS-IV GAI = –0.9656 × NART error + 126.5
Predicted WAIS-IV VCI = –1.0745 × NART error + 126.81
Predicted WAIS-IV PRI = –0.6242 × NART error + 120.18
Predicted WAIS-IV WMI = –0.7901 × NART error + 120.53
Predicted WAIS-IV PSI = –0.5285 × NART error + 114.53

New Zealand data, aged 18–84 using NART-2 to predict WAIS-III (Barker-Collo et al., 2011)

NZ–Predicted WAIS–III FSIQ = 145.716 + (–1.063 × NART error score) + (1.31 × years of education) + (–11.98 × ethnicity) + (-8.2 × gender). The SE_E is 7.21.
NZ–Predicted WAIS–III VIQ = 152.471 + (–1.267) (NART total score) + (–0.390) (age in years) + (1.009) (years of education) + (–9.343) (ethnicity) + (–6.923) (gender). The SE_E is 7.23.
NZ–Predicted WAIS–III PIQ = 125.632 + (–.595) (NART total score) + (1.379) (years of education) + (–13.788) (ethnicity) + (–5.804)(gender). The SE_E is 9.20.
where ethnicity Pakeha/NZ European = 1, Other = 2; gender male = 1, female = 2

NZART equations to predict WASI (Starkey & Halliday, 2011)

Predicted WASI FSIQ = 124.18 – 0.903 (NZART error). The SE_E is 8.99.
Predicted WASI VIQ = 123.07 – 1.025 (NZART error). The SE_E is 8.56.
Predicted WASI PIQ = 119.616 – 0.535 (NZART error). The SE_E is 10.09.

The equation can also be downloaded from Dr. Crawford's site, https://homepages.abdn.ac.uk/j.crawford/pages/dept/psychom.htm. The equation allows the clinician to compare a current NART score against a predicted score to determine whether the NART score is valid. A large discrepancy between the predicted and obtained scores (i.e., obtained error score more than 11.4 points over the predicted score) suggests impaired NART performance and alerts the clinician to the fact that the NART will not provide an accurate estimate of premorbid ability.

TABLE 4–3 Predicted Wechsler Adult Intelligence Scale-Third Edition (WAIS-III) Full Scale IQ (FSIQ) Scores Based on the Word Accentuation Test (WAT) for European Spanish Speakers

WAT SCORE	PREDICTED WAIS-III FSIQ	WAT SCORE	PREDICTED WAIS-III FSIQ
1	60	16	89
2	62	17	91
3	64	18	93
4	66	19	95
5	67	20	97
6	69	21	98
7	71	22	100
8	73	23	102
9	75	24	104
10	77	25	106
11	79	26	108
12	81	27	110
13	83	28	112
14	85	29	114
15	87	30	116

SOURCE: From Gomar et al. (2011).

DEMOGRAPHIC EFFECTS

As might be expected, NART (NART-2, NAART) errors systematically decrease with increasing FSIQ (Wiens et al., 1993). NART (NAART, AMNART) performance is correlated with years of education and social class. Age, gender, and ethnicity (Caucasian vs. African American) have little effect on performance (Anstey et al., 2001; Beardsall, 1998; Boekamp et al., 1995; Cockburn et al., 2000; Crawford, Stewart et al., 1988; Freeman & Godfrey, 2000; Graf & Uttl, 1995; Grober & Sliwinski, 1991; Krueger et al., 2006; Ivnik et al., 1996; Nelson, 1982; Nelson & Willison, 1991; Starr et al., 1992; Storandt et al., 1995; Wiens et al., 1993), although when a wide age range is studied (well-educated healthy individuals aged 16–84 years), an age-related increase in "correct" NAART scores appears to emerge (Graf & Uttl, 1995; Parkin & Java, 1999; Uttl, 2002; Uttl & Graf, 1997) due largely to the relatively weak performance of young adults. In a New Zealand sample, the NART failed to correlate with FSIQ and Verbal IQ (VIQ) among the

TABLE 4–4 National Adult Reading Test (NART) Equations to Predict FAS Verbal Fluency, Paced Auditory Serial Addition Test (PASAT), and Raven's Progressive Matrices

Estimated premorbid FAS verbal fluency task (Crawford et al., 1992)

Estimated FAS = 57.5 – (0.76 × NART errors). The SE_E is 9.09; also see https://homepages.abdn.ac.uk/j.crawford/pages/dept/psychom.htm

Estimated premorbid PASAT (Crawford et al., 1998)

Estimated PASAT Total = 215.74 – (1.85 × NART errors) – (.77 × Age). The SE_E is 34.87; also see https://homepages.abdn.ac.uk/j.crawford/pages/dept/psychom.htm

Estimated premorbid Raven's Standard Progressive Matrices (Freeman & Godfrey, 2000; Van den Broek & Bradshaw, 1994)

Estimated RSPM = 66.65 + (–.462 × NART errors) + (–.254 × age)

Maori, whereas correlation with Performance IQ (PIQ) was significant but low (Barker-Collo et al., 2008).

With regard to aging, cross-sectional studies suggest that the NART scores do not decline significantly (all versions) in older adults; however, a longitudinal study (Deary et al., 1998) revealed evidence of decline with aging. In that study, 387 healthy older adults were tested with the NART-2 at baseline and followed-up four years later. NART-estimated IQ fell by a mean of 2.1 points over four years. However, the amount of decline is differentially related to initial cognitive status, social class, and education. Those with higher baseline ability, in higher social groups, with more education, and who were younger were relatively protected from decline. These findings suggest that aging effects on NART-estimated IQ may be modified by other psychosocial factors at baseline.

EVIDENCE FOR RELIABILITY

EVIDENCE FOR INTERNAL RELIABILITY

The NART is among the most reliable tests in clinical use. Reliability estimates are above .90 for the various versions, including the Swedish version (NART-SWE; Rolstad et al., 2008), the Japanese version (JART; Matsuoka et al., 2006), and the Spanish version (WAT-C; Krueger et al., 2006; WAT-BA; Burin et al., 2000).

EVIDENCE FOR TEST-RETEST RELIABILITY, MEASURING CHANGE, AND PRACTICE EFFECTS

A test-retest reliability of .98 has been reported for the NART, with practice effects emerging over the short term (10 days; Crawford, Stewart, Besson, Parker, & De Lacey, 1989). However, the mean change is less than one word, suggesting that practice effects are of little clinical significance. Test-retest reliability over 11 days ($n = 10$) is very high ($r = .94$) for the WAT-C. One-year test-retest coefficients were high for the NART-2 and NART-R ($r = .89$; Deary et al., 2004; $r = .92$; Raguet et al., 1996); practice effects are minimal. Test-retest reliability over two years is very high for the NART-SWE ($r = .92$) and AMNART ($r = .93$ for healthy individuals, $r = .94$ for individuals with prodromal Huntington's disease; Carlozzi et al., 2011). With longer retest intervals (e.g., four years), reliability is lower, though still respectable (.67 to .72; Deary et al., 1998; Kondel et al., 2003).

EVIDENCE FOR INTERRATER RELIABILITY

The NART-2 (and other versions) also has high interrater reliability (above .88; Crawford, Stewart, Besson et al., 1989; O'Carroll, 1987; Riley & Simmonds, 2003; Sharpe & O'Carroll, 1991). Some NART-2 words, however, have a disproportionately high rate of interrater disagreement (*aeon, puerperal, aver, sidereal,* and *prelate*) and particular care should be taken when scoring these words (Crawford, Stewart, Besson et al., 1989). Training by an experienced examiner and use of the pronunciation guide appears to improve accuracy for these items (Alcott et al., 1999).

EVIDENCE FOR VALIDITY

RELATIONSHIP WITH IQ TESTS

Researchers generally report moderate to high correlations (.40 to .80) between NART (NAART, AMNART, WAT) performance and concurrently given measures of general intellectual status (Blair & Spreen, 1989; Bright et al., 2016; Carswell et al., 1997; Cockburn et al., 2000; Crawford, Stewart, Besson et al., 1989, Crawford, Deary et al., 2001; Freeman & Godfrey, 2000; Grober & Sliwinski, 1991; Johnstone et al., 1996; Paolo et al., 1997; Raguet et al., 1996; Sharpe & O'Carroll, 1991; Uttl, 2002; Wiens et al., 1993; Willshire et al., 1991). In the standardization sample, the NART-2 predicted 55%, 60%, and 30% of the variance in prorated WAIS FSIQ, VIQ, and PIQ, respectively (Nelson, 1982). Similar results have been reported by others for the various versions (e.g., Blair & Spreen, 1989; Crawford, Stewart, Besson et al., 1989; Ryan & Paolo, 1992; Starkey & Halliday, 2011; Wiens et al., 1993). Findings for the JART were notably higher, with correlations between predicted and actual scores ranging from marginal to very high (WAIS-R FSIQ, $r = .88$; VIQ, $r = .91$; PIQ, $r = .68$), accounting for 78% (FSIQ), 84% (VIQ), and 46% (PIQ) of the actual scores (Matsuoka et al., 2006). In short, the test is a good predictor of VIQ and FSIQ but is relatively poor at predicting PIQ. With the WAIS-IV, correlations with the General Ability Index (GAI) and Verbal Comprehension Index (VCI) are high, and with Perceptual Reasoning Index (PRI) and Working Memory Index (WMI), moderate ($r = .64$, .66, .50, and .45, respectively). Correlation with the Processing Speed Index (PSI) is low ($r = .36$) indicating that the NART is not a reliable estimate for PSI (Bright et al., 2016). Among verbal subtests, NAART errors correlate most highly with Vocabulary and Information (Wiens et al., 1993). The NAART appears to measure verbal intelligence with the same degree of accuracy in various age groups (Uttl, 2002). Estimates of IQ over a two-year period also appear more stable with the AMNART compared to a two-subtest WASI (Carlozzi et al., 2011).

The test has good accuracy in the retrospective estimation of IQ (Berry et al., 1994; Carswell et al., 1997; Moss & Dowd, 1991; Raguet et al., 1996). A study by Crawford et al. (2001) followed-up 177 individuals who had been administered an IQ test (Moray House Test, MHT) at age 11. They found a correlation of .73 between these scores and NART scores at age 77.

RELATIONSHIP WITH OTHER PREMORBID IQ ESTIMATION METHODS

The NAART and NART-R show high correlation with the Wide Range Achievement Test-Revised (WRAT-R) Reading ($r = .87$; Johnstone et al., 1996). The Schonell, a single-word reading test originally developed to measure reading level in children, is also very strongly correlated with the NART-2 (r = .91; Kiely et al., 2011). When compared to the Spot-the-Word test (STW), a promising premorbid estimate of performance intelligence which requires examinees to decide which word in a word pair is real and which is not, the NART-2 is very accurate in predicting the FSIQ of those in the high-average and average range, whereas the STW is better for estimating those in the average range only (Barker-Collo et al., 2008). Moreover, patients with mild Alzheimer's disease (AD) perform worse than healthy controls on NART-2, but there is no difference in their performance on the STW, suggesting STW may provide a more accurate estimate of premorbid functioning (McFarlane, Welch, & Rodgers, 2006).

Mathias, Bowden, and Barrett-Woodbridge (2007) reported that the NART-2 underestimates WAIS-III FSIQ and VIQ by as much as 36 IQ points when current IQ was above average but overestimates the same by as much as 30 IQ points for those with below-average IQ in a healthy Australian sample. However, the margin of discrepancy between predicted and current IQ is smaller with the NART-2 than the Wechsler Test of Adult Reading (WTAR), a prior version of the Test of Premorbid Functioning (TOPF). The authors recommended the use of both measures to estimate premorbid IQ in Australians. Bright et al. (2016) reported similar findings of overestimation or underestimation of premorbid intelligence in the extremes of the distribution using the NART and WAIS-IV in their healthy British sample.

For a discussion on the NART/NART-2 comparison with the TOPF, see TOPF discussed later in this chapter.

RELATIONSHIPS WITH OTHER TESTS

The NART exhibits a relationship with cognitive domains other than IQ, although the association appears modest and inconsistent. For example, Frick and colleagues (2011) reported that NART-2 errors obtained in 2005 show moderate correlations (range = −.19 to −.41) with Wechsler Memory Scale-Third Edition (WMS-III) Logical Memory, Letter-Number Sequencing (LNS), and Spatial Span measured in 2001, 2005, and 2008. NART-2 errors also predicted seven-year Logical Memory and LNS changes; a higher number of NART errors and older age are associated with greater memory and working memory declines over time (Frick et al., 2011). The Italian version of the NART, however, did not provide reliable estimates of memory (RAVLT; Isella et al., 2005).

The NART-R has also been found to correlate modestly with most cognitive domains (r = −.24 [Trails A], r = −.53 [Trails B], r = .31 [WCST categories], r = .38 [BNT), r = .39 to .48 [Verbal Fluency], r = .40 [Design Fluency], r = .33 [RCFT copy]) but not to sustained attention as measured using the Continuous Performance Test (CPT). Overall, NART-R accounted for only a mean 10% of variance for cognitive measures (Schretlen et al., 2005). The correlation with the Mini-Mental State Examination (MMSE) among patients with AD is also modest (r = .41; Starr & Lonie, 2007). Once childhood IQ is entered into the prediction model, the NART–MMSE correlation falls to near zero (Crawford et al., 2001). These results provide some support for the claim that NART scores estimate premorbid rather than current cognitive functioning (Crawford et al., 2001), but it is a weak cognitive predictor (Schretlen et al., 2005).

PREDICTION USING COMBINED DEMOGRAPHICS AND NART

Whether combining demographic and NART (or NAART/AMNART) estimates increases predictive accuracy is of some debate. Bright et al. (2002) found that an equation combining NART scores with demographic variables did not significantly increase the amount of variance in WAIS/WAIS-R IQ explained by NART only, either in patients (e.g., with AD, Korsakoff's syndrome) or healthy controls. By contrast, other authors have concluded that the addition of NART to demographic information improves prediction (Carswell et al., 1997; Gladsjo et al., 1999; Grober & Sliwinski, 1991; Watt & O'Carroll, 1999; Willshire et al., 1991). For example, Watt et al. (2017) reported that the NART/NART-2 accounted for about 39% of variance on the WAIS-IV FSIQ. Once demographic variables were added to the NART/NART-2 errors model, the variance increased to about 47%. When the regression equations were validated on a traumatic brain injury sample, the difference between actual and predicted scores without demographic variables was 8.21, as opposed to the 4.35-point difference between actual and predicted scores with demographic variables (Watt et al., 2017). The use of the AMNART with demographic information appeared particularly useful in those examinees who have unusual combinations of lower than expected reading ability given their educational achievement.

CLINICAL STUDIES

Dementia. Patients with mild dementia who have accompanying linguistic or semantic memory deficits perform poorly on this test (Grober & Sliwinski, 1991; Stebbins, Gilley et al., 1990; Storandt et al., 1995). Patients with moderate to severe levels of dementia also perform poorly (Boekamp et al., 1995; Fromm et al., 1991; Grober & Sliwinski, 1991; Paolo et al., 1997; Stebbins et al., 1988; Stebbins, Gilley et al., 1990), even when obviously aphasic or alexic patients are excluded (Taylor, 1999). Patterson, Graham, and Hodges (1994) found a dramatic decrease in NART performance as a function of AD severity, possibly due to the deterioration of semantic memory in AD. Compared to other conventional tests, NART performance declines in dementia, but the deterioration of VIQ and PIQ may be more rapid and severe (Paque & Warrington, 1995). Patients whose reading declined tended to have a lower VIQ than PIQ, raising the concern that verbal skills may have already been compromised by disease. Similar results have been reported by others, particularly if the initial MMSE score was low (Taylor et al., 1996; Cockburn et al., 2000). Cockburn et al. also found that lower frequency words disappear faster from the lexicon than do higher frequency words. However, in dementia, performance may vary so that words might be recognized at one visit, not recognized a year later, but then correctly recognized in later visits. NART scores may also be used to predict treatment response. Among patients with AD treated with either donepezil or rivastigmine and retested over 78 weeks, Starr and Lonie (2008) found that, over time, initial NART did not predict memory performance, but higher initial NART was associated with improved letter fluency.

Other Neurological Conditions. The test is generally thought to be resistant to neurological insults such as brain injury (Crawford, Parker et al., 1988; Watt & O'Carroll, 1999) and is one of the few cognitive measures that is relatively robust against the effects of disease and decline in old age (Anstey et al., 2001). However, the test is not insensitive to neurological compromise, and deterioration in reading test performance does occur in some patients. One study suggests that NART underestimates FSIQ but improvements in performance are seen in the first year after mild brain injury (Skilbeck et al., 2013). Deterioration in reading test performance has also been seen among patients with multiple sclerosis (MS), particularly those with a chronic-progressive course (Friend & Grattan, 1998), among patients with severe traumatic brain injury tested within 12 months of injury (Riley & Simmonds, 2003), and among depressed patients who have suffered head injuries (Watt & O'Carroll, 1999), although the association could be related to socioeconomic conditions (Rajput et al., 2011). Although some (O'Carroll et al., 1992) have reported that NART scores are low in patients with Korsakoff's syndrome or frontal lobe disturbance, others (Bright et al., 2002; Crawford & Warrington, 2002) have not found that NART performance is affected in these patients.

Psychiatric Conditions. NART performance has been studied in a number of psychiatric disorders, predominantly in schizophrenia. Among patients with schizophrenia, the NART does not appear to be a reliable estimate of IQ. For example, findings by Kondel et al. (2003) suggest that the NART provided a reasonable estimate of premorbid IQ in younger patients (20–51 years), but not necessarily in older ones (52–85 years). In fact, the NART overestimated IQ by as much as 15 IQ points (O'Connor et al., 2012; Russell et al., 2000). In mood disorders, some have reported that NART performance is not affected by depression (Crawford et al., 1987) whereas others have found that NART scores are influenced by a number of mental disorders, most notably depression and anxiety disorders (Rajput et al., 2011).

PERFORMANCE VALIDITY

This has not been well studied. Until more research is available, clinicians may use the Crawford et al. (1990) regression equation to estimate NART scores using demographic variables to determine the validity of current NART scores.

COMMENT

Administration of this measure is relatively straightforward and takes little time. The test has high levels of internal, test-retest, and interrater reliability. It correlates moderately well with measures of intelligence (particularly VIQ and FSIQ) and is less related to demographic variables than various other measures of cognitive functioning such as Wechsler tests (Bright et al., 2002). Although the reading ability assessed by the NART may not be entirely insensitive to brain disease, the available evidence suggests that it may be less vulnerable than many other cognitive measures, such as the MMSE and Wechsler tests (Berry et al., 1994; Christensen et al., 1991; Cockburn et al., 2000; Maddrey et al., 1996). Thus, although far from perfect, tests like the NART may be the instruments of choice for assessing premorbid IQ.

The test, however, should not be used with patients who have compromised language or reading ability, with those who have VIQs less than PIQs, or with those who have significant articulatory or visual acuity problems. Use of the NART (or its variants) within 12 months of a severe brain injury is also not recommended since doing so runs the risk of significantly underestimating premorbid IQ (Riley & Simmonds, 2003). Furthermore, while the test may provide an acceptable premorbid index in the early stages of a dementing disorder, it is susceptible to changes that occur with disease progression. The potential confounding effect of depression requires additional study.

It is also important to bear in mind that use of regression procedures has some limitations, including regression toward the mean and limited range of scores. These limitations suggest that two types of errors may occur when the equations are applied to individuals with suspected dementia. In the case of superior premorbid ability, the predicted IQ will represent an underestimate of the amount of cognitive deterioration present. On the other hand, in individuals whose premorbid abilities are relatively low, the estimated IQ might suggest cognitive deterioration when, in actuality, it has not occurred. Note, too, that a fairly large loss in cognitive ability (about 15–21 IQ points) may need to occur before the NART (NAART) can reliably identify potential abnormality. Accordingly, the clinician needs to be cautious in inferring an absence of decline when cutoff discrepancies are not met.

These limitations underscore the need to supplement NART estimates of premorbid functioning with clinical observations and information about a patient's educational and occupational accomplishments as well as other performance-based data (e.g., MMSE, Vocabulary). Watt et al. (2017) have attempted to address the problem by developing regression equations to predict whether a given NART/NART-2 score is valid and interpretable using demographic variables. A similar procedure has been developed for use with the TOPF.

The majority of research on the NART has focused on estimating premorbid intelligence. NART equations are also available for estimating premorbid performance on other cognitive tasks. Some (Schlosser & Ivison, 1989) have speculated that NART equations based on memory test performance may be capable of assessing dementia earlier than the NART/WAIS-R combination. However, findings by Gladsjo et al. (1999) and Isella et al. (2005) suggest that the NART (or its variants) does not improve accuracy of prediction of premorbid memory abilities beyond that accomplished by demographic correction of performance on memory tests.

Although the rationale for developing various versions of the NART appears sound, there is no empirical comparison of their relative efficacy. The various forms and equations should not be used interchangeably, and the exact version should be specified in clinical or research reports. Furthermore, many of the local/other language versions of the NART (e.g., WAT-C, WAT-BA) do not provide interpretive guidelines or information to estimate IQ scores. Until a method of converting these scores to IQ scores is available, their use in clinical settings may be limited.

One major limitation deserves attention. The various NART versions have been developed for use with the WAIS, WAIS-R, and WAIS-III. We do not recommend using NART versions that predict older WAIS versions because estimates are likely impacted by the Flynn effect. To date, only limited studies have validated the NART against the WAIS-IV in Australian and British samples. To predict WAIS-IV scores in American samples, use the TOPF or Oklahoma Premorbid Intelligence Estimate-IV (OPIE-IV), discussed later in this chapter.

REFERENCES

Alcott, D., Swann, R., & Grafhan, A. (1999). The effect of training on rater reliability on the scoring of the NART. *British Journal of Clinical Psychology, 38,* 431–434.

Anstey, K. J., Luszcz, M. A., Giles, L. C., & Andrews, G. R. (2001). Demographic, health, cognitive, and sensory variables as predictors of mortality in very old adults. *Psychology and Aging, 16,* 3–11.

Barker-Collo, S., Bartle, H., Clarke, A., van Toledo, A., Vykopal, H., & Willetts, A. (2008). Accuracy of the National Adult Reading Test and Spot the Word estimates of premorbid intelligence in a non-clinical New Zealand sample. *New Zealand Journal of Psychology, 37*(3), 53–61.

Barker-Collo, S. L., Thomas, K., Riddick, E., & de Jager, A. (2011). A New Zealand regression formula for premorbid estimation using the National Adult Reading Test. *New Zealand Journal of Psychology, 40*(2), 47–55.

Beardsall, L. (1998). Development of the Cambridge Contextual Reading Test for improving the estimation of premorbid verbal intelligence in older persons with dementia. *British Journal of Clinical Psychology, 37,* 229–240.

Beardsall, L., & Brayne, C. (1990). Estimation of verbal intelligence in an elderly community: A prediction analysis using a shortened NART. *British Journal of Clinical Psychology, 29,* 83–90.

Beardsall, L., & Huppert, F. A. (1994). Improvement in NART word reading in demented and normal older persons using the Cambridge Contextual Reading Test. *Journal of Clinical and Experimental Neuropsychology, 16,* 232–242.

Berry, D. T. R., Carpenter, G. S., Campbell, D. A., Schmitt, F. A., Helton, K., & Lipke-Molby, T. (1994). The New Adult Reading Test-Revised: Accuracy in estimating WAIS-R IQ scores obtained 3.5 years earlier from normal older persons. *Archives of Clinical Neuropsychology, 9,* 239–250.

Blair, J. R., & Spreen, O. (1989). Predicting premorbid IQ: A revision of the National Adult Reading Test. *The Clinical Neuropsychologist, 3,* 129–136.

Boekamp, J. R., Strauss, M. E., & Adams, N. (1995). Estimating premorbid intelligence in African-American and white elderly veterans using the American version of the National Adult Reading Test. *Journal of Clinical and Experimental Neuropsychology, 17,* 645–653.

Bright, P., Hale, E., Gooch, V. J., Myhill, T., & van der Linde, I. (2016). The National Adult Reading Test: restandardisation against the Wechsler Adult Intelligence Scale—Fourth edition. *Neuropsychological Rehabilitation,* 1–9. https://doi.org/10.1080/09602011.2016.1231121

Bright, P., Jadlow, E., & Kopelman, M. D. (2002). The National Adult Reading Test as a measure of premorbid intelligence: A comparison with estimates derived from premorbid levels. *Journal of the International Neuropsychological Society, 8,* 847–854.

Burin, D. I., Jorge, R. E., Arizaga, R. A., & Paulsen, J. S. (2000). Estimation of premorbid intelligence: The Word Accentuation Test-Buenos Aires version. *Journal of Clinical and Experimental Neuropsychology, 22*(5), 677–685.

Carlozzi, N. E., Stout, J. C., Mills, J. A., Duff, K., Beglinger, L. J., Aylward, E. H., & Paulsen, J. S. (2011). Estimating premorbid IQ in the prodromal phase of a neurodegenerative disease. *The Clinical Neuropsychologist, 25*(5), 757–777.

Carswell, L. M., Graves, R. E., Snow, W. G., & Tierney, M. C. (1997). Postdicting verbal IQ of elderly individuals. *Journal of Clinical and Experimental Neuropsychology, 19,* 914–921.

Christensen, H., Hadzi-Pavlovic, D., & Jacomb, P. (1991). The psychometric differentiation of dementia from normal aging: A meta-analysis. *Psychological Assessment, 3,* 147–155.

Cockburn, J., Keene, J., Hope, T., & Smith, P. (2000). Progressive decline in NART scores with increasing dementia severity. *Journal of Clinical and Experimental Neuropsychology, 22,* 508–517.

Colombo, L., Sartori, G., & Brivio, C. (2002). Stima del quoziente intellettivo tramite l'applicazione del TIB (Test Breve di Intelligenza). *Giornale Italiano di Psicologia, 3,* 613–637.

Conway, S. C., & O'Carroll, R. E. (1997). An evaluation of the Cambridge Contextual Reading Test (CCRT) in Alzheimer's disease. *British Journal of Clinical Psychology, 36,* 623–625.

Crawford, J. R., Allan, K. M., Cochrane, R. H. B., & Parker, D. M. (1990). Assessing the validity of NART-estimated premorbid IQs in the individual case. *British Journal of Clinical Psychology, 29,* 435–436.

Crawford, J. R., Besson, J. A. O., Parker, D. M., Sutherland, K. M., & Keen, P. L. (1987). Estimation of premorbid intellectual status in depression. *British Journal of Clinical Psychology, 26,* 313–314.

Crawford, J. R., Deary, I. J., Starr, J., & Whalley, L. J. (2001). The NART as an index of prior intellectual functioning: A retrospective validity study covering a 66-year interval. *Psychological Medicine, 31,* 451–458.

Crawford, J. R., Moore, J. W., & Cameron, I. M. (1992). Verbal fluency: A NART-based equation for the estimation of premorbid performance. *British Journal of Clinical Psychology, 31,* 327–329.

Crawford, J. R., Obansawin, M. C., & Allan, K. M. (1998). PASAT and components of WAIS-R performance: Convergent and discriminant validity. *Neuropsychological Rehabilitation, 8,* 255–272.

Crawford, J. R., Parker, D. M., & Besson, J. A. O. (1988). Estimation of premorbid intelligence in organic conditions. *British Journal of Psychiatry, 153,* 178–181.

Crawford, J. R., Stewart, L. E., Besson, J. A. O., Parker, D. M., & De Lacey, G. (1989). Prediction of WAIS IQ with the National Adult Reading Test: Cross-validation and extension. *British Journal of Clinical Psychology, 28,* 267–273.

Crawford, J. R., Stewart, L. E., Cochrane, R. H. B., Parker, D. M., & Besson, J. A. O. (1989). Construct validity of the National Adult Reading Test: A factor analytic study. *Personality and Individual Differences, 10,* 585–587.

Crawford, J. R., Stewart, L. E., Garthwaite, P. H., Parker, D. M., & Besson, J. A. O. (1988). The relationship between demographic variables and NART performance in normal subjects. *British Journal of Clinical Psychology, 27,* 181–182.

Crawford, J. R., & Warrington, E. K. (2002). The Homophone Meaning Generation Test: Psychometric properties and a method for estimating premorbid performance. *Journal of the International Neuropsychological Society, 8,* 547–554.

Deary, I. J., MacLennan, W. J., & Starr, J. M. (1998). Is age kinder to the initially more able?: Differential ageing of a verbal ability in the healthy old people in Edinburgh study. *Intelligence, 26,* 357–375.

Deary, I. J., Whalley, L. J., & Crawford, J. R. (2004). An "instantaneous" estimate of a lifetime's cognitive change. *Intelligence, 32,* 113–119.

Del Ser, T., González-Montalvo, J., Martínez-Espinosa, S., Delgado-Villapalos, C., & Bermejo, F. (1997). Estimation of premorbid intelligence in Spanish people with the Word Accentuation Test and its application to the diagnosis of dementia. *Brain and Cognition, 33*(3), 343–356.

Freeman, J., & Godfrey, H. (2000). The validity of the NART-RSPM index in detecting intellectual declines following traumatic brain injury: A controlled study. *British Journal of Clinical Psychology, 39,* 95–103.

Frick, A., Wahlin, T., Pachana, N. A., & Byrne, G. J. (2011). Relationships between the National Adult Reading Test and memory. *Neuropsychology, 25*(3), 397–403.

Friend, K. B., & Grattan, L. (1998). Use of the North American Adult Reading Test to estimate premorbid intellectual function in patients with multiple sclerosis. *Journal of Clinical and Experimental Neuropsychology, 20,* 846, 851.

Fromm, D., Holland, A. L., Nebes, R. D., & Oakley, M. A. (1991). A longitudinal study of word-reading ability in Alzheimer's disease: Evidence from the National Adult Reading Test. *Cortex, 27,* 367–376.

Gladsjo, J. A., Heaton, R. K., Palmer, B. W. M. Taylor, M. J., & Jeste, D. V. (1999). Use of oral reading to estimate premorbid intellectual and neuropsychological functioning. *Journal of the International Neuropsychological Society, 5,* 247–254.

Gomar, J. J., Ortiz-Gil, J., McKenna, P. J., Salvador, R., Sans-Sansa, B., Sarró, S., & Guerrero, A. (2011). Validation of the Word Accentuation Test (TAP) as a means of estimating premorbid IQ in Spanish speakers. *Schizophrenia Research, 128*(1–3), 175–176.

Graf, P., & Uttl, B. (1995). Component processes of memory: Changes across the adult lifespan. *Swiss Journal of Psychology, 54,* 113–130.

Grober, E., & Sliwinski, M. (1991). Development and validation of a model for estimating premorbid verbal intelligence in the elderly. *Journal of Clinical and Experimental Neuropsychology, 13,* 933–949.

Isella, V., Villa, M. L., Forapani, F., Piamarta, A., Russo, I. M., & Appolonio, I. M. (2005). Ineffectiveness of an Italian NART-equivalent for the estimation of verbal learning ability in normal elderly. *Journal of Clinical and Experimental Neuropsychology, 27,* 618–623.

Ivnik, R. J., Malec, J. F., Smith, G. E., Tangalos, E. G., & Petersen, R. C. (1996). Neuropsychological tests norms above age 55: COWAT, BNT, token, WRAT-R reading, AMNART, Stroop, TMT, JLO. *The Clinical Neuropsychologist, 10,* 262–278.

Johnstone, B., Callahan, C. D., Kapila, C. J., & Bouman, D. E. (1996). The comparability of the WRAT-R reading test and NAART as estimates of premorbid intelligence in neurologically impaired patients. *Archives of Clinical Neuropsychology, 11,* 513–519.

Kiely, K. M., Luszcz, M. A., Piguet, O., Christensen, H., Bennett, H., & Anstey, K. J. (2011). Functional equivalence of the National Adult Reading Test (NART) and Schonell reading tests and NART norms in the Dynamic Analyses to Optimise Ageing (DYNOPTA) project. *Journal of Clinical and Experimental Neuropsychology, 33*(4), 410–421.

Kondel, T. K., Mortimer, A. M., Leeson, M. C., Laws, K. R., & Hirsch, S. R. (2003). Intellectual differences between schizophrenic patients and normal controls across the adult lifespan. *Journal of Clinical and Experimental Neuropsychology, 25,* 1045–1056.

Krueger, K. R., Lam, C. S., & Wilson, R. S. (2006). The Word Accentuation Test-Chicago. *Journal of Clinical and Experimental Neuropsychology, 28*(7), 1201–1207.

Lucas, S. K., Carstairs, J. R., & Shores, E. A. (2003). A comparison of methods to estimate premorbid intelligence in an Australian sample: Data from the Macquarie University Neuropsychological Normative Study (MUNNS). *Australian Psychologist, 38,* 227–237.

Maddrey, A. M., Cullum, C. M., Weiner, M. F., & Filley, C. M. (1996). Premorbid intelligence estimation and level of dementia in Alzheimer's disease. *Journal of the International Neuropsychological Society, 2,* 551–555.

Mathias, J. L., Bowden, S. C., & Barrett-Woodbridge, M. (2007). Accuracy of the Wechsler Test of Adult Reading (WTAR) and National Adult Reading Test (NART) when estimating IQ in a healthy Australian sample. *Australian Psychologist, 42*(1), 49–56.

Matsuoka, K., Uno, M., Kasai, K., Koyama, K., & Kim, Y. (2006). Estimation of premorbid IQ in individuals with Alzheimer's disease using Japanese ideographic script (Kanji) compound words: Japanese version of National Adult Reading Test. *Psychiatry and Clinical Neurosciences, 60*(3), 332–339.

McFarlane, J., Welch, J., & Rodgers, J. (2006). Severity of Alzheimer's disease and effect on premorbid measures of intelligence. *British Journal of Clinical Psychology, 45*(4), 453–464.

Moss, A. R., & Dowd, T. (1991). Does the NART hold after head injury: A case report. *British Journal of Clinical Psychology, 30,* 179–180.

Nelson, H. E. (1982). *National Adult Reading Test (NART): Test manual.* Windsor, UK: NFER Nelson.

Nelson, H. E., & O'Connell, A. (1978). Dementia: The estimation of pre-morbid intelligence levels using the New Adult Reading Test. *Cortex, 14,* 234–244.

Nelson, H. E., & Willison, J. (1991). *National Adult Reading Test (NART): Test manual* (2nd Ed.). Windsor, UK: NFER Nelson.

O'Carroll, R. E. (1987). The inter-rater reliability of the National Adult Reading Test (NART): A pilot study. *British Journal of Clinical Psychology, 26,* 229–230.

O'Carroll, R. E., Moffoot, A., Ebmeier, K. P., & Goodwin, G. M. (1992). Estimating pre-morbid intellectual ability in the alcoholic Korsakoff syndrome. *Psychological Medicine, 22,* 903–909.

O'Connor, J. A., Wiffen, B. D. R., Reichenberg, A., Aas, M., Falcone, M. A., Russo, M., . . . David, A. S. (2012). Is deterioration of IQ a feature of first episode psychosis and how can we measure it? *Schizophrenia Research, 137*(1–3), 104–109.

Paque, L., & Warrington, E. K. (1995). A longitudinal study of reading ability in patients suffering from dementia. *Journal of the International Neuropsychological Society, 1,* 517–524.

Paolo, A. M., Troster, A. I., Ryan, J. J., & Koller, W. C. (1997). Comparison of NART and Barona demographic equation premorbid IQ estimates in Alzheimer's disease. *Journal of Clinical Psychology, 53,* 713–722.

Parkin, A. J., & Java, R. I. (1999). Deterioration of frontal lobe function in normal aging: Influences of fluid intelligence versus perceptual speed. *Neuropsychology, 13,* 539–545.

Patterson, K., Graham, N., & Hodges, J. R. (1994). Reading in dementia of the Alzheimer type: A preserved ability? *Neuropsychology, 8,* 395–407.

Raguet, M. L., Campbell, D. A., Berry, D. T. R., Schmitt, F. A., & Smith, G. T. (1996). Stability of intelligence and intellectual predictors in older persons. *Psychological Assessment, 8,* 154–160.

Rajput, S. S., Hassiotis, A. A., Richards, M. M., Hatch, S. L., & Stewart, R. R. (2011). Associations between IQ and common mental disorders: The 2000 British National Survey of Psychiatric Morbidity. *European Psychiatry, 26*(6), 390–395.

Riley, G. A., & Simmonds, L. V. (2003). How robust is performance on the National Adult Reading Test following traumatic brain injury? *British Journal of Clinical Psychology, 42,* 319–328.

Rolstad, S., Nordlund, A., Gustavsson, M., Eckerström, C., Klang, O., Hansen, S., & Wallin, A. (2008). The Swedish National Adult Reading Test (NART-SWE): A test of premorbid IQ. *Scandinavian Journal of Psychology, 49*(6), 577–582.

Russell, A. J., Munro, J., Jones, P. B., Hayward, P., Hemsley, D. R., & Murray, R. M. (2000). The National Adult Reading Test as a measure of premorbid IQ in schizophrenia. *British Journal of Clinical Psychology, 39,* 297–305.

Ryan, J. J., & Paolo, A. M. (1992). A screening procedure for estimating premorbid intelligence in the elderly. *The Clinical Neuropsychologist, 6,* 53–62.

Schlosser, D., & Ivison, D. (1989). Assessing memory deterioration with the Wechsler Memory Scale, the National Adult Reading Test, and the Schonell Graded Word Reading Test. *Journal of Clinical and Experimental Neuropsychology, 11,* 785–792.

Schretlen, D. J., Buffington, A. H., Meyer, S. M., & Pearlson, G. D. (2005). The use of word-reading to estimate "premorbid" ability in cognitive domains other than intelligence. *Journal of the International Neuropsychological Society, 11*(6), 784–787.

Sharpe, K., & O'Carroll, R. (1991). Estimating premorbid intellectual level in dementia using the National Adult Reading Test: A Canadian study. *British Journal of Clinical Psychology, 30,* 381–384.

Skilbeck, C., Dean, T., Thomas, M., & Slatyer, M. (2013). Impaired National Adult Reading Test (NART) performance in traumatic brain injury. *Neuropsychological Rehabilitation, 23*(2), 234–255.

Starkey, N. J., & Halliday, T. (2011). Development of the New Zealand Adult Reading Test (NZART): Preliminary findings. *New Zealand Journal of Psychology, 40*(3), 129–141.

Starr, J. M., & Lonie, J. (2007). The influence of pre-morbid IQ on Mini-Mental State Examination score at time of dementia presentation. *International Journal of Geriatric Psychiatry, 22*(4), 382–384.

Starr, J. M., & Lonie, J. (2008). Estimated pre-morbid IQ effects on cognitive and functional outcomes in Alzheimer disease: A longitudinal study in a treated cohort. *BMC Psychiatry, 8.* doi:10.1186/1471-244X-8-27

Starr, J. M., Whalley, L. J., Inch, S., & Shering, P. A. (1992). The quantification of the relative effects of age and NART-predicted IQ on cognitive function in healthy old people. *International Journal of Geriatric Psychiatry, 7,* 153–157.

Stebbins, G. T., Gilley, D. W., Wilson, R. S., Bernard, B. A., & Fox, J. H. (1990). Effects of language disturbances on premorbid estimates of IQ in mild dementia. *The Clinical Neuropsychologist, 4,* 64–68.

Stebbins, G. T., Wilson, R. S., Gilley, D. W., Bernard, B. A., & Fox, J. H. (1988). Estimation of premorbid intelligence in dementia. *Journal of Clinical and Experimental Neuropsychology, 10,* 63–64.

Stebbins, G. T., Wilson, R. S., Gilley, D. W., Bernard, B. A., & Fox, J. H. (1990). Use of the National Adult Reading Test to estimate premorbid IQ in dementia. *The Clinical Neuropsychologist, 4,* 18–24.

Storandt, M., Stone, K., & LaBarge, E. (1995). Deficits in reading performance in very mild dementia of the Alzheimer type. *Neuropsychology, 9,* 174–176.

Taylor, K. I., Salmon, D. P., Rice, V. A., Bondi, M. W., Hill, L. R., Ernesto, C. R., & Butters, N. (1996). A longitudinal examination of American National Adult Reading Test (AMNART) performance in dementia of the Alzheimer type (DAT): Validation and correction based on rate of cognitive decline. *Journal of Clinical and Experimental Neuropsychology, 18,* 883–891.

Taylor, R. (1999). National Adult Reading Test performance in established dementia. *Archives of Gerontology and Geriatrics, 29,* 291–296.

Uttl, B. (2002). North American Reading Test: Age norms, reliability, and validity. *Journal of Clinical and Experimental Neuropsychology, 24,* 1123–1137.

Uttl, B., & Graf, P. (1997). Color Word Stroop test performance across the life span. *Journal of Clinical and Experimental Neuropsychology, 19,* 405–420.

Van den Broek, M. D., & Bradshaw, C. M. (1994). Detection of acquired deficits in general intelligence using the National Adult Reading Test and Raven's Standard Progressive Matrices. *British Journal of Clinical Psychology, 33,* 509–515.

Watt, K. J., & O'Carroll, R. E. (1999). Evaluating methods for estimating premorbid intellectual ability in closed head injury. *Journal of Neurology, Neurosurgery, and Psychiatry, 66,* 474–479.

Watt, S., Ong, B., & Crowe, S. F. (2017). Developing a regression equation for predicting premorbid functioning in an Australian sample using the National Adult Reading Test: Predicting premorbid functioning. *Australian Journal of Psychology.* https://doi.org/10.1111/ajpy.12188

Wiens, A. N., Bryan, J. E., & Crossen, J. R. (1993). Estimating WAIS-R FSIQ from the National Adult Reading Test-Revised in normal subjects. *The Clinical Neuropsychologist, 7,* 70–84.

Willshire, D., Kinsella, G., & Prior, M. (1991). Estimating WAIS-R from the National Adult Reading Test: A cross-validation. *Journal of Clinical and Experimental Neuropsychology, 13,* 204–216.

OKLAHOMA PREMORBID INTELLIGENCE ESTIMATE-IV (OPIE-IV)

TEST NAME	**Oklahoma Premorbid Intelligence Estimate-IV (OPIE-IV)**
DOMAIN	Premorbid intellectual functioning
AGE RANGE	20 to 90 years
ADMINISTRATION TIME	5 minutes
SCORING FORMAT	Hand scored
REFERENCE	Holdnack, J. A., Schoenberg, M. R., Lange, R. T., & Iverson, G. L. (2013). Predicting premorbid ability for WAIS-IV, WMS-IV and WASI-II. In J. A. Holdnack, L. Drozdick, L. G. Weiss, & G. L., Iverson (Eds.), *WAIS-IV, WMS-IV, and ACS: Advanced clinical interpretation* (pp. 217–278). San Diego, CA: Elsevier Science.

DESCRIPTION

The Oklahoma Premorbid Intelligence Estimate-IV (OPIE-IV) is a formula that combines select WAIS-IV subtests that are relatively insensitive to neurological dysfunction and demographic information to predict premorbid WAIS-IV scores. The OPIE-IV aims to increase the power of prediction, producing less range restriction and less over- and underestimation of premorbid ability seen in other prediction methods by pairing test behavior with data from demographic variables. The addition of demographics serves to buffer some of the effects of clinical status impacting cognitive performance; the inclusion of current performance indicators can improve predictive accuracy, particularly in those with unusual combinations (e.g., lower than expected reading ability given their educational achievement; Gladsjo et al., 1999).

The OPIE-IV equations were developed using hierarchical regression models, entering the WAIS-IV subtests typically not affected by neurological compromise (i.e., Vocabulary, Matrix Reasoning) first, before entering demographic variables (i.e., age, education, sex, region, and ethnicity). By contrast, on the TOPF (Pearson, 2009), demographic variables were entered into the prediction equation before the TOPF Word Reading score. Therefore, compared to the TOPF, the OPIE-IV is more affected by individual current performance than by demographic variables because the latter were entered in the prediction equation after the WAIS-IV subtest scores.

The OPIE was initially developed by Krull, Scott, and Schere (1995) and Vanderploeg, Schinka, and Axelrod (1996) for use with the WAIS-R and was shown to correlate highly with premorbid ability (Hoofien et al., 2000). Formulas have also been generated for the WAIS-III (Schoenberg et al., 2002, 2004). With the WAIS-IV, a total of 24 OPIE-IV algorithms were developed using the WAIS-IV standardization sample to predict WAIS-IV FSIQ, GAI, VCI, and PRI, including prorated and alternate indices. Unlike the OPIE-3, which included more subtests, only WAIS-IV Vocabulary and Matrix Reasoning subtests were used in the algorithm. A worksheet for computing FSIQ, VCI, PRI, and GAI is included in Table 4–5. Similar to the TOPF, statistical significance levels and base rates for actual versus predicted scores are provided (Tables 4–6 to 4–8).

ADMINISTRATION

Users apply WAIS-IV Vocabulary and/or Matrix Reasoning raw scores as well as demographic information of the examinee to the appropriate equation as shown in Table 4–5.

SCORING

A number of predicted scores can be generated, including FSIQ, GAI, VCI, and PRI, using either both or one of WAIS-IV Vocabulary and Matrix Reasoning raw scores. Predicted IQ can be generated for standard WAIS-IV indexes or for prorated WAIS-IV indexes. The scores are calculated using the equations found in Table 4–5. Significance of the difference between actual IQ and predicted IQ, as well as base rates of the difference, are determined by referring to Tables 4–6 to 4–8.

DEMOGRAPHIC EFFECTS

Effects of age, gender, and ethnicity have not been reported.

TABLE 4–5 Oklahoma Premorbid Intelligence Estimate-IV (OPIE-IV) Calculation Worksheet

OPIE-IV FOR STANDARD WAIS-IV INDEXES

Using VC/MR

Predicted FSIQ = 57.84718185 + (0.706570548 * VC raw) + (1.38658557 * MR raw) + (−0.204106431 * Age in years) + (0.0000415057 * Age^3) + (−4.213630131 * Kinder CAT) + (−1.880854304 * 8–10th grade CAT) + (1.765273315 * bachelor's degree CAT) + (1.568961576 * Sex CAT) + (1.061002858 * Midwest region CAT) + (−5.143182795 * African American CAT)

Predicted GAI = 52.97658443 + (0.789874 * VC raw) + (1.406248 * MR raw) + (−0.224896406 * Age in years) + (0.0000441068 * Age^3) + (1.49458 * bachelor's degree CAT) + (3.234337 * Sex CAT) + (−4.46367 * African American CAT)

Using VC only

Predicted FSIQ = 82.86006918 + (0.931060376 * VC raw) + (−0.376169362 * Age in years) + (0.0000392298 * Age^3) + (−5.891117334 * Kinder CAT) + (−4.073450564 * 8–10th grade CAT) + (−2.830601142 * 11th grade CAT) + (4.241005492 * bachelor's degree CAT) + (2.526538833 * post bachelor's/master's degree CAT) + (4.743247729 * post master's, no doctorate CAT) + (2.538945816 * Sex CAT) + (−7.390687749 * African American CAT)

Using MR only

Predicted FSIQ = 57.42662034 + (2.006596115 * MR raw) + (0.0000318464 * Age^3) + (−10.46845904 * Kinder CAT) + (−7.351663122 * 8–10th grade CAT) + (−2.781401808 * 11th grade CAT) + (2.899985431 * one year of college CAT) + (2.537006071 * associate's degree or two years of college CAT) + (4.201333866 * 3–5 years of college, no degree CAT) + (6.294217609 * bachelor's degree CAT) + (5.960155042 * post bachelor's/master's degree CAT) + (6.502111716 * post master's, no degree CAT) + (1.38533733 * Sex CAT) + (2.084914692 * West region CAT)

OPIE-IV FOR PRORATED WAIS-IV INDEXES

Using VC/MR

Predicted FSIQ = 65.77827122 + (0.646258435 * VC raw) + (1.182068623 * MR raw) + (−0.197692558 * Age in years) + (0.0000373292 * Age^3) + (−5.753441804 * Kinder CAT) + (−2.889407206 * 8–10th grade CAT) + (2.196080965 * bachelor's degree CAT) + (1.955504838 * Sex CAT) + (−6.408803891 * African American CAT)

Predicted GAI = 60.14203956 + (0.763136717 * VC raw) + (1.127062322 * MR raw) + (−0.246247784 * Age in years) + (0.0000416209 * Age^3) + (4.708926488 * Sex CAT) + (−6.115458508 * African American CAT)

Using VC only

Predicted FSIQ = 86.63733022 + (0.825479066 * VC raw) + (−0.355783733 * Age in years) + (0.0000373292 * Age^3) + (−6.680477054 * Kinder CAT) + (−4.662311507 * 8–10th grade CAT) + (−3.186323014 * 11th grade CAT) + (4.726126229 * bachelor's degree CAT) + (2.633221566 * post bachelor's/master's degree CAT) + (5.499588668 * post master's, no doctorate CAT) + (2.795447219 * Sex CAT) + (−8.310210877 * African American CAT)

Using MR only

Predicted FSIQ = 62.02281403 + (1.719384768 * MR raw) + (0.0000275723 * Age^3) + (−11.56620904 * Kinder CAT) + (−7.947319233 * 8–10th grade CAT) + (−2.809230427 * 11th grade CAT) + (3.53868906 * one year of college CAT) + (3.007371787 * associate's degree/two years of college CAT) + (4.87775878 * 3–5 years of college, no degree CAT) + (7.134143065 * bachelor's degree CAT) + (6.727414092 * post bachelor's/master's degree CAT) + (7.370474506 * post master's, no doctorate CAT) + (6.439956971 * Doctorate CAT) + (1.509479923 * Sex CAT) + (2.265782512 * West region CAT)

NOTE: VC = Vocabulary subtest; MR = Matrix Reasoning subtest; Kinder CAT = Kindergarten–7th grade; Sex CAT: 0 = Female, 1 = Male; CAT = category: 0 = does not belong to category, 1 = belongs to category (for education, ethnicity, and region variables); FSIQ = Full Scale IQ; GAI = General Ability Index.

SOURCE: Adapted from Holdnack et al. (2013).

TABLE 4–6 Critical Values Required for Statistical Significance of Oklahoma Premorbid Intelligence Estimate-IV (OPIE-IV) Predicted Premorbid vs. Current Wechsler Adult Intelligence Scale-Fourth Edition (WAIS-IV) Indexes

	SIG. LEVEL	STANDARD FSIQ	PRORATED FSIQ	STANDARD GAI	PRORATED GAI
Vocabulary and Matrix Reasoning Predicted Indexes					
	0.05	6.90	7.15	5.88	7.94
	0.01	9.01	9.66	7.68	10.73
Vocabulary Only Predicted Indexes					
	0.05	8.00	7.48	6.93	8.35
	0.01	10.45	10.11	9.05	11.28
Matrix Reasoning Only Predicted Indexes					
	0.05	9.63	9.42	6.47	9.93
	0.01	12.58	12.73	8.45	13.42
Vocabulary or Matrix Reasoning Only Predicted Indexes					
	0.05	6.76	9.08	7.96	10.02
	0.01	8.83	12.26	10.46	13.54

SOURCE: Adapted from Holdnack et al. (2013).

NORMATIVE DATA

The OPIE-IV regression equations were developed using the WAIS-IV standardization sample. Please refer to the description of the WAIS-IV in Chapter 5 for more information about the standardization sample.

EVIDENCE FOR VALIDITY

The only validation study to date was conducted during the development of the OPIE-IV algorithm using a subgroup of the WAIS-IV standardization sample. The development sample and validation sample generated similar results, providing support for the validity of the OPIE-IV to estimate IQ. The correlations between the actual and predicted scores in the validation sample ranged from .70 to .90 (Holdnack et al., 2013).

The accuracy of the estimates obtained by the OPIE-IV equations was verified by comparing the predicted scores with the actual WAIS-IV scores. The equations using both Vocabulary and Matrix Reasoning generated predicted standard scores that are within ±5 points for more than 93% of the sample and within ±10 points for about 98% of the sample. The equations using Vocabulary only and Matrix Reasoning only were less accurate in predicting FSIQ/GAI, at about 87% and 76%, respectively, of predicted scores within ±5 points of actual scores and about 95% and about 91%, respectively, of predicted scores within ±10 points of actual scores. The accuracy data for prorated scores were in the same trend but lower than the standard scores. Overall, more than 90% of predicted scores were in the same category as the actual scores for all equations except prorated PRI (Holdnack et al., 2013).

COMPARISONS WITH OTHER PREDICTION METHODS

To date, limited studies have compared the OPIE-IV to other prediction methods. The authors of the OPIE-IV compared the WAIS-IV predicted scores obtained by the OPIE-IV to that of the TOPF and found that the OPIE-IV generated higher R^2 values for the FSIQ and GAI when using the Vocabulary and Matrix Reasoning equations. They indicated that the R^2 values for the TOPF are generally similar compared to Vocabulary-only OPIE-IV and somewhat higher than the Matrix Reasoning-only equations.

CLINICAL STUDIES

None have been published as of the writing of this chapter.

COMMENT

The OPIE-IV is relatively new, and no independent validation studies have been carried out as of this writing. An advantage of the OPIE-IV is that a premorbid estimate can be obtained without having to administer additional tests. Moreover, equations to obtain IQ estimates and base rate comparisons for prorated indices are available in the event the whole WAIS-IV was not administered. Compared to word-reading prediction methods such as the TOPF, another advantage of the OPIE-IV is that it can be used to estimate premorbid functioning among examinees whose reading and/or pronunciation is negatively affected by their conditions, including developmental or acquired reading or language disturbances, all of which preclude use of tests such as the TOPF and the NART. Users are encouraged to include both Vocabulary and Matrix Reasoning scores in their prediction model because inclusion of these two subtests

TABLE 4–7 Base Rates of Actual Versus Predicted Standard Wechsler Adult Intelligence Scale-Fourth Edition (WAIS-IV) Full Scale IQ, General Ability Index, Verbal Comprehension Index, and Perceptual Reasoning Index

	FSIQ FROM VC/MR		FSIQ FROM VC		FSIQ FROM MR		GAI FROM VC/MR		GAI FROM VC		GAI FROM MR		VCI FROM VC		PRI FROM MR	
	ACT <PRED	ACT >PRED	ACT <PRED	ACT >PRED	ACT <PRED	ACT >PRED	ACT <PRED	ACT >PRED	ACT <PRED	ACT >PRED	ACT <PRED	ACT >PRED	ACT <PRED	ACT >PRED	ACT <PRED	ACT >PRED
35	–	–	–	0.20	–	–	–	–	–	–	–	–	–	–	–	–
34	–	–	–	0.29	–	–	–	–	–	–	–	–	–	–	–	–
33	–	–	–	0.29	–	–	–	–	–	–	–	–	–	–	–	0.10
32	–	–	–	0.29	–	–	–	–	–	–	–	–	–	–	–	0.29
31	–	–	–	0.29	–	–	–	–	–	–	–	–	–	–	–	0.29
30	–	–	–	0.29	–	0.10	–	–	–	–	–	0.10	–	–	–	0.29
29	–	–	–	0.29	–	0.29	–	–	0.10	–	–	0.29	–	–	–	0.29
28	–	–	–	0.29	–	0.29	–	–	0.20	0.20	–	0.29	–	–	–	0.29
27	–	–	0.10	0.29	–	0.29	–	–	0.29	0.29	–	0.39	–	–	–	0.29
26	–	0.10	0.29	0.29	–	0.39	–	–	0.29	0.29	–	0.59	–	–	–	0.29
25	–	0.20	0.49	0.29	0.20	0.49	–	–	0.39	0.29	–	0.79	–	0.10	–	0.69
24	–	0.20	0.59	0.49	0.29	0.69	–	–	0.79	0.29	0.10	0.98	–	0.20	–	0.69
23	–	0.29	0.59	0.79	0.49	0.98	–	0.10	0.79	0.39	0.29	0.98	–	0.20	–	0.69
22	–	0.29	0.79	0.88	0.59	1.28	–	0.20	0.79	0.49	0.39	1.38	–	0.20	0.10	0.98
21	0.10	0.29	0.79	1.08	0.98	1.47	–	0.20	0.88	0.69	0.49	1.67	–	0.20	0.20	1.28
20	0.20	0.29	1.18	1.96	1.18	2.06	–	0.29	1.28	0.88	0.88	2.06	–	0.29	0.29	1.67
19	0.20	0.39	1.57	1.96	1.57	2.85	0.10	0.29	1.38	1.38	1.08	2.36	0.10	0.29	0.59	1.67
18	0.49	0.39	2.06	2.55	2.16	3.63	0.29	0.39	1.96	1.77	1.38	3.05	0.39	0.29	0.79	2.36
17	0.69	0.88	3.05	3.34	3.24	4.42	0.39	0.39	2.26	2.36	1.96	3.24	0.39	0.39	1.47	3.54
16	0.98	1.57	4.03	3.93	4.62	5.11	0.69	0.69	3.05	3.44	2.85	4.13	0.39	0.88	2.75	4.52
15	1.87	1.87	4.81	4.91	5.21	6.39	1.08	1.28	3.83	4.22	3.63	5.21	0.39	1.28	3.63	5.89
14	2.75	2.95	5.70	5.80	6.58	7.56	1.38	1.57	4.22	5.11	4.72	6.68	0.88	1.77	4.52	7.47
13	3.54	3.63	6.78	7.66	7.86	8.74	1.87	2.26	5.70	6.78	6.97	8.35	1.67	2.26	5.80	8.64
12	4.72	4.72	8.74	9.33	10.12	10.61	2.55	2.85	7.56	8.45	9.63	9.92	2.36	3.05	7.96	9.72
11	5.89	5.80	10.90	10.90	12.38	12.48	4.03	4.03	9.43	10.22	11.69	12.08	3.24	4.52	10.31	11.89
10	7.66	7.96	13.06	12.38	14.54	14.34	5.30	5.40	11.20	12.38	13.75	13.85	5.21	6.19	12.48	14.05
9	10.31	9.92	16.40	14.83	18.07	16.99	7.07	6.88	13.46	15.23	17.88	17.19	6.19	7.37	15.42	16.31
8	13.46	13.56	18.57	17.98	20.73	19.94	9.72	9.63	16.31	18.27	21.12	20.63	9.04	9.43	19.25	19.35
7	16.80	16.70	21.02	21.51	24.56	22.79	13.26	13.06	20.43	21.81	24.56	22.89	12.77	12.67	23.08	22.99
6	20.92	19.94	25.15	24.95	28.49	26.52	17.19	18.07	24.07	24.75	28.29	26.33	16.11	16.11	28.19	26.33
5	25.25	25.25	28.98	29.47	31.63	30.16	22.20	22.99	28.19	28.00	32.81	30.26	21.12	20.92	32.71	29.57
4	30.55	30.94	33.10	33.69	34.77	33.79	27.41	27.80	32.91	32.22	37.52	34.68	26.23	26.52	37.13	33.50
3	36.84	36.64	37.82	37.92	38.31	37.33	33.60	33.40	37.72	36.44	40.96	38.70	32.71	31.34	41.94	36.74
2	41.45	41.45	43.81	42.83	44.30	42.83	40.28	39.39	43.03	40.28	44.89	41.75	40.67	37.23	46.17	39.59
1	47.54	46.17	48.13	46.37	49.31	45.97	47.45	45.28	47.64	45.38	49.02	46.07	48.43	44.50	49.71	44.40
M	5.72	5.89	7.30	7.03	7.34	7.84	4.97	5.21	6.70	7.10	7.28	7.74	4.70	5.12	6.93	7.75
SD	3.96	4.09	5.35	5.17	5.19	5.70	3.53	3.64	4.96	5.05	4.67	5.58	3.33	3.81	4.36	5.46

NOTE: FSIQ = Full Scale IQ; GAI = General Ability Index; VCI = Verbal Comprehension Index; PRI = Perceptual Reasoning Index; VC = Vocabulary; MR = Matrix Reasoning; ACT = Actual; PRED = Predicted.

SOURCE: From Holdnack et al. (2013).

TABLE 4–8 Base Rates of Actual Versus Predicted Prorated Wechsler Adult Intelligence Scale-Fourth Edition (WAIS-IV) Full Scale IQ, General Ability Index, Verbal Comprehension Index, and Perceptual Reasoning Index

	FSIQ FROM VC/MR		FSIQ FROM VC		FSIQ FROM MR		GAI FROM VC/MR		GAI FROM VC		GAI FROM MR		VCI FROM VC		PRI FROM MR	
	ACT <PRED	ACT >PRED	ACT <PRED	ACT >PRED	ACT <PRED	ACT >PRED	ACT <PRED	ACT >PRED	ACT <PRED	ACT >PRED	ACT <PRED	ACT >PRED	ACT <PRED	ACT >PRED	ACT <PRED	ACT >PRED
>40	–	–	–	–	–	–	–	–	–	–	–	0.10	–	–	–	0.10
40	–	–	–	–	–	–	–	–	–	–	–	0.39	–	–	–	0.15
39	–	–	–	–	–	–	–	–	–	–	–	0.39	–	–	–	0.15
38	–	–	–	–	–	–	–	0.10	–	–	–	0.39	–	–	–	0.20
37	–	–	0.10	–	–	–	–	0.20	–	–	–	0.39	–	–	–	0.20
36	–	–	0.20	–	–	–	–	0.20	–	–	–	0.39	–	–	–	0.20
35	–	–	0.49	–	–	–	–	0.20	0.10	–	–	0.39	–	0.10	–	0.25
34	–	–	0.49	–	–	–	–	0.20	0.20	–	–	0.39	–	0.20	0.05	0.25
33	–	–	0.49	–	–	0.10	–	0.20	0.20	–	–	0.49	–	0.20	0.15	0.25
32	–	–	0.49	–	–	0.20	–	0.29	0.20	–	–	0.59	–	0.20	0.15	0.25
31	–	0.10	0.49	–	–	0.20	–	0.29	0.29	0.20	–	0.69	–	0.20	0.25	0.30
30	–	0.20	0.49	0.10	–	0.29	–	0.29	0.29	0.29	–	0.79	–	0.20	0.30	0.54
29	–	0.20	0.49	0.20	–	0.39	–	0.39	0.29	0.29	–	0.79	–	0.29	0.30	0.79
28	–	0.20	0.49	0.39	–	0.49	–	0.39	0.29	0.29	0.10	0.98	–	0.49	0.34	1.03
27	–	0.29	0.49	0.49	0.29	0.69	0.10	0.39	0.39	0.29	0.20	1.08	0.10	0.49	0.44	1.23
26	–	0.29	0.69	0.59	0.39	0.79	0.20	0.39	0.59	0.39	0.39	1.47	0.49	0.59	0.64	1.53
25	0.10	0.29	0.79	0.59	0.39	1.18	0.20	0.39	0.59	0.39	0.88	1.77	0.49	0.69	0.98	1.82
24	0.20	0.29	0.98	1.08	0.49	1.38	0.20	0.88	0.88	0.59	0.88	2.26	0.49	0.69	1.13	2.41
23	0.20	0.39	1.08	1.08	0.98	1.77	0.39	0.88	0.88	0.79	1.38	2.55	0.49	0.88	1.53	2.85
22	0.49	0.59	1.08	1.08	1.18	2.16	0.59	0.88	1.08	0.79	1.38	2.85	0.49	1.18	2.02	3.30
21	0.59	0.88	1.77	1.47	1.37	2.65	0.69	1.28	1.47	1.38	1.77	3.24	0.59	1.18	2.76	3.89
20	0.98	1.47	2.16	1.96	2.16	3.44	0.98	1.47	1.96	1.77	2.16	3.93	0.88	1.67	3.30	5.07
19	1.38	1.96	2.95	2.65	2.65	4.03	1.67	1.96	2.36	1.87	2.55	4.81	1.18	2.26	3.89	6.25
18	1.87	2.36	3.73	3.73	4.32	4.32	2.16	2.75	3.14	2.55	3.24	5.50	1.87	2.85	5.07	6.89
17	2.95	2.65	4.62	4.13	5.01	5.40	3.14	3.14	3.54	3.63	4.52	6.19	2.46	3.34	6.40	7.73
16	3.54	3.34	5.70	5.11	6.19	6.78	3.93	3.63	4.52	4.72	6.29	7.27	3.14	4.13	7.63	8.56
15	4.32	3.73	6.68	5.99	6.78	8.06	4.72	4.32	5.30	5.89	7.47	8.55	4.13	4.52	8.91	9.69
14	5.11	5.01	7.96	7.07	8.06	9.33	5.80	5.21	6.29	6.97	9.43	10.31	5.11	5.21	10.68	11.12
13	6.39	6.29	9.72	9.23	9.92	11.10	6.97	6.48	7.56	8.35	11.69	12.18	6.68	6.48	12.16	12.84
12	8.15	7.76	11.30	10.81	11.98	12.37	8.55	7.96	9.14	10.22	12.97	13.16	7.96	7.36	14.37	14.71
11	9.82	9.92	12.77	13.06	13.95	14.24	10.51	10.22	10.81	12.77	16.11	15.72	10.12	9.72	16.98	16.88
10	13.06	12.57	14.83	15.52	17.39	16.80	13.06	12.67	12.97	14.83	18.96	18.76	12.38	11.59	20.13	19.29
9	15.91	15.32	17.09	18.27	20.04	19.16	15.91	15.32	15.82	17.68	22.79	20.83	14.73	13.75	23.43	21.65
8	19.06	18.57	20.73	20.33	23.38	22.20	19.45	19.06	19.16	20.33	25.25	22.79	17.58	17.68	26.48	24.51
7	22.30	21.51	23.87	24.46	26.92	24.85	22.79	21.91	22.69	23.08	28.98	25.93	20.92	21.02	29.33	27.81
6	24.95	26.03	27.41	27.21	30.16	28.09	26.03	25.93	25.93	25.74	31.93	29.17	25.44	24.75	32.09	30.36
5	30.55	30.65	31.04	30.75	33.60	31.14	30.75	29.17	30.06	28.49	35.36	33.30	29.76	28.98	34.84	33.76
4	34.38	33.99	34.48	34.18	36.44	35.07	35.66	33.50	34.38	33.60	39.19	35.56	33.40	31.83	38.29	37.16
3	38.11	38.21	37.72	39.69	39.98	38.80	39.49	38.02	38.90	37.52	43.03	38.70	37.92	35.85	41.93	41.68
2	43.22	42.73	42.93	44.89	44.80	43.03	43.81	41.94	43.81	41.06	45.48	42.04	43.22	41.36	45.28	44.69
1	48.82	46.86	47.25	48.72	49.71	47.25	48.82	46.17	48.13	46.56	48.82	45.58	47.94	46.46	48.08	48.33
M	6.89	7.13	7.91	7.69	8.02	8.43	7.09	7.30	7.34	7.58	8.65	9.23	6.85	7.05	8.68	9.16
SD	4.92	5.03	5.99	5.70	5.69	6.36	5.01	5.37	5.56	5.59	5.55	6.92	4.86	5.51	5.84	7.12

NOTE: FSIQ = Full Scale IQ; GAI = General Ability Index; VCI = Verbal Comprehension Index; PRI = Perceptual Reasoning Index; VC = Vocabulary; MR = Matrix Reasoning; ACT = Actual; PRED = Predicted.

SOURCE: From Holdnack et al. (2013).

yields the highest prediction accuracy. In the event of an examinee with severe language disturbance, users may decide to utilize the Matrix Reasoning-only equation, although the use of prorated PRI is discouraged. Unlike the OPIE-3, the OPIE-IV uses only the Vocabulary and Matrix Reasoning subtests in the prediction equations. By including only the subtests most resistant to neurological insults, the susceptibility of the premorbid estimates to neurological effects seen in previous clinical studies on the OPIE-3 are likely minimized (Langeluddecke & Lucas, 2004). At this time, however, this method requires additional independent validation studies, including studies in clinical populations such as traumatic brain injury and dementia, as well as against an actual premorbid criterion. The OPIE-3 is susceptible to relatively large errors of prediction (standard errors of estimation, SEEs) and may under- or overestimate FSIQ in various age groups, but whether or not these issues apply to the OPIE-IV has not been reported.

REFERENCES

Gladsjo, J. A., Heaton, R. K., Palmer, B. W., Taylor, M. J., & Jeste, D. V. (1999). Use of oral reading to estimate premorbid intellectual and neuropsychological functioning. *Journal of the International Neuropsychological Society*, *5*(03), 247–254.

Holdnack, J. A., Schoenberg, M. R., Lange, R. T., & Iverson, G. L. (2013). Predicting premorbid ability for WAIS-IV, WMS-IV and WASI-II. In J. A. Holdnack, L. Drozdick, L. G. Weiss, & G. L., Iverson (Eds.), *WAIS-IV, WMS-IV, and ACS: Advanced clinical interpretation* (pp. 217–278). San Diego, CA: Elsevier Science.

Hoofien, D., Vakil, E., & Gilboa, A. (2000). Criterion validation of premorbid intelligence estimation in persons with traumatic brain injury: "Hold/don't hold" versus "best performance" procedures. *Journal of Clinical and Experimental Neuropsychology*, *22*(3), 305–315.

Krull, K. R., Scott, J. G., & Sherer, M. (1995). Estimation of premorbid intelligence from combined performance and demographic variables. *The Clinical Neuropsychologist*, *9*(1), 83–88.

Langeluddecke, P. M., & Lucas, S. K. (2004). Evaluation of two methods for estimating premorbid intelligence on the WAIS-III in a clinical sample. *The Clinical Neuropsychologist*, *18*(3), 423–432.

Pearson, N. C. S. (2009). *Advanced Clinical Solutions for WAIS-IV and WMS-IV: Administration and scoring manual.* San Antonio, TX: The Psychological Corporation.

Schoenberg, M., Duff, K., Dorfman, K., & Adams, R. (2004). Differential estimation of verbal intelligence and performance intelligence scores from combined performance and demographic variables: The OPIE-3 Verbal and Performance Algorithms. *The Clinical Neuropsychologist*, *18*(2), 266–276.

Schoenberg, M. R., Scott, J. G., Duff, K., & Adams, R. L. (2002). Estimation of WAIS-III intelligence from combined performance and demographic variables: Development of the OPIE-3. *The Clinical Neuropsychologist*, *16*(4), 426–438.

Vanderploeg, R. D., Schinka, J. A., & Axelrod, B. N. (1996). Estimation of WAIS-R premorbid intelligence: Current ability and demographic data used in a best-performance fashion. *Psychological Assessment*, *8*(4), 404.

TEST OF PREMORBID FUNCTIONING (TOPF)

TEST NAME	**Test of Premorbid Functioning (TOPF)**
DOMAIN	Premorbid intellectual and memory functioning
AGE RANGE	16 to 90 years
ADMINISTRATION TIME	10 minutes
SCORING FORMAT	Computer scored
REFERENCE	Pearson, N. C. S. (2009). *Advanced Clinical Solutions for WAIS-IV and WMS-IV: Administration and scoring manual.* The Psychological Corporation, San Antonio. www.pearsonclinical.com

DESCRIPTION

The Test of Premorbid Functioning (TOPF; Pearson, 2009) provides an estimate of premorbid intellectual and memory functioning using one of three methods: (1) demographic variables, (2) performance on a word reading test of irregular words (i.e., atypical grapheme-to-phoneme translation), or (3) combinations of both approaches. As such, it includes features of other estimation methods such as the NART and the OPIE-IV, with the added component of premorbid memory estimation and the use of a large normative dataset from the WAIS-IV/WMS-IV standardization sample (all reviewed in this volume). It is a revision of the Wechsler Test of Adult Reading (WTAR; PsychCorp, 2001), but the name was changed to better reflect the purpose of the measure: to estimate premorbid functioning rather than to measure reading ability (Pearson, 2009).

Like other reading-based premorbid estimation methods, the TOPF uses irregular words to assess premorbid functioning because standard pronunciation rules cannot be applied to read the words correctly; accurate performance therefore depends on prior learning. The utility of the method relies on (a) the relatively strong correlation between reading ability and intellectual functioning in healthy people and (b) the fact that word reading is relatively resistant to the cognitive decline associated with normal aging and brain insult. As a consequence, word reading tends to result in a fairly reasonable estimate of premorbid ability. However, the TOPF should not be used to diagnose reading proficiency or reading disability.

Similar to its predecessor, the WTAR, the TOPF is co-normed with the WAIS-IV and WMS-IV, allowing for direct comparison between predicted and actual functioning with regard to general intellectual status and memory. This feature is an advantage over other word-reading prediction methods such as the NART (but see "Comment" section). Several updates were made to address shortcomings of the WTAR and of other prediction methods (e.g., OPIE-IV) such as restricted range due to regression to the mean. Modifications to the WTAR regression equations were made to improve the prediction range and accuracy of the TOPF by (1) expanding the education levels through to the doctorate; (2) adding other demographic information, including occupation, geographic region, and other personal and developmental factors to the prediction model; (3) equating scores on the TOPF with the WAIS-IV and WMS-IV scores prior to entry into the equation; (4) increasing the number of items, especially difficult items, to raise the ceiling of the TOPF; and (5) changing the order of entry for the hierarchical regression model by entering education and occupation before the TOPF Word Reading scores to reduce the latter's impact on the prediction score in the event that the word reading score is affected by brain injury (Pearson, 2009). In addition, *equipercentile equating* was used to transform TOPF Word Reading age-adjusted standard scores. It is a statistical method to ensure that the TOPF has an equivalent percentile to the Wechsler tests. This method purportedly reduces some of the effects of regression to the mean. To account for differences in calculating education and occupation variables for those aged 16–19, two separate regression equations for ages 16–19 and 20–90 are provided.

ADMINISTRATION

The TOPF Word Reading comprises 70 words. This word reading test is administered by the examiner, who presents the word card and asks the examinee to pronounce each word. If the examinee does not respond within 30 seconds, a score of 0 is given for that item. The criterion for discontinuation is 5 consecutive scores of 0.

SCORING

The TOPF is part of the Advanced Clinical Solutions (ACS) software. An audio clip with various accepted pronunciation is included in the software. Scoring must be completed by the scoring software. The administration manual provides a table to convert TOPF Word Reading raw scores to standard scores stratified by age; however, the ACS software is needed to obtain comparison data and the estimate of premorbid functioning based on different prediction models.

A number of prediction models are available to estimate the premorbid functioning of the examinee. For the 16–19 age group, only the simple demographic equation is available. In this age group, parent education and race/ethnicity are used. For the 20–90 age group, the prediction models are:

1. Demographic prediction models:
    a. Simple demographic equation uses education, occupation, region, and race/ethnicity
    b. Complex demographic equation uses education, occupation, region, race/ethnicity, and personal and developmental factors
2. TOPF Word Reading only
3. Combined TOPF Word Reading and demographic prediction models:
    a. TOPF Word Reading + simple demographic prediction model
    b. TOPF Word Reading + complex demographic prediction model

Personal factors assess achievement, personal success, activity level, and socioeconomic status. Developmental factors assess factors such as quality of elementary school, wealth of neighborhood, parents' level of education, and parents' occupation while growing up.

The examiner decides on the prediction model to estimate premorbid functioning based on a number of factors. Holdnack et al. (2013) recommend using background factors such as representativeness of the examinees' demographic variables and history of conditions that can affect academic achievement or employment.

In cases where the acquisition of reading skills is interrupted by illnesses, learning disability, medical or neurological conditions, English as a second language, or illiteracy, the TOPF Word Reading test may not be appropriate for estimating premorbid functioning. In order to quantitatively assess whether the current TOPF Word Reading performance is affected by injury or illness, the examiner may estimate expected TOPF Word Reading score using demographic variables to determine the significance and base rate of the obtained-predicted word reading discrepancy. Such information is useful in determining whether the current word reading performance has been compromised and also allows the clinician to determine which prediction model (e.g., word reading and/or demographics) is most appropriate for estimating the premorbid functioning of an individual examinee.

The ACS software provides base rates of the discrepancy between the actual TOPF Word Reading score and demographically predicted word reading score. If the base rate of the discrepancy is low (e.g., <10%), the examiner may choose to use the demographic-only model to estimate premorbid functioning. However, unless the TOPF Word Reading performance is severely compromised, the preferred methodology suggested in the manual is the combined TOPF word-reading-demographics prediction of premorbid functioning.

The examiner follows the steps outlined here to make an estimate of the examinee's premorbid functioning. Users are encouraged to refer to Holdnack et al. (2013) for details on the decision matrix.

1. Administer the word reading test to the examinee.
2. Assess whether the obtained word reading test score is an accurate representation of the examinee's ability by:
    a. Using the examinee's demographic background to predict the word reading score.
    b. Comparing the obtained word reading score to the demographically predicted word reading score.
    c. Determining if the obtained-predicted word reading score discrepancy is statistically significant.
    d. If it is significant, determining if the discrepancy occurs at a low base rate (i.e., <10%).
3. Choose a prediction model for estimating the examinee's premorbid functioning based on the outcome of steps 2a to 2d.

PREDICTION OF TOPF WORD READING USING DEMOGRAPHIC DATA

The TOPF Word Reading score can also be estimated using demographic data. The predicted word reading score can then be compared with the obtained TOPF Word Reading score to determine if the obtained score aligns with the expected word reading score based on the demographic background of the examinee. Base rates of the discrepancy between the obtained and the predicted word reading score are provided to determine the frequency of the score difference.

The simple demographic model shows low predictive power for 16–19 year-olds ($R^2 = .16$). As such, the manual cautions against the use of demographic variables to estimate TOPF Word Reading in this group. The predictive power of the simple demographic model is much better for the adult group ($R^2 = .42$); addition of other variables (i.e., the complex demographic model) did not improve the predictive power, but the variance accounted for by each variable changed with the addition of personal and developmental factors. Given the power of the simple demographic model to predict TOPF Word Reading, the predicted score may be used to assess whether or not the obtained TOPF score is unusually low in the adult group. If so, the TOPF Word Reading score may have been influenced by factors unrelated to premorbid functioning and may not be suitable as a premorbid intellectual estimate for the individual. Use of the demographic-only prediction model for estimating premorbid functioning is encouraged in this case.

PREDICTION OF INTELLECTUAL AND MEMORY FUNCTIONING

The manual provides a number of different prediction equations based on demographic variables alone, TOPF score alone, or combinations of demographics and TOPF scores. As seen in Table 4–9, in the age 16–19 group, both simple demographics and the combined simple demographics and TOPF Word Reading models obtain the best prediction accuracy for FSIQ and VCI, although the predictive accuracy is low with the simple demographics only model. It is important to note that the prediction error in this age group is relatively large. For example, using the combined model, which explains the largest variance of the two models, 49% of the sample's predicted score is within 5 points of the actual VCI score, while 74% have predicted scores within 10 points. Predictive accuracy is in the low to very low range for other WAIS-IV and WMS-IV indices using either model. Correlations between demographics and WMS-IV Immediate Memory Index (IMI), Delayed Memory Index (DMI), and Visual Working Memory Index (VWMI) are too low to provide adequate predictions and are not presented (Pearson, 2009).

In the 20–90 group, all the prediction models (i.e., simple demographics only, complex demographics only, simple demographics and TOPF Word Reading, and complex demographics and TOPF Word Reading) obtain the best prediction accuracy and in the moderate range for FSIQ and VCI (Table 4–10). Addition of the TOPF Word Reading score to the demographic variables improves the predictive accuracy substantially. For example, using simple demographics only, predictive accuracies are $R^2 = .47$ and .46 for FSIQ and VCI, respectively. With the addition of the TOPF Word Reading score, the predictive accuracies increase to $R^2 = .68$ (VCI) and .63 (FSIQ). Although these scores have the smallest prediction errors, they are still rather large. For example, VCI had the highest overall prediction accuracy for both the combined models, with about 48% of the sample's predicted scores within 5 points of the actual score, and about 78% have predicted scores within 10 points. Correlations between demographics and WMS-IV IMI and DMI are too low to provide adequate predictions and are not presented.

With regard to accuracy of classification based on TOPF Word Reading alone, in about 66% of the cases, predicted FSIQ is within ±10 points (39% are within ±5 points); similar percentages are observed for VCI. However, estimates for WMS-IV memory performance are poor (about 50% within ±10 points). In short, TOPF Word Reading performance appears to be a reasonable predictor of premorbid intellectual functioning (particularly VCI) but should only be considered a modest predictor of premorbid memory ability.

RELIABLE CHANGE

The Reliable Change method can also be used to determine the significance of the difference in a reassessment. Using the reliable change method for reassessment, levels of statistical significance between predicted Time 2 score and actual Time 2 score are provided to determine if the Time 2 score represents a significant decline from Time 1. If the Time 2 TOPF Word Reading score is significantly

TABLE 4–9 Prediction Accuracy of the Simple Demographics and Combined Simple Demographics and Test of Premorbid Functioning (TOPF) Word Reading Scores for Ages 16 to 19

PREDICTION MODEL	INDEX	R^2	PERCENTAGE OF CASES WITHIN ±5 POINTS OF ACTUAL SCORE	PERCENTAGE OF CASES WITHIN ±10 POINTS OF ACTUAL SCORE	RANGE OF PREDICTED INDEX SCORES
Simple demographics	FSIQ	.26	38	66	85–119
	VCI	.27	36	61	74–123
	PRI	.17	34	56	82–113
	WMI	.16	34	58	87–111
	PSI	.16	37	64	87–121
Simple demographics and TOPF Word Reading	FSIQ	.46	42	71	57–138
	VCI	.52	49	74	59–146
	PRI	.27	33	60	70–126
	WMI	.31	42	65	71–129
	PSI	.20	37	67	78–125
	IMI	.29	38	66	68–133
	DMI	.23	35	64	76–129
	VWMI	.24	33	61	72–125

NOTE: Values are rounded. FSIQ = Full Scale IQ; VCI = Verbal Comprehension Index; PRI = Perceptual Reasoning Index; WMI = Working Memory Index; PSI = Processing Speed Index; IMI = Immediate Memory Index; DMI = Delayed Memory Index; VWMI = Visual Working Memory Index.

SOURCE: Adapted from Pearson Assessment (2009).

TABLE 4–10 Prediction Accuracy of the Simple Demographics Only, Complex Demographics Only, Combined Simple Demographics and Test of Premorbid Functioning (TOPF) Word Reading Scores, and Combined Complex Demographics and TOPF Word Reading Scores for Ages 20 to 90

PREDICTION MODEL	INDEX	R^2	PERCENTAGE OF CASES WITHIN ±5 POINTS OF ACTUAL SCORE	PERCENTAGE OF CASES WITHIN ±10 POINTS OF ACTUAL SCORE	RANGE OF PREDICTED INDEX SCORES
Simple demographics	FSIQ	.47	37	66	67–121
	VCI	.46	37	65	71–123
	PRI	.30	34	59	74–115
	WMI	.34	36	62	74–117
	PSI	.22	33	57	78–116
	VWMI	.23	30	55	79–112
Complex demographics	FSIQ	.49	40	69	64–130
	VCI	.47	38	67	63–134
	PRI	.32	34	61	68–123
	WMI	.33	36	62	74–119
	PSI	.23	33	59	70–126
	VWMI	.20	29	54	80–119
Simple demographics and TOPF Word Reading	FSIQ	.63	46	75	53–141
	VCI	.68	48	78	57–142
	PRI	.38	36	62	65–126
	WMI	.49	38	67	62–133
	PSI	.25	34	59	71–124
	IMI	.27	33	58	66–129
	DMI	.21	32	57	68–125
	VWMI	.30	32	56	66–126
Complex demographics and TOPF Word Reading	FSIQ	.61	45	77	50–145
	VCI	.67	49	78	56–142
	PRI	.36	35	63	65–131
	WMI	.48	39	68	64–133
	PSI	.24	34	60	67–129
	IMI	.26	33	58	66–130
	DMI	.20	33	57	70–127
	VWMI	.29	32	58	68–127

NOTE: Values are rounded. FSIQ = Full Scale IQ; VCI = Verbal Comprehension Index; PRI = Perceptual Reasoning Index; WMI = Working Memory Index; PSI = Processing Speed Index; IMI = Immediate Memory Index; DMI = Delayed Memory Index; VWMI = Visual Working Memory Index.

SOURCE: From Pearson (2009).

lower than the Time 1 score, the manual recommends using the Time 1 score or demographic data to predict premorbid cognitive functioning. If the Time 1 score is significantly lower than the Time 2 score, the manual indicates that the Time 1 measurement may underestimate the examinee's ability, and use of the Time 2 score is suggested instead.

DEMOGRAPHIC EFFECTS

AGE

Age has minimal effects on TOPF Word Reading by about age 20 to 25 (Pearson, 2009).

GENDER

Gender has little effect on TOPF Word Reading across all ages (Pearson, 2009).

EDUCATION

In those age 20–90, education shows moderate correlation with TOPF Word Reading ($r = .55$). Of all the demographic variables, education accounts for the most variance on TOPF Word Reading (Pearson, 2009).

Among 16- to 19-year-olds, parent education shows the highest correlation among all demographic variables ($r = .36$; Pearson, 2009).

ETHNICITY, NATIONALITY, AND LINGUISTIC EFFECTS

In those age 20–90, correlations between TOPF Word Reading and race/ethnicity range from .05 (Asian) to .36 (white) while correlations between TOPF Word Reading and region ranges from −.20 (South) to .06 (Midwest). Among 16- to 19-year-olds, race/ethnicity/region reveals minimal correlations (Pearson, 2009).

NORMATIVE SAMPLE

The TOPF prediction equations are developed using the WAIS-IV standardization sample plus the race/ethnicity and education oversample. Please refer to the description of WAIS-IV in Chapter 5 for the composition of the standardization sample and oversample. The complete sample is not US census-based in order to ensure examinees from African American, Hispanic, and Asian background, as well as those with very low or very high scholastic attainment are adequately represented for developing the regression equations.

EVIDENCE FOR RELIABILITY

EVIDENCE FOR INTERNAL RELIABILITY

As reported in the manual, internal consistency based on the split-half method for TOPF Word Reading is very high across all age groups and clinical groups (r_{SB} = .96 to .99 and .97 to .99, respectively; Pearson, 2009).

EVIDENCE FOR TEST-RETEST RELIABILITY, MEASURING CHANGE, AND PRACTICE EFFECTS

Test-retest stability was examined in a subset of 293 examinees retested about three weeks apart. Test-retest reliability coefficients for the TOPF Word Reading score ranged from high to very high across the age groups (corrected r = .89 to .95; Pearson, 2009).

Regarding reliable change, Time 1 predicts Time 2 performance highly accurately (R = .93, R^2 = .86, SEE = 5.67). No further information regarding measuring change and practice effects are provided in the manual.

EVIDENCE FOR VALIDITY

COMPARISONS WITH OTHER MEASURES OF PREMORBID INTELLECTUAL FUNCTIONING

Norton, Watt, Gow, and Crowe (2016) reported that in a healthy Australian sample, scores were lowest on the TOPF Word Reading (Mean [*M*] = 102.2, standard deviation [*SD*] = 10.45) compared to the WTAR (*M* = 104.4, *SD* = 6.37), the NART-2 (*M* = 104.25, *SD* = 6.47), and the NART (*M* = 110.08, *SD* = 4.25). There is a difference of 2.3 to 7.9 IQ points between the TOPF Word Reading and other measures, with the largest difference seen between the TOPF Word Reading and the NART. As the NART is the oldest of all the measures, the authors concluded that the Flynn effect applies to measures of premorbid estimates. Use of the most recent measure (i.e., the TOPF Word Reading) to estimate premorbid functioning may be recommended to combat Flynn effects, though it is unclear from this study whether the TOPF Word Reading is the most accurate estimate of FSIQ.

In a follow-up study, Watt, Gow, Norton, and Crowe (2016) reported that, compared to other word reading measures of estimated premorbid functioning, the TOPF Word Reading appears to underestimate FSIQ on the WAIS-IV, although the accuracy of the estimation also depends on the actual IQ band of the individual. They examined the accuracy of the NART, NART-2, WTAR, and TOPF Word Reading in predicting the WAIS-IV scores in a healthy Australian sample. Differences between the obtained FSIQ and the NART, NART-2, WTAR, and TOPF Word Reading were −5.39 (overestimated), .44, .27, and 2.53 IQ points, respectively. According to this study, the TOPF Word Reading score accurately estimates the FSIQ of those with average and low-average IQ but underestimates those with high-average IQ. As well, the WTAR and NART-2 overestimate low-average IQ, are accurate in average IQ, and underestimate high-average IQ. Last, the NART overestimates low-average IQ but accurately estimates average and high-average IQ. However, the TOPF Word Reading shows the largest standard deviations across all IQ groups compared to the other measures. In short, all the measures have shortcomings as tests of premorbid functioning, and the TOPF may not be the most accurate measure for estimating premorbid functioning.

The combined TOPF Word Reading and simple demographic prediction model was compared to the WRAT-4 Reading as a measure of premorbid functioning in a neurodegenerative disorder clinic sample (Berg et al., 2016). Correlation between the WRAT-4 and the combined TOPF was strong, and stronger between the WRAT-4 and TOPF Word Reading (r = .72 and .81, respectively). About 32% of the sample obtained lower scores on the combined TOPF than on the WRAT-4, about 11% showed equivalent scores, and about 57% obtained lower scores on the WRAT-4 than the combined TOPF. Analysis also showed that the WRAT-4 consistently generated a lower premorbid estimate (on average 1.78 points) than the TOPF, except in older adults with neurological conditions, though the differences in the two measures were generally not due to differences in demographic background or neuropsychological functioning. It is unknown which measure is a more accurate estimate of actual FSIQ. Regardless, the results indicate that these two tests should not be used interchangeably.

CORRELATIONS WITH MEASURES OF INTELLIGENCE, MEMORY, AND ACADEMIC ACHIEVEMENT

TOPF Word Reading appears to adequately predict intellectual functioning but to only modestly predict memory. According to the manual, correlations with the WAIS-IV are highest for the VCI (r = .75), FSIQ, and GAI (both r = .70), but lower for other indices (PRI, r = .50; WMI, r = .61; PSI, r = .37). Among the subtests, the highest correlation is seen with Vocabulary and the lowest with Cancellation (r = .73 and .24, respectively). Correlations with the WMS-IV indices are moderate (Auditory Memory Index [AMI], r = .41; Visual Memory Index [VMI], r = .36; VWMI, r = .47; IMI, r = .46; DMI, r = .41); correlations with the WMS-IV subtests range from moderate to low.

TABLE 4–11 Test of Premorbid Functioning (TOPF) Sensitivity and Specificity for Alzheimer's Disease vs. Healthy Controls with One, Two, Three, or Four Unusually Low Actual–Predicted Discrepancy Scores at Various Base Rates

	25% BASE RATE		15% BASE RATE		10% BASE RATE		5% BASE RATE		2% BASE RATE	
	SENS (%)	SPEC (%)	SENS (%)	SPEC (%)	SENS (%)	SPEC (%)	SENS (%)	SPEC (%)	SENS (%)	SPEC (%)
≥1	92	46	92	65	92	69	88	85	85	96
≥2	88	77	88	85	88	92	81	96	77	100
≥3	88	81	85	96	81	100	65	100	62	100
≥4	81	85	77	100	69	100	65	100	50	100

NOTE: Sens = Sensitivity, Spec = Specificity.
SOURCE: Adapted from Pearson (2009).

TOPF Word Reading is highly correlated with academic achievement, not surprisingly given the impact of education on this test. High correlations have been reported for Weschler Individual Achievement Test-Second Edition (WIAT-II) Total Composite, Reading Composite, and Written Language Composite ($r = .80$, .82, and .70, respectively). Among the WIAT-II subtests, correlations are highest for the Word Reading and Spelling subtests while moderate with other subtests ($r = .77$, .79, and .50 to .66, respectively; Pearson, 2009).

Regarding measures of general cognitive functioning, lower Addenbrooke Cognitive Examination-III (ACE-III) scores are predictive of lower TOPF Word Reading scores in older adults with or without dementia (Stott et al., 2017).

CLINICAL STUDIES

TOPF Word Reading performance appears relatively resistant to neurological compromise. However, it is not insensitive to such impairment. As reported in the manual, TOPF Word Reading performance was evaluated in patients with mild AD, mild cognitive impairment (MCI), traumatic brain injury (TBI), Asperger's disorder, Attention Deficit/Hyperactivity Disorder (ADHD), and persons with epilepsy who had undergone temporal lobectomy (Pearson, 2009). Base rates of unusually low scores indicated that Asperger's disorder and ADHD groups obtained similar rates of low TOPF Word Reading scores as the healthy premorbid prediction sample (base rates of 26%, 19%, and 25%, respectively). In contrast, the other groups obtained much higher base rates of low scores. Base rates were 39% for AD, 38% for MCI, 40% for TBI, and as high as 62% for temporal lobectomy. This indicates that the TOPF Word Reading should not be used in some clinical groups, particularly people who have undergone temporal lobectomy, as this procedure is not associated with decrements in IQ. The other three groups could conceivably have decrements in IQ, in contrast. As such, TOPF Word Reading scores must be assessed in the latter clinical groups; should the TOPF Word Reading score be unexpectedly low (e.g., the difference between actual and predicted TOPF score is at or below a 25% base rate in the prediction model per the manual), use of demographics only to predict premorbid functioning is recommended. A separate study found that dementia is independently predictive of lower TOPF Word Reading even after controlling for education and age but the type of dementia (AD vs. others) does not affect TOPF performance (Stott et al., 2017). As such, TOPF Word Reading may not be suitable for estimating the premorbid functioning of those suspected of dementia.

Tables 4–11 to 4–14 present sensitivity and specificity data using simple demographics with or without TOPF Word Reading for actual–obtained discrepancy for distinguishing mild AD, MCI, TBI, and temporal lobectomy from healthy controls. The prediction models appear to differentiate mild AD from healthy controls most accurately. Having one or more discrepant actual–predicted scores at a 2% base rate, or three or more discrepant actual–predicted scores at a 15% base rate generated the best combination of sensitivity (85%) and specificity (96%). The prediction models are less accurate for identifying MCI (maximum sensitivity, 87%; specificity, 34%), TBI (maximum sensitivity, 92%; specificity, 52%), and temporal lobectomy (maximum sensitivity, 91%; specificity, 30%).

TABLE 4–12 Test of Premorbid Functioning (TOPF) Sensitivity and Specificity for Mild Cognitive Impairment vs. Healthy Controls with One, Two, Three, or Four Unusually Low Actual–Predicted Discrepancy Scores at Various Base Rates

	25% BASE RATE		15% BASE RATE		10% BASE RATE		5% BASE RATE		2% BASE RATE	
	SENS (%)	SPEC (%)	SENS (%)	SPEC (%)	SENS (%)	SPEC (%)	SENS (%)	SPEC (%)	SENS (%)	SPEC (%)
≥1	87	34	79	45	74	66	58	84	39	97
≥2	76	53	66	74	58	84	42	97	26	100
≥3	71	63	53	79	42	92	29	100	13	100
≥4	53	82	37	89	26	100	18	100	11	100

NOTE: Sens = Sensitivity, Spec = Specificity.
SOURCE: Adapted from Pearson (2009).

TABLE 4–13 Test of Premorbid Functioning (TOPF) Sensitivity and Specificity for Traumatic Brain Injury vs. Healthy Controls with One, Two, Three, or Four Unusually Low Actual–Predicted Discrepancy Scores at Various Base Rates

	25% BASE RATE		15% BASE RATE		10% BASE RATE		5% BASE RATE		2% BASE RATE	
	SENS (%)	SPEC (%)	SENS (%)	SPEC (%)	SENS (%)	SPEC (%)	SENS (%)	SPEC (%)	SENS (%)	SPEC (%)
≥1	92	28	92	44	88	64	80	80	76	84
≥2	92	52	76	64	72	84	68	88	56	96
≥3	80	68	64	88	56	92	56	92	32	100
≥4	76	76	60	92	56	92	36	96	24	100

NOTE: Sens = Sensitivity, Spec = Specificity.
SOURCE: Adapted from Pearson (2009).

The combined simple demographics with TOPF Word Reading prediction model shows the best classification for mild AD relative to MCI and major depressive disorder at 88% accuracy rate to identify cognitive decline (Table 4–15). Classification rates are lower for differentiating TBI and autistic disorder (63% and 80%, respectively) from other conditions with varying degrees of cognitive impairments (i.e., temporal lobectomy, depression, Asperger's disorder, and ADHD).

Among the developmental disorders of Asperger's disorder and ADHD, the sensitivity and specificity data are low. At the best combination, sensitivity is 33% at a specificity of 90% for the Asperger's disorder group. The specificity never exceeded 86% in the autistic disorder group, and the data for the ADHD group are even lower. This makes sense because these disorders are not associated with acquired decrements in IQ or memory.

PERFORMANCE VALIDITY

The use of the TOPF as a performance validity indicator shows some promise. For example, the relationship between performance validity and rate of abnormally low TOPF Word Reading scores was examined in an outpatient neuropsychology clinic sample (Martin et al., 2016). Individuals with dementia, intellectual disability, or left-hemisphere stroke were excluded in the study due to the impact of these conditions on TOPF Word Reading performance. Invalid performance was defined as failure on two or more of these performance validity tests (PVTs): Test of Memory Malingering (TOMM), Word Memory Test (WMT), Sentence Repetition, Word Choice Test, Dot Counting Test, Finger Tapping, and the Coin-in-the-Hand Test. In this study, a base rate of 10% or less for the discrepancy between obtained TOPF Word Reading standard score and demographically predicted word reading standard score was considered abnormally low. PVT failure accounted for about 8% of variance in TOPF Word Reading even after controlling for education. The invalid performance group obtained lower TOPF Word Reading and combined TOPF Word Reading and simple demographic FSIQ estimates than did the valid performance group. The invalid group also scored, on average, 9 points lower on TOPF Word Reading than their demographically predicted word reading standard score, even though the scores were in the average range. By contrast, the valid group scored, on average, 3 standard score points lower on TOPF Word Reading than the demographically predicted word reading standard score. The Invalid group had a higher proportion of patients with abnormally low TOPF reading score (33%) than the Valid group (16%). The proportion showing abnormally low TOPF reading score in the Invalid group was similar to that of those with AD, and twice that of those with moderate/severe TBI. In order to achieve a specificity of 90% or higher for valid performance, the cutoff for the normative base rate of discrepancy between obtained and demographically predicted word reading standard score was adjusted to 7.2% (i.e., 7.2% showed a specific difference between obtained and demographically predicted word reading score). However, at this cutoff, the sensitivity was only 19%. In sum, while individuals who feign cognitive impairments may obtain abnormality low TOPF Word

TABLE 4–14 Test of Premorbid Functioning (TOPF) Sensitivity and Specificity for Temporal Lobectomy vs. Healthy Controls with One, Two, Three, or Four Unusually Low Actual-Predicted Discrepancy Scores at Various Base Rates

	25% BASE RATE		15% BASE RATE		10% BASE RATE		5% BASE RATE		2% BASE RATE	
	SENS (%)	SPEC (%)	SENS (%)	SPEC (%)	SENS (%)	SPEC (%)	SENS (%)	SPEC (%)	SENS (%)	SPEC (%)
≥1	91	30	83	43	74	52	70	61	52	78
≥2	78	57	70	61	61	78	39	91	26	100
≥3	74	57	65	78	52	91	35	96	13	100
≥4	65	70	52	87	48	96	17	96	9	100

NOTE: Sens = Sensitivity, Spec = Specificity.
SOURCE: Adapted from Pearson (2009).

TABLE 4–15 Test of Premorbid Functioning (TOPF) Classification Accuracy for Differentiating Mild Alzheimer's Disease, Mild Cognitive Impairment, and Major Depressive Disorder

PREDICTED DIAGNOSIS	ACTUAL DIAGNOSIS AD	MCI	MDD	ANY DIAGNOSIS	BASE RATE IN PREMORBID PREDICTION SAMPLE
AD	88	16	0	35	1.52
MCI	8	39	8	20	8.34
MDD	0	3	4	2	0.66
Any diagnosis	96	58	13	57	10.53
PPV (%)	100	91	0		
NPV (%)	93	69	50		

NOTE: AD, Alzheimer's disease; MCI, mild cognitive impairment; MDD, major depressive disorder; PPV, positive predictive value; NPV, negative predictive value.

SOURCE: A Table from the Advanced Clinical Solutions for WAIS-IV and WMS-IV (ACS). Copyright © 2009 NCS Pearson, Inc. Reproduced with permission. All rights reserved.

Reading scores, the use of abnormally low TOPF Word Reading is insufficient as an embedded validity indicator (Martin et al., 2016).

Martin, Hunter, Rach, Heinrichs, and Schroeder (2017) developed three performance indicators using the TOPF simple demographic equation alone: namely, the Excessive Decline from Premorbid Functioning (EDPF) indicators. EDPF identifies an atypical discrepancy between predicted premorbid estimate and current test performance in individuals with true cognitive impairments. The three indicators are:

EDPF-FSIQ
 = TOPF demographically predicted FSIQ minus obtained WAIS-IV FSIQ

EDPF-Verbal/Working Memory (EDPF-VW)
 = (TOPF demographically predicted WMI minus WAIS-IV WMI) + (TOPF demographically predicted VCI minus WAIS-IV VCI)

EDPF-Perceptual Reasoning/Processing Speed (EDPF-PP)
 = (TOPF demographically predicted PRI minus WAIS-IV PRI) + (TOPF demographically predicted PSI minus WAIS-IV PSI)

Using an outpatient neuropsychology clinic sample excluding those with dementia, intellectual disability, or left-hemisphere stroke, and invalid performance defined as failures on two or more PVTs (TOMM, WMT, Sentence Repetition, Word Choice Test, Dot Counting Test, Finger Tapping, and the Coin-in-the-Hand Test), they found that the Invalid group had greater WAIS-IV obtained versus predicted index score discrepancies than the Valid group. The area under the curve (AUC) for the various WAIS-IV index discrepancy scores ranged from .65 (PRI) to .84 (WMI). To achieve a specificity of 90% or greater for performance validity, a VCI index discrepancy score cutoff of 13 yielded a sensitivity of 49%; a WMI index discrepancy

TABLE 4–16 Test of Premorbid Functioning (TOPF) Cutoff and Sensitivity of Excessive Decline from Premorbid Functioning (EDPF) Indicators for Neurocognitive, Psychiatric, and Traumatic Brain Injury Groups at ≥90% Specificity

	N	AUC	CUTOFF	SENSITIVITY (%)
EDPF-VW				
Neurocognitive	54	.82	31	54
Psychiatric	63	.82	28	61
TBI	14	.87	20	68
EDPF-PP				
Neurocognitive	54	.66	48	32
Psychiatric	63	.82	25	61
TBI	14	.80	36	39
EDPF-FSIQ				
Neurocognitive	54	.78	20	51
Psychiatric	63	.87	16	61
TBI	14	.84	20	51

NOTE: EDPF-VW, Excessive Decline from Premorbid Functioning—Verbal/Working Memory; EDPF-PP, Excessive Decline from Premorbid Functioning—Perceptual Reasoning/Processing Speed; EDPF-FSIQ, Excessive Decline from Premorbid Functioning—Full Scale Intelligence Quotient, AUC, area under the curve; TBI, moderate or severe traumatic brain injury. The neurocognitive group was comprised of ADHD, brain tumor, cognitive disorder NOS, epilepsy, hypoxia/anoxia, MCI, MS, and other neurologic conditions.

SOURCE: Adapted from Martin et al. (2017).

score cutoff of 20 yielded a sensitivity of 54%; the PRI index discrepancy score cutoff of 20 yielded a sensitivity of 27%; and the PSI index discrepancy score cutoff of 22 yielded a sensitivity of 49%. In comparison, a Reliable Digit Span (RDS) cutoff of 6 yielded a sensitivity of 37%.

Using the EDPF equations to classify performance validity at 90% or greater specificity, a EDPF-VW cutoff of 28 yielded a sensitivity of 61%, a EDPF-PP cutoff of 36 yielded a sensitivity of 39%, and a EDPF-FSIQ cutoff of 18 yielded a sensitivity of 56%. As seen in Table 4–16, the EDPF-VW and EDPF-FSIQ are adequate in specific diagnoses, whereas the EDPF-PP is suitable for psychiatric and moderate-severe TBI groups, although note that the sample size of the TBI group is small. In short, the EDPFs appear to be useful as embedded indicators of performance and an improvement over the RDS.

COMMENT

The TOPF is a sophisticated and complicated measure that appears to provide a reasonable estimate of general intellectual functioning, particularly verbal ability, and is co-normed with the WAIS-IV and WMS-IV. The increased prediction range of the demographic-TOPF Word Reading models is an improvement over the WTAR and other prediction methods. The availability of a number of different prediction models with and without demographic variables is advantageous. While the combined TOPF Word Reading and simple demographics prediction model provides adequate performance predictions using basic background information and its use is recommended, other options (i.e., demographics only, reading only) are available to the examiner based on the individual characteristics of the examinee being seen. For example, if there is any concern that reading ability could be compromised by a neurological condition (e.g., aphasia), the demographics-only prediction model may be used to obtain premorbid estimates. However, the TOPF should not be used in those younger than 20 given its weak predictive power. Several equations (EDPFs) have been developed to examine the validity of the examinee's test performance and show promise as embedded performance validity indicators.

Based on the information presented in the manual, the test should be used for estimation of FSIQ and VCI only. The prediction models also appear most useful for neurological conditions with acute or progressive cognitive decline such as AD or TBI.

However, several limitations remain. The regression equations have only been validated in a US population and so are not necessarily appropriate for use in other countries. Use to estimate premorbid functions for developmental disorders or chronic neurological disorders that can affect educational opportunities or reading, such as epilepsy, is also not supported. Moreover, the TOPF Word Reading score underestimates high IQ and may be suitable only for those with average and low-average IQ, at least among Australians (Watt et al., 2016).

Its ability to predict other domains of functioning, including memory, appears limited. Given the very low correlations between demographic variables and WMS-IV indices, demographic data alone should not be used to predict premorbid memory functioning. The complex demographic prediction model (with or without TOPF Word Reading) does not appear to provide additional predictive power over the simple demographic prediction model; its routine use is not necessary. Finally, the TOPF is part of the ACS software that is linked to the WAIS-IV and WMS-IV platform and therefore cannot be purchased separately. Other public domain or stand-alone tests or tests such as the OPIE-IV (reviewed in this volume) or WRAT-4 Reading may therefore be preferable to some users (but see the section "Comparisons with Other Measures of Premorbid Intellectual Functioning").

The TOPF should not be used to diagnose learning disorders, nor should it be employed in those with a preexisting learning disorder, in those who suffer language and perceptual disorders (e.g., aphasia and alexia), or in those who have not had lengthy exposure to English reading. Like other performance-based methods (e.g., NART, WRAT-4 Reading), it is also not impervious to the effects of significant cognitive dysfunction (e.g., moderate dementia). If TOPF Word Reading performance is severely compromised, as determined by a comparison of actual and predicted scores, the examiner should use demographics-predicted scores only. It should be noted that demographics-only prediction models may under- or overestimate scores in extreme ability levels. Finally, this updated version is relatively new. Its relationship with other neuropsychological tests has not yet been reported. Because the majority of the existing information on the test is from the publishers, additional independent large-scale clinical studies are also needed, especially with respect to the accuracy of the demographic-only prediction models.

REFERENCES

Berg, J.-L., Durant, J., Banks, S. J., & Miller, J. B. (2016). Estimates of premorbid ability in a neurodegenerative disease clinic population: comparing the Test of Premorbid Functioning and the Wide Range Achievement Test, 4th Edition. *The Clinical Neuropsychologist, 30*(4), 547–557. https://doi.org/10.1080/13854046.2016.1186224

Holdnack, J. A., Drozdick, L., Weiss, L. G., & Iverson, G. L. (Eds.). (2013). *WAIS-IV, WMS-IV, and ACS: Advanced clinical interpretation*. New York: Academic Press.

Martin, P. K., Hunter, B. P., Rach, A. M., Heinrichs, R. J., & Schroeder, R. W. (2017). Excessive decline from premorbid functioning: detecting performance invalidity with the WAIS-IV and demographic predictions. *The Clinical Neuropsychologist, 31*(5), 829–843. https://doi.org/10.1080/13854046.2017.1284265

Martin, P. K., Schroeder, R. W., Wyman-Chick, K. A., Hunter, B. P., Heinrichs, R. J., & Baade, L. E. (2016). Rates of abnormally low TOPF word reading scores in individuals failing versus passing performance validity testing. *Assessment, 25*(5), 640–652. https://doi.org/10.1177/1073191116656796

Norton, K., Watt, S., Gow, B., & Crowe, S. F. (2016). Are Tests of premorbid functioning subject to the Flynn effect?: Accuracy of premorbid functioning tests. *Australian Psychologist, 51*(5), 374–379. https://doi.org/10.1111/ap.12235

Pearson Assessment (2009). *Advanced Clinical Solutions for the WAIS-IV/WMS-IV*. San Antonio, TX: Author.

PsychCorp (2001). *Wechsler Test of Adult Reading manual*. San Antonio, TX: The Psychological Corporation.

Stott, J., Scior, K., Mandy, W., & Charlesworth, G. (2017). Dementia screening accuracy is robust to premorbid IQ variation: Evidence from the Addenbrooke's Cognitive Examination-III and the Test of Premorbid Function. *Journal of Alzheimer's Disease, 57*(4), 1293–1302. https://doi.org/10.3233/JAD-161218

Watt, S., Gow, B., Norton, K., & Crowe, S. F. (2016). Investigating discrepancies between predicted and observed Wechsler Adult Intelligence Scale-Version IV Full-Scale Intelligence Quotient scores in a non-clinical sample: Discrepancies between predicted and observed. *Australian Psychologist, 51*(5), 380–388. https://doi.org/10.1111/ap.12239

5 | INTELLIGENCE

KAUFMAN BRIEF INTELLIGENCE TEST, SECOND EDITION (KBIT-2)

TEST NAME	**Kaufman Brief Intelligence Test, Second Edition (KBIT-2)**
DOMAIN	Intellectual function
AGE RANGE	In adults, to 90 years
ADMINISTRATION TIME	30 minutes
SCORING FORMAT	Hand scored
REFERENCE	Kaufman, A. S., & Kaufman, N. L. (2004). *Kaufman Brief Intelligence Test, Second Edition*. Bloomington, MN: Pearson, Inc. www.pearsonclinical.com

DESCRIPTION

The purpose of the Kaufman Brief Intelligence Test, Second Edition (KBIT-2; Kaufman & Kaufman, 2004) is to measure verbal, nonverbal, and composite intelligence in a brief manner. The Verbal Score is comprised of two subtests (Verbal Knowledge and Riddles), and the Nonverbal Score is comprised of the Matrices subtest. See Table 5–1 for a description of the subtests and the manual for specific details regarding content derivation. The KBIT-2 is interpreted with reference to the Cattell-Horn-Carrol (CHC) theory of intelligence, which focuses on fluid and crystallized intelligence (see manual). It may be of interest to readers that in adult samples (aged 26 to 90), the KBIT-2 was co-normed with the Kaufman Test of Educational Achievement, Second Edition (KTEA-II, Brief Form).

The KBIT-2 offers the following improvements compared to its predecessor: a new Verbal Score comprised of two subtests, the same content administered across age ranges, updated Matrices subtest with inclusion of new items, colored stimuli for subtest, and updated normative data (see also Bain & Jaspers, 2010). In addition to its use as a screening measure of intelligence, the test may be used when time or practical constraints preclude lengthy test administration.

ADMINISTRATION

Detailed administration instructions are provided in the manual. Examiners are able to support examinees in understanding the task on Matrices and Riddles (e.g., rephrase, use another language, use gestures). The emphasis while supporting the examinee should be on modifying task instructions as needed, rather than teaching a strategy or problem solving. The option to support examinees can be particularly useful with examinees who may be challenged to understand instructions immediately, such as those who are very young or examinees who have an intellectual disability. Verbal subtests do not require reading and, as indicated in Table 5–1, pointing can be used to indicate a response. Comparability of eye tracking technology compared to conventional administration has also been examined (Desideri et al., 2016).

SCORING

Raw scores are converted to age-based standard scores with a mean of 100 and a standard deviation (*SD*) of 15. A score of 0 or 1 is provided for each item. Scoring, interpretation guidelines, confidence intervals, and age equivalents are also provided (manual).

TABLE 5–1 Description of Kaufman Brief Intelligence Test, Second Edition (KBIT-2) Subtests

DOMAIN	SUBTEST NAME	SUBTEST DESCRIPTION	EXAMINEE'S TASK
Verbal	Verbal Knowledge	60-item measure that includes two types of information: receptive vocabulary and general information.	The examinee is presented with six full color illustrations or photographs. The examiner asks a word or general information question, and the examinee points to the correct answer.
	Riddles	48 items that measure verbal comprehension, reasoning, and vocabulary knowledge. Two or three clues are provided.	The examiner asks a riddle, and the examinee either points to a picture that shows the answer or says a single word that answers the riddle.
Nonverbal	Matrices	46 items that are made of visual stimuli, both familiar, such as people and objects, and abstract, such as symbols. All require understanding of relationships between stimuli. All are multiple choice.	The examinee selects, among five response options, which picture goes best with a stimulus picture.

NOTE: Due to basals, ceilings, and differential start points based on age, all the items for one subtest would not be administered to a single examinee (e.g., fewer than 46 items would be administered to an examinee on Matrices).

SOURCE: Adapted from Kaufman and Kaufman (2004).

DEMOGRAPHIC EFFECTS

AGE

In adults, performance on Riddles and Verbal Knowledge peaks at 30 years of age, plateaus until age 60, then declines. Riddles shows a more noticeable decline in the 60s than Verbal Knowledge. Matrices peaks at 18 years of age, plateaus until age 40, and then steadily declines (see also Kaufman et al., 2008).

GENDER

Gender differences are small (less than 1–2 points on composite scores) and not significant.

ETHNICITY, NATIONALITY, AND LINGUISTIC EFFECTS

No information is provided on the effect of these variables. However, it should be noted that the sample is Census stratified, and the test includes Spanish instructions for Matrices and Spanish responses to the Riddles subtest.

NORMATIVE DATA

The KBIT-2 was normed on a sample of 2,120 children and adults. Data were collected over a year-long interval (2002–2003). Consent procedures and quality control procedures are described in the manual. Participants excluded from the standardization sample were those who did not speak English; were institutionalized; had significant physical, medical, perceptual, or psychological conditions; or were taking medication with cognition-interfering effects. A screening checklist that was used is provided in the manual.

The normative sample targets were set to match the 2001 US Census. The sample includes 23 age groups with equal numbers of males and females matching the US population in terms of education level, ethnicity, and geographic region. The sample characteristics are summarized in Table 5–2. Proportions closely matched Census targets, with the exception of some minor differences in geographical representation.

Each subtest was analyzed in terms of reliability, item discrimination, and statistical item bias. Weak items were omitted. Refer to the manual for decisions regarding rationale for item inclusion for each subtest, procedures for sequencing items, and determining discontinuation and starting points (informed via Rasch calibration). In the process of norm smoothing, a standard score (M = 100, SD = 15) that corresponded to the mid-interval percentile rank for each raw score value at each age was calculated. Norms were then smoothed within ages and across ages using a statistical program designed for that purpose. The IQ composite was based on the summation of Verbal and Nonverbal standard scores.

TABLE 5–2 Demographic Characteristics of the Adult Standardization Sample for the Kaufman Brief Intelligence Test, Second Edition (KBIT-2)

Sample size	695[a]
Age	17 to 90
Geographic region	16% Northeast 25% North Central 39% South 20% West
Education	18% ≤11th grade 30% High school 24% College 29% University degree[b]
Gender	45% Male 55% Female
Ethnicity	74% White 12% African American 10% Hispanic 4% Other

[a]Adult sample only.

[b]Education levels were calculated differently for 18- to 25-year-olds compared to 26- to 90-year-olds.

Education categorizations for 26- to 90-year-olds are listed in the table. Categorizations for 18- to 25-year-olds were: in high school or dropped out, high school, began a two-year postsecondary program, and began a four-year postsecondary program.

SOURCE: Adapted from Kaufman and Kaufman (2004).

As discussed in the section "Administration," responses provided via eye tracking technology have been compared to those provided via the conventional paper-based version of the test (Desideri et al., 2016). Descriptive statistics (mean, *SD*) are provided in Table 5–3. The sample was comprised of 43 right-handed undergraduate volunteers at a University in Italy (age $M = 23.8$, $SD = 1.1$; 67% female). Anxiety and attention were screened via psychometric tests and reported to be within the average range.

A regression equation was calculated that significantly predicted performance on the conventional test in a sample of undergraduates (Desideri et al., 2016). The regression equation for Vocabulary is

Predicted eye-controlled KBIT-2 (Vocabulary) raw score = 37.4 + 0.3 × [KBIT-2 (Vocabulary) standard version raw score]

The regression equation to predict performance on the Matrices subtest is

Predicted eye-controlled KBIT-2 (Matrices) raw score = 12 + 0.7 × [KBIT-2 (Matrices) standard version raw score]

Of note, results suggested somewhat higher scores, fewer errors, and lower administration time on the Vocabulary subtest using the conventional (paper-based) version compared to the eye-tracking version, without differences between versions on the Matrices subtest.

EVIDENCE FOR RELIABILITY

EVIDENCE FOR INTERNAL RELIABILITY

Split-half reliability coefficients across adult age groups are high to very high for adults for Matrices ($r = .87$ to .96). Riddles and Verbal Knowledge have somewhat lower but still generally high internal reliabilities ($r = .77$ to .94).

TABLE 5–3 Descriptive Statistics (Means and *SDs*) for Kaufman Brief Intelligence Test, Second Edition (KBIT-2) Performance in Standard and Eye-Controlled Versions of the KBIT-2

	TOTAL	
	STANDARD	EYE-CONTROLLED
Raw scores		
Vocabulary	55.9 (1.3)	55.1 (2)[a]
Matrices	41 (3.2)	41.2 (2.9)
Errors		
Vocabulary	4 (1.3)	4.7 (1.9)[a]
Matrices	5.1 (3.1)	4 (2.9)
Time		
Vocabulary	1.9 (5.7)	4.2 (8.8)[a]
Matrices	4.8 (2.1)	5.3 (1.7)

[a]Significant difference with $p < 0.05$ between Paper/Eye-controlled versions.
SOURCE: Desideri et al. (2016).

Standard errors of measurement (*SEMs*) are relatively small for composite scores (range is from 2.8 to 5.7 points) and subtests (range of .8 to 1.3; manual).

EVIDENCE FOR TEST-RETEST RELIABILITY, MEASURING CHANGE, AND PRACTICE EFFECTS

Test-retest reliability of composite scores in a subsample of adults is strong over a test-retest interval of approximately 1 month ($r = .84$ to .92). See the manual for demographic details pertaining to the subsamples on which these estimates are based. A gain was noted on second administration (range of 1.2–5.3 points), with somewhat smaller gains for Nonverbal scores and older adults.

EVIDENCE FOR VALIDITY

WITHIN-TASK RELATIONSHIPS

Verbal and Nonverbal composite scores show moderate to large correlations in the adult subsample ($r = .58$; manual).

FACTOR-ANALYTIC STUDIES AND RELATIONSHIPS WITH OTHER TESTS

The manual reports correlations between the KBIT-2 and a number of intelligence tests, including the first edition of the test, the Wechsler Abbreviated Scales of Intelligence (WASI), and the Wechsler Adult Intelligence Scale-Third Edition (WAIS-III). Generally, large correlations are found between scores assessing similar abilities. Scores on the KBIT-2 tend to be lower than scores on other screening measures, particularly for Nonverbal composites.

Compared to the K-BIT, scores on the KBIT-2 are somewhat lower in an adult subsample ($n = 74$, 16- to 45-year-olds), ranging from 1 point for the Verbal Score to 3 points for the Nonverbal Score. Note that the K-BIT included different subtests than the KBIT-2 (i.e., Vocabulary and Matrices) and a general IQ composite, so comparisons were made between approximate counterparts on each test. Verbal counterparts correlated highly at $r = .80$, with lower correlations between the KBIT-2 Verbal composite and the K-BIT Matrices ($r = .44$). Nonverbal counterparts are also highly correlated ($r = .78$), with lower correlations between the KBIT-2 Nonverbal composite and K-BIT Vocabulary ($r = .47$). IQ composites from both tests are correlated highly ($r = .85$), and also show strong relationships with all subtests ($r = .72$ to .75; manual).

Similarly, in another adult subsample (age 35 to 52), the Verbal composite on the KBIT-2 was strongly correlated with WASI verbal subtests and composite scores (range $r = .77$ to .86), and highly correlated with WASI visual subtests (range $r = .62$ to .76). Correlations between visual subtests were large but somewhat more disparate, ranging from $r = .59$ to $r = .81$. Large correlations were also obtained with verbal subtests (range $r = .62$ to .67). As may be expected, the overall IQ composite generally correlates highly with each WASI subtest and composite score, with the lowest correlation with Block Design ($r = .66$) and the highest correlation with Full-Scale IQ (FSIQ) based on four subtests ($r = .90$). Overall, lower scores were found on the KBIT-2 than the WASI, with a difference of approximately 1 point for verbal scores and 7 points for nonverbal scores (manual).

The KBIT-2 and WAIS-III were also completed by a sample of examinees 20–48 years of age. Correlations between counterparts were large (e.g., Verbal composites were correlated at $r = .81$ to .82 and Nonverbal composites at $r = .79$ to .83). IQ composites were also highly correlated at $r = .89$, and the KBIT-2 IQ composite was correlated with a number of other scores in the large range overall (e.g., $r = .37$ to $r = .84$). The KBIT-2 Verbal composite was correlated to a lesser degree with the WAIS-III visual scores, with large correlations overall ($r = .61, .66$). Similarly, the KBIT-2 Nonverbal composite was correlated to a lesser degree with the WAIS-III Verbal scores ($r = .64, .58$) than the Nonverbal composites. Overall, scores on the KBIT-2 were 5 to 7 points lower than scores on the WAIS-III (manual). Other research has reported moderate correlations between the KBIT-2 and a measure of adaptive behavior, the Vineland Adaptive Behaviour scales, in young male prisoners ($r = .39$; Herrington, 2009).

CLINICAL STUDIES

The manual describes a number of clinical studies, including child and youth samples. In general, clinical groups perform lower than healthy controls. Specifically, a sample of participants from 4 to 38 years of age with intellectual disability performed worse than a reference group after controlling for demographic variables. As may be expected, the largest score discrepancies were found between persons with intellectual disability and the reference group relative to comparisons with other clinical groups (manual).

Similarly, a sample of persons with speech and language difficulties 4–38 years of age performed lower than a reference group after demographic effects (e.g., gender, ethnicity, education) were controlled for. Finally, a dementia group also obtained lower scores than a reference group when demographic factors were controlled for (manual).

In other research, the test has been used as an intelligence screen in a number of groups, including young male prisoners (Herrington, 2009), persons appearing before the courts in Australia (Vanny, Levy, Greenberg, & Hayes, 2009), people with schizophrenia (Kessler et al., 2007), persons with autism spectrum disorder (ASD; Kirvovski et al., 2015, 2016), people with Williams syndrome (Ito & Martens, 2017), and deaf readers (Emmorey et al., 2016). The test was used in a study of depression and reassurance-seeking in persons with intellectual disability (Hartley et al., 2008). Intelligence, as measured by the KBIT-2, does not relate to money mismanagement among adults with severe mental illness and substance abuse (Moore et al., 2016) or measures of day-to-day function in persons with schizophrenia (Thornton et al., 2010).

NEUROANATOMICAL CORRELATES AND IMAGING STUDIES

No information is available.

PERFORMANCE VALIDITY

No information is available.

COMMENT

The KBIT-2 is a screening test of intelligence that has many strengths. The test is well-founded theoretically and appears to be suitable for examinees presenting at a range of ability levels. In terms of demographic effects, the test follows the expected trajectory of age-related development of intellectual abilities, including disparate trajectories for crystallized and fluid intelligence. Gender differences are negligible. The normative database is Census-stratified and well-defined.

Reliability is strong. Practice effects are relatively small. The test shows strong relationships with similar scores from other intelligence tests (e.g., WASI, WAIS-III). However, standard scores on the KBIT-2 tend to be lower than other intelligence tests. As expected, clinical groups tend to score lower than controls, with the largest discrepancies between clinical groups and controls in a study of persons with intellectual disability. In independent research, the test has been used as a screener of intelligence in diverse groups.

In light of its considerable strengths, there are select weaknesses that bear mention. More research in clinical samples is needed. Although the normative sample was Census-stratified according to ethnicity and other demographic factors, and some test modifications have been made to use the test in Spanish, the effects of ethnicity and linguistic variables are not well understood. The normative data were collected in 2002–2003; thus, at the time of this writing, the test is over 20 years old. No information is available on neuroanatomical correlates and performance validity.

It should be noted that this test was designed as a screening instrument and provides a relatively gross estimate of intellectual function. In addition, the test does not include processing speed or working memory subtests, important aspects of cognitive assessment particularly in neuropsychological populations. The majority of clinical situations will call for administration of a full-length intelligence battery that reflects multiple aspects of intelligence.

REFERENCES

Bain, S. K., & Jaspers, K. E. (2010). Test review: Review of Kaufman Brief Intelligence Test, Second Edition. *Journal of Psychoeducational Assessment, 28*(2), 167–174. https://doi.org/10.1177/0734282909348217

Desideri, L., Tarabelloni, G., Nanni, I., Malavasi, M., Nori, R., & Bonifacci, P. (2016). An eye-controlled version of the Kaufman

Brief Intelligence Test 2 (KBIT-2) to assess cognitive functioning. *Computers in Human Behavior, 63*, 502–508. https://doi.org/10.1016/j.chb.2016.05.077

Emmorey, K., McCullough, S., & Weisberg, J. (2016). The neural underpinnings of reading skill in deaf adults. *Brain and Language, 160*, 11–20. https://doi.org/10.1016/j.bandl.2016.06.007

Hartley, S. L., Lickel, A. H., & MacLean Jr., W. E. (2008). Reassurance seeking and depression in adults with mild intellectual disability. *Journal of Intellectual Disability Research, 52*(11), 917–929. https://doi.org/10.1111/j.1365-2788.2008.01126.x

Herrington, V. (2009). Assessing the prevalence of intellectual disability among young male prisoners. *Journal of Intellectual Disability Research, 53*(5), 397–410. https://doi.org/10.1111/j.1365-2788.2008.01150.x

Ito, K., & Martens, M. A. (2017). Contrast-marking prosodic emphasis in Williams syndrome: results of detailed phonetic analysis: Prosodic emphasis in Williams syndrome. *International Journal of Language & Communication Disorders, 52*(1), 46–58. https://doi.org/10.1111/1460-6984.12250

Kaufman, A. S., Johnson, C. K., & Xin, L. (2008). A CHC theory-based analysis of age differences on cognitive abilities and academic skills at ages 22 to 90 years. *Journal of Psychoeducational Assessment, 26*(4), 350–381. https://doi.org/10.1177/0734282908314108

Kaufman, A. S., & Kaufman, N. L. (2004). *Kaufman Brief Intelligence Test, Second Edition*. Bloomington, MN: Pearson, Inc.

Kessler, R. K., Giovannetti, T., & MacMullen, L. R. (2007). Everyday action in schizophrenia: Performance patterns and underlying cognitive mechanisms. *Neuropsychology, 21*(4), 439–447. https://doi.org/10.103§7/0894-4105.21.4.439

Kirkovski, M., Enticott, P. G., Hughes, M. E., Rossell, S. L., & Fitzgerald, P. B. (2016). Atypical neural activity in males but not females with autism spectrum disorder. *Journal of Autism and Developmental Disorders, 46*(3), 954–963. https://doi.org/10.1007/s10803-015-2639-7

Kirkovski, M., Enticott, P. G., Maller, J. J., Rossell, S. L., & Fitzgerald, P. B. (2015). Diffusion tensor imaging reveals no white matter impairments among adults with autism spectrum disorder. *Psychiatry Research: Neuroimaging, 233*(1), 64–72. https://doi.org/10.1016/j.pscychresns.2015.05.003

Moore, B. A., Black, A. C., & Rosen, M. I. (2016). Factors associated with money mismanagement among adults with severe mental illness and substance abuse. *International Journal of Mental Health and Addiction, 14*(4), 400–409. https://doi.org/10.1007/s11469-015-9625-3

Thornton, A. E., Kristinsson, H., DeFreitas, V. G., & Thornton, W. L. (2010). The ecological validity of everyday cognition in hospitalized patients with serious mental illness. *Journal of Clinical and Experimental Neuropsychology, 32*(3), 299–308. https://doi.org/10.1080/13803390903002209

Vanny, K. A., Levy, M. H., Greenberg, D. M., & Hayes, S. C. (2009). Mental illness and intellectual disability in Magistrates Courts in New South Wales, Australia. *Journal of Intellectual Disability Research, 53*(3), 289–297. https://doi.org/10.1111/j.1365-2788.2008.01148.x

RAVEN'S PROGRESSIVE MATRICES

TEST NAME	**Raven's Progressive Matrices**
DOMAIN	Intellectual function
AGE RANGE	In adults, up to 85, depending on version
ADMINISTRATION TIME	25 to 60 minutes depending on version
SCORING FORMAT	Hand scored
REFERENCES	Raven, J., Raven, J. C., & Court, J. H. (1998a). *Raven manual: Section 1. General overview.* Oxford: Oxford Psychologists Press Ltd. Raven, J., Raven, J. C., & Court, J. H. (1998b). *Raven manual: Section 2. Colored Progressive Matrices.* Oxford: Oxford Psychologists Press Ltd. Raven, J., Raven, J. C., & Court, J. H. (1998c). *Raven manual: Section 4. Advanced Progressive Matrices.* Oxford: Oxford Psychologists Press Ltd. Raven, J., Raven, J. C., & Court, J. H. (2000). *Raven manual: Section 3. Standard Progressive Matrices.* Oxford: Oxford Psychologists Press Ltd.

DESCRIPTION

Raven's Progressive Matrices (Raven et al., 2000a) requires inductive reasoning (Alderton & Larson, 1990) and has been used to gauge the ability of the examinee to become more efficient by learning from experience with the items as the task progresses (Mills et al., 1993). According to the authors, the test was constructed to measure the "educative" component of *g* as defined in Spearman's theory of cognitive ability. They define educative ability as "the ability to forge new insights, the ability to discern meaning in confusion, the ability to perceive, and the ability to identify relationships" (Raven et al., 2000a, p. 1). The test is posited as being a relatively pure reflection of Spearman's *g* and fluid intelligence (Llabre, 1984; Neisser, 1998). The test is often used to study reasoning processes (e.g., Kubricht et al., 2017; Lovett & Forbus, 2017; Rasmussen & Eliasmith, 2011).

Three forms of this test have been developed, and they vary in difficulty. The Standard Progressive Matrices (also known as the Classic SPM or CPM-C) was originally published in 1938 (Raven, 1938/1996). Normative studies, linkage to a measure of word knowledge (the Mill Hill Vocabulary Scale), and the development of the Colored Progressive Matrices (CPM) and Advanced Progressive Matrices (APM) followed in the 1940s. In 1956, the SPM items were resequenced, and the CPM and APM were revised (McCallum et al., 2000). In 1998, several new versions (Parallel CPM, Parallel SPM, and SPM+) were introduced. Item difficulty on the test may be related to a number of dimensions (e.g., quantity of rules, complexity of the rules, and element salience; see Meo, Roberts, & Marucci, 2007).

STANDARD PROGRESSIVE MATRICES AND VARIANTS

The SPM (Raven et al., 2000a) consists of 60 items grouped into five sets (A to E), with each set containing 12 items. Each item contains a pattern with one part removed and six to eight pictured inserts, one of which contains the correct pattern (see Figure 5–1). Each set involves different

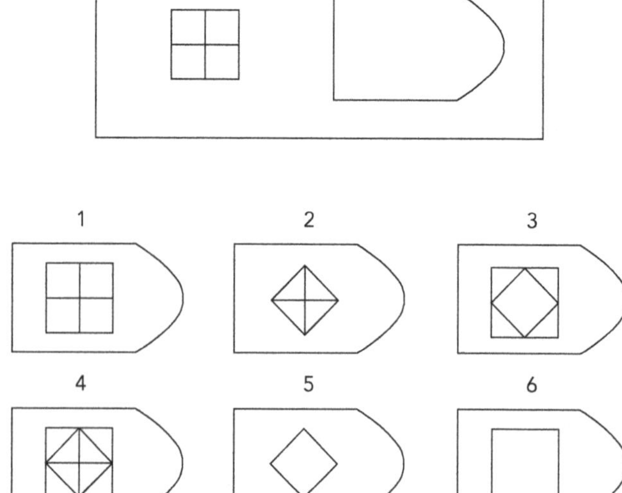

Figure 5–1 *Standard Progressive Matrices (SPM) sample item.*

SOURCE: Raven's Progressive Matrices (Standard, Sets A-E). Copyright © 1998, 1976, 1958, 1938 NCS Pearson, Inc. Reproduced with permission. All rights reserved.

principles of matrix transformation, and, within each set, the items become increasingly more difficult.

All examinees, regardless of their age or ability, are given the same series of items in the same order and asked to work at their own speed, without interruption from the beginning to the end. Persons with cognitive impairment may not be able to solve problems beyond Sets A and B of the scale and the easier problems of Sets C and D, where reasoning by analogy is not essential. A parallel version has been developed (SPM-P; Raven et al., 2000a). The original version (1938) is limited in its ability to differentiate different ability levels as a result of the worldwide increase in intellectual ability over the years (Raven et al., 2000a). In fact, ceiling effects are quite noticeable in adolescence (Pind et al., 2003). An Extended Plus version (SPM+) has been developed, which contains more difficult items but retains the 60-item format (Raven et al., 2000a).

COLORED PROGRESSIVE MATRICES AND VARIANTS

The CPM (Classic CPM or CPM-C; Raven, 1947; Raven et al., 1998b) provides a shorter and simpler form of the test. The test consists of 36 items, grouped into three sets (A, Ab, B) of 12 items each. Sets C, D, and E of the Standard series have been omitted, and an additional set of 12 problems (Ab) has been added between Sets A and B. The last few problems in Set B are printed in the Colored version exactly as they appear in the Standard version. In this way, an examinee who succeeds in solving these problems can proceed without interruption to Sets C, D, and E of the SPM so that intellectual function can be more accurately assessed (Raven et al., 1998a). By omitting an examinee's score on Set Ab, the total score on Sets A, B, C, D, and E can be used to determine the percentile score on the SPM. Set A consists of items in the form of a continuous pattern or gestalt continuation (see Figure 5–2). As one progresses in the set, the perceptual difficulty of items increases. Items in the Ab and B series are made up of four elements or parts, three of which are given and one of which is to be selected among the response alternatives (see Figure 5–1). There is a gradual shift through the Ab and B sets from four parts, which form a coherent whole or gestalt, to problems in which each part is a symbol in an analogies test and there is no perceptual gestalt per se (Costa, 1976).

The CPM was developed for use with children and older people, and it can reportedly be used with people with limited English-language comprehension, motor or sensory difficulties, and people with intellectual disabilities. The items are printed on colored backgrounds. The scale is arranged so that it can be presented in the form of illustrations in a book or as boards with movable pieces. The board form makes the nature of the task even clearer to the examinee. If the examinee is thought to be able to reason by analogy, the SPM is the more suitable scale to use. A parallel form (CPM-P) has also been developed (Raven et al., 1998b).

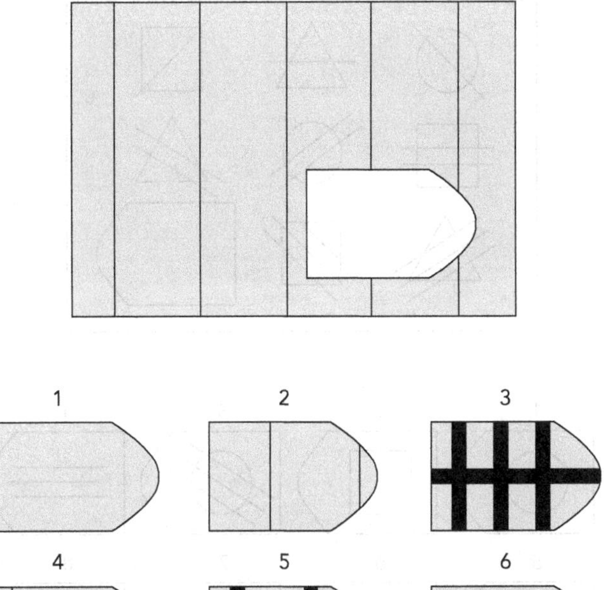

Figure 5–2 *Colored Progressive Matrix (CPM) sample item.*

SOURCE: Raven's Progressive Matrices (Standard, Sets A-E). Copyright © 1998, 1976, 1958, 1938 NCS Pearson, Inc. Reproduced with permission. All rights reserved.

ADVANCED PROGRESSIVE MATRICES

The APM (Raven, 1965/1994; Raven et al., 1998c) was constructed as a test of intellectual ability that could be used with people with above-average intellectual ability (see Figure 5–3) for whom the SPM is too easy (i.e., for persons obtaining a raw score above about 50 on the SPM). It consists of two sets of items. In Set I, there are 12 problems designed to introduce a person to the method and to cover the intellectual processes assessed by the SPM. It can be used as a short 10-minute test or as a practice test before starting Set II. The 36 items in Set II are identical in presentation and reasoning to those in Set I. However, they increase in difficulty more steadily and become considerably more complex.

ADMINISTRATION

Administration details are provided in the manual. Briefly, the examinee points to a response or writes the corresponding number on an answer sheet. There is some evidence that computerized forms yield similar outcomes as paper-and-pencil forms (Raven, 1938/1996; Raven et al., 2000a). Raven cautions that, in order to obtain equivalence with the printed version, the answer selected by the examinee should be shown on the screen and be alterable and that the examinee should be required to make a second, separate response to move the display to the next item. Of note, Matzen et al. (2010) provide software that combines relationships found in the SPM to provide a number of matrices that cover the dimensions of the test and provide the

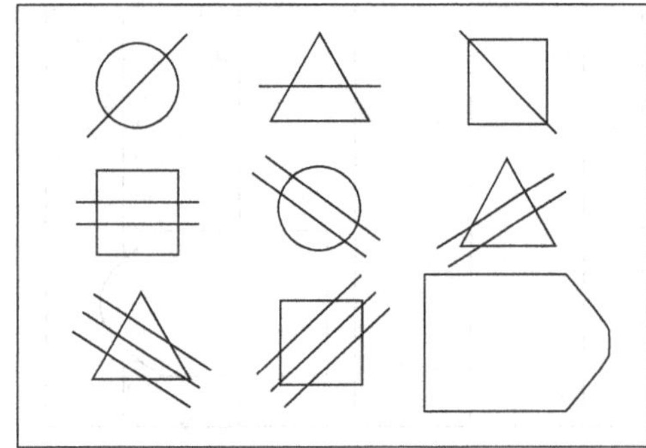

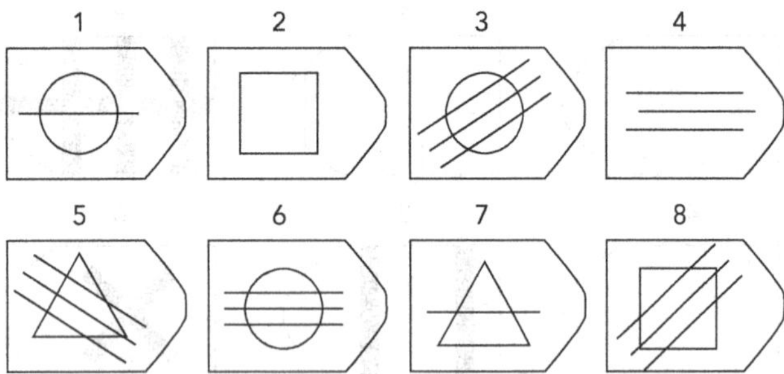

Figure 5–3 *Advanced Progressive Matrix (APM) sample item.*

SOURCE: Raven's Progressive Matrices (Standard, Sets A-E). Copyright © 1998, 1976, 1958, 1938 NCS Pearson, Inc. Reproduced with permission. All rights reserved.

ability to expand the difficulty level of problems; as part of development, the authors also provide detailed analysis of the nature of each item of the SPM.

Both the SPM and CPM are untimed tests. The SPM takes about 40 minutes, and the CPM requires about 25 minutes. Some administer the APM under time constraints while others do not. Set II of the APM can be used without a time limit to assess total reasoning capacity. In that case, the examinee should be shown Set I as examples to explain the principles of the test. About one hour should be allowed to complete the task. The most common time limit for Set II is 40 minutes. Note that responses do not require verbalization, skilled manipulative ability, or subtle differentiation of visuospatial information, and minimal verbal instruction is involved, so the test can be used with a range of ability levels. The test can be given in individual or group format.

SCORING

The total number correct is recorded. Scores are converted to percentiles. The answer sheets and scoring keys must correspond to the test used because different items are provided across forms and versions. Tables provided in the manual provide conversion of scores from one test to the other (e.g., transformation of CPM scores to SPM scores, and vice versa; Raven et al., 1998b, 2000a). One can also convert SPM-C/SPM-P to SPM+ scores (Raven et al., 2000) as well as to APM scores (Raven et al., 1998c). Supplemental information regarding error classification on the SPM is available (see Kunda et al., 2016).

DEMOGRAPHIC EFFECTS

AGE

Age is related to performance (Borella et al., 2006; Brouwers et al., 2009; Locascio et al., 2003; Marcopulos & McLain, 2003; Raven et al., 2000b; Salthouse, 1993), with performance declining with advancing age (e.g., 0.6 *SD* from 79 to 89 years; Der, Allerhand, Starr, Hofer, & Deary, 2009).

GENDER

Evidence for gender effects is mixed. Some have reported that gender has minimal impact on performance (Flynn & Rossi-Casé, 2011; Raven et al., 1998c; Savage-McGlynn, 2012). However, others have reported gender-related differences at least in various age groups (e.g., Lynn et al., 2004) and subsets of the test (e.g., male advantage on Set II of the APM; Bors & Stokes, 1998). Gender differences may be attributable to sample characteristics (Flynn & Rossi-Casé, 2011; Savage-McGlynn, 2012) or the nature of specific items. For example, the visuospatial nature of the test (Abad et al., 2004) or the specific type of rule required to solve the problem may account for gender-related differences (Mackintosh & Bennett, 2005).

ETHNICITY, NATIONALITY, AND LINGUISTIC EFFECTS

Historically, the test was generally considered more "culture fair" than other tests for measuring reasoning ability (O'Leary et al., 1991). One approach to demonstrating test fairness is to compare the item difficulty calibrations across ethnic groups. Overall, such studies reveal that the test has similar psychometric properties across various groups (McCallum et al., 2000). It also has relatively low correlations with tests of academic achievement (Esquivel, 1984; Llabre, 1984; see manual), which has been interpreted to suggest that it may be a fairer measure than other intelligence tests or specific ability measures (Mills et al., 1993; Raven et al., 1990).

However, the test performs differently across groups and is not impervious to demographic and cultural effects. Like many other tests, scores are affected by sociodemographic factors and show a significant increase with increasing years of education and socioeconomic status (Burke, 1958; Freeman & Godfrey, 2000; Marcopulos et al., 1997; Measso et al., 1993; O'Leary et al., 1991; Smits et al., 1997; also see manual).

Ethnicity and nationality can also impact performance (Raven et al., 2000b). In their meta-analysis, Brouwers et al. (2009) analyzed data from nearly 800 samples from 45 countries from studies published between 1944 and 2003. The number of years of education and publication year were related to performance. The authors concluded that the Flynn effect is found across countries examined, with education and country moderating the size of the Flynn effect. The largest Flynn effects were found in India, Iran, and Poland, with increasing country affluence related to a smaller Flynn effect. Overall, based on publication date, a Flynn effect of 2.01 points per decade on the test was reported independent of education. Wicherts, Dolan, Carlson, and van der Maas (2010) provide a review of normative data for sub-Saharan African samples. The authors note an average score of 80 in African samples when using US norms. In addition to the lower mean score obtained in African samples, the test behaved differently in other ways (e.g., weaker correlations with other cognitive tests, lower *g* loadings, and loadings of the test on factors in addition to *g*).

NORMATIVE DATA

Normative data were originally derived from studies conducted in the 1930s and 1940s. Since that time, there has been an upward shift in level of performance (Daley et al., 2003; Raven et al., 1998a, 1998b, 2000b), and the test is often involved in studies describing the Flynn effect (e.g., Brouwers et al., 2009; Flynn & Rossi-Casé, 2012, see also the section "Demographic Effects"). For example, one study reported an increase of approximately 21 points over 34 years in Argentina (to 1998; Flynn & Rossi-Casé, 2012). Consequently, recent normative data are preferable to older normative data.

International and local norms are provided in the manual. In general, norms for high socioeconomic status regions are higher than others and rural areas lower than others (Raven et al., 1998b, 2000a). Although local norms may be preferable for clinical use, they can be problematic when used to make comparative judgments across populations (Mills et al., 1993).

STANDARD PROGRESSIVE MATRICES AND VARIANTS

American norms for ages 18 and older have been developed by Raven et al. (2000a, 2000b). By early adolescence, ceiling effects begin to emerge, suggesting that it is not a suitable measure of intellectual ability for all age groups (see also Pind et al., 2003). Because the SPM+ does not have independent norms, it can only be interpreted by converting its scores to Classic SPM scores (SPM-C; Raven et al., 2000a), which minimizes many of the benefits of its increased ceiling (McCallum et al., 2000).

COLORED PROGRESSIVE MATRICES AND VARIANTS

This test is quite easy, and Raven et al.'s (1998b, 2000b) data suggest ceiling effects at approximately 9 years of age. Yeudall, Fromm, Reddon, and Stefanyuk (1986) tested 225 healthy Canadians (aged 15 to 40) with the CPM. Few errors were found within age groupings (e.g., 15–20, 21–25, etc.). The mean number correct for the combined group (aged 15 to 40) was 34.9 ($SD = 1.25$). Norms for the older participants (55- to 85-year-olds) are provided by Smits et al. (1997). Note that, in this study, only Sets A and B were given (Ab was omitted). Because section Ab correlated strongly (>.90) with the sum of sections A and B, estimated total scores were derived (Raven et al., 1998b). Marcopulos et al. (1997) report a mean of 17.5 ($SD = 6.0$) for 110 community-dwelling older adults (age, $M = 76.48$ years, $SD = 7.87$) with an average educational level of 6.65 years ($SD = 2.14$). Marcopulos and McLain (2003) retested this sample four years later, with data available in their paper.

ADVANCED PROGRESSIVE MATRICES

Raven et al. (1998c) provide North American norms for adults (18 to 68 years and older; Sets I and II) for untimed (aged 12 to 70 years and older) and timed (aged 17 to 28 years old) versions.

EVIDENCE FOR RELIABILITY

STANDARD PROGRESSIVE MATRICES AND VARIANTS

Raven et al. (2000a) summarized numerous studies and reported that split-half reliability is high (>.80). Likewise, Borella et al. (2006) reported excellent internal reliability (Cronbach's alpha = .94). Test-retest reliability is high (>.80) with retest intervals of less than a year. With longer intervals (i.e., years), values tend to be lower. Practice effects are not reported in the manual. The two forms appear to be interchangeable based on Rasch analysis (Raven et al., 2000a).

COLORED PROGRESSIVE MATRICES AND VARIANTS

Test-retest reliability is high ($r > .80$) following intervals of days or weeks. Over longer intervals (six months to one year), however, values decline (.59 to .79; Raven et al., 1998b). Practice effects are not reported in the manual. Original and parallel items in the CPM appear to be similar (i.e., the item difficulties of both forms expressed in Rasch logits were very similar; Raven et al., 1998b).

ADVANCED PROGRESSIVE MATRICES

APM Set II has high internal reliability, with split-half reliability coefficients varying between .83 and .87 (Bors & Stokes, 1998; Raven et al., 1998c). Set I, which has only 12 items, yields lower reliability estimates. Data on retest reliability were originally collected for a 48-item version of the test that was in use from 1947 to 1962. There were 109 children and 243 adults who took the test (with a 40-minute time limit), and they were retested after six to eight weeks. The test was highly reliable for those over 11 years of age ($r > .80$). Overall, Set II scores increased by about 3 points on retest (Raven et al., 1998c). Scores on Set I correlate moderately well with those of Set II (.53; Bors & Stokes, 1998).

EVIDENCE FOR VALIDITY

FACTOR-ANALYTIC STUDIES AND RELATIONSHIPS WITH OTHER TESTS

Studies show moderately strong correlations (generally $r = .50$ to .70) between Raven tests and conventional tests of intelligence such as the Wechsler and Stanford-Binet scales, the National Adult Reading Test, and the Test of Nonverbal Intelligence, Second Edition (Bölte et al., 2009; Bostantjopoulou et al., 2001; Burke, 1985; Deary et al., 2004; Jensen et al., 1988; O'Leary et al., 1991; also see manual). Although the test is thought to reflect *g* (see the section "Description"), a number of authors have contended that it also involves other skills (e.g., Lynn et al., 2004), including an incremental, reiterative strategy for encoding and inducing the regularities in each problem, inducing abstract relations, and dynamically managing a large set of problem-solving goals in working memory (Carpenter et al., 1990). Spatial reasoning is a component of performance with strong relationships between the test and Block Design (Dawson et al., 2007; Mills et al., 1993). There is also a strong working memory component (Borella et al., 2006; Gabrieli, 1996; Harrison et al., 2015; Salthouse, 1993), especially as item difficulty increases (Little et al., 2014). Speed of processing (e.g., inspection time) also correlates with test performance, with high scores associated with more rapid processing (Bates & Rock, 2004).

CLINICAL STUDIES

CPM and SPM performance is reportedly impaired in various neurologic and neuropsychiatric conditions, including dementia (Ambra et al., 2016; Court et al., in Raven et al., 2000b), schizophrenia (Parnas et al., 2001), and severe depression (Naismith et al., 2003). Some research has suggested specific error types are more typical of Alzheimer's disease than vascular dementia (e.g., Gainotti et al., 1992) or amnestic mild cognitive impairment (Ambra et al., 2016). Amyloid beta deposition is correlated with test performance in older adults without dementia (Snitz et al., 2013). In patients with Parkinson's disease without dementia, impairment on the CPM appears to be related to visuospatial difficulties (Cronin-Golomb & Braun, 1997). The CPM items show some degree of sensitivity to hemispheric differences when items are categorized based on cognitive abilities that underlie their solution (i.e., gestalt or visuospatial compared to analogical reasoning; Denes et al., 1978; Villardita, 1985; Zaidel et al., 1981).

Visual field defects and visual neglect impact performance (Court et al., in Raven et al., 2000b). Costa et al. (1969) developed criteria for assessing the presence of unilateral spatial inattention from CPM protocols. The number of answers chosen from the right side of the page (options 3 and 6) is subtracted from the number of answers from the left side of the page (options 1 and 4). The probability of this score, called the *position preference score* (PP), being 7 or greater, or −7 or less, is less than .01 in the healthy population. A positive score of 7 or greater suggests right-sided neglect, whereas a negative score of 7 or less suggests left-sided neglect. Constructional apraxia is associated with lower test scores (Court et al., in Raven et al., 2000b), and the evidence from patients with aphasia is mixed regarding the role of verbal mediation in the task (see Court et al., in Raven et al., 2000b). Performance on the test improves after cardiovascular intervention in older adults (Iuliano et al., 2015). Test performance also correlates with personality variables, such as confidence ratings of performance and neuroticism (see Birney et al., 2017; Double & Birney, 2017).

NEUROANATOMICAL CORRELATES AND IMAGING STUDIES

Neuroimaging studies of the test and variants have implicated a widespread frontoparietal network (Geake & Hansen, 2010; Golde et al., 2010; Vakhtin et al., 2014). It has been suggested that anterior prefrontal cortex is relatively more engaged in integration whereas premotor cortex is more engaged in linking relations sequentially (Golde et al., 2010). Studies using regional cerebral blood flow or positron emission tomography suggest that performance is associated with posterior regions important in visual cognition and gestalt integration (e.g., parietal-temporal-occipital; Abe et al., 2003; Esposito et al., 1999; Haier et al., 1988). A functional magnetic resonance imaging (fMRI) study suggested that performance activates an extensive network of brain regions associated with working memory (Prabhakaran et al., 1997), consistent with studies suggesting a link between working memory and performance. Crone et al. (2009) also reported engagement of both prefrontal cortex and parietal cortex in fMRI. As the task increases in difficulty, cerebral activation patterns increasingly involve somatosensory areas and Wernicke's area, likely related to processing demands reflective of synthesis and analysis of complex information (Mazhirina et al., 2016). In healthy young adults, hippocampal subfields volume, particularly of the right CA1, are associated with performance (Zhu, Chen, Dang, Dong, & Lin, 2017).

Neural correlates of performance may also differ between clinical and nonclinical groups. For example, fMRI studies suggest that as item complexity increased, activity in the left superior occipital gyrus and the left middle occipital gyrus increase for autistic participants, but control participants show increased activity in the left middle frontal gyrus and bilateral precuneus, which may indicate that different cognitive processes underlie performance in different groups (Simard et al., 2015).

PERFORMANCE VALIDITY

A performance validity formula has been developed for the SPM (Gudjonsson & Shackleton, 1986; McKinzey et al., 1999). The formula compares the number of correct

TABLE 5–4 Standard Progressive Matrices (SPM) Performance Validity Cutoff Values

TOTAL SCORE	CUTOFF	TOTAL SCORE	CUTOFF
2	1	32	12
3	2	33	10
4	3	34	10
5	4	35	10
6	5	36	10
7	6	37	10
8	7	38	8
9	7	39	8
10	7	40	8
11	7	41	8
12	7	42	8
13	9	43	7
14	9	44	7
15	9	45	7
16	9	46	7
17	9	47	7
18	10	48	6
19	10	49	6
20	10	50	6
21	10	51	6
22	10	52	6
23	11	53	2
24	11	54	2
25	11	55	2
26	11	56	2
27	11	57	0
28	12	58	0
29	12	59	–1
30	12	60	–1
31	12		

NOTE: The rate of decay is calculated by comparing the number of correct answers in each subset according to the formula ([2A + B] – [D + 2E]). The cutoff is determined by the total score. The SPM is considered invalid if the rate of decay is below the cutoff listed for each total score.

SOURCE: From McKinzey et al. (1999).

answers for the first 24 items against the number of correct answers for the last 24 items (i.e., the "rate of decay") using a set of cutoff numbers derived from the expected, theoretical rate of decay (see Table 5–4). The rate of decay is calculated by comparing the number of correct answers in each subset according to the formula ([2A + B] – [D + 2E]). The cutoff is determined by the total score. The SPM is considered invalid if the rate of decay is below the cutoff listed for each total score. In 46 simulators and 381 people from the adult standardization sample (Raven et al., 2000a), the formula yielded a 26% false-negative rate and 5% false-positive rate (McKinzey et al., 1999). The indices remain to be cross-validated in neurologic and forensic samples.

COMMENT

Historically, the Raven's Progressive Matrices was a commonly used test to measure IQ, specifically fluid intelligence. The test has strengths, including the simple requirements of the task and its nonverbal nature, as well as modified versions for high (APM), low (CPM), or moderate (SPM) levels of ability. Consistent with cognitive demands of the test, neuroimaging studies suggest that an extensive network in both posterior and frontal regions is involved in performance. However, as an IQ test, the test is circumscribed in that it assesses only fluid intelligence and inductive reasoning, and, in this way, it is dissimilar to contemporary, multifaceted conceptualizations of intelligence. As a unidimensional measure of cognitive function, strengths and weaknesses are unlikely to be detected, and multidimensional measures provide intelligence estimates that better reflect current conceptualizations of intelligence and may have better predictive validity at predicting school achievement or occupational achievement. Thus, the test may provide additional information, but alternative measures are needed to gain a true picture of an individual's intellectual abilities.

The test can be used with examinees with language and physical limitations because it does not require an oral response or complex motor functions. However, the test is affected by visual field defects, neglect, and constructional apraxia. The position preference score (Court et al., in Raven et al., 2000b) can be used to assess the validity of administration, although more research on its utility would be beneficial. There is some evidence that the test can be used cross-culturally; however, other evidence suggests that the test performs differently in different cultural contexts and casts doubt on the notion that the test is culturally fair and impervious to the effects of sociodemographic factors. There are age, education, and other sociodemographic effects and mixed data regarding gender effects.

In terms of normative data, international norms are presented in the manual; however, details regarding the normative samples are not well-defined and are dated. The dated nature of norms is a significant limitation given the well-documented Flynn effect on this test (e.g., Hiscock et al., 2002). That is, like other cognitive tests, scores have been increasing over time (Raven et al., 2000a). The magnitude of the increase for the test is about 6 IQ points or 0.4 *z*-score units per decade (Hiscock et al., 2002). For example, on the classic SPM, people born in 1877 and tested in 1942 averaged 24 raw score points on the test, while people born in 1947 and tested in 1992 averaged 54 raw score points. Accordingly, newer normative data are recommended because use of older norms diminish the test's ability to detect impairment (Hiscock et al., 2002). Users should also be aware that there are ceiling effects on the tests, which are particularly evident on the CPM and the SPM.

In terms of psychometric information, internal reliability is high (SPM, CPM, APM), as is test-retest reliability for intervals of less than a year (SPM), months, or days (CPM), with lower coefficients at longer test-retest intervals. The test shows strong correlations with other intelligence measures and also shows relationships with working memory and processing speed.

The clinical research is scant and not well-defined, showing group differences between some patient populations and controls but limited information regarding functional and clinical correlates, responsivity to treatment, and diagnostic value. There is also limited evidence for use of this test for performance validity assessment. Most importantly, the test is quite long to administer, and although the matrices-type items were a fairly unique aspect of the Raven's scales when they were first published, most standard intelligence batteries including the Wechsler scales and other tests such as the Reynolds Intellectual Assessment Scales (RIAS) and dedicated nonverbal IQ batteries now also include matrices-type subtests in formats requiring considerably less administration time.

REFERENCES

Abad, F. J., Colom, R., Rebollo, I., & Escorial, S. (2004). Sex differential item functioning in the Raven's Advanced Progressive Matrices: Evidence for bias. *Personality and Individual Differences, 36,* 1459–1470.

Abe, Y., Kachi, T., Kato, T., Arahata, Y., Vamada, T., Washimi, Y., . . . Sobue, G. (2003). Occipital hypoperfusion in Parkinson's disease without dementia: Correlation to impaired cortical visual processing. *Journal of Neurology, Neurosurgery & Psychiatry, 74,* 419–422.

Alderton, D. L., & Larson, G. E. (1990). Dimensionality of Raven's Advanced Progressive Matrices items. *Educational and Psychological Measurement, 50,* 887–900.

Ambra, F. I., Iavarone, A., Ronga, B., Chieffi, S., Carnevale, G., Iaccarino, L., . . .Garofalo, E. (2016). Qualitative patterns at Raven's Colored Progressive Matrices in mild cognitive impairment and Alzheimer's disease. *Aging Clinical and Experimental Research, 28*(3), 561–565. https://doi.org/10.1007/s40520-015-0438-9

Bates, T. C., & Rock, A. (2004). Personality and information processing speed: Independent influences on intelligent performance. *Intelligence, 32,* 33–46.

Birney, D. P., Beckmann, J. F., Beckmann, N., & Double, K. S. (2017). Beyond the intellect: Complexity and learning trajectories in Raven's Progressive Matrices depend on self-regulatory processes and conative dispositions. *Intelligence, 61,* 63–77. https://doi.org/10.1016/j.intell.2017.01.005

Bölte, S., Dziobek, I., & Poustka, F. (2009). Brief report: The level and nature of autistic intelligence revisited. *Journal of Autism and Developmental Disorders, 39*(4), 678–682. https://doi.org/10.1007/s10803-008-0667-2

Borella, E., Carretti, B., & Mammarella, I. (2006). Do working memory and susceptibility to interference predict individual differences in fluid intelligence? *European Journal of Cognitive Psychology, 18*(1), 51–69. https://doi.org/10.1080/09541440500215962

Bors, D. A., & Stokes, T. L. (1998). Raven's Advanced Progressive Matrices: Norms for first-year university students and the development of a short form. *Educational and Psychological Measurement, 58,* 382–398.

Bostantjopoulou, S., Kiosseoglou, G., Katsarou, Z., & Alevriadou, A. (2001). Concurrent validity of the Test of Nonverbal Intelligence in Parkinson's disease patients. *Journal of Psychology, 135,* 205–212.

Brouwers, S. A., Van de Vijver, F. J. R., & Van Hemert, D. A. (2009). Variation in Raven's Progressive Matrices scores across time and place. *Learning and Individual Differences, 19*(3), 330–338. https://doi.org/10.1016/j.lindif.2008.10.006

Burke, H. R. (1985). Raven's Progressive Matrices: More on norms, reliability, and validity. *Journal of Clinical Psychology, 41,* 231–235.

Carpenter, P. A., Just, M. A., & Shell, P. (1990). What one intelligence test measures: A theoretical account of the processing in the Raven Progressive Matrices test. *Psychological Review, 97,* 404–431.

Costa, L. D. (1976). Interset variability on the Raven Colored Progressive Matrices as an indicator of specific ability deficit in brain-lesioned patients. *Cortex, 12,* 31–40.

Costa, L. D., Vaughan, H. G., Horwitz, M., & Ritter, W. (1969). Patterns of behavioral deficit associated with visual spatial neglect. *Cortex, 5,* 242–263.

Crone, E. A., Wendelken, C., van Leijenhorst, L., Honomichl, R. D., Christoff, K., & Bunge, S. A. (2009). Neurocognitive development of relational reasoning. *Developmental Science, 12*(1), 55–66. https://doi.org/10.1111/j.1467-7687.2008.00743.x

Cronin-Golomb, A., & Braun, A. E. (1997). Visuospatial dysfunction and problem-solving in Parkinson's disease. *Neuropsychology, 11,* 44–52.

Daley, T. C., Whaley, S. E., Sigman, M. D., Espinosa, M. P., & Neuumann, C. (2003). IQ on the rise: The Flynn effect in rural Kenyan children. *Psychological Science, 14,* 215–219.

Dawson, M., Soulières, I., Gernsbacher, M. A., & Mottron, L. (2007). The level and nature of autistic intelligence. *Psychological Science, 18*(8), 657–662.

Deary, I. J., Whalley, L. J., & Crawford, J. R. (2004). An "instantaneous" estimate of a lifetime's cognitive change. *Intelligence, 32,* 113–119.

Denes, F., Semenza, C., & Stoppa, E. (1978). Selective improvement by unilateral brain-damaged patients on Raven Coloured Matrices. *Neuropsychologia, 16,* 749–752.

Der, G., Allerhand, M., Starr, J. M., Hofer, S. M., & Deary, I. J. (2009). Age-related changes in memory and fluid reasoning in a sample of healthy old people. *Aging, Neuropsychology, and Cognition, 17*(1), 55–70. https://doi.org/10.1080/13825580903009071

Double, K. S., & Birney, D. P. (2017). Are you sure about that? Eliciting confidence ratings may influence performance on Raven's Progressive Matrices. *Thinking & Reasoning, 23*(2), 190–206. https://doi.org/10.1080/13546783.2017.1289121

Esposito, G., Kirkby, B. S., Van Horn, J. D., Ellmore, T. M., & Berman, K. F. (1999). Context-dependent, neural system-specific neurophysiological concomitants of ageing: Mapping PET correlates during cognitive activation. *Brain, 122,* 963–979.

Esquivel, G. B. (1984). Coloured Progressive Matrices. In D. J. Keyser & R. C. Sweetland (Eds.), *Test critiques, Vol. 1* (pp. 206–213). Kansas City, MO: Test Corporation of America.

Flynn, J. R., & Rossi-Casé, L. (2011). Modern women match men on Raven's Progressive Matrices. *Personality and Individual Differences, 50*(6), 799–803. https://doi.org/10.1016/j.paid.2010.12.035

Flynn, J. R., & Rossi-Casé, L. (2012). IQ gains in Argentina between 1964 and 1998. *Intelligence, 40*(2), 145–150. https://doi.org/10.1016/j.intell.2012.01.006

Freeman, J., & Godfrey, H. (2000). The validity of the NART-RSPM index in detecting intellectual decline following traumatic brain injury: A controlled study. *British Journal of Clinical Psychology, 39,* 95–103.

Gabrieli, J. D. E. (1996). Memory systems analyses of mnemonic disorders in aging and age-related disease. *Proceedings of the New York Academy of Sciences of the United States of America, 93,* 13534–13540.

Gainotti, G., Parlato, V., Monteleone, D., & Carlomagno, S. (1992). Neuropsychological markers of dementia on visual-spatial tasks: A comparison between Alzheimer's type and vascular forms of dementia. *Journal of Clinical and Experimental Neuropsychology, 14,* 239–252.

Geake, J. G., & Hansen, P. C. (2010). Functional neural correlates of fluid and crystallized analogizing. *NeuroImage, 49*(4), 3489–3497. https://doi.org/10.1016/j.neuroimage.2009.09.008

Golde, M., von Cramon, D. Y., & Schubotz, R. I. (2010). Differential role of anterior prefrontal and premotor cortex in the processing of relational information. *NeuroImage, 49*(3), 2890–2900. https://doi.org/10.1016/j.neuroimage.2009.09.009

Gudjonsson, G., & Schackleton, H. (1986). The pattern of scores on Raven's Matrices during "faking bad" and "non-faking" performance. *British Journal of Clinical Psychology, 25*, 35–41.

Haier, R., Seigel, B., Nuechterlein, K., & Hazlett, E. (1988). Cortical glucose metabolic rate correlates of abstract reasoning and attention studied with positron emission tomography. *Intelligence, 12*, 199–217.

Harrison, T. L., Shipstead, Z., & Engle, R. W. (2015). Why is working memory capacity related to matrix reasoning tasks? *Memory & Cognition, 43*(3), 389–396. https://doi.org/10.3758/s13421-014-0473-3

Hiscock, M., Inch, R., & Gleason, A. (2002). Raven's Progressive Matrices performance in adults with traumatic brain injury. *Applied Neuropsychology, 9*, 129–138.

Iuliano, E., di Cagno, A., Aquino, G., Fiorilli, G., Mignogna, P., Calcagno, G., & Di Costanzo, A. (2015). Effects of different types of physical activity on the cognitive functions and attention in older people: A randomized controlled study. *Experimental Gerontology, 70*, 105–110. https://doi.org/10.1016/j.exger.2015.07.008

Jensen, A. R., Saccuzzo, D. P., & Larsen, G. E. (1988). Equating the Standard and Advanced forms of the Raven Progressive Matrices. *Educational and Psychological Measurement, 48*, 1091–1095.

Kubricht, J. R., Lu, H., & Holyoak, K. J. (2017). Individual differences in spontaneous analogical transfer. *Memory & Cognition, 45*(4), 576–588. https://doi.org/10.3758/s13421-016-0687-7

Kunda, M., Soulières, I., Rozga, A., & Goel, A. K. (2016). Error patterns on the Raven's Standard Progressive Matrices Test. *Intelligence, 59*, 181–198. https://doi.org/10.1016/j.intell.2016.09.004

Little, D. R., Lewandowsky, S., & Craig, S. (2014). Working memory capacity and fluid abilities: The more difficult the item, the more is better. *Frontiers in Psychology, 5*, 239. https://doi.org/10.3389/fpsyg.2014.00239

Llabre, M. M. (1984). Standard Progressive Matrices. In D. J. Keyser & R. C. Sweetland (Eds.), *Test critiques, Vol. 1* (pp. 595–602). Kansas City, MO: Test Corporation of America.

Locascio, J. J., Corkin, S., & Growde, J. H. (2003). Relation between clinical characteristics of Parkinson's disease and cognitive decline. *Journal of Clinical and Experimental Neuropsychology, 25*, 94–109.

Lovett, A., & Forbus, K. (2017). Modeling visual problem solving as analogical reasoning. *Psychological Review, 124*(1), 60–90. https://doi.org/10.1037/rev0000039

Lynn, R., Allik, J., & Irwing, P. (2004). Sex differences on three factors identified in Raven's Standard Progressive Matrices. *Intelligence, 32*, 411–424.

Mackintosh, N. J., & Bennett, E. S. (2005). What do Raven's Matrices measure? An analysis in terms of sex differences. *Intelligence, 33*(6), 663–674. https://doi.org/10.1016/j.intell.2005.03.004

Marcopulos, B. A., & McLain, C. A. (2003). Are our norms "normal"? A 4-year follow-up study of a biracial sample of rural elders with low education. *The Clinical Neuropsychologist, 17*, 19–33.

Marcopulos, B. A., McLain, C. A., & Giuliano, A. J. (1997). Cognitive impairment or inadequate norms? A study of healthy, rural, older adults with limited education. *The Clinical Neuropsychologist, 11*, 111–131.

Matzen, L. E., Benz, Z. O., Dixon, K. R., Posey, J., Kroger, J. K., & Speed, A. E. (2010). Recreating Raven's: Software for systematically generating large numbers of Raven-like matrix problems with normed properties. *Behavior Research Methods, 42*(2), 525–541. https://doi.org/10.3758/BRM.42.2.525

Mazhirina, K. G., Mel'nikov, M. E., Pokrovskii, M. A., Petrovskii, E. D., Savelov, A. A., & Shtark, M. B. (2016). Raven's Progressive Matrices in the lexicon of dynamic mapping of the brain (MRI). *Bulletin of Experimental Biology and Medicine, 160*(6), 850–856. https://doi.org/10.1007/s10517-016-3325-2

McCallum, S., Bracken, B., & Wasserman, J. (2000). *Essentials of nonverbal assessment.* New York: John Wiley & Sons.

McKinzey, R. M., Podd, M. H., Krehbiel, M. A., & Raven, J. (1999). Detection of malingering on Raven's Standard Progressive Matrices: A cross-validation. *British Journal of Clinical Psychology, 38*, 435–439.

Measso, G., Zaooala, G., Cavarzeran, F., Crook, T. H., Romani, L., Pirozzolo, F. J., Grigoletto, F., Amaducci, L., Massari, D., & Lebowitz, B. D. (1993). Raven's Colored Progressive Matrices: A normative study of a random sample of healthy adults. *Acta Neurologica Scandinavia, 88*, 70–74.

Mills, C. J., Ablard, K. E., & Brody, L. E. (1993). The Raven's Progressive Matrices: Its usefulness for identifying gifted/talented students. *Roeper Review, 15*, 183–186.

Naismith, S. L., Hickie, I. B., Turner, K., Little, C. L., Winter, V., Ward, P. B., Wilhelm, K., Mitchell, P., & Parker, G. (2003). Neuropsychological performance in patients with depression is associated with clinical, etiological and genetic risk factors. *Journal of Clinical and Experimental Neuropsychology, 25*, 866–877.

Neisser, U. (1998). Introduction: Rising test scores and what they mean. In U. Neisser (Ed.), *The rising curve: Long-term gains in IQ and related measures* (pp. 3–22). Washington, DC: American Psychological Association.

O'Leary, U-M., Rusch, K. M., & Guastello, S. J. (1991). Estimating age-stratified WAIS-R IQs from scores on the Raven's Standard Progressive Matrices. *Journal of Clinical Psychology, 47*, 277–284.

Parnas, J., Vianin, P., Saebye, D., Jansson, L., Volmer-Larsen, A., & Bovet, P. (2001). Visual binding abilities in the initial and advanced stages of schizophrenia. *Acta Psychiatrica Scandinavia, 103*, 171–189.

Pind, J., Gunnarsdottir, E. K., & Johannesson, H. S. (2003). Raven's Standard Progressive Matrices: New school age norms and a study of the test's validity. *Personality and Individual Differences, 34*, 375–386.

Prabhakaran, V., Smith, J. A. L., Desmond, J. E., Glover, G. H., & Gabrieli, J. D. E. (1997). Neural substrates of fluid reasoning: An fMRI study of neocortical activation during performance of the Raven's Progressive Matrices. *Cognitive Psychology, 33*, 43–63.

Rasmussen, D., & Eliasmith, C. (2011). A neural model of rule generation in inductive reasoning. *Topics in Cognitive Science, 3*(1), 140–153. https://doi.org/10.1111/j.1756-8765.2010.01127.x

Raven, J., Raven, J. C., & Court, J. H. (1998a). *Raven manual: Section 1. General overview.* Oxford: Oxford Psychologists Press Ltd.

Raven, J., Raven, J. C., & Court, J. H. (1998b). *Raven manual: Section 2. Colored Progressive Matrices.* Oxford: Oxford Psychologists Press Ltd.

Raven, J., Raven, J. C., & Court, J. H. (1998c). *Raven manual: Section 4. Advanced Progressive Matrices.* Oxford: Oxford Psychologists Press Ltd.

Raven, J., Raven, J. C., & Court, J. H. (2000a). *Raven manual: Section 3. Standard Progressive Matrices.* Oxford: Oxford Psychologists Press Ltd.

Raven, J., Summers, B., Birchfield, M., Brosier, G., Burciaga, L., Byrkit, B., et al. (1990). (2000b). Manual for Raven's Progressive Matrices and Vocabulary scales. *Research supplement no. 3: A compendium of North American normative and validity studies.* Oxford: Oxford Psychologists Press.

Raven, J., Summers, B., Birchfield, M., et al. (1990). Manual for Raven's Progressive Matrices and Vocabulary scales. *Research Supplement No. 3: A Compendium of North American Normative and Validity Studies.* Oxford: Oxford Psychologists Press Ltd.

Raven, J. C. (1938/1996). *Progressive Matrices: A perceptual test of intelligence. Individual Form.* Oxford: Oxford Psychologists Press Ltd.

Raven, J. C. (1947). *Colored Progressive Matrices Sets A, Ab, B.* Oxford: Oxford Psychologists Press Ltd.

Raven, J. C. (1965/1994). *Advanced Progressive Matrices Sets I and II.* Oxford: Oxford Psychologists Press Ltd.

Salthouse, T. A. (1993). Influence of working memory on adult age differences in matrix reasoning. *British Journal of Psychology, 84,* 171–179.

Savage-McGlynn, E. (2012). Sex differences in intelligence in younger and older participants of the Raven's Standard Progressive Matrices Plus. *Personality and Individual Differences, 53*(2), 137–141. https://doi.org/10.1016/j.paid.2011.06.013

Simard, I., Luck, D., Mottron, L., Zeffiro, T. A., & Soulières, I. (2015). Autistic fluid intelligence: Increased reliance on visual functional connectivity with diminished modulation of coupling by task difficulty. *NeuroImage. Clinical, 9,* 467–478. https://doi.org/10.1016/j.nicl.2015.09.007

Smits, C. H. M., Smit, J. H., van den Heuvel, N., & Jonker, C. (1997). Norms for an abbreviated Raven's Coloured Progressive Matrices in an older sample. *Journal of Clinical Psychology, 53,* 687–697.

Snitz, B. E., Weissfeld, L. A., Lopez, O. L., Kuller, L. H., Saxton, J., Singhababu, D. M., . . . Dekosky, S. T. (2013). Cognitive trajectories associated with β-amyloid deposition in the oldest-old without dementia. *Neurology, 80*(15), 1378–1384. https://doi.org/10.1212/WNL.0b013e31828c2fc8

Vakhtin, A. A., Ryman, S. G., Flores, R. A., & Jung, R. E. (2014). Functional brain networks contributing to the Parieto-Frontal Integration Theory of Intelligence. *NeuroImage, 103,* 349–354.

Villardita, C. (1985). Raven's Colored Progressive Matrices and intellectual impairment in patients with focal brain damage. *Cortex, 21,* 627–634.

Wicherts, J. M., Dolan, C. V., Carlson, J. S., & van der Maas, H. L. J. (2010). Raven's test performance of sub-Saharan Africans: Average performance, psychometric properties, and the Flynn effect. *Learning and Individual Differences, 20*(3), 135–151. https://doi.org/10.1016/j.lindif.2009.12.001

Yeudall, L. T., Fromm, D., Reddon, J. R., & Stefanyuk, W. O. (1986). Normative data stratified by age and sex for 12 neuropsychological tests. *Journal of Clinical Psychology, 42,* 920–946.

Zaidel, E., Zaidel, D. W., & Sperry, R. W. (1981). Left and right intelligence: Case studies of Raven's Progressive Matrices following brain bisection and hemidecortication. *Cortex, 17,* 167–186.

Zhu, B., Chen, C., Dang, X., Dong, Q., & Lin, C. (2017). Hippocampal subfields' volumes are more relevant to fluid intelligence than verbal working memory. *Intelligence, 61,* 169–175. https://doi.org/10.1016/j.intell.2017.02.003

REYNOLDS INTELLECTUAL ASSESSMENT SCALES, SECOND EDITION (RIAS-2) AND REYNOLDS INTELLECTUAL SCREENING TEST, SECOND EDITION (RIST-2)

TEST NAME	**Reynolds Intellectual Assessment Scales, Second Edition (RIAS-2) and Reynolds Intellectual Screening Test, Second Edition (RIST-2)**
DOMAIN	Intellectual function
AGE RANGE	In adults, to 94 years
ADMINISTRATION TIME	25 minutes (RIAS-2), 15 minutes (RIST-2)
SCORING FORMAT	Hand scored
REFERENCE	Reynolds, C. R., & Kamphaus, R. W. (2015). *RIAS-2: Reynolds Intellectual Assessment Scales, Second Edition professional manual and RIST-2: Reynolds Intellectual Screening Test, Second Edition professional manual.* Lutz, FL: PAR. www.parinc.com

DESCRIPTION

The purpose of the Reynolds Intellectual Assessment Scales, Second Edition (RIAS-2; Reynolds & Kamphaus, 2015) is to measure general intelligence as well as verbal intelligence, nonverbal intelligence, memory, and processing speed. The test is comprised of a two-subtest Verbal Intelligence Index (VIX) and a two-subtest Nonverbal Intelligence Index (NIX), which sum to a Composite Intelligence Index (CIX). Two supplementary memory subtests form the Composite Memory Index (CMX). Two supplementary processing speed subtests form the Speeded Processing Index (SPI). See Table 5–5 for subtests and structure of the RIAS-2.

The nine primary goals for the RIAS-2 are detailed at length in the manual. In brief, the test aims to provide a reliable measurement of *g* (including verbal and nonverbal intelligence), provide a practical tool to evaluate intelligence, provide continuity of measurement across the life span, minimize motor and visuomotor demands, minimize reliance on reading as a confound in the measurement of intelligence, accurately predict basic academic achievement, use familiar and common concepts with simple administration and scoring, eliminate items that are shown to be associated with gender or ethnicity, and provide both a verbal and a nonverbal assessment of memory. Although the test is relatively brief, the authors

TABLE 5–5 Subtests and Structure of the Reynolds Intellectual Assessment Scales, Second Edition (RIAS-2)

	COMPOSITE	SUBTEST	DESCRIPTION
Composite Intelligence Index (CIX)	Verbal Intelligence Index (VIX)	Guess What (GWH)	Examinee is provided with clues and asked to deduce the object or concept being described.
		Verbal Reasoning (VRZ)	Examinee hears a statement that forms a verbal analogy and is asked to respond with one or two words that complete the idea or proposition.
	Nonverbal Intelligence Index (NIX)	Odd-Item Out (OIO)	Examinee is presented with a picture card and is asked to designate which picture among an array does not belong with the others.
		What's Missing (WHM)	Examinee is shown a picture with an element missing and is asked to identify the missing element.
	Composite Memory Index (CMX)	Verbal Memory (VRM)	Sentences or brief stories are read aloud by the examiner and recalled by the examinee.
		Nonverbal Memory (NVM)	A stimulus picture is presented for five seconds, and then an array of pictures is presented, from which the examinee must identify the target picture shown.
	Speeded Processing Index (SPI)	Speeded Naming Task (SNT)	Examinee is asked to quickly name common objects presented in a grid format.
		Speeded Picture Search (SPS)	Examinee is asked to find three target pictures within an array of pictures.

SOURCE: Adapted from Reynolds and Kamphaus (2015). Reproduced by special permission of the Publisher, Psychological Assessment Resources, Inc. (PAR), 16204 North Florida Avenue, Lutz, Florida 33549, from the Reynolds Intellectual Assessment Scales, Second Edition by Cecil R. Reynolds, PhD and Randy W. Kamphaus, PhD, Copyright 1998, 1999, 2002, 2003, 2007, 2015 by PAR. Further reproduction is prohibited without permission from PAR.

view it as a comprehensive measure of intelligence and useful with assessment of learning disability, intellectual disability, and so on.

CHANGES FROM RIAS TO RIAS-2

New to the second edition of the test is the incorporation of the processing speed subtests. Additional changes include removal of controversial items, addition of new content, extension of floors and ceilings, modification of ceiling rules, and updated norms that correspond with current US Census data.

According to the manual, test development began in 2011, by surveying purchasers of the RIAS regarding user satisfaction and revisions needed, which subsequently informed the revisions as described in the manual. Prototype data were collected for the novel processing speed tests. The existing items were also revised based on feedback and author input. The test was then piloted in 2012 on a sample of 160 participants across four age bands, reflecting a broad representation in terms of educational and ethnic background. Both classical test theory and Rasch analysis were employed, which also included evaluation of item bias (partial point-biserial correlations and Mantel-Haenszel procedure). Expert review with a culturally and linguistically diverse panel was also completed. Details regarding sample characteristics, specific items removed, and additional procedures are provided in the manual.

REYNOLDS INTELLECTUAL SCREENING TEST, SECOND EDITION (RIST-2)

The Reynolds Intellectual Screening Test, Second Edition (RIST-2) is a screening measure of intelligence provided either as part of the RIAS-2 or which can be purchased separately. The RIST-2 is a two-subtest version of the RIAS-2. It is comprised of only the Guess What and the Odd-Item Out subtests to yield a single composite called the RIST-2 Index and is not intended for clinically impactful decisions such as diagnosis or high-stakes assessments. The authors describe the purpose of the RIST-2 as answering the question "Should I refer this individual for a comprehensive intellectual assessment?" (manual, p. 131). If a full assessment is required, an advantage of using the RIST-2 initially is that the remaining subtests from the RIAS-2 could be administered without having to administer an entirely different IQ battery. The authors recommend an interval of no more than three weeks between the RIST-2 and subsequent administration of the remaining RIAS-2 subtests. If the interval is longer than three weeks, the RIAS-2 should instead be administered in its entirety.

ADMINISTRATION

See manual. The RIST-2 uses the same administration as the RIAS-2 for the Guess What and the Odd-Item Out subtests. Like most IQ tests, the RIAS-2 has limited use in severe intellectual disability (IQs below 45). It is noted that the extent of hearing impairment may impact the ability to complete the verbal subtests. The nonverbal subtests should not be administered to those with visual impairment. Thus, administration of the nonverbal intelligence, nonverbal memory, and speeded processing subtests may not be appropriate for examinees with significant visual problems.

SCORING

Detailed scoring rules and interpretation guidelines are provided in the manual. Index scores have a mean of 100 and an *SD* of 15. The RIAS-2 subtests are scaled to a mean of 50 and an *SD* of 10. Other scores are also available, such as percentile ranks, T scores, z scores, normal curve equivalents, and stanines. Detailed interpretative steps, including case vignettes, are presented in the manual.

The RIST-2 follows similar scoring procedures as the RIAS-2, with both subtest scores summed to a composite score called the RIS-2 Index. The composite score is recommended as the only RIST-2 score used for screening decisions.

DEMOGRAPHIC EFFECTS

AGE

Performance on the RIAS-2 is related to age in a manner similar to other intelligence tests. Specifically, performance tends to begin to plateau in late adolescence, with some continued growth in verbal abilities with age. Performance begins to decline in older years. The decline is steeper for nonverbal intelligence.

GENDER

At test development, items were reviewed by an expert panel for biased or offensive content. Identified items were eliminated or modified. The impact of gender was also investigated using classical test theory and item response theory procedures at the item level. As well, the sample was stratified according to the US Census for gender. The test appears to have similar underlying structure in males and females (see the section "Evidence for Validity").

ETHNICITY, NATIONALITY, AND LINGUISTIC EFFECTS

At the test development stage, items that were biased or offensive were eliminated or modified following review by an expert panel that varied in terms of ethnic background. The standardization sample was Census-stratified according to a number of variables, including ethnicity, to increase the diversity of the sample and minimize test bias. The impact of ethnicity was also investigated using classical test theory and item response theory procedures at the item level. The test appears to show similar underlying structure in various ethnic groups (see the section "Evidence for Validity").

NORMATIVE DATA

The RIAS-2 was normed on a sample of 2,154 examinees from 32 US states from 2013 to 2014, reflecting the 2012 US Census. Participants were screened for color blindness, uncorrected hearing or visual impairment, history of neurologic or psychiatric condition (i.e., traumatic brain injury [TBI], epilepsy, Attention Deficit Hyperactivity Disorder [ADHD], and schizophrenia), and prescription medication use. Some conditions, such as depression, were not excluded.

Characteristics of the adult sample are provided in Table 5–6. Data closely matched Census figures across the sample, with the exception of some slight disparities in terms of regional representation (e.g., slightly greater representation from Northeast and Midwest regions). However, no significant score differences were found regionally on statistical analysis, suggesting minimal impact of region on performance. After the final items were determined, the raw scores were weighted on the basis of age, gender, ethnicity, and education in the proportions found in the US 2012 Census.

Items were scaled using a continuous norming procedure, a regression-based procedure to correct for irregularities in the distributions of scores (see manual). The RIST-2 subtests were extracted from the RIAS-2 and have the same normative sample and followed the same procedure in terms of standardization as the RIAS-2.

TABLE 5–6 Demographic Characteristics of the Adult Standardization Sample for the Reynolds Intellectual Assessment Scales, Second Edition (RIAS-2)

Sample size	783
Age	18 to 94 years
Sample type	2012 US Census-based
Education	12% ≤ High school 31% High school 27% Some college 29% College
Gender	48% Men 52% Women
Ethnicity	68% Caucasian 11% African American 15% Hispanic 6% Other

NOTE: Estimates are approximate.

Age bands: 18 years, 19 years, 20 to 29 years, 30 to 39 years, 40 to 49 years, 50 to 59 years, 60 to 69 years, 70 to 79 years, 80 to 94 years.

SOURCE: Adapted from Reynolds and Kamphaus (2015). Reproduced by special permission of the Publisher, Psychological Assessment Resources, Inc. (PAR), 16204 North Florida Avenue, Lutz, Florida 33549, from the Reynolds Intellectual Assessment Scales, Second Edition by Cecil R. Reynolds, PhD and Randy W. Kamphaus, PhD, Copyright 1998, 1999, 2002, 2003, 2007, 2015 by PAR. Further reproduction is prohibited without permission from PAR.

EVIDENCE FOR RELIABILITY

EVIDENCE FOR INTERNAL RELIABILITY

Cronbach's alpha coefficients are high to very high for RIAS-2 subtest and index scores (*rs* ≥ .80, *rs* ≥ .86, respectively). When subdivided according to age by demographic grouping variable (e.g., gender, ethnicity), reliability coefficients remain high to very high overall. *SEMs* are presented for index scores and are relatively small, ranging from under 2 points to approximately 5 points. Reliability coefficients are similarly high when the sample is subgrouped according to gender and ethnicity, with estimates in excess of .86. In terms of the RIST-2, the composite score has a very high median internal reliability coefficient (.92), with a median *SEM* of 4.37.

EVIDENCE FOR TEST-RETEST RELIABILITY, MEASURING CHANGE, AND PRACTICE EFFECTS

According to the manual, RIAS-2 test-retest reliability after a median retest interval of 18 days (range of 7 to 43 days) is generally high to very high for subtests (*rs* ≥ .86, with the exception of Speeded Picture Search, which has a reliability coefficient of .72). Index scores are also high (*rs* ≥ .83) in a healthy sample of 97 participants (age $M = 22.3$, $SD = 19.4$, range = 3 to 72; see manual for additional demographic information). Coefficients are also provided separately for age groupings, again showing high to very high estimates overall with some exceptions for subtest scores, which were in the adequate range in the adult subgroup (e.g., *rs* = .70 to .77 for memory scores and Speeded Picture Search). Overall, the indices are associated with the strongest reliability and the speeded subtests with somewhat lower, but still adequate, reliability coefficients.

In the overall sample, practice effects on the RIAS-2 subtests range from approximately 2 to 5 points, and practice effects on the indices range from approximately 3 points (Speeded Processing Index) to 6 points (Nonverbal Intelligence Index, Composite Intelligence Index). In adults, practice effects generally range from 2 to 5 points for the subtest scores and 2 to 9 points for the indices (Composite Memory Index, 18- to 30-year-olds). Practice effects on most indices approximate a change of 4 to 5 points. Of note, the manual provides tables for calculating reliable change for the RIAS-2. RIST-2 test-retest reliability is very high (.99 in adult samples). No information on practice effects or reliable change is available.

EVIDENCE FOR INTERRATER RELIABILITY

Two independent raters scored 35 protocols that were randomly selected from the normative sample. Interrater reliability was excellent, with correlations of .99 and 1.00 reported (manual).

EVIDENCE FOR VALIDITY

FACTOR-ANALYTIC STUDIES

The test authors first conducted exploratory factor analyses, then confirmatory factor analyses to evaluate goodness-of-fit. Exploratory factor analyses were conducted with four separate age groupings, two of which were adult groups (aged 18 to 30, aged 31 to 94). Subtest loadings suggested that a three-factor structure best fits the data, consisting of verbal IQ/memory (Guess What, Verbal Reasoning, Verbal Memory), nonverbal IQ/memory (Odd-Item Out, What's Missing, Nonverbal Memory), and processing speed (Speeded Naming Task, Speeded Picture Search).

Factor analyses were also conducted separately by gender (male, female) and ethnicity (Caucasian, African American, Hispanic). The factor structures in these groups were broadly consistent with the factor structure reported in the age groupings, suggesting similar task structure across age, gender, and ethnicity.

In confirmatory factor analyses, the following types of models were evaluated: one-factor (*g*), two-factor (verbal and nonverbal ability), three-factor (verbal, nonverbal, and either memory or processing speed), and a four-factor model (verbal, nonverbal, memory, processing speed). The best fitting model according to confirmatory factor analysis was a three-factor model that reflected verbal IQ (Guess What, Verbal Reasoning), nonverbal IQ (Odd-Item Out, What's Missing), and processing speed (Speeded Naming Task, Speeded Picture Search).

RELATIONSHIP WITH THE RIAS

The manual reports that the RIAS-2 and RIAS subtests and index scores are highly correlated, ranging from $r = .71$ (Odd-Item Out) to $r = .93$ (Guess What, Verbal Memory).

RELATIONSHIP BETWEEN RIAS-2 AND RIST-2

The RIST-2 composite score (RIST-2 Index) is highly correlated with the RIAS-2 indices in the adult sample, ranging from $r = .60$ for CMX to $r = .96$ for the CIX. However, correlations with the Speeded Processing Index are relatively small ($r = .25$).

RELATIONSHIPS WITH THE OTHER IQ TESTS

The RIAS-2 indices show weak to strong correlations with the WAIS-IV index scores, ranging from .23 (SPI with WAIS-IV Perceptual Reasoning) to .77 (VIX with WAIS-IV Verbal Comprehension). Correlation between SPI and WAIS-IV Processing Speed Index is moderate ($r = .38$). Subtest correlations are mostly in the moderate range, with some in the high range (e.g., Verbal Reasoning with WAIS-IV Information, .70). Overall, the pattern of relationships between the RIAS-2 and the WAIS-IV suggests that the nonverbal and verbal reasoning measures on both tests show stronger correlations than those between WAIS-IV reasoning and RIAS-2 processing speed scores.

The RIST-2 composite score is highly correlated with the WAIS-IV FSIQ ($r = .62$). Correlations with the index scores are generally moderate ($r = .45$ to .59) except with the Processing Speed Index ($r = .27$).

RELATIONSHIPS WITH ACHIEVEMENT

Correlations between the RIAS-2 and Academic Achievement Battery (AAB), a comprehensive achievement battery by the same publisher, are weak to moderate. Processing speed scores from the RIAS-2 show the weakest correlations with the achievement battery.

The RIAS-2 and the Feifer Assessment of Reading (FAR), a measure of reading ability, generally yield moderate correlations, except for the RIAS-2 processing speed scores, which generally show weak correlations with the reading measure. Similarly, tests on the reading measure related to fluency and visual perception also show weak correlations with reasoning scores on the RIAS-2. Correlations between the RIST-2 and academic achievement tests are moderate ($r = .53$ and $r = .40$ with the AAB composite and the FAR Total Index, respectively).

CLINICAL STUDIES

The manual provides data on a number of clinical groups that generally perform as expected on the test. In adults, this includes patients with stroke, dementia, hearing impairment, intellectual disability, TBI, learning disability, and ADHD. Samples range in size from 22 to 31 people. The data for these groups were collected in the course of standardization, and the diagnoses were from the referral sources and were not independently verified by the test developers.

Patients with stroke, dementia, or hearing impairment obtained significantly lower scores on all RIAS-2 subtests and indices compared to demographically matched controls. As expected, the dementia group showed the lowest performance. Patients with TBI scored lower than a demographically matched sample on all RIAS-2 indices, with the VIX broadly in the average range. Adults with intellectual disability generally obtained low RIAS-2 index scores (range of 45–55). Among adults with learning disabilities, scores were lower compared to demographically matched controls on the CMX and the SPI, and specific subtests (Verbal Reasoning, Nonverbal Memory, and Speeded Naming). Scores of adults with ADHD did not differ significantly from demographically matched controls.

In terms of the RIST-2, adult patients with stroke, dementia, hearing impairment, TBI, and intellectual disability obtained lower scores than demographically matched controls, with the intellectual disability group showing the largest differences. No differences in performance were found between adults with learning disability or ADHD and matched controls (manual). At this writing, no independent studies on the RIAS-2/RIST-2 have been published to our knowledge.

NEUROANATOMICAL CORRELATES AND IMAGING STUDIES

No information is available.

PERFORMANCE VALIDITY

Unique to measures assessing intellectual functioning, the RIAS-2 manual provides information on the impact of feigned impairment. The manual presents data from a sample of 40 examinees coached to simulate impairment on the RIAS-2. To confirm that the examinees followed the instructions to feign, the Test of Memory Malingering (TOMM) was given and all examinees performed in the invalid range. Simulators showed significantly worse performance on each RIAS-2 score compared to matched controls; however, no embedded validity indices are provided for the RIAS-2, and thus to assess performance validity a performance validity test must be co-administered.

COMMENT

The RIAS-2 provides a measure of general intelligence and is quicker to administer and more affordable than the more popular WAIS-IV. Moreover, its most recent iteration also includes memory and processing speed measures. The RIST-2 is a shorter two-subtest version of the RIAS-2 that can be easily administered in cases where a screening evaluation is indicated. The normative database is impressive in that it is large and Census-stratified on a number of variables.

The test is reliable, with generally high to very high coefficients across different types of reliability. Factor-analytic studies generally support a verbal reasoning and a nonverbal reasoning component, with processing speed reflecting a relatively independent construct. The RIAS-2 demonstrates convergent and divergent validity with other measures. Overall, the test also shows expected effects in specific clinical groups. For example, persons with intellectual disability or dementia score well below demographically matched controls.

However, at this writing, independent research is needed on the RIAS-2 and the RIST-2. The clinical data available are provided by the test developers and include small samples that are heterogeneous in demographic characteristics. This latest version includes memory measures, but it does not include a delayed memory component. It also does not have any embedded validity indicators. As such, use of the RIAS-2 should not replace more comprehensive IQ tests. Finally, information on neuroanatomical correlates would be desirable. Given these limitations, the WAIS-IV or other comprehensive IQ tests are preferred for high-stakes assessment.

REFERENCE

Reynolds, C. R., & Kamphaus, R. W. (2015). *RIAS-2: Reynolds Intellectual Assessment Scales, Second Edition professional manual, RIST-2: Reynolds Intellectual Screening Test, Second Edition professional manual.* Lutz, FL: PAR.

TEST OF NONVERBAL INTELLIGENCE, FOURTH EDITION (TONI 4)

TEST NAME	**Test of Nonverbal Intelligence, Fourth Edition (TONI 4)**
DOMAIN	Intellectual function
AGE RANGE	In adults, to 89 years
ADMINISTRATION TIME	20 minutes
SCORING FORMAT	Hand scored
REFERENCE	Brown, L., Sherbenou, R. J., & Johnsen, S. K. (2010). *Test of Nonverbal Intelligence, Fourth Edition.* Austin, TX: PRO-ED.

DESCRIPTION

The purpose of the Test of Nonverbal Intelligence, Fourth Edition (TONI 4; Brown et al., 2010) is to measure general intelligence in a nonverbal format with minimal linguistic and motor skill requirements. The test measures abstract reasoning and figural problem solving, including intellectual abilities in people who present with language or motor challenges. The test was originally designed "to fill a gap, not to test a theory" (p. 1, manual), but the authors state that the test conforms to the theoretical construct of *g* and fluid intelligence.

The test has two equivalent 60-item forms. Each item is comprised of an abstract figure, which eliminates advantages that may be conferred by displaying familiar objects. Item difficulty is manipulated by salient characteristics of the items (e.g., shape, position), as well as by the type and number of problem-solving rules required to correctly solve the problem. The items are broadly categorized as Matching, Analogy, Progression, Classification, and Intersection.

This is the fourth iteration of the test, which was originally published in 1982. According to the manual, many items remain unchanged across editions, therefore research from previous editions is relevant to the current edition. The research based on previous editions is synthesized by Johnsen, Brown, and Sherbenou (2010) for the interested reader, including reliability data in various populations.

A number of improvements were made to the fourth edition based on previous research and reviews, including inclusion of new Census-stratified normative data (see the section "Normative Data"), analysis of bias in test items related to demographic characteristics (see "Demographic Effects"), and augmented reliability and validity data. New items were added to improve floors and ceilings; additional data analysis (e.g., item analytic and differential item functioning analysis) and data were reported (e.g., means and *SD*s for validity studies, correlations between forms across ages and versions, and equivalency data for individuals without linguistic or motor impairments). Finally, items were reordered and sorted to balance Form A and B in terms of difficulty, and modifications to instructions were completed (e.g., inclusion of both verbal and nonverbal directions and instructions in languages other than English). Of note, the TONI 4 has also been reviewed elsewhere (Ritter et al., 2011).

ADMINISTRATION

Detailed administration instructions are provided in the manual. The test is intended for use with examinees with linguistic, hearing, or motor impairments, as well as persons with limited English proficiency. Instructions can be provided nonverbally or verbally, and only nonverbal responses are required. Note that the addition of oral instructions is a major change relative to previous editions. The test instructions can be provided verbally in English, Spanish, French, German, simplified Chinese, Vietnamese, Korean, and Tagalog.

According to a study reported in the manual, performance does not appear to differ when verbal compared to nonverbal instructions are provided, and performance in both conditions is highly correlated (r = .79). However, the nonverbal format is typically the preferred mode of administration in order to minimize linguistic or sensory confounds.

SCORING

Detailed scoring rules and interpretation guidelines are provided in the manual. Each of the 60 items is scored as correct or incorrect, and they progress in levels of difficulty. Basal and ceiling rules apply. Raw scores are converted to standard scores and can also be converted to percentile rankings. Qualitative terms are assigned to index scores in a conventional manner; for example, an "Average" descriptor corresponds to a standard score ranging from 90 to 110. See manual for additional qualitative descriptors.

DEMOGRAPHIC EFFECTS

AGE

Performance is related to age in a manner similar to other intelligence tests. Specifically, performance tends to plateau from approximately 17 to 60 years of age, then gradually declines.

GENDER

Gender differences are small (2 points) when males and females of the normative sample are compared, with females obtaining slightly higher scores. Bias in reference to gender was found to be minimal via differential item functioning analysis (see also "Normative Data").

ETHNICITY, NATIONALITY, AND LINGUISTIC EFFECTS

The sample was Census-stratified according to a number of variables, including ethnic characteristics. This serves to increase the diversity of the sample and minimize test bias. When the normative sample was subdivided into ethnic groups, each group scored in the average range. However, white and Asian/Pacific Islander examinees obtained mean index scores of 99 to 101 (across Forms A and B), whereas Hispanic and African-American examinees obtained mean index scores ranging from 93 to 97. It is not clear whether these differences were statistically significant. Bias in reference to ethnicity was found to be minimal via differential item functioning analysis (as discussed in "Normative Data"). Of note, instruction is available in a number of languages (see "Administration").

NORMATIVE DATA

The TONI 4 was normed on a sample of 2,272 children and adults, Census-stratified according to gender, education, income, ethnicity, and geographic region. Data provided in the manual indicate that the adult normative sample closely approximated the Census data on relevant variables. Demographic characteristics of the adult sample are provided in Table 5–7. Data were collected over a three-year interval (2005 to 2008). Thirty-one states were represented; however, 87% of the normative data were collected at major sites in the South, West, Northeast, and Midwest United States. The majority of the sample was tested using English language instructions (77%), and the remainder of participants were tested using nonverbal instructions (23% of the sample).

Item discriminating power (i.e., the degree to which an item differentiates among examinees) and item difficulty (i.e., percentage of examinees who passed a specific item) were evaluated and were reported to be within target range by the authors. Minimal item bias based on gender and ethnicity was identified via differential item functioning. Differential item functioning evaluates whether examinees from identified subgroups (e.g., subdivided by gender or ethnicity) perform differently despite similar ability level. This analysis is described in the manual but, in brief, involves comparison of regression models. One model uses the subtest score (i.e., ability) alone to predict item performance and is compared to a second, broader model that uses both ability and group membership (e.g., based on gender, ethnicity, etc.) to predict item performance. If the test is minimally biased, these models should yield similar results. If the test is biased, the models would yield discrepant results. According to this analysis, items are non-biased with respect to gender and ethnicity (e.g., African American, Hispanic).

TABLE 5–7 Demographic Characteristics of the Adult Standardization Sample for the Test of Nonverbal Intelligence, Fourth Edition (TONI 4)

Sample size	696[a]
Age	19 to 89 years
Geographic location	21% Northeast 38% South 20% Midwest 21% West
Education	70% ≤ Bachelor's degree 20% Bachelor's degree 10% Graduate degree
Gender	48% Men 52% Women
Ethnicity	83% Caucasian 11% African American 3% Asian/Pacific Islander 2% Two or more or other
Hispanic	89% No 11% Yes
Family income (dollars)	11% <$15,000 9% $15,000 to $24,999 10% $25,000 to $34,999 15% $35,000 to $49,999 20% $50,000 to $74,999 34% >$75,000
Exceptionality status	75% No disability 2% Specific learning disability 0% Speech language disorder 3% Intellectual disability 2% Other disability

[a]The majority of *ns* provided for adults for each demographic variable is $n = 696$.

EVIDENCE FOR RELIABILITY

EVIDENCE FOR INTERNAL RELIABILITY

Cronbach's alpha coefficients across adult age groups are very high for Form A and Form B ($r = .96$ to $.97$). When subdivided according to grouping variable (e.g., by gender, ethnicity, diagnosis, etc.), reliability coefficients remain high for both forms ($r = .92$ to $.97$). *SEMs* are relatively small, ranging from 2 to 3 points for each form.

EVIDENCE FOR TEST-RETEST RELIABILITY, MEASURING CHANGE, AND PRACTICE EFFECTS

According to the manual, test-retest reliability after a 1- to 2-week test-retest interval is high for Form A and Form B (r = .82, .83, respectively) in a sample of healthy people (n = 63, 9 to 72 years of age, 50% adult; manual).

EVIDENCE FOR ALTERNATE FORMS RELIABILITY

Forms completed in the same session are highly correlated in adult subsamples (r = .75 to r = .89, manual). The correlations between Form A at first testing and Form B at second testing, as well as Form B at first testing and Form A at second testing, also yield high coefficients (r = .82, .83).

EVIDENCE FOR INTERRATER RELIABILITY

Two independent raters scored 50 pairs of Form A and B protocols that were randomly selected from the normative sample, with agreement coefficients approximating r = .99 (manual).

EVIDENCE FOR VALIDITY

FACTOR-ANALYTIC STUDIES AND RELATIONSHIPS WITH OTHER TESTS

As would be expected due to its unidimensional structure, TONI 4 items load on a single factor (manual). Correlations between the TONI 4 and TONI-3 in a mixed child and adult sample are high (r = .74; manual). Furthermore, the sensitivity and specificity associated with identifying intellectual disability with the TONI-3 as the reference standard were 83% and 92%, respectively. Of note, correlations between the TONI 4 and other tests of intelligence and tests of achievement are reported in the manual for child samples only.

CLINICAL STUDIES

The manual provides data to indicate that gifted and talented individuals score approximately 1.8 *SD* above the mean (mean = 121, 125, Form A and Form B), while examinees with intellectual disability score 2 *SD* below the mean (mean = 78, 77, Form A and Form B). Other groups (e.g., ADHD, learning disability, physical impairment, speech and language disorder) perform broadly within the average range. Of note, the authors state that due to the shared item content of the TONI-3 and TONI 4, much validity research that applies to the TONI-3 can be generalized to the TONI 4. The test has also been used as a screener in studies involving adults with learning disabilities (Bourgoyne & Alt, 2017), as well as in electrophysiological (Kaganovich & Schumaker, 2016) and neuroimaging studies (Newsome et al., 2016).

NEUROANATOMICAL CORRELATES AND IMAGING STUDIES

To our knowledge, the test has been used in one neuroimaging study (i.e., Newsome et al., 2016).

PERFORMANCE VALIDITY

No information is available.

COMMENT

The TONI 4 provides a measure of general intelligence in a nonverbal format, thus minimizing confounds of linguistic or motor impairments. A major strength of the TONI 4 is the attempt by the developers to minimize test bias and render the test a fair and accurate estimate of intelligence for examinees who may be challenged to complete verbally based or complex measures. The test can be administered verbally or nonverbally (although nonverbal is generally preferred, see "Administration") and is available for use in a number of languages.

In terms of demographic effects, as would be expected, age is related to performance. Gender differences are negligible. Ethnic characteristics appear to not significantly affect performance according to differential item function analysis. The normative database is quite impressive in that it is large and Census-stratified on a number of variables.

The test is reliable, with high to very high coefficients across different types of reliability. The TONI 4 demonstrates strong relationships with similar measures and shows expected effects in specific groups (e.g., gifted individuals score well above the mean, persons with intellectual disability score well below the mean).

Additional research is needed on the TONI 4. However, the test has a near 40-year history, and, according to the manual, many items remain unchanged across editions. Thus, research from previous editions may be relevant to the current edition to an extent, although it should be noted that there are significant revisions to the current edition, including changes to normative data and format. The interested reader is referred to Johnsen et al. (2010) for summary data on previous editions.

REFERENCES

Bourgoyne, A., & Alt, M. (2017). The effect of visual variability on the learning of academic concepts. *Journal of Speech, Language, and Hearing Research*, *60*(6), 1568–1576. https://doi.org/10.1044/2017_JSLHR-L-16-0271

Brown, L., Sherbenou, R. J., & Johnsen, S. K. (2010). *Test of Nonverbal Intelligence*, Fourth Edition. Austin, TX: PRO-ED.

Johnsen, S. K., Brown, L., & Sherbenou, R. J. (2010). *Test of Nonverbal Intelligence: Critical reviews and research findings, 1982–2009*. Austin, TX: PRO-ED.

Kaganovich, N., & Schumaker, J. (2016). Electrophysiological correlates of individual differences in perception of audiovisual temporal asynchrony. *Neuropsychologia, 86,* 119–130. https://doi.org/10.1016/j.neuropsychologia.2016.04.015

Newsome, M. R., Mayer, A. R., Lin, X., Troyanskaya, M., Jackson, G. R., Scheibel, R. S., . . . Levin, H. S. (2016). Chronic effects of blast-related TBI on subcortical functional connectivity in Veterans. *Journal of the International Neuropsychological Society, 22*(6), 631–642. https://doi.org/10.1017/S1355617716000448

Ritter, N., Kilinc, E., Navruz, B., & Bae, Y. (2011). Test Review: L. Brown, R. J. Sherbenou, & S. K. Johnsen Test of Nonverbal Intelligence-4 (TONI-4). Austin, TX: PRO-ED, 2010. *Journal of Psychoeducational Assessment, 29*(5), 484–488. https://doi.org/10.1177/0734282911400400

WECHSLER ABBREVIATED SCALE OF INTELLIGENCE—SECOND EDITION (WASI-II)

TEST NAME	**Wechsler Abbreviated Scale of Intelligence—Second Edition (WASI-II)**
DOMAIN	Intellectual function
AGE RANGE	In adults, to 90 years
ADMINISTRATION TIME	30 minutes
SCORING FORMAT	Computerized or hand scored
REFERENCE	Wechsler, D. (2011). *Wechsler Abbreviated Scale of Intelligence—Second Edition (WASI-II)*. San Antonio, TX: NCS Pearson. www.pearsonclinical.com

DESCRIPTION

The Wechsler Abbreviated Scale of Intelligence—Second Edition (WASI-II; Wechsler, 2011) is a brief measure of intelligence. The test may be used in situations that include: obtaining an IQ estimate when administration of a full battery is not possible or desired, screening to determine the need for further assessment, re-evaluation when time constraints do not permit full battery administration, and obtaining estimates of IQ for research purposes (manual). The test is co-linked with the Wechsler Intelligence Scale for Children—Fourth Edition (WISC-IV) and the WAIS-IV, and provides tables for converting WASI-II scores to IQ scores on these tests. The WASI-II is comprised of four subtests: Block Design, Vocabulary, Matrix Reasoning, and Similarities. Of note, these subtests are not comprised of the same items as their WISC-IV and WAIS-IV counterparts and are thus not directly interchangeable. Vocabulary and Matrix Reasoning alone can be given to provide an estimate of cognitive function. See also Irby and Floyd (2013) and McCrimmon and Smith (2013) for test reviews.

A number of revisions were made to the WASI-II to update the test. These changes include: enhancing the linkages between the WISC-IV and WAIS-IV, enhancing user-friendliness, and improving psychometric properties. Strengthening links with the other Wechsler tests involved increasing consistency of items and administration rules and administering the WAIS-IV and WASI-II to a sample of 182 adults. This enabled norm equivalence to be investigated and also facilitated conversion of WASI-II subtest scores to WAIS-IV scores. For example, if screening results via the WASI-II prompt the clinician to conduct a more comprehensive assessment, the WASI-II subscales can be used in place of the WAIS-IV counterparts.

A second revision category involved increasing user-friendliness, which included reduction of verbal instructions, simplification of discontinue and reversal rules, and easier-to-use test materials. A third type of revision involved improving psychometric properties. This was done in a number of ways. First, norms were updated. Data were collected between 2010 and 2011, and norms were stratified based on demographic factors (age, gender, ethnicity, education, geographic region) according to 2008 US Census data. Second, reliability and validity data were updated, including test-retest data for four different age groups and investigation of convergent and discriminant validity with the first edition, the WISC-IV, WAIS-IV, and KBIT-2. Factor analysis and clinical studies with matched control samples were also done. Furthermore, floors and ceilings were extended. Finally, a subsample of examinees aged 6 to 50 years was administered the WASI-II and the Wechsler Fundamentals: Academic Skills, an academic achievement battery. Psychometric qualities of the WASI-II are addressed in more detail later in this review.

ADMINISTRATION

Administration instructions are provided in the manual.

SCORING

Unlike the WAIS-IV, T scores are the standardized score metric on the WASI-II (mean of 50, *SD* of 10, and a range of 20–80). Tables are provided to convert raw scores to T-score equivalents, as well as for comparing the WASI-II subtest scores to their WAIS-IV counterparts.

Composite scores are also available, including the Verbal Comprehension Index (VCI; comprised of the two verbal subtests), the Perceptual Reasoning Index (PRI; comprised of the two non-verbal subtests), the FSIQ-4 (a four-subtest composite), and an FSIQ-2 (a two-subtest composite). The composite scores are in standard score metric (M = 100, SD = 15). A table to convert raw scores to age equivalents, critical values (discrepancy between Index scores required for statistical significance), and base rate data (frequency of score differences in normative sample) is also provided.

DEMOGRAPHIC EFFECTS

Detailed information regarding the effect of age, gender, education, ethnicity and other sociodemographic variables is not available.

NORMATIVE DATA

Normative data were stratified based on 2008 US Census data along demographic variables, including age, gender, ethnicity, educational level, and geographic region. The sample was comprised of 2,300 individuals 6 to 90 years of age. Adult normative data are presented across 12 age bands, with band length ranging from two years (i.e., 17- to 19-year-olds) to nine years (e.g., 35 to 44, 45 to 54, 55 to 64). Most data are presented in four-year intervals. There were 100 participants in each of the 23 age groupings across the normative sample.

Exclusion criteria were extensive, and participants who met one or more of the following criteria were excluded: unable to speak or understand English, nonverbal or aphasic, uncorrected visual or hearing impairment, unable to understand and participate in testing, lack of compliance, uncorrected fine or gross motor disability, substance abuse or dependence within one year of testing, admission to a hospital or psychiatric facility at the time of testing, taking medication that could impact cognitive test performance, change in functional ability related to cognitive decline, neurologic condition, testing on an intelligence measure over the last six months, graduate-level training in psychology, twin of another examinee, or relative of an examiner.

In people older than 19 years, additional exclusion criteria included current diagnosis of a neurologic condition such as ADHD, dementia, Parkinson's disease and so on; a diagnosis of psychosis, mood, or anxiety disorder; chemotherapy; history of electroconvulsive therapy (ECT) or radiation; and a period of unconsciousness lasting longer than 20 minutes that was related to a medical condition.

In terms of gender distribution, equal numbers of males and females were included in each age group. For individuals 65 years and older, there was a female majority, consistent with Census data. Ethnic composition was according to Census data, as was education level. Education groupings were divided into the following categories: 8 years or less, 9 to 11 years, 12 years, 13 to 15 years, and 16 years or more. Geographic regions in the US were categorized as Northeast, Midwest, South, and West. Exact figures relating to education and geographic region of examinees are not provided in the manual, although a bar graph is provided. Specific percentages of people in the normative sample subdivided by age, ethnicity, and gender are presented in tables.

Normative data were derived via inferential norming (see Wilkins, Rolfhus, Weiss, & Zhu, 2005 as cited by Wechsler, 2011). This involved calculation of "moments" (means, *SD*s, skewness) for each subtest for each age group, plotted across age, with regressions fit to moment data. Functions for each moment were chosen based on consistency with theory and the observed trajectory of performance within each age group. Functions were then used to derive estimates of the moments, with estimated moments then used to generate theoretical distributions for each age group, resulting in percentiles for each raw score. Smoothing was used to eliminate minor deviations in the distribution.

EVIDENCE FOR RELIABILITY

EVIDENCE FOR INTERNAL RELIABILITY

Split-half reliability coefficients across age groups are very high for composite scores (*rs* = .90 to .97) and high to very high for subtest scores (*rs* = .83 to .95 across subtests and ages). In the adult sample alone, *SEM*s are low and range from 2.77 (FSIQ-4) to 3.75 (FSIQ-2). Confidence interval tables are provided in the manual.

EVIDENCE FOR TEST-RETEST RELIABILITY, MEASURING CHANGE, AND PRACTICE EFFECTS

Test-retest reliability is strong overall. Test-retest data are reported in the manual based on 215 participants tested within a test-retest interval of 12 to 88 days (*M* interval = 10 days). Participants were predominantly female (58%) and Caucasian (55%), with 82% achieving high school education or higher (see manual for additional details regarding demographic composition).

Reliabilities are high for composite scores ($r \geq .89$). Test-retest reliability is high to very high for most subtests (Block Design $r = .89$, Vocabulary $r = .93$, Similarities $r = .86$), with the exception of Matrix Reasoning, which was in the adequate range ($r = .75$) due apparently to relatively weak test-retest reliability in 17- to 54-year-olds ($r = .65$). Estimates were in the high range when coefficients adjusting for variability in the normative sample were used. Practice effects are found. In terms of composite scores, the increase on retest is 2.5 to 5.4 points, with PRI showing the greatest gains. Subtest scores are 1.2 to 3.5 points higher on retest. Matrix Reasoning was associated with the greatest gains.

EVIDENCE FOR INTERRATER RELIABILITY

Interrater reliability is excellent. All WASI-II protocols from the normative sample were scored by two independent raters. Block Design and Matrix Reasoning yielded correlation coefficients of $r \geq .98$. Verbal subtests from 60 protocols were scored by two raters, with reliabilities of $r = .95$ for Vocabulary and $r = .94$ for Similarities (manual).

EVIDENCE FOR VALIDITY

FACTOR-ANALYTIC STUDIES AND WITHIN-TEST RELATIONSHIPS

Factor-analytic and intercorrelation studies presented in the manual suggest that overall, the WASI-II reflects verbal and perceptual components rather than simply a general intelligence factor. Across the sample, most subtests show moderate to large intercorrelations (e.g., *rs* = .40 to .70), which is fairly typical for intelligence batteries and is thought to reflect a common factor of intelligence (general intelligence factor, *g*). Vocabulary and Similarities show large correlations with one another across groups ($r = .64$ to $r = .82$), and in the majority of age groups Block Design correlated moderately to highly with Matrix Reasoning ($r = .44$ to $r = .66$).

Exploratory and confirmatory factor analyses of data from the WASI-II/WISC-IV and WASI-II/WAIS-IV correlation studies indicate that, in the adult sample, a verbal comprehension factor was comprised of WASI-II Vocabulary and Similarities and WAIS-IV Information. A perceptual reasoning factor had loadings from WASI-II Block Design, WASI-II Matrix Reasoning, and WAIS-IV Visual Puzzles. Information regarding relationships between other WAIS-IV verbal and perceptual subtests is not reported in the manual. Working memory and processing speed factors had loadings from the WAIS-IV working memory and processing speed subtests. In confirmatory factor analysis, a two-factor (verbal comprehension vs. perceptual reasoning) model was compared against a one-factor model, with a two-factor model best fitting the data (see manual for additional details).

RELATIONSHIPS WITH OTHER TESTS

Overall, correlations between the WASI-II and other measures are moderate to large in magnitude. Correlational studies were done between the WASI-II and WASI ($n = 142$), WAIS-IV ($n = 182$), KBIT-2 ($n = 81$), and Wechsler Fundamentals: Academic Skills ($n = 104$ adults), with demographic details provided in the manual. Overall, uncorrected correlation coefficients between WASI-II and WASI subtests were high ($r = .66$ to $r = .85$). In terms of differences between tests, composite score differences ranged from 4.2 standard score points (VCI) to 5.5 standard scores points (FSIQ-2). For subtest scores, Matrix Reasoning showed the largest difference, and Block Design the smallest (4.3 T-score points vs. 2.3 T-score points, respectively).

Correlations between the WASI-II and WAIS-IV showed a similar pattern. Uncorrected correlation coefficients for subtest scores were high ($r = .67$ to $r = .85$). To facilitate comparisons, the WASI-II subtest scores were converted to scaled scores. Differences between scaled scores were small (≤.40 scaled score points). Composite scores similarly showed small differences (≤1.5 standard score points; manual).

Correlations between the KBIT-2 IQ Composite and WASI-II composite scores were high ($r = .69$ to $r \geq .80$) Correlations between the Reading Composite on the Wechsler Fundamentals: Academic Skills and WASI-II composite scores were also large ($r = .68$ to $r \geq .76$, PRI, VCI, FISIQ-2, FSIQ-4; manual).

CLINICAL STUDIES

Studies on WASI-II performance in people with intellectual disabilities, giftedness, ADHD, learning disability, and TBI are reported in the WASI-II manual. Independent examiners and researchers conducted these studies in a variety of settings, so although inclusion criteria were met to ensure appropriate age range and diagnosis (see manual), samples and settings were heterogeneous. The mean age across groups ranged from adolescence to young adulthood (range of mean ages 12–27 years). The majority were Caucasian (ranging from 56% to 81%). Gender, educational level, and region represented also varied. WASI-II performance of clinical groups were compared with demographically matched controls (similar in terms of age, gender, ethnicity, education, and geographic region).

Overall, group differences were observed in the anticipated direction. Individuals 16 to 64 years with mild intellectual disability ($n = 36$) or moderate intellectual disability ($n = 31$) performed significantly worse than matched controls, with WASI-II composite scores ranging from 63.9 (FSIQ-4) to 66.7 (VCI; vs. scores of controls that ranged from 97.7 for FSIQ-2 to 98.8 for VCI). Persons with a moderate intellectual disability performed worse than matched controls, ranging from 51.4 (FSIQ-4) to 55.6 (PRI), with controls performing from 100.2 (PRI, FSIQ-4) to 100.6 (VCI). Subtest scores followed a similar pattern. *SD*s were also noted to be comparatively smaller than in demographically matched controls (see manual). In the sample of individuals with mild intellectual disability, 94% of people had FSIQ-4 scores 75 standard score points or lower. In the sample of individuals with moderate intellectual disability, all had FSIQ-4 scores lower than 70, and 84% had FSIQ-4 scores lower than 60.

Individuals with learning disabilities 6 to 24 years of age also completed the WASI-II. As predicted by the test authors, individuals with Reading Disorder obtained lower scores than matched controls on Vocabulary, Similarities, and VCI; they also scored lower on FSIQ-4 and FSIQ-2. Individuals with Mathematics Disorder performed worse than matched controls on all subtests and composite scores, with Matrix Reasoning showing the largest effect size among the subtests, and all composite scores showing large effect sizes. The WASI-II was also administered to 36 gifted participants, age 6–64, and matched controls. Gifted persons scored significantly higher than matched controls, with FSIQ-4 scores of 125 or higher in 69% in this sample (manual).

The WASI-II was completed by 54 people with ADHD, ranging in age from 6 to 24 years, who did not differ from matched controls on the WASI-II. The WASI-II was completed by 21 persons, aged 16 to 40, who sustained a TBI 6 to 18 months prior to testing. This sample obtained lower scores on all subtests and composite scores compared to demographically matched controls. Group mean composite scores were 12.5 to 15 points lower, and subtest scores were 6.4 to 8.7 points lower, reflecting moderate to large effect sizes.

NEUROANATOMICAL CORRELATES AND IMAGING STUDIES

No information is available.

PERFORMANCE VALIDITY

No information is available.

COMMENT

The WASI-II has several strengths. However, it should be noted that the test was designed as a screening instrument and does not provide a comprehensive evaluation of intellectual function, does not include processing speed or working memory subtests, and would yield scores discrepant from the WAIS-IV if an individual has a fair amount of variability in their profile. However, the test also includes more subtests than briefer measures of intellectual function, although this is concomitant with a longer administration time.

Like most Wechsler tests, the normative database is exceptional, with several strengths, including a large sample size, Census stratification, and multiple age bands. Reliability coefficients are strong. Based on material presented in the manual, construct validity is supported via moderate to large within-task correlations and a two-factor structure, as well as sizable correlations with other measures. The limited clinical data from the manual show group differences in the expected direction, supporting validity.

There is important information lacking from the manual, including demographic effects (e.g., age, gender, ethnicity) and clinical classification accuracy (e.g., percent classification agreement between WAIS-IV and WASI-II regarding classification of individuals into specific IQ ranges). Additional inclusion of information pertaining to demographic effects would be useful, given the otherwise notable strengths of this test, and the well-established effects of demographic variables for other Wechsler tests. Research investigating demographic effects on the WASI-II and provision of normative adjustments if demographic effects are found would be a valuable addition for neuropsychologists who wish to use this test in practice.

Although some information regarding performance in clinical populations is presented, sample sizes are small and generally focused on group differences. More clinical and demographic research is needed, as well as more independent research. Additionally, limited information is available on neuroanatomical correlates and performance validity.

REFERENCES

Irby, S. M., & Floyd, R. G. (2013). *Test Review: Wechsler Abbreviated Scale of Intelligence*. Los Angeles, CA: Sage. Retrieved from http://journals.sagepub.com/doi/full/10.1177/0829573513493982

McCrimmon, A. W., & Smith, A. D. (2013). Review of the Wechsler Abbreviated Scale of Intelligence, Second Edition (WASI-II). *Journal of Psychoeducational Assessment, 31*(3), 337–341. https://doi.org/10.1177/0734282912467756

Wechsler, D. (2011). *Wechsler Abbreviated Scale of Intelligence—Second Edition*. San Antonio, TX: Pearson.

WECHSLER ADULT INTELLIGENCE SCALE—FOURTH EDITION (WAIS-IV)

TEST NAME	**Wechsler Adult Intelligence Scale–Fourth Edition (WAIS-IV)**
DOMAIN	Intellectual function
AGE RANGE	16 to 90 years
ADMINISTRATION TIME	67 minutes
SCORING FORMAT	Computerized or hand scored
REFERENCE	Wechsler, D. (2008). *Wechsler Adult Intelligence Scale–Fourth Edition.* San Antonio, TX: Pearson. www.pearsonclinical.com

DESCRIPTION

The Wechsler Adult Intelligence Scale–Fourth Edition (WAIS-IV; Wechsler, 2008) is the fourth iteration of the Wechsler Scales of Intelligence, which have been successively refined since the original publication of the Wechsler-Bellevue scales and the WAIS-Revised in 1981 (see the manual for a detailed overview, including major research stages of WAIS-IV development). The Advanced Clinical Solutions (ACS) is also published by Pearson and is designed to extend the utility of the WAIS-IV and the Wechsler Memory Scale–Fourth Edition (WMS-IV). The ACS provides supplemental scores, performance validity, reliable change estimates, premorbid IQ, social perception, and demographically adjusted norms (see the section "Demographic Effects").

The WAIS-IV includes the VCI, PRI, Working Memory Index (WMI), and Processing Speed Index (PSI), which represent different intellectual domains. These scores are summed into a composite measure of FSIQ. Users will note that the Verbal and Performance composites of the WAIS-III no longer exist in the WAIS-IV, as factor-analytic studies and theory were supportive of a four-factor structure (see the section "Factor–Analytic Studies"). The manual indicates that VCI and PRI should be used for clinical decision-making in place of Verbal IQ (VIQ) and Performance IQ (PIQ). The index scores and their composite subscales are as described in Table 5–8. Supplemental subtests are intended to provide additional clinical information and act as substitutions for core subtests in the calculation of composite scores if necessary (e.g., in the event of a spoiled core subtest due to examinee responses or administrator errors). Note that many of the supplemental scores can only be administered to a truncated age range, as noted in Table 5–8.

The General Ability Index (GAI), reflecting only VCI and PRI, may be also be used. Process scores are also available, which do not contribute to the calculation of composite scores but can provide additional insight into how the examinee completed the test. Process scores are included for Block Design (performance without time bonus points), Digit Span (number of digits recalled on last correctly completed trial for Forward, Backward, and Sequencing conditions), and Letter-Number Sequencing (number of digits and letters on the last correctly completed trial of Sequencing).

The WAIS-IV is a sophisticated instrument with a long history, and, concomitantly, there is a multitude of psychometric and interpretive information associated with this test. Readers are referred to additional resources to enhance understanding, administration, and interpretation of the WAIS-IV, in addition to manuals included with the test itself. Resources include Holdnack, Drozdick, Weiss, and Iverson (2013), Lichtenberger and Kaufman (2009), and Sattler and Ryan (2009). Test reviews have also been published that offer useful information (e.g., Climie & Rostad, 2011; Hartman, 2009).

TABLE 5–8 Wechsler Adult Intelligence Scale-Fourth Edition (WAIS-IV) Subtests and Index Scores

INDEX SCORE	CORE SUBTESTS COMPRISING INDEX SCORE	SUPPLEMENTAL SUBTESTS COMPRISING INDEX SCORE
Verbal Comprehension	Similarities Vocabulary Information	Comprehension
Perceptual Reasoning	Block Design Matrix Reasoning Visual Puzzles	Figure Weights* Picture Completion
Working Memory	Digit Span Arithmetic	Letter-Number Sequencing*
Processing Speed	Symbol Search Coding	Cancellation*

*Administered to age 16 to 69.

SOURCE: Adapted from Wechsler (2008).

WAIS-III VERSUS WAIS-IV

According to the manual, the WAIS-IV was revised with the goals of updating theory, enhancing developmental appropriateness, improving user-friendliness, improving clinical utility, and enhancing psychometric properties. Theoretical foundations were improved by adding a number of subtests (see later discussion), revising Arithmetic items, and adding a sequencing condition to Digit Span.

Developmental appropriateness was enhanced by modifications that adjusted for sensory changes in aging (e.g., hearing, vision, and speed). These modifications include explicit instructions on each item (regardless of the accuracy of performance on the sample items), reduction or elimination of time bonuses on some subtests (i.e., Block Design, Arithmetic), limited use of phonetically similar stimuli on Digits and Letter-Number Sequencing to reduce demands on auditory discrimination, enlargement and simplification of visual stimuli, and minimization of motor demands on perceptual reasoning subtests (see manual for additional changes).

To enhance user-friendliness, testing time was reduced (10 subtests vs. 13 subtests; the average administration time was reduced from 80 minutes to 67 minutes), the number of items required for discontinuation was reduced, and specific changes were made to the design of the test materials (see manual).

Revisions made to enhance clinical utility and psychometric properties are a primary focus of later sections in this review so are only briefly mentioned here. To enhance clinical utility, a number of group studies were included, involving 13 different clinical groups. The WAIS-IV was co-normed with the WMS-IV, and the Wechsler Individual Achievement Test–Second Edition (WIAT-II) and ACS were administered to a subsample of WAIS-IV examinees. To enhance psychometric properties, item and scoring rules were updated, normative data were collected from 2007 to 2008 and were Census-stratified, reliability and validity data were collected, and floors and ceilings were updated. In addition, items were reviewed for bias and excluded when appropriate, based on expert review and statistical analyses. See manual for additional details.

A number of subtest changes were made from the WAIS-III to the WAIS-IV. Picture Arrangement and Object Assembly were eliminated to reduce motor demands and bonuses based on time. Digit Symbol Incidental Learning and Digit Symbol Copy were also eliminated. Item content, administration, and/or scoring were changed in the retained subtests (see the manual for specific details). Visual Puzzles, Figure Weights, and Cancellation were added as new subtests (see Figure 5–4 for representative examples of these subtests). Visual Puzzles requires the examinee to view a finished puzzle and choose three pieces that recreate the puzzle when they are combined. Figure Weights involves viewing a scale with an omitted weight and selecting the weight that balances the scale. Cancellation involves scanning an array and marking a target. Each new subtest has a time limit.

In addition to information reported in the manual, some additional research has been completed comparing the WAIS-III and the WAIS-IV. The WAIS-IV was found via structural equation modeling to provide a more accurate measurement of FSIQ than the WAIS-III (see Taub & Benson, 2013, for discussion). When the Incidental Learning Procedure from the Coding subtests of the WAIS-III was applied to the WAIS-IV Coding subtest, the Pairing procedure was found to be more difficult in a mixed outpatient sample. Additionally, some items were recalled more frequently than others (Ashendorf, 2012).

ADMINISTRATION

Detailed administration instructions are provided in the manual. Unlike many cognitive tests, there are also published models available regarding effective ways to teach WAIS-IV administration and scoring procedures given the high frequency of examiner errors on Wechsler intelligence tests.

For example, a meta-analysis of studies of examiner errors on Wechsler intelligence tests (Styck & Walsh, 2016) reported that 41% of protocols included an examinee error (not including failure to record a response), with 73% of FSIQ indices affected as a result of these errors, and 16% (PRI) to 77% (VCI) of index scores rendered inaccurate. These errors tended to result in an overestimation of FSIQ and an underestimation of VCI. In light of the finding that high error rates have been found in learners, involvement of an expert in WAIS-IV training is desirable (see Roberts & Davis, 2015). Lichtenberger and Kaufman (2009) provide an excellent resource for administration and scoring, as do Sattler and Ryan (2009).

Minor variances in administration that may occur do not have a substantial effect on performance. For example, in a sample of college students, responding with an "X" rather than a slash mark on Symbol Search did not affect performance, and neither did administration of Block Design with red surfaces pointing upward (Ryan et al., 2015).

SCORING

Raw scores are converted into age-corrected standard scores. Subtest scores are converted to scaled scores (M = 10, SD = 3) and composite scores to standard scores (M = 100, SD = 15). Scores are also presented according to percentile rankings, confidence intervals, and descriptive labels (i.e., Very Superior to Extremely Low).

Profile analysis and score interpretation are provided in the manual and discussed in the literature regarding variability and base rates of low scores in the healthy population (e.g., Brooks et al., 2013; Oakes et al., 2013; see also later

Visual Puzzles. Which three of these pieces go together to make this puzzle?

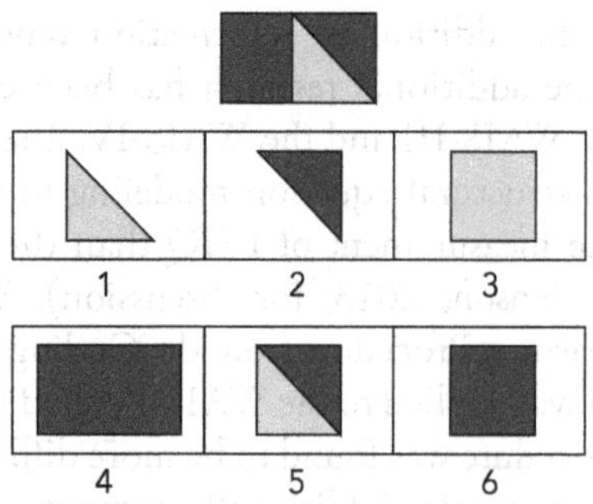

Figure Weights. Which one of these goes here to balance the scale?

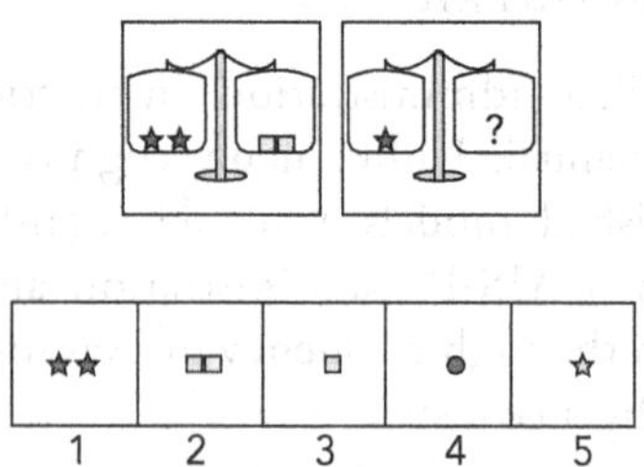

Cancellation. When I say go, draw a line through each *red* square and *yellow* triangle.

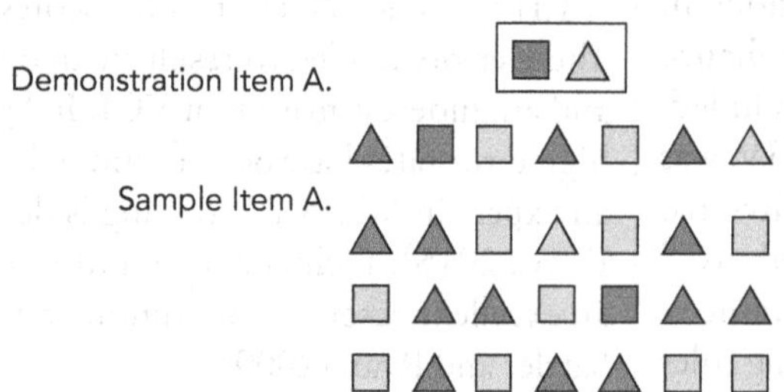

Figure 5–4 *Sample items from Visual Puzzles, Figure Weights, and Cancellation.*

SOURCE: Simulated items similar to those found in the Wechsler Adult Intelligence Scale–Fourth Edition (WAIS-IV). Copyright © 2008 NCS Pearson, Inc. Reproduced with permission. All rights reserved.

discussion). Resources to aid in the interpretation of profiles are available for a number of groups and clinical situations. For example, interpretive resources relate to predicting premorbid ability (Holdnack, Schoenberg, Lange, & Iverson, 2013), use in older adults (Drozdick et al., 2013), profile analysis in moderate to severe TBI (Iverson et al., 2013), and psychiatric and developmental disorders (Goldstein et al., 2013).

Critical values, or the differences between index scores required for statistical significance, are presented in the manual and are also provided for subtest scaled score differences. The frequency of observed score differences in the general population is also provided, as are base rates relative to the overall sample and by FSIQ (see also Brooks et al., 2013, for interpretation of base rates of low scores in the context of the WAIS-IV).

Other interpretation methods for difference scores, including differences relative to subtest scores and process score differences, are discussed in the manual. Index and subtest scatter is also discussed in Oakes, Lovejoy, Tartar, and Holdnack (2013) and Binder and Binder (2011). Overall, it is important to consider not only statistical significance of score differences, but also base rates of low scores in the normative population, which can be large in some cases (see "Normative Data" for discussion of base rates). A special issue of the journal *Assessment* has also been dedicated to WAIS-IV/WMS-IV interpretation (see Frazier, 2011, for overview).

Of note, a novel incidental learning measure has also been developed based on Similarities and Vocabulary subtests. This novel measure was highly correlated with conventional memory measures (Hammers et al., 2017; Spencer et al., 2016), and patients with probable Alzheimer's disease (AD) showed lower performance on this measure compared to patients with mild cognitive impairment (MCI; Hammers et al., 2017).

DEMOGRAPHIC EFFECTS

Demographically adjusted norms are available via use of the ACS in conjunction with the WAIS-IV.

AGE

Age affects performance, and age-corrected scores are provided in the manual. See also Whipple Drozdick, Holdnack, Salthouse, and Cullum (2013) for a discussion of age effects. Baxendale (2011) plotted age-related changes on the WAIS-IV based on different FSIQ levels using data from the standardization sample (see Figure 5–5). Results showed relative stability in verbal skills compared to nonverbal skills. Specifically, VCI develops into the fifth decade, with only a mild decline in the seventh decade. In contrast, PRI and PSI show a peak in adolescence, with decreasing performance into the third decade. A large discrepancy was noted when youngest and oldest cohorts were compared. Research suggests processing speed may be highly contributory to age-related decline in reasoning (Scheiber et al., 2017).

In terms of age interactions with FSIQ, trends are less pronounced in lower FSIQ groups and more pronounced in higher FSIQ groups. PRI and FSIQ decline somewhat later in the higher FSIQ cohort. Using the coefficient of variation (*SD*/mean ×100), Wisdom, Mignogna, and Collins (2012) reported that, across the standardization sample, increased variability was noted for PRI and PSI subtests, with less heterogeneity across age on VCI and WMI subtests.

GENDER

Overall, gender differences in performance are small. Using data from the standardization sample, Holdnack and Weiss (2013) reported a male advantage on VCI, PRI, and WMI and a female advantage on PSI. However, effect sizes tend to be small in magnitude. In terms of gender differences on subtests, men perform better on Similarities, Information, Block Design, Visual Puzzles, and Arithmetic. Women perform better on processing speed subtests. The largest effect size is for Coding, which amounts to a difference of approximately 1 scaled score point.

EDUCATION

Education affects test scores, especially at extremes of the education distribution and especially for verbal scores. Using standardization sample data and comparing three subgroups consisting of examinees with 12 years of education, 13 to 15 years of education, and more than 18 years of education, Holdnack and Weiss (2013) reported sizable effect sizes when other groups were compared to the most highly educated group, especially for VCI. When the 12- and 13- to 15-year education groups were compared, the effect sizes were smaller. When the VCI–PRI discrepancy of the high-education group was examined, the VCI was 10 points greater than the PRI, with abilities approximately equal in the other education groups.

A number of differences were noted at the subtest level, especially when other groups were compared to the highest education group, again with the smallest difference on PSI subtests and the largest differences on the verbal subtests. When the lower education groups were compared, smaller differences were noted, some of which were not statistically significant. Education-adjusted scores for Vocabulary are provided in Holdnack and Weiss (2013).

ETHNICITY, NATIONALITY, AND LINGUISTIC EFFECTS

Overall, differences found between Caucasian and African-American participants on composite scores are large in terms of effect size. Differences between subtests are statistically significant. After controlling for other demographic variables (i.e., education, occupation, income, region, gender) in the standardization sample, Holdnack and Weiss (2013) reported that ethnicity accounts for 9% of the variance in scores of African-American compared to Caucasian examinees and 4% of the variance in scores from Hispanic compared to Caucasian examinees. Shuttleworth-Edwards (2012) provide a mechanism for converting WAIS-IV scores to WAIS-III profile scores for use of norms when working with Xhosa-speaking individuals with low education levels. Interested readers are referred to their paper for details.

Canadians tend to obtain higher raw scores on the WAIS-IV compared to US examinees (Bowden et al., 2011; Chevalier et al., 2016; Harrison et al., 2014). This finding has implications for the identification of intellectual disabilities (Chevalier et al., 2016) and learning disabilities because scores using US and Canadian normative data may differ significantly.

For example, although scores from both normative sets were highly correlated, a high percent agreement (+/− 5 points) was found only between 49% (WMI) and 76% (PRI) of composite scores. There were large mean differences and altered educational classifications for a large proportion of students depending on which normative set was used (Harrison et al., 2014). Harrison, Holme, Silvestri, and Armstrong (2015) reported in subsequent research that 45% of their sample who scored in the Average range and 85% who scored Below Average on American norms were classified into lower categories when IQ was interpreted via Canadian norms. Chevalier et al. (2016) similarly report that scores of persons with Extremely Low or Borderline FSIQs are particularly affected, with nearly 53% of FSIQs yielding different clinical classifications depending on the norm set used. Miller et al. (2015) caution against using US norms in Canadian samples, and they provide rationale and practice guidelines regarding comprehensive assessment of intellectual and learning disabilities, which will be

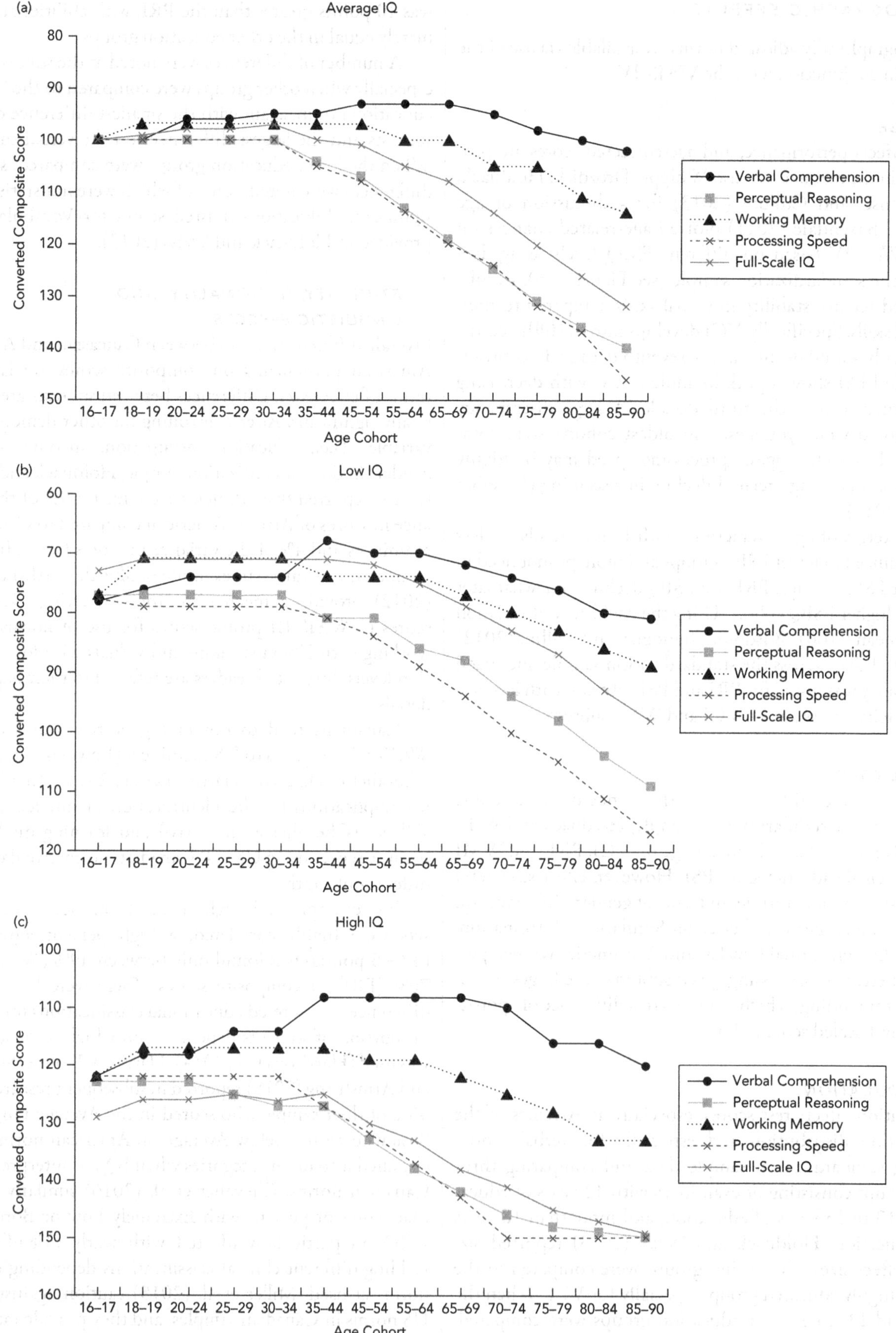

Figure 5–5 *Trajectories of age-related change in Wechsler Adult Intelligence Scale–Fourth Edition (WAIS-IV) composite scores.*

NOTE: The scale has been reversed on the IQ axis so that the orientation of graph lines reflects the development (up) and decline (down) in ability across the age ranges in an intuitive way. (a) Average IQ: Start point FSIQ = 100. (b) Low IQ: Start point FSIQ = 73. (c) High IQ: Start point FSIQ = 129.

SOURCE: From Baxendale (2011).

familiar to neuropsychologists (see their paper for details). Chevalier et al. (2016) similarly provide clinical guidelines for practice.

NORMATIVE DATA

The standardization sample consists of 2,200 examinees 16 to 90 years of age, with stratification along demographic variables including age, gender, ethnicity, education level, and geographic region, based on 2005 US Census data. Normative development is detailed in the Technical Manual, including derivation of specific start and discontinue points, standard scores, and time bonus points.

Subtest scaled scores (and scaled process scores) were devised via inferential norming, which involved a number of steps. Moments (means, *SD*, skewness) of each score were created for each age group. Moments were plotted across age, and polynomial regressions were fitted to the moment data. Functions were selected based on theoretical consistency and pattern of growth curves observed in the normative sample. Functions were then used to derive estimates of midpoint population moments for each age group, which were in turn used to create theoretical distributions for each group, yielding percentiles. Smoothing was then done to eliminate irregularities. See manual for additional details.

Scaled scores range from 1 to 19. In addition to age-corrected subtest scaled scores, "reference group" subtest scaled scores are based on the performance of participants 20 to 34 years of age in the normative sample, with demographic characteristics representative of US Census data. The manual describes that these norms are provided for research purposes, with age-corrected scaled scores preferable in most clinical situations. Of note, due to a restricted range, Digit Span and Letter-Number Sequencing process scores are reported as raw scores and base rates. Composite scores are calculated as summations of age-corrected scaled scores. Variances of sums of scaled scores were not different by age group, and the sum of scaled scores were normally distributed.

A variety of recruitment methods were used that employed trained recruiters, marketing research firms, and independent examiners. Sources of recruitment included community organization sites, staffed booths in shopping centers, neighborhood flyers, self-referral via internet, and referrals via existing examinees. See the manual for additional recruitment details. Examiners and examinees were paid for participation.

Exclusion criteria were comprehensive and included primary language not English, primarily nonverbal, unable to understand instructions and participate in testing, insufficient compliance, previous testing with intelligence measure over the past six months, graduate training or familiarity with intelligence tests, family member or close friend of examinee, twin of examinee, uncorrected sensory impairment (hearing, vision), upper extremity disability, currently in hospital, taking medication that could impact cognition, recent functional change related to cognition, current chemotherapy or chemotherapy in the previous 2 months, electroconvulsive therapy (ECT) or central nervous system radiation treatment, unconsciousness duration greater than 20 minutes, or the presence of a physical condition or illness (e.g., neurologic, psychiatric).

Thirteen age groups were used, with band lengths ranging from 1:11 years (e.g., 16 to 17:11, 18 to 19:11), 4:11 years (most adult age bands), to 9:11 years (35 to 44:11, 45 to 54:11, 55 to 64:11). Each of the youngest age group bands was comprised of 200 participants, and each of the four older groups was comprised of 100 participants.

For 65- to 90-year-olds, the normative sample had an equal number of female and male examinees. The five oldest groups had more women (consistent with Census data). Ethnicity was categorized as White, African American, Hispanic, Asian, and other groups. Education levels were categorized into five categories, ranging from 8 years or less, 9 to 11 years, 12 years, 13 to 15 years, and 16 years or more. Parental education level was used for adolescents. Geographic region was classified as Northeast, Midwest, South, and West. Overall proportions of the sample according to demographic variables are not presented, but proportions relative to age group and other characteristics (e.g., ethnicity, gender, education) are presented in a number of tables in the manual.

BASE RATES OF LOW SCORES

Base rates of low scores are another important source of interpretation of examinee data. Research has suggested that obtaining some low scores on the WAIS-IV is not uncommon. Even those with high-average intelligence and education levels have some low scores in their profiles, with nearly 60% of people in this subgroup demonstrating one or more cognitive score that is one to 1.5 *SD* below the mean (Heyanka et al., 2013).

A number of studies have further examined and quantified base rates of low scores on the WAIS-IV. Crawford, Garthwaite, Longman, and Batty (2012) provide supplementary methods to analyze performance on the WAIS-IV, including further elaboration of confidence interval calculations and quantification of the prevalence of low scores. The authors provide tables in the paper and a computer program online (visit https://homepages.abdn.ac.uk/j.crawford/pages/dept/WAIS4Supp.htm).

Brooks, Holdnack, and Iverson (2011) provide base rates for the WAIS-IV and WMS-IV based on 900 healthy adults from the standardization sample, with subsequent validation on a sample of 28 patients who sustained a moderate to severe TBI. Base rates of low scores increase with less education (<8 years) and lower IQ (<80). For example, when a low score is defined as 80 standard score points or lower, 73% of the sample of patients with premorbid ability scores 80 or less on the Test of Premorbid

TABLE 5–9 Percent of Wechsler Adult Intelligence Scale-Fourth Edition (WAIS-IV) Normative Sample with Significant Index Score Discrepancy

	OVERALL SAMPLE	MALE	FEMALE
|VCI – AI| ≥ 6.89	41.4	42.8	40.1
|PRI – AI| ≥ 7.74	35.2	37.7	32.8
|WMI – AI| ≥ 8.01	30.8	34.0	27.8
|PSI – AI| ≥ 9.67	32.8	34.1	31.5

NOTE: VCI = Verbal Comprehension Index; PRI = Perceptual Reasoning Index; WMI = Working Memory Index; PSI = Processing Speed Index; AI = Average Index.

SOURCE: Grégoire et al. (2011).

Function (TOPF) have one or more low scores, compared to less than 5% with a TOPF score of 120 or more. The TBI patients were 13 times more likely to have a low cognitive profile than controls. Base rate data that consider base rates of low scores on both the WMS-IV and WAIS-IV in the context of the TOPF score and education are presented in their paper. See also Brooks, Iverson, and Holdnack (2013).

Grégoire et al. (2011) present the mean of the four index scores as a baseline for estimating variability among scores in the standardization sample. Although having one discrepancy score was common (see Table 5–9), having four was uncommon (31–42%, compared to 3%). In their paper, they also provide discrepancy information based on IQ. Of note, Carrasco et al. (2015) provide base rate data for discrepancies between WAIS-IV and WMS-IV scores.

SHORT FORMS

Norms have also been developed for WAIS-IV short forms. Users should note that short forms should be used in limited circumstances because short forms do not reflect the accuracy or comprehensiveness provided by conventional versions of the test (see van Ool et al., 2017).

Dyad short forms have been examined. Girard, Axelrod, Patel, and Crawford (2015) reported that the Coding and Information dyad was the most reliable and valid in a mixed clinical sample. Denney et al. (2015) provide nine dyad short forms of the WAIS-IV, based on clinical samples. The test sample included 113 examinees with known or suspected neurologic disorders evaluated at a neuropsychology service, with a mean age of 60 years (*SD* = 13.0; range 25 to 86 years). Mean education level was 14 years (*SD* = 3.2). The sample was 48% female and predominantly Caucasian (86%). The short forms were subsequently validated on a mixed sample of 50 patients. The Vocabulary/Block Design dyad was identified as providing the best estimate of IQ. Tables for converting short form scores to FSIQ and GAI are presented in Table 5–10 and 5–11, respectively. Regression formulas for conversion are also presented in Table 5–12.

Ryan, Kreiner, Gontovsky, and Umfleet (2015) present short forms based on the completion of two, three, four, or five subtests in a mixed clinical sample, predominantly comprised of patients with neurologic disorders evaluated as part of routine clinical care for outpatient rehabilitation (n = 121; age M = 53.03 years, *SD* = 14.17; education M = 13.93 years, *SD* = 2.59; 87% Caucasian; 89% right-handed). Short forms were calculated via Tellegen and Briggs's (1967) formula as reported in Sattler and Ryan (2009; see paper). In general, specificity was excellent for all short forms at cutoffs examined (94% to 99%). Sensitivity was more variable (53% to 90%). The four and five subtest forms were also associated with high sensitivity at the 79 or lower cutoff (88%). False-positive rates were low for all short forms (<1% to 4%), but false-negative rates ranged from 3% to 13%.

Ryan, Umfleet, and Gontkovsy (2016) also presented prorated composites based on two, six, and eight WAIS-IV subtests in outpatients with multiple sclerosis (MS). No statistically significant differences were found between prorated and standard scores, with high correlations between each composite ($r \geq .89$). A similar pattern of correlations was noted between standard and prorated composites with demographic and clinical variables (e.g., education and disability status) and WMS-IV performance. Similarly, Umfleet, Ryan, Gontkovsky, and Morris (2012) reported high correlations between prorated and linear scaled index scores in a mixed clinical sample; in patients with evidence of neurologic involvement (e.g., MS, TBI, stroke, dementia), significant differences were found when actual and estimated composites were compared. However, differences did not exceed 3 points. No significant advantages were noted for use of either the prorated or linear scaling methods.

Other research has suggested that WAIS-IV short forms correspond reasonably well with WAIS-IV FSIQs. For example, Meyers, Zellinger, Kockler, Wagner, and Miller (2013) reported that a prorated seven-subtest short form (comprised of Block Design, Similarities, Digit Span, Arithmetic, Information, Coding, and Picture Completion) was significantly correlated with the FSIQ. Similarly, the FSIQ was correctly identified within ±7 points in 87% of a mixed clinical sample (van Ool et al., 2017).

ADDITIONAL NORMATIVE DATA

Saklofske et al. (2012) provide normative data for a novel composite, the Cognitive Proficiency Index (CPI, comprised of the WMI and PSI), based on the Canadian WAIS-IV standardization sample. The CPI is to be used in a complementary manner with the GAI (which is comprised of the VCI and PRI). CPI conversion is provided in Table 5–13, and GAI-CPI discrepancy base rate data are provided in Table 5–14.

Ryan, Townsend, and Kreiner (2014) provide data for administration of Digit Span via nonverbal response (writing, pointing). They included 78 healthy participants, and the sample was 78% female and predominantly Caucasian. Mean age was 22.91 (*SD* = 10.2) with a mean education level of 13.39 (*SD* = 1.7). All participants spoke

TABLE 5–10 Conversion Table for Wechsler Adult Intelligence Scale-Fourth Edition (WAIS-IV) Short Form Scores to Full Scale IQ (FSIQ) Scores

SUM OF AGE-SCALED SCORES	V/BD	V/MR	V/VP	I/BD	I/MR	I/VP	S/BD	S/MR	S/VP
2	*45*	*50*	*43*	*50*	*51*	*49*	*49*	*52*	*48*
3	*48*	*52*	*46*	*53*	*53*	*52*	*51*	*55*	*51*
4	*51*	*55*	*49*	*56*	*56*	*54*	54	*57*	*53*
5	*54*	*57*	*51*	*58*	*58*	*57*	57	*60*	*56*
6	*56*	*60*	*54*	61	*61*	60	59	62	59
7	*59*	*62*	*57*	63	*63*	62	62	64	61
8	62	*64*	60	66	66	65	65	67	64
9	65	67	63	69	68	68	67	69	67
10	67	69	66	71	71	71	70	71	70
11	70	72	69	74	73	73	73	74	72
12	73	74	72	76	76	76	75	76	75
13	76	77	75	79	78	79	78	79	78
14	78	79	78	82	81	81	81	81	80
15	81	81	80	84	83	84	83	83	83
16	84	84	83	87	86	87	86	86	86
17	87	86	86	90	88	89	89	88	88
18	89	89	89	92	91	92	91	90	91
19	92	91	92	95	93	95	94	93	94
20	95	94	95	97	96	97	97	95	97
21	98	96	98	100	98	100	99	98	99
22	100	98	101	103	101	103	102	100	102
23	103	101	104	105	103	106	105	102	105
24	106	103	107	108	106	108	107	105	107
25	109	106	109	110	108	111	110	107	110
26	111	108	112	113	111	114	113	109	113
27	114	111	115	116	113	116	115	112	115
28	117	113	118	118	116	119	118	114	118
29	120	116	121	121	118	122	121	117	121
30	122	118	124	123	121	124	123	119	124
31	125	120	127	126	123	127	126	121	126
32	128	123	130	*129*	126	130	129	*124*	*129*
33	*131*	*125*	133	*131*	128	*132*	*131*	*126*	*132*
34	*133*	*128*	*136*	*134*	*131*	*135*	*134*	*129*	*134*
35	*136*	*130*	*138*	*136*	*133*	*138*	*137*	*131*	*137*
36	*139*	*133*	*141*	*139*	*136*	*140*	*139*	*133*	*140*
37	*142*	*135*	*144*	*142*	*138*	*143*	*142*	*136*	*142*
38	*144*	*137*	*147*	*144*	*141*	*146*	*145*	*138*	*145*

NOTE: The italicized scores in the table were not derived from actual data, and thus the Full Scale IQ estimates outside of these boundaries are suspect.

V/BD = Vocabulary/Block Design; V/MR = Vocabulary/Matrix Reasoning; V/VP = Vocabulary/Visual Puzzles; I/BD = Information/Block Design; I/MR = Information/Matrix Reasoning; I/VP = Information/Visual Puzzles; S/BD = Similarities/Block Design; S/MR = Similarities/Matrix Reasoning; S/VP = Similarities/Visual Puzzles.

SOURCE: Denney et al. (2015).

English as a primary language and had intact hearing and vision. Twenty-six participants completed Digit Span as conventionally administered, 26 wrote responses to each item, and 26 pointed on a stimulus board. Means and *SD*s are presented in Table 5–15.

EVIDENCE FOR RELIABILITY

EVIDENCE FOR INTERNAL RELIABILITY

In the manual, internal reliability is high to excellent for most subtests in most age groups, with average internal reliabilities generally exceeding .81. Overall, somewhat lower reliability coefficients were obtained for Cancellation (average .78). Composite scores had excellent reliabilities, with averages exceeding .90. Internal reliability estimates in special groups/clinical groups also yield high to very high coefficients overall.

Other research has also reported strong internal reliability coefficients. Internal reliability estimates are reported to be high to very high for most scores (FSIQ, VCI, PRI, WMI), and slighter lower for PSI (≥.72; Gignac & Watkins, 2013). Glass, Ryan, and Charter (2010) reported high to very high (.80 to .91) internal reliabilities for the WAIS-IV Index discrepancy scores, with lower reliabilities for subtest discrepancy scores (range of .55 to .88). The GAI in a Canadian sample had excellent reliabilities across age groups (≥.95), as did the CPI (≥.91).

*SEM*s ranged from 2.12 to 3.35 for the GAI, and 3.35 to 4.50 for the CPI (Saklofske et al., 2012). Of note, replacement of core subtests with supplementary subtests

TABLE 5–11 Conversion Table for Wechsler Adult Intelligence Scale-Fourth Edition (WAIS-IV) Short Form Scores to General Ability Index (GAI) Scores

SUM OF AGE-SCALED SCORES	V/BD	V/MR	V/VP	I/BD	I/MR	I/VP	S/BD	S/MR	S/VP
2	*49*	*52*	*46*	*54*	*54*	*52*	*53*	*56*	*52*
3	*52*	*55*	*49*	*57*	*56*	*55*	*56*	*58*	*55*
4	*54*	*57*	*52*	*59*	*59*	*58*	58	*60*	*57*
5	*57*	*60*	*54*	*62*	*61*	60	61	*63*	*60*
6	*60*	*62*	*57*	64	*64*	63	63	65	63
7	*63*	*65*	*60*	67	*66*	66	66	68	65
8	65	*67*	63	70	69	68	69	70	68
9	68	70	66	72	71	71	71	72	71
10	71	72	69	75	74	74	74	75	73
11	74	75	72	77	76	76	76	77	76
12	76	77	75	80	79	79	79	79	79
13	79	80	78	82	81	82	82	82	81
14	82	82	81	85	84	84	84	84	84
15	84	84	83	88	87	87	87	86	87
16	87	87	86	90	89	90	89	89	89
17	90	89	89	93	92	93	92	91	92
18	93	92	92	95	94	95	95	94	95
19	95	94	95	98	97	98	97	96	97
20	98	97	98	101	99	101	100	98	100
21	101	99	101	103	102	103	102	101	102
22	103	102	104	106	104	106	105	103	105
23	106	104	107	108	107	109	108	105	108
24	109	107	110	111	109	111	110	108	110
25	112	109	112	113	112	114	113	110	113
26	114	112	115	116	114	117	115	112	116
27	117	114	118	119	117	119	118	115	118
28	120	116	121	121	119	122	120	117	121
29	122	119	124	124	122	125	123	119	124
30	125	121	127	126	124	128	126	122	126
31	128	124	130	129	127	130	128	124	129
32	131	126	133	*131*	130	133	131	*127*	*132*
33	*133*	*129*	136	*134*	132	*136*	*133*	*129*	*134*
34	*136*	*131*	*139*	*137*	*135*	*138*	*136*	*131*	*137*
35	*139*	*134*	*141*	*139*	*137*	*141*	*139*	*134*	*140*
36	*142*	*136*	*144*	*142*	*140*	*144*	*141*	*136*	*142*
37	*144*	*139*	*147*	*144*	*142*	*146*	*144*	*138*	*145*
38	*147*	*141*	*150*	*147*	*145*	*149*	*146*	*141*	*148*

NOTE: The italicized scores in the table were not derived from actual data, and thus the General Ability Index estimates outside of these boundaries are suspect.

V/BD = Vocabulary/Block Design; V/MR = Vocabulary/Matrix Reasoning; V/VP = Vocabulary/Visual Puzzles; I/BD = Information/Block Design; I/MR = Information/Matrix Reasoning; I/VP = Information/Visual Puzzles; S/BD = Similarities/Block Design; S/MR = Similarities/Matrix Reasoning; S/VP = Similarities/Visual Puzzles.

SOURCE: Denney et al. (2015).

for one composite does not appear to significantly alter index score reliabilities (Ryan & Glass, 2010). *SEM*s tend to be small in magnitude, as may be expected given strong reliabilities. *SEM*s range from .73 (Vocabulary) to 1.43 (Cancellation) for subtest and process scores. The *SEM*s for composite scores are also small, ranging from 2.16 (FSIQ) to 4.78 (PSI).

TEST-RETEST RELIABILITY, MEASURING CHANGE, AND PRACTICE EFFECTS

Test-retest reliability was derived from a subsample of participants in the standardization sample, with a test-retest mean interval of 22 days (range 8–82 days). Overall, correlation coefficients are strong. Most exceed $r = .80$, with the exception of process scores and scores from a few subtests, which are lower but still adequate ($r = .71$ to .78; Matrix Reasoning, Visual Puzzles, Figure Weights, Cancellation, Picture Completion). Reliability for composite scores range from high to very high ($r = .87$ to $r = .96$). Reliability coefficients are also presented in tables according to four age groups. Overall, these scores are also quite strong, with the exception of some isolated lower scores (see manual).

As is the case for most tests, performance on the WAIS-IV improves with prior exposure. Practice effects for the WAIS-IV vary depending on composite scores and age groups examined, but tend to be relatively larger for processing speed measures (e.g., 2.7 to 5.3 standard score points). For most age groups in the test-retest sample, practice effects were smallest for VCI (2.1–3.3; see Holdnack et al., 2013).

WAIS-IV reliable change calculations are included in the ACS software. Holdnack et al. (2013) also provide data to calculate significance of change on repeat assessments,

TABLE 5–12 Regression Formulas for Predicting Wechsler Adult Intelligence Scale-Fourth Edition (WAIS-IV) Full Scale IQ (FSIQ) and General Ability Index (GAI) Based on Short Forms

DYAD	PREDICTED FSIQ EQUATION	PREDICTED GAI EQUATION
V/BD	(V + BD) 2.75 + 39.94	(V + BD) 2.72 + 43.66
V/MR	(V + MR) 2.43 + 45.03	(V + MR) 2.46 + 47.55
V/VP	(V + VP) 2.90 + 36.95	(V + VP) 2.90 + 39.98
I/BD	(I + BD) 2.61 + 45.13	(I + BD) 2.58 + 48.91
I/MR	(I + MR) 2.50 + 45.94	(I + MR) 2.53 + 48.59
I/VP	(I + VP) 2.69 + 43.64	(I + VP) 2.69 + 46.82
S/BD	(S + BD) 2.67 + 43.37	(S + BD) 2.59 + 47.93
S/MR	(S + MR) 2.38 + 47.61	(S + MR) 2.36 + 51.02
S/VP	(S + VP) 2.70 + 42.57	(S + VP) 2.66 + 46.62

NOTE: n = 113 for FSIQ and n = 113 for GAI. Dyads are sums of age scaled scores.

V/BD = Vocabulary/Block Design; V/MR = Vocabulary/Matrix Reasoning; V/VP = Vocabulary/Visual Puzzles; I/BD = Information/Block Design; I/MR = Information/Matrix Reasoning; I/VP = Information/Visual Puzzles; S/BD = Similarities/Block Design; S/MR = Similarities/Matrix Reasoning; S/VP = Similarities/Visual Puzzles.

SOURCE: Denney et al. (2015).

including comparability of WAIS-III and WAIS-IV on retest and WISC-IV and WAIS-IV on retest.

Estevis, Basso, and Combs (2012) provide test-retest data at three- and six-month intervals for a sample of 54 healthy participants (age, $M = 20.9$; education, $M = 14.9$; initial FSIQ = 111.6). All scores improved on retest (WMI, 4 points to PSI, 9 points). Regression methods were superior to simple difference methods in estimating change. Data to calculate change are provided in Table 5–16 (composites) and Table 5–17 (subtests). Values outside the confidence intervals provided indicate significant change.

EVIDENCE FOR INTERRATER RELIABILITY

The manual describes that intrarater reliability was calculated via scoring by two independent scorers, with very high agreement for the majority of subtests ($r = .98$ to $r = .99$). A random sample of 60 verbal subtests was selected from the normative sample (see manual for demographic characteristics) and independently scored by three raters. Intraclass correlation coefficients (ICCs) were excellent (ranging from Comprehension $ICC = .91$ to Information $ICC = .97$).

EVIDENCE FOR VALIDITY

Correlations within the WAIS-IV and between the WAIS-IV and other measures are provided in the manual. As may be expected for a test measuring an overarching construct such as intelligence, the WAIS-IV tends to correlate moderately with many other tests. Within those correlations, some divergence is noted, such that tests of the same ability tend to correlate more highly than tests of relatively more disparate abilities. Results from within-test correlations and correlations with other tests are summarized here.

TABLE 5–13 Conversion of Wechsler Adult Intelligence Scale-Fourth Edition (WAIS-IV) Scaled Scores to Cognitive Proficiency Index (CPI)

SUM OF SCALED SCORES	CPI	PERCENTILE RANK	CONFIDENCE LEVEL 90%	95%
4	40	<0.1	38–49	37–50
5	41	<0.1	39–50	38–51
6	43	<0.1	41–52	40–53
7	45	<0.1	43–54	42–55
8	47	<0.1	44–56	43–57
9	48	<0.1	45–57	44–58
10	50	<0.1	47–59	46–60
11	52	0.1	49–61	48–62
12	54	0.1	51–62	50–64
13	55	0.1	52–63	51–64
14	57	0.2	54–65	53–66
15	59	0.3	56–67	55–68
16	60	0.4	57–68	56–69
17	62	1	59–70	58–71
18	64	1	60–72	59–73
19	66	1	62–74	61–75
20	68	2	64–76	63–77
21	69	2	65–77	64–78
22	71	3	67–78	66–80
23	72	3	68–79	67–80
24	73	4	69–80	68–81
25	75	5	71–82	70–83
26	76	5	72–83	71–84
27	78	7	74–85	73–86
28	79	8	75–86	73–87
29	81	10	76–88	75–89
30	82	12	77–89	76–90
31	84	14	79–91	78–92
32	85	16	80–92	79–93
33	87	19	82–93	81–95
34	89	23	84–95	83–96
35	91	27	86–97	85–98
36	93	32	88–99	87–100
37	95	37	90–101	89–102
38	97	42	91–103	90–104
39	99	47	93–105	92–106
40	100	50	94–106	93–107
41	102	55	96–108	95–109
42	103	58	97–109	96–110
43	105	63	99–110	98–111
44	106	66	100–111	99–112
45	107	68	101–112	100–113
46	109	73	103–114	102–115
47	111	77	105–116	104–117
48	113	81	107–118	105–119
49	114	82	107–119	106–120
50	116	86	109–121	108–122
51	118	88	111–123	110–124
52	120	91	113–124	112–126
53	122	93	115–126	114–127
54	124	95	117–128	116–129
55	125	95	118–129	117–130
56	127	96	120–131	119–132
57	129	97	122–133	120–134
58	131	98	123–135	122–136
59	133	99	125–137	124–138
60	134	99	126–138	125–139
61	136	99	128–140	127–141
62	138	99	130–141	129–142

(continued)

TABLE 5–13 Continued

SUM OF SCALED SCORES	CPI	PERCENTILE RANK	CONFIDENCE LEVEL 90%	95%
63	140	99.6	132–143	131–144
64	142	99.7	134–145	133–146
65	144	99.8	136–147	135–148
66	146	99.9	138–149	136–150
67	148	99.9	139–151	138–152
68	151	>99.9	142–154	141–155
69	153	>99.9	144–156	143–157
70	155	>99.9	146–157	145–158
71	157	>99.9	148–159	147–160
72	160	>99.9	151–162	150–163
73	160	>99.9	151–162	150–163
74	160	>99.9	151–162	150–163
75	160	>99.9	151–162	150–163
76	160	>99.9	151–162	150–163

NOTE: CPI = Cognitive Proficiency Index.
SOURCE: Saklofske et al. (2012).

FACTOR-ANALYTIC STUDIES

The intercorrelations of subtest, process, and composite scores are provided for each age group in the manual. Intercorrelations are statistically significant and tend to be moderate overall (range, $r = .21$ for Comprehension with Cancellation to $r = .74$ for Similarities with Vocabulary). On inspection, most subtests appear to correlate more highly with other subtests from within their domain than with others. Correlations between process scores and other scores are also moderate overall, and process scores are moderately to highly correlated with their subtest counterparts. Composite scores are highly correlated with the subtests that comprise them, and FSIQ is moderately to highly correlated with subtests.

In terms of factor structure, confirmatory factor analysis suggests four first-order factors best fit the data (see manual for additional details regarding results of other models that were evaluated). Other research also supports a four-factor structure. For example, this structure has been replicated in both US and Canadian standardization samples (Bowden et al., 2011), a Census-stratified sample in Spain (Abad et al., 2016), people with intellectual disability and matched controls (Reynolds et al., 2013), and a sample of persons referred for psychoeducational evaluations (Nelson et al., 2013).

Others have reported that a five-factor model best fits WAIS-IV data (Sudarshan et al., Weiss, 2016), consistent with a Cattell-Horn-Carroll framework that includes crystallized ability, fluid reasoning, visual processing, short-term memory, and processing speed (Benson et al., 2010; Niileksela et al., 2013; Weiss et al., 2013). The five-factor structure is similar to the four-factor structure but subdivides PRI into a perceptual organization factor consisting of Block Design, Visual Puzzles, and Picture Completion, and a fluid reasoning factor consisting of Matrix Reasoning, Arithmetic, and Figure Weights (Weiss et al., 2013). Benson et al. (2010) provide formulas for calculating alternative composite scores based on a five-factor model from Wechsler subtests. Although a four- or five-factor model fits the data in various groups, some have argued that the practical impact in day-to-day practice of conceptualizing one model over the other is unclear (see Schwartz, 2013).

CORRELATIONS WITH INTELLIGENCE TESTS AND NEUROPSYCHOLOGICAL BATTERIES

Overall, the WAIS-III and WAIS-IV perform similarly, although WAIS-III scores tend to be somewhat higher, which may reflect the Flynn effect. The WAIS-III and WAIS-IV were administered to 240 participants in the standardization sample. Corresponding subtests were generally highly correlated (range $r = .65$ for Picture Completion to $r = .90$ for Information), as were corresponding composite scores ($r \geq .83$).

In a group of participants with mild intellectual disability ($n = 25$), WAIS-III scores were also somewhat higher than WAIS-IV scores. Subtest correlations ranged from $r = .46$ (Information) to $r = .87$ (Coding). Composite scores were also highly related, ranging from $r = .76$ (WMI) to $r = .89$ (PSI). All participants in the sample were classified according to both instruments as FSIQ 75 or lower, suggesting diagnostic accuracy was maintained regardless of test used. Similar diagnostic accuracy was reported in a sample with borderline intellectual function (see manual).

A sample of 157 examinees 16 years of age were administered the WAIS-IV and the WISC-IV. WISC-IV scores were overall somewhat higher than WAIS-IV scores (except PSI). Correlations were moderate to large overall (ranging from $r = .51$ to $r = .82$), and high overall for composite scores ($r = .77$ to $r = .91$). In regard to neuropsychological test batteries, the Repeatable Battery for the Assessment of Neuropsychological Status (RBANS) and WAIS-IV indices were moderately correlated in 82 examinees, with the FSIQ showing large correlations with the RBANS Total Scale score ($r = .75$).

CORRELATIONS WITH MEMORY TESTS

Relationships with memory tests are variable. The WAIS-IV and WMS-III were administered to 97 examinees as described in the manual. Correlations were overall moderate, although some were very low, especially between Cancellation and memory scores (range $r = .06$ to $r = .31$). WMI subtests were highly correlated ($r = .60$), and, on visual inspection of the correlation matrix, verbal and working memory indices from the WAIS-IV appear to be more highly correlated with auditory WMS-III counterparts.

TABLE 5-14 Base Rates of General Ability Index (GAI)–Cognitive Proficiency Index (CPI) Discrepancy Scores by Full Scale IQ (FSIQ)

	OVERALL SAMPLE		FSIQ ≤ 79		FSIQ = 80–89		FSIQ = 90–109		FSIQ = 110–119		FSIQ ≥ 120	
AMOUNT OF DISCREPANCY	GAI < CPI	GAI > CPI	GAI < CPI	GAI > CPI	GAI < CPI	GAI > CPI	GAI < CPI	GAI > CPI	GAI < CPI	GAI > CPI	GAI < CPI	GAI > CPI
40	0.1	0.0	0.0	0.0	0.0	0.0	0.3	0.0	0.0	0.0	0.0	0.0
39	0.1	0.0	0.0	0.0	0.0	0.0	0.3	0.0	0.0	0.0	0.0	0.0
38	0.1	0.0	0.0	0.0	0.0	0.0	0.3	0.0	0.0	0.0	0.0	0.0
37	0.3	0.1	0.0	0.0	0.0	0.0	0.3	0.3	0.8	0.0	0.0	0.0
36	0.3	0.3	0.0	0.0	0.0	0.0	0.3	0.6	0.8	0.0	0.0	0.0
35	0.3	0.3	0.0	0.0	0.0	0.0	0.3	0.6	0.8	0.0	0.0	0.0
34	0.6	0.3	0.0	0.0	1.0	0.0	0.6	0.6	0.8	0.0	0.0	0.0
33	0.7	0.4	0.0	0.0	1.0	0.0	0.9	0.6	0.8	0.8	0.0	0.0
32	0.9	0.7	0.0	0.0	1.0	0.0	0.9	1.2	1.7	0.8	0.0	0.0
31	1.0	1.0	0.0	0.0	1.0	0.0	0.9	1.5	2.5	0.8	0.0	1.6
30	1.2	1.3	0.0	0.0	2.0	0.0	0.9	1.8	2.5	1.7	0.0	1.6
29	1.3	1.5	0.0	0.0	2.0	0.0	0.9	1.8	3.3	2.5	0.0	1.6
28	1.8	2.1	0.0	0.0	2.0	0.0	1.5	2.7	4.2	3.3	0.0	1.6
27	2.3	2.2	1.5	0.0	4.1	0.0	1.8	2.7	4.2	4.2	0.0	1.6
26	2.3	2.8	1.5	0.0	4.1	0.0	1.8	3.0	4.2	5.8	0.0	3.2
25	3.1	3.1	3.0	0.0	5.1	0.0	2.7	3.3	4.2	6.7	0.0	3.2
24	3.7	3.2	4.5	0.0	5.1	0.0	3.3	3.6	4.2	6.7	1.6	3.2
23	4.6	3.8	4.5	0.0	7.1	0.0	4.2	4.5	4.2	6.7	3.2	4.8
22	5.1	4.8	4.5	1.5	8.2	1.0	5.1	5.4	4.2	8.3	3.2	4.8
21	5.1	5.1	4.5	1.5	8.2	1.0	5.1	5.7	4.2	9.2	3.2	4.8
20	6.0	5.7	6.1	1.5	9.2	1.0	5.4	6.6	6.7	9.2	3.2	6.3
19	6.5	6.5	6.1	3.0	10.2	2.0	6.0	6.9	6.7	10.0	3.2	7.9
18	7.6	7.9	7.6	3.0	12.2	2.0	6.9	9.3	7.5	10.8	4.8	9.5
17	8.5	9.3	7.6	3.0	13.3	3.1	8.1	11.1	8.3	10.8	4.8	12.7
16	10.3	10.4	7.6	3.0	15.3	3.1	10.2	12.3	10.8	14.2	4.8	12.7
15	12.5	12.5	12.1	3.0	17.3	7.1	12.0	14.4	14.2	16.7	4.8	12.7
14	13.5	14.7	12.1	3.0	20.4	7.1	13.2	17.1	14.2	19.2	4.8	17.5
13	15.7	16.2	16.7	6.1	21.4	8.2	15.6	17.7	15.8	20.8	6.3	22.2
12	17.2	19.1	16.7	12.1	23.5	11.2	17.4	19.8	17.5	23.3	6.3	27.0
11	19.5	21.1	21.2	16.7	27.6	12.2	18.9	21.0	20.0	27.5	7.9	28.6
10	20.9	23.2	25.8	19.7	30.6	13.3	19.8	23.1	20.0	30.0	7.9	30.2
9	23.6	25.3	28.8	21.2	31.6	15.3	22.8	24.9	22.5	34.2	12.7	30.2
8	27.2	27.9	30.3	21.2	33.7	21.4	26.9	27.5	26.7	35.8	15.9	31.7
7	29.5	29.2	31.8	24.2	34.7	23.5	29.9	28.1	26.7	37.5	22.2	33.3
6	33.9	32.7	40.9	28.8	37.8	25.5	33.8	31.7	29.2	41.7	30.2	36.5
5	37.7	35.5	43.9	31.8	45.9	26.5	36.8	34.1	32.5	45.8	33.3	41.3
4	40.4	38.0	47.0	36.4	49.0	30.6	39.5	35.6	35.0	47.5	34.9	46.0
3	43.2	41.1	48.5	39.4	51.0	34.7	43.4	38.9	37.5	48.3	34.9	50.8
2	47.0	44.5	51.5	43.9	55.1	38.8	47.9	41.9	40.0	52.5	38.1	52.4
1	49.8	46.8	53.0	43.9	57.1	38.8	51.2	46.1	43.3	53.3	39.7	54.0
M	10.2	10.7	10.2	8.4	11.4	8.4	9.7	11	11.1	12.1	8.4	11
SD	7.6	7.6	6.6	5	8.1	5.2	7.5	8.2	8.7	7.9	5.8	7.3
Median	8	9	9	7	10	8	8	9.5	9	11	7	11.5

NOTE: FSIQ = Full Scale IQ; GAI = General Ability Index; CPI = Cognitive Proficiency Index.

SOURCE: Saklofske et al. (2012).

A small sample (n = 20) of 16-year-old examinees also completed the Children's Memory Scale (CMS) and the WAIS-IV. When examining index score relationships, the correlation matrix is somewhat variable. The lowest correlations are between PSI and Delayed Recognition (r = .13) and the highest between PRI and Attention/Concentration (r = .78). The California Verbal Learning Test, Second Edition (CVLT-II) was administered to 331 participants as described in the manual, with small to moderate correlations generally reported for WAIS-IV indices and primary CVLT-II variables.

CORRELATIONS WITH ATTENTION AND EXECUTIVE FUNCTION TESTS

As described in the manual, The WAIS-IV and the Brown Attention-Deficit Disorder Scales were administered to 41 adults (aged 18–29) with ADHD. Overall, small to negligible correlations were obtained, and the largest correlations were between Cancellation and ADD cluster scores (r = −.06 to −.49).

Moderate to large correlations were obtained between WAIS-IV indices and Trail Making and Verbal Fluency scores from the Delis-Kaplan Executive Function System

TABLE 5–15 Means and Standard Deviations for Nonverbal Responses on Digit Span

	ADMINISTRATION CONDITION					
	STANDARD		WRITING		POINTING	
SCORE	*M*	*SD*	*M*	*SD*	*M*	*SD*
DS Raw	30.12	5.71	30.19	3.80	29.42	3.82
DS Scaled	11.04	3.18	11.04	2.16	10.65	2.15
DSF Raw	11.00	2.08	10.77	1.82	9.92	1.67
DSB Raw	9.08	2.45	9.65	2.12	9.15	1.54
DSS Raw	10.04	2.16	9.77	1.24	10.35	2.00
Longest DSF	6.96	1.25	7.00	1.30	6.42	1.10
Longest DSB	5.19	1.42	5.27	1.19	4.96	0.87
Longest DSS	6.65	1.13	6.38	0.70	6.85	1.19

NOTE: DS = Digit Span; DSF = Digit Span Forward; DSB = Digit Span Backward; DSS = Digit Span Sequencing.

SOURCE: Ryan et al. (2014).

(D-KEFS; $r = .22$ to $r = .72$). Moderate to large correlations between the D-KEFS subtests and the WAIS-IV were also found in patients who had sustained a moderate to severe brain injury.

Buczylowska and Petermann (2017) also reported correlations between executive function tests, particularly the Judgment task from the Neuropsychological Assessment Battery (NAB), and composite WAIS-IV IQ measures. Logue et al. (2015) reported that the CPI is generally highly correlated with other measures demanding attention and processing speed (e.g., Trail Making Test A [TMT], Paced Auditory Serial Addition Task [PASAT] errors, Continuous Performance Test, Second Edition [CPT II], Symbol Digit Modalities Test [SDMT], Dementia Rating Scale, Second Edition [DRS-2] Attention Index, and the RBANS Attention Index). Divergent validity was also shown, with small and non-significant correlations between the CPI and less related variables.

TABLE 5–16 Standard Error and Confidence Intervals for Wechsler Adult Intelligence Scale-Fourth Edition (WAIS-IV) Composite Scores for Calculating Change

INDEX	r_{xx}	SEP	95% CI (SEP)	SEM_{T1}	SEM_{T2}	SED	95% CI (SED)
FSIQ	.91	5.82	±11	3.63	4.20	5.55	±11
VCI	.85	7.88	±15	5.38	5.77	7.88	±16
PRI	.83	6.90	±14	5.44	5.11	7.46	±15
WMI	.92	5.70	±11	3.84	4.10	5.62	±11
PSI	.72	10.28	±20	7.24	7.83	10.66	±21
GAI	.86	7.06	±14	4.86	5.16	7.09	±14

NOTE: FSIQ = Full Scale IQ; VCI = Verbal Comprehension Index; PRI = Perceptual Reasoning Index; WMI = Working Memory Index; PSI = Processing Speed Index; GAI = General Ability Index; CI = Confidence Interval; SEP = Standard Error of Prediction; SEM_{T1} = Standard Error of Measurement during the initial evaluation; SEM_{T2} = Standard Error of Measurement during re-evaluation; SED = Standard Error of Difference. r_{xx} reflects average test-retest coefficient for the entire sample. All confidence intervals are rounded to the nearest whole digit. To use the confidence intervals, the desired confidence band should be summed with an individual's estimated true score. Significant changes reflect the frequency of obtained scores that fell above or below the confidence interval.

SOURCE: Estevis et al. (2012).

CORRELATIONS WITH ACADEMIC ACHIEVEMENT

The WIAT-II was administered to a subset of youth as a part of standardization. The sample ranged in age from 16 to 19 years ($n = 93$). In terms of index scores from the two measures, correlations tended to be moderate to large overall (range of $r = .26$ to $r = .80$). On qualitative examination, generally more visually based scores correlated on both measures, as did verbally based scores. Data are provided in tabular format in the manual to calculate ability–achievement discrepancies.

CORRELATIONS WITH OTHER NEUROPSYCHOLOGICAL TESTS

Other research has provided support for the convergent and divergent validity of WAIS-IV subtests. In a mixed outpatient sample, WAIS-IV Coding was found to be moderately correlated with both conditions of the TMT and the Grooved Pegboard (absolute value *rs* = .42 to .53), but not CVLT-II or the Rey-Osterreith Complex Figure Test (RCFT; Ashendorf, 2012). As may be expected, Coding and Symbol Search were reportedly highly related ($r = .74$, Ashendorf, 2012).

In a sample of patients with MS, the Mini Mental State Examination (MMSE) was highly correlated with the WAIS-IV, even after correcting for education (Gontkovsy, 2014). Fallows and Hilsabeck (2012) reported that Visual Puzzles was moderately correlated with measures of verbal and visual memory (CVLT-II, RCFT, respectively), mental flexibility (TMT, Stroop), processing speed (Stroop, TMT), and naming (Boston Naming Test [BNT]) in a mixed clinical sample of veterans. Measures accounted for 50% of the variance in Visual Puzzles performance. Soble et al. (2016) reported that the VCI correlated with the BNT, Visual Naming Test, and the NAB Naming test, as did PRI, in a mixed clinical sample of veterans (range *rs* = .37 to .72).

CLINICAL STUDIES

Most clinical research on the WAIS-IV is contained within the manual. The manual describes a number of group difference studies involving an intellectually gifted group as well as persons with intellectual disability (mild, moderate), borderline intellectual function, learning disorders (reading, mathematics), ADHD, TBI, autism spectrum, major depressive disorder, MCI, and mild dementia. Sample sizes range from 16 (autism) to 73 participants (mild intellectual disability). Overall, group differences are in the expected directions and will be briefly described here (refer to the manual for additional details). Unless otherwise noted, the research presented here is from the manual.

Intellectually Gifted. Gifted adults outperform matched controls on each index (i.e., simple difference scores ranging from 10.28 for PSI to 21.06 for VCI, and 21.15 for FSIQ).

Intellectual Disability. Persons with intellectual disability obtain lower scores than matched controls, with

TABLE 5–17 Standard Error and Confidence Intervals for Wechsler Adult Intelligence Scale-Fourth Edition (WAIS-IV) Subtest Scores for Calculating Change

SUBTEST	r_{XX}	SEP	95%CI	(SEP)	SEM_{T1}	SEM_{T2} SED	95%CI (SED)
Vocabulary	.80	1.56	+3	1.09	1.17	1.60	±3
Similarities	.65	2.12	+4	1.79	1.66	2.44	±5
Arithmetic	.81	1.59	+3	1.20	1.16	1.66	±3
Digit Span	.88	1.51	+3	.98	1.11	1.48	±3
Information	.86	1.63	+3	1.16	1.19	1.66	±3
Comprehension	.73	1.91	+4	1.42	1.44	2.02	±4
Letter-Number	.80	1.62	+3	1.41	1.22	1.86	±4
Picture Completion	.55	2.00	+4	1.47	1.58	2.16	±4
Coding	.78	1.93	+4	1.24	1.43	1.89	±4
Block Design	.80	1.74	+3	1.33	1.31	1.87	±4
Matrix Reasoning	.46	2.30	+5	1.86	1.87	2.64	±5
Visual Puzzles	.71	2.04	+4	1.45	1.44	2.04	±4
Symbol Search	.52	2.65	+5	1.79	2.13	2.78	±5
Figure Weights	.73	1.85	+4	1.64	1.42	2.17	±4
Cancellation	.72	1.80	+4	1.71	1.37	2.19	±4

NOTE: CI = Confidence Interval; SEP = Standard Error of Prediction; SEM_{T1} = Standard Error of Measurement during the initial evaluation; SEM_{T2} = Standard Error of Measurement during re-evaluation; SED = Standard Error of Difference. r_{xx} reflects average test-retest coefficient for the entire sample. All confidence intervals are rounded to the nearest whole digit. To use the confidence intervals, the desired confidence band should be summed with an individual's estimated true score. Significant changes reflect the frequency of obtained scores that fell above or below the confidence interval.

SOURCE: Estevis et al. (2012).

simple difference scores reflecting the continuum of the expected discrepancy (i.e., persons with mild intellectual disability show smaller differences than persons with moderate intellectual disability). The mean FSIQ for the mild intellectual disability group was 58.5 (*SD* = 7.5), and the mean FSIQ for the moderate intellectual disability was 48.2 (*SD* = 4.7). Relatively high classification accuracy was reported, especially for mild and moderate intellectual disability compared to borderline intellectual function (100% of mild intellectual disability examinees had FSIQ ≤75 vs. 7% of matched controls; 97% of moderate intellectual disability examinees had FSIQ ≤60 vs. 3% of matched controls; 96% borderline intellectual function examinees had FSIQ ≤84 points vs. 22% of matched controls).

Learning Disorder. The performance of patients with Reading Disorder significantly differed from matched controls on VCI, WMI, and FSIQ, with moderate to large effect sizes reported. No differences were noted on PRI and PSI. In terms of subtests, large effect size differences were found on Letter-Number Sequencing, Arithmetic, and Vocabulary. In terms of Mathematics Disorder, patients significantly differed from matched controls on VCI, PRI, WMI, and FSIQ, but not PSI. In terms of subtests, the largest differences were reported on Arithmetic, Figure Weights, and Letter-Number Sequencing.

ADHD. An ADHD group performed lower than matched controls on all indices except VCI, with a small effect size noted. Coding, Arithmetic, Matrix Reasoning, and Figure Weights showed the largest effects in terms of subtests. Theiling and Petermann (2016) reported that people with ADHD showed worse performance on WMI and PSI than matched controls, with effect sizes moderate to large in magnitude. As may be expected, GAI was higher than FSIQ. Digit Span on the WAIS-IV has also been used to evaluate outcome of working memory training in ADHD (Mawjee, Woltering, & Tannock, 2015).

TBI. A moderate and severe TBI group was tested as described in the manual, as were matched controls. Differences in favor of matched controls were found on all index scores as well as on FSIQ (moderate to large effect sizes). At the subtest level, moderate to large effect sizes were found on subtests comprising PRI, PSI, and WMI, with verbal subtests yielding the smallest effects.

Other research has also suggested that the WAIS-IV has clinical utility in differentiating TBI and controls, with PSI reported to be especially useful. For example, Carlozzi, Kirsch, Kisala, and Tulsky (2015) reported that a mild to moderate TBI group performed lower than controls on WMI, PSI, and FSIQ, as well as on specific subtests (those comprising PSI, those comprising WMI, and Block Design). In turn, patients with severe TBI were found to perform worse than the mild to moderate TBI group on PSI, processing speed subtests, and Visual Puzzles. PSI had high sensitivity (75%) and specificity (84%) in classification of severe TBI from controls. Donders and Strong (2015) reported that PSI was the only index score that could accurately differentiate moderate to severe TBI from less severe TBI or demographically matched healthy controls.

ASD. Persons with ASD perform significantly worse than matched controls across indices (large effect sizes), with a pattern overall of weakest performance on VCI and PSI and their constituent subtests and relatively better PRI performance (manual). Persons with Asperger's showed higher levels of performance than persons with ASD, but obtained lower scores than matched controls on WMI, PSI, and FSIQ (moderate to large effect sizes). See also

Holdnack, Goldstein, and Drozdick (2011). In contrast, Bucaille et al. (2016) reported that adults with Asperger's disorder performed worse than controls on PSI, without other significant differences noted at the composite score level.

MCI and Dementia. Examinees with MCI perform worse than matched controls on all indices, with moderate effect sizes for each composite except for VCI. Subtest differences are somewhat variable (see manual). Similarly, a group of participants with probable AD performed worse than matched controls on all composite scores and subtests, with the largest effect sizes for Symbol Search, Information, Coding, and Arithmetic. Kessels, Overbeek, and Bouman (2015) reported that patients with MCI and AD perform worse than controls on Digit Span.

Psychiatric Conditions. People with major depressive disorder do not perform significantly differently on index scores than matched controls, with also generally null findings at the subtest level (manual). Michel et al. (2013) reported that people with schizophrenia showed greatest impairment on PSI and WMI, with relatively intact performance on VCI. Normative data for Canadian individuals with schizophrenia and low-average intelligence are included in this paper for the interested reader.

Other Populations. Baxendale, McGrath, and Thompson (2014) reported that 44% of their sample of patients with epilepsy had a significant GAI–FSIQ discrepancy, which was related to the number of antiepileptic medications taken and the duration of epilepsy. The authors concluded that reduced WMI and PSI can cause underestimation of intelligence in epilepsy when FSIQ, rather than GAI, is used.

Ryan, Gontkovsky, Kreiner, and Tree (2012) reported that patients with MS scored lower than a group of healthy controls with similar demographics who were part of the WAIS-IV standardization sample. In addition, 78% of patients with MS had FSIQ scores that were lower than pre-illness demographically based IQ estimates.

In a mixed clinical sample that scored below an MMSE cutoff, Logue et al. (2015) identified optimal cutoff scores in the identification of cognitive impairment. These cutoffs included a CPI standard score of 84 (sensitivity, 95%, specificity, 84%), a PSI cutoff score of 82 (sensitivity, 76%, specificity, 95%), and a WMI cutoff score of 87 (sensitivity, 80%, specificity, 95%).

In a sample of undergraduates, Buelow and Frakey (2013) demonstrated that math anxiety influenced performance on WAIS-IV Arithmetic but not Digit Span or Letter-Number Sequencing, even after gender, generalized test anxiety, and math performance were considered.

NEUROANATOMICAL CORRELATES AND IMAGING STUDIES

In a large sample of healthy adults, bilateral caudate volume, controlling for age, gender, and brain volume, was significantly correlated with a four-subtest WAIS-IV short form IQ estimate (Grazioplene et al., 2015).

PERFORMANCE VALIDITY

A number of performance validity indices have been derived from the WAIS-IV, but Digit Span indices are most common, with Reliable Digit Span (RDS) the most well-known metric of all. RDS is calculated as the sum of the longest digit string repeated without error over two trials. Overall, research suggests that RDS sensitivity is low to moderate, with relatively high specificity; in many studies, the RDS is not as accurate at prediction than are stand-alone performance validity tests (PVTs) (see reviews in Chapter 15).

The ACS can be used to derive combined validity indices consisting of RDS and other embedded PVTs from the WMS-IV (see "Word Choice," in Chapter 15, for information on the general approach to these indices, and also Holdnack, Millis, Larrabee, & Iverson, 2013). Non-Digit Span WAIS performance validity indices have also been derived, for instance, based on Vocabulary or other subtests, the majority for the prior edition of the test (WAIS-III) and not yet validated for the WAIS-IV; these are reviewed elsewhere (e.g., Carone & Bush, 2013).

A number of studies have examined Digit Span variables in veteran samples. Spencer et al. (2013) compared the diagnostic accuracy statistics of various RDS scores relative to the TOMM in 138 veterans evaluated in a TBI clinic. Sensitivities ranged from 33% to 39%, and specificities ranged from 82% to 91%. The highest accuracy was associated with a revised RDS score of 11 or lower and an age-corrected scale score of 6 or lower.

In another study, Digit Span Sequencing Total was found to yield the highest diagnostic accuracy among Digit Span variables examined in a veteran sample; however, sensitivity was poor (Whitney, Shepard, & Davis, 2013). Young, Sawyer, Roper, and Baughman (2012) examined a number of RDS indices in a sample of 259 veterans, with the Word Memory Test as the reference standard. Sensitivity values varied from 10% to 49% depending on the validity index and cutoff score used. Specificity was generally moderate to high (78% to 98%). Overall, the scores yielding highest sensitivity were RDS 7 or less and a revised RDS score of 11 or less (sensitivity range of 48% to 49%, specificity range of 78% to 81%).

In a mixed sample of clinically referred veterans, all indices examined (RDS, RDS-Revised [RDS-R], age-corrected scaled score [ACSS]) predicted group membership (credible vs. noncredible; optimal cutoffs of RDS ≤5, RDS-R ≤9, and ACSS ≤5). The ACSS was associated with the highest sensitivity and specificity (i.e., total sample ACSS ≤ 5; 62%, 87% respectively). In a cognitively unimpaired subsample, an ACSS of 5 or less was associated with a sensitivity of 62% and a specificity of 95%, and in a cognitively impaired sample, an ACSS of 4 or less was associated with a sensitivity of 39% and specificity of 86% (Webber & Soble, 2017).

Glassmire, Ross, Kinney, and Nitch (2016) provided normative scores on RDS measures in a sample of patients with schizophrenia spectrum disorders who did not have external incentives for poor performance and who performed within the adequate range on other PVTs (e.g., TOMM, Dot Counting, Validity Indicator Profile, Rey Fifteen-Item Test, CVLT-II embedded indices). A 90% specificity rate or greater was maintained. Cutoff scores were then validated on a sample of patients with schizophrenia spectrum disorders who were deemed incompetent to stand trial. The sensitivities for RDS measures were low to modest, ranging from 18% to 41%. When compared with higher-IQ groups, patients performing credibly with lower FSIQ scores were more likely to be erroneously deemed as noncredible. This study highlights the need for caution in using the RDS in patients with lower IQ.

Other Digit Span-type indices have been derived based on simulation studies involving the Digit Span Sequencing score (e.g., Reese, Suhr, & Riddle, 2012). Of note, the RDS does not appear to effectively detect feigning in ADHD (Williamson et al., 2014).

COMMENT

The WAIS-IV is a sophisticated instrument that has a long history of use in neuropsychology and in many ways represents a psychometric gold standard for the measurement of cognition. As discussed, there are useful resources published in addition to the manual to aid in use and interpretation of the measure (e.g., Holdnack, Drozdick, Weiss, & Iverson, 2013; Lichtenberger & Kaufman, 2009; Sattler & Ryan, 2009).

There are a number of substantive changes from the WAIS-III to the WAIS-IV that aimed to update theory, enhance developmental appropriateness, improve user-friendliness, improve clinical utility, and enhance psychometric properties. The WAIS-IV measures multiple domains of intelligence and aligns with current theoretical conceptualizations of intelligence. The test provides rich data and enables the clinician to obtain a multidimensional view of intellectual function.

There are demographic effects on performance, some quite sizeable, which should be taken into account. Although the WAIS-IV norms offer only age correction, in appropriate situations demographically adjusted norms can be calculated via the ACS. Normative data for this test are exceptional, offering a large, Census-stratified sample of examinees covering a broad age range in narrow age bands for most ages, with comprehensive exclusion criteria. Extensive base rate data are also available, and, given that the prevalence of low scores varies by a number of factors (e.g., IQ, education), it is important to consider base rate data when interpreting whether or not an examinee meets criteria for actual impairment on this test.

Short forms are also available; users should note that although short forms afford the advantage of reduced testing time, they do compromise accuracy and are not interchangeable with the standard version of the test, particularly for determining intellectual disability or in other high-stakes assessments. Norms have also been extended for different clinical situations. For example, Saklofske et al. (2012) provide data for the CPI, an analogue to the GAI. Ryan et al. (2014) provide data for Digit Span when a nonverbal response is provided.

Reliability is a strength of this test. Internal reliability is generally high to excellent. Test-retest reliability is generally also strong, with somewhat lower scores reported for process scores and some subtests. Practice effects tend to be largest for PSI and smaller for VCI. Reliable change calculations are provided with ACS software and in Holdnack, Drozdick, Iverson, and Chelune (2013) and Estevis et al. (2012). Intrarater and interrater reliability are excellent.

In terms of test validity, most of the research as of this writing that evaluates the WAIS-IV in relation to other measures comes from the manual. As expected for an overarching construct like intelligence that subsumes many abilities, the WAIS-IV tends to correlate moderately with most other tests from various cognitive domains. When the pattern of correlations is examined, tests of similar purported ability tend to correlate more with one another than tests of disparate abilities. In terms of factor structure, data published in the manual and in other research studies generally suggest a four-factor structure, whereas others suggest that a five-factor model best reflects the data, with perceptual reasoning subdivided into two factors.

Most clinical research on the test to date is found in the manual, with findings reported generally in the expected direction. For example, gifted adults significantly outperform matched controls, and patients with intellectual disability score lower than matched controls. The magnitude of the difference corresponds to the intellectual disability classification. In many clinical groups, PSI appears to be particularly sensitive. Overall, most research as of this writing consists of group differences, with few research findings on intervention effects, diagnostic accuracy statistics, and other clinical correlates.

Variables derived from Digit Span, most notably RDS, have been used as an indication of performance validity. Overall, sensitivity is low to moderate with relatively high specificity; in many studies, the RDS is not as accurate at prediction as are stand-alone PVTs. However, the test appears useful when used in conjunction with other PVTs, as in the ACS.

The WAIS-IV is an exceptional instrument with a large number of strengths. However, more information is needed on neuroanatomical correlates of WAIS-IV performance, and there is a need for more independent research on relationships between the WAIS-IV with other measures and in a variety of clinical populations.

REFERENCES

Abad, F. J., Sorrel, M. A., Román, F. J., & Colom, R. (2016). The relationships between WAIS-IV factor index scores and educational level: A bifactor model approach. *Psychological Assessment, 28*(8), 987–1000. https://doi.org/10.1037/pas0000228

Ashendorf, L. (2012). An exploratory study of the use of the Wechsler Digit–Symbol Incidental Learning Procedure with the WAIS-IV. *Applied Neuropsychology, 19*(4), 272–278. https://doi.org/10.1080/09084282.2012.670151

Baxendale, S. (2011). IQ and ability across the adult life span. *Applied Neuropsychology, 18*(3), 164–167. https://doi.org/10.1080/09084282.2011.595442

Baxendale, S., McGrath, K., & Thompson, P. J. (2014). Epilepsy & IQ: The clinical utility of the Wechsler Adult Intelligence Scale–Fourth Edition (WAIS–IV) indices in the neuropsychological assessment of people with epilepsy. *Journal of Clinical and Experimental Neuropsychology, 36*(2), 137–143. https://doi.org/10.1080/13803395.2013.870535

Benson, N., Hulac, D. M., & Kranzler, J. H. (2010). Independent examination of the Wechsler Adult Intelligence Scale—Fourth Edition (WAIS-IV): What does the WAIS-IV measure? *Psychological Assessment, 22*(1), 121–130. https://doi.org/10.1037/a0017767

Binder, L. M., & Binder, A. L. (2011). Relative subtest scatter in the WAIS-IV standardization sample. *The Clinical Neuropsychologist, 25*(1), 62–71. https://doi.org/10.1080/13854046.2010.533195

Bowden, S. C., Saklofske, D. H., & Weiss, L. G. (2011). Augmenting the core battery with supplementary subtests: Wechsler Adult Intelligence Scale--IV measurement invariance across the United States and Canada. *Assessment, 18*(2), 133–140. https://doi.org/10.1177/1073191110381717

Brooks, B. L., Holdnack, J. A., & Iverson, G. L. (2011). Advanced clinical interpretation of the WAIS-IV and WMS-IV: Prevalence of low scores varies by level of intelligence and years of education. *Assessment*, 18(2), 156–167.

Brooks, B. L., Iverson, G. L., & Holdnack, J. A. (2013). Understanding and using multivariate base rates with the WAIS-IV/WMS-IV. In J. A. Holdnack, L. Whipple Drozdick, L. G. Weiss, & G. Iverson (Eds.), *WAIS-IV, WMS-IV, and ACS: Advanced clinical interpretation* (pp. 75–102). Waltham, MA: Academic Press.

Bucaille, A., Grandgeorge, M., Degrez, C., Mallégol, C., Cam, P., Botbol, M., & Planche, P. (2016). Cognitive profile in adults with Asperger syndrome using WAIS-IV: Comparison to typical adults. *Research in Autism Spectrum Disorders, 21*, 1–9. https://doi.org/10.1016/j.rasd.2015.09.001

Buczylowska, D., & Petermann, F. (2017). Age-related commonalities and differences in the relationship between executive functions and intelligence: Analysis of the NAB executive functions module and WAIS-IV scores. *Applied Neuropsychology. Adult, 24*(5), 465–480. https://doi.org/10.1080/23279095.2016.1211528

Buelow, M. T., & Frakey, L. L. (2013). Math anxiety differentially affects WAIS-IV arithmetic performance in undergraduates. *Archives of Clinical Neuropsychology, 28*(4), 356–362. https://doi.org/10.1093/arclin/act006

Carlozzi, N. E., Kirsch, N. L., Kisala, P. A., & Tulsky, D. S. (2015). An examination of the Wechsler Adult Intelligence Scales, Fourth Edition (WAIS-IV) in individuals with complicated mild, moderate and severe traumatic brain injury (TBI). *The Clinical Neuropsychologist, 29*(1), 21–37. https://doi.org/10.1080/13854046.2015.1005677

Carone, D. A., & Bush, S. S. (2013). *Mild traumatic brain injury: Symptom validity assessment and malingering.* New York: Springer.

Carrasco, R. M., Grups, J., Evans, B., Simco, E., & Mittenberg, W. (2015). Apparently abnormal Wechsler Memory Scale Index score patterns in the normal population. *Applied Neuropsychology: Adult, 22*(1), 1–6. https://doi.org/10.1080/23279095.2013.816702

Chevalier, T. M., Stewart, G., Nelson, M., McInerney, R. J., & Brodie, N. (2016). Impaired or not impaired, that is the question: Navigating the challenges associated with using Canadian normative data in a comprehensive test battery that contains American tests. *Archives of Clinical Neuropsychology, 31*(5), 446–455. https://doi.org/10.1093/arclin/acw031

Climie, E. A., & Rostad, K. (2011). *Test review: Wechsler Adult Intelligence Scale.* Los Angeles, CA: Sage. Retrieved from http://journals.sagepub.com/doi/full/10.1177/0734282911408707

Crawford, J. R., Garthwaite, P. H., Longman, R. S., & Batty, A. M. (2012). Some supplementary methods for the analysis of WAIS-IV index scores in neuropsychological assessment: Supplementary methods for the analysis of WAIS-IV. *Journal of Neuropsychology, 6*(2), 192–211. https://doi.org/10.1111/j.1748-6653.2011.02022.x

Denney, D. A., Ringe, W. K., & Lacritz, L. H. (2015). Dyadic short forms of the Wechsler Adult Intelligence Scale-IV. *Archives of Clinical Neuropsychology, 30*(5), 404–412. https://doi.org/10.1093/arclin/acv035

Donders, J., & Strong, C. A. H. (2015). Clinical utility of the Wechsler Adult Intelligence Scale–Fourth Edition after traumatic brain injury. *Assessment*, 22(1), 17–22.

Estevis, E., Basso, M. R., & Combs, D. (2012). Effects of practice on the Wechsler Adult Intelligence Scale-IV across 3- and 6-month intervals. *The Clinical Neuropsychologist, 26*(2), 239–254. https://doi.org/10.1080/13854046.2012.659219

Fallows, R. R., & Hilsabeck, R. C. (2012). WAIS-IV Visual Puzzles in a mixed clinical sample. *The Clinical Neuropsychologist, 26*(6), 942–950. https://doi.org/10.1080/13854046.2012.697193

Frazier, T. W. (2011). Introduction to the Special Section on Advancing WAIS-IV and WMS-IV clinical interpretation. *Assessment, 18*(2), 131–132. https://doi.org/10.1177/1073191111408581

Gignac, G. E., & Watkins, M. W. (2013). Bifactor modeling and the estimation of model-based reliability in the WAIS-IV. *Multivariate Behavioral Research, 48*(5), 639–662. https://doi.org/10.1080/00273171.2013.804398

Girard, T. A., Axelrod, B. N., Patel, R., & Crawford, J. R. (2015). Wechsler Adult Intelligence Scale-IV dyads for estimating global intelligence. *Assessment, 22*(4), 441–448. https://doi.org/10.1177/1073191114551551

Glass, L. A., Ryan, J. J., & Charter, R. A. (2010). Discrepancy score reliabilities in the WAIS-IV standardization sample. *Journal of Psychoeducational Assessment, 28*(3), 201–208. https://doi.org/10.1177/0734282909346710

Glassmire, D. M., Ross, P. T., Kinney, D. I., & Nitch, S. R. (2016). Derivation and cross-validation of cutoff scores for patients with schizophrenia spectrum disorders on WAIS-IV Digit Span–based performance validity measures. *Assessment, 23*(3), 292–306.

Goldstein, G., Oakes, H., Lovejoy, D., & Holdnack, J. A. (2013). Assessing individuals with psychiatric and developmental disorders. In J. A. Holdnack, L. Whipple Drozdick, L. G. Weiss, & G. Iverson (Eds.), *WAIS-IV, WMS-IV, and ACS: Advanced clinical interpretation* (pp. 545–599). Waltham, MA: Academic Press.

Gontkovsky, S. T. (2014). Influence of IQ in interpreting MMSE scores in patients with multiple sclerosis. *Aging, Neuropsychology, and Cognition, 21*(2), 214–221. https://doi.org/10.1080/13825585.2013.795515

Grazioplene, R. G., G. Ryman, S., Gray, J. R., Rustichini, A., Jung, R. E., & DeYoung, C. G. (2015). Subcortical intelligence: Caudate volume predicts IQ in healthy adults: Caudate Volume and Intelligence. *Human Brain Mapping, 36*(4), 1407–1416. https://doi.org/10.1002/hbm.22710

Grégoire, J., Coalson, D. L., & Zhu, J. (2011). Analysis of WAIS-IV index score scatter using significant deviation from the mean index score. *Assessment, 18*(2), 168–177.

Hammers, D. B., Kucera, A. M., Card, S. J., Tolle, K. A., Atkinson, T. J., Duff, K., & Spencer, R. J. (2017). Validity of a verbal incidental learning measure from the WAIS-IV in older adults. *Applied Neuropsychology. Adult*, 1–8. https://doi.org/10.1080/23279095.2017.1295968

Harrison, A. G., Armstrong, I. T., Harrison, L. E., Lange, R. T., & Iverson, G. L. (2014). Comparing Canadian and American normative scores on the Wechsler Adult Intelligence Scale-Fourth Edition. *Archives of Clinical Neuropsychology, 29*(8), 737–746. https://doi.org/10.1093/arclin/acu048

Harrison, A. G., Holmes, A., Silvestri, R., & Armstrong, I. T. (2015). Implications for educational classification and psychological diagnoses using the Wechsler Adult Intelligence Scale–Fourth Edition with Canadian versus American norms. *Journal of Psychoeducational Assessment*, 734282915573723.

Hartman, D. E. (2009). Wechsler Adult Intelligence Scale IV (WAIS IV): Return of the gold standard. *Applied Neuropsychology, 16*(1), 85–87. https://doi.org/10.1080/09084280802644466

Heyanka, D. J., Holster, J. L., & Golden, C. J. (2013). Intraindividual neuropsychological test variability in healthy individuals with high average intelligence and educational attainment. *International Journal of Neuroscience, 123*(8), 526–531. https://doi.org/10.3109/00207454.2013.771261

Holdnack, J., Goldstein, G., & Drozdick, L. (2011). Social perception and WAIS-IV performance in adolescents and adults diagnosed with Asperger's syndrome and autism. *Assessment, 18*(2), 192–200. https://doi.org/10.1177/1073191110394771

Holdnack, J. A., Millis, S., Larrabee, G. J., & Iverson, G. L. (2013). Assessing performance validity with the ACS. In J. A. Holdnack, L. Whipple Drozdick, L. G. Weiss, & G. Iverson (Eds.), *WAIS-IV, WMS-IV, and ACS: Advanced clinical interpretation* (pp. 331–365). Waltham, MA: Academic Press.

Holdnack, J. A., Schoenberg, M. R., Lange, R. T., & Iverson, G. L. (2013). Predicting premorbid ability for WAIS-IV, WMS-IV, and WASI-II. In J. A. Holdnack, L. Whipple Drozdick, L. G. Weiss, & G. Iverson (Eds.), *WAIS-IV, WMS-IV, and ACS: Advanced clinical interpretation* (pp. 217–278). Waltham, MA: Academic Press.

Holdnack, J. A., & Weiss, L. G. (2013). Demographic adjustments to WAIS-IV/WMS-IV norms. In J. A. Holdnack, L. Whipple Drozdick, L. G. Weiss, & G. Iverson (Eds.), *WAIS-IV, WMS-IV, and ACS: Advanced clinical interpretation* (pp. 171–216). Waltham, MA: Academic Press.

Holdnack, J. A., Whipple Drozdick, L., Iverson, G. L., & Chelune, G. J. (2013). Serial assessment with WAIS-IV and WMS-IV. In J. A. Holdnack, L. Whipple Drozdick, L. G. Weiss, & G. Iverson (Eds.), *WAIS-IV, WMS-IV, and ACS: Advanced clinical interpretation.* (pp. 279–329). Waltham, MA: Academic Press.

Holdnack, J. A., Whipple Drozdick, L., Weiss, L. G., & Iverson, G. (Eds.) (2013). *WAIS-IV, WMS-IV, and ACS: Advanced clinical interpretation.* Waltham, MA: Academic Press.

Iverson, G. L., Holdnack, J. A., & Lange, R. T. (2013). Using the WAIS-IV/WMS-IV/ACS following moderate-severe traumatic brain injury. In J. A. Holdnack, L. Whipple Drozdick, L. G. Weiss, & G. Iverson (Eds.), *WAIS-IV, WMS-IV, and ACS: Advanced clinical interpretation* (pp. 485–544). Waltham, MA: Academic Press.

Kessels, R. P. C., Overbeek, A., & Bouman, Z. (2015). Assessment of verbal and visuospatial working memory in mild cognitive impairment and Alzheimer's dementia. *Dementia & Neuropsychologia, 9*(3), 301–305. https://doi.org/10.1590/1980-57642015dn93000014

Lichtenberger, E. O., & Kaufman, A. S. (2009). *Essentials of WAIS-IV assessment.* Hoboken, NJ: Wiley.

Logue, E., Scarisbrick, D. M., Thaler, N. S., Mahoney, J. J., Block, C. K., Adams, R., & Scott, J. (2015). Criterion Validity of the WAIS-IV Cognitive Proficiency Index (CPI). *The Clinical Neuropsychologist, 29*(6),777–787. https://doi.org/10.1080/13854046.2015.1101490

Mawjee, K., Woltering, S., & Tannock, R. (2015). Working memory training in post-secondary students with ADHD: A randomized controlled study. *PLOS ONE, 10*(9), e0137173. https://doi.org/10.1371/journal.pone.0137173

Meyers, J. E., Zellinger, M. M., Kockler, T., Wagner, M., & Miller, R. M. (2013). A validated seven-subtest Short Form for the WAIS-IV. *Applied Neuropsychology. Adult.* https://doi.org/10.1080/09084282.2012.710180

Michel, N. M., Goldberg, J. O., Heinrichs, R. W., Miles, A. A., Ammari, N., & Vaz, S. M. (2013). WAIS-IV profile of cognition in schizophrenia. *Assessment, 20*(4), 462–473.

Miller, J. L., Weiss, L. G., Beal, A. L., Saklofske, D. H., Zhu, J., & Holdnack, J. A. (2015). Intelligent use of intelligence tests empirical and clinical support for Canadian WAIS–IV norms. *Journal of Psychoeducational Assessment*, 734282915578577.

Nelson, J. M., Canivez, G. L., & Watkins, M. W. (2013). Structural and incremental validity of the Wechsler Adult Intelligence Scale–Fourth Edition with a clinical sample. *Psychological Assessment, 25*(2), 618–630. https://doi.org/10.1037/a0032086

Niileksela, C. R., Reynolds, M. R., & Kaufman, A. S. (2013). An alternative Cattell–Horn–Carroll (CHC) factor structure of the WAIS-IV: Age invariance of an alternative model for ages 70–90. *Psychological Assessment, 25*(2), 391–404. https://doi.org/10.1037/a0031175

Oakes, H., Lovejoy, D., Tartar, S., & Holdnack, J. (2013). Understanding index and subtest scatter in healthy adults. In J. A. Holdnack, L. Whipple Drozdick, L. G. Weiss, & G. Iverson (Eds.), *WAIS-IV, WMS-IV, and ACS: Advanced clinical interpretation* (pp. 103–169). Waltham, MA: Academic Press.

Peters, M., Servos, P., & Day, R. (1990). Marked sex differences on a fine motor skill task disappear when finger size is used as a covariate. *Journal of Applied Psychology, 75,* 87–90.

Reese, C. S., Suhr, J. A., & Riddle, T. L. (2012). Exploration of malingering indices in the Wechsler Adult Intelligence Scale-Fourth Edition Digit Span subtest. *Archives of Clinical Neuropsychology, 27*(2), 176–181. https://doi.org/10.1093/arclin/acr117

Reynolds, M. R., Ingram, P. B., Seeley, J. S., & Newby, K. D. (2013). Investigating the structure and invariance of the Wechsler Adult Intelligence Scales, Fourth Edition in a sample of adults with intellectual disabilities. *Research in Developmental Disabilities, 34*(10), 3235–3245. https://doi.org/10.1016/j.ridd.2013.06.029

Roberts, R. M., & Davis, M. C. (2015). Assessment of a model for achieving competency in administration and scoring of the WAIS-IV in post-graduate psychology students. *Frontiers in Psychology, 6.* https://doi.org/10.3389/fpsyg.2015.00641

Ryan, J. J., & Glass, L. A. (2010). Substitution of supplementary subtests for core subtests on composite reliability of WAIS–IV indexes. *Psychological Reports, 106*(1), 13–18. https://doi.org/10.2466/PR0.106.1.13-18

Ryan, J. J., Gontkovsky, S. T., Kreiner, D. S., & Tree, H. A. (2012). Wechsler Adult Intelligence Scale–Fourth Edition performance in relapsing–remitting multiple sclerosis. *Journal of Clinical and Experimental Neuropsychology, 34*(6), 571–579. https://doi.org/10.1080/13803395.2012.666229

Ryan, J. J., Kreiner, D. S., Gontkovsky, S. T., & Glass Umfleet, L. (2015). Classification accuracy of sequentially administered WAIS-IV short forms. *Applied Neuropsychology: Adult, 22*(6), 409–414. https://doi.org/10.1080/23279095.2014.953677

Ryan, J. J., Swopes-Willhite, N., Franklin, C., & Kreiner, D. S. (2015). WAIS-IV administration errors: effects of altered response requirements on Symbol Search and violation of standard surface-variety patterns on Block Design. *Applied Neuropsychology: Adult, 22*(1), 42–45. https://doi.org/10.1080/23279095.2013.828726

Ryan, J. J., Townsend, J. M., & Kreiner, D. S. (2014). Comparison of oral, written, and pointing responses to WAIS-IV Digit Span. *Applied Neuropsychology: Adult, 21*(2), 94–97. https://doi.org/10.1080/09084282.2012.753076

Ryan, J. J., Umfleet, L. G., & Gontkovsky, S. T. (2016). Prorating WAIS—IV summary scores for patients with relapsing-remitting multiple sclerosis. *International Journal of Neuroscience, 126*(11), 1025–1029. https://doi.org/10.3109/00207454.2015.1101596

Saklofske, D. H., Zhu, J., Miller, J. L., Weiss, L. G., Babcock, S. E., Cayton, T. G., . . . Coalson, D. L. (2012). The Cognitive Proficiency Index for the Canadian edition of the Wechsler Adult Intelligence Scale–Fourth Edition. *Canadian Journal of Behavioural Science/ Revue Canadienne Des Sciences Du Comportement, 44*(2), 117–123. https://doi.org/10.1037/a0026734

Sattler, J. M., & Ryan, J. J. (2009). *Assessment with the WAIS-IV.* San Diego, CA: Jerome M. Sattler, Publisher Inc.

Scheiber, C., Chen, H., Kaufman, A. S., & Weiss, L. G. (2017). How much does WAIS-IV Perceptual Reasoning decline across the 20- to 90-year lifespan when processing speed is controlled? *Applied Neuropsychology. Adult, 24*(2), 116–131. https://doi.org/10.1080/23279095.2015.1107564

Schwartz, D. M. (2013). A four-and five-factor structural model for Wechsler tests: Does it really matter clinically? *Journal of Psychoeducational Assessment, 31*(2), 175–185.

Shuttleworth-Edwards, A. B. (2012). Guidelines for the use of the WAIS-IV with WAIS-III cross-cultural normative indications. *South African Journal of Psychology, 42*(3), 399–410.

Soble, J. R., Sordahl, J. A., Critchfield, E. A., Highsmith, J. M., González, D. A., Ashish, D., Marceaux, J. C., O'Rourke, J. J. F., & McCoy, K. J. M. (2016). Slow and steady does not always win the race: Investigating the effect of processing speed across five naming tests. *Archives of Clinical Neuropsychology.* https://doi.org/10.1093/arclin/acw073

Spencer, R. J., Axelrod, B. N., Drag, L. L., Waldron-Perrine, B., Pangilinan, P. H., & Bieliauskas, L. A. (2013). WAIS-IV Reliable Digit Span is no more accurate than age corrected scaled score as an indicator of invalid performance in a veteran sample undergoing evaluation for mTBI. *The Clinical Neuropsychologist, 27*(8), 1362–1372. https://doi.org/10.1080/13854046.2013.845248

Spencer, R. J., Reckow, J., Drag, L. L., & Bieliauskas, L. A. (2016). Incidental learning: A brief, valid measure of memory based on the WAIS-IV Vocabulary and Similarities subtests. *Cognitive and Behavioral Neurology, 29*(4), 206–211. https://doi.org/10.1097/WNN.0000000000000108

Styck, K. M., & Walsh, S. M. (2016). Evaluating the prevalence and impact of examiner errors on the Wechsler scales of intelligence: A meta-analysis. *Psychological Assessment, 28*(1), 3–17. https://doi.org/10.1037/pas0000157

Sudarshan, N. J., Bowden, S. C., Saklofske, D. H., & Weiss, L. G. (2016). Age-related invariance of abilities measured with the Wechsler Adult Intelligence Scale-IV. *Psychological Assessment, 28*(11), 1489–1501. https://doi.org/10.1037/pas0000290

Taub, G. E., & Benson, N. (2013). Matters of Consequence: An empirical investigation of the WAIS-III and WAIS-IV and implications for addressing the Atkins intelligence criterion. *Journal of Forensic Psychology Practice, 13*(1), 27–48. https://doi.org/10.1080/15228932.2013.746913

Tellegen, A., & Briggs, P. F. (1967). Old wine in new skins: Grouping Wechsler subtests into new scales. *Journal of Consulting Psychology,* 31(5), 499.

Theiling, J., & Petermann, F. (2016). Neuropsychological profiles on the WAIS-IV of adults with ADHD. *Journal of Attention Disorders, 20*(11), 913–924. https://doi.org/10.1177/1087054713518241

Umfleet, L. G., Ryan, J. J., Gontkovsky, S. T., & Morris, J. (2012). Estimating WAIS-IV indexes: Proration versus linear scaling on WAIS-IV. *Journal of Clinical Psychology, 68*(4), 390–396. https://doi.org/10.1002/jclp.21827

van Ool, J. S., Hurks, P. P. M., Snoeijen-Schouwenaars, F. M., Tan, I. Y., Schelhaas, H. J., Klinkenberg, S., . . . Hendriksen, J. G. M. (2017). Accuracy of WISC-III and WAIS-IV short forms in patients with neurological disorders. *Developmental Neurorehabilitation,* 1–7. https://doi.org/10.1080/17518423.2016.1277799

Webber, T. A., & Soble, J. R. (2017). Utility of various WAIS-IV Digit Span indices for identifying noncredible performance validity among cognitively impaired and unimpaired examinees. *The Clinical Neuropsychologist,* 1–14. https://doi.org/10.1080/13854046.2017.1415374

Wechsler D. (2008). *Wechsler Adult Intelligence Scale–Fourth Edition.* San Antonio, TX: Pearson.

Weiss, L. G., Keith, T. Z., Zhu, J., & Chen, H. (2013). WAIS-IV and clinical validation of the four-and five-factor interpretative approaches. *Journal of Psychoeducational Assessment, 31*(2), 94–113.

Whipple Drozdick, L., Holdnack, J. A., Salthouse, T., & Munro Cullum, C. (2013). Assessing cognition in older adults with the WAIS-IV, WMS-IV, and ACS. In J. A. Holdnack, L. Whipple Drozdick, L. G. Weiss, & G. Iverson (Eds.), *WAIS-IV, WMS-IV, and ACS: Advanced clinical interpretation* (pp. 407–483). Waltham, MA: Academic Press.

Whitney, K. A., Shepard, P. H., & Davis, J. J. (2013). WAIS-IV Digit Span variables: Are they valuable for use in predicting TOMM and MSVT failure? *Applied Neuropsychology, 20*(2), 83–94. https://doi.org/10.1080/09084282.2012.670167

Williamson, K. D., Combs, H. L., Berry, D. T. R., Harp, J. P., Mason, L. H., & Edmundson, M. (2014). Discriminating among ADHD alone, ADHD with a comorbid psychological disorder, and feigned ADHD in a college sample. *The Clinical Neuropsychologist, 28*(7), 1182–1196. https://doi.org/10.1080/13854046.2014.956674

Wisdom, N. M., Mignogna, J., & Collins, R. L. (2012). Variability in Wechsler Adult Intelligence Scale-IV subtest performance across age. *Archives of Clinical Neuropsychology, 27*(4), 389–397. https://doi.org/10.1093/arclin/acs041

Yeudall, L. T., Fromm, D., Reddon, J. R., & Stefanyk, W. O. (1986). Normative data stratified by age and sex for 12 neuropsychological tests. *Journal of Clinical Psychology, 42,* 918–946.

Young, J. C., Sawyer, R. J., Roper, B. L., & Baughman, B. C. (2012). Expansion and re-examination of Digit Span effort indices on the WAIS-IV. *The Clinical Neuropsychologist, 26*(1), 147–159. https://doi.org/10.1080/13854046.2011.647083

WOODCOCK-JOHNSON IV TESTS OF COGNITIVE ABILITIES (WJ IV COG)

TEST NAME	**Woodcock-Johnson IV Tests of Cognitive Abilities (WJ IV COG)**
DOMAIN	Intellectual function
AGE RANGE	In adults, to 90 years
ADMINISTRATION TIME	35 minutes for standard battery, 5 minutes for each additional subtest
SCORING FORMAT	Computerized or hand scored
REFERENCES	McGrew, K. S., LaForte, E. M., & Schrank, F. A. (2014). *Technical manual. Woodcock-Johnson IV.* Rolling Meadows, IL: Riverside. Schrank, F. A., McGrew, K. S., & Mather, N. (2014c). *Woodcock-Johnson IV Tests of Cognitive Abilities.* Rolling Meadows, IL: Riverside.

DESCRIPTION

The Woodcock-Johnson IV (WJ IV; McGrew et al., 2014; Schrank et al., 2014c) is comprised of three co-normed batteries: the Woodcock-Johnson IV Tests of Cognitive Abilities (WJ IV COG; Schrank et al., 2014c), the Woodcock-Johnson IV Tests of Achievement (WJ IV ACH; Schrank et al., 2014a), and the Woodcock-Johnson IV Tests of Oral Language (WJ IV OL; Schrank et al., 2014b). These tests measure general intelligence (*g*) and specific cognitive abilities, academic achievement, and oral language, respectively. The WJ IV COG is the focus of this review. Major content is discussed in this review, and the interested reader is referred to the manual for additional discussion.

The WJ IV COG is based on the Cattell-Horn-Carroll (CHC) theory of intelligence, with neuropsychological and developmental research used to inform the revision. It is comprised of 18 tests that measure general intellectual ability, broad and narrow cognitive abilities, aptitudes specific to academic domains, and related aspects of cognitive functioning. The tests are subdivided into a Standard Battery (Tests 1–10) and an Extended Battery (Tests 11–18). Table 5–18 summarizes the way the tests are organized. Note that some tests measure a narrowly defined cognitive ability whereas others focus on cognitive complexity. Each test within the Standard Battery was chosen because it met the following criteria: (a) strongly reflective of the identified CHC ability domain, (b) high loadings on the general intelligence (*g*) factor, (c) high loadings on the dimension of cognitive complexity, and (d) one of the best predictors of WJ IV ACH scores. Tests were organized so they involved the least amount of testing needed while still maximizing interpretive possibilities.

The theoretical basis for the WJ IV is discussed at length in the manual. A number of revisions were made to the WJ IV COG relative to its predecessors. Broadly speaking, changes include an updated measurement model to conform to the most recent iteration of CHC theory (e.g., addition of new tests, enhanced complexity, and addition of a fluid-crystallized [*Gf-Gc*] cognitive composite across domains), increased comparison options within and between batteries (e.g., identification of relative strengths and weaknesses across batteries, improved organization of tests), and updated psychometric qualities (e.g., new norming sample, updated items and simplified administration and interpretation, improved scaling of speeded tests, and use of sophisticated data collection and analytic methods to develop the tests).

The most significant changes to the WJ IV interpretive model are to the constructs of working memory, speed of lexical access, and memory for sound patterns. As with its predecessors, the WJ IV COG includes the dimension of cognitive complexity, whereby tasks range from simple cognitive operations to complex cognitive processes. Of note, however, there are substantive differences in content and theory between the third edition of the cognitive test and the WJ IV COG, including the General Intellectual Ability (GIA) cluster; the user is cautioned that "many of the WJ III and WJ IV clusters are not identical in test composition despite having similar or identical names in the two batteries. In fact, all of the major WJ IV COG cognitive composite clusters and CHC factor clusters are different, to varying degrees, from how they were in the WJ III" (p. 31, manual). The specific changes are detailed in the manual, and only an example will be provided here. The WJ IV Auditory Processing (*Ga*) cluster is made of two new *Ga* tests (COG Test 5: Phonological Processing and Test 12: Nonword Repetition); however, the WJ III *Ga* cluster was comprised of COG Test 14: Auditory Attention (eliminated in WJ IV COG) and COG Test

TABLE 5–18 Woodcock-Johnson IV Tests of Cognitive Abilities (WJ IV COG) with Composites, CHC Factors, and Narrow Ability and Other Clinical Clusters

			Cognitive Composites			CHC Factors							Narrow Ability and Other Clinical Clusters					
			General Intellectual Ability (GIA)	Brief Intellectual Ability (BAI)	Gf-Gc Composite	Comprehension-Knowledge (Gc)	Fluid Reasoning (Gf)	Short-Term Working Memory (Gwm)	Cognitive Processing Speed (Gs)	Auditory Processing (Ga)	Long-Term Retrieval (Glr)	Visual Processing (Gv)	Quantitative Reasoning (RQ)	Auditory Memory Span (MS)	Number Facility (N)	Perceptual Speed (P)	Vocabulary (VL/LD)	Cognitive Efficiency
Standard Battery	COG 1	Oral Vocabulary	■	■	■	■											■	
Standard Battery	COG 2	Number Series	■	■	■		■						■					
Standard Battery	COG 3	Verbal Attention	■	■				■										□
Standard Battery	COG 4	Letter-Pattern Matching	■						■							■		■
Standard Battery	COG 5	Phonological Processing	■							■								
Standard Battery	COG 6	Story Recall	■								■							
Standard Battery	COG 7	Visualization	■									■						
Standard Battery	COG 8	General Information			■	■												
Standard Battery	COG 9	Concept Formation			■		■											
Standard Battery	COG 10	Numbers Reversed						■							■			■
Extended Battery	COG 11	Number-Pattern Matching													■	■		□
Extended Battery	COG 12	Nonword Repetition								■								
Extended Battery	COG 13	Visual-Auditory Learning									■							
Extended Battery	COG 14	Picture Recognition										■						
Extended Battery	COG 15	Analysis-Synthesis					□						■					
Extended Battery	COG 16	Object-Number Sequencing						□										
Extended Battery	COG 17	Pair Cancellation							■									
Extended Battery	COG 18	Memory for Words												■				
Oral Language Battery	OL 1	Picture Vocabulary				□											■	
Oral Language Battery	OL 5	Sentence Repetition												■				

■ Tests required to create the cluster listed.
□ Additional tests required to create an extended version of the cluster listed.

SOURCE: From Woodcock-Johnson IV™ (WJ IV™). Copyright 2014 © Houghton Mifflin Harcourt Publishing Company. All rights reserved. Used by permission of the publisher. Any further duplication is strictly prohibited unless written permission is obtained from Houghton Mifflin Harcourt Publishing Company.

4: Sound Blending (now part of the Oral Language battery). Therefore, the WJ III and WJ IV Auditory Processing (*Ga*) cluster scores, like other composite scores, are not directly comparable.

The specific details for each subtest are described in Table 5–19. New subtests added to the WJ IV COG include Verbal Attention, Letter-Pattern Matching, Phonological Processing, and Nonword Repetition. These tests underwent pilot testing as described in the manual, including administration to a convenience sample to evaluate if further item modification was needed prior to the tryout phase. In addition to these new tests, items from many subtests were rewritten. Expert reviewers reviewed item content, sensitivity, and bias.

All of the WJ IV item pools were calibrated into a common scale (W scale) using Rasch analyses. After Rasch

TABLE 5–19 Description, Stimuli, Task Requirements, Cognitive Processes, and Responses of Woodcock-Johnson IV Tests of Cognitive Abilities (WJ IV COG) Subtests

COGNITIVE TEST	PRIMARY BROAD CHC ABILITY *NARROW ABILITY*	STIMULI	TASK REQUIREMENTS	COGNITIVE PROCESSES	RESPONSE
1: Oral Vocabulary A: Synonyms B: Antonyms	Comprehension-Knowledge (*Gc*) *Lexical knowledge* (VL) *Language development* (LD)	Auditory (words)	Listening to a word and providing a synonym; listening to a word and providing an antonym	Semantic activation, access, and matching	Oral (words)
2: Number Series	Fluid Reasoning (*Gf*) *Quantitative reasoning* (RQ) *Induction* (I)	Visual (numeric)	Determining a numerical sequence	Representation and manipulation of points on a mental number line; identifying and applying an underlying rule/ principle to complete a numerical sequence	Oral (numbers)
3: Verbal Attention	Short-Term Working Memory (*Gwm*) *Working memory capacity* (WM) *Attentional control* (AC)	Auditory (words, numbers)	Listening to a series of numbers and animals intermingled and answering a specific question regarding the sequence	Controlled executive function; working memory capacity; recoding of acoustic, verbalized stimuli held in immediate awareness; selective auditory attention; attentional control	Oral (words)
4: Letter-Pattern Matching	Processing Speed (GS) *Perceptual speed* (P)	Visual (letters)	Rapidly locating and circling identical letters or letter patterns	Speeded visual perception and matching; visual discrimination; orthographic processing; divided attention	Motoric (circling)
5: Phonological Processing A: Word Access B: Word Fluency C: Substitution	Auditory Processing (*Ga*) *Phonetic coding* (PC) *Word fluency* (*Glr-FW*) *Speed of lexical access* (*Glr-LA*)	Auditory (words)	Providing a word with a specific phonic element; naming as many words as possible that begin with a specified sound; substituting part of a word to make a new word	Semantic activation, access; speed of lexical access	Oral (words)
6: Story Recall	Long-Term Retrieval (*Glr*) *Meaningful memory* (MM) *Listening ability* (*Gc-LS*)	Auditory (text)	Listening to and recalling details of stories	Construction of prepositional representations and recoding	Oral (passages)
7: Visualization A: Spatial Relations B: Block Rotation	Visual Processing (*Gv*) *Visualization* (Vz)	Visual (shapes, designs)	Identifying two-dimensional pieces that form a shape; identifying two three-dimensional rotated block patterns that match a target	Visual feature detection; manipulation (mental rotation) of visual images in space; matching	Oral (letters) or Motoric (pointing)
8: General Information A: Where B: What	Comprehension-Knowledge (*Gc*) *General (verbal) information* (KO)	Auditory (questions)	Identifying where an object is found and what people typically do with an object	Semantic activation and access to declarative generic knowledge	Oral (phrases, sentences)
9: Concept Formation	Fluid Reasoning (*Gf*) *Induction* (I)	Visual (drawings)	Identifying, categorizing, and determining rules	Rule-based categorization; rule switching; induction/ inference	Oral (words)
10: Numbers Reversed	Short-Term Working Memory (*Gwm*) *Working memory capacity* (WM) *Attentional control* (AC)	Auditory (numbers)	Listening to and recalling a sequence of digits in reversed order	Span of apprehension and recoding in working memory; working memory capacity, attentional capacity	Oral (numbers)

(continued)

TABLE 5–19 Continued

COGNITIVE TEST	PRIMARY BROAD CHC ABILITY *NARROW ABILITY*	STIMULI	TASK REQUIREMENTS	COGNITIVE PROCESSES	RESPONSE
11: Number-Pattern Matching	Processing Speed (*Gs*) *Perceptual speed* (P)	Visual (numbers)	Rapidly locating and circling identical numerals from a defined set	Speeded visual perception and matching; visual discrimination; divided attention	Motoric (circling)
12: Nonword Repetition	Auditory Processing (*Ga*) *Phonetic coding* (PC) *Memory for sound patterns* (UM) *Memory span* (Gwn-MS)	Auditory (nonsense words)	Listening to a nonsense word and repeating it exactly	Analysis of a sequence of acoustic phonological elements in immediate awareness; efficiency of the phonological loop	Oral (words)
13: Visual-Auditory Learning	Long-Term Retrieval (*Glr*) *Associative memory* (MA)	Visual (rebuses) Auditory (words)	Learning and recalling pictographic representations of words	Paired-associative encoding via directed spotlight attention; storage and retrieval	Oral (sentences)
14: Picture Recognition	Visual Processing (*Gv*) *Visual memory* (MV)	Visual (pictures)	Recognizing a subset of previously presented pictures within a field of similar distracting pictures	Formation of iconic memories and matching of visual stimuli to stored visual representations	Oral (words) or Motoric (pointing)
15: Analysis-Synthesis	Fluid Reasoning (*Gf*) *General sequential reasoning* (RG)	Visual (drawings)	Analyzing puzzles (using symbolic formulations) to determine missing components	Algorithmic reasoning; deduction	Oral (words)
16: Object-Number Sequencing	Short-Term Working Memory (*Gwm*) *Working memory capacity* (WM)	Auditory (words, numbers)	Listening to a series of numbers and words intermingled and recalling in two reordered sequences	Recoding of acoustic, verbalized stimuli held in immediate awareness; working memory capacity	Oral (words, numbers)
17: Pair Cancellation	Processing Speed (*Gs*) *Perceptual speed* (P) *Spatial scanning* (Gv-SS) *Attentional control* (AC)	Visual (drawings)	Rapidly locating and marking a repeated pattern	Executive processing; attentional control; inhibition and interference control; sustained attention	Motoric (circling)
18: Memory for Words	Short-Term Working Memory (*Gwm*) *Memory span* (MS)	Auditory (words)	Listening to and repeating a sequence of unrelated words	Formation of echoic memories and verbal same span of echoic store	Oral (words)

SOURCE: From Woodcock-Johnson IV™ (WJ IV™). Copyright 2014 © Houghton Mifflin Harcourt Publishing Company. All rights reserved. Used by permission of the publisher. Any further duplication is strictly prohibited unless written permission is obtained from Houghton Mifflin Harcourt Publishing Company.

calibration, item difficulty and examinee ability are placed on a logit scale that quantifies the examinee's ability compared to the difficulty of items above and below the examinee's ability on the scale, with each logit being equidistant from the other. The W scale is a modification of the logit scale. Item tryouts were completed to further develop item pools and evaluate the psychometric qualities and usability of new test items. Convenience samples (ranging from $n = 100$ to $n = 500$) were used in this phase, specifically aimed at sampling a variety of age and ability levels. See manual for further specifications regarding item development.

ADMINISTRATION

Detailed administration instructions are provided in the manual. A number of features were incorporated to enhance the test's usability across ability levels, including clear and concise administration instructions, artwork with pictures and text, and flexibility in test order and administration.

SCORING

Table 5–18 outlines specific scores available, including composite scores and specific CHC factors. In brief, Tests 1 through 3 comprise the Brief Intellectual Ability (BIA) score, including one test from the comprehension-knowledge (*Gc*), fluid reasoning (*Gf*), and short-term working memory (*Gwm*) factors. These tests are strongly correlated with general intellectual ability and do not include a processing speed (*Gs*) measure. The GIA score is comprised of tests from the comprehension-knowledge (*Gc*), fluid reasoning (*Gf*), short-term working memory (*Gwm*), processing speed (*Gs*), auditory processing (*Ga*), long-term retrieval (*Glr*), and visual processing (*Gv*) CHC ability domains. When Test 1–10 are combined, the following additional clusters are measured: comprehension-knowledge

(*Gc*), fluid reasoning (*Gf*), short-term working memory (*Gwm*), cognitive efficiency, and the *Gf-Gc* composite. The extended battery scores augment the information available from the core battery, and, when selectively added, can provide enough information for cluster scores that reflect broad and narrow cognitive abilities.

Of note, Scholastic Aptitude (SAPT) cluster scores are also available. These are derived from WJ IV COG scores and serve to predict academic achievement scores. In brief, each SAPT cluster score is derived from four WJ IV COG tests that best predict a specific achievement area. For the most part, WJ IV cluster scores are the arithmetic average of the W scores of the tests comprising the cluster score (see the section "Description" for a discussion of W scores). The manual provides additional details regarding the derivation of the GIA cluster score, which was derived via principal components analysis of data from the normative sample.

DEMOGRAPHIC EFFECTS

AGE

Growth curves based on normative data are provided in the manual. Broadly speaking, the pattern of growth curves is consistent with research on developmental changes of intelligence. For example, processing speed (*Gs*) develops quickly, peaks at approximately 20 to 30 years of age, then declines. In contrast, the *Gc* factor shows growth into adulthood (i.e., ages 55 to 70) and shows a slower decline. Other trajectories are as illustrated in Figures 5–6 and 5–7 and detailed in the manual.

GENDER

A gender bias was identified for some subtests via differential item functioning (see discussion in "Ethnicity, Nationality, and Linguistic Effects"), with the majority of these items subsequently removed.

ETHNICITY, NATIONALITY, AND LINGUISTIC EFFECTS

A Spanish version of the test is available, and items were developed according to Rasch analysis (see "Description" and manual for details). Items were examined for bias via differential item functioning, which, in brief, entails examining whether an item is more or less difficult for a specific subgroup despite similar overall ability. The specific subgrouping variables examined were gender (male, female), race (white, non-white), and ethnicity (Hispanic, non-Hispanic). The median percentage of flagged items across subgroups for subtests was 0–9%. In most cases, flagged items were removed (manual).

NORMATIVE DATA

Normative data were collected over a two-year period in 2009. Examiner training was quite rigorous and additional efforts (i.e., use of a marketing firm) were made to recruit more difficult to reach participants, such as older and rural participants. As the WJ IV COG was co-normed with other tests, 51 tests would have to have been administered to all examinees. Due to the impracticalities of this method and the error that can be introduced by administering lengthy batteries over multiple sessions, a multiple matrix sampling

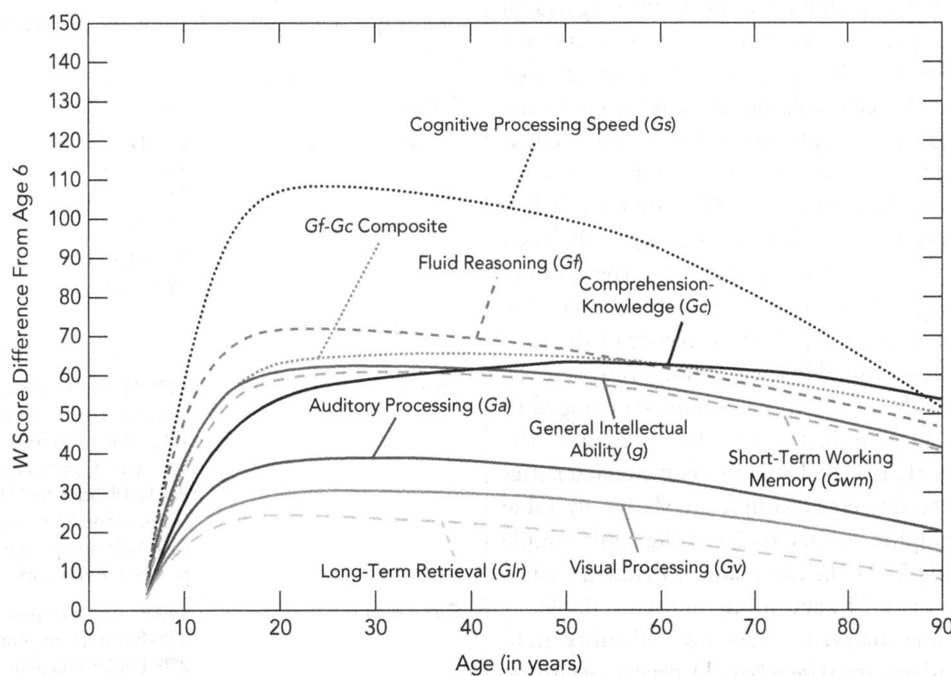

Figure 5–6 *Growth curves of Woodcock-Johnson IV (WJ IV) COG General Intellectual Ability (GIA), Cattell-Horn-Carrol (CHC) Factor Clusters, and Gf-Gc composite scores based on age.*

SOURCE: From Woodcock-Johnson IV™ (WJ IV™). Copyright 2014 © Houghton Mifflin Harcourt Publishing Company. All rights reserved. Used by permission of the publisher. Any further duplication is strictly prohibited unless written permission is obtained from Houghton Mifflin Harcourt Publishing Company.

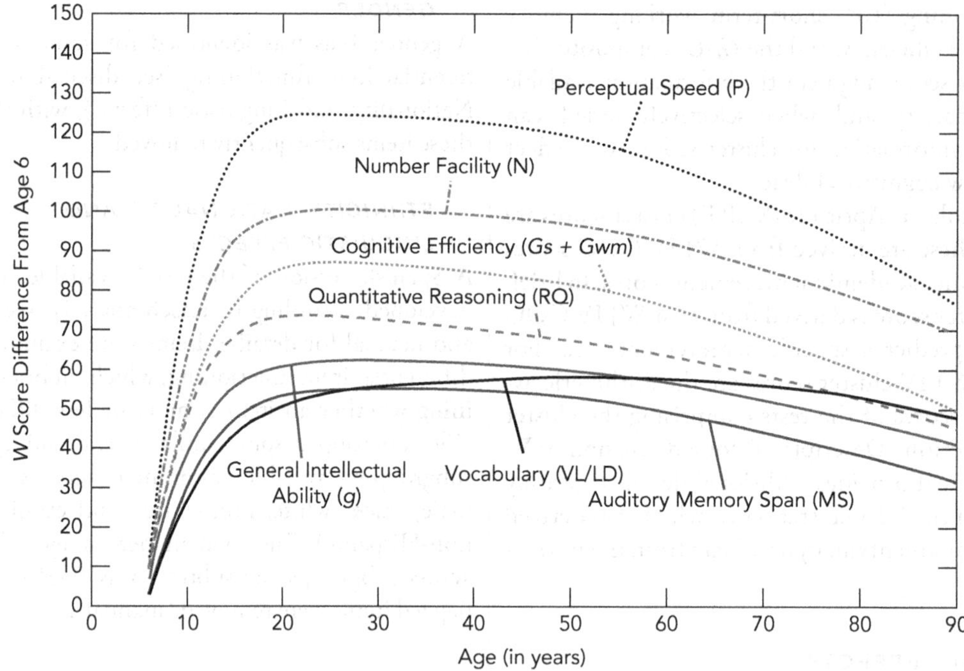

Figure 5–7 Growth curves of Woodcock-Johnson IV (WJ IV) COG General Intellectual Ability (GIA), Narrow Cognitive Ability, and Clinical cluster scores based on age.

SOURCE: From Woodcock-Johnson IV™ (WJ IV™). Copyright 2014 © Houghton Mifflin Harcourt Publishing Company. All rights reserved. Used by permission of the publisher. Any further duplication is strictly prohibited unless written permission is obtained from Houghton Mifflin Harcourt Publishing Company.

design was used to collect data. In brief, this involves administering a core set of tests to each examinee in the normative sample and matrix sampling others.

The normative sample was large (N = 7,416) and predominantly comprised of children and youth (61%) from 46 states and the District of Columbia in the United States. The remainder of the sample included 775 college/university participants and 2,860 adult examinees. Participants were randomly selected within a stratified sampling design and were broadly representative of the US population on a number of variables, including geographical region, gender, country of birth, ethnicity, community type, educational attainment, college type, employment status, and occupational level. Overall, the representativeness of the normative sample on these variables approximated Census data. When this was not the case, partial weights were assigned. In brief, a weight for each participant was calculated as the product of many partial weights that corresponded to a demographic variable. If an examinee belonged to a category of the variable that was overrepresented in the norming study sample, the weight was less than 1.00; if the examinee belonged to a category of the variable that was underrepresented, the weight was greater than 1.00. Demographic characteristics of the adult college/university sample are shown in Table 5–20, and demographic characteristics of the adult sample are shown in Table 5–21. In the manual, detailed demographic data are provided by age group for each variable.

Each subtest was analyzed in terms of reliability, item discrimination, and statistical item bias. Decisions regarding inclusion of specific items are described in the manual, as are steps regarding sequencing of items and selection of specific discontinuation and starting points (informed via Rasch calibration). Of note, timed tests were calibrated via a rate-based calibration method, which was derived from a Rasch model.

In the process of norm smoothing, the first step was calculation of a standard score (mean = 100, SD = 15)

TABLE 5–20 Demographic Characteristics of the College/University Standardization Sample for the Woodcock-Johnson IV (WJ IV)

Sample size	775
Geographic region	19% Northeast 20% Midwest 31% South 29% West
Gender	45% Men 55% Women
Country of birth	95% US 5% Other
Ethnicity	68% White, Not Hispanic 14% Black, Not Hispanic 12% White, Hispanic 4% Asian, Native, Hawaiian, or other Pacific Islander, Not Hispanic Note: other 2% broken down into six ethnic groups, each 1% or smaller proportion of sample
College type	45% Public, four-year 32% Private, four-year 22% Public, two-year <1% Private, two-year

SOURCE: Adapted from McGrew et al. (2014).

TABLE 5–21 Demographic Characteristics of the Adult Standardization Sample for the Woodcock-Johnson IV (WJ IV)

Sample size	2,860
Geographic region	18% Northeast 23% Midwest 32% South 27% West
Education	<1% <9th grade 9% <High school 31% High school 28% Some college 15% Bachelor's degree 15% Master's degree or higher
Gender	46% Men 54% Women
Country of birth	93% USA 7% Other
Race/Ethnicity	67% White, Not Hispanic 14% Black, Not Hispanic 13% White, Hispanic 4% Asian, Native, Hawaiian, or other Pacific Islander, Not Hispanic Note: other 2% broken down into six racial and ethnic groups, each 1% or smaller proportion of sample
Employment status	60% Employed 10% Unemployed 30% Not in labor force
Occupational level	44% Management/Professional 26% Sales/Office 19% Service 6% Production/Transportation/Material moving 5% Natural resources/Construction/Maintenance

SOURCE: Adapted from McGrew et al. (2014).

that corresponded to the mid-interval percentile rank for each raw score value at each age. Norms were then smoothed within age and across age using a computer program designed for smoothing. Additional details regarding norm construction, including bootstrapping, resampling, and normative curve fitting, as well as calculation of age equivalents and difference scores, are outlined in detail in the manual. The IQ composite was based on summation of verbal and nonverbal standard scores.

EVIDENCE FOR RELIABILITY

EVIDENCE FOR INTERNAL RELIABILITY

Split-half reliabilities and *SEMs* for untimed subtests are presented in the manual by age group. Median reliabilities in the adult subsample are high overall, with most exceeding $r = .84$. The median reliability of Picture Recognition was somewhat lower ($r = .74$). Cluster scores are associated with median reliabilities in the very high range overall, with most exceeding $r = .90$ in adult samples (with the exception of Visual Processing, with a median of $r = .86$). The authors recommend cluster scores, rather than subtest scores, for clinical decision making (manual).

EVIDENCE FOR TEST-RETEST RELIABILITY, MEASURING CHANGE, AND PRACTICE EFFECTS

An adult subgroup of 50 examinees was administered the speeded tests twice, within a 1-day test-retest interval. The median test-retest reliability was $r = .92$ (manual).

EVIDENCE FOR VALIDITY

FACTOR-ANALYTIC STUDIES AND WITHIN-TEST RELATIONSHIPS

In terms of the WJ IV COG in adult samples, the subtests generally correlate within the moderate range, with a wide range noted (i.e., *rs* = .18 to .77). Overall, subtests measuring similar constructs tend to correlate more highly with one another than subtests measuring disparate abilities. In addition, correlations between cognitive and achievement measures are generally lower than within-domain correlations.

Multidimensional scaling (MDS) was used to evaluate relationships among all subtests within the WJ IV batteries and is used as an alternative to factor analysis when working with multidimensional data sets (manual). Similarity of stimuli is represented spatially, with conceptually similar stimuli closer together and distinct stimuli farther apart. Most relevant for the current discussion is that the WJ IV COG subtests tended to be classified as expected based on content, such that verbal subtests were found to be part of auditory linguistic groupings and spatial subtests were reported to be part of the figural-visual groupings. Consistency in grouping was reflected across age subgroups, with the exception of Numbers Reversed. In support of convergent validity, tasks that shared common content across WJ IV batteries were reflected in similar groupings. In support of divergent validity, none of the WJ IV COG subtests were aligned with the reading-writing grouping.

A factor analysis was used to evaluate the complexity of the WJ IV COG subtests (manual). Specifically, the first unrotated factor was interpreted to reflect a general intelligence factor (*g*) and cognitive complexity. Most subtests reportedly load on this factor, with the tests with the highest loadings including Oral Vocabulary, Phonological Processing, and Object-Number Sequencing. To further evaluate the internal validity of the test, exploratory, factor, and confirmatory factor analyses were completed (manual). The process followed is as depicted in Figure 5–8.

The process and findings are detailed at length in the manual and will be only briefly described here. During Stage 1, six age groups were differentiated, and each subgroup was split into model development (MD) and cross validation (MCV) samples ($n = 208–843$). Data from a subsample of children (9–13 years of age) were subjected to the three-stage structural validity process, and the results generated from these data were used as a starting model (Stage 2b) for each age group. Because of the importance

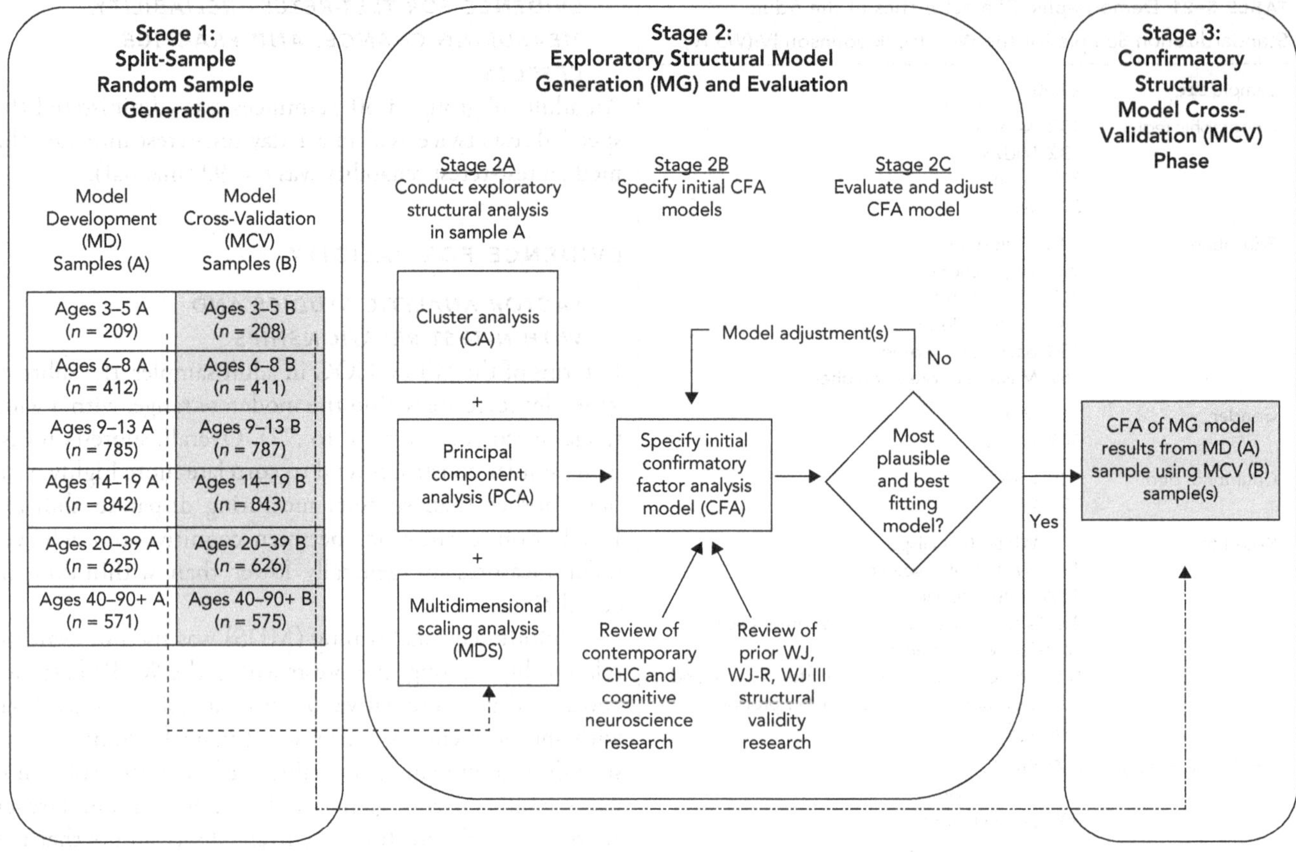

Figure 5–8 *Staged validity procedures for evaluation of Cattell-Horn-Carrol (WJ IV) construct validity.*

SOURCE: From Woodcock-Johnson IV™ (WJ IV™). Copyright 2014 © Houghton Mifflin Harcourt Publishing Company. All rights reserved. Used by permission of the publisher. Any further duplication is strictly prohibited unless written permission is obtained from Houghton Mifflin Harcourt Publishing Company.

of this group to the analyses, the manual focuses most explicitly on the results from this sample. As depicted in Figure 5–8, cross-validation following model generation via structural equation modeling confirmatory factor analysis (CFA) was completed in the MCV sample.

Data from the MD sample were analyzed via cluster analysis (CA), exploratory principal components analysis (PCA), and multidimensional scaling analysis (see Stage 2a in Figure 5–8). Cluster analysis yields classification via clusters/groups of similar entities. Results overall supported CHC factor clusters (*Gwm, Ga, Gv, Gf, Glr, Gq, Gc, Grw,* and *Gs*). A PCA was completed with all tests in the WJ IV batteries using varimax rotation. The test developers chose a priori to retain at least eight to ten factors, given the cluster analysis results. It is noteworthy that, across all PCA solutions, five broad CHC components were found, including *Gc, Gs, Grw, Gq+Gf,* and *Gwm*. MDS, as previously described, was also used to evaluate internal validity, such that tests in close proximity on the MDS map reflected measurement of similar constructs. The MDS map is similar to the results of the cluster analysis and the PCA, providing support for *Ga, Gc, Grw, Gq/Gf*-RQ, *Gwm, Gf,* and *Gv* (manual).

Two models were identified as best fitting the data, with the most parsimonious model selected and subsequently cross-validated. The model was termed a broad CHC factor top-down CFA model and included a higher order *g* factor and nine broad CHC factors (*Gc, Grw, Gf, Gs, Gq, Gv, Glr, Gwm,* and *Ga*). Figure 5–9 provides factor loading of most relevance to the WJ IV COG. Overall, the CFA pattern loading generally supported the model across age groups. For example, there were high loadings of broad CHC ability factors (generally ranging from .79 to .95) on the *g* factor, as would be expected (manual).

RELATIONSHIPS WITH OTHER TESTS

The manual presents data regarding correlations between the WJ IV COG and other measures; comparisons were generally made at the cluster or composite score level. Of note, data are reported in a number of child samples for intelligence tests that will not be reviewed here. As well, oral language and achievement measures are also included in child samples (manual).

The WAIS-IV and WJ IV study involved 177 adolescents and adults (16–82 years of age; M = 37.1 years, SD = 14.3 years). The mean composite IQ scores from both measures were similar, with a difference of 2.8 standard score points for global composites (i.e., WJ IV GIA and WAIS-IV FSIQ). The WJ IV COG clusters (GIA, BIA, and *Gf-Gc*) were highly correlated with the WAIS-IV FSIQ

	Battery & Test Number	Test Name	Cognitive Composite Clusters			CHC Factors & Clusters							Other CHC Factors
			General Intellectual Ability (GIA)	Brief Intellectual Ability (BIA)	Gf-Gc Composite	Comprehension-Knowledge (Gc)	Fluid Reasoning (Gf)	Short-Term Working Memory (Gwm)	Cognitive Processing Speed (Gs)	Auditory Processing (Ga)	Long-Term Retrieval (Glr)	Visual Processing (Gv)	Quantitative Knowledge (Gq)
Cognitive Standard Battery	COG 1	Oral Vocabulary	**0.72**	**0.72**	**0.72**	**0.87**							
	COG 2	Number Series	**0.62**	**0.62**	**0.62**		**0.79**						
	COG 3	Verbal Attention	**0.64**	**0.64**				**0.77**					
	COG 4	Letter-Pattern Matching	**0.57**						**0.74**				
	COG 5	Phonological Processing	**0.71**			0.27				**0.62**			
	COG 6	Story Recall	**0.58**								**0.57**		
	COG 7	Visualization	**0.61**									**0.74**	
	COG 8	General Information			**0.59**	**0.78**							
	COG 9	Concept Formation			**0.66**		**0.69**						
	COG 10	Numbers Reversed						**0.48**					**0.25**
Cognitive Extended Battery	COG 11	Number-Pattern Matching											
	COG 12	Nonword Repetition						0.59		**0.18**			
	COG 13	Visual-Auditory Learning									**0.51**		
	COG 14	Picture Recognition										**0.49**	
	COG 15	Analysis-Synthesis					*0.63*						
	COG 16	Object-Number Sequencing						*0.75*					
	COG 17	Pair Cancellation							**0.58**			0.22	
	COG 18	Memory for Words											
Other Tests	DL 1	Picture Vocabulary				*0.82*							
	DL 5	Sentence Repetition											

Note: Gray shading designates loadings on other CHC factors not listed in CHC Factors and Clusters section. Bold font designates tests required to create the primary cluster listed. Italic font designates tests required to create the extended cluster listed. Regular font designates loading on other nontarget CHC factors.

Figure 5–9 *Median broad Cattell-Horn-Carrol (CHC) factor loadings.*

SOURCE: From Woodcock-Johnson IV™ (WJ IV™). Copyright 2014 © Houghton Mifflin Harcourt Publishing Company. All rights reserved. Used by permission of the publisher. Any further duplication is strictly prohibited unless written permission is obtained from Houghton Mifflin Harcourt Publishing Company."

($r = .74$ to $r = .84$). Correlations between the WJ IV COG composite scores and achievement clusters on the WJ IV ACH were also large ($r = .65$ to $r = .81$).

CLINICAL STUDIES

The interested reader is referred to the manual for details regarding a number of clinical studies completed with various child diagnostic groups, including gifted, intellectual disabilities, learning disabilities (reading, math, and writing), language delay, ADHD, TBI, and ASD. To our knowledge, there is limited information on adult clinical groups.

NEUROANATOMICAL CORRELATES AND IMAGING STUDIES

No information is available.

PERFORMANCE VALIDITY

No information is available.

COMMENT

The WJ IV COG is the most recent iteration in the WJ series of tests. Building on an existing strong psychometric approach, the development of the WJ IV COG was sophisticated and technically rigorous. The test is well-founded from a theoretical perspective, based on the CHC theory of intelligence and updates from contemporary neuropsychological and developmental research. The scores available reflect both broad and specific cognitive abilities, as well as cognitive complexity and achievement predictor scores across a wide range of domains. On a practical level, users should note that the revisions in the fourth edition are substantive, and direct comparisons of subtests between the WJ III and WJ IV may be difficult. As well, a number of subtests require an oral response and thus would likely not be the most appropriate for use with examinees with linguistic or verbal communication impairments.

In terms of technical development, the test items appear to have been developed and refined with a considerable amount of research, including pilot testing, content reviews, and item tryouts. Furthermore, item development was extended from classical test theory alone to item response theory, with items calibrated according to Rasch analyses. Effects of age are well-defined and follow expected patterns (e.g., most prominent rise and fall in processing speed, relatively maintained crystallized intelligence across age groups). Bias based on gender and ethnicity was systematically examined via differential item function analyses, and the majority of items that reflected bias were removed. Normative data are exceptional, with a sample of 3,635 adults that was Census-stratified on a number of demographic variables. One significant advantage of the WJ IV COG is that it was co-normed with tests of achievement (WJ IV ACH) and oral language (WJ IV OL).

In terms of reliability and validity, reliability is generally high to very high, and the test authors recommend cluster scores be used for clinical decision-making, rather than individual subtests. Within-task construct validity is supported by correlations between subtests and both model generation and cross-validation approaches involving a series of both exploratory and confirmatory statistical analyses. The manual reports results of a WAIS-IV and WJ IV study suggesting large correlations and small score differences between counterpart scores on the WJ IV COG and the WAIS-IV. The manual presents data regarding relationships between the WJ IV COG and a number of child and youth intelligence tests, as well as clinical studies in pediatric populations. Research regarding performance in adult populations, concordance with adult-oriented measures, neuroanatomical correlates, and performance validity is lacking, and these are limitations compared to other IQ batteries typically used with adults in neuropsychological assessment.

REFERENCES

McGrew, K. S., LaForte, E. M., & Schrank, F. A. (2014). *Technical manual. Woodcock-Johnson IV*. Rolling Meadows, IL: Riverside.

Schrank, F. A., & Dailey, D. (2014). *Woodcock-Johnson Online Scoring and Reporting* [Online format]. Rolling Meadows, IL: Riverside.

Schrank, F. A., Mather, N., & McGrew, K. S. (2014a). *Woodcock-Johnson IV Tests of Achievement*. Rolling Meadows, IL: Riverside.

Schrank, F. A., Mather, N., & McGrew, K. S. (2014b). *Woodcock-Johnson IV Tests of Oral Language*. Rolling Meadows, IL: Riverside.

Schrank, F. A., McGrew, K. S., & Mather, N. (2014c). *Woodcock-Johnson IV Tests of Cognitive Abilities*. Rolling Meadows, IL: Riverside.

Schrank, F. A., McGrew, K. S., & Mather, N. (2014d). *Woodcock-Johnson IV*. Rolling Meadows, IL: Riverside.

6 | NEUROPSYCHOLOGICAL BATTERIES AND RELATED SCALES

CNS VITAL SIGNS (CNS VS)

TEST NAME	**CNS Vital Signs (CNS VS)**
DOMAIN	Neuropsychological functioning
AGE RANGE	In adults, to 90 years
ADMINISTRATION TIME	30 minutes
SCORING FORMAT	Computerized
REFERENCE	www.cnsvs.com

DESCRIPTION

CNS Vital Signs (CNS VS) is a computer-administered test designed for use as a clinical battery for assessing neuropsychological functioning. The test is comprised of seven core subtests specifically modeled after traditional neuropsychological tests. These are Verbal Memory, Visual Memory, the Finger Tapping Test, Symbol Digit Coding, the Stroop Test, the Shifting Attention Test, and the Continuous Performance Test (Table 6–1), modeled after the Rey Auditory Verbal Learning Test (RAVLT), Rey Visual Design Learning Test, Stroop, finger tapping, go/no-go and flanker-task type switching paradigms, and traditional continuous performance paradigms, respectively (e.g., Gualtieri & Johnson, 2006).

The test provides an overall score, the Neurocognition Index (NCI), as well as five original core domain scores based on the seven core subtests. These five original core domains are the Verbal Memory, Visual Memory, Psychomotor Speed, Complex Attention, and Cognitive Flexibility domains (Table 6–2). Later versions added an additional five core domain scores derived from the same original seven subtests; these additional core domain scores are Reaction Time, Processing Speed, Executive Function, Simple Attention, and Motor Speed. An additional three subtests were added later, in 2005 (C. Gualtieri, personal communication, March 2017), providing an additional four new domain scores ("Expanded Clinical Domains"). These Expanded Clinical Domains are Working Memory, Sustained Attention, Social Acuity, and Nonverbal Reasoning. Depending on the version used, these expanded domains may or may not be included. See www.cnsvs.com for Expanded subtests descriptions.

The NCI is the average of the original five domain scores (i.e., Composite Memory, Psychomotor Speed, Reaction Time, Complex Attention, and Cognitive Flexibility). Cognitive domain scores were constructed based on theoretical grounds by the authors. Some of these domain scores for the CNS VS are based on calculations involving single tests (e.g., Verbal Memory, Visual Memory, Processing Speed, Executive Function, Simple Attention, and Motor Speed), whereas others are based on combining scores from two or more subtests (Composite Memory, Psychomotor Speed, Reaction Time, Complex Attention, Cognitive Flexibility; see Table 6–2).

It is important for users to not assume the content of the domain based on its label. For example, a domain score that appears to measure a broad domain such as the Executive Function score is actually based solely on a single subtest (Shifting Attention Test), whereas another domain score reflecting what appears to be a more specific aspect of the general category of executive functioning, such as Cognitive Flexibility, is based on a broader set of scores (i.e., Shifting Attention Test scores combined with Stroop). As well, some scores relating to "speed" actually measure accuracy, not speed per se; Reaction Time is based on reaction time variables (although technically decision-making speed, not reaction time, as based on the Stroop task), Processing Speed measures Symbol Digit Coding accuracy, and Psychomotor

TABLE 6–1 Core CNS Vital Signs (CNS VS) Subtests

SUBTEST	CONSTRUCT MEASURED	DESCRIPTION
Core Subtests		
Verbal Memory	Recognition memory for words	Immediate and delayed recognition of 15 words drawn from a reservoir of 100 words, with one learning trial
Visual Memory	Recognition memory for geometric designs	Immediate and delayed recognition of 15 geometric designs drawn from a reservoir of 45 designs, with one learning trial
Finger Tapping Test	Fine motor speed (bimanual)	Examinee presses the space bar with the index finger as fast as possible, with three separate trials for right and left hands
Symbol Digit Coding	Visual processing speed	Examinee types in the numbers that correspond to eight different symbols presented on the screen, as fast as possible, drawn from an item bank of 32 symbols
Stroop Test	Standard Stroop paradigm measuring cognitive flexibility and speed	Contains three parts that involve responding to words and colors. Part one involves pressing the space bar as soon as the word RED, YELLOW, BLUE, or GREEN is shown on the screen (printed in black). Part two involves pressing the space bar when the color of the word matches the word (e.g., the word RED in red ink) but not responding when the color of the word does not match the word (e.g., the word RED in blue ink). Part three involves pressing the space bar when the color of the word does not match the word (e.g., the word RED in blue ink) but not responding when the color of the word matches the word (e.g., the word RED in red ink).
Shifting Attention Test	Cognitive flexibility and speed	Examinee must match geometric objects either by shape or by color, in response to cues corresponding to an alternating matching rule
Continuous Performance Test	Standard continuous performance paradigm measuring sustained attention and impulse control	Examinee must respond to a target stimulus ("B") while ignoring other distractor stimuli over a five-minute interval

NOTE: For definitions of subtests contributing to the Expanded Domains such as Working Memory, Sustained Attention, Social Acuity, and Non-Verbal Reasoning, see www.cnsvs.com

SOURCE: Adapted from Brooks and Sherman (2012).

Speed measures Symbol Digit Coding accuracy combined with Finger Tapping.

The CNS VS records timing with millisecond accuracy, requires only a fourth-grade reading level, and has been translated into more than 50 languages (Gualtieri & Johnson, 2006).

The CNS VS is designed for a wide range of examinees, with the goal of assisting in screening and detection of clinical conditions affecting cognition. Nevertheless, the authors note that the CNS VS does not have the specificity to be a stand-alone diagnostic tool, but it is highly sensitive to clinical conditions, which makes it suitable for brief clinical evaluation (Gualtieri & Johnson, 2006), and that the test is not the same as a formal neuropsychological evaluation. As well, although the test appears branded as a tool suitable for administration and interpretation in

TABLE 6–2 Corresponding Single- and Multi-Subtest Domain Scores for the CNS Vital Signs (CNS VS) for the Seven Core Subtests

SINGLE-SUBTEST DOMAINS	SCORE DEFINITION	MULTI-SUBTEST DOMAINS	SCORE DEFINITION
Verbal Memory	Verbal Memory Hits Immediate + Correct Passes Immediate + Hits Delayed + Correct Passes Delayed	*Composite Memory*	Verbal Memory + Visual Memory scores
Visual Memory	Visual Memory Hits Immediate + Correct Passes Immediate + Hits Delayed + Correct Passes Delayed	*Psychomotor Speed*	Symbol Digit Coding Correct + Finger Tapping
Processing Speed	Symbol Digit Coding Correct – Symbol Digit Coding Errors	*Cognitive Flexibility*	Shifting Attention Test Correct – Shifting Attention Test Errors – Stroop Commission Errors
Executive Function	Shifting Attention Test Correct – Shifting Attention Test Errors	*Complex Attention*	CPT Commission Errors + CPT Omission Errors + Stroop Commission Errors + Shifting Attention Test Errors
Simple Attention	CPT Correct – CPT Commission Errors		
Reaction Time	(Stroop Test Complex Reaction Time Correct + Stroop Test Reaction Time Correct)/2		
Motor Speed	Finger Tapping Right + Finger Tapping Left		

NOTE: The Neurocognitive Index (NCI) is an average of five core domain scores: Composite Memory, Psychomotor Speed, Reaction Time, Complex Attention, and Cognitive Flexibility.

SOURCE: Adapted from Interpretation Guide, http://www.cnsvs.com/WhitePapers/CNSVS-BriefInterpretationGuide.pdf.

medical clinics by non-psychologists, early publications by the authors note that physicians are not always able to interpret test results and that the test requires the active participation of consulting neuropsychologists when used in the medical setting (Gualtieri & Johnson, 2006).

One of the features of the CNS VS is that each of the original seven subtests has an embedded validity indicator designed to determine whether performance is valid and which is automatically generated. Embedded validity indicators are not available for newer subtests (C. Gualtieri, personal communication, March 2017). Invalid scores may occur for several reasons, such as the examinee misreading instructions or giving up on the test, and therefore invalid scores should not automatically be interpreted as an attempt to feign impairment. See the section "Performance Validity" for more information on embedded validity indicators.

The CNS VS can also be administered along with a number of specific computer-administered behavioral, medical, and quality-of-life scales, including fairly well known scales (e.g., the Neurobehavioral Symptom Inventory [NSI], useful for tracking concussion symptoms, the Patient Health Questionnaire [PHQ-9], a gold-standard depression inventory, and the Adult ADHD Self-Report Scale [ASRS-v1.1]), although these are not necessarily based on the same normative sample (see www.cnsvs.com for details). Although some of these scales are freely available, being able to set up automatic administration as part of the CNS VS would be an asset in many settings. There are also CNS VS versions designed for specific clinical groups such as concussion, which include additional scales. For example, the Concussion Vital Signs retains the standard CNS VS subtests but also includes a self-report section for demographic and health history relevant to concussion.

There is also a version called the Computerized Neurocognitive Test (CNT), which appears to be the original test battery recoded with more modern platforms and renormed using a more recent and larger normative dataset, which derives scores based on age and education and which has three different domain scores based on factor analysis (C. Gualtieri, personal communication, March 2017). Although this test is purported to be different from the CNS VS, existing publications reveal that it appears to be the original CNS VS test. Based on these similarities, it does appear that findings on the CNT should generally apply to the CNS VS (e.g., Gualtieri & Hervey, 2015a; 2015b).

ADMINISTRATION

The test is computer-administered, and responses are obtained via keyboard to maximize reaction time precision. An online Test Administration Guide (www.cnsvs.com) outlines exact instructions to give examinees. According to the test authors, "a medical office assistant can initiate the test" (Gualtieri & Johnson, 2006), "and a child with a fourth-grade reading level can take the test battery, unassisted." We highly discourage both these practices as examinees may misread or skip through instructions and need assistance. In our opinion, the test should be given by an experienced examiner familiar with testing procedures, one who remains in the room with the examinee during the test.

Notably, proctors in a reliability study involving military personnel reported a high number of participants asking about task instructions, often mid-task (Cole et al., 2013). The website now provides more precise instructions in addition to those presented as part of the test. Because some examinees start the test before reading instructions carefully, it is important for the examiner to make sure the examinee reads these instructions, particularly the instructions regarding the memory tests, as these begin fairly abruptly. These instructions caution examinees to be prepared because they will immediately have to remember a series of words. We also find that some examinees misread or skip the instructions for Shifting Attention Test and Symbol Digit Coding, and need redirection from the examiner.

People with more computer familiarity do better on the CNS VS than those with less familiarity, and effect sizes can be medium to large, comparable to the effects of traumatic brain injury (TBI), cannabis, depression, attention deficit hyperactivity disorder (ADHD), and other conditions (Iverson et al., 2009). Therefore, the examiner should always enquire as to how often the examinee uses the computer in daily life and use this information during interpretation, particularly when scores are unexpectedly low. Older adults and adults with significant cognitive impairments can find the test challenging. However, the Interpretation Guide suggests that older adults with Mini-Mental State Examination (MMSE) scores higher than 22 can complete the test.

SCORING

The CNS VS core domain scores are standard scores (mean [*M*] = 100, standard deviation [*SD*] = 15) derived from performance on the subtests as per Table 6–2; percentiles and classification ratings are also provided on the results summary for domains and individual subtest scores. According to the authors, scores are normally distributed except for Continuous Performance Test responses and error scores (Gualtieri & Johnson, 2006).

There are a large number of possible scores. Altogether, there are 23 possible subtest scores based on the seven core subtests automatically calculated by the program, as well as additional scores if the three expanded subtests are also administered. These include multiple scores for various aspects of accuracy (hits, false positives) and timing (simple and choice reaction time).

TABLE 6–3 CNS Vital Signs (CNS VS) Impairment Classifications

STANDARD SCORES	PERCENTILES	CLASSIFICATION	INTERPRETATION
>110	>74	Above Average	High function and high capacity
90–110	25–74	Average	Normal function and normal capacity
80–89	9–24	Low Average	Slight deficit and slight impairment
70–79	2–8	Low	Moderate deficit and impairment possible
<70	<2	Very Low	Deficit and impairment likely

SOURCE: Adapted from the CNS Vital Signs Interpretation Guide (www.cnsvs.com).

Scores are categorized according to impairment classifications, where a standard score of less than 70 is considered very low and a standard score greater than 110 is indicative of above-average scores (see Table 6–3).

The online Interpretation Guide (www.cnsvs.com) indicates that the pattern of scores across domains may be helpful for evaluating results and provides patterns suggestive of different pathology, including ADHD, mild cognitive impairment (MCI; amnestic and nonamnestic), early dementia, depression, mild TBI/concussion, multiple sclerosis (MS), and "chemo brain." For example, according to these patterns, the Memory domains along with Complex Attention and Cognitive Flexibility would be the most sensitive to Amnestic MCI, whereas Complex Attention, Cognitive Flexibility and Executive Function would be most sensitive to mild TBI; Psychomotor Speed, Reaction Time, Processing Speed and Motor Speed would be most sensitive to MS. It is not clear on which specific research studies these patterns are based, and, although these make general sense and have intuitive appeal based on the literature (see "Clinical Studies"), these general patterns would clearly be of limited utility used in isolation in diagnosis.

DEMOGRAPHIC EFFECTS

AGE

According to the authors, peak performance is achieved during the third decade of life, with slow declines after this point (Gualtieri & Johnson, 2006). Accordingly, age-based standard scores are provided based on 10 age groupings in the normative dataset (see Table 6–4).

GENDER

Gender effects are minimal and not likely of clinical significance. These consist of men having better scores on Finger Tapping and women showing a nonsignificant trend for better Symbol Digit Coding and Verbal Memory (Iverson et al., 2014).

EDUCATION AND IQ

The Interpretive Guide states that education may affect test performance but does not indicate the degree to which education and scores are related. It is likely that performance is dependent to a non-negligible degree on education, as per the Iverson et al. (2011) study, which showed that healthy people with lower education have a higher base rate of low scores. In one study involving patients with MS, associations with education were minimal (Papathanasiou et al., 2014). Similarly, in college athletes, high-school GPA and Scholastic Achievement Test (SAT) scores predict only 12% and 11% of scores on Processing Speed and Complex Attention, respectively, and do not predict performance on any other CNS VS scores (Trinidad et al., 2013).

IQ appears to be related to scores on the CNT, a computerized battery that uses the same paradigms as the CNS VS; specifically, Wechsler Adult Intelligence Scale (WAIS) IQ scores are moderately to highly related to Verbal Memory, Visual Memory, Symbol Digit Coding, and Shifting Attention (Gualtieri & Hervey, 2015a).

ETHNICITY, NATIONALITY, AND LINGUISTIC EFFECTS

To our knowledge, there are no studies on ethnicity apart from one study showing that a history of non-European ancestry is related to poorer CNS VS outcome after TBI (Theadom et al., 2016), although this is likely due to socioeconomic effects rather than to differential ethnicity effects on the test.

NORMATIVE DATA

Features of the standardization sample are summarized in Table 6–4, based on Gualtieri and Johnson (2006). Overall, the standardization sample was large. Specifics of recruitment and education level are not specified, and sample size, gender composition, and ethnicity are somewhat uneven depending on the age band. Of the 10 different age bands, there are 150 to more than 200 people per age band between ages 20 to 29 and 50 to 59, but only 48 individuals in the 15 to 19 age band, and 26 in the 80 to 90 age band. Males are underrepresented in each adult age band except for the 15 to 19 age band (56% male), ranging from 32% (20 to 29 age band) to 42% (60 to 69 age band). For some tests, gender composition may not matter, but for tests that tap executive functioning (particularly indices of false alarm responding, which tends to be higher in males), this may be problematic (but see "Demographic Effects"). Caucasians are overrepresented, particularly in the older age bands. Computer familiarity decreases with age, with frequent computer use reported in only approximately 30% of the 70 to 79 age band and in only 7% of the 80+ age band, consistent with the expected computer familiarity in those age cohorts.

TABLE 6–4 Characteristics of the CNS Vital Signs Standardization Sample

	STANDARDIZATION SAMPLE
Sample size	1,069
Recruitment	Not reported
Age	8 to 90
Education	Not reported
Gender	Varies by age band, but female overrepresentation in most age bands
Ethnicity	Varies by age group, with most age bands 80% white or higher, particularly in the older age groups (i.e., 96% in the 70 to 79 and 80+ age bands)
Inclusion criteria	In good health, without past or present psychiatric or neurological disorder, head injury, or learning disability, and free of centrally acting medications

NOTE: Norms based on 10 age groups: <10, 10 to 14, 15 to 19, 20 to 29, 30 to 39, 40 to 49, 50 to 59, 60 to 69, 70 to 79, and 80+, with a maximum age of 90 noted. Values are rounded.

SOURCE: Adapted from Gualtieri and Johnson (2006).

Notably, the normative sample has expanded over time since it was first published to include more subjects (now at $N = 1{,}906$; personal communication, A. Boyd, April 2017); its demographics are not specified.

BASE RATES OF LOW SCORES IN HEALTHY PEOPLE

As is the case for all other neuropsychological test batteries, healthy people do obtain some low scores on the CNS VS, and so base rate data on the prevalence of low scores is important for interpretation in order to avoid overpathologizing performance. Iverson et al. (2011) present base rates of low scores in healthy adults, calculated from the normative sample ($n = 659$; see Table 6–5) and based on five core domains. These data show that it is common for healthy people to obtain one low CNS VS domain scores when five core domains are examined, with 23% of the sample obtaining one or more low domain score below the 5th percentile. A single low domain score should therefore not automatically be interpreted as evidence of deficit. Instead, according to Iverson et al., two domain scores below the 5th percentile is a reasonable psychometric criterion for identifying cognitive impairment. Table 6–5 can be used to determine the base rate of low scores in a given case. Note that these base rates are based on adding up the number of low scores in five domain scores only: Memory, Psychomotor Speed, Reaction Time, Complex Attention, and Cognitive Flexibility. To use these tables, low scores in other domains (e.g., Executive Function, Motor Speed) should not be counted.

EVIDENCE FOR RELIABILITY

EVIDENCE FOR INTERNAL RELIABILITY

Not available.

EVIDENCE FOR TEST-RETEST RELIABILITY, MEASURING CHANGE, AND PRACTICE EFFECTS

Test-retest reliability was originally reported by the authors for a mixed sample of 99 participants from the standardization sample comprised of healthy volunteers and neuropsychiatric patients, with median interval of approximately one month (range 1 to 282 days; Gualtieri & Johnson, 2006). Of the index scores, Psychomotor Speed and Reaction Time had the highest reliability ($r = .87$ and .80, respectively); Memory and Cognitive Flexibility had adequate reliability ($r = .73$ and .74, respectively), and Complex Attention had marginal reliability ($r = .65$). At the subtest level, coefficients ranged from high for reaction time estimates (e.g., Continuous Performance Test Reaction Time, Shifting Attention Test Reaction Time, Stroop Test Reaction Time) to low (Stroop Test Errors, Continuous Performance Test Correct and Errors). According to the authors, test-retest reliabilities are better for clinical groups than controls and are similar across age groups, but decrease slightly with increasing interval (Gualtieri & Johnson, 2006).

In other studies, estimates of test-retest reliability are lower. For example, in military service personnel, only one-third of scores from the CNS VS had adequate or better reliability (Cole et al., 2013). Notably, Psychomotor Speed, Reaction Time, and Complex Attention all had adequate reliability ($r = .77$ to .79), but memory scores in particular had poor reliabilities. Test-retest reliabilities in a college-age

TABLE 6–5 Base Rates (%) of Low Domain Scores on the CNS Vital Signs (CNS VS) for Healthy Adults Based on Age and Education

NUMBER OF CNS VS DOMAIN SCORES FALLING BELOW THE 5TH PERCENTILE	AGE				EDUCATION		
	20–29	30–39	40–49	50–54	12	13–15	16+
0	80.0	74.0	77.3	78.7	77.8	73.4	76.1
1 or more	20.0	26.0	22.7	21.3	22.2	26.6	23.9
2 or more	9.7	7.3	7.6	9.0	7.4	8.5	9.7
3 or more	1.9	1.1	1.3	4.5	–	2.1	2.7
4 or more	–		0.4	1.1	–	–	0.4

NOTE: To find the applicable base rate for an examinee, add up the number of low scores in the following five domain scores: (Composite) Memory, Psychomotor Speed, Reaction Time, Complex Attention, and Cognitive Flexibility. Values based on an overall *N* of 659 healthy individuals.

SOURCE: Adapted from Iverson et al. (2011).

sample of healthy people have been reported as excellent for Psychomotor Speed (Intraclass Coefficient [ICC] = .85), but poor for Verbal Memory, Visual Memory, Processing Speed, Reaction Time and Reasoning (ICC = .10, .52, .58, .54, and .54, respectively; $N = 40$; Littleton, Schmidt et al., 2015).

The CNS VS provides reliabilities for many scores that are ignored or unreported by conventional tests tapping similar constructs. For example, error scores for tests such as the Stroop tend to yield low reliabilities versus reaction time measures for the same paradigm. It may be prudent therefore to use only domain scores for clinical interpretation as reliabilities for individual scores at the subtest level are not as well researched.

EVIDENCE FOR RELIABILITY OF ALTERNATE, SHORT, OR COMPUTER FORMS

This is not reported. According to the authors, the CNS VS generates a unique auto-randomized algorithm that provides the ability to generate an unlimited number of alternate forms for repeat testing. However, not all subtests provide unique forms—for each administration, Verbal Memory, Visual Memory, and Symbol Digit Coding retrieve a set of items from an item bank: this means that their test-retest coefficients and those of related index scores such as the NCI, Composite Memory, and Processing Speed actually reflect both test-retest stability and alternate forms reliability. Other subtests presumably present a standard set of test items each time they are administered.

Practice effects are present on some subtests and are most evident from the first session to the second session when examinees are tested more than twice. Specifically, healthy people tested serially at one-week intervals perform better on Psychomotor Speed, Cognitive Flexibility, Processing Speed, and Reaction Time on the second administration compared to the first; practice effects appear to level out after this, with no significant changes from the second administration to the third (Littleton, Schmidt et al., 2015). In terms of relative size of practice effects, in a study using a small group of controls ($N = 22$), the largest effects were found for Processing Speed (30% improvement), with moderate effects for Psychomotor Speed, Cognitive Flexibility, and Executive Function (18 to 14% improvement), and negligible practice effects for Reaction Time and the NCI (5% and 9% improvement, respectively; Turner et al., 2015). As such, a lack of practice effects in some clinical groups is indicative of impairment, particularly on domains where these would be expected (i.e., Processing Speed, Psychomotor Speed, Cognitive Flexibility).

Reliable change values are recommended for interpreting change. Values are provided based on a variety of samples and time intervals using 80% and 90% confidence intervals in Table 6–6. Note that these values are not adjusted for practice effects. Also note how large changes need to be to be indicative of real change on the Verbal Memory score (i.e., requiring a 1.5 *SD* increase to represent real change; see Table 6–6). Practice effects should therefore be considered so as not to misinterpret practice effects as real change.

TABLE 6–6 Reliable Change Index (RCI) Domain Values for One-Week Test-Retest Intervals for the CNS Vital Signs for Different Samples

	HEALTHY CONTROLS[a]	HEALTHY CONTROLS[a]	UNMEDICATED ADHD[b]
	INTERVAL: 1 WEEK	INTERVAL: 1 WEEK	INTERVAL: 1 WEEK
	RCI 90% CI	RCI 80% CI	RCI 80% CI
Verbal Memory	25.94	20.22	21.36
Visual Memory	22.32	17.49	14.55
Psychomotor Speed	12.11	9.44	9.50
Reaction Time	12.50	9.74	15.90
Complex Attention	15.35	11.96	19.02
Cognitive Flexibility	13.66	10.65	15.24
Processing Speed	17.88	13.93	11.63
Executive Function	13.73	10.70	14.37
Nonverbal Reasoning	19.92	15.52	16.66

[a]Adapted from Littleton, Schmidtt, Register-Mihalik et al. (2015a); $N = 40$, *M* age = 21.05 (*SD* = 2.17); test-retest interval = 1 week.

[b]Adapted from Littleton, Register-Mihalik, and Guskiewicz (2015b); $N = 22$ individuals with ADHD.

NOTE: Change values exceeding the RCI value likely represent meaningful change.

EVIDENCE FOR VALIDITY

CNS VS DOMAIN AND SUBTEST INTERCORRELATIONS

There are few studies showing patterns of correlations between CNS VS domains and subtests. For instance, in MS, only some CNS VS domains are intercorrelated, with medium to large correlations between Processing Speed and Executive Function ($r = .69$), Complex Attention and Cognitive Flexibility ($r = -.58$), and Complex Attention and Reaction Time ($r = -.42$). Correlations between reaction time and speed measures (Processing Speed, Reaction Time, Psychomotor Speed) are only modest and sometimes in opposite directions of expected relationships (Papathanasiou et al., 2014).

FACTOR-ANALYTIC STUDIES

CNS VS domain scores were constructed based on theoretical grounds by the authors, not based on factor analysis. To our knowledge, no factor-analytic studies of the original CNS VS exist. However, the CNT, which includes all the original seven CNS VS subtests, was factor analyzed, yielding three main factors: Memory, Attention and Information Speed, with the Finger Tapping Test not loading on any of these factors. Memory was comprised of scores on the Verbal and Visual Memory subtests; Attention from scores on the Stroop Test and Continuous Performance Test; and

Processing Speed, of Symbol Digit Coding, Stroop Test, and Shifting Attention Test scores. A superordinate processing speed factor accounted for 30% of variance in the memory and attention factors (Gualtieri & Hervey, 2015b), suggesting that processing speed is a significant predictor of performance on all the CNS VS subtests.

CORRELATIONS WITH OTHER NEUROPSYCHOLOGICAL TESTS

Correlations between CNS VS scores and conventional neuropsychological tests were reported as moderate in the original study on this question (Gualtieri & Johnson, 2006). More recently, one of the original CNS VS authors has specified that correlations ranged from −.13 to .79 (Gualtieri & Hervey, 2015b), correlations that suggest less than optimal correspondence between CNS VS and some corresponding neuropsychological tests. For example, correlations between CNS VS Verbal Memory and verbal memory tests such as the RAVLT and Logical Memory were reported as moderate to strong (r = .45 to .56), but were also in the moderate range with visual memory tests such as the Facial Recognition Test (r = .30 to. 35). Likewise, Visual Memory had high correlations with RAVLT (r = .49 to .50), but demonstrated only modest correlations with visual memory tests (r = .06 to .21; Facial Recognition). CNS VS Finger Tapping demonstrated only minimal correlations with performance on the mechanical Finger Tapping tapper (r = .13 to .24). In contrast, CNS VS Symbol Digit Coding and WAIS Digit Symbol were highly related (r = .79), demonstrating good construct validity for this subtest. The CNS VS Stroop Test and conventional Stroop are highly related when the Reaction Time score is examined (r = .51), but error scores show lower convergence. The Shifting Attention Test also shows moderate to high correlations with the conventional Stroop, likely due to the common requirement for cognitive flexibility.

In MS, the test shows good convergence with similar measures. For example, Cognitive Flexibility shows moderate to high correlations with Trail Making Test (TMT)-A and TMT-B (rs = −.47, −.65), as well as with verbal fluency (r = .49 to .62). Psychomotor Speed also correlates with TMT-A and TMT-B (rs = −.44, −.51, respectively). However, Executive Dysfunction does not correlate with measures of executive dysfunction such as TMT and verbal fluency (Papathanasiou et al., 2014). CNS VS scores appear much more sensitive to detection of MS-related impairments than conventional neuropsychological tests such as TMT and verbal fluency, with more than 83% of progressive MS cases showing impairments on Reaction Time (vs. 50 to 63% on conventional tests), and 58% of relapsing-remitting cases showing Reaction Time impairments (vs. 24 to 34%) on conventional neuropsychological tests (Papathanasiou et al., 2014). Of course, Reaction Time reflects performance on Finger Tapping, which would be expected to show deficits compared to other nonmotor tasks in this population.

In women with breast cancer, CNS VS Processing Speed reliably loads with WAIS-III Digits Symbol and Symbol Search in principal components analyses with traditional neuropsychological tests, with the TMT also loading on the same factor. Similarly, CNS Verbal Memory loads on the same factor as the Hopkins Verbal Learning Test (HVLT), and Visual Memory loads on a factor with the Brief Visuospatial Memory Test, Revised (BVMT-R) (Collins et al., 2013).

CNS VS Psychomotor Speed appears to have modest correlations with subjective ratings of cognition such as the Cognitive Failures Questionnaire (CFQ), but other scores appear unrelated (Barker-Collo et al., 2015). Measures of depression also show modest correlations with Psychomotor Speed, but not to other scores (Barker-Collo et al., 2015).

CLINICAL STUDIES

There are an impressively large number of studies on the use of the CNS VS in a variety of clinical groups, showing generally good evidence for clinical validity.

Alzheimer's Disease (AD), Mild Cognitive Impairment (MCI), and other Dementias. According to a study by the authors, Memory, Processing Speed, and Cognitive Flexibility are the most effective at discriminating between healthy controls and MCI, but also between MCI and mild dementia (Gualtieri & Johnson, 2005). In addition to tests of memory, Processing Speed and Cognitive Flexibility were best at discriminating between groups, consistent with the view that executive dysfunction is an early precursor of dementia, not only memory dysfunction. In terms of sensitivity and specificity based on raw score cutoffs, two primary subtests had 90% sensitivity with acceptable specificity (75%) for differentiating controls from MCI patients: Symbol Digit Coding and the Shifting Attention Test. Using the same levels of sensitivity/specificity, tests and scores able to effectively differentiate MCI from mild dementia included Reaction Time, Symbol Digit Coding, and the Shifting Attention Test (Gualtieri & Johnson, 2005).

Postmenopausal women obtain lower scores on average compared to normative levels, especially on Processing Speed, which some attribute to a "reversible MCI" associated with menopause (Bojar et al., 2012; N = 109). In postmenopausal women, polymorphisms of the APOE gene are linked to CNS VS scores, with the presence of e2/e3 polymorphism associated with better CNS VS scores and e3/e4 and e4/e4 with lower scores (Bojar et al., 2012), including very low Cognitive Flexibility, Complex Attention, and Executive Function along with a very low NCI. Of note, Verbal Memory is not clearly associated with APOE polymorphisms, raising questions about the validity of Verbal Memory for predicting MCI.

Other Neurological Conditions. The CNS VS has been used as an effective outcome measure in clinical trials on the tolerability and side-effect profile of several medications, including antiepileptic drugs (Meador et al., 2016). With regard to MS, Reaction Time appears to have high sensitivity to detecting deficits (Papathanasiou et al., 2014). Other CNS VS measures also differentiate MS patients from controls, but with only medium to small effect sizes. Within MS groups, large effect sizes are found between relapsing-remitting and secondary progressive patients on Psychomotor Speed, with the latter demonstrating lower scores overall (Papathanasiou et al., 2014). Similarly, Psychomotor Speed appears to be related to functional outcomes in MS as measured by instrumental activities of daily living, and CNS VS Memory is associated with employment status (Papathanasiou et al., 2015). The CNS VS also appears useful for tracking cognitive improvements after meningioma surgery, with test performance improving in all domains except Psychomotor Speed and Reaction Time (Meskal et al., 2015).

TBI. CNS VS scores show sensitivity to tracking improvements in cognition after concussion in some studies. In one important study that tracked concussion cases in the community as opposed to in hospital (since the vast majority of concussion cases are not seen in hospital), although the majority of cases scored in the average range, more than 20% had very low scores on Executive Function, Complex Attention, and Cognitive Flexibility. At one- and six-month follow-up, more than 20% continued to have very low scores on Complex Attention, with 16% remaining so at 12-month follow-up (Barker-Collo et al., 2015). Processing Speed was the one domain that continued to improve from the 6- to 12-month testing period. CNS VS Psychomotor Speed scores in particular were moderately correlated with postconcussion symptom ratings, as well as mood and self-reported cognition after mild TBI (Barker-Collo et al., 2015). Notably, the Memory scores did not show changes over time, nor any association with postconcussive symptoms, suggesting reduced sensitivity to track changes after mild TBI for these scores. The NCI appears to be impaired in 13%, 10%, 11%, and 11% of community-based mild TBI cases at baseline, 1-month, 6-month, and 12-month intervals, respectively, after injury (Theadom et al., 2016), with a history of non-European ancestry related to poorer CNS VS outcome.

The CNS VS has also been used to track concussion effects in active-duty army soldiers, where no significant score differences are found based on number of concussions despite concomitant increases in postconcussive symptom scales after three or more concussions (Dretsch et al., 2015). In a study by the authors, CNS VS scores were related to severity of brain injury and degree of recovery after severe or mild brain injury, with Psychomotor Speed and Cognitive Flexibility most related to injury severity, and with recovered mild TBI cases scoring almost as well as healthy people (Gualtieri & Johnson, 2008). In contrast, Lynall et al. (2016) demonstrated little change between pre-injury, post-injury, and repeat baseline CNS VS scores in college athletes using an 80% Reliable Change Index (RCI) criterion, with no score differences over time exceeding RCIs. In college athletes, CNS VS appears to be unaffected by moderate sleep restriction, even though postconcussive symptom ratings increase in severity in moderately sleep-restricted athletes, providing some validity for its use in baseline testing (Mihalik et al., 2013). Lynall et al. (2016) found no support for routine re-baselining athletes after concussion (i.e., routinely retesting athletes who have sustained a concussion to obtain a new baseline test), reporting better scores after concussion than after re-baseline evaluation, with no differences exceeding RCIs.

In professional boxers and mixed martial arts (MMA) fighters, lower Processing Speed is associated with increased fight exposure, and boxers have lower CNS VS scores overall than MMA fighters. The proportion of fighters with impaired CNS VS Verbal Memory and Psychomotor Speed increases with fight exposure history, an estimate of repetitive head trauma (Bernick et al., 2015). In addition, the test has been used to test the cognitive reserve hypothesis in professional fighters, where less education is associated with lower Psychomotor Speed. Of note, Verbal Memory scores do not differ in this population, contrary to hypotheses regarding expected cognitive precursors of chronic traumatic encephalopathy in athletes exposed to repetitive head trauma (Banks et al., 2014), raising some questions about the sensitivity of CNS VS memory scores to detect early changes in athletes exposed to repetitive head trauma.

ADHD. Individuals with ADHD perform worse than controls on Psychomotor Speed; after stimulant medication treatment, Reaction Time scores improve (Littleton et al., 2015a; see www.cnsvs.com for more ADHD studies).

Psychiatric Disorders. Studies indicate that the CNS VS is able to detect a distinct subgroup of people with depression or bipolar disorder who demonstrate widespread cognitive impairments (Iverson et al., 2009a; Iverson et al., 2009b; Iverson et al., 2011; Levy, 2014). In bipolar patients, Memory measures (particularly Verbal Memory) demonstrate the smallest effect sizes in terms of differences versus matched controls, with the largest effect sizes found for Complex Attention and Cognitive Flexibility (Iverson et al., 2009a). In contrast, in depressed patients, the largest effect sizes are found for Complex Attention and Memory (Iverson et al., 2009b). However, substantially higher deficits on CNS VS memory measures compared with other cognitive domains are not found, and this is in contrast to other studies that show very high effect sizes for memory as measured by other tests. This may relate to the type of memory testing employed on the CNS VS—namely, recognition versus free recall—and that the CNS VS has low sensitivity but very high positive predictive power, an expected finding when only a subgroup of the sample has cognitive impairment, as is the case in depression (Iverson et al., 2009a).

The CNS VS is sensitive to an acceleration of age-related cognitive decline in individuals with depression, with depressed persons declining more rapidly than controls after age 65 (Gualtieri & Johnson, 2008). The CNS VS appears sensitive to improved cognition after antidepressant treatment, with patients who improve on CNS VS more likely to show greater improvement in clinical and work functioning (Lam et al., 2016). Medication trials for schizophrenia have also used the CNS VS as a critical outcome measure for drug-related adverse events (e.g., Tsai et al., 2016).

Other Conditions. Adult survivors of severe congenital heart disease show impairments on Psychomotor Speed, Processing Speed, Complex Attention, Reaction Time, and the NCI, with number of surgeries related to worse Executive Function (Klouda et al., 2017). Persons with sickle cell disease perform lower than controls on CNS VS Processing Speed (Crawford & Jonassaint, 2016). The CNS VS shows promise as a tool for detecting and tracking hepatic encephalopathy (Kappus & Bajaj, 2012).

In persons with schizophrenia, lipid and glucose abnormalities predict performance on the CNS VS, particularly Reaction Time, Cognitive Flexibility, Executive Function, Verbal Memory, and Complex Attention, but hypertension, unexpectedly, is related to better CNS VS performance (Wysokinski et al., 2013). Visual Memory is not related to these indicators of metabolic syndrome. CNS VS has also shown to be of use in tracking cognitive effects of chemotherapy in breast cancer treatment, in combination with standard neuropsychological scores (Collins et al., 2014).

The CNS VS also appears to be a relevant tool for measuring health outcomes in healthy people. A randomized control trial involving 10 weeks of exercise improved performance on CNS VS Cognitive Flexibility in a dose-response pattern, with the most frequent exercisers obtaining the most benefits on cognition (Masley et al., 2009). Another study found that higher levels of omega-3 fatty acid intake are related to higher Cognitive Flexibility and Executive Function on the CNS VS, particularly in those with poor sleep quality, suggesting that omega-3 intake may confer resilience to poor sleep (Johnston et al., 2013).

In postmenopausal women, the level of homocysteine, a marker for inflammation, is related to CNS VS performance, with low levels associated with higher NCI, Executive Function, Complex Attention, and Cognitive Flexibility, but not with Visual or Verbal Memory (Raszewksi et al., 2015).

Hypoxia also affects CNS VS scores, with the largest declines evident on Processing Speed and Verbal Memory, in the range of 34 to 36% reduced performance, with the least effect on Reaction Time (10% decrement; Turner et al., 2015). Last, the CNS VS shows sensitivity to detecting marijuana-related effects on cognition in heavy users, with abstinence associated with improvements in Verbal Memory in particular, as well as on Psychomotor Speed (Roten et al., 2015).

NEUROANATOMICAL CORRELATES AND IMAGING STUDIES

CNS VS Memory and Psychomotor Speed are related to thalamic area in MS and to magnetic resonance imaging (MRI)-based atrophy, but more weakly with lesion volume (Papathanasiou et al., 2015). In repetitive brain injury, CNS VS scores are related to brain volume in professional boxers and MMA fighters, with lower Processing Speed associated with decreased thalamus, amygdala, and left hippocampus volume (Bernick et al., 2015).

PERFORMANCE VALIDITY

One asset of the CNS VS is that it contains embedded validity indicators for each of the seven core subtests automatically calculated by the test. However, the method for the development of these validity indicators is not well described and appears mainly based on theoretical or logical grounds (e.g., number of correct targets being higher than chance, based on the number of correct targets possible in a subtest; having more correct responses than errors; doing better on complex reaction time tasks than simple ones). These are shown in Table 6–7.

On standard CNS VS scores, simulated malingerers and clinically verified malingerers score lower than both healthy controls and patients with brain injury (Gualtieri & Hervey, 2015a). In a reliability and validity study on the normative sample, the authors reported that 18 malingerers performed worse on standard CNS VS scores than did patients with dementia, severe TBI, mild intellectual disability, or conversion disorder. No information was provided on this sample other than that the

TABLE 6–7 CNS Vital Signs (CNS VS) Subtest Embedded Validity Indicators Based on Raw Scores

CNS VS SUBTEST	CRITERIA FOR VALID SCORES
Verbal Memory	Total of all four raw scores > 30
Visual Memory	Total of all four raw scores > 30
Finger Tapping Test	Right Taps Average + Left Taps Average ≥ 40
Symbol Digit Coding Test	Correct Responses ≥ 20 *and* Correct Responses > Errors
Stroop Test	[Simple RT < ((Complex RT Correct × 0.1) + Complex RT Correct)] *and* [Complex RT Correct < ((RT Correct × 0.1) + RT Correct)] *and* (Complex Correct > Complex Errors) *and* (Correct > Errors)
Shifting Attention Test	Correct Responses > Errors
Continuous Performance Test	Correct Responses ≥ 30 *and* Correct Responses > Commission Errors

NOTE: Domain scores are invalid if any subtest contributing to the domain score is invalid. Adapted from FAQ section of cnsvs.com diagnoses were obtained independently via formal neuropsychological/neuropsychiatric assessment (Gualtieri & Johnson, 2006).

Gualtieri and Hervey (2015a) provided the most detailed study on validity indicators relevant to the CNS VS, based on the CNT. Based on a large overall sample comprised of clinically confirmed malingerers meeting Slick, Sherman, and Iverson (1999) criteria for malingered neurocognitive dysfunction, along with patients with TBI and healthy controls ($N = 60$, $N = 40$, $N = 589$, and $N = 2{,}172$, respectively), they identified four important criteria for invalid performance:

1. NCI score <45
2. Six or more standard scores <70
3. Five or more raw scores below validity indicator cutoffs, as per the Validity Indicator rating provided by the CNS VS computer scoring, as defined in Table 6–7 (resulting in a 97% likelihood of invalid performance)
4. Performance of raw score of <30 on the total Verbal Memory or Visual Memory subtests (both of which are akin to a four-trial 60-item forced-choice memory test comprised of a score out of 15 for each of Immediate Hits, Immediate Passes, Delay Hits, and Delay Passes, with a score of 25 projected to occur randomly only 4.5% of the time)

Importantly, the authors noted that the sensitivity of individual validity indicators is relatively low as a single validity indicator is unlikely to capture more than 40% of invalid responders. However, combining validity indicators increases confidence in identifying invalid responding. They note, however, that, for example, using only two validity indicator criteria (say, validity indicator 3 and validity indicator 4), only 65% of the simulated malingers were correctly identified. The authors encouraged the use of additional stand-alone validity indicators to increase sensitivity, in addition to the use of the embedded validity indicators. Notably, these levels of sensitivity are generally consistent with that of most performance validity tests (PVTs) when optimal specificity is maintained, and also fare well compared to most embedded PVTs.

Approximately 12% of healthy college student volunteers fail at least one CNS VS embedded validity indicator, 11% fail on repeat administration, and 15% fail at least one validity indicator on either administration (Deright & Jorgensen, 2015). Failure appears more frequent when examinees are tested in the morning, and validity indicator failure was related to worse performance on the test, particularly for the Continuous Performance Test. Failure on validity indicators was related to self-reported poor effort (r = −.32 to −.39), providing evidence for validity. These authors provide revised embedded validity cut-scores relevant to the undergraduate population (see Deright & Jorgensen, 2015). They found that the optimal diagnostic results were obtained when at least two embedded validity indicators were failed, equivalent to a healthy college student scoring below the 3rd percentile on at least two domain scores, equivalent to 70% sensitivity and 97% specificity, and twice the failure rate expected in pediatric neurological populations (Brooks et al., 2014).

In concussion baseline testing, intentionally performing poorly on a baseline concussion test ("sandbagging") is unlikely to be detected when using the standard CNS VS validity indicators (Hill et al., 2015). Consequently, Hill et al. (2015) developed a regression equation to more accurately identify feigning on the CNS VS, where the probability of feigning is calculated as follows:

$$\text{Probability of Feigning} = \frac{e\,[6.051 - .286\,(\text{Verbal Memory Immediate Hits raw}) - .574\,(\text{Verbal Memory Immediate Passes raw})] + .007\,(\text{Stroop Test Complex Reaction Time raw})}{1 + e\,[6.051 - .286\,(\text{Verbal Memory Immediate Hits raw}) - .574\,(\text{Verbal Memory Immediate Passes raw})] + .007\,(\text{Stroop Test Complex Reaction Time raw})}$$

where e = natural log

Based on this equation, if the obtained probability is greater than .70, feigning is suspected. Table 6–8 shows positive and negative predictive values for different estimates of base rates of feigning in the population that best matches the examinee, for use with this equation.

COMMENT

Computerized testing ensures standardized testing parameters, accurate reaction times, portability, instant scoring, and, most often, cost efficiency. Among computerized test batteries, the CNS VS is appealing because of all these reasons, but also because it is specifically modeled on traditional neuropsychological paradigms such as verbal list-learning, finger tapping, continuous performance tasks,

TABLE 6–8 Positive and Negative Predictive Values for a CNS Vital Signs (CNS VS) Regression Method to Identify Feigning

	POSITIVE AND NEGATIVE PREDICTIVE VALUES FOR DIFFERENT ESTIMATED BASE RATES OF FEIGNING		
Base Rate	15%	30%	45%
PPV (%)	79	90	95
NPV (%)	94	87	77

NOTE: PPV = positive predictive value; NPV = negative predictive value.
SOURCE: Adapted from Hill et al. (2015).

and the Stroop—all paradigms with ample evidence of validity in neuropsychological populations and familiar to most practitioners. As well, because of the way it is administered and the importance of speed in most of the subtests, processing speed appears to be a significant predictor of performance on all the CNS VS subtests. This makes it particularly suited to assessment in some conditions (e.g., concussion, MS). The availability of translations in multiple languages, base rate data, and reliable change data is also an advantage for practitioners compared to many other tests.

Compared to some other computerized batteries, the test has been used in an impressively large number of studies in clinical populations, showing generally good evidence for clinical validity. The embedded validity indicators are also an asset, particularly when used with some of the additional validity cutoffs and equations reviewed here (e.g., Hill et al., 2015).

Of note, the CNS VS battery is sometimes seen more as a battery of separate tests than as a measure of overall function based on several clinical studies reviewed that omitted mention of the NCI, the overall composite score. Not interpreting the NCI may make sense given the modest intercorrelations between subtests found in some studies.

The test can also be given with a number of standardized scales such as the PHQ-9 and NSI; although some of these scales are freely available elsewhere, the ability to administer them via computer as part of the CNS VS platform would be an asset in many circumstances.

Importantly, a single low domain score on the CNS VS is insufficient to infer deficits (Iverson et al., 2011); rather, two or more domain scores should be used as sufficient evidence of cognitive deficits. Practice effects inflate retest scores at retesting from the initial to second testing session and may interfere with interpretation of change in conditions requiring tracking over time, such as concussion. Reliable change scores are recommended for interpretation of repeat testing results, as some subtests (e.g., Verbal Memory) have practice effects that are large enough to mimic clinically significant change. Practice effects over longer intervals would be of benefit.

Anecdotally, we find that some examinees with anxiety do poorly on Verbal Memory because it is the first subtest administered. As well, examinees with impulse control problems may rush through the instructions and invalidate some subtests as they tend to begin subtests before fully understanding task demands. For this reason, it is important to have an examiner present who can observe and intervene as needed to prevent rushing through instructions, some of which are somewhat complex.

Notably, the memory subtests involve recognition memory only, which limits sensitivity to memory deficits. Supplementing with additional memory tests with recall requirements and multiple learning trials is recommended when memory needs to be assessed, particularly in conditions such as MCI, AD, and dementia. Simply relying on the CNS VS for memory assessment would be insufficient in most cases.

Norms for older adults are not optimal, and the test yields overestimates of impairment in computer-naïve subjects, as would be the case for most computerized test batteries. Like some computer test batteries, the test may cause anxiety and stress for older examinees unfamiliar with computers (Wild et al., 2008). Information on the test's use in minorities or in non–English speaking countries is unknown, although the test is available in several languages.

Test-retest reliabilities are not optimal for all domain scores and are not well reported for individual subtest scores. Although the scoring printout includes a large number of scores—including multiple scores for various aspects of accuracy (hits, false positives), and timing (simple and choice reaction time)—the domain scores should form the basis for interpretation for most clinical purposes.

The test also has an overwhelming number of derived composites, with new composites having appeared over time as the test evolved, as well as entirely new subtests developed without much supportive development literature. Earlier research is based on the initial five domain scores, but more recent studies are based on seven domain scores; as well, there are now three new subtests with their own new "Expanded" domain scores. This results in a large number of composites arising from the seven core subtests (now increased to 10 with the new subtests), with many domains having overlapping content—specifically, Processing Speed, Psychomotor Speed, and Motor Speed; Complex Attention, Simple Attention, and Sustained Attention; and Cognitive Flexibility and Executive Function, which can be confusing for users. In addition, the domain scores are not intuitive; for instance, Cognitive Flexibility and Complex Attention are virtually identical, and some seemingly broad domains (Executive Function) actually only measure performance on a single subtest (Shifting Attention Test), whereas others combine scores from two subtests (Cognitive Flexibility = Shifting Attention and Stroop). Fully understanding how the test works is not a straightforward task. The test would benefit from having an actual test manual, as some information such as validity indicators, normative sample composition, reliability, and validity is difficult to track down easily because it appears on different website pages or in various clinical studies or posters rather than in one easily accessed reference.

Last, evidence for the validity of the separate domains, such as factor analysis, is currently lacking. Domain score patterns suggestive of specific disorders (see www.cnsvs.com) have not been empirically verified and should not be used for diagnosis of individual examinees.

REFERENCES

Banks, S. J., Obuchowski, N., Shin, W., Lowe, M., Phillips, M., Modic, M., & Bernick, C. (2014). The protective effect of education on cognition in professional fighters. *Archives of Clinical Neuropsychology, 29*(1), 54–59. https://doi.org/10.1093/arclin/act079

Barker-Collo, S., Jones, K., Theadom, A., Starkey, N., Dowell, A., McPherson, K., . . . BIONIC Research Group. (2015). Neuropsychological outcome and its correlates in the first year after adult mild traumatic brain injury: A population-based New Zealand study. *Brain Injury, 29*(13–14), 1604–1616. https://doi.org/10.3109/02699052.2015.1075143

Bernick, C., Banks, S. J., Shin, W., Obuchowski, N., Butler, S., Noback, M., . . . Modic, M. (2015). Repeated head trauma is associated with smaller thalamic volumes and slower processing speed: the Professional Fighters' Brain Health Study. *Br J Sports Med*, bjsports-2014-093877. https://doi.org/10.1136/bjsports-2014-093877

Bojar, I., Wojcik-Fatla, A., Owoc, A., & Lewinski, A. (2012). Polymorphisms of apolipoprotein E gene and cognitive functions of postmenopausal women, measured by battery of computer tests—Central Nervous System Vital Signs. *Neuro Endocrinology Letters, 33*(4), 385–392.

Brooks, B. L., & Sherman, E. M. S. (2012). Computerized neuropsychological testing to rapidly evaluate cognition in pediatric patients with neurologic disorders. *Journal of Child Neurology, 27*(8), 982–991. https://doi.org/10.1177/0883073811430863

Brooks, B. L., Sherman, E. M. S., & Iverson, G. L. (2014). Embedded validity indicators on CNS Vital Signs in youth with neurological diagnoses. *Archives of Clinical Neuropsychology, 29*, 422–431.

Cole, W. R., Arrieux, J. P., Schwab, K., Ivins, B. J., Qashu, F. M., & Lewis, S. C. (2013). Test-retest reliability of four computerized neurocognitive assessment tools in an active duty military population. *Archives of Clinical Neuropsychology, 28*(7), 732–742. https://doi.org/10.1093/arclin/act040

Collins, B., MacKenzie, J., Tasca, G. A., Scherling, C., & Smith, A. (2013). Cognitive effects of chemotherapy in breast cancer patients: a dose-response study. *Psycho-Oncology, 22*(7), 1517–1527. https://doi.org/10.1002/pon.3163

Collins, B., Mackenzie, J., Tasca, G. A., Scherling, C., & Smith, A. (2014). Persistent cognitive changes in breast cancer patients 1 year following completion of chemotherapy. *Journal of the International Neuropsychological Society, 20*(4), 370–379. https://doi.org/10.1017/S1355617713001215

Crawford, R. D., & Jonassaint, C. R. (2016). Adults with sickle cell disease may perform cognitive tests as well as controls when processing speed is taken into account: A preliminary case-control study. *Journal of Advanced Nursing, 72*(6), 1409–1416. https://doi.org/10.1111/jan.12755

DeRight, J., & Jorgensen, R. S. (2015). I just want my research credit: Frequency of suboptimal effort in a non-clinical healthy undergraduate sample. *The Clinical Neuropsychologist, 29*(1), 101–117. https://doi.org/10.1080/13854046.2014.989267

Dretsch, M. N., Silverberg, N. D., & Iverson, G. L. (2015). Multiple past concussions are associated with ongoing post-concussive symptoms but not cognitive impairment in active-duty army soldiers. *Journal of Neurotrauma, 32*(17), 1301–1306. https://doi.org/10.1089/neu.2014.3810

Gualtieri, C. T., & Hervey, A. S. (2015a). A computerized neurocognitive test to detect malingering. *Frontiers, 4*(1), 1–10.

Gualtieri, C. T., & Hervey, A. S. (2015b). The structure and meaning of a computerized neurocognitive test battery. *Frontiers, 4*(2), 11–21.

Gualtieri, C., & Johnson, L. (2005). Neurocognitive testing supports a broader concept of mild cognitive impairment. *American Journal of Alzheimer's Disease and Other Dementias, 20*(6), 359–366.

Gualtieri, C., & Johnson, L. (2006). Reliability and validity of a computerized neurocognitive test battery, CNS Vital Signs. *Archives of Clinical Neuropsychology, 21*(7), 623–643. https://doi.org/10.1016/j.acn.2006.05.007

Gualtieri, C. T., & Johnson, L. G. (2008). Age-related cognitive decline in patients with mood disorders. *Progress in Neuro-Psychopharmacology and Biological Psychiatry, 32*(4), 962–967. https://doi.org/10.1016/j.pnpbp.2007.12.030

Hill, B. D., Womble, M. N., & Rohling, M. L. (2015). Logistic regression function for detection of suspicious performance during baseline evaluations using concussion vital signs. *Applied Neuropsychology. Adult, 22*(3), 233–240. https://doi.org/10.1080/23279095.2014.910215

Iverson, G. L., Brooks, B. L., & Ashton Rennison, V. L. (2014). Minimal gender differences on the CNS Vital Signs computerized neurocognitive battery. *Applied Neuropsychology. Adult, 21*(1), 36–42. https://doi.org/10.1080/09084282.2012.721149

Iverson, G. L., Brooks, B. L., Ashton, V. L., Johnson, L. G., & Gualtieri, C. T. (2009). Does familiarity with computers affect computerized neuropsychological test performance? *Journal of Clinical and Experimental Neuropsychology, 31*(5), 594–604. https://doi.org/10.1080/13803390802372125

Iverson, G. L., Brooks, B. L., Langenecker, S. A., & Young, A. H. (2011). Identifying a cognitive impairment subgroup in adults with mood disorders. *Journal of Affective Disorders, 132*(3), 360–367. https://doi.org/10.1016/j.jad.2011.03.001

Iverson, G. L., Brooks, B. L., & Young, A. H. (2009a). Identifying neurocognitive impairment in depression using computerized testing. *Applied Neuropsychology, 16*(4), 254–261. https://doi.org/10.1080/09084280903297594

Iverson, G. L., Brooks, B. L., & Young, A. H. (2009b). Rapid computerized assessment of neurocognitive deficits in bipolar disorder. *Applied Neuropsychology, 16*(3), 207–213. https://doi.org/10.1080/09084280903098778

Johnston, D. T., Deuster, P. A., Harris, W. S., Macrae, H., & Dretsch, M. N. (2013). Red blood cell omega-3 fatty acid levels and neurocognitive performance in deployed US servicemembers. *Nutritional Neuroscience, 16*(1), 30–38. https://doi.org/10.1179/1476830512Y.0000000025

Kappus, M. R., & Bajaj, J. S. (2012). Covert hepatic encephalopathy: Not as minimal as you might think. *Clinical Gastroenterology and Hepatology:, 10*(11), 1208–1219. https://doi.org/10.1016/j.cgh.2012.05.026

Klouda, L., Franklin, W. J., Saraf, A., Parekh, D. R., & Schwartz, D. D. (2017). Neurocognitive and executive functioning in adult survivors of congenital heart disease. *Congenital Heart Disease, 12*(1), 91–98. https://doi.org/10.1111/chd.12409

Lam, R. W., Iverson, G. L., Evans, V. C., Yatham, L. N., Stewart, K., Tam, E. M., . . . Woo, C. (2016). The effects of desvenlafaxine on neurocognitive and work functioning in employed outpatients with major depressive disorder. *Journal of Affective Disorders, 203*, 55–61. https://doi.org/10.1016/j.jad.2016.05.074

Levy, B. (2014). Illness severity, trait anxiety, cognitive impairment and heart rate variability in bipolar disorder. *Psychiatry Research, 220*(3), 890–895. https://doi.org/10.1016/j.psychres.2014.07.059

Littleton, A. C., Register-Mihalik, J. K., & Guskiewicz, K. M. (2015b). Test-retest reliability of a computerized concussion test: CNS Vital Signs. *Sports Health, 7*(5), 443–447. https://doi.org/10.1177/1941738115586997

Littleton, A. C., Schmidt, J. D., Register-Mihalik, J. K., Gioia, G. A., Waicus, K. M., Mihalik, J. P., & Guskiewicz, K. M. (2015a). Effects of attention deficit hyperactivity disorder and stimulant medication on concussion symptom reporting and computerized neurocognitive test performance. *Archives of Clinical Neuropsychology:, 30*(7), 683–693. https://doi.org/10.1093/arclin/acv043

Lynall, R. C., Schmidt, J. D., Mihalik, J. P., & Guskiewicz, K. M. (2016). The clinical utility of a concussion rebaseline protocol after concussion recovery. *Clinical Journal of Sport Medicine:, 26*(4), 285–290. https://doi.org/10.1097/JSM.0000000000000260

Masley, S., Roetzheim, R., & Gualtieri, T. (2009). Aerobic exercise enhances cognitive flexibility. *Journal of Clinical Psychology in Medical Settings, 16*(2), 186–193. https://doi.org/10.1007/s10880-009-9159-6

Meador, K. J., Loring, D. W., Boyd, A., Echauz, J., LaRoche, S., Velez-Ruiz, N., . . . Webster, E. (2016). Randomized double-blind comparison of cognitive and EEG effects of lacosamide and carbamazepine. *Epilepsy & Behavior:, 62,* 267–275. https://doi.org/10.1016/j.yebeh.2016.07.007

Meskal, I., Gehring, K., van der Linden, S. D., Rutten, G.-J. M., & Sitskoorn, M. M. (2015). Cognitive improvement in meningioma patients after surgery: Clinical relevance of computerized testing. *Journal of Neuro-Oncology, 121*(3), 617–625. https://doi.org/10.1007/s11060-014-1679-8

Mihalik, J. P., Lengas, E., Register-Mihalik, J. K., Oyama, S., Begalle, R. L., & Guskiewicz, K. M. (2013). The effects of sleep quality and sleep quantity on concussion baseline assessment. *Clinical Journal of Sport Medicine:, 23*(5), 343–348. https://doi.org/10.1097/JSM.0b013e318295a834

Papathanasiou, A., Messinis, L., Georgiou, V. L., & Papathanasopoulos, P. (2014). Cognitive impairment in relapsing remitting and secondary progressive multiple sclerosis patients: Efficacy of a computerized cognitive screening battery. *ISRN Neurology, 2014,* 151379. https://doi.org/10.1155/2014/151379

Papathanasiou, A., Messinis, L., Zampakis, P., Panagiotakis, G., Gourzis, P., Georgiou, V., & Papathanasopoulos, P. (2015). Thalamic atrophy predicts cognitive impairment in relapsing remitting multiple sclerosis. Effect on instrumental activities of daily living and employment status. *Journal of the Neurological Sciences, 358*(1–2), 236–242. https://doi.org/10.1016/j.jns.2015.09.001

Raszewski, G., Loroch, M., Owoc, A., Łukawski, K., Filip, R., & Bojar, I. (2015). Homocysteine and cognitive disorders of postmenopausal women measured by a battery of computer tests: Central Nervous System Vital Signs. *Archives of Women's Mental Health, 18*(4), 623–630. https://doi.org/10.1007/s00737-015-0518-z

Roten, A., Baker, N. L., & Gray, K. M. (2015). Cognitive performance in a placebo-controlled pharmacotherapy trial for youth with marijuana dependence. *Addictive Behaviors, 45,* 119–123. https://doi.org/10.1016/j.addbeh.2015.01.013

Slick, D. J., Sherman, E. M., & Iverson, G. L. (1999). Diagnostic criteria for malingered neurocognitive dysfunction: Proposed standards for clinical practice and research. *The Clinical Neuropsychologist, 13*(4), 545–561. https://doi.org/10.1076/1385-4046(199911)13:04;1-Y;FT545

Theadom, A., Parag, V., Dowell, T., McPherson, K., Starkey, N., Barker-Collo, S., . . . BIONIC Research Group. (2016). Persistent problems 1 year after mild traumatic brain injury: A longitudinal population study in New Zealand. *British Journal of General Practice:, 66*(642), e16-23. https://doi.org/10.3399/bjgp16X683161

Trinidad, K. J., Schmidt, J. D., Register-Mihalik, J. K., Groff, D., Goto, S., & Guskiewicz, K. M. (2013). Predicting clinical concussion measures at baseline based on motivation and academic profile. *Clinical Journal of Sport Medicine:, 23*(6), 462–469. https://doi.org/10.1097/JSM.0b013e318295e425

Tsai, M., Chrones, L., Xie, J., Gevorkyan, H., & Macek, T. A. (2016). A phase 1 study of the safety, tolerability, pharmacokinetics, and pharmacodynamics of TAK-063, a selective PDE10A inhibitor. *Psychopharmacology, 233*(21–22), 3787–3795. https://doi.org/10.1007/s00213-016-4412-9

Turner, C. E., Barker-Collo, S. L., Connell, C. J. W., & Gant, N. (2015). Acute hypoxic gas breathing severely impairs cognition and task learning in humans. *Physiology & Behavior, 142,* 104–110. https://doi.org/10.1016/j.physbeh.2015.02.006

Wild, K., Howieson, D., Webbe, F., Seelye, A., & Kaye, J. (2008). Status of computerized cognitive testing in aging: A systematic review. *Alzheimer's and Dementia, 4*(6), 428–437. doi: 10.1016/j.jalz.2008.07.003.

Wysokiński, A., Dzienniak, M., & Kloszewska, I. (2013). Effect of metabolic abnormalities on cognitive performance and clinical symptoms in schizophrenia. *Archives of Psychiatry and Psychotherapy, 4,* 13–25.

KAPLAN BAYCREST NEUROCOGNITIVE ASSESSMENT (KBNA)

TEST NAME	**Kaplan Baycrest Neurocognitive Assessment (KBNA)**
DOMAIN	Neuropsychological functioning
AGE RANGE	20 to 89 years
ADMINISTRATION TIME	1.5 to 2 hours
SCORING FORMAT	Hand scored
REFERENCE	Leach, L., Kaplan, E., Rewilak, D., Richards, B., & Proulx, G.B. (2000). *Kaplan Baycrest Neurocognitive Assessment.* San Antonio, TX: The Psychological Corporation. www.pearsonclinical.com

DESCRIPTION

The Kaplan Baycrest Neurocognitive Assessment (KBNA; Leach et al., 2000) was designed as a comprehensive neuropsychological battery to identify and characterize mild as well as severe forms of cognitive dysfunction in adults, including older examinees. The KBNA is intended to capture within a reasonable time period (<2 hours) the full range of neuropsychological functioning using tasks that derive from both behavioral neurology and psychometric approaches.

The KBNA has one overall index, the Total Index, along with seven core indices measuring attention and working memory, episodic memory, language, judgment, reasoning, visual-spatial skills, and constructional skills (see Table 6–9; Leach et al., 2000). Note that only half of the subtests contribute to the indices. Other tests not in the indices are those with highly skewed distributions.

TABLE 6–9 Kaplan Baycrest Neurocognitive Assessment (KBNA) Indices and Contributing Scores

INDEX	SCORES
Attention/Concentration	Sequences Total score Spatial Location Adjusted score
Immediate Memory—Recall	Word Lists 1—Recall Total score Complex Figure 1—Recall Total score
Delayed Memory—Recall	Word Lists 2—Recall Total score Complex Figure 2—Recall Total score
Delayed Memory—Recognition	Word Lists 2—Recognition Total score Complex Figure 2—Recognition Total score
Spatial Processing	Complex Figure 1—Copy/Clocks Combined score
Verbal Fluency	Verbal Fluency—Phonemic score Verbal Fluency—Semantic score
Reasoning/Conceptual Shifting	Practical Problem Solving/Conceptual Shifting Combined score
Total	Attention/Concentration Index Memory—Immediate Recall Index Memory—Delayed Recall Index Memory—Delayed Recognition Index Spatial Processing Index Verbal Fluency Index Reasoning/Conceptual Shifting Index

The KBNA has 25 subtests similar in format to those found in neuropsychological batteries with widespread clinical use, including subtests such as Orientation, Sequences, Numbers, Word Lists, Complex Figure, Motor Programming, Auditory Signal Detection, Symbol Cancellation, Clocks, Picture Naming, Sentence Reading, Reading Single Words, Spatial Location, Verbal Fluency, Praxis, Picture Recognition, Expression of Emotion, Practical Problem Solving, Conceptual Shifting, Picture Description—Oral, Auditory Comprehension, Repetition, and Picture Description—Written. See Table 6–10 for subtest descriptions. The subtests were designed to measure specific aspects of functioning and to yield multiple scores (including error analyses) so that the clinician can evaluate the processes with which the person completed the tasks.

ADMINISTRATION

Directions for administering the items, time limits, and correct responses are in the test manual. Instructions for recording information for each subtest are also provided on the record form. The subtests should be given in the numbered order in which they appear in the subtest instructions because the duration of the delay intervals are determined by the administration of the intervening tasks. The authors recommend that the test be given in one test session. However, not all subtests need be given to each client (L. Leach, personal communication, November 7, 2002); the choice depends on whether specific problems need more elaborate testing. In addition, the authors caution that circumstances may warrant deviations from the order and time frame. For example, in cases of suspected aphasia, it is suggested that the examiner begin with the Picture Naming subtest since doing so may allow the examiner to assess the impact of language disturbance on tests of memory and comprehension.

TABLE 6–10 Description of Kaplan Baycrest Neurocognitive Assessment (KBNA) Subtests

SUBTEST	DESCRIPTION
Orientation	Declarative memory for personally relevant information (e.g., date of birth, age)
Sequences	Mental control tasks (e.g., recite months of year in normal and reverse sequence, name letters that rhyme with word key)
Numbers	Recalling a set of telephone numbers in two oral-response trials and one written-response trial
Word Lists 1	Learning and remembering a list of 12 words on four list-learning trials; the list is categorized with four words representing each of three categories
Complex Figure 1	Copy of a complex figure
Motor Programming	Examinee performs five alternating movements with hands
Auditory Signal Detection	Examinee listens to a recording of alphabet letters and signals, by tapping, each time the letter A appears; subtest lasts for 195 seconds
Symbol Cancellation	Examinee is presented with a page containing more than 200 geometric figures and asked to circle the figures that match a designated target; time limit is two minutes
Clocks	Consists of five components: free drawing (with clock hands set at 10 after 11), predrawn clock, copy, reading without numbers, and reading with numbers
Word Lists 2	Free recall, cued recall, and recognition of target words from Word List 1
Complex Figure 2	Recall and recognition of Complex Figure 1
Picture Naming	Naming of 20 black-and-white line drawings; semantic and phonemic cues are provided if examinee cannot name item
Sentence Reading—Arithmetic	One task requires examinee to read two word problems out loud and calculate the answers, using paper and pencil. The second task requires solving nine calculations involving addition, subtraction, or multiplication
Reading Single Words	Examinee reads aloud a set of 10 words and five nonsense words
Spatial Location	Examinee is shown a series of figures, each consisting of a rectangle in which are arrayed three to seven dots. The design is hidden and the examinee is asked to place response chips on a response grid in the corresponding locations
Verbal Fluency	Consists of three components: "c" words, animals, and first names; one minute for each
Praxis	Tests of ideomotor praxis for intransitive (e.g., waving), transitive (e.g., turning a key), and buccofacial (e.g., blowing out a candle) movements. If examinee fails to perform any movement, the examinee is asked to imitate the examiner's performance
Picture Recognition	Examinee is presented with a series of 40 pictures including those from the Picture Naming task and is asked to indicate if each picture was presented before
Expression of Emotion	Examinee must demonstrate a series of facial expressions (angry, happy, surprised, sad); if examinee fails, they are asked to imitate the examiner's expression
Practical Problem Solving	Examiner reads aloud scenarios representing situations of urgency (e.g., if smelled smoke) and examinee has to indicate how they would respond
Conceptual Shifting	Examinee is presented with a set of four line drawings that can be variously grouped and must indicate the three drawings that are alike and in what way. The examinee must then select three of the same four designs according to another shared attribute and state or describe the attribute
Picture Description—Oral	Examinee must describe orally events depicted in a line drawing
Auditory Comprehension	Examinee is read five questions (e.g., "Do you put on your shoes after your socks?") and must respond with yes or no
Repetition	Examinee is asked to repeat five orally presented items, ranging from single words (e.g., president) to complete sentences (e.g., "If he comes, I will go")
Picture Description—Written	Examinee is asked to describe events depicted in a line-drawn scene

SCORING

Most of the subtests require little interpretation of scoring criteria. However, detailed scoring criteria are provided (see Appendix A of the test manual) for Complex Figure 1, Picture Description—Oral, Picture Description—Written, and the Free Drawing Component of Clocks.

The record form provides space to note responses, to convert raw scores to age-based scaled scores (1–19, $M = 10$, $SD = 3$), and to index scores (T score, $M = 50$, $SD = 10$) using tables in Appendices B and C of the Examiner's Manual. Percentile-rank equivalents and confidence intervals at the 90% and 95% levels are also provided for the index scores (Appendix C of the manual). A graph is also available to plot the index scores. The various process scores can also be converted to percentile ranges (<2, 2–16, >16) using age-based tables in Appendix D of the manual. These bands correspond to Below Average, Equivocal, and Average, respectively. Subtest and index discrepancy criteria are also provided (Appendix E). The difference between pairs of subtest or index scores required for statistical significance (.05 level) ranges from about four to six points. Discrepancies between indices of about 20 points or more would be considered rare, although this varies considerably depending on the particular indices selected.

DEMOGRAPHIC EFFECTS

AGE

The test authors noted that age impacts performance, with scores declining with advancing age. Accordingly, performance is evaluated relative to age-based norms.

EDUCATION

The authors report that level of education may also impact performance, and they provide some data (table 5.2 in the test manual) showing that performance across the various indices increases with increasing education. However, the various subtest and index scores are not broken down by age as well as education.

ETHNICITY, NATIONALITY, AND LINGUISTIC EFFECTS

No information is available.

NORMATIVE DATA

STANDARDIZATION SAMPLE

Norms presented in the KBNA Manual are based on a sample of 700 healthy individuals, aged 20 to 89 years, considered representative of the US population (see Table 6–11).

EVIDENCE FOR RELIABILITY

EVIDENCE FOR INTERNAL RELIABILITY

Split-half reliability coefficients for the subtests vary depending on the age group. Considering the average reliability coefficients, they range from marginal (Sequences, $r = .67$) to high (Word Lists 2-Recall, $r = .90$; see Table 6–12). The average reliability coefficients for the index scores are reported by the authors to be in the .70s to .80s. The average reliability for the total scale score is .81.

TABLE 6–11 Characteristics of the Kaplan Baycrest Neurocognitive Assessment (KBNA) Normative Sample

Sample size	700
Age	20 to 89 years
Geographic location	Proportional representation from northeast, north central, south, and west regions of the United States
Sample type	Stratified sample according to 1999 US Census data
Education	≤8 to ≥16 years
Gender	Approximate Census proportions of males and females in each age group, with 53% female overall
Race/ethnicity	For each age group, based on racial/ethnic proportions of individuals in those age bands in the US population according to Census data, with 78% Caucasian
Screening	Screened by self-report for medical and psychiatric conditions that could affect cognitive functioning

Broken down into seven age groups: 20 to 29, 30 to 39, 40 to 49, 50 to 59, 60 to 69, 70 to 79, and 80 to 89, each consisting of 100 participants.

EVIDENCE FOR TEST-RETEST RELIABILITY, MEASURING CHANGE, AND PRACTICE EFFECTS

The stability of KBNA scores was evaluated in 94 adults from the normative sample (L. Leach, personal communication, November 15, 2004) who were retested following an interval ranging from two to eight weeks. Reliability coefficients were high for the total scale ($r = .85$), but lower for the individual subtests (see Table 6–12). Many of these stability coefficients are low due to truncated distributions. Clinical classification of scores according to the three categorical dimensions in the manual (Below Average, Equivocal, Average) for many subtests is, however, relatively consistent from test to retest (see KBNA manual).

Mean retest scores are generally higher than initial scores (particularly in the areas of memory and spatial processing, where gains of about 8 to 10 standard score points were evident); however, on two of the indices (Memory—Delayed Recognition, Verbal Fluency), scores decline by about one point on retest (see manual).

EVIDENCE FOR INTERRATER RELIABILITY

Interscorer agreement for some of the subtests that require interpretation (e.g., Complex Figure; Picture Description—Oral, Written; and the Free Drawing Component of Clocks) is not provided, raising concern about the reliability of these scores.

EVIDENCE FOR VALIDITY

INDEX AND SUBTEST INTERCORRELATIONS

The subtests comprising each index were determined by the authors in part on theoretical grounds. However, intercorrelations between subtests comprising indexes are low (see Table 6–13), raising questions regarding the meaning of these indices in individual examinees. The manual provides some evidence of construct validity by examining the pattern of intercorrelations among the various indices. The authors note that the correlations between related KBNA indices (i.e., Immediate, Delayed, and Recognition Memory) are relatively high ($r = .60$ to $.80$), while correlations with other indices are relatively lower. However, in light of the low correlations between subtests, further research is needed to determine whether these index scores are measuring distinct cognitive constructs.

CORRELATIONS WITH OTHER NEUROPSYCHOLOGICAL TESTS

The authors report correlational data suggesting that the KBNA is broadly consistent with the results of other global measures of cognitive status. For example, the KBNA Total

TABLE 6–12 Magnitude of Reliability Coefficients of Kaplan Baycrest Neurocognitive Assessment (KBNA) Subtests and Indices

MAGNITUDE OF COEFFICIENT	INTERNAL CONSISTENCY	TEST-RETEST
Very high (.90+)	Word List 2–Recall	
High (.80–.89)	Word Lists 1 Word Lists 2–Recognition Complex Figure 1–Recall Complex Figure 2–Recognition Attention/Concentration Index Memory–Immediate Recall Index Memory–Delayed Recall Index Spatial Processing Index Total Index	Sequences Attention/Concentration Index Total Index
Adequate (.70–.79)	Complex Figure 2–Recall Complex Figure 1–Copy/Clocks Spatial Location Practical Problem Solving/Conceptual Shifting Memory–Delayed Recognition Index Verbal Fluency Index Reasoning/Conceptual Shifting Index	Word Lists 1 Word Lists 2–Recall Verbal Fluency–Semantic Memory-Immediate Recall Index Memory–Delayed Recall Index Memory–Delayed Recognition Index
Marginal (.60–.69)	Sequences Verbal Fluency–Phonemic Verbal Fluency–Semantic	Complex Figure 1–Recall Complex Figure 2–Recognition Spatial Location Spatial Processing Index
Low (≤.59)		Word Lists 2–Recognition Complex Figure 2–Recall Complex Figure 1–Copy/Clocks Practical Problem Solving/Conceptual Shifting Verbal Fluency Index Reasoning/Conceptual Shifting Index

Index score correlated .67 with the Wechsler Abbreviated Scale of Intelligence (WASI) Full-Scale IQ (FSIQ) in about 500 nonimpaired people who participated in the standardization sample. In a very small ($N = 14$) mixed clinical sample, the KBNA total index score correlated strongly ($r = .82$) with the total score on the Dementia Rating Scale (DRS). The KBNA Index score was also highly correlated with the DRS in a study on individuals with dementia ($r = .70$; Leach, 2010).

The authors provide some evidence of convergent validity for some of the KBNA indices in small, clinically mixed samples. Thus, correlations between the KBNA Attention/Concentration Index and various measures of attention on the WAIS-R (Digit Symbol, $r = .64$; Digit Span, $r = .76$) and Wechsler Memory Scale (WMS-III Spatial Span, $r = .71$) were high, with one exception (WMS-III Mental Control, $r = .24$). With regard to the memory indices, verbal memory (CVLT) scores showed a moderate to high degree of association with the relevant memory indices of the KBNA ($r = .48$ to .77); however, correlations were low between Rey-Osterrieth Complex Figure Test (RCFT) Delayed Recall and the delayed measures of the KBNA ($r = -.03$ to $-.12$). As might be expected, the KBNA Spatial Processing Index correlated most strongly with the RCFT Copy score, and the KBNA Reasoning/Conceptual Shifting Index showed a strong relation to WAIS-R measures of crystallized and fluid ability (Vocabulary, $r = .80$; Block Design, $r = .81$). While FAS verbal fluency correlated highly with the KBNA Verbal Fluency-Phonemic score ($r = .91$), associations between KBNA Verbal Fluency and the Boston Naming Test were lower, as would be expected ($r = .49$).

It should also be noted that no information is provided in the manual regarding the construct validity of subtests not included in the indices or of any of the process scores.

TABLE 6–13 Intercorrelations Between Subtests Comprising Indices for Ages 20–89

INDEX	CORRELATION BETWEEN INDEX SUBTESTS
Attention/Concentration	.42
Memory–Immediate Recall	.20
Memory–Delayed Recall	.24
Memory–Delayed Recognition	.22
Verbal Fluency	.57

Note that the Spatial Processing and Reasoning/Conceptual Shifting Index scores are direct linear transformations of their respective contributing scaled scores.

CLINICAL STUDIES

The authors compared a mixed sample, consisting mostly of examinees (size of sample not reported) with dementia or head injury, with a matched group of controls and found that the patients scored significantly below the nonimpaired individuals on all indices except the Reasoning/Conceptual Shifting Index. Unfortunately, no information is provided regarding the severity of impairments in the clinical sample (see manual). However, the test appears effective at differentiating MCI from depression, with a 96% correct classification rate (Monette & Leach, 2013).

In dementia, the KBNA has a 96% correct classification rate (Leach, 2010), with memory subtests showing the largest between-group effect sizes. The three subtests of Complex Figure 1 Recall, Word List 2 Recognition, and Verbal Fluency-Semantic are particularly effective at correctly classifying dementia cases. According to the authors, the Total Index Sum score (as opposed to the Total Index score) is the most useful score in terms of clinical cutoffs for determining the likelihood of dementia. A KNBA Index Sum cutoff score of 305 was found to give an optimal classification rate, with a cut-score of 295 preferable when minimizing false positives and a cut-score of 330 when minimizing false negatives (Monette & Leach, 2013). Replication of these cut-scores in larger, independent samples would be beneficial, but these do provide an initial benchmark by which to interpret scores. The authors also recommend examining scores on the three subtests with best discrimination as low scores on these are most predictive of a dementia diagnosis (Complex Figure 1 Recall, Word Lists 2 Recognition, and Verbal Fluency-Semantic). The KBNA Index is also moderately correlated with ratings of functional decline in dementia (Leach, 2010).

A subtest of the KBNA, the Spatial Location task, differentiates between individuals at high risk of schizophrenia and healthy controls (Chung et al., 2008).

NEUROANATOMICAL CORRELATES AND IMAGING STUDIES

No information is available.

PERFORMANCE VALIDITY

No information is available.

COMMENT

Unlike rapid screening tools, the KBNA provides an entire battery with potential to identify domain-specific disorders while maintaining a reasonable administration time. Thus, it has the potential to provide considerably more information than brief screens while still providing a more streamlined and efficient testing approach than a full neuropsychological battery assembled from diverse tests with different normative sets. In addition to assessing a wide array of traditional areas using well-known paradigms (e.g., verbal fluency, complex figure drawing, clock drawing), it measures behaviors commonly overlooked by neuropsychologists (e.g., praxis, emotion expression) and thus provides a more comprehensive evaluation than many other similar batteries. Furthermore, the battery approach facilitates cross-subtest comparisons afforded by a common normative sample.

The quantification of process scores (e.g., intrusions, repetitions, perseverations, semantic errors) may be an asset for some examiners, although these scores are not supported psychometrically and should not be used for clinical diagnostic purposes. Other aspects of its psychometric properties are also less than optimal. Although age-based normative data are provided, users cannot evaluate test performance in the context of both age and education. Furthermore, information on the impact of other demographic variables (e.g., gender, ethnicity/culture) is not reported. The lack of data on the impact of ethnicity suggests considerable caution in the use of the test with members of minority groups or in countries with cultural and ethnic composition different from the US.

Many subtests (except Word Lists 1 and Phonemic and Semantic Fluency) have truncated floors and ceilings. For example, an 80-year-old who recalls nothing of the Complex Figure following the delay obtains a scaled score of 5. Similarly, a 20-year-old who recognizes all of the items from the Complex Figure only achieves a scaled score of 12. Accordingly, scores from the various subtests must be interpreted with care as they offer limited discrimination at the ends of the distribution for very high or very low functioning individuals.

Information on interrater reliability for scores requiring subjective judgment is lacking. Some of the subtests have reliabilities necessitating considerable caution in interpretation—particularly when the issue of change is of concern. Apart from studies conducted by the authors, there are few data to inform on how effective the test is at identifying and characterizing different disorders. Whether it is more sensitive to impairment than other tests (e.g., DRS, Repeatable Battery for the Assessment of Neuropsychological Status [RBANS]) remains to be determined, and until suitable research is conducted, these tests may be preferred. Its sensitivity to change/progression of disorder, its association with neurological markers and brain imaging indices, and its relation to functional capacity also needs study. The lack of independent clinical studies is a major limitation in a battery designed for use in older adults where tracking of progression of potential degenerative disorders is often needed. Research on feigning and exaggeration is also needed to help users identify invalid profiles.

Of note, the KBNA yields a variety of scores, including index scores, subtest scaled scores, process scores, and discrepancy scores. Given the large number of scores that are evaluated in this battery, the process of score conversion/

recording is cumbersome. A computerized scoring program would be beneficial.

REFERENCES

Chung, Y. S., Kang, D. H., Shin, N. Y., Yoo, S. Y., & Kwon, J. S. (2008). Deficit of theory of mind in individuals at ultra-high-risk for schizophrenia. *Schizophrenia Research, 99*(1–3), 111–118.

Leach, L. (2010). The diagnostic prediction of the Kaplan-Baycrest Neurocognitive Assessment for identification of mild dementia. *Archives of Clinical Neuropsychology, 25*(5), 359–370. doi: 10.1093/arclin/acq034. Epub 2010 May 25.

Leach, L., Kaplan, E., Rewilak, D., Richards, B., & Proulx, G. B. (2000). *Kaplan Baycrest Neurocognitive Assessment.* San Antonio, TX: The Psychological Corporation.

Monette, M. C., & Leach, L. (2013). Discrimination of the cognitive profiles of MCI and depression using the KBNA. *Canadian Journal of Neurological Science, 40*(5), 670–677.

NEUROPSYCHOLOGICAL ASSESSMENT BATTERY (NAB)

TEST NAME	**Neuropsychological Assessment Battery (NAB)**
DOMAIN	Neuropsychological functioning
AGE RANGE	18 to 97 years
ADMINISTRATION TIME	75 minutes
SCORING FORMAT	Computerized or hand scored
REFERENCE	Stern, R. A., & White, T. (2003). *Neuropsychological Assessment Battery: Administration, scoring, and interpretation manual.* Lutz, FL: Psychological Assessment Resources. www.parinc.com

DESCRIPTION

The Neuropsychological Assessment Battery (NAB; Stern & White, 2003) is a modular battery of neuropsychological tests with Attention, Language, Memory, Spatial, and Executive Functions domains. A Screening Module (NAB-SM) is also available. The NAB-SM measures the same functional domains and can be administered alone or as a means to identify the need to administer the main NAB modules. For example, examinees who perform very poorly or very well on sections of the NAB-SM may not require administration of the main module(s).

The NAB has coordinated norms with a screening measure of intelligence (Reynolds Intellectual Screening Test [RIST]; Reynolds & Kamphaus, 2003; note, however, that there is now a revised version of the RIST, the RIST-2, reviewed elsewhere in this volume). This enables the examiner to use a single set of normative tables that allow for within- and between-examinee score comparisons across the NAB and enables comparison between these measures and estimated IQ level. Additional features include the provision of demographically corrected norms, the availability of two equivalent parallel forms, and the inclusion in each module of tasks that evaluate activities of daily living (ADLs). The organization of the NAB is shown in Table 6–14, and descriptions of the individual tests are provided in Table 6–15.

The NAB-SM is based on a limited range of items. NAB-SM tests are either (a) similar to the main module tests but with different stimuli and tasks parameters (e.g., Shape Learning, Story Learning), (b) shorter versions of the same tests included in the main modules (e.g., Numbers & Letters, Mazes), or (c) identical to the main module tests (e.g., Orientation, Digits Forward).

The types of testing paradigms found on the NAB are familiar to most neuropsychologists. For example, the Attention Module includes measures of forward and backward digit span. The Language Module includes measures of picture naming and comprehension of commands of increasing complexity. The Memory Module incorporates measures of list, story, and shape learning. The Spatial Module includes tests of design construction and complex figure drawing. The Executive Functions Module contains tasks such as mazes, categorization, and word generation. A novel feature is that each NAB module (except Screening) also includes one Daily Living test that is designed to be congruent with real-life behavior.

ADMINISTRATION

See the Source for details. Instructions for administration are provided on the record form. The recording, discontinue rules, and time limits are clearly displayed to examiners on the record form, so the manual is not needed during administration. Based on recommended cutoffs on the NAB-SM record form, a judgment is made regarding whether the corresponding main module should be given. Examinees who achieve very low (e.g., standard scores <74 or 75) or very high (e.g., standard scores >115) scores on a NAB-SM module may not require administration of the corresponding main module (see the section "Evidence for Validity"). If used, the NAB-SM should be administered before any other NAB modules or tests. The suggested order of domain-specific module administration is Attention, Language, Memory, Spatial, and Executive Functions.

SCORING

There are three types of NAB scores: primary, secondary, and descriptive (see Table 6–16). Primary scores represent the most important scores for interpreting performance and are also used to compute composite scores (Module

TABLE 6–14 Neuropsychological Assessment Battery (NAB) Modules, Tests, and Administration Time

MODULE	TESTS	ADMINISTRATION TIME (MIN)	INDEX SCORES
Screening Modules		45	Total Screening Index (S-NAB)
Attention	Orientation Digits Forward Digits Backward Numbers & Letters		Screening Attention Domain (S-ATT)
Language	Auditory Comprehension Naming		Screening Language Domain (S-LAN)
Memory	Shape Learning Story Learning		Screening Memory Domain (S-MEM)
Spatial	Visual Discrimination Design Construction		Screening Spatial Domain (S-SPT)
Executive Functions	Mazes Word Generation		Screening Executive Functions Domain (S-EXE)
Main Modules			Total NAB Index (T-NAB)
Attention	Orientation Digits Forward Digits Backward Dots Numbers & Letters *Driving Scenes*	45	Attention Index (ATT)
Language	Oral Production Auditory Comprehension Naming Reading Comprehension Writing *Bill Payment*	35	Language Index (LAN)
Memory	List Learning Shape Learning Story Learning *Daily Living Memory*	45	Memory Index (MEM)
Spatial	Visual Discrimination Design Construction Figure Drawing *Map Reading*	45	Spatial Index (SPT)
Executive Functions	Mazes *Judgment* Categories Word Generation	30	Executive Functions Index (EXE)

NOTE: Italicized subtests refer to Daily Living tests designed to be congruent with analogous real-world behavior.

SOURCE: Adapted from Stern and White (2003).

Index scores, Screening Domain/Index scores), which contribute equally to their respective composites (Total NAB and Screening NAB indices).

Overall, primary scores have a relatively large range of possible raw scores and approximately normal distributions. Secondary scores have skewed distributions and/or limited score ranges. All secondary scores are scaled so that higher percentiles reflect better performance. Descriptive scores have highly skewed score distributions and/or limited score ranges. Higher cumulative percentages reflect better performance for all scores except List Learning Perseverations and List Learning Intrusions; for these two scores, higher cumulative percentages reflect poorer performance. Secondary and descriptive scores are provided as sources of qualitative information.

For the Screening Module, selected primary T scores are summed to obtain each Screening Domain score, and the five Screening Domain scores are summed to obtain the Total Screening Index (S-NAB). Similarly, for each of the main domain-specific modules, a Module Index score is calculated as the sum of selected primary T scores in that module. The Total NAB Index (T-NAB) is based on the sum of the five Module Index scores and represents the examinee's overall performance.

TABLE 6–15 Description of Neuropsychological Assessment Battery (NAB) Tasks

MODULE	TEST	DESCRIPTION
Attention	Orientation	Examinee asked to answer questions about orientation to self, time, place, and situation (e.g., name, year, city, why here).
Attention	Digits Forward	Examinee asked to repeat digits spoken by the examiner (span length is three to nine).
Attention	Digits Backward	Examinee asked to orally reverse digits spoken by the examiner (span length is three to nine).
Attention	Dots	An array of dots is briefly exposed, followed by a blank interference page, followed by a new array with one additional dot that the examinee is asked to identify.
Attention	Numbers & Letters	Part A: a letter-cancellation task requiring the examinee to mark target Xs in 24 rows of numbers and letters Part B: examinee asked to count the number of Xs in each row and write the total at the end of each row. Part C: examinee asked to add the numbers in each row and write the sum at the end of each row. Part D: examinee asked to mark a slash through each X and simultaneously add the numbers and write the sum at the end of each row.
Attention	Driving Scenes	Examinee presented with a base stimulus depicting a driving scene as viewed from behind the steering wheel of a car. Examinee is presented with additional scenes and must identify modifications.
Language	Oral Production	Examinee asked to orally describe a scene in a picture.
Language	Auditory Comprehension	Six separate subtests that require the examinee to listen to orally presented commands and to respond by pointing to stimuli such as (a) colored rectangles, (b) geometric shapes, and (c) colored geometric shapes with numbers printed on them; or to respond (d) by pointing to body parts or places in the room; (e) by answering orally presented pairs of yes/no questions; or (f) by folding paper according to one- to four-step commands.
Language	Naming	The examinee is asked to name pictured items.
Language	Reading Comprehension	The examinee is asked to select the target word or sentence from a set of foils that best matches a photograph of an object or a scene.
Language	Writing	A narrative writing sample depicted in a stimulus picture.
Language	Bill Payment	The examinee is presented with a bill statement, a blank check, a check ledger, and an envelope and is asked to respond to questions based on the available information.
Memory	List Learning	Three learning trials of a 12-word list, followed by an interference list, then short-delay free recall, long-delay free recall, and long-delay forced-choice recognition task. The word list includes three semantic categories with four words in each category.
Memory	Shape Learning	Three learning trials of nine target nonsense shapes, each learning trial followed by nine, four-stimulus, multiple-choice recognition items (target and three foils). After a 15-minute delay, there is another multiple-choice recognition trial, followed by an 18-item forced-choice, yes/no recognition trial composed of nine targets and nine foils.
Memory	Story Learning	Includes two learning trials of a passage, separate measures of verbatim and gist recall, and both immediate and delayed recall trials.
Memory	Daily Living Memory	The examinee is asked to learn a name, address, and phone number as well as medication dosing instructions; involves immediate free recall, delayed free recall, and delayed multiple-choice recognition trials.
Spatial	Visual Discrimination	Requires matching of nonsense shapes to one of four choices (target and three foils).
Spatial	Design Construction	Examinee uses shapes to reproduce designs of increasing difficulty.
Spatial	Figure Drawing	Requires copying and immediate free recall of a complex figure; the scoring system includes an overall summary score (based on presence, accuracy, and placement of elements) as well as an evaluation of qualitative features: fragmentation, planning, and organization. A pen-switching procedure is used.
Spatial	Map Reading	Examinee is asked to respond to a number of questions regarding map locations/directions.
Executive Functions	Mazes	Examinee is asked to trace a route through mazes of increasing difficulty.
Executive Functions	Judgment	Examinee is asked to answer a series of questions about home safety, health, and medical issues.
Executive Functions	Concept Formation	Two panels of photographs of six adults with identifying information are presented. For each panel, the examinee is asked to indicate as many ways as possible to sort the photos into two categories.
Executive Functions	Word Generation	Examinee is presented with a set of letters from which to generate as many three-letter words as possible within a specific time limit.

SOURCE: Adapted from Stern and White (2003). Reproduced by special permission of the Publisher, Psychological Assessment Resources, Inc. (PAR), 16204 North Florida Avenue, Lutz, Florida 33549, from the Neuropsychological Assessment Battery by Robert A. Stern, PhD and Travis White, PhD, Copyright 2001, 2003 by PAR. Further reproduction is prohibited without permission from PAR.

TABLE 6–16 Types of Neuropsychological Assessment Battery (NAB) Test Scores

SCORE TYPE	DESCRIPTION	NORMATIVE METRIC
Primary	Most important; in most cases, there is only one primary score per test; but some tests yield multiple primary scores. Select primary scores contribute to composites: Module Index, Screening Domain/Index scores.	Primary test scores are converted to T scores (*M* = 50, *SD* = 10). Module Indices, Screening Domain scores, S-NAB and T-NAB indices have a mean of 100 and *SD* of 15.
Secondary	Less important but can provide significant information; have lower reliability and nonparametric distributions; do not contribute to Module Index and T-NAB Index scores.	Percentiles by nine age groups.
Descriptive	Have poor reliability and/or highly skewed distributions in healthy people; provide qualitative indicators of performance; do not contribute to Module Index and T-NAB Index scores.	Cumulative percentages for the overall sample.

DEMOGRAPHIC EFFECTS

AGE

Age affects performance (White & Stern, 2003b; Yochim et al., 2009; Yochim et al., 2015). Buczylowska and Petermann (2016) reported age effects on a German adaptation of the NAB Executive Functions subtests in a large sample (n = 484) of healthy adults 18 to 99 years of age. In general, the subtests that showed the most age-related decline also showed the greatest score heterogeneity (e.g., Mazes, Categories), whereas Letter Fluency (a subtest that is unique to the German adaptation), Word Generation, and Judgment showed less decline and score heterogeneity.

GENDER

Gender tends to have a small effect on performance (White & Stern, 2003a; NAB Naming, Yochim et al., 2009). Buczylowska and Petermann (2016) reported that men outperform women on Mazes and women outperform men on Letter Fluency.

EDUCATION AND IQ

Education and IQ also impact test scores, although typically less so than age (White & Stern, 2003a). Yochim et al. (2009) found moderate correlations between education and Naming in older adults.

ETHNICITY, NATIONALITY, AND LINGUISTIC EFFECTS

The impact of ethnicity is not reported, although the authors indicate that all items were reviewed for bias, and the items with the highest biases were eliminated. Of note, the NAB has been translated into German (Buczylowska et al., 2013), and many NAB subtests have been translated into many other languages (contact Psychological Assessment Resources, who publishes the NAB, for additional details regarding translated versions).

NORMATIVE DATA

The NAB standardization data were collected in 2001 to 2002 at five sites selected to provide representation in each of four geographic regions of the United States, including Rhode Island, Florida, Indiana, and Los Angeles (California). The NAB provides both demographically corrected norms (n = 1,448) and age-based, US Census-matched norms (n = 950), consisting of a subsample of the overall NAB standardization sample selected to closely match the US population with respect to education, gender, ethnicity, and geographic region.

The demographically corrected norms are the primary normative standard and facilitate interpretation of an individual's NAB performance relative to healthy individuals of the same age, gender, and educational level. The characteristics of the demographically corrected standardization sample are shown in Table 6–17. Of the 1,448 participants, 711 were administered Form 1 and 737 were administered Form 2 as part of the standardization study. None of the examinees completed both forms.

TABLE 6–17 Characteristics of the Neuropsychological Assessment Battery (NAB) Demographically Corrected Normative Sample

Sample size	1,448
Age	18 to 97[a]
Geographic location	21% Northeast 23% Midwest 33% South 23% West
Sample type	Community-dwelling individuals
Education	21%[b] ≤11 years 23% 12 years 27% 13–15 years 29% ≥16 years
Gender	47% Men 54% Women
Ethnicity	85% Caucasian 7% African American 5% Hispanic 4% Other
Screening	Screened for substance abuse and medical, psychiatric, motor, or sensory conditions that could potentially affect performance; in addition, 14 participants judged to be disoriented on the basis of their Orientation scores were excluded.

[a]The sample was divided into the following age groups: 18 to 29, 30 to 39, 40 to 49, 50 to 59, 60 to 64, 65 to 69, 70 to 74, 75 to 79, and 80 to 97. Note that a majority of the participants in the oldest age group were less than 90 years of age.

[b]A graduate equivalency degree (GED) was coded as 11 years.

Raw primary scores for each test are converted to *z* scores, which are then converted to T scores (e.g., by gender, age group, and education level) and percentiles. In general, T scores less than 40 are categorized as impaired. Secondary raw scores are converted to percentiles, and descriptive raw scores are converted to cumulative percentages. Secondary score percentiles less than the 16th percentile are categorized as impaired.

Selected primary T scores are used to obtain Module Domain/Index scores, and the latter are used to obtain Total Index scores. These summary scores are converted to standard scores ($M = 100$, $SD = 15$). The T-NAB Index represents the sum of the five module indices, with each module contributing equally to the T-NAB Index. Similarly, the S-NAB reflects the sum of the five Screening Domain scores. Index scores below 85 are classified as impaired.

Tables are also provided in the manual to determine the significance and rarity of between-score differences, frequencies of score differences, and comparisons of raw scores and intelligence scores (i.e., as measured by the RIST). Brooks, Iverson, and White (2009) presented RIST-NAB discrepancy scores (see Table 6–18). Fewer than 20% of participants had NAB index scores more than 16 to 18 points below their RIST Index scores.

BASE RATES OF LOW SCORES

The importance of attending to base rates of low scores, specifically the proportion of low scores among healthy people, is illustrated in research involving the NAB. For example, Brooks, Iverson, and White (2007) examined base rates of low memory scores in more than 700 older adults from the standardization sample using memory scores from the Memory Module of the NAB. Of the 10

TABLE 6–18 Cumulative Percentages of Sample with Uncommon RIST-NAB Discrepancies

	CUMULATIVE PERCENTAGE OF SAMPLE WITH RIST–NAB DISCREPANCY SCORES				
GROUPS AND DISCREPANCY SCORES	<20%	<15%	<10%	<5%	<1%
All older adults					
RIST-Attention Index	18–21	22–24	25–31	32–41	42+
RIST-Language Index	17–19	20–23	24–27	28–41	42+
RIST-Memory Index	17–19	20–23	24–28	29–37	38+
RIST-Spatial Index	18–20	21–23	24–28	29–36	37+
RIST-Executive Functions Index	17–19	20–23	24–27	28–35	36+
RIST-Total Index	16–18	19–22	23–25	26–33	34+
Low average intellectual abilities					
RIST-Attention Index	13–14	15–16	17–18	19–23	24+
RIST-Language Index	11	12–14	15–18	19–34	35+
RIST-Memory Index	12–13	14	15	16–19	20+
RIST-Spatial Index	12–13	14–15	16–17	18–23	24+
RIST-Executive Functions Index	11–12	13–14	15–16	17–21	22+
RIST-Total Index	11–13	14–16	17–18	19–26	27+
Average intellectual abilities					
RIST-Attention Index	12–14	15–17	18–21	22–32	33+
RIST-Language Index	12–13	14–16	17–21	22–32	33+
RIST-Memory Index	12–14	15–17	18–19	20–30	31+
RIST-Spatial Index	12–13	14–17	18–21	22–32	33+
RIST-Executive Functions Index	12–15	16–17	18–22	23–29	30+
RIST-Total Index	12–13	14–15	16–21	22–25	26+
High average intellectual abilities					
RIST-Attention Index	24–26	27–29	30–32	33–43	44+
RIST-Language Index	20–22	23–25	26	27–35	36+
RIST-Memory Index	22–24	25–26	27–29	30–40	41+
RIST-Spatial Index	22–25	26–28	29–30	31–36	37+
RIST-Executive Functions Index	21–22	23–26	27–30	31–36	37+
RIST-Total Index	21–22	23–24	25–27	28–34	35+
Superior/very superior intellectual abilities					
RIST-Attention Index	32	33–39	40–44	45–49	50+
RIST-Language Index	34	35–37	38–43	44–62	63+
RIST-Memory Index	30–32	33–35	36–40	41–49	50+
RIST-Spatial Index	28–30	31–34	35–37	38–47	48+
RIST-Executive Functions Index	28–29	30–32	33–36	37–49	50+
RIST-Total Index	26–28	29–30	31–36	37–49	50+

NOTE: %ile, percentile. RIST = Reynolds Intellectual Screening Test; NAB = Neuropsychological Assessment Battery. The difference scores were created by subtracting the NAB Index score from the RIST score. Intellectual abilities are based on the RIST Index and comprise the following scores: Low average, RIST = 80-89; Average, RIST = 90-109; High average, RIST = 110–119; Superior/very superior, RIST = 120+.

SOURCE: Brooks et al. (2009). Reproduced by special permission of the Publisher, Psychological Assessment Resources, Inc. (PAR), 16204 North Florida Avenue, Lutz, Florida 33549, from the Neuropsychological Assessment Battery by Robert A. Stern, PhD and Travis White, PhD, Copyright 2001, 2003 by PAR. Further reproduction is prohibited without permission from PAR.

TABLE 6–19 Neuropsychological Assessment Battery (NAB) Base Rates of Low Memory Index Scores (Age 55 to 79 Years)

		CUTOFF SCORES			
	N	<1 *SD*	<10TH %ILE	≤5TH %ILE	<2 *SD*
Total Sample	742	14.4	8.8	4.4	1.5
Age Groups					
55–59	80	12.5	7.5	5.0	2.5
60–64	162	13.6	7.4	3.7	0.6
65–69	171	14.0	8.8	4.7	1.2
70–74	173	12.1	8.1	4.0	1.7
75–79	156	19.2	11.5	5.1	1.9
Education Groups					
≤11 years	172	14.5	9.3	5.8	2.3
12 years	184	13.6	8.7	4.3	1.1
13–15 years	183	19.1	9.8	4.4	2.2
16+ years	203	10.8	7.4	3.4	0.5
RIST Score Groups					
80–89	85	44.7	28.2	21.2	8.2
90–109	382	13.1	7.6	2.9	0.8
110–119	166	4.8	3.0	0.0	0.0
120+	100	5.0	2.0	0.0	0.0

NOTE: %ile, percentile; *SD*, standard deviation; RIST = Reynolds Intellectual Screening Test.
SOURCE: Brooks et al. (2007).

demographically corrected T scores, nearly 31% of the healthy sample obtained one or more memory scores 1.5 *SD* or more below the mean, with low-average intellectual ability associated with a higher base rate of impairment (i.e., approximately 56% of the sample compared to approximately 21% in participants with high-average intellectual ability). Base rates of low Memory Index scores (i.e., percent of participants scoring below cutoffs) are depicted in Table 6–19. Cumulative percentages and percentages of low scores by age, education, and RIST score are shown in Tables 6–20 to 6–22.

As can be seen in the tables, obtaining one low score is not unusual, especially a low score defined as 1 *SD* or lower. However, examination of the data indicates that the probability of obtaining a low score interacts with specific variables, such as age (older age is related to higher base rates of low scores) and intellectual function (higher intelligence is related to fewer low scores, lower intelligence is related to more low scores). The information provided by Brooks et al. therefore suggests that demographic characteristics (age, education, intelligence) should be considered when evaluating the clinical significance of low scores to avoid overidentification of impairment.

EVIDENCE FOR RELIABILITY

EVIDENCE FOR INTERNAL RELIABILITY

Many of the NAB primary subtests were excluded from internal reliability analyses due to the use of a unique item presentation format with inter-item dependency issues that would artificially inflate the reliability estimate and the use of speeded performance formats for a number of test measures (White & Stern, 2003b). The range of alpha coefficients in the normative sample is quite diverse for selected primary scores for the six modules when averaged for both forms across the age groups. As shown in Table 6–23, coefficients range from high (e.g., Oral Production; Story Learning Phrase Unit, Immediate and Delayed Recall) to inadequate, likely in part due to the limited range of scores on some tests (e.g., Auditory Comprehension, Screening Naming) and construct heterogeneity (e.g., Judgment).

Generalizability coefficients were used to calculate the reliability estimates of the Screening Domain, S-NAB, Module Index, and T-NAB Index scores. The reliabilities for the Screening Domain scores varied (e.g., $r = .55$ for the Screening Language Domain score to $r = .91$ for the Screening Attention Domain score). The S-NAB reliability coefficient was .80. The Module Index scores reliabilities tended to be higher ($r = .79$ for the Language Index score to $r = .93$ for both the Attention and Memory Index scores). The reliability coefficient of the T-NAB Index score was very high ($r = .96$).

Internal reliability in clinical groups varies by group and by subtest. For example, internal reliability of the Judgment subtest was high in a sample of older adults from assisted living facilities referred for neuropsychological assessment in a memory disorders clinic (Cronbach's alpha = .83; MacDougall & Mansbach, 2013). Sachs, Rush, and Pedraza (2016) reported adequate internal reliability of the Naming subtest in a sample of patients consecutively referred for neuropsychological assessment (Cronbach's alpha = .78, .77). Zgaljardic and Temple (2010b) reported poor internal reliability for scores comprising the Screening Module in their sample of patients with moderate to severe brain injury in residential rehabilitation (Cronbach's alpha for Memory = .42 to Executive Functions = −.37) and marginal internal reliability for the composite score from the NAB (Cronbach's alpha = .60).

Tables are provided in the manual (White & Stern, 2003b) that summarize the various reliability estimates and the standard errors of measurement (*SEMs*). Note that the *SEMs* are quite large. For the Screening Module, *SEMs* range from 4.5 to 10.06 (Screening Attention, Screening Language, respectively). For scores derived from the main modules, *SEMs* range from 3.00 to 6.87 (T-NAB Index, Language Index, respectively). Because *SEMs* are large, confidence intervals are also sizable.

Users should note that Pearson correlations and associated *SEMs* are presented to evaluate the stability of primary scores and Module indices for each form separately. In contrast, generalizability coefficients (and associated *SEMs*) are provided with regard to equivalent forms reliability. *SEMs* based on generalizability coefficients appear smaller than those based on Pearson correlations.

TABLE 6–20 Neuropsychological Assessment Battery (NAB) Base Rates of Low Memory Index Scores by Age Group

# OF LOW SCORES	TOTAL SAMPLE (N = 742)		AGE GROUPS 55–59 (N = 80)		60–64 (N = 162)		65–69 (N = 171)		70–74 (N = 173)		75–79 (N = 156)		# OF LOW SCORES
	P	CP	P	CP	P	CP	P	CP	P	CP	P	CP	
<1 SD													*<1 SD*
9	0.4	0.4	2.5	2.5	–	–	–	–	–	–	0.6	0.6	9
8	0.7	1.1	0.0	2.5	–	–	1.2	1.2	0.6	0.6	1.3	1.9	8
7	1.3	2.4	2.5	5.0	0.6	0.6	1.8	3.0	1.2	1.8	1.3	3.2	7
6	2.6	5.0	0.0	5.0	2.5	3.1	1.2	4.2	4.0	5.8	3.8	7.0	6
5	2.6	7.6	1.3	6.3	2.5	5.6	1.8	6.0	2.9	8.7	3.8	10.8	5
4	4.6	12.2	2.5	8.8	5.6	11.2	5.3	11.3	2.3	11.0	6.4	17.2	4
3	6.3	18.5	7.5	16.3	5.6	16.8	7.0	18.3	7.5	18.5	4.5	21.7	3
2	11.5	30.0	12.5	28.8	10.5	27.3	17.5	35.8	10.4	28.9	6.4	28.1	2
1	25.5	55.5	25.0	53.8	27.2	54.5	22.2	58.0	28.9	57.8	23.7	51.8	1
0	44.6	100	46.3	100	45.7	100	42.1	100	42.2	100	48.1	100	0
<10th %ile													<10th %ile
9	0.1	0.1	1.3	1.3	–	–	–	–	–	–	–	–	9
8	0.0	0.1	0.0	1.3	–	–	–	–	–	–	–	–	8
7	0.5	0.6	1.3	2.6	–	–	1.2	1.2	–	–	0.6	0.6	7
6	1.3	1.9	0.0	2.6	0.6	0.6	0.6	1.8	2.3	2.3	2.6	3.2	6
5	1.5	3.4	1.3	3.9	1.9	2.5	2.3	4.1	0.0	2.3	1.9	5.1	5
4	3.2	6.6	1.3	5.2	2.5	5.0	1.8	5.9	4.6	6.9	5.1	10.2	4
3	4.2	10.8	5.0	10.2	6.8	11.8	1.8	7.7	3.5	10.4	4.5	14.7	3
2	7.8	18.6	11.3	21.5	6.8	18.6	11.7	19.4	6.9	17.3	3.8	18.5	2
1	20.2	38.8	16.3	37.8	18.5	37.1	22.8	42.2	21.4	38.7	19.9	38.4	1
0	61.1	100	62.5	100	63.0	100	57.9	100	61.3	100	61.5	100	0
≤5th %ile													≤5th %ile
6+	0.6	0.6	1.3	1.3	0.6	0.6	–	–	–	–	1.2	1.2	6+
5	1.5	2.1	2.5	3.8	0.0	0.6	2.3	2.3	2.3	2.3	0.6	1.8	5
4	2.6	4.7	0.0	3.8	3.1	3.7	0.6	2.9	2.9	5.2	5.1	6.9	4
3	3.2	7.9	3.8	7.6	4.3	8.0	3.5	6.4	1.7	6.9	3.2	10.1	3
2	5.5	13.4	7.5	15.1	5.6	13.6	5.8	12.2	5.2	12.1	4.5	14.6	2
1	17.4	30.8	15.0	30.1	16.0	29.6	17.5	29.7	19.7	31.8	17.3	31.9	1
0	69.3	100	70.0	100	70.4	100	70.2	100	68.2	100	67.9	100	0
<2 SDs													*<2 SDs*
6+	0.1	0.1	1.3	1.3	–	–	–	–	–	–	–	–	6+
5	0.0	0.1	0.0	1.3	–	–	–	–	–	–	–	–	5
4	0.3	0.4	0.0	1.3	–	–	0.6	0.6	0.6	0.6	–	–	4
3	1.3	1.9	1.3	2.6	1.2	1.2	2.3	2.9	1.2	1.8	1.3	1.3	3
2	3.4	5.3	3.8	6.4	1.9	3.1	2.3	5.2	4.6	6.4	4.5	5.8	2
1	11.1	16.4	12.5	18.9	13.0	16.1	11.1	16.3	9.2	15.6	10.3	16.1	1
0	83.7	100	81.3	100	84.0	100	83.6	100	84.4	100	84.0	100	0

NOTE: %ile, percentile; *SD*, standard deviation; P, Percentage; CP, Cumulative Percentage.

SOURCE: Brooks et al. (2007).

EVIDENCE FOR TEST-RETEST RELIABILITY, MEASURING CHANGE, AND PRACTICE EFFECTS

The authors (White & Stern, 2003b) indicate that the stability of both NAB forms was assessed with an average test-retest interval of more than six months (M = 193.1 days, SD = 20.3) sampled across a wide age range (20 to 97 years). Healthy individuals (n = 45) were given Form 1 on two occasions, and 50 healthy people were administered Form 2 on two occasions. Reliability coefficients for Form 2 tend to be somewhat higher than those for Form 1 (e.g., S-NAB coefficient for Form 1 is r = .66, and r = .85 for Form 2; T-NAB coefficient for Form 1 is r = .74, r = .89 for Form 2). As Table 6–23 shows, test-retest correlations of the primary scores tend to be marginal or low. As might be expected, composite scores tend to be more stable than the individual test scores. However, reliabilities of some of the domains (e.g., Language, Screening Spatial, Executive Functions) are weak. Of note, the retest interval is longer than that of most published tests.

To examine the temporal stability of the secondary and descriptive scores, a percentage agreement coefficient was calculated with test and retest scores divided into three categories based on standard deviation units (≤−2.0 SD, −1.9 to +1.9 SD, ≥2.0 SD). The test and retest ranges were then evaluated to determine the percentage agreement of each category from test to retest. Using this method, the authors reported a high classification agreement (based on the

TABLE 6–21 Neuropsychological Assessment Battery (NAB) Base Rates of Low Memory Index Scores by Education

	EDUCATION								
# OF LOW SCORES	≤11 YEARS (*N* = 172)		12 YEARS (*N* = 184)		13–15 YEARS (*N* = 183)		16+ YEARS (*N* = 203)		# OF LOW SCORES
	P	CP	P	CP	P	CP	P	CP	
<1 *SD*									<1 *SD*
9	0.6	0.6	0.5	0.5	0.5	0.5	–	–	9
8	0.6	1.2	0.0	0.5	1.1	1.6	1.0	1.0	8
7	2.3	3.5	0.5	1.0	1.6	3.2	1.0	2.0	7
6	3.5	7.0	3.3	4.3	2.2	5.4	1.5	3.5	6
5	1.7	8.7	2.7	7.0	3.3	8.7	2.5	6.0	5
4	2.9	11.6	4.9	11.9	6.0	14.7	4.4	10.4	4
3	5.8	17.4	6.5	18.4	8.7	23.4	4.4	14.8	3
2	11.0	28.4	13.6	32.0	10.9	34.3	10.3	25.1	2
1	27.9	56.3	21.2	53.2	23.5	57.8	29.1	54.2	1
0	43.6	100	46.7	100	42.1	100	45.8	100	0
<10th %ile									<10th %ile
9	–	–	0.5	0.5	–	–	–	–	9
8	–	–	0.0	0.5	–	–	–	–	8
7	0.6	0.6	0.0	0.5	1.1	1.1	0.5	0.5	7
6	1.2	1.8	0.5	1.0	1.6	2.7	2.0	2.5	6
5	2.3	4.1	2.2	3.2	1.1	3.8	0.5	3.0	5
4	3.5	7.6	3.3	6.5	3.3	7.1	3.0	6.0	4
3	3.5	11.1	4.3	10.8	6.0	13.1	3.0	9.0	3
2	7.6	18.7	7.1	17.9	8.7	21.8	7.9	16.9	2
1	22.7	41.4	17.4	35.3	19.1	40.9	21.7	38.6	1
0	58.7	100	64.7	100	59.0	100	61.6	100	0
≤5th %ile									≤5th %ile
7	-	–	–	–	0.5	0.5	0.5	0.5	7
6	–	–	0.5	0.5	0.0	0.5	0.5	1.0	6
5	1.7	1.7	0.5	1.0	1.6	2.1	2.0	3.0	5
4	3.5	5.2	3.3	4.3	2.2	4.3	1.5	4.5	4
3	4.1	9.3	3.8	8.1	3.8	8.1	1.5	6.0	3
2	4.1	13.4	6.0	14.1	7.1	15.2	4.9	10.9	2
1	20.9	34.3	15.8	29.9	14.8	30.0	18.2	29.1	1
0	65.7	100	70.1	100	69.9	100	70.9	100	0
<2 *SDs*									<2 *SDs*
6	–	–	–	–	0.5	0.5	–	–	6
5	–	–	–	–	0.0	0.5	–	–	5
4	0.6	0.6	–	–	0.5	1.0	–	–	4
3	1.2	1.8	0.5	0.5	1.1	2.1	3.0	3.0	3
2	2.3	4.1	3.8	4.3	4.9	7.0	2.5	5.5	2
1	13.4	17.5	10.9	15.2	9.3	16.3	10.8	16.3	1
0	82.6	100	84.8	100	83.6	100	83.7	100	0

NOTE: %ile, percentile; *SD*, standard deviation; P, Percentage; CP, Cumulative Percentage.

SOURCE: Brooks et al. (2007).

average correct classification performance for all ages; see Table 6–24).

Practice effects are evident for most of the NAB tasks; however, gains are small (≤2 T-score points) across a six-month interval (White & Stern, 2003b). With the exception of the Screening Memory Domain score, the NAB Screening Domain scores demonstrate relatively small practice effects (less than half of a standard deviation). A similar pattern of practice effects is seen for the Module Index scores and the T-NAB Index score. Of note, healthy controls and people with MCI show practice effects on NAB memory measures, whereas persons with AD tend to show stability or decline across testing sessions (Gavett et al., 2016).

Brooks et al. (2009) provide test-retest data (test-retest interval, *M* = 6.7 months, *SD* = 6.9 months) for 742 older adults from the standardization sample (age, *M* = 67.3 years, *SD* = 8.3 years). Difference scores (Time 2 – Time 1) were calculated, and frequency distributions were created for each difference score. Cutoffs for interpreting change were determined using cumulative percentile ranks corresponding to the 20th and 10th percentiles, and cutoff scores are presented in Table 6–25. Cutoff scores for declines vary depending on the domain scores used. For example, declines range from 3 to 14 points for the Attention tests and improvements on Attention tests range from 7 to 17 points.

TABLE 6–22 Neuropsychological Assessment Battery (NAB) Base Rates of Low Memory Index Scores by Intellectual Function (RIST)

# OF LOW SCORES	RIST SCORE 80–89 (*N* = 85) P	CP	90–109 (*N* = 382) P	CP	110–119 (*N* = 166) P	CP	120 + (*N* = 100) P	CP	# OF LOW SCORES
<1 *SD*									<1 *SD*
9	1.2	1.2	0.3	0.3	–	–	–	–	9
8	3.5	4.7	0.5	0.8	–	–	–	–	8
7	7.1	11.8	0.5	1.3	–	–	–	–	7
6	12.9	24.7	1.6	2.9	0.6	0.6	–	–	6
5	7.1	31.8	2.6	5.5	0.6	1.2	2.0	2.0	5
4	5.9	37.7	5.5	11.0	1.8	3.0	4.0	6.0	4
3	9.4	47.1	8.1	19.1	3.0	6.0	1.0	7.0	3
2	10.6	57.7	11.5	30.6	12.7	18.7	10.0	17.0	2
1	22.4	80.1	25.4	56.0	27.7	46.4	27.0	44.0	1
0	20.0	100	44.0	100	53.6	100	56.0	100	0
<10th %ile									<10th %ile
7	4.7	4.7	–	–	–	–	–	–	7
6	3.5	8.2	1.3	1.3	–	–	–	–	6
5	9.4	17.6	0.8	2.1	–	–	–	–	5
4	8.2	25.8	3.4	5.5	0.6	0.6	2.0	2.0	4
3	4.7	30.5	4.7	10.2	1.8	2.4	3.0	5.0	3
2	14.1	44.6	8.4	18.6	4.2	6.6	6.0	11.0	2
1	21.2	65.8	20.2	38.8	24.7	31.3	14.0	25.0	1
0	34.1	100	61.3	100	68.7	100	75.0	100	0
≤5th %ile									≤5th %ile
7	2.4	2.4	–	–	–	–	–	–	7
6	1.2	3.6	–	–	–	–	–	–	6
5	8.2	11.8	0.5	0.5	–	–	–	–	5
4	10.6	22.4	2.4	2.9	–	–	1.0	1.0	4
3	4.7	27.1	3.7	6.6	0.6	0.6	1.0	2.0	3
2	5.9	33.0	6.8	13.4	2.4	3.0	6.0	8.0	2
1	23.5	56.5	17.8	31.2	18.1	21.1	10.0	18.0	1
0	43.5	100	68.8	100	78.9	100	82.0	100	0
<2 *SDs*									<2 *SDs*
6	1.2	1.2	–	–	–	–	–	–	6
5	0.0	1.2	–	–	–	–	–	–	5
4	2.4	3.6	–	–	–	–	–	–	4
3	5.9	9.5	0.8	0.8	0.6	0.6	1.0	1.0	3
2	3.5	13.0	3.7	4.5	1.2	1.8	3.0	4.0	2
1	20.0	33.0	11.8	16.3	6.6	8.4	7.0	11.0	1
0	67.1	100	83.8	100	91.6	100	89.0	100	0

NOTE: %ile, percentile; *SD*, standard deviation; P, Percentage; CP, Cumulative Percentage.

SOURCE: Brooks et al. (2007).

EVIDENCE FOR RELIABILITY OF ALTERNATE, SHORT, OR COMPUTER FORMS

The manual reports a generalizability study in which 100 participants (age 18–84 years, $M = 57.9$ years, $SD = 19.5$) were given Forms 1 and 2 in a counterbalanced design. The mean interval between administrations was 25 days ($SD = 6.3$). Median generalizability coefficients for the Screening Module and for the primary scores tended to exceed .60, suggesting adequate reliability. Yochim et al. (2009) reported slightly lower alternate forms reliability for the Naming subtest (Spearman's rho = .45). Use of Spearman's rho rather than Pearson correlations may have lowered the estimate. Sachs et al. (2016) reported adequate alternate forms reliability ($r = .78$) in a sample of adults referred for neuropsychological assessment.

EVIDENCE FOR INTERRATER RELIABILITY

Thirty Form 1 and 30 Form 2 standardization protocols were independently scored by two raters (White & Stern, 2003b), with interrater reliability evaluated for the following subtests that require some subjectivity: Writing, Story Learning, Figure Drawing, Judgment, and Categories. Scoring reliability was high for all subtests evaluated.

EVIDENCE FOR VALIDITY

WITHIN-TEST CORRELATIONS

The intercorrelations between the primary scores of subtests that comprise a module domain tend to be positive and of modest to moderate strength. In general, the module primary scores correlate most highly with

TABLE 6–23 Magnitude of Reliability Coefficients for Neuropsychological Assessment Battery (NAB) Primary Scores and Domains and Total Index Scores for the Demographically Corrected Standardization Sample for All Age Groups

	INTERNAL RELIABILITY[a]	TEST-RETEST PRIMARY SCORES	TEST-RETEST DOMAIN AND TOTAL INDEX SCORES
Very high (.90+)			
High (.80–.89)	Oral Production Story Learning Phrase Unit IR Story Learning Phrase Unit DR	Numbers & Letters Part A Speed Numbers & Letters Part A Efficiency	Attention Index T-NAB Index
Adequate (.70–.79)	Screening Digits Forward Screening Digits Backward Screening Story Learning DR Naming Mazes	Screening Numbers & Letters Part A Efficiency Naming	Screening Attention Domain S-NAB Spatial Index
Marginal (.60–.69)	Screening Story Learning IR Bill Payment Shape Learning IR Visual Discrimination Design Construction Map Reading	Screening Digits Forward Screening Digits Backward Screening Numbers & Letters Part A Speed Screening Mazes Screening Word Generation Numbers & Letters Part D Efficiency Driving Scenes Story Learning Phrase Unit DR Design Construction Word Generation	Screening Language Domain Screening Executive Functions Domain Memory Index Executive Functions Index
Low (≤.59)	Screening Auditory Comprehension Screening Naming Screening Visual Discrimination Screening Design Construction Screening Mazes Auditory Comprehension Shape Learning DR Judgment	Screening Numbers & Letters Part A Errors Screening Numbers & Letters Part B Efficiency Screening Auditory Comprehension Screening Naming Screening Shape Learning IR & DR Screening Story Learning IR & DR Screening Visual Discrimination Screening Design Construction Dots Numbers & Letters Part A Errors Numbers & Letters Part B Efficiency Numbers & Letters Part C Efficiency Numbers & Letters Part D Disruption Oral Production Auditory Comprehension Writing Bill Payment List Learning List A IR List Learning List B IR List Learning List A Short DR List Learning List A Long DR Shape Learning IR Shape Learning DR Story Learning Phase Unit IR Daily Living Memory IR Daily Living Memory DR Visual Discrimination Figure Drawing Copy Figure Drawing Copy Organization Figure Drawing IR Map Reading Mazes Judgment Categories	Screening Memory Domain Screening Spatial Domain Language Index

NOTE: IR, Immediate Recall; DR, Delayed Recall.

[a]Internal reliability estimates were not computed for all subtests.

the Module Index score that subsumes them. Screening Domain scores also tend to have the highest correlations with their respective Index score counterparts. The correlations range from .35 (Screening Language Domain and the Language Index) to .78 (Screening Attention Domain and the Attention Index). The S-NAB score and the T-NAB Index score are highly correlated (r = .79; White & Stern, 2003b).

TABLE 6–24 Median Percentage Agreement Coefficients for Correct Classifications for Secondary and Descriptive Scores

MODULE	SECONDARY SCORES (%)	DESCRIPTIVE (%)
Screening	86	99
Attention	90	100
Language	99	98
Memory	92	83
Spatial	85	—
Executive Functions	82	—

NOTE: Test and retest scores were divided into three categories (≤−2.0 *SD*, −1.9 *SD* to +1.9 *SD*, ≥2.0 *SD*), and the test and retest ranges were then evaluated to determine the percentage agreement of each category from test to retest. Percentages are rounded to the nearest whole.

As discussed in the "Description" section of this review, one use of the Screening Module is to predict performance on the main module. The ability of the Screening Domain scores to predict performance on the corresponding Module Index scores was evaluated in the standardization sample as well as in a number of clinical groups (White & Stern, 2003b). Three groupings were formed on the basis of each of the five Module Index scores: moderate to severely impaired (index score of 45–61), moderately impaired to average (index score of 62–106), and above average and better (index score of 107–155). For each module, the cumulative score distribution of the Screening Domain score was computed for each of the three Index score ranges and a conservative criterion was selected to identify at least 95% of the individuals who are recommended to receive the full module. This criterion was based on the concept that it is more desirable to give the main module unnecessarily than to screen out an individual who may, in fact, require the main module.

As Table 6–26 shows, only 5% of the individuals who obtained Index scores in the 62–106 range (i.e., who are judged to require administration of the main module) were missed by the respective cutoff scores. However, the false-positive rates were found to be high, with many intact individuals falsely flagged for main module administration. For example, the above-average and higher cutoff scores correctly identify only between 3% (Language Domain) and 43% (Attention Domain) of individuals who obtained Index scores in the 107 to 155 range (i.e., who were judged not to require administration of the main module). Overall, the cutoffs appear more useful for lower, as opposed to higher, functioning individuals. The above-average and higher cutoffs are of limited utility in identifying cognitively healthy individuals who do not require administration of the main module.

FACTOR-ANALYTIC STUDIES AND RELATIONSHIPS WITH OTHER TESTS

Exploratory and confirmatory factor-analytic studies are presented in the manual (White & Stern, 2003b). The models that were derived are somewhat different from the models originally hypothesized (e.g., psychomotor speed tended to emerge as a separate factor with loadings from Mazes and Numbers & Letters Efficiency).

Overall, patterns of correlations support convergent and divergent validity of the NAB. A subset of 50 unimpaired individuals (aged 20 to 85 years, $M = 59.5$, $SD = 17.5$ years) who participated in the NAB standardization study also completed a number of standard cognitive measures (White & Stern, 2003b). The T-NAB Index moderately correlated with the Modified Mini-Mental State Test (3MS), Mini-Mental State Examination (MMSE), Repeatable Battery for the Assessment of Neuropsychological Status (RBANS), and the RIST ($r = .40$ to $r = .65$), suggesting that this composite has substantial overlap with overall intellectual ability, yet its structure also reflects other cognitive domains.

The manual also reported comparisons of NAB scores with other frequently used measures of cognitive function (e.g., WMS-III; California Verbal Learning Test [CVLT], Second Edition; TMT; RBANS; Ruff 2 & 7 Test; Boston Naming Test [BNT]; Token Test; Controlled Oral Word Association Test; Rey-Osterreith Complex Figure Test; and so on). Correlational analyses based on unimpaired and impaired samples (e.g., patients with dementia, patients with aphasia) tend to show the expected pattern of relationships, with criterion measures correlating more highly with those NAB scores that reflect similar, as opposed to different, cognitive processes.

Other research has also supported convergent validity of the NAB in clinical groups. Specifically, NAB subtests have been shown to moderately correlate with measures of similar constructs in patients with epilepsy (Hill et al., 2012), older adults referred to a memory clinic (MacDougall & Mansbach, 2013), and patients with moderate to severe TBI (Zgaljardic & Temple, 2010a). Zgaljardic and Temple also reported lower correlations between the NAB subtests and measures from disparate cognitive domains, providing support for the test's divergent validity. Of note, modest correlations were reported between Judgement of Line Orientation and NAB Visual Discrimination in patients with Parkinson's disease (PD), suggesting that the tests may measure different constructs (Renfroe et al., 2017).

The NAB Naming test has been the subject of a number of studies. Overall, NAB Naming and the BNT are highly correlated (e.g., Soble, Sordahl, et al., 2016; Yochim et al., 2015). The NAB appears to be less affected by visual abilities than the BNT (Soble, Marceaux, et al., 2016; Yochim et al., 2009). Yochim et al. (2009) further reported that the BNT showed stronger correlations with gender and education than the NAB. The range of obtained scores appears to differ as well, with NAB Naming scores relatively evenly distributed about the mean (i.e., +1.5 *SD* to −1.5 *SD*) and a greater proportion of BNT scores falling below the mean (i.e., +.7SD to −2.2 *SD*). There is support for convergent and divergent validity of NAB Naming, with overall stronger correlations with confrontation naming

TABLE 6–25 Neuropsychological Assessment Battery (NAB) Change Scores (Index and Primary Scores)

NAB INDEXES AND SUBTESTS	MEAN CHANGE SCORE	PERCENTAGE OF SAMPLE WITH DECLINE ON RETEST		PERCENTAGE OF SAMPLE WITH IMPROVEMENT ON RETEST	
		≤20%	≤10%	≤20%	≤10%
Indexes					
Attention Index	2.6	6–7	8+	10–12	13+
Language Index	4.8	5–10	11+	12–20	21+
Memory Index	4.8	4–11	12+	13–17	18+
Spatial Index	–3.3	13–18	19+	7–11	12+
Executive Functions Index	5.4	5–7	8+	17–20	21+
Total Index	3.7	5–6	7+	11–15	16+
Attention module subtests					
Digits Forward	–0.4	8–12	13+	8–12	13+
Digits Backward	1.6	5–10	11+	7–10	11+
Dots	1.9	8–11	12+	12–15	16+
Numbers & Letters Part A Speed	0.1	6–7	8+	6–7	8+
Numbers & Letters Part A Errors	–0.3	8–14	15+	8–12	13+
Numbers & Letters Part A Efficiency	–0.5	6–7	8+	5	6+
Numbers & Letters Part B Efficiency	–0.1	8–12	13+	5–9	10+
Numbers & Letters Part C Efficiency	2.8	3–6	7+	8–11	12+
Numbers & Letters Part D Efficiency	1.5	6–9	10+	10–12	13+
Numbers & Letters Part D Disruption	3.0	6–8	9+	12–16	17+
Driving Scenes	2.0	7–8	9+	11–14	15+
Language module subtests					
Oral Production	4.4	6–8	9+	14–18	19+
Auditory Comprehension	3.2	1–3	4+	11–18	19+
Naming	0.3	1–10	11+	2–9	10+
Writing	1.8	3–13	14+	10–21	22+
Bill Payment	–0.8	2–19	20+	2–11	12+
Memory module subtests					
List Learning A Immediate Recall	1.6	7–14	15+	11–13	14+
List Learning B Immediate Recall	–0.9	9–13	14+	8–13	14+
List Learning A Short Delayed	1.8	6–9	10+	10–14	15+
List Learning A Long Delayed	3.3	4–5	6+	10–13	14+
Shape Learning Immediate Recall	3.9	7	8+	12–17	18+
Shape Learning Delayed	1.4	8–14	15+	13–14	15+
Story Learning Immediate Recall	0.5	8–9	10+	7–11	12+
Story Learning Delayed	0.5	7–8	9+	7–13	14+
Daily Living Memory Immediate Recall	4.2	5–9	10+	12–13	14+
Daily Living Memory Delayed	1.5	6–9	10+	10–12	13+
Spatial module subtests					
Visual Discrimination	1.1	10–19	20+	8–13	14+
Design Construction	2.5	4–8	9+	11–13	14+
Figure Drawing Copy	–7.8	20–24	25+	4–10	11+
Figure Drawing Organization	–0.6	10–13	14+	8–9	10+
Figure Drawing Immediate Recall	–2.1	9–10	11+	5–11	12+
Map Reading	–0.2	10–14	15+	7–10	11+
Executive functions module subtests					
Mazes	2.0	6–8	9+	10–12	13+
Judgment	–0.2	12–14	15+	12–13	14+
Categories	5.9	2–6	7+	14–16	17+
Word Generation	2.2	5–6	7+	9–11	12+

NOTE: The cutoff scores were derived based on statistical consideration. The frequency distribution of difference scores for each variable was examined, and for the majority of scores the cutoff presented is *less* than the 20% or 10% percentile rank in each tail of the distribution. Index scores have a mean = 100 and *SD* = 15. Subtests scores have a mean = 50 and a *SD* = 10.

SOURCE: Brooks et al. (2009).

and semantic tasks than tests of other abilities (see Yochim et al., 2009, 2015). The test correlates moderately with intelligence, and relationships between visual reasoning and naming remain after demographic and other variables are controlled (see Soble et al., 2016). Processing speed also contributes to performance (Soble et al., 2016).

CLINICAL STUDIES

NAB performance across a number of clinical groups is presented in the manual, including individuals with dementia, aphasia, TBI, human immunodeficiency virus (HIV) and acquired immunodeficiency syndrome (AIDS), MS, conditions requiring inpatient rehabilitation, and

TABLE 6–26 Recommendations for Administering Neuropsychological Assessment Battery (NAB) Modules Based on Screening Domain Scores: Decision Accuracy Rates

SCREENING DOMAIN	CUTOFF	FALSE-POSITIVE RATE	FALSE-NEGATIVE RATE
Attention	Moderate-severely impaired (≤74)	.41	.05
	Above average (≥114)	.57	.05
Language	Moderate-severely impaired (≤75)	.25	.05
	Above average (≥126)	.97	.04
Memory	Moderate-severely impaired (≤75)	.29	.05
	Above average (≥119)	.79	.05
Spatial	Moderate-severely impaired (≤74)	.56	.05
	Above average (≥120)	.78	.05
Executive	Moderate-severely impaired (≤73)	.33	.05
	Above average (≥115)	.62	.05

SOURCE: From White and Stern (2003b). Reproduced by special permission of the Publisher, Psychological Assessment Resources, Inc. (PAR), 16204 North Florida Avenue, Lutz, Florida 33549, from the Neuropsychological Assessment Battery by Robert A. Stern, PhD and Travis White, PhD, Copyright 2001, 2003 by PAR. Further reproduction is prohibited without permission from PAR.

adult Attention-Deficit/Hyperactivity Disorder (ADHD). Overall, the findings are consistent with the expected neuropsychological profile associated with the clinical conditions. For example, almost 90% of the patients with dementia score in the impaired range on the Memory Index. Similarly, a sizable percentage of mild to moderate TBI patients (screened for performance validity) show impairments on variables from the Attention, Memory, and Executive Functions domains.

MCI and Dementia. AD is associated with lower performance on the NAB (Gavett et al., 2012), and the test has shown utility in differentiating between healthy controls, patients with MCI, and patients with AD. For instance, Gavett et al. (2009) reported that specific cutoffs on NAB List Learning were associated with strong sensitivity and specificity estimates when consensus diagnosis via a multidisciplinary team was used as the reference standard. At a cutoff T score of 37 or lower on List A Short Delay Recall or 40 or lower on List A Long Delay Recall, AD patients were differentiated from controls at more than 90% sensitivity and specificity. AD was differentiated from Amnestic MCI (aMCI) with greater than 70% sensitivity and greater than 80% specificity using a cutoff T score of 30 or lower on List A Short Delay Recall. Patients with aMCI were differentiated from controls using a List A Short Delay Recall cutoff T score of 48 or lower at a sensitivity of 86% and specificity of 72%. A regression model classified individuals with 80% accuracy, with List B Immediate Recall and List A Short Delay Recall the most influential in the equation. When base rates were considered, the positive predictive power (PPP) and negative predictive power (NPP) were high for base rates of AD ranging from 10% to 50% (PPP range, 71% to 96%; NPP range, 73% to 96%) and somewhat lower for aMCI (highest at base rates of 20% to 50%, ranging from PPP of 57% to 84%, NPP of 63% to 87%).

Findings suggest that in clinical settings with base rates of aMCI and AD of 20% or lower, good performance on NAB List Learning suggests the patient would not be diagnosed with aMCI according to the reference standard used in the study (consensus diagnosis). In settings with base rates of 50% or higher (i.e., memory disorder clinic), however, poor performance on NAB List Learning suggests that there is a high probability a patient would be given a diagnosis of aMCI according to the reference standard (consensus diagnosis).

In a subsequent study, Gavett et al. (2010) used the diagnostic algorithm generated from the NAB List Learning test to predict the clinical course on other cognitive measures in AD, aMCI, and control groups. The NAB List Learning algorithm was predictive of more rapid decline in language (Animal Fluency), attention/processing speed (WAIS, Revised, Digit Symbol), and overall cognitive functioning (MMSE), relative to controls, as well as shorter time to consensus diagnosis of AD. The NAB algorithm classifying MCI was predictive of a faster decline in language (Animal Fluency) and episodic memory (Consortium to Establish a Registry for Alzheimer's Disease [CERAD] Word List Recall Trial 3) and shorter time to consensus diagnosis. Discrimination between AD and MCI was less accurate. However, the AD group was reported to show a more rapid rate of decline in overall cognitive functioning (MMSE) and visuospatial functioning (Hooper Visual Organization Test) compared to people with MCI.

Gavett et al. (2012) further reported that Daily Living Memory was associated with the highest sensitivity and specificity estimates in detecting AD (Immediate Recall sensitivity of 86%, Delayed Recall sensitivity of 97%, Immediate Recall specificity of 90%, Delayed Recall specificity of 88%) and had correspondingly high PPVs and NPVs (exceeding .80 at 33% and 50% base rates). The NAB has shown value in predicting ADLs in dementia populations. List Learning Delayed Recall and Daily Living Memory Delayed Recall were associated with the highest sensitivity rates in terms of predicting ADLs at a 95% specificity rate (71%, 88%, respectively; Ashendorf et al., 2017).

TBI. The NAB shows strong utility in TBI, including sensitivity to impairment, and correlates with day-to-day function. Donders and Levitt (2012) reported that patients with complicated mild to severe TBI perform worse on the Attention, Executive Functions, and Memory modules of the NAB compared to demographically matched controls, with moderate to large effect sizes (Cohen's d = .77 to 1.07). Patients were four to eight times more likely than matched controls to have scores lower than the 10th percentile. Furthermore, performance was related to coma duration, with Executive Functions explaining the greatest amount of variance (24%). Hacker et al. (2017) similarly reported that patients with TBI perform worse than controls on the Attention Index and the Executive Functions Index, with degree of impairment related to injury severity. The Screening Module also shows good utility in inpatients with mild to severe TBI, as does a novel shortened index.

Zgaljardic and Temple (2010a) reported that patients with moderate to severe TBI admitted to a residential post-acute rehabilitation program perform more poorly relative to normative values on the NAB-SM on Total Score, Attention, Memory, and Executive Functions, without significant difference on Language scores. Spatial Domain Index scores were reported to be above average. In terms of base rates of low scores, 35% of patients performed below the 10th percentile on two or more scores, and approximately 10% performed below the 10th percentile on four index scores.

Temple et al. (2009) reported that the NAB-SM correlated with ADLs in patients with moderate or severe TBI, and the NAB Total score accounted for 26% of the variance in the ADL score after demographic factors were taken into account. Specific relationships between NAB domains and the ADL measure were also found. Zgaljardic, Yancy, Temple, Watford, and Miller (2011) reported relationships between the NAB-SM, Daily Living, and a clinician-rated measure of function in patients following brain injury (Mayo-Portland Adaptability Inventory-4 [MPAI-4]).

Stroke. Pulsipher, Stricker, Sadek, and Haaland (2013) reported that both left and right hemisphere stroke groups performed worse than controls on Attention, Spatial, and Executive Functions modules, with the left hemisphere group showing greater impairment on Language and Memory. Modality of impairment also corresponded to some degree to area of damage. For example, patients with aphasia due to left hemisphere stroke showed greater impairment on all NAB domains, and right hemisphere patients with spatial impairment performed worse than controls only on the Spatial Domain.

Stricker, Tybur, Sadek, and Haaland (2010) reported that a group of patients with stroke performed worse than demographically matched controls on NAB Total and Domain scores (large effect sizes). Sensitivity and specificity were also high (range of 86% to 89% sensitivity, with the exception of the Spatial Domain score, which was lower; specificity ranged from 75% to 86%, except for the Memory Domain score, which was 62%). Of note, the cutoff scores for optimal diagnostic accuracy estimates in this study were quite high for Domain scores, ranging from 83.50 (NAB Attention) to 101.50 (NAB Spatial).

The NAB also relates to everyday function in stroke. Sadek, Stricker, Adair, and Haaland (2011) reported that NAB composite scores were correlated with a performance-based battery of daily living skills in stroke patients ($rs > .70$), with the NAB Total score predicting impairment on a measure of daily living with 92% sensitivity and 84% specificity.

Other Populations. The NAB has utility in a number of additional clinical populations, including mixed neurologic samples, epilepsy, and dysnomia. Correlates with functional activities have also been reported (e.g., driving).

Iverson, Williamson, Ropacki, and Reilly (2007) found that in a mixed sample of neurologic patients, a number of patients obtained low scores on the Attention Index and the Executive Functions Index. Patients performed broadly within typical limits across other index scores.

High diagnostic accuracy has been reported in various clinical groups. When combined with a verbal memory measure, the Shape Learning subtest predicted side of seizure onset in patients with unilateral temporal lobe epilepsy with 80% accuracy, and NAB Shape Learning showed higher diagnostic accuracy than Visual Reproduction of the WMS-III (Hill et al., 2012). The Shape Learning Delayed Recall condition accounted for the largest area under the curve according to receiver operating characteristic (ROC) analyses and provided the most accurate discriminator between right and left temporal lobe epilepsy of variables examined. Using a BNT score of −1 *SD* as the reference standard for dysnomia in patients consecutively referred for neuropsychological assessment, NAB Naming demonstrated sensitivities of 80% (Form 1) and 79% (Form 2), as well as specificities of 73% (Form 1) and 78% (Form 2; Yochim et al., 2015). Grohman and Fals-Stewart (2004) reported that the NAB-SM showed strong sensitivity and specificity (81%, 92%), PPV (87%), and NPV (88%) when compared with the Neuropsychological Screening Battery as the reference standard in the diagnosis of cognitive impairment in a sample of patients in a residential program for substance abuse treatment.

There is some evidence of the ecological validity of NAB scores, especially with respect to driving. Brown et al. (2005) reported moderate correlations between Driving Scenes and on-road performance in persons with mild dementia. People rated as safe drivers performed better on Driving Scenes than those rated as marginal or unsafe. NAB Mazes, along with the TMT-A, was found to be the best predictor of failure on a road driving test in a sample of individuals with impairment referred to a driving clinic (Niewoehner et al., 2012). Similarly, NAB Driving Scenes was one of the best predictors of at-risk driving in older adults (Stern et al., 2016).

Patients who show capacity for consent perform better on the NAB Judgment task than those who do not demonstrate consent capacity (Cohen's $d = .75$), and Judgment scores predict a significant portion of variance in ADLs, even when MMSE and TMT are considered (MacDougall & Mansbach, 2013). Last, the Memory score from the NAB-SM correlates moderately well with therapists' ratings of memory functioning of inpatients in a rehabilitation hospital (White & Stern, 2003b).

NEUROANATOMICAL CORRELATES AND IMAGING STUDIES

No information is available.

PERFORMANCE VALIDITY

There are very few studies on the use of the NAB to detect noncredible performance deficits. However, a simulation paradigm was used to examine the impact of feigned or exaggerated impairment on NAB performance (White & Stern, 2003b). Simulators performed significantly worse than controls on most primary and module scores. Simulators could be distinguished from controls as well as patients with TBI by their pattern of very poor scores on 11 NAB indicators: Driving Scenes, Auditory Comprehension, Visual Discrimination, Figure Drawing Immediate Recall, Daily Living Immediate and Delayed Recall, Judgment, Categories, and the Attention Index, Language Index, and Memory Index. Low to moderately high correlations were obtained between these NAB scores and three criterion measures of performance validity: the Test of Memory Malingering (TOMM), the Word Memory Test (WMT), and the Victoria Symptom Validity Test.

Lange, Iverson, Brooks, and Rennison (2010) investigated the effects of noncredible performance on NAB Screening performance in patients referred to a concussion clinic evaluated within five months post-injury who were receiving workers' compensation. Patients who failed the TOMM scored worse on the NAB-SM than those who passed, particularly on the Attention, Memory, and Executive Functions modules (large effect sizes; range Cohen's $d = .70$ to 1.26).

COMMENT

The NAB has been reviewed favorably (Hartman, 2006; Iverson et al., 2008; Lynch, 2004) due to its many strengths, including flexibility of administration, wide breadth of coverage of cognitive domains (e.g., attention, executive functions, language, memory, spatial), co-norming with an intelligence screen, strong normative base, inclusion of a screening module, and the inclusion of purportedly ecologically valid subtests and alternate forms.

In terms of demographic effects, age appears to be the most influential, with education and IQ also impacting performance. On the Executive Functions Module, a pattern of less resistance to age-related change and more homogeneity across the age range is noted for subtests that emphasize crystallized skills, with the opposite pattern noted on subtests relating more to fluid abilities. Gender does not significantly affect performance for most subtests. The impact of ethnicity and other sociodemographic variables is unclear, although the NAB has been translated into other languages (e.g., German).

The standardization sample has many strengths, including that it is large, demographically adjusted, and distributed regionally and by gender and education. Note, however, that the normative sample is predominantly Caucasian (85%), and the generalizability to other groups is thus not clear.

In terms of score interpretation, the Language Module does not have a normal distribution, so most healthy adults and patients with mild language problems would be expected to perform within typical limits on these tests (Brooks et al., 2007). Although domain and index scores, as well as primary test scores, are demographically corrected for age, education, and gender, users should note that secondary test scores are corrected for age alone, and descriptive scores (cumulative percentage) are highly skewed and are not demographically corrected (see Table 6–16 in this review). Primary scores are thus the most important for interpretation, with secondary and descriptive scores providing supplemental information. The availability of base rate data of low scores on the NAB is a significant advantage of this test. This enables the clinician to evaluate the relative significance of low scores obtained clinically. Base rate data suggest that low scores are not overly unusual and interact with demographic variables (e.g., age and intelligence).

In terms of reliability, internal reliability coefficients are variable, ranging from high to modest. Test-retest reliability is quite weak overall, with somewhat higher reliability for composite scores. Form 2 composite scores tend to be higher than Form 1 scores. Practice effects are small overall, and Brooks et al. (2007) provide data for older adults from the standardization sample regarding base rates of uncommon change (see Table 6–20). Interrater reliability is high. *SEMs* are fairly large, as are confidence intervals.

The task shows relatively strong coherence among measures. For example, the primary scores tend to demonstrate highest correlations with their Module Index score, and the screening composite and total NAB composite scores are highly correlated. The procedure for decision-making in the context of screening score results is well-described.

Screening is more likely to result in false-positive errors than false-negative errors, with higher functioning individuals incorrectly identified as in need of the main module administration. On the other hand, only 5% of individuals in the low range who were identified as in need of administration of the full module were missed (false negatives). Because the NAB screening modules are intended to identify the need for additional testing, it may be viewed clinically as a more serious error to miss people who actually need additional testing compared to including people erroneously for additional testing. Thus, relatively higher false-positive rates may be acceptable in this regard. Overall, the cutoffs appear more useful for lower, as opposed to higher functioning patients. The above-average and higher cutoffs perform with limited accuracy in identifying cognitively intact individuals who do not require administration of the full module.

The NAB Total Score correlates moderately with other broad measures of overall cognitive function, and NAB scores show an overall pattern of divergent and convergent relationships with measures of specific cognitive function. NAB Naming has been subject to additional research, which supports the convergent and divergent validity of the subtest and suggests that it shares similarities with the BNT but is not identical to it. Clinically, the NAB is useful in a number of populations, including TBI, dementia, stroke, neurologic groups, and substance use populations. In addition to group differences and impairments in clinical groups, research has also provided some support for diagnostic accuracy statistics (e.g., sensitivity, specificity, predictive power), within-group differentiation, and functional correlates (e.g., driving).

The NAB provides measures of many domains of cognition, but users should note that it does not include measures of intelligence, fine motor, sensory, personality or behavioral functioning, or performance validity. Iverson et al. (2008) also point out there is not a repetition task in the Language Module. There is limited information pertaining to neurologic correlates. As with most neuropsychological tests, patients with suspect presentation perform worse on many NAB modules (Attention, Memory, Executive Functions), and although the NAB has some research on the detection of noncredible performance, additional research in clinical groups is needed.

REFERENCES

Ashendorf, L., Alosco, M. L., Bing-Canar, H., Chapman, K. R., Martin, B., Chaisson, C. E., . . . Stern, R. A. (2017). Clinical utility of select Neuropsychological Assessment Battery tests in predicting functional abilities in dementia. *Archives of Clinical Neuropsychology:*, 1–11. https://doi.org/10.1093/arclin/acx100

Brooks, B. L., Iverson, G. L., & White, T. (2007). Substantial risk of "accidental MCI" in healthy older adults: Base rates of low memory scores in neuropsychological assessment. *Journal of the International Neuropsychological Society, 13*(3), 490–500.

Brooks, B. L., Iverson, G. L., & White, T. (2009). Advanced interpretation of the Neuropsychological Assessment Battery with older adults: Base rate analyses, discrepancy scores, and interpreting change. *Archives of Clinical Neuropsychology, 24*(7), 647–657. https://doi.org/10.1093/arclin/acp061

Brown, L. B., Stern, R. A., Cahn-Weiner, D. A., Rogers, B., Messer, M. A., Lannon, M. C., . . . Ott, B. R. (2005). Driving Scenes test of the Neuropsychological Assessment Battery (NAB) and on-road driving performance in aging and very mild dementia. *Archives of Clinical Neuropsychology, 20,* 209–216.

Buczylowska, D., Bornschlegl, M., Daseking, M., Jäncke, L., & Petermann, F. (2013). Zur deutschen Adaptation der Neuropsychological Assessment Battery (NAB) [German adaption of the Neuropsychological Assessment Battery (NAB)]. *Zeitschrift für Neuropsychologie, 24,* 217–227.

Buczylowska, D., & Petermann, F. (2016). Age-related differences and heterogeneity in executive functions: Analysis of NAB Executive Functions module scores. *Archives of Clinical Neuropsychology, 31*(3), 254–262. https://doi.org/10.1093/arclin/acw005

Donders, J., & Levitt, T. (2012). Criterion validity of the Neuropsychological Assessment Battery after traumatic brain injury. *Archives of Clinical Neuropsychology, 27*(4), 440–445. https://doi.org/10.1093/arclin/acs043

Gavett, B. E., Gurnani, A. S., Saurman, J. L., Chapman, K. R., Steinberg, E. G., Martin, B., . . . Stern, R. A. (2016). Practice effects on Story Memory and List Learning tests in the neuropsychological assessment of older adults. *PloS One, 11*(10), e0164492. https://doi.org/10.1371/journal.pone.0164492

Gavett, B. E., Lou, K. R., Daneshvar, D. H., Green, R. C., Jefferson, A. L., & Stern, R. A. (2012). Diagnostic accuracy statistics for seven Neuropsychological Assessment Battery (NAB) test variables in the diagnosis of Alzheimer's disease. *Applied Neuropsychology, 19*(2), 108–115. https://doi.org/10.1080/09084282.2011.643947

Gavett, B. E., Ozonoff, A., Doktor, V., Palmisano, J., Nair, A. K., Green, R. C., . . . Stern, R. A. (2010). Predicting cognitive decline and conversion to Alzheimer's disease in older adults using the NAB List Learning test. *Journal of the International Neuropsychological Society, 16*(4), 651–660. https://doi.org/10.1017/S1355617710000421

Gavett, B. E., Poon, S. J., Ozonoff, A., Jefferson, A. L., Nair, A. K., Green, R. C., & Stern, R. A. (2009). Diagnostic utility of the NAB List Learning test in Alzheimer's disease and amnestic mild cognitive impairment. *Journal of the International Neuropsychological Society, 15*(1), 121. https://doi.org/10.1017/S1355617708090176

Grohman, K., & Fals-Stewart, W. (2004). The detection of cognitive impairment among substance-abusing patients: The accuracy of the Neuropsychological Assessment Battery-Screening Module. *Experimental and Clinical Psychopharmacology, 12*(3), 200–207. https://doi.org/10.1037/1064-1297.12.3.200

Hacker, D., Jones, C. A., Clowes, Z., Belli, A., Su, Z., Sitaraman, M., . . . Pettigrew, Y. (2017). The development and psychometric evaluation of a supplementary index score of the Neuropsychological Assessment Battery Screening Module that is sensitive to traumatic brain injury. *Archives of Clinical Neuropsychology:, 32*(2), 215–227. https://doi.org/10.1093/arclin/acw087

Hartman, D. E. (2006). Test review. *Applied Neuropsychology, 13*(1), 58–61.

Hill, S. W., Strutt, A. M., Uber-Zak, L., Fogel, T. G., & Ropacki, M. T. (2012). The NAB shape learning subtest as a predictor of lateralized seizure onset. *Epilepsy & Behavior, 24*(1), 59–64. https://doi.org/10.1016/j.yebeh.2012.02.021

Iverson, G. L., Brooks, B. L., White, T., & Stern, R. A. (2008). Neuropsychological Assessment Battery (NAB): Introduction and advanced interpretation. In J. A. M. Horton, & D. Wedding (Eds.), *The neuropsychology handbook* (3rd ed., pp. 279–343). New York: Springer.

Iverson, G. L., Williamson, D. J., Ropacki, M., & Reilly, K. J. (2007). Frequency of abnormal scores on the Neuropsychological Assessment Battery Screening Module (S-NAB) in a mixed neurological sample. *Applied Neuropsychology, 14*(3), 178–182.

Lange, R. T., Iverson, G. L., Brooks, B. L., & Ashton Rennison, V. L. (2010). Influence of poor effort on self-reported symptoms and neurocognitive test performance following mild traumatic brain injury. *Journal of Clinical and Experimental Neuropsychology, 32*(9), 961–972. https://doi.org/10.1080/13803391003645657

Lynch, W. J. (2004). A new neuropsychological test battery: The NAB. *The Journal of Head Trauma Rehabilitation, 19*(2), 180–183.

MacDougall, E. E., & Mansbach, W. E. (2013). The Judgment test of the Neuropsychological Assessment Battery (NAB): Psychometric considerations in an assisted-living sample. *The Clinical Neuropsychologist, 27*(5), 827–839. https://doi.org/10.1080/13854046.2013.786759

Niewoehner, P. M., Henderson, R. R., Dalchow, J., Beardsley, T. L., Stern, R. A., & Carr, D. B. (2012). Predicting road test performance in adults with cognitive or visual impairment referred to a Veterans

Affairs medical center driving clinic. *Journal of the American Geriatrics Society*. https://doi.org/10.1111/j.1532-5415.2012.04201.x

Pulsipher, D. T., Stricker, N. H., Sadek, J. R., & Haaland, K. Y. (2013). Clinical utility of the Neuropsychological Assessment Battery (NAB) after unilateral stroke. *The Clinical Neuropsychologist, 27*(6), 924–945. https://doi.org/10.1080/13854046.2013.799714

Renfroe, J. B., Turner, T. H., & Hinson, V. K. (2017). Assessing visuospatial skills in Parkinson's: Comparison of Neuropsychological Assessment Battery Visual Discrimination to the Judgment of Line Orientation. *Archives of Clinical Neuropsychology:, 32*(1), 123–127. https://doi.org/10.1093/arclin/acw102

Reynolds, C. R., & Kamphaus, R. W. (2003). *Reynolds Intellectual Screening Test.* Lutz, FL: Psychological Assessment Resources.

Sachs, B. C., Rush, B. K., & Pedraza, O. (2016). Validity and reliability of the NAB Naming test. *The Clinical Neuropsychologist, 30*(4), 629–638. https://doi.org/10.1080/13854046.2016.1149618

Sadek, J. R., Stricker, N., Adair, J. C., & Haaland, K. Y. (2011). Performance-based everyday functioning after stroke: Relationship with IADL questionnaire and neurocognitive performance. *Journal of the International Neuropsychological Society, 17*(5), 832–840. https://doi.org/10.1017/S1355617711000841

Soble, J. R., Marceaux, J. C., Galindo, J., Sordahl, J. A., Highsmith, J. M., O'Rourke, J. J. F., ... McCoy, K. J. M. (2016). The effect of perceptual reasoning abilities on confrontation naming performance: An examination of three naming tests. *Journal of Clinical and Experimental Neuropsychology, 38*(3), 284–292. https://doi.org/10.1080/13803395.2015.1107030

Soble, J. R., Sordahl, J. A., Critchfield, E. A., Highsmith, J. M., González, D. A., Ashish, D., . . . McCoy, K. J. M. (2016). Slow and steady does not always win the race: Investigating the effect of processing speed across five naming tests. *Archives of Clinical Neuropsychology:*. https://doi.org/10.1093/arclin/acw073

Stern, R. A., Abularach, L. M., Seichepine, D. R., Alosco, M. L., Gavett, B. E., & Tripodis, Y. (2016). Office-based assessment of at-risk driving in older adults with and without cognitive impairment. *Journal of Geriatric Psychiatry and Neurology*. https://doi.org/10.1177/0891988716666378

Stern, R. A., & White, T. (2003). *Neuropsychological Assessment Battery: Administration, scoring, and interpretation manual.* Lutz, FL: Psychological Assessment Resources.

Stricker, N. H., Tybur, J. M., Sadek, J. R., & Haaland, K. Y. (2010). Utility of the Neuropsychological Assessment Battery in detecting cognitive impairment after unilateral stroke. *Journal of the International Neuropsychological Society, 16*(5), 813–821. https://doi.org/10.1017/S1355617710000652

Temple, R. O., Zgaljardic, D. J., Abreu, B. C., Seale, G. S., Ostir, G. V., & Ottenbacher, K. J. (2009). Ecological validity of the neuropsychological assessment battery screening module in post-acute brain injury rehabilitation. *Brain Injury, 23*(1), 45–50. https://doi.org/10.1080/02699050802590361

White, T., & Stern, R.A. (2003a). *Neuropsychological Assessment Battery: Demographically corrected norms manual.* Lutz, FL: Psychological Assessment Resources.

White, T., & Stern, R.A. (2003b). *Neuropsychological Assessment Battery: Psychometric and technical manual.* Lutz, FL: Psychological Assessment Resources.

White, T., & Stern, R. A. (2003c). *US Census-matched norms manual.* Lutz, FL: Psychological Assessment Resources.

Yochim, B. P., Beaudreau, S. A., Kaci Fairchild, J., Yutsis, M. V., Raymond, N., Friedman, L., & Yesavage, J. (2015). Verbal naming test for use with older adults: Development and initial validation. *Journal of the International Neuropsychological Society:, 21*(3), 239–248. https://doi.org/10.1017/S1355617715000120

Yochim, B. P., Kane, K. D., & Mueller, A. E. (2009). Naming test of the Neuropsychological Assessment Battery: Convergent and discriminant validity. *Archives of Clinical Neuropsychology:, 24*(6), 575–583. https://doi.org/10.1093/arclin/acp053

Zgaljardic, D. J., & Temple, R. O. (2010a). Neuropsychological Assessment Battery (NAB): Performance in a sample of patients with moderate-to-severe traumatic brain injury. *Applied Neuropsychology, 17*(4), 283–288. https://doi.org/10.1080/09084282.2010.525118

Zgaljardic, D. J., & Temple, R. O. (2010b). Reliability and validity of the Neuropsychological Assessment Battery-Screening Module (NAB-SM) in a sample of patients with moderate-to-severe acquired brain injury. *Applied Neuropsychology, 17*(1), 27–36. https://doi.org/10.1080/09084280903297909

Zgaljardic, D. J., Yancy, S., Temple, R. O., Watford, M. F., & Miller, R. (2011). Ecological validity of the screening module and the Daily Living tests of the Neuropsychological Assessment Battery using the Mayo-Portland Adaptability Inventory-4 in postacute brain injury rehabilitation. *Rehabilitation Psychology, 56*(4), 359–365. https://doi.org/10.1037/a0025466

REPEATABLE BATTERY FOR THE ASSESSMENT OF NEUROPSYCHOLOGICAL STATUS (RBANS UPDATE)

TEST NAME	**Repeatable Battery for the Assessment of Neuropsychological Status (RBANS Update)**
DOMAIN	Neuropsychological functioning
AGE RANGE	Up to 89 years
ADMINISTRATION TIME	30 minutes
SCORING FORMAT	Hand scored
REFERENCE	Randolph, C. (2012). *Repeatable Battery for the Assessment of Neuropsychological Status (RBANS Update)*. Bloomington: MN. PsychCorp. www.pearsonclinical.com

DESCRIPTION

The Repeatable Battery for the Assessment of Neuropsychological Status (RBANS; Randolph, 1998) was originally designed as a brief test to identify and characterize mild to severe forms of dementia in older adults, with the most recent version, the RBANS Update (Randolph, 2012), expanding the test's purpose to include screening in acute care settings and tracking recovery during rehabilitation. The test is comprised of 12 subtests that contribute to one of five domain indices: Immediate Memory (List Learning, Story Memory), Visuospatial/Constructional (Figure Copy, Line Orientation), Language (Picture Naming, Semantic Fluency), Attention (Digit Span, Coding), and Delayed Memory (List Recall, List Recognition, Story Memory, Figure Recall). In addition, a Total Scale score can be computed and is comprised of a combination of the five domain scores. Descriptions of the subtests and indices are shown in Table 6–27. Four parallel forms are offered (Forms A through D).

The RBANS Update includes an inclusion of adolescent to young adult normative data (12 to 20 years of age), equating of Forms C and D to Form A, improved retranslations of Form A and B Spanish versions, inclusion of subtest scaled scores (vs. only index scores), and color coding of stimulus and response booklets to increase user friendliness. Items remain unchanged from the original RBANS, as do normative data for the adult age group (i.e., ≥20 years). The test is also designed to be used as a screening tool by non-neuropsychologists (i.e., clinical psychologists and allied health professionals). However, the authors state that "Although any of these individuals may engage in some initial interpretation of performance on RBANS, the test results should ultimately be interpreted only by individuals with appropriate professional training in neuropsychological assessment for diagnostic purposes" (manual, p. 9).

ADMINISTRATION

Directions for administering the items, discontinuation rules, correct responses, time limits, prompts, and instructions for recording information appear on the record form. The subtests should be administered in the numbered order in which they appear on the record form because the duration of the delay interval is determined by the administration of the intervening tasks. An alternate form is available so that the test can be repeated on another occasion.

When used in conjunction with other measures, it should be noted that order effects may occur. For example, Mossbarger, Whitney, Herman, and Mariner (2012) reported that when veterans were administered other instruments prior to RBANS administration, more than one-third of participants showed carryover on subsequently administered RBANS verbal memory tests. Calamia, Roye, and Lemke (2017) reported administering the RBANS prior to additional tests did not affect performance on subsequent tests; however, when the RBANS was administered after other tests, performance was worse on delayed memory measures from the RBANS. The mechanism of this performance decrement was likely proactive interference (i.e., information to be recalled from memory measures administered initially presented as intrusions on subsequent administration). These results suggest that administering the RBANS initially as a screen prior to subsequent administration of tests is unlikely to impact performance; however, care in administering multiple memory measures is needed due to the potential for interference effects. There is some evidence that time of testing can impact Story Memory performance in older adults, with higher recall scores at the examinees' preferred time of day (Paradee et al., 2005).

TABLE 6–27 Description of Repeatable Battery for the Assessment of Neuropsychological Status Update (RBANS) Indices and Subtests

INDEX	SUBTEST	DESCRIPTION
Immediate Memory	List Learning	Ten semantically unrelated words are presented orally and the examinee is asked to recall words; four learning trials are provided.
	Story Memory	Short story is orally presented and the examinee must retell the story; two learning trials are provided.
Visuospatial/ Constructional	Figure Copy	The examinee must draw a complex figure.
	Line Orientation	The examinee is presented with pattern of 13 equal lines radiating from a single point. Below are two lines and the examinee must identify which two lines they match in the pattern.
Language	Picture Naming	The examinee must name line drawings; a semantic cue is provided if an object is obviously misperceived.
	Semantic Fluency	The examinee is given one minute to generate fruits and vegetables (Form A) and animals found in a zoo (Form B).
Attention	Digit Span	A forward digit span task.
	Coding	The examinee must code numbers to symbols in 90 seconds.
Delayed Memory	List Recall	The examinee must recall the list of 10 words from the List Learning subtest.
	List Recognition	The examinee is read 20 words and asked to indicate the words from the word list.
	Story Memory	The examinee is asked to recall a story learned earlier.
	Figure Recall	The examinee redraws the figure shown earlier.
Total Scale		Sum of Indices: Immediate Memory Visuospatial/Constructional Language Attention Delayed Memory

SOURCE: Adapted from Randolph (2012).

SCORING

Subtest raw scores are converted to age-based index scores via tables included in the Stimulus Booklet. Index scores range from 40 to 160 ($M = 100$, $SD = 15$). The manual also provides the subtest and index *M*s and *SD*s subdivided by age group (20 to 49, 50 to 69, and 70 to 89) and educational level (less than high school, high school, more than high school).

Note that the raw total scores from two subtests are needed for the conversion to an index score for the domains of Immediate Memory, Visuospatial/Constructional, Language, and Attention. The List Recall, List Recognition, Story Recall, and Figure Recall total scores are summed for the Delayed Memory Index. That sum, along with the List Recognition total score, is used for the conversion to an index score. Percentile equivalents, confidence intervals (90% and 95%), and index discrepancy criteria are also provided. The difference between pairs of index scores required for statistical significance varies (see Source), with differences of 30 points or greater in magnitude considered rare.

Supplemental scores are available in the literature. A novel percent retention score derived from the verbal memory subtests was associated with excellent diagnostic discriminability between people with AD, MCI, and controls (see Clark et al., 2010). However, other research has suggested little enhanced diagnostic utility in AD and MCI with use of percent retention scores compared to use of standard RBANS memory scores alone (Jodouin et al., 2017). Duff, Leber, Patton, Schoenberg, Mold, Scott, and Adams (2007) evaluated a set of modified scoring criteria for the Figure Copy and Recall subtests. In a community-dwelling sample of older adults and a mixed clinical sample, conventional scoring criteria led to lower scores than the modified criteria. Interrater reliability was high, and no age effects were found for the modified criteria. Detailed scoring criteria are presented in their paper.

Crawford, Garthwaite, Morrice, and Duff (2011) provide a computer program for supplementary analysis of RBANS scores that enables the clinician to estimate the percentage of the normative population that would be expected to show a specific number of low scores and the base rate of differences between scores (https://homepages.abdn.ac.uk/j.crawford/pages/dept/Programs/RBANS_Supplementary_Analysis.exe). Monte Carlo simulation procedures to estimate base rates of scores suggested that low scores are not unusual, with 21% of the population expected to exhibit one index score below the 5th percentile. However, this number drops to 4% of the population when the probability of obtaining two index scores below the 5th percentile is considered. Differences between scores are also not unusual, with 28% of the normative population expected to have abnormal pairwise differences at a criterion of less than 5%.

DEMOGRAPHIC EFFECTS

AGE

Scores decline with age (Duff et al., 2003; Gontkovsky et al., 2002; Green et al., 2008; Lim et al., 2010; Randolph, 2012; but see Gold et al., 1999; Hobart et al., 1999; Wilk et al., 2004).

GENDER

Modest gender effects are reported. Men tend to perform better on subtests that have visuospatial demands (Gold et al., 1999; Iverson et al., 2009; Wilk et al., 2004; but see Gogos et al., 2010), and women tend to perform better on language and memory subtests (see Beatty et al., 2003a; Duff, Schoenberg, Mold, Scott, & Adams, 2011c; Wilk et al., 2004). Mean differences between men and women are small (i.e., one to two raw score points; Duff et al., 2011c). Duff et al. provide gender-adjusted normative data in their paper.

EDUCATION

Performance improves with educational achievement (Duff et al., 2003; Gold et al., 1999; Gontkovsky et al., 2002; Hobart et al., 1999; Iverson et al., 2009; Lim et al., 2010; Mooney et al., 2007; Randolph, 1998; Wilk et al., 2004). Green et al. (2008) reported that education was more influential than age in their normative study of Australians.

ETHNICITY, NATIONALITY, AND LINGUISTIC EFFECTS

The RBANS has been translated into a number of languages. A Spanish translation demonstrated convergent validity, group differences between clinical patients and healthy controls, and strong internal reliability (Sanz et al., 2009). Normative data are available for the Australian population (Green et al., 2008) and older Chinese people (Lim et al., 2010; see the section "Normative Data").

Ethnic differences in performance among groups have been described, generally with Caucasian patients obtaining higher scores than other groups, including Hispanic (Mooney et al., 2007) and African-American patients (Gold et al., 1999; Patton et al., 2003). Some research indicates that these effects are secondary to reading ability (Gold et al., 1999), whereas other research has indicated differences remain after controlling for demographic factors (Patton et al., 2003).

NORMATIVE DATA

STANDARDIZATION SAMPLE

Normative data are based on a sample of 540 individuals, 20–89 years of age, with demographic factors broadly consistent with 1995 US Census data (see Table 6–28). The sample is overrepresented by individuals in the North Central regions and underrepresented by individuals in the West and Northeast. However, subsequent analysis did not suggest any significant regional differences with regard to the Total Scale score.

OTHER NORMATIVE DATA

Duff et al. (2003) calculated age- and education-adjusted scaled scores for individual subtests, index, and total scores. The data are based on a group of 718 community-dwelling older adults (65 years or older), predominantly Caucasian, recruited from an outpatient primary care setting in Oklahoma and participating in a broader study (the Oklahoma Longitudinal Assessment of Health Outcomes in Mature Adults [OKLAHOMA]). Participants with significant medical conditions likely to affect performance were excluded (e.g., stroke, TBI, seizures, PD, macular degeneration).

TABLE 6–28 Characteristics of the Repeatable Battery for the Assessment of Neuropsychological Status Update (RBANS) Normative Sample

Sample size	540
Age	20 to 89[a]
Geographic location	7% Northeast 24% South 62% North Central 77% West
Sample type	Standardization sample considered representative of the US adult population in terms of gender, educational level, and ethnicity based on 1995 US Census data.
Education	20% <High school 35% High school 45% >High school
Gender	Not reported
Ethnicity	81% White 13% African American 7% Hispanic
Screening	Screened to exclude participants with medical and psychiatric conditions.

[a]Based on several age groupings: 20 to 39, 40 to 49, 50 to 59, 60 to 69, 70 to 79, 80 to 89. *N* = 90 per age group. Age groups 12 to 19 are not included in this table.

SOURCE: Adapted from Randolph (2012).

TABLE 6–29 Repeatable Battery for the Assessment of Neuropsychological Status (RBANS) Raw Score Conversions to Age-Corrected Scaled Scores for Midpoint Age = 70

SCALED SCORE	LIST LEARN	STORY MEM	FIGURE COPY	LINE ORIENT	PICT NAM	SEM FLUEN	DIGIT SPAN	COD	LIST RECALL	LIST RECOG	SCORE RECALL	FIGURE RECALL	%ILE RANGE
2	0–7	0–3	0–10	0	0–4	0–4	0–4	0–3	—	0–11	—	—	<1
3	8–13	4	11	1–5	5–6	5–8	5	4–14	—	12–13	0	0–1	1
4	14	5–6	12	6	7	9	6	15–18	—	14	1	2–3	2
5	15	7–8	13–14	7–8	—	10	7	19–22	0	15	2	4–5	3–5
6	16–17	9–10	15	9–10	8	11	—	23–26	1	16	3–4	6–7	6–10
7	18–19	11	16	11–12	—	12–13	8	27–29	2	17	5	8–9	11–18
8	20–21	12–13	17	13–14	9	14	9	30–32	3	18	6	10	19–28
9	22–23	14–15	18	15	—	15–16	10	33–35	4	—	7	11–12	29–40
10	24–26	16–17	—	16–17	10	17–18	11	36–40	5	19	8–9	13–14	41–59
11	27–28	18	19	18	—	19–20	12	41–43	6	20	—	15	60–71
12	29	19	20	—	—	21	13	44–46	7	—	10	16	72–81
13	30–31	20	—	19	—	22–23	14	47–50	8	—	—	17	82–89
14	32–33	21	—	20	—	24–25	15	51–52	—	—	11	18	90–94
15	34–35	22	—	—	—	26	16	53–58	9	—	12	19	95–97
16	36–38	23	—	—	—	27	—	59–60	10	—	—	20	98
17	39	24	—	—	—	28–30	—	61–65	—	—	—	—	99
18	40	—	—	—	—	≥31	—	≥66	—	—	—	—	>99

NOTE: Age Range = 65–75, *N* = 495; %ile, percentile.; Learn, Learning; Mem, Memory; Orient, Orientation; Pict Nam, Picture Naming; Sem Fluen, Semantic Fluency; Cod, Coding; Recog, Recognition.

SOURCE: From Duff et al. (2003).

Tables 6–29 to 6–32 provides conversions of subtest raw scores to age-corrected scaled scores based on four midpoint age groups (70, 75, 80, 85). Tables 6–33 to 6–36 provide conversions of subtest age-corrected scaled scores to age- and education-adjusted scaled scores based on four education groups (i.e., ≤11 years, 12 years, 13–15 years, ≥16 years). Table 6–37 provides conversions of age-corrected scaled scores to age-corrected index scores and total scores, and Table 6–38 provides conversions of age- and education-corrected index and total scores. Of note, scoring criteria for Figure Copy and Figure Recall were relaxed (e.g., discouraging the use of a ruler or protractor measuring elements) because it was noted that when the original scoring criteria were applied, the resulting data were significantly below expectation.

The sample studied by Duff et al. (2003) performed slightly lower than the original RBANS standardization sample and demonstrated greater variability in their scores. The sample studied by Duff et al. (2003) may be considered more representative of a population of older adults living in the Midwest who regularly visit their primary care physicians.

TABLE 6–30 Repeatable Battery for the Assessment of Neuropsychological Status (RBANS) Raw Score Conversions to Age-Corrected Scaled Scores for Midpoint Age = 75

SCALED SCORE	LIST LEARN	STORY MEM	FIGURE COPY	LINE ORIENT	PICT NAM	SEM FLUEN	DIGIT SPAN	COD	LIST RECALL	LIST RECOG	STORY RECALL	FIGURE RECALL	%ILE RANGE
2	0–7	0–2	0–6	0	0–3	0–5	0–4	0–3	—	0–11	—	0–1	<1
3	8–11	3–5	7–11	1–5	4–6	6	5	4–6	—	12	—	2	1
4	12	—	12	6	7	—	—	7–13	—	13	0	—	2
5	13–14	6–7	13	7–8	—	7–9	6	14–18	—	14	1–2	3–4	3–5
6	15–16	8–9	14–15	9–10	8	10–11	7	19–20	0	15	3	5–6	6–10
7	17–18	10–11	16	11–12	—	12	8	21–25	1	16–17	4	7–8	11–18
8	19–20	12	17	13	—	13	9	26–28	2	—	5–6	9	19–28
9	21–22	13–14	—	14–15	9	14–15	—	29–32	3	18	7	10–11	29–40
10	23–25	15–17	18	16	10	16–17	10–11	33–37	4–5	19	8	12–13	41–59
11	26–27	18	19	17–18	—	18–19	12	38–40	—	20	9	14	60–71
12	28–29	19	20	—	—	20	13	41–43	6–7	—	10	15–16	72–81
13	30	20	—	19	—	21–22	14–15	44–46	—	—	—	17	82–89
14	31–33	21	—	20	—	23–25	16	47–51	8	—	11	18	90–94
15	34	22	—	—	—	26	—	52–54	9	—	12	19	95–97
16	35	23	—	—	—	27–28	—	55–56	10	—	—	20	98
17	36	24	—	—	—	29–31	—	57–59	—	—	—	—	99
18	37–40	—	—	—	—	≥32	—	≥60	—	—	—	—	>99

NOTE: Age Range = 70–80, *N* = 396; %ile, percentile; Learn, Learning; Mem, Memory; Orient, Orientation; Pict Nam, Picture Naming; Sem Fluen, Semantic Fluency; Cod, Coding; Recog, Recognition.

SOURCE: From Duff et al. (2003).

TABLE 6–31 Repeatable Battery for the Assessment of Neuropsychological Status (RBANS) Raw Score Conversions to Age-Corrected Scaled Scores for Midpoint Age = 80

SCALED SCORE	LIST LEARN	STORY MEM	FIGURE COPY	LINE ORIENT	PICT NAM	SEM FLUEN	DIGIT SPAN	COD	LIST RECALL	LIST RECOG	STORY RECALL	FIGURE RECALL	%ILE RANGE
2	0–7	0–1	0–6	0–1	0–5	0–5	—	0–5	—	0–11	—	—	<1
3	8–9	2–4	7–10	2–5	6	6–7	0–3	6–7	—	12	—	0–1	1
4	10–12	5	11–12	6	—	—	4	8–11	—	13	—	2	2
5	13–14	—	13	7–8	7	8	5–6	12–15	—	14	0	3	3–5
6	15	6–7	14	9–10	8	9–10	7	16–18	0	15	1–2	4–6	6–10
7	16–17	8–10	15	11	—	11–12	8	19–21	1	16	3	7	11–18
8	18–19	11	16	12–13	—	13	9	22–25	2	17	4	8–9	19–28
9	20–21	12–13	17	14	9	14	—	26–29	—	18	5–6	10	29–40
10	22–23	14–16	18	15–16	10	15–17	10–11	30–33	3–4	19	7–8	11–13	41–59
11	24–25	17	—	17	—	18	12–13	34–37	5	20	—	14	60–71
12	26–28	18–19	19	18	—	19	—	38–39	6	—	9	15	72–81
13	29	20	20	19	—	20–21	14–15	40–42	7	—	10	16	82–89
14	30–31	21	—	20	—	22–24	16	43–44	8	—	—	17	90–94
15	32–34	22	—	—	—	25–26	—	45–48	—	—	11	18–19	95–97
16	35	—	—	—	—	27–28	—	49–50	9	—	12	20	98
17	36–37	23	—	—	—	29–31	—	51–53	10	—	—	—	99
18	38–40	24	—	—	—	≥32	—	≥54	—	—	—	—	>99

NOTE: Age Range = 75–85, *N* = 239; %ile, percentile; Learn, Learning; Mem, Memory; Orient, Orientation; Pict Nam, Picture Naming; Sem Fluen, Semantic Fluency; Cod, Coding; Recog, Recognition.

SOURCE: From Duff et al. (2003).

Comparison of the use of norms from the original standardization sample versus Duff et al. (2003) sample norms suggests that use of the original standardization sample norms in older behavioral health inpatients (70 to 89 years of age) resulted in higher classification of impairment (i.e., 1 to 11 times more likely to indicate impairment, depending on subtest; Martin et al., 2017). Coding was associated with the largest discrepancy (65% impaired with original standardization norms vs. 8% with OKLAHOMA norms in the 80- to 89-year-old sample).

Demographic adjustments based on the OKLAHOMA project are also available from other sources and include regression-based adjustments for education on index scores (Gontovsky et al., 2002), regression-based adjustments for gender (Beatty et al., 2003a), demographically adjusted normative data based on 61 African Americans (Patton et al., 2003), and base rate data for RBANS discrepancy scores in a large sample of community-dwelling older adults (Patton et al., 2006).

Duff et al. (2011b) provide base rate data for discrepancy scores for a sample of 718 people from the OKLAHOMA

TABLE 6–32 Repeatable Battery for the Assessment of Neuropsychological Status (RBANS) Raw Score Conversions to Age-Corrected Scaled Scores for Midpoint Age = 85

SCALED SCORE	LIST LEARN	STORY MEM	FIGURE COPY	LINE ORIENT	PICT NAM	SEM FLUEN	DIGIT SPAN	COD	LIST RECALL	LIST RECOG	STORY RECALL	FIGURE RECALL	%ILE RANGE
2	0–8	0–3	0–7	0	—	0–3	—	0–5	—	0–12	—	—	<1
3	9	4	8	1	0–4	4	—	6	—	13	—	—	1
4	10	—	9–11	2–5	5	5–6	0–3	7	—	—	—	—	2
5	11–12	5	12–13	6	6	7–8	4	8–10	—	14	—	0	3–5
6	13	—	14	7–10	7	9	5–6	11–15	—	15	0	1–4	6–10
7	14–15	6–8	—	11	8	10	7	16–18	0–1	16	1	5–6	11–18
8	16–17	9–10	15–16	12	—	11–12	8–9	19–21	2	17	2–4	7–8	19–28
9	18–20	11–12	17	13–14	—	13	—	22–25	—	18	5	9	29–40
10	21–22	13–15	—	15–16	9	14–16	10–11	26–30	3–4	—	6–7	10–12	41–59
11	23–24	16	18	17	10	17–18	—	31–32	—	19	8	13	60–71
12	25–27	17–18	19	18	—	19	12–13	33–36	5	20	9	14	72–81
13	28–29	19	20	—	—	20	14	37–39	6	—	—	15	82–89
14	30	20	—	19	—	21	15	40–41	7	—	10	16	90–94
15	31–37	21	—	20	—	22–24	16	42–44	8	—	11	17–18	95–97
16	38–40	22	—	—	—	25	—	45	—	—	12	—	98
17	—	23–24	—	—	—	26–27	—	46–50	9	—	—	19	99
18	—	—	—	—	—	≥28	—	≥51	10	—	—	20	>99

NOTE: Age Range = 80–94, *N* = 116; %ile, percentile; Learn, Learning; Mem, Memory; Orient, Orientation; Pict Nam, Picture Naming; Sem Fluen, Semantic Fluency; Cod, Coding; Recog, Recognition.

SOURCE: From Duff et al. (2003).

TABLE 6–33 Repeatable Battery for the Assessment of Neuropsychological Status (RBANS) Age-Corrected Scaled Score Conversions to Age- and Education-Corrected Scaled Scores for ≤ 11 Years of Education (N = 100)

SCALED SCORE	LIST LEARN	STORY MEM	FIGURE COPY	LINE ORIENT	PICT NAM	SEM FLUEN	DIGIT SPAN	COD	LIST RECALL	LIST RECOG	STORY RECALL	FIGURE RECALL	%ILE RANGE
2	—	—	2	—	—	—	—	—	—	—	—	—	<1
3	2	2	3	2	2	2	2	2	—	2	—	3	1
4	3	3	—	3	—	3	—	—	2–4	3	2–3	—	2
5	4–5	—	4	4	3	4–5	3–4	3	5	4–5	4	—	3–5
6	—	4	5	5	4–5	6	5	4	6	6	—	4–5	6–10
7	6	5	6	—	—	—	6	5	7	—	5–6	6	11–18
8	7	6	7	6–7	6	7–8	7	6	—	7	7	7	19–28
9	8	7	8	—	7	—	8	7	8	8	8	8	29–40
10	9	8	9–10	8–9	8	9	9	8	9	9	9	9	41–59
11	—	9	—	—	9	10	—	9	10	10	—	10	60–71
12	10–11	10	11	10	—	11	10	—	—	—	10–11	11	72–81
13	12	11	—	11	10	12	11–12	10	11–12	11	—	12	82–89
14	13–14	12	12	12	11	13	13	11–12	13	12	12–13	13–14	90–94
15	15–17	—	13	13	12–18	14–16	14	—	—	13–18	14	—	95–97
16	18	13	14–18	14	—	17	15	13	14	—	15	15	98
17	—	14	—	15–18	—	18	16–18	14	15	—	16–18	16–18	99
18	—	15–18	—	—	—	—	—	15–18	16–18	—	—	—	>99

NOTE: Age-scaled scores were taken from tables 6-29 to 6-32. Learn, Learning; Mem, Memory; Orient, Orientation; Pict Nam, Picture Naming; Sem Fluen, Semantic Fluency; Cod, Coding; Recog, Recognition.

SOURCE: From Duff et al. (2003).

study, derived from Duff et al. (2003) scores as provided in Tables 6–29 to 6–38. Participants were an average age of 73 years (SD = 5.8). The sample was 58% female and predominantly Caucasian (86%). The majority of participants completed high school and some college (58%; see paper for additional details regarding educational levels). Subtest discrepancy scores are presented in Tables 6–39 to 6–41 according to age and subdivided by total composite score.

Based on relatively consistent findings of a two-factor structure underlying the RBANS (see "Factor-Analytic Studies and Within-Test Relationships"), Duff et al. (2009) provided age- and education-adjusted normative data to calculate Verbal and Visual RBANS indices (see also "Evidence for Reliability"). Normative data for the Verbal and Visual indices are based on 718 healthy community-dwelling adults who were participating in the broader

TABLE 6–34 Repeatable Battery for the Assessment of Neuropsychological Status (RBANS) Age-Corrected Scaled Score Conversions to Age- and Education-Corrected Scaled Scores for 12 Years of Education (N = 188)

SCALED SCORE	LIST LEARN	STORY MEM	FIGURE COPY	LINE ORIENT	PICT NAM	SEM FLUEN	DIGIT SPAN	COD	LIST RECALL	LIST RECOG	STORY RECALL	FIGURE RECALL	%ILE RANGE
2	—	2	2	2–3	—	2–3	—	2–4	—	2	2	2–3	<1
3	2–3	3	3	—	—	—	—	—	—	3	3	—	1
4	4	4	—	4	—	4	2–3	—	2–4	—	4	—	2
5	5	5	4	5	2–5	5	4–5	5	5	4–5	5	4–5	3–5
6	6	6	5–6	6	6	6	6	6	6	6	—	6	6–10
7	7	7	7	7	—	7	7	—	7	7	6	7	11–18
8	8	8	8	—	7–8	8	8	7–8	8	8–9	7	8	19–28
9	9	—	9	8–9	9	9	9	—	9	—	8–9	9	29–40
10	10	9	10	—	—	10	10	9	10	10	—	10	41–59
11	—	10–11	11	10	10	11	11	10	11	—	10–11	11	60–71
12	11–12	12	—	11–12	11	12	12	11	12	11	12	12	72–81
13	—	13	12	—	12–18	—	13	12	13	12	13	13	82–89
14	13	—	13	13	—	13	14	13	14	13–18	14	—	90–94
15	14	14	14–18	—	—	14	15	14	15	—	—	14–15	95–97
16	15	15	—	14	—	15	16	15	—	—	15	16–18	98
17	16	16–17	—	15–18	—	16–17	17–18	16	16	—	16–18	—	99
18	17–18	18	—	—	—	18	—	17–18	17–18	—	—	—	>99

NOTE: Age-scaled scores were taken from tables 6-29 to 6-32; %ile, percentile; Learn, Learning; Mem, Memory; Orient, Orientation; Pict Nam, Picture Naming; Sem Fluen, Semantic Fluency; Cod, Coding; Recog, Recognition.

SOURCE: From Duff et al. (2003).

TABLE 6–35 Repeatable Battery for the Assessment of Neuropsychological Status (RBANS) Age-Corrected Scaled Score Conversions to Age- and Education-Corrected Scaled Scores for 13–15 Years of Education (N = 230)

SCALED SCORE	LIST LEARN	STORY MEM	FIGURE COPY	LINE ORIENT	PICT NAM	SEM FLUEN	DIGIT SPAN	COD	LIST RECALL	LIST RECOG	STORY RECALL	FIGURE RECALL	%ILE RANGE
2	—	—	2	2	2	—	2–3	2	—	2	2–3	2	<1
3	2	2–3	3–4	—	3–4	2	4	—	2–4	3–4	4	3	1
4	3	—	5	3–4	—	3	5	3–5	5	—	5	4	2
5	4–5	5	6	5	6–7	5–6	6	6	—	5	—	5–6	3–5
6	6	6	7	6	—	—	—	—	6	6	6	—	6–10
7	7	7	8	7	8	7	7	7	7	7	7–8	7	11–18
8	8	8	—	8	9	8	8	8	8	8–9	9	8	19–28
9	9	9	9–10	9	—	9	9	9	9	—	—	9	29–40
10	10	10	—	10	10	10	10	10	10–11	10	10–11	10	41–59
11	11	11	11	11–12	11	11–12	11–12	11	—	—	—	11	60–71
12	12	12	—	—	12–18	—	—	12	12	11	12–13	12	72–81
13	13	13	12	13	—	13	13	13	13–14	12	—	13	82–89
14	14	14	13	14	—	14	14	14	15	13–18	14–16	14	90–94
15	—	15	14–18	15	—	15–16	15	15	—	—	—	15	95–97
16	15	16	—	16–18	—	—	16–18	16	16	—	—	16	98
17	16–17	17	—	—	—	17	—	17	17–18	—	17	17–18	99
18	18	18	—	—	—	18	—	18	—	—	18	—	>99

NOTE: Age-scaled scores were taken from tables 6-29 to 6-32; %ile, percentile; Learn, Learning; Mem, Memory; Orient, Orientation; Pict Nam, Picture Naming; Sem Fluen, Semantic Fluency; Cod, Coding; Recog, Recognition.

SOURCE: From Duff et al. (2003).

OKLAHOMA study. These participants were as described by Duff et al. (2003). Normative data are provided in Table 6–42, along with formulas for calculation of indices.

Duff, Schoenberg, Beglinger, Moser, Bayless, Culp, et al. (2008) provide normative data for the discrepancy scores between premorbid function (Barona equation) and the Total Scale score on the RBANS, derived from a community-dwelling sample of older adults as part of the OKLAHOMA study. The demographic characteristics were similar to those already described. The mean age of the sample was 73.4 years (SD = 5.9 years). The sample was 57% female, predominantly Caucasian (88%), and the majority of participants had more than 12 years of education (<12 years, 15%, 12 years, 26%; >12 years, 59%). The estimated IQ was in the average range (M = 104.4, SD = 6.7). As may be expected, premorbid IQ was similar to the RBANS score in the community-dwelling sample, with larger discrepancies reported between estimated premorbid

TABLE 6–36 Repeatable Battery for the Assessment of Neuropsychological Status (RBANS) Age-Corrected Scaled Score Conversions to Age- and Education-Corrected Scaled Scores for ≥16 Years of Education (N = 200)

SCALED SCORE	LIST LEARN	STORY MEM	FIGURE COPY	LINE ORIENT	PICT NAM	SEM FLUEN	DIGIT SPAN	COD	LIST RECALL	LIST RECOG	STORY RECALL	FIGURE RECALL	%ILE RANGE
2	2	2	2	2	2–4	—	—	2	—	2–3	2–3	2	<1
3	3	3	—	3	—	2–4	2	3	2–4	4	4	—	1
4	—	—	3	—	—	5	3	4	5	—	—	3	2
5	4–6	4–6	4–6	4–6	5–6	—	4–6	5	—	5–6	—	4–5	3–5
6	—	7	7	7	7	6	—	6–7	6	7	6–7	6	6–10
7	7	8	8	8	8–9	7–8	7–8	8	7	8	8	7–8	11–18
8	8	9	9	9	—	—	9	9	8	9	9	—	19–28
9	9	—	10	—	10	9	—	—	9	10	—	9	29–40
10	10–11	10–11	11	10–12	11	10	10–11	10	10–11	—	10–11	10–11	41–59
11	12	12	—	—	12–18	11	12	11	—	11	12–13	—	60–71
12	13	13	12	13	—	12	13	12	12–13	12	—	12	72–81
13	14	14	13	—	—	13	—	13	14	13–18	14	13–14	82–89
14	—	15	14–18	14	—	14	14	14	15	—	—	15	90–94
15	15	16	—	15	—	15	15	15	—	—	15	—	95–97
16	16	17	—	16–18	—	16	16–18	16	16	—	16	16	98
17	17	18	—	—	—	17	—	17	17–18	—	17–18	17–18	99
18	18	—	—	—	—	18	—	18	—	—	—	—	>99

NOTE: Age-scaled scores were taken from tables 6-29 to 6-32; %ile, percentile; Learn, Learning; Mem, Memory; Orient, Orientation; Pict Nam, Picture Naming; Sem Fluen, Semantic Fluency; Cod, Coding; Recog, Recognition.

SOURCE: From Duff et al. (2003).

TABLE 6–37 Repeatable Battery for the Assessment of Neuropsychological Status (RBANS) Age-Corrected Scaled Score Conversions to Age-Corrected Index Scores

INDEX SCORE	IM	VC	LANG	ATTN	DM	TOTAL	%ILE	INDEX SCORE	IM	VC	LANG	ATTN	DM	TOTAL	%ILE
≤62	≤6	≤6	≤7	≤9	≤14	≤74	<1	100				20		124	50
65	7–9	7–10	8–10	10–11	15–21	75–78	1	101					42	125	53
70	10	11	11		22–23	79–85	2	102	21	21				126	55
71	11		12	12	24–25	86	3	103			20	21	43	127–128	58
72		12	13		26	87	3	104						129	61
73				13	27	88	4	105	22				44	130	63
74						89	4	106				22		131–132	66
75	12		14		28	90	5	107		22			45	133	68
76		13				91–92	5	108	23					134	70
77						93	6	109			21	23	46	135	73
78	13				29	94–95	7	110		23				136	75
79		14		14		96	8	111	24					137	77
80					30	97	9	112			22		47	138	79
81			15			98	10	113		24		24	48	139	81
82	14	15		15	31	99–100	12	114	25						82
83						101	13	115						140	84
84			16		32	102	14	116					49	141–142	86
85	15	16		16	33	103	16	117	26			25			87
86						104–105	18	118					50	143–144	88
87					34	106	19	119	27		23		51	145	90
88	16					107	21	120		25		26		146	91
89		17		17	35	108	23	121					52	147	92
90	17		17		36	109–110	25	122						148	93
91						111	27	123	28		24	27		149	94
92		18		18		112–113	30	124					53	150–151	95
93	18		18		37	114	32	126	29		25		54	152–154	96
94					38	115–116	34	128				28		155	97
95		19				117	37	130	30		26		55	156	98
96	19			19	39	118	39	132		26		29	56	157–158	98
97					40	119–120	42	134	31			30		159–161	99
98			19			121–122	45	137	32	27	27	31	57–58	162–164	99
99	20	20			41	123	47	≥138	≥33	≥28	≥28	≥32	≥59	≥165	>99

NOTE: %ile, percentile; IM, Immediate Memory; VC, Visuospatial/Constructional; Lang, Language; Attn, Attention; DM, Delayed Memory. To determine the Index (standard) scores, add up the age-corrected scaled scores of the subtests that comprise the Index (i.e., IM, List Learning + Story Memory; VC, Figure Copy + Line Orientation; Lang, Picture Naming + Semantic Fluency; Attn, Digit Span + Coding; DM, List Recall + List Recognition + Story Recall + Figure Recall), and refer to the appropriate column in the table above. To determine the Total Score, add up the age-corrected scaled scores of all the subtests of the RBANS, and refer to the appropriate column in the table.

SOURCE: From Duff et al. (2003).

IQ and RBANS in a sample of adults referred to neuropsychological service in an academic health centre as well as a nursing home sample. The normative data for discrepancy data, along with accompanying equations, are presented in their paper.

Schoenberg et al. (2008) reported normative data based on a novel retention rate score in healthy older controls (n = 718) who were part of the OKLAHOMA study. A clinical group was included for comparison purposes, and scored lower than the community-dwelling sample. Demographic characteristics of the sample were similar to those described by Duff et al. (2011b). The clinical sample was drawn from referrals to a neuropsychology service at an academic health center (see paper for details). Retention score formulas are provided in Tables 6–43 to 6–45, along with normative data.

Green et al. (2008) provided RBANS demographically adjusted normative data for 172 Australians. Participants were community-dwelling and enrolled in a separate study. Exclusion criteria included a history of neurologic or psychiatric condition or substance abuse. The sample was 58% female, predominantly Caucasian (90%), with an age range of 20 to 89 years and an average age of 58 years (SD = 18). The sample had a mean of 14 years of education (SD = 4).

TABLE 6–38 Repeatable Battery for the Assessment of Neuropsychological Status (RBANS) Age- and Education-Corrected Scaled Score Conversions to Age- and Education-Corrected Index Scores

INDEX SCORE	IM	VC	LANG	ATTN	DM	TOTAL	%ILE	INDEX SCORE	IM	VC	LANG	ATTN	DM	TOTAL	%ILE
≤62	≤8	≤9	≤8	≤10	≤18	≤77	<1	100			24		44	132	50
65	9–10	10	9–11	11	20–21	78–84	1	101				21		133	53
70	11	11	12	12	22–23	85–89	2	102	21	22			45	134	55
71		12	13	13	24–25	90–91	3	103					46	135	58
72	12					92	3	104	22	23	25			136–137	61
73					26	93	4	105				22	47	138–139	63
74						94	4	106						140	66
75		13		14	27	95	5	107					48	141	68
76			14		28	96	5	108	23	24	26	23	49	142	70
77	13				29	97–98	6	109						143	73
78		14	15			99–101	7	110					50	144	75
79					30	102	8	111	24	25		24		145	77
80				15		103	9	112						146	79
81	14				31	104	10	113					51	147–148	81
82		15	16		32	105–107	12	114	25		27			149	82
83				16		108	13	115		26	28		52	150	84
84	15		17				14	116	26			25		151	86
85		16			33	109	16	117					53	152	87
86	16		18		34	110–111	18	118		27			54	153	88
87				17			19	119	27			26		154–155	90
88		17	19		35	112–113	21	120					55	156	91
89	17					114	23	121			29				92
90			20		36	115–116	25	122	28	28		27	56	157–158	93
91	18	18		18	37	117–118	27	123		29			57	159–160	94
92			21		38	119–120	30	124						161	95
93					39	121	32	126	29		30	28	58	162	96
94	19	19	22	19	40	122	34	128	30					163–165	97
95						123–124	37	130		30		29	59	166	98
96					41	125	39	132	31		31		60–61	167–168	98
97		20	23	20	42	126–127	42	134		31	32	30	62	169–170	99
98	20					128–129	45	137		32	33	31	63–64	171–174	99
99		21			43	130–131	47	≥138	≥32	≥33	≥34	≥32	≥65	≥175	>99

NOTE: %ile, percentile; IM, Immediate Memory; VC, Visuospatial/Constructional; Lang, Language; Attn, Attention; DM, Delayed Memory. To determine the Index (Standard) Scores, add up the age- and education-corrected scaled scores of the subtests that comprise the Index (i.e., IM, List Learning + Story Memory; VC, Figure Copy + Line Orientation; Lang, Picture Naming + Semantic Fluency; Attn, Digit Span + Coding; DM, List Recall + List Recognition + Story Recall + Figure Recall), and refer to the appropriate column in the table above. To determine the Total Score, add up the age- and education-corrected scaled scores of all the subtests of the RBANS, and refer to the appropriate column in the table.

SOURCE: From Duff et al. (2003).

Overall, participants were reported to score higher compared to normative data from the United States, especially on language-based tasks. Age- and education-adjusted norms are presented in Table 6–46.

Lim et al. (2010) provided normative data on 352 community-dwelling older Chinese participants enrolled in the Singapore Longitudinal Ageing Study (SLAS; Table 6–47). Exclusion criteria included neurologic or psychiatric condition, substance abuse, and MMSE cutoff. The sample was 60% female and ranged in age from 55 to 84 years (M = 65 years). Most of the sample had 6 or fewer years of education (52%), and 13% had no formal education. Participants primarily spoke Cantonese, Hokkien, Teochew, or Mandarin, with some English speakers (18%). Age- and education-adjusted normative data are provided in their paper. Note that some cell sizes are very small, for example n = 2 for people older than 75 with 7 to 10 years of education.

Wilk et al. (2004) provided normative data for a large sample (n = 575, aged 18 to 59 years) of patients with schizophrenia or schizoaffective disorder. Such data are particularly useful when the clinician wishes to determine whether the pattern or severity of impairment is unusual relative to expectations based on the diagnosis. The

TABLE 6–39 Frequencies of Repeatable Battery for the Assessment of Neuropsychological Status (RBANS) Discrepancy Scores (Age Corrected, Total Scale Score < 90)

	CUMULATIVE PERCENTAGES					
DISCREPANCY SCORES	≤1%	2%	5%	10%	20%	50%
Age-Corrected						
List Learning – Story Memory	−7/+9	−6/+6	−5/+4	−4/+3	+3/+1	0
Figure Copy – Line Orientation	−9/+9	−7/+8	−6/+5	−5/+4	−3/+2	0
Picture Naming – Semantic Fluency	−9/+7	−8/+6	−6/+5	−5/+3	−3/+2	0
Digit Span – Coding	−8/+9	−7/+8	−6/+7	−4/+6	−3/+4	0
List Recall – List Recognition	−6/+4	−5/+3	−4/+3	−3/+2	−2/+1	−1
List Recall – Story Recall	−6/+5	−5/+4	−4/+3	−3/+3	−2/+2	0
List Recall – Figure Recall	−7/+5	−6/+4	−5/+3	−3/+3	−2/+2	0
List Recognition – Story Recall	−7/+6	−6/+5	−4/+4	−3/+3	−2/+2	0
List Recognition – Figure Recall	−7/+7	−6/+6	−5/+4	−3/+3	−2/+2	0
Story Recall – Figure Recall	−8/+6	−7/+5	−5/+4	−4/+3	−3/+1	0
List Learning – List Recall	−7/+5	−6/+4	−5/+3	−4/+2	−3/+1	−1
List Learning – List Recognition	−8/+7	−7/+6	−6/+3	−4/+2	−3/+1	−1
Story Memory – Story Recall	−5/+4	−4/+3	−4/+2	−3/+2	−2/+1	−1
Figure Copy – Figure Recall	−6/+8	−5/+7	−5/+6	−4/+5	−2/+3	0
Age- and Education-Corrected						
List Learning – Story Memory	−7/+5	−6/+4	−5/+3	−4/+2	−3/+2	−1
Figure Copy – Line Orientation	−10/+9	−9/+7	−7/+5	−5/+4	−4/+2	−1
Picture Naming – Semantic Fluency	−8/+7	−7/+6	−5/+5	−4/+4	−3/+3	0
Digit Span – Coding	−8/+10	−7/+9	−6/+7	−5/+6	−4/+4	0
List Recall – List Recognition	−7/+5	−6/+4	−5/+3	−3/+3	−2/+2	0
List Recall – Story Recall	−7/+6	−5/+5	−4/+4	−3/+3	−2/+2	0
List Recall – Figure Recall	−7/+7	−7/+5	−6/+4	−4/+3	−2/+2	0
List Recognition – Story Recall	−7/+7	−5/+6	−4/+5	−3/+4	−2/+2	0
List Recognition – Figure Recall	−7/+8	−6/+7	−5/+5	−4/+4	−3/+3	0
Story Recall – Figure Recall	−5/+5	−5/+5	−6/+4	−4/+3	−3/+2	0
List Learning – List Recall	−7/+6	−6/+5	−5/+3	−4/+2	−3/+1	−1
List Learning – List Recognition	−7/+7	−6/+6	−6/+4	−5/+2	−3/+1	−1
Story Memory – Story Recall	−5/+5	−5/+4	−4/+3	−3/+2	−2/+1	0
Figure Copy – Figure Recall	−7/+9	−6/+8	−5/+7	−4/+5	−3/+3	0

NOTE: Subtest discrepancy scores are based on age- or age- and education-corrected scores based on the OKLAHOMA normative studies (Duff et al., 2003). In determining which table to use, calculate the age-corrected Total Scale score based on Duff et al. (2003) normative data.

SOURCE: Duff et al. (2011b).

interested reader is referred to normative tables provided in their article. Iverson et al. (2009) replicated and extended Wilk et al.'s normative data. A high base rate of impairment was noted. For example, it was not unusual for three or more index scores to be impaired (<2nd percentile) in patients with schizophrenia spectrum disorders. Normative data by diagnosis, gender, and education are found in their paper.

EVIDENCE FOR RELIABILITY

EVIDENCE FOR INTERNAL RELIABILITY

Internal reliability is high overall for both subtests (*rs* = .78 to .85) and indices (*r* > .75). Total Scale reliability is consistently high to very high (*rs* = .86 to .94; Chianetta et al., 2008; Gontkovsky et al., 2004; Hobart et al., 1999; Randolph, 1998; Sanz et al., 2009, see also manual). Note, however, that internal reliability of the Verbal and Visual RBANS indices derived by Duff et al. (2009) was quite poor (Verbal Index = .58, Visual Index = .40). However, the original indices also had weak reliability coefficients (.21 to .58). The average *SEMs* for subscale scores are generally one to 2 points. Index scores have average *SEMs* that are relatively large, about 5 to 6 points across the age range.

EVIDENCE FOR TEST-RETEST RELIABILITY, MEASURING CHANGE, AND PRACTICE EFFECTS

Test-retest reliability is variable. The stability of Form A index scores was evaluated in 40 older adults (*M* = 70.7 years of age) who were retested following an interval of about 39 weeks (Randolph, 2012). At the subtest level, List Recognition had the weakest reliability (*r* = .27), and Coding the strongest (*r* = .83), with most subtests showing poor reliability (*r* ≤ .50). Reliability coefficients were high for the Total Scale score (*r* = .88), but lower for the individual indices (Language, *r* = .55; Immediate Memory, *r* = .78). Similar findings were reported by Duff, Beglinger, Schoenberg, Patton, Mold, Scott, and Adams (2005) in their sample of older adults. Duff et al. (2009) also reported adequate reliability for derived Verbal and Visual indices at a one-year retest interval (.74 for each index).

TABLE 6–40 Frequencies of Repeatable Battery for the Assessment of Neuropsychological Status (RBANS) Discrepancy Scores (Age-Corrected, Total Score 90 to 109)

	CUMULATIVE PERCENTAGES					
DISCREPANCY SCORES	≤1%	2%	5%	10%	20%	50%
Age-Corrected						
List Learning – Story Memory	−7/+7	−6/+6	−5/+4	−4/+3	−3/+2	0
Figure Copy – Line Orientation	−8/+7	−7/+6	−5/+4	−4/+3	−3/+2	0
Picture Naming – Semantic Fluency	−8/+4	−7/+3	−6/+3	−5/+2	−4/+1	−1
Digit Span – Coding	−8/+7	−7/+6	−6/+5	−4/+4	−3/+2	0
List Recall – List Recognition	−5/+5	−4/+4	−4/+3	−3/+3	−2/+2	0
List Recall – Story Recall	−7/+6	−6/+5	−5/+4	−4/+3	−3/+1	0
List Recall – Figure Recall	−8/+6	−7/+5	−6/+4	−5/+3	−3/+2	−1
List Recognition – Story Recall	−8/+5	−7/+4	−6/+3	−5/+2	−3/+1	−1
List Recognition – Figure Recall	−8/+5	−7/+4	−6/+3	−5/+2	−3/+1	−1
Story Recall – Figure Recall	−8/+7	−7/+6	−6/+4	−5/+3	−3/+2	−1
List Learning – List Recall	−6/+7	−5/+6	−4/+4	−3/+2	−2/+1	−1
List learning – List Recognition	−6/+8	−5/+6	−4/+4	−3/+3	−2/+1	0
Story Memory – Story Recall	−6/+4	−5/+3	−4/+3	−3/+2	−2/+1	−1
Figure Copy – Figure Recall	−7/+6	−6/+5	−5/+4	−4/+3	−3/+2	−1
Age- and Education-Corrected						
List Learning – Story Memory	−7/+7	−6/+5	−5/+4	−4/+3	−3/+2	−1
Figure Copy – Line Orientation	−8/+7	−7/+6	−6/+4	−5/+3	−3/+2	−1
Picture Naming – Semantic Fluency	−8/+5	−7/+4	−6/+3	−5/+2	−4/+1	−1
Digit Span – Coding	−8/+8	−7/+7	−6/+5	−5/+4	−4/+2	−1
List Recall – List Recognition	−5/+5	−4/+4	−4/+3	−3/+2	−2/+1	−1
List Recall – Story Recall	−7/+6	−6/+5	−5/+4	−4/+3	−3/+1	−1
List Recall – Figure Recall	−8/+7	−7/+6	−6/+4	−4/+3	−3/+2	−1
List Recognition – Story Recall	−8/+6	−7/+5	−6/+4	−5/+3	−3/+2	0
List Recognition – Figure Recall	−8/+6	−7/+5	−6/+4	−5/+3	−3/+2	0
Story Recall – Figure Recall	−9/+7	−8/+6	−6/+4	−5/+3	−3/+2	0
List Learning – List Recall	−6/+7	−5/+6	−4/+4	−3/+2	−2/+1	−1
List Learning – List Recognition	−6/+7	−5/+6	−4/+4	−3/+3	−2/+2	−1
Story Memory – Story Recall	−5/+5	−4/+4	−4/+3	−3/+2	−2/+1	−1
Figure Copy – Figure Recall	−7/+6	−6/+5	−5/+4	−4/+3	−3/+2	−1

NOTE: Subtest discrepancy scores are based on age- or age and education-corrected scores based on the OKLAHOMA normative studies (Duff et al. 2003). In determining which table to use, calculate the age-corrected Total Scale score based on Duff et al. (2003) normative data.

SOURCE: Duff et al. (2011b).

On retest, most subtest scores slightly increased between testing intervals, with some showing a slight decrease on repeat testing (e.g., List Learning, Picture Naming, Digit Span, List Recall). Mean retest scores were generally higher than initial scores (range of one point for Immediate Memory to 10 points for Visuospatial/Constructional). However, on the Language Index, scores declined by about 2 points on retest. In their sample of healthy older adults, Duff, Beglinger, Schoenberg, Patton, Mold, Scott, and Adams (2005) reported that practice effects were largely absent, with most scores slightly decreased at retest.

Test-retest reliability was good overall for the French translation of the RBANS in a sample of patients with schizophrenia spectrum disorders tested twice within two weeks, with the exception of Picture Naming, Digit Span, and List Recognition, which showed weak reliability (Chianetta et al., 2008). Significant practice effects were found for List Learning. See also Wilk et al. (2002).

Duff et al. (2004; Duff, Schoenberg, Patton, Paulsen, Bayless, Mold, Scott, & Adams, 2005) provide regression-based equations to assess change across time in older adults. The equations were developed on a sample of 223 adults and subsequently cross-validated in a separate sample of 222 adults. Of note, Figure Copy and Figure Recall were scored with revised scoring criteria (see Duff et al., 2003). Prediction equations for each of the indices and the Total Scale score are shown in Table 6–48. Algorithms for the 12 subtests are shown in Table 6–49.

The data (Duff, Schoenberg, Patton, Paulsen, Bayless, Mold, Scott, & Adams, 2005) suggest that initial performance is the best predictor of follow-up performance, with demographic variables also influencing performance. As noted by the authors, these equations are susceptible to regression to the mean effects and will thus tend to under- or overestimate the performance of individuals whose scores fall at extremes (e.g., <2nd percentile or >98th percentile).

Error is also likely to be introduced if formulas are applied to examinees with demographic characteristics outside of parameters in the model (i.e., <64 or >90 years old) or when the retest interval is shorter or longer than the retest interval in the model. Of note, Duff, Schoenberg, Patton, Mold, Scott, and Adams (2008), provide prediction

TABLE 6–41 Frequencies of Repeatable Battery for the Assessment of Neuropsychological Status (RBANS) Discrepancy Scores (Age-Corrected, Total Scale Score ≥ 110)

	CUMULATIVE PERCENTAGES					
DISCREPANCY SCORES	≤1%	2%	5%	10%	20%	50%
Age-Corrected						
List Learning – Story Memory	−8/+5	−7/+4	−5/+4	−4/+3	−3/+2	−1
Figure Copy – Line Orientation	−7/+4	−6/+3	−5/+2	−4/+2	−3/+1	−1
Picture Naming – Semantic Fluency	−9/+3	−8/+2	−7/+2	−6/+1	−5/+0	−3
Digit Span – Coding	−11/+7	−10/+6	−7/+4	−5/+3	−3/+2	−1
List Recall – List Recognition	−4/+6	−3/+5	−2/+5	−1/+4	0/+4	2
List Recall – Story Recall	−7/+6	−5/+5	−4/+4	−3/+3	−2/+1	0
List Recall – Figure Recall	−7/+7	−6/+6	−5/+5	−4/+4	−3/+3	0
List Recognition – Story Recall	−7/+3	−6/+2	−5/+1	−5/+0	−4/+1	−3
List Recognition – Figure Recall	−7/+4	−6/+3	−6/+2	−5/+1	−4/+0	−2
Story Recall – Figure Recall	−8/+7	−6/+6	−5/+5	−4/+4	−2/+3	0
List Learning – List Recall	−5/+5	−4/+4	−4/+3	−3/+2	−2/+1	−1
List Learning – List Recognition	−4/+7	−3/+6	−2/+5	−1/+4	0/+3	2
Story Memory – Story Recall	−6/+5	−5/+4	−5/+4	−4/+3	−3/+2	0
Figure Copy – Figure Recall	−7/+4	−6/+3	−5/+2	−5/+1	−4/+0	−2
Age- and Education-Corrected						
List Learning – Story Memory	−7/+5	−6/+4	−5/+4	−4/+3	−3/+2	−1
Figure Copy – Line Orientation	−7/+5	−6/+4	−5/+3	−4/+2	−3/+2	−1
Picture Naming – Semantic Fluency	−10/+4	−9/+3	−8/+2	−6/+1	−5/+0	−3
Digit Span – Coding	−13/+8	−11/+7	−8/+4	−6/+3	−4/+2	−1
List Recall – List Recognition	−4/+5	−3/+5	−3/+4	−2/+4	0/+3	1
List Recall – Story Recall	−7/+6	−6/+5	−4/+4	−3/+3	−2/+2	−1
List Recall – Figure Recall	−7/+8	−6/+7	−5/+5	−4/+4	−3/+3	0
List Recognition – Story Recall	−7/+4	−6/+3	−5/+1	−5/+1	−4/+0	−2
List Recognition – Figure Recall	−8/+5	−7/+4	−6/+3	−5/+2	−4/+1	−2
Story Recall – Figure Recall	−7/+7	−6/+6	−5/+5	−4/+4	−3/+3	0
List Learning – List Recall	−6/+6	−4/+5	−3/+3	−3/+2	−2/+1	−1
List Learning – List Recognition	−4/+7	−3/+6	−3/+5	−2/+4	−1/+3	1
Story Memory – Story Recall	−6/+5	−5/+4	−4/+4	−3/+3	−2/+2	0
Figure Copy – Figure Recall	−7/+4	−6/+3	−5/+3	−5/+2	−4/+1	−2

NOTE: Subtest discrepancy scores are based on age- or age- and education-corrected scores based on the OKLAHOMA normative studies (Duff et al., 2003). In determining which table to use, calculate the age-corrected Total Scale score based on Duff el al. (2003) normative data.

SOURCE: Duff et al. (2011b).

equations based on 146 community-dwelling older adults across two years, with validation in another older adult sample of $n = 145$. Predicted and observed scores showed a high degree of concordance, with details provided in their paper. Reliable change indices derived from a sample of patients with medically managed PD are also available (see Schoenberg et al., 2012).

One alternative to reliable change algorithms is the use of base rate data for discrepancy scores across a clinically meaningful period of time. According to this method, if a discrepancy between two scores at two testing points exceeds a predetermined threshold (<10th percentile), this change in performance is interpreted to be clinically significant. Patton et al. (2005) provided base rate data for RBANS scores using Form A in a cognitively healthy community-dwelling sample of older adults over one- and two-year retest intervals. Base rates of discrepancies were calculated and organized into three groups (i.e., below average, average, and above average) with respect to the age- and education-corrected RBANS Total Scale score. The below average group was comprised of participants who obtained age- and education-corrected Total Scale scores less than 90, the average group scored between 90 and 109, and the above average group scored 110 or above. Base rate data were drawn from three sources: OKLAHOMA age-corrected index scores, OKLAHOMA age- and education-corrected index scores, and age-corrected index scores based on the original RBANS normative sample (Randolph, 1998). The data suggest that relatively large differences across time are common.

EVIDENCE FOR RELIABILITY OF ALTERNATE, SHORT, OR COMPUTER FORMS

Overall, alternate forms reliability suggests high reliability for the Total Scale score ($r \geq .82$) and weaker reliability for index scores, with the exception of the Attention Index, which tends to show high to very high reliability over various intervals (see manual).

EVIDENCE FOR INTERRATER RELIABILITY

Interscorer agreement for Figure Copy is high (intraclass correlation coefficient = .85; Randolph, 1998).

TABLE 6–42 Age- and Education-Adjusted Repeatable Battery for the Assessment of Neuropsychological Status (RBANS) Verbal and Visual Factor Scores

INDEX SCORE	VERBAL	VISUAL	%ILE	INDEX SCORE	VERBAL	VISUAL	%ILE
≤62	≤22	≤18	<1	100			50
65	23–28	19–24	1	101	53	43	53
70	29–30	25	2	102	54		55
71	31	26	3	103	55	44	58
72	32	27	3	104			61
73	33		4	105	56	45	63
74		28	4	106			66
75	34		5	107	57		68
76	35		5	108		46	70
77		29	6	109	58		73
78	36	30	7	110		47	75
79			8	111	59		77
80	37	31	9	112	60	48	79
81	38		10	113			81
82	39	32	12	114	61		82
83			13	115		49	84
84	40	33	14	116			86
85	41	34	16	117	64	50	87
86	42		18	118			88
87	43	35	19	119	65	51	90
88			21	120	66		91
89	44	36	23	121			92
90	45		25	122	67	52	93
91		37	27	123	68		94
92	46	38	30	124	69	53	95
93	47		32	126		54	96
94	48	39	34	128	70	55	97
95	49		37	130	71	56	98
96	50	40	39	132	72	57	98
97	51	41	42	134	73	58	99
98			45	137	74	59	99
99	52	42	47	≥138	≥75	≥60	>99

NOTE: %ile, percentile. These age- and education-corrected scores were obtained from Duff et al. (2003). To determine the Index Scores, add up the age- and education-corrected scale scores of the subtests that comprise the Index (i.e., Verbal = List Learning + Story Memory + List Recall + List Recognition + Story Recall; Visual = Figure Copy + Line Orientation + Coding + Figure Recall), and refer to the appropriate column in the table above.

SOURCE: Duff et al. (2009).

EVIDENCE FOR VALIDITY

FACTOR-ANALYTIC STUDIES AND WITHIN-TEST RELATIONSHIPS

Factor-analytic studies have generally supported a two-factor solution (i.e., memory and visuospatial processing; although see Garcia, Leahy, Corradi, & Forchetti, 2008, and Thaler, Scott, Duff, Mold, & Adams, 2013, who reported three- and four-factor solutions, respectively). Samples in which a two-factor solution has been found include community-dwelling older adults (Duff et al., 2006), veterans (Carlozzi et al., 2008), patients with schizophrenia spectrum disorders (King et al., 2012), patients with dementia (Schmitt et al., 2010), people with stroke (Wilde, 2006), and in a reanalysis of multiple datasets (Vogt et al., 2017).

RBANS scores generally show moderate correlations with one another (Carlozzi et al., 2008, Gontovsky et al., 2004, manual; Wilde, 2006), with the largest correlations between Immediate and Delayed Memory Indices (range $r = .63$ to $r = .75$; Carlozzi et al., 2008; manual; Wilde, 2006) and Total Scale score with Index scores ($r = .64$ to $r = .87$; Carlozzi et al., 2008; Wilde, 2006).

RELATIONSHIPS WITH OTHER TESTS

The RBANS Total Scale score is highly correlated with Wechsler FSIQ estimates (*rs* = .75 to .77; Gold et al., 1999; manual), composite scores based on various measures ($r = .79$, Hobart et al., 1999), and memory scores (WMS-III; *rs* = .67 to .69, Gold et al., 1999). Of note, Wechsler FSIQ and memory index scores tend to be higher on average than the RBANS Total Scale score. The RBANS Total Scale score and the MMSE are also correlated (*rs* = .41 to 65; Schmitt et al., 2016).

Correlations between individual RBANS indices with domain counterparts on Wechsler intelligence and memory tests, the Rey Complex Figure Test (RCFT), Judgment of Line Orientation, BNT, Controlled Oral Word Association Test, and other neuropsychological tests, tend to show variable correlations, ranging from modest to large in magnitude ($r = .21$ to .82; Source). Gold et al. (1999) similarly provided evidence of convergent validity for some of the RBANS scales in a sample of patients with schizophrenia, with three out of five indices (Immediate Memory, Attention, Delayed Memory) correlating with similar indices on the WMS-III and WAIS-III.

RBANS indices have also shown evidence of convergent and discriminant validity in stroke patients, with all RBANS indices also correlating moderately with language measures (Larson et al., 2005). In a mixed clinical sample, the Language Index showed moderate correlations overall with other language tests (*rs* = .38 to .79; Verbal Fluency, Multilingual Aphasia Examination, Boston Naming Test; Merz et al., 2017).

Pachet (2007) similarly reported correlations between RBANS scores and other neuropsychological tests in a small sample of 37 post-acute adults with moderate to severe brain injury. Large correlations overall were observed between RBANS subtests and comparable tests (e.g., *rs* = .61 to .78; RBANS List Learning with CVLT; RBANS Story Memory with WMS Logical Memory; Digit Span with Wechsler Digit Span; Coding with the Symbol Digit Modalities Test [SDMT]), with the exception of RBANS Figure and the RCFT. Moderate to large correlations were generally observed between RBANS indices and comparable tests (e.g., *rs* = .47 to .79; RBANS Attention with Digit Span, Immediate Memory with CVLT and Wechsler Logical Memory, Visuospatial/Constructional with Block

TABLE 6–43 Repeatable Battery for the Assessment of Neuropsychological Status (RBANS) List Retention Novel Score Age-Corrected Scaled Scores for Midpoint Age Ranges

SCALED SCORE	MIDPOINT 70 (RANGE, 65–75)	MIDPOINT 75 (RANGE, 70–80)	MIDPOINT 80 (RANGE, 75–85)	MIDPOINT 85 (RANGE, 80–94)	PERCENTILE
2	—	—	—	—	<1
3	—	—	—	—	1
4	0	—	—	—	2
5	0.01–0.04	0	0	0	3–5
6	0.05–0.09	0.01–0.05	0.01–0.04	0.01–0.03	6–10
7	0.10–0.13	0.06–0.11	0.05–0.10	0.04–0.09	11–18
8	0.14–0.16	0.12–0.15	0.11–0.13	0.10–0.13	19–28
9	0.17–0.19	0.16–0.18	0.14–0.16	0.14–0.15	29–40
10	0.20–0.24	0.19–0.22	0.17–0.21	0.16–0.19	41–59
11	0.25–0.26	0.23–0.24	0.22–0.24	0.20–0.24	60–71
12	0.27–0.28	0.25–0.28	0.25–0.26	0.25–0.27	72–81
13	0.29–0.30	0.29–0.30	0.27–0.29	0.28–0.29	82–89
14	0.31	0.31	0.30–0.31	0.30–0.31	90–94
15	0.32	0.32–0.33	0.32	0.32–0.33	95–97
16	0.33–0.34	0.34–0.35	0.33–0.35	0.34–0.37	98
17	0.35–0.38	0.36–0.43	0.36–0.39	0.38	99
18	0.39–1.0	0.44–1.0	0.40–1.0	0.39–1.0	>99

NOTE: Retention rate = List Recall raw score (range, 0–10)/List Learning Total raw score (range, 0–40).

SOURCE: Schoenberg et al. (2008).

Design and RCFT), without relations between RBANS indices and the RCFT, SDMT, and the TMT. The RBANS Memory subscales were related to the Somatic Complaints scale of the Personality Assessment Inventory (PAI); however, the PAI scales did not differentiate high and low scoring groups on the RBANS (Aikman & Souheaver, 2008).

CLINICAL STUDIES

Dementia. Given that the RBANS' original purpose was to screen dementia, it is perhaps not surprising that there is a fairly large literature on use of this test in that population. In summary, the test has utility in differentiating between patients with dementia and controls, mixed utility in differentiation of dementia types, and somewhat weaker discriminability in differentiating MCI from other groups. The RBANS appears to be more sensitive than the MMSE or Dementia Rating Scale (DRS) in detecting cognitive impairment (manual).

The RBANS has shown utility in differentiating patients with AD from controls. Duff et al. (2008) reported that patients with AD scored lower on the RBANS than demographically matched controls. Diagnostic accuracy statistics

TABLE 6–44 Repeatable Battery for the Assessment of Neuropsychological Status (RBANS) Story Retention Novel Score Age-Corrected Scaled Scores for Midpoint Age Ranges

SCALED SCORE	MIDPOINT 70 (RANGE 65–75)	MIDPOINT 75 (RANGE, 70–80)	MIDPOINT 80 (RANGE, 75–85)	MIDPOINT 85 (RANGE, 80–94)	PERCENTILE
2	0–0.09	—	—	—	<1
3	0.10–0.17	0	—	—	1
4	0.18–0.21	0.01–0.09	0	—	2
5	0.22–0.27	0.10–0.24	0.01–0.09	0	3–5
6	0.28–0.36	0.25–0.31	0.10–0.16	0.01–0.10	6–10
7	0.37–0.42	0.32–0.38	0.17–0.32	0.11–0.29	11–18
8	0.43–0.45	0.39–0.43	0.33–0.40	0.30–0.37	19–28
9	0.46–0.49	0.44–0.47	0.41–0.44	0.38–0.43	29–40
10	0.50–0.54	0.48–0.53	0.45–0.52	0.44–0.48	41–59
11	0.55–0.57	0.54–0.57	0.53–0.55	0.49–0.55	60–71
12	0.58–0.60	0.58–0.59	0.56–0.58	0.56–0.58	72–81
13	0.61–0.65	0.60–0.65	0.59–0.62	0.59	82–89
14	0.66–0.69	0.66–0.69	0.63–0.67	0.60–0.67	90–94
15	0.70–0.75	0.70–0.71	0.68–0.70	0.68–0.71	95–97
16	0.76–0.82	0.72–0.73	0.71–0.72	0.72–0.73	98
17	0.83–0.90	0.74–0.82	0.73–0.75	0.74–0.75	99
18	0.91–1.0	0.83–1.0	0.76–1.0	0.76–1.0	>99

NOTE: Retention rate = Story Recall raw score (range, 0–12)/Story Memory Total score (range, 0–24).

SOURCE: Schoenberg et al. (2008).

TABLE 6-45 Repeatable Battery for the Assessment of Neuropsychological Status (RBANS) Figure Retention Novel Score Age-Corrected Scaled Scores for Midpoint Age Ranges

SCALED SCORE	MIDPOINT 70 (RANGE, 65–75)	MIDPOINT 75 (RANGE, 70–80)	MIDPOINT 80 (RANGE, 75–85)	MIDPOINT 85 (RANGE, 80–94)	PERCENTILE
2	0–0.10	0–0.11	0	—	<1
3	0.11–0.16	0.12–0.16	0.01–0.10	—	1
4	0.17–0.21	0.17–0.19	0.11–0.14	0	2
5	0.22–0.35	0.20–0.29	0.15–0.25	0.01–0.13	3–5
6	0.36–0.47	0.30–0.43	0.26–0.37	0.14–0.28	6–10
7	0.48–0.55	0.44–0.47	0.38–0.47	0.29–0.41	11–18
8	0.56–0.63	0.48–0.59	0.48–0.55	0.42–0.53	19–28
9	0.64–0.69	0.60–0.66	0.56–0.63	0.54–0.60	29–40
10	0.70–0.79	0.67–0.75	0.64–0.74	0.61–0.75	41–59
11	0.80–0.85	0.76–0.82	0.75–0.79	0.76–0.80	60–71
12	0.86–0.89	0.83–0. 89	0.80–0.83	0.81–0.83	72–81
13	0.90–0.95	0.90–0.94	0.84–0.89	0.84–0.87	82–89
14	0.96–0.99	0.95	0.90–0.95	0.88–0.93	90–94
15	1.0	0.96–0.99	0.96–0.99	0.94–0.95	95–97
16	—	1.0	1.0	0.96–0.99	98
17	—	—	—	1.0	99
18	—	—	—	—	>99

NOTE: Retention rate = Figure Copy raw score (range, 0–20)/Figure Recall raw score (range, 0–20).

SOURCE: Schoenberg et al. (2008).

suggested optimal sensitivity and specificity at 1.5 *SD*s below the mean. All index scores were associated with high specificity (≥91%), although most index scores were associated with lower sensitivity (e.g., 26% for the Language Index to 46% for the Attention Index). However, both sensitivity and specificity for Immediate and Delayed Memory index scores were excellent (Immediate Memory sensitivity of 82%, specificity of 93%; Delayed Memory sensitivity of 92%, specificity of 92%).

Research has also examined the utility of the RBANS in differentiating between AD and other dementias. For example, McDermott and DeFillipis (2010) reported that a vascular dementia group performed better on Delayed Memory than an AD group (Cohen's d = 1.3). No other differences were found between groups on index scores. Although the sensitivity was excellent, the specificity was comparatively weaker (92% vs. 61%). The manual reported that patients with probable AD perform most poorly on Language and Delayed Memory, and patients with Huntington's disease (HD) obtain lowest scores on Attention and Visuospatial/Constructional subtests.

Similar findings differentiating patients with primarily cortical versus subcortical disorders have been reported by Beatty et al. (2003b). They found that the profile of patients with AD resembled that of HD (i.e., relatively more impairment on the Language and Delayed Memory indices), but patients with PD showed greater impairment on the Attention Index. Classification accuracy using an algorithm termed the Cortical Subcortical Index (CSI) provided in the manual (i.e., CSI = (Visuospatial/Construction + Attention)/(2) – (Language + Delayed Memory)/(2)) showed low accuracy in classifying patients with PD who did not have dementia. Duff, Schoenberg, Mold, Scott, and Adams (2007) examined the utility of the CSI in n = 793 older primary care patients. If the resulting value of CSI is greater than 0, the score is deemed "Cortical." If CSI is 0 or less, then the value is deemed "Subcortical." Duff et al., however, reported that the "Cortical" profiles were common in their sample of healthy older adults, with 37% of their sample scoring 10 or more points on the CSI. The stability of the scores was moderate over one- and two-year periods (r = .58 to .61). These data suggest that a discrepancy in scores based on RBANS indices may actually be common in healthy older adults.

A percent retention score derived from verbal memory subtests shows strong sensitivity and specificity in differentiating between groups of AD, MCI, and controls (Clark et al., 2010). For example, optimal cutoff scores of less than 60% on List Retention and less than 70% on Story Retention effectively classified individuals with AD versus controls with sensitivity and specificity values exceeding 90%. Diagnostic accuracy was somewhat lower for AD compared to MCI groups.

The utility of RBANS verbal and visual processing factors, such as proposed by Duff et al. (2009; see "Normative Data") in differentiating MCI, AD, and PD have also been examined (see Morgan et al., 2010). Controls and the AD group differed from all other groups on the factors. MCI and PD patients did not differ. Sensitivity of differentiating the AD participants from the healthy participants using both factors was excellent (92%), and specificity was strong (79%). Diagnostic accuracy when classifying healthy versus other groups was somewhat lower (i.e., MCI sensitivity of 79%; specificity of 72%; PD sensitivity of 66%, specificity of 66%). Differentiation between clinical groups was also comparatively lower (i.e., MCI vs. AD sensitivity of 66%, specificity of 75%; AD vs. PD sensitivity of 73%, specificity of 60%).

TABLE 6–46 Australian Normative Data for the Repeatable Battery for the Assessment of Neuropsychological Status (RBANS) Stratified by Age and Education

	20–39		40–49		50–59		60–69		70–79		80–89	
SUBTEST	<12 EDU	≥12 EDU	<12 EDU	≥12 EDU	<12 EDU	≥12 EDU	<12 EDU	≥12 EDU	<12 EDU	≥12 EDU	<12 EDU	≥12 EDU
List Learning	29.6 (4.0)	33.0 (4.0)	33.0 (3.7)	32.5 (3.2)	29.4 (5.0)	30.8 (3.2)	28.3 (5.2)	30.1 (3.3)	26.5 (6.4)	25.4 (4.6)	23.7 (53)	25.6 (3.2)
Story Memory	19.8 (1.3)	20.0 (2.3)	21.5 (1.7)	20.7 (2.3)	17.8 (3.0)	18.8 (2.6)	19.2 (3.8)	19.0 (2.3)	16.9 (3.5)	17.4 (2.6)	14.7 (5.7)	16.9 (4.3)
Figure Copy	17.8 (1.4)	18.6 (1.7)	15.7 (2.9)	17.5 (12)	18.6 (1.9)	17.8 (2.9)	17.0 (3.3)	17.9 (2.3)	16.0 (2.8)	16.9 (2.7)	16.7 (2.2)	15.4 (3.8)
Line Orientation	19.1 (.93)	18.4 (2.8)	16.8 (3.3)	18.0 (2.4)	18.0 (1.7)	17.3 (4.0)	18.0 (2.7)	19.2 (1.1)	17.3 (2.5)	17.7 (2.5)	14.0 (6.5)	18.8 (1.0)
Picture Naming	10.0 (0)	9.9 (.2)	10.0 (0)	10.0 (0)	10.0 (0)	9.9 (.21)	10.0 (0)	9.9 (.32)	9.9 (.30)	9.8 (.41)	9.9 (.11)	9.9 (.35)
Semantic Fluency	23.7 (4.9)	24.0 (6.0)	25.0 (5.6)	28.5 (4.9)	23.0 (6.0)	24.0 (5.9)	23.0 (6.6)	23.3 (4.8)	22.4 (6.2)	22.0 (5.1)	19.0 (2.3)	22.8 (5.5)
Digit Span	12.0 (2.4)	11.8 (2.7)	13.3 (3.1)	13.8 (1.7)	12.2 (1.9)	12.1 (2.4)	11.6 (2.4)	12.1 (2.3)	9.7 (1.8)	11.5 (3.2)	10.4 (2.5)	11.5 (3.0)
Coding	58.6 (7.7)	59.6 (7.6)	53.0 (5.4)	57.0 (7.0)	45.0 (4.0)	51.0 (6.2)	46.1 (8.9)	49.0 (5.4)	35.0 (11.6)	38.7 (12)	24.9 (8.4)	38.0 (7.9)
List Recall	7.3 (1.4)	8.3 (1.8)	7.8 (2.7)	8.2 (1.8)	5.4 (1.9)	6.8 (2.2)	6.9 (2.3)	6.8 (2.1)	6.8 (2.1)	5.5 (2.3)	5.1 (2.8)	6.0 (1.9)
List Recognition	19.8 (.67)	19.8 (.53)	19.3 (.96)	19.4 (1.0)	19.5 (.52)	18.8 (3.3)	19.4 (1.3)	19.3 (1.2)	19.4 (.81)	18.8 (1.6)	18.7 (.95)	18.8 (1.8)
Story Recall	11.2 (.44)	11.2 (.86)	10.8 (.96)	10.8 (1.2)	9.6 (2.0)	11.0 (2.4)	10.6 (1.5)	10.4 (1.7)	9.0 (2.1)	9.7 (1.8)	7.6 (2.9)	9.3 (1.6)
Figure Recall	13.6 (4.4)	16.3 (3.4)	12.0 (3.9)	14.0 (3.7)	14.0 (4.1)	13.6 (.82)	12.2 (4.9)	14.3 (4.3)	12.1 (3.3)	11.9 (3.5)	10.3 (2.8)	9.4 (.11)
	(*n* = 3)	(*n* = 34)	(*n* = 2)	(*n* = 12)	(*n* = 9)	(*n* = 24)	(*n* = 9)	(*n* = 22)	(*n* = 11)	(*n* = 30)	(*n* = 6)	(*n* = 10)

NOTE: EDU = Education in years.

SOURCE: Green et al. (2008).

TABLE 6–47 Chinese Normative Data for the Repeatable Battery for the Assessment of Neuropsychological Status (RBANS)

SUBTESTS	55–59 YEARS (N = 97)	60–64 YEARS (N = 93)	65–69 YEARS (N = 80)	70–74 YEARS (N = 58)	75 YEARS AND ABOVE (N = 24)
List Learning	28.6 (3.8)	27.0 (4.4)	27.0 (3.8)	25.7 (4.9)	23.0 (4.6)
Story Memory	16.6 (3.5)	16.7 (3.5)	16.0 (3.7)	15.8 (3.4)	14.8 (4.1)
Figure Copy	17.4 (2.7)	16.7 (2.8)	16.7 (2.6)	16.5 (2.8)	14.8 (3.4)
Line Orientation	16.3 (3.2)	14.9 (3.7)	14.2 (3.6)	13.8 (3.6)	12.4 (4.3)
Picture Naming	9.8 (1.0)	9.8 (0.5)	9.9 (0.3)	9.8 (0.4)	9.6 (0.6)
Semantic Fluency	17.0 (3.0)	16.2 (3.0)	15.5 (3.0)	15.7 (3.0)	14.4 (3.2)
Digit Span	13.5 (2.6)	13.8 (1.8)	13.7 (2.4)	13.6 (1.9)	13.3 (2.5)
Coding	40.5 (12.1)	33.3 (13.2)	27.2 (10.5)	26.6 (10.6)	19.2 (13.2)
List Recall	7.7 (1.7)	7.2 (2.0)	6.5 (2.5)	5.8 (2.5)	5.1 (2.0)
List Recognition	19.7 (0.7)	19.6 (0.9)	19.3 (1.3)	19.1 (1.0)	19.0 (1.0)
Story Recall	9.3 (2.0)	9.2 (1.9)	8.7 (2.0)	8.7 (2.1)	7.3 (2.5)
Figure Recall	12.9 (4.1)	11.9 (4.6)	11.1 (4.5)	10.5 (4.3)	8.3 (3.8)

SOURCE: Lim et al. (2010).

Although research suggests strong discriminability between AD and controls, the RBANS appears to have decreased accuracy in differentiating between MCI and controls. Duff, Hobson, Beglinger, and O'Bryant (2010) reported that patients with MCI perform worse than controls on the RBANS Total Scale score, three of five indices, and half of the subtests. Although specificity was good, sensitivity was weak, in the poor to moderate range overall.

The RBANS has correlates with day-to-day life in dementia. Informant report correlates with language and memory variables from the RBANS (Hobson, Hall, Humphreys-Clark, Schrimsher, & O'Bryant, 2010). The RBANS correlates with measures of ADLs in patients with dementia, with RBANS, MMSE, depressive symptoms, and demographic and clinical variables (age, education, years since onset), accounting for 50% of the variance in ADLs (Freilich & Hyer, 2007). Immediate Memory and Attention were identified as particularly important predictors.

TABLE 6–48 Algorithms to Predict Time 2 Repeatable Battery for the Assessment of Neuropsychological Status (RBANS) Index Scores in Older Adults Who Were Administered Form A

INDEX	R^2	SE^a_{EST}	C^b	B^c	B^d	B^e	B^f
Immediate Memory	.56	11.08	53.76	.63	−.37	2.58	
Visuospatial/ Construction	.43	12.50	35.89	.57		2.81	
Language	.39	8.79	35.28	.63			
Attention	.60	9.65	37.04	.75	−.30		.03
Delayed Memory	.51	11.46	30.60	.71			
Total Score	.72	7.81	37.65	.75	−.23	1.47	

NOTE: Based on older adults, aged 65+, retested following about one year. To calculate the Predicted Time 2 score based on the formulas above, use the age-corrected scaled score from the RBANS Manual for the Time 1 score; use age in years; use the education coding listed below; and use the number of days for the retest interval.

Education Coding:
11 years or less = 1
12 years = 2
13–15 years = 3
16 years or more = 4

Change indices can be calculated as follows:
Observed Time 2 score–Predicted Time 2 score = Predicted Difference score
Predicted Difference score/Standard error of the estimate = *z* score of difference
If *z* score of difference > 1.64, then significant change at 90% confidence.

[a]Standard error of the estimate.
[b]Constant.
[c]Unstandardized beta weight for Time 1 Index score.
[d]Unstandardized beta weight for age.
[e]Unstandardized beta weight for education.
[f]Unstandardized beta weight for retest interval.

SOURCE: From Duff et al. (2004).

PD and HD. Patients with HD demonstrated deficits on 11 of 12 RBANS subtests in one study (Duff, Beglinger, Theriault, Allison, & Paulsen, 2010). In addition, patients with HD showed decline over a 16-month period on the Attention Index and specific RBANS subtests (Beglinger et al., 2010).

However, in another study, the RBANS was not found to be predictive of change in PD patients over a 12- to 18-month period (Schneider, Elm, Parashos, Ravina, & Galpern, 2010). More patients in a group that underwent deep brain stimulation showed change in RBANS scores than did patients in medically managed groups (Rinehardt et al., 2010; Schoenberg et al., 2012). Patients with PD and MS show distinct patterns of recall and recognition on verbal memory subtests (Beatty et al., 2003b; Beatty, 2004). See also the "Dementia" section.

Stroke. Group differences based on conceptualizations of hemispheric specialization have been reported in stroke, with left hemisphere stroke associated with verbal impairments and right hemisphere stroke associated with visual impairments (see "Factor-Analytic Studies and Within-Test Relationships"; Wilde, 2006).

The RBANS has been used as a measure of outcome in stroke (e.g., Wagle et al., 2009, 2010), and research suggests evidence of predictive validity. Improvement was noted on the Total Scale score and Delayed Memory scores in stroke patients following treatment with escitalopram (Jorge, Acion, Moser, Adams, & Robinson, 2010). The RBANS was one factor predicting institutionalization at

TABLE 6–49 Algorithms to Predict Time 2 Repeatable Battery for the Assessment of Neuropsychological Status (RBANS) Subtests in Older Adults Who Were Administered Form A

SUBTEST	R^2	SE^a_{EST}	C[b]	B[c]	OTHER VARIABLES IN EQUATION[d]
List Learning	.52	3.74	19.34	.55	(ed × 1.18) – (age × .16)
Story Memory	.43	3.48	18.25	.61	– (age × .17)
Figure Copy	.25	1.65	8.50	.53	
Line Orientation	.46	2.28	11.23	.45	(gender × .69) – (age × .07) + (ed × .56) + (race × 1.73)
Picture Naming	.42	0.59	3.45	.62	(gender × .21)
Semantic Fluency	.35	3.60	6.48	.53	(ed × .59)
Digit Span	.39	1.90	8.25	.51	– (age × .07) + (interval × .01)
Coding	.75	5.45	18.86	.86	– (age × 19)
List Recall	.47	1.96	6.78	.64	– (age × .07)
List Recognition	.33	1.22	11.88	.51	– (age × .04)
Story Recall	.45	2.10	2.03	.63	(ed × .34)
Figure Recall	.39	3.16	10.31	.57	– (age × .08) + (ed × .59)

NOTE: ed = Education in years.
Based on older adults, aged 65+, retested following about one year.
[a]Standard error of the estimate.
[b]Constant.
[c]Unstandardized beta weight for the same Time 1 subtest.
[d]Unstandardized beta weights for other variables in the equation.

To calculate the Predicted Time 2 score, use the subtest raw scores; use age in years; use the demographic listed below; use the number of days for the retest interval. Use the following formula: (Constant value for the subtest) + (Unstandardized beta weight for the subtest at Time 1 × raw score for the subtest at Time 1) + (Other variables in equation as noted in the table).

ed = Education Coding:
11 years or less = 1
12 years = 2
13–15 years = 3
16 years or more = 4

Gender Coding:
Female = 0
Male = 1

Race Coding:
Non-white/Non-Caucasian = 0
White/Caucasian = 1

Change indices can be calculated as follows:
Observed Time 2 score – Predicted Time 2 score = Predicted Difference score
Predicted Difference score/Standard error of the estimate = *z score* of difference
If *z* of difference >1.64, then significant change at 90% confidence. Contact author for computer program.

SOURCE: Duff et al. (2005).

13-month follow-up, with Delayed Memory predicting depression (Farner et al., 2010). Coding and Figure Copy predicted a significant amount of variance in long-term functional outcome (Wagle et al., 2011). Larson et al. (2005) reported that the RBANS predicted self-report of cognitive disability as well as instrumental ADLs at 12-month follow-up.

TBI. Individuals with TBI perform worse than controls on RBANS indices, with modest to strong sensitivity and high specificity (McKay et al., 2008). In an acute TBI sample, patients were tested six days after resolution of posttraumatic amnesia (PTA), with mean index scores in excess of 1.5 *SD* below the standardization sample. After controlling for demographic factors, Delayed Memory and Total Scale scores were significantly predicted by length of PTA (Lippa et al., 2013).

Psychiatric Conditions. The RBANS also appears to be a useful screening instrument in psychiatric patients (Gold et al., 1999; Hobart et al., 1999; Wilk et al., 2002, 2004). Patients with schizophrenia demonstrate marked impairment on the test, despite showing relatively adequate performance on a measure of premorbid function (Wide Range Achievement Test, Third Edition, Reading; e.g., Gold et al., 1999; Wilk et al., 2002, 2004). Iverson et al. (2009) reported that the median performance of patients with schizophrenia was one to two *SD*s below the mean. The RBANS Total Scale score is associated with high sensitivity and specificity in this population (sensitivity from 88% to 90%; specificity from 86% to 100%; De la Torre et al., 2016; Sanz et al., 2009).

Patients with schizophrenia tend to show more impairment on the RBANS than patients with bipolar disorder (Gogos et al., 2010; Hobart et al., 1999). In terms of functional correlates, the Immediate Memory Index shows accurate differentiation with respect to employment status (Gold et al., 1999). The RBANS has been used to evaluate treatment outcome in schizophrenia (e.g., Boggs et al., 2012; Chouinard et al., 2007), and performance has shown to be related to biological correlates (e.g., elevated infectious and inflammatory factors, Dickerson et al., 2012; brain-derived neurotropic factor, Zhang et al, 2012). Negative symptom change predicted the RBANS Total Scale score in patients with psychosis (Anda et al., 2016).

Research on patients with depression suggests some group differences and relations between RBANS performance and symptom severity. Depressed individuals perform worse on the RBANS than healthy controls, with individuals who were previously depressed also showing impairments on specific domains relative to healthy controls (Baune et al., 2010). Mild to moderate depression is related to RBANS scores reflecting attention, memory, and visuospatial/constructional abilities (Faust et al., 2017). Severity of depression relates to Immediate Memory Index scores (Hook et al., 2010). In patients diagnosed with depression, psychiatric comorbidity is associated with decreased visuospatial/constructional and language function (Baune et al., 2009). Bipolar patients perform worse than controls on the RBANS Total Scale score and most subtests (Gerber et al., 2012).

Other Populations. Decrements in RBANS performance have been reported in a number of patient groups, including patients with asymptomatic carotid artery stenosis (Landgraff et al., 2010), chronic pain (Weiner et al., 2006), and end-stage liver disease (Mooney et al., 2007). The test has also shown utility in patients with brain tumor (Lageman et al., 2010), heart failure (Bauer et al., 2012), and fragile X syndrome (Berry-Kravis et al., 2008).

The RBANS has been used to evaluate treatment outcome, including following a computerized cognitive training program in community-dwelling older adults (Smith et al., 2009; Zelinski et al., 2011), following cancer treatment (e.g., Jansen, Cooper, Dodd, & Miaskowski, 2011), after treatment of carotid artery stenosis (Takaiwa et al., 2009), after treatment in fragile X syndrome (Berry-Kravis et al., 2008), and following substance use treatment (Schrimsher, & Parker, 2008). In psychosis and substance use disorders, patients classified as showing good recovery perform significantly better on Delayed Memory (deVille et al., 2011).

NEUROANATOMICAL CORRELATES AND IMAGING STUDIES

Commensurate with its emphasis on providing an overall estimate of cognitive function, the Total Scale score correlates with total brain volume in older adults (Paul et al., 2011). Lower RBANS scores are associated with shorter whole brain white fiber length, with the relationship between the RBANS and fiber length moderated by cognitive reserve (Baker et al., 2017). Hippocampal volume and specific hippocampal subfields are related to Figure Recall (Zammit et al., 2017). As discussed, relationships have also been reported between laterality of hemispheric damage in stroke and performance (see "Clinical Studies").

PERFORMANCE VALIDITY

Overall, performance validity indices derived from the RBANS appear to be associated with relatively strong classification accuracy in patients with TBI (e.g., Jones, 2016) and are moderately correlated with other PVTs. The Effort Index (EI) in particular shows promise, and an alternative measure, the Effort Scale (ES), has been developed, but more research is needed to validate its use in clinical populations. Considerable caution is required in using these indexes in geriatric populations, other clinical populations with significant impairment, and people who are in the low range of cognitive and adaptive function.

EFFORT INDEX

Silverberg, Wertheimer, and Fichtenberg (2007) devised the Effort Index (EI) comprised of RBANS List Recognition and RBANS Digit Span based on the purported insensitivity of these subtests to veritable cognitive dysfunction. Their sample included 103 participants who completed neuropsychological assessments at a neurorehabilitation outpatient clinic; all had a neurologic disorder (e.g., TBI, stroke, dementia, epilepsy, MS, anoxia) or psychiatric disorder, and 24% were involved in litigation or a compensation claim. However, none met Slick et al.'s (1999) criteria for malingering. Raw scores were converted to weighted scores, which corresponded to percentile ranges, such that higher percentile ranges were associated with lower weighted scores (see Table 6–50). The weighted scores were then added to form an EI. Silverberg et al. (2007) then applied the EI in identified malingerers with mild TBI, nonmalingerers with mild TBI, and groups of simulated malingerers. The patients with documented TBIs performed better than both clinical and simulated malingerer groups. A cutoff score of greater than zero was identified as the point of optimal classification accuracy (87%), whereas a score of greater than 3 was deemed to reflect potentially invalid performance.

Using an EI cutoff score of greater than 3, sensitivity was low to moderate (24% to 31%) with a high specificity of 96–97% in an active military sample (Armistead-Jehle & Hansen, 2011). Similarly, Young, Baughman, and Roper

TABLE 6–50 Repeatable Battery for the Assessment of Neuropsychological Status (RBANS) Conversion from Raw Scores to Weighted Scores to Provide an Effort Index

DIGIT SPAN (RAW SCORE)	LIST RECOGNITION (RAW SCORE)	WEIGHTED SCORE
8–16	18–20	0
–	17	1
7	15–16	2
6	13–14	3
–	11–12	4
5	10	5
0–4	0–9	6

SOURCE: Silverberg et al. (2007).

(2012) reported modest EI sensitivity (31%) despite excellent specificity (94%) in a nongeriatric veteran sample. Notably, List Recognition of less than 17 was associated with an acceptable sensitivity of 52% at a 90% specificity. Using combined RBANS scores, Barker, Horner, and Bachman (2010) reported that cutoff scores of less than 15 on List Recognition, less than 8 on Digit Span, and more than 3 on the EI in a geriatric veteran sample evaluated in a memory disorders clinic were associated with better sensitivity (51–64%) at a specificity of 85%. Similarly, use of an EI cutoff score of 1 or greater yielded acceptable sensitivities of 53% to 62% with high specificities (92% to 96%).

In populations with cognitive deficits, a high rate of false positives may occur, as is the case for most PVTs. For example, Hook, Marquine, and Hoelzle (2009) reported that 31% of their sample of nonlitigating older adults were classified as demonstrating invalid performance (EI >3). No one in their sample who obtained a RBANS Total Scale score of 70 or lower or an MMSE score of 23 or lower obtained a passing EI score, suggesting that persons who are low functioning may be more likely to be erroneously identified as performing invalidly using the EI. Similar results are reported by Duff et al. (2011), who provided base rate failures of the EI in geriatric samples comprised of participants representing a wide range of function, including cognitively healthy, nursing home-dwelling, and probable AD. In cognitively healthy and mildly impaired samples, only 3% met criteria on the RBANS for invalid performance. However, older patients and those with lower education levels were more likely to have scores consistent with invalid performance. In patients with greater impairment, a high number had EI scores above suggested cutoff scores (i.e., 37% in a nursing home sample, 33% in a probable AD sample). Overall, lower education was associated with failure on the EI in the majority of participants, as was lower cognitive level.

On the positive side, the EI demonstrates moderate to high correlations with other PVTs. Armistead-Jehle and Hansen (2011) reported that the EI was correlated with other PVTs in an active duty military sample, including the TOMM, Medical Symptom Validity Test (MSVT), and the Non-Verbal Medical Symptom Validity Test (NV-MSVT; *rs* = .32 to .58).

The test-rest reliability of the EI is apparently not strong. For example, O'Mahar et al. (2012) reported that the one-year test-retest reliability of the EI was poor (Spearman's rho .32 to .36) in both cognitively healthy older adults and those with amnestic MCI. Older adults who performed worse on retesting tended to have lower Total Scale scores.

EFFORT SCALE

In recognition of previous research suggesting a high number of EI false positives in patients with dementia, Novitski, Steele, Karantzoulis, and Randolph (2012) created a new performance validity scale, the Effort Scale (ES), for the RBANS. The RBANS ES is calculated from RBANS Recognition and Digit Span subtest raw scores, to be used when a patient performs poorly on List Recognition and/or Digit Span subtests (i.e., List Recognition scores of <19 or Digit Span scores of <9).

$$\text{RBANS ES} = [(\text{List Recognition} - (\text{List Recall} + \text{Story Recall} + \text{Figure Recall})] + \text{Digit Span}$$

Scores of less than 12 on the ES are considered suggestive of invalid performance. The ES showed good discriminability between a sample of patients with amnestic disorders and a sample of mild TBI patients who failed the WMT. In one study that applied both the EI and the ES, the majority of patients with HD passed the EI (82% of patients). However, poorer cognitive, adaptive, and motor function was associated with failure on the EI (Sieck et al., 2013). Fewer than one-third of patients passed the ES, suggesting limited utility in this population.

COMMENT

The RBANS Update was designed as a brief screen of neuropsychological functioning. It offers a means to evaluate major neuropsychological domains via tests that will be familiar to most neuropsychologists (e.g., list learning and memory, story memory and recall, figure copy and recall, line orientation, confrontation naming, fluency, digit span, coding). Alternate forms are also included, and the test is available in Spanish and other languages. Ease of administration is facilitated via portable administration materials, with administration details provided on the record form. The RBANS Update has apparent utility as a brief screen, but in most high-stakes clinical situations, a more comprehensive assessment will be preferred.

In terms of demographic effects, age and education affect performance, with small effects of gender reported (i.e., men better on visual spatial/constructional tests, women better on delayed memory and language). Differences with respect to ethnicity have been reported, although this variable may be a proxy for other variables, such as education.

The normative sample is of decent size (N = 500) and is Census-stratified. Age- and education-corrected supplemental norms are also available, as well as some cross-cultural norms. There is a particularly robust supplemental normative set for older adults. Notably, significant differences in interpretation can result depending on which normative dataset is used in older adult populations. Some of the subtests have a restricted range in the healthy population (e.g., Figure Copy, Line Orientation, Picture Naming, List Recognition). That is, most healthy individuals obtain raw scores that approach the maximum possible for the subtest, with few individuals scoring below a perfect score. It is also worth bearing in mind that the test was designed to be used with healthy adults as well as individuals who may have moderate to severe dementia. As a consequence, it may have limited utility in detecting impairment at the higher end of the intellectual distribution.

In terms of reliability, internal reliability is generally high. Test-retest reliability is generally poor for most subtests and slightly better for composite scores, such as the index scores and the Total Scale score. Given weak reliability for subtest scores, it is recommended that the entire battery be administered and the composite scores be given relative importance compared to the other scores for clinical decision-making purposes. Practice effects appear quite small with the exception of Visuospatial/Constructional scores. In addition to age- and education-corrected normative data, Duff and colleagues have also provided algorithms to estimate significant change. Because these are vulnerable to regression to the mean, base rate data for discrepancy scores may be useful for individuals likely to be at the extreme scores of the distribution (e.g., Patton et al., 2005).

The RBANS has considerable evidence of test validity. The test correlates with more extensive batteries; however, there is evidence for a two-factor, rather than five-factor solution, suggesting that the indices are not entirely separate. In clinical populations, research suggests that the test is useful in differentiating between patients with dementia and controls. However, there is mixed evidence with respect to differentiation between dementia subtypes. Although group differences are typically found, the accuracy of scores such as the Cortical/Subcortical Index may be of limited utility given high base rates in healthy populations. The clinical research is predominantly concentrated in dementia populations; however, the test has also been used in a number of clinical groups, including HD, PD, schizophrenia, and mood disorders, among others. The RBANS has also demonstrated predictive validity in stroke, utility as a measure to aid in diagnosis in psychiatric populations, and as an outcome measure.

In terms of performance validity assessment, the EI shows promise in TBI samples but considerable caution is required in geriatric populations, other clinical populations with significant impairment, and people who are in the low range of cognitive and adaptive function , as is true of most PVTs. An alternative measure, the ES, has been developed, but more research is needed to validate its use in clinical populations.

REFERENCES

Aikman, G. G., & Souheaver, G. T. (2008). Use of the Personality Assessment Inventory (PAI) in neuropsychological testing of psychiatric outpatients. *Applied Neuropsychology, 15*(3), 176–183. https://doi.org/10.1080/09084280802324283

American Psychiatric Association, (Eds.). (2000). *Diagnostic and statistical manual of mental disorders: DSM-IV-TR* (4th ed., text revision). American Psychiatric Association.

Anda, L., Brønnick, K. S., Johnsen, E., Kroken, R. A., Jørgensen, H., & Løberg, E.-M. (2016). The course of neurocognitive changes in acute psychosis: Relation to symptomatic improvement. *PloS One, 11*(12), e0167390. https://doi.org/10.1371/journal.pone.0167390

Armistead-Jehle, P., & Hansen, C. L. (2011). Comparison of the Repeatable Battery for the Assessment of Neuropsychological Status Effort Index and stand-alone symptom validity tests in a military sample. *Archives of Clinical Neuropsychology:, 26*(7), 592–601. https://doi.org/10.1093/arclin/acr049

Baker, L. M., Laidlaw, D. H., Cabeen, R., Akbudak, E., Conturo, T. E., Correia, S., . . . Paul, R. H. (2017). Cognitive reserve moderates the relationship between neuropsychological performance and white matter fiber bundle length in healthy older adults. *Brain Imaging and Behavior, 11*(3), 632–639. https://doi.org/10.1007/s11682-016-9540-7

Barker, M. D., Horner, M. D., & Bachman, D. L. (2010). Embedded indices of effort in the Repeatable Battery for the Assessment of Neuropsychological Status (RBANS) in a geriatric sample. *The Clinical Neuropsychologist, 24*(6), 1064–1077. https://doi.org/10.1080/13854046.2010.486009

Bauer, L., Pozehl, B., Hertzog, M., Johnson, J., Zimmerman, L., & Filipi, M. (2012). A brief neuropsychological battery for use in the chronic heart failure population. *European Journal of Cardiovascular Nursing, 11*(2), 223–230. https://doi.org/10.1016/j.ejcnurse.2011.03.007

Baune, B. T., McAfoose, J., Leach, G., Quirk, F., & Mitchell, D. (2009). Impact of psychiatric and medical comorbidity on cognitive function in depression. *Psychiatry and Clinical Neurosciences, 63*(3), 392–400. https://doi.org/10.1111/j.1440-1819.2009.01971.x

Baune, B. T., Miller, R., McAfoose, J., Johnson, M., Quirk, F., & Mitchell, D. (2010). The role of cognitive impairment in general functioning in major depression. *Psychiatry Research, 176*(2–3), 183–189. https://doi.org/10.1016/j.psychres.2008.12.001

Beatty, W. W. (2004). RBANS analysis of verbal memory in multiple sclerosis. *Archives of Clinical Neuropsychology, 19,* 825–834.

Beatty, W. W., Mold, J. W., & Gontkovsky, S. T. (2003a). RBANS performance: Influences of sex and education. *Journal of Clinical and Experimental Neuropsychology, 25,* 1065–1069.

Beatty, W. W., Ryder, K. A., Gontkovsky, S. T., Scott, J. G., McSwan, K. L., & Bharucha, K. J. (2003b). Analyzing the subcortical dementia syndrome of Parkinson's disease using the RBANS. *Archives of Clinical Neuropsychology, 18,* 509–520.

Beglinger, L. J., Duff, K., Allison, J., Theriault, D., O'Rourke, J. J. F., Leserman, A., & Paulsen, J. S. (2010). Cognitive change in patients with Huntington disease on the Repeatable Battery for the Assessment of Neuropsychological Status. *Journal of Clinical and Experimental Neuropsychology, 32*(6), 573–578. https://doi.org/10.1080/13803390903313564

Berry-Kravis, E., Sumis, A., Kim, O.-K., Lara, R., & Wuu, J. (2008). Characterization of potential outcome measures for future clinical trials in fragile X syndrome. *Journal of Autism and Developmental Disorders, 38*(9), 1751–1757. https://doi.org/10.1007/s10803-008-0564-8

Boggs, D. L., Kelly, D. L., McMahon, R. P., Gold, J. M., Gorelick, D. A., Linthicum, J., . . . Buchanan, R. W. (2012). Rimonabant for neurocognition in schizophrenia: A 16-week double blind randomized placebo controlled trial. *Schizophrenia Research, 134*(2–3), 207–210. https://doi.org/10.1016/j.schres.2011.11.009

Calamia, M., Roye, S., & Lemke, A. (2017). Does prior administration of the RBANS influence performance on subsequent neuropsychological testing? *Applied Neuropsychology. Adult,* 1–4. https://doi.org/10.1080/23279095.2017.1299736

Carlozzi, N. E., Horner, M. D., Yang, C., & Tilley, B. C. (2008). Factor analysis of the Repeatable Battery for the Assessment of

Neuropsychological Status. *Applied Neuropsychology, 15*(4), 274–279. https://doi.org/10.1080/09084280802325124

Chianetta, J.-M., Lefebvre, M., LeBlanc, R., & Grignon, S. (2008). Comparative psychometric properties of the BACS and RBANS in patients with schizophrenia and schizoaffective disorder. *Schizophrenia Research, 105*(1–3), 86–94. https://doi.org/10.1016/j.schres.2008.05.024

Chouinard, S., Stip, E., Poulin, J., Melun, J.-P., Godbout, R., Guillem, F., & Cohen, H. (2007). Rivastigmine treatment as an add-on to antipsychotics in patients with schizophrenia and cognitive deficits. *Current Medical Research and Opinion, 23*(3), 575–583. https://doi.org/10.1185/030079906X167372

Clark, J. H., Hobson, V. L., & O'Bryant, S. E. (2010). Diagnostic accuracy of percent retention scores on RBANS verbal memory Subtests for the diagnosis of Alzheimer's disease and mild cognitive impairment. *Archives of Clinical Neuropsychology, 25*(4), 318–326. https://doi.org/10.1093/arclin/acq023

Crawford, J. R., Garthwaite, P. H., Morrice, N., & Duff, K. (2011). Some supplementary methods for the analysis of the RBANS. *Psychological Assessment, 24*(2), 365–374. https://doi.org/10.1037/a0025652

De la Torre, G. G., Perez, M. J., Ramallo, M. A., Randolph, C., & González-Villegas, M. B. (2016). Screening of cognitive impairment in schizophrenia: Reliability, sensitivity, and specificity of the Repeatable Battery for the Assessment of Neuropsychological Status in a Spanish sample. *Assessment, 23*(2), 221–231. https://doi.org/10.1177/1073191115583715

deVille, M., Baker, A., Lewin, T. J., Bucci, S., & Loughland, C. (2011). Associations between substance use, neuropsychological functioning and treatment response in psychosis. *Psychiatry Research, 186*(2–3), 190–196. https://doi.org/10.1016/j.psychres.2010.08.025

Dickerson, F., Stallings, C., Origoni, A., Vaughan, C., Khushalani, S., & Yolken, R. (2012). Additive effects of elevated C-reactive protein and exposure to Herpes Simplex Virus type 1 on cognitive impairment in individuals with schizophrenia. *Schizophrenia Research, 134*(1), 83–88. https://doi.org/10.1016/j.schres.2011.10.003

Duff, K., Beglinger, L. J., Schoenberg, M. R., Patton, D. E., Mold, J., Scott, J. G., & Adams, R. L. (2005). Test-retest stability and practice effects of the RBANS in a community-dwelling elderly sample. *Journal of Clinical and Experimental Neuropsychology, 27,* 565–575.

Duff, K., Beglinger, L. J., Theriault, D., Allison, J., & Paulsen, J. S. (2010). Cognitive deficits in Huntington's disease on the Repeatable Battery for the Assessment of Neuropsychological Status. *Journal of Clinical and Experimental Neuropsychology, 32*(3), 231–238. https://doi.org/10.1080/13803390902926184

Duff, K., Hobson, V. L., Beglinger, L. J., & O'Bryant, S. E. (2010). Diagnostic accuracy of the RBANS in mild cognitive impairment: Limitations on assessing milder impairments. *Archives of Clinical Neuropsychology, 25*(5), 429–441. https://doi.org/10.1093/arclin/acq045

Duff, K., Humphreys-Clark, J., Obryant, S., Mold, J., Schiffer, R., & Sutker, P. (2008). Utility of the RBANS in detecting cognitive impairment associated with Alzheimer's disease: Sensitivity, specificity, and positive and negative predictive powers. *Archives of Clinical Neuropsychology, 23*(5), 603–612. https://doi.org/10.1016/j.acn.2008.06.004

Duff, K., Langbehn, D. R., Schoenberg, M. R., Moser, D. J., Baade, L. E., Mold, J., . . . Adams, R. L. (2006). Examining the Repeatable Battery for the Assessment of Neuropsychological Status: Factor analytic studies in an elderly sample. *American Journal of Geriatric Psychiatry, 14*(11), 976–979.

Duff, K., Langbehn, D. R., Schoenberg, M. R., Moser, D. J., Baade, L. E., Mold, J. W., . . . Adams, R. L. (2009). Normative data on and psychometric properties of Verbal and Visual Indexes of the RBANS in older adults. *The Clinical Neuropsychologist, 23*(1), 39–50. https://doi.org/10.1080/13854040701861391

Duff, K., Leber, W. R., Patton, D. E., Schoenberg, M. R., Mold, J. W., Scott, J. G., & Adams, R. L. (2007). Modified scoring criteria for the RBANS figures. *Applied Neuropsychology, 14*(2), 73–83.

Duff, K., Patton, D., Schoenberg, M. R., Mold, J., Scott, J. G., & Adams, R. L. (2003). Age- and education-corrected independent normative data for the RBANS in a community-dwelling elderly sample. *The Clinical Neuropsychologist, 17,* 351–366.

Duff, K., Patton, D. E., Schoenberg, M. R., Mold, J., Scott, J. G., & Adams, R. L. (2011b). Intersubtest discrepancies on the RBANS: Results from the OKLAHOMA study. *Applied Neuropsychology, 18*(2), 79–85. https://doi.org/10.1080/09084282.2010.523359

Duff, K., Schoenberg, M. R., Beglinger, L. J., Moser, D. J., Bayless, J. D., Culp, K. R., . . . Adams, R. L. (2008). Premorbid intellect and current RBANS performance: Discrepancy scores in three geriatric samples. *Applied Neuropsychology, 15*(4), 241–249. https://doi.org/10.1080/09084280802325041

Duff, K., Schoenberg, M. R., Mold, J. W., Scott, J. G., & Adams, R. L. (2007). Normative and retest data on the RBANS cortical/subcortical index in older adults. *Journal of Clinical and Experimental Neuropsychology, 29*(8), 854–859. https://doi.org/10.1080/13803390601147629

Duff, K., Schoenberg, M. R., Mold, J. W., Scott, J. G., & Adams, R. L. (2011c). Gender differences on the Repeatable Battery for the Assessment of Neuropsychological Status subtests in older adults: Baseline and retest data. *Journal of Clinical and Experimental Neuropsychology, 33*(4), 448–455. https://doi.org/10.1080/13803395.2010.533156

Duff, K., Schoenberg, M. R., Patton, D., Mold, J., Scott, J. G., & Adams, R. L. (2004). Predicting change with the RBANS in an elderly sample. *Journal of the International Neuropsychological Society, 10,* 828–834.

Duff, K., Schoenberg, M. R., Patton, D. E., Mold, J. W., Scott, J. G., & Adams, R. L. (2008). Predicting cognitive change across 3 years in community-dwelling elders. *The Clinical Neuropsychologist, 22*(4), 651–661. https://doi.org/10.1080/13854040701448785

Duff, K., Schoenberg, M. R., Patton, D., Paulsen, J. S., Bayless, J. D., Mold, J., Scott, J. G., & Adams, R. L. (2005). Regression-based formulas for predicting change in RBANS subtests with older adults. *Archives of Clinical Neuropsychology, 20,* 281–290.

Duff, K., Spering, C. C., O'Bryant, S. E., Beglinger, L. J., Moser, D. J., Bayless, J. D., . . . Scott, J. G. (2011). The RBANS Effort Index: Base rates in geriatric samples. *Applied Neuropsychology, 18*(1), 11–17. https://doi.org/10.1080/09084282.2010.523354

Farner, L., Wagle, J., Engedal, K., Flekkøy, K. M., Wyller, T. B., & Fure, B. (2010). Depressive symptoms in stroke patients: A 13-month follow-up study of patients referred to a rehabilitation unit. *Journal of Affective Disorders, 127*(1–3), 211–218. https://doi.org/10.1016/j.jad.2010.05.025

Faust, K., Nelson, B. D., Sarapas, C., & Pliskin, N. H. (2017). Depression and performance on the Repeatable Battery for the Assessment of Neuropsychological Status. *Applied Neuropsychology. Adult, 24*(4), 350–356. https://doi.org/10.1080/23279095.2016.1185426

Freilich, B. M., & Hyer, L. A. (2007). Relation of the Repeatable Battery for Assessment of Neuropsychological Status to measures of daily functioning in dementia. *Psychological Reports, 101*(1), 119–129. https://doi.org/10.2466/pr0.101.1.119-129

Garcia, C., Leahy, B., Corradi, K., & Forchetti, C. (2008). Component structure of the Repeatable Battery for the Assessment of Neuropsychological Status in dementia. *Archives of Clinical Neuropsychology, 23*(1), 63–72. https://doi.org/10.1016/j.acn.2007.08.008

Gerber, S. I., Krienke, U. J., Biedermann, N.-C., Grunze, H., Yolken, R. H., Dittmann, S., & Langosch, J. M. (2012). Impaired functioning in euthymic patients with bipolar disorder—HSV-1 as a predictor. *Progress in Neuro-Psychopharmacology and Biological Psychiatry, 36*(1), 110–116. https://doi.org/10.1016/j.pnpbp.2011.09.003

Gogos, A., Joshua, N., & Rossell, S. L. (2010). Use of the Repeatable Battery for the Assessment of Neuropsychological Status (RBANS) to investigate group and gender differences in schizophrenia and bipolar disorder. *Australian and New Zealand Journal of Psychiatry, 44*(3), 220–229. https://doi.org/10.3109/00048670903446882

Gold, J. M., Queern, C., Iannone, V. N., & Buchanan, R. B. (1999). Repeatable Battery for the Assessment of Neuropsychological Status as a screening test in schizophrenia, I: Sensitivity, reliability, and validity. *American Journal of Psychiatry, 158,* 1944–1950.

Gontkovsky, S. T., Beatty, W. W., & Mold, J. W. (2004). Repeatable Battery for the Assessment of Neurological Status in a normal, geriatric sample. *Clinical Gerontologist, 27,* 79–86.

Gontkovsky, S. T., Mold, J. W., & Beatty, E. E. (2002). Age and educational influences on RBANS index scores in a nondemented geriatric sample. *The Clinical Neuropsychologist, 16,* 258–263.

Green, A., Garrick, T., Sheedy, D., Blake, H., Shores, A., & Harper, C. (2008). Repeatable Battery for the Assessment of Neuropsychological Status (RBANS): Preliminary Australian normative data. *Australian Journal of Psychology, 60*(2), 72–79. https://doi.org/10.1080/00049530701656257

Hobart, M. P., Goldberg, R., Bartko, J. J., & Gold, J. M. (1999). Repeatable Battery for the Assessment of Neuropsychological Status as a screening test in schizophrenia, II: Convergent/discriminant validity and diagnostic group comparisons. *American Journal of Psychiatry, 156,* 1951–1957.

Hobson, V. L., Hall, J. R., Humphreys-Clark, J. D., Schrimsher, G. W., & O'Bryant, S. E. (2010). Identifying functional impairment with scores from the repeatable battery for the assessment of neuropsychological status (RBANS). *International Journal of Geriatric Psychiatry, 25*(5), 525–530. https://doi.org/10.1002/gps.2382

Hook, J. N., Han, D. Y., & Smith, C. A. (2010). Repeatable Battery for the Assessment of Neuropsychological Status (RBANS) and depressive complaints in older adults. *Clinical Gerontologist, 33*(2), 84–91. https://doi.org/10.1080/07317110903552164

Hook, J. N., Marquine, M. J., & Hoelzle, J. B. (2009). Repeatable Battery for the Assessment of Neuropsychological Status Effort Index performance in a medically ill geriatric sample. *Archives of Clinical Neuropsychology:, 24*(3), 231–235. https://doi.org/10.1093/arclin/acp026

Iverson, G. L., Brooks, B. L., & Haley, G. M. T. (2009). Interpretation of the RBANS in inpatient psychiatry: Clinical normative data and prevalence of low scores for patients with schizophrenia. *Applied Neuropsychology, 16*(1), 31–41. https://doi.org/10.1080/09084280802644128

Jansen, C. E., Cooper, B. A., Dodd, M. J., & Miaskowski, C. A. (2011). A prospective longitudinal study of chemotherapy-induced cognitive changes in breast cancer patients. *Supportive Care in Cancer, 19*(10), 1647–1656. https://doi.org/10.1007/s00520-010-0997-4

Jodouin, K. A., O'Connell, M. E., & Morgan, D. G. (2017). RBANS memory percentage retention: No evidence of incremental validity beyond RBANS scores for diagnostic classification of mild cognitive impairment and dementia and for prediction of daily function. *Applied Neuropsychology. Adult, 24*(5), 420–428. https://doi.org/10.1080/23279095

Jones, A. (2016). Repeatable Battery for the Assessment of Neuropsychological Status: Effort Index cutoff scores for psychometrically defined malingering groups in a military sample. *Archives of Clinical Neuropsychology:, 31*(3), 273–283. https://doi.org/10.1093/arclin/acw006

Jorge, R. E., Acion, L., Moser, D., Adams, H. P., & Robinson, R. G. (2010). Escitalopram and enhancement of cognitive recovery following stroke. *Archives of General Psychiatry, 67*(2), 187–196. https://doi.org/10.1001/archgenpsychiatry.2009.185

King, L. C., Bailie, J. M., Kinney, D. I., & Nitch, S. R. (2012). Is the Repeatable Battery for the Assessment of Neuropsychological Status factor structure appropriate for inpatient psychiatry? An exploratory and higher-order analysis. *Archives of Clinical Neuropsychology, 27*(7), 756–765. https://doi.org/10.1093/arclin/acs062

Lageman, S. K., Cerhan, J. H., Locke, D. E. C., Anderson, S. K., Wu, W., & Brown, P. D. (2010). Comparing neuropsychological tasks to optimize brief cognitive batteries for brain tumor clinical trials. *Journal of Neuro-Oncology, 96*(2), 271–276. https://doi.org/10.1007/s11060-009-9960-y

Landgraff, N. C., Whitney, S. L., Rubinstein, E. N., & Yonas, H. (2010). Cognitive and physical performance in patients with asymptomatic carotid artery disease. *Journal of Neurology, 257*(6), 982–991. https://doi.org/10.1007/s00415-009-5449-z

Larson, E. B., Kirschner, K., Bode, R., Heinemann, A., & Goodman, R. (2005). Construct and predictive validity of the Repeatable Battery for the Assessment of Neuropsychological Status in the evaluation of stroke patients. *Journal of Clinical and Experimental Neuropsychology, 27,* 16–32.

Lim, M.-L., Collinson, S. L., Feng, L., & Ng, T.-P. (2010). Cross-cultural application of the Repeatable Battery for the Assessment of Neuropsychological Status (RBANS): Performances of elderly Chinese Singaporeans. *The Clinical Neuropsychologist, 24*(5), 811–826. https://doi.org/10.1080/13854046.2010.490789

Lippa, S. M., Hawes, S., Jokic, E., & Caroselli, J. S. (2013). Sensitivity of the RBANS to acute traumatic brain injury and length of post-traumatic amnesia. *Brain Injury, 27*(6), 689–695. https://doi.org/10.3109/02699052.2013.771793

Martin, P. K., Schroeder, R. W., & Baade, L. E. (2017). A tale of two norms: The impact of normative sample selection criteria on standardized scores in older adults. *The Clinical Neuropsychologist, 31*(6–7), 1204–1218. https://doi.org/10.1080/13854046.2017.1349182

McDermott, A. T., & DeFilippis, N. A. (2010). Are the indices of the RBANS sufficient for differentiating Alzheimer's disease and subcortical vascular dementia? *Archives of Clinical Neuropsychology, 25*(4), 327–334. https://doi.org/10.1093/arclin/acq028

McKay, C., Wertheimer, J. C., Fichtenberg, N. L., & Casey, J. E. (2008). The Repeatable Battery for the Assessment of Neuropsychological Status (RBANS): Clinical utility in a traumatic brain injury sample. *The Clinical Neuropsychologist, 22*(2), 228–241. https://doi.org/10.1080/13854040701260370

Merz, Z. C., Hurless, N., & Wright, J. D. (2017). Examination of the construct validity of the Repeatable Battery for the Assessment of Neuropsychological Status Language Index in a mixed neurological sample. *Archives of Clinical Neuropsychology:,* 1–6. https://doi.org/10.1093/arclin/acx115

Mooney, S., Hasssanein, T., Hilsabeck, R., Ziegler, E., Carlson, M., Maron, L., & Perry, W. (2007). Utility of the Repeatable Battery for the Assessment of Neuropsychological Status (RBANS) in patients with end-stage liver disease awaiting liver transplant. *Archives of Clinical Neuropsychology, 22*(2), 175–186. https://doi.org/10.1016/j.acn.2006.12.005

Morgan, D. R., Linck, J., Scott, J., Adams, R., & Mold, J. (2010). Assessment of the RBANS Visual and Verbal Indices in a sample of neurologically impaired elderly participants. *The Clinical Neuropsychologist, 24*(8), 1365–1378. https://doi.org/10.1080/13854046.2010.516769

Mossbarger, B., Whitney, K. A., Herman, S. M., & Mariner, J. E. (2012). Evidence of carry-over in memory test batteries using RBANS and screening measures. *Applied Neuropsychology, 19*(1), 38–41. https://doi.org/10.1080/09084282.2011.643939

Novitski, J., Steele, S., Karantzoulis, S., & Randolph, C. (2012). The Repeatable Battery for the Assessment of Neuropsychological Status Effort Scale. *Archives of Clinical Neuropsychology:, 27*(2), 190–195. https://doi.org/10.1093/arclin/acr119

O'Mahar, K. M., Duff, K., Scott, J. G., Linck, J. F., Adams, R. L., & Mold, J. W. (2012). Brief report: the temporal stability of the Repeatable Battery for the Assessment of Neuropsychological Status Effort

Index in geriatric samples. *Archives of Clinical Neuropsychology*:, *27*(1), 114–118. https://doi.org/10.1093/arclin/acr072

Pachet, A. K. (2007). Construct validity of the Repeatable Battery of Neuropsychological Status (RBANS) with acquired brain injury patients. *The Clinical Neuropsychologist, 21*(2), 286–293. https://doi.org/10.1080/13854040500376823

Paradee, C. V., Rapport, L. J., Hanks, R. A., & Levy, J. A. (2005). Circadian preference and cognitive functioning among rehabilitation inpatients. *The Clinical Neuropsychologist, 19,* 55–72.

Patton, D. E., Duff, K., Schoenberg, M. R., Mold, J., Scott, J. G., & Adams, R. L. (2003). Performance of cognitively normal African Americans on the RBANS in community-dwelling older adults. *The Clinical Neuropsychologist, 17,* 515–530.

Patton, D. E., Duff, K., Schoenberg, M. R., Mold, J., Scott, J. G., & Adams, R. L. (2005). Base rates of longitudinal RBANS discrepancies at one- and two-year intervals in community-dwelling older adults. *The Clinical Neuropsychologist, 19,* 27–44.

Patton, D., Duff, K., Schoenberg, M., Mold, J., Scott, J., & Adams, R. (2006). RBANS index discrepancies: Base rates for older adults. *Archives of Clinical Neuropsychology, 21*(2), 151–160. https://doi.org/10.1016/j.acn.2005.08.005

Paul, R., Lane, E. M., Tate, D. F., Heaps, J., Romo, D. M., Akbudak, E., . . . Conturo, T. E. (2011). Neuroimaging signatures and cognitive correlates of the Montreal Cognitive Assessment screen in a nonclinical elderly sample. *Archives of Clinical Neuropsychology, 26*(5), 454–460. https://doi.org/10.1093/arclin/acr017

Randolph, C. (1998). *RBANS manual.* San Antonio, TX: Psychological Corporation.

Randolph, C. (2012). *Repeatable Battery for the Assessment of Neuropsychological Status (RBANS Update).* Bloomington, MN: PsychCorp.

Rinehardt, E., Duff, K., Schoenberg, M., Mattingly, M., Bharucha, K., & Scott, J. (2010). Cognitive change on the Repeatable Battery for the Assessment of Neuropsychological Status (RBANS) in Parkinson's disease with and without bilateral subthalamic nucleus deep brain stimulation surgery. *The Clinical Neuropsychologist, 24*(8), 1339–1354. https://doi.org/10.1080/13854046.2010.521770

Sanz, J. C., Vargas, M. L., & Marín, J. J. (2009). Repeatable Battery for the Assessment of Neuropsychological Status (RBANS) in schizophrenia: A pilot study in the Spanish population. *Acta Neuropsychiatrica, 21*(1), 18–25. https://doi.org/10.1111/j.1601-5215.2008.00341.x

Schmitt, A. L., Livingston, R. B., Goette, W. F., & Galusha-Glasscock, J. M. (2016). Relationship between the Mini-Mental State Examination and the Repeatable Battery for the Assessment of Neuropsychological Status in patients referred for a dementia evaluation. *Perceptual and Motor Skills, 123*(3), 606–623. https://doi.org/10.1177/0031512516667674

Schmitt, A. L., Livingston, R. B., Smernoff, E. N., Reese, E. M., Hafer, D. G., & Harris, J. B. (2010). Factor analysis of the Repeatable Battery for the Assessment of Neuropsychological Status (RBANS) in a large sample of patients suspected of dementia. *Applied Neuropsychology, 17*(1), 8–17. https://doi.org/10.1080/09084280903297719

Schneider, J. S., Elm, J. J., Parashos, S. A., Ravina, B. M., Galpern, W. R., & NET-PD Investigators. (2010). Predictors of cognitive outcomes in early Parkinson disease patients: The National Institutes of Health Exploratory Trials in Parkinson Disease (NET-PD) experience. *Parkinsonism & Related Disorders, 16*(8), 507–512. https://doi.org/10.1016/j.parkreldis.2010.06.001

Schoenberg, M. R., Duff, K., Beglinger, L. J., Moser, D. J., Bayless, J. D., Mold, J., . . . Adams, R. L. (2008). Retention rates on RBANS Memory subtests in elderly adults. *Journal of Geriatric Psychiatry and Neurology, 21*(1), 26–33. https://doi.org/10.1177/0891988707311030

Schoenberg, M. R., Rinehardt, E., Duff, K., Mattingly, M., Bharucha, K. J., & Scott, J. G. (2012). Assessing Reliable Change using the Repeatable Battery for the Assessment of Neuropsychological Status (RBANS) for patients with Parkinson's disease undergoing deep brain stimulation (DBS) surgery. *The Clinical Neuropsychologist, 26*(2), 255–270. https://doi.org/10.1080/13854046.2011.653587

Schrimsher, G. W., & Parker, J. D. (2008). Changes in cognitive function during substance use disorder treatment. *Journal of Psychopathology and Behavioral Assessment, 30*(2), 146–153. https://doi.org/10.1007/s10862-007-9054-0

Sieck, B. C., Smith, M. M., Duff, K., Paulsen, J. S., & Beglinger, L. J. (2013). Symptom validity test performance in the Huntington disease clinic. *Archives of Clinical Neuropsychology, 28*(2), 135–143. https://doi.org/10.1093/arclin/acs109

Silverberg, N. D., Wertheimer, J. C., & Fichtenberg, N. L. (2007). An effort index for the Repeatable Battery for the Assessment of Neuropsychological Status (RBANS). *The Clinical Neuropsychologist, 21*(5), 841–854. https://doi.org/10.1080/13854040600850958

Slick, D. J., Sherman, E. M. S., & Iverson, G. L. (1999). Diagnostic criteria for Malingered Neurocognitive Dysfunction: Proposed standards for clinical practice and research. *The Clinical Neuropsychologist, 13*(4), 545–561. https://doi.org/10.1076/1385-4046(199911)13:04;1-Y;FT545

Smith, G. E., Housen, P., Yaffe, K., Ruff, R., Kennison, R. F., Mahncke, H. W., & Zelinski, E. M. (2009). A Cognitive training program based on principles of brain plasticity: Results from the Improvement in Memory with Plasticity-based Adaptive Cognitive Training (IMPACT) study: Results from the impact study. *Journal of the American Geriatrics Society, 57*(4), 594–603. https://doi.org/10.1111/j.1532-5415.2008.02167.x

Takaiwa, A., Hayashi, N., Kuwayama, N., Akioka, N., Kubo, M., & Endo, S. (2009). Changes in cognitive function during the 1-year period following endarterectomy and stenting of patients with high-grade carotid artery stenosis. *Acta Neurochirurgica, 151*(12), 1593–1600. https://doi.org/10.1007/s00701-009-0420-4

Thaler, N. S., Scott, J. G., Duff, K., Mold, J., & Adams, R. L. (2013). RBANS cluster profiles in a geriatric community-dwelling sample. *The Clinical Neuropsychologist, 27*(5), 794–807. https://doi.org/10.1080/13854046.2013.783121

Vogt, E. M., Prichett, G. D., & Hoelzle, J. B. (2017). Invariant two-component structure of the Repeatable Battery for the Assessment of Neuropsychological Status (RBANS). *Applied Neuropsychology. Adult, 24*(1), 50–64. https://doi.org/10.1080/23279095.2015.1088852

Wagle, J., Farner, L., Flekkøy, K., Wyller, T. B., Sandvik, L., Eiklid, K. L., Fure, B., Stensrød, B., & Engedal, K. (2009). Association between ApoE ε4 and Cognitive Impairment after Stroke. *Dementia and Geriatric Cognitive Disorders, 27*(6), 525–533. https://doi.org/10.1159/000223230

Wagle, J., Farner, L., Flekkøy, K., Wyller, T. B., Sandvik, L., Eiklid, K. L., . . . Engedal, K. (2010). Cognitive impairment and the role of the ApoE epsilon4-allele after stroke: A 13 months follow-up study. *International Journal of Geriatric Psychiatry, 25*(8), 833–842. https://doi.org/10.1002/gps.2425

Wagle, J., Farner, L., Flekkøy, K., Bruun Wyller, T., Sandvik, L., Fure, B., Stensrød, B., & Engedal, K. (2011). Early post-stroke cognition in stroke rehabilitation patients predicts functional outcome at 13 months. *Dementia and Geriatric Cognitive Disorders, 31*(5), 379–387. https://doi.org/10.1159/000328970

Weiner, D. K., Rudy, T. E., Morrow, L., Slaboda, J., & Lieber, S. (2006). The relationship between pain, neuropsychological performance, and physical function in community-dwelling older adults with chronic low back pain. *Pain Medicine, 7*(1), 60–70. https://doi.org/10.1111/j.1526-4637.2006.00091.x

Wilde, M. (2010). Lesion location and Repeatable Battery for the Assessment of Neuropsychological Status performance in acute ischemic stroke. *The Clinical Neuropsychologist, 24*(1), 57–69. https://doi.org/10.1080/13854040902984505

Wilde, M. C. (2006). The validity of the Repeatable Battery of Neuropsychological Status in acute stroke. *The Clinical Neuropsychologist, 20*(4), 702–715. https://doi.org/10.1080/13854040500246901

Wilk, C. M., Gold, J. M., Bartko, J. J., Dickerson, F., Fenton, W. S., Knable, M., Randolph, C., & Buchanaan, R. W. (2002). Test-retest stability of the Repeatable Battery for the Assessment of Neuropsychological Status in schizophrenia. *American Journal of Psychiatry, 159,* 838–844.

Wilk, C. M., Gold, J. M., Humber, K., Dickerson, F., Fenton, W. S., & Buchanan, R. W. (2004). Brief cognitive assessment in schizophrenia: Normative data for the Repeatable Battery for the Assessment of Neuropsychological Status. *Schizophrenia Research, 70,* 175–186.

Young, J. C., Baughman, B. C., & Roper, B. L. (2012). Validation of the Repeatable Battery for the Assessment of Neuropsychological Status: Effort Index in a veteran sample. *The Clinical Neuropsychologist, 26*(4), 688–699. https://doi.org/10.1080/13854046.2012.679624

Zammit, A. R., Ezzati, A., Zimmerman, M. E., Lipton, R. B., Lipton, M. L., & Katz, M. J. (2017). Roles of hippocampal subfields in verbal and visual episodic memory. *Behavioural Brain Research, 317,* 157–162. https://doi.org/10.1016/j.bbr.2016.09.038

Zelinski, E. M., Spina, L. M., Yaffe, K., Ruff, R., Kennison, R. F., Mahncke, H. W., & Smith, G. E. (2011). Improvement in memory with plasticity-based adaptive cognitive training: Results of the 3-month follow-up. *Journal of the American Geriatrics Society, 59*(2), 258–265. https://doi.org/10.1111/j.1532-5415.2010.03277.x

Zhang, X. Y., Liang, J., Chen, D. C., Xiu, M. H., Yang, F. D., Kosten, T. A., & Kosten, T. R. (2012). Low BDNF is associated with cognitive impairment in chronic patients with schizophrenia. *Psychopharmacology, 222*(2), 277–284. https://doi.org/10.1007/s00213-012-2643-y

RUFF NEUROBEHAVIORAL INVENTORY (RNBI)

TEST NAME	**Ruff Neurobehavioral Inventory (RNBI)**
DOMAIN	Neuropsychological functioning, self-reported
AGE RANGE	18 to 75 years
ADMINISTRATION TIME	30 to 45 minutes
SCORING FORMAT	Computerized or hand scored
REFERENCE	Ruff, R.M., & Hibbard, K.M. (2003). *Ruff Neurobehavioral Inventory.* Lutz, FL: PAR. www.parinc.com

DESCRIPTION

The RNBI is a 243-item self-report rating scale designed to measure cognitive, emotional, physical, and psychosocial problems before and after a specific event such as an injury or neuropsychiatric illness (Ruff & Hibbard, 2003). Both premorbid and postmorbid ratings are completed in relation to the event. The RNBI was constructed within a constructivist, holistic assessment framework, meaning that the instrument reflects consideration of multiple dimensions of function, including intrapersonal (e.g., emotional, cognitive, physical) and interpersonal domains (e.g., spirituality, financial and vocational aspects, social and recreational functioning). The RNBI is a unique instrument in that it assesses an examinee's subjective impressions of premorbid and postmorbid function in a number of domains, many of which are often not evaluated empirically in neuropsychological evaluations despite their importance. In the RNBI, the examinee's perception of outcome is emphasized (see p. 3 in the manual for theoretical model).

The RNBI consists of 243 items distributed among four Composite scales and 18 Basic scales; each scale is further subdivided into Premorbid and Postmorbid scales (see Table 6–51 for description). Items from Basic scales are based on diagnostic criteria from the *Diagnostic and Statistical Manual of Mental Disorders* (DSM-IV; American Psychiatric Association, 1994), although, as with all standardized instruments, scales should not be the exclusive basis for rendering a diagnosis in clinical practice. The Abuse scale contains critical items that require follow-up if endorsed so should be examined individually on an item-to-item basis by the clinician. In addition, the RNBI has four Validity scales to assist in detecting invalid profiles (Table 6–52).

SCORING

RNBI raw scores are transformed into linear T scores (M = 50; SD = 10). RNBI scales tend to be skewed; transformation procedures that normalize distributions (e.g., normalized scores of uniform T scores) were reportedly considered but not used because many constructs included in the RNBI are not normally distributed in the population. Percentile ranges are provided for Composite scales in the manual, but not Basic scales, due to limited range.

Interpretive cutoffs are similar to most standardized questionnaires, with Composite and Basic Scale T scores of 60 to 69 defined as Moderately Elevated, and T scores 70 or higher suggestive of clinically significant difficulty. Validity scales with T scores 70 or higher suggest an unusual response style that may affect validity.

Interpretive steps include first examining Validity scales to elucidate the respondent's approach in answering questions. Weaknesses in premorbid function according to interpretive cutoffs for Premorbid scores are then examined, with conjoint consideration of reliability of reporting. Similarly, Postmorbid scores are then examined according to interpretive cutoffs. The discrepancy between Postmorbid and Premorbid scores is next examined, first qualitatively (e.g., T scores of <60 both premorbidly and postmorbidly suggest long-standing absence of impairment in that area), then according to the magnitude of T-score discrepancy (Difference scores). Table A5 in Appendix A of the manual provides difference score values that are statistically significant for the standardization sample; discrepancies yielded by a respondent in excess of these values can be interpreted as clinically significant. The final step in interpretation is examination of 17 critical items that may prompt clinical follow-up. Case studies illustrating the interpretation process are provided in the manual.

NORMATIVE DATA

Features of the standardization sample are summarized in Table 6–53. Overall, the standardization sample is large, equally distributed between gender and age, predominantly Caucasian, and well-educated. The normative sample is

TABLE 6–51 Ruff Neurobehavioral Inventory (RNBI) Composite and Basic Scales

COMPOSITE SCALES	DESCRIPTION	BASIC SCALES	DESCRIPTION
Cognitive Domain	Self-perceived neuropsychological function	Attention & Concentration	ADHD symptoms (Premorbid); difficulty in attention and concentration (Postmorbid)
		Executive Functions	Problem-solving, adaptation, concentration, multi-tasking
		Learning & Memory	Learning and academic difficulties (Premorbid); difficulty with learning and memory (Postmorbid)
		Speech & Language	Difficulty with expression and comprehension (Premorbid); aspects of aphasia (Postmorbid)
Emotional Domain	Emotional dimensions most frequently affected by neuropsychiatric illness or catastrophic events	Anger & Aggression	Antisocial behaviors (Premorbid); anger-related adjustment difficulty (Postmorbid)
		Anxiety	Generalized anxiety and panic
		Depression	Mood, interest, sleep, concentration, libido, suicidal ideation
		Paranoia & Suspicion	Suspicion about friends and associates
		Posttraumatic Stress Disorder	Experience of extreme event with threat of death or injury, intense feelings elicited, recurrent recollections, avoidance, persistence of hyperarousal
		Substance Abuse	Drug and alcohol use and associated social and occupational difficulties
Physical Domain	Self-perceived physical function	Neurological Status	Sensory, motor, and seizure disorders
		Pain	Chronic pain (Premorbid); pain due to accident/illness (Postmorbid)
		Somatic Complaints	Non-neurological physical difficulties (e.g., poor health, back or neck, digestive)
Quality of Life Domain	Interpersonal dimensions relevant to quality of life	Abuse	Mistreatment of respondent via physical or sexual abuse
		Activities of Daily Living	Level of assistance required with activities of daily living
		Psychosocial Integration & Recreation	Degree of social interaction
		Vocation & Finances	Vocational identity and financial need
		Spirituality[a]	Spiritual beliefs and meaning

[a]Spirituality was retained only in Postmorbid items due to psychometric viability. Spirituality is part of the Quality of Life domain, but it does not comprise part of the Quality of Life Composite.

SOURCE: Adapted from Ruff and Hibbard (2003). Reproduced by special permission of the Publisher, Psychological Assessment Resources, Inc. (PAR), 16204 North Florida Avenue, Lutz, Florida 33549, from the Ruff Neurobehavioral Inventory by Ronald M. Ruff, PhD and Kristin M. Hibbard, PhD, Copyright 2000, 2003 by PAR. Further reproduction is prohibited without permission from PAR.

apparently not Census-based. The standardization sample completed an online version of the RNBI, and the clinical sample completed an in-person version. The authors compared the reliability estimates derived from the two samples, with general concordance (see pp. 49–50 in the manual).

DEMOGRAPHIC EFFECTS

AGE

Age is correlated with multiple RNBI scales, with older participants having lower levels of problems than younger participants. Therefore, the authors recommend considering age-corrected T scores as well as total sample T scores.

GENDER

Gender accounts for less than 5% of the variance in RNBI scale scores in the standardization sample (i.e., correlations below .20) and thus there are not gender-based scores.

EDUCATION AND IQ

The relationship between scores and education is small (i.e., accounted for <5% of the variance; see manual). There is scarce information on IQ effects.

ETHNICITY, NATIONALITY, AND LINGUISTIC EFFECTS

Comparisons between Caucasian and a combined minority group suggest that the minority group endorsed significantly less difficulty on the Postmorbid Physical Composite score, with a number of differences emerging on basic scales (pp. 34 to 35 in the manual). Users should therefore be aware of differences when interpreting the RNBI with clients from minority groups.

EVIDENCE FOR RELIABILITY

EVIDENCE FOR INTERNAL RELIABILITY

Internal consistency estimates are based on the standardization sample. Overall, internal consistency estimates are generally similar for the clinical sample. As seen in Table 6–54, internal consistency estimates for some Composite scales are marginal (e.g., Quality of Life), but most Composite scores are in the adequate to very high range, especially the Cognitive Composite and the Emotional Composite. Basic scales have more variable reliabilities ranging from very low to high, but with most scales demonstrating satisfactory reliability.

TABLE 6–52 Ruff Neurobehavioral Inventory (RNBI) Validity Scales

VALIDITY SCALE	DESCRIPTION
Inconsistency	Extent to which similar pairs of items are answered consistently
Infrequency	Items that were endorsed in an extreme manner by few respondents across standardization and clinical samples
Negative Impression	"Fake bad"; tendency to exaggerate complaints
Positive Impression	"Fake good"; tendency to deny flaws or difficulties

SOURCE: Adapted from Ruff and Hibbard (2003). Reproduced by special permission of the Publisher, Psychological Assessment Resources, Inc. (PAR), 16204 North Florida Avenue, Lutz, Florida 33549, from the Ruff Neurobehavioral Inventory by Ronald M. Ruff, PhD and Kristin M. Hibbard, PhD, Copyright 2000, 2003 by PAR. Further reproduction is prohibited without permission from PAR.

EVIDENCE FOR TEST-RETEST RELIABILITY, MEASURING CHANGE, AND PRACTICE EFFECTS

Test-retest reliability was evaluated on 94 college students, most of whom were between 18 and 25 years of age, female (59%), and Caucasian (65%), over a two- to four-week interval (manual). Test-retest reliability coefficients for Composite scores ranged from marginal (e.g., Physical Composite) to very high (e.g., Cognitive Composite), but for Basic scales ranged from low to very high (see Table 6–54). Thus, while the Composite scales tend to have at least adequate reliability overall, some of the Basic scales have unacceptably low reliability for clinical use so interpretation of Composite scales, rather than Basic scales, may be preferable clinically. Reliability estimates for Validity scales range from low to high (see Table 6–55).

TABLE 6–53 Characteristics of Standardization and Clinical Samples for the Ruff Neurobehavioral Inventory (RNBI)

	STANDARDIZATION SAMPLE	CLINICAL SAMPLE
Sample size	N = 1,024 community-dwelling via online recruitment	N = 195
Age	45% 18–45 years 54% 46–75 years	38% 18–45 years 55% 46–75 years
Sample type	Private internet research company	In/outpatient settings where undergoing assessment or treatment
Education	4% ≤11 years 19% 12 years 38% 13 to 15 years 39% ≥16 years	8% ≤11years 23% 12 years 27% 13 to 15 years 33% ≥16 years
Gender	47% Men 53% Women	58% Men 42% Women
Ethnicity	81% Caucasian 7% African American 7% Hispanic <1% Asian 3% Other	73% Caucasian 8% African American 3% Hispanic 4% Asian 5% Other

NOTE: Values are rounded. Age distribution shown according to distribution in age-corrected normative tables. Groups for clinical sample included: n = 52 pain disorders; n = 43 cerebral vascular accident; n = 52 traumatic brain injury; n = 37 spinal cord injury. Clinical samples had a proportion of missing demographic data (6–8%); no missing data in standardization samples were reported.

SOURCE: Data from the *Ruff Neurobehavioral Inventory professional manual*, by R. M. Ruff & K. M. Hibbard, 2003, Lutz, FL: PAR. Reproduced by special permission of the Publisher, Psychological Assessment Resources, Inc. (PAR), 16204 North Florida Avenue, Lutz, Florida 33549, from the Ruff Neurobehavioral Inventory by Ronald M. Ruff, PhD and Kristin M. Hibbard, PhD, Copyright 2000, 2003 by PAR. Further reproduction is prohibited without permission from PAR.

EVIDENCE FOR VALIDITY

Support for content validity is reflected in the test development process, which included literature review for construct conceptualization and expert raters for quality, appropriateness, bias, and theoretical relevance. Beginning with a pool of 1,000 items, items were subsequently eliminated through steps in the process. Expert raters rated initial items for quality and appropriateness, specificity to construct, length, reading level, and absence of colloquialisms or slang. Experts reviewed items for bias or unfairness to minority groups, followed by experts in rehabilitation and neuropsychology for content appropriateness (only items reaching 85% agreement levels were included). A subsample of patients then completed a 570-item questionnaire in the rehabilitation unit of a major hospital; 230 healthy adults without history of illness were also included. The authors selected items for theoretical relevance and psychometric functioning, reaching a final version. Important aspects of content validity were thus addressed, including wording, literature review, correspondence to construct, and expert review.

FACTOR-ANALYTIC STUDIES

Factor analyses of the standardization sample data yield factors paralleling the theoretical construct of the RNBI, specifically reflecting emotional, cognitive, and physical domains; factor analysis with Premorbid scales yields a three-factor solution accounting for 60% of the variance (manual). Factor loadings were interpreted to indicate an Emotional/Quality of Life factor, a Cognitive factor, and a Physical Dysfunction factor. Factor analysis with Postmorbid scales indicated a three-factor solution accounting for 70% of the variance, interpreted as reflecting Emotional/Quality of Life, Physical Dysfunction, and Cognitive domains.

CORRELATIONS WITH OTHER NEUROPSYCHOLOGICAL TESTS

There is some evidence of an association between subjective RNBI cognitive ratings and performance-based neuropsychological tests. Specifically, Jamora, Young, and Ruff (2012) reported that self-rated cognitive function on the RNBI predicted performance on neuropsychological measures in a sample of patients with TBI. In mild TBI, a predictive relationship was found between RNBI Attention and Concentration difference scores and a neuropsychological attention composite comprised of the Ruff 2 & 7, TMT, and Digit Symbol. In moderate to severe

TABLE 6–54 Magnitude of Reliability Coefficients of Ruff Neurobehavioral Inventory (RNBI) Indices and Subtests

MAGNITUDE OF COEFFICIENT	INTERNAL CONSISTENCY		TEST-RETEST	
	PREMORBID	POSTMORBID	PREMORBID	POSTMORBID
Very high (.90+)		Cognitive Composite Pain	Cognitive Composite Emotional Composite Attention & Concentration Learning & Memory Anger & Aggression Substance Abuse Abuse	
High (.80–.89)	Cognitive Composite Emotional Composite Attention & Concentration Learning & Memory Anger & Aggression Anxiety Depression Pain Abuse Psychosocial Integration & Recreation	Emotional Composite Physical Composite Attention & Concentration Learning & Memory Speech & Language Anger & Aggression Anxiety Somatic Complaints	Anxiety Paranoia & Suspicion	Cognitive Composite Attention & Concentration Learning & Memory Physical Composite Neurological Status Pain
Adequate (.70–.79)	Speech & Language Paranoia & Suspicion Posttraumatic Stress Disorder Substance Abuse Physical Composite Somatic Complaints	Executive Functions Depression Paranoia & Suspicion Posttraumatic Stress Disorder Substance Abuse Neurological Status Quality of Life Composite Abuse Activities of Daily Living Psychosocial Integration & Recreation Vocation & Finances	Executive Functions Posttraumatic Stress Disorder Somatic Complaints Quality of Life Composite	Emotional Composite Anxiety Depression Substance Abuse Somatic Complaints Psychosocial Integration & Recreation
Marginal (.60–.69)	Executive Functions Quality of Life Composite Activities of Daily Living Vocation and Finances	Spirituality	Speech & Language Depression Physical Composite Psychosocial Integration & Recreation Physical Composite	Executive Functions Speech & Language Anger & Aggression Paranoia & Suspicion Posttraumatic Stress Disorder Quality of Life Composite Spirituality
Low (≤.59)	Neurological Status		Neurological Status Pain Activities of Daily Living Vocation & Finances	Abuse Activities of Daily Living Vocation & Finances

SOURCE: Reproduced by special permission of the Publisher, Psychological Assessment Resources, Inc. (PAR), 16204 North Florida Avenue, Lutz, Florida 33549, from the Ruff Neurobehavioral Inventory by Ronald M. Ruff, PhD & Kristin M. Hibbard, PhD, Copyright 2000, 2003 by PAR. Further reproduction is prohibited without permission from PAR.

TABLE 6–55 Validity Scale Reliabilities

COMPOSITE SCALES	BASIC SCALES	INTERNAL CONSISTENCY		TEST-RETEST RELIABILITY	
		PREMORBID	POSTMORBID	PREMORBID	POSTMORBID
Validity[a]	Inconsistency	.19		.38	
	Infrequency	–		.80	
	Negative Impression	.63	.82	.78	.59
	Positive Impression	.58	.71	.79	.69

[a]Note that validity scales do not form an overall Composite.

SOURCE: Data from the *Ruff Neurobehavioral Inventory professional manual*, by R. M. Ruff & K. M. Hibbard, 2003, Lutz, FL: PAR. Reproduced by special permission of the Publisher, Psychological Assessment Resources, Inc. (PAR), 16204 North Florida Avenue, Lutz, Florida 33549, from the Ruff Neurobehavioral Inventory by Ronald M. Ruff, PhD and Kristin M. Hibbard, PhD, Copyright 2000, 2003 by PAR. Further reproduction is prohibited without permission from PAR.

TBI, a predictive relationship was found between RNBI Difference Memory and Learning scores and a neuropsychological memory and learning composite comprised of Buschke Selective Reminding, Wechsler Logical Memory, RCFT, and Ruff Light Trail Learning Test (RULIT). However, the mild TBI group rated themselves as comparatively more impaired than the moderate to severe group, a finding that has been replicated in other studies using different instruments and which may relate to the mild TBI group being more cognitively able to notice and recall deficits or to overextending themselves more in daily life with consequent negative effects on cognitive difficulties (Jamora et al., 2013). Note that malingering and exaggeration were excluded in this study using established performance validity tests in addition to symptom validity scales in the RBNI, so this is unlikely to account for elevated reporting in mild TBI.

Jamora, Schroeder, and Ruff (2013) found that there were no differences on neuropsychological test composites comprised of well-known tests such as Digit Symbol, TMT, WMS, RCFT, Controlled Oral Word Association Test (COWAT), or Stroop for patients with mild TBI categorized with either high or low pain based on the RNBI Pain score. However, differences emerged when the RBNI was used; high-pain individuals with TBI tended to report higher RNBI Anger & Aggression, Anxiety, Depression, and Paranoia & Suspicion, and worse Cognition, Physical, and Quality of Life difference scores.

CORRELATIONS WITH OTHER QUESTIONNAIRES

Correlations between the RNBI and the Millon Clinical Multiaxial Inventory-III (MCMI-III) and Quality of Life Enjoyment and Satisfaction Questionnaire (Q-LES-Q) were computed in a subsample of college students (see manual). Comparisons with the RNBI scales and the questionnaires suggested broad patterns of relations, which were generally in the expected direction but nonspecific. This led the authors to suggest that many RNBI scales may reflect a general dimension of psychopathology. For example, correlations between the RNBI and MCMI-III ranged from −.44 (RNBI Substance Use with MCMI-II Compulsive) to .73 (RNBI Postmorbid Depression with MCMI-III Borderline). Correlations between the RNBI and Q-LES-Q ranged from −.20 (RNBI Pain with Q-LES-Q Work; RNBI Somatic Complaints with Q-LES-Q Household Duties; and RNBI Activities of Daily Living with Q-LES-Q Leisure Time) to −.55 (RNBI Speech & Language with Q-LES-Q Work, and RNBI Activities of Daily Living with Q-LES-Q Household Duties). In terms of validity scales, a pattern of divergent and convergent findings was obtained generally in the expected direction (e.g., RNBI Negative Impression scale correlating positively with Disclosure scales from the MCMI and negatively with Desirability). A subset of the clinical sample (n = 40) also completed the Mayo-Portland Adaptability Inventory (MPAI) designed to capture outcome for patients with mild to moderate brain injuries. As expected, the MPAI scales showed significant correlations with many RNBI Postmorbid scales, although a number of significant correlations also emerged between the MPAI scales and RNBI Premorbid scales.

CLINICAL STUDIES

Overall, a high number of postmorbid difficulties were endorsed across clinical groups in the manual, which to some extent paralleled what would be expected, including predominant cognitive difficulties in cerebrovascular accident (CVA) and TBI, and physical difficulties in spinal cord injury and pain. However, for some scales and clinical samples, a high degree of premorbid complaints was also endorsed.

Notably, research on the RNBI in other clinical samples is scant, and most of the studies were conducted by the test authors. For example, Jamora, Young, and Ruff (2012) administered the RNBI to a compensation-seeking TBI sample, with the mild TBI group reporting more cognitive symptoms than the moderate and severe TBI group; mild TBI patients also reported more posttraumatic stress disorder (PTSD). Johansson, Jamora, Ruff, and Pack (2008) also administered the RNBI to a TBI sample, with correspondence found between clinical ratings of aggression and the RNBI Postmorbid Anger scale, and post/premorbid differences found between aggression groups. Murray et al. (2007) administered the RNBI to a spinal cord injury sample, with significant differences found between pre/post morbid function in a number of domains, with post-spinal cord injury pain a significant predictor of multiple areas of function as assessed by the RNBI.

In one study, comparisons between mild TBI patients and orthopedic controls showed no differences on the RNBI Pain scale at one month, six months, and 12 months post-injury, with 96% of patients returning to work after injury; individual trajectories indicated that pain plateaued after six months post-injury (Losoi et al., 2016).

PERFORMANCE VALIDITY

Research focused on specific symptom validity indicators in RNBI samples has not been conducted apart from a study by Young, Merali, and Ruff (2009), which found concordance between validity scales from the RNBI, MCMI-III, and the Detailed Assessment of Posttraumatic Stress (DAPS), suggesting some concurrent validity between validity scales in a private practice sample of motor vehicle accident pain patients without neurologic injury. Results point to the unique value of the RNBI in being able to capture both symptom exaggeration (postmorbid symptoms) and symptom minimization (premorbid symptoms), a common pattern in litigating examinees exaggerating claims of personal injury.

Importantly, in the context of the test development process, identification of validity items with the best psychometric properties was completed by administering the RNBI to samples instructed to "fake good," "fake bad," or "fake litigation." Based on these respondents, items were analyzed to identify those with optimal reliability, a more sophisticated approach to developing validity indicators than in most standardized scales developed for neuropsychology. As depicted in Table 6–54, users of the RNBI should note that some of the validity scales have low levels of reliability, but most are quite adequate for use. Most manuals do not report the reliability of validity indicators, and this is certainly an asset for the RNBI.

COMMENT

The RNBI is a unique instrument in that it assesses an examinee's subjective impressions of premorbid and postmorbid function in a number of domains, many of which are often not assessed empirically despite their importance in neuropsychological assessment. This is a formidable feat for a single instrument, and more so for an instrument that demonstrates generally strong reliability across scales. Notably, while the Composite scales tend to have at least adequate reliability overall, some of the Basic scales have unacceptably low reliability for clinical use, and judicious interpretation of scores with adequate reliabilities is preferable clinically (see Table 6–54). Note that specific Basic scales (e.g., Abuse) are important to evaluate qualitatively because clinical follow-up is indicated with item endorsement.

A strength of the RNBI is its inclusion of multiple validity scales validated on feigning groups as part of the standardization process, a clear asset—particularly in compensation or litigation contexts—but also useful for most clinicians to help identify invalid responding in uncooperative, disengaged, distracted, or very low-ability examinees. Another strength of the RNBI is the large clinical sample: the authors report interesting differentiations on a number of scales across clinical samples, particularly in terms of cognitive vs. physical problems. However, given broad relations that are obtained between other questionnaires and the RNBI, as well as a significant proportion of clinical samples reporting both premorbid and postmorbid difficulties, many of the RNBI scales may reflect more general dimensions than specific dimensions. In particular, data on the concordance between the Emotional Composite and Basic scores with established DSM diagnoses is needed. Of note, the test should not be used to estimate activities of daily living, given low reliabilities generally for this domain. Additional use of established standardized questionnaires for assessing psychiatric status and activities of daily living is recommended to supplement diagnostic impressions gleaned from the RNBI. Importantly, the RNBI is designed to assess subjective impression of premorbid function and should be used in conjunction with objective records of premorbid function (e.g., premorbid employment, school, and medical records).

Overall, the RNBI is a promising, carefully constructed, compelling, and unique questionnaire that would be useful in the neuropsychological assessment of patients with neurobehavioral impairments, particularly those with brain injury seen in workers' compensation or litigation contexts, given the important information the RNBI provides on the subjective impact of injury on the examinee in daily life. Nevertheless, more clinical research generally is needed on the RNBI, including on pre/postmorbid difference scores, neuropsychological test correlates of the Cognitive Composite, exaggeration and feigning, sensitivity to treatment effects, and psychometric properties in minority groups. As well, although the RNBI emphasizes patients' self-perception, an informant version of the RNBI would be a useful addition to the instrument, as would a short form, as the questionnaire is fairly lengthy for some examinees.

REFERENCES

American Psychiatric Association (1994). *Diagnostic and statistical manual of mental disorders: DSM-IV*. Washington, DC: American Psychiatric Association.

Jamora, C. W, Schroeder, S. C., & Ruff, R. M. (2013). Pain and mild traumatic brain injury: The implications of pain severity on emotional and cognitive functioning. *Brain Injury, 27,* 1134–1140.

Jamora, C. W., Young, A., & Ruff, R. M. (2012). Comparison of subjective cognitive complaints with neuropsychological tests in individuals with mild vs. more severe traumatic brain injuries. *Brain Injury, 26,* 36–47.

Johansson, S. H., Jamora, C. W., Ruff, R. M., & Pack, N. M. (2008). A biopsychosocial perspective of aggression in the context of traumatic brain injury. *Brain Injury, 22,* 999–1006.

Losoi, H., Silverberg, N. D., Wäljas, M., Turunen, S., Rosti-Otajärvi, E., Helminen, M., . . . Iverson, G. L. (2016). Recovery from mild traumatic brain injury in previously healthy adults. *Neurotrauma, 33*(8), 766–776. doi: 10.1089/neu.2015.4070.

Murray, R. F. et al. (2007). Impact of spinal cord injury on self-perceived pre- and postmorbid cognitive, emotional and physical functioning. *Spinal Cord, 45,* 429–436.

Ruff, R. M., & Hibbard, K. M. (2003). *Ruff Neurobehavioral Inventory*. Lutz, FL: PAR.

Young, G., Merali, N. L., & Ruff, R. M. (2009). The Ruff Neurobehavioral Inventory: Validity indicators and validity. *Psychological Injury and Law, 2,* 53–60.

7 | DEMENTIA SCREENING

7 MINUTE SCREEN (7MS)

TEST NAME	**7 Minute Screen (7MS)**
DOMAIN	Dementia screening
AGE RANGE	65+ years
ADMINISTRATION TIME	7 minutes, up to 15 minutes in individuals with dementia
SCORING FORMAT	Hand scored
REFERENCES	Budson, A. E., & Price B. H. (2005). Memory dysfunction [Supplementary material]. *New England Journal of Medicine, 352,* 692–699. Solomon, P. R., Hirschoff, A., Kelly, B. Relin, M., Brush, M., DeVeaux, R. D., & Pendlebury, W. W. (1998). A 7 minute neurocognitive screening battery highly sensitive to Alzheimer's Disease. *Archives of Neurology, 55,* 349–355.

DESCRIPTION

The 7 Minute Screen (7MS) is a dementia screen specifically designed to screen for Alzheimer's disease (AD). It comprises four modified versions of well-established tests that are sensitive to AD, including temporal orientation, memory, verbal fluency, and visuospatial/visuoconstruction. A paper-and-pencil version for group administration is also available (Ijuin et al., 2008). In the original study, Solomon and colleagues (1998) reported a mean administration time of less than eight minutes (Solomon et al., 1998). Follow-up studies by other authors have reported longer administration time of more than eight minutes for cognitively intact older adults, and 12 to 16 minutes for AD or other cognitively impaired patients (Meulen et al., 2004; Tsolaki et al., 2002; Skjerve et al., 2007). Different translations in languages including Greek (Tsolaki et al., 2002), Polish (Sobów & Kloszewska, 2001), Thai (Sungkarat et al., 2011), and Spanish (Del Ser et al., 2006) are available.

ADMINISTRATION

See the manual for the original test materials and administration instructions. The group-administered paper-and-pencil version follows a very similar procedure as the original version except for the verbal fluency subtest. In this subtest, the examinee is given 180 seconds to write down as many different animals as they can (Ijuin et al., 2008).

SCORING

The 7MS uses a formula to estimate the probability of dementia:

$$\begin{aligned} \text{7MS Total score} &= \text{Ln}\,[P \div (1-P)] \\ &= 35.59 - 1.303 \times ECR - 1.378 \\ &\quad \times VF + 3.298 \times BTO - 0.838 \times CD \end{aligned}$$

where P = Probability of having dementia, ECR = Enhanced Cued Recall score, VF = Verbal Fluency, BTO = Benton Temporal Orientation, and CD = Clock Drawing.

The BTO raw score is calculated based on the degree of error. For each year deviation, 10 error points are assigned; five points are given for each month deviation; one point for the wrong date; one point for the wrong day of the week; and one point for each 30-minute deviation in time up to a maximum error score of 113. In the ECR, the raw score is based on the number of pictures remembered spontaneously or with cue, up to a maximum possible score of 16. The CD item is scored to a maximum score of 7, while each animal given within 60 seconds in the VF subtest is awarded one point to a maximum score of 45. In general, *p* greater than .70 suggests a high probability of AD. The authors categorized those who obtained *p* between .30 and .70 as needing further testing. Scoring can also be completed on the website to obtain a probability (high vs. low) that the examinee has AD: http://www.memorydoc.org/7minutescreen.

To reduce the scoring complexity, Del Ser and colleagues (2006) developed a different algorithm based on the sum of *z* scores. Scoring for each subtest is similar to the original version except for BTO where the raw score is reversed scored (i.e., 113 minus error score). For ease of scoring, Table 7–1 presents the conversion from raw scores to *z* scores. To obtain the standardized Total score, the sum of *z* scores is transformed to S scores (mean [*M*] = 50, standard deviation [*SD*] = 20). This algorithm is based on a European Spanish-speaking sample.

DEMOGRAPHIC EFFECTS

Effects of age, gender, and education are minimal on the Total score (Del Ser et al., 2006; Ijuin et al., 2008; Skjerve et al., 2007; Solomon et al., 1998; Tsolaki et al., 2002). Performance is also consistent across samples from different countries and languages, suggesting stability of the test across ethnicities and languages (Skjerve et al., 2007). However, it has been noted that for Indians with low education or from rural areas, Clock Drawing and Orientation may not be suitable but Memory appeared appropriate (De Jager et al., 2008).

NORMATIVE DATA

The original study was comprised of 60 community-dwelling older adults (age mean = 77.5, range = 67 to 91; 46% females; education mean = 14.4, range = 6 to 23) screened for history of psychiatric or neurological disorder and current use of antidepressant or psychoactive medications. In addition, 60 patients seen at a memory disorders clinic who meet the National Institute of Neurological Disorders and Stroke-Alzheimer's Disease and Related Disorders Association (NINCDS-ARDA) diagnostic criteria for AD (age mean = 77.6, range = 66 to 89; 50% females; education mean = 13.3, range = 8 to 20) were also included. As a screening measure, the test yields a probability score to identify at-risk older adults for further comprehensive assessment (see "Scoring"). Probability scores have been reported in Greek, Japanese, Norwegian, and Spanish dementia samples (see "Clinical Studies").

EVIDENCE FOR RELIABILITY

EVIDENCE FOR INTERNAL RELIABILITY

Not available.

EVIDENCE FOR TEST-RETEST RELIABILITY, MEASURING CHANGE, AND PRACTICE EFFECTS

The original study reported very high one- to two-month test-retest reliability (*r* = .91; Solomon et al., 1998).

EVIDENCE FOR RELIABILITY OF ALTERNATE FORMS

Not available.

EVIDENCE FOR INTERRATER RELIABILITY

Interrater reliability was very high in the original study (*r* = .93; Solomon et al., 1998).

EVIDENCE FOR VALIDITY

RELATIONSHIPS WITH OTHER TESTS

Few studies have reported on the relationship of the original 7MS with other tests. One study compared the 7MS to the Mini-Mental State Examination (MMSE). The authors found higher sensitivity (89 to 93%), specificity (94%), positive predictive value (PPV; 98%), and negative predictive value (NPV; 75%) compared to the MMSE (sensitivity 60 to 71%; PPV, 99%; and NPV, 44%) in their sample of mixed dementia in The Netherlands (Meulen et al., 2004). The group-administered version showed high correlations with other dementia measures including the MMSE (*r* = −.72), Hasegawa's Dementia Scale-Revised, and MIS (both *r* = −.70) in a Japanese sample (Ijuin et al., 2008).

CLINICAL STUDIES

Only one study examining the utility of the 7MS as a screening measure in primary care has been published to date (Solomon et al., 2000). In this study, screening of older adults seen in primary care identified by the 7MS as having a high probability of dementia yielded a PPV of 91% for dementia based on NINCDS-ARDA criteria (NPV was 96%). While the 7MS appears suitable as a screening measure for population studies because older adults in a large-scale community screening program found the 7MS highly acceptable (Lawrence et al., 2003), only a small percent (1.5%) of those who were screened were eventually diagnosed with probable AD. The study authors remarked that this form of screening appears inefficient, partly because of multiple obstacles to follow-up care, which may include denial on the part of those who screen positive or forgetting to follow-up with their physicians. Physicians who did follow-up with the participants did not conduct further cognitive testing or they ordered inappropriate tests and dismissed the concerns (Lawrence et al., 2003).

TABLE 7–1 The Conversion from Raw Scores to *z* Scores for Use with Del Ser et al. (2006) Sum of *z* Scores Algorithm to Obtain 7 Minute Screen (7MS) Total Score

CT		TOTAL RECALL		CF		OT		TOTAL 7MS	
RAW SCORE	*Z* SCORE	RAW SCORE	*Z* SCORE	RAW SCORE	*Z* SCORE	RAW SCORE	*Z* SCORE	SUM *Z*	S SCORE
7	0.88	16	0.82	30	3.48	113	0.34	5.52	89
6	0.47	15	0.26	29	3.25	112	0.27	4.88	84
5	0.06	14	-0.30	28	3.02	111	0.20	4.65	83
4	-0.36	13	-0.85	27	2.79	110	0.14	4.61	82
3	-0.77	12	-1.41	26	2.56	109	0.07	4.38	81
2	-1.18	11	-1.97	25	2.34	108	0.01	4.15	79
		10	-2.57	24	2.11	107	-0.01	3.93	78
		9	-3.09	23	1.88	106	-0.06	3.70	76
		8	-3.65	22	1.65	105	-0.16	3.43	74
		7	-4.21	21	1.43	104	-0.26	3.24	73
		6	-4.77	20	1.20	103	-0.33	3.16	72
		5	-5.32	19	0.97	102	-0.39	2.98	71
		4	-5.88	18	0.74	101	-0.46	2.83	70
				17	0.51	100	-0.53	2.68	69
				16	0.20	99	-0.59	2.56	68
				15	0.06	98	-0.66	2.39	67
				14	-0.17	97	-0.73	2.26	66
				13	-0.40	96	-0.79	2.13	65
				12	-0.62	95	-0.86	2.00	64
				11	-0.85	94	-0.92	1.87	63
				10	-1.08	93	-0.99	1.68	62
				9	-1.31	84	-1.51	1.57	61
				8	-1.54	81	-1.79	1.44	60
						78	-1.99	1.27	59
						77	-2.06	1.15	58
						73	-2.32	1	57
						72	-2.39	0.85	56
						63	-2.99	0.72	55
						53	-3.65	0.57	54
						52	-3.72	0.41	53
						50	-3.85	0.31	52
						48	-3.99	0.10	51
						47	-4.05	-0.01	50
						43	-4.32	-0.13	49
								-0.29	48
								-0.43	47
								-0.55	46
								-0.70	45
								-0.87	44
								-0.98	43
								-1.16	42
								-1.25	41
								-1.45	40
								-1.59	39
								-1.73	38
								-1.84	37
								-1.96	36
								-2.14	35
								-2.27	34
								-2.42	33
								-2.56	32
								-2.68	31
								-2.85	30
								-3.01	29
								-3.08	28
								-3.24	27
								-3.43	26
								-3.56	25
								-3.70	24
								-3.87	23
								-4	22

TABLE 7–1 Continued

CT		TOTAL RECALL		CF		OT		TOTAL 7MS	
RAW SCORE	*Z* SCORE	RAW SCORE	*Z* SCORE	RAW SCORE	*Z* SCORE	RAW SCORE	*Z* SCORE	SUM *Z*	S SCORE
				7	−1.76	41	−4.45	−4.27	20
		3	−6.44					−4.38	19
				6	−1.99	38	−4.65	−4.85	16
1	−1.60					34	−4.92	−5.02	15
				5	−2.22	33	−4.98	−5.09	14
						32	−5.05	−5.21	13
		2	−7.00			27	−5.38	−5.35	12
				4	−2.45	18	−5.98	−5.59	11
						15	−6.18	−5.77	9
				3	−2.67	14	−6.25	−5.97	8
		1	−7.56			13	−6.32	−6.21	6
				2	−2.90	7	−6.71	−6.37	5
0	−2.01					5	−6.85	−6.50	4
				1	−3.13	3	−6.98	−6.67	3
		0	−8.12			1	−7.11	−6.81	2
				0	−3.36	0	−7.18	−7.14	0

NOTE: CT, Clock Drawing Test; CF, Category Fluency; OT, Orientation Test. S score has a mean of 50 and a standard deviation of 20.

SOURCE: From Del Ser et al. (2006). Copyright © 2006, © 2006 S. Karger AG, Basel.

Within specialty clinics, the 7MS shows high sensitivity and specificity for detecting mild AD from healthy controls (Solomon et al., 1998; Tsolaki et al., 2002), including with the group-administered version (Ijuin et al., 2008) and using Total scores based on sum of *z* scores (Del Ser et al., 2006). However, its utility in differentiating between mild cognitive impairment (MCI) and mild dementia is weaker, as seen in Table 7–2 (Skjerve et al., 2008). When Parkinson's disease (PD) and AD patients were compared, AD patients did worse than PD patients on ECR, but no differences were seen in other subscales in a Czech Republic sample (Rasovska & Rektorova, 2011).

NEUROANATOMICAL CORRELATES AND IMAGING STUDIES

Not available.

PERFORMANCE VALIDITY

Not reported.

TABLE 7–2 Sensitivity, Specificity, Positive Predictive Value, and Negative Predictive Value of the 7 Minute Screen (7MS) as Reported in Different Studies for Various Dementia Base Rates

STUDY	SAMPLE	CUTOFF	BASE RATE OF DEMENTIA (%)	SENSITIVITY (%)	SPECIFICITY (%)	PPV (%)	NPV (%)
Del Ser et al. (2006)	Spanish population sample of mixed dementia	<−5.84 or <9 S score based on z-score method (see Table 7–1)	11	100	95	79	100
		<−6.11 or <8 S score (see Table 7–1)		100	96	48	100
Ijuin et al. (2008)	Japanese AD sample from a specialty clinic and healthy controls from the community	$p > .50$	5	90	92	68	99
			10			82	99
			15			88	98
			20			91	98
Skjerve et al. (2008)	Norwegian MCI and mild dementia from a specialty clinic	$p > .70$	Not reported	73	69	Not reported	Not reported
Solomon et al. (1998)	AD and healthy control from a specialty clinic	$p < .10$ for cognitively intact and $p > .90$ for AD	5	98	98	55	99
			10			72	99
			20			85	98
			50			96	92
Tsolaki et al. (2002)	Greek AD and healthy control in specialty clinic	$p > .50$	Not reported	93	98	98	90

NOTE: PPV, positive predictive value; NPV, negative predictive value; MCI, mild cognitive impairment; AD, Alzheimer's disease.

COMMENT

The 7MS is a psychometrically sound dementia screen that is made up of four shortened versions of well-established tests that are sensitive to AD. It appears to have high sensitivity for AD within specialty clinic settings, and its utility for identifying AD in different countries and languages has been established in multiple studies. Moreover, with the exception of low-education and rural samples, demographic background including age, education, and gender appear to have minimal impact on the 7MS.

Calculation and interpretation of the 7MS can be confusing because it uses an equation that is not easily understood by users who are not statistically savvy, though a web-based calculator is available to aid in the calculation and interpretation. Del Ser and colleagues (2006) attempted to reduce the scoring complexity by developing a different formula. However, this formula has not been cross-validated in other languages and settings. Furthermore, many studies have reported that the 7MS can take up to 15 minutes to administer if the patient is severely impaired despite what its name suggests (Meulan et al., 2004; Tsolaki et al., 2002; Skjerve et al., 2007). Finally, although the 7MS may be feasible as a measure for large-scale screening in population studies, the yield is low and multiple obstacles to follow-up care have been reported.

Based on reviews of available cognitive screens, a number of review studies including one by the US Preventive Task Force indicated that the 7MS as a publicly available test appears to have adequate psychometric properties; however, evidence for primary care screening is limited as it has only been studied once in English (Lin et al., 2013; Velayudhan et al., 2014). Further validation including identifying neuroanatomical/imaging correlates and examining its utility within primary care settings is therefore needed. Based on the validation evidence to date, the MoCA is recommended over the 7MS.

REFERENCES

Budson, A. E., & Price B. H. (2005). Memory dysfunction [Supplementary material]. *New England Journal of Medicine, 352*, 692–699.

de Jager, C. A., Thambisetty, M., Praveen, K. V., Sheeba, P. D., Ajini, K. N., Sajeev, A., . . . David, S. A. (2008). Utility of the Malayalam translation of the 7 Minute Screen for Alzheimer's disease risk in an Indian community. *Neurology India, 56*(2), 161–166.

del Ser, T., Sánchez-Sánchez, F., García, d. Y., Otero, A., & Munoz, D. G. (2006). Validation of the 7 Minute Screen neurocognitive battery for the diagnosis of dementia in a Spanish population-based sample. *Dementia and Geriatric Cognitive Disorders, 22*(5–6), 454–464.

Ijuin, M., Homma, A., Mimura, M., Kitamura, S., Kawai, Y., Imai, Y., & Gondo, Y. (2008). Validation of the 7 Minute Screen for the detection of early stage Alzheimer's disease. *Dementia and Geriatric Cognitive Disorders, 25*(3), 248–255.

Lawrence, J. M., Davidoff, D. A., Katt-Lloyd, D., Connell, A., Berlow, Y. A., & Savoie, J. A. (2003). Is large-scale community memory screening feasible? Experience from a regional memory-screening day. *Journal of the American Geriatrics Society, 51*(8), 1072–1078.

Lin, J. S., O'Connor, E., Rossom, R. C., Perdue, L. A., & Eckstrom, E. (2013). Screening for cognitive impairment in older adults: A systematic review for the US preventive services task force. *Annals of Internal Medicine, 159*(9), 601–612.

Meulen, E. F. J., Schmand, B., van Campen, J. P., de Koning, S. J., Ponds, R. W., Scheltens, P., & Verhey, F. R. (2004). The 7 Minute Screen: A neurocognitive screening test highly sensitive to various types of dementia. *Journal of Neurology, Neurosurgery & Psychiatry, 75*(5), 700–705.

Rasovska, H., & Rektorova, I. (2011). Instrumental activities of daily living in Parkinson's disease dementia as compared with Alzheimer's disease: Relationship to motor disability and cognitive deficits: A pilot study. *Journal of the Neurological Sciences, 310*(1–2), 279–282.

Skjerve, A., Nordhus, I. H., Engedal, K., Brækhus, A., Nygaard, H. A., Pallesen, S., & Haugen, P. K. (2008). Validation of the Seven Minute Screen and Syndrome Kurztest among elderly Norwegian outpatients. *International Psychogeriatrics, 20*(4), 807–814.

Skjerve, A., Nordhus, I. H., Engedal, K., Pallesen, S., Braekhus, A., & Nygaard, H. A. (2007). Seven Minute Screen performance in a normal elderly sample. *International Journal of Geriatric Psychiatry, 22*(8), 764–769.

Sobów, T. M., & Kloszewska, I. (2001). ["7 Minute Screen." part I: A new tool in the diagnosis of Alzheimer's disease—polish translation and description of its clinical application]. *Psychiatria Polska, 35*(3), 467–473.

Solomon, P. R., Brush, M., Calvo, V., Adams, F., DeVeaux, R. D., Pendlebury, W. W., & Sullivan, D. M. (2000). Identifying dementia in the primary care practice. *International Psychogeriatrics, 12*(4), 483–493.

Solomon, P. R., Hirschoff, A., Kelly, B., Relin, M., Brush, M., DeVeaux, R. D., & Pendlebury, W. W. (1998). A 7 minute neurocognitive screening battery highly sensitive to Alzheimer's disease. *Archives of Neurology, 55*(3), 349–355.

Sungkarat, S., Methapatara, P., Taneyhill, K., & Apiwong, R. (2011). Sensitivity and specificity of 7 Minute Screen (7MS) Thai version in screening Alzheimer's disease. *Journal of the Medical Association of Thailand [Chotmaihet Thangphaet], 94*(7), 842–848.

Tsolaki, M., Iakovidou, V., Papadopoulou, E., Aminta, M., Nakopoulou, E., Pantazi, T., & Kazis, A. (2002). Greek validation of the seven-minute screening battery for Alzheimer's disease in the elderly. *American Journal of Alzheimer's Disease and Other Dementias, 17*(3), 139–148.

Velayudhan, L., Ryu, S., Raczek, M., Philpot, M., Lindesay, J., Critchfield, M., & Livingston, G. (2014). Review of brief cognitive tests for patients with suspected dementia. *International Psychogeriatrics, 26*(8), 1247–1262.

ALZHEIMER'S DISEASE ASSESSMENT SCALE-COGNITIVE (ADAS-COG)

TEST NAME	**Alzheimer's Disease Assessment Scale-Cognitive (ADAS-Cog)**
DOMAIN	Dementia screening
AGE RANGE	60+ years
ADMINISTRATION TIME	45 minutes
SCORING FORMAT	Hand scored
REFERENCE	Rosen, W. G., Mohs, R. C., & Davis, K. L. (1984). A new rating scale for Alzheimer's disease. *American Journal of Psychiatry, 141,* 1356–1364.

DESCRIPTION

The Alzheimer's Disease Assessment Scale-Cognitive (ADAS-Cog) is the cognitive section of the Alzheimer's Disease Assessment Scale (ADAS) specifically developed to identify cognitive dysfunction due to AD. Its development was guided by the major features of AD. The aims of the test development were to (1) reliably identify the features of AD, (2) measure a wide range of cognitive dysfunction from mild to severe, (3) be relatively quick to administer, and (4) be suitable to use with patients in different environments. The ADAS-Cog includes items assessing orientation, memory recall, recognition, naming, commands, and comprehension, as well as constructional and ideational praxis. Because of subsequent studies highlighting the insensitivity of the ADAS-Cog to mild cognitive dysfunction, delayed recall, cancellation and mazes tasks were added to increase sensitivity to a broad range of dementia severity, including mild AD. Since its initial development, the ADAS-Cog has become the most widely used measure to assess the efficacy of anti-dementia drugs in clinical trials. Linguistically validated translations are available for simplified Chinese (for mainland China), Traditional Chinese (for Taiwan, Hong Kong, and Singapore), English (for Hong Kong and Singapore), and Korean (Shen et al., 2014).

ADMINISTRATION

See the manual. The original reference contains the original administration and scoring protocol for the ADAS. Administration has been standardized by the Alzheimer's Disease Cooperative Study and can be obtained by contacting the publisher (Prepress Type and Graphics; PrepressType@cox.net).

SCORING

See Source. Points are given for errors in each subscale to a maximum total of 70 points. Higher scores represent greater severity of cognitive dysfunction.

DEMOGRAPHIC EFFECTS

The ADAS-Cog total score appears to be correlated with age (Liu et al., 2001; Mavioglu et al., 2006; Pyo et al., 2006; Weyer et al., 1997; Ylikoski et al., 2007). The effect of education is less clear, with some studies suggesting an impact of education (Ylikoski et al., 2007) but only among those with less than six years of education (Liu et al., 2001), and other studies indicating minimal education effects (Mavioglu et al., 2006; Pyo et al., 2006).

EVIDENCE FOR RELIABILITY

EVIDENCE FOR INTERNAL RELIABILITY

Internal consistency for the whole scale and language subscale as measured by Cronbach's alpha is adequate to high (Cano et al., 2010; Hobart et al., 2013a; Karin et al., 2014; Liu et al., 2001; Mavioglu et al., 2006; Weyer et al., 1997). Internal consistency is marginal for memory and praxis subscales (Karin et al., 2014).

EVIDENCE FOR TEST-RETEST RELIABILITY, MEASURING CHANGE, AND PRACTICE EFFECTS

Test-retest reliability over one to two months is generally very high (Cano et al., 2010; Karin et al., 2014; Liu et al., 2001; Mavioglu et al., 1997; Rosen et al., 1984; Weyer et al., 1997) and acceptable for the Asian version (Shen et al., 2014). In a sample of mild and moderate PD dementia patients, four-week test-retest reliability was marginal to adequate (Harvey et al., 2010).

Meaningful change has been defined by a four-point change in most studies based on the recommendation of the US Food and Drug Administration's Peripheral and Central Nervous System Drugs Advisory Committee. However, empirical studies suggest that meaningful change in ADAS-Cog scores may depend on baseline cognitive status and measurement period. In studies that examined meaningful change, actual change is reflected by a seven-point change over three to four weeks (Weyer et al., 1997) or a four to five-point change over 12 months for those with baseline AD (Hobart et al., 2013b; Rosen et al., 1984). A decrease of three ADAS-Cog scores over six months appeared appropriate for assessing change in clinical trials with early AD patients based on anchor-based minimal clinically relevant change method (i.e., clinician judgment on relevant worsening on memory, non-memory cognitive function, functional status, and Clinical Dementia Rating (CDR); Schrag & Schott, 2012). In the Asian version of the ADAS-Cog, the change score over 78 weeks failed to find any difference between the AD (ADAS-Cog change score = 3.86) and healthy control (change score = 2.99) groups (Shen et al., 2014).

One study using the placebo arm of a drug trial found that the rate of decline over 26 weeks differed depending on the severity of dementia at baseline: the moderate dementia group (ADAS-Cog change score = 4.03) experienced 84% greater change in ADAS-Cog than the mild dementia group (change score = 2.19). In this sample, word recognition items showed a large measurement error variability, whereas word recall items showed a large improvement of 154%, suggesting a "placebo" effect. Results suggest that the ADAS-Cog may not be useful for short-term studies of patients with mild cognitive dysfunction (Doraiswamy et al., 2001).

Some researchers suggest that a combination of ADAS-Cog with standard neuropsychological and functional measures is more sensitive than the ADAS-Cog alone for measuring change in clinical drug trials for MCI (Raghavan et al., 2013). A combination of three ADAS-Cog items (Word Recall, Delayed Recall, Orientation) with the Auditory Verbal Learning Test (AVLT), MMSE/CDR-SB, and Functional Activities Questionnaire (FAQ) appeared to increase the power to detect target treatment effects in MCI over the ADAS-Cog alone. Moreover, the standardized response mean, in the moderate to large range for the novel composites, was superior to the ADAS-Cog used alone.

EVIDENCE FOR RELIABILITY OF ALTERNATE FORMS

No studies have been conducted to evaluate the alternate form reliability of parallel versions. This is of particular concern in a survey of ADAS-Cog used in an international cooperative study in eight European countries. When local versions were compared, differences were found in the items for object naming (real vs. pictures), verbal memory (number of trials and imagery value of words used), and number of parallel versions used (Verhey et al., 2004).

EVIDENCE FOR INTERRATER RELIABILITY

Interrater reliability is generally very high (Liu et al., 2001; Mavioglu et al., 2006; Rosen et al., 1984; Shen et al., 2014). However, in a survey evaluating the variance in test administration among different clinical trials using the ADAS-Cog, significant intrarater differences in administration procedures (e.g., exposure time for word list, number of trials for word recognition), scoring rules (e.g., criteria for scoring "place" and "rhombus"), and materials used in clinical trials (e.g., length of worksheet, words on word list) were found, indicating threats to interrater reliability (Connor & Sabbagh, 2008).

EVIDENCE FOR VALIDITY

FACTOR-ANALYTIC STUDIES

Based on a sample of AD and amnestic MCI patients, exploratory factor analysis yielded a single factor explaining 62% of the variance indicating unidimensionality; follow-up confirmatory factor analysis confirmed unidimensionality (Benge et al., 2009). ADAS-Cog total score also showed a continuum for measuring cognitive performance and not a defined point. The items are a conformable set, allowing summation to a total score while maintaining meaning (Hobart et al., 2013b).

STUDIES USING ITEM RESPONSE THEORY

One study reported that participants with the same ADAS-Cog total score may exhibit a wide range of latent cognitive dysfunction. Different ADAS-Cog total scores also demonstrate a large overlap in latent cognitive dysfunction. For example, an ADAS-Cog total score of 22 and 23 showed an overlap of .52 *SD* of latent cognitive dysfunction. The fact that there is overlap suggests that ADAS-Cog total scores may be imprecise indicators of cognitive dysfunction (Balsis et al., 2012). A separate study also found a poor match between the range of performance measured by ADAS-Cog and the sample's range in that the scale showed a large standard error and therefore was less able to discriminate cognitive dysfunction precisely (Hobart et al., 2013b).

The ability of the ADAS-Cog to measure cognitive dysfunction may depend on the degree of dementia, with the best utility at the moderate stage of dementia. Benge and colleagues (2009) found that the ADAS-Cog showed the highest level of latent cognitive dysfunction in the moderate level of dementia (−1.00 and 1.75 *SD* of cognitive dysfunction), suggesting good discrimination of degrees of cognitive dysfunction in this range, especially in memory, language, and praxis. As expected, memory subscales showed best discrimination at lower levels of cognitive dysfunction, with the word recall test being most sensitive to milder levels of dysfunction. The language and praxis subscales demonstrated large overlap, indicating that similar information about cognitive dysfunction can be obtained from either one of these subscales. The ADAS-Cog subscales and the measure as a whole was poor in discriminating among cognitive dysfunction in the mild and severe levels of dementia. Interestingly, at milder and more severe stages of dementia, small changes in raw scores are associated with large changes in latent cognitive dysfunction. In the moderate range of dementia, each raw score point reflects a smaller change in latent cognitive dysfunction. For example, a three-point raw score change can reflect .36 *SD* of cognitive dysfunction (raw score of 12 to 9) to .71 *SD* of cognitive dysfunction (raw score of 69 to 66). These findings have also been reported by Hobart and colleagues (2013b), who concluded that changes in raw score at the extremes have greater implications than changes in the center of the scale.

When the individual items were considered, Hobart and colleagues (2013a) reported that only the word recall, word recognition, and orientation items measured degree of impairment as intended (i.e., a higher score does not necessary reflect more cognitive impairment). A separate study also found that the other items did not adequately match the cognitive range in a sample of mild to moderate AD patients (Cano et al., 2010). Moreover, studies have found ceiling/floor effects on all but the same three items, especially with mild cognitive dysfunction (Cano et al., 2010; Hobart et al., 2013a; Karin et al., 2014). These findings raise concern that the components of the ADAS-Cog may be insensitive to mild cognitive changes such as those that may be seen with short-term drug trials for MCI/mild AD.

RELATIONSHIPS WITH OTHER TESTS

The ADAS-Cog appears to demonstrate good convergent validity. It yields high correlations with global cognitive screeners, including the MMSE (Cano et al., 2010; Harvey et al., 2010; Hobart et al., 2013a; Liu et al., 2001; Mavioglu et al., 2006; Pyo et al., 2006; Weyer et al., 1997; Wouters et al., 2010); Memory-Information-Concentration Test (Mavioglu et al., 2006; Rosen et al., 1984); Sandoz Clinical Assessment-Geriatric score (Rosen et al., 1984); Global Deterioration Scale (Mavioglu et al., 2006); Cognitive Assessment Screening Instrument (Liu et al., 2001); DRS (Rosen et al., 1984); CDR (Liu et al., 2001); and the Cambridge Cognitive Examination (CAMCOG) (Wouters et al., 2010). The ADAS-Cog also correlates with other neuropsychological test batteries comprising attention, executive function, and memory (Karin et al., 2014; Shen et al., 2014; Weyer et al., 1997). However, it was reported that the relationship with the MMSE was mostly carried by the ADAS-Cog memory items (word recall, delayed recall, and word recognition) but not by the nonmemory items (Pyo et al., 2006).

By contrast, an earlier study reported high correlations with the noncognitive section of the ADAS, as well as with the mood and disruptive behavior items on the NOSGER (Weyer et al., 1997).

CLINICAL STUDIES

It is well-established that the ADAS-Cog differentiates cognitively healthy individuals from those with mild to moderate AD (e.g., Mavioglu et al., 2006; Shen et al., 2014; Weyer et al., 1997). One study suggested that ADAS-Cog total score in the 15 to 61 range predicted mild to moderate dementia (Weyer et al., 1997). Evidence for MCI or very early AD is less clear. For example, in a study that investigated the utility of the ADAS-Cog to identify MCI (based on CDR .5 but not meeting the diagnostic criteria for AD as defined by NINCDS-ADRDA), the authors found that the MCI group was better than those of AD CDR .5 on most subtests, but there was significant overlap between these groups, suggesting that the ADAS-Cog may not be useful to differentiate between MCI and early AD.

The unresponsiveness of the ADAS-Cog to mild cognitive changes has been reported by Karin and colleagues (2014) in a post-hoc analysis using data from a clinical drug trial in mild to moderate AD. After 12 weeks, small effect sizes were obtained in both donepezil and placebo groups as measured by the ADAS-Cog, but clear differences between the groups' effect sizes were seen when neuropsychological test measures were used.

To improve the sensitivity of the ADAS-Cog, some researchers suggested adding other items to the ADAS-Cog (Sano et al., 2011; Skinner et al., 2012). For example, the benefits of adding delayed recall to the ADAS-Cog was examined using a sample of MCI and AD patients in the placebo arm of a drug study. AD patients showed floor effect with minimal change over one year, whereas the MCI participants improved by .20±1.7 over one year. The addition of the delayed recall item provided 18% improvement in standardized change for the MCI but no measureable difference in the AD participants, even when matched for MMSE scores (Sano et al., 2011). Similarly, addition of executive function (vegetable fluency, Trail Making Test [TMT]-A and -B, Digit Symbol) and functional ability (items from FAQ) improved prediction of conversion from MCI to dementia over 12 months (Skinner et al., 2012).

Although most studies have established the use of ADAS-Cog in AD, Harvey and colleagues (2010) reported that the ADAS-Cog was also able to distinguish PD dementia patients of mild and moderate severity level. The ADAS-Cog did not correlate with the Neuropsychiatric Inventory (NPI-10). Coupled with weak correlation with TMT-A and CDR, moderate correlation with the Delis-Kaplan Executive Function System (DKEFS) verbal fluency, Ten-Point Clock Test (TPCT), and ADCS-ADL, and strongest correlation with MMSE, these results support the convergent and discriminant validity of the ADAS-Cog. Taken together, the ADAS-Cog appears adequate for assessing PD with dementia.

NEUROANATOMICAL CORRELATES AND IMAGING STUDIES

The limited studies that have examined the neuroanatomic correlates of the ADAS-Cog found relationships with white matter hyperintensity (WMH), brain volume, and APOE E4 status. In one study, ADAS-Cog was only able to differentiate between the mild and severe WMH groups in a community-dwelling sample of older adults. However, with addition of digit cancellation and verbal fluency tests, the extended ADAS-Cog was more sensitive to white matter load (Ylikoski et al., 2007). Skinner et al. (2012) also reported that an extended version comprising executive function and functional ability tests (ADAS-plus-EF & FA) was strongly related to baseline ventricular volume and total brain volume, but not p-tau; the scale was not strongly related to hippocampal volume or entorhinal thickness. Similarly, when considering ADAS-Cog delayed recall change score over 12 months, this item alone appeared to differentiate between MCI patients who are APOE E4 negative and those who are APOE E4 negative; no effect of E4 status in AD was observed (Sano et al., 2011).

PERFORMANCE VALIDITY

Not reported.

COMMENT

The ADAS-Cog is a brief dementia screen developed primarily to identify AD. It is one of the most well-studied dementia screening tools and the most commonly used tool to monitor response in clinical drug trials for AD. It appears to demonstrate good psychometric properties for assessing cognitive functioning based on classical test theory and is clearly adequate for discriminating between healthy individuals and those with AD. It is useful for measuring cognitive change in clinical drug trials, at least for moderate AD.

Although the ADAS-Cog demonstrated utility in moderate AD, it is insensitive to mild cognitive changes that may be seen in MCI/early AD. Studies have also reported on the large overlap between the performance of those with MCI and early AD, such that the ADAS-Cog is unable to distinguish between these two groups. Its lack of sensitivity in the early stages may be because the original ADAS-Cog did not include a delayed recall item, a hallmark of amnesia in early AD. The delayed recall item was included in some recent studies, but this is not consistent across all studies. It also does not have items assessing visual memory, psychomotor speed, and attention/concentration. The language subscale is heavily dependent on clinician rating and therefore lacks objective assessment of language. Accordingly, use of the ADAS-Cog in clinical drug trials for MCI/early AD is not recommended, and the ADAS-Cog cannot be considered a comprehensive diagnostic tool.

It may be important to note that most clinical drug trials have utilized a four-point change to signify clinically significant change, but the rationale for this value is unclear. When Oremus (2014) attempted to verify the source of this recommendation by conducting a literature review, the author found that all secondary sources cited a single FDA meeting proceeding source, which did not provide justification for the four-point threshold. According to relevant research, baseline cognitive status and measurement period must be taken into consideration when interpreting meaningful change using the ADAS-Cog.

REFERENCES

Balsis, S., Unger, A. A., Benge, J. F., Geraci, L., & Doody, R. S. (2012). Gaining precision on the Alzheimer's disease assessment scale-cognitive: A comparison of item response theory-based scores and total scores. *Alzheimer's & Dementia, 8*(4), 288–294.

Benge, J. F., Balsis, S., Geraci, L., Massman, P. J., & Doody, R. S. (2009). How well do the ADAS-cog and its subscales measure cognitive dysfunction in Alzheimer's disease? *Dementia and Geriatric Cognitive Disorders, 28*(1), 63–69.

Cano, S. J., Posner, H. B., Moline, M. L., Hurt, S. W., Swartz, J., Hsu, T., & Hobart, J. C. (2010). The ADAS-cog in Alzheimer's disease clinical trials: Psychometric evaluation of the sum and its parts. *Journal of Neurology, Neurosurgery & Psychiatry, 81*(12), 1363–1368.

Connor, D. J., & Sabbagh, M. N. (2008). Administration and scoring variance on the ADAS-cog. *Journal of Alzheimer's Disease, 15*(3), 461–464.

Doraiswamy, P. M., Kaiser, L., Bieber, F., & Garman, R. L. (2001). The Alzheimer's disease assessment scale: Evaluation of psychometric properties and patterns of cognitive decline in multicenter clinical trials of mild to moderate Alzheimer's disease. *Alzheimer Disease and Associated Disorders, 15*(4), 174–183.

Harvey, P. D., Ferris, S. H., Cummings, J. L., Wesnes, K. A., Hsu, C., Lane, R. M., & Tekin, S. (2010). Evaluation of dementia rating scales in Parkinson's disease dementia. *American Journal of Alzheimer's Disease and Other Dementias, 25*(2), 142–148.

Hobart, J., Cano, S., Posner, H., Selnes, O., Stern, Y., Thomas, R., & Zajicek, J. (2013a). Putting the Alzheimer's cognitive test to the test I: Traditional psychometric methods. *Alzheimer's & Dementia, 9*(1), S4–S9.

Hobart, J., Cano, S., Posner, H., Selnes, O., Stern, Y., Thomas, R., & Zajicek, J. (2013b). Putting the Alzheimer's cognitive test to the test II: Rasch measurement theory. *Alzheimer's & Dementia, 9*(1), S10–S20.

Karin, A., Hannesdottir, K., Jaeger, J., Annas, P., Segerdahl, M., Karlsson, P., . . . Miller, F. (2014). Psychometric evaluation of ADAS-Cog and NTB for measuring drug response. *Acta Neurologica Scandinavica, 129*(2), 114–122.

Liu, H. C., Teng, E. L., Chuang, Y. Y., Lin, K. N., Fuh, J. L., & Wang, P. N. (2001). The Alzheimer's Disease Assessment Scale: Findings from a low-education population. *Dementia and Geriatric Cognitive Disorders, 13*(1), 21–26.

Mavioglu, H., Gedizlioglu, M., Akyel, S., Aslaner, T., & Eser, E. (2006). The validity and reliability of the Turkish version of Alzheimer's Disease Assessment Scale-Cognitive Subscale (ADAS-Cog) in patients with mild and moderate Alzheimer's disease and normal subjects. *International Journal of Geriatric Psychiatry, 21*(3), 259–265.

Oremus, M. (2014). Does the evidence say a 4-point change in ADAS-Cog score is clinically significant? *Alzheimer's & Dementia, 10*(3), 416–417.

Pyo, G., Elble, R. J., Ala, T., & Markwell, S. J. (2006). The characteristics of patients with uncertain/mild cognitive impairment on the Alzheimer's Disease Assessment Scale-Cognitive subscale. *Alzheimer Disease & Associated Disorders, 20*(1), 16–22.

Raghavan, N., Samtani, M. N., Farnum, M., Yang, E., Novak, G., Grundman, M., . . . the Alzheimer's Disease Neuroimaging Initiative (2013). The ADAS-cog revisited: Novel composite scales based on ADAS-cog to improve efficiency in MCI and early AD trials. *Alzheimer's & Dementia, 9*(1), S21–S31.

Rosen, W. G., Mohs, R. C., & Davis, K. L. (1984). A new rating scale for Alzheimer's disease. *American Journal of Psychiatry, 141*(11), 1356–1364.

Sano, M., Raman, R., Emond, J., Thomas, R. G., Petersen, R., Schneider, L. S., & Aisen, P. S. (2011). Adding delayed recall to the Alzheimer

Disease Assessment Scale is useful in studies of mild cognitive impairment but not Alzheimer disease. *Alzheimer Disease and Associated Disorders, 25*(2), 122–127.

Schrag, A., & Schott, J. M. (2012). What is the clinically relevant change on the ADAS-cog? *Journal of Neurology, Neurosurgery & Psychiatry, 83*(2), 171–173. doi:10.1136/jnnp-2011-300881

Shen, J. H., Shen, Q., Yu, H., Lai, J. S., Beaumont, J. L., Zhang, Z., . . . Cummings, J. (2014). Validation of an Alzheimer's disease assessment battery in Asian participants with mild to moderate Alzheimer's disease. *American Journal of Neurodegenerative Diseases, 3*(3), 158–169.

Skinner, J., Carvalho, J. O., Potter, G. G., Thames, A., Zelinski, E., Crane, P. K., & Gibbons, L. E. (2012). The Alzheimer's Disease Assessment Scale (ADAS-cog-plus): An expansion of the ADAS-cog to improve responsiveness in MCI. *Brain Imaging and Behavior, 6*(4), 489–501.

Verhey, F. R., Houx, P., van Lang, N., Huppert, F., Stoppe, G., Saerens, J., . . . Jolles, J. (2004). Cross-national comparison and validation of the Alzheimer's Disease Assessment Scale: Results from the European Harmonization Project for Instruments in Dementia (EURO-HARPID). *International Journal of Geriatric Psychiatry, 19*(1), 41–50.

Weyer, G., Erzigkeit, H., Kanowski, S., Ihl, R., & Hadler, D. (1997). Alzheimer's Disease Assessment Scale: Reliability and validity in a multicenter clinical trial. *International Psychogeriatrics, 9*(2), 123–138.

Wouters, H., van Gool, W. A., Schmand, B., Zwinderman, A. H., & Lindeboom, R. (2010). Three sides of the same coin: Measuring global cognitive impairment with the MMSE, ADAS-cog and CAMCOG. *International Journal of Geriatric Psychiatry, 25*(8), 770–779.

Ylikoski, R., Jokinen, H., Andersen, P., Salonen, O., Madureira, S., Ferro, J., . . . Erkinjuntti, T. (2007). Comparison of the Alzheimer's Disease Assessment Scale cognitive subscale and the Vascular Dementia Assessment Scale in differentiating elderly individuals with different degrees of white matter changes. *Dementia and Geriatric Cognitive Disorders, 24*, 73–81.

CLINICAL DEMENTIA RATING (CDR)

TEST NAME	**Clinical Dementia Rating (CDR)**
DOMAIN	Dementia staging
AGE RANGE	Older adults
ADMINISTRATION TIME	90 minutes
SCORING FORMAT	Hand scored or computer scored
REFERENCE	Hughes, C. P., Berg, L., Danziger, W. L., Coben, L. A., & Martin, R. L. (1982). A new clinical scale for the staging of dementia. *The British Journal of Psychiatry, 140*, 566–572.

DESCRIPTION

The Clinical Dementia Rating (CDR; Hughes et al., 1982) is a semi-structured, clinician-rated interview widely used to stage the progression of dementia. The CDR was originally developed at the Washington University School of Medicine in 1979 to evaluate the progression of AD. Using information provided by the patient and an informant, the clinician rates the patient's functioning in six domains commonly affected in AD: memory, orientation, judgment and problem solving, community affairs, home and hobbies, and personal care. A protocol that includes language and behavior domains has also been developed to better characterize the symptoms seen in frontotemporal dementia (FTD; Knopman et al., 2011; Russo et al., 2014). The CDR is based solely on clinical information obtained from the patient and informant; performance on psychometric tests is not considered. A variety of scoring methods is available to stage the severity of dementia or quantify the severity of dementia in longitudinal studies. The global CDR is widely used primarily for the staging of AD. It has also been used to stage other dementing disorders such as PD and FTD. In recent years, the CDR has been used to characterize MCI, though it appears to capture a different entity from MCI (see "Clinical Studies").

The original focus of the CDR was to assess community-dwelling older adults since its anchor points probe for examples of one's engagement with the home and community. Since its initial purpose, the CDR has been used in clinical practice and multicenter clinical trials. It has also been adapted for use in chronic long-term care facilities (Marin et al., 2001). Available in more than 60 languages and dialects, the CDR is used in cross-cultural dementia studies around the world. The translations can be downloaded free of cost for clinical and research use on the CDR website (https://knightadrc.wustl.edu/professionals-clinicians/cdr-dementia-staging-instrument).

ADMINISTRATION

Live, in-person training is recommended by the authors prior to using the CDR. If such an arrangement is not possible, an online training video on the use of the CDR is available free for registered individual users and takes about eight to nine hours to complete. Individual users must submit an application in order to receive password access to the free training. Group or corporate users may request tailored protocols on a case-by-case basis with a fee.

Only impairments due to cognitive deficits and not physical disability are to be rated. Table 7–3 summarizes the CDR domains and their respective scoring elements, including the expanded domains. The CDR takes about 90 minutes to administer.

To use the CDR in chronic care facilities, other questions relevant to activities in a chronic care facility may be asked in place of the standard questions without compromising its psychometric property. Table 7–4 presents the modifications to use the CDR in chronic care facilities (CDR-CC; Marin et al., 2001).

SCORING

An online scoring worksheet and detailed scoring algorithms, including "tie-break" rules, are available on the CDR website. Depending on the assessment purpose, users may choose from a number of scoring methods. Briefly, a box score ranging from 0 to 3, representing "none" to "severe" impairment, is generated for each of the six domains (see Table 7–3). The expanded domains sensitive to FTD are also presented in Table 7–3.

Global CDR is used to stage the severity of dementia. One of five possible stages based on a scoring algorithm is derived from the individual box scores: CDR 0 (no dementia); CDR 0.5 (questionable dementia); CDR 1 (mild dementia); CDR 2 (moderate dementia); CDR 3 (severe

TABLE 7–3 Summary of Clinical Dementia Rating (CDR) and CDR for Frontotemporal Dementia Domains

	CDR 0	CDR 0.5	CDR 1	CDR 2	CDR 3
Memory	No memory loss or slight inconstant forgetfulness	Mild consistent forgetfulness; "benign" forgetfulness	Moderate memory loss, more marked for recent events; interferes with everyday activities	Only highly learned material retained; new material rapidly lost	Only fragments remain
Orientation	Fully oriented		Some difficulty with time relationships; oriented to place and person at examination but may have geographic disorientation	Usually disoriented in time, often to place	Oriented to person only
Judgment and Problem Solving	Solves everyday problems well; judgment good relative to past	Only doubtful impairment in solving problems	Moderate difficulties in handling complex problems; social judgment usually maintained	Severely impaired in handling problems; social judgment usually impaired	Unable to make judgments or solve problems
Community Affairs	Independent function at usual level	Only doubtful or mild impairment, if any	Unable to function independently but may still engage in some; may still appear normal to casual inspection	No pretense of independent function outside of home	
Home and Hobbies	Life at home, hobbies, intellectual interests well maintained	Life at home, hobbies, intellectual interests well maintained or only slightly impaired	Mild but definite impairment of function at home; more difficult chores and more complicated hobbies or interests abandoned	Only simple chores preserved; very restricted interests	No significant function in home outside of own room
Personal Care	Fully capable of self-care		Needs occasional prompting	Requires assistance in dressing, hygiene, keeping of personal effects	Requires much help with personal care; often incontinent
Behavior, Comportment, and Personality	Socially appropriate behavior	Questionable changes in comportment, empathy	Mild but definite changes in behavior	Moderate behavioral changes affecting interpersonal relationships and interactions in a significant manner	Severe behavioral changes making interpersonal interactions all unidirectional
Language	No language difficulty or occasional mild tip-o-the tongue	Consistent mild word finding difficulties; simplification of word choice; circumlocutions; decreased phrase length; and/or mild comprehension difficulties	Moderate word finding difficulty in speech; cannot name objects in environment; reduced phrase length and/or agrammatical speech; and/or reduced comprehension in conversation and reading	Moderate to severe impairments in either speech or comprehension; has difficulty communicating thoughts; writing may be slightly more effective	Severe comprehension deficits; no intelligible speech

SOURCE: Adapted from Hughes et al. (1982) and Knopman et al. (2011).

TABLE 7–4 Modifications for Using the Clinical Dementia Rating in Chronic Care Facilities (CDR-CC)

DOMAIN	MODIFICATION
Memory	Assess ability to recall daily schedule of activities
Orientation	Assess orientation to institution and unit
Judgment and Problem Solving	Assess interactions with staff and request for self-care or transport
Community Affairs	Assess participation and performance in activities
Home and Hobbies	Assess participation in hobbies such as reading, watching TV or listening to music as well as concern for maintenance of room
Personal Care	Unchanged

SOURCE: From Marin et al. (2001).

dementia). An extension of this scale to include CDR 4 (profound) and CDR 5 (terminal) may also be used to classify the later stages.

Sum of Boxes (CDR-SB) is generally used to quantify severity of dementia in clinical trials. CDR-SB is generated by adding all the box scores to form a total score that ranges from 0 to 18.

The Item Response Theory (IRT)-based scoring method is used when precise measurement of dementia severity is needed. Please see Lowe et al. (2012) for the item parameters for IRT-based scoring using Multilog software.

If only the Global Deterioration Scale (GDS) is given, conversion between CDR and GDS can also be made by using Table 7–5.

TABLE 7–5 Conversion of Clinical Dementia Rating into Global Deterioration Scale (GDS), and Conversion of GDS into CDR and CDR-SB

	CDR 0	CDR 0.5	CDR 1	CDR 2	CDR 3	CDR 4	CDR 5
GDS							
Total subjects (*N* = 112)	1.30	3.27	4.25	5.40	6.12	6.66	7.08
Group A (*N* = 75)	1.33	3.16	4.16	5.38	6.17	6.75	7.22
Group B (*N* = 71)	1.32	3.12	4.10	5.29	6.06	6.63	7.09
	GDS 1	**GDS 2**	**GDS 3**	**GDS 4**	**GDS 5**	**GDS 6**	**GDS 7**
CDR							
Total subjects (*N* = 112)	–0.04	0.13	0.40	0.85	1.59	2.80	4.80
Group A (*N* = 75)	–0.05	0.14	0.44	0.90	1.63	2.75	4.50
Group B (*N* = 71)	–0.05	0.14	0.45	0.94	1.70	2.91	4.79
CDR-SB							
Total subjects (*N* = 112)	–0.24	0.52	1.86	4.24	8.49	16.04	29.49
Group A (*N* = 75)	–0.22	0.53	1.85	4.19	8.31	15.58	28.41
Group B (*N* = 71)	–0.32	0.41	1.74	4.17	8.60	16.70	31.48

NOTE: Group A = Alzheimer's disease, group B = vascular dementia. Based on 41 AD patients, 37 VD patients, and 34 healthy older adults.

SOURCE: From Choi et al. (2003).

DEMOGRAPHIC EFFECTS

Because the CDR is based on clinician rating of changes relative to prior level of functioning and is easily adapted to local contexts, demographic effects are minimized, though it has been reported that the rate of cognitive decline is higher in those who have low education and are CDR 1 at baseline (Adak et al., 2004). The interview may be modified for illiteracy or adjusted for cultural factors (e.g., Homma et al., 2006; Lim et al., 2005). As such, the use of the CDR has also been accepted as an appropriate comprehensive measure for studies of dementia patients in Asian populations (Lim et al., 2005; Senanarong et al., 2006), although empirical validation of various translations is needed.

EVIDENCE FOR RELIABILITY

FACTOR-ANALYTIC STUDIES

The CDR-SB yields a two-factor solution with a Cognitive factor consisting of Memory, Orientation, and Judgment and Problem Solving box scores, and a Functional factor consisting of Community Affairs, Home and Hobbies, and Personal Care box scores (Cedarbaum et al., 2013; Coley et al., 2011). When used to track disease progression over two years in a sample of older adults with very mild cognitive dysfunction, both Cognitive and Functional factors contributed equally to cognitive outcome.

EVIDENCE FOR INTERNAL RELIABILITY

The CDR-SB has excellent internal reliability. Cronbach's alphas are generally greater than .90 in healthy older adults and mild AD patients and greater than .85 in AD patients (Cedarbaum et al., 2013; Coley et al., 2011).

EVIDENCE FOR TEST-RETEST RELIABILITY, MEASURING CHANGE, AND PRACTICE EFFECTS

The CDR-CC for chronic care facility residents has excellent one-month test-retest reliability (Intraclass Correlation Coefficient = .92; Marin et al., 2001). The annual rate of change of CDR-SB in symptomatic AD is 1.43 points (SE = .05) for CDR 0.5 at baseline and 1.91 points (SE = .07) for CDR 1 at baseline (Williams et al., 2013).

EVIDENCE FOR INTERRATER RELIABILITY

Most of the psychometric studies on the CDR have focused on interrater reliability in multicenter clinical trials. These studies have concluded that experience using the CDR increases reliability estimates, although adequately trained inexperienced raters may also demonstrate a high level of agreement (kappa = .83 or higher; Schafer et al., 2004; Tractenberg, Schafer, & Morris, 2001). The CDR also shows good reliability among raters of various qualifications. There are no major differences in reliability among physicians, nurses, PhDs, social workers, psychometrists, research assistant raters, or trained community health workers (85% for non-MDs and 82% for MDs; Chaves et al., 2007; Han et al., 2013; McCulla et al., 1989; Oremus et al., 2000). Kappas between physician raters range from .75 to .94 for the six individual domain scores and CDR-SB score (Oremus et al., 2000). Kappas among psychiatrists and neurologists is .87, with agreement lowest for Judgment and Problem Solving at 68%; all other boxes have agreement greater than 80% (Burke et al., 1988). Kappas between nurses, or between nurses and physicians, range from 0.66 to 0.77 (McCulla et al., 1989; Oremus et al., 2000).

The CDR has also been used to rate impairment in traumatic brain injury (TBI). In TBI, overall concordance is moderate to strong (Kendall's W = .53), with interrater reliability greater than .70 for Global CDR. Domain interrater reliabilities are generally in the .49 (Judgment and Problem Solving) to .79 (Orientation) range (Webber et al., 2013).

EVIDENCE FOR VALIDITY

RELATIONSHIPS WITH OTHER TESTS

Evidence for construct validity of the CDR appears solid. The CDR shows high agreement with various dementia gold standards (e.g., 87% with NINCDS-ADRDA and 86% with DSM-III; Chaves et al., 2007). In the original study, the CDR had strong correlations with the Blessed Dementia Scale (BDS; r = .74) and the Pfeiffer Short Portable Mental Status Questionnaire (SPMSQ; r = .84) among individuals with CDR ratings between no dementia and very mild dementia (Hughes et al., 1982). Correlations of CDR and CDR-SB with various global cognitive measures range from small to large in community-dwelling or chronic care facility samples (ADAS-Cog, r = .53; MMSE, r = .33 to −.94; BDS, r = .74 to .98; GDS, r = .97; PMSQ, r = .84; e.g., Cedarbaum et al., 2013; Chaves et al., 2007; Choi et al., 2003; Marin et al., 2001). However, Reisberg (2007) concluded in his review of various dementia staging instruments that the GDS appears better than the CDR because it has more specific staging descriptors than the CDR.

Similar correlations are found with neuropsychological measures such as the Consortium to Establish a Registry for Alzheimer's Disease (CERAD) Boston Naming Test (BNT), list learning, and verbal fluency (Oremus et al., 2000) or functional measures such as the FAQ (Cedarbaum et al., 2013). Moreover, the CDR remains stable over a 30-year period relative to psychometric cognitive test scores despite variations in participants' demographic background over the time span (Williams et al., 2009).

Studies have shown that the CDR taps into both cognitive and functional skills independently. The CDR Cognitive factor correlates with ADAS-Cog, MMSE, and FAQ, with the CDR Functional factor correlating more with FAQ than cognitive measures (Cedarbaum et al., 2013). The relationship of CDR severity and cognitive/functional measures is also evident when IRT-based scoring is used. Greater dementia severity on the CDR is correlated with functional outcome except at the CDR 0.5 stage because of the lack of functional dependency at this stage (Miller et al., 2011).

CLINICAL STUDIES

The global CDR is widely used primarily for the staging of AD. It has also been used to stage other dementing disorders such as PD and FTD (Russo et al., 2014). The CDR 0.5 has been used to characterize MCI; however, there is evidence that a large proportion (30%) of individuals at CDR 0.5 also meet ICD-10 criteria for mild dementia (Lynch et al., 2006). Use of CDR 0.5 interchangeably with MCI has also been brought into question by Meguro et al. (2004). The authors suggest that CDR 0.5 may be more relevant for community samples than for MCI following comparisons between various CDR 0.5 and MCI subtypes using a Japanese population-based sample. About 30% of the sample was classified as CDR 0.5 of various subtypes (incipient dementia, AD, uncertain dementia, others), whereas 5% were classified as MCI (Petersen criteria). More than 40% of CDR 0.5/AD were classified as MCI, whereas the ratio between MCI subtypes and CDR 0.5 subtypes was similar. The low prevalence rate based on MCI (Petersen criteria) may be due to the subjective memory complaints criteria; in a community-based sample, memory decline may be perceived as aging-related, whereas those with memory complaints are more likely to be seen in memory clinics.

Of the two scoring methods, the CDR-SB is more commonly used in clinical drug trials because it is sensitive to changes within 12 months following baseline measurement in donepezil drug trials, whereas the global CDR is not (e.g., Petersen et al., 2005). There is also evidence that the CDR-SB is more useful than the global CDR in distinguishing mild cognitive deficits from dementia (Lynch et al., 2006).

PREDICTIVE VALIDITY

Both global CDR and CDR-SB show high predictive utility for dementia. Trained community health workers' CDR rating are consistent with physician diagnosed MCI/dementia in community-dwelling older adults, suggesting that the CDR may be effective in identifying older adults living in the community who require follow-up assessment and care (Han et al., 2013). Indeed, use of the CDR as a screening tool for dementia revealed a sensitivity of 92% and specificity of 94% for mild dementia in a community sample of adults older than 75 (Juva et al., 1995). In a Brazilian sample, global CDR yielded a sensitivity of 86% and a specificity of 80% for detection of dementia (all types) in relation to NINCDS-ADRDA as a gold standard (Chaves et al., 2007). The CDR-SB yielded an overall 94% classification rate for a heterogeneous sample of dementia cases in the National Alzheimer's Coordinating Center (NACC) database (O'Bryant et al., 2010). However, the CDR-SB does not discriminate AD from behavioral variant FTD (bvFTD) or primary progressive aphasia (PPA; Knopman et al., 2011). When the expanded CDR-SB is used to classify AD and FTLD (PPA and bvFTD), the addition of Language as well as Behavior domains improves the classification accuracy from 65% to 94% compared to the Memory domain alone (Knopman et al., 2011; Russo et al., 2014). For example, a one-point increase on the Language domain increased the odds of PPA by three times. Although the bvFTD and PPA patients obtained very mild CDR-SB ratings, they were rated as abnormal on the Language or Behavior domains, whereas the other patients obtained generally questionable ratings on these domains (Knopman et al., 2011).

In terms of longitudinal studies of AD progression, both the global CDR and the CDR-SB appear useful for tracking cognitive changes over a two- to three-year period (e.g., Cortes et al., 2008; Meguro et al., 2004). Poor scores on Memory and Orientation at baseline are predictive of decliners. In general, higher CDR at baseline predicts a higher rate of cognitive decline over two to six years, though the relationship is modified by age and presence of the APOE E4 allele at least in the CDR 0 group (Adak et al., 2004; Cedarbaum et al., 2013). The rate of decline appears higher in those with a baseline global CDR of greater than 0.5 than in those with CDR 0.5 (Cedarbaum et al., 2013), especially in CDR 1 with lower education (Adak et al., 2004).

There is evidence that individuals with higher CDR-SB scores are more likely to develop dementia in the future (Lynch et al., 2006). Those who are CDR 0.5 with impaired CDR items related to instrumental activities of daily living (IADL) are also more likely to progress to AD over two years than those with intact IADL (Chang et al., 2011). Among those with symptomatic AD who are CDR 0.5 at baseline, it takes about 3.75 years to progress to the next CDR stage, whereas those who are CDR 1 at baseline take 2.98 years (Williams et al., 2013). Among CDR 0.5, predictors of progression are age at diagnosis and APOE E4 genotype. In addition, CDR scores predict survival in individuals with suspected dementia. Using survival as outcome, the median survival was one year for CDR 5, two years for CDR 4, 2.5 years for CDR 3, three years for CDR 2, and 3.5 years for CDR 1 (Dooneief et al., 1996).

CDR AS AN OUTCOME MEASURE IN CLINICAL TRIALS

Studies have shown that the CDR-SB is more sensitive than the global CDR to cognitive changes associated with drug treatment for MCI and AD. In a 36-month treatment trial for MCI, it was observed that, of CDR-SB, GDS, ADAS-Cog, MMSE, and a battery of tests, all but the global CDR were sensitive to the treatment effect of donepezil in MCI, suggesting that the global CDR may not be a useful outcome measure for MCI treatment trials (Petersen et al., 2005). When the psychometric properties of the CDR-SB as an endpoint in clinical trials or AD was examined, the authors found excellent internal responsiveness with large effect sizes (1.2) and standardized response mean (1.17) at two years. External responsiveness was most highly correlated with two-year MMSE and ADL changes but was of modest magnitude. When compared to clinically meaningful changes on the ADAS-Cog and IADL, external responsiveness was borderline acceptable (Coley et al., 2011). Similarly, Cedarbaum and colleagues (2013) found that effect sizes for two-year change for CDR-SB were higher than all other measures, suggesting that the CDR-SB may require smaller sample sizes than ADAS-Cog, MMSE, or FAQ as an outcome measure in clinical studies, particularly in early AD. Accordingly, the CDR-SB appears appropriate as an endpoint measure in MCI and AD treatment trials.

NEUROANATOMICAL CORRELATES AND IMAGING STUDIES

In terms of neuropathology, there are differences in regional brain volumes depending on the global CDR. For example, total brain, ventricular, subarachnoid CSF, and temporal lobe volumes were different between CDR 0 and CDR 1, as well as CDR 0.5 and CDR 1, though the differences disappeared when stratified by gender in a sample with and without early AD. Only hippocampal volume was different for the baseline CDR 0 and CDR 0.5 groups (Adak et al., 2004).

Even at a mild level, CDR 0.5 has been associated with multiple pathological signs including those related to AD, dementia with Lewy bodies (DLB), and vascular dementia, as well as nonspecific pathology (Saito & Murayama, 2007). Specifically, CDR items assessing daily tasks are associated with widespread gray matter loss in the frontal and parietal regions (Chang et al., 2011). Furthermore, increased microglia activation, an inflammatory biomarker of AD, is seen with advancing CDR stages (Xiang et al., 2006). A negative association is also found between the CDR-SB score and glucose metabolism in the right posterior cingulate gyrus (Perneczky et al., 2007).

PERFORMANCE VALIDITY

Not reported.

COMMENT

The flexibility of the structured interview format of the CDR presents several advantages over psychometric tests. First, it is an assessment option for patients who are illiterate or have limited English-language proficiency. Moreover, it can also be used in the presence of aphasia, a condition common among patients with dementing disorders. Last, the administration of the CDR does not require a standardized set of instructions but depends on a set of guidelines; the semi-structured nature of the interview, therefore, allows easy adaptation to local cultural and ethnic contexts. The interview may be modified for illiteracy or adjusted for the cultural factors that give rise to a restricted lifestyle. That is, older adults in some cultural groups are less likely to participate in cognitively demanding daily activities that are evaluated by the original CDR (e.g., Homma et al., 2006; Lim et al., 2005). Given these advantages and its excellent psychometric properties, the CDR is considered one of the best scales for staging AD compared to other clinical dementia staging instruments (Rikkert et al., 2011). A disadvantage of the CDR is that it takes a long time to administer. Studies verifying the expanded CDR-SB for FTD and translated versions, as well as the IRT-based scoring method are also lacking.

REFERENCES

Adak, S., Illouz, K., Gorman, W., Tandon, R., Zimmerman, E. A., Guariglia, R., . . . Kaye, J. A. (2004). Predicting the rate of cognitive decline in aging and early Alzheimer disease. *Neurology, 63*(1), 108–114.

Burke, W. J., Miller, J. P., Rubin, E. H., Morris, J. C., Coben, L. A., Duchek, J., . . . Berg, L. (1988). Reliability of the Washington University Clinical Dementia Rating. *Archives of Neurology, 45*(1), 31–32.

Cedarbaum, J. M., Jaros, M., Hernandez, C., Coley, N., Andrieu, S., Grundman, M., & Vellas, B. (2013). Rationale for use of the Clinical Dementia Rating sum of boxes as a primary outcome measure for Alzheimer's disease clinical trials. *Alzheimer's & Dementia, 9*(1), S45–S55.

Chang, Y. L., Bondi, M. W., McEvoy, L. K., Fennema-Notestine, C., Salmon, D. P., Galasko, D., . . . Alzheimer's Disease Neuroimaging Initiative. (2011). Global clinical dementia rating of 0.5 in MCI masks variability related to level of function. *Neurology, 76*(7), 652–659.

Chaves, M. L. F., Camozzato, A. L., Godinho, C., Kochhann, R., Schuh, A., De Almeida, V. L., & Kaye, J. (2007). Validity of the Clinical Dementia Rating scale for the detection and staging of dementia in Brazilian patients. *Alzheimer Disease & Associated Disorders, 21*(3), 210–217.

Choi, S. H., Lee, B. H., Kim, S., Hahm, D. S., Jeong, J. H., Yoon, S. J., . . . Nab, D. L. (2003). Interchanging scores between Clinical Dementia Rating scale and Global Deterioration Scale. *Alzheimer Disease & Associated Disorders, 17*(2), 98–105.

Coley, N., Andrieu, S., Jaros, M., Weiner, M., Cedarbaum, J., & Vellas, B. (2011). Suitability of Clinical Dementia Rating Sum of Boxes as a single primary endpoint for Alzheimer's disease trials. *Alzheimer's & Dementia, 7*(6), 602–610.

Cortes, F., Nourhashémi, F., Guérin, O., Cantet, C., Gillette-Guyonnet, S., Andrieu, S., . . . Group, R. F. (2008). Prognosis of Alzheimer's disease today: A two-year prospective study in 686 patients from the REAL-FR Study. *Alzheimer's & Dementia, 4*(1), 22–29.

Dooneief, G., Marder, K., Tang, M. X., & Stern, Y. (1996). The Clinical Dementia Rating Scale Community-based validation of "profound" and "terminal" stages. *Neurology, 46*(6), 1746–1749.

Han, H., Park, S., Song, H., Kim, M., Kim, K. B., & Lee, H. B. (2013). Feasibility and validity of dementia assessment by trained community health workers based on Clinical Dementia Rating. *Journal of the American Geriatrics Society, 61*(7), 1141–1145.

Homma, A., Meguro, K., Dominguez, J., Sahadevan, S., Wang, Y. H., & Morris, J. C. (2006). Clinical Dementia Rating workshop: The Asian experience. *Alzheimer Disease & Associated Disorders, 20*(4), 318–321.

Hughes, C. P., Berg, L., Danziger, W. L., Coben, L. A., & Martin, R. L. (1982). A new clinical scale for the staging of dementia. *The British Journal of Psychiatry, 140*(6), 566–572.

Juva, K., Sulkava, R., Erkinjuntti, T., Ylikoski, R., Valvanne, J., & Tilvis, R. (1995). Usefulness of the Clinical Dementia Rating scale in screening for dementia. *International Psychogeriatrics, 7*(01), 17–24.

Knopman, D. S., Weintraub, S., & Pankratz, V. S. (2011). Language and behavior domains enhance the value of the Clinical Dementia Rating scale. *Alzheimer's & Dementia, 7*(3), 293–299.

Lim, W. S., Chin, J. J., Lam, C. K., Lim, P. I. P. J., & Sahadevan, S. (2005). Clinical Dementia Rating: Experience of a multi-racial Asian population. *Alzheimer Disease & Associated Disorders, 19*(3), 135–142.

Lowe, D. A., Balsis, S., Miller, T. M., Benge, J. F., & Doody, R. S. (2012). Greater precision when measuring dementia severity: Establishing item parameters for the Clinical Dementia Rating scale. *Dementia and Geriatric Cognitive Disorders, 34*(2), 128–134.

Lynch, C. A., Walsh, C., Blanco, A., Moran, M., Coen, R. F., Walsh, J. B., & Lawlor, B. A. (2006). The Clinical Dementia Rating Sum of Box score in mild dementia. *Dementia and Geriatric Cognitive Disorders, 21*(1), 40–43.

Marin, D. B., Flynn, S., Mare, M., Lantz, M., Hsu, M. A., Laurans, M., . . . Mohs, R. C. (2001). Reliability and validity of a chronic care facility adaptation of the Clinical Dementia Rating scale. *International Journal of Geriatric Psychiatry, 16*(8), 745–750.

McCulla, M. M., Coats, M., Van Fleet, N., Duchek, J., Grant, E., & Morris, J. C. (1989). Reliability of clinical nurse specialists in the staging of dementia. *Archives of Neurology, 46*(11), 1210–1211.

Meguro, K., Shimada, M., & Yamaguchi, S. (2005). Neuropsychosocial Features of Very Mild Alzheimer's Disease (CDR 0.5) and Progression to Dementia in a Community: The Tajiri Project. *Journal of Geriatric Psychiatry and Neurology, 14*(1), 139–145.

Miller, T. M., Balsis, S., Lowe, D. A., Benge, J. F., & Doody, R. S. (2011). Item Response Theory reveals variability of functional impairment within Clinical Dementia Rating scale stages. *Dementia and Geriatric Cognitive Disorders, 32*(5), 362–366.

O'Bryant, S. E., Lacritz, L. H., Hall, J., Waring, S. C., Chan, W., Khodr, Z. G., . . . Cullum, C. M. (2010). Validation of the new interpretive guidelines for the Clinical Dementia Rating scale Sum of Boxes score in the National Alzheimer's Coordinating Center database. *Archives of Neurology, 67*(6), 746–749.

Oremus, M., Perrault, A., Demers, L., & Wolfson, C. (2000). Review of outcome measurement instruments in Alzheimer's disease drug trials: Psychometric properties of global scales. *Journal of Geriatric Psychiatry and Neurology, 13*(4), 197–205.

Perneczky, R., Hartmann, J., Grimmer, T., Drzezga, A., & Kurz, A. (2007). Cerebral metabolic correlates of the Clinical Dementia Rating scale in mild cognitive impairment. *Journal of Geriatric Psychiatry and Neurology, 20*(2), 84–88.

Petersen, R. C., Thomas, R. G., Grundman, M., Bennett, D., Doody, R., Ferris, S., . . . Pfeiffer, E. (2005). Vitamin E and donepezil for the treatment of mild cognitive impairment. *New England Journal of Medicine, 352*(23), 2379–2388.

Reisberg, B. (2007). Global measures: Utility in defining and measuring treatment response in dementia. *International Psychogeriatrics, 19*(03), 421–456.

Rikkert, O. M. G., Tona, K. D., Janssen, L., Burns, A., Lobo, A., Robert, P., . . . Waldemar, G. (2011). Validity, reliability, and feasibility of clinical staging scales in dementia: A systematic review. *American Journal of Alzheimer's Disease & Other Dementias®, 26*(5), 357–365.

Russo, G., Russo, M. J., Buyatti, D., Chrem, P., Bagnati, P., Suarez, M. F., . . . Knopman, D. S. (2014). Utility of the Spanish version of the FTLD-modified CDR in the diagnosis and staging in frontotemporal lobar degeneration. *Journal of the Neurological Sciences, 344*(1–2), 63–68.

Saito, Y., & Murayama, S. (2007). Neuropathology of mild cognitive impairment. *Neuropathology, 27*(6), 578–584.

Schafer, K. A., Tractenberg, R. E., Sano, M., Mackell, J. A., Thomas, R. G., Gamst, A., . . . Morris, J. C. (2004). Reliability of monitoring the Clinical Dementia Rating in multicenter clinical trials. *Alzheimer Disease and Associated Disorders, 18*(4), 219.

Senanarong, V., Chen, C. P., Orgogozo, J. M., & Program Committee. (2006). Third Asia-Pacific Regional Meeting of the International Working Group on Harmonization of Dementia Drug Guidelines: Meeting report summary. *Alzheimer Disease & Associated Disorders, 20*(4), 311–312.

Tractenberg, R. E., Schafer, K., & Morris, J. C. (2001). Interobserver disagreements on Clinical Dementia Rating assessment: Interpretation and implications for training. *Alzheimer Disease & Associated Disorders, 15*(3), 155–161.

Webber, D., Collins, M., DeFilippis, N., & Hill, F. (2013). Reliability of the Clinical Dementia Rating with a traumatic brain injury population: A preliminary study. *Applied Neuropsychology: Adult, 20*(2), 145–151.

Williams, M. M., Roe, C. M., & Morris, J. C. (2009). Stability of the Clinical Dementia Rating, 1979–2007. *Archives of Neurology, 66*(6), 773–777.

Williams, M. M., Storandt, M., Roe, C. M., & Morris, J. C. (2013). Progression of Alzheimer's disease as measured by Clinical Dementia Rating Sum of Boxes scores. *Alzheimer's & Dementia, 9*(1), S39–S44.

Xiang, Z., Haroutunian, V., Ho, L., Purohit, D., & Pasinetti, G. M. (2006). Microglia activation in the brain as inflammatory biomarker of Alzheimer's disease neuropathology and clinical dementia. *Disease Markers, 22*(1–2), 95–102.

DEMENTIA RATING SCALE-2 (DRS-2)

TEST NAME	**Dementia Rating Scale-2 (DRS-2)**
DOMAIN	Dementia screening
AGE RANGE	56 to 105 years
ADMINISTRATION TIME	10 to 15 minutes for healthy older adults; may take 30 to 45 minutes with examinees with dementia
SCORING FORMAT	Hand scored
REFERENCE	Jurica, P. J., Leitten, C. L., & Mattis, S. (2004). *DRS-2 Dementia Rating Scale-2: Professional manual.* Psychological Assessment Resources. www.parinc.com

DESCRIPTION

The purpose of the Dementia Rating Scale (DRS) is to provide an index of cognitive function in people with known or suspected dementia. It was specifically developed to quantify the mental status of patients with profound cognitive impairments who may not generate enough responses to assess the magnitude of their mental impairments (Mattis, 1976, 1988). The Dementia Rating Scale-2 (DRS-2; Jurica et al., 2004) is the same test but with an updated manual, improved scoring booklet, and new norms. In addition, an alternate form (DRS-2: Alternate Form), consisting of new item content, has been provided (Schmidt & Mattis, 2004).

The items on the test are similar to those employed by neurologists in bedside mental status examinations. They are arranged hierarchically, from difficult to easier items, so that adequate performance on an initial item allows the examiner to discontinue testing within that section and to assume that credit can be given for adequate performance on the subsequent tasks. A global measure of dementia severity is derived from subscales of specific cognitive capacities. See Table 7–6 for the composition of each subscale.

ADMINISTRATION

See Source. The DRS-2 subtests are presented in a fixed order generally corresponding to the Attention (ATT), Initiation/Perseveration (I/P), Construction (CONST), Conceptualization (CONCEPT), and Memory (MEM) subscales; however, not all Attention tasks are presented in a sequence because some also serve as time-filling distracters between presentations of memory tasks. Generally, if the first one or two tasks in a subscale are performed well, subsequent (easier) tasks are credited with a correct performance, and the examiner proceeds to the next subscale.

The item "name items examiner is wearing" may cause discomfort for some people (Dean et al., 2013). To evaluate the effect of skipping this item, the authors re-examined some data that included this item by giving full credit for this item to all patients. The majority (97%) of dementia-severity ratings did not change despite the adjustment, suggesting that this item may be skipped without endangering the psychometric properties of the measure.

TABLE 7–6 Subscales and Subtests of the Dementia Rating Scale-2 (DRS-2)

SUBSCALE	SUBTESTS	MAXIMUM POINTS
Attention	Digit Span Two Successive Commands Single Command Imitation Counting Distraction 1 and 2 Verbal Recognition–Presentation Visual Matching	37
Initiation/ Perseveration	Complex Verbal Initiation/ Perseveration Consonant Perseveration Vowel Perseveration Double Alternating Movements Alternate Tapping Graphomotor Design	37
Construction	Construction Designs	6
Conceptualization	Identities and Oddities Similarities Priming Inductive Reasoning Differences Similarities–Multiple Choice	39
Memory	Orientation Verbal Recall–Reading Verbal Recall–Sentence Initiation Verbal Recognition Visual Recognition	25

SOURCE: Adapted from Jurica et al. (2004). Reproduced by special permission of the Publisher, Psychological Assessment Resources, Inc. (PAR), 16204 North Florida Avenue, Lutz, Florida 33549, from the Dementia Rating Scale-2 by Steven Mattis, PhD, Copyright 1973, 1988, 2001 by PAR. Further reproduction is prohibited without permission from PAR.

SCORING

See Source. One point is given for each item performed correctly. Maximum score is 144.

If a patient has been given a different mental status test (e.g., MMSE), one can translate the score on the test into scale-free units such as a *z* score or percentile score, or one can use a conversion formula. Equations have been developed to convert Total scores from one test to the other (Bobholz & Brandt, 1993; Meiran et al., 1996; Salmon et al., 1990), but given the mixed results in the literature (see the section "Evidence for Validity"), these should be used with caution. The equations are shown in Table 7–7. The formulas should be applied to similar patients.

DEMOGRAPHIC EFFECTS

AGE

Age affects performance, with younger adults obtaining higher scores than older ones (e.g., Bank et al., 2000; Foss et al., 2013; Katsarou et al., 2010; Lavoie et al., 2013; Lucas et al., 1998; Rilling et al., 2005; Smith et al., 1994; Strutt et al., 2012).

GENDER

Gender has little impact on test scores (Bank et al., 2000; Chan et al., 2001; Katsarou et al., 2010; Lavoie et al., 2013; Lucas et al., 1998; Monsch et al., 1995; Rilling et al., 2005; Schmidt et al., 1994; Strutt et al., 2012). One study noted that gender is only correlated with performance on the Attention subscale (Foss et al., 2013).

EDUCATION AND IQ

Numerous authors have reported that performance varies not only by age, but also by education and IQ (Bank et al., 2000; Chan et al., 2001, 2003; Foss et al., 2013; Freidl et al., 1996, 1997; Kantarci et al., 2002; Katsarou et al., 2010; Lavoie et al., 2013; Lucas et al., 1998; Marcopulos & McLain, 2003; Marcopulos et al., 1997; Monsch et al., 1995; Rilling et al., 2005; Schmidt et al., 1994; Smith et al., 1994; Strutt et al., 2012). Accordingly, normative data broken down by age and education are preferred.

TABLE 7–7 Conversion Formulas to Derive Dementia Rating Scale-2 (DRS-2) Scores from the Mini-Mental State Examination (MMSE)

TEST	FORMULA	REFERENCE
DRS	41.53 + 3.26 (MMSE)	Salmon et al. (1990) Based on a sample of 92 patients with probable AD
DRS	33.86 + 3.39 (MMSE)	Bobholz and Brandt (1993) Based on a sample of 50 patients with suspected cognitive impairment
DRS	45.5 + 3.01 (MMSE)	Meiran et al. (1996) Based on a sample of 466 patients in a memory disorders clinic; the expected error associated with this formula is ±11.1

ETHNICITY, NATIONALITY, AND LINGUISTIC EFFECTS

African Americans tend to obtain lower scores than Caucasians (Rilling et al., 2005), suggesting the need for ethnicity-specific norms. Cultural factors also appear to have an impact (see "Evidence for Validity"). For example, healthy Spanish speakers living in the United States perform significantly worse than English speakers on the Total score and on the Attention, Conceptualization, and Memory subscales, particularly on Counting Distraction 1, Identities and Oddities, and Verbal Recall–Reading and Verbal Recognition (Lyness et al., 2006; Strutt et al., 2012). The largest difference is seen on the Memory subscale, where more than half of English speakers have perfect scores compared to almost no Spanish speakers (Strutt et al., 2012). When performance on the translated version is compared to the original norms, about a third of the sample is misclassified.

Years of residence in the United States are not associated with DRS performance (Lyness et al., 2006), though level of acculturation is, particularly on the Attention and Initiation/Perseveration subscales (Strutt et al., 2012). No differences are seen between Spanish-English bilinguals and monolinguals except on the Memory subscales, where bilinguals score higher than monolinguals (Lyness et al., 2006). Given the discrepancy in scores among Spanish and English speakers, norms from English speakers should not be applied to Spanish speakers (see "Clinical Studies" for further discussion).

Attempts to develop other language versions of the DRS have met with varying success, perhaps because of cultural bias inherent in the subscales or individual subscale items. For example, Hohl et al. (1999) found that Hispanic AD patients performed significantly worse than non-Hispanics in terms of DRS Total score (on a translated version), despite being matched by MMSE score. This difference was accounted for primarily by poorer performance of the Hispanic patients, relative to the non-Hispanic patients, on the Memory and Conceptualization subtests. A Chinese version (Chan et al., 2001, 2003) has also been developed that shows similar sensitivity and specificity as the English version. Comparison of age- and education-matched groups in Hong Kong and San Diego revealed differences in the pattern of subtest performance, even though groups did not differ in DRS Total scores. Individuals in Hong Kong scored significantly higher than the San Diego participants on the Construction scale, whereas the opposite pattern was observed on the Initiation/Perseveration and Memory subscales.

Woodard et al. (1998) investigated possible racial bias in the test by comparing 40 pairs of African-American and Caucasian dementia patients matched for age, years of education, and gender. Principal component analysis revealed similar patterns and magnitudes across component loadings for each racial group, suggesting no evidence of test bias. In addition, they identified only four of the 36 items of the DRS that showed differential item functioning: "palm up/palm down, fist clenched/fist extended, point out and count the As, and visual recognition." The implication is that the DRS may be used in both African-American and Caucasian populations to assess dementia severity. Another study (Teresi et al., 2000) found that most items of the Attention subscale of the DRS performed in an education-fair manner. Strutt et al. (2012) reported that once three items were omitted (current president, governor, and mayor), the rate of perfect scores became comparable between their groups of healthy English- and Spanish-speaking older adults living in the United States.

NORMATIVE DATA

Mattis (1976; cited in Montgomery, 1982) initially recommended a cutoff score of 137 for identifying impairment. However, this cutoff is of limited value since the sample sizes on which the score is based (Coblentz et al., 1973) were extremely small (i.e., 20 brain-damaged patients, 11 healthy individuals). Different cutoff scores (e.g., DRS <123) have been provided by others (e.g., Montgomery, 1982). However, the clinical utility of these scores is also limited because sample sizes were small and the participants were relatively well educated (see Table 7–32 for additional information about cutoff scores). Because studies have demonstrated significant relationships among age, education, and DRS performance (see previous discussion as well as DRS-2 Manual), simple cutoff scores are considered inappropriate. Some studies have provided data stratified by both age and education.

Lucas et al. (1998; see also DRS-2 Manual) presented norms for 623 community-dwelling adults over the age of 55 years (age, $M = 79.2$ years, $SD = 7.6$). The participants were predominantly Caucasian with a relatively high level of education ($M = 13.1$ years, $SD = 7.6$) and were reported by their physician to have no active medical disorder with potential to affect cognition. These data were collected as part of Mayo's Older Americans Normative Studies (MOANS) and afford the clinician the advantage of being able to compare DRS scores to scores on other tests with MOANS norms (e.g., Rey Auditory Verbal Learning Test [RAVLT]; Lucas et al., 1998). Please refer to Lucas et al. (1998) for information about the MOANS normative characteristics. The DRS data are shown in Tables 7–8 through 7–16. Age-corrected MOANS scaled scores ($M = 10$, $SD = 3$) are presented in the left-hand column of the table while corresponding percentile ranks are given in the right-hand column. To further adjust for the effects of education, a standard linear regression was used to derive age- and education-corrected MOANS Total scaled scores. This formula is presented in Table 7–17. Efforts to provide adjustment for education at the subtest level resulted in scaling problems due to the highly skewed nature of some subtests. Therefore, education corrections are applied only to the Total score. Note, however, that the underrepresentation of participants with limited educational backgrounds (i.e., <8 years) cautions against the application of this formula in such individuals.

TABLE 7–8 Dementia Rating Scale-2 (DRS-2) Mayo's Older Americans Normative Studies (MOANS) Scaled Scores for Persons Under Age 69 Years

	DEMENTIA RATING SCALE SUBTESTS						
SCALED SCORES	ATTENTION	INITIATION/ PERSEVERATION	CONSTRUCTION	CONCEPTUALIZATION	MEMORY	TOTAL	PERCENTILE RANGES
2	<27	<24	0–2	<25	<17	<115	<1
3	27–28	24–26	3	25–26	17	115–119	1
4	29–30	27–28	–	27	18–19	120–121	2
5	31	29–30	4	28–29	20	122–127	3–5
6	32	31–33	–	30–32	21	128–130	6–10
7	33	34	5	33	22	131–132	11–18
8	34	35	–	34–35	–	133–134	19–28
9	–	–	–	36	23	135–136	29–40
10	35	36	6	37	24	137–139	41–59
11	36	37	–	38	–	140	60–71
12	–	–	–	39	–	141	72–81
13	37	–	–	–	25	142	82–89
14	–	–	–	–	–	143	90–94
15	–	–	–	–	–	144	95–97
16	–	–	–	–	–	–	98
17	–	–	–	–	–	–	99
18	–	–	–	–	–	–	>99

SOURCE: From Lucas et al. (1998).

TABLE 7–9 Dementia Rating Scale-2 (DRS-2) Mayo's Older Americans Normative Studies (MOANS) Scaled Scores for Persons Aged 69 to 71 Years

SCALED SCORES	DEMENTIA RATING SCALE SUBTESTS: ATTENTION	INITIATION/ PERSEVERATION	CONSTRUCTION	CONCEPTUALIZATION	MEMORY	TOTAL	PERCENTILE RANGES
2	<27	<24	0–2	<25	<17	<110	<1
3	27–28	24–26	3	25–26	17	110–119	1
4	29–30	27–28	–	27	18–19	120–121	2
5	31	29–30	4	28–29	20	122–126	3–5
6	32	31–32	–	30–31	21	127–129	6–10
7	33	33–34	5	32–33	22	130–132	11–18
8	34	35	–	34	–	133–134	19–28
9	–	–	–	35	23	135–136	29–40
10	35	36	6	36–37	24	137–139	41–59
11	36	37	–	38	–	140	60–71
12	–	–	–	–	–	141	72–81
13	37	–	–	39	25	142	82–89
14	–	–	–	–	–	143	90–94
15	–	–	–	–	–	144	95–97
16	–	–	–	–	–	–	98
17	–	–	–	–	–	–	99
18	–	–	–	–	–	–	>99

SOURCE: From Lucas et al. (1998).

Although the MOANS (Lucas et al., 1998) data represent a very important contribution to the normative base, the sample consists largely of Caucasian adults living in economically stable regions of the United States. As a result, the norms will likely overestimate cognitive impairment in those with limited education and different cultural or health-related experiences (Bank et al., 2000; Yochim et al., 2003). A number of authors (Bank et al., 2000; Vangel & Lichtenberg, 1995) have attempted to address the issue by increasing African-American representation in the normative samples. Rilling et al. (2005) provide age- and education-adjusted normative data based on 307 African-American community-dwelling participants from the Mayo's Older African Americans Normative Studies (MOAANS) project in Jacksonville, Florida. Participants were predominantly female (75%), ranged in age from 56 to 94 years ($M = 69.6$ years, $SD = 6.87$), and varied in education from 0 to 20 years of formal education ($M = 12.2$ years, $SD = 3.48$). They were screened to exclude those with active neurological, psychiatric, or other conditions that might

TABLE 7–10 Dementia Rating Scale-2 (DRS-2) Mayo's Older Americans Normative Studies (MOANS) Scaled Scores for Persons Aged 72 to 74 Years

SCALED SCORES	DEMENTIA RATING SCALE SUBTESTS: ATTENTION	INITIATION/ PERSEVERATION	CONSTRUCTION	CONCEPTUALIZATION	MEMORY	TOTAL	PERCENTILE RANGES
2	<27	<24	0–2	<25	<17	<110	<1
3	27–28	24–26	3	25–26	17	110–119	1
4	29	27–28	–	27	18–19	120–121	2
5	30	29–30	4	28–29	20	122–126	3–5
6	31	31	–	30–31	21	127–129	6–10
7	32	32–33	5	32–33	–	130–131	11–18
8	33–34	34–35	–	34	22	132–133	19–28
9	–	–	–	35	–	134–135	29–40
10	35	36	6	36–37	23–24	136–138	41–59
11	36	–	–	38	–	139	60–71
12	–	37	–	–	–	140–141	72–81
13	37	–	–	39	25	142	82–89
14	–	–	–	–	–	–	90–94
15	–	–	–	–	–	143–144	95–97
16	–	–	–	–	–	–	98
17	–	–	–	–	–	–	99
18	–	–	–	–	–	–	>99

SOURCE: From Lucas et al. (1998).

TABLE 7–11 Dementia Rating Scale-2 (DRS-2) Mayo's Older Americans Normative Studies (MOANS) Scaled Scores for Persons Aged 75 to 77 Years

	DEMENTIA RATING SCALE SUBTESTS						
SCALED SCORES	ATTENTION	INITIATION/ PERSEVERATION	CONSTRUCTION	CONCEPTUALIZATION	MEMORY	TOTAL	PERCENTILE RANGES
2	<27	<24	0–2	<23	<17	<109	<1
3	27–28	24–26	3	23–26	17	109–119	1
4	29	27–28	–	27	18	120–121	2
5	30	29–30	4	28–29	19–20	122–125	3–5
6	31	31	–	30–31	–	126–128	6–10
7	32	32–33	5	32	21	129–130	11–18
8	33–34	34	–	33–34	22	131–132	19–28
9	–	35	–	35		133–134	29–40
10	35	36	6	36–37	23	135–137	41–59
11	–	–	–	–	24	138–139	60–71
12	36	37	–	38	–	140	72–81
13	37	–	–	39	25	141–142	82–89
14	–	–	–	–	–	–	90–94
15	–	–	–	–	–	143	95–97
16	–	–	–	–	–	144	98
17	–	–	–	–	–	–	99
18	–	–	–	–	–	–	>99

SOURCE: From Lucas et al. (1998).

affect cognition. Age-corrected MOAANS scaled scores and percentile ranks for the DRS-2 Total and subtest scores are presented in Tables 7–18 through 7–24. The computational formula to calculate age- and education-corrected MOAANS scaled scores ($MSS_{A\&E}$) for the DRS Total score is shown in Table 7–25.

The MOAANS normative data are similar to normative estimates provided by others (Bank et al., 2000; Marcopulos & McLain, 2003), based on mixed-ethnic samples with significant proportions of older African-American participants. Of note, norms for the DRS were developed in conjunction with norms for other tests (e.g., BNT, RAVLT, Judgment of Line Orientation [JLO], verbal fluency, Multilingual Aphasia Examination [MAE] Token Test; see descriptions elsewhere in this volume), allowing the clinician to compare an individual's performance across tasks included in the MOANS/MOAANS battery.

Foss et al. (2013) present normative data from 502 healthy Brazilians from Caete, Riberao, and Sao Paulo, aged 50 years and older (62% females; mean age = 71.00,

TABLE 7–12 Dementia Rating Scale-2 (DRS-2) Mayo's Older Americans Normative Studies (MOANS) Scaled Scores for Persons Aged 78 to 80 Years

	DEMENTIA RATING SCALE SUBTESTS						
SCALED SCORES	ATTENTION	INITIATION/ PERSEVERATION	CONSTRUCTION	CONCEPTUALIZATION	MEMORY	TOTAL	PERCENTILE RANGES
2	<26	<24	0–2	<19	<17	<108	<1
3	26–28	24–26	3	19–25	17	108–115	1
4	29	27–28	–	26	18	116–119	2
5	30	29–30	4	27–28	19–20	120–122	3–5
6	31	31	–	29–30	–	123–126	6–10
7	32	32	5	31–32	21	127–129	11–18
8	33	33–34	–	33–34	22	130–131	19–28
9	34	–	–	35	–	132–134	29–40
10	35	35–36	6	36	23	135–136	41–59
11	–	–	–	37	24	137–138	60–71
12	36	37	–	38	–	139–140	72–81
13	–	–	–	–	25	141	82–89
14	37	–	–	39	–	142	90–94
15	–	–	–	–	–	143	95–97
16	–	–	–	–	–	144	98
17	–	–	–	–	–	–	99
18	–	–	–	–	–	–	>99

SOURCE: From Lucas et al. (1998).

TABLE 7–13 Dementia Rating Scale-2 (DRS-2) Mayo's Older Americans Normative Studies (MOANS) Scaled Scores for Persons Aged 81 to 83 Years

	DEMENTIA RATING SCALE SUBTESTS						
SCALED SCORES	ATTENTION	INITIATION/ PERSEVERATION	CONSTRUCTION	CONCEPTUALIZATION	MEMORY	TOTAL	PERCENTILE RANGES
2	<26	<24	0–2	<19	<16	<108	<1
3	26–28	24–25	3	19–24	16	108–114	1
4	29	26–27	–	25	17–18	115–117	2
5	30	28–29	4	26–27	19	118–121	3–5
6	31	30	–	28–30	20	122–126	6–10
7	32	31–32	5	31–32	21	127–128	11–18
8	33	33–34	–	33	22	129–130	19–28
9	34	–	–	34	–	131–133	29–40
10	35	35	6	35–36	23	134–136	41–59
11	–	36	–	37	–	137	60–71
12	36	–	–	38	24	138–139	72–81
13	–	37	–	–	–	140–141	82–89
14	37	–	–	39	25	–	90–94
15	–	–	–	–	–	142	95–97
16	–	–	–	–	–	143	98
17	–	–	–	–	–	144	99
18	–	–	–	–	–	–	>99

SOURCE: From Lucas et al. (1998).

SD = 8.70; mean education = 8.00, *SD* = 5.28). A strength of the norms is the inclusion of a wide range of education levels from illiterates (i.e., 0 year of education) to 13+ years. Examinees' DRS-2 Total and subscale raw scores can be converted to percentiles as a function age and education levels. Please refer to original paper for details.

Katsarou et al. (2010) provide norms for a Greek translation of the DRS-2 (DRS-GR). Norms are presented in Table 7–26.

Lavoie et al. (2013) provide normative data for 432 French-Canadian older adults (mostly from Quebec City, Montreal, and Sherbrooke) using the French version of the DRS-2. Several items were modified for the local Quebec context. The items "supermarket" were replaced with "grocery store," "who is the president?" with "who is the prime minister of Canada?," and "who is the prime minister" with "who is the premier of Quebec?" Percentile ranks are presented in Tables 7–27 to 7–31 as a function of age and education. The authors suggested the

TABLE 7–14 Dementia Rating Scale-2 (DRS-2) Mayo's Older Americans Normative Studies (MOANS) Scaled Scores for Persons Aged 84 to 86 Years

	DEMENTIA RATING SCALE SUBTESTS						
SCALED SCORES	ATTENTION	INITIATION/ PERSEVERATION	CONSTRUCTION	CONCEPTUALIZATION	MEMORY	TOTAL	PERCENTILE RANGES
2	<26	<24	0–2	<19	<15	<107	<1
3	26–28	24–25	3	19–23	15	107–112	1
4	29	26	–	24	16	113	2
5	30	27–28	4	25–26	17–19	114–120	3–5
6	31	29–30	–	27–29	20	121–124	6–10
7	32	31	–	30–31	–	125–127	11–18
8	33	32–33	5	32–33	21	128–129	19–28
9	–	34	–	34	22	130–132	29–40
10	34–35	35	6	35–36	23	133–135	41–59
11	–	36	–	37	–	136–137	60–71
12	36	–	–	38	24	138	72–81
13	–	37	–	–	–	139–140	82–89
14	37	–	–	39	25	141	90–94
15	–	–	–	–	–	142	95–97
16	–	–	–	–	–	–	98
17	–	–	–	–	–	143–144	99
18	–	–	–	–	–	–	>99

SOURCE: From Lucas et al. (1998).

TABLE 7–15 Dementia Rating Scale-2 (DRS-2) Mayo's Older Americans Normative Studies (MOANS) Scaled Scores for Persons Aged 87 to 89 Years

	DEMENTIA RATING SCALE SUBTESTS						
SCALED SCORES	ATTENTION	INITIATION/ PERSEVERATION	CONSTRUCTION	CONCEPTUALIZATION	MEMORY	TOTAL	PERCENTILE RANGES
2	<26	<19	0–1	<19	<14	<104	<1
3	26–28	19–21	2	19–22	14–15	104–109	1
4	29	22–23	3	23–24	–	110–112	2
5	30	24–26	–	25–26	16	113–115	3–5
6	31	27–29	4	27–28	17–19	116–122	6–10
7	32	30–31	–	29–30	20	123–126	11–18
8	–	32–33	5	31–32	21	127–129	19–28
9	33	34	–	33–34	22	130–131	29–40
10	34–35	35	6	35–36	23	132–134	41–59
11	–	36	–	37	–	135–136	60–71
12	36	–	–	–	24	137–138	72–81
13	–	37	–	38	–	139	82–89
14	37	–	–	39	25	140–141	90–94
15	–	–	–	–	–	142	95–97
16	–	–	–	–	–	–	98
17	–	–	–	–	–	143	99
18	–	–	–	–	–	144	>99

SOURCE: From Lucas et al. (1998).

following interpretations of cognitive impairment for the percentiles: ≤5 = significant; 10 = mild; 15 = borderline; 50 = median of the population.

EVIDENCE FOR RELIABILITY

EVIDENCE FOR INTERNAL RELIABILITY

High internal consistencies have been reported in a sample of nursing home patients with neurological disorders for the DRS-2 (split-half r = .90; Gardner et al., 1981) and for the Greek version (Cronbach's alpha = .82; Katsarou et al., 2010). In a small sample of individuals with probable AD, alpha coefficients were adequate to high for the subscales of Attention (.95), Initiation/Perseveration (.87), Conceptualization (.95), and Memory (.75; Vitaliano et al., 1984). Smith et al. (1994) found mixed support for the reliability of DRS scales in a sample of 274 older patients with cognitive impairment. Internal consistency (Cronbach's alpha) was greater than .70 for Construction, Conceptualization, Memory, and Total

TABLE 7–16 Dementia Rating Scale-2 (DRS-2) Mayo's Older Americans Normative Studies (MOANS) Scaled Scores for Persons Over Age 89 Years

	DEMENTIA RATING SCALE SUBTESTS						
SCALED SCORES	ATTENTION	INITIATION/ PERSEVERATION	CONSTRUCTION	CONCEPTUALIZATION	MEMORY	TOTAL	PERCENTILE RANGES
2	<26	<19	0–1	<19	<14	<104	<1
3	26–28	19–20	2	19–21	14	104–108	1
4	29	21	3	22	15	109–112	2
5	30	22–25	–	23–25	16	113–114	3–5
6	31	26–27	4	26–27	17	115–118	6–10
7	32	28–29	–	28–30	18–19	119–123	11–18
8	–	30–32	5	31	20	124–126	19–28
9	33	33	–	32–33	21	127–129	29–40
10	34–35	34	6	34–36	22	130–133	41–59
11	–	35	–	37	23	134–135	60–71
12	36	36	–	–	–	136–137	72–81
13	–	–	–	38	24	138–139	82–89
14	37	37	–	–	–	140–141	90–94
15	–	–	–	39	25	142	95–97
16	–	–	–	–	–	–	98
17	–	–	–	–	–	143	99
18	–	–	–	–	–	144	>99

SOURCE: From Lucas et al. (1998).

TABLE 7–17 Regression Formula for Age- and Education-Corrected Mayo's Older Americans Normative Studies (MOANS) Scaled Scores for Dementia Rating Scale-2 (DRS-2) Total

Age- and education-corrected MOANS scaled scores (AEMSS) can be calculated for DRS-2 Total scores by using age-corrected MOANS scaled scores (AMSS) and education (expressed in years completed) in the following formula:

AEMSS = 2.56 + (1.11 × AMSS) – (0.30 × EDUC).

SOURCE: From Lucas et al. (1998).

score; greater than .65 for Attention; and only about .45 for Initiation/Perseveration. Interpretation of the Initiation/Perseveration subscale as measuring a single construct is, therefore, hazardous.

EVIDENCE FOR TEST-RETEST RELIABILITY, MEASURING CHANGE, AND PRACTICE EFFECTS

Smith et al. (1994) retested a sample of 154 healthy older individuals following an interval of about one year and found that DRS Total score declines of 10 points or greater occurred in less than 5% of healthy individuals. Not surprisingly, over this comparable interval, 61% of 110 dementia patients displayed a decline in DRS Total scores of 10 or more points.

In a sample of nondemented PD patients, three-week test-retest reliability of the Greek version was very high (Intraclass Correlation Coefficient [ICC] = .97) for Total score and marginal to adequate for all subscales (range = .61 to .75) except Construction, which was modest (Katsarou et al., 2010).

EVIDENCE FOR RELIABILITY OF ALTERNATE FORMS

The alternate form developed by Schmidt and Mattis (DRS-2: Alternate Form; 2004) shows high alternate-form reliability in community-dwelling older adults (r = .82 for the Total score and r = .66 to .80 for the subscales). In addition, no significant differences are found between Total and subscale scores of the two forms (Schmidt et al., 2005).

EVIDENCE FOR INTERRATER RELIABILITY

Not reported.

EVIDENCE FOR VALIDITY

FACTOR-ANALYTIC STUDIES

Factor-analytic studies suggest that the five subscales do not reflect exclusively the constructs with which they are labeled (Colantonio et al., 1993; Kessler et al., 1994; Woodard et al., 1996). For example, a two-factor model specifying separate verbal and nonverbal functions was obtained in a heterogeneous sample comprising primarily psychiatric (depression) or dementia (AD-type) diagnoses (Kessler et al., 1994), and in a sample of individuals with intellectual disability of moderate to severe degree (Das et al., 1995). In patients with probable AD, three factors labeled as Conceptualization/Organization, Visuospatial, and Memory have been reported (Colantonio et al., 1993; Woodard et al., 1996). Moderate correlations are found between these factors and supplementary neuropsychological measures, supporting the validity of these factors. On the other hand, Hofer et al. (1996) found

TABLE 7–18 Dementia Rating Scale-2 (DRS-2) Mayo's Older African Americans Normative Studies (MOAANS) Scaled Scores for Persons Aged 56 to 62 Years (Midpoint Age = 61, Age Range for Norms = 56 to 66, N = 108)

	DEMENTIA RATING SCALE SUBTESTS						
SCALED SCORES	ATTENTION	INITIATION/ PERSEVERATION	CONSTRUCTION	CONCEPTUALIZATION	MEMORY	TOTAL	PERCENTILE RANGES
2	0–23	0–27	0–1	0–23	0–15	0–110	<1
3	24–29	28–29	2	24–25	16–17	111–115	1
4	–	30	–	26	18	116	2
5	30	31	–	27–28	–	117–121	3–5
6	31	32	3	29	19–20	122–123	6–10
7	32	33–34	–	30–31	21	124–126	11–18
8	33	35	4	32	22	127–129	19–28
9	34	36	5	33–34	23	130–132	29–40
10	35	–	–	35	24	133–135	41–59
11	36	–	–	36	–	136–137	60–71
12	–	37	6	37	25	138	72–81
13	–	–	–	38	–	139–141	82–89
14	37	–	–	–	–	142	90–94
15	–	–	–	39	–	143	95–97
16	–	–	–	–	–	–	98
17	–	–	–	–	–	144	99
18	–	–	–	–	–	–	>99

SOURCE: From Rilling et al. (2005).

TABLE 7–19 Dementia Rating Scale-2 (DRS-2) Mayo's Older African Americans Normative Studies (MOAANS) Scaled Scores for Persons Aged 63 to 65 Years (Midpoint Age = 64, Age Range for Norms = 59 to 69, *N* = 130)

	DEMENTIA RATING SCALE SUBTESTS						
SCALED SCORES	ATTENTION	INITIATION/ PERSEVERATION	CONSTRUCTION	CONCEPTUALIZATION	MEMORY	TOTAL	PERCENTILE RANGES
2	0–23	0–27	0–1	0–21	0–15	0–102	<1
3	24–27	28–29	2	22–23	16–17	103–107	1
4	28–29	30	–	24	–	108–114	2
5	–	31	–	25–27	18	115–118	3–5
6	30–31	32	3	28–29	19	119–122	6–10
7	32	33–34	–	30	20	123–125	11–18
8	33	35	4	31–32	21–22	126–129	19–28
9	34	36	5	33	23	130–131	29–40
10	35	–	–	34–35	–	132–134	41–59
11	–	–	–	36	24	135–136	60–71
12	36	37	6	–	–	137–138	72–81
13	–	–	–	37–38	25	139–140	82–89
14	37	–	–	–	–	141	90–94
15	–	–	–	39	–	142–143	95–97
16	–	–	–	–	–	–	98
17	–	–	–	–	–	144	99
18	–	–	–	–	–	–	>99

SOURCE: From Rilling et al. (2005).

five factors, which they labeled Long-term Memory (Recall)/Verbal Fluency, Construction, Memory (Short-term), Initiation/Perseveration, and Simple Commands in patients with dementia and older healthy controls grouped together. The contrasting results (Hofer et al., 1996; Kessler et al., 1994 vs. Colantonio et al., 1993; Woodard et al., 1996) highlight the fact that the resulting factor structure depends critically on the characteristics of the population studied, including the severity of their impairment.

RELATIONSHIPS WITH OTHER TESTS

The test correlates well with the Wechsler Memory Scale (WMS) Memory Quotient (r = .70), the Wechsler Adult Intelligence Scale (WAIS) Full Scale IQ (FSIQ; r = .67), and composite scores derived from standard neuropsychological tests (Knox et al., 2003), supporting its use as a global assessment measure. Smith et al. (1994) found that in older adults who were cognitively impaired, DRS Total score shared 54% of its variance with FSIQ and 57% with Verbal IQ (VIQ). In individuals with mental deficiency,

TABLE 7–20 Dementia Rating Scale-2 (DRS-2) Mayo's Older African Americans Normative Studies (MOAANS) Scaled Scores for Persons Aged 66 to 68 Years (Midpoint Age = 67, Age Range for Norms = 62 to 72, *N* = 167)

	DEMENTIA RATING SCALE SUBTESTS						
SCALED SCORES	ATTENTION	INITIATION/ PERSEVERATION	CONSTRUCTION	CONCEPTUALIZATION	MEMORY	TOTAL	PERCENTILE RANGES
2	0–23	0–27	0–1	0–21	0–15	0–102	<1
3	24–27	28	2	22–23	16	103–107	1
4	28–29	29	–	24	17	108–113	2
5	–	30	–	25–26	18	114–117	3–5
6	30–31	31–32	3	27–28	19	118–121	6–10
7	32	33–34	–	29	20	122–125	11–18
8	33	35	4	30–31	21	126–128	19–28
9	34	36	–	32–33	22	129–130	29–40
10	35	–	5	34–35	23	131–133	41–59
11	–	–	–	–	24	134–135	60–71
12	36	37	6	36	–	136–137	72–81
13	–	–	–	37	25	138–139	82–89
14	37	–	–	38	–	140	90–94
15	–	–	–	39	–	141–142	95–97
16	–	–	–	–	–	143	98
17	–	–	–	–	–	144	99
18	–	–	–	–	–	–	>99

SOURCE: From Rilling et al. (2005).

TABLE 7-21 Dementia Rating Scale-2 (DRS-2) Mayo's Older African Americans Normative Studies (MOAANS) Scaled Scores for Persons Aged 69 to 71 Years (Midpoint Age = 70, Age Range for Norms = 65 to 75, N = 182)

	DEMENTIA RATING SCALE SUBTESTS						
SCALED SCORES	ATTENTION	INITIATION/ PERSEVERATION	CONSTRUCTION	CONCEPTUALIZATION	MEMORY	TOTAL	PERCENTILE RANGES
2	0–23	0–24	0–1	0–21	0–15	0–100	<1
3	24–27	25–28	2	22–23	16	101–106	1
4	28–29	29	–	24	–	107	2
5	30	30	–	25	17–18	108–116	3–5
6	31	31	3	26–27	19	117–119	6–10
7	32	32–33	–	28–29	20	120–123	11–18
8	33	34–35	4	30	21	124–127	19–28
9	34	36	–	31–32	22	128–130	29–40
10	35	–	5	33–35	23	131–133	41–59
11	–	–	–	–	24	134–135	60–71
12	36	37	6	36	–	136–137	72–81
13	–	–	–	37	25	138	82–89
14	37	–	–	38	–	139–140	90–94
15	–	–	–	–	–	141	95–97
16	–	–	–	39	–	142	98
17	–	–	–	–	–	143	99
18	–	–	–	–	–	144	>99

SOURCE: From Rilling et al. (2005).

the test loads on the same factor as the Peabody Picture Vocabulary Test-Revised (Das et al., 1995). Moreover, the test correlates highly (about r = .70 to .80) with other commonly used standardized mental status examinations, such as the MMSE and the Information-Memory-Concentration test, suggesting that they evaluate overlapping mental abilities (e.g., Bobholz & Brandt, 1993; Katsarou et al., 2010; Salmon et al., 1990). Freidl et al. (1996, 2002), however, found only a weak relationship between the DRS and MMSE (r = .29) and low agreement with regard to cognitive impairment in a community sample. Conversion formulas are available (see "Comparing Scores on Different Tests") but, given their lack of precision, should be used with considerable caution.

In designing the test, Mattis grouped the tasks according to their face validity into five subsets: Memory, Construction, Initiation and Perseveration, Conceptualization, and Attention. Although there are generally high correlations

TABLE 7-22 Dementia Rating Scale-2 (DRS-2) Mayo's Older African Americans Normative Studies (MOAANS) Scaled Scores for Persons Aged 72 to 74 Years (Midpoint Age = 73, Age Range for Norms = 68 to 78, N = 157)

	DEMENTIA RATING SCALE SUBTESTS						
SCALED SCORES	ATTENTION	INITIATION/ PERSEVERATION	CONSTRUCTION	CONCEPTUALIZATION	MEMORY	TOTAL	PERCENTILE RANGES
2	0–23	0–22	–	0–21	0–15	0–100	>1
3	24–27	23–25	0–1	22–23	16	101–106	1
4	28	26–27	2	24	–	107	2
5	29	28–30	–	25	17–18	108–114	3–5
6	30–31	31	3	26	19	115–118	6–10
7	32	32	–	27–28	20	119–121	11–18
8	33	33–34	4	29	21	122–126	19–28
9	34	35	–	30–32	22	127–129	29–40
10	–	36	5	33–34	23	130–133	41–59
11	35	–	–	35	24	134–135	60–71
12	36	37	6	36	–	136–137	72–81
13	–	–	–	37	25	138	82–89
14	37	–	–	38	–	139–140	90–94
15	–	–	–	–	–	141	95–97
16	–	–	–	39	–	142	98
17	–	–	–	–	–	143	99
18	–	–	–	–	–	144	>99

SOURCE: From Rilling et al. (2005).

TABLE 7–23 Dementia Rating Scale-2 (DRS-2) Mayo's Older African Americans Normative Studies (MOAANS) Scaled Scores for Persons Aged 75 to 77 Years (Midpoint Age = 76, Age Range for Norms = 71 to 81, *N* = 119)

	DEMENTIA RATING SCALE SUBTESTS						
SCALED SCORES	ATTENTION	INITIATION/ PERSEVERATION	CONSTRUCTION	CONCEPTUALIZATION	MEMORY	TOTAL	PERCENTILE RANGES
2	0–23	0–22	–	0–21	0–15	0–100	<1
3	24–27	23–24	0–1	22–23	16	101–106	1
4	28	25–26	–	–	–	107	2
5	29	27–29	2	24	17	108–111	3–5
6	30–31	30	3	25–26	18	112–117	6–10
7	32	31–32	–	27	19–20	118–121	11–18
8	33	33–34	4	28–29	21	122–125	19–28
9	34	35	–	30–31	22	126–128	29–40
10	–	36	5	32–34	23	129–132	41–59
11	35	–	–	35	24	133–134	60–71
12	36	37	6	36	–	135–137	72–81
13	–	–	–	37	25	138	82–89
14	–	–	–	38	–	139–140	90–94
15	37	–	–	–	–	141	95–97
16	–	–	–	39	–	142	98
17	–	–	–	–	–	143	99
18	–	–	–	–	–	144	>99

SOURCE: From Rilling et al. (2005).

between DRS and MMSE Total scores, subscales of the DRS do not always show the expected relationships with items of the MMSE. For example, Bobholz and Brandt (1993) reported that the Attention item of the MMSE (serial sevens) was not significantly correlated with the Attention subscale of the DRS. In another study on AD, Davidson et al. (2010) found overlapping results between the DRS-2 and MMSE subscales when they submitted both measures to latent class analysis. They found a four-class solution labeled Mild, Attention/Construction, Memory, and Severe. The Mild and Severe classes each represent the lowest scoring and highest scoring halves, respectively, of the sample across all cognitive domains on the DRS-2 and MMSE. DRS-2 Attention and Conceptualization subscales loaded with MMSE Attention and Construction subscales to form the Attention/Construction class. The Memory class comprised mostly DRS-2 Conceptualization, Memory,

TABLE 7–24 Dementia Rating Scale-2 (DRS-2) Mayo's Older African Americans Normative Studies (MOAANS) Scaled Scores for Persons Aged 78 + (Midpoint Age = 79, Age Range for Norms = 74 to 94, *N* = 79)

	DEMENTIA RATING SCALE SUBTESTS						
SCALED SCORES	ATTENTION	INITIATION/ PERSEVERATION	CONSTRUCTION	CONCEPTUALIZATION	MEMORY	TOTAL	PERCENTILE RANGES
2	0–23	0–17	–	0–17	0–3	0–78	<1
3	24–27	18–23	0–1	18–22	4–12	79–103	1
4	28	24	–	23	13–16	104–106	2
5	29	25–27	2	24	17	107–110	3–5
6	30	28–30	3	25–26	18	111–115	6–10
7	31	31	–	27	19	116–118	11–18
8	32	32	4	28	20	119–121	19–28
9	33	33–34	–	29–30	21	122–126	29–40
10	34	35–36	5	31–33	22–23	127–130	41–59
11	35	–	–	34–35	–	131–133	60–71
12	36	–	6	36	24	134–135	72–81
13	–	37	–	37	25	136–138	82–89
14	–	–	–	38	–	139	90–94
15	37	–	–	–	–	140	95–97
16	–	–	–	39	–	141	98
17	–	–	–	–	–	142–143	99
18	–	–	–	–	–	144	>99

SOURCE: From Rilling et al. (2005).

TABLE 7–25 Regression Formula for Age- and Education-Corrected Mayo's Older African Americans Normative Studies (MOAANS) Scaled Scores for Dementia Rating Scale-2 (DRS-2) Total

Age- and education-corrected MOAANS scaled scores ($MSS_{A\&E}$) can be calculated for DRS Total scores by using aged-corrected MOAANS scaled scores (MSS_A) and education (expressed in years completed) in the following formula:

$$MSS_{A\&E} = 3.01 + (1.19 + MSS_A) - (0.41 \times EDUC)$$

SOURCE: From Rilling et al. (2005).

and Initiation/Perseveration subscales, as well as MMSE Memory and Orientation subscales.

Smith et al. (1994) provided evidence of convergent validity for some of the DRS scales. In a sample of 234 older patients with cognitive impairment, DRS subscale scores for Memory, Attention, and Conceptualization were significantly correlated with appropriate indices (General Memory, Attention/Concentration, and VIQ, respectively) from the WAIS-R and Wechsler Memory Scale-Revised (WMS-R), as assessed in the MOANS. Support for the convergent validity of the Construction scale was more problematic. Smith et al. found that this scale correlated more highly with VIQ and the Attention/Concentration Index than with Performance IQ (PIQ), raising the concern that it may provide a better index of attention and general cognitive status than of visual-perceptual/visual-constructional skills per se. Marson et al. (1997) reported that in a sample of 50 patients with mild to moderate AD, four of the five DRS subscales correlated most strongly with their assigned criterion variables (Attention with WMS-R Attention, Initiation/Perseveration with Controlled Oral Word Association Test (COWA), Conceptualization with WAIS-R Similarities, Memory with WMS-R Verbal Memory). However, the Construction scale correlated as highly with Block Design as with WMS-R Attention. Brown et al. (1999) found that in a sample of patients with PD, some DRS subscales correlated significantly with conceptually related measures from other tests (Attention with WAIS-R Digit Span Forward, Initiation/Perseveration with Wisconsin Card Sorting Test (WCST) perseverative responses, Conceptualization with WAIS-R Similarities, Memory with WMS Immediate Logical Memory). No signification correlation was observed between the Construction subscale and other tests. Thus, the available literature suggests that the DRS does not assess aspects of visual-constructional/visual-spatial functioning and that additional measures will need to be supplemented to adequately examine this domain.

The DRS-2: Alternate Form shows strong correlation with the MMSE ($r = .81$) in older adults with and without dementia (Schmidt et al., 2006). Overlapping findings are seen on the subscales, with the Attention subscale moderately to highly correlated with WAIS-III Digit Span ($r = .67$), Animal Fluency ($r = .51$), and Hopkins Verbal Learning Test-Revised (HVLT-R) delayed recall ($r = .46$). Additionally, the Initiation/Perseveration subscale was highly correlated with Animal Fluency ($r = .58$). The Conceptualization subscale was correlated with WAIS-III Similarities ($r = .51$) and HVLT-R Delayed Recall ($r = .39$). The Memory subscale was strongly correlated with HVLT-R delayed recall ($r = .75$) and had lower correlations with Animal Fluency ($r = .51$) and WAIS-III Similarities ($r = .39$).

TABLE 7–26 Mean Raw Scores of Healthy Older Adults as a Function of Age and Education Level for the Greek Translation of the Dementia Rating Scale (DRS-GR)

EDUCATION LEVEL	TOTAL DRS-GR SCORE	ATTENTION	INITIATION / PERSEVERATION	CONSTRUCTION	CONCEPTUALIZATION	MEMORY
Age 50–59 yrs						
Elementary (*N* = 20)	135.25 (4.55)	35.30 (1.03)	36.3 (1.62)	5.8 (0.52)	36.0 (1.26)	21.85 (2.45)
Middle (*N* = 37)	138.24 (3.68)	35.89 (0.96)	36.04 (1.46)	6[a]	36.56 (1.36)	23.37 (2.39)
High (*N* = 22)	141.14 (1.72)	36.54 (1.06)	37[a]	6[a]	37.82 (1.53)	23.77 (1.11)
Age 60–69 yrs						
Elementary (*N* = 30)	134.8 (4.77)	35.7 (1.05)	34.67 (2.3)	5.96 (0.18)	35.8 (1.6)	22.67 (2.25)
Middle (*N* = 40)	137.17 (5.2)	35.82 (0.95)	36.15 (1.71)	5.8 (0.88)	36.3 (1.67)	23.1 (2.51)
High (*N* = 20)	139.05 (2.76)	36.1 (0.71)	35.65 (2.0)	6[a]	37.9 (1.25)	23.4 (1.9)
Age 70–79 yrs						
Elementary (*N* = 46)	130.78 (4.75)	35.35 (0.97)	33.84 (3.1)	5.86 (0.34)	34.17 (2.39)	21.54 (2.59)
Middle (*N* = 25)	134.92 (4.48)	35.76 (1.16)	34.08 (3.38)	5.84 (0.47)	35.84 (3.18)	23.44 (1.73)
High (*N* = 14)	135.78 (3.21)	35.57 (0.94)	35.64 (1.86)	6[a]	36.14 (1.41)	22.42 (1.95)

NOTE: Values in parenthesis represent *SD*. Elementary level = 4–8 years of education; middle level = 9–12 years of education; high level = 13+ years of education. Based on *N* = 254, 57% females, mean age = 64.28 (*SD* = 8.5), mean education = 10 (*SD* = 3.1).

[a]Constant value.

SOURCE: From Katsarou et al. (2010).

TABLE 7–27 Dementia Rating Scale-2 (DRS-2) Raw Scores to Percentile Conversion for French-Canadian Older Adults Aged 50 to 60

FEWER THAN 12 YEARS OF EDUCATION							MORE THAN 12 YEARS OF EDUCATION						
DRS SUBTEST SCORES													
ATT	INIT/ PERS	CONSTRUCT	CONCEPT	MEM	TOTAL	PERCENTILE RANGES	ATT	INIT/ PERS	CONSTRUCT	CONCEPT	MEM	TOTAL	PERCENTILE RANGES
33	30–33	5	32	21	124–128	1	31	26–28	5	30–33	19–20	127–130	1
–	–	–	–	–	–	2	32–33	29–32	–	–	21–22	131–133	2
34	–	–	–	–	129–135	5	34	33	6	34	23	134–136	5
35	34–35	6	33–34	22–23	136–137	10	35	34–35	–	35	–	137	10
36	–	–	35–36	–	–	15	–	36	–	36	24	138–139	15
–	36	–	37–38	24	138–141	25	36	–	–	37–38	–	140	25
37	37	–	39	25	142–143	50	37	37	–	39	25	141–143	50
–	–	–	–	–	144	95	–	–	–	–	–	144	95

NOTE: Age range used = 50–64, *n* =153; Mean = 57.67, *SD* = 3.76. Fewer than 12 years of education, *n* = 30; more than 12 years of education, *n* = 123; Mean = 15. 86, *SD* = 3.75.

Att, Attention; Init/Pers, Initiation/Perseveration; Construct, Construction; Concept, Conceptualization; Mem, Memory. The sample was screened for neurological disease, psychiatric illness, head injury, or stroke, Montreal Cognitive Assessment (MoCA) or Mini-Mental State Examination (MMSE) <26.

SOURCE: From Lavoie et al. (2013).

TABLE 7–28 Dementia Rating Scale-2 (DRS-2) Raw Scores to Percentile Conversion for French-Canadian Older Adults Aged 61 to 65

FEWER THAN 12 YEARS OF EDUCATION							MORE THAN 12 YEARS OF EDUCATION						
DRS SUBTEST SCORES													
ATT	INIT/ PERS	CONSTRUCT	CONCEPT	MEM	TOTAL	PERCENTILE RANGES	ATT	INIT/ PERS	CONSTRUCT	CONCEPT	MEM	TOTAL	PERCENTILE RANGES
30–32	25	5	30–31	21	119	1	31–32	27–29	5	31–33	19–20	127–130	1
–	26–29	–	–	–	120–123	2	33	30–31	–	34	21	131–133	2
33	30–32	–	32–33	22	124–133	5	–	32–33	6	35	22	134–135	5
34	33	6	34	–	134–135	10	34	34	–	36	23	136	10
35	34	–	35	23–24	136–137	15	35	35	–	–	–	137	15
36	35–36	–	36–37	–	138–139	25	–	36	–	37–38	24	138–140	25
37	37	.	38	25	140–143	50	36	37	–	39	25	141–143	50
–	–	–	39	–	144	95	37	–	–	–	–	144	95

NOTE: Age range = 57–69, *n* = 185; Mean= 63.58, *SD* = 3.80. Fewer than 12 years of education, *n* = 57; more than 12 years of education, *n* = 128; Mean = 14.92, *SD* = 3.77. Att, Attention; Init/Pers, Initiation/Perseveration; Construct, Construction; Concept, Conceptualization; Mem, Memory. The sample was screened for neurological disease, psychiatric illness, head injury, or stroke, Montreal Cognitive Assessment (MoCA) or Mini-Mental State Examination (MMSE) <26.

SOURCE: From Lavoie et al. (2013).

TABLE 7–29 Dementia Rating Scale-2 (DRS-2) Raw Scores to Percentile Conversion for French-Canadian Older Adults Aged 66 to 70

FEWER THAN 12 YEARS OF EDUCATION							MORE THAN 12 YEARS OF EDUCATION						
DRS SUBTEST SCORES													
ATT	INIT/ PERS	CONSTRUCT	CONCEPT	MEM	TOTAL	PERCENTILE RANGES	ATT	INIT/ PERS	CONSTRUCT	CONCEPT	MEM	TOTAL	PERCENTILE RANGES
30–31	25	5	30–31	19–21	119–121	1	32	31	5	33	18–19	130	1
32	26–29	–	–	–	122–125	2	33	–	–	34	20	131–133	2
33	30–31	–	32–33	22	126–132	5	34	32–33	–	35	21	134–135	5
34	32–33	6	34	–	133	10	–	34	6	36	22	136	10
–	34–35	–	35	23	134–136	15	35	35	–	37–38	23	137	15
35	36	–	36	–	137–139	25	36	36	–	–	24	138–140	25
36	37	–	37–38	24	140–143	50	–	37	–	39	25	141–143	50
37	–	–	39	25	144	95	37	–	–	–	–	144	95

NOTE: Age range used = 62–74, *n* = 223; Mean = 68.59, *SD* = 3.41. Fewer than 12 years of education, *n* = 89; more than 12 years of education, *n* = 134; Mean = 14.14, *SD* = 3.81. Att, Attention; Init/Pers, Initiation/Perseveration; Construct, Construction; Concept., Conceptualization; Mem, Memory. The sample was screened for neurological disease, psychiatric illness, head injury, or stroke, Montreal Cognitive Assessment (MoCA) or Mini-Mental State Examination (MMSE) <26.

SOURCE: From Lavoie et al. (2013).

TABLE 7–30 Dementia Rating Scale-2 (DRS-2) Raw Scores to Percentile Conversion for French-Canadian Older Adults Aged 71 to 75

FEWER THAN 12 YEARS OF EDUCATION							MORE THAN 12 YEARS OF EDUCATION						
DRS SUBTEST SCORES													
ATT	INIT/ PERS	CONSTRUCT	CONCEPT	MEM	TOTAL	PERCENTILE RANGES	ATT	INIT/ PERS	CONSTRUCT	CONCEPT	MEM	TOTAL	PERCENTILE RANGES
32–33	26–28	5	30–31	19–21	125	1	30–31	31	4	33–34	17–18	129–131	1
–	29–30	–	–	–	126–128	2	32–33	–	5	–	19–20	132–133	2
34	31–32	6	32–33	22	129–132	5	34	32–33	–	35	21	134–135	5
–	33	–	34	23–24	133	10	–	34	6	36	22	136	10
35	34–35	–	35	–	134–136	15	35	35	–	37–38	23	137	15
–	36	–	36	–	137–139	25	–	36	–	–	24	138–139	25
36	37	–	37–38	25	140–142	50	36	37	–	39	25	140–143	50
37	–	–	39	–	143	95	37	–	–	–	–	144	95

NOTE: Age range used = 67–79, *n* = 212; Mean = 72.03, *SD* = 3.53. Fewer than 12 years of education, *n* = 92; more than 12 years of education, *n* = 120; Mean = 13.84, *SD* = 3.99. Att, Attention; Init/Pers, Initiation/Perseveration; Construct., Construction; Concept., Conceptualization; Mem, Memory. The sample was screened for neurological disease, psychiatric illness, head injury, or stroke, Montreal Cognitive Assessment (MoCA) or Mini-Mental State Examination (MMSE) <26.

SOURCE: From Lavoie et al. (2013).

CLINICAL STUDIES

The DRS is useful in detecting cognitive impairment in older adults (e.g., Yochim et al., 2003). It can differentiate patients with AD from healthy older adults (Chan et al., 2003; Monsch et al., 1995; Salmon et al., 2002; Springate et al., 2014); it is sensitive to MCI, PD-MCI (Matteau et al., 2011, 2012; Pirogovsky et al., 2014; Springate et al., 2014), and early stages of dementia (Knox et al., 2003; Monsch et al., 1995; Salmon et al., 2002), including in individuals with intellectual disability (Das et al., 1995); and it is useful in identifying stages (severity) of impairment (Chan et al., 2003; Shay et al., 1991). Furthermore, the DRS has demonstrated the ability to predict cognitive decline in patients with PD (Pigott et al., 2015) and accurately track progression of cognitive decline, even in the later stages of AD (Salmon et al., 1990). Although the DRS tends to be highly correlated with other mental status exams such as the Information Memory Concentration and MMSE, it shows equal sensitivity to dementia (Chan et al., 2003; van Gorp et al., 1999) and provides more precise estimates of change than these tests, likely due to its wider sampling of item difficulty (Gould et al., 2001; Salmon et al., 1990). Therefore, to follow progression in severely demented patients, the DRS is clearly the instrument of choice.

Unlike other standardized mental status examinations that were developed as screening instruments (e.g., MMSE), the DRS was designed with the intention to discriminate among patients with dementia. There is evidence that pattern analysis of the DRS can distinguish the dementias associated with AD from those associated with Huntington's disease (HD), PD, and vascular dementia (e.g., Cahn-Weiner et al., 2002; Kertesz & Clydesdale, 1994; Lukatela et al., 2000; Matteau et al., 2011, 2012;

TABLE 7–31 Dementia Rating Scale-2 (DRS-2) Raw Scores to Percentile Conversion for French-Canadian Older Adults 76 to 85

FEWER THAN 12 YEARS OF EDUCATION							MORE THAN 12 YEARS OF EDUCATION						
DRS SUBTEST SCORES													
ATT	INIT/ PERS	CONSTRUCT	CONCEPT	MEM	TOTAL	PERCENTILE RANGES	ATT	INIT/ PERS	CONSTRUCT	CONCEPT	MEM	TOTAL	PERCENTILE RANGES
31	29	3	30	21	126–128	1	30–31	31	4	32–33	17	129	1
32	30	4	31	22	–	2	32–33	–	–	–	18–19	130–132	2
33	31–32	5	32–33	–	129–132	5	34	32	5	34	20–21	133	5
34	33–35	–	34	–	133	10	–	33	6	35–36	22	134–135	10
–	–	6	35	23	134	15	35	34	–	37	23–24	136–137	15
35	36	–	36	–	135–138	25	–	35–36	–	–	–	138	25
36	37	–	37–38	24	139–142	50	36	37	–	38	25	139–143	50
37	–	–	39	25	143	95	37	–	–	39	–	144	95

NOTE: Age range used = 72–85, *n* = 143; Mean = 76.24, *SD* = 3.61. Fewer than 12 years of education, *n* = 74; more than 12 years of education, *n* = 69; Mean = 13.08, *SD* = 4.24. Att, Attention; Init/Pers, Initiation/Perseveration; Construct, Construction; Concept, Conceptualization; Mem, Memory. The sample was screened for neurological disease, psychiatric illness, head injury, or stroke, Montreal Cognitive Assessment (MoCA) or Mini-Mental State Examination (MMSE) <26.

SOURCE: From Lavoie et al. (2013).

Paolo et al., 1994; Paulsen et al., 1995; Porto et al., 2007). Patients with AD display more severe memory impairment; patients with HD are more severely impaired on items that involve the programming of motor sequences (Initiation/Perseveration subtest), while patients with PD or vascular dementia display more severe constructional problems. Patients with PD may also show memory impairment on the DRS, although this may also reflect the effects of depression (Norman et al., 2002). Furthermore, patients with FTD are less impaired on the Memory subscale than AD patients (Rascovsky et al., 2002). It is worth noting that these various distinctions among patient groups emerge even when patients are similar in terms of overall level of cognitive impairment.

In direct comparisons of various MCI and dementia types (Parkinson's dementia, AD, vascular dementia) groups, specific DRS-2 subscales appear to be somewhat useful to discriminate among different patient groups. Matteau et al. (2011) reported that the DRS-2 is useful to distinguish among patients with amnestic MCI (aMCI) and dementia, but not between MCI types or between dementia types. In their sample of aMCI, PD-MCI, Parkinson's dementia, and AD patients, both MCI groups performed similarly on the Total and subscale scores, as did both dementia groups. As expected, the AD group scored higher than the Parkinson's dementia group on Conceptualization but lower on Memory subscales. The PD-MCI group scored lower than healthy controls on Initiation/Perseveration and Memory subscales, whereas the aMCI group scored lower than healthy controls on the Memory subscale only. Discriminant function using Conceptualization, Initiation/Perseveration, Memory, and age yielded a classification accuracy of 82% for differentiating healthy controls and dementia groups, with 100% classification for healthy controls, 86% for AD, and 50% for Parkinson's dementia. Memory appeared to be the best variable to differentiate between healthy controls and the MCI groups, although only yielding an overall classification accuracy of 50% (68% for healthy controls, 50% for aMCI, and 32% for PD-MCI). When only PD patients were considered, using the same three subscale scores yielded an overall classification accuracy of 75%, with 86% for healthy controls, 64% for PD-MCI, and 75% for Parkinson's dementia (Matteau et al., 2012). Porto et al. (2007) reported that Initiation/Perseveration, Memory, Conceptualization, and Attention subscales best discriminated vascular dementia from healthy controls, while only the Initiation/Perseveration subscale discriminated vascular dementia (lower score) from AD (higher score). Cutoff scores for detecting MCI and dementia groups are presented in Table 7–32.

There is evidence that depression impairs DRS performance, at least to some extent (Harrell et al., 1991; van

TABLE 7–32 Dementia Rating Scale-2 (DRS-2) Cutoff Scores, AUC, Sensitivity, Specificity, PPV, and NPV to Identify Amnestic MCI, PD Dementia, PD-MCI, VaD, and Other Dementias

REFERENCE	PURPOSE/POPULATION	CUTOFF	AUC	SENS (%)	SPEC (%)	PPV (%)	NPV (%)
Matteau et al. (2011)	Amnestic MCI (*N* = 22), PD-MCI (*N* = 22), PDD (*N* = 16), AD (*N* = 22), healthy controls (*N* = 22)	<140 to detect MCI from healthy controls	.81	80	68	–	–
		<133 to detect dementia only from healthy controls	1.0	100	100		
Matteau et al. (2012)	PDD (*N* = 16), PD-MCI (*N* = 22), healthy controls (*N* unknown)	≤140 to detect PD-MCI from healthy controls	.82	86	54	–	–
		≤132 to detect PDD from healthy controls	1.0	100	100		
Pirogovsky et al. (2014)	PD-normal cognition (*N* = 68), PD-MCI (*N* = 30)	≤139 for screening purpose	.76	77	65	–	–
		≤137 for diagnostic purpose		57	82		
Villeneuve et al. (2011)	PD-MCI (*N* = 18), PD-noMCI (*N* = 22) idiopathic REM sleep behavior disorder and MCI (iRBD-MCI; *N* = 20), iRBD-noMCI; (*N* = 14)	≤138 for identifying PD-MCI out of all PD cases	.80	72	86	81	79
		≤141 for identifying iRBD-MCI out of all iRBD cases	.86	90	71	82	83
Pontone et al. (2013)	PD with cognitive disorder NOS without dementia as defined by DSM-IV-TR (PD-CD; *N* = 21), PD-no dementia (*N* = 77), PDD (*N* = 27)	≤132 to identify PDD from all PD cases	.93	89	87	65	97
		≤137 to identify PD-CD from PD-ND	.59	62	70	36	87
Porto et al. (2007)	VaD (*N* = 12), AD (*N* = 56), healthy controls (*N* = 60)	<124 to identify VaD from controls	.99	93	92	–	–
		DRS-2 Total score not useful to differentiate between VaD and AD					
Springate et al. (2014)	AD (*N* = 49), MCI (*N* = 98), healthy controls (*N* = 50)	>136 to identify healthy controls from MCI	.87	71	86	–	–
		<124 to identify AD from MCI	.87	82	78		
		>136 to identify healthy controls from MCI and AD	.91	81	86		

NOTE: Sens = sensitivity; Spec = specificity; PPV = positive predictive value; NPV = negative predictive value; MCI = mild cognitive impairment; PD = Parkinson's disease; PD MCI = Parkinson's disease-mild cognitive impairment; iRBD-MCI = idiopathic REM sleep behavior disorder and MCI; iRBD-noMCI = idiopathic REM sleep behavior disorder and no MCI; PD-CD = Parkinson's disease with cognitive disorder NOS without dementia; PDD = Parkinson's disease dementia; VaD = vascular dementia; AD = Alzheimer's disease.

Reekum et al., 2000), although some studies do not find any correlation between DRS-2 scores and Geriatric Depression Scale (GDS) scores (Kane et al., 2010). For example, one group of investigators (Butters et al., 2000) studied 45 nondemented, older depressed patients before and after successful treatment with pharmacotherapy. Among depressed patients with concomitant cognitive impairment at baseline, successful treatment of depression was associated with gains on the DRS measures of Conceptualization and Initiation/Perseveration. Nonetheless, the overall level of cognitive functioning in these patients remained mildly impaired, especially in the Memory and Initiation/Perseveration domains.

The relationship between objective memory functioning as measured by the DRS-2 and subjective memory complaints appears to be moderated by negative affect, especially anxiety sensitivity. Dux et al. (2008) reported that in their healthy older adult sample, DRS-2 Total and Memory subscale scores were positively correlated with subjective memory complaints as measured by the Memory Functioning Questionnaire (MFQ), whereas a negative correlation was seen between the MFQ and GDS scores. Individuals with better objective cognitive functioning had fewer subjective memory complaints, but those with higher negative affect had more subjective memory complaints.

Interestingly, personality traits may be associated with DRS-2 performance. Williams et al. (2013) gave the NEO Personality Inventory-Revised and the DRS-2 to 75 healthy community dwelling older adults. They found that only Neuroticism and Agreeableness were correlated with DRS-2 scores at baseline, whereas all but Extraversion were correlated with one-year follow-up DRS-2 scores. Low scores on Openness to Experience was associated with cognitive decline over one year and accounted for 13% of unique variance over age, education, and cognitive baseline score. The authors suggested that low Openness to Experience may represent the point of nearly depleted cognitive reserve and ensuing cognitive decline.

Although the DRS is typically used with older adults, it has found use in other groups as well. Thus, it has been given to adolescents and adults with intellectual disability (spanning the spectrum from mild to severe; Das et al., 1995; McDaniel & McLaughlin, 2000). However, it should not be used to diagnose intellectual disability.

ACTIVITIES OF DAILY LIVING AND OTHER FUNCTIONAL OUTCOME VARIABLES

DRS scores show modest correlations with measures of functional competence (the ability to perform ADLs as well as engage in complex recreational activities; e.g., Baird, 2006; Cahn et al., 1998; LaBuda & Lichtenberg, 1999; Lemsky et al., 1996; Loewenstein et al., 1992; Smith et al., 1994). Lower DRS-2 scores are related to greater problems in ADLs (Fields et al., 2010). In particular, the Initiation/Perseveration and Memory subtests have proved valuable as indicators of functional status in older adults (Fields et al., 2010; Greenaway et al., 2012; Nadler et al., 1993; Plehn et al., 2004). Specifically, those with borderline DRS scores (Total DRS = 123 to 129) differ from those with normal DRS scores (Total DRS ≥130) on the Independent Living Scale (ILS) Money Management and Memory subscales. Those with borderline DRS scores differ from those with mild dementia (Total DRS = 103 to 122) on the Health and Safety subscale, who then differ from those with moderate dementia (Total DRS <103) on all ILS subscales except Memory (Baird, 2006). Similar findings were reported in another study, where those in the mild range of DRS-2 scores (i.e., 126–131) were likely to have difficulties on instrumental ADLs (IADLs) such as household upkeep and functioning outside a familiar environment, with almost half of this group showing impairment on driving and financial management. Moderate DRS-2 scores (i.e., 105–116) were additionally associated with difficulty with washing/grooming and dressing, and a large proportion of this group had impairments in IADLs. Severe DRS-2 scores (i.e., 54–89) were associated with difficulty with all basic ADLs, and the majority reported impairment in IADLs. These findings suggest that while some difficulties on basic ADLs may be seen with mildly impaired cognitive functioning (i.e., DRS Total score of 121), difficulties with driving may be seen even in those with scores in the normal range (i.e., DRS Total score of 139; Fields et al., 2010).

However, the DRS-2 may explain less variance on functional measures than more specific tests. For example, Triebel et al. (2010) reported that global cognitive measures (DRS-2 and MMSE) explained only 14% of variance over race on the Financial Capacity Instrument among older adults with amnestic MCI, compared to the Wide Range Achievement Test (WRAT-3) Arithmetic scores, which accounted for 54% of variance.

The DRS may be useful in predicting functional decline (Hochberg et al., 1989) and survival (Kane et al., 2010; Smith et al., 1994). Higher depressive symptoms and lower DRS-2 scores at admission to long-term care have been found to be predictive of all-cause mortality 12 months after admission (Kane et al., 2010). Smith et al. (1994) reported that in a sample of 274 persons over age 55 with cognitive impairment, DRS Total scores supplemented age information and provided a better basis for estimating survival than did gender or duration of disease. Median survival for those with DRS Total scores lower than 100 was 3.7 years.

NEUROANATOMICAL CORRELATES AND IMAGING STUDIES

Fama et al. (1997) found that Memory subscale scores in patients with AD were related to magnetic resonance imaging (MRI)-derived hippocampal volumes, while Initiation/Perseveration scores were related to prefrontal sulcal widening. Among older adults with AD-related alteration in central olfactory system neural activity, DRS-2 Total and Memory subscale scores were correlated with functional magnetic resonance imaging (fMRI) activation in the left primary olfactory cortex, left hippocampus, and left insula at the lowest odorant level (Wang et al., 2010). Others have also observed that scores on select subscales are related to the integrity of specific brain regions. In patients with vascular dementia, performance on the Memory subscale is associated with whole brain volume, whereas the Initiation/Perseveration and Construction subscales are related to subcortical hyperintensities (Paul et al., 2001). Even in the absence of dementia, subcortical ischemic vascular disease is associated with subtle declines in executive functioning, as measured by the Initiation/Perseveration subscale (Kramer et al., 2002).

In PD, baseline cerebrospinal fluid (CSF) biomarker levels have been associated with DRS-2 scores over time (Siderowf et al., 2010). Specifically, those with lower baseline $A\beta_{1-42}$ show more rapid cognitive decline, with an average of 5.85 DRS-2 points per year more so than those with higher baseline levels after adjusting for age, disease duration, and baseline stage. After two years, those with low baseline $A\beta_{1-42}$ have DRS-2 scores of less than 123, whereas those with high baseline $A\beta_{1-42}$ remain above a DRS-2 score of 130. The most notable declines are seen on the Attention subscale, followed by Conceptualization and Memory subscales. CSF total tau and p-tau_{181p} levels are not associated with cognitive decline on the DRS-2 (Siderowf et al., 2010).

PERFORMANCE VALIDITY

Not available.

COMMENT

The DRS is a fairly comprehensive screening test, evaluating aspects of cognition not well assessed by tests such as the MMSE (e.g., verbal conceptualization, verbal fluency). It also appears to be more useful than other measures such as the MMSE in identifying milder level of cognitive dysfunction, including changes related to amnestic MCI, PD-MCI, and early dementia, as well as tracking change. Scores on the DRS-2 may also translate into functional disability and predict functional decline over time. On the other hand, the DRS takes about four times longer to administer than rapid screening tests and may be susceptible to cultural or educational factors in some populations (Bobholz & Brandt, 1993; Hohl et al., 1999; Lyness et al., 2006; Strutt et al., 2012). In particular, even though the Total scores may be equivalent, non-English speakers perform differently on the subscales, and, therefore, pattern analysis should not be used to differentiate among various dementias in minority groups.

The summary score appears to have relatively good concurrent and predictive validity. Given that the DRS may also be helpful in distinguishing among dementing disorders even in later stages of disease, the focus should also be on specific cognitive dimensions that the test offers. However, the subscales were created via face validity, and factor-analytic studies suggest that each subscale does not represent a unitary construct but may tap into other cognitive domains. In this context, it is worth bearing in mind that the Conceptualization and Memory subscales appear fairly reliable and seem to represent discrete constructs. Construction, Initiation/Perseveration, and Attention items should also be administered, but, given concerns regarding reliability and validity, their interpretation is more problematic. Supplementing the screening battery with visuospatial/visuoconstructional and attention tasks may be helpful.

It is also important to note that the test is a screening device and the clinician may need to follow-up with a more in-depth investigation. Furthermore, although sensitive to differences at the lower end of functioning, the DRS may not detect impairment in the higher ranges of intelligence (Jurica et al., 2001; Teresi et al., 2001). This is because the DRS was developed to avoid floor effects in clinically impaired populations rather than ceiling effects in high-functioning individuals (Jurica et al., 2001).

Some (Chan et al., 2003; Monsch et al., 1995) have suggested that an abbreviated version composed only of the Memory and Initiation/Perseveration subscales may be useful as a quick screening for individuals suspected of AD. This focus is consistent with literature suggesting that deterioration of memory is an early, prominent symptom of the disease. However, with use of such a shortened procedure, the comprehensive data on different aspects of cognitive functioning will be lost (Chan et al., 2003). Derivation of performance validity indicators would be of benefit.

REFERENCES

Baird, A. (2006). Fine tuning recommendations for older adults with memory complaints: Using the Independent Living Scales with the Dementia Rating Scale. *The Clinical Neuropsychologist, 20*(4), 649–661.

Bank, A. L., Yochim, B. P., MacNeill, S. E., & Lichtenberg, P. A. (2000). Expanded normative data for the Mattis Dementia Rating Scale for use with urban, elderly medical patients. *The Clinical Neuropsychologist, 14,* 149–156.

Bobholz, J. H., & Brandt, J. (1993). Assessment of cognitive impairment: Relationship of the Dementia Rating Scale to the Mini-Mental State Examination. *Journal of Geriatric Psychiatry and Neurology, 6,* 210–213.

Brown, G. G., Rahill, A. A., Gorell, J. M., McDonald, C., Brown, S. J., Sillanpaa, M., & Shults, C. (1999). Validity of the Dementia Rating Scale in assessing cognitive function in Parkinson's disease. *Journal of Geriatric Psychiatry and Neurology, 12,* 180–188.

Butters, M. A., Becker, J. T., Nebes, R. D., Zmuda, M. D., Mulsant, B. H., Pollock, B. G., & Reynolds, C. F., III. (2000). Changes in cognitive functioning following treatment of late-life depression. *American Journal of Psychiatry, 157,* 1949–1954.

Cahn, D. A., Sullivan, E. V., Shear, P. K., Pfefferbaum, A., Heit, G., & Silverberg, G. (1998). Differential contributions of cognitive and motor component processes to physical and instrumental activities of daily living in Parkinson's disease. *Archives of Clinical Neuropsychology, 13,* 575–583.

Cahn-Weiner, D. A., Grace, J., Ott, B. R., Fernandez, H. H., & Friedman, J. H. (2002). Cognitive and behavioural features discriminate between Alzheimer's and Parkinson's disease. *Neuropsychiatry, Neuropsychology, & Behavioural Neurology, 15,* 79–87.

Chan, A. S., Choi, A., Chiu, H., & Liu, L. (2003). Clinical validity of the Chinese version of Mattis Dementia Rating Scale in differentiating dementia of Alzheimer's type in Hong Kong. *Journal of the International Neuropsychological Society, 9,* 45–55.

Chan, A. S., Salmon, D. P., & Choi, M-K. (2001). The effects of age, education, and gender on the Mattis Dementia Rating Scale performance of elderly Chinese and American individuals. *Journal of Gerontology: Series B: Psychological Sciences & Social Sciences, 56B,* 356–363.

Coblentz, J. M., Mattis, S., Zingesser, L. H., Kasoff, S. S., Wisniewski, H. M., & Katzman, R. (1973). Presenile dementia. *Archives of Neurology, 29,* 299–308.

Colantonio, A., Becker, J. T., & Huff, F. J. (1993). Factor structure of the Mattis Dementia Rating Scale among patients with probable Alzheimer's disease. *The Clinical Neuropsychologist 7,* 313–318.

Das, J. P., Mishra, R. K., Davison, M., & Naglieri, J. A. (1995). Measurement of dementia in individuals with mental retardation: Comparison based on PPVT and Dementia Rating Scale. *The Clinical Neuropsychologist, 9,* 32–37.

Davidson, J. E., Irizarry, M. C., Bray, B. C., Wetten, S., Galwey, N., Gibson, R., . . . Monsch, A. U. (2010). An exploration of cognitive subgroups in Alzheimer's disease. *Journal of the International Neuropsychological Society,16*(2), 233–243.

Dean, P. M., & Cerhan, J. H. (2013). Correction for a potentially biased item on the Mattis Dementia Rating Scale. *American Journal of Alzheimer's Disease and Other Dementias, 28*(8), 734–737.

Dux, M. C., Woodard, J. L., Calamari, J. E., Messina, M., Arora, S., Chik, H., & Pontarelli, N. (2008). The moderating role of negative affect on objective verbal memory performance and subjective memory complaints in healthy older adults. *Journal of the International Neuropsychological Society, 14*(2), 327–336.

Fama, R., Sullivan, E. V., Shear, P. K., Marsh, L., Yesavage, J., Tinklenberg, J. R., Lim, K. O., & Pfefferbaum, A. (1997). Selective cortical and hippocampal volume correlates of Mattis Dementia Rating Scale in Alzheimer disease. *Archives of Neurology, 54,* 719–728.

Fields, J. A., Machulda, M., Aakre, J., Ivnik, R. J., Boeve, B. F., Knopman, D. S., . . . Smith, G. E. (2010). Utility of the DRS for predicting problems in day-to-day functioning. *The Clinical Neuropsychologist, 24*(7), 1167–1180.

Foss, M. P., Carvalho, V. A. D., Machado, T. H., Reis, G. C. D., Tumas, V., Caramelli, P., . . . Porto, C. S. (2013). Mattis Dementia Rating Scale (DRS): Normative data for the Brazilian middle-age and elderly populations. *Dementia & Neuropsychologia, 7*(4), 374–379.

Freidl, W., Schmidt, R., Stronegger, W. J., Fazekas, F., & Reinhart, B. (1996). Sociodemographic predictors and concurrent validity of the Mini Mental State Examination and the Mattis Dementia Rating Scale. *European Archives of Psychiatry and Clinical Neuroscience, 246,* 317–319.

Freidl, W., Schmidt, R., Stronegger, W. J., & Reinhart, B. (1997). The impact of sociodemographic, environmental, and behavioural factors, and cerebrovascular risk factors as potential predictors on the Mattis Dementia Rating Scale. *Journal of Gerontology, 52A,* M111–M116.

Freidl, W., Stronegger, W.-J., Berghold, A., Reinhart, B., Petrovic, K., & Schmidt, R. (2002). The agreement of the Mattis Dementia Rating Scale with the Mini-Mental State Examination. *International Journal of Psychiatry, 17,* 685–686.

Gardner, R., Oliver-Munoz, S., Fisher, L., & Empting, L. (1981). Mattis Dementia Rating Scale: Internal reliability study using a diffusely impaired population. *Journal of Clinical Neuropsychology, 3,* 271–275.

Gould, R., Abramson, I., Galasko, D., & Salmon, D. (2001). Rate of cognitive change in Alzheimer's disease: Methodological approaches using random effects models. *Journal of the International Neuropsychological Society, 7,* 813–824.

Greenaway, M. C., Duncan, N. L., Hanna, S., & Smith, G. E. (2012). Predicting functional ability in mild cognitive impairment with the Dementia Rating Scale-2. *International Psychogeriatrics, 24*(6), 987–993.

Harrell, L. E., Duvall, E., Folks, D. G., Duke, L., Bartolucci, A., Conboy, T., . . . Kerns, D. (1991). The relationship of high-intensity signals on magnetic resonance images to cognitive and psychiatric state in Alzheimer's disease. *Archives of Neurology, 48,* 1136–1140.

Hochberg, M. G., Russo, J., Vitaliano, P. P., Prinz, P. N., Vitiello, M. V., & Yi, S. (1989). Initiation and perseveration as a subscale of the Dementia Rating Scale. *Clinical Gerontologist, 8,* 27–41.

Hofer, S. M., Piccinin, A. M., & Hershey, D. (1996). Analysis of structure and discriminative power of the Mattis Dementia Rating Scale. *Journal of Clinical Psychology, 52,* 395–409.

Hohl, U., Grundman, M., Salmon, D. P., Thomas, R. G., & Thal, L. J. (1999). Mini-Mental State Examination and Mattis Dementia Rating Scale performance differs in Hispanic and non-Hispanic Alzheimer's disease patients. *Journal of the International Neuropsychological Society, 5,* 301–307.

Jurica, P. J., Leitten, C. L., & Mattis, S. (2001). *Dementia Rating Scale—2.* Odessa, FL: Psychological Assessment Resources.

Jurica, P. J., Leitten, C. L., & Mattis, S. (2004). *DRS-2 Dementia Rating Scale—2: Professional manual.* Psychological Assessment Resources.

Kane, K. D., Yochim, B. P., & Lichtenberg, P. A. (2010). Depressive symptoms and cognitive impairment predict all-cause mortality in long-term care residents. *Psychology and Aging, 25*(2), 446–452.

Kantarci, K., Smith, G. E., Ivnik, R. J., Petersen, R. C., Boeve, B. F., Knopman, D. S., . . . Jack, C. R. (2002). H magnetic resonance spectroscopy, cognitive function, and apolipoprotein E genotype in normal aging, mild cognitive impairment and Alzheimer's disease. *Journal of the International Neuropsychological Society, 8,* 934–942.

Katsarou, Z., Bostantjopoulou, S., Zikouli, A., Kazazi, E., Kafantari, A., Tsipropoulou, V., . . . Peitsidou, E. (2010). Performance of Greek demented and nondemented subjects on the Greek version of the Mattis Dementia Rating Scale. A validation study. *International Journal of Neuroscience, 120*(11), 724–730.

Kertesz, A., & Clydesdale, S. (1994). Neuropsychological deficits in vascular dementia vs Alzheimer's disease. *Archives of Neurology, 51,* 1226–1231.

Kessler, H. R., Roth, D. L., Kaplan, R. F., & Goode, K. T. (1994). Confirmatory factor analysis of the Mattis Dementia Rating Scale. *The Clinical Neuropsychologist, 8,* 451–461.

Knox, M. R., Lacritz, L. H., Chandler, M. J., & Cullum, C. M. (2003). Association between Dementia Rating Scale performance and neurocognitive domains in Alzheimer's disease. *The Clinical Neuropsychologist, 17,* 216–219.

Kramer, J. H., Reed, B. R., Mungas, D., Weiner, N. W., & Chui, H. C. (2002). Executive dysfunction in subcortical ischaemic vascular disease. *Journal of Neurology, Neurosurgery and Psychiatry, 72,* 217–220.

LaBuda, J., & Lichtenberg, P. (1999). The role of cognition, depression, and awareness of deficit in predicting geriatric rehabilitation patients' IADL performance. *The Clinical Neuropsychologist, 13,* 258–267.

Lavoie, M., Callahan, B., Belleville, S., Simard, M., Bier, N., Gagnon, L., . . . Macoir, J. (2013). Normative data for the Dementia Rating Scale-2 in the French-Quebec population. *The Clinical Neuropsychologist, 27*(7), 1150–1166.

Lemsky, C. M., Smith, G., Malec, J. F., & Ivnik, R. J. (1996). Identifying risk for functional impairment using cognitive measures: An application of CART modeling. *Neuropsychology, 10,* 368–375.

Loewenstein, D. A., Rupert, M. P., Berkowitz-Zimmer, N., Guterman, A., Morgan, R., Hayden, S. (1992) Neuropsychological test performance and prediction of functional capacities in dementia. *Behavior, Health, and Aging, 2,* 149–158.

Lucas, J. A., Ivnick, R. J., Smith, G. E., Bohac, D. L., Tangalos, E. G., Kokmen, E., . . . Petersen, R. C. (1998). Normative data for the Mattis Dementia Rating Scale. *Journal of Clinical and Experimental Neuropsychology, 20,* 536–547.

Lukatela, K., Cohen, R. A., Kessler, H., Jenkins, M. A., Moser, D. J., Stone, W. F., . . . Kaplan, R. F. (2000). Dementia Rating Scale performance: A comparison of vascular and Alzheimer's dementia. *Journal of Clinical and Experimental Neuropsychology, 22,* 445–454.

Lyness, S. A., Hernandez, I., Chui, H. C., & Teng, E. L. (2006). Performance of Spanish speakers on the Mattis Dementia Rating Scale (MDRS). *Archives of Clinical Neuropsychology, 21*(8), 827–836.

Marcopulos, B. A., & McLain, C. A. (2003). Are our norms "normal"? A 4-year follow-up study of a biracial sample of rural elders with low education. *The Clinical Neuropsychologist, 17,* 19–33.

Marcopulos, B. A., McLain, C. A., & Giuliano, A. J. (1997). Cognitive impairment or inadequate norms? A study of healthy, rural, older adults with limited education. *The Clinical Neuropsychologist, 11,* 111–113.

Marson, D. C., Dymek, M. P., Duke, L. W., & Harrell, L. E. (1997). Subscale validity of the Mattis Dementia Rating Scale. *Archives of Clinical Neuropsychology, 12,* 269–275.

Matteau, E., Dupré, N., Langlois, M., Jean, L., Thivierge, S., Provencher, P., & Simard, M. (2011). Mattis Dementia Rating Scale 2 screening for MCI and dementia. *American Journal of Alzheimer's Disease and Other Dementias, 26*(5), 389–398.

Matteau, E., Dupré, N., Langlois, M., Provencher, P., & Simard, M. (2012). Clinical validity of the Mattis Dementia Rating Scale-2 in Parkinson disease with MCI and dementia. *Journal of Geriatric Psychiatry and Neurology, 25*(2), 100–106.

Mattis, S. (1976). Mental status examination for organic mental syndrome in the elderly patient. In L. Bellak & T. B. Karasu (Eds.), *Geriatric Psychiatry* (pp. 77–121). New York: Grune and Stratton.

Mattis, S. (1988). *Dementia Rating Scale: Professional manual.* Odessa, FL: Psychological Assessment Resources.

McDaniel, W. F., & McLaughlin, T. (2000). Further support for using the Dementia Rating Scale in the assessment of neuro-cognitive functions of individuals with mental retardation. *The Clinical Neuropsychologist, 14,* 72–75.

Meiran, N., Stuss, D. T., Guzman, D. A., Lafleche, G., & Willmer, J. (1996). Diagnosis of dementia: Methods for interpretation of scores of 5 neuropsychological tests. *Archives of Neurology, 53,* 1043–1054.

Monsch, A. U., Bondi, M. W., Salmon, D. P., Butters, N., Thal, L. J., Hansen, L. A., . . . Klauber, M. R. (1995). Clinical validity of the Mattis Dementia Rating Scale in detecting dementia of the Alzheimer type. *Archives of Neurology, 52,* 899–904.

Montgomery, K. M. (1982). *A normative study of neuropsychological test performance of a normal elderly sample* (unpublished Master's thesis). University of Victoria, Victoria, British Columbia.

Nadler, J. D., Richardson, E. D., Malloy, P. F., Marran, M. E., & Hostetler Brinson, M. E. (1993). The ability of the Dementia Rating Scale to predict everyday functioning. *Archives of Clinical Neuropsychology, 8,* 449–460.

Norman, S., Troster, A. I., Fields, J. A., & Brooks, R. (2002). Effects of depression and Parkinson's disease on cognitive functioning. *Journal of Neuropsychiatry and Clinical Neurosciences, 14,* 31–36.

Paolo, A. M., Troster, A. I., Glatt, S. L., Hubble, J. P., & Koller, W. C. (1994). *Utility of the Dementia Rating Scale to differentiate the dementias of Alzheimer's and Parkinson's disease.* Paper presented to the International Neuropsychological Society, Cincinnati, OH.

Paul, R. H., Cohen, R. A., Moser, D., Ott, B. R., Zawacki, T., Gordon, N., Bell, S., & Stone, W. (2001). Performance on the Mattis Dementia Rating Scale in patients with vascular dementia: Relationships to neuroimaging findings. *Journal of Geriatric Psychiatry & Neurology, 14,* 33–36.

Paulsen, J. S., Butters, N., Sadek, B. S., Johnson, B. S., Salmon, D. P., Swerdlow, N. R., & Swenson. M. R. (1995). Distinct cognitive profiles of cortical and subcortical dementia in advanced illness. *Neurology, 45,* 951–956.

Pigott, K., Rick, J., Xie, S. X., Hurtig, H., Chen-Plotkin, A., Duda, J. E., . . . Siderowf, A. (2015). Longitudinal study of normal cognition in Parkinson disease. *Neurology, 85*(15), 1276–1282.

Pirogovsky, E., Schiehser, D. M., Litvan, I., Obtera, K. M., Burke, M. M., Lessig, S. L., . . . Filoteo, J. V. (2014). The utility of the Mattis Dementia Rating Scale in Parkinson's disease Mild Cognitive Impairment. *Parkinsonism & Related Disorders, 20*(6), 627–631.

Plehn, K., Marcopulos, B. A., & McLain, C. A. (2004). The relationship between neuropsychological test performance, social functioning, and instrumental activities of daily living in a sample of rural older adults. *The Clinical Neuropsychologist, 18,* 101–113.

Pontone, G. M., Palanci, J., Williams, J. R., & Bassett, S. S. (2013). Screening for DSM-IV-TR cognitive disorder NOS in Parkinson's disease using the Mattis Dementia Rating Scale. *International Journal of Geriatric Psychiatry, 28*(4), 364–371.

Porto, C. S., Caramelli, P., & Nitrini, R. (2007). The Dementia Rating Scale (DRS) in the diagnosis of vascular dementia. *Dementia & Neuropsychologia, 3,* 282–287.

Rascovsky, K., Salmon, D. P., Hi, G. J., Galasko, D., Peavy, G. M., Hansen, L. A., & Thal, L. J. (2002). Cognitive profiles differ in autopsy-confirmed frontotemporal dementia and AD. *Neurology,* 1801–1807.

Rilling, L. M., Lucas, J. A., Ivnik, R. J., Smith, G. E., Willis, F. B., Ferman, T. J., Petersen, R. C., & Graff-Radford, N. R. (2005). Mayo's Older African American Normative Studies: Norms for the Mattis Dementia Rating Scale. *The Clinical Neuropsychologist, 19,* 229–242.

Salmon, D. P., Thal, L. J., Butters, N., & Heindel, W. C. (1990). Longitudinal evaluation of dementia of the Alzheimer's type: A comparison of 3 standardized mental status examinations. *Neurology, 40,* 1225–1230.

Salmon, D. P., Thomas, R. G., Pay, M. M., Booth, A., Hofstetter, C. R., Thal, L. J., & Katzman, R. (2002). Alzheimer's disease can be accurately diagnosed in very mildly impaired individuals. *Neurology, 59,* 1022–1028.

Schmidt, R., Freidl, W., Fazekas, F., Reinhart, P., Greishofer, P., Koch, M., . . . Petersen, R. C. (1994). Psychometric properties of the Mattis Dementia Rating Scale. *Assessment, 1,* 123–131.

Schmidt, K. S., Lieto, J. M., Kiryankova, E., & Salvucci, A. (2006). Construct and concurrent validity of the Dementia Rating Scale-2 alternate form. *Journal of Clinical and Experimental Neuropsychology, 28*(5), 646–654.

Schmidt, K., & Mattis, S. (2004). *Dementia Rating Scale-2: Alternate form.* Lutz, FL: PAR.

Schmidt, K. S., Mattis, P. J., Adams, J., & Nestor, P. (2005). Alternate-form reliability of the Dementia Rating Scale-2. *Archives of Clinical Neuropsychology, 20,* 435–441.

Shay, K. A., Duke, L. W., Conboy, T., Harrell, L. E., Callaway, R., & Folks, D. G. (1991). The clinical validity of the Mattis Dementia Rating Scale in staging Alzheimer's dementia. *Journal of Geriatric Psychiatry and Neurology, 4,* 18–25.

Siderowf, A., Xie, S. X., Hurtig, H., Weintraub, D., Duda, J., Chen-Plotkin, A., . . . Clark, C. (2010). CSF amyloid β1-42 predicts cognitive decline in Parkinson disease. *Neurology, 75*(12), 1055–1061.

Smith, G. E., Ivnik, R. J., Malec, J. F., Kokmen, E., Tangalos, E. G., & Petersen, R. C. (1994). Psychometric properties of the Mattis Dementia Rating Scale. *Assessment, 1,* 123–131.

Springate, B. A., Tremont, G., Papandonatos, G., & Ott, B. R. (2014). Screening for mild cognitive impairment using the Dementia Rating Scale-2. *Journal of Geriatric Psychiatry and Neurology, 27*(2), 139–144.

Strutt, A. M., Ayanegui, I. G., Scott, B. M., Mahoney, M. L., York, M. K., & Montes, L. E. S. M. (2012). Influence of socio-demographic characteristics on DRS-2 performance in Spanish-speaking older adults. *Archives of Clinical Neuropsychology, 27*(5), 545–556.

Teresi, J. A., Holmes, D., Ramirez, M., Gurland, B. J., & Lantigua, R. (2001). Performance of cognitive tests among different racial/ethnic and education groups: Findings of differential item functioning and possible item bias. *Journal of Mental Health and Aging, 17,* 79–89.

Teresi, J. A., Kleinman, M., & Ocepek-Welikson, K. (2000). Modern psychometric methods for detection of differential item functioning: Application to cognitive assessment measures. *Statistics in Medicine, 19,* 1651–1683.

Triebel, K. L., Okonkwo, O. C., Martin, R., Griffith, H. R., Crowther, M., & Marson, D. C. (2010). Financial capacity of older African Americans with amnestic mild cognitive impairment. *Alzheimer Disease and Associated Disorders, 24*(4), 365–371.

Van Gorp, W. G., Marcotte, T. D., Sultzer, D., Hinkin, C., Mahler, M., & Cummings, J. L. (1999). Screening for dementia: Comparison of three commonly used instruments. *Journal of Clinical and Experimental Neuropsychology, 21,* 29–38.

Van Reekum, R., Simard, M., Clarke, D., Conn, D., Cohen, T., & Wong, J. (2000). The role of depression severity in the cognitive functioning of elderly subjects with central nervous system disease. *Journal of Psychiatry and Neuroscience, 25,* 262–268.

Vangel Jr., S. J., & Lichtenberg, P. A. (1995) Mattis Dementia Rating Scale: Clinical utility and relationship with demographic variables. *The Clinical Neuropsychologist, 9,* 209–213.

Villeneuve, S., Rodrigues-Brazète, J., Joncas, S., Postuma, R. B., Latreille, V., & Gagnon, J. (2011). Validity of the Mattis Dementia Rating Scale to detect mild cognitive impairment in Parkinson's disease and REM sleep behavior disorder. *Dementia and Geriatric Cognitive Disorders, 31*(3), 210–217.

Vitaliano, P. P., Breen, A. R., Russo, J., Albert, M., Vitiello, M., & Prinz, P. N. (1984). The clinical utility of the Dementia Rating Scale for assessing Alzheimer's patients. *Journal of Chronic Disabilities, 37*(9/10), 743–753.

Wang, J., Eslinger, P. J., Doty, R. L., Zimmerman, E. K., Grunfeld, R., Sun, X., . . . Yang, Q. X. (2010). Olfactory deficit detected by fMRI in early Alzheimer's disease. *Brain Research, 1357,* 184–194.

Williams, P. G., Suchy, Y., & Kraybill, M. L. (2013). Preliminary evidence for low openness to experience as a pre-clinical marker of incipient cognitive decline in older adults. *Journal of Research in Personality, 47*(6), 945–951.

Woodard, J. L., Auchus, A. P., Godsall, R. E., & Green, R. C. (1998). An analysis of test bias and differential item functioning due to race on the Mattis Dementia Rating Scale. *Journal of Gerontology: Psychological Sciences, 53B,* 370–374.

Woodard, J. L., Salthouse, T. A., Godsall, R. E., & Green, R. C. (1996). Confirmatory factor analysis of the Mattis Dementia Rating Scale in patients with Alzheimer's disease. *Psychological Assessment, 8,* 85–91.

Yochim, B. P., Bank, A. L., Mast, B. T., MacNeill, S. E., & Lichtenberg, P. A. (2003). Clinical utility of the Mattis Dementia Rating Scale in older, urban medical patients: An expanded study. *Aging, Neuropsychology and Cognition, 10,* 230–237.

GENERAL PRACTITIONER ASSESSMENT OF COGNITION (GPCOG)

TEST NAME	**General Practitioner Assessment of Cognition (GPCOG)**
DOMAIN	Dementia screening
AGE RANGE	50+ years
ADMINISTRATION TIME	4 to 6 minutes
SCORING FORMAT	Hand scored and web-based scoring
REFERENCE	Brodaty, H., Pond, D., Kemp, N. M., Luscombe, G., Harding, L., Berman, K., & Huppert, F. (2002). The GPCOG: A new screening test for dementia designed for general practice. *Journal of the American Geriatrics Society, 50,* 530–534.

DESCRIPTION

The General Practitioner Assessment of Cognition (GPCOG) is a brief dementia screen for use specifically in the primary care setting. It includes a Patient Examination section and an Informant Interview section. The Patient Examination section comprises items measuring orientation, current affairs, memory, and clock drawing. An informant provides a report of the examinee's everyday functioning in the Informant Interview section. Translations are available in 22 languages and can be downloaded for free at http://www.gpcog.com.au.

ADMINISTRATION

The English version of the GPCOG is reproduced in Figure 7–1. Users may refer to the figure for specific test administration instructions. The two sections can be administered together or sequentially. It may be more time efficient to administer the sections sequentially because the informant section need not be administered unless the examinee scored between 5 and 8. The Patient Examination section takes less than four minutes to administer, while the Informant Interview section takes no more than two additional minutes. An interactive web-based administration and scoring is also available at http://www.gpcog.com.au.

SCORING

One point is given to each correct response to a maximum score of 9 on the Patient Examination section. The Informant Interview section is scored based on the number of "no" responses to a maximum of 6 points. In this section, only examinee difficulties that are changed compared to a few years ago are to be scored. When summed together, higher scores represent better performance. A cutoff score of 10/11 or less is used to screen for dementia.

DEMOGRAPHIC EFFECTS

Age and education effects on GPCOG patient scores are small, whereas no demographic effects have been reported on the informant scores (Brodaty et al., 2004), including in multicultural samples (Basic et al., 2009). Most studies do not find age and education effects on GPCOG total scores (Brodaty et al., 2002; Basic et al., 2009; Pirani et al., 2010), although one study showed that age has the greatest effects on the total score, with those older than 80 obtaining the highest rate of misclassification for dementia (22%) compared to those younger than 80 (1 to 8%) (Brodaty et al., 2004). GPCOG scores are not affected by gender (Basic et al., 2009; Brodaty et al., 2002, 2004; Pirani et al., 2010).

EVIDENCE FOR RELIABILITY

EVIDENCE FOR INTERNAL RELIABILITY

Evidence for internal consistency is high for both Patient Examination and Informant Interview sections (Cronbach's alpha = .84 for Patient Examination section, and .80 for Informant Interview section) (Brodaty et al., 2002).

EVIDENCE FOR TEST-RETEST RELIABILITY, MEASURING CHANGE, AND PRACTICE EFFECTS

Evidence for test-retest reliability ranges from high to very high. The two-week test-retest reliability of the Chinese version is excellent (r = .98) (Li et al., 2013). The original version has high test-retest reliability (r = .87 for Patient Examination section and .84 for Informant Interview section) over five weeks (Brodaty et al., 2002).

EVIDENCE FOR RELIABILITY OF ALTERNATE FORMS

Not available.

GPCOG Patient Examination

Unless specified, each question should only be asked once.

Name and address for subsequent recall test

1. *"I am going to give you a name and address. After I have said it, I want you to repeat it. Remember this name and address because I am going to ask you to tell it to me again in a few minutes: John Brown, 42 West Street, Kensington."* (Allow a maximum of 4 attempts but do not score yet)

	Correct	Incorrect
Time Orientation		
2. *What is the date?* (exact only)	☐	☐
Clock Drawing (visuospatial functioning) - use page with printed circle		
3. *Please mark in all the numbers to indicate the hours of a clock* (correct spacing required)	☐	☐
4. *Please mark in hands to show 10 minutes past eleven o'clock* (11:10)	☐	☐
Information		
5. *Can you tell me something that happened in the news recently?* (recently = in the last week)	☐	☐
Recall		
6. *What was the name and address I asked you to remember?*		
John	☐	☐
Brown	☐	☐
42	☐	☐
West (St)	☐	☐
Kensington	☐	☐

Scoring guidelines

Clock drawing: For a correct response to question 3, the numbers 12, 3, 6, and 9 should be in the correct quadrants of the circle and the other numbers should be approximately correctly placed. For a correct response to question 4, the hands should be pointing to the 11 and the 2, but do not penalize if the respondent fails to distinguish the long and short hands.

Information: Respondents are not required to provide extensive details, as long as they demonstrate awareness of a recent news story. If a general answer is given, such as "war," "a lot of rain," ask for details—if unable to give details, the answer should be scored as incorrect.

GPCOG Informant Interview

Ask the informant: *"Compared to a few years ago,*

		Yes	No	Don't Know	N/A
I.	*Does the patient have more trouble remembering things that have happened recently?*	☐	☐	☐	
II.	*Does he or she have more trouble recalling conversations a few days later?*	☐	☐	☐	
III.	*When speaking, does the patient have more difficulty in finding the right word or tend to use the wrong words more often?*	☐	☐	☐	
IV.	*Is the patient less able to manage money and financial affairs (e.g., paying bills, budgeting)?*	☐	☐	☐	☐
V.	*Is the patient less able to manage his or her medication independently?*	☐	☐	☐	☐
VI.	*Does the patient need more assistance with transport (either private or public)?*	☐	☐	☐	☐

Figure 7–1 *Administration and scoring guidelines for the General Practitioner Assessment of Cognition (GPCOG).*
SOURCE: Brodaty et al. (2002).

EVIDENCE FOR INTERRATER RELIABILITY

Interrater reliability among general practitioners is adequate for the Patient Examination section (r = .75) and low (r = .56) for the Informant Interview section (Brodaty et al., 2002). The Chinese version has very high interrater reliability (Li et al., 2013).

EVIDENCE FOR VALIDITY

RELATIONSHIPS WITHIN-TEST

The correlation between Patient Examination and Informant Interview sections is moderate (r = .57; Basic et al., 2009).

RELATIONSHIPS WITH OTHER TESTS

The GPCOG total and subsections show strong to very strong correlations with the MMSE and Rowland Universal Dementia Assessment Scale (RUDAS; r = .55 to .83), with the Informant Interview section showing the lesser correlation coefficient (Basic et al., 2009). The Italian version also shows strong to very strong correlations with the MMSE, CAMCOG, ADAS-Cog, and CDR-SB (r = −.55 to .84; Pirani et al., 2010).

The GPCOG Patient Examination section but not the Informant Interview section is minimally correlated with Geriatric Depression Scale (GDS) scores (r = −.13).

Frequency of contact with the physician has no impact on the scores (Basic et al., 2009; Brodaty et al., 2004).

CLINICAL STUDIES

The GPCOG has been tested within a primary care setting with good results. At a 29% dementia base rate, the total score yielded reasonably good sensitivity (82%), specificity (83%), PPV (67%), NPV (92%), and overall misclassification rate (17%) for dementia, although the two-stage method (where only patient section scores of 5–8 out of 9 required completion of the informant interview) was slightly better (sensitivity = 85%, specificity = 86%, PPV = 71%, NPV = 93%, and misclassification rate = 14%). Both scoring methods obtained lower misclassification rates than the MMSE (23%) and Abbreviated Mental Test (22%), supporting the GPCOG's utility for dementia detection in the primary care setting (Brodaty et al., 2002).

Within community samples, the original as well as the translated versions are generally adequate at identifying dementia (Basic et al., 2009; Li et al., 2013; Pirani et al., 2010). Table 7–33 shows the sensitivity, specificity, PPV, and NPV of the various translations. Misclassification rates for the Italian version were 9% for the total score and 17% for the two-stage method (Pirani et al., 2010). The GPCOG outperformed the RUDAS and MMSE for identifying dementia in community samples (Basic et al., 2009).

Depression has been found to affect performance on the GPCOG. Those who are depressed have a 20% rate of being misclassified. In a sample of primary care patients at a dementia base rate of 29%, the GPCOG yielded a sensitivity of 92%, specificity of 71%, PPV of 71%, and NPV of 92% for depression (Brodaty et al., 2004). Therefore, caution must be practiced when interpreting GPCOG scores in those who are depressed, as is the case for most dementia screeners.

NEUROANATOMICAL CORRELATES AND IMAGING STUDIES

Not available.

PERFORMANCE VALIDITY

Not available.

COMMENT

The GPCOG was developed as a brief screen to detect dementia within primary care settings. It is unique in that it includes an informant section to enhance the sensitivity of dementia identification. Studies to date have shown good psychometric properties for dementia screening. Primary care physicians have been surveyed about their use of GPCOG, with the majority surveyed finding the GPCOG highly practical, economically viable, and acceptable to patient. The majority of the primary care physicians surveyed also said they were satisfied or very satisfied with the GPCOG and would continue to use it (Brodaty et al., 2002). The GPCOG is free to use, and a web-based interactive administration is available for ease of administration and scoring. Many translated versions are available and have been validated in separate studies.

In general, reviews of the cognitive screens used in primary care or community samples reported in the literature have concluded that while the MMSE continues to be the most widely utilized cognitive screening test, the GPCOG, Memory Impairment Screen (MIS), and Mini-Cog appear equally or better suited than the MMSE as a cognitive screen in primary care (Brodaty et al., 2006; Culverwell et al., 2008; Ismail et al., 2010; Lorentz et al., 2002; Milne et al., 2008; Yokomizo et al., 2014). These tests have been found to be brief, easy to administer, acceptable to primary care physicians, psychometrically sound, and not affected by education, ethnicity, and gender (Brodaty et al., 2006; Culverwell et al., 2008; Lorentz et al., 2002; Milne et al., 2008). It is also of note that the GPCOG yielded the highest predictive utility for dementia within community samples among all tests in a systematic review (Yokomizo et al., 2014).

Although the GPCOG is an effective dementia screen, caution is needed when using the GPCOG with adults age 80 and older, or in older adults who are depressed because of the high misclassification rate (Brodaty et al., 2004). Furthermore, there is limited evidence on the etiology of dementia when an individual performs below the cut-score. The studies conducted to date have depended on clinical diagnosis of dementia, and no studies using autopsy-confirmed dementia cases have been carried out. Information on neuroanatomical/imaging correlates is also lacking. Regardless,

TABLE 7–33 Sensitivity, Specificity, PPV, NPV, and AUC of Different GPCOG Translated Versions

	SENSITIVITY (%)	SPECIFICITY (%)	PPV (%)	NPV (%)	AUC	DEMENTIA BASE RATE
English (Basic et al., 2009)	98	77	–	–	.97	Not reported
Chinese (Li et al., 2013)	97	86	53 (88)*	100 (98)*	.97	51%
Italian (Pirani et al., 2010)	92	88	92	88	.96	Not reported

NOTE: Cutoff score of 10 for English version, 10/11 for translated versions.

*Values in parenthesis are based on 51% dementia base rate.

PPV, positive predictive value; NPV, negative predictive value; AUC, area under the curve.

the GPCOG appears to show promise as a primary care dementia screening measure to identify older adults who may benefit from further comprehensive dementia workup.

REFERENCES

Basic, D., Khoo, A., Conforti, D., Rowland, J., Vrantsidis, F., LoGiudice, D., . . . Prowse, R. (2009). Rowland Universal Dementia Assessment Scale, Mini-Mental State Examination and General Practitioner Assessment of Cognition in a multicultural cohort of community-dwelling older persons with early dementia. *Australian Psychologist, 44*(1), 40–53.

Brodaty, H., Kemp, N. M., & Low, L. (2004). Characteristics of the GPCOG, a screening tool for cognitive impairment. *International Journal of Geriatric Psychiatry, 19*(9), 870–874.

Brodaty, H., Low, L., Gibson, L., & Burns, K. (2006). What is the best dementia screening instrument for general practitioners to use? *The American Journal of Geriatric Psychiatry, 14*(5), 391–400.

Brodaty, H., Pond, D., Kemp, N. M., Luscombe, G., Harding, L., Berman, K., & Huppert, F. A. (2002). The GPCOG: A new screening test for dementia designed for general practice. *Journal of the American Geriatrics Society, 50*(3), 530–534.

Culverwell, A., Milne, A., Guss, R., & Tuppen, J. (2008). Screening for dementia in primary care: how is it measuring up? *Quality in Ageing and Older Adults, 9* (3), 39–44.

Ismail, Z., Rajji, T. K., & Shulman, K. I. (2010). Brief cognitive screening instruments: An update. *International Journal of Geriatric Psychiatry, 25*(2), 111–120.

Li, X., Xiao, S., Fang, Y., Zhu, M., Wang, T., Seeher, K., & Brodaty, H. (2013). Validation of the General Practitioner Assessment of Cognition-Chinese version (GPCOG-C) in China. *International Psychogeriatrics, 25*(10), 1649–1657.

Lorentz, W. J., Scanlan, J. M., & Borson, S. (2002). Brief screening tests for dementia. *The Canadian Journal of Psychiatry/La Revue Canadienne De Psychiatrie, 47*(8), 723–733.

Milne, A., Culverwell, A., Guss, R., Tuppen, J., & Whelton, R. (2008). Screening for dementia in primary care: A review of the use, efficacy and quality of measures. *International Psychogeriatrics, 20*(5), 911–926.

Pirani, A., Brodaty, H., Martini, E., Zaccherini, D., Neviani, F., & Neri, M. (2010). The validation of Italian version of the GPCOG (GPCOG-it): A contribution to cross-national implementation of a screening test for dementia in general practice. *International Psychogeriatrics, 22*(1), 82–90.

Yokomizo, J. E., Simon, S. S., & de Campos, B. (2014). Cognitive screening for dementia in primary care: A systematic review. *International Psychogeriatrics / IPA, 26*(11), 1783–1804.

MINI-MENTAL STATE EXAMINATION (MMSE), MINI-MENTAL STATE EXAMINATION, 2ND EDITION (MMSE-2), AND MODIFIED MINI-MENTAL STATE (3MS)

TEST NAME	**Mini-Mental State Examination (MMSE), Mini-Mental State Examination, 2nd Edition (MMSE-2), and Modified Mini-Mental State (3MS)**
DOMAIN	Dementia screening
AGE RANGE	18 to 100 years
ADMINISTRATION TIME	10 minutes
SCORING FORMAT	Hand scored
REFERENCES	Folstein, M. F., Folstein, S. E., & McHugh, P. R. (1975). "Mini-Mental State". A practical method for grading the cognitive state of patients for the clinician. *Journal of Psychiatric Research, 12,* 189–198. Folstein, M. F., Folstein, S. E., White, T., Messer, M. (2010). *MMSE-2 Manual.* Lutz, FL: PAR. Teng, E. L., & Chui, H. C. (1987). The Modified Mini-Mental State (3MS) examination. *Journal of Clinical Psychiatry, 48,* 314–318. www.parinc.com

DESCRIPTION

The Mini-Mental State Examination (MMSE) is a popular measure to screen for cognitive impairment, to track cognitive changes that occur with time, and to assess the effects of potential therapeutic agents on cognitive functioning. It is attractive because it is brief, easily administered, and easily scored. Most studies report that the MMSE summary score is sensitive to the presence of dementia, particularly in those with moderate to severe forms of cognitive impairment. However, it is less than ideal in those with mild cognitive deficits.

Because of the shortcomings of the original version, an updated version, the Mini-Mental State Examination, 2nd Edition (MMSE-2; Folstein et al., 2010), is now commercially available via PAR, which now holds the copyright to the MMSE, although limited independent studies have been done at this time. The clinician can choose from three versions of the MMSE-2 depending on the purpose of the screen. This includes a brief version (MMSE-2:BV) for rapid administration, designed for screening purposes in population studies; a standard version (MMSE-2:SV; referred to as MMSE-2 in this chapter) similar to the original; and an expanded version (MMSE-2:EV) that is purportedly sensitive to mild cognitive dysfunction and subcortical dementia. The items have been modified to allow for easy translation to other languages. As such, the MMSE-2 is available in many different languages, including Dutch, French, German, Hindi, Italian, Russian, simplified Chinese, and Spanish. Moreover, each version has an equivalent alternate form to minimize practice effects on serial examination.

MMSE AND MMSE-2

The MMSE-2 retains the same structure as the original MMSE. The items assess orientation to time and place, attention and calculation (serial 7s), language (naming, repetition, comprehension, reading, writing, copying), and registration and delayed recall. In the MMSE-2, the words for the registration and delayed recall items were changed based on grammatical usage, imagery, number of syllables, and familiarity in most languages. The selection process resulted in words that are slightly more challenging than the original MMSE words. Spelling "world" backward was eliminated as an alternate item. Modifications were also made to the repetition and comprehension items to allow for easily translation to other languages and to make it easier for those with physical limitations to complete, respectively.

The Brief Version (MMSE-2:BV) is comprised of MMSE-2 items assessing registration and delayed recall, as well as orientation to time and place. For the Expanded Version (MMSE-2:EV), two items that measure story memory and processing speed are added to the standard version to reduce ceiling effects and increase sensitivity to mild cognitive dysfunction and subcortical dementia.

To date, almost all studies have employed the original MMSE.

MODIFIED MINI-MENTAL STATE (3MS)

The 3MS is a popular expansion of the original MMSE that has been in use for more than 30 years (Teng & Chui, 1987). Four additional questions that assess temporal and spatial orientation, the ability to see relations between objects, and verbal fluency (i.e., date and place of birth, word fluency, similarities, and delayed recall of words) were added. In addition, the 3MS includes items that assess different aspects of memory including cued recall, recognition memory, delayed free and cued recall, and delayed recognition memory. One of the advantages of the 3MS is that both a 3MS and an MMSE score can be derived from a single administration.

The 3MS has been modified (3MS-R; Tschantz et al., 2002). The modifications are primarily in the area of assessing remote memory where the authors substituted the recall of personal demographic information (date and place of birth) with the recall of current and past prominent politicians to make the information easier to verify. They also changed some of the item scaling in the orientation section and shortened the time allotted for the verbal fluency item (from 30 to 20 seconds).

SHORT FORMS

A short form of the MMSE (Short MMSE) comprising the three-word registration and three-word delayed recall has been tested as a dementia screen for use in primary care (Haubois et al., 2013; Stein et al., 2015). A simpler version of the MMSE, the Severe-MMSE (SMMSE), has been developed to monitor the cognitive functioning of those with moderate to severe AD. The SMMSE has simpler commands and questions such as birthdate and complete name, constructional praxis, spelling, and animal fluency (Wajman et al., 2014).

ADMINISTRATION AND SCORING

See Source. The MMSE/MMSE-2 is generally straightforward to administer and can be scored rapidly. All correct items are summed together to a maximum total of 30 points, with higher points representing better cognitive functioning. A cutoff score of less than 24 is typically used to identify dementia on the MMSE. However, age- and education-adjusted cut-scores are preferred (see the section "Normative Data").

The MMSE-2:BV total score yields a maximum of 16 points. The expanded MMSE-2 (MMSE-2:EV) takes about 20 minutes to administer and has a 0–90 point range. The MMSE-2 provides T scores corrected for age and education, as well as reliable change scores for serial testing. Use of a standard cut-score is not recommended on the MMSE-2. Rather, users are instructed to use age- and education-adjusted T scores provided in the Manual.

For the 3MS, the maximum score is 100 points. A modified scoring procedure was introduced that allows partial credit for some items (see Figure 7–2).

A qualitative scoring approach for the pentagon item on the MMSE has been proposed to differentiate AD from DLB based on five criteria (Caffarra et al., 2013). The criteria include (1) number of angles, (2) distance/intersection between the two figures, (3) closing/opening of the contour, (4) rotation of one or both pentagons, and (5) closing-in and a total score corresponding to the sum of individual scores of each parameter. For specific scoring criteria, see Table 7–34.

USING MMSE TO PREDICT WAIS-IV FSIQ

The MMSE can be used to predict WAIS-IV FSIQ using a regression-based prediction equation (Sugarman & Axelrod, 2014). The equations were generated from a sample of older veterans age 60+ who were referred by their physicians for neuropsychological evaluation:

$$\text{FSIQ} = 2.32 \times \text{MMSE} + 26.16,$$
$$\text{error in prediction} = 8.5\ (SD = 6.3)$$

This equation is accurate to within 5 FSIQ points in 34% of the sample, within 10 points in 63% of the sample, and within 15 points in 87% of the sample. Raw scores of 23 or less predict borderline FSIQ or lower, and an MMSE of less than 25 predicts less than 85 FSIQ.

USING MMSE AND TEST OF PREMORBID FUNCTIONING (TOPF) TO PREDICT WAIS-IV FSIQ

The prediction can be improved with the addition of the TOPF score, accounting for 49% of the variance in obtained FSIQ (Sugarman & Axelrod, 2014).

$$\text{FSIQ} = (.44 \times \text{R-TOPF}) + (.23 \times \text{D-TOPF}) + (1.61 \times \text{MMSE}) - 17.37,$$
$$\text{error in prediction} = 7.0\ (SD = 5.4)$$

where R-TOPF = TOPF Word Reading; D-TOPF = TOPF demographic variables.

This equation is accurate to within 5 points in 40% of the sample, within 10 points for 75%, and within 15 points for 90% of the sample.

DEMOGRAPHIC EFFECTS

AGE

MMSE/3MS scores decrease with advancing age in adults (Anderson et al., 2007; Ansari et al., 2010; Antsey et al., 2000; Bravo & Hebert, 1997; Brown et al., 2003; Crum et al., 1993; Dufouil et al., 2000; Freidl et al., 1996; Mokri et al., 2013; Mystakidou et al., 2007; O'Connell et al., 2004; Tombaugh & McIntyre, 1992; Tombaugh et al., 1996). Most of the age-related change in adults begins at about age 55 to 60 and then dramatically accelerates at the age of 75 to 80. Healthy centenarians could score as low as 12 points compared to near centenarians, who score about 19 points. These age effects persist even when individuals are stratified by educational level (Dai et al., 2013). Limited information is available on the MMSE-2. The MMSE-2 Manual reports that about 6% of the variance on the Brief and Standard Versions was accounted for by age while 14% was accounted for on the Expanded Version.

GENDER

Gender has little impact on the total score (e.g., Ansari et al., 2010; Antsey et al., 2000; Besson & Labbe, 1997; Bravo & Hebert, 1997), except among centenarians, with men scoring higher than women (Dai et al., 2013). There are suggestions that the gender effect varies as a function of education. For example, healthy women with primary or lower education obtain the lowest scores of all (Ibrahim et al., 2009). Gender may also influence performance on some items. For example, Jones and Gallo (2002) reported that women are more likely to err on serial subtractions and men on spelling and other language tasks; however, the magnitude of the effect tends to be quite small. Gender effects are not seen on individual items among centenarians (Dai et al., 2013). Gender effects are not reported on the MMSE-2.

EDUCATION AND IQ

MMSE/3MS scores are related to premorbid intelligence and educational attainment: individuals with higher premorbid ability and/or more education tend to score higher than those with lower IQs and/or few years of schooling (Anderson et al., 2007; Ansari et al., 2010; Antsey et al., 2000; Bravo & Hebert, 1997; Brown et al., 2003; Crum et al., 1993; de Silva et al., 2009; Dufouil et al., 2000; Fountoulakis et al., 2000; Freidl et al., 1996; Ishizaki et al., 1998; Marcopulos et al., 1997; Mokri et al., 2013; O'Connell et al., 2004; Ouvrier et al., 1993; Tombaugh et al., 1996). Over a span of more than 10 years, those with more education outperform those with less education in Total and non-memory scores; memory items appear less affected by education (Matallana et al., 2011). However, IQ has a stronger relationship to MMSE scores than education (Bieliauskas et al., 2000). On the MMSE-2, education effects accounted for about 5 to 8%

Modified Mini-Mental State Examination (3MS)

Name: ____________________ Date: __________ Age: ______ Education: ________ Gender: ________

Total Score: ________/100 Administered by: _______________

___ **Date & Place of Birth**
5

- What is your date of birth? Date: year _____(1) month ______(1) day _____(1)
- What is your place of birth? Place: town __________(1) state/province __________(1)

___ **Registration** (no. of trials needed to repeat all three words ______)
3

- I shall say three words for you to remember. Repeat them after I have said all three words.
  SHIRT (1), BROWN (1), HONESTY (1) [or SHOES, BLACK, MODESTY; or SOCKS, BLUE, CHARITY]
- Remember what they are because I am going to ask you to name them again in a few minutes.

___ **Mental Reversal**
7

- Can you count from 1 to 10? Like this, 1, 2, 3, all the way to 10. Go. (no score)
- If correct: Now, can you count backwards from 5? Go. Accurate (2); 1 or 2 misses (1)
- Now I am going to spell a word forwards and I want you to spell it backwards. The word is "world." W-O-R-L-D. Spell "world" backwards.

______________ (D L R O W) Each correctly placed letter (5)

___ **First Recall**
9

- What are the three words that I asked you to remember? (If not recalled, provide a category prompt; if not recalled, ask them to choose one of the three multiple-choice options; if correct answer not given, score 0 and provide the correct answer.)

Spontaneous Recall	SHIRT (3) BROWN (3) HONESTY (3)
Category Prompt	Something to wear (2) a color (2) a good personal quality (2)
Multiple Choice	Shoes, Shirt, Socks (1) Blue, Black, Brown (1) Honesty, Charity, Modesty (1)

___ **Temporal Orientation**
15

• What is the year?	______	Accurate (8); miss by 1 year (4); miss by 2-5 years (2)
• What is the season?	______	Accurate or within 1 month (1)
• What is the month?	______	Accurate within 5 days (2); miss by 1 month (1)
• What is the date?	______	Accurate (3); miss by 1-2 days (2); miss by 3-5 days (1)
• What is the day of the week?	______	Accurate (1)

Figure 7–2 *Modified Mini-Mental State (3MS) Examination.*

SOURCE: Reproduced by special permission of the Publisher, Psychological Assessment Resources, Inc. (PAR), 16204 North Florida Avenue, Lutz, Florida 33549, from Teng, E. L., & Chui, H. C. (1987). The Modified Mini-Mental State (3MS) Examination. *Journal of Clinical Psychiatry, 48*, 314-318. Further reproduction is prohibited without permission of PAR.

___ **Spatial Orientation**
5

- Can you tell me where we are right now? E.g., what state/province are we in? ________ (2)
- What city are we in? _______________ (1)
- Are we in a hospital or office building or home? _______________ (1)
- What is the name of this place? _____________________ (1)
- What floor of the building are we on? _____________(1)

___ **Naming**
5

- What is this called? (show wristwatch) _________ (no points)
- What is this called? (show pencil) _________ (no points)
- What is this called? (point to a part of your own body: score 0 if client cannot readily name)
  Shoulder (1) Chin (1) Forehead (1) Elbow (1) Knuckle (1)

___ **Four-Legged Animals**
10

- What animals have four legs? Allow 30 seconds (record responses). If no response after 10 seconds, repeat the question once. Prompt after only the first incorrect answer by saying: I want four-legged animals.

___ **Similarities**
6

- In what way are an arm and a leg alike? Body parts; limbs (2) Less accurate answer (1 or 0)
  If incorrect, this time only, prompt with: An arm and leg are both limbs or parts of the body.
- In what way are laughing and crying alike? Feelings; emotions (2) Less accurate answer (1 or 0)
- In what way are eating and sleeping alike? Essential for life (2) Less accurate answer (1 or 0)

___ **Repetition**
5

- Repeat what I say: I would like to go home/out. Accurate (2) 1-2 missed/wrong words (1 or 0)
- Now repeat: No ifs, ands, or buts. Accurate (3) One point each (1 or 2)
  (no credit if "s" is left off a word)

___ **Read & Obey** (Hold up paper on which the command is printed "Close your eyes")
3

- Please do this. (wait 5 seconds; if no response provide next prompt)
- Read and do what this says. (if already said or reads the sentence only provide next prompt)
- Do what this says.

Obeys without prompting (3) Obeys after prompting (2) Reads aloud only (no eye closure) (1 or 0)

___ **Writing**
5

- Provide pencil with eraser and say: Please write this down "I would like to go home/out." Repeat sentence word by word, if necessary. Allow one minute. Do not penalize self-corrections. (1) point for each word, except "I"

___ **Copying Two Pentagons**
10

- Here is a drawing. Please copy the drawing on the same paper. Allow one minute. If longer time is needed, document how much of design was complete in one minute and allow to finish.

	Pentagon 1	Pentagon 2
5 approximately equal sides	(4)	(4)
5 unequal sides (>2:1)	(3)	(3)
Other enclosed figure	(2)	(2)
2 or more lines	(1)	(1)
Less than 2 lines	(0)	(0)

Intersection: 4 corners (2) Not-4-corner enclosure (1) No enclosure (0)

___ **Three-Stage Command**
3

Hold up a sheet of plain paper and say:
- Take this paper with your left hand (1), fold it in half (1), and hand it back to me (1).

(Note: use right hand for left-handed clients; do not repeat any part of the command or give visual cues to return the paper, such as keeping hand in ready to receive posture.)

___ **Second Recall**
9

- What are the three words that I asked you to remember? (If not recalled, provide a category prompt; if not recalled, ask them to choose one of the three multiple-choice options; if correct answer not given, score 0).

Spontaneous Recall	SHIRT (3) BROWN (3) HONESTY (3)
Category Prompt	Something to wear (2) a color (2) a good personal quality (2)
Multiple Choice	Shoes, Shirt, Socks (1) Blue, Black, Brown (1) Honesty, Charity, Modesty (1)

Figure 7–2 *Continued*

CLOSE YOUR EYES

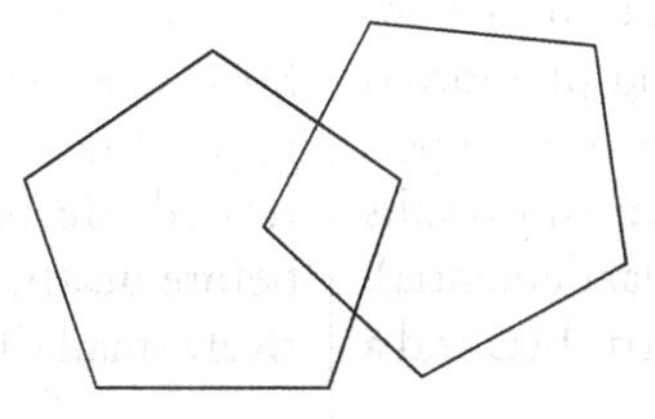

Figure 7–2 Continued

TABLE 7–34 Qualitative Scoring Method for Mini-Mental State Examination (MMSE) Pentagon Copy

PARAMETERS	SCORE	CRITERIA
Number of angles	4	10
	3	10±1
	2	10±2
	1	7–5
	0	<5 or >13
Distance/ Intersection	4	Correct intersection
	3	Wrong intersection
	2	Contact without intersection
	1	No contact, distance <1 cm
	0	No contact, distance >1 cm
Closure/ Opening*	2	Closing both figures
	1	Closing only one figure
	0	Opening both figures
Rotation**	2	Correct orientation of both figures
	1	Rotation of one figure (either one figure is absent or it is not a Pentagon—not assessable)
	0	Rotation of both figures (or both not assessable-like pentagons
Closing in	1	Absent
	0	Present
Total	Sum of 1 + 2 + 3 + 4 + 5	

*Figure is considered closed even if two sides do not touch each other but the distance is ≤ 1 mm.

**When there is not a figure or figure is not a pentagon (then rotation is not assessable) score is 0. When rotation is less than 45°, figure is not considered a rotation. Tremor is ignored.

SOURCE: From Caffarra et al. (2013).

of the variance on the Brief and Expanded Versions and 15% on the Standard Version.

There is evidence that low educational or intelligence levels increase the likelihood of misclassifying healthy people as cognitively impaired, while higher ability and educational levels may mask mild impairment. For example, in one Brazilian study, using the MMSE to identify dementia resulted in four times more dementia diagnoses than when using DSM-IV criteria for dementia among illiterate older adults. The use of different thresholds based on education still resulted in significant rates of misclassification: those with one or more years of education were 42% less likely to be misclassified by MMSE than those with no formal education (Scazufca et al., 2009). Education and premorbid ability, however, may reflect etiological factors (e.g., hypertension, obesity) critical in the process that eventually results in some form of dementia (e.g., ischemic vascular dementia). In short, education may represent a psychometric bias and a risk factor.

ETHNICITY, NATIONALITY, AND LINGUISTIC EFFECTS

No information is available on the MMSE-2. There is some evidence that MMSE scores are affected by ethnicity and social class (e.g., Anderson et al., 2007; Espino et al., 2004; Mulgrew et al., 1999). MMSE scores tend to be decreased in individuals of non-white ethnicity (Espino et al., 2001, 2004; Shadlen et al., 1999; Tappen et al., 2012; but see Ford et al., 1996; Marcopulos et al., 1997; Marcopulos & McLain, 2003) and lower social class. The ethnic differences appear to attenuate when the MMSE is combined with the FAQ for cognitive status classification (Tappen et al., 2012). Ethnic differences, at least in the case of Mexican Americans, appear related to educational differences and location of residence (neighborhood), with barrio residents scoring considerably lower than Mexican Americans living in transitional neighborhoods and the suburbs (Espino et al., 2001). Espino and colleagues (2001) have speculated that regional differences reflect cultural and social factors (e.g., differences in familiarity with the kinds of skills measured by the MMSE, daily stress, and assimilation).

Some of the items appear to be biased with respect to ethnicity and education (Jones & Gallo, 2002; Mulgrew et al., 1999; Teresi et al., 2001). For example, the sentence production item appears easier for Caucasians than for African Americans. The items "Close your eyes" and serial 7s are also problematic, having different results for various ethnic and education groups. Among healthy centenarians, the concentration item was affected by race, while the orientation item was affected by residential status (Dai et al., 2013).

There is also some evidence that language of testing may impact performance. For example, Bravo and Hebert (1997) noted that English-speaking older adults performed slightly better than their French-speaking counterparts, although the effect was very small (less than one point for the MMSE and about two points for the 3MS). In another study, Spanish-speaking Mexican Americans obtained higher scores than their English-speaking counterparts once scores were adjusted for education (Matallana et al., 2011). When Japanese speakers were compared to Americans, recall and auditory comprehension were easier for the Japanese, but reading comprehension and sentence construction were easier for the Americans. Registration, naming, and constructional praxis showed no difference (Dodge et al., 2009).

OTHER

Health status (e.g., history of heart disease) impacts performance (Antsey et al., 2000). There is also evidence that impending mortality lowers performance. The mortality-related effects appear most pronounced within three years before death; however, the magnitude of the effect is relatively small (Tan, 2004).

NORMATIVE DATA

MMSE

Extensive norms by age (18 to approximately 85 years) and education (no formal schooling to one or more college degrees) have been reported (Crum et al., 1993), based on probability sampling of more than 18,000 community-dwelling adults. The sample includes individuals, regardless of their physical or mental health status, from five US metropolitan areas: New Haven, Baltimore, Durham, St. Louis, and Los Angeles. The data are presented in Table 7–35. Iverson (1998) derived age- and education-corrected cutoff scores for individuals aged 60 and older in this dataset. The cutoffs, also shown in Table 7–35, are greater than 1.64 *SD*s below the sample mean (if normally distributed, 90% of all scores should fall within ±1.64 *z* score units from the mean). Note that the MMSE scores were based on either the response to serial 7s or spelling "world" backward, whichever yielded the higher score. Also note the wider range of scores in the lowest educational groups and at the oldest ages. MMSE scores ranged from a median of 29 for those aged 18 to 24 years to 25 for individuals aged 80 years and older. The median MMSE score was 29 for individuals with at least nine years of schooling, 26 for those with five to eight years of schooling, and 22 for those with zero to four years of schooling.

Schretlen, Testa, and Pearlson (2010) provide norms for 325 adults on the MMSE; these use the Calibrated Neuropsychological Normative System (CNNS) scoring to derive T scores and discrepancies, based on a large sample of older adults from the north-eastern US. Characteristics of the normative sample are shown in Table 7–36. The norms are available through Psychological Assessment Resources (PAR; www.parinc.com). A major advantage of these norms is the option to correct for demographic variables such as age, sex, education, and ethnicity. Several other commonly used neuropsychological tests are co-normed using this sample, which facilitates cross-test comparisons.

Similar data have been reported for rural US older adults (ages 55+; Marcopulos & McLain, 2003), participants (ages 65+) drawn from various geographical regions in Canada who were classified as cognitively intact on the basis of an extensive battery of neuropsychological and medical tests (Bravo & Hebert, 1997; Tombaugh et al., 1996), older adults (aged 62–95) living in retirement villages and institutions in Australia (Antsey et al., 2000), Spanish-speaking noninstitutionalized older Mexican adults (Table 7–37; Mokri et al., 2013), and Sri Lankans with low education (Table 7–38; de Silva et al., 2009). About 95% of nondemented older adults score greater than 23 on the MMSE (Bravo & Hebert, 1997; Meiran et al., 1996).

Because of the age and education impact on the MMSE, age- and education-adjusted MMSE scores are available based on a Mexican sample of healthy older adults and older adults with dementia due to vascular disease or AD aged 50+ (Table 7–39). Adjusted-MMSE (AMMSE) scores are highly correlated with original values (r = .89). The sensitivity/specificity of the AMMSE is higher at a cutoff of less than 25 than that of the MMSE at a cutoff of less than 24 for dementia (Villasenor-Cabrera et al., 2010). To obtain the age- and education-corrected AMMSE score, the respective value in Table 7–39 is added to the MMSE raw score.

MMSE-2

As seen in Table 7–40, the MMSE-2 was normed using 1,531 adults recruited mostly from 26 states. Cognitively impaired (dementia) samples were recruited from academic medical centers and private psychology clinics in the United States. Age- and education-corrected normative data are presented in Appendix A to C of the manual. A standard cutoff score is not used, but users are referred to tables 2–4 to 2–12 in the manual for cut-scores and their respective sensitivities, specificities, PPVs, and NPVs for dementia, AD, and subcortical dementia.

3MS

Bravo and Hebert (1997) provide data based on 7,754 adults, aged 65+, randomly chosen to take part in the Canadian Study of Health and Aging (CSHA). Individuals classified as cognitively impaired or demented following a clinical and neuropsychological examination were excluded. The reference values, stratified by age and education, are shown in Table 7–41. About 95% of the sample obtained a score greater than 76.

Other smaller normative sets have also been provided. Tombaugh et al. (1996) report percentile scores derived from a select subsample of the CSHA, judged to be cognitively intact on the basis of an extensive clinical examination. The normative data were stratified across two age groups (65–79 and 80–89) and two educational levels (0–8 and 9+ years). Jones et al. (2002) present normative data on the 3MS for a sample of 393 US community-dwelling, primarily Caucasian, older adults. Their sample of individuals aged 80+ or with less than 12 years of education is relatively small (N = 44).

Brown et al. (2003) provide normative data based on a sample of 238 African-American, community-dwelling older adults, aged 60 to 84. Tables 7–42 and 7–43 provide these data along with the score adjustments for education and gender. Brown et al. (2003) caution that the quality of education varies greatly within the population of African Americans and that matching on years of education does not necessarily mean that the quality of education is comparable.

EVIDENCE FOR RELIABILITY

EVIDENCE FOR INTERNAL RELIABILITY

MMSE

With regard to the original version, estimates of internal consistency range from .31 for community-based samples to .89 in advanced cancer patients to .96 for mixed medical patients (Espino et al., 2004; Hopp et al., 1997; Lopez et al.,

TABLE 7–35 Age- and Education-Weighted Norms for the Mini-Mental State Examination (MMSE)

	EDUCATION (YEARS)									
	0 TO 4		5 TO 8		9 TO 12		13+		ALL EDUCATION	
AGE	M	*SD*	M	*SD*	M	*SD*	M	*SD*	M	*SD*
18 to 24	22	2.9	27	2.7	29	2.2	29	1.3	29	2.0
	N = 17		*N* = 94		*N* = 1326		*N* = 783		*N* = 2220	
25 to 29	25	2.0	27	2.5	29	1.3	29	0.9	29	1.3
	N = 23		*N* = 83		*N* = 958		*N* = 1012		*N* = 2076	
30 to 34	25	2.4	26	1.8	29	1.3	29	1.0	29	1.3
	N = 41		*N* = 74		*N* = 822		*N* = 989		*N* = 1926	
35 to 39	23	2.5	26	2.8	28	1.8	29	1.0	29	1.8
	N = 33		*N* = 101		*N* = 668		*N* = 641		*N* = 1443	
40 to 44	23	2.5	27	1.8	28	1.9	29	1.7	28	2.0
	N = 36		*N* = 100		*N* = 489		*N* = 354		*N* = 979	
45 to 49	23	3.7	26	2.5	28	2.4	29	1.6	28	2.5
	N = 28		*N* = 121		*N* = 423		*N* = 259		*N* = 831	
50 to 54	23	2.6	27	2.4	28	2.2	29	1.5	28	2.4
	N = 34		*N* = 154		*N* = 462		*N* = 220		*N* = 870	
55 to 59	22	2.7	26	2.9	28	2.2	29	1.5	28	2.5
	N = 49		*N* = 208		*N* = 525		*N* = 231		*N* = 1013	
60 to 64	23	1.9	26	2.3	28	1.7	29	1.3	28	2.0
	N = 88		*N* = 310		*N* = 626		*N* = 270		*N* = 1294	
Abnormal cutoff	*19*		*22*		*25*		*26*		*24*	
65 to 69	22	1.9	26	1.7	28	1.4	29	1.0	27	1.6
	N = 126		*N* = 633		*N* = 814		*N* = 358		*N* = 1931	
Abnormal cutoff	*18*		*23*		*25*		*27*		*24*	
70 to 74	22	1.7	26	1.8	27	1.6	28	1.6	27	1.8
	N = 139		*N* = 533		*N* = 550		*N* = 255		*N* = 1477	
Abnormal cutoff	*19*		*23*		*24*		*25*		*24*	
75 to 79	21	2.0	25	2.1	27	1.5	28	1.6	26	2.1
	N = 112		*N* = 437		*N* = 315		*N* = 181		*N* = 1045	
Abnormal cutoff	*17*		*21*		*24*		*25*		*22*	
80 to 84	20	2.2	25	1.9	25	2.3	27	0.9	25	2.2
	N = 105		*N* = 241		*N* = 163		*N* = 96		*N* = 605	
Abnormal cutoff	*16*		*21*		*21*		*25*		*21*	
85+	19	2.9	23	3.3	26	2.0	27	1.3	24	2.9
	N = 61		*N* = 134		*N* = 99		*N* = 52		*N* = 346	
Abnormal cutoff	*14*		*17*		*22*		*24*		*19*	
All ages	22	2.3	26	2.2	28	1.9	29	1.3	28	2.0
	N = 892		*N* = 3223		*N* = 8240		*N* = 5701		*N* = 18056	

NOTE: Abnormal cutoff scores reflect greater than 1.64 *SD* below the sample means for those aged 60+; Iverson (1998).

N, number of individuals; M, Mean MMSE score; *SD*, Standard Deviation.

SOURCE: From Crum et al. (1993).

TABLE 7–36 Characteristics of the Mini-Mental State Examination (MMSE) Normative Sample from the Calibrated Neuropsychological Normative System (CNNS)

Sample size	325
Age	18 to 92 years
Geographic location	Baltimore, MD, and Hartford, CT, USA
Sample type	Community sample
Education	14.2 (*SD* = 3.0), range 3 to 20 years
Gender	56% Women 44% Men
Ethnicity	80% Caucasian 18% African American 2% Hispanic, Asian, or Other
Screening	History of Alzheimer's disease, Parkinson's disease, stroke, brain injury, bipolar disorder, or substance abuse

SOURCE: Adapted from Schretlen, Testa, and Pearlson (2010).

2005; Mystakidou et al., 2007; Tombaugh et al., 1996). The lower reliability in some samples likely reflects the reduced variability in healthy and better-educated samples.

The MMSE can be scored using three strategies: serial 7s or spelling (using the greater number of correct responses from either item), serial 7s only, and spelling only. In another study, the serial 7s-only method maximized variability and yielded the highest alpha coefficient ($r = .81$) in a community-based sample. The serial-7s or spelling method yielded a marginally adequate level ($r = .68$), while the alpha coefficient for the spelling-only method was less than optimal ($r = .59$; Espino et al., 2004).

Internal consistency of the Short MMSE was poor (Cronbach's alpha = .45; .49 at follow-up), though it is predictive of dementia at follow-up (Haubois et al., 2013; Stein et al., 2015).

MMSE-2

The internal consistency of the MMSE-2 is generally adequate but less so for the Brief Version ($r = .54$ to .79 and $r = .36$ to .73, respectively).

3MS

In studies comparing these directly, the internal consistency of the 3MS tends to be higher than that of the MMSE. For example, Tombaugh et al. (1996) reported that, in healthy individuals, Cronbach's alpha was .82 for the 3MS and .62 for the MMSE. For patients with AD, Cronbach's alpha was .88 for the 3MS and .81 for the MMSE. The consistently higher alphas for the 3MS reflect, at least in part, its larger number of items.

TABLE 7–37 Mini-Mental State Examination (MMSE) Normative Data for Noninstitutionalized Mexican Older Adults Aged >70 Stratified By Age, Gender, and Education Level

	MALE (*N* = 466) EDUCATION			FEMALE (*N* = 581) EDUCATION			TOTAL (*N* = 1,047) EDUCATION		
AGE	0	1–5	6+	0	1–5	6+	0	1–5	6+
70–79									
N	32	74	187	57	98	229	89	172	416
5th percentile	13	14	18	13	16	19	13	16	19
10th percentile	15	18	20	14	17	20	14	17	20
25th percentile	17	20	23	17	19	22	17	19	22
50th percentile	19	22	25	19	21	25	19	21	25
75th percentile	21	25	27	21	23	27	21	24	27
90th percentile	24	28	29	23	25	28	23	26	28
Mean	19	22.1	24.6	18.7	21.1	24.2			
SD	3.5	3.9	3.4	3.2	3.2	3.3			
Range	10–27	11–30	11–30	10–25	11–29	10–30			
80+									
N	29	39	105	35	53	109	64	92	214
5th percentile	10	11	13	10	10	14	10	11	14
10th percentile	12	12	16	11	13	16	11	13	16
25th percentile	15	16	19	14	14	19	15	14	19
50th percentile	17	19	22	18	18	23	18	18	22
75th percentile	21	22	25	19	21	25	20	21	25
90th percentile	23	23	27	21	24	27	22	24	27
Mean	17.5	18.3	21.9	16.7	17.7	22.2			
SD	4.3	3.9	4.6	3.7	4.5	4.2			
Range	10–26	10–27	10–30	10–23	10–29	10–29			

NOTE: Norms from a population-based cohort study (Coyoacán Cohort Study) sample of 1,047 Spanish-speaking non-institutionalized older adults age >70 living in Coyoacán, a district of Mexico City.

SOURCE: From Mokri et al. (2013).

TABLE 7–38 Sri Lankan Norms for Those Aged 75+ Living in Elderly Care Homes in the Western Province of Sri Lanka Based on the Sinhalese Version of the Mini-Mental State Examination (MMSE)

GENDER	LEVEL OF EDUCATION	N (%)	PERCENTILE 10	50 (MEDIAN)	20
Male	<5 years	68 (50.00)	14.00	22.00	21.85
	6–10 years	42 (30.88)	14.30	24.00	21.60
	>10 years	26 (19.12)	22.00	26.50	23.00
	Total	136 (29.82)	14.00	24.00	18.00
Female	<5 years	148 (46.25)	11.00	18.00	14.00
	6–10 years	93 (29.06)	16.00	22.00	18.00
	>10 years	79 (24.69)	16.00	25.00	21.00
	Total	320 (70.18)	13.00	21.00	16.00
Total		456	14.00	22.00	16.00

NOTE: *N* = 456; illiterate elders were verbally asked to perform "close your eyes" and articulate a spontaneous sentence (instead of writing). Significant effects of education and gender but not age were reported. Median score for those with <5 years education was 19 and for >5 years education was 24.

SOURCE: From de Silva et al. (2009).

EVIDENCE FOR TEST-RETEST RELIABILITY, MEASURING CHANGE, AND PRACTICE EFFECTS

MMSE

Test-retest reliability estimates for intervals of less than two months generally fall between .80 and .95 (see Clark et al., 1999; Folstein et al., 1975; Mystakidou et al., 2007; Tombaugh & McIntyre, 1992). In one study, among healthy community-dwelling older adults, however, three-month test-retest reliability was poor (r_s = .35; Spencer et al., 2013).

In patients with probable AD retested within a two-week period, slight improvement is noted (.2 to ± 2.1 points), with most patients (95%) showing a short-term change of four points or less (Doraiswamy & Kaiser, 2000). Following retest intervals of about three months, nondemented individuals tend to show slight improvement (<1 point; Tombaugh, 2005), while individuals with dementia or MCI tend not to benefit from prior exposure to the test (Helkala et al., 2002).

TABLE 7–39 Values to Be Added to the Mini-Mental State Examination (MMSE) Raw Score in Order to Obtain the Adjusted-MMSE Score

	AGE ≤ 59	60 TO 69	70 TO 79	80 TO 89	AGE ≥ 90
Up to 6 years in school	0	1	2	3	3
More than 6 years in school	0	0	1	2	3

NOTE: AMMSE, Adjusted Mini-Mental State Examination.

NOTE: Based on Mexican sample.

SOURCE: From Villaseñor-Cabrera et al. (2010).

With lengthier retest intervals (e.g., one to two years), healthy individuals typically show a small amount of change (less than two points), and retest correlations are lower (<.80; Hopp et al., 1997; Mitrushina & Satz, 1991), perhaps due in part to the inclusion at one time of individuals with MCI (Tombaugh, 2005). Recall and attention items tend to be the least reliable (Olin & Zelinski, 1991).

In patients with probable AD, the average annual change in MMSE score is about four points, although there is high measurement error (which almost equals the average annual score change) and there is striking variability among individuals (Clark et al., 1999; Doody et al., 2001). The implication of these findings is that clinicians monitoring change in older adults should be cautious in interpreting small changes in scores. Iverson (1998) has reported that, depending on the age and education of the examinee, changes of about two points may be statistically reliable. However, Clark et al. (1999) have suggested that to be clinically meaningful (rather than merely reflecting testing imprecision), a change in MMSE score must exceed three points. Doody et al. (2001) recommend a drop of five or more points to reflect clinically meaningful decline.

Over intervals of five years, test-retest correlations are modest for older adults (65–99 years) who remain healthy on both test occasions (r = .55) as well as for individuals who were reclassified as showing MCI on the second test session (r = .59; Tombaugh, 2005). In part, the modest correlation for intact individuals is due to regression to the mean (high scores tend to decline whereas low scores tend to increase on subsequent testing). However, there is also considerable variability among older individuals over a five-year period. On average, MMSE scores remain relatively stable among intact older adults, changing less than one point (+.08) over a five-year interval, but declining (−1.38) in those with MCI.

Tombaugh (2005) used reliable change methodology to provide a better estimate of whether an individual's retest score has changed significantly from the initial test score over both short (<3 months) and long (five years) retest intervals on the MMSE and 3MS. Table 7–44 shows the regression formulas, the percent of variance explained by all variables (e.g., test one score, age, education, gender), and the amount of change needed to exceed the .05 level (one-tailed). Note that most of the variance is accounted for by the score on the first test occasion. A normative table containing the percentile equivalents for various change scores is also provided (see Table 7–45). The data are based on a sample of 232 older adults who were retested following both short and long intervals and who received consensus diagnoses of no cognitive impairment on both examinations. The values needed for clinically meaningful change agree fairly well with those suggested by Clark et al. (1999), Doody et al. (2001), and Eslinger et al. (2003).

TABLE 7–40 Characteristics of Mini-Mental State Examination, 2nd Edition (MMSE-2) Standardization Sample

CHARACTERISTIC	STANDARDIZATION SAMPLE	TOTAL CLINICAL SAMPLE	AD	SUBCORTICAL DEMENTIA
Sample size	1531	232	136	96
Age	18 to 100	23 to 98	52 to 98	23 to 92
Geographical location	16% Northeast 44% Midwest 38% South 3% West			
Education	3% ≤6 years 19% 7 to 8 years 23% 9 to 11 years 42% 12 to 15 years 14% ≥16 years	M = 13.34 (*SD* = 3.47) 3 to 24 years	M = 13.07 (*SD* = 3.74) 3 to 20 years	M = 13.71 (*SD* = 3.03) 6 to 24 years
Gender	54% Women 46% Men	57% Women 43% Men	63% Women 37% Men	51% Men 49% Women
Ethnicity	66% Caucasian 23% African American 8% Hispanic 3% Other	91% Caucasian 2% African American 6% Hispanic 1% Other	90% Caucasian 6% Hispanic 3% African American 1% Other	93% Caucasian 5% Hispanic 1% African American 1% Other
Exclusion/Inclusion criteria	Exclusion criteria: Uncorrected sensory impairment that will impact ability to complete assessment; inability to understand or read fourth-grade level English; inability to provide informed consent; dementia, or acute/severe psychiatric disorder	Exclusion criteria: Younger than 18 years of age; non-English-speaking; history of other neuropsychiatric disease; DSM-IV alcohol-related or drug-dependence disorder; administration of original MMSE within a month of participation	Inclusion criteria: Diagnostic criteria include presence of a memory and cognitive impairment in one or more of language, perceptual skills, attention, construction, orientation, problem solving, or functional abilities confirmed by neuropsychological testing; no disturbance of consciousness	Inclusion criteria: Parkinson's disease, Huntington's disease, or vascular dementia

NOTE: Values are rounded. With the exception of characteristics that are relatively uniformly distributed, only the percentage of the majority is shown.

SOURCE: Adapted from Folstein et al. (2010). Reproduced by special permission of the Publisher, Psychological Assessment Resources, Inc. (PAR), 16204 North Florida Avenue, Lutz, Florida 33549, from the Mini-Mental State Examination, by Marshal F. Folstein, MD and Susan E. Folstein, MD, Copyright 1975, 1998, 2001 and the Mini-Mental State Examination-2, Copyright 2010 by Mini Mental LLC, Inc. Published 2001, 2010 by PAR. Further reproduction is prohibited without permission of PAR.

TABLE 7–41 Age- and Education-Specific Reference Values for the Modified Mini-Mental State Examination (3MS) Based on a Sample of 7,754 Healthy Older Adults in Canada

	AGE (YEARS)				
EDUCATION	65 TO 69	70 TO 74	75 TO 79	80 TO 84	85+
0 to 4 years	*N* = 78 82.0 (8.7) (70, 79, 82)	*N* = 85 82.6 (7.5) (71, 78, 83)	*N* = 93 81.0 (5.4) (70, 77, 83)	*N* = 78 79.6 (8.1) (65, 76, 81)	*N* = 65 77.0 (8.8) (50, 74, 80)
5 to 8 years	*N* = 495 87.1 (7.7) (76, 83, 88)	*N* = 422 87.1 (8.1) (78, 83, 87)	*N* = 556 85.7 (5.8) (75, 81, 86)	*N* = 277 84.0 (6.0) (70, 79, 85)	*N* = 239 82.6 (5.1) (66, 78, 83)
9 to 12 years	*N* = 942 91.7 (6.5) (81, 89, 93)	*N* = 752 90.7 (6.3) (80, 87, 92)	*N* = 921 89.8 (4.7) (79, 86, 90)	*N* = 455 87.5 (5.1) (76, 83, 88)	*N* = 332 85.6 (4.3) (72, 81, 86)
13 years and over	*N* = 581 93.9 (5.7) (85, 92, 95)	*N* = 375 92.9 (6.4) (82, 91, 94)	*N* = 535 91.3 (5.2) (80, 88, 92)	*N* = 236 89.8 (5.3) (79, 86, 91)	*N* = 208 88.0 (4.2) (75, 84, 89)

NOTE: Data reported as sample size, mean (standard deviation), and (5th, 25th, 50th) percentiles.

SOURCE: Bravo and Hebert (1997a).

TABLE 7–42 Percentile Scores for Modified Mini-Mental State Examination (3MS) Raw Scores Based on a Sample of Older African-American Adults

RAW SCORE	AGE GROUP 60 TO 71	AGE GROUP 72 TO 84
100		
99	97	99
98	94	98
97	89	98
96	87	94
95	84	92
94	80	89
93	75	81
92	69	78
91	60	76
90	54	73
89	48	69
88	46	63
87	41	60
86	38	58
85	34	52
84	28	50
83	23	47
82	20	43
81	16	38
80	13	36
79	12	33
78	10	32
77	8	32
76	8	29
75	7	26
74	6	26
73	5	25
72	4	23
71	3	21
70	3	21
69	2	18
68	2	17
67	1	15
66	1	15
65	1	14
64	1	13
63	<1	10
62	<1	9
61	<1	7
60	<1	6
59	<1	6
58	<1	6
57	<1	3
56	<1	2
55	<1	2
54	<1	1

NOTE: *N* = 238 African Americans who reported no history of neurological disorder. The sample was not screened for psychiatric disorder.

SOURCE: From Brown et al. (2003).

MMSE-2

Three-week test-retest reliability is high for the standard MMSE-2 and MMSE-2:EV but low for the Brief Version (r = .80, .86, and .44, respectively). To determine reliable change over serial assessments, a raw score difference of 5 or greater, 14 or greater, and 4 or greater for MMSE-2:SV, MMSE-2:EV, and MMSE-2:BV, respectively, at a .01 significance level are needed (or see table D.1 in the manual for raw score difference at other significance level).

TABLE 7–43 Adjustments for Modified Mini-Mental State Examination (3MS) Raw Scores for Older African Americans

YEARS OF EDUCATION	AGE GROUP 60 TO 71 MALE	60 TO 71 FEMALE	72 TO 84 MALE	72 TO 84 FEMALE
<12	+4	0	+7	−3
12	0	−2	−1	−11
>12	−4	−7	−13	−12

SOURCE: From Brown et al. (2003).

3MS

Test-retest reliability for the 3MS is reported to be high for intervals of about three months in individuals diagnosed with dementia (intraclass correlation of .85; Correa et al., 2001).

One study (Correa et al., 2001) showed that, under conditions of repeat testing (<90 days but >14 days) with two different assessors in a setting compatible with no change in cognitive status, the discrepancy between repeat 3MS scores of people with dementia can be as large as ±16 points. This suggests that the smallest individual change in score that can be reliably detected must exceed 16 points. With lengthier retest intervals (five years), declines of about seven points are unusual in healthy older adults (Tombaugh, 2005; see Table 7–44). See Tables 7–44 and 7–45 for information on how to derive reliable change values for the 3MS.

EVIDENCE FOR RELIABILITY OF ALTERNATE FORMS

The alternate form for the MMSE-2 is highly correlated with the standard MMSE-2 (Generalizability coefficient >.96). No other information is available on other forms (Folstein et al., 2010).

EVIDENCE FOR INTERRATER RELIABILITY

MMSE

Scoring of some items (e.g., overlapping polygons) is somewhat subjective, and there is no suggested time limit for any item. Interrater reliability is marginal (>.65; Folstein et al., 1975) and could be enhanced with more precise administration and scoring criteria (Molloy et al., 1991; Olin & Zelinski, 1991).

MMSE-2

As the instructions have been standardized in this version, interrater reliability is consistently high across all items (ICC >.94; see Manual).

TABLE 7–44 Regression Formulas for Detecting Reliable Change on the Mini-Mental State Examination (MMSE) and Modified Mini-Mental State Examination (3MS)

	PERCENT OF VARIANCE EXPLAINED BY ALL VARIABLES (R^2) TOTAL	FORMULA FOR OBTAINING PREDICTED SCORE	VALUE NEEDED FOR DETECTING RELIABLE CHANGE
MMSE Short Interval	.41	.38 (test 1) – .07 (age) + .10 (educ) + 21.65	±2.73
3MS Short Interval	.60	.53 (test 1) – .27 (age) + .20 (educ) + 62.60	±7.41
MMSE Long Interval	.37	.45 (test 1) – .09 (age) + 1.06 (sex) + 19.12	±3.60
3MS Long Interval	.53	.52 (test 1) – .23 (age) + .30 (educ) + 1.93 (sex) + 53.86	±9.82

NOTE: Based on a sample of 232 older adults who were retested following three-month and five-year intervals and who received consensus diagnoses of no cognitive impairment on both examination. RCI-Reg, Reliable Change Index-Regression: After the predicted retest score is obtained, it is subtracted from the observed test score. If this change score exceeds the Value Needed for Reliable Change, it is considered to represent a significant change at .05 (one-tailed). Age and education are expressed in years. Sex was coded as male = 1 and female = 2.

SOURCE: From Tombaugh (2005).

3MS

The interrater reliability of the 3MS is moderate when measured by agreement of clinician categorization of cognitive impairment versus no cognitive impairment based on 3MS scores (kappa = 0.67; Lamarre & Patten, 1991). Interrater reliability is reported to be high (r = .98) for the overlapping figures (Teng & Chui, 1987).

EVIDENCE FOR VALIDITY

FACTOR-ANALYTIC STUDIES

MMSE

Folstein et al. (1975) grouped the items into discrete subsections (e.g., orientation, registration, attention and calculation, recall, language); however, these categories were derived without empirical justification, and it is not clear whether the MMSE subsections and individual items can be viewed as measures of specific aspects of cognition (Giordani et al., 1990; Mitrushina & Satz, 1994). Concordance rates between individual MMSE tasks and neuropsychological tests addressing corresponding cognitive domains can be quite low (Benedict & Brandt, 1992; Giordani et al., 1990; Jefferson et al., 2002; Mitrushina & Satz, 1994).

TABLE 7–45 Percentiles for the Difference Between Obtained Retest Scores and Regression-Predicted Retest Scores for the Mini-Mental State Examination (MMSE) and Modified Mini-Mental State Examination (3MS) for Short and Long Time Intervals

	MMSE	MMSE	3MS	3MS
PERCENTILES	SHORT INTERVAL (<3 MONTHS)	LONG INTERVAL (5 YEARS)	SHORT INTERVAL (<3 MONTHS)	LONG INTERVAL (5 YEARS)
98 (+2 *SD*)	3.08	4.26	11.27	12.06
95	2.53	3.79	7.48	8.90
90	2.05	3.44	4.90	7.05
84 (+1 *SD*)	1.43	3.16	3.99	4.62
75	1.06	2.55	2.66	3.45
50 (0 *SD*)	0.13	1.18	0.21	0.47
25	–0.78	0.01	–1.54	–3.12
16 (–1 *SD*)	–1.50	–0.84	–2.96	–5.47
10	–2.16	–1.67	–5.40	–7.79
05	–3.20	–2.99	–8.47	–10.15
02 (–2 *SD*)	–4.22	–4.67	–10.28	–17.31

NOTE: Based on a sample of 232 older adults who were retested following three-month and five-year intervals and who received consensus diagnosis of no cognitive impairment on both examinations.

SOURCE: Tombaugh (2005).

Factor-analytic studies of the MMSE often yield a two-factor solution (Braekhus et al., 1992; Giordani et al., 1990; Tombaugh & McIntyre, 1992), although other solutions have also been found. For example, a study with a large sample (N = 8,556) of community-dwelling older adults suggested the presence of five separate dimensions (concentration, language and praxis, orientation, memory, and attention), although the MMSE also satisfied criteria of unidimensionality (Jones & Gallo, 2000). Similar findings have been reported by Banos and Franklin (2002) in 339 adult inpatients at a nonforensic state psychiatric hospital. Two studies (Banos & Franklin, 2002; Jones & Gallo, 2000) provide empirical support for some of the traditional categories, such as orientation (time and place), attention (serial 7s), and memory (recall of three words). There is less empirical support for the categories of registration, language, and construction.

The stability of the MMSE factor structure over 10 years was examined by Castro-Costa and colleagues (2014) in a community-based Brazilian sample with low education. Similar to past studies, the first factor (concentration) comprised serial 5s; the language/praxis factor comprised repetition, write a sentence, read and follow instruction, pentagon copy, and period of the day; the orientation factor comprised orientation to time and place; the attention factor comprised registration; and, last, the memory factor comprised delayed recall (Castro-Costa et al., 2014). In this sample, the five-factor structure of the MMSE based on confirmatory factor analysis (principal component analysis) remained unchanged across the measurement periods.

3MS

The 3MS by Teng et al. (1987) added four additional items (date and place of birth, word fluency, similarities, and delayed recall of words), included items that assess different aspects of memory, and increased the maximum score to permit greater differentiation among individuals. A factor analysis of the 3MS yielded the following five domains: psychomotor skills, memory, identification and association, orientation, and concentration and calculation (Abraham et al., 1993).

RELATIONSHIPS BETWEEN ITEMS

MMSE

Analyses of individual items reveal that errors rarely occur on questions related to orientation to place and language; for both healthy and demented individuals, most errors occur for the recall of three words, serial 7s/"world," pentagon, and orientation to time. In short, these latter items are the most sensitive to normal aging and a variety of diseases (e.g., diabetes, cardiovascular disease) including dementing processes (Hill & Backman, 1995; Nilsson et al., 2002; Tombaugh & McIntyre, 1992; Tombaugh et al., 1996; Wells et al., 1992). For example, risk of AD with two errors on orientation and three-word recall generates a sensitivity of 95% and a specificity of 71%. Loss of one point on the items showed twice the risk of incident AD than loss of one point on the other MMSE scores (Carcaillon et al., 2009).

There is evidence that serial 7s and reverse spelling of "world" represent different tasks. Spelling "world" backward consistently produces higher scores than does counting backward by sevens (Tombaugh & McIntyre, 1992). Serial 7s maximizes variability, increases internal consistency, and reduces measurement error, thus increasing the likelihood of discriminating between individuals in their level of cognitive ability (Espino et al., 2004). In fact, Espino et al. (2004) have argued that only serial 7s should be given. As the "world" item was found to be easier than the serial 7s item and was difficult to translate, spelling of "world" has been removed from the MMSE-2 (Folstein et al., 2010). However, users should bear in mind that performance on the serial 7s task appears heavily influenced by basic arithmetic skills and therefore should be used with caution as a measure of concentration (Karzmark, 2000).

The results from the factor-analytic studies reported previously imply that the individual subsection scores of the MMSE should not be used in lieu of more comprehensive assessments if a detailed diagnostic profile is desired (Banos & Franklin, 2002; Giordani et al., 1990). This does not mean that the MMSE cannot provide useful information in differentiating among patients with dementia. For example, Jefferson et al. (2002) found that patients with AD scored lower than patients with ischemic vascular dementia or PD on temporal orientation and recall tasks, while those with vascular dementia obtained lower scores than patients with AD on motor/constructional tasks (copying, writing) and an index comprising items requiring working memory (spelling "world" backward, carrying out three-step commands). The vascular dementia and PD groups also made more errors in writing a sentence and copying intersecting polygons.

MMSE-2

On the MMSE-2, correlations between the repetition, comprehension, and drawing items with other items are weakest ($r < .30$) in the normative sample but much higher in the clinical samples. Similarly, inter-item correlations for all other items tend to be higher in the clinical than normative samples (see manual). Correlations with the total scores of all MMSE-2 versions are generally in the moderate to high range (Folstein et al., 2010).

COMPARISONS WITH THE MoCA

The MoCA is more sensitive than the MMSE for identifying subtle cognitive impairment (see Table 7–46; Damian et al., 2011; Gluhm et al., 2013; Whitney et al., 2012), post-stroke vascular cognitive impairment (Cumming et al., 2013; Dong et al., 2010), Korsakoff's syndrome (Oudman et al., 2014), PD dementia, and MCI (Hoops et al., 2009). It is also better at identifying potential to return to work after aneurysmal subarachnoid hemorrhage (Schweizer et al., 2012) and in differentiating between AD, DLB, and healthy controls (Wang et al., 2013). For example, about 14 days post-stroke, 32% of those with unimpaired MMSE scores have impaired MoCA whereas only 5% with unimpaired MoCA have impaired MMSE. MMSE subtest scores could not differentiate between groups with mild, moderate, and no vascular cognitive impairment or no dementia, whereas the MoCA visuospatial-executive, attention, and recall scores were different for all three groups (Dong et al., 2010). Similarly, among those who have aneurysmal subarachnoid hemorrhage, 42% more patients are impaired on the MoCA than on the MMSE, and the MMSE is not related to impairment on any neuropsychological tests (Schweizer et al., 2012).

The MoCA also appears to detect age-related cognitive decline better than the MMSE. In one cross-sectional study, neurologically healthy community-dwelling adults across the life span (age 20–89) were administered the MMSE and MoCA. Modest worsening across the life span was seen on the MMSE, whereas the MoCA showed greater decline. MMSE and MoCA scores were statistically different, as were the visuospatial, language, and memory items. When examined by the decade, there were no consistent differences in the 30–49 age ranges, but memory and language scores on the MMSE and MoCA were different by the 50–89 age range. These results suggest that ceiling effects are less of an issue on the MoCA than the MMSE (Gluhm et al., 2013).

COMPARISONS WITH OTHER SCREENERS

Based on a meta-analysis comparing the Addenbrooke's Cognitive Examination (ACE), MoCA, and MMSE in identifying dementia, the ACE yielded higher effectiveness than the MMSE and MoCA and was a better cognitive screen than the MMSE and 3MS (Queally et al., 2011). The MMSE also pales in comparison to the Mini-Cog for

TABLE 7–46 Studies Comparing the Mini-Mental State Examination (MMSE) and Montreal Cognitive Assessment (MoCA), and Their Respective Cutoff, Sensitivity, Specificity, Positive Predictive Value, and Negative Predictive Value

REFERENCE	PURPOSE/POPULATION	OPTIMAL CUTOFF	AUC	SENS (%)	SPEC (%)	PPV (%)	NPV (%)
Cumming, Churilov, Linden, and Bernhradt (2013)	Post-stroke cognitive impairment at three months	MoCA ≤ 23	.87	92	67	84	82
		MMSE ≤ 26	.84	82	76	86	70
Damian, Jacobson, Hentz, et al. (2011)	Cognitive impairment with varying etiologies and healthy controls	MoCA ≤ 23	.90	87	75	38	97
		MMSE ≤ 27	.82	76	75	35	95
Hoops, Nazem, Siderowf, et al. (2009)	Parkinson's disease dementia and PD-MCI	Screening:					
		MoCA ≤ 26	.79	90	53	46	92
		MMSE ≤ 29	.76	90	38	39	90
		Diagnostic:					
		MoCA ≤ 17		18	99	88	73
		MMSE ≤ 24		20	99	89	74
Oudman, Postma, Van der Stigchel, et al. (2014)	Korsakoff's syndrome vs. healthy controls	MoCA ≤ 26	1.00	100	63	73	100
		MMSE ≤ 27	.92	100	73	77	88
Wang, Pai, Chen, et al. (2013)	AD and DLB	For AD:					
		MoCA ≤ 21	.95	95	82	85	94
		MMSE ≤ 24	.92	88	86	87	87
		For DLB:					
		MoCA ≤ 22	.93	92	81	73	94
		MMSE ≤ 24	.90	78	86	76	87

NOTE: Sens, sensitivity; Spec, specificity; PPV, positive predictive value; NPV, negative predictive value; AD, Alzheimer's disease; DLB, dementia with Lewy bodies; PD-MCI, Parkinson's disease with mild cognitive impairment.

differentiating between dementia and healthy controls but is comparably poor for identification of MCI (Kaufer et al., 2008; Milian et al., 2012). In one study based on a German memory clinic patient sample, Mini-Cog (sensitivity 87%, specificity 100%) was better than MMSE (sensitivity 73% at ≤24 or 79% at ≤25, specificity 100%) and CDT (sensitivity 78%, specificity 97%) at discriminating people with dementia from healthy controls. The Mini-Cog also showed lesser education effects than the MMSE (Milian et al., 2012). However, among assisted living/residential care residents, Mini-Cog and MMSE showed similarly high sensitivity (96% at <28 cutoff for MMSE; 87% at 0 for Mini-Cog) and NPV (96% for MMSE; 88% for Mini-Cog) for dementia. The discriminatory power for MCI was, however, poor (sensitivity 37% at <27 cutoff for MMSE; 50% at 0 for Mini-Cog; NPV 21% for MMSE; 22% for Mini-Cog; Kaufer et al., 2008). The MMSE has moderate to strong correlations with the CDR-SB ($r = -.76$) in a sample of healthy individuals and people with aMCI and AD (Malek-Ahmadi et al., 2014).

Combining the MMSE and CDT to identify MCI and mild AD appears to yield good results (Cacho et al., 2010; Kato et al., 2013). For example, in a memory disorder clinic sample, the combination was able to differentiate between MCI, mild AD, and controls better than the MMSE or CDT alone (Cacho et al., 2010; Kato et al., 2013). The MMSE-CDT combination was also more effective at differentiating AD from MCI and healthy controls at similar rates as the ADAS-Cog Japanese version (Kato et al., 2013).

The MMSE appears insensitive to change over five years compared to the Short Test of Mental Status (STMS; Tang-Wai et al., 2003). At baseline, the STMS was better than MMSE in differentiating people with MCI from healthy controls, with the MMSE demonstrating poor sensitivity using a standard cutoff. Over a five-year period, the MMSE was not able to differentiate between those who remained cognitively healthy from those who developed incident MCI or AD, whereas the STMS did, suggesting insensitivity to change for the MMSE.

The ADAS-Cog, CAMCOG, and MMSE have been tested for a common dimension of global cognitive impairment using IRT to evaluate their equivalence/comparability. It was found that mean level of global cognitive impairment corresponded to 11.4 on the ADAS-Cog, 72.6 on the CAMCOG, and 22.2 on the MMSE. The authors noted that the MMSE appeared to be too easy even for individuals with dementia (Wouters et al., 2010).

3MS

Although some studies have found the sensitivity and specificity of the 3MS and MMSE to be similar (Nadler et al., 1995; Tombaugh et al., 1996), others have found the 3MS to be more sensitive in detecting cognitive deficits and to be a better predictor of functional outcome (Grace et al., 1995). In these studies, the criterion validity of the 3MS was high. For example, Tombaugh et al. (1996) reported that the sensitivity of the 3MS was 93% when screening for AD versus no cognitive impairment at a cutoff score of 77/78 (i.e., those who scored 77 or lower were classed as impaired, whereas those who scored 78 or higher were classed as normal).

OTHER BRIEF VERSIONS

When the MMSE and Short MMSE are compared (Stein et al., 2015), every one-point increase in MMSE is associated with a 65% decrease in likelihood of dementia diagnosis; a one-point increase in Short MMSE is associated with an 86% decrease in likelihood of dementia diagnosis. For the MMSE, an optimal cutoff of 24 or lower yields a sensitivity of 93%, a specificity of 96%, and correct classification rate of 96%. An optimal cutoff of 4 or less for the Short MMSE yields a sensitivity of 98%, a specificity of 71%, and a correct classification rate of 72%. In sum, the Short MMSE shows poor psychometric properties for identification of dementia when compared to the MMSE.

On the Severe-MMSE (SMMSE), each one-year increase in educational level resulted in an additional .29 points. The SMMSE and MMSE are correlated, with 63% shared variability (Wajman et al., 2014).

RELATIONSHIPS WITH OTHER TESTS

MMSE

The MMSE is highly correlated with the WAIS-IV, especially FSIQ (r = .51 to .80), at least among multiple sclerosis (MS) patients and older veterans (Gontkovsky, 2014; Sugarman & Axelrod, 2014). PSI shows the weakest correlation with the MMSE (r = .65), though once education is partialled out, VCI shows the weakest correlation (r = .48; Gontkovsky, 2014). The MMSE has moderate to strong correlations with the CASI and FAQ in illiterate Brazilians with dementia (Rezende et al., 2013).

The MMSE is correlated with some neuropsychological measures but not others. For example, the MMSE did not correlate with any tests except the BNT in a sample of patients who had aneurysmal subarachnoid hemorrhage (Schweizer et al., 2012). In a sample of healthy community-dwelling older adults, small to medium correlations were found with WMS-R Visual Reproduction-Delayed, TMT B, Golden Stroop, and the computer-based Subtle Cognitive Impairment Test (SCIT). There was a gradient of number of errors made on the SCIT associated with lower MMSE scores, with those who scored 25–27 on the MMSE making the most errors on the SCIT. Insignificant correlations were found with WMS-R Logical Memory, Trails A, WMS-R Digit Span, WMS-R Visual Span, WAIS-R Block Design, and JLO (Friedman et al., 2012; Spencer et al., 2013).

MMSE-2

In AD, the MMSE-2 is weakly correlated with JLO and TMT-A, and moderately correlated with WMS-III Digit Span, BNT, FAS, TMT-B, WAIS-R Digit Symbol and Block Design, Stroop Test, and HVLT-R. Strong correlation is seen with category fluency (Folstein et al., 2010). There is to our knowledge no independent research on correlations with other tests.

3MS

The 3MS has moderate to high correlations with neuropsychological tests that assess similar domains (Grace et al., 1995), providing evidence for its concurrent validity.

CLINICAL STUDIES

Neurodegenerative Disorders. Most studies report that the MMSE total score is sensitive to the presence of dementia, particularly in those with moderate to severe forms of cognitive impairment. The MMSE also appears useful in predicting who will develop AD or vascular dementia (Small et al., 1997a; Jones et al., 2004). For example, Jones et al. (2004) found that lower baseline scores on the MMSE in nondemented persons were associated with an increased risk of AD or vascular dementia after a three-year follow-up period. Delayed memory was the best predictor in both preclinical vascular dementia and preclinical AD.

A number of investigators report an average annual rate of decline of about two to four points on the MMSE for patients with AD (Clark et al., 1999; Doody et al., 2001; Salmon et al., 1990; Small et al., 1997b). However, progression rates of AD are nonlinear and quite variable between persons (Clark et al., 1999; Doody et al., 2001). Nonetheless, there is some consistency in that patients who begin with progression rates that are more rapid than average (≥5 MMSE points per year) continue to decline sooner than patients who begin at slow (≤1.9 points per year) or average rates (2.0–4.9 points per year; Doody et al., 2001). Furthermore, individuals with AD decline at a faster rate than patients with vascular dementia (Nyenhuis et al., 2002) or FTD (Pasquier et al., 2004).

The MMSE may be useful to differentiate between patients with AD or DLB based on qualitative analysis of item performance. Using the qualitative scoring approach (see Table 7–34; Caffarra et al., 2013), DLB was associated with low scores on opening/closure, repetition, number of angles, and language (naming, written comprehension). As expected, AD was associated with poor delayed recall, temporal orientation, and constructional apraxia. The DLB group performed worse than the AD group on number of angles, distance/intersection, closure/opening, rotation, and total score; no difference was seen on closing-in phenomenon (Caffarra et al., 2013).

In early-onset PD, various genetic mutations found in PD did not differ on the MMSE even though glucocerebrosidase (GBA) carriers reported more cognitive complaints than other carrier groups (Alcalay et al., 2010).

The test is somewhat sensitive to mortality-related effects with declines in scores evident about three to five years prior to death (e.g., Nguyen et al., 2003; Tan, 2004). The greatest risk is for those with moderate to severe cognitive impairment, although mild impairment (e.g., MMSE scores 18–23) is also associated with increased risk (Nguyen et al., 2003). A decline of at least four points over two years is also predictive of an increased risk of mortality, perhaps reflecting symptoms of medical diseases that carry with them long-term risk of mortality (Nguyen et al., 2003). It is worth bearing in mind, however, that although a large proportion (more than two-thirds) of cognitively impaired individuals became demented or died within three years in a separate study, a substantial proportion improved over the same period without a higher risk of later progressing to dementia (Palmer et al., 2002). Stern et al. (1997) have developed an equation to predict the estimated time to nursing home care and death in people with AD.

Interestingly, obtaining full points on the MMSE does not entirely rule out dementia. Shiroky and colleagues (2007) reported on eight memory disorder clinic patients with diagnosis of probable AD based on NINCDS-ADRDA criteria. These patients achieved 30/30 on the MMSE even though they performed very poorly on full neuropsychological assessment. The authors indicated that education could be a confounding factor because all had at least 11 years of education (Shiroky et al., 2007), rendering the MMSE less sensitive for these patients than other neuropsychological tests.

MMSE scores show modest relations with measures of functional capacity (e.g., driving, cooking, caring for finances, consent to participate in studies), functional outcome after stroke, and time to nursing home care and death (e.g., Adunsky et al., 2002; Bigler et al., 2002; Burns et al., 1991; Kim & Caine, 2002; Lemsky et al., 1996; Marcopulos et al., 1997; Stern et al., 1997; see also Ruchinskas & Curyto, 2003, for a review). For example, Gallo et al. (1998) reported that poor performance on the polygons task is associated with an increase in motor vehicle crashes.

The MMSE appears less than ideal when those with aphasia or MCI are evaluated, or when focal neurological deficits are present (e.g., poststroke; Benedict & Brandt, 1992; Feher et al., 1992; Grut et al., 1993; Kupke et al., 1993; Kuslansky et al., 2004; Meyer et al., 2001; Nys et al., 2005; Shah et al., 1992; Tombaugh & McIntyre, 1992; Wells et al., 1992). There are a number of possible explanations for this decreased sensitivity and specificity in these groups. One possibility rests on the fact that the MMSE is biased toward verbal items and does not adequately measure other functions such as ability to attend to relevant input, ability to solve abstract problems, ability to retain information over prolonged time intervals, visual-spatial ability, constructional praxis, and mood. Accordingly, it may overestimate dementia in aphasic patients. At the same time, it may be relatively insensitive to various dysexecutive and amnestic syndromes as well as to disturbances of the right hemisphere, resulting in an increase in false negatives. In addition, the language items are very simple, and mild impairments may go undetected.

MMSE-2. To our knowledge, no independent clinical studies of the MMSE-2 have been conducted as of this writing. The manual reported that the Standard Version and Expanded Version yielded similar diagnostic sensitivity for dementia when the whole range of MMSE-2 scores was examined. Using only those with MMSE-2 raw score of more than 22, the Expanded Version appeared superior to the Standard Version due to improved classification accuracy in a subcortical dementia group (Folstein et al., 2010). Better performance on an ADL questionnaire is also associated with better performance on the MMSE-2 (Folstein et al., 2010).

Medical Conditions. Use of the MMSE to screen for delirium has also been reported. For instance, Ringdal and colleagues reported that use of the MMSE to screen for delirium in older adults with hip fracture based on standard cutoff of less than 24 yielded a sensitivity of 88% and a specificity of 54% (Ringdal et al., 2011). A meta-analysis yielded overall sensitivity of 84% and specificity of 73%; if the cutoff of less than 24 was used, the sensitivity was unchanged but specificity decreased to 68%. Using a base rate of 25% for delirium, the authors reported a PPV of 51% and an NPV of 93% (Mitchell et al., 2014). The MMSE appears adequate as a screen to identify those who likely do not have delirium but not for detecting those who in fact do have delirium.

Medical patients have also been evaluated using the MMSE. In a sample of patients with advanced cancer, the MMSE differentiated among subgroups of patients: those with worse disease status obtained higher MMSE scores than those with better disease status as defined by the Eastern Cooperative Oncology Group (Mystakidou et al., 2007). Within a one-year timeframe, patients receiving hemodialysis showed greater decline in MMSE (24 to 21) than healthy controls (26 to 25), and a higher number of the former group than the latter switched from normal to mild-moderate or severe MMSE classification. The MMSE showed negative correlation with hypertension, angina, and Beck Depression Inventory (Bossola et al., 2011).

Psychiatric Conditions. In older adults with severe psychiatric conditions receiving services at community mental health centers, the MMSE had a sensitivity of 43% and a specificity of 90% for cognitive impairment at a cutoff of 25 (Mackin et al., 2010). The MMSE has been used to predict short-term memory impairments in those undergoing electroconvulsive therapy (ECT) for severe depression. MMSE scores dropped during the ECT course but improved after a one-week and one-month follow-up after cessation of ECT. MMSE score changes predicted 97% of the changes in memory scores from pre-ECT to a month after treatment (Nehra et al., 2006).

Because cognitive deficits can render self-report (e.g., including responses on the Geriatric Depression Scale, Beck Depression Inventory) invalid, interpretation of self-reported scales is considered hazardous once MMSE scores decline below 20 (Bedard et al., 2003). In such cases, reports from informants and observations are critical.

Medical Decision Making. A threshold of 20 may also apply to patient involvement in medical decision making (Hirschman et al., 2003). However, Kim and Caine (2002) noted that in a sample of patients with mild to moderate AD, a fairly wide range of MMSE scores (21 to 25, which includes an often-used cutoff for normal) did not discriminate consent capacity status well. Similarly, in a sample of patients with dementia, acquired brain injury, or psychiatric illness, at a cutoff of 22, the MMSE yielded extremely poor sensitivity (38%) but excellent specificity (91%) for decision-making ability (Pachet et al., 2010). As such, Kim and Caine (2002) recommend that if there are strong ethical reasons to select only patients who are clearly capable of providing consent, then the researcher/practitioner is advised to use a higher MMSE cutoff score (e.g., 26). Indeed, cutoff scores of less than 28/29 yield sensitivities of 67% to 74% and specificities of 76% to 84% on existing health literacy scales ("health literacy" refers to the ability to obtain and understand basic health information and services to make appropriate decisions about healthcare; Dahlke et al., 2014).

NEUROANATOMICAL CORRELATES AND IMAGING STUDIES

MMSE scores correlate with histopathological findings in in-vivo brain images and event-related potentials (Aylward et al., 1996; Bigler et al., 2002; DeKoskey et al., 1990; Stout et al., 1996). In mild to moderate AD, proton spectroscopy shows that, in the posterior cingulate, MMSE scores may be associated with neuronal density (Lee et al., 2007). Past studies (e.g., Bigler et al., 2002; Stout et al., 1996) have reported an association between MRI white matter lesions and impaired cognitive function as measured by the MMSE. Clinical-pathological study of patients with AD reveal that the best predictors of MMSE scores are the total counts of neurofibrillary tangles (NFT) in the entorhinal cortex and Area 9, as well as the degree of neuronal loss in the CA1 field of the hippocampus (Giannakapoulos et al., 2003). However, it has been shown that while some areas of atrophy related to AD are correlated with MMSE, other areas affected by AD (such as temporal pole and parahippocampal cortex) are not associated with MMSE scores in patients with mild to moderate AD (Fjell et al., 2009). When healthy community-dwelling older adults are examined, MMSE serial 7s and word recall yield minimal correlations ($r_s = -.22$) with MRI-derived indices of white matter disease and brain atrophy, whereas the total score does not show association with any MRI measures (Spencer et al., 2013). These results suggest that the MMSE may be sensitive, but not exclusively, to AD-related atrophy.

One study reported that the 10-minute delayed recall, but not the one-minute recall on baseline 3MS obtained five years before death predicted pathology-confirmed AD. Using a cutoff of 4 or less on the 10-minute delayed recall item, sensitivity and specificity for AD pathology were comparable to that of consensus clinical diagnosis (sensitivity 87% and 82%, specificity 47% and 47%, respectively; Lyness et al., 2014).

PERFORMANCE VALIDITY

There are few studies examining this question. In one study, the utility of the MMSE to identify individuals who may be malingering was tested in a sample of homicide pretrial defendants, of which about 17% were independently determined to be malingering. MMSE and Rey Fifteen-Item Test (FIT) scores were highly correlated ($r = .74$), and malingerers and nonmalingers obtained significantly different MMSE scores (22.5 vs. 27.3, respectively). Using a cutoff of less than 24, more malingerers than nonmalingerers scored below the cutoff, giving rise to a sensitivity of 67%, specificity of 93%, PPV of 67%, and NPV of 93% for malingering. FIT fared slightly worse, yielding a sensitivity of 50%, specificity of 86%, PPV of 43%, and NPV of 89% for malingering. The authors concluded that both the MMSE and FIT appear limited as tools to detect malingering in this population; however, they may be useful in identifying true-negative cases rather than true-positive cases for malingering (Myers et al., 2012).

COMMENT

The MMSE has been used widely to detect dementia for more than 40 years. Part of its popularity can be attributed to its ease of administration, its brevity, and the large volume of literature that has accumulated on its use. The MMSE is also available in many languages, many of which have been validated in independent studies over the past decade. The choice of screening measure for identifying dementia will depend on the goals of the examination and on the sample studied. However, it is important to bear in mind that agreement between dementia screening tests is not assured.

As a result of the popularity of the MMSE, Folstein et al. (2010) provided an updated version, the MMSE-2, which offers several advantages over the original MMSE. One of the criticisms of the original MMSE is the lack of clear administration and scoring guidelines. Clear administration and scoring instructions for the MMSE-2 are readily accessed in an easy-to-read manual, which improves interrater reliability. Psychometric information on the various MMSE-2 versions is also found in the manual. A pocket norms guide is also included as a quick normative reference. Finally, the MMSE-2 has an equivalent alternate form to minimize practice effects in serial assessment.

Users should be aware of the test's limitations. The MMSE lacks diagnostic specificity: low scores signal that there *may* be important changes in cognition and health. Analysis of some of the items (particularly those related to orientation, attention, and memory) may generate more targeted questions and offer clues with regard to the type of disorder. In short, the presence and nature of cognitive impairment should not be diagnosed on the basis of MMSE scores alone. The examiner needs to follow-up suspicions of impairment with a more in-depth evaluation. In head-to-head comparisons with the MoCA, the MMSE is weaker as a screening tool for most medical/neurological conditions examined (e.g., Cumming et al., 2013; Damian et al., 2011; Hoops et al., 2009). Moreover, some of the MMSE norms are fairly old and not stratified or population-based (e.g., Crum et al., 1993; Iverson, 1998). This issue is addressed in the MMSE-2.

In geriatric or neurological samples with a high prevalence of patients with illiteracy or language or motor disorders, the MMSE may not be ideal and may lead to an overestimation of dementia (e.g., Kuslansky et al., 2004; Tombaugh & McIntyre, 1992). At the same time, it may miss a significant proportion of individuals who have mild memory or other cognitive losses (e.g., Wang et al., 2013).

The use of age- and education-stratified normative variables when screening for dementia or cognitive impairment has been questioned. O'Connell et al. (2004) reported that correcting for demographic influences (age, education, gender) failed to improve the accuracy of the 3MS. Similar findings have been reported with regard to the MMSE (Kraemer et al., 1998). Because age and education are in themselves apparent risk factors for dementia, removal of the effects of these demographic variables might remove some of the predictive power of the screening measure (Sliwinski et al., 1997). However, adjusting for age and education improves the sensitivity/specificity of identifying vascular dementia (Villaseñor-Cabrera et al., 2010). Whether this is applicable in other contexts remains to be seen.

Finally, while there have been several modifications of the MMSE, including the MMSE-2 and 3MS, the latter of which has promising psychometric characteristics, these modifications have not yet gained widespread use. The few studies on the 3MS are outdated. Moreover, the psychometric characteristics of the MMSE-2 and its Brief and Expanded Versions have not yet been demonstrated in independent studies. The cost of using the MMSE-2 may be a limiting factor and could be prohibitive in many clinical settings, particularly compared to the free and psychometrically superior MoCA. On the other hand, MMSE/MMSE-2 norms are much more extensive than those of the MoCA at least as of this writing, which may be a distinct advantage.

REFERENCES

Abraham, I. L., Manning, C. A., Boyd, M. R., Neese, J. B., Newman, M. C., Plowfield, L. A., & Reel, S. J. (1993). Cognitive screening of nursing home residents: Factor structure of the modified mini-mental state (3MS) examination. *International Journal of Geriatric Psychiatry, 8*(2), 133–138.

Adunsky, A., Fleissig, Y., Levenkrohn, S., Arad, M., & Noy, S. (2002). Clock drawing task, Mini-Mental State Examination and cognitive-functional independence measure: Relation to functional outcome of stroke patients. *Archives of Gerontology and Geriatrics, 35,* 153–160.

Alcalay, R. N., Mejia-Santana, H., Tang, M. X., Rakitin, B., Rosado, L., Ross, B., . . . Colcher, A. (2010). Self-report of cognitive impairment and Mini-Mental State Examination performance in PRKN, LRRK2, and GBA carriers with early onset Parkinson's disease. *Journal of Clinical and Experimental Neuropsychology, 32*(7), 775–779.

Anderson, T. M., Sachdev, P. S., Brodaty, H., Trollor, J. N., & Andrews, G. (2007). Effects of sociodemographic and health variables on Mini-Mental State Exam scores in older Australians. *The American Journal of Geriatric Psychiatry, 15*(6), 467–476.

Ansari, N. N., Naghdi, S., Hasson, S., Valizadeh, L., & Jalaie, S. (2010). Validation of a Mini-Mental State Examination (MMSE) for the Persian population: A pilot study. *Applied Neuropsychology, 17*(3), 190–195.

Antsey, K. J., Matters, B., Brown, A. K., & Lord, S. R. (2000). Normative data on neuropsychological tests for very old adults living in retirement villages and hostels. *The Clinical Neuropsychologist, 14,* 309–317.

Aylward, E. H., Rasmussen, D. X., Brandt, J., Raimundo, L., Folstein, M., & Pearlson, G. D. (1996). CT measurement of supracellar cistern predicts rate of cognitive decline in Alzheimer's disease. *Journal of the International Neuropsychological Society, 2,* 89–95.

Banos, J. H., & Franklin, L. M. (2002). Factor structure of the Mini-Mental State Examination in adult psychiatric inpatients. *Psychological Assessment, 14,* 397–400.

Bedard, M., Molloy, D. W., Squire, L., Minthorn-Biggs, M-B., Dubois, S., Lever, J. A., & O'Donnell, M. (2003). Validity of self-reports in dementia research: The Geriatric Depression Scale. *Clinical Gerontologist, 26,* 155–163.

Benedict, R. H. B., & Brandt, J. (1992). Limitation of the Mini-Mental State Examination for the detection of amnesia. *Journal of Geriatric Psychiatry and Neurology,* 5233–5237.

Besson, P. S., & Labbe, E. E. (1997). Use of the modified Mini-Mental State Examination with children. *Journal of Child Neurology, 12,* 455–460.

Bieliauskas, L. A., Depp, C., Kauszler, M. L., Steinberg, B. A., & Lacy, M. (2000). IQ and scores on the Mini-Mental State Examination (MMSE). *Aging, Neuropsychology, and Cognition, 7,* 227–229.

Bigler, E. D., Kerr, B., Victoroff, J., Tate, D. F., & Breitmner, J. C. S. (2002). White matter lesions, quantitative magnetic resonance imaging and dementia. *Alzheimer Disease and Associated Disorders, 16,* 161–170.

Bossola, M., Antocicco, M., Di Stasio, E., Ciciarelli, C., Luciani, G., Tazza, L., . . . Onder, G. (2011). Mini Mental State Examination over time in chronic hemodialysis patients. *Journal of Psychosomatic Research, 71*(1), 50–54.

Braekhus, A., Laake, K., & Engedal, K. (1992). The Mini-Mental State Examination: Identifying the most efficient variables for detecting cognitive impairment in the elderly. *Journal of the American Geriatrics Society, 40,* 1139–1145.

Bravo, G., & Hebert, R. (1997). Age- and education-specific references values for the Mini-Mental and Modified Mini-Mental State Examinations derived from a non-demented elderly population. *International Journal of Geriatric Psychiatry, 12,* 1008–1018.

Brown, L. M., Schinka, J. A., Mortimer, J. A., & Graves, A. B. (2003). 3MS normative data for elderly African Americans. *Journal of Clinical and Experimental Neuropsychology, 25,* 234–241.

Burns, A., Jacoby, R., & Levy, R. (1991). Progression of cognitive impairment in Alzheimer's disease. *Journal of the American Geriatric Society, 39,* 39–45.

Cacho, J., Benito-León, J., García-García, R., Fernández-Calvo, B., Vicente-Villardón, J. L., & Mitchell, A. J. (2010). Does the combination of the MMSE and clock drawing test (mini-clock) improve the detection of mild Alzheimer's disease and mild cognitive impairment?. *Journal of Alzheimer's Disease, 22*(3), 889–896.

Caffarra, P., Gardini, S., Dieci, F., Copelli, S., Maset, L., Concari, L., . . . Grossi, E. (2013). The qualitative scoring MMSE pentagon test (QSPT): a new method for differentiating dementia with Lewy body from Alzheimer's disease. *Behavioural Neurology, 27*(2), 213–220.

Carcaillon, L., Amieva, H., Auriacombe, S., Helmer, C., & Dartigues, J. F. (2009). A subtest of the MMSE as a valid test of episodic memory? Comparison with the Free and Cued Selective Reminding Test. *Dementia and Geriatric Cognitive Disorders, 27*(5), 429–438.

Castro-Costa, É., Dewey, M. E., Uchôa, E., Firmo, J. O., Lima-Costa, M. F., & Stewart, R. (2014). Construct validity of the Mini Mental State Examination across time in a sample with low education levels: 10-year follow-up of the Bambuí Cohort Study of Ageing. *International Journal of Geriatric Psychiatry, 29*(12), 1294–1303.

Clark, C. M., Sheppard, L., Fillenbaum, G. G., Galasko, D., Morris, J. C., Koss, E., . . . the CERAD Investigators. (1999). Variability in annual Mini-Mental State Examination score in patients with probable Alzheimer disease. *Archives of Neurology, 56,* 857–862.

Correa, J. A., Perrault, H., & Wolfson, C. (2001). Reliable individual change scores on the 3MS in older persons with dementia: Results from the Canadian Study of Health and Aging. *International Psychogeriatrics, 13,* 71–78.

Crum, R. M., Anthony, J. C., Bassett, S. S., & Folstein, M. F. (1993). Population-based norms for the Mini-Mental State Examination by age and educational level. *Journal of the American Medical Association, 269,* 2386–2391.

Cumming, T. B., Churilov, L., Lindén, T., & Bernhardt, J. (2013). Montreal Cognitive Assessment and Mini–Mental State Examination are both valid cognitive tools in stroke. *Acta Neurologica Scandinavica, 128*(2), 122–129.

Dahlke, A. R., Curtis, L. M., Federman, A. D., & Wolf, M. S. (2014). The Mini-Mental State Examination as a surrogate measure of health literacy. *Journal of General Internal Medicine, 29*(4), 615–620.

Damian, A. M. Jacobson, S. A., Hentz, J. G., Belden, C. M., Shill, H. A., Sabbagh, M. N., Caviness, J. N., & Alder, C. H. (2011). The Montreal Cognitive Assessment and the Mini-Mental State Examination as screening instruments for cognitive impairment: Item analyses and threshold scores. *Dementia and Geriatric Cognitive Disorders, 31,* 126–131.

Dai, T., Davey, A., Woodard, J. L., Miller, L. S., Gondo, Y., Kim, S. H., & Poon, L. W. (2013). Sources of variation on the Mini-Mental State Examination in a population-based sample of centenarians. *Journal of the American Geriatrics Society, 61*(8), 1369–1376.

De Silva, R., Disanayaka, S., De Zoysa, N., Sanjeewanie, N., Somaratne, S., Foster, J., . . . Martins, R. M. (2009). Norms for the Mini-Mental State Examination from a sample of Sri Lankan older people. *International Journal of Geriatric Psychiatry: A Journal of the Psychiatry of Late Life and Allied Sciences, 24*(7), 666–670.

DeKosky, S. T., Shih, W. J., Schmitt, F. A., Coupal, J., & Kirkpatrick, C. (1990). Assessing utility of single photon emission computed tomography (SPECT) scan in Alzheimer disease: Correlation with cognitive severity. *Alzheimer Disease and Associated Disorders, 4,* 14–23.

Dodge, H. H., Meguro, K., Ishii, H., Yamaguchi, S., Saxton, J. A., & Ganguli, M. (2009). Cross-cultural comparisons of the Mini-mental State Examination between Japanese and US cohorts. *International Psychogeriatrics, 21*(01), 113–122.

Dong, Y., Sharma, V. K., Chan, B. P. L., Venketasubramanian, N., Teoh, H. L., Seet, R. C. S., . . . Chen, C. (2010). The Montreal Cognitive Assessment (MoCA) is superior to the Mini-Mental State Examination (MMSE) for the detection of vascular cognitive impairment after acute stroke. *Journal of the Neurological Sciences, 299*(1–2), 15–18.

Doody, R. S., Massman, P., & Dunn, J. K. (2001). A method for estimating progression rates in Alzheimer disease. *Archives of Neurology, 58,* 449–454.

Doraiswamy, P. M., & Kaiser, L. (2000). Variability of the Mini-Mental State Examination in dementia. *Neurology, 54,* 1538–1539.

Dufouil, C., Clayton, D., Brayne, C., Chi, L. Y., Dening, T. R., Paykel, E. S., . . . Huppert, F. A. (2000). Population norms for the MMSE in the very old. *Neurology, 55,* 1609–1612.

Eslinger, P. J., Swan, G. E., & Carmelli, D. (2003). Changes in the Mini-Mental State Examination in community-dwelling older persons over 6 years: Relationships to health and neuropsychological measures. *Neuroepidemiology, 22,* 23–30.

Espino, D. V., Lichtenstein, M. J., Palmer, R. F., & Hazuda, H. P. (2001). Ethnic differences in Mini-Mental State Examination (MMSE) scores: Where you live makes a difference. *Journal of the American Geriatric Society, 49,* 538–548.

Espino, D. V., Lichtenstein, M. J., Palmer, R. F., & Hazuda, H. P. (2004). Evaluation of the Mini-Mental State Examination's internal consistency in a community-based sample of Mexican-American and European-American elders: Results from the San Antonio Longitudinal Study of Aging. *Journal of the American Geriatrics Society, 52,* 822–827.

Feher, E. P., Mahurin, R. K., Doody, R. S., Cooke, N., Sims, J., & Pirozzolo, F. J. (1992). Establishing the limits of the Mini-Mental State. *Archives of Neurology, 49,* 87–92.

Fjell, A. M., Amlien, I. K., Westlye, L. T., & Walhovd, K. B. (2009). Mini-Mental State Examination is sensitive to brain atrophy in Alzheimer's disease. *Dementia and Geriatric Cognitive Disorders, 28*(3), 252–258.

Folstein, M. F., Folstein, S. E., & McHugh, P. R. (1975). "Mini-Mental State." A practical method for grading the cognitive state of patients for the clinician. *Journal of Psychiatric Research, 12,* 189–198.

Folstein, M. F., Folstein, S. E., McHugh, P. R., & Fanjiang, G. (2001). *Mini-Mental State Examination: User's guide.* Odessa, FL: PAR.

Folstein, M. F., Folstein, S. E., White, T., Messer, M. (2010). *MMSE-2 Manual.* Lutz, FL: PAR.

Ford, G. R., Haley, W. E., Thrower, S. L., West, C. A. C., & Harrell, L. E. (1996). Utility of Mini-Mental State Exam scores in predicting functional impairment among White and African American dementia patients. *Journal of Gerontology: Medical Sciences, 51A,* M185–M188.

Fountoulakis, K. N., Tsolaki, M., Chantzi, H., & Kazis, A. (2000). Mini Mental State Examination (MMSE): A validation study in Greece. *American Journal of Alzheimer's Disease and Other Dementias, 15,* 342–345.

Freidl, W., Schmidt, R., Stronegger, W. J., Fazekas, F., & Reinhart, B. (1996). Sociodemographic predictors and concurrent validity of the Mini Mental State Examination and the Mattis Dementia Rating Scale. *European Archives of Psychiatry and Clinical Neuroscience, 246,* 317–319.

Friedman, T. W., Yelland, G. W., & Robinson, S. R. (2012). Subtle cogni ive impairment in elders with Mini-Mental State Examination scores within the 'normal' range. *International Journal of Geriatric Psychiatry, 27*(5), 463–471.

Gallo, J. J., Rebok, G., & Lesikar, S. (1998). The driving habits of adults aged 60 years and older. *Journal of the American Geriatrics Society, 47,* 335–341.

Giannakopoulos, P., Herrmann, F. R., Bussiere, T., Bouras, C., Kovari, E., Perl, D. P., . . . Hof, P. R. (2003). Tangle and neuron numbers, but not amyloid load, predict cognitive status in Alzheimer's disease. *Neurology, 60,* 1495–1500.

Giordani, B., Boivin, M. J., Hall, A. L., Foster, N. L., Lehtinen, S. J., Bluemlein, M. S., & Berent, S. (1990). The utility and generality of Mini-Mental State Examination scores in Alzheimer's disease. *Neurology, 40,* 1894–1896.

Gluhm, S., Goldstein, J., Loc, K., Colt, A., Van Liew, C., & Corey-Bloom, J. (2013). Cognitive performance on the Mini-Mental State Examination and the Montreal Cognitive Assessment across the healthy adult lifespan. *Cognitive and Behavioral Neurology, 26*(1), 1.

Gontkovsky, S. T. (2014). Influence of IQ in interpreting MMSE scores in patients with multiple sclerosis. *Aging, Neuropsychology, and Cognition, 21*(2), 214–221.

Grace, J., Nadler, J. D., White, D. A., Guilmette, T. J., et al. (1995). Folstein vs modified Mini-Mental State Examination in geriatric stroke: Stability, validity, and screening utility. *Archives of Neurology, 52,* 477–484.

Grut, M., Fraiglioni, L., Viitanen, M., & Winblad, B. (1993). Accuracy of the Mini-Mental Status Examination as a screening test for dementia in a Swedish elderly population. *Acta Neurologica Scandinavica, 87,* 312–317.

Haubois, G., Decker, L., Annweiler, C., Launay, C., Allali, G., Herrmann, F. R., & Beauchet, O. (2013). Derivation and validation of a Short Form of the Mini-Mental State Examination for the screening of dementia in older adults with a memory complaint. *European Journal of Neurology, 20*(3), 588–590.

Helkala, E-L., Kivipelto, M., Hallikainen, M., Alhainene, K., Heinonen, H., Tuomilehto, J., . . . Nissines, A. (2002). Usefulness of repeated presentation of Mini-Mental State Examination as a diagnostic procedure—a population-based study. *Acta Neurologica Scandinavica, 106,* 341–346.

Hill, R. D., & Backman, L. (1995). The relationships between the Mini-Mental State Examination and cognitive functioning in normal elderly adults: A componential analysis. *Age Aging, 24,* 440–446.

Hirschman, K. B., Xie, S. X., Feudtner, C., & Karlawish, J. H. T. (2003). How does Alzheimer's disease patient's role in medical decision making change over time? *Journal of Geriatric Psychiatry & Neurology, 17,* 55–60.

Hoops, S., Nazem, S., Siderowf, A. D., Duda, J. E., Xie, S. X., Stern, M. B., & Weintraub, D. (2009). Validity of the MoCA and MMSE in the detection of MCI and dementia in Parkinson disease. *Neurology, 73*(21), 1738–1745.

Hopp, G. A., Dixon, R. A., Backman, I., & Grut, M. (1997). Stability of two measures of cognitive functioning in nondemented old-old adults. *Journal of Clinical Psychology, 53,* 673–686.

Ibrahim, N. M., Shohaimi, S., Chong, H. T., Rahman, A. H. A., Razali, R., Esther, E., & Basri, H. B. (2009). Validation study of the Mini-Mental State Examination in a Malay-speaking elderly population in Malaysia. *Dementia and Geriatric Cognitive Disorders, 27,* 247–53.

Ishizaki, J., Meguro, K., Ambo, H., Shimada, M., Yamaguchi, S., Hayasaka, C., Komatsu, H., Sekita, Y., & Yamadori, A. (1998). A normative, community-based study of Mini-Mental State in elderly adults: The effect of age and educational level. *Journal of Gerontology: Psychological Sciences, 53B,* P359–P363.

Iverson, G. L. (1998). Interpretation of Mini-Mental State Examination scores in community-dwelling elderly and geriatric neuropsychiatry patients. *International Journal of Geriatric Psychiatry, 13,* 661–666.

Jefferson, A. L., Consentino, S. A., Ball, S. K., Bogdanoff, B., Kaplan, E., & Libon, D. J. (2002). Errors produced on the Mini-Mental State Examination and neuropsychological test performance in Alzheimer's disease, ischemic vascular dementia, and Parkinson's disease. *Journal of Neuropsychiatry and Clinical Neurosciences, 14,* 311–320.

Jones, R. N., & Gallo, J. J. (2000). Dimensions of the Mini-Mental State Examination among community dwelling older adults. *Psychological Medicine, 30,* 605–618.

Jones, R. N., & Gallo, J. J. (2002). Education and sex differences in the Mini-Mental State Examination: Effects of differential item functioning. *Journals of Gerontology: Series B: Psychological Sciences & Social Sciences, 57B,* P548–P558.

Jones, S., Laukka, E. J., Small, B. J., Fratiglioni, L., & Backman, L. (2004). A preclinical phase in vascular dementia: Cognitive impairment three years before diagnosis. *Dementia & Geriatric Cognitive Disorders, 18,* 233–239.

Jones, T. G., Schinka, J. A., Vanderploeg, R. D., Small, B. J., Graves, A. B., & Mortimer, J. A. (2002). 3MS normative data for the elderly. *Archives of Clinical Neuropsychology, 17,* 171–177.

Karzmark, P. (2000). Validity of the serial seven procedure. *International Journal of Geriatric Psychiatry, 15,* 677–679.

Kato, Y., Narumoto, J., Matsuoka, T., Okamura, A., Koumi, H., Kishikawa, Y., . . . Fukui, K. (2013). Diagnostic performance of a combination of Mini-Mental State Examination and Clock Drawing Test in detecting Alzheimer's disease. *Neuropsychiatric Disease and Treatment, 9,* 581.

Kaufer, D. I., Williams, C. S., Braaten, A. J., Gill, K., Zimmerman, S., & Sloane, P. D. (2008). Cognitive screening for dementia and Mild Cognitive Impairment in assisted living: Comparison of 3 tests. *Journal of the American Medical Directors Association, 9*(8), 586–593.

Kim, S. Y. K., & Caine, E. D. (2002). Utility and limits of the Mini Mental State Examination in evaluating consent capacity in Alzheimer's disease. *Psychiatric Services, 53,* 1322–1324.

Kraemer, H. C., Moritz, D. J., & Yesavage, J. (1998). Adjusting Mini-Mental State Examination scores for age and education level to screen for dementia: Correcting bias or reducing variability. *International Psychogeriatrics, 10,* 43–51.

Kupke, T., Revis, E. S., & Gantner, A. B. (1993). Hemispheric bias of the Mini-Mental State Examination in elderly males. *The Clinical Neuropsychologist, 7,* 210–214.

Kuslansky, G., Katz, M., Verhese, J., Hall, C. B., Lapuerta, P., LaRuffa, G., & Lipton, R. B. (2004). Detecting dementia with the Hopkins learning test and the Mini-Mental State Examination. *Archives of Clinical Neuropsychology, 19,* 89–104.

Lamarre, C. J., & Patten, S. B. (1991). Evaluation of the modified Mini-Mental State Examination in a general psychiatric population. *Canadian Journal of Psychiatry, 36,* 507–511.

Lee, H. W., Caramelli, P., Otaduy, M. C. G., Nitrini, R., & da Costa Leite, C. (2007). Mini-Mental State Examination and proton spectroscopy of the posterior cingulate in Alzheimer disease. *Dementia Neuropsychologia, 3,* 248–252.

Lemsky, C. M., Smith, G., Malec, J. R., & Ivnik, R. J. (1996). Identifying risk for functional impairment using cognitive measures: An application of CART modeling. *Neuropsychology, 10,* 368–375.

Lopez, M. N., Charter, R. A., Mostafavi, B., Nibut, L. P., & Smith, W. E. (2005). Psychometric properties of the Folstein Mini-Mental State Examination. *Assessment, 12,* 137–144.

Lyness, S. A., Lee, A. Y., Zarow, C., Teng, E. L., & Chui, H. C. (2014). 10-minute delayed recall from the Modified Mini-Mental State Test predicts Alzheimer's disease pathology. *Journal of Alzheimer's Disease, 39*(3), 575–582.

Mackin, R. S., Ayalon, L., Feliciano, L., & Areán, P. A. (2010). The sensitivity and specificity of cognitive screening instruments to detect cognitive impairment in older adults with severe psychiatric illness. *Journal of Geriatric Psychiatry and Neurology, 23*(2), 94–99.

Malek-Ahmadi, M., Davis, K., Belden, C. M., & Sabbagh, M. N. (2014). Comparative Analysis of the Alzheimer's Questionnaire (AQ) with the CDR Sum of Boxes, MoCA, and MMSE. *Alzheimer Disease and Associated Disorders, 28*(3), 296.

Malek-Ahmadi, M., Powell, J. J., Belden, C. M., O'Connor, K., Evans, L., Coon, D. W., & Nieri, W. (2015). Age-and education-adjusted normative data for the Montreal Cognitive Assessment (MoCA) in older adults age 70–99. *Aging, Neuropsychology, and Cognition, 22*(6), 755–761.

Matallana, D., De Santacruz, C., Cano, C., Reyes, P., Samper-Ternent, R., Markides, K. S., . . . Reyes-Ortiz, C. A. (2011). The relationship between education level and Mini-Mental State Examination domains among older Mexican Americans. *Journal of Geriatric Psychiatry and Neurology, 24*(1), 9–18.

Marcopulos, B. A., & McLain, C. A. (2003). Are our norms "normal"? A 4-year follow-up study of a biracial sample of rural elders with low education. *The Clinical Neuropsychologist, 17,* 19–33.

Marcopulos, B. A., McLain, C. A., & Giuliano, A. J. (1997). Cognitive impairment or inadequate norms? A study of healthy, rural, older adults with limited education. *The Clinical Neuropsychologist, 11,* 111–131.

Meiran, N., Stuss, D. T., Guzman, A., Lafleche, G., & Willmer, J. (1996). Diagnosis of dementia: Methods for interpretation of scores of 5 neuropsychological tests. *Archives of Neurology, 53,* 1043–1054.

Meyer, J. S., Li, Y-S., & Thornby, J. (2001). Validating Mini-Mental Status, cognitive capacity screening and Hamilton Depression Scales utilizing subjects with vascular headaches. *International Journal of Geriatric Psychiatry, 16,* 430–435.

Milian, M., Leiherr, A. M., Straten, G., Müller, S., Leyhe, T., & Eschweiler, G. W. (2012). The Mini-Cog versus the Mini-Mental State Examination and the Clock Drawing Test in daily clinical practice: screening value in a German Memory Clinic. *International Psychogeriatrics, 24*(5), 766.

Mitchell, A. J., Shukla, D., Ajumal, H. A., Stubbs, B., & Tahir, T. A. (2014). The Mini-Mental State Examination as a diagnostic and screening test for delirium: systematic review and meta-analysis. *General Hospital Psychiatry, 36*(6), 627–633.

Mitrushina, M., & Satz, P. (1991). Reliability and validity of the Mini-Mental State Exam in neurologically intact elderly. *Journal of Clinical Psychology, 47,* 537–543.

Mitrushina, M., & Satz, P. (1994). Utility of Mini-Mental State Examination in assessing cognition in the elderly. Paper presented to the International Neuropsychological Society, Cincinnati, OH.

Mokri, H., Ávila-Funes, J. A., Meillon, C., Gutiérrez Robledo, L. M., & Amieva, H. (2013). Normative data for the Mini-Mental State Examination, the Free and Cued Selective Reminding Test and the Isaacs Set Test for an older adult Mexican population: The Coyoacán Cohort Study. *The Clinical Neuropsychologist, 27*(6), 1004–1018.

Molloy, D. W., Alemayehu, E., & Roberts, R. (1991). Reliability of a standardized Mini-Mental State Examination compared with the traditional Mini-Mental State Examination. *American Journal of Psychiatry, 148,* 102–105.

Mulgrew, C. L., Morgenstern, N., Shtterly, S. M., Baxter, J., Baron, A. E., & Hamman, R. F. (1999). Cognitive functioning and impairment among rural elderly Hispanics and non-Hispanic Whites as assessed by the Mini-Mental State Examination. *Journal of Gerontology: Psychological Sciences, 54B,* P223–230.

Myers, W. C., Hall, R. C., & Tolou-Shams, M. (2012). Prevalence and assessment of malingering in homicide defendants using the Mini-Mental State Examination and the Rey 15-Item Memory Test. *Homicide Studies,* 1088767912465609.

Mystakidou, K., Tsilika, E., Parpa, E., Galanos, A., & Vlahos, L. (2007). Brief cognitive assessment of cancer patients: Evaluation of the Mini-Mental State Examination (MMSE) psychometric properties. *Psycho-Oncology, 16*(4), 352–357.

Nadler, J. D., Relkin, N. R., Cohen, M. S., Hodder, R. A., Reingold, J., & Plum, F. (1995). Mental status testing in the elderly nursing home populations. *Journal of Geriatric Neurology, 8,* 177–183.

Nehra, R. Chakrabarti, S. Sharma, R., & Painuly, N. (2006) Can Mini-Mental State Examination scores predict short-term impairments in memory during Electroconvulsive Therapy (ECT)? *German Journal of Psychiatry,* 8–10.

Nilsson, E., Fastbom, J., & Wahlin, A. (2002). Cognitive functioning in a population-based sample of very old non-demented and non-depressed persons: The impact of diabetes. *Archives of Gerontology and Geriatrics, 35,* 95–105.

Nguyen, H. T., Black, S. A., Ray, L., Espino, D. V., & Markides, K. S. (2003). Cognitive impairment and mortality in older Mexican Americans. *Journal of the American Geriatrics Society, 51,* 178–183.

Nyenhuis, D. L., Gorelick, P. B., Freels, S., & Garron, D. C. (2002). Cognitive and functional decline in African Americans with VaD, AD, and stroke without dementia. *Neurology, 58,* 56–61.

Nys, G. M. S., van Zandvoort, M. J. E., de Kort, P. L. M., Jansen, B. P. W., Kappelle, L. J., & de Haan, E. H. F. (2005). Restrictions of the Mini-Mental State Examination in acute stroke. *Archives of Clinical Neuropsychology, 20,* 623–629.

O'Connell, M. E., Tuokko, H., Graves, R. E., & Kadlec, H. (2004). Correcting the 3MS for bias does not improve accuracy when screening for cognitive impairment or dementia. *Journal of Clinical and Experimental Neuropsychology, 26,* 970–980.

Olin, J. T., & Zelinski, E. M. (1991). The 12-month stability of the Mini-Mental State Examination. *Psychological Assessment, 3,* 427–432.

Oudman, E., Postma, A., Van der Stigchel, S., Appelhof, B., Wijnia, J. W., & Nijboer, T. C. (2014). The Montreal Cognitive Assessment (MoCA) is superior to the Mini Mental State Examination (MMSE) in detection of Korsakoff's syndrome. *The Clinical Neuropsychologist, 28*(7), 1123–1132.

Ouvrier, R. A., Goldsmith, R. F., Ouvrier, S., & Williams, I. C. (1993). The value of the Mini-Mental State Examination in childhood: A preliminary study. *Journal of Child Neurology, 8,* 145–149.

Pachet, A., Astner, K., & Brown, L. (2010). Clinical utility of the Mini-Mental State Examination when assessing decision-making capacity. *Journal of Geriatric Psychiatry and Neurology, 23*(1), 3–8.

Palmer, K., Wang, H-X., Backman, L., Winblad, B., & Fratiglioni, L. (2002). Differential evolution of cognitive impairment in nondemented older persons: Results from the Kungsholmen project. *American Journal of Psychiatry, 159,* 436–442.

Pasquier, F., Richard, F., & Lebert, F. (2004). Natural history of frontotemporal dementia: Comparison with Alzheimer's disease. *Dementia & Geriatric Cognitive Disorders, 17,* 253–257.

Queally, V. R., Evans, J. J., & McMillan, T. M. (2011). A meta-analysis of studies comparing the effectiveness of three cognitive screening tests in the detection of dementia populations. *International Journal of Geriatric Psychiatry, 26*(5), 548–549.

Rezende, G. P., Cecato, J., & Martinelli, J. E. (2013). Cognitive Abilities Screening Instrument-short form, Mini-Mental State Examination and Functional Activities Questionnaire in the illiterate elderly [Triagem de habilidades cognitivas em idosos analfabetos: CASI-S, mini-exame do estado mental e questionário de atividades funcionais]. *Dementia Neuropsychology, 7*(4).

Ringdal, G. I., Ringdal, K., Juliebø, V., Wyller, T. B., Hjermstad, M. J., & Loge, J. H. (2011). Using the Mini-Mental State Examination to screen for delirium in elderly patients with hip fracture. *Dementia and Geriatric Cognitive Disorders, 32*(6), 394–400.

Ruchinskas, R. A., & Curyto, K. J. (2003). Cognitive screening in geriatric rehabilitation. *Rehabilitation Psychology, 48,* 14–22.

Salmon, D. P., Thal, L. J., Butters, N., & Heindel, W. C. (1990). Longitudinal evaluation of dementia of the Alzheimer type: A comparison of 3 standardized mental status examinations. *Neurology, 40,* 1225–1230.

Scazufca, M., Almeida, O. P., Vallada, H. P., Tasse, W. A., & Menezes, P. R. (2009). Limitations of the Mini-Mental State Examination for screening dementia in a community with low socioeconomic status. *European Archives of Psychiatry and Clinical Neuroscience, 259*(1), 8–15.

Schretlen, D. J., Testa, S. M., & Pearlson, G. D. (2010). *Calibrated Neuropsychological Normative System.* Lutz, FL: PAR.

Schweizer, T. A., Al-Khindi, T., & Macdonald, R. L. (2012). Mini-Mental State Examination versus Montreal Cognitive Assessment: Rapid assessment tools for cognitive and functional outcome after aneurysmal subarachnoid hemorrhage. *Journal of the Neurological Sciences, 316*(1), 137–140.

Shadlen, M-F., Larson, E. B., Gibbons, L., McCormick, W. C., & Teri, L. (1999). Alzheimer's disease symptom severity in blacks and whites. *Journal of the American Geriatrics Society, 47,* 482–486.

Shah, A., Phongsathorn, V., George, C., Bielawska, C., & Katona, C. (1992). Psychiatric morbidity among continuing care geriatric inpatients. *International Journal of Geriatric Psychiatry, 7,* 517–525.

Shiroky, J. S., Schipper, H. M., Bergman, H., & Chertkow, H. (2007). Can you have dementia with an MMSE score of 30?. *American Journal of Alzheimer's Disease and Other Dementias, 22*(5), 406–415.

Sliwinski, M., Buschke, H., Stewart, W. F., Masur, D., & Lipton, R. D. (1997). The effect of dementia risk factors on comparative and diagnostic selective reminding norms. *Journal of the International Neuropsychological Society, 3,* 317–326.

Small, B. J., Herlitz, A., Fratiglioni, L., Almkvist, O., & Bäckman, L. (1997a). Cognitive predictors of incident Alzheimer's disease: A prospective longitudinal study. *Neuropsychology, 11,* 413–420.

Small, B. J., Viitanen, M., Winblad, B., & Bäckman, L. (1997b). Cognitive changes in very old persons with dementia: The influence of demographic, psychometric, and biological variables. *Journal of Clinical and Experimental Neuropsychology, 19,* 245–260.

Spencer, R. J., Wendell, C. R., Giggey, P. P., Katzel, L. I., Lefkowitz, D. M., Siegel, E. L., & Waldstein, S. R. (2013). Psychometric limitations of the Mini-Mental State Examination among nondemented older adults: An evaluation of neurocognitive and magnetic resonance imaging correlates. *Experimental Aging Research, 39*(4), 382–397.

Stein, J., Luppa, M., Kaduszkiewicz, H., Eisele, M., Weyerer, S., Werle, J., . . . Pentzek, M. (2015). Is the Short Form of the Mini-Mental State Examination (MMSE) a better screening instrument for dementia in older primary care patients than the original MMSE? Results of the German study on ageing, cognition, and dementia in primary care patients (AgeCoDe). *Psychological Assessment, 27*(3), 895.

Sugarman, M. A., & Axelrod, B. N. (2014). Utility of the Montreal Cognitive Assessment and Mini-Mental State Examination in predicting general intellectual abilities. *Cognitive and Behavioral Neurology, 27*(3), 148–154.

Stern, Y., Tang, M-X., Albert, M. S., Brandt, J., Jacobs, D. M., Bell, K., . . . Tsai, W-Y. (1997). Predicting time to nursing home care and death in individuals with Alzheimer disease. *Journal of the American Medical Association, 277,* 806–812.

Stout, J. C., Jernigan, T. L., Archibald, S. L., & Salmon, D. P. (1996). Association of dementia severity with cortical gray matter and abnormal white matter volumes in dementia of the Alzheimer type. *Archives of Neurology, 53,* 742–749.

Tan, J. (2004). *Influence of impending death on the MMSE.* MSc Thesis, University of Victoria.

Tang-Wai, D. F., Knopman, D. S., Geda, Y. E. Edland, S. D., Smith, G. E., Ivnik, R. J., . . . Petersen, R. C. (2003). Comparison of the Short Test of Mental Status and the Mini-Mental State Examination in Mild Cognitive Impairment. *Archives of Neurolology, 60,* 1777–1781.

Tappen, R. M., Rosselli, M., & Engstrom, G. (2012). Use of the MC-FAQ and MMSE-FAQ in cognitive screening of older African Americans, Hispanic Americans, and European Americans. *The American Journal of Geriatric Psychiatry, 20*(11), 955–962.

Teng, E. L., & Chui, H. C. (1987). The modified Mini-Mental State (3MS) Examination. *Journal of Clinical Psychiatry, 48,* 314–318.

Teng, E. L., Chiu, H. C., Schneider, L. S., & Metzger, L. E. (1987). Alzheimer's dementia: Performance on the Mini-Mental State Examination. *Journal of Consulting and Clinical Psychology, 55,* 96–100.

Teresi, J. A., Holmes, D., Ramirez, M., Gurland, B. J., & Lantigua, R. (2001). Performance of cognitive tests among different racial/ethnic and education groups: Findings of differential item functioning and possible item bias. *Journal of Mental Health and Aging, 7,* 79–89.

Tombaugh, T. N. (2005). Test-retest reliable coefficients and 5-year change scores for the MMSE and the 3MS. *Archives of Clinical Neuropsychology, 20,* 485–503.

Tombaugh, T. N., McDowell, I., Krisjansson, B., & Hubley, A. M. (1996). Mini-Mental State Examination (MMSE) and the modified MMSE (3MS): A psychometric comparison and normative data. *Psychological Assessment, 8,* 48–59.

Tombaugh, T. N., & McIntyre, N. J. (1992). The Mini-Mental State Examination: A comprehensive review. *Journal of the American Geriatric Society, 40,* 922–935.

Tschanz, J. T., Welsh-Bohmer, K. A., Plassman, B. L., Norton, M. C., Wyse, B. W., & Breitner, J. C. S. (2002). An adaptation of the modified Mini-Mental State Examination: Analysis of demographic influences and normative data. *Neuropsychiatry, Neuropsychology, and Behavioral Neurology, 15,* 28–38.

Villaseñor-Cabrera, T., Guàrdia-Olmos, J., Jiménez-Maldonado, M., Rizo-Curiel, G., & Peró-Cebollero, M. (2010). Sensitivity and specificity of the Mini-Mental State Examination in the Mexican population. *Quality & Quantity, 44*(6), 1105–1112.

Wajman, J. R., Oliveira, F. F. D., Schultz, R. R., Marin, S. D. M. C., & Bertolucci, P. H. F. (2014). Educational bias in the assessment of severe dementia: Brazilian cutoffs for severe Mini-Mental State Examination. *Arquivos de Neuro-psiquiatria, 72*(4), 273–277.

Wang, C. S. M., Pai, M. C., Chen, P. L., Hou, N. T., Chien, P. F., & Huang, Y. C. (2013). Montreal Cognitive Assessment and Mini-Mental State Examination performance in patients with mild-to-moderate dementia with Lewy bodies, Alzheimer's disease, and normal participants in Taiwan. *International Psychogeriatrics, 25*(11), 1839–1848.

Wells, J. C., Keyl, P. M., Aboraya, A., Folstein, M. F., & Anthony, J. C. (1992). Discriminant validity of a reduced set of Mini-Mental State Examination items for dementia and Alzheimer's disease. *Acta Psychiatrica Scandinavica, 86,* 23–31.

Whitney, K. A., Mossbarger, B., Herman, S. M., & Ibarra, S. L. (2012). Is the Montreal Cognitive Assessment superior to the Mini-Mental State Examination in detecting subtle cognitive impairment among middle-aged outpatient US Military veterans?. *Archives of Clinical Neuropsychology, 27*(7), 742–748.

Wouters, H., van Gool, W. A., Schmand, B., Zwinderman, A. H., & Lindeboom, R. (2010). Three sides of the same coin: Measuring global cognitive impairment with the MMSE, ADAS-Cog and CAMCOG. *International Journal of Geriatric Psychiatry, 25*(8), 770–779.

MONTREAL COGNITIVE ASSESSMENT (MOCA)

TEST NAME	**Montreal Cognitive Assessment (MoCA)**
DOMAIN	Dementia screening
AGE RANGE	20 to 99 years
ADMINISTRATION TIME	10 minutes
SCORING FORMAT	Hand scored
REFERENCE	Nasreddine, Z. S., Phillips, N. A., Bédirian, V., Charbonneau, S., Whitehead, V., Collin, I., et al. (2005). The Montreal Cognitive Assessment, MoCA: A brief screening tool for Mild Cognitive Impairment. *Journal of the American Geriatrics Society*, *53*(4), 695–699. www.mocatest.org

DESCRIPTION

The Montreal Cognitive Assessment (MoCA; Nasreddine et al., 2005) is a brief measure of global cognitive functioning that has gained tremendous popularity since its publication in 2005. It is freely available for clinical and academic use. The availability of multiple alternate forms also allows repeat testing in short intervals without concern for practice effects. Many studies have been done to validate its usefulness as a cognitive screen in different countries, and it has been translated into many languages with validation studies completed based on local samples.

The MoCA assesses six cognitive domains including orientation, attention/concentration, memory, visuospatial skills, language, and executive functions. Because of its inclusion of complex executive items and a five-word list, it is sensitive to mild cognitive dysfunction despite its brevity. As such, it is a useful screen for cognitive impairment in several neurologic and medical conditions, as well as in psychiatric conditions. Given its established superiority over the MMSE in detecting mild cognitive dysfunction, the MoCA has been recommended by the Canadian Cardiovascular Society and the National Institute of Neurological Disorders and Stroke-Canadian Stroke Network (NINDS-CSN) to screen for cognitive impairments in patients with heart failure (Arnold et al., 2007) and vascular diseases (Hachinski et al., 2006), respectively.

Since its initial development, three additional simplified versions have been created for various purposes. The MoCA-Basic allows assessment of cognitive impairment in those who are illiterate or with low education (<5 years of education). The MoCA-Basic assesses the same cognitive domains as the original version except for visuoperception instead of visuoconstructional skills. MoCA-Mini is a five-minute protocol comprising four items assessing memory, executive function/language, and orientation that can be administered over the telephone. Finally, the MoCA-Blind relies entirely on auditory items to assess individuals who have visual impairments.

A computerized version, the MoCA-CC, based on the Beijing version is also available (Yu et al., 2015). The website also offers an electronic version, although details about its equivalence to the paper test are scarce as of the writing of this review.

ADMINISTRATION

Full instructions are available on the website for free download (https://mocatest.org).

SCORING

Item scores are added to a total of 30 points. Higher points reflect better cognitive functioning. Based on the original study, those with 12 years or less of education are given +1 point. Follow-up studies suggested +1 point for those with six or less years of education when using the MoCA in Asia and/or developing countries (Hu et al., 2013; Tan et al., 2015; Wong et al., 2009). The original authors have also provided evidence for a revised education correction: +1 point for 10–12 years of education and +2 points for 4–9 years of education (Chertkow et al., 2011). When using the Peking MoCA, it has been suggested that two points be added for those with six years or less of education and one point be added for those with more than six and 12 or less years of education (Tan et al., 2015). However, see the sections "Demographic Effects" and "Normative Data" for discussions advising against correcting for education. Typically, a cutoff score of less than 26 represents cognitive impairment requiring further detailed testing, but this cutoff has been criticized for being too high, resulting in a high false-positive error rate (Rossetti et al., 2012). Other cutoffs have been suggested for different populations and disorders (see Tables 7–55 to 7–58).

MoCA-Basic retains a total of 30 points. One point is added for those with less than four years of education. An additional point is added for those who are illiterate, defined as the inability to read or write fluently in daily living. MoCA-Mini also is scored out of 30 points, although no information regarding cutoff scores for cognitive dysfunction is available at the writing of this review. MoCA-Blind is scored out of 22. Scores of 18 or less reflect cognitive dysfunction requiring further investigation.

USING MOCA TO PREDICT WAIS-IV FSIQ

The MoCA can be used to predict WAIS-IV FSIQ using regression-based prediction equations (Sugarman & Axelrod, 2014). The equations were generated from a sample of older veterans age 60+ who were referred by their physicians for neuropsychological evaluation.

$$\text{FSIQ} = (2.01 \times \text{MoCA} + 43.23)$$

Error in prediction = 7.5 (*SD* = 6.0) points.

This equation is accurate to within 5 FSIQ points in 45%, within 10 points in 69%, and within 15 points in 87% of the sample. A raw score of less than 19 predicts borderline FSIQ or lower, and less than 21 predicts less than 85 FSIQ.

USING MOCA AND TOPF TO PREDICT WAIS-IV FSIQ

The prediction can be improved with the addition of the TOPF score, which in total accounted for 58% of the variance on obtained FSIQ.

$$\text{FSIQ} = (.39 \times \text{R-TOPF}) + (.20 \times \text{D-TOPF}) + (1.5 \times \text{MoCA}) + .19$$

where R-TOPF = TOPF Word Reading ability; D-TOPF = TOPF demographic variables.

Error in prediction was 6.6 (*SD* = 4.9) points.

This equation is accurate to within 5 FSIQ points for 45% of the sample, within 10 points for 78%, and within 15 points for 94% of the sample. Both of these equations are calculated *without* applying education correction on the MoCA.

DEMOGRAPHIC EFFECTS

AGE

MoCA scores appear to remain stable throughout adulthood and decrease with increasing age in older adults (Bernstein et al., 2011; Conti et al., 2015; Freitas et al., 2011, 2014; Gluhm et al., 2013; Hu et al., 2013; Wong et al., 2009, 2012; Wu et al., 2014). In general, weak to moderate correlations with age have been reported (Bernstein et al., 2011; Musso et al., 2014; Roalf et al., 2009; Tan et al., 2015; Tsai et al., 2012; Waldron-Perrine & Axelrod, 2012).

GENDER

Gender effects appear minimal (Bernstein et al., 2011; Conti et al., 2015; Freitas et al., 2011, 2014; Hu et al., 2013; Tsai et al., 2012; Wong et al., 2009).

EDUCATION

Education appears to have the strongest impact on MoCA performance, with generally moderate correlations reported in many studies (Bernstein et al., 2011; Tan et al., 2015; Tsai et al., 2012; Waldron-Perrine et al., 2012; Wu et al., 2014). Given the education effects on the MoCA, the original authors recommended an education adjustment for those with 12 years or less education. However, follow-up studies have indicated the inadequacy of this education correction given the high education attainment of the original sample (e.g., Hu et al., 2013; Mai et al., 2013). As such, follow-up studies have recommended education adjustment at a much lower level (e.g., ≤6 years of education; Wong et al., 2009; Hu et al., 2013). Based on the revised education corrections suggested by the original authors (see "Scoring"), the correction for 10–12 education years yields a specificity of 69% and a sensitivity of 90% for MCI (100% for AD); the correction for 4–9 education years yields a specificity of 74% and a sensitivity of 88% for MCI (100% for AD; Chertkow et al., 2011).

However, some authors have shown that any education correction may compromise sensitivity with a minimal increase in specificity in both dementia/MCI and stroke prevention clinic patients (Gagnon et al., 2013; Mai et al., 2013). In one study, the adjustment yielded more false negatives (Gagnon et al., 2013). These authors suggested that correcting for low education without consideration of cognitive reserve may artificially inflate performance. As such, instead of education correction, they recommended the use of normative data to guide interpretation.

ETHNICITY, NATIONALITY, AND LINGUISTIC EFFECTS

Cultural impacts have been noted on abstraction, fluency, naming, and word-list items when examinees have a lack of familiarity with the concept/item or if there are linguistic differences (Dominguez et al., 2013; Fujiwara et al., 2010; Hu et al., 2013; Ozdilek & Kenangil, 2014; Sahathevan et al., 2014). Thus, most of the translated versions have modified these items according to the local context. Likewise, regional differences have been reported in a Portuguese and a Beijing study; however, the regional effects appear to attenuate once age and education are accounted for (Freitas et al., 2011; Yu et al., 2015).

NORMATIVE DATA

Cutoff scores have typically been used to identify those who can benefit from detailed neuropsychological testing. Given concerns about artificial inflation of performance by education correction (Gagnon et al., 2013), use of normative data has been suggested to guide interpretation. Tables 7–47 and 7–48 present normative data from American community samples stratified by age and education (Malek-Ahmadi et al., 2015; Rossetti et al., 2011). While the Rossetti et al. norms are larger, the Malek-Ahmadi et al. norms provide data on individuals with 13 to 16 years of

TABLE 7–47 American Montreal Cognitive Assessment (MoCA) Norms for Older Adults Ages 70 to 99 Stratified by Age and Education

	EDUCATION (YEARS)								
	≤12			13 TO 15			≥16		
AGE (YEARS)	N	MEAN	*SD*	N	MEAN	*SD*	N	MEAN	*SD*
70 to 79	4	25.25	4.11	27	27.78	2.24	22	27.59	2.04
80 to 89	15	23.47	2.97	40	25.08	3.13	34	25.82	2.75
90 to 99	14	23.00	2.63	26	23.35	3.43	23	24.61	2.59

NOTE: Based on healthy participants drawn from an ongoing study on longevity in Phoenix, Arizona. *N* = 205 (65 males; 140 females); mean age = 84.67, *SD* = 7.88.

SOURCE: From Malek-Ahmadi et al. (2015).

education. Normative data based on a community sample from all geographical regions of Portugal are presented in Table 7–49. The sample distribution is reportedly comparable to target Portuguese population and is comprised of individuals age 25+, about 63% females, 84% from coastal (vs. 16% inland) areas, and are predominantly from urban (69%) and moderately urban (17%) areas (Freitas et al., 2011). Italian samples are presented in Table 7–50 (Santangelo et al., 2015) and Table 7–51 (Conti et al., 2015). Note that cell sizes for certain age and education levels are very small.

Regression-based equations to adjust for demographic impact have also been reported in the literature to simplify interpretation (Santangelo et al., 2015). Table 7–52 shows cumulative frequencies of different scores after adjustment for age, education, and gender. Memory was not reported because the outer tolerance limit was negative and did not allow for correction. Domain scores were based on (1) visuospatial abilities (clock drawing and cube copy; range 0–4), (2) executive functions (trail making, phonemic fluency, and verbal abstraction; range 0–4), (3) attention, concentration, and working memory (sustained attention, serial subtraction, and digit span; range 0–6), (4) language (naming, repetition, and phonemic fluency; range 0–6), and (5) orientation (range 0–6). Conti and colleagues (2015) presented similar information based on healthy participants drawn from a memory disorders clinic and a senior center in Bologna, Italy (Table 7–53).

EVIDENCE FOR RELIABILITY

EVIDENCE FOR INTERNAL RELIABILITY

Internal consistency is at least fair to excellent in most clinical studies (Cronbach's alpha >.70; Bezdicek et al., 2013; Dominguez et al., 2013; Freitas et al., 2011, 2012a, 2013; Fujiwara et al., 2010; Hu et al., 2013; Lee et al., 2008; Memória et al., 2013; Nasreddine et al., 2005; Ozdilek & Kenangil, 2014; Rahman & El Gaafary, 2009; Tan et al., 2015; Tsai et al., 2012; Wong et al., 2009; Wong et al., 2013; Yu et al., 2012, 2015). In clinical groups, Cronbach's alpha ranges from .72 in older adults with cerebral small-vessel disease to .95 in MCI and dementia. The internal consistency tends to be low with healthy controls, especially those who are young and highly educated (Bezdicek et al., 2013; Freitas et al., 2012a; McLennan et al., 2011).

TABLE 7–48 American Montreal Cognitive Assessment (MoCA) Norms Stratified by Age and Education

	EDUCATION (YEARS)															
	<12				12				>12				TOTAL			
AGE	*N*	MEAN	*SD*	MEDIAN	*N*	MEAN	*SD*	MEDIAN	*N*	MEAN	*SD*	MEDIAN	*N*	MEAN	*SD*	MEDIAN
<35	20	22.80	3.38	23	65	24.46	3.49	25	122	25.93	2.48	26	207	25.16	3.08	26
30–40	37	22.84	3.18	23	106	23.99	2.93	24	264	25.81	2.64	26	408	25.07	2.95	25
35–45	55	22.11	3.33	23	177	23.02	3.67	24	355	25.38	3.05	26	588	24.37	3.51	25
40–50	77	21.36	3.73	22	227	22.26	3.94	23	418	25.09	3.16	26	723	23.8	3.80	24
45–55	77	20.75	3.80	21	216	21.87	3.95	22	461	24.70	3.24	25	755	23.48	3.84	24
50–60	62	19.94	4.34	20	172	22.25	3.46	22	424	24.34	3.38	25	659	23.37	3.78	24
55–65	60	19.60	4.14	20	143	21.58	3.93	22	369	24.43	3.31	25	573	23.20	3.96	23
60–70	57	19.30	3.79	19	113	20.89	4.50	21	246	24.32	3.04	25	418	22.69	4.12	23
65–75	38	18.37	3.87	19	67	20.57	4.79	21	122	24.00	3.35	24	228	22.05	4.48	23
70–80	14	16.07	3.17	17	23	20.35	4.91	20	42	23.60	3.47	24	79	21.32	4.78	22
Total	230	20.55	4.04	21	608	22.34	3.97	23	1306	24.81	3.20	25	2148	23.65	3.84	24

NOTE: Norms based on community-sample from the Dallas Heart Study. *N* = 2653, 60% Females. Sample comprised of Black (54%), White (33%), Hispanic (11%), and Other (2%). Age mean = 50.30, *SD* = 11.20; Education mean = 13.35, *SD* = 2.50.

SOURCE: Rossetti et al. (2011).

TABLE 7–49 Normative Data for the Portuguese Montreal Cognitive Assessment (MoCA) Stratified by Age and Education Level

	EDUCATION (YEARS)														
	PRIMARY (1 TO 4)			MIDDLE (5 TO 9)			HIGH (10 TO 12)			UNIVERSITY (>12)			ALL EDUCATION		
AGE	*N*	MEAN	*SD*	*N*	MEAN	*SD*	*N*	MEAN	*SD*	*N*	MEAN	*SD*	*N*	MEAN	*SD*
25–49	29	23.55 [a](21, 20, 18)	2.56	66	26.42 [a](24, 23, 22)	2.18	59	27.39 [a](26, 25, 24)	1.86	60	28.83 [a](28, 27, 26)	1.38	214	26.98 [a](24, 23, 22)	2.55
50–64	91	21.78 [a](19, 18, 16)	2.86	59	25.58 [a](23, 22, 21)	2.25	33	26.61 [a](24, 23, 22)	2.28	35	27.51 [a](25, 24, 23)	2.13	218	24.46 [a](21, 19, 18)	3.43
>65	136	21.27 [a](18, 16, 15)	3.37	45	24.60 [a](22, 20, 19)	2.87	20	25.11 [a](23, 22, 21)	1.94	17	26.35 [a](25, 24, 23)	1.87	218	22.71 [a](19, 17, 16)	3.6
All ages	256	21.71 [a](19, 17, 15)	3.18	170	25.65 [a](23, 22, 21)	2.5	112	26.77 [a](25, 24, 23)	2.15	112	28.04 [a](26, 25, 24)	1.94	650	24.70 [a](21, 19, 17)	3.67

NOTE: Healthy community-based sample living in all geographical regions of the Portuguese continental territory who speaks Portuguese as their native language, and educated in Portugal. *N* = 650, Mean age = 55.84, *SD* = 15.12, range = 25–91; mean education = 8.16, *SD* = 4.72, range = 2–27. Distribution is comparable to target Portuguese population.

[a]Numbers in parentheses represent 1SD, 1.5SD, 2SD below mean.

SOURCE: From Freitas et al. (2011).

EVIDENCE FOR TEST-RETEST RELIABILITY, MEASURING CHANGE, AND PRACTICE EFFECTS

Estimates of test-retest reliability appear to be affected more by the population than the retest interval. Overall, estimates are at least adequate in community-based samples (ICC = .75 for intervals of four weeks to three months) to very high in neurology clinic patients (ICC = .97 for two-week interval; Lee et al., 2008; Dominguez et al., 2013; Fujiwara et al., 2010; Hu et al., 2013; Memória et al., 2013; Nasreddine et al., 2005; Ozdilek & Kenangil, 2014; Pirrotta et al., 2015; Rahman et al., 2009; Tan et al., 2015; Tsai et al., 2012; Wong et al., 2009; Yu et al., 2015). At an 18-month retest interval, reliability remains high (ICC = .88; Freitas et al., 2013).

Mean change on the MoCA over short periods appears minimal, less than one point. Over two weeks, a community sample of older adults showed a mean change of −.74 (*SD* = 2.26; Dominguez et al., 2013). In a MCI/AD sample, four-week mean change ranged from −.54 to 1.23 (Lee et al., 2008). Over 35 days, a MCI/AD sample demonstrated a mean change of .90 (*SD* = 2.50; Nasreddine et al., 2005; Rahman et al., 2009).

EVIDENCE FOR RELIABILITY OF ALTERNATE FORMS

Information on alternate form reliability is limited. One study reported no significant differences between all three English alternate forms in a sample of AD, MCI, and healthy controls (*N* = 79). Total scores were within .80 points of all three forms. In the MCI group, a 1.3 point difference between version 1 and 3 was reported (Chertkow et al., 2011).

The German alternate forms showed moderate correlations with the original MoCA in a healthy group (*r* = .52 to .69), and strong correlations with the original MoCA in MCI and AD samples (*r* = .83 to .95). No significant differences between the raw scores on all forms were found (Costa et al., 2012).

MoCA-Mini completed over the phone is highly correlated with the original MoCA (*r* = .87). Cronbach's alpha in a sample of patients with transient ischemic attack (TIA) or ischemic stroke was .79. One-month test-retest reliability was excellent (ICC = .89; Wong et al., 2015).

A computerized version, MoCA-CC, appears to be equivalent to the regular version (*r* = .93 with

TABLE 7–50 Italian Montreal Cognitive Assessment (MoCA) Raw Scores Stratified by Age and Education

	AGE (YEARS)																							
EDUCATION (YEARS)	20–29			30–39			40–49			50–59			60–69			70–79			80+			TOTAL		
	N	*M*	*SD*	*N*	*M*	*SD*	*N*	*M*	*SD*	*N*	*M*	*SD*	*N*	*M*	*SD*	*N*	*M*	*SD*	*N*	*M*	*SD*	*N*	*M*	*SD*
1 to 3	–			–			–			–			1	22		3	16.6	1.1	8	12.5	2.6	12	14.3	3.7
4 to 5	–			1	13.0		3	16.6	3.7	6	19.8	3.6	12	18.8	4.3	22	17.6	4.1	19	16.2	2.9	63	17.5	3.8
6 to 8	14	21.2	3.3	19	21.5	3.7	12	22.1	3.0	9	21.6	3.4	24	21.2	3.4	31	20.4	3.0	12	18.5	3.5	121	20.9	3.4
9 to 13	15	23.9	2.5	11	25.4	1.8	18	23.9	2.3	20	22.8	3.2	24	23.8	2.4	23	21.4	2.9	4	24.7	2.0	115	23.4	2.8
>13	17	25.7	2.4	22	25.6	2.3	20	25.7	1.7	22	24.5	2.2	14	24.0	3.2	4	25.5	1.0	5	25.2	2.2	104	25.2	2.3
Total	46	23.7	3.2	53	23.9	3.7	53	23.7	3.2	57	23.0	3.3	75	22.2	3.7	83	20.0	3.7	48	17.8	4.9	415	21.9	4.2

NOTE: Based on healthy community-based sample drawn from different districts of Italy (mostly Naples, Milan, and Siena). *N* = 415, Mean age = 56.82, *SD* = 18.8, median = 59, range = 21–95; mean education = 11.13, *SD* = .76, median = 13, range = 1–21; 252 women, 163 men.

SOURCE: Adapted from Santangelo et al. (2015).

TABLE 7–51 Montreal Cognitive Assessment (MoCA) Raw Scores of an Italian Sample Stratified by Age and Education

	EDUCATION (YEARS)														
	5			6 TO 8			9 TO 13			14+			TOTAL		
AGE (YEARS)	N	M	SD	N	M	SD	N	M	SD	N	M	SD	N	M	SD
60 to 64	8	23.50	2.27	11	25.09	2.12	13	25.08	2.60	10	26.70	1.95	42	25.17	2.43
65 to 70	15	19.47	3.54	27	23.59	2.34	17	26.00	1.54	12	25.42	1.88	71	23.61	3.36
71 to 75	24	21.04	3.07	13	23.31	2.98	15	24.47	2.53	11	24.73	1.95	63	22.97	3.14
76 to 80	18	20.67	3.09	9	21.67	2.74	11	22.09	2.88	11	22.55	2.07	49	21.59	2.80
Total	65	20.88	3.25	60	23.52	2.65	56	24.61	2.69	44	24.82	2.41	225	23.28	3.22

NOTE: N = 225 (111 males, 114 females) healthy participants drawn from memory disorders clinic and senior centers. Mean age = 70.1, *SD* = 5.7, range = 60–80; mean education = 9.9 years, *SD* = 4.6, range = 5–23.

SOURCE: Adapted from Conti et al. (2015).

TABLE 7–52 Equivalent Scores (ES) for Total Adjusted Montreal Cognitive Assessment (MoCA) Values and Its Cognitive Domains in an Italian Sample

ES	INTERVAL	CUMULATIVE FREQUENCY
Total MoCA score		
0	≤15.5	14
1	15.51–18.28	46
2	18.29–20.25	112
3	20.26–22.23	208
4	>22.23	415
Visuospatial Abilities		
0	≤0.76	14
1	0.77–1.35	46
2	1.36–1.96	112
3	1.97–2.52	208
4	>2.52	415
Executive Functions		
0	≤0.44	14
1	0.45–1.10	46
2	1.11–1.92	112
3	1.93–2.53	208
4	>2.53	415
Language		
0	<3.08	14
1	3.09–3.87	46
2	3.88–4.42	112
3	4.43–5.12	208
4	>5.12	415
Orientation		
0	≤5.03	24
1	5.04–5.92	61
2	5.93–5.94	124
3	5.95–5.98	208
4	>5.98	415
Attention		
0	≤2.42	19
1	2.43–3.56	54
2	3.57–4.46	119
3	4.47–5.21	208
4	>5.21	415

NOTE: Based on Italian community-based sample drawn from different districts of Italy. *N* = 415, Mean age = 56.82, *SD* = 18.8, median = 59, range = 21–95; Mean education = 11.13, *SD* = .76, median = 13, range = 1–21; 252 women, 163 men.

ES, Equivalent Score. 0 = scores equal or lower than the outer tolerance limit (5%); 4 = scores higher than the median value of the whole sample; 1, 2, and 3 were obtained by dividing the area of distribution between 0 and 4 into three equal parts. Based on 95% tolerance limits using nonparametric procedure.

SOURCE: From Santangelo et al. (2015).

MoCA-Beijing), at least in a sample of older Chinese who are relatively highly educated (Yu et al., 2015). The MoCA-CC yielded adequate internal consistency (Cronbach's alpha = .72) and high six-week test-retest reliability (ICC = .82).

EVIDENCE FOR INTERRATER RELIABILITY

Interrater reliability is excellent (.87 to .99), likely because of the clear instructions and scoring criteria that accompany the test protocols (Dominguez et al., 2013; Freitas et al., 2013; Hu et al., 2013; Wong et al., 2009).

EVIDENCE FOR VALIDITY

RELATIONSHIPS WITH OTHER TESTS

As a screen of global cognitive functioning, the MoCA shows moderate to strong correlation with the gold-standard brief cognitive screen MMSE. Correlation coefficients range from .55 in community samples to .91 in memory clinic samples (Lee et al., 2008; Dominguez et al., 2013; Lam et al., 2013; Memória et al., 2013; Tsai et al., 2012; Waldron-Perrine et al., 2012; Wong et al., 2009). The MoCA is also correlated with other global cognitive measures such as the Clinical Dementia Rating-Sum of Boxes (CDR-SB; $r = -.62$), Clinical Dementia

TABLE 7–53 Equivalent Scores (ES) Classification of Adjusted Scores in an Italian Sample

EQUIVALENT SCORES	SCORE INTERVAL	DENSITY	CUMULATIVE FREQUENCY
ES = 0	0 → 17.362	6	6
ES = 1	17.363 → 19.500	16	22
ES = 2	19.501 → 21.562	36	58
ES = 3	21.563 → 23.361	54	112
ES = 4	>23.361	113	225

NOTE: Based on healthy participants drawn from memory disorders clinic and senior centers in Italy. *N* = 225; mean age = 70.1, *SD* = 5.7, range = 60–80; mean education = 9.9 years, *SD* = 4.6, range = 5–23; 111 males, 114 females.

ES = 0 corresponds to an inferentially controlled judgment of being below the norm; 4 is equal or better than the 50th percentile; 1, 2, and 3 are intermediate between 0 and 4 on a quasi-interval scale. Based on 95% tolerance limits using nonparametric procedure.

SOURCE: From Conti et al. (2015).

Rating (CDR; $r = -.79$), Dementia Rating Scale (DRS; $r = .77$), as well as the Hasegawa's Dementia Scale-Revised (HDS-R; $r = .79$) in AD/MCI samples (Dagenais et al., 2013; Fujiwara et al., 2010; Lee et al., 2008). See "Clinical Studies" for clinical sensitivity of the MoCA versus the MMSE. For more information about the correlations between the MMSE and MoCA, see the MMSE review in this chapter.

Modest to high correlations have also been reported between MoCA total score and specific neuropsychological tests measuring a wide variety of cognitive functions, including CVLT-II, FCSRT, Rey-Osterrieth Complex Figure Test (RCFT), Stroop, COWA, TMT-B, BNT, Symbol Digit Modalities Test (SDMT), and Grooved Pegboard (Bezdicek et al., 2013; Dagenais et al., 2013; Schweizer et al., 2012; Tsai et al., 2012; Waldron-Perrine et al., 2012). Thus, the MoCA total score seems to measure a broad range of cognitive ability.

All MoCA subscales appear to have at least modest correlation with most neuropsychological measures (Bezdicek et al., 2013; Dagenais et al., 2013; Lam et al., 2013; McLennan et al., 2011; Schweizer et al., 2012). For example, Lam and colleagues (2013) reported domain-specific correlations with the respective MoCA subscales, with the highest correlation found for the memory domain ($r_s = .73$) and lowest for the language domain ($r_s = .42$; see Table 7–54).

The MoCA has minimal correlation with noncognitive measures. For example, the MoCA was not correlated with the Unified Huntington's Disease Rating Scale-Motor score or medication status among individuals with HD (Bezdicek et al., 2013) or BDI-Fast Screen among patients with MS (Dagenais et al., 2013). It was also minimally correlated with the Epworth Sleepiness Scale ($r = -.23$), Clinical Global Impression Scale (CGI; $r = -.23$), and Positive and Negative Symptom Scale (PANSS; $r = -.27$; Dominguez et al., 2013; Wu et al., 2014), suggesting only modest overlap.

CLINICAL STUDIES

Clinical Sensitivity Versus the MMSE. To examine sensitivity to aging effects on the MMSE and MoCA, neurologically healthy community-dwelling adults across the life span (ages 20 to 89) were administered both screening tests. Modest worsening across the life span was seen on the MMSE whereas the MoCA showed greater decline. When examined by the decade, there were no consistent differences in the 30 to 49 age ranges, but memory and language scores on the MMSE and MoCA were different by the 50 to 89 age range. These results suggest that the MoCA is less affected by ceiling effects and more sensitive to normal aging than the MMSE (Gluhm et al., 2013).

The identification of cognitive impairments, especially in mild cases, is highly affected by the choice of cognitive screener as reported in many studies (e.g., Nasreddine et al., 2005; Sweet et al., 2011; Wang et al., 2013; Whitney et al., 2012). For example, Sweet et al. (2011) reported that at the time of admission to a geriatric rehabilitation center for orthopedic injury, 25% of patients obtained a MoCA score of greater than 25 versus 80% who obtained a MMSE score of greater than 23 (i.e., traditional cutoff scores for cognitive impairment). At discharge, 82% obtained normal MMSE scores whereas only 39% were cognitively normal according to the MoCA. Similarly, a seminal paper reported that 73% of persons with MCI obtained abnormal MoCA scores but had normal scores on the MMSE (Nasreddine et al., 2005). However, the sensitivity of the measures may depend on the diagnosis. For example, Wang and colleagues (2013) noted that in their study of older adults recruited from neurologic or geropsychiatric clinics, 9% of AD and 19% of DLB patients obtained a normal MoCA despite an abnormal MMSE score; about 6% of DLB patient obtained a normal MMSE but an abnormal MoCA. For sensitivity/specificity comparisons between MoCA and MMSE, please refer to the MMSE review in this chapter.

Among those who sustained aneurysmal subarachnoid hemorrhage, 42% more patients were impaired on the

TABLE 7–54 Spearman Correlations Between Montreal Cognitive Assessment (MoCA) Subscales and Neuropsychological Domains

	NEUROPSYCHOLOGY DOMAIN				
MoCA SUBSCALE	MEMORY	VISUOSPATIAL	LANGUAGE	ATTENTION	EXECUTIVE
Memory	.73***	.14	.19*	.16	.29**
Visuospatial	.29**	.56***	.42***	.50***	.53***
Language	.33**	.27**	.46***	.34***	.41***
Attention	.36***	.50***	.18	.51***	.45***
Executive	.40***	.53***	.41***	.59***	.60***

NOTE: Tests contributing to memory (CVLT, DRS memory); visuospatial (RCFT Copy, Benton JLO, DRS construction); language (BNT, animal fluency); attention (TMT-A, WAIS-R backward span, DRS attention); executive (TMT-B, WCST, letter fluency, DRS conceptualization).

***$p < .001$ **$p < .01$ *$p < .05$.

CVLT, California Verbal Learning Test; DRS, Dementia Rating Scale; RCFT, Rey-Osterrieth Complex Figure Test; JLO, Judgment of Line Orientation; BNT, Boston Naming Test; TMT, Trail Making Test; WAIS-R, Wechsler Adult Intelligence Scale-Revised; WCST, Wisconsin Card Sorting Test.

SOURCE: From Lam et al. (2013).

MoCA than on the MMSE (Schweizer et al., 2012). All who obtained a normal MoCA had normal MMSE, whereas among those with MoCA of less than 26, 45% had normal MMSE (defined as ≥27; Wong et al., 2012). In general, the MoCA is more sensitive than the MMSE to identify vascular cognitive impairment at two weeks post-stroke. Of those with unimpaired MMSE scores, 32% had impaired MoCA scores, whereas only 5% of those who were unimpaired on the MoCA had impaired MMSE scores (Dong et al., 2010). Given these findings, the original authors suggested that if a patient presents with cognitive complaints and functional dependency, the MMSE can be administered first; if the patient obtains an MMSE score of 26 or higher, then the MoCA can be administered. In the case of a patient with cognitive complaints but no functional impairment, the MoCA can be administered first (Nasreddine et al., 2005).

AD/MCI. As seen in Table 7–55, the MoCA is sensitive to AD and MCI, though the cutoff score to identify cognitive impairment appears to be lower for samples outside of North America (Lifshitz et al., 2012; Malek-Ahmadi et al., 2014; Nasreddine et al., 2005; Tsai et al., 2012; Roalf et al., 2103; Yu et al., 2012). In general, most items differentiate AD, MCI, and healthy controls, but the AD and MCI/controls appear to differ on the attention subscale (Nasreddine et al., 2005). The delayed recall item seems most sensitive to MCI compared to other items (Nasreddine et al., 2005; Yu et al., 2012). Interestingly, one study based on IRT indicated that while the utility of MoCA-Taiwanese peaks at mild cognitive dysfunction, the subscales show different discriminating power at different cognitive ranges. Frontal and language subscales showed high discriminating power and information across

TABLE 7–55 Cutoff Scores, AUC, Sensitivity, Specificity, PPV, and NPV for Various Versions of the Montreal Cognitive Assessment (MoCA) to Identify MCI and/or AD

REFERENCE	POPULATION	CUTOFF	AUC	SENS (%)	SPEC (%)	PPV (%)	NPV (%)
Freitas et al. (2013)	Portuguese MoCA for MCI (*N* = 90), AD (*N* = 90), matched controls (*N* = 180)	MCI <22 AD <17	MCI: .85 AD: .98	MCI: 81 AD: 88	MCI: 77 AD: 98	MCI: 78 AD: 98	MCI: 80 AD: 89
Fujiwara et al. (2010)	Japanese MoCA for MCI (*N* = 30), AD (*N* = 30), healthy controls (*N* = 36)	<26	MCI: .95 AD: .99	MCI: 93 AD: 100	MCI: 89 AD: 89	MCI: 88 AD: 88	MCI: 94 AD: 100
Hu et al. (2013)	Chinese MoCA for AD (*N* = 72), MCI (*N* = 84), healthy controls (*N* = 146) in eastern China	<26	MCI: .92 AD: .96	MCI: 92 AD: 96	MCI: 85 AD: 85		
Lee et al. (2008)	Korean MoCA for MCI (*N* = 37), mild AD (*N* = 44), healthy older adults (*N* = 115)	<23	MCI: .94 AD: .98	MCI: 89 AD: 98	MCI: 84 AD: 84	MCI: 65 AD: 70	MCI: 96 AD: 99
Lifshitz et al. (2012)	Hebrew MoCA for MCI (*N* = 74) and healthy controls (*N* = 80) from memory clinic and community centers, respectively	<26	.96	95	76	79	94
Luis et al. (2009)	Southeastern US community-dwelling older adults with AD (*N* = 20), amnestic MCI (*N* = 24), healthy controls (*N* = 74)	≤26 Optimal cutoff: ≤23	MCI: .97 MCI/AD: .96	MCI: 100 MCI/AD: 97 MCI: 96	MCI: 35 MCI/AD: 35 MCI: 95		
Memoria et al. (2013)	Brazilian MoCA for AD (*N* = 28), MCI (*N* = 43), healthy controls (*N* = 41)	MCI <25 AD <22	MCI: .82 AD: .99	MCI: 81 AD: 91	MCI: 77 AD: 100		
Nasreddine et al. (2005)	MCI (*N* = 94), AD (*N* = 93), healthy community controls (*N* = 90)	<26		MCI: 90 AD: 100	MCI: 87 AD: 87	MCI: 89 AD: 89	MCI: 97 AD: 100
Roalf et al. (2013)	AD (*N* = 321), MCI (*N* = 126), healthy controls (*N* = 140)	Control vs AD: <23 Control vs MCI: <25 MCI vs AD: <19	Control vs AD: .99 Control vs MCI: .89 MCI vs AD: .85	94 84 77	96 79 80		
Tsai et al. (2012)	Taiwanese MoCA (MoCA-T) for AD (*N* = 97), MCI (*N* = 70), healthy controls (*N* = 40) from memory clinic	MCI: <24 AD: <22	MCI: .91 AD: .99	MCI: 92 AD: 98	MCI: 78 AD: 95	MCI: 88 AD: 88	MCI: 94 AD: 100

NOTE: AUC, area under the curve; Sens, sensitivity; Spec, specificity; PPV, positive predictive value; NPV, negative predictive value; MCI, mild cognitive impairment; AD, Alzheimer's disease.

all cognitive ranges; the memory subscale showed high discriminating power and was most informative in the mild cognitive dysfunction range. The orientation subscale was best in the moderate to severe range, but poor at lower ranges. Finally, the language and visual-spatial subscales were not discriminative in the severe cognitive dysfunction range (Tsai et al., 2012).

Performance on the MoCA may indicate conversion of MCI to AD over 18 months. Julayanont and colleagues (2014) reported that their retrospective chart review of a community-dwelling memory clinic sample revealed a mean rate of decline of 2.19 ± 0.39 points per year on the MoCA for the converters, and 1.72 ± 0.45 points/year for the nonconverters. On the MoCA Memory Index Score (MoCA-MIS), the mean rate of decline was 1.08 ± 0.37 points/year for converters and 0.90 ± 0.57 points/year for nonconverters. Over 18 months, the majority (91%) of those with MoCA of less than 20 (education adjusted) *and* MoCA-MIS less than 7 progressed to AD; only half of those above these cutoff scores converted to AD (Julayanont et al., 2014). Note that MoCA-MIS = free delayed recall, category-cued recall, and multiple choice-cued recall multiplied by 3, 2, and 1, respectively, with score ranging from 0 to 15.

AD may be differentiated from other neurodegenerative disorders such as FTD, vascular dementia, or DLB using the MoCA, but FTD and vascular dementia do not differ in their MoCA scores (Freitas et al., 2014; Wang et al., 2013). However, based on subscale performance, DLB and AD may be distinguished (Wang et al., 2013). For example, DLB is associated with higher naming scores than AD, and AD is associated with lower scores on the orientation and memory subscales (Wang et al., 2013). The MoCA is also useful to identify cognitive impairments in various degenerative disorders, including very mild cognitive dysfunction in PD and HD (see Table 7–56; Hoops et al., 2009; Ozdilek & Kenangil, 2014; Bezdicek et al., 2013).

Stroke. The MoCA is sensitive to cognitive impairments at two weeks to three months post-stroke (Cumming et al., 2013; Dong et al., 2010; Wong et al., 2012; see Tables 7–56 and 7–57). Specifically, visuospatial-executive, attention, and recall scores are different for mild or moderate vascular cognitive impairment groups and those without vascular cognitive impairment or dementia (Dong et al., 2010). Interestingly, the MoCA showed greater predictive validity for right than left hemisphere stroke (Cumming et al., 2013).

Other Medical/Psychiatric Conditions. The MoCA can also be used to identify cognitive impairments in MS, epilepsy, Korsakoff's syndrome, schizophrenia, and severe affective disorders (Dagenais et al., 2013; Musso et al., 2014; Oudman et al., 2014a, b; Phabphal et al., 2011; Wester et al., 2013; see Table 7–58). For example, Korsakoff's patients can be differentiated from patients with non-Korsakoff alcohol-related cognitive impairment and healthy controls on the MoCA (Oudman et al., 2014a, b; Wester et al., 2013). Although the two clinical groups perform equally on the executive function subscale compared to the healthy controls, the memory subscale differentiates the groups, with the Korsakoff's group performing the worst. Korsakoff's patients also obtain lower scores than the other group on the orientation subscale. The groups do not differ on attention and language subscales (Wester et al., 2013).

Predicting Outcome After Acquired Brain Injury. The MoCA is useful to predict outcome after acquired brain injuries such as aneurysmal hemorrhage or hemorrhage due to TBI, as well as to predict potential for rehabilitation in geriatric orthopedic patients (see Tables 7–56 and 7–58). For example, among older adults admitted to a geriatric rehabilitation center for orthopedic injuries, the MoCA attention subscale at admission was a unique predictor of rehabilitation success once other subscales were controlled for (Sweet et al., 2011). When the subscales were examined, MoCA naming and abstraction items were associated with return to work following aneurysmal subarachnoid hemorrhage (Schweizer et al., 2012). At one-year post aneurysmal subarachnoid hemorrhage, excellent outcome on the modified Rankin Scale (assessing return to work, family responsibilities, and participation in social activities) was associated with MoCA delayed recall and sustained attention; excellent IADL outcome was associated with delayed recall and orientation (Wong et al., 2014). At three to five years post-injury with intracranial hemorrhage, baseline MoCA of less than 24 had a threefold increase in poor outcome based on Glasgow Outcome Scale-Extended (Wong et al., 2013).

NEUROANATOMICAL CORRELATES AND IMAGING STUDIES

Among a sample of healthy, highly educated, community-dwelling older adults, the MoCA total score was not correlated with MRI-derived indices of whole brain volume, subcortical hyperintensities, frontal gray matter, and hippocampal volume (Paul et al., 2011). However, among those with low education, global cortical atrophy, medial temporal atrophy, and diffusion tensor imaging-derived indices of small-vessel disease were associated with MoCA total scores, even after controlling for demographic and depression variables (del Brutto et al., 2015; Pasi et al., 2015). No association with white matter hyperintensities and lacunar infarcts was found (Pasi et al., 2015). When subscales were examined, higher visuospatial/executive, attention, and memory scores were correlated with larger whole-brain volume. As well, naming scores were associated with total hippocampal and frontal volumes (Paul et al., 2011).

PERFORMANCE VALIDITY

Not available.

TABLE 7–56 Cutoff Scores, AUC, Sensitivity, Specificity, PPV, and NPV for Various Versions of the MoCA to Identify Cognitive Impairments in Neurological Conditions

REFERENCE	PURPOSE/ POPULATION	CUTOFF	AUC	SENS (%)	SPEC (%)	PPV (%)	NPV (%)
Bezdicek et al. (2013)	HD (*N* = 20) and healthy controls (*N* = 23)	<26 (optimal screening and diagnostic cutoff)	.90	94	84	81	95
Dalrymple-Alford (2010)	PDD, PD-MCI, healthy controls with PD	For screening: PDD: <21 PD-MCI: <26	PDD: .97 PD-MCI: .90	PDD: 81 PD-MCI: 90	PDD: 95 PD-MCI: 75	PDD: 87 PD-MCI: 61	PD: 92 PD-MCI: 95
		For diagnostic: PDD: <22 PD-MCI: <24		PDD: 90 PD-MCI: 62	PDD: 91 PD-MCI: 94	PDD: 82 PD-MCI: 79	PDD: 96 PD-MCI: 85
Ozdilek and Kenangil (2014)	PD (*N* = 50) and healthy controls (*N* = 50)	<21	.79	59	89	81	73
Pirrotta et al. (2014)	Italian MoCA (*N* = 287), patients in neurology clinic and healthy controls	<16	.96	83	97	98	83
Wang et al. (2013)	AD (*N* = 67), DLB (*N* = 36), and healthy controls (*N* = 62) recruited from neurologic or geropsychiatric clinics	AD: <22 DLB: <23	.95 .93	95 92	82 81	85 73	94 94
Freitas et al. (2012)	Portuguese MoCA to identify bvFTD (*N* = 50) and matched healthy controls (*N* = 50)	<17	.93	78	98	98	82
Wong et al. (2009)	Hong Kong MoCA, patients with cerebral small vessel disease (*N* = 40) and matched controls (*N* = 40)	<22	.81	73	75	74	73
Wong et al. (2012)	Hong Kong MoCA for identifying favorable outcome (modified Rankin Scale) or IADL following aneurysmal subarachnoid hemorrhage at three-month post-stroke (*N* = 90)	<20	mRS: .91 IADL: .83	86 87	78 70	94 89	73 65
Wong et al. (2013)	Hong Kong MoCA, TBI with intracranial hemorrhage (*N* = 48) and healthy controls (*N* = 40)	<26	.70	75	48	61	63

NOTE: AUC, area under the curve; Sens, sensitivity; Spec, specificity; PPV, positive predictive value; NPV, negative predictive value; AD, Alzheimer's disease; bvFTD, behavioral-variant frontotemporal dementia; HD, Huntington's disease; PD, Parkinson's disease; PD-MCI, Parkinson's disease with mild cognitive impairment; PDD, Parkinson's disease dementia; mRS, modified Rankin Scale; IADL, instrumental activities of daily living; TBI, traumatic brain injury.

TABLE 7–57 Cutoff Scores, AUC, Sensitivity, Specificity, PPV, and NPV for Various Versions of the MoCA to Identify Vascular Cognitive Impairment

REFERENCE	POPULATION	CUTOFF	AUC	SENS (%)	SPEC (%)	PPV (%)	NPV (%)
Freitas, Simões, Alves, Vincente, and Santana (2012)	Portuguese MoCA, Vascular Dementia (*N* = 34)	Standard: <17 Short[a]: <8	Standard: .95 Short: .93	Standard: 77 Short: 85	Standard: 97 Short: 88	Standard: 96 Short: 88	Standard: 81 Short: 86
Mai et al. (2013)	Stroke prevention clinic patients (*N* = 102)	≤7 (subset of three items out of 10 points)		99	78	86	97
McLennan et al. (2011)	Cardiovascular outpatient clinic (*N* = 110) to identify MCI	<24		aMCI: 100 mMCI: 83	aMCI: 50 mMCI: 52	aMCI: 5 mMCI: 18	aMCI: 100 mMCI: 96

NOTE: AUC, area under the curve; Sens, sensitivity; Spec, specificity; PPV, positive predictive value; NPV, negative predictive value; MCI, mild cognitive impairment; aMCI, amnestic mild cognitive impairment; mMCI, multidomain mild cognitive impairment.

[a]Short MoCA comprises 12 items: five-word immediate and delayed recall, six-item orientation, and phonemic fluency.

TABLE 7–58 Cutoff Scores, AUC, Sensitivity, Specificity, PPV, and NPV for Various Versions of the MoCA in Psychiatric and Other Medical Conditions

REFERENCE	POPULATION	CUTOFF	AUC	SENS (%)	SPEC (%)	PPV (%)	NPV (%)
Musso et al. (2014)	Severe mental illness (schizophrenia, mood/affective; *N* =28) and non-psychiatric controls (*N* = 18)	<26		89	61	78	79
Overton et al. (2013)	HIV-infected virologically suppressed with HAART (*N* = 200); 64% cognitively impaired	≤27	.66	90	42	73	70
		≤26	.65	75	55	74	56
		≤25	.67	63	71	79	52
		≤24	.68	53	82	84	50
		≤23	.66	38	94	92	46
Oudman et al. (2014)	Korsakoff's syndrome (*N* = 30), healthy controls (*N* = 30)	<23	1.00	100	100	100	91
Wester et al. (2013)	Dutch MoCA, Korsakoff's syndrome (*N* = 20), non-Korsakoff alcohol-related cognitive impairment (*N* = 26), and healthy controls (*N* = 33)	KS: ≤23	.97	88	95		
		Non-KS: ≤24	.85	85	69		
		KS vs non-KS: ≤20* *best possible cutoff	.73	73	75		
Sweet et al. (2011)	MoCA in geriatric rehabilitation for orthopedic injury to predict relative functional efficacy/potential for improvement (*N* = 47)	Total <26		80	30		
		Attention <5		40	90		

NOTE: AUC, area under the curve; Sens, sensitivity; Spec, specificity; PPV, positive predictive value; NPV, negative predictive value; KS, Korsakoff's syndrome; HAART, highly active antiretroviral therapy.

COMMENT

The MoCA is a very popular global cognitive screen that has gained international attention because of its brevity, free access, clear instructions, and ease of administration. Instructions and test protocols have been translated into many languages and modified for local contexts. Validation studies have been completed on local versions demonstrating excellent psychometric properties similar to the original version. There is a growing body of research supporting its use over the gold-standard MMSE, especially in conditions where sensitivity to mild cognitive dysfunction is pivotal. The MoCA is sensitive not only to memory dysfunction but also to executive dysfunction. Thus, the MoCA is useful to detect cognitive dysfunction in a wide variety of neurological, medical, and psychiatric illnesses.

A major criticism that has been raised in the research literature relates to the cutoff score for cognitive impairment. Researchers are concerned that the cutoff score (<26) suggested by the original authors is too high, possibly because of their "supernormal" sample (Coen et al., 2011). Studies that included cognitively healthy participants with common diseases of old age (e.g., high blood pressure, high cholesterol) or those with very low education have resulted in a high false-positive rate for cognitive dysfunction when the suggested cutoff score (<26) was used (e.g., Freitas et al., 2012c, 2013; Lee et al., 2008; Luis et al., 2009; Pirrotta et al., 2015; Rossetti et al., 2012). The debate is still ongoing (e.g., Nasreddine et al., 2012; Rosetti et al., 2012). Users may wish to choose the cutoff score based on the purpose of their evaluation with reference to Tables 7–55 to 7–58.

Another debate surrounds the application of education corrections. Similar to the criticism related to the cutoff score, the amount of points to be added remains unclear. Some suggest that +1 point be applied to those with six years of education or less, while others apply +2 or +1 points depending on the level of education (Chertkow et al., 2011; Tan et al., 2015). Some researchers note that correcting for education improved sensitivity by very little at the expense of specificity (Gagnon et al., 2013; Mai et al., 2013). To address both criticisms, use of normative data to guide interpretation may be a possible solution; however, few sets of norms have been published in the literature.

Regardless of the limitations, the MoCA appears to be a pychometrically superior global cognitive screen over the MMSE. It is a useful tool to identify possible cognitive dysfunction that may require in-depth neuropsychological evaluation. Given its brevity, the MoCA cannot replace a comprehensive assessment to determine the etiology or severity of the cognitive dysfunction.

REFERENCES

Arnold, J. M. O., Howlett, J. G., Dorian, P., Ducharme, A., Giannetti, N., Haddad, H., . . . White, M. (2007). Canadian Cardiovascular Society Consensus Conference recommendations on heart failure update 2007: Prevention, management during intercurrent illness or acute decompensation, and use of biomarkers. *Canadian Journal of Cardiology, 23*(1), 21–45.

Bernstein, I. H., Lacritz, L., Barlow, C. E., Weiner, M. F., & DeFina, L. F. (2011). Psychometric evaluation of the Montreal Cognitive Assessment (MoCA) in three diverse samples. *The Clinical Neuropsychologist, 25*(1), 119–126.

Bezdicek, O., Majerova, V., Novak, M., Nikolai, T., Ruzicka, E., & Roth, J. (2013). Validity of the Montreal Cognitive Assessment in the detection of cognitive dysfunction in Huntington's disease. *Applied Neuropsychology: Adult, 20*(1), 33–40.

Chertkow, H., Nasreddine, Z., Johns, E., Phillips, N., & McHenry, C. (2011). The Montreal Cognitive Assessment (MoCA): Validation of alternate forms and new recommendations for education corrections. *Alzheimer's & Dementia, 7*(4), S157.

Coen, R. F., Cahill, R., & Lawlor, B. A. (2011). Things to watch out for when using the Montreal Cognitive Assessment (MoCA). *International Journal of Geriatric Psychiatry, 26*(1), 107–108.

Conti, S., Bonazzi, S., Laiacona, M., Masina, M., & Coralli, M. V. (2015). Montreal Cognitive Assessment (MoCA)-Italian version: Regression based norms and equivalent scores. *Neurological Sciences, 36*(2), 209–214.

Costa, A. S., Fimm, B., Friesen, P., Soundjock, H., Rottschya, C., Gross, T., . . . Reetz, K. (2012). Alternate-form reliability of the Montreal Cognitive Assessment screening test in a clinical setting. *Dementia and Geriatric Cognitive Disorders, 33*(6), 379–384.

Cumming, T. B., Churilov, L., Linden, T., & Bernhardt, J. (2013). Montreal Cognitive Assessment and Mini–Mental State Examination are both valid cognitive tools in stroke. *Acta Neurologica Scandinavica, 128*(2), 122–129.

Dagenais, E., Rouleau, I., Demers, M., Jobin, C., Roger, É., Chamelian, L., & Duquette, P. (2013). Value of the MoCA test as a screening instrument in multiple sclerosis. *The Canadian Journal of Neurological Sciences/Le Journal Canadien Des Sciences Neurologiques, 40*(3), 410–415.

Dalrymple-Alford, J., MacAskill, M. R., Nakas, C. T., Livingston, L., Graham, C., Crucian, G. P., . . . Anderson, T. J. (2010). The MoCA: Well-suited screen for cognitive impairment in Parkinson disease. *Neurology, 75*(19), 1717–1725.

Del Brutto, O. H., Mera, R. M., Zambrano, M., Soriano, F., & Lama, J. (2015). Global cortical atrophy (GCA) associates with worse performance in the Montreal Cognitive Assessment (MoCA). A population-based study in community-dwelling elders living in rural Ecuador. *Archives of Gerontology and Geriatrics, 60*(1), 206–209.

Dominguez, J. C., Orquiza, M. G. S., Soriano, J. R., Magpantay, C. D., Esteban, R. C., Corrales, M. L., & Ampil, E. R. (2013). Adaptation of the Montreal Cognitive Assessment for elderly filipino patients. *East Asian Archives of Psychiatry, 23*(3), 80–85.

Dong, Y., Sharma, V. K., Chan, B. P., Venketasubramanian, N., Teoh, H. L., Seet, R. C. S., . . . Chen, C. (2010). The Montreal Cognitive Assessment (MoCA) is superior to the Mini-Mental State Examination (MMSE) for the detection of vascular cognitive impairment after acute stroke. *Journal of the Neurological Sciences, 299*(1–2), 15–18.

Freitas, S., Prieto, G., Simões, M. R., & Santana, I. (2014). Psychometric properties of the Montreal Cognitive Assessment (MoCA): An analysis using the Rasch model. *The Clinical Neuropsychologist, 28*(1), 65–83.

Freitas, S., Simo˜es, M. R., Marôco, J., Alves, L., & Santana, I. (2012a). Construct validity of the Montreal Cognitive Assessment (MoCA). *Journal of the International Neuropsychological Society, 18*(2), 242–250.

Freitas, S., Simões, M. R., Alves, L., Duro, D., & Santana, I. (2012b). Montreal Cognitive Assessment (MOCA): Validation study for frontotemporal dementia. *Journal of Geriatric Psychiatry and Neurology, 25*(3), 146–154.

Freitas, S., Simões, M. R., Alves, L., & Santana, I. (2011). Montreal Cognitive Assessment (MoCA): Normative study for the Portuguese population. *Journal of Clinical and Experimental Neuropsychology, 33*(9), 989–996.

Freitas, S., Simões, M. R., Alves, L., & Santana, I. (2012c). Montreal Cognitive Assessment: Influence of sociodemographic and health variables. *Archives of Clinical Neuropsychology, 27*(2), 165–175.

Freitas, S., Simões, M. R., Alves, L., Vicente, M., & Santana, I. (2012d). Montreal Cognitive Assessment (MoCA): Validation study for vascular dementia. *Journal of the International Neuropsychological Society, 18*(6), 1031–1040.

Freitas, S., Simões, M. R., Alves, L., & Santana, I. (2013). Montreal Cognitive Assessment: Validation study for Mild Cognitive Impairment and Alzheimer disease. *Alzheimer Disease and Associated Disorders, 27*(1), 37–43.

Fujiwara, Y., Suzuki, H., Yasunaga, M., Sugiyama, M., Ijuin, M., Sakuma, N., . . . Shinkai, S. (2010). Brief screening tool for Mild Cognitive Impairment in older Japanese: Validation of the Japanese version of the Montreal Cognitive Assessment. *Geriatrics & Gerontology International, 10*(3), 225–232.

Gagnon, G., Hansen, K. T., Woolmore-Goodwin, S., Gutmanis, I., Wells, J., Borrie, M., & Fogarty, J. (2013). Correcting the MoCA for education: effect on sensitivity. *The Canadian Journal of Neurological Sciences, 40*(05), 678–683.

Gluhm, S., Goldstein, J., Loc, K., Colt, A., Van Liew, C., & Corey-Bloom, J. (2013). Cognitive performance on the Mini-Mental State Examination and the Montreal Cognitive Assessment across the healthy adult lifespan. *Cognitive and Behavioral Neurology, 26*(1), 1–5.

Hachinski, V., Iadecola, C., Petersen, R. C., Breteler, M. M., Nyenhuis, D. L., Black, S. E., . . . Leblanc, G. G. (2006). National Institute of Neurological Disorders and Stroke–Canadian Stroke Network Vascular Cognitive Impairment harmonization standards. *Stroke, 37*(9), 2220–2241.

Hoops, S., Nazem, S., Siderowf, A. D., Duda, J. E., Xie, S. X., Stern, M. B., & Weintraub, D. (2009). Validity of the MoCA and MMSE in the detection of MCI and dementia in Parkinson disease. *Neurology, 73*(21), 1738–1745.

Hu, J., Zhou, W., Hu, S., Huang, M., Wei, N., Qi, H., . . . Xu, Y. (2013). Cross-cultural difference and validation of the Chinese version of Montreal Cognitive Assessment in older adults residing in eastern China: Preliminary findings. *Archives of Gerontology and Geriatrics, 56*(1), 38–43.

Julayanont, P., Brousseau, M., Chertkow, H., Phillips, N., & Nasreddine, Z. S. (2014). Montreal Cognitive Assessment Memory Index Score (MoCA-MIS) as a predictor of conversion from Mild Cognitive Impairment to Alzheimer's disease. *Journal of the American Geriatrics Society, 62*(4), 679–684.

Lam, B., Middleton, L. E., Masellis, M., Stuss, D. T., Harry, R. D., Kiss, A., & Black, S. E. (2013). Criterion and convergent validity of the Montreal Cognitive Assessment with screening and standardized neuropsychological testing. *Journal of the American Geriatrics Society, 61*(12), 2181–2185.

Lee, J., Lee, D. W., Cho, S., Na, D. L., Jeon, H. J., Kim, S., . . . Cho, M. J. (2008). Brief screening for Mild Cognitive Impairment in elderly outpatient clinic: Validation of the Korean version of the Montreal Cognitive Assessment. *Journal of Geriatric Psychiatry and Neurology, 21*(2), 104–110.

Lifshitz, M., Dwolatzky, T., & Press, Y. (2012). Validation of the Hebrew version of the MOCA test as a screening instrument for the early detection of Mild Cognitive Impairment in elderly individuals. *Journal of Geriatric Psychiatry and Neurology, 25*(3), 155–161.

Luis, C. A., Keegan, A. P., & Mullan, M. (2009). Cross validation of the Montreal Cognitive Assessment in community dwelling older adults residing in the southeastern US. *International Journal of Geriatric Psychiatry, 24*(2), 197–201.

Mai, L. M., Oczkowski, W., Mackenzie, G., Shuster, A., Wasielesky, L., Franchetto, A., . . . Sahlas, D. J. (2013). Screening for cognitive impairment in a stroke prevention clinic using the MoCA. *The Canadian Journal of Neurological Sciences/Le Journal Canadien Des Sciences Neurologiques, 40*(2), 192–197.

Malek-Ahmadi, M., Davis, K., Belden, C. M., & Sabbagh, M. N. (2014). Comparative analysis of the Alzheimer questionnaire (AQ) with the CDR sum of boxes, MoCA, and MMSE. *Alzheimer Disease and Associated Disorders, 28*(3), 296–298.

Malek-Ahmadi, M., Powell, J. J., Belden, C. M., O'Connor, K., Evans, L., Coon, D. W., & Nieri, W. (2015). Age-and education-adjusted normative data for the Montreal Cognitive Assessment (MoCA) in older adults age 70–99. *Aging, Neuropsychology, and Cognition, 22*(6), 755–761.

McLennan, S. N., Mathias, J. L., Brennan, L. C., & Stewart, S. (2011). Validity of the Montreal Cognitive Assessment (MoCA) as a screening test for Mild Cognitive Impairment (MCI) in a cardiovascular population. *Journal of Geriatric Psychiatry and Neurology, 24*(1), 33–38.

Memória, C. M., Yassuda, M., Nakano, E. Y., & Forlenza, O. V. (2013). Brief screening for Mild Cognitive Impairment: Validation of the Brazilian version of the Montreal Cognitive Assessment. *International Journal of Geriatric Psychiatry, 28*(1), 34–40.

Musso, M. W., Cohen, A. S., Auster, T. L., & McGovern, J. E. (2014). Investigation of the Montreal Cognitive Assessment (MoCA) as a cognitive screener in severe mental illness. *Psychiatry Research, 220*(1–2), 664–668.

Nasreddine, Z. S., Phillips, N. A., Bédirian, V., Charbonneau, S., Whitehead, V., Collin, I., . . . Chertkow, H. (2005). The Montreal Cognitive Assessment, MoCA: A brief screening tool for mild cognitive impairment. *Journal of the American Geriatrics Society, 53*(4), 695–699.

Nasreddine, Z. S., Phillips, N., & Chertkow, H. (2012). Normative data for the Montreal Cognitive Assessment (MoCA) in a population-based sample. *Neurology, 78*(10), 765–766.

Oudman, E., Postma, A., Van, d. S., Appelhof, B., Wijnia, J. W., & Nijboer, T. C. W. (2014a). The Montreal Cognitive Assessment (MoCA) is superior to the Mini-Mental State Examination (MMSE) in detection of Korsakoff's syndrome. *The Clinical Neuropsychologist, 28*(7), 1123–1132.

Oudman, E., Postma, A., Van, d. S., Appelhof, B., Wijnia, J. W., & Nijboer, T. C. W. (2014b). "The Montreal Cognitive Assessment (MoCA) is superior to the Mini-Mental State Examination (MMSE) in detection of Korsakoff's syndrome": Erratum. *The Clinical Neuropsychologist, 28*(8), 1398–1399.

Overton, E. T., Azad, T. D., Parker, N., Demarco Shaw, D., Frain, J., Spitz, T., . . . Ances, B. M. (2013). The Alzheimer's disease-8 and Montreal Cognitive Assessment as screening tools for neurocognitive impairment in HIV-infected persons. *Journal of Neurovirology, 19*(1), 109–116.

Ozdilek, B., & Kenangil, G. (2014). Validation of the Turkish version of the Montreal Cognitive Assessment scale (MOCA-TR) in patients with Parkinson's disease. *The Clinical Neuropsychologist, 28*(2), 333–343.

Pasi, M., Salvadori, E., Poggesi, A., Ciolli, L., Del Bene, A., Marini, S., . . . Pantoni, L. (2015). White matter microstructural damage in small vessel disease is associated with Montreal Cognitive Assessment but not with Mini Mental State Examination Performances Vascular Mild Cognitive Impairment Tuscany Study. *Stroke, 46*(1), 262–264.

Paul, R., Lane, E. M., Tate, D. F., Heaps, J., Romo, D. M., Akbudak, E., . . . Conturo, T. E. (2011). Neuroimaging signatures and cognitive correlates of the Montreal cognitive assessment screen in a nonclinical elderly sample. *Archives of Clinical Neuropsychology, 26*(5), 454–460.

Phabphal, K., & Kanjanasatien, J. (2011). Montreal Cognitive Assessment in cryptogenic epilepsy patients with normal Mini-Mental State Examination scores. *Epileptic Disorders, 13*(4), 375–381.

Pirrotta, F., Timpano, F., Bonanno, L., Nunnari, D., Marino, S., Bramanti, P., & Lanzafame, P. (2015). Italian validation of Montreal Cognitive Assessment. *European Journal of Psychological Assessment, 31*(2), 131–137.

Rahman, T. T. A., & El Gaafary, M. M. (2009). Montreal Cognitive Assessment Arabic version: Reliability and validity prevalence of Mild Cognitive Impairment among elderly attending geriatric clubs in Cairo. *Geriatrics & Gerontology International, 9*(1), 54–61.

Roalf, D. R., Moberg, P. J., Xie, S. X., Wolk, D. A., Moelter, S. T., & Arnold, S. E. (2013). Comparative accuracies of two common screening instruments for classification of Alzheimer's disease, Mild Cognitive Impairment, and healthy aging. *Alzheimer's & Dementia, 9*(5), 529–537.

Rossetti, H. C., Lacritz, L. H., Cullum, C. M., & Weiner, M. F. (2011). Normative data for the Montreal Cognitive Assessment (MoCA) in a population-based sample. *Neurology, 77*(13), 1272–1275.

Rossetti, H., Lacritz, L., Cullum, M., & Weiner, M. (2012). "Normative data for the Montreal Cognitive Assessment (MoCA) in a population-based sample": Author response. *Neurology, 78*(10), 766–766.

Sahathevan, R., Mohd Ali, K., Ellery, F., Mohamad, N. F., Hamdan, N., Ibrahim, N. M., . . . Cumming, T. B. (2014). *A Bahasa Malaysia version of the Montreal Cognitive Assessment: Validation in stroke.* Cambridge: Cambridge University Press.

Santangelo, G., Siciliano, M., Pedone, R., Vitale, C., Falco, F., Bisogno, R., . . . Trojano, L. (2015). Normative data for the Montreal Cognitive Assessment in an Italian population sample. *Neurological Sciences, 36*(4), 585–591.

Schweizer, T. A., Al-Khindi, T., & Macdonald, R. L. (2012). Mini-Mental State Examination versus Montreal Cognitive Assessment: Rapid assessment tools for cognitive and functional outcome after aneurysmal subarachnoid hemorrhage. *Journal of the Neurological Sciences, 316*(1–2), 137–140.

Sugarman, M. A., & Axelrod, B. N. (2014). Utility of the Montreal Cognitive Assessment and Mini-Mental State Examination in predicting general intellectual abilities. *Cognitive and Behavioral Neurology, 27*(3), 148–154.

Sweet, L., Van Adel, M., Metcalf, V., Wright, L., Harley, A., Leiva, R., & Taler, V. (2011). The Montreal Cognitive Assessment (MoCA) in geriatric rehabilitation: Psychometric properties and association with rehabilitation outcomes. *International Psychogeriatrics, 23*(10), 1582–1591.

Tan, J., Li, N., Gao, J., Wang, L., Zhao, Y., Yu, B., . . . Zhou, P. (2015). Optimal cutoff scores for dementia and Mild Cognitive Impairment of the Montreal Cognitive Assessment among elderly and oldest-old Chinese population. *Journal of Alzheimer's Disease, 43*(4), 1403–1412.

Tsai, C., Lee, W., Wang, S., Shia, B., Nasreddine, Z., & Fuh, J. (2012). Psychometrics of the Montreal Cognitive Assessment (MoCA) and its subscales: Validation of the Taiwanese version of the MoCA and an Item Response Theory analysis. *International Psychogeriatrics, 24*(4), 651–658.

Waldron-Perrine, B., & Axelrod, B. N. (2012). Determining an appropriate cutting score for indication of impairment on the Montreal Cognitive Assessment. International *Journal of Geriatric Psychiatry, 27*(11), 1189–1194.

Wang, C. S., Pai, M., Chen, P., Hou, N., Chien, P., & Huang, Y. (2013). Montreal Cognitive Assessment and Mini-Mental State Examination performance in patients with mild-to-moderate dementia with Lewy bodies, Alzheimer's disease, and normal participants in Taiwan. *International Psychogeriatrics, 25*(11), 1839–1848.

Wester, A. J., Westhoff, J., Kessels, R. P. C., & Egger, J. I. M. (2013). The Montreal Cognitive Assessment (MoCA) as a measure of severity of amnesia in patients with alcohol-related cognitive impairments and Korsakoff syndrome. *Clinical Neuropsychiatry: Journal of Treatment Evaluation, 10*(3–4), 134–141.

Whitney, K. A., Mossbarger, B., Herman, S. M., & Ibarra, S. L. (2012). Is the Montreal Cognitive Assessment superior to the Mini-Mental State Examination in detecting subtle cognitive impairment among middle-aged outpatient US military veterans? *Archives of Clinical Neuropsychology, 27*(7), 742–748.

Wong, A., Xiong, Y. Y., Kwan, P. W. L., Chan, A. Y. Y., Lam, W. W. M., Wang, K., . . . Mok, V. C. T. (2009). The validity, reliability and clinical utility of the Hong Kong Montreal Cognitive Assessment (HK-MoCA) in patients with cerebral small vessel disease. *Dementia and Geriatric Cognitive Disorders, 28*(1), 81–87.

Wong, G. K. C., Lam, S. W., Wong, A., Lai, M., Siu, D., Poon, W. S., & Mok, V. (2014). MoCA-assessed cognitive function and excellent outcome after aneurysmal subarachnoid hemorrhage at 1 year. *European Journal of Neurology, 21*(5), 725–730.

Wong, G. K. C., Lam, S., Ngai, K., Wong, A., Mok, V., & Poon, W. S. (2012). Evaluation of cognitive impairment by the Montreal Cognitive Assessment in patients with aneurysmal subarachnoid haemorrhage: Prevalence, risk factors and correlations with 3 month outcomes. *Journal of Neurology, Neurosurgery & Psychiatry, 83*(11), 1112–1117.

Wong, G. K. C., Ngai, K., Lam, S. W., Wong, A., Mok, V., & Poon, W. S. (2013). Validity of the Montreal Cognitive Assessment for traumatic brain injury patients with intracranial haemorrhage. *Brain Injury, 27*(4), 394–398.

Wong, A., Nyenhuis, D., Black, S. E., Law, L. S., Lo, E. S., Kwan, P. W., . . . Mok, V. (2015). Montreal Cognitive Assessment 5-Minute Protocol is a brief, valid, reliable, and feasible cognitive screen for telephone administration. *Stroke, 46*(4), 1059–1064.

Wu, C., Dagg, P., & Molgat, C. (2014). A pilot study to measure cognitive impairment in patients with severe schizophrenia with the Montreal Cognitive Assessment (MoCA). *Schizophrenia research, 158*(1), 151–155.

Yu, J., Li, J., & Huang, X. (2012). The Beijing version of the Montreal Cognitive Assessment as a brief screening tool for mild cognitive impairment: A community-based study. *BMC Psychiatry, 12*(1), 156.

Yu, K., Zhang, S., Wang, Q., Wang, X., Qin, Y., Wang, J., . . . Lin, H. (2015). Development of a computerized tool for the Chinese version of the Montreal Cognitive Assessment for screening Mild Cognitive Impairment. *International Psychogeriatrics, 27*(2), 213–219.

8 | ATTENTION

BRIEF TEST OF ATTENTION (BTA)

TEST NAME	**Brief Test of Attention (BTA)**
DOMAIN	Attention
AGE RANGE	17 to 82
ADMINISTRATION TIME	10 minutes
SCORING FORMAT	Hand scored
REFERENCE	Schretlen, D. (1997). *Brief Test of Attention professional manual.* Odessa, FL: Psychological Assessment Resources. www.parinc.com

DESCRIPTION

The Brief Test of Attention (BTA) is a test of auditory divided attention. The BTA was developed following the attentional model proposed by Cooley and Morris (1990), and the test was designed specifically to reduce the influence of confounding factors that complicate the interpretation of attention tests (e.g., motor speed, visual scanning, memory; Schretlen, Bobholz, & Brandt, 1996). Note that the test is designed to detect attentional impairments rather than differentiating levels of intact attention (Schretlen, 1997).

The test consists of two lists of alphanumeric strings (e.g., "M-6-3-R-2"), presented via audio format, that increase in length from 4 to 18 characters across 10 items. In the first list (Form N, where N signifies numbers), the examinee's task is to disregard the letters and count how many numbers are presented aloud. In the second list (Form L, where L signifies letters), the same items are presented, but this time the examinee is instructed to disregard the numbers and count the number of letters.

ADMINISTRATION

Detailed administration instructions are provided in the manual (Schretlen, 1997).

SCORING

Correct responses are credited a score of one. For each form, the score range is 0 to 10 (entire test 0 to 20). Discontinuation rules apply, described in the manual, that enable administration of the first form only. Abnormal performance is considered 3/10 correct. This degree of poor performance is rare in the normative sample (<1% of healthy adults), and considerably more frequent in the clinical sample (nearly 17%). Raw scores are converted to percentiles based on age (see manual). During standardization, slight inconsistencies in the percentile distribution across age were corrected. Percentiles above the 74th are interpreted as Above Average, 25th to 74th as Average, 10th to 24th as Low Average, 2nd to 9th as Borderline Impaired, and 2nd or below as Impaired. The highest possible score should thus be reported as ">74th percentile."

DEMOGRAPHIC EFFECTS

Demographic variables account for nearly 18% of variance in performance, with age the most influential and gender the least influential (i.e., 9% for age, 5% for ethnicity, 4% for education, and 1% for gender; Schretlen, 1997). Standardized scores are provided based only on age because of the minimal association with other demographic variables. Rivera et al. (2015) reported that demographic effects jointly explained 11–41% of the variance in performance.

AGE

In healthy adults, age is correlated with performance, with performance decrements most notable at approximately 60 years of age (Schretlen, 1997). This trend was also reported by Rivera et al. (2015) in most countries included in a large-scale normative study involving 11 Latin American countries.

GENDER

Gender is not highly influential. Schretlen (1997) reported that women scored slightly higher than men (a difference of 0.8 points). No significant gender differences were reported in a large-scale normative study across 11 countries, with the exception of Honduras, where men performed slightly better than women (Rivera et al., 2015).

EDUCATION

There are significant education effects on the test, which account for a small amount of variance (Rivera et al., 2015; Schretlen, 1997; see later discussion).

ETHNICITY, NATIONALITY, AND LINGUISTIC EFFECTS

African Americans reportedly score somewhat lower than Caucasians by approximately 2 points. However, African Americans slightly outperform Caucasians in the highest age group (0.4 points) and score slightly lower in the lower education groups (2 points). Ojeda, Aretouli, Pena, and Schretlen (2016) reported that the BTA did not vary between a group of Americans and Spaniards.

Socioeconomic status may be an influential factor. For example, Dore, Waldstein, Evans, and Zonderman (2015) reported that among African Americans below the poverty level, people with diabetes performed worse on the BTA and other cognitive tests, despite the finding that consistent differences were not found between diabetic and nondiabetic participants above the poverty level.

NORMATIVE DATA

The adult sample described in the manual consists of a combined sample of the standardization sample (n = 462), research controls (n = 187), and participants in a hypertension study (n = 92). Participants ranged in age from 17 to 82 years [mean age = 13.8 years (standard deviation [SD] = 2.6 years)], with data divided into 13 age groups. The sample was 63% female, with ethnic composition as 82% Caucasian, 18% African American, and fewer than 1% classified as "other" ethnicity. Adults were screened for dementia, severe psychiatric disorders, and substance dependence. Data regarding ethnicity were not recorded for 33 individuals in the adult normative sample, and 45 of the adults in the adult normative sample were not screened. A child sample and a clinical sample are also described in detail in the manual.

Schretlen, Testa, and Pearlson (2010) provide norms for 322 adults as part of the Calibrated Neuropsychological Normative System (CNNS) available through Psychological Assessment Resources (PAR; www.parinc.com). These provide T scores and discrepancies based on a large sample of older adults from the northeastern United States. A major advantage of these norms is the option to correct for demographic variables such as age, sex, education, and ethnicity. Several other commonly used neuropsychological tests are co-normed using this sample, which facilitates cross-test comparisons.

Rivera et al. (2015) present normative data for 3,970 healthy people recruited from 11 Latin American countries, including Argentina, Bolivia, Chile, Cuba, El Salvador, Guatemala, Honduras, Mexico, Paraguay, Peru, and, Puerto Rico. Participants were 18–95 years old, spoke Spanish as their native language, completed one or more years of formal education, could read and write, scored 23 or higher on the Mini-Mental State Examination (MMSE), 4 or less on the Patient Health Questionnaire–9 (PHQ-9; depressive symptom scale), and 90 or more on the Barthel Index (a measure of activities of daily living [ADLs]). People with neurologic or psychiatric conditions were excluded, as were individuals presenting with substance abuse, active systemic or unmanaged disease affecting cognition, those with severe sensory deficits, and those who were using medications that could impact cognition. Demographic characteristics are shown in Table 8–1. Normative data for each country are presented in Tables 8–2 to 8–12.

EVIDENCE FOR RELIABILITY

EVIDENCE FOR INTERNAL RELIABILITY

Based on the normative data for adult and child samples combined, internal reliability for the entire BTA is high (r = .80), with marginal coefficients for the separate forms (r = .69 and .65, respectively, for Forms L and N). When both the normative and clinical samples are combined, reliability estimates for the entire test and separate forms are high to very high (r = .90 for the BTA, and r = .82 and .81, respectively, for Forms L and N; Schretlen, 1997).

EVIDENCE FOR TEST-RETEST RELIABILITY, AND PRACTICE EFFECTS

Test-retest reliability is reportedly adequate in a sample of older healthy adults with mild hypertension retested after a nine-month interval (r = .70; Schretlen, 1997) and low for adolescent girls receiving iron supplementation retested over a three-month interval as described in the manual (r = .45). The authors suggest that restriction of range may have lowered the coefficient in this case (only 14% of the group had scores lower than 15 of 20 on the BTA).

Practice effects are minimal, with less than 5% of individuals showing retest changes exceeding ±4 or 5 points

TABLE 8–1 Characteristics of the Rivera et al. (2015) BTA Normative Samples for Latin-American Countries

			EDUCATION		GENDER	
	N TOTAL	AGE MEAN (SD)	1 TO 12 *N* (%)	>12 *N* (%)	MALE *N* (%)	FEMALE *N* (%)
Argentina	320	45.7 (19.5)	148 (46.3)	172 (53.8)	96 (30.0)	224 (70.0)
Bolivia	274	55.8 (22.0)	226 (82.5)	48 (17.5)	99 (36.1)	175 (63.9)
Chile	320	55.1 (19.6)	241 (75.3)	79 (24.7)	134 (41.9)	186 (58.1)
Cuba	306	53.0 (19.7)	234 (76.5)	72 (23.5)	142 (46.4)	164 (53.6)
El Salvador	257	56.0 (20.7)	203 (79.0)	54 (21.0)	100 (38.9)	157 (61.1)
Guatemala	214	53.2 (17.4)	133 (62.1)	81 (37.9)	95 (44.4)	119 (55.6)
Honduras	184	48.6 (18.8)	140 (76.1)	44 (23.9)	67 (36.4)	117 (63.6)
Mexico	1300	52.5 (20.5)	1005 (77.3)	295 (22.7)	431 (33.2)	869 (66.8)
Paraguay	263	53.0 (14.8)	216 (82.1)	47 (17.9)	101 (38.4)	162 (61.6)
Peru	245	43.4 (20.6)	87 (35.5)	158 (64.5)	87 (35.5)	158 (64.5)
Puerto Rico	294	50.9 (18.5)	160 (54.4)	134 (45.6)	126 (42.9)	168 (57.1)

SOURCE: From Guàrdia-Olmos et al. (2015).

(Schretlen, 1997). However, ceiling effects may restrict the extent of practice effects. There are no significant order or practice effects between Forms N and L in healthy controls (Schretlen, 1997) or in patients with Huntington's disease (HD; Schretlen, Brandt, & Bobholz, 1996).

EVIDENCE FOR VALIDITY

CORRELATIONS BETWEEN FORMS L AND N

Correlations between Forms L and N are .65 for the normative sample and .79 for the combined normative and clinical sample. Forms L and N differ by less than 0.20 points in healthy people (Schretlen, 1997), with nearly 95% of participants in the standardization sample obtaining Form L and N scores within 3 points of each other.

FACTOR-ANALYTIC STUDIES AND RELATIONSHIPS WITH OTHER TESTS

The BTA correlates slightly more with Digits Backward than with Digits Forward ($r = .53$ vs. $r = .43$), and with the Trail Making Test (TMT)-B than the TMT-A ($r = .-55$ vs. $-.48$; Schretlen, 1997; see also Busse & Whiteside, 2012;

TABLE 8–2 BTA Normative Data for Argentina

		AGE (YEARS)												
	PERCENTILE	18 TO 22	23 TO 27	28 TO 32	33 TO 37	38 TO 42	43 TO 47	48 TO 52	53 TO 57	58 TO 62	63 TO 67	68 TO 72	73 TO 77	>77
>12 years of education	95	–	–	–	–	–	–	20.0	20.0	20.0	20.0	20.0	19.9	19.7
	90	–	–	20.0	20.0	20.0	20.0	19.8	19.7	19.5	19.3	19.1	19.0	18.8
	85	20.0	20.0	19.9	19.7	19.6	19.4	19.2	19.0	18.8	18.7	18.5	18.3	18.1
	80	19.8	19.6	19.4	19.2	19.0	18.9	18.7	18.5	18.3	18.1	18.0	17.8	17.6
	70	18.9	18.7	18.5	18.4	18.2	18.0	17.8	17.6	17.5	17.3	17.1	16.9	16.8
	60	18.2	18.0	17.8	17.6	17.5	17.3	17.1	16.9	16.7	16.6	16.4	16.2	16.0
	50	17.5	17.3	17.2	17.0	16.8	16.6	16.4	16.3	16.1	15.9	15.7	15.5	15.4
	40	16.9	16.7	16.5	16.3	16.1	16.0	15.8	15.6	15.4	15.2	15.1	14.9	14.7
	30	16.1	16.0	15.8	15.6	15.4	15.2	15.1	14.9	14.7	14.5	14.3	14.2	14.0
	20	15.3	15.1	14.9	14.7	14.6	14.4	14.2	14.0	13.9	13.7	13.5	13.3	13.1
	15	14.8	14.6	14.4	14.2	14.0	13.9	13.7	13.5	13.3	13.1	13.0	12.8	12.6
	10	14.1	13.9	13.8	13.6	13.4	13.2	13.0	12.9	12.7	12.5	12.3	12.1	12.0
	5	13.2	13.0	12.8	12.6	12.4	12.3	12.1	11.9	11.7	11.5	11.4	11.2	11.0
1 to 12 years of education	95	20.0	20.0	20.0	19.9	19.7	19.5	19.4	19.2	19.0	18.8	18.6	18.5	18.3
	90	19.5	19.3	19.1	18.9	18.8	18.6	18.4	18.2	18.1	17.9	17.7	17.5	17.3
	85	18.8	18.7	18.5	18.3	18.1	17.9	17.8	17.6	17.4	17.2	17.1	16.9	16.7
	80	18.3	18.1	18.0	17.8	17.6	17.4	17.2	17.1	16.9	16.7	16.5	16.3	16.2
	70	17.5	17.3	17.1	16.9	16.7	16.6	16.4	16.2	16.0	15.9	15.7	15.5	15.3
	60	16.7	16.6	16.4	16.2	16.0	15.8	15.7	15.5	15.3	15.1	15.0	14.8	14.6
	50	16.1	15.9	15.7	15.5	15.4	15.2	15.0	14.8	14.6	14.5	14.3	14.1	13.9
	40	15.4	15.2	15.1	14.9	14.7	14.5	14.3	14.2	14.0	13.8	13.6	13.4	13.3
	30	14.7	14.5	14.3	14.2	14.0	13.8	13.6	13.4	13.3	13.1	12.9	12.7	12.5
	20	13.8	13.7	13.5	13.3	13.1	13.0	12.8	12.6	12.4	12.2	12.1	11.9	11.7
	15	13.3	13.1	13.0	12.8	12.6	12.4	12.2	12.1	11.9	11.7	11.5	11.3	11.2
	10	12.7	12.5	12.3	12.1	12.0	11.8	11.6	11.4	11.2	11.1	10.9	10.7	10.5
	5	11.7	11.5	11.4	11.2	11.0	10.8	10.6	10.5	10.3	10.1	9.9	9.8	9.6

SOURCE: From Rivera et al. (2015).

TABLE 8–3 BTA Normative Data for Bolivia

		AGE (YEARS)												
	PERCENTILE	18 TO 22	23 TO 27	28 TO 32	33 TO 37	38 TO 42	43 TO 47	48 TO 52	53 TO 57	58 TO 62	63 TO 67	68 TO 72	73 TO 77	>77
>12 years of education	95	–	–	–	20.0	20.0	20.0	20.0	19.9	19.6	19.3	19.0	18.7	18.4
	90	20.0	20.0	20.0	19.7	19.4	19.1	18.8	18.5	18.2	17.9	17.6	17.3	17.0
	85	19.6	19.4	19.1	18.8	18.5	18.2	17.9	17.6	17.3	17.0	16.7	16.4	16.1
	80	18.9	18.6	18.3	18.0	17.7	17.4	17.1	16.8	16.5	16.3	16.0	15.7	15.4
	70	17.7	17.4	17.1	16.8	16.5	16.2	15.9	15.6	15.3	15.0	14.7	14.5	14.2
	60	16.7	16.4	16.1	15.8	15.5	15.2	14.9	14.6	14.3	14.0	13.7	13.4	13.1
	50	15.7	15.4	15.1	14.8	14.5	14.2	14.0	13.7	13.4	13.1	12.8	12.5	12.2
	40	14.8	14.5	14.2	13.9	13.6	13.3	13.0	12.7	12.4	12.1	11.8	11.5	11.2
	30	13.7	13.5	13.2	12.9	12.6	12.3	12.0	11.7	11.4	11.1	10.8	10.5	10.2
	20	12.5	12.2	11.9	11.7	11.4	11.1	10.8	10.5	10.2	9.9	9.6	9.3	9.0
	15	11.8	11.5	11.2	10.9	10.6	10.3	10.0	9.7	9.4	9.1	8.8	8.6	8.3
	10	10.9	10.6	10.3	10.0	9.7	9.4	9.1	8.8	8.5	8.2	7.9	7.6	7.3
	5	9.5	9.2	8.9	8.6	8.3	8.0	7.7	7.5	7.2	6.9	6.6	6.3	6.0
1 to 12 years of education	95	20.0	19.7	19.4	19.1	18.8	18.5	18.2	17.9	17.6	17.3	17.0	16.8	16.5
	90	18.6	18.3	18.0	17.7	17.4	17.1	16.9	16.6	16.3	16.0	15.7	15.4	15.1
	85	17.7	17.4	17.1	16.8	16.5	16.2	15.9	15.7	15.4	15.1	14.8	14.5	14.2
	80	16.9	16.7	16.4	16.1	15.8	15.5	15.2	14.9	14.6	14.3	14.0	13.7	13.4
	70	15.7	15.4	15.2	14.9	14.6	14.3	14.0	13.7	13.4	13.1	12.8	12.5	12.2
	60	14.7	14.4	14.1	13.8	13.5	13.2	13.0	12.7	12.4	12.1	11.8	11.5	11.2
	50	13.8	13.5	13.2	12.9	12.6	12.3	12.0	11.7	11.4	11.1	10.8	10.5	10.3
	40	12.8	12.5	12.2	11.9	11.7	11.4	11.1	10.8	10.5	10.2	9.9	9.6	9.3
	30	11.8	11.5	11.2	10.9	10.6	10.3	10.0	9.7	9.5	9.2	8.9	8.6	8.3
	20	10.6	10.3	10.0	9.7	9.4	9.1	8.8	8.5	8.2	8.0	7.7	7.4	7.1
	15	9.8	9.5	9.2	9.0	8.7	8.4	8.1	7.8	7.5	7.2	6.9	6.6	6.3
	10	8.9	8.6	8.3	8.0	7.8	7.5	7.2	6.9	6.6	6.3	6.0	5.7	5.4
	5	7.6	7.3	7.0	6.7	6.4	6.1	5.8	5.5	5.2	4.9	4.6	4.3	4.0

SOURCE: From Rivera et al. (2015).

TABLE 8–4 BTA Normative Data for Chile

		AGE (YEARS)												
	PERCENTILE	18 TO 22	23 TO 27	28 TO 32	33 TO 37	38 TO 42	43 TO 47	48 TO 52	53 TO 57	58 TO 62	63 TO 67	68 TO 72	73 TO 77	>77
>12 years of education	95	–	–	–	–	–	–	–	20.0	20.0	20.0	20.0	19.8	19.5
	90	–	–	–	–	20.0	20.0	20.0	19.7	19.4	19.1	18.8	18.5	18.1
	85	–	–	20.0	20.0	19.8	19.5	19.2	18.8	18.5	18.2	17.9	17.6	17.3
	80	20.0	20.0	19.7	19.4	19.1	18.7	18.4	18.1	17.8	17.5	17.2	16.8	16.5
	70	19.2	18.8	18.5	18.2	17.9	17.6	17.3	16.9	16.6	16.3	16.0	15.7	15.3
	60	18.2	17.8	17.5	17.2	16.9	16.6	16.3	15.9	15.6	15.3	15.0	14.7	14.4
	50	17.2	16.9	16.6	16.3	16.0	15.7	15.3	15.0	14.7	14.4	14.1	13.8	13.4
	40	16.3	16.0	15.7	15.4	15.1	14.7	14.4	14.1	13.8	13.5	13.2	12.8	12.5
	30	15.3	15.0	14.7	14.4	14.1	13.7	13.4	13.1	12.8	12.5	12.2	11.8	11.5
	20	14.1	13.8	13.5	13.2	12.9	12.6	12.2	11.9	11.6	11.3	11.0	10.7	10.3
	15	13.4	13.1	12.8	12.5	12.1	11.8	11.5	11.2	10.9	10.6	10.2	9.9	9.6
	10	12.5	12.2	11.9	11.6	11.3	10.9	10.6	10.3	10.0	9.7	9.4	9.0	8.7
	5	11.2	10.9	10.6	10.3	9.9	9.6	9.3	9.0	8.7	8.4	8.0	7.7	7.4
1 to 12 years of education	95	20.0	20.0	20.0	20.0	19.8	19.5	19.2	18.8	18.5	18.2	17.9	17.6	17.2
	90	19.7	19.4	19.1	18.8	18.5	18.1	17.8	17.5	17.2	16.9	16.6	16.2	15.9
	85	18.8	18.5	18.2	17.9	17.6	17.3	16.9	16.6	16.3	16.0	15.7	15.4	15.0
	80	18.1	17.8	17.5	17.2	16.8	16.5	16.2	15.9	15.6	15.3	14.9	14.6	14.3
	70	16.9	16.6	16.3	16.0	15.7	15.3	15.0	14.7	14.4	14.1	13.8	13.4	13.1
	60	15.9	15.6	15.3	15.0	14.7	14.4	14.0	13.7	13.4	13.1	12.8	12.5	12.1
	50	15.0	14.7	14.4	14.1	13.8	13.4	13.1	12.8	12.5	12.2	11.8	11.5	11.2
	40	14.1	13.8	13.5	13.1	12.8	12.5	12.2	11.9	11.6	11.2	10.9	10.6	10.3
	30	13.1	12.8	12.5	12.2	11.8	11.5	11.2	10.9	10.6	10.3	9.9	9.6	9.3
	20	11.9	11.6	11.3	11.0	10.7	10.3	10.0	9.7	9.4	9.1	8.8	8.4	8.1
	15	11.2	10.9	10.6	10.2	9.9	9.6	9.3	9.0	8.7	8.3	8.0	7.7	7.4
	10	10.3	10.0	9.7	9.4	9.0	8.7	8.4	8.1	7.8	7.5	7.1	6.8	6.5
	5	9.0	8.7	8.4	8.0	7.7	7.4	7.1	6.8	6.4	6.1	5.8	5.5	5.2

SOURCE: From Rivera et al. (2015).

TABLE 8-5 BTA Normative Data for Cuba

		AGE (YEARS)												
	PERCENTILE	18 TO 22	23 TO 27	28 TO 32	33 TO 37	38 TO 42	43 TO 47	48 TO 52	53 TO 37	58 TO 62	63 TO 67	68 TO 72	73 TO 77	>77
>12 years of education	95	–	–	–	–	–	–	–	–	–	20.0	20.0	20.0	20.0
	90	–	–	–	–	–	–	20.0	20.0	20.0	19.8	19.5	19.2	18.9
	85	–	–	–	–	20.0	20.0	19.9	19.6	19.3	19.0	18.7	18.4	18.1
	80	–	20.0	20.0	20.0	19.8	19.5	19.2	18.9	18.6	18.3	18.0	17.7	17.4
	70	20.0	19.7	19.4	19.1	18.8	18.4	18.1	17.8	17.5	17.2	16.9	16.6	16.3
	60	19.1	18.8	18.5	18.2	17.9	17.6	17.2	16.9	16.6	16.3	16.0	15.7	15.4
	50	18.2	17.9	17.6	17.3	17.0	16.7	16.4	16.1	15.8	15.5	15.2	14.9	14.6
	40	17.4	17.1	16.8	16.5	16.2	15.9	15.6	15.3	15.0	14.7	14.4	14.1	13.8
	30	16.5	16.2	15.9	15.6	15.3	15.0	14.7	14.4	14.1	13.8	13.5	13.2	12.9
	20	15.4	15.1	14.8	14.5	14.2	13.9	13.6	13.3	13.0	12.7	12.4	12.1	11.8
	15	14.8	14.5	14.2	13.9	13.6	13.3	13.0	12.6	12.3	12.0	11.7	11.4	11.1
	10	14.0	13.7	13.4	13.1	12.8	12.5	12.2	11.8	11.5	11.2	10.9	10.6	10.3
	5	12.8	12.5	12.2	11.9	11.6	11.3	11.0	10.6	10.3	10.0	9.7	9.4	9.1
1 to 12 years of education	95	20.0	20.0	20.0	19.9	19.6	19.3	19.0	18.7	18.4	18.1	17.8	17.5	17.2
	90	19.6	19.3	19.0	18.7	18.4	18.1	17.8	17.5	17.2	16.9	16.6	16.3	16.0
	85	18.8	18.5	18.2	17.9	17.6	17.3	17.0	16.7	16.4	16.1	15.8	15.5	15.2
	80	18.2	17.9	17.6	17.3	17.0	16.7	16.3	16.0	15.7	15.4	15.1	14.8	14.5
	70	17.1	16.8	16.5	16.2	15.9	15.6	15.3	15.0	14.7	14.4	14.1	13.8	13.5
	60	16.2	15.9	15.6	15.3	15.0	14.7	14.4	14.1	13.8	13.5	13.2	12.9	12.6
	50	15.4	15.1	14.8	14.5	14.2	13.9	13.5	13.2	12.9	12.6	12.3	12.0	11.7
	40	14.5	14.2	13.9	13.6	13.3	13.0	12.7	12.4	12.1	11.8	11.5	11.2	10.9
	30	13.6	13.3	13.0	12.7	12.4	12.1	11.8	11.5	11.2	10.9	10.6	10.3	10.0
	20	12.6	12.3	12.0	11.7	11.4	11.1	10.8	10.4	10.1	9.8	9.5	9.2	8.9
	15	11.9	11.6	11.3	11.0	10.7	10.4	10.1	9.8	9.5	9.2	8.9	8.6	8.3
	10	11.1	10.8	10.5	10.2	9.9	9.6	9.3	9.0	8.7	8.4	8.1	7.8	7.5
	5	9.9	9.6	9.3	9.0	8.7	8.4	8.1	7.8	7.5	7.2	6.9	6.6	6.3

SOURCE: From Rivera et al. (2015).

TABLE 8-6 BTA Normative Data for El Salvador

		AGE (YEARS)												
	PERCENTILE	18 TO 22	23 TO 27	28 TO 32	33 TO 37	38 TO 42	43 TO 47	48 TO 52	53 TO 57	58 TO 62	63 TO 67	68 TO 72	73 TO 77	>77
>12 years of education	95	–	–	–	–	–	–	–	–	–	20.0	20.0	20.0	20.0
	90	–	–	–	–	–	–	20.0	20.0	20.0	19.9	19.6	19.3	19.0
	85	–	–	–	20.0	20.0	20.0	19.8	19.5	19.3	19.0	18.7	18.4	18.1
	80	20.0	20.0	20.0	19.9	19.6	19.4	19.1	18.8	18.5	18.2	18.0	17.7	17.4
	70	19.6	19.3	19.0	18.7	18.5	18.2	17.9	17.6	17.3	17.1	16.8	16.5	16.2
	60	18.6	18.3	18.0	17.8	17.5	17.2	16.9	16.6	16.4	16.1	15.8	15.5	15.2
	50	17.7	17.4	17.1	16.8	16.6	16.3	16.0	15.7	15.4	15.2	14.9	14.6	14.3
	40	16.8	16.5	16.2	15.9	15.6	15.4	15.1	14.8	14.5	14.2	14.0	13.7	13.4
	30	15.8	15.5	15.2	14.9	14.6	14.4	14.1	13.8	13.5	13.2	13.0	12.7	12.4
	20	14.6	14.3	14.0	13.8	13.5	13.2	12.9	12.6	12.4	12.1	11.8	11.5	11.2
	15	13.9	13.6	13.3	13.0	12.7	12.5	12.2	11.9	11.6	11.3	11.1	10.8	10.5
	10	13.0	12.7	12.4	12.1	11.9	11.6	11.3	11.0	10.7	10.5	10.2	9.9	9.6
	5	11.7	11.4	11.1	10.8	10.5	10.3	10.0	9.7	9.4	9.1	8.9	8.6	8.3
1 to 12 years of education	95	18.7	18.5	18.2	17.9	17.6	17.3	17.1	16.8	16.5	16.2	15.9	15.7	15.4
	90	17.4	17.1	16.9	16.6	16.3	16.0	15.7	15.5	15.2	14.9	14.6	14.3	14.1
	85	16.5	16.3	16.0	15.7	15.4	15.1	14.9	14.6	14.3	14.0	13.7	13.5	13.2
	80	15.8	15.5	15.2	15.0	14.7	14.4	14.1	13.8	13.6	13.3	13.0	12.7	12.4
	70	14.6	14.3	14.1	13.8	13.5	13.2	12.9	12.7	12.4	12.1	11.8	11.5	11.3
	60	13.6	13.4	13.1	12.8	12.5	12.2	12.0	11.7	11.4	11.1	10.8	10.6	10.3
	50	12.7	12.4	12.2	11.9	11.6	11.3	11.0	10.8	10.5	10.2	9.9	9.6	9.4
	40	11.8	11.5	11.2	11.0	10.7	10.4	10.1	9.8	9.6	9.3	9.0	8.7	8.4
	30	10.8	10.5	10.2	10.0	9.7	9.4	9.1	8.8	8.6	8.3	8.0	7.7	7.4
	20	9.6	9.4	9.1	8.8	8.5	8.2	8.0	7.7	7.4	7.1	6.8	6.5	6.3
	15	8.9	8.6	8.3	8.1	7.8	7.5	7.2	6.9	6.7	6.4	6.1	5.8	5.5
	10	8.0	7.7	7.5	7.2	6.9	6.6	6.3	6.1	5.8	5.5	5.2	4.9	4.7
	5	6.7	6.4	6.1	5.9	5.6	5.3	5.0	4.7	4.5	4.2	3.9	3.6	3.3

SOURCE: From Rivera et al. (2015).

TABLE 8-7 BTA Normative Data for Guatemala

PERCENTILE	1–12 YEARS OF EDUCATION	>12 YEARS OF EDUCATION
95	19.5	–
90	18.3	–
85	17.5	20.0
80	16.8	19.5
70	15.7	18.4
60	14.8	17.5
50	13.9	16.6
40	13.1	15.8
30	12.1	14.8
20	11.1	13.7
15	10.4	13.1
10	9.6	12.2
5	8.3	11.0

SOURCE: From Rivera et al. (2015).

Wong, 1999). In healthy people, the BTA is highly correlated with all parts of the Stroop, not just the interference trial (r = .66 to .68), suggesting that speed may be an important component of the task. However, in patient samples, the BTA correlates most highly with the Stroop interference trial (Schretlen, 1997). The BTA correlates moderately with Continuous Performance Test (CPT) omission and commission errors in a TBI sample (rs = −.37, −.36; Busse & Whiteside, 2012). In a study involving principal components analysis with psychiatric patients, the BTA emerged on an attention factor along with Digit Span, Digit Symbol, and Stroop components when examined with a number of other neuropsychological tests (Schretlen, 1997). Correlation analyses and principal components analyses (Schretlen, Bobholz, & Brandt, 1996) show that the BTA correlates more strongly with measures of attention than with other cognitive tasks such as the Rey Osterrieth Complex Figure, Boston Naming Test (BNT), Wechsler Memory Scale, Revised (WMS-R) Logical Memory, General Memory, and Delayed Memory indices.

CLINICAL STUDIES

People with HD without dementia perform more poorly on the BTA compared with healthy adults (Schretlen, Brandt, & Bobholtz, 1996). Amnesic patients, however, are not impaired compared with controls, suggesting that memory is not an integral component of performance (Schretlen, 1997). In a group of adults with traumatic brain injury (TBI), BTA scores were significantly related to psychosocial outcome (Schretlen, 1992); BTA scores, along with scores from the Cognitive Estimation Test, accounted for nearly 40% of the variance in psychosocial outcome. Rao et al. (2010), however, reported that the BTA did not differ between patients with mild TBI who were depressed compared to those who were not.

TABLE 8-8 BTA Normative Data for Honduras

		AGE (YEARS)												
	PERCENTILE	18 TO 22	23 TO 27	28 TO 32	33 TO 37	38 TO 42	43 TO 47	48 TO 52	53 TO 57	58 TO 62	63 TO 67	68 TO 72	73 TO 77	>77
>12 years of education	95	–	–	20.0	20.0	20.0	20.0	19.6	19.2	18.7	18.2	17.8	17.3	16.8
	90	20.0	20.0	19.8	19.4	18.9	18.4	18.0	17.5	17.0	16.6	16.1	15.6	15.1
	85	19.6	19.2	18.7	18.2	17.8	17.3	16.8	16.4	15.9	15.4	15.0	14.5	14.0
	80	18.7	18.2	17.8	17.3	16.8	16.4	15.9	15.4	15.0	14.5	14.0	13.6	13.1
	70	17.2	16.7	16.3	15.8	15.3	14.9	14.4	13.9	13.5	13.0	12.5	12.1	11.6
	60	15.9	15.5	15.0	14.5	14.1	13.6	13.1	12.7	12.2	11.7	11.3	10.8	10.3
	50	14.8	14.3	13.8	13.4	12.9	12.4	12.0	11.5	11.0	10.6	10.1	9.6	9.2
	40	13.6	13.1	12.7	12.2	11.7	11.3	10.8	10.3	9.9	9.4	8.9	8.5	8.0
	30	12.3	11.9	11.4	10.9	10.5	10.0	9.5	9.1	8.6	8.1	7.7	7.2	6.7
	20	10.8	10.4	9.9	9.4	9.0	8.5	8.0	7.6	7.1	6.6	6.2	5.7	5.2
	15	9.9	9.4	9.0	8.5	8.0	7.6	7.1	6.6	6.2	5.7	5.2	4.8	4.3
	10	8.8	8.3	7.8	7.4	6.9	6.4	6.0	5.5	5.0	4.6	4.1	3.6	3.2
	5	7.1	6.6	6.2	5.7	5.2	4.8	4.3	3.8	3.4	2.9	2.4	1.9	1.5
1 to 12 years of education	95	19.9	19.4	18.9	18.5	18.0	17.5	17.0	16.6	16.1	15.6	15.2	14.7	14.2
	90	18.2	17.7	17.2	16.8	16.3	15.8	15.4	14.9	14.4	14.0	13.5	13.0	12.6
	85	17.0	16.6	16.1	15.6	15.2	14.7	14.2	13.8	13.3	12.8	12.4	11.9	11.4
	80	16.1	15.6	15.2	14.7	14.2	13.8	13.3	12.8	12.4	11.9	11.4	11.0	10.5
	70	14.6	14.1	13.7	13.2	12.7	12.3	11.8	11.3	10.9	10.4	9.9	9.5	9.0
	60	13.3	12.9	12.4	11.9	11.5	11.0	10.5	10.1	9.6	9.1	8.7	8.2	7.7
	50	12.2	11.7	11.2	10.8	10.3	9.8	9.4	8.9	8.4	8.0	7.5	7.0	6.6
	40	11.0	10.5	10.1	9.6	9.1	8.7	8.2	7.7	7.3	6.8	6.3	5.9	5.4
	30	9.7	9.3	8.8	8.3	7.9	7.4	6.9	6.5	6.0	5.5	5.1	4.6	4.1
	20	8.2	7.8	7.3	6.8	6.4	5.9	5.4	5.0	4.5	4.0	3.6	3.1	2.6
	15	7.3	6.8	6.4	5.9	5.4	5.0	4.5	4.0	3.6	3.1	2.6	2.2	1.7
	10	6.2	5.7	5.3	4.8	4.3	3.9	3.4	2.9	2.4	2.0	1.5	1.0	0.6
	5	4.5	4.0	3.6	3.1	2.6	2.2	1.7	1.2	0.8	0.3	–	–	–

SOURCE: From Rivera et al. (2015).

TABLE 8–9 BTA Normative Data for Mexico

		AGE (YEARS)												
	PERCENTILE	18 TO 22	23 TO 27	28 TO 32	33 TO 37	38 TO 42	43 TO 47	48 TO 52	53 TO 57	58 TO 62	63 TO 67	68 TO 72	73 TO 77	>77
>12 years of education	95	–	–	–	–	–	–	–	20.0	20.0	20.0	20.0	20.0	19.8
	90	–	–	–	–	20.0	20.0	20.0	19.8	19.5	19.3	19.0	18.8	18.5
	85	–	20.0	20.0	20.0	19.7	19.4	19.2	18.9	18.7	18.4	18.1	17.9	17.6
	80	20.0	19.8	19.5	19.2	19.0	18.7	18.5	18.2	17.9	17.7	17.4	17.1	16.9
	70	18.8	18.6	18.3	18.1	17.8	17.5	17.3	17.0	16.8	16.5	16.2	16.0	15.7
	60	17.9	17.6	17.3	17.1	16.8	16.6	16.3	16.0	15.8	15.5	15.3	15.0	14.7
	50	16.9	16.7	16.4	16.2	15.9	15.6	15.4	15.1	14.9	14.6	14.3	14.1	13.8
	40	16.0	15.8	15.5	15.2	15.0	14.7	14.5	14.2	13.9	13.7	13.4	13.2	12.9
	30	15.0	14.8	14.5	14.3	14.0	13.7	13.5	13.2	13.0	12.7	12.4	12.2	11.9
	20	13.9	13.6	13.4	13.1	12.8	12.6	12.3	12.1	11.8	11.5	11.3	11.0	10.7
	15	13.1	12.9	12.6	12.4	12.1	11.8	11.6	11.3	11.1	10.8	10.5	10.3	10.0
	10	12.3	12.0	11.7	11.5	11.2	11.0	10.7	10.4	10.2	9.9	9.7	9.4	9.1
	5	11.0	10.7	10.4	10.2	9.9	9.6	9.4	9.1	8.9	8.6	8.3	8.1	7.8
1 to 12 years of education	95	20.0	20.0	20.0	20.0	20.0	20.0	20.0	19.9	19.7	19.4	19.1	18.9	18.6
	90	20.0	20.0	19.9	19.6	19.4	19.1	18.9	18.6	18.3	18.1	17.8	17.6	17.3
	85	19.5	19.3	19.0	18.8	18.5	18.2	18.0	17.7	17.5	17.2	16.9	16.7	16.4
	80	18.8	18.6	18.3	18.0	17.8	17.5	17.3	17.0	16.7	16.5	16.2	15.9	15.7
	70	17.6	17.4	17.1	16.9	16.6	16.3	16.1	15.8	15.6	15.3	15.0	14.8	14.5
	60	16.7	16.4	16.1	15.9	15.6	15.4	15.1	14.8	14.6	14.3	14.1	13.8	13.5
	50	15.7	15.5	15.2	15.0	14.7	14.4	14.2	13.9	13.7	13.4	13.1	12.9	12.6
	40	14.8	14.6	14.3	14.0	13.8	13.5	13.3	13.0	12.7	12.5	12.2	12.0	11.7
	30	13.8	13.6	13.3	13.1	12.8	12.5	12.3	12.0	11.8	11.5	11.2	11.0	10.7
	20	12.7	12.4	12.2	11.9	11.6	11.4	11.1	10.9	10.6	10.3	10.1	9.8	9.5
	15	11.9	11.7	11.4	11.2	10.9	10.6	10.4	10.1	9.9	9.6	9.3	9.1	8.8
	10	11.1	10.8	10.5	10.3	10.0	9.8	9.5	9.2	9.0	8.7	8.5	8.2	7.9
	5	9.8	9.5	9.2	9.0	8.7	84	8.2	7.9	7.7	7.4	7.1	6.9	6.6

SOURCE: From Rivera et al. (2015).

TABLE 8–10 BTA Normative Data for Paraguay

		AGE (YEARS)												
	PERCENTILE	18 TO 22	23 TO 27	28 TO 32	33 TO 37	38 TO 42	43 TO 47	48 TO 52	53 TO 57	58 TO 62	63 TO 67	68 TO 72	73 TO 77	>77
>12 years of education	95	17.1	16.9	16.7	16.4	16.2	16.0	15.8	15.5	15.3	15.1	14.9	14.7	14.4
	90	16.1	15.9	15.7	15.5	15.3	15.0	14.8	14.6	14.4	14.1	13.9	13.7	13.5
	85	15.5	15.3	15.1	14.8	14.6	14.4	14.2	14.0	13.7	13.5	13.3	13.1	12.8
	80	15.0	14.8	14.5	14.3	14.1	13.9	13.6	13.4	13.2	13.0	12.8	12.5	12.3
	70	14.1	13.9	13.7	13.5	13.2	13.0	12.8	12.6	12.4	12.1	11.9	11.7	11.5
	60	13.4	13.2	13.0	12.7	12.5	12.3	12.1	11.9	11.6	11.4	11.2	11.0	10.7
	50	12.7	12.5	12.3	12.1	11.9	11.6	11.4	11.2	11.0	10.8	10.5	10.3	10.1
	40	12.1	11.9	11.6	11.4	11.2	11.0	10.8	10.5	10.3	10.1	9.9	9.6	9.4
	30	11.4	11.2	10.9	10.7	10.5	10.3	10.0	9.8	9.6	9.4	9.2	8.9	8.7
	20	10.5	10.3	10.1	9.9	9.6	9.4	9.2	9.0	8.7	8.5	8.3	8.1	7.9
	15	10.0	9.8	9.6	9.3	9.1	8.9	8.7	8.4	8.2	8.0	7.8	7.6	7.3
	10	9.4	9.1	8.9	8.7	8.5	8.2	8.0	7.8	7.6	7.4	7.1	6.9	6.7
	5	8.4	8.2	8.0	7.7	7.5	7.3	7.1	6.9	6.6	6.4	6.2	6.0	5.7
1 to 12 years of education	95	12.3	12.1	11.9	11.6	11.4	11.2	11.0	10.7	10.5	10.3	10.1	9.9	9.6
	90	11.3	11.1	10.9	10.7	10.5	10.2	10.0	9.8	9.6	9.4	9.1	8.9	8.7
	85	10.7	10.5	10.3	10.0	9.8	9.6	9.4	9.2	8.9	8.7	8.5	8.3	8.0
	80	10.2	10.0	9.7	9.5	9.3	9.1	8.9	8.6	8.4	8.2	8.0	7.7	7.5
	70	9.3	9.1	8.9	8.7	8.4	8.2	8.0	7.8	7.6	7.3	7.1	6.9	6.7
	60	8.6	8.4	8.2	8.0	7.7	7.5	7.3	7.1	6.8	6.6	6.4	6.2	6.0
	50	8.0	7.7	7.5	7.3	7.1	6.8	6.6	6.4	6.2	6.0	5.7	5.5	5.3
	40	7.3	7.1	6.9	6.6	6.4	6.2	6.0	5.7	5.5	5.3	5.1	4.9	4.6
	30	6.6	6.4	6.1	5.9	5.7	5.5	5.2	5.0	4.8	4.6	4.4	4.1	3.9
	20	5.7	5.5	5.3	5.1	4.8	4.6	4.4	4.2	4.0	3.7	3.5	3.3	3.1
	15	5.2	5.0	4.8	4.5	4.3	4.1	3.9	3.6	3.4	3.2	3.0	2.8	2.5
	10	4.6	4.3	4.1	3.9	3.7	3.5	3.2	3.0	2.8	2.6	2.3	2.1	1.9
	5	3.6	3.4	3.2	2.9	2.7	2.5	2.3	2.1	1.8	1.6	1.4	1.2	0.9

SOURCE: From Rivera et al. (2015).

TABLE 8–11 BTA Normative Data for Peru

		AGE (YEARS)												
	PERCENTILE	18 TO 22	23 TO 27	28 TO 32	33 TO 37	38 TO 42	43 TO 47	48 TO 52	53 TO 57	58 TO 62	63 TO 67	68 TO 72	73 TO 77	>77
>12 years of education	95	–	–	–	–	–	20.0	20.0	20.0	20.0	20.0	19.8	19.7	19.5
	90	–	–	20.0	20.0	20.0	19.8	19.6	19.4	19.2	19.0	18.8	18.6	18.4
	85	20.0	20.0	19.7	19.5	19.3	19.1	18.9	18.7	18.5	18.3	18.1	17.9	17.7
	80	19.6	19.4	19.2	19.0	18.8	18.6	18.4	18.2	18.0	17.8	17.6	17.4	17.2
	70	18.6	18.4	18.2	18.0	17.8	17.6	17.4	17.2	17.0	16.8	16.7	16.5	16.3
	60	17.9	17.7	17.5	17.3	17.1	16.9	16.7	16.5	16.3	16.1	15.9	15.7	15.5
	50	17.2	17.0	16.8	16.6	16.4	16.2	16.0	15.8	15.6	15.4	15.2	15.0	14.8
	40	16.4	16.2	16.0	15.8	15.6	15.4	15.2	15.0	14.8	14.7	14.5	14.3	14.1
	30	15.7	15.5	15.3	15.1	14.9	14.7	14.5	14.3	14.1	13.9	13.7	13.5	13.3
	20	14.8	14.6	14.4	14.2	14.0	13.8	13.6	13.4	13.2	13.0	12.8	12.6	12.4
	15	14.2	14.0	13.8	13.6	13.4	13.2	13.0	12.8	12.6	12.4	12.2	12.0	11.8
	10	13.5	13.3	13.1	12.9	12.7	12.5	12.3	12.1	11.9	11.7	11.5	11.3	11.1
	5	12.5	12.3	12.1	11.9	11.7	11.5	11.3	11.1	10.9	10.7	10.5	10.3	10.1
1 to 12 years of education	95	19.1	18.9	18.7	18.5	18.3	18.1	17.9	17.7	17.5	17.3	17.1	16.9	16.7
	90	18.0	17.8	17.7	17.5	17.3	17.1	16.9	16.7	16.5	16.3	16.1	15.9	15.7
	85	17.4	17.2	17.0	16.8	16.6	16.4	16.2	16.0	15.8	15.6	15.4	15.2	15.0
	80	16.8	16.6	16.4	16.2	16.0	15.8	15.6	15.4	15.2	15.0	14.8	14.6	14.4
	70	15.9	15.7	15.5	15.3	15.1	14.9	14.7	14.5	14.3	14.1	13.9	13.7	13.5
	60	15.1	14.9	14.7	14.5	14.3	14.1	13.9	13.7	13.5	13.3	13.1	12.9	12.7
	50	14.4	14.2	14.0	13.8	13.6	13.4	13.2	13.0	12.8	12.6	12.4	12.2	12.0
	40	13.7	13.5	13.3	13.1	12.9	12.7	12.5	12.3	12.1	11.9	11.7	11.5	11.3
	30	12.9	12.7	12.5	12.3	12.1	11.9	11.7	11.5	11.3	11.1	10.9	10.7	10.5
	20	12.0	11.8	11.6	11.4	11.2	11.0	10.8	10.6	10.4	10.2	10.0	9.8	9.6
	15	11.4	11.2	11.0	10.8	10.6	10.4	10.2	10.0	9.8	9.6	9.4	9.2	9.0
	10	10.7	10.5	10.3	10.1	9.9	9.7	9.5	9.3	9.1	8.9	8.7	8.5	8.3
	5	9.7	9.5	9.3	9.1	8.9	8.7	8.5	8.3	8.1	7.9	7.7	7.5	7.3

SOURCE: From Rivera et al. (2015).

TABLE 8–12 BTA Normative Data for Puerto Rico

		AGE (YEARS)												
	PERCENTILE	18 TO 22	23 TO 27	28 TO 32	33 TO 37	38 TO 42	43 TO 47	48 TO 52	53 TO 57	58 TO 62	63 TO 67	68 TO 72	73 TO 77	>77
>12 years of education	95	–	–	–	–	–	–	–	–	–	20.0	20.0	20.0	20.0
	90	–	–	–	–	–	–	20.0	20.0	20.0	19.7	19.4	19.2	18.9
	85	–	–	–	–	20.0	20.0	19.8	19.5	19.2	19.0	18.7	18.5	18.2
	80	20.0	20.0	20.0	20.0	19.7	19.4	19.2	18.9	18.7	18.4	18.1	17.9	17.6
	70	19.8	19.5	19.3	19.0	18.8	18.5	18.3	18.0	17.7	17.5	17.2	17.0	16.7
	60	19.0	18.8	18.5	18.2	18.0	17.7	17.5	17.2	16.9	16.7	16.4	16.2	15.9
	50	18.3	18.0	17.8	17.5	17.3	17.0	16.7	16.5	16.2	16.0	15.7	15.4	15.2
	40	17.6	17.3	17.0	16.8	16.5	16.3	16.0	15.7	15.5	15.2	15.0	14.7	14.4
	30	16.8	16.5	16.3	16.0	15.7	15.5	15.2	15.0	14.7	14.4	14.2	13.9	13.7
	20	15.8	15.6	15.3	15.1	14.8	14.5	14.3	14.0	13.8	13.5	13.2	13.0	12.7
	15	15.3	15.0	14.7	14.5	14.2	14.0	13.7	13.4	13.2	12.9	12.7	12.4	12.1
	10	14.6	14.3	14.0	13.8	13.5	13.3	13.0	12.7	12.5	12.2	12.0	11.7	11.4
	5	13.5	13.2	13.0	12.7	12.5	12.2	11.9	11.7	11.4	11.2	10.9	10.6	10.4
1 to 12 years of education	95	–	–	–	–	–	20.0	20.0	20.0	20.0	19.7	19.5	19.2	18.9
	90	–	–	20.0	20.0	20.0	19.7	19.4	19.2	18.9	18.7	18.4	18.1	17.9
	85	20.0	20.0	19.8	19.5	19.3	19.0	18.7	18.5	18.2	18.0	17.7	17.4	17.2
	80	19.7	19.5	19.2	18.9	18.7	18.4	18.2	17.9	17.6	17.4	17.1	16.9	16.6
	70	18.8	18.5	18.3	18.0	17.7	17.5	17.2	17.0	16.7	16.4	16.2	15.9	15.7
	60	18.0	17.7	17.5	17.2	17.0	16.7	16.4	16.2	15.9	15.7	15.4	15.1	14.9
	50	17.3	17.0	16.7	16.5	16.2	16.0	15.7	15.4	15.2	14.9	14.7	14.4	14.1
	40	16.5	16.3	16.0	15.8	15.5	15.2	15.0	14.7	14.5	14.2	13.9	13.7	13.4
	30	15.7	15.5	15.2	15.0	14.7	14.4	14.2	13.9	13.7	13.4	13.1	12.9	12.6
	20	14.8	14.5	14.3	14.0	13.8	13.5	13.2	13.0	12.7	12.5	12.2	11.9	11.7
	15	14.2	14.0	13.7	13.4	13.2	12.9	12.7	12.4	12.1	11.9	11.6	11.4	11.1
	10	13.5	13.3	13.0	12.7	12.5	12.2	12.0	11.7	11.4	11.2	10.9	10.7	10.4
	5	12.5	12.2	12.0	11.7	11.4	11.2	10.9	10.7	10.4	10.1	9.9	9.6	9.4

SOURCE: From Rivera et al. (2015).

The BTA has been used in conjunction with physical measures to differentiate Parkinson's disease (PD) from related disorders (e.g., Parkinsonian variant of multiple system atrophy, progressive supranuclear palsy), with high sensitivity and specificity reported (Neely et al., 2013). BTA scores are related to aspects of physical function in persons with PD (Kluger et al., 2014). Improved BTA scores have also been reported following exercise intervention in patients with PD (David et al., 2015) and treatment with donepezil (Dubois et al., 2012).

In psychiatric patients, the BTA has been found to correlate highly with and account for more variance in ADLs than other tests of cognitive ability (e.g., verbal and performance IQ, phonemic fluency, the Hooper Visual Learning Test; Schretlen, Jayaram, Maki, Robinson, & Devilliers, 1997). The BTA also appears to have potential as a screening instrument for driving capacity (Keyl et al., 1996). The BTA has been used with tests of vision, cognition, health status, and self-reported distress to predict lane change errors in older drivers, with BTA emerging, along with the Developmental Test of Visual-Motor Integration, as significantly predicting lane change errors (Munro et al., 2010).

NEUROANATOMICAL CORRELATES AND IMAGING STUDIES

Schretlen, Pearlson, and Anthony (1997) reported that BTA scores were related to individual differences in cerebral volume as measured via magnetic resonance imaging (MRI); the effects of age on BTA performance may be mediated in part by age-related differences in cerebral volume.

PERFORMANCE VALIDITY

There are few studies on the detection of exaggerated deficits using the BTA. Busse and Whiteside (2012) conducted an informative study regarding performance validity using the BTA. Consecutive neuropsychological assessments from a private practice comprised primarily of TBI patients were divided based on Test of Memory Malingering (TOMM) cutoffs, with an 8% sample failure rate of the TOMM in the sample. A cutoff of 15 on the BTA yielded a sensitivity of 54% and specificity of 91%. Positive predictive power (PPP) at an 8% base rate (assumed for clinical populations) was 24%, with negative predictive power (NPP) 96%. A 40% base rate (assumed for forensic populations) yielded a PPP of 80% and a NPP of 75%. Thus, the BTA is associated with modest sensitivity and high specificity, with, unsurprisingly, the positive predictive power increased substantially in high versus low base-rate settings (i.e., forensic vs. clinical). Note that this cutoff also needs to be validated using a two-performance validity test (PVT)-failure criterion, as failure on a single PVT is insufficient to infer invalid performance.

Whiteside et al. (2015) calculated a logistically derived performance validity measure using multiple measures in addition to the BTA, including the California Verbal Learning Test, Second Edition (CVLT-II, Trial 5, Total Hits, False Positives), the BNT, and Animal Fluency. Participants were patients who sustained moderate to severe TBI or possible mild TBI who failed at least two independent PVTs. Logistic regression and receiver operating characteristic (ROC) analyses were conducted indicating that the BTA, along with the CVLT-II Total Hits and False Positives, best differentiated between those failing versus passing PVTs. A BTA cutoff of 10 was associated with a 42% sensitivity rate and at a 91% specificity rate.

COMMENT

The BTA is theory-based and brief to administer and score, with strong internal reliability, some evidence of validity, and research suggesting some relationships with day-to-day function (e.g., driving). Because recall of stimuli, visual scanning, and motor response are not required, the BTA can be used with patients with impairments in these areas. Because the test is designed to detect presence or absence of attention deficit and has ceiling effects and a restricted range, the BTA may be most appropriate for use as a screening measure for attentional deficits.

Users should note that although large, the standardization normative sample was collected many years ago, is heterogeneous (e.g., comprised of participants from a standardization sample, research controls, and a hypertension study), largely Caucasian, and regionally based, thus limiting generalizability. Education levels are not described, nor are screening procedures. There is no information provided on whether sample sizes and gender distribution in each age band are equivalent, and overall sex distribution is uneven (i.e., 63% female). Of note, a large normative study involving Latin American countries provides normative data, adjusted for age and education, for a number of countries (Rivera et al., 2015); see also the norms provided by Shretlen et al. (2010) for the northeastern United States.

Studies of the BTA as a measure of performance validity indicate moderate sensitivity of this test as an indicator of performance validity, suggesting that it should not be used in isolation but rather in conjunction with other measures and indicators and that it requires further validation. Last, publications in clinical populations are limited, and, overall, more current research on this measure is desirable.

REFERENCES

American Psychiatric Association (Eds.). (2000). *Diagnostic and statistical manual of mental disorders: DSM-IV-TR* (4th ed., text revision). American Psychiatric Association.

Busse, M., & Whiteside, D. (2012). Detecting suboptimal cognitive effort: Classification accuracy of the Conner's Continuous Performance Test-II, Brief Test of Attention, and Trail Making

Test. *The Clinical Neuropsychologist, 26*(4), 675–687. http://doi.org/10.1080/13854046.2012.679623

Cooley, E. L., & Morris, R. D. (1990). Attention in children: A neuropsychologically based model for assessment. *Developmental Neuropsychology, 6,* 239–274.

David, F. J., Robichaud, J. A., Leurgans, S. E., Poon, C., Kohrt, W. M., Goldman, J. G., . . . Corcos, D. M. (2015). Exercise improves cognition in Parkinson's disease: The PRET-PD randomized, clinical trial: Exercise Improves Cognition IN PD. *Movement Disorders, 30*(12), 1657–1663. https://doi.org/10.1002/mds.26291

Dore, G. A., Waldstein, S. R., Evans, M. K., & Zonderman, A. B. (2015). Associations between diabetes and cognitive function in socioeconomically diverse African American and White men and women. *Psychosomatic Medicine, 77*(6), 643–652. http://doi.org/10.1097/PSY.0000000000000196

Dubois, B., Tolosa, E., Katzenschlager, R., Emre, M., Lees, A. J., Schumann, G., . . . Moline, M. L. (2012). Donepezil in Parkinson's disease dementia: A randomized, double-blind efficacy and safety study. *Movement Disorders, 27*(10), 1230–1238. https://doi.org/10.1002/mds.25098

Guàrdia-Olmos, J., Peró-Cebollero, M., Rivera, D., & Arango-Lasprilla, J. C. (2015). Methodology for the development of normative data for ten Spanish-language neuropsychological tests in eleven Latin American countries. *NeuroRehabilitation, 37,* 493–499.

Keyl, P. M., Rebok, G. W., & Gallo, J. J. (1996). *Screening elderly drivers in general medical settings: Toward the development of a valid and feasible assessment procedure (final report).* Andrus Foundation of the NRTA/AARP.

Kluger, B. M., Brown, R. P., Aerts, S., & Schenkman, M. (2014). Determinants of objectively measured physical functional performance in early to mid-stage Parkinson disease. *PM&R, 6*(11), 992–998. https://doi.org/10.1016/j.pmrj.2014.05.013

Munro, C. A., Jefferys, J., Gower, E. W., Muñoz, B. E., Lyketsos, C. G., Keay, L., . . . West, S. K. (2010). Predictors of lane-change errors in older drivers. *Journal of the American Geriatrics Society, 58*(3), 457–464. http://doi.org/10.1111/j.1532-5415.2010.02729.x

Neely, K. A., Planetta, P. J., Prodoehl, J., Corcos, D. M., Comella, C. L., Goetz, C. G., . . . Vaillancourt, D. E. (2013). Force control deficits in individuals with Parkinson's disease, multiple systems atrophy, and progressive supranuclear palsy. *PLoS ONE, 8*(3), e58403. https://doi.org/10.1371/journal.pone.0058403

Ojeda, N., Aretouli, E., Peña, J., & Schretlen, D. J. (2016). Age differences in cognitive performance: A study of cultural differences in Historical Context. *Journal of Neuropsychology, 10*(1), 104–115. http://doi.org/10.1111/jnp.12059

Rao, V., Bertrand, M., Rosenberg, P., Makley, M., Schretlen, D. J., Brandt, J., & Mielke, M. M. (2010). Predictors of New-Onset Depression After Mild Traumatic Brain Injury. *Journal of Neuropsychiatry, 22*(1), 100–104. https://doi.org/10.1176/appi.neuropsych.22.1.100

Rivera, D., Perrin, P. B., Aliaga, A., Garza, M. T., Saracho, C. P., Rodríguez, W., . . . Arango-Lasprilla, J. C. (2015). Brief Test of Attention: Normative data for the Latin American Spanish speaking adult population. *NeuroRehabilitation, 37*(4), 663–676. http://doi.org/10.3233/NRE-151283

Schretlen, D. (1992). Accounting for variance in long-term recovery from traumatic brain injury with executive abilities and injury severity [Abstract]. *Journal of Clinical and Experimental Neuropsychology, 14,* 77.

Schretlen, D. (1997). *Brief Test of Attention professional manual.* Odessa, FL: Psychological Assessment Resources.

Schretlen, D., Bobholz, J. H., & Brandt, J. (1996). Development and psychometric properties of the Brief Test of Attention. *The Clinical Neuropsychologist, 10,* 80–89.

Schretlen, D., Brandt, J., & Bobholz, J. H. (1996). Validation of the Brief Test of Attention in patients with Huntington's disease and amnesia. *The Clinical Neuropsychologist, 10,* 90–95.

Schretlen, D., Jayaram, G., Maki, P., Robinson, H., & Devilliers, C. (1997). Functional correlates of neurocognitive deficits in adults with severe mental disorders [Abstract]. *Journal of the International Neuropsychological Society, 3,* 25.

Schretlen, D., Pearlson, G., & Anthony, J. (1997). *Individual differences in cerebral volume and BTA performance.* Unpublished data.

Schretlen, D. J., Testa, S. M., & Pearlson, G. D. (2010). Calibrated Neuropsychological Normative System. Lutz, FL: PAR.

Whiteside, D. M., Gaasedelen, O. J., Hahn-Ketter, A. E., Luu, H., Miller, M. L., Persinger, V., . . . Basso, M. R. (2015). Derivation of a cross-domain embedded performance validity measure in traumatic brain injury. *The Clinical Neuropsychologist, 29*(6), 788–803. http://doi.org/10.1080/13854046.2015.1093660

Wong, T. M. (1999). Validity and sensitivity of the Brief Test of Attention with acute brain injury and mild head injury patients. [Abstract]. *Archives of Clinical Neuropsychology, 14*(8), 617–818.

CONNERS CONTINUOUS PERFORMANCE TEST 3RD EDITION (CPT 3)

TEST NAME	**Conners Continuous Performance Test 3rd Edition (CPT 3)**
DOMAIN	Attention
AGE RANGE	In adults, to 89 years
ADMINISTRATION TIME	14 minutes
SCORING FORMAT	Computerized
REFERENCE	Conners, C. K. (2014). *Conners Continuous Performance Test 3rd Edition (Conners CPT 3) & Conners Continuous Auditory Test of Attention (Conners CATA)*. Toronto, ON: Multi-Health Systems. www.mhs.com

DESCRIPTION

The Conners Continuous Performance Test 3rd Edition (CPT 3) is a computerized test of sustained attention in which the examinee is asked to respond when any letter, except the letter X, appears on the monitor (Conners, 2014). The Conners CPT 3 is the newest edition in the Conners CPT series, with the original Conners CPT introduced in 1994. Of note, the Conners Continuous Auditory Test of Attention (Conners CATA) was also introduced in this iteration. The reader is referred to the test publisher for additional information on the CATA.

Objectives of the CPT 3 revision included improving usability, representativeness of the normative sample, and psychometric properties (see manual). A summary of differences between the current version and the previous version is described in Table 8–13. As illustrated graphically in Figure 8–1, the CPT 3 consists of 360 trials comprised of six blocks, with three subblocks consisting of 20 trials. Within each block, subblocks have different interstimulus intervals (ISIs; 1, 2, and 4 seconds), and the order of ISI presentation systematically varies between blocks.

ADMINISTRATION

Detailed administration instructions are found in the manual. The CPT 3 software for administration and scoring is on a portable USB drive and can be administered on a desktop computer or laptop. The examinee can respond via space bar or computer mouse. A quiet environment is important; the administrator should be in the same room as the sole examinee, but at a distance (see manual). The manual describes severe cognitive impairment, visual impairment, agitation, severe psychotic symptoms, and failure to understand instructions during the practice trials as exclusionary for administration.

The authors explored the effect of input device (i.e., mouse vs. keyboard) and computer type (i.e., laptop vs. desktop) on scores. A comparison of demographically matched samples of 700 mouse administrations and 700 keyboard assessments indicated that differences across most scores were not significant, with the exception of Detectability (d') and Omissions, with higher d' scores for keyboard users (−2.6 vs. −2.4), and more Omissions for mouse users (2.7 vs. 2.2). However, effect sizes were small. No significant differences were found across comparisons of demographically matched samples of 86 laptop and 86 desktop administrations.

TABLE 8–13 Differences Between the CPT II and CPT 3

	CPT II	CPT 3
Age range	6 and older	8 and older[a]
Stimuli presentation[b]	White letter, black background	Black letter, white background
Trial number[c]	360 trials	361 trials
Target proportion[d]	9 target: 1 non-target	8 target: 2 non-target
Score changes[e]	Beta HRT SE Confidence Index	*C* HRT *SD* Clinical Likelihood Statement
Dimensions of attention	Inattentiveness, Impulsivity, Vigilance	Inattentiveness, Impulsivity, Sustained Attention, Vigilance
Additional normative groups	General population ADHD Neurologically impaired	General population
Oldest age group	55+	60+

NOTE: C, Response Style; HRT, Hit Reaction Time; SE, Standard Error.

[a]The minimum age for the CPT 3 was raised from six years to eight years, given reportedly comparable results in the pilot study between CPT 3 and Kiddie CPT II performance for six- and seven-year-olds.

[b]To reduce glare and increase visibility.

[c]Unscored trial at outset of test to prepare respondent for trials.

[d]The non-target proportion was increased to improve reliability of the Commissions variable (commissions are calculated based on responses to nontargets).

[e]Scoring changes as described in the section "Scoring."

SOURCE: Adapted based on Conners, C.K. (2014). Conners Continuous Performance Test 3rd Edition (Conners CPT 3) & Conners Continuous Auditory Test of Attention (Conners CATA). Toronto, ON: Multi-Health Systems, p. 48.

60 trials		
20 trials	20 trials	20 trials
ISI of 1, 2, or 4	ISI of 1, 2, or 4	ISI of 1, 2, or 4

Figure 8–1 *Structure of each Continuous Performance Test (CPT 3) block.*

NOTE: One block is shown; there are a total of 6 blocks in the CPT 3. Figure adapted from the Manual (Conners, 2014). Specific order of ISI presentation varies by block.

SOURCE: Adapted based on Conners, C.K. (2014). *Conners Continuous Performance Test 3rd Edition (Conners CPT 3) & Conners Continuous Auditory Test of Attention (Conners CATA).* Toronto, ON: Multi-Health Systems, p. 2.

SCORING

The majority of data from the CPT 3 are converted to T scores (mean [*M*] = 50, *SD* = 10; range from 0 to 90) and percentiles, and raw data are used in profile analyses for select measures (e.g., Hit Reaction Time or HRT). An Assessment Report, indicating details of a single CPT 3 administration, and a Progress Report, indicating change over time from two to three CPT 3 administrations, are available. Report sections include an overview of CPT 3 scores (i.e., all scores in tabular and graphical format), scores for factors comprising each dimension of attention (dimensions include Inattentiveness, Impulsivity, Sustained Attention, and Vigilance), and raw scores. An introduction, including the purpose and validity of the administration, is provided initially, and the report concludes with a glossary of each variable.

Score descriptions are presented in Table 8–14, with broad dimensions of attention measured by the CPT 3 depicted in Table 8–15. In general, higher T scores on the CPT 3 indicate worse performance (e.g., ranging from a T score of 70+ as Very Elevated, suggesting poor performance, to a T score of <45 as Low, suggesting good performance). Response Style (*C*) and HRT are exceptions, as scores reflect qualitative information. For instance, based on the T score, Response Style (*C*) is classified into one of five categories ranging from Very Conservative (T score of 70+; much emphasis on accuracy over speed) to Very Liberal (T score of ≤30; much emphasis on speed over accuracy). The Response Style (*C*) influences the interpretation of specific scores; for example, a respondent who is Very Liberal in their Response Style is more likely to have faster reaction times and relatively more commission errors (see manual). HRT is classified in one of six categories ranging from Atypically Slow (T score of 70+; very slow response speed) to Atypically Fast (T score of ≤40; very fast response speed).

The CPT 3 also provides qualitative information regarding the validity of the administration in terms of timing, missing scores, and pattern of responding, as detailed in Table 8–14. The suggested order of interpretation of the CPT 3 data includes examination of validity first, followed by Response Style (*C*), score overview, the overall summary

TABLE 8–14 Description of CPT 3 Scores

SCORE		DESCRIPTION
Validity		Timing (actual runtime exceeding expected runtime) Missing Score (one or more scores could not be computed due to too few responses) Unusual response pattern (highly unusual number of omission errors)
Response Style	*C*	Signal detection statistic assessing response style dimensions of speed vs. accuracy[a]
Clinical Likelihood	Clinical Likelihood Statement	Probability (very high, high, moderate, or minimal) that the respondent has a disorder characterized by attention deficits (e.g., ADHD)[b]
Detectability	D prime (*d'*)	Signal detection statistic describing how well a respondent discriminates nontargets from targets[c]
Error Types	Omissions[d] Commissions[e] Perseverations	Missed targets Incorrect response to nontargets Responses made in less than 100 ms after stimulus presentation
Reaction Time Statistics	Hit Reaction Time (HRT) HRT Standard Deviation (HRT *SD*) HRT Block Change HRT Inter-Stimulus Interval (HRT ISI Change) Variability	Mean response speed (ms) for all non-perseverative responses during test Consistency of response speed to targets during test Slope of change in HRT across blocks of the test[f] Slope of change in reaction time across the three ISIs (1, 2, and 4 seconds) Amount of variability respondent shows in 18 separate subblocks of administration in relation to respondent's overall HRT *SD* score

NOTE: ADHD, Attention-Deficit/Hyperactivity Disorder; HRT, Hit Reaction Time; ISI, Inter-Stimulus Interval.

[a]Classification into one of five categories including: Very Conservative (emphasis on Accuracy over Speed) to Very Liberal (emphasis on Speed over Accuracy).

[b]Ranging from Minimal (less than 2 atypical or very atypical scores) to Very High (4 or more atypical scores, or a combination of 8 or more atypical or very atypical scores).

[c]Measures differences between signal (targets) and noise (nontargets) distributions. Higher raw score and T scores indicate worse performance (reverse-scored).

[d]Omissions by block are also calculated, which is a raw score metric indicating the rate of missed targets in each of the six blocks. Omissions by ISI are also calculated, which is a raw score metric indicating the rate of missed targets in each of the three ISI trial types.

[e]Commissions by block are also calculated, which is a raw score metric indicating the rate of incorrect responses to nontargets in each of the six blocks. Commissions by ISI are also calculated, which is a raw score metric indicating the rate of incorrect responses to non-targets in each of the three ISI trial types.

[f]Positive slope indicates decelerating HRT as test progresses, negative slope accelerating HRT, and flat slope no HRT change.

SOURCE: Adapted based on Conners, C.K. (2014). Conners Continuous Performance Test 3rd Edition (Conners CPT 3) & Conners Continuous Auditory Test of Attention (Conners CATA). Toronto, ON: Multi-Health Systems, p. 53.

TABLE 8–15 Dimensions of Attention Measured by the CPT 3

	INATTENTIVENESS	SUSTAINED ATTENTION	VIGILANCE	IMPULSIVITY
Detectability	x			
Omissions	x	By block	By ISI	
Commissions	x	By block	By ISI	x
Perseverations				x
HRT	x			x
HRT *SD*	x			
HRT Block Change		x		
HRT ISI Change			x	
Variability	x			

NOTE: HRT, Hit Reaction Time; ISI, Inter-Stimulus Interval.

SOURCE: Adapted from Conners, C. K. (2014). *Conners Continuous Performance Test 3rd Edition (Conners CPT 3) & Conners Continuous Auditory Test of Attention (Conners CATA)*. Toronto, ON: Multi-Health Systems.

and clinical likelihoods, and individual scores. Detailed interpretation guidelines are provided in the manual, along with illustrative examples and a case study.

Of note, many CPT 3 scores are not normally distributed, with violations to normality most pronounced for Omissions and Perseverations due to the low occurrence of these errors in the normative sample (e.g., Omissions were made <5% of the time, Perseverations <1% of the time). Log transformations of raw scores for HRT Standard Deviation (HRT *SD*), Variability, HRT Block Change, and HRT ISI Change were undertaken.

Scoring Changes Compared to the CPT II. It bears mention that there are a number of score changes from the CPT II. The manual states that the rationale for scoring changes was to improve psychometric properties of scores. For example, *C* replaced *B* as a measure of Response Style, as it is less affected by Detectability. Perseverative responses now include both target and nontarget trials (vs. only target trials in the CPT II). Perseverative responses were removed from Detectability and Commission scores, which now only include responses over 100 ms.

Consistency of response speed was based on HRT Standard Error (HRT SE) in the CPT II, which was subsequently changed to HRT *SD* in the CPT 3. This was reportedly done to avoid the metric being affected by the number of hits, as well as *SD* reportedly easier to interpret due to user familiarity. Other variables involving HRT SE (e.g., HRT Block Change, HRT SE ISI Change) were removed due to weak reliability. The Confidence Index from the CPT II was eliminated and replaced by the Clinical Likelihood variable. This was done to simplify interpretation for users and limit overreliance on a probabilistic index score.

The difference between Vigilance and Sustained Attention is now distinctly evaluated. The dimension of Sustained Attention was added to the conceptualization of attention. This was reportedly done to better reflect the factor structure of the CPT II. Sustained Attention reflects performance across blocks and was renamed Sustained Attention rather than Vigilance. Vigilance now reflects ISI statistics.

DEMOGRAPHIC EFFECTS

AGE

Age influences performance on CPT 3 scores in the normative sample, with the exception of HRT Block Change. Effect sizes are generally medium to large. Response Style (*C*) increases with age, suggesting that respondents adopt a more conservative Response Style with age. Other scores tend to decrease, indicating better performance. The HRT displays a U-shaped curve, with response speed decreasing in youth and increasing in adults.

GENDER

Overall, gender effects on the CPT 3 are minimal, with many not reaching significance and others small in size. The largest effect is found for Perseverations, with males making more errors than females. Males also make more Commissions than females and have lower rates of Detectability. There is a small trend for females to respond more slowly than males (HRT). Gender-specific norms, as well as gender combined norms, are available.

EDUCATION

Information regarding the effects of education on performance is not available.

ETHNICITY, NATIONALITY, AND LINGUISTIC EFFECTS

Data from African-American (n = 182), Hispanic (n = 261), and white (n = 844) groups from the normative sample were analyzed. Significant differences between groups were found on Omissions, Commissions, and HRT ISI Change. Specifically, the Hispanic sample made more Omissions than the white sample. The white sample made more Commissions and performed higher on HRT ISI change than the African-American sample. Effect sizes were minimal.

The effects of nationality were also examined, specifically by comparing 205 Canadians to 205 demographically matched Americans. Significant score differences were found on variables including HRT, HRT *SD*, Variability, and HRT ISI Change, overall suggesting longer reaction times and greater reaction time variability in the American sample. Effect sizes ranged from Cohen's *d* of .26 (HRT ISI Change) to .35 (Variability).

NORMATIVE DATA

Characteristics of the normative sample are described in Table 8–16. Note that a youth normative sample (aged 8–17) also exists but is not reported here. Data for the normative sample were collected between 2011 and 2013 and were Census-stratified, with age, gender, ethnicity, education level, and region matching the 2010 US Census targets within .3%. In brief, the normative sample was predominantly Caucasian (approximately 55% to 67%), with a large proportion attaining some college education or higher. Gender was equally represented.

Of note, the CPT 3, unlike the CPT II, does not provide Attention-Deficit/Hyperactivity Disorder (ADHD) or neurological norms for comparison. This change was reportedly made based on research indicating a low likelihood of a typical ADHD or neurological profile on the CPT. However, a clinical sample is included in the manual for test development purposes, including investigation of reliability and validity.

Inclusion criteria for the clinical sample were a single primary diagnosis, a diagnosis made by a professional (e.g., psychiatrist, psychologist), diagnosis according to the *Diagnostic and Statistical Manual of Mental Disorders* (DSM-IV-R; American Psychological Association, 1994) or the International Statistical Classification of Diseases and Related Health Problems, 10th revision (ICD-10), and use of multiple methods in diagnosis (e.g., record review, rating scales, observation, interview). Approximately 64% of the adult clinical sample was comprised of persons with ADHD, with the remainder classified as "other." In the adult clinical sample, gender was approximately equally represented (55% female) and the sample was predominantly Caucasian (73%), with most of the sample attaining some college education or higher (76%), and most participants from the Southern US (63%).

TABLE 8–16 Characteristics of the Normative Sample for the CPT 3

Sample size	600[a]
Age	18 to 60+
Region	18% Northeast 22% Midwest 37% South 23% West
Education	45% High school or less 30% Some college 25% University or higher
Gender	50% female
Ethnicity	67% Caucasian 14% Hispanic 12% African American 7% Other

[a]Groups included ages 18 to 34, 35 to 59, and 60+. Each age group was approximately equally represented.

EVIDENCE FOR RELIABILITY

EVIDENCE FOR INTERNAL RELIABILITY

Internal reliability is high to very high for most scores across normative and clinical samples (see manual), with split-half reliability exceeding r = .90 for the majority of variables. Reliability data based on adult subsamples are depicted in Table 8–17. Adequate reliability was reported for Variability (r = .73) and Preservations (r = .73) in the adult normative sample.

EVIDENCE FOR TEST-RETEST RELIABILITY, MEASURING CHANGE, AND PRACTICE EFFECTS

A sample of 120 individuals (57 youth, 63 adults) from the general population participated in a study evaluating test-retest reliability. The sample was 51% female, and 53% of the sample was 18 years of age or older. The sample was 68% Caucasian, and 40% had some high school or less (or equivalent parental education). Test-retest intervals averaged 18 (*SD* = 5) days, and coefficients ranged from low (r = .12, HRT Block Change) to high (r = .89, HRT), with median test-retest reliability estimates of r = .67.

As shown in Table 8–18, variables in the low to marginal range included Response Style, Perseverations, HRT *SD*, Variability, HRT Block Change, and HRT ISI Change. Means of differences between administrations were small overall (median absolute values of Cohen's d = .15, with a range from Response Style C = .36 to Commissions = −.31).

TABLE 8–17 Magnitude of Internal Reliability Coefficients for the CPT 3

MAGNITUDE OF COEFFICIENT	TEST-RETEST RELIABILITY
Very high (.90+)	Detectability (d′) Omissions Commissions HRT HRT *SD* HRT Block Change HRT ISI Change
High (.80 to .89)	Response style (C) Perseverations
Adequate (.70 to .79)	Variability
Marginal (.60 to .69)	
Low (<.59)	

NOTE: HRT, Hit Reaction Time; ISI, Inter-Stimulus Interval.

TABLE 8–18 Magnitude of Test-Retest Reliability Coefficients for the CPT 3

MAGNITUDE OF COEFFICIENT	TEST-RETEST RELIABILITY
Very high (.90+)	
High (.80 to .89)	Omissions Commissions HRT
Adequate (.70 to .79)	Detectability (d′) HRT ISI Change
Marginal (.60 to .69)	Response style (C) HRT SD
Low (<.59)	Perseverations Variability HRT Block Change

NOTE: HRT, Hit Reaction Time; ISI, Inter-Stimulus Interval.

EVIDENCE FOR VALIDITY

FACTOR-ANALYTIC STUDIES AND RELATIONSHIPS WITH OTHER TESTS

There are few studies as yet on this question. The authors compared the Conners CPT 3 with the Wechsler Intelligence Scale for Children, Fourth Edition (WISC-IV) and the Comprehensive Executive Function Inventory Parent Form (CEFI-Parent Form) in a sample of youth with ADHD, controlling for age and gender. Significant correlations were reported between the WISC-IV Full Scale IQ score and HRT ($r = -.32$) and HRT *SD* ($r = -.28$), without other significant correlations reported.

In a sample of youths with ADHD who completed both the CEFI and CPT 3, significant relationships were found between the CEFI-P and d' ($r = -.32$), Perseverations ($r = -.31$), and HRT *SD* ($r = -.33$). In terms of rating scales, correlations between the Conners CPT 3 and Conners 3 Parent Scale (Conners 3-P) were small ($rs = -.20$ to .30), as were relations between the CPT 3 and Conners' Adult ADHD Rating Scales (CAARS-S:L; $rs = -.17$ to .24).

CLINICAL STUDIES

The test authors examined the ability of the CPT 3 to discriminate between ADHD and the general population in three ways: group differences, prediction of likelihood of ADHD diagnosis, and effectiveness of CPT 3 in combination with other measures. A sample of participants with ADHD (73% 17 years and younger; 38% female; 73% Caucasian; 41% Southern US; 50% university or higher) and a general population sample were matched on age, gender, ethnicity, (parental) education level, and region. The ADHD sample had significantly worse scores on the most variables, with the exception of HRT which revealed no significant differences. Effect sizes of significant differences ranged from Cohen's *d* of .21 (HRT Block Change) to .49 (HRT *SD*).

More individuals with a diagnosis of ADHD were found to have a Clinical Likelihood labeled "Very High," compared to those with a Clinical Likelihood of "Minimal" (85% vs. 41%, respectively). Likewise, more individuals with a diagnosis of ADHD were classified as showing a Strong Indication of attention problems across dimensions of Inattentiveness, Impulsivity, Sustained Attention, and Vigilance (62–71%) than No Indication (42–48%). When combined across dimensions (i.e., Strong Indications of attention problems in three to four dimensions of attention), the probability of an ADHD diagnosis was 88%.

The CPT 3 improved the ability of rating scales to predict ADHD, particularly when used with the Conners CATA. The diagnostic accuracy of the Conners 3rd Edition Parent Rating Scale increased from approximately 84% to 88% (sensitivity of 90%, specificity of 87%) when used with the CPT 3, and nearly 94% (sensitivity 95%, specificity 93%) when used in conjunction with the CATA and CPT 3. When used with the Conners Adult ADHD Rating Scales, diagnostic accuracy increased from 89% to 93% (sensitivity 73%, specificity 97%) when the CPT 3 was added as a predictor.

In addition to ADHD groups, other clinical groups have been examined. Specifically, a mixed clinical sample of 148 individuals with learning disabilities, mood disorders, autism, anxiety, and other conditions were compared with controls matched on age, gender, ethnicity, (parental) education level, and region. Results suggested that the clinical group performed worse than controls on nearly all variables, with the exception of Commissions and HRT ISI change, which did not reach significance. Effect sizes (Cohen's *d*) for significant differences were small to moderate overall, ranging from .21 (HRT) to .49 (Omissions).

NEUROANATOMICAL CORRELATES AND IMAGING STUDIES

No information is available regarding neuroanatomical correlates or imaging studies for the CPT 3.

PERFORMANCE VALIDITY

No independent research is available regarding detecting noncredible performance on the CPT 3. However, there is some information regarding validity provided in the scoring program regarding timing, missing scores, or patterns that may indicate limited validity.

COMMENT

The CPT 3 is the latest edition in a long-standing line of Conners sustained attention tests. The structure of the Conners CPTs is described as a non-X paradigm in the CPT literature as it requires responding to all letters except for the letter X (Epstein et al., 2003). This structure is generally associated with a higher proportion of targets to nontargets, which may result in increased sensitivity to attention problems due to a higher rate of possible errors and increased variability compared to CPTs that involve responding to X alone (Conners, 2014). The newest edition includes some substantive revisions aimed at increasing usability and psychometric properties, including normative data and reliability.

The test yields rich data concerning the nature of the examinee's attention over the course of the CPT, which is provided to the assessor in a usable report format. Data generated include a number of variables that are likely to be familiar to users of CPTs, including reaction time statistics, accuracy data, validity of administration, and response style metrics. Of note, score interpretation is not intuitive (e.g., higher scores typically mean poorer performance and some scores are interpreted bidirectionally), and there is a suggested sequence of interpretation. Thus, although the test is computerized and relatively simple to administer, it is important that the user be well-versed in the CPT data generated.

CPTs can be quite demanding for the examinee and, as the test authors suggest, are not appropriate for examinees with severe cognitive impairment, significant psychiatric symptoms, or visual impairment. Of note, data presented in the manual suggest that keyboard and mouse administrations are equivalent for most but not all scores, with worse Detectability for keyboard users and more Omissions for mouse users; note that these differences are relatively negligible from a clinical standpoint. Laptop and desktop administrations do not differ.

The normative sample is impressive, large, and Census-stratified (age, gender, ethnicity, education level and region matching 2010 US Census targets). Sex and ethnicity differences are reported for some scores but are small overall. Age shows expected effects, with better performance overall with age and a U-shaped curve for HRT. The effects of education are not reported, although effects of education are reportedly minimal on most CPTs (Riccio et al., 2001).

Internal reliability is strong. Test-retest reliability is somewhat variable across scores, ranging from low to high, with scores in the low to marginal range for Response Style, Perseverations, and many reaction time scores (e.g., HRT *SD*, Variability, HRT Block Change, and HRT ISI Change). Although practice effects are quite small, some are sizable, including those for Response Style and Commissions which are small to medium in magnitude.

In terms of clinical studies, data presented in the manual suggest that persons with ADHD perform worse than controls on the majority of scores and that the CPT 3 provides a small degree of incremental validity of an ADHD diagnosis when used in conjunction with parental rating scales. Of note, as the authors suggest and is commonly known, the CPT should not be used in isolation to diagnose ADHD, but should be part of multidimensional clinical assessment. Poor performance on CPTs is not specific to ADHD, and attention may be impaired in a wide range of conditions. Due to the relative newness of this test, information regarding neuroanatomical correlates, performance validity, and greater information regarding clinical studies is needed; however, it bears mention that there is research on previous editions of the CPT on these topics (see prior edition of this volume and Conners, 2014).

REFERENCES

Conners, C. K. (2014). *Conners Continuous Performance Test 3rd Edition (Conners CPT 3) & Conners Continuous Auditory Test of Attention (Conners CATA)*. Toronto, ON: Multi-Health Systems.

Epstein, J. N., Erkanli, A., Conners, C. K., Klaric, J., Costello, J. E., & Angold, A. (2003). Relations between continuous performance test performance measures and ADHD behaviors. *Journal of Abnormal Child Psychology, 31*, 543–554.

Riccio, C. A., Reynolds, C. R., & Lowe, P. A. (2001). *Clinical applications of continuous performance tests: Measuring attention and impulsive responding in children and adults*. New York: John Wiley & Sons.

INTEGRATED VISUAL AND AUDITORY CONTINUOUS PERFORMANCE TEST, SECOND EDITION (IVA-2)

TEST NAME	**Integrated Visual and Auditory Continuous Performance Test, Second Edition (IVA-2)**
DOMAIN	Attention
AGE RANGE	In adults, to 99 years
ADMINISTRATION TIME	20 minutes
SCORING FORMAT	Computerized
REFERENCE	Sandford, J. A., & Sandford, S.E. (2016). *IVA-2™: Integrated Visual and Auditory Continuous Performance Test.* Richmond, VA: Brain Train, Inc. www.braintrain.com

DESCRIPTION

The Integrated Visual and Auditory Continuous Performance Test, Second Edition (IVA-2; Sandford & Sandford, 2016) is a computerized sustained attention test that evaluates both visual and auditory attention as well as impulse control. The major purpose of the test is for clinical screening, diagnosis, and staging of symptom severity in ADHD) including subtype differentiation (see manual). A secondary purpose is to evaluate therapeutic effects and attention difficulties more generally.

During the IVA-2, a series of 1s and 2s are presented pseudorandomly in both visual and auditory domains. The examinee is asked to respond (via mouse click) to 1s (target) and ignore 2s (foils). At specific intervals, the test places relatively more demand on impulse control by creating a response set that demands constant responding and an infrequent demand to inhibit the response, resulting in more errors of commission. At other intervals, errors of omission are more likely, with the test presenting a large number of foils and infrequently requiring a response.

The IVA-2 is the newest iteration in the series of IVAs (e.g., Sandford & Turner, 1995, 2004a, 2004b). The IVA-2 incorporates a number of additional features relative to previous editions, including additional interpretative reports, integration of ADHD rating scale data, an enhanced interface, refinement and expansion of analyses to detect invalid performance, inclusion of a report processor, a researcher tool kit, and a diagnostic flowchart. These were reportedly incorporated to accommodate changes in the DSM-5. The IVA+Plus and IVA-2 do not differ in terms of task procedure, age range, scores calculated, normative database, and reliability estimates (V. Sandford, Personal Communication, May 26, 2016).

The IVA-2 is designed based on attention models and historical features of CPTs (Sandford & Sandford, 2016). Benefits of the IVA-2 include the automated and standardized presentation of stimuli and measurement of attention, as well as inclusion of both auditory and visual stimuli, which may not be interchangeable (Sandford & Sandford, 2016). Measurements of both response control/impulsivity and attention/inattention are additional benefits.

There are four stages in the IVA-2: a warm-up period, a practice period, the main test, and a cool-down period. The warm-up section includes a 1-minute visual only condition and a 1-minute auditory-only condition that each consist of 10 test items. The practice section combines the visual and auditory targets and foils for 1.5 minutes. The main test is 12 minutes in duration, and the cool-down section mirrors the warm-up with a 1-minute visual-only and a 1-minute auditory-only section. Although the majority of the test is automated, the examiner moves the test from one stage to the next.

The main section consists of five sets of 100 trials. Each set is then comprised of two blocks of 50 trials, with each trial 1.56 seconds in duration. The visual targets (1s) and foils (2s) are approximately 1.5 inches in height and presented for 167 milliseconds (ms). The spoken auditory targets (1s) and foils (2s) are 500 ms in duration. During the first 50 trials of each block, 84% of the trials consist of targets (1), with only eight trials consisting of foils (2). During the second set of 50 trials, only 16% of the trials consist of targets, and the remaining 42 trials are foils.

ADMINISTRATION

See the manual for specific administration details (Sandford & Sandford, 2016).

SCORING

Raw scores are converted to standard scores (M = 100, SD = 15) based on age and gender. Overall, the IVA-2 generates numerous scores. The IVA-2 Standard Analysis provides eight Composite, Quotient and 19 other scales subdivided into four groups termed: Response Control, Attention, Sustained Attention, and Symptomatic. The primary diagnostic scores are (a) the Full-Scale Response Control Quotient score and (b) the Full Attention Quotient score, which are derived from six primary visual and six primary auditory scales. Modality-specific scores are also provided (i.e., Visual Response Control Quotient, Visual Attention Quotient, Auditory Response Control Quotient, and Auditory Attention Quotient).

Primary scales make up the Quotient scores. In the case of Response Control, these include Prudence, Consistency, and Stamina. Primary scales for the Attention Quotients include Vigilance, Focus, and Speed. Attribute and Symptomatic scores are designed to provide information on test-taking characteristics. The Attribute scales measure the examinee's optimum performance (i.e., visual vs. auditory, high vs. low target load), whereas the Symptomatic scales assess adherence to task requirements (e.g., as indicated by random responding, motor speed impairments, and so on).

Table 8–19 describes basic scores. Table 8–20 depicts formulas for computing scores, automatically calculated by the scoring program. In addition to the main scores, the test yields additional optional analyses and reports. For example, the Special Analyses Report provides further detailing of examinee performance according to additional scores such as Mental Concentration Analysis (Reliability, Accuracy, Quickness, Stability), High and Low Demand Analysis, and Malingering Analysis. The Investigator module allows the user to determine whether IVA-2 Quotient scores from test to retest are significantly different. The criterion for significant change is set at one SD (i.e., 15 points). Guidelines for describing change are provided (<8 points = No Significant Change; 8–10 points = Slight Change; 11–18 points = Mild Change; 19–27 points = Moderate Change; 28+ points = Major Change; Sandford & Sandford, 2016, p. 75). Questionnaires are also included, such as a health screener and self- and assessor rating of qualitative behavior during the test (see Sandford & Sandford, 2016).

TABLE 8–19 Summary of IVA-2 Scores

IVA-2 QUOTIENT	IVA-2 SCALE	DESCRIPTION
Response Control[a]	Prudence	Assesses impulsivity/response inhibition; combines three types of commission errors
	Consistency	Assesses ability to stay on task; involves reliability and variability of response times
	Stamina	Assesses sustained attention; compares the mean reaction time of correct responses during the first 200 responses to that during the last 200 responses
Attention[a]	Vigilance	Measures attention; combines two different types of omission errors
	Focus	Assesses variability of response speed
	Speed	Provides information on the average reaction time for all correct responses
Attribute	Balance	Indicates the examinee's most efficient modality (i.e., auditory, visual, or both)
	Readiness	Indicates whether the examinee processes information more quickly under rapid conditions or under slower conditions
Symptomatic	Comprehension	Identifies random responding; is reportedly the most sensitive scale to ADHD
	Persistence	Assesses motivation or motor or mental fatigue
	Sensory/Motor	Identifies slow reaction that may impair performance
	Fine Motor Regulation	Measures fine motor hyperactivity via off-task mouse clicks; quantifies restlessness and fidgetiness

[a]Full Scale, Auditory, and Visual Quotients; Full-Scale Response Control Quotient is based on both the Auditory Response Control Quotient and Visual Response Control Quotient; Full-Scale Attention Quotient is based on the Auditory Attention Quotient and the Visual Attention Quotient.

SOURCE: Adapted from Sandford and Sandford (2016).

DEMOGRAPHIC EFFECTS

AGE

According to the manual, reaction time (Speed scale) shows optimal performance in young adults, stability through adulthood, and then a slight slowing beginning at age 45. In adults with ADHD, performance is also moderately related to age (r = .38; Tinius, 2003).

GENDER

The manual describes faster reaction times and higher commission error rates in men than in women (Sandford & Sandford, 2016), which supports the need for gender-based normative data. In their sample of 70-year-old adults, Berginström, Johansson, Nordström, and Nordström (2015) reported small gender differences in six scales in a highly educated group and in two scales for the lower educated group, although these were not consistently in favor of men or women.

EDUCATION AND IQ

The manual does not provide information on the test's relationship to education in the normative sample. Tinius (2003) found conflicting results: performance was not correlated with education in controls or in adults with TBI, but performance was moderately related to education in ADHD. Berginström et al. (2015) reported education effects for half of the scales examined, with participants with more than

TABLE 8–20 List of Formulas for Deriving IVA-2 Scores

AAQ	Auditory Attention Quotient Based on: VIA% + FOCA + MNA
ARCQ	Auditory Response Control Quotient Based on: PRA% + CONA + STMA
CONA	Consistency Auditory Scale (Quartile 1 + 2 RT / Quartile 4 + 5 RT) * 100
CONV	Consistency Visual Scale (Quartile 1 + 2 RT / Quartile 4 + 5 RT) * 100
CMPA	Comprehension Auditory (Co + Om) Scale 100 – (IDIOERR# / ((50+80) * 100))
CMPV	Comprehension Visual (Co + Om) Scale 100 – (IDIOERR# / ((60+80) * 100))
FAQ	Full scale Attention Quotient Based on: AAQ + VAQ
FOCA	Focus Auditory Scale (1 – (SD / MN)) * 100
FOCV	Focus Visual Scale (1 – (SD/MN)) * 100
FRCQ	Full scale Response Control Quotient Based on: ARCQ + VRCQ
HYP	Hyperactivity Scale (XCL + LRT + ZRT + SCL) off-task behaviors
MNA	Mean Auditory reaction time for all trials (Speed Scale)
MNV	Mean Visual reaction time for all trials (Speed Scale)
PRA%	Prudence Auditory Scale Percent 100 – ((PRA# / 75) * 100)
PRV%	Prudence Visual Scale Percent 100 – ((PRV# / 65) * 100)
SAAQ	Sustained Auditory Attention Quotient Based on: DEPA, SWFA, POA, IAA, ECAR, & EOAF
RWCA	Ratio Warm-Up/Cool-Down Auditory RT * 100 (Persistence Scale)
RWCV	Ratio Warm-Up/Cool-Down Visual RT * 100 (Persistence Scale)
SMA	Sensory/Motor Auditory Scale (better of Warm-Up or Cool-Down RT)
SMV	Sensory/Motor Visual Scale (better of Warm-Up or Cool-Down RT)
STMA	Stamina Auditory Scale RT ((Set 1 + 2)/(Set 4 + 5) * 100)
STMV	Stamina Visual Scale RT ((Set 1 + 2)/(Set 4 + 5) * 100)
SVAQ	Sustained Visual Attention Quotient Based on: DEPV, SWFV, POV, IAV, ECVR, & EOVF
VAQ	Visual Attention Quotient Based on: VIV% + FOCV + MNV
VIA %	Vigilance Auditory Scale Percent 100 – ((VIA# / 45) * 100)
VIV%	Vigilance Visual Scale Percent 100 – ((VIV# / 45) * 100)
VRCQ	Visual Response Control Quotient Based on: PRV% + CONV + STMV

Common Code Conventions:

# = Number of errors	A = Auditory mode
% = Percent of errors	V = Visual mode

F = High demand block - 42 targets/block of 50 trials
R = Low demand block - 8 targets/block of 50 trials
Sets = Two blocks of 50 trials each

MN = Mean of reaction times
SD = Standard Deviation of reaction times (N-1 correction factor)

N = Number of cases used to compute MN and SD
R = Ratio (used for visual/auditory, high demand/low demand)
RT = Reaction Time in milliseconds

SOURCE: From Sandford and Sandford (2016).

12 years of education performing better than participants with less than 12 years of education. Performance is not correlated with IQ in controls or in adults with mild TBI (Tinius, 2003). However, in adults with ADHD, performance is highly related to IQ ($r = .64$; Tinius, 2003).

ETHNICITY, NATIONALITY, AND LINGUISTIC EFFECTS

Information on the effects of ethnicity and other sociodemographic variables is not available.

NORMATIVE DATA

The standardization sample consists of 1,700 individuals. Information regarding participant characteristics, such as education, regional distribution, and ethnicity, is not provided. See Table 8–21 for other sample characteristics. Cell sizes for adults based on age and gender are not entirely uniform, but range from 18 to 89 participants, with most in the 30- to 40-participant range.

Berginström et al. (2015) provide gender- and education-stratified normative data for more than 600 Swedish 70-year-old adults. Sample characteristics are described in Table 8–22. Due to the skewed distribution of some scales, normative data are provided in percentiles as presented in Tables 8–23 to 8–28. Note that these norms were collected in the Swedish language and so may not be generalizable to English-speakers, particularly for the auditory scales.

EVIDENCE FOR RELIABILITY

EVIDENCE FOR INTERNAL RELIABILITY

No information is available.

EVIDENCE FOR TEST-RETEST RELIABILITY, MEASURING CHANGE, AND PRACTICE EFFECTS

The manual presents data on 70 healthy participants tested twice over an interval of 1 to 44 weeks (age, $M = 22$ years,

TABLE 8–21 Characteristics of the IVA-2 Normative Sample

Sample size	1,700
Age	6 to 99 years[a]
Sample type	Not reported
Geographic location	US sample, unspecified location
Education	Not reported
Gender	Varies by age band
Ethnicity	Not reported
Screening	Exclusion criteria included participation in therapy, history of learning disability, hyperactivity or attention problems, medication usage, history of neurological problems, or inability to complete the test.

[a]Based on age groupings: 6, 7, 8, 9, 10, 11, 12, 13, 14, 15, 16, 17 to 18, 19 to 21, 22 to 24, 25 to 29, 30 to 34, 35 to 39, 40 to 44, 45 to 54, 55 to 65, and 66 to 99.

SOURCE: Adapted from Sandford and Sandford (2016).

TABLE 8–22 Characteristics of the IVA-2 Berginström et al. (2015) Swedish Normative Sample of 70-Year-Olds

Sample size	640
Age	70 years
Geographic location	Sweden
Sample type	Part of ongoing study
Education	51% >12 years
Gender	48% female
Race/ethnicity	>99% Caucasian
Screening	Data collected as part of a Healthy Aging Initiative Study to examine risk factors for dementia, heart disease, and injurious falls in 70-year-olds. Participants had to be 70 years old at the time of contact and had to reside in the municipality of Umeå, Sweden.

SOURCE: Adapted from Berginström et al. (2015).

range = 5 to 70 years; Sandford & Sandford, 2016). As shown in Table 8–29, reliability is marginal to adequate for the Attention Quotient scores (i.e., *rs* = .66 to .75) but limited for all of the Response Control scores (i.e., *rs* = .37 to .41). Reliability of primary scores is generally high. Overall, reliability coefficients vary across scores, with several well below clinical standards. The Manual indicates that variability in the sample is small (i.e., error rates of 1–6%), which likely attenuated some correlations due to ceiling effects.

Practice effects are small overall. For Quotient scores, mean score changes are 3% or less (i.e., ≤3 standard score points; see Sandford & Sandford, 2016). A heuristic presented in the manual is that a change is considered significant if a Quotient score changes by at least 8 points, which equates to one half of a *SD*. Changes greater than 8 points are graded on a continuum from slight change to major change (see "Scoring").

EVIDENCE FOR VALIDITY

WITHIN-TASK CORRELATIONS

Correlations for the six primary scales (i.e., Prudence, Consistency, Stamina, Vigilance, Focus, and Speed) are high in a subset of the normative sample (*rs* = .53 to .86; Sandford & Sandford, 2016). Berginström et al. (2015) reported correlations among primary scores to be significant overall. Visual-based scales show correlations with auditory counterparts (*rs* > .34), with correlations also reported between most scales on the test irrespective of modality (Berginström et al., 2015).

FACTOR-ANALYTIC STUDIES AND RELATIONSHIPS WITH OTHER TESTS

The factor structure of the IVA-2 is not reported in the manual. There are few studies on adults. The test is not related to self-ratings of neuropsychological symptoms in adults

TABLE 8–23 Swedish IVA-2 Norms for 70-Year-Olds with High Education (>12 Years; Total Sample)

PERCENTILE	PRUDENCE AUD	PRUDENCE VIS	CONSISTENCY AUD	CONSISTENCY VIS	STAMINA AUD	STAMINA VIA	VIGILANCE AUD	VIGILANCE VIS	FOCUS AUD	FOCUS VIA	SPEED AUD	SPEED VIA
10	92.00	86.80	63.80	73.08	88.10	91.94	97.80	97.80	65.80	71.60	408.20	380.40
20	94.70	89.20	67.44	76.20	91.68	95.10	100.00	100.00	68.90	74.72	431.80	399.80
30	96.00	92.30	70.00	77.92	94.02	97.72	100.00	100.00	71.00	77.00	453.20	411.20
40	96.00	93.80	72.00	79.40	96.20	99.60	100.00	100.00	72.60	78.40	471.60	423.60
50	97.30	95.40	74.20	80.70	98.20	101.40	100.00	100.00	74.60	79.70	486.00	434.00
60	97.30	95.40	75.80	81.90	99.84	103.62	100.00	100.00	76.24	81.30	507.40	446.00
70	98.70	96.90	77.80	82.70	101.86	106.08	100.00	100.00	78.08	82.30	525.00	463.00
80	98.70	98.50	79.50	83.90	103.80	107.92	100.00	100.00	79.70	83.54	542.20	479.20
90	100.00	100.00	81.80	85.60	107.80	111.46	100.00	100.00	81.96	85.46	591.00	507.60
100	100.00	100.00	95.70	90.00	125.40	128.70	100.00	100.00	86.50	89.50	897.00	662.00

PERCENTILE	HYPERACTIVE EVENTS	BALANCE	READINESS AUD	READINESS VIS	COMPREHENSION AUD	COMPREHENSION VIS	PERSISTENCE AUD	PERSISTENCE VIS	SENSORY/ MOTOR AUD	SENSORY/ MOTOR VIS
10	3.00	79.76	89.13	87.84	98.50	97.90	74.00	75.90	173.00	209.50
20	4.00	83.22	92.70	89.90	99.20	99.30	83.40	82.38	183.00	219.00
30	5.20	85.50	95.20	92.40	100.00	99.30	88.00	86.52	188.00	229.00
40	7.00	87.42	97.12	93.46	100.00	100.00	91.70	89.58	194.00	234.00
50	9.00	89.85	99.00	94.50	100.00	100.00	95.00	92.10	201.50	239.00
60	11.00	91.50	101.06	95.90	100.00	100.00	97.60	95.80	209.00	249.00
70	13.00	94.11	103.90	97.90	100.00	100.00	102.60	100.00	220.00	255.10
80	15.00	97.10	107.00	100.22	100.00	100.00	106.60	104.00	236.00	267.60
90	20.00	101.92	110.70	103.46	100.00	100.00	121.30	111.63	256.00	289.50
100	300.00	129.40	147.70	122.10	100.00	100.00	220.80	191.00	522.00	390.00

NOTE: *N* = 323. Aud = auditory, Vis = visual.

SOURCE: Adapted from Berginström et al. (2015).

TABLE 8–24 Swedish IVA-2 Norms for 70-Year-Olds with Low Education (<12 Years; Total Sample)

PERCENTILE	PRUDENCE AUD	PRUDENCE VIS	CONSISTENCY AUD	CONSISTENSY VIS	STAMINA AUD	STAMINA VIS	VIGILANCE AUD	VIGILANCE VIS	FOCUS AUD	FOCUS VIS	SPEED AUD	SPEED VIS
10	88.00	87.25	58.24	70.37	85.56	91.82	97.80	95.60	60.77	68.30	411.10	395.00
20	92.00	89.84	63.80	74.20	90.02	95.42	100.00	97.80	65.40	72.20	432.00	412.00
40	94.70	92.30	66.61	76.40	92.98	97.50	100.00	100.00	68.10	74.40	457.00	423.10
40	94.70	93.80	68.88	78.20	95.40	100.04	100.00	100.00	69.80	75.90	475.80	436.80
50	96.00	95.40	71.15	79.40	97.10	102.00	100.00	100.00	71.85	77.95	490.50	450.50
60	97.30	96.90	73.12	81.10	99.30	103.56	100.00	100.00	73.42	79.70	509.00	465.00
70	97.30	96.90	75.10	82.20	102.14	105.52	100.00	100.00	75.30	80.99	530.00	485.90
80	98.00	98.50	77.50	83.12	105.60	108.40	100.00	100.00	77.56	82.06	558.00	507.00
90	100.00	100.00	80.43	84.70	109.24	111.30	100.00	100.00	80.93	84.30	605.90	539.60
100	100.00	100.00	85.60	90.90	132.30	123.00	100.00	100.00	87.00	90.90	773.00	708.00

PERCENTILE	HYPERACTIVE EVENTS	BALANCE	READINESS AUD	READINESS VIS	COMPREHENSION AUD	COMPREHENSION VIS	PERSISTENCE AUD	PERSISTENCE VIS	SENSORY/ MOTOR AUD	SENSORY/ MOTOR VIS
10	4.00	80.74	87.76	87.05	96.90	95.70	71.82	74.44	173.00	213.00
20	6.00	84.20	90.84	91.20	98.50	97.90	80.04	80.40	183.00	229.00
30	7.00	87.90	94.48	92.65	99.20	98.60	87.10	84.84	193.00	234.00
40	8.20	90.26	97.44	94.30	99.20	99.30	91.06	89.32	195.60	239.00
50	10.00	92.40	99.90	96.30	100.00	99.30	95.00	93.20	204.00	244.00
60	12.00	95.20	102.20	98.10	100.00	100.00	99.62	97.64	210.00	250.00
70	14.00	97.60	104.72	99.90	100.00	100.00	102.30	100.20	215.80	260.00
80	17.00	101.32	107.70	102.80	100.00	100.00	105.50	106.44	230.00	276.00
90	22.20	105.76	114.34	106.30	100.00	100.00	114.96	117.58	256.00	291.30
100	372.00	153.40	139.40	127.50	100.00	100.00	349.80	358.10	449.00	1108.00

NOTE: *N* = 317; Aud = auditory, Vis = visual.

SOURCE: Adapted from Berginström et al. (2015).

TABLE 8–25 Swedish IVA-2 Norms for 70-Year-Old Males with High Education (>12 Years)

PERCENTILE	PRUDENCE AUD	PRUDENCE VIS	CONSISTENCY AUD	CONSISTENCY VIS	STAMINA AUD	STAMINA VIS	VIGILANCE AUD	VIGILANCE VIS	FOCUS AUD	FOCUS VIS	SPEED AUD	SPEED VIS
10	92.00	87.70	63.14	74.10	86.78	92.14	97.80	97.80	64.22	71.22	405.20	377.80
20	94.70	90.80	65.80	76.70	90.10	95.10	100.00	100.00	68.08	73.88	429.80	397.60
30	96.00	93.80	67.72	78.72	93.84	97.12	100.00	100.00	70.00	77.04	449.00	407.00
40	97.30	94.76	70.36	79.92	96.30	98.90	100.00	100.00	71.66	78.96	471.20	420.60
50	97.30	95.40	72.20	81.40	97.80	100.20	100.00	100.00	73.10	80.30	486.00	433.00
60	97.30	96.90	73.64	82.20	99.90	101.74	100.00	100.00	75.24	81.80	508.40	445.00
70	98.70	96.90	75.84	83.28	101.46	104.50	100.00	100.00	77.22	82.50	524.60	455.80
80	98.96	98.50	78.84	84.50	103.40	107.18	100.00	100.00	78.54	83.32	550.80	473.60
90	100.00	100.00	81.88	85.66	106.14	110.38	100.00	100.00	81.10	85.60	601.00	509.80
100	100.00	100.00	85.20	90.00	123.00	128.70	100.00	100.00	86.50	88.80	747.00	618.00

PERCENTILE	HYPERACTIVE EVENTS	BALANCE	READINESS AUD	READINESS VIS	COMPREHENSION AUD	COMPREHENSION VIS	PERSISTENCE AUD	PERSISTENCE VIS	SENSORY/ MOTOR AUD	SENSORY/ MOTOR VIS
10	2.00	78.60	88.10	87.20	98.50	98.60	75.86	75.41	173.00	213.00
20	4.00	81.70	92.46	89.16	99.20	99.30	84.90	80.42	178.00	224.00
30	5.00	85.14	94.64	91.80	100.00	99.30	89.42	85.23	188.00	229.00
40	7.00	86.74	96.76	92.80	100.00	100.00	91.68	87.60	199.00	234.00
50	9.00	89.10	98.10	93.80	100.00	100.00	94.30	91.05	204.00	244.00
60	10.00	92.06	100.34	94.70	100.00	100.00	97.34	94.30	208.20	255.00
70	12.00	94.52	103.66	95.98	100.00	100.00	101.04	97.25	220.00	265.00
80	14.00	97.42	106.28	98.02	100.00	100.00	106.46	103.48	232.40	271.80
90	19.00	102.16	109.90	101.72	100.00	100.00	124.92	109.49	261.70	291.00
100	300.00	115.80	135.10	112.90	100.00	100.00	219.90	191.00	365.00	390.00

NOTE: *N* = 180. Aud = auditory, Vis = visual.

SOURCE: Adapted from Berginström et al. (2015).

TABLE 8–26 Swedish IVA-2 Norms for 70-Year-Old Females with High Education (>12 Years)

PERCENTILE	PRUDENCE AUD	PRUDENCE VIS	CONSISTENCY AUD	CONSISTENCY VIA	STAMINA AUD	STAMINA VIS	VIGILANCE AUD	VIGILANCE VIA	FOCUS AUD	FOCUS VIS	SPEED AUD	SPEED VIS
10	90.70	86.20	65.89	71.21	88.87	91.71	97.80	97.80	66.72	72.21	411.30	384.00
20	93.30	89.20	68.94	75.62	92.60	95.12	100.00	98.24	69.92	74.94	438.00	403.00
30	94.70	90.80	71.10	77.70	94.13	98.23	100.00	100.00	71.66	76.80	458.30	415.00
40	96.00	92.30	74.20	79.28	95.78	100.40	100.00	100.00	73.28	77.98	471.40	425.00
50	97.30	93.80	75.55	80.10	98.20	102.60	100.00	100.00	75.40	79.25	486.00	435.50
60	97.30	95.40	76.86	81.50	99.80	104.96	100.00	100.00	77.12	80.96	504.00	448.20
70	98.70	96.90	78.40	82.30	102.20	107.17	100.00	100.00	78.30	82.04	525.70	469.70
80	98.70	98.50	79.98	83.62	104.36	108.20	100.00	100.00	80.48	83.90	539.80	484.80
90	100.00	98.50	81.80	85.60	108.97	112.08	100.00	100.00	82.29	85.39	586.00	506.80
100	100.00	100.00	95.70	89.40	125.40	126.40	100.00	100.00	85.40	89.50	897.00	662.00

PERCENTILE	HYPERACTIVE EVENTS	BALANCE	READINESS AUD	READINESS VIS	COMPREHENSION AUD	COMPREHENSION VIS	PERSISTENCE AUD	PERSISTENCE VIS	SENSORY/ MOTOR AUD	SENSORY/ MOTOR VIS
10	3.00	81.10	89.40	88.51	98.57	97.90	70.60	76.79	168.50	208.00
20	4.00	84.00	92.80	90.32	99.20	98.60	80.98	83.06	183.00	218.00
30	6.00	86.20	95.70	92.60	100.00	99.30	86.41	87.70	189.00	224.00
40	8.00	87.80	97.60	94.24	100.00	100.00	91.46	90.92	194.00	234.00
50	10.00	89.90	100.00	95.50	100.00	100.00	95.30	93.70	199.00	235.00
60	12.00	91.40	101.90	97.00	100.00	100.00	98.72	96.88	209.00	245.00
70	14.00	94.00	104.10	98.87	100.00	100.00	102.70	100.09	220.00	254.00
80	16.00	96.60	107.70	101.74	100.00	100.00	107.06	105.08	236.00	265.00
90	23.90	101.50	111.80	105.23	100.00	100.00	118.42	114.49	256.00	281.00
100	126.00	129.40	147.70	122.10	100.00	100.00	220.80	179.60	522.00	374.00

NOTE: *N* = 143. Aud = auditory, Vis = visual.

SOURCE: Adapted from Berginström et al. (2015).

TABLE 8–27 Swedish IVA-2 Norms for 70-Year-Old Males with Low Education (<12 Years)

PERCENTILE	PRUDENCE AUD	PRUDENCE VIS	CONSISTENCY AUD	CONSISTENCY VIS	STAMINA AUD	STAMINA VIS	VIGILANCE AUD	VIGILANCE VIS	FOCUS AUD	FOCUS VIS	SPEED AUD	SPEED VIS
10	88.00	87.70	57.20	73.30	84.79	91.90	97.80	95.60	59.76	68.54	409.00	398.00
20	92.78	90.80	62.38	75.70	90.04	95.66	97.80	97.80	63.76	71.98	428.80	413.00
30	94.70	92.30	65.04	77.42	92.73	97.70	100.00	100.00	67.14	74.44	455.80	426.00
40	96.00	93.80	67.60	79.32	95.48	100.14	100.00	100.00	69.32	75.62	471.20	437.20
50	96.00	95.40	70.50	80.60	97.30	102.00	100.00	100.00	71.40	78.30	487.00	452.00
60	97.30	96.90	72.90	82.06	99.72	103.36	100.00	100.00	73.46	79.70	510.80	463.00
70	98.70	97.86	74.36	82.70	102.58	105.50	100.00	100.00	75.30	81.16	530.00	480.00
80	98.70	98.50	76.88	83.48	105.66	107.54	100.00	100.00	77.40	82.60	557.40	499.00
90	100.00	100.00	79.50	85.60	108.31	110.44	100.00	100.00	80.90	84.56	602.20	523.00
100	100.00	100.00	85.30	90.90	127.30	119.20	100.00	100.00	85.30	90.90	676.00	708.00

PERCENTILE	HYPERACTIVE EVENTS	BALANCE	READINESS AUD	READINESS VIS	COMPREHENSION AUD	COMPREHENSION VIS	PERSISTENCE AUD	PERSISTENCE VIS	SENSORY/ MOTOR AUD	SENSORY/ MOTOR VIS
10	3.00	80.01	87.34	87.15	97.70	96.40	74.50	72.68	178.00	218.00
20	5.00	83.74	90.30	90.92	99.20	98.32	82.16	80.26	184.00	229.00
30	6.00	86.82	94.44	92.01	99.20	98.60	88.30	84.44	194.00	234.00
40	8.00	89.44	97.74	94.00	99.20	99.30	91.64	88.70	199.00	244.00
50	10.00	92.15	99.90	95.60	100.00	99.30	97.00	91.60	209.00	250.00
60	11.80	95.72	101.48	97.10	100.00	100.00	100.00	96.38	214.00	260.00
70	14.00	99.66	104.42	98.69	100.00	100.00	102.52	100.00	220.00	270.00
80	15.40	102.24	107.82	101.88	100.00	100.00	106.96	106.64	235.00	281.00
90	22.00	106.39	115.04	106.20	100.00	100.00	120.10	119.60	266.20	301.20
100	372.00	153.40	139.40	118.70	100.00	100.00	164.80	358.10	381.00	364.00

NOTE: *N* = 150. Aud = auditory, Vis = visual.

SOURCE: Adapted from Berginström et al. (2015).

TABLE 8–28 Swedish IVA-2 Norms for 70-Year-Old Females with Low Education (<12 Years)

PERCENTILE	PRUDENCE AUD	PRUDENCE VIS	CONSISTENCY AUD	CONSISTENCY VIS	STAMINA AUD	STAMINA VIS	VIGILANCE AUD	VIGILANCE VIS	FOCUS AUD	FOCUS VIS	SPEED AUD	SPEED VIS
10	88.00	86.20	59.70	69.10	86.70	90.49	97.80	95.60	62.60	67.90	417.00	391.00
20	92.00	89.20	65.10	71.60	90.00	95.36	100.00	97.80	67.10	72.40	434.00	407.00
30	94.70	90.80	68.30	75.00	93.10	96.97	100.00	97.80	69.20	74.40	460.00	419.00
40	94.70	92.30	69.80	76.70	95.00	99.90	100.00	100.00	70.50	76.10	479.00	436.00
50	96.00	93.80	71.50	78.50	96.90	102.20	100.00	100.00	72.10	77.80	494.00	450.00
60	97.30	95.40	73.80	79.50	99.20	103.80	100.00	100.00	73.40	79.40	507.00	471.00
70	97.30	96.90	76.00	81.50	101.70	106.21	100.00	100.00	75.30	80.80	530.00	494.00
80	98.70	96.90	78.00	82.60	105.60	108.90	100.00	100.00	77.90	81.90	562.00	518.00
90	100.00	100.00	81.10	83.80	110.00	114.01	100.00	100.00	81.70	83.00	618.00	557.00
100	100.00	100.00	85.60	87.40	132.30	123.00	100.00	100.00	87.00	88.60	773.00	703.00

PERCENTILE	HYPERACTIVE EVENTS	BALANCE	READINESS AUD	READINESS VIS	COMPREHENSION AUD	COMPREHENSION VIS	PERSISTENCE AUD	PERSISTENCE VIS	SENSORY/ MOTOR AUD	SENSORY/ MOTOR VIS
10	4.00	81.36	87.79	86.50	96.90	95.00	66.84	74.98	173.00	213.00
20	7.00	85.00	91.54	91.58	98.50	97.10	75.80	80.56	183.00	223.00
30	8.00	88.28	94.65	92.90	99.20	98.11	84.42	85.83	188.00	234.00
40	9.00	90.92	97.32	95.16	99.20	99.30	89.56	90.74	194.00	237.00
50	11.00	92.70	99.60	97.40	100.00	99.30	93.75	95.05	199.00	244.00
60	12.60	95.06	103.20	99.22	100.00	100.00	97.90	97.72	206.60	245.00
70	15.70	96.36	105.63	101.03	100.00	100.00	101.92	102.07	215.00	251.00
80	18.00	99.18	107.62	103.90	100.00	100.00	104.90	106.52	230.00	260.00
90	23.00	105.36	111.77	107.43	100.00	100.00	112.84	114.76	251.00	287.00
100	326.00	130.90	125.50	127.50	100.00	100.00	349.80	316.50	449.00	1108.00

NOTE: N = 167. Aud = auditory, Vis = visual.

SOURCE: Adapted from Berginström et al. (2015).

with ADHD or mild TBI using the Neuropsychological Impairment Scale (Tinius, 2003). In their sample of 70-year-olds, Berginström et al. (2015) reported that the MMSE was modestly correlated with the majority of primary scales (all rs ≤ .21). When participants were divided on the basis of MMSE scores, those who scored lower performed worse on Visual Focus and Auditory Focus. The Geriatric Depression Scale (GDS) was also significantly correlated with the majority of primary scales, but correlations were small (rs < .18).

CLINICAL STUDIES

The majority of adult clinical studies using this test have been conducted in ADHD samples. Adults with ADHD perform more poorly than controls on the IVA+Plus (Quinn, 2003; Tinius, 2003; White et al., 2005), although differences on Response Control scores, which are used to support ADHD subtype diagnoses (see manual), are not always found (Quinn, 2003).

Adults with ADHD and mild TBI perform similarly on the test (Tinius, 2003). Although individuals with mild TBI perform more poorly than controls, performance is not related to markers of injury severity, such as time since injury (Tinius, 2003). Adults with schizophrenia and those with bipolar disorder show dissimilar patterns in terms of auditory compared to visual modalities on the test, with both groups showing decrements in processing speed (Baerwald et al., 2001). Berginström et al. (2015) reported that patients with stroke or myocardial infarction did not differ from healthy controls, whereas people with diabetes performed worse on three scales (Auditory Consistency, Auditory Focus, Visual Focus).

NEUROANATOMICAL CORRELATES AND IMAGING STUDIES

In adults with ADHD, an increased quantitative electroencephalography (QEEG) theta-to-beta ratio has been reported to relate to poorer performance (White et al., 2005).

PERFORMANCE VALIDITY

Analyses focused on detecting noncredible performance on the IVA-2 are based on the concept that standard scores of malingerers are likely to be in the extreme range, beyond the level typically found in adults with ADHD or TBI. Cutoff scores for the prior version are described in Quinn (2003). Simulated malingerers perform more poorly on the IVA+Plus than do adults with ADHD, with 81% of scales showing significant group differences, especially the Vigilance and Comprehension scales (Quinn, 2003). Scores in the auditory modality are particularly sensitive, demonstrating excellent PPP and NPP (see Table 8–30). Unusually low scores, such as T scores of 50 or below, may therefore suggest exaggeration. Note that examinees in this study were also able to successfully simulate symptoms on

TABLE 8–29 Magnitude of Test-Retest Reliability Coefficients for the Integrated Visual and Auditory Continuous Performance Test (IVA-2)

MAGNITUDE OF COEFFICIENT	TEST-RETEST RELIABILITY
Very high (.90+)	—
High (.80 to .89)	Hyperactivity Comprehension Visual Scale Mean Auditory RT Mean Visual RT
Adequate (.70–.79)	*Full-Scale Attention Quotient* *Visual Attention Quotient* Comprehension Auditory Scale Sensory/Motor Visual Scale Vigilance Visual Scale Percent
Marginal (.60 to .69)	*Auditory Attention Quotient* Prudence Visual Scale Percent Prudence Auditory Scale Percent Focus Visual Scale Focus Auditory Scale Consistency Auditory Scale Ratio Visual/Auditory Combined RT
Low (<.59)	*Full-Scale Response Control Quotient* *Auditory Response Control Quotient* *Visual Response Control Quotient* Ratio Warm-up/Cool-down Auditory RT Stamina Visual Scale RT Stamina Auditory Scale RT Vigilance Auditory Scale Percent Ratio Warm-up/Cool-down Visual RT Ratio Frequent/Rare Auditory RT Ratio Frequent/Rare Visual RT Consistency Visual Scale Sensory/Motor Auditory Scale

NOTE: Composite Quotient Scores are presented in italics.

ADHD rating scales (Quinn, 2003; see also Leppma et al., 2018). To our knowledge, there are no studies on verified malingerers to validate these possible cutoffs. The manual also describes Malingering Analyses, but, to our knowledge, there has been no independent research on these indices.

TABLE 8–30 Detection of Noncredible Performance on the IVA-2: Diagnostic Utility of Impairment Indices

IMPAIRMENT INDEX	SENSITIVITY (%)	SPECIFICITY (%)	PPV (%)	NPV (%)
Full-Scale Response Control >75 and Full-Scale Attention Quotient >37	81	91	88	87
Auditory Response Control >74 and Auditory Attention Quotient >44	94	91	88	95
Visual Response Control >76 and Visual Attention Quotient >40	81	74	68	85

NOTE: PPV, positive predictive value; NPV, negative predictive value.
SOURCE: From Quinn (2003).

In an update using a clinical sample, Leppma et al. (2018) re-examined the IVA+Plus cutoff score for identifying invalid performance in a sample of university students who requested for ADHD screening in the university counseling center. Using the same analysis procedures as Quinn (2003), the new cutoff scores are as follow: Full Scale Response Control Quotient (FSRCQ) less than 48.7, Full Scale Attention Quotient (FSAQ) less than 20.8, and combined score less than 69.5. Using the new cutoff, 48% of the sample performed below the IVA+Plus validity marker, compared to 67% using the Quinn cutoff. However, when a combination of failure on the Non-Verbal Medical Symptom Validity Test and Quinn cutoff was used to establish possible feigners in this sample, both the original and revised cutoff yielded similar rates for identifying feigners (17% vs. 16%).

COMMENT

Several features of the IVA-2 make it a compelling measure. It presents stimuli in both auditory and visual modalities, which aids in the detection of attention deficits in different populations (e.g., Baerwald et al., 2001; Reed & McCarthy, 2012). Attention in day-to-day life is multimodal, requiring attention to stimuli from multiple senses, potentially rendering the IVA-2 ecologically valid in this regard.

The IVA-2 combines several features of different CPTs. It provides variable interstimulus intervals designed to capture both impulse control and vigilance deficits, requiring the examinee to respond almost continuously at times (i.e., similar to "response"-type CPTs or "not-X" CPTs such as the Conners CPT 3) or, alternatively, to respond infrequently, like the "X" CPT (e.g., Test of Variables of Attention [T.O.V.A.]; Sandford & Sandford, 2016). Other features are its ability to provide screening for simple reaction time deficits, including pre- and post-test reaction time to assess for fatigue, and its provision of validity indicators. Additionally, its discrimination task is simpler than some other CPTs because only a single nontarget ("2") is presented (Riccio et al., 2001). The test may also be of utility in detecting exaggeration of attention symptoms (Quinn, 2003; Leppma et al., 2018), but more validation is needed for cutoffs.

As is commonly known, a CPT such as the IVA-2 should not be used in isolation to diagnose ADHD but should be viewed only within the context of multidimensional clinical assessment. Although CPTs may be useful in ruling out ADHD (Riccio et al., 2001), they are not diagnostic of ADHD. Of note, although the test is computerized and relatively simple to administer, it is important that the user be well-versed in the data generated and limit overreliance on the interpretive reports.

The IVA-2 has some drawbacks. Test-retest reliability is marginal to adequate for some scores, but limited for some scores of interpretive significance (e.g., Response Control scores). Second, there are a great number of scores. The multitude of variables can be confusing for the user, render interpretation difficult, and make it difficult to decipher research findings. Older versions of the test (e.g., Sandford & Turner, 1995) were criticized on several fronts, including lack of norm stratification; unclear date of norming; unspecified ethnicity, education, and socioeconomic status of the normative sample; and lack of internal reliability information (Riccio et al., 2001). Many of these criticisms remain for the current edition.

There is a lack of comprehensive research on this test in clinical groups, performance across the life span, and reliable change methodology to provide data on meaningful change in performance. Research on ADHD is somewhat limited as well, particularly in terms of subtype differentiation, sensitivity to treatment effects, and detecting invalid performance.

REFERENCES

Baerwald, J. P., Tryon, W., & Sandford, J. (2001). Modal attention asymmetry in patients with schizophrenia and bipolar disorder. *Neuropsychology, 15*(4), 535–543.

Berginström, N., Johansson, J., Nordström, P., & Nordström, A. (2015). Attention in older adults: A normative study of the Integrated Visual and Auditory Continuous Performance Test for persons aged 70 years. *The Clinical Neuropsychologist, 29*(5), 595–610. http://doi.org/10.1080/13854046.2015.1063695

Leppma, M., Long, D., Smith, M., & Lassiter, C. (2018). Detecting symptom exaggeration in college students seeking ADHD treatment: Performance validity assessment using the NV-MSVT and IVA-Plus. *Applied Neuropsychology: Adult, 25*(3), 210–218.

Quinn, C. A. (2003). Detection of malingering in assessment of adult ADHD. *Archives of Clinical Neuropsychology, 18,* 379–395.

Reed, P., & McCarthy, J. (2012). Cross-modal attention-switching is impaired in autism spectrum disorders. *Journal of Autism & Developmental Disorders, 42,* 947–953.

Riccio, C. A., Reynolds, C. R., & Lowe, P. A. (2001). *Clinical applications of continuous performance tests: Measuring attention and impulsive responding in children and adults.* New York: John Wiley & Sons.

Sandford, J. A., & Sandford, S. E. (2016). *IVA-2TM: Integrated Visual and Auditory Continuous Performance Test.* Richmond, VA: Brain Train, Inc.

Sandford, J. A., & Turner, A. (1995). *Integrated Visual and Auditory Continuous Performance Test.* Richmond, VA: Brain Train.

Sandford, J. A., & Turner, A. (2004a). *IVA+PlusTM: Integrated Visual and Auditory Continuous Performance Test administration.* Richmond, VA: Brain Train, Inc.

Sandford, J. A., & Turner, A. (2004b). *IVA+PlusTM: Integrated Visual and Auditory Continuous Performance Test interpretation.* Richmond, VA: Brain Train, Inc.

Tinius, T. P. (2003). The Intermediate [*sic*] Visual and Auditory Continuous Performance Test as a neuropsychological measure. *Archives of Clinical Neuropsychology, 18,* 199–214.

White, J. N., Hutchens, T. A., & Lubar, J. F. (2005). Quantitative EEG assessment during neuropsychological task performance in adults with attention deficit hyperactivity disorder. *Journal of Adult Development, 12*(2–3), 113–121. http://doi.org/10.1007/s10804-005-7027-7

PACED AUDITORY SERIAL ADDITION TEST (PASAT)

TEST NAME	**Paced Auditory Serial Addition Test (PASAT)**
DOMAIN	Attention
AGE RANGE	In adults, up to 74 years
ADMINISTRATION TIME	6 to 20 minutes depending on version
SCORING FORMAT	Computerized or hand scored
REFERENCES	Gronwall, D., & Wrightson, P. (1974). Delayed recovery of intellectual function after minor head injury. *Lancet, 2,* 605–609. Levin, H. S., Mattis, S., Ruff, R. M., Eisenberg, H. M., et al. (1987). Neurobehavioral outcome following minor head injury: A three center study. *Journal of Neurosurgery, 66,* 234–243.

DESCRIPTION

The Paced Auditory Serial Addition Test (PASAT) was devised by Gronwall and colleagues (Gronwall, 1977; Gronwall & Sampson, 1974; Gronwall & Wrightson, 1974), based on a procedure originally developed by Sampson (1956). The basic PASAT task structure consists of a random series of numbers from 1 to 9, and the examinee consecutively adds pairs of numbers such that each number is added to the one that immediately preceded it (i.e., the second number is added to the first, the third number to the second, etc.). For example, if the stimulus "1" followed by "9" is presented, the examinee must respond "10"; if the next stimulus is "4," the examinee must respond "13" (i.e., by adding the "4" to the previous digit "9"), and so on. This response requirement is sustained over numerous items until the end of the trial. The interstimulus interval (ISI) is then decreased, and the same process is repeated.

The PASAT is a multifactorial task. It demands divided attention, sustained attention, and working memory because of the requirement to switch between two ongoing tasks (adding two digits and encoding the next presented digit) over several trials. The task's rapid, paced responding also requires information processing speed (Shucard et al., 2004) as well as basic arithmetic skills and numeracy.

Several different versions of the PASAT exist. Most are auditory, but visual versions also exist (e.g., Paced Visual Serial Addition Test [PVSAT]; Fos et al., 2000). Some versions are computerized. The number of items and length of ISIs also differ across PASAT versions, as may other task parameters. Most versions are modeled on either the Gronwall (61 items per trial; Gronwall & Sampson, 1974) or Levin (50 items per trial; Levin et al., 1987) version. Short forms of the audio PASAT have also been developed based on one-trial (PASAT-50) and two-trial (PASAT-100) administrations (Diehr et al., 2003).

Other versions exist as well, including computer versions (auditory or visual stimuli), versions modified for use in functional magnetic resonance imaging (fMRI) paradigms (see the section "Neuroanatomical Correlates and Imaging Studies"), multiple sclerosis (MS) studies (see "Clinical Studies"), and adaptive testing PASATs, which adjust ISIs based on examinee performance level (e.g., Adjusting-PSAT; Tombaugh, 1999). In the Self-Paced Auditory Serial Addition Task (SPASAT) variant, digits are presented after every response, as opposed to at fixed intervals as in the conventional versions. If the response latency is longer than 5 seconds or the examinee forgets the last digit, four new digits are presented (Van Gerven et al., 2007). Non-numerical variants have also been developed, including the Paced Auditory Serial Opposites Task (PASOT; see Deary & Der, 2005). Regional variations are present across forms. Gronwall's original audio was created in New Zealand, and the majority of the Levin/50-item-per-trial versions were created in the United States (e.g., Diehr et al., 2003; Wiens et al., 1997), with other versions created in Canada (e.g., Stuss et al., 1988).

The PASAT can be sourced in various ways. Email and web addresses are provided here, with postal addresses given in the footnote.[1] The original PASAT (ISIs 2.4, 2.0, 1.6, and 1.2; 61 items per trial), the Gronwall version, is auditory and can be purchased from the University of Victoria Psychology Test sales office (psyctest@uvic.ca), and a computerized version is available via Dr. McInerney (www.mcinerney.ca/software.html). A Levin modification also

[1] Additional Contact Information for the PASAT: Dr. Bruce J. Diamond; William Paterson University; Neuropsychology, Cognitive and Clinical Neuroscience Lab; Wayne, NJ 07470; 973-720-3400. Donald Franklin, Jr.; 220 Dickinson Street, Suite B; San Diego, CA 92103; Office: 619-543-5007; Fax: 619-543-1235. Dr. Carl W. Lejuez, Dean, College of Liberal Arts and Sciences; University of Kansas; Strong Hall, Room 200; 1450 Jayhawk Boulevard; Lawrence, KS 66049; 240-535-0467.

exists (ISIs 2.4, 2.0, 1.6, and 1.2; 50 items per trial), with norms provided by Brittain, la Marche, Reeder, Roth, and Boll (1991); Roman, Edwall, Buchanan, and Patton (1991); and Wiens et al. (1997). Diehr and colleagues (Diehr et al., 1998, 2003) use different ISIs than the Levin version (3.0, 2.4, 2.0, 1.6), and this version is available by contacting dofranklin@ucsd.edu. Diamond, DeLuca, Kim, and Kelley (1997; DiamondB@wpunj.edu) provide a visual version. The PASAT 3″ and 2″ uses 3- and 2- second ISI trials and is used in MS research, with forms and instructions available from the MS Society (http://www.nationalmssociety.org/For-Professionals/Researchers/Resources-for-Researchers/Clinical-Study-Measures/Paced-Auditory-Serial-Addition-Test-(PASAT)). Lejuez, Kahler, and Brown (2003) provide a version intended for distress tolerance research (clejuez@ku.edu). Most of these versions have no cost for use at the time of writing, with the exception of the Gronwall version ($150). The fee for the Diamond visual PASAT is as yet undetermined as of this writing.

ADMINISTRATION

Administration instructions for the Gronwall version and the Diehr version are presented in Figures 8–2 and 8–3.

SCORING

Common scores yielded by the PASAT are described in Table 8–31. Correct responses and errors are conventional measures. A number of other measures derived from consideration of dyad and chunking responses have also been devised. Responding to alternate items significantly reduces the working memory requirements of the task and enables the examinee a longer response time per correct item and thus may be an adaptive strategy from an examinee's perspective. Both control and clinical populations tend to use chunking strategies as task difficulty increases. Some authors have reported that the mean number of dyads is more clinically sensitive than traditional PASAT scores (e.g., Snyder & Cappelleri, 2001).

Importantly, chunking reflects use of a compensatory strategy to compensate for difficulties keeping up with the task, and dyad scores do not reflect performance accuracy, but rather reflect adherence to task demands (Shucard et al., 2004). For example, an examinee with a high percent dyad score followed task instructions well (i.e., did not revert to responding to alternate items only), even if performance level was poor (as evidenced by few correct responses overall). This examinee may actually have better information processing capacity than another examinee who achieved a high overall performance (i.e., a high number correct) by circumventing the test's imposed pace by chunking.

Dyad scores and scores based on correct responses may reflect different processes. For example, Gonzalez et al. (2006b; PASAT-200) compared dyad and total correct scores in their sample of nearly 400 predominantly male (60%) and African American (65%) healthy adults (mean age 36.6 years; mean education 13.8 years). Although scores were highly correlated overall ($r = .96$), the magnitude of the relationship was decreased in faster trials (i.e. those with shorter ISIs), particularly for individuals with poorer working memory.

The scores listed in Table 8–31 are not exhaustive, and a number of other scores are available (Figure 8–4). For example, Gonzalez et al. (2006b) report *Average Percent Change in Dyads* (change in percent of dyads across trials; APCid) and *Score of Intermittent Performance* (the number of times an examinee stops providing responses; ScIP). APCid was found to demonstrate high variability across scores and was not related to demographic factors (Gonzalez et al., 2006b). According to Gonzalez and colleagues, very high ScIP scores (scaled scores ≤2 or T scores ≤25) are suggestive of excess skipping and may represent invalid PASAT performance. Note, however, that these scores were not validated against measures of performance validity. The PASAT has also been used as a measure of cognitive fatigue, whereby fatigue is determined to influence performance if correct responses in the second half are fewer than in the first half (e.g., Kozora et al., 2013). See also the section "Stress Induction and Psychiatric Conditions."

Computer versions typically provide more scoring options; however, less is known about psychometric properties of these scores than conventional PASAT versions. The Adjusting-PSAT uses the temporal threshold (the shortest ISI yielding a correct response) in addition to the number of correct responses (Tombaugh, 1999). Among possible PASAT scores, it may be the variable that most closely captures the construct of information processing speed (see "Comment").

DEMOGRAPHIC EFFECTS

Demographic effects are found on the PASAT. For example, in one normative study, a combination of ethnicity, education, and age were found to account for 24% of the variance in dyad scores (Gonzalez et al., 2006a).

AGE

Overall, age is related to PASAT performance (Barker-Collo et al., 2010a; Brittain et al., 1991; Deary & Der, 2005; Gonzalez et al., 2006a; Obradovic et al., 2012; Roman et al., 1991; Stuss et al., 1988; Thompson et al., 2011; Whelan et al., 2010; Wiens et al., 1997). Processing speed is found to significantly account for age-related differences on the PASAT (e.g., Deary & Der, 2005; Van Gerven et al., 2007), especially in middle age (e.g., Deary & Der, 2005; Roman et al., 1991).

Instructions for the PASAT (Gronwall Version)

Oral and Written Demonstration

I am going to ask you to add together pairs of single-digit numbers. You will hear a tape-recorded list of numbers read one after the other. I will ask you to add the numbers in pairs and give your answers out loud. Although this is really a concentration task, and not a test to see how well you can add, it might help to do a little adding before I explain the task in more detail. Please add the following pairs of numbers together as fast as you can and give your answers out loud: 3, 8 (11); 4, 9 (13); 7, 8 (15); 8, 6 (14); 8, 9 (17); 5, 7 (12); 6, 5 (11); 6, 9 (15); 4, 7(11); 7, 6 (13). Good. The task that I want you to do involves adding together pairs of numbers, just like you have done, except that the numbers will be read as a list, one after the other. Let me give you an example with a short, easy list. Suppose I gave you the following: 1, 2, 3, 4. Here is what you would do. After hearing the first two numbers on the list, which were 1 and 2, you would add these together and give your answer, 1 + 2 = 3. The next number on the list is 3, so when you heard it, you would add this number to the number right before it on the list, which was 2, and give your answer, 2 + 3 = 5. Are you following so far? The last number you heard is 4 (remember the list is 1, 2, 3, 4), so you would add 4 to the number right before it, which was 3, and give your answer, 3 + 4 = 7. The important thing to remember is that you must add each number on the list to the number right before it on the list, and <u>not</u> to the answer you have just given. You can forget your answers as soon as you have said them. All you have to remember is the last digit that you have heard and add it to the next digit that you hear. OK? Let's try that short list again, only this time you say the answers. Ready? 1, 2, (3), 3, (5), 4, (7). Now let's try another, longer practice list of numbers. This time the numbers on the list won't be in any particular order. Ready? 4, 6, (10), 1, (7), 8, (9), 8, (16), 4, (12), 3, (7), 8, (11), 2, (10), 7, (9). Good.

If the subject has difficulty understanding the oral instruction, then provide a written demonstration. Say: *That sounds complicated. Let me show you what I mean.*

Write down a list of five numbers: *5, 3, 7, 4, 2. You see, you add the 5 and the 3 together, and say 8, then you have to forget the 8 and remember the 3. When the 7 comes along you add it to the 3, and say 10, and you have to remember the 7. All right, what do you say after 4?*

Continue until the subject understands what they are to do. Say: *It's very easy when all the numbers are written down for you. Try it with me saying some numbers to you.*

See above list. Discontinue if the subject is unable to get at least the first three answers from the unpaced practice list correct, after two trials.

Paced Practice

Remember that I said the numbers would be tape-recorded? The task is not easy and no one is expected to get all of the answers right. The hard part is keeping up with the speed of the recording. However, if you can't answer in time, don't worry; just wait until you hear two more numbers, add them together and go on from there. OK? Any questions? I'll play a practice list of numbers and get you to give the answers.

Play to the end of the first practice list.

Test Trials

You see what I meant about the task measuring how well you can concentrate. It doesn't have anything to do with how smart you are. Now we'll try the first real trial. This trial is just the same as the practice trial you've just done, except that it is six times as long, so it goes on for almost two and a half minutes. Don't worry if you make adding mistakes or miss some answers. This is a difficult task. I want to see not only how long you can keep going without stopping, but also how quickly you can pick up again if you do stop. No one is expected to get all the answers. After this trial, we will take a break and then do another trial at a faster speed.

Instructions for the PASAT (Diehr version)

On the tape recording, you will hear a man's voice say numbers from 1 to 9. Add the first number that you hear to the second number that you hear and tell me the sum out loud. Then add the second number that you hear to the third number that you hear and tell me the sum out loud. Let's do some examples.

The examinee is given four sample sequences of four digits each orally. The instructions are repeated as needed, and participants who have trouble with the practice items are given additional practice items written on a piece of paper to clarify which digits are to be added together. Then the examinee is told: *The tape moves quickly so be sure to get your answer in before you hear the next number. If you get lost, be sure to pick up the addition as quickly as you can.*

The examinee is given encouragement to perform at their best and is given brief rests between the four sample sets of numbers if they appear frustrated. In addition, if an examinee initially uses a strategy of adding every other pair of numbers, the tape is stopped, the instructions repeated, and the tape restarted.

Figure 8–2 Instructions for the Paced Auditory Serial Addition Test (PASAT) (Gronwall Version; Diehr version).

PASAT—Gronwall Version

Name ______________ Date ______________ Tested by ______________

	2.4"	2.0"	1.6"	1.2"		2.4"	2.0"	1.6"	1.2"		2.4"	2.0"	1.6"	1.2"
7 (9)					8 (12)					5 (13)				
5 (12)					7 (15)					4 (9)				
1 (6)					1 (8)					8 (12)				
4 (5)					6 (7)					2 (10)				
9 (13)					3 (9)					1 (3)				
6 (15)					5 (8)					7 (8)				
5 (11)					9 (14)					5 (12)				
3 (8)					2 (11)					9 (14)				
8 (11)					7 (9)					1 (10)				
4 (12)					5 (12)					3 (4)				
3 (7)					3 (6)					6 (9)				
2 (5)					4 (7)					2 (8)				
6 (8)					7 (11)					9 (11)				
9 (15)					1 (8)					7 (16)				
3 (12)					5 (6)					8 (15)				
4 (7)					8 (13)					2 (10)				
5 (9)					3 (11)					4 (6)				
8 (13)					4 (7)					7 (11)				
6 (14)					6 (10)					6 (13)				
4 (10)					8 (14)					3 (9)				

	Total Correct	z	%ile
2.4"Pacing	________	________	________
2.0"Pacing	________	________	________
1.6"Pacing	________	________	________
1.2"Pacing	________	________	________

Figure 8–3 *Gronwall Paced Auditory Serial Addition Test (PASAT) Form.*

TABLE 8–31 Description of Paced Auditory Serial Addition Test (PASAT) Scores

SCORE	CALCULATION	NOTES
Correct Responses	Number of correct responses by trial and across trials.	Most commonly reported variable; presentation must be made before presentation of the next stimulus[a] to be considered correct.
Errors	Omissions, as well as incorrect responses, across trials.	As a heuristic, the proportion of errors would be expected to be less than 10%; if errors are >20%, the PASAT may be invalid; for example, only one participant in the study by Wingenfeld, Holdwich, Davis, and Hunter (1999) met the exclusion criterion of more than 20% errors. Omissions are the most common errors, and incorrect responses are less common.
Dyad	Two consecutive correct answers provided by the examinee.	Derived to account for a strategy used that decreases the difficulty of the task by "chunking"; i.e., responding to alternate items rather than consecutive items (e.g., Fisk & Archibald, 2001; Snyder, Cappelleri, Archibald, & Fisk, 1993).
Percent Dyad	Percentage of total correct responses accounted for by dyads.	See Fisk and Archibald, 2001; Snyder et al., 1993.
Chunking[b]	Number of correct responses that follow a skipped response.	Note that the examiner must write down incorrect, correct, and omitted responses to derive dyad/ chunking scores.

[a]Balzano, Chiaravalloti, Lengenfelder, Moore, and DeLuca (2006) evaluated whether considering late responses (i.e., responses made after the next number was presented) on the PASAT as accurate would affect the test outcome in individuals with multiple sclerosis. When scores were penalized for late responses, significantly more scores were classified as impaired on the 2-second trial of the PASAT. The authors argue that considering late responses as incorrect increases the sensitivity of the task to processing speed, whereas considering late responses as correct increases the sensitivity of the task to working memory.

[b]Note that some renditions of the PASAT disallow chunking. For example, in Diehr et al.'s (2003) PASAT-200, examiners halt the testing session and repeat instructions if examinees begin engaging in chunking.

Dyad Score

- A correct response that is preceded by a correct response. The response to the first pair of numbers at each presentation rate, if correct, is scored as a dyad.
- Dyad scores are tallied to yield a total dyad score for each presentation rate. (Fisk and Archibald, 2001).

Chunking Score

- A correct response that is preceded by a skipped response.
- Chunking scores are tallied to yield a total chunking score for each presentation rate.

Other Score

- A correct response that is preceded by an incorrect response.
- Other scores are tallied to yield a total other score for each presentation rate.

Total dyad score + total chunking score + total other score = total correct.
Percent dyad = (total dyad score/total correct score) x 100
Percent chunking = (total chunking score/total correct score) x 100

PASAT Dyad/Chunking Scoring Example:

Stimulus Sequence	Correct Response	Response given by participant	Scoring
2			
7	9	9 (correct)	Dyad
3	10	No response	No score
4	7	7 (correct)	Chunking
8	12	No response	No score
1	9	9 (correct)	Chunking
5	6	6 (correct)	Dyad
9	14	14 (incorrect)	No score
1	10	10 (correct)	Other*
3	4	4 (correct)	Dyad
2	5	5 (correct)	Dyad

*Not a dyad or chunking; this response is considered a correct score according to the standard PASAT scoring and is included in the total correct score.

Figure 8–4 *Dyad and chunking scoring for the Paced Auditory Serial Addition Test (PASAT).*
SOURCE: Shucard et al. (2004).

GENDER

Overall, gender effects are small to minimal, but in some studies men perform better than women (Brittain et al., 1991; Deary & Der, 2005; Obradovic et al., 2012; Schweitzer et al., 2006; Wiens et al., 1997). One study estimated that gender accounted for less than 1% of the variance in PASAT scores (Diehr et al., 2003). Another study (Gonzalez et al., 2006a) reported that gender had relatively weak associations with a dyad measure and omission errors (*rs* = .10, .11).

EDUCATION

Across most studies, performance is correlated with education. The higher the educational level, the better the performance (Gonzalez et al., 2006a; Stuss et al., 1989; Obradovic et al., 2012).

ETHNICITY, NATIONALITY, AND LINGUISTIC EFFECTS

Overall, effects of ethnicity have been reported in large-scale normative studies. For example, Diehr et al. (2003) reported that age, education, and ethnicity were all significant predictors of short-form PASAT scores. Demographically adjusted scores are therefore provided for this PASAT version (see later discussion).

Gonzalez et al. (2006a) reported that ethnicity was significantly associated with total dyads, incorrect responses, and omission errors (*rs* = −.27 to −.34), with Caucasian participants performing better than African-American participants. Demographic variables such as age, gender, and education accounted for relatively more variance overall in PASAT scores in an African-American sample than a Caucasian sample.

TABLE 8–32 Characteristics of the Stuss et al. (1988) Normative Sample for the Gronwall Version of the Paced Auditory Serial Addition Test (PASAT)

Sample size	90
Age	16 to 69 years
Geographic location	Ottawa, Canada
Sample type	Community Volunteers
Education	Approximately 14 years
Gender	49% Men 51% Women
Ethnicity	Not reported
Screening	No history of neurological or psychiatric disorder

Brittain et al. (1991) found no significant effects of ethnicity. However, ethnicity was unequally represented across ages in the study (particularly in older participants), which complicates interpretation. Note that in a large normative study using the Levin version, Wiens et al. (1997) found that differences on the PASAT were actually due to the effects of IQ, age, and education, rather than to ethnicity per se.

NORMATIVE DATA

GRONWALL VERSION

The original Gronwall norms are based on a sample of 80 people from New Zealand (Gronwall & Wrightson, 1974). Because this sample was predominantly male, not well-described demographically, and is dated, alternate norms are preferred.

Table 8–32 shows the demographic characteristics for the Gronwall version collected by Stuss et al. (1988). Normative data are shown in Table 8–33. The normative data are based on a sample of healthy North-American adults. The data shown for young adults are similar to those reported by others (e.g., Gronwall, 1977) but somewhat lower than those provided by Crawford, Obonsawin, and Allan (1998) in a UK sample.

The Crawford et al. (1998) sample characteristics and normative data are presented in Tables 8–34 to 8–35. Crawford et al.'s regression equations to determine whether PASAT performance is discrepant with premorbid IQ (National Adult Reading Test [NART]) or current IQ (Wechsler Adult Intelligence Scale, Revised [WAIS-R]) is provided in Table 8–36. The regression-based scoring program can be downloaded at Crawford's website (https://homepages.abdn.ac.uk/j.crawford/pages/dept/psychom.htm).

PASAT-50, PASAT-100, PASAT-200

Diehr et al.'s PASAT (1998, 2003) is an adaptation of the Levin version, using different ISIs (3.0, 2.4, 2.0, and 1.6 seconds). Diehr et al.'s (1998) demographically corrected norms allow for correction for age, education, and ethnicity, based on a large (n = 560), ethnically diverse sample. The composition of the normative sample and procedures for score derivation are presented in Table 8–37. Diehr

TABLE 8–33 Stuss et al. (1988) Norms for the Gronwall Version of the Paced Auditory Serial Addition Test (PASAT)

	AGE IN YEARS					
	16 TO 29 (N = 30)		30 TO 49 (N = 30)		50 TO 69 (N = 30)	
PRESENTATION	*M*	*SD*	*M*	*SD*	*M*	*SD*
2.4	47.4	10.1	43.4	10.2	43.5	13.6
2.0	42.0	12.5	41.9	10.2	35.6	14.6
1.6	36.0	13.0	33.1	12.2	30.8	15.9
1.2	27.4	9.9	24.6	10.6	21.2	14.4

Data derived from a sample of healthy, relatively well-educated adults.
SOURCE: From Stuss et al. (1988).

TABLE 8–34 Characteristics of the Crawford et al. (1998) Normative Sample for the Gronwall Version of the Paced Auditory Serial Addition Test (PASAT)

Sample size	152
Age	16 to 74 years (M = 40.2, SD = 13.9)
Geographic location	United Kingdom
Sample type	Community Volunteers
SES	Social class based on occupation did not differ from a Census-derived social class of the adult UK population
Education	M = 13.0 (SD = 2.9)
Gender	51% Men 49% Women
Ethnicity	Not reported
Screening	Via interview, for neurological, psychiatric, or major systemic disorder

TABLE 8–35 Normative Data from Crawford et al. (1998) for the Gronwall Version of the Paced Auditory Serial Addition Test (PASAT) for Adults

	AGE		
	16–29 YEARS	30–49 YEARS	50–74 YEARS
N	38	78	36
Total PASAT	169.2	149.8	136.9
PASAT *SD*	30.12	40.29	43.79
PASAT *SEM*	9.38	12.54	13.63

Based on a UK sample (education, M = 13 years, SD = 2.9).
SOURCE: From Crawford et al. (1998).

TABLE 8–36 Predicted Paced Auditory Serial Addition Test (PASAT) Scores Based on a Premorbid IQ Estimate (NART[a]) and Current IQ (WAIS-R) at Different Ages

PREDICTORS	EQUATIONS	MULTIPLE R^2	SE_{EST}	DISCREPANCY REQUIRED FOR ONE-TAILED SIGNIFICANCE .15	.10	.05
NART errors and age	215.74 – (1.85 × NART) – (.77 × Age)	.52	34.87	35.9	44.6	57.2
WAIS-R FSIQ and age	12.87 + (1.65 × FSIQ) – (.87 × Age)	.66	30.66	31.6	39.3	50.3

NOTE: These are one-tailed because only discrepancies suggesting that an examinee's PASAT performance is *below* their IQ are typically required in clinical practice. (FSIQ, Full Scale IQ).

[a]National Adult Reading Test (NART), Nelson (1982); WAIS-R, Wechsler Adult Intelligence Scale, Revised.

SOURCE: From Crawford et al. (1998).

et al. (1998) argue that, in most contexts, demographically adjusted scores are preferred to IQ-corrected scores because, like PASAT performance, IQ may also be adversely affected by neurologic conditions.

Diehr et al. (2003) also provide demographically corrected PASAT scores for two short forms, based on either administering only the first trial (PASAT-50), the first two trials (PASAT-100), or the full-length version (PASAT-200). These short forms are based on normative data collected for the full-length administration. Procedures for calculating demographically corrected scores are presented in Table 8–37. The two-trial version (i.e., 100-item form) appears to be particularly promising. See also Gonzalez et al. (2006a) for normative data for the PASAT-200.

DYAD AND CHUNKING NORMS

Normative data for these scores can be found in Gonzalez et al. (2006a), with preliminary data in Shucard et al. (2004) and Snyder and Cappelleri (2001). Characteristics of the Gonzalez et al. normative sample are provided in Table 8–38, with normative data and equations for adjustment for demographic variables provided in Table 8–39. Additional supplemental scores are also described (see also "Scoring").

PASAT 3″ AND 2″

Drake et al. (2010) provide normative data for a sample of 400 patients with MS, as well as demographically matched controls for the PASAT version that is part of the Multiple Sclerosis Functional Composite version (3-second ISI only). The majority of patients were part of the study for routine clinical monitoring or were referred due to suspected cognitive impairment. Data were collected at an MS clinic in Buffalo, New York. Exclusion criteria were a history of psychiatric or medical condition that could affect cognitive function or neurologic system functioning, substance abuse or current major depression, neurologic impairment, or an MS relapse or acute corticosteroid treatment within six weeks of testing. Mean age was 44.6 (*SD* = 9.2 years), and the sample was predominantly female (78%) and Caucasian (92%). Participants attained a mean education level of 14.6 (*SD* = 2.2) years. The majority of patients presented with relapsing-remitting MS (78%), with smaller proportions reflecting secondary progressive MS (18%), relapsing progressive MS (3%), and primary progressive MS (3%).

A sample of 100 healthy controls was also included, matched to patients with respect to age (*M* = 43.7, *SD* = 9.8), education (mean = 14.8, *SD* = 2.0), gender (78% female), and ethnicity (90% Caucasian). The mean for the PASAT 3″ for controls was 48 (*SD* = 10.7) and for patients was 40.2 (*SD* = 12.8).

TABLE 8–37 Characteristics of the Diehr et al. (1998, 2003) Normative Sample and Procedure for Deriving Demographically Corrected Paced Auditory Serial Addition Test PASAT-200, PASAT-100, and PASAT-50 Scores

Sample size	566
Age	20 to 68 years (*M* = 39.7, *SD* = 12.1)
Geographic location	Not specified, but presumably Southwestern US/California
Sample type	Mixed (one group from a normative study, the remainder consisting of controls from three different research studies)
Education	9 to 20 years (*M* = 14.2, *SD* = 2.6)[a]
Gender	61% Men 39% Women
Ethnicity	45% Caucasian 55% African American
Screening	History of neuropsychiatric condition (e.g., psychosis, developmental disability, substance abuse, traumatic brain injury)

[a]Educational composition: 12% = <12 years; 21% = 12 years; 33% = 13 to 15 years; 34% = 16 to 20 years.

To obtain demographically corrected T scores, use the following values in the regression equations that follow. (Note that these values correspond to a PASAT version that employs interstimulus intervals [ISIs] of 3.0, 2.4, 2.0, and 1.6 seconds per digit.)

Obtain the scaled score from the conversion table, using the appropriate version. Then enter the appropriate values for education, age, and ethnicity using the values shown below in the regression equation.

Scaled scores corresponding to total number of correct responses summed across trials for full-length and abbreviated PASAT versions (i.e., PASAT-200, PASAT-100, and PASAT-50), for use with demographic correction equations.

TABLE 8–37 Continued

PASAT-200 TOTAL			PASAT-100 TOTAL			PASAT-50 TOTAL		
MIN	MAX	SCALED SCORE	MIN	MAX	SCALED SCORE	MIN	MAX	SCALED SCORE
24	33	2	0	19	2	0	10	2
34	44	3	20	21	3	11	12	3
45	55	4	22	29	4	13	16	4
56	66	5	30	39	5	17	19	5
67	77	6	40	46	6	20	24	6
78	88	7	47	52	7	25	29	7
89	99	8	53	59	8	30	33	8
100	110	9	60	68	9	34	37	9
111	121	10	69	73	10	38	41	10
122	132	11	74	79	11	42	44	11
133	142	12	80	84	12	45	46	12
143	153	13	85	89	13	47	47	13
154	164	14	90	92	14	48	48	14
165	175	15	93	94	15	49	49	15
176	186	16	95	96	16			
187	192	17	97	98	17			

NOTE: Min and Max values refer to total raw score across all trials.

Ethnicity: Caucasian = 0 African American = 1

Education: I.e., grade level of formal education completed; technical/vocational training are not counted as years of education,

Maximum values as follows:

High school = 12

GED = last high school grade completed

Two-year college = 14

Four-year college = 16

Master's/JD = 18

PhD/MD = 20

Regression Equations for Demographically Corrected T Scores

PASAT-200 T Score = 50.0 + (3.33 × *Scaled Score* – 10) + (0.1894 × *Age*) – (0.8217 × *Education*) + (7.314 × *Ethnicity*)

PASAT-100 T Score = 12.52 + (3.81 × *Scaled Score*) + (0.24 × *Age*) – (0.97 × *Education*) + (6.72 × *Ethnicity*)

PASAT-50 T Score = 12.93 + (4.0 × *Scaled Score*) + (0.23 × *Age*) – (1.06 × *Education*) + (5.87 × *Ethnicity*)

*PASAT-200 = four-trial, 50-item/trial version; PASAT-100 = two-trial, 15-item/trial version; PASAT-50 = one-trial, 50-item/trial version. All trials with ISIs = 3.0, 2.4, 2.0, and 1.6 seconds per digit. Each trial of 50 digits unique. Max raw score per trial = 49.

NOTE: As the authors report, these formulas should be used with caution in individuals who have less than nine years of education, are of a different ethnicity, or are younger than 20 years of age or older than 68 years of age.

SOURCE: From Diehr et al. (1998, 2003).

TABLE 8–38 Characteristics of the Gonzalez et al. (2006a) Normative Sample for the Paced Auditory Serial Addition Test (PASAT-200)

Sample size	500
Age	18 to 69 (M = 36.6, *SD* = 13.1)
Geographic location	San Diego, California
Sample type	Controls in three studies (i.e., the HIV Neurobehavioral Research Center, the African American Norms Project, and the Alcohol Abuse and Neuropsychological Impairment Project)
Education	13.8 (*SD* = 2.4; range 8–20 years)
Gender	60% Men 40% Women
Ethnicity	65% African American
Screening	No history of medical, neurological or psychiatric disorder

Obradovic et al. (2012) also provided normative data for 140 Serbian individuals for the PASAT that is part of the Serbian translation of the Brief Repeatable Battery of tests used in MS studies. Participants were community-dwelling, with intact vision and hearing. Exclusion criteria included the presence of neurologic and psychiatric conditions, substance abuse, or major medical illness. The sample was predominantly female (64%), with a mean age of 37 years (*SD* = 2 years). Most of the sample had attained an education level of 9 to 12 years (47%) or more (44%). Normative data are provided in Table 8–40.

EVIDENCE FOR RELIABILITY

EVIDENCE FOR INTERNAL RELIABILITY

Cronbach's alpha for the four PASAT trials is very high (i.e., $r = .90$; Crawford et al., 1998).

EVIDENCE FOR INTERRATER RELIABILITY

High intrarater and interrater reliability coefficients (intraclass correlation coefficients [ICCs] ranging from .87 to .90) were reported in a small Finnish sample of patients with MS (Rosti-Otaja et al., 2008).

EVIDENCE FOR TEST-RETEST RELIABILITY, MEASURING CHANGE, AND PRACTICE EFFECTS

Test-retest correlations are generally high to very high for test-retest intervals measured in days (e.g., $r > .90$; McCaffrey et al., 1995) and months (e.g., *rs* > .83, Edgar et al. 2011; Sjøgren et al., 2000). Others have reported slightly lower reliabilities; however, coefficients are still in the adequate to high range (i.e., *rs* = .73 to .83; Baird et al., 2007; Schächinger et al., 2003).

There are significant practice effects on the PASAT (Baird et al., 2007; Gronwall, 1977; López-Góngora et al., 2015; Schächinger et al., 2003; Tomporowski et al., 2005). Healthy individuals who complete the PASAT on two occasions spaced one week apart perform about 18% (6 points) higher on the second administration (Stuss et al., 1988). Significant practice effects are reported across versions including the Adjusting-PASAT (Baird et al., 2007), the Gronwall version (Barker-Collo, 2005), and the PASAT 3" (Edgar et al., 2011; Rosti-Otaja et al., 2008), and in multiple clinical samples including TBI (Stuss et al., 1989), MS (Barker-Collo, 2005), and human immunodeficiency virus (HIV; McCaffrey et al., 1995).

The most prominent gains occur over the first trials. For example, Baird et al. (2007) reported significant practice effects on the Adjusting-PASAT, with the largest gains occurring on the first retest trial, regardless of the length of the test-retest interval (e.g., 20 minutes, one week, or three months), with maintenance of gains for up to six months. Barker-Collo (2005; Gronwall version)

TABLE 8–39 Gonzalez et al. (2006a) Normative Data for the Paced Auditory Serial Addition Test (PASAT-200) and the Procedure for Deriving Demographically-Corrected PASAT-200 and Supplemental Scores

SCALED SCORE	TOTAL DYADS	APCID	ScIP	OMISSION ERRORS	INCORRECT RESPONSES
0	–	>70.1	>78.1	–	>87
1	0	69.6–70.1	76.7–78.1	>152	79–87
2	1	61.3–69.5	75.3–76.6	142–152	66–78
3	2–3	58.6–61.2	68.8–75.2	136–141	51–65
4	4–8	54.9–58.5	63.0–68.7	123–135	44–50
5	9–16	50.6–54.8	57.8–62.9	111–122	38–43
6	17–28	46.1–50.5	53.7–57.7	99–110	32–37
7	29–39	39.9–46.0	50.0–53.6	89–98	26–31
8	40–52	36.1–39.8	46.4–49.9	77–88	22–25
9	53–63	31.1–36.0	42.2–46.3	68–76	18–21
10	64–80	26.6–31.0	38.0–42.1	58–67	14–17
11	81–94	21.7–26.5	33.9–37.9	48–57	11–13
12	95–110	15.6–21.6	30.8–33.8	36–47	9–10
13	111–124	8.9–15.5	26.6–30.7	26–35	7–8
14	125–145	1.8–8.8	21.4–26.5	21–25	5–6
15	146–153	–10.3 to 1.7	17.2–21.3	15–20	4
16	154–162	–34.4 to –10.4	14.1–17.1	10–14	3
17	163–170	–57.4 to –34.5	9.9–14.0	8–9	2
18	171–180	–76.4 to –57.5	4.7–9.8	3–7	1
19	181–188	–83.3 to –76.5	3.1–4.6	0–2	0
20	>188	<–83.3	<3.1	–	–

NOTE: Table based on data from the normative sample (n = 500; see Table 8-38); APCID, Average Percent Change in Dyads; ScIP, Score of Intermittent Performance.
Total dyads (TD) = Add the number of correct responses in each of the four trial blocks that were immediately preceded by a correct response. Dyad scores for each trial range from 0 to 48 (maximum TD = 192).
APCID (Average Percent Change in Dyads) = where Dx is the number of dyads in each trial (e.g., D1 = dyads in Trial 1).

$$\text{APCID} = \left(1 - \left\{\left[(D_2 + 1)/(D_1 + 1) + (D_3 + 1)/(D_2 + 1) + (D_4 + 1)/(D_3 + 1)\right]/3\right\}\right) * 100$$

ScIP (Score of Intermittent Performance) = where TC is Total Correct and TD is Total Dyads

$$\text{ScIP} = \left[(TC - TD - 1)/96\right] * 100$$

Computing Demographically-Adjusted T Scores from Scaled Scores

Refer to the appropriate formula depending on the participant's race (i.e., African American or Caucasian) and the measure of interest (i.e., TD, APCID, ScIP, omission errors, or incorrect responses). Replace the variables in the formula with the appropriate value, as indicated below:

SS = Scaled score for the respective measure
Age = participant's age in years
Edu = successfully completed years of regular academic schooling (as described below)
Sex = 0, male; 1, female

Education is calculated as actual number of years of regular academic schooling the subject successfully completed; vocation/trade school years are not counted, and no additional credit is given for completion of a general equivalency diploma (GED). Also, partial years are not counted (e.g., 11 1/2 = 11), nor are years that were not passed (exclude if subject obtained an overall failing grade point average). Finally, credit for 12 years requires awarding of a high school diploma (otherwise, count as 11), credit for 16 years must be associated with a bachelor's degree (otherwise, count as 15). Credit for 18 years must be associated with a master's degree (otherwise, count as 17), and credit for 20 years requires completing of a doctoral level degree (otherwise, count as 19). (This paragraph is adapted from Heaton et al., 1991.)

Formulas for African-American Participants

Total dyads T score = 24.0008 + (3.74883 * SS) + (0.226485 * age) – (1.23297 * edu) + (0.15266 * sex)
APCID T score = 14.0038 + (3.19387 * SS) – (0.00446247 * age) + (0.237812 * edu + (2.21303 * sex)
ScIP T score = 15.9826 + (3.60205 * SS) + (0.151293 * age) – (0.489618 * edu) + (0.896863 * sex)
Incorrect responses T score = 7.05654 + (3.75375 * SS) + (0.240777 * age) – (0.0122173 * edu) – (1.63897 * sex)
Omission errors T score = 28.7469 + (3.64708 * SS) + (0.113499 * age) – (1.29595 * edu) + (1.72647 * sex)

Formulas for Caucasian Participants

Total dyads T score = 12.064 + (4.15593 *SS) + (0.0365655* age) – (0.850036 *edu) + (3.43551 * sex)
APCID T score = 20.165 + (3.77245 * SS) – (0.0264618 * age) – (0.503023 *edu) + (1.415* sex)
ScIP T score = 20.9409 + (3.30251 * SS) + (0.029432 * age) – (0.566886 * edu) + (1.7278 * sex)
Commission errors = 13.698 + (3.61559 * SS) + (0.0924167 * age) – (0.4674 *edu) – (1.03459* sex)
Omission errors T score = 15.1429 + (4.03965 * SS) + (0.000759858 * age) – (0.858218 *edu) + (5.05657 * sex)

NOTE: These formulas are based on a sample of 323 African-American and 177 Caucasian participants.
Caution is warranted when generating T scores for individuals whose age, education, or race is not represented.

reported significant practice effects on all trials except the slowest trials within the session. Rosti-Otaja et al. (2008) reported significant practice effects on the PASAT 3″, with MS patients improving over the first four sessions (of five; tested over a four-week period) and healthy controls exhibiting the most improvement between the first two sessions.

EVIDENCE FOR VALIDITY

RELATIONSHIPS BETWEEN VERSIONS

Although more research is needed, computerized and audio versions appear comparable (Wingenfeld et al., 1999). Additionally, short and long forms are highly correlated in healthy individuals (e.g., r = .86 for the PASAT-50

TABLE 8–40 Normative Data for PASAT 3″ and 2″

		N	MEAN (SD) PASAT 3	PASAT 2
Gender	Male	51	38.5 (10.21)	46.35 (9.94)
	Female	89	35.17 (11.17)	42.29 (11.60)
Age	<30	45	40.96 (10.4.)	47.47 (11.17)
	30–39	33	40.42 (9.43)	47.08 (9.05)
	40–49	38	35.23 (8.22)	35.78 (9.40)
	>50	24	24.17 (7.27)	26.66 (9.40)
Education	≤8	12	26.33 (6.71)	26.67 (5.74)
	9–12	66	34.34 (9.16)	42.72 (9.36)
	>12	62	39.94 (11.72)	47.28 (11.11)
Total		140	36.39 (10.91)	43.77 (11.16)

SOURCE: From Obradovic et al. (2012).

and $r = .95$ for the PASAT-100) and in people with HIV (Diehr et al., 2003). In a sample of patients with MS, dyad scores for each trial of the PASAT and the total score were highly correlated (*rs* ≥ .94; Lynch et al., 2010). Gow and Deary (2004) reported that the non-numerical variant (PASOT) was correlated with the PASAT in a sample of healthy controls ($r = .71$).

The auditory (Gronwall) PASAT and the visual PVSAT are also highly correlated (i.e., *rs* = .63 to .73; Fos et al., 2000). The PASAT and PVSAT also appear to have similar factor structures when evaluated with other attention tests (see later discussion). However, there may be differences in performance on auditory and visual versions. This may potentially relate to an increased interference effect in the auditory version (Fos et al., 2000; Royan et al., 2004). This interference effect, when combined with demands on processing speed, is thought to underlie the PASAT's sensitivity in conditions such as TBI (Royan et al., 2004) and renders the visual version easier. The visual version may be a purer measure of processing speed due to the lack of an interference effect and consequent demands on working memory (Tombaugh et al., 2004). When versions are compared, the type of modality appears to be a larger moderating variable for PASAT performance than math skills (Tombaugh et al., 2004).

Ceiling effects may occur on trials with longer ISIs. This makes single-trial short forms based on longer ISIs (e.g., Diehr et al., 2003) less appropriate for higher functioning individuals. In the visual modality, Fos et al. (2000) found ceiling effects for the first two trials of the PVSAT, but no floor effects in a mixed sample of healthy college students and those with TBI. Performance on the PASAT 3″ differed between MS patients and controls, whereas no differences were found on the Adjusting-PASAT. The authors suggested that the Adjusting-PASAT is not of sufficient sensitivity to detect processing speed deficits common in relapsing-remitting MS (Tombaugh et al., 2010).

FACTOR-ANALYTIC STUDIES

In most factor-analytic studies involving clinical groups, the PASAT loads with attention and processing speed tests, such as working memory measures from the Wechsler scales, the Symbol Digit Modalities Test (SDMT), and the TMT (see Crawford et al., 1998; Deary et al., 1991; Haslam et al., 1995; Larrabee & Curtiss, 1995; O'Donnell et al., 1994; Townsend et al., 2002). A principal components analysis (PCA) involving the PASAT and Stroop scores yielded a single factor that accounted for 66% of the variance in scores in an MS sample (Lynch et al., 2010). Parmenter et al. (2006) reported that the PASAT, *n*-back, and TMT loaded together.

RELATIONSHIPS WITH TESTS OF ATTENTION, EXECUTIVE FUNCTION, AND PROCESSING SPEED

The Stroop is correlated with the PASAT, with most correlations moderate in magnitude, including in studies of people with PD (Spearman's rho ranging from −.59 to −.82), MS (correlations approximating $r = .50$; Lynch et al., 2010), and healthy controls ($r = .40$, Morrow, 2013).

The PASAT shows moderate to large correlations with the SDMT in MS patients (Belenguer, Parcet-Ibars, & Avila, 2008; Berrigan et al., 2014; Chiaravalloti, Wylie, Leavitt, & Deluca, 2012; López-Góngora et al., 2015), patients with PD (Dujardin et al., 2007) and healthy controls (Morrow, 2013). When Forn et al. (2008) covaried out SDMT performance, group differences on the PASAT between MS patients and healthy controls were no longer significant, leading the authors to suggest that speed of processing is the major factor differentiating the two groups. Similar findings were reported in patients with PD (Dujardin et al., 2007).

In a healthy sample, the PASAT correlated more highly with Digit Span Backward than did a simpler non-numerical PASAT version ($r = .65$ vs. $r = .36$, respectively; Gow & Deary, 2004). Parmenter, Shucard, Benedict, and Shucard (2006) reported that the PASAT and *n*-back tasks were highly correlated (generally in the .50 to .60 range), with a high degree of shared variance accounted for by information processing speed demands. In their sample of patients with schizotypal personality disorder, Mitropoulou et al. (2005) reported significant correlations between the PASAT and the TMT-B ($r = -.46$). In their longitudinal study of reaction time in aging, Deary and Der (2005) reported that the PASAT correlated with choice reaction time (*rs* = −.19 to −.42), with low correlations between the PASAT and simple reaction time (*rs* = −.09 and −.26).

Edgar et al. (2011) reported significant relations between the PASAT and the Cognitive Drug Research (CDR) battery ($r = .49$). There is also some evidence that different PASAT speeds may involve different types of cognitive processing. Deary, Langnan, Hepburn, and Frier (1991) found that slower rates of presentation correlated moderately with verbal memory scores, whereas a faster rate showed little correlation with memory measures.

In addition to measuring a degree of common variance, the PASAT appears to measure unique aspects of attentional functioning not measured by other paradigms. For instance, both the PASAT and PVSAT load on a factor separate from other measures such as Digit Span, TMT, and Stroop (Fos et al., 2000).

CORRELATIONS WITH IQ

Performance is significantly related to IQ (Brittain et al., 1991; Crawford et al., 1998; Deary et al., 1991; Hirvikoski et al., 2011; Sherman et al., 1997; Wiens et al., 1997). Crawford et al. (1998) gave the PASAT and the WAIS-R to a sample of healthy individuals. A PCA suggested that the PASAT loaded on general intelligence, with loadings that exceeded that of many WAIS-R subtests. In MS, cognitive reserve as measured by Wechsler Vocabulary moderates the effect of pathology on information processing efficiency (PASAT and SDMT), with greater neuropathology required to show cognitive impairment in patients with higher cognitive reserve (Sumowski et al., 2009). The North American Adult Reading Test (NAART) accounted for approximately 8% of PASAT score variance in healthy controls (Morrow et al., 2015). In their sample of patients with schizotypal personality disorder, Mitropoulou et al. (2005) reported moderate correlations between the PASAT and WAIS Vocabulary ($r = .36$).

CORRELATION WITH MATHEMATICAL ABILITY

The PASAT is moderately correlated with numerical ability in both healthy and clinical samples (e.g., .41 to .68, Crawford et al., 1998; Sherman et al., 1997), and in numerical and non-numerical variants (Gow & Deary, 2004). For example, arithmetic tests were the strongest unique predictors of PASAT performance in a TBI sample (Sherman et al., 1997). Performance is also strongly related to math scores in the Adjusting-PSAT test, particularly when the auditory modality is used ($r = -.74$), with math accounting for 26% of the variance in threshold scores (i.e., the shortest ISI with a correct response; Royan et al., 2004).

Sandry, Paxton, and Sumowski (2016) found that in patients with MS, mathematical ability was not only related to PASAT performance, but fully mediated the relationship between intelligence and PASAT performance and the relationship between education and PASAT performance. The authors argued that although the PASAT involves only simple, single-digit arithmetic, better math skills may confer an advantage by enabling faster retrieval of single-digit math facts.

Other research also indicates that PASAT performance is related to reaction time in simple addition problems and to attainment in school mathematics examinations and self-ratings of mental arithmetic skills (Chronicle & MacGregor, 1998). Intelligence (Shipley Institute of Living Scale) and arithmetic ability (WAIS-R Arithmetic) accounted for 46% of the variance in PASAT scores in healthy controls, with intelligence and arithmetic contributing roughly equally (Wills & Leathem, 2004).

Even though the addition skills involved in the PASAT appear basic, the degree of difficulty of the addition problem affects performance. Royan et al. (2004) and Tombaugh et al. (2004) found that item pairs yielding simple sums yielded a higher proportion of correct responses compared to those requiring complex sums (e.g., sums of 2 to 10 compared to sums of 11 to 18).

There may also be cohort effects of PASAT performance related to mathematical ability. Ward (1997) reported that the task was less easily accomplished by younger adults than by older adults, which was similar to a finding by Wills and Leathem (2004) who found that older adults performed better than younger adults at a 2-second ISI. Ward concluded that cross-generational effects on numeracy favoring automaticity of memorized sums in older individuals may differentially affect PASAT performance depending on the age cohort examined.

CLINICAL STUDIES

MS. There is a large body of literature on PASAT performance in persons with MS. The test is commonly used in this population because the rate of information processing depends on subcortical brain systems and white matter tracts, areas that are particularly affected in this demyelinating disease (Fisk & Archibald, 2001). Because of its sensitivity to MS-related cognitive impairment, the PASAT has been recommended as a core measure in clinical trials involving MS patients. A 3-second-per-item, 60-item version constitutes part of the Multiple Sclerosis Functional Composite (MSFC) Score, which has been used in several multicenter MS outcome studies (Cohen et al., 2002; Fischer et al., 1999; Rudick et al., 1997). It is also a component of the Neuropsychological Screening Battery for Multiple Sclerosis (Rao et al., 1991). One study reported that the PASAT was associated with relatively good overall accuracy and high specificity in identifying cognitive impairment in MS (Portaccio et al., 2009). For example, the PASAT 3″ was associated with a 79% accuracy rate, with 58% sensitivity and 95% specificity (PPP = 91%; NPP = 74%). The PASAT 2″ was associated with a 78% accuracy rate, with a 52% sensitivity and 98% specificity (PPP = 96%, NPP = 72%).

People with MS perform worse on the PASAT than healthy controls (Parmenter et al., 2006), with large differences according to Cohen's conventions (e.g., Cohen's d of .76 to .91, Lynch et al., 2010; see also Niccolai et al., 2015). Some have reported that dyad scores are especially sensitive (Fisk & Archibald, 2001). The test is also sensitive to MS subtypes (e.g., Aupperle et al., 2002, and Snyder et al., 2001). Huijbregts, Kalkers, de Sonneville, de Groot and Polman (2006) reported that people with progressive

MS did not improve on the PASAT on two-year follow-up, whereas controls showed improvement. Barker-Collo (2005) reported relapsing-remitting MS patients showed more improvement on retest compared to those with progressive MS, with the exception of the slowest trials, which did not show practice effects.

Akbar, Honarmand, and Feinstein (2011) reported that, after controlling for demographic variables, significant predictors of self-reported cognitive dysfunction in patients with MS included anxiety, conscientiousness, and PASAT performance. Disease duration in MS correlates with PASAT 2″ performance. Five years after disease onset, performance declined by about 10%, with change most notable on the PASAT seven years after disease onset (Achiron et al., 2005). Edgar et al. (2011) reported moderate correlations between the PASAT 3″ and the Expanded Disability Status Scale in their sample of patients with relapsing-remitting MS. The PASAT is related to accident rates in driving simulations in people with MS (Kotterba et al., 2003).

The PASAT is reportedly sensitive to treatment effects in MS (Cohen et al., 2002), including computer rehabilitation (Mattioli, Stampatori, Zanotti, Parrinello, & Capra, 2010), autologous nonmyeloblative hemopoietic stem cell transplantation in patients with relapsing-remitting MS who had not responded to treatment with interferon beta (Burt et al., 2009), and treatment via methylphenidate (Harel et al., 2009).

The PASAT and SDMT are both frequently used in MS research. A shortened version of Rao's Brief Repeatable Battery, a widely used battery for cognitive screening in MS, comprised of selective reminding tests, PASAT 3″, and the SDMT, was able to detect cognitive impairment in MS patients with a sensitivity equal to 94% and a specificity of 84% (Portaccio et al., 2009). Research suggests that the SDMT may be comparatively more sensitive at identifying impairment and also better tolerated by patients. López-Góngora et al. (2015) reported that the PASAT 3″ demonstrated a sensitivity of 78% (the SDMT was associated with sensitivity of 81%) in classifying patients with MS as cognitively impaired. At one-year follow-up, the PASAT 3″ and the SMDT were associated with comparable sensitivity rates (80%, 82%, respectively). The PASAT 3″ was completed by approximately 87% of patients and 95% of healthy controls, and the SDMT was completed by all participants.

TBI. The PASAT is sensitive to mild concussion (Gronwall & Sampson, 1974; Gronwall & Wrightson, 1974), and some research has suggested it may be a more sensitive indicator of information processing capacity in TBI than other standard measures of attention, such as working memory subtests from the Wechsler scales (Cicerone, 1997; Crossen & Wiens, 1988). Some research has suggested the test is sensitive to time since injury (Bate et al., 2001).

In contrast to these findings, null relationships have also been found between the PASAT and measures of injury severity in TBI (e.g., Sherman et al., 1997; Stuss et al., 1989). In addition, no significant relationships between PASAT performance and vocational status in TBI has been found (Nolin & Heroux, 2006). Aspects of the test may account for some discrepancies in findings, such as the length of the ISI (e.g., shorter ISIs are more likely to lead to group differences; Bate et al., 2001). Some have also reported that the nature of neuropathological involvement in the injury may influence findings. For example, persons who sustain marked acceleration/deceleration forces and subcortical involvement (e.g., motor vehicle accident) may be more likely to perform more poorly on the PASAT than other types of injury characterized by less diffuse pathology (Roman et al., 1991). Similarly, Mendez et al. (2013) reported that veterans who sustained pure blast force TBI performed worse on the PASAT than a veteran group who sustained pure blunt force TBI. Authors also reported that PASAT scores were correlated only in the blast group with regional metabolic changes (hypometabolism in the right superior parietal region), which the authors suggested may indicate comparatively greater disruption to attention networks after blast force mild TBI.

Of note, the test has also been used to evaluate postconcussion syndrome (PCS) in patients screened for performance validity (Cicerone & Azulay, 2002) with a sensitivity of 38% and specificity of 84%. Thus, the test is better able to rule out than rule in PCS.

ADHD. People with ADHD perform worse than controls on the PASAT (Hirvikoski et al., 2011; Schweitzer et al., 2006; White et al., 2005). Hirvikoski et al. (2011) reported that the PASAT correctly classified 53% of an ADHD group and 77% of controls. The PASAT has also been reported to be sensitive to methylphenidate treatment in adults with ADHD (Schweitzer et al., 2004).

Systemic Lupus Erythematosus (SLE). Patients with SLE perform worse than controls (Kozora et al., 2013), with 29% showing impaired performance. Patients with SLE, even without neurological impairment, perform below expectations when chunking scoring is used (Shucard et al., 2004). Worse performance was reported in patients with SLE who had elevated levels of C-reactive protein (a marker for atherosclerosis) compared with those who did not have elevated levels (Shucard et al., 2007). See also "Neuroanatomical Correlates and Imaging Studies."

Other Populations. Dujardin et al. (2007) reported that compared with healthy controls, patients with PD were impaired on the PASAT. The PASAT has been reported to correlate with aspects of quality of life post-stroke (Barker-Collo et al., 2010a). The PASAT is sensitive to moderate hypoglycemia (Schächinger et al., 2003), first-episode psychosis (Townsend et al., 2002), and schizotypal personality disorder (Mitropolou et al., 2002, 2005). The PASAT has also been used to examine cognitive function in chronic fatigue syndrome (mixed results; see Johnson et al., 1997; Cockshell & Mathias,

2007), sleep quality (Draganich & Erdal, 2014), and the effects of exercise on cognition (Martins et al., 2013; Tomporowski et al., 2005).

The PASAT has been used to assess cognitive fatigue in people with mild TBI (O'Jile et al., 2006) and MS (Morrow et al., 2015; Tartaglia et al., 2008), often by comparing performance on the first and second halves of the test. Berard, Bowman, Atkins, Freedman, and Walker (2014) examined PASAT performance at baseline and at subsequent six-month intervals for three years in patients with MS undergoing high-dose immunosuppression and hematopoietic stem cell transplantation, reporting consistent and high levels of cognitive fatigue at each time point across PASAT scores. Other studies report percent dyad is more sensitive to cognitive fatigue than other variables (Walker et al., 2012). Although it may be expected that fatigue would adversely impact performance, Johnson et al. (1997) found no evidence for fatigue effects in healthy controls and patients (e.g., MS, depression, chronic fatigue syndrome) when the PASAT was readministered four times within the same testing session. Performance continued to improve over administrations, presumably due to practice effects (see "Evidence for Reliability").

Stress Induction and Psychiatric Conditions. There is considerable evidence the PASAT is experienced as an aversive task, even in healthy individuals (e.g., 74% of participants rated moderate to high levels of anxiety during the PASAT; Wills & Leathem, 2004). Even in high-functioning samples (e.g., a sample of medical students), dislike of the task and relatively poor performance has been reported, although normative values were not provided (Brooks et al., 2011). Increased dysphoria and physical discomfort compared to baseline have also been reported (Brown et al., 2009; Daughters et al., 2005). Physiological responses to the PASAT include increased skin conductance and blood pressure (Brown et al., 2009).

The PASAT was found to increase negative mood in healthy individuals who were in a neutral or positive mood prior to the task. Furthermore, those who were in a sad mood had poorer performance at the most rapid ISI (1.2 seconds) compared to those in a neutral mood (Holdwick & Wingenfeld, 1999). Diehr et al. (2003) reported that several participants in their HIV longitudinal research preferred the lumbar puncture to the PASAT. In this study, more than half of the sample reported significant discomfort associated with the full-length PASAT compared to 30% who took an abbreviated version.

As a result, there is a sizable body of literature that has used the PASAT to induce stress in diverse populations (Ellis et al., 2010; Feldner et al., 2006; Gorka et al., 2012; Lejuez et al., 2003; VanderKaay & Patterson, 2006), including substance use (Brown et al., 2009; Daughters et al., 2005; VanderKaay & Patterson, 2006), ADHD (Hirvikowski et al., 2011), borderline personality disorder and people with borderline personality disorder traits (Iverson et al., 2012; Sauer & Baer, 2012), and studies of menstrual phase effects (Lustyk et al., 2010, 2012).

Studies are mixed with respect to the effect of depression symptoms on performance. Johnson et al. (1997) found no relationship between depression ratings and PASAT performance in patients with chronic fatigue, MS, and depression. However, other studies indicate that depression is related to PASAT performance (e.g., Shawaryn et al., 2002). In the context of MS, Demaree, Gaudino, and DeLuca (2003) concluded that depression increases the severity of processing speed deficits as measured by the PASAT.

Discontinuation Rates. High levels of refusal or discontinuation have been noted in clinical studies, ranging from 6% to 70% (e.g., post-stroke, Barker-Collo et al., 2010a; substance abuse, Daughters et al., 2005; Gorka et al., 2012; borderline personality disorder spectrum, Iverson et al., 2012; mild TBI, Vanderploeg et al., 2005; MS, Aupperle et al., 2002; Warlop et al., 2009). Locke, Stonnington, Thomas, and Caselli (2011) reported a somewhat lower refusal rate of approximately 5% in a sample of 606 healthy older adult participants. They further examined factors related to premature discontinuation versus completion of the PASAT. Personality variables (high on depression and low on excitement-seeking), older age, and lower WAIS-R Arithmetic scores classified participants who discontinued with a relatively high degree of accuracy (approximately 76%).

The high rate of persons unable to complete the PASAT can also contribute to restriction of range, specifically that only a select group within the sample may be able to complete the task (Barker-Collo et al., 2010a, 2010b; Deary & Der, 2005). In their eight-year follow-up cross-sectional study of veterans who sustained a mild TBI, Vanderploeg et al. (2005) reported that on the first trial nearly all participants continued the PASAT, with continuation rates decreasing in a linear fashion to within the range of a 60 to 70 percentage continuation rate by the third trial. Although all groups showed this trend, the mild TBI group was significantly more likely to discontinue by the third trial of the PASAT than the other groups. Some authors have further suggested that the decision to participate in research studies may be impacted by desire to avoid the PASAT (Lynch et al., 2010).

NEUROANATOMICAL CORRELATES AND IMAGING STUDIES

Imaging studies suggest that the PASAT activates a broad range of brain networks, including those important for attention and working memory (i.e., frontal and parietal areas; Forn et al., 2011; Kiiski et al., 2011a, 2011b; Whelan et al., 2010), with some studies also implicating temporal regions (Schweitzer et al., 2004). White matter in the left frontal lobe has been associated with PASAT performance in SLE (Filley et al., 2009; Kozora et al., 2013).

When considering fMRI research on the PASAT, there may be departures from parameters of the task that may alter the demands associated with it. Important considerations in this regard are the modality type (visual vs. auditory) and the response type (e.g., use of paradigms that require a covert response to minimize movement artifact vs. the standard approach that requires an overt response). As discussed previously, the difficulty of the PASAT may be reduced when input/output modalities are incongruent (e.g., visual/verbal). Some modifications used in fMRI studies to limit movement artifacts associated with speaking (e.g., pressing a button rather than providing a verbal response, indicating a response only when digits sum to 10; Chiaravolloti et al., 2005) may thus render the task easier than the conventional version, which involves congruent response modalities (i.e., auditory/verbal). However, it should be noted that Forn et al. (2008) reported that both overt (aloud) and covert (silent) versions of the PASAT were associated with parietal and frontal activation, with increased activation of the left superior and inferior frontal gyrus, bilateral occipital cortex, caudate nucleus, and cerebellum in the overt version.

Much of the research on the neural correlates of PASAT performance is from studies involving patients with MS. The PASAT is strongly correlated to total lesion volume (e.g., Hohol et al., 1997; Snyder & Cappelleri, 2001). Vollmer et al. (2016) conducted a systematic review of the relationship between cognition and whole-brain volume in people with MS. Of those conducted with the PASAT, 86% of studies reported significant associations between brain volume loss and lower PASAT scores.

Audoin et al. (2005) reported that the white matter magnetization transfer ratio correlated with PASAT scores in patients with clinically isolated syndrome (CIS) suggestive of MS, suggesting that neuroanatomical correlates of performance can be observed early in the disease course. Ranjeva et al. (2006) provided a model that explained 90% of the variance in PASAT scores in patients with CIS, based on seven MRI/fMRI parameters that reflected the extent of local tissue damage, brain activation, and the functional connectivity between regions. D'haeseleer et al. (2013) reported that performance on the PASAT in people with MS correlates with cerebral blood flow to the left centrum semiovale, implicating left frontoparietal white matter tracts.

fMRI studies suggest that different brain systems are activated in MS patients compared with controls. Increased effort on the part of MS patients to maintain performance levels and/or compensatory mechanisms recruiting other brain systems are thought to account for activation differences (Audoin et al., 2003, 2005; Lesage et al., 2010). In controls, a visual version of the test activated the right cingulate gyrus, whereas, in MS patients, the right frontal cortex was activated along with areas in the left frontal lobe (Staffen et al., 2002). Similarly, Rachbauer, Kronbichler, Ropele, Enzinger, and Fazekas (2006) reported recruitment of a frontoparietal network in healthy controls using fMRI and a visual variant of the PASAT, with persons with MS showing greater activation of hippocampal and parahippocampal areas, and patients with CIS showing greater anterior cingulate activation. Chiaravalotti et al. (2005) investigated fMRI patterns in people with MS with and without deficits on neuropsychological testing, compared with healthy controls. Patterns of cerebral activation were similar in the MS nonimpaired group and healthy controls (left hemisphere frontal regions), whereas the impaired group demonstrated more right frontal and parietal activation than controls. PASAT performance was correlated with regional cerebellar gray matter volume (Grothe et al., 2017). Lesage et al. (2010) reported that in patients with relapsing-remitting MS, the cerebellum was involved to a larger extent than in matched controls, despite similar performance. Interestingly, increased activation sites compared to healthy controls have also been reported via positron emission tomography in people with ADHD (Schweitzer et al., 2004).

The PASAT and the SDMT are frequently used in MS research, and both involve processing speed and attention. Both the PASAT and SDMT activate frontal and parietal areas, most prominently in the left, as well as cerebellar and occipital areas. As may be expected given the demanding executive nature of the PASAT, the test has been associated with greater activation in frontal regions (e.g., right medial frontal gyrus, right anterior cingulate gyrus, bilateral middle frontal gyrus, and the left precentral gyrus) compared with the SDMT (Forn et al., 2011). However, Yu et al. (2012) reported greater associations between white matter involvement (i.e., fractional anisotropy reductions as measured by diffusion tensor imaging [DTI]) and the SDMT, rather than the PASAT, in patients with relapsing-remitting MS. Similarly, Riccitelli et al. (2017) reported that the PASAT was more associated with gray matter atrophy, while the SDMT was more associated with microstructural damage in white matter regions.

PERFORMANCE VALIDITY

There is limited information on this topic. Unsurprisingly, persons attempting to feign the effects of brain injury perform more poorly than nonmalingerers on the PASAT, at least at the 2-second interval (Strauss et al., 1994).

COMMENT

There are a number of variations of the PASAT, but all employ the same basic structure and task requirements. In addition to the classically computed scores of number correct and errors, a number of authors have devised other scoring variables. Chunking and dyad scoring have proved especially beneficial to elucidating examinee strategy and providing qualitative information with respect to the actual processes used by examinees to complete the task and may in fact be more sensitive to impairment than conventionally computed scores. Consideration of these variables is especially important given the multifactorial demands of the PASAT, which involve not only complex attention and working memory, but also processing speed.

Internal reliability and interrater reliability are strong. Test-retest reliability is adequate to high, even across lengthy intervals. Practice effects are significant on the PASAT. Clinically, it is important to note that the greatest practice effect appears to occur from initial to second administration, with lower practice effects at subsequent sessions. This has led some authors (e.g., Baird et al., 2007) to recommend that if the PASAT is to be administered repeatedly, implementation of a dual baseline procedure, using only the second testing session as a baseline measurement, may be useful.

Versions appear to be highly correlated. However, high correlations do not indicate that the versions are interchangeable. In fact, the degree to which input/output modalities are congruent may influence difficulty, as does ISI length. Evidence from relationships with other tests suggests that the PASAT measures what it was designed to measure: specifically, attention, executive function, and processing speed. Arithmetic ability and IQ also exert a significant effect on performance. The test is associated with frontal and parietal activation in many different groups, as would be expected for a task demanding complex attention.

There is a sizable literature on the PASAT in patients with MS, including group differences between MS and controls, clinical and functional correlates, sensitivity to disease severity, and relationships with neuroimaging. The test has also been used in other populations, including those with brain injury, ADHD, and SLE, among others.

Age and education affect PASAT scores, whereas gender does not appear to be highly influential. Ethnicity effects have been reported, with demographic factors found to be particularly influential in African-American individuals in some studies. Whenever possible, demographic influences should be considered in norm selection.

Despite some psychometric strengths, there is now a substantial body of literature indicating that the task is aversive. In fact, many researchers have capitalized on this aspect of the PASAT and have utilized it in ways not originally intended, such as for induction of negative mood and assessment of fatigue. Not only is the test often experienced negatively by examinees, but this experience may influence the quality of data collected, with high levels of discontinuation rates and contributing to restriction of range and limited generalizability to the population of interest. Research studies using the PASAT should report continuation or termination rates in their samples, as well as factors that differentiate people who complete the PASAT compared to those who do not.

This task may not be appropriate for all examinees. Although many individuals reportedly find the task aversive regardless of cognitive ability or functional level, research has suggested that there are a number of factors that may be associated with discontinuation, including poorer arithmetic abilities, less education, older age, and increased clinical severity. Other recommendations for avoiding the PASAT include high anxiety levels and patients for whom speech and language impairment renders rapid oral responding impossible. Of course, in a clinical setting many of these factors may be present.

Modifications of the traditional PASAT, such as short forms or use of the Adjusting-PSAT, may be helpful in reducing discomfort by shortening the task. Bosnes, Dahl, and Almkvist (2015) reported that an examinee-paced version of the PASAT was correlated with an experimenter-paced version. Both tests demonstrated a similar pattern of correlations with other measures of attention, executive function, and processing speed. There is also a version that employs words instead of numbers ("day/night") to avoid the confound of mathematical skill level (PASOT). Although the test is less aversive to examinees, it is a less challenging task than the standard version and therefore may not be as sensitive in some populations.

Other tasks that retain the essential constructs underlying the PASAT, while being more tolerable for examinees, may also be of benefit to consider. The SDMT correlates highly with the PASAT and measures similar abilities; in head-to-head comparisons it may fare somewhat better than the PASAT in terms of classification accuracy, at least in MS samples. Note, however, that neuroimaging research has suggested that the PASAT is associated with greater frontal activation than the SDMT, suggesting that it may be more sensitive to executive abilities. The computerized test of information processing (CTIP) incorporates simple, choice, and semantic reaction time components and was introduced as an alternative to the PASAT, with nearly 50% of MS patients performing below the 10th percentile on this test (Tombaugh et al., 2010).

If the PASAT is administered clinically, it is recommended that participants be screened for arithmetic ability prior to administration. The PASAT may also be particularly well-suited to higher functioning individuals who may encounter ceiling effects on other attention tests. Specifically, because of its requirements for mathematical ability and its relationship to IQ and education, the test may best be conceptualized as a measure appropriate for individuals of average to above average cognitive ability (Wiens et al., 1997). More research is needed in terms of performance validity as well as reliable change methodology.

REFERENCES

Achiron, A., Polliack, M., Rao, S. M., Barak, Y., Lavie, M., Appelboim, N., & Harel, Y. (2005). Cognitive patterns and progression in multiple sclerosis: Construction and validation of percentile curves.

Journal of Neurology, Neurosurgery & Psychiatry, 76(5), 744–749. http://doi.org/10.1136/jnnp.2004.045518

Akbar, N., Honarmand, K., & Feinstein, A. (2011). Self-assessment of cognition in multiple sclerosis: The role of personality and anxiety. *Cognitive and Behavioral Neurology, 24*(3), 115–121. http://doi.org/10.1097/WNN.0b013e31822a20ae

Audoin, B., Ibarrola, D., Ranjeva, J.–P., Confort-Gouny, S., Malikova, I., Ali-Chérif, A., . . . Cozzone, P. (2003). Compensatory cortical activation observed by fMRI during a cognitive task at the earliest stage of MS. *Human Brain Mapping, 20*(2), 51–58. http://doi.org/10.1002/hbm.10128

Audoin, B., Van Au Duong, M., Ranjeva, J.–P., Ibarrola, D., Malikova, I., Confort-Gouny, S., . . . Cozzone, P. J. (2005). Magnetic resonance study of the influence of tissue damage and cortical reorganization on PASAT performance at the earliest stage of multiple sclerosis. *Human Brain Mapping, 24*(3), 216–228. http://doi.org/10.1002/hbm.20083

Aupperle, R. L., Beatty, W. W., Shelton, F., & Gontkovsky, S. T. (2002). Three screening batteries to detect cognitive impairment in multiple sclerosis. *Multiple Sclerosis, 8*, 382–389.

Baird, B. J., Tombaugh, T. N., & Francis, M. (2007). The effects of practice on speed of information processing using the Adjusting-Paced Serial Addition Test (Adjusting-PSAT) and the Computerized Tests of Information Processing (CTIP). *Applied Neuropsychology, 14*(2), 88–100. http://doi.org/10.1080/09084280701319912

Balzano, J., Chiaravalloti, N., Lengenfelder, J., Moore, N., & DeLuca, J. (2006). Does the scoring of late responses affect the outcome of the paced auditory serial addition task (PASAT)? *Archives of Clinical Neuropsychology, 21*(8), 819–825. http://doi.org/10.1016/j.acn.2006.09.002

Barker-Collo, S. L. (2005). Within session practice effects on the PASAT in clients with multiple sclerosis. *Archives of Clinical Neuropsychology, 20*(2), 145–152. http://doi.org/10.1016/j.acn.2004.03.007

Barker-Collo, S., Feigin, V., Lawes, C., Senior, H., & Parag, V. (2010a). Natural history of attention deficits and their influence on functional recovery from acute stages to 6 months after stroke. *Neuroepidemiology, 35*(4), 255–262. http://d oi.org/10.1159/000319894

Barker-Collo, S. L., Feigin, V. L., Lawes, C. M. M., Parag, V., & Senior, H. (2010b). Attention deficits after incident stroke in the acute period: Frequency across types of attention and relationships to patient characteristics and functional outcomes. *Topics in Stroke Rehabilitation, 17*(6), 463–476. http://doi.org/10.1310/tsr1706-463

Bate, A. J., Mathias, J. L., & Crawford, J. R. (2001). Performance on the Test of Everyday Attention and standard tests of attention Paced Auditory Serial Addition Test (PASAT) and Children's Paced Auditory Serial Addition Test (CHIPASAT) following severe traumatic brain injury. *The Clinical Neuropsychologist, 15*(3), 405–422.

Berard, J. A., Bowman, M., Atkins, H. L., Freedman, M. S., & Walker, L. A. S. (2014). Cognitive fatigue in individuals with multiple sclerosis undergoing immunoablative therapy and hematopoietic stem cell transplantation. *Journal of the Neurological Sciences, 336*(1–2), 132–137. http://doi.org/10.1016/j.jns.2013.10.023

Berrigan, L. I., Fisk, J. D., Walker, L. A. S., Wojtowicz, M., Rees, L. M., Freedman, M. S., & Marrie, R. A. (2014). Reliability of regression-based normative data for the oral Symbol Digit Modalities Test: An evaluation of demographic influences, construct validity, and impairment classification rates in multiple sclerosis samples. *The Clinical Neuropsychologist, 28*(2), 281–299. https://doi.org/10.1080/13854046.2013.871337

Bosnes, O., Dahl, O.–P., & Almkvist, O. (2015). Including a subject-paced trial may make the PASAT more acceptable for MS patients. *Acta Neurologica Scandinavica, 132*(4), 219–225. http://doi.org/10.1111/ane.12385

Brittain, J. L., la Marche, J. A., Reeder, K. P., Roth, D. L., & Boll, T. J. (1991). Effects of age and IQ on Paced Auditory Serial Addition Task (PASAT) performance. *The Clinical Neuropsychologist, 5*(2), 163–175. http://doi.org/10.1080/13854049108403300

Brooks, J. B., Giraud, V. O., Saleh, Y. J., Rodrigues, S. J., Daia, L. A., & Fragoso, Y. D. (2011). Paced auditory serial addition test (PASAT): A very difficult test even for individuals with high intellectual capability. *Arquivos de Neuro-Psiquiatria, 69*(3), 482–484. http://doi.org/10.1590/S0004-282X2011000400014

Brown, R. A., Lejuez, C. W., Strong, D. R., Kahler, C. W., Zvolensky, M. J., Carpenter, L. L., . . . Price, L. H. (2009). A prospective examination of distress tolerance and early smoking lapse in adult self-quitters. *Nicotine & Tobacco Research, 11*(5), 493–502. http://doi.org/10.1093/ntr/ntp041

Burt, R. K., Loh, Y., Cohen, B., Stefoski, D., Balabanov, R., Katsamakis, G., . . . Burns, W. H. (2009). "Autologous non-myeloablative haemopoietic stem cell transplantation in relapsing-remitting multiple sclerosis: A phase I/II study": Erratum. *Lancet Neurology, 8*(4), 309–309. http://doi.org/10.1016/S1474-4422(09)70071-7

Burt, R. K., Loh, Y., Cohen, B., Stefosky, D., Balabanov, R., Katsamakis, G., . . . Burns, W. H. (2009). Autologous non-myeloablative haemopoietic stem cell transplantation in relapsing-remitting multiple sclerosis: A phase I/II study. *Lancet Neurology, 8*(3), 244–253. http://doi.org/10.1016/S1474-4422(09)70017-1

Chiaravalloti, N. D., Hillary, F. G., Ricker, J. H., Christodoulou, C., Kalnin, A. J., Liu, W.–C., . . . Deluca, J. (2005). Cerebral activation patterns during working memory performance in multiple sclerosis using fMRI. *Journal of Clinical and Experimental Neuropsychology, 27*(1), 33–54. http://doi.org/10.1080/138033990513609

Chiaravalloti, N. D., Wylie, G., Leavitt, V., & Deluca, J. (2012). Increased cerebral activation after behavioral treatment for memory deficits in MS. *Journal of Neurology, 259*(7), 1337–1346. https://doi.org/10.1007/s00415-011-6353-x

Chronicle, E. P., & MacGregor, N. A. (1998). Are PASAT scores related to mathematical ability? *Neuropsychological Rehabilitation, 8*(3), 273–282. http://doi.org/10.1080/713755571

Cicerone, K. D. (1997). Clinical sensitivity of four measures of attention to mild traumatic brain injury. *The Clinical Neuropsychologist, 11*(3), 266–272. http://doi.org/10.1080/13854049708400455

Cicerone, K. D., & Azulay, J. (2002). Diagnostic utility of attention measures in postconcussion syndrome. *The Clinical Neuropsychologist, 16*(3), 280–289. http://doi.org/10.1076/clin.16.3.280.13849

Cockshell, S. J., & Mathias, J. L. (2014). Cognitive functioning in people with chronic fatigue syndrome: A comparison between subjective and objective measures. *Neuropsychology, 28*(3), 394–405. http://doi.org/10.1037/neu0000025

Cohen, J. A., Cutter, G. R., Fischer, J. S., Goodman, A. D., Heidenreich, F. R., Kooijmans, M. F., . . . Whitaker, J. N. (2002). Benefit of interferon β-1a on MSFC progression in secondary progressive MS. *Neurology, 59*(5), 679–687. http://doi.org/10.1212/WNL.59.5.679

Crawford, J. R., Obonsawin, M. C., & Allan, K. M. (1998). PASAT and components of WAIS-R performance: Convergent and discriminant validity. *Neuropsychological Rehabilitation, 8*(3), 255–272. http://doi.org/10.1080/713755575

Crossen, J. R., & Wiens, A. N. (1988). Residual neuropsychological deficits following head-injury on the Wechsler Memory Scale—Revised. *The Clinical Neuropsychologist, 2*(4), 393–399. http://doi.org/10.1080/13854048808403276

Daughters, S. B., Lejuez, C. W., Kahler, C. W., Strong, D. R., & Brown, R. A. (2005). Psychological distress tolerance and duration of most recent abstinence attempt among residential treatment-seeking substance abusers. *Psychology of Addictive Behaviors, 19*(2), 208–211. http://doi.org/10.1037/0893-164X.19.2.208

Deary, I. J., & Der, G. (2005). Reaction time, age, and cognitive ability: Longitudinal findings from age 16 to 63 years in representative population samples. *Aging, Neuropsychology, and Cognition, 12*(2), 187–215. http://doi.org/10.1080/13825580590969235

Deary, I. J., Langan, S. J., Hepburn, D. A., & Frier, B. M. (1991). Which abilities does the PASAT test? *Personality and Individual Differences, 12*(10), 983–987. http://doi.org/10.1016/0191-8869(91)90027-9

Demaree, J. A., Gaudino, E., & DeLuca, J. (2003). The relationship between depressive symptoms and cognitive dysfunction in multiple sclerosis. *Cognitive Neuropsychiatry, 8*(3), 161–171.

D'haeseleer, M., Steen, C., Hoogduin, J. M., van Osch, M. J. P., Fierens, Y., Cambron, M., . . . De Keyser, J. (2013). Performance on Paced Auditory Serial Addition Test and cerebral blood flow in multiple sclerosis. *Acta Neurologica Scandinavica, 128*(5), e26–e29.

Diamond, B. J., DeLuca, J., Kim, H., & Kelley, S. M. (1997). The question of disproportionate impairments in visual and auditory information processing in multiple sclerosis. *Journal of Clinical and Experimental Neuropsychology, 19*(1), 34–42. http://doi.org/10.1080/01688639708403834

Diehr, M. C., Cherner, M., Wolfson, T. J., Miller, S. W., Grant, I., & Heaton, R. K. (2003). The 50 and 100-item short forms of the Paced Auditory Serial Addition Test (PASAT): Demographically corrected norms and comparisons with the full PASAT in normal and clinical samples. *Journal of Clinical and Experimental Neuropsychology, 25*(4), 571–585. http://doi.org/10.1076/jcen.25.4.571.13876

Diehr, M. C., Heaton, R. K., Miller, W., & Grant, I. (1998). The Paced Auditory Serial Addition Task (PASAT): Norms for age, education, and ethnicity. *Assessment, 5*(4), 375–387. http://doi.org/10.1177/107319119800500407

Diehr, M. C., Heaton, R. K., Miller, W., & Grant, I. (1999). "The Paced Auditory Serial Addition Task (PASAT): Norms for age, education, and ethnicity": Erratum. *Assessment, 6*(1), 101–101. http://doi.org/10.1177/107319119900600111

Draganich, C., & Erdal, K. (2014). Placebo sleep affects cognitive functioning. *Journal of Experimental Psychology: Learning, Memory, and Cognition, 40*(3), 857–864. http://doi.org/10.1037/a0035546

Drake, A. S., Weinstock-Guttman, B., Morrow, S. A., Hojnacki, D., Munschauer, F. E., & Benedict, R. H. B. (2010). Psychometrics and normative data for the Multiple Sclerosis Functional Composite: Replacing the PASAT with the Symbol Digit Modalities Test. *Multiple Sclerosis (Houndmills, Basingstoke, England), 16*(2), 228–237. https://doi.org/10.1177/1352458509354552

Dujardin, K., Denève, C., Ronval, M., Krystkowiak, P., Humez, C., Destée, A., & Defebvre, L. (2007). Is the Paced Auditory Serial Addition Test (PASAT) a valid means of assessing executive function in Parkinson's disease? *Cortex, 43*(5), 601–606. http://doi.org/10.1016/S0010-9452(08)70490-8

Edgar, C., Jongen, P. J., Sanders, E., Sindic, C., Goffette, S., Dupuis, M., . . . Wesnes, K. (2011). Cognitive performance in relapsing remitting multiple sclerosis: A longitudinal study in daily practice using a brief computerized cognitive battery. *BMC Neurology, 11*. http://doi.org/10.1186/1471-2377-11-68

Ellis, A. J., Fischer, K. M., & Beevers, C. G. (2010). Is dysphoria about being red and blue? Potentiation of anger and reduced distress tolerance among dysphoric individuals. *Cognition and Emotion, 24*(4), 596–608. http://doi.org/10.1080/13803390902851176

Feldner, M. T., Leen-Feldner, E. W., Zvolensky, M. J., & Lejuez, C. W. (2006). Examining the association between rumination, negative affectivity, and negative affect induced by a paced auditory serial addition task. *Journal of Behavior Therapy and Experimental Psychiatry, 37*(3), 171–187. http://doi.org/10.1016/j.jbtep.2005.06.002

Filley, C. M., Kozora, E., Brown, M. S., Miller, D. E., West, S. G., Arciniegas, D. B., . . . Zhang, L. (2009). White matter microstructure and cognition in non-neuropsychiatric systemic lupus erythematosus. *Cognitive and Behavioral Neurology, 22*(1), 38–44. http://doi.org/10.1097/WNN.0b013e318190d174

Fischer, J. S., Rudick, R. A., Cutter, G. R., & Reingold, S. C. (1999). The Multiple Sclerosis Functional Composite measure (MSFC): An integrated approach to MS clinical outcome assessment. *Multiple Sclerosis, 5*, 244–250.

Fisk, J. D., & Archibald, C. J. (2001). Limitations of the Paced Auditory Serial Addition Test as a measure of working memory in patients with multiple sclerosis. *Journal of the International Neuropsychological Society, 7*(3), 363–372. http://doi.org/10.1017/S1355617701733103

Flavia, M., Stampatori, C., Zanotti, D., Parrinello, G., & Capra, R. (2010). Efficacy and specificity of intensive cognitive rehabilitation of attention and executive functions in multiple sclerosis. *Journal of the Neurological Sciences, 288*(1–2), 101–105. https://doi.org/10.1016/j.jns.2009.09.024

Forn, C., Belenguer, A., Parcet-Ibars, M. A., & Ávila, C. (2008). Information-processing speed is the primary deficit underlying the poor performance of multiple sclerosis patients in the Paced Auditory Serial Addition Test (PASAT). *Journal of Clinical and Experimental Neuropsychology, 30*(7), 789–796. https://doi.org/10.1080/13803390701779560

Forn, C., Belenguer, A., Belloch, V., Sanjuan, A., Parcet, M. A., & Ávila, C. (2011). Anatomical and functional differences between the Paced Auditory Serial Addition Test and the Symbol Digit Modalities Test. *Journal of Clinical and Experimental Neuropsychology, 33*(1), 42–50. http://doi.org/10.1080/13803395.2010.481620

Forn, C., Belenguer, A., Parcet-Ibars, M. A., & Ávila, C. (2008). Information-processing speed is the primary deficit underlying the poor performance of multiple sclerosis patients in the Paced Auditory Serial Addition Test (PASAT). *Journal of Clinical and Experimental Neuropsychology, 30*(7), 789–796. http://doi.org/10.1080/13803390701779560

Forn, C., Ventura-Campos, N., Belenguer, A., Belloch, V., Parcet, M. A., & Ávila, C. (2008). A comparison of brain activation patterns during covert and overt Paced Auditory Serial Addition Test tasks. *Human Brain Mapping, 29*(6), 644–650. http://doi.org/10.1002/hbm.20430

Fos, L. A., Greve, K. W., South, M. B., Mathias, C., & Benefield, H. (2000). Paced Visual Serial Addition Test: An alternative measure of information processing speed. *Applied Neuropsychology, 7*(3), 140–146. http://doi.org/10.1207/S15324826AN0703_4

Gonzalez, R., Grant, I., Miller, S. W., Taylor, M. J., Schweinsburg, B. C., Carey, C. L., . . . Heaton, R. K. (2006a). Demographically adjusted normative standards for new indices of performance on the Paced Auditory Serial Addition Task (PASAT). *The Clinical Neuropsychologist, 20*(3), 396–413. http://doi.org/10.1080/13854040590967559

Gonzalez, R., Miller, S. W., Carey, C. L., Woods, S. P., Rippeth, J. D., Schweinsburg, B. C., . . . Heaton, R. K. (2006b). Association between dyads and correct responses on the Paced Auditory Serial Addition Task (PASAT). *Assessment, 13*(4), 381–384. http://doi.org/10.1177/1073191106286567

Gorka, S. M., Ali, B., & Daughters, S. B. (2012). The role of distress tolerance in the relationship between depressive symptoms and problematic alcohol use. *Psychology of Addictive Behaviors, 26*(3), 621–626. http://doi.org/10.1037/a0026386

Gow, A. J., & Deary, I. J. (2004). Is the PASAT past it? Testing attention and concentration without numbers. *Journal of Clinical and Experimental Neuropsychology, 26*(6), 723–736. http://doi.org/10.1080/13803390490509295

Gronwall, D. M. (1977). Paced auditory serial-addition task: A measure of recovery from concussion. *Perceptual and Motor Skills, 44*(2), 367–373.

Gronwall, D., & Wrightson, P. (1974). Delayed recovery of intellectual function after minor head injury. *Lancet, 2*, 605–609.

Gronwall, D., & Wrightson, P. (1981). Memory and information processing capacity after closed head injury. *Journal of Neurology, Neurosurgery & Psychiatry, 44*(10), 889–895. https://doi.org/10.1136/jnnp.44.10.889

Gronwall, D. M. A., & Sampson, H. (1974). *The psychological effects of concussion*. New Zealand: Auckland University Press.

Grothe, M., Lotze, M., Langner, S., & Dressel, A. (2017). Impairments in walking ability, dexterity, and cognitive function in multiple sclerosis are associated with different regional cerebellar gray matter loss. *Cerebellum (London, England), 16*(5–6), 945–950. https://doi.org/10.1007/s12311-017-0871-8

Harel, Y., Appleboim, N., Lavie, M., & Achiron, A. (2009). Single dose of methylphenidate improves cognitive performance in multiple sclerosis patients with impaired attention process. *Journal of the*

Neurological Sciences, 276(1-2), 38–40. http://doi.org/10.1016/j.jns.2008.08.025

Haslam, C., Batchelor, J., Fearnside, M. R., Haslam, A. S., & Hawkins, S. (1995). Further examination of post-traumatic amnesia and post-coma disturbance as non-linear predictors of outcome after head injury. *Neuropsychology, 9*, 599–605.

Hirvikoski, T., Olsson, E. M. G., Nordenström, A., Lindholm, T., Nordström, A.–L., & Lajic, S. (2011). Deficient cardiovascular stress reactivity predicts poor executive functions in adults with attention-deficit/hyperactivity disorder. *Journal of Clinical and Experimental Neuropsychology, 33*(1), 63–73. http://doi.org/10.1080/13803395.2010.493145

Hohol, M. J., Guttman, C. R., Orav, J., Mackin, G. A., Kikinis, R., Khoury, S. J., Jolesz, F. A., & Weiner, H. L. (1997). Serial neuropsychological assessment and magnetic resonance imaging analysis in multiple sclerosis. *Archives of Neurology, 54*, 1018–1025.

Holdwick, D. J. J., & Wingenfeld, S. A. (1999). The subjective experience of PASAT testing: Does the PASAT induce negative mood? *Archives of Clinical Neuropsychology, 14*(3), 273–284. http://doi.org/10.1093/arclin/14.3.273

Huijbregts, S. C. J., Kalkers, N. F., de Sonneville, L. M. J., de Groot, V., & Polman, C. H. (2006). Cognitive impairment and decline in different MS subtypes. *Journal of the Neurological Sciences, 245*(1-2), 187–194. http://doi.org/10.1016/j.jns.2005.07.018

Iverson, K. M., Follette, V. M., Pistorello, J., & Fruzzetti, A. E. (2012). An investigation of experiential avoidance, emotion dysregulation, and distress tolerance in young adult outpatients with borderline personality disorder symptoms. *Personality Disorders: Theory, Research, and Treatment, 3*(4), 415–422. http://doi.org/10.1037/a0023703

Johnson, S. K., Lange, G., DeLuca, J., Korn, L. R., & Natelson, B. (1997). The effects of fatigue on neuropsychological performance in patients with chronic fatigue syndrome, multiple sclerosis, and depression. *Applied Neuropsychology, 4*(3), 145–153. http://doi.org/10.1207/s15324826an0403_1

Kiiski, H., Reilly, R. B., Lonergan, R., Kelly, S., O'Brien, M., Kinsella, K., . . . Whelan, R. (2011a). Change in PASAT performance correlates with change in P3 ERP amplitude over a 12-month period in multiple sclerosis patients. *Journal of the Neurological Sciences, 305*(1–2), 45–52. http://doi.org/10.1016/j.jns.2011.03.018

Kiiski, H., Whelan, R., Lonergan, R., Nolan, H., Kinsella, K., Hutchinson, M., . . . Reilly, R. B. (2011b). Preliminary evidence for correlation between PASAT performance and P3a and P3b amplitudes in progressive multiple sclerosis. *European Journal of Neurology, 18*(5), 792–795. http://doi.org/10.1111/j.1468-1331.2010.03172.x

Kotterba, S., Orth, M., Eren, E., Fangerau, T., & Sindern, E. (2003). Assessment of driving performance in patients with relapsing-remitting multiple sclerosis by a driving simulator. *European Neurology, 50*(3), 160–164. http://doi.org/10.1159/000073057

Kozora, E., Arciniegas, D. B., Duggan, E., West, S., Brown, M. S., & Filley, C. M. (2013). White matter abnormalities and working memory impairment in systemic lupus erythematosus. *Cognitive and Behavioral Neurology, 26*(2), 63–72. http://doi.org/10.1097/WNN.0b013e31829d5c74

Larrabee, G. J., & Curtiss, G. (1995). Construct validity of various verbal and visual memory tests. *Journal of Clinical and Experimental Neuropsychology, 17*, 536–547.

Lejuez, C. W., Kahler, C. W., & Brown, R. A. (2003). A modified computer version of the Paced Auditory Serial Addition Task (PASAT) as a laboratory-based stressor. *Behavior Therapist, 26*(4), 290–293.

Lesage, E., Apps, M. A. J., Hayter, A. L., Beckmann, C. F., Barnes, D., Langdon, D. W., & Ramnani, N. (2010). Cerebellar information processing in relapsing-remitting multiple sclerosis (RRMS). *Behavioural Neurology, 23*(1–2), 39–49. http://doi.org/10.1155/2010/482139

Levin, H. S., Mattis, S., Ruff, R. M., Eisenberg, H. M., et al. (1987). Neurobehavioral outcome following minor head injury: A three center study. *Journal of Neurosurgery, 66*, 234–243.

Locke, D. E. C., Stonnington, C. M., Thomas, M. L., & Caselli, R. J. (2011). Correlates of quitting the Paced Auditory Serial Addition Test in cognitively normal older adults participating in a study of normal cognitive aging. *Journal of Clinical and Experimental Neuropsychology, 33*(8), 937–943. http://doi.org/10.1080/13803395.2011.578571

López-Góngora, M., Querol, L., & Escartín, A. (2015). A one-year follow-up study of the Symbol Digit Modalities Test (SDMT) and the Paced Auditory Serial Addition Test (PASAT) in relapsing-remitting multiple sclerosis: an appraisal of comparative longitudinal sensitivity. *BMC Neurology, 15*, 40. https://doi.org/10.1186/s12883-015-0296-2

Lustyk, M. K. B., Douglas, H. A. C., Shilling, E. A., & Woods, N. F. (2012). Hemodynamic and psychological responses to laboratory stressors in women: Assessing the roles of menstrual cycle phase, premenstrual symptomatology, and sleep characteristics. *International Journal of Psychophysiology, 86*(3), 283–290. http://doi.org/10.1016/j.ijpsycho.2012.10.009

Lustyk, M. K. B., Olson, K. C., Gerrish, W. G., Holder, A., & Widman, L. (2010). Psychophysiological and neuroendocrine responses to laboratory stressors in women: Implications of menstrual cycle phase and stressor type. *Biological Psychology, 83*(2), 84–92. http://doi.org/10.1016/j.biopsycho.2009.11.003

Lynch, S. G., Dickerson, K. J., & Denney, D. R. (2010). Evaluating processing speed in multiple sclerosis: A comparison of two rapid serial processing measures. *The Clinical Neuropsychologist, 24*(6), 963–976. http://doi.org/10.1080/13854046.2010.502128

Martins, A. Q., Kavussanu, M., Willoughby, A., & Ring, C. (2013). Moderate intensity exercise facilitates working memory. *Psychology of Sport and Exercise, 14*(3), 323–328. http://doi.org/10.1016/j.psychsport.2012.11.010

Mattioli, F., Stampatori, C., & Capra, R. (2011). The effect of natalizumab on cognitive function in patients with relapsing-remitting multiple sclerosis: Preliminary results of a 1-year follow-up study. *Neurological Sciences, 32*(1), 83–88. http://doi.org/10.1007/s10072-010-0412-4

McCaffrey, R. J., Cousins, J. P., Westervelt, H. J., Martynowicz, M., Remick, S. C., Szebenyi, S., . . . Haase, R. F. (1995). Practice effects with the NIMH AIDS abbreviated neuropsychological battery. *Archives of Clinical Neuropsychology, 10*(3), 241–250. http://doi.org/10.1016/0887-6177(94)00048-U

Mendez, M. F., Owens, E. M., Berenji, G. R., Peppers, D. C., Liang, L.–J., & Licht, E. A. (2013). Mild traumatic brain injury from primary blast vs. blunt forces: Post-concussion consequences and functional neuroimaging. *NeuroRehabilitation, 32*(2), 397–407.

Mitropoulou, V., Harvey, P. D., Maldari, L. A., Moriarty, P. J., New, A. S., Silverman, J. M., & Siever, L. J. (2002). Neuropsychological performance in schizotypal personality disorder: Evidence regarding diagnostic specificity. *Biological Psychiatry, 52*(12), 1175–1182. http://doi.org/10.1016/S0006-3223(02)01426-9

Mitropoulou, V., Harvey, P. D., Zegarelli, G., New, A. S., Silverman, J. M., & Siever, L. J. (2005). Neuropsychological performance in schizotypal personality disorder: Importance of working memory. *American Journal of Psychiatry, 162*(10), 1896–1903. http://doi.org/10.1176/appi.ajp.162.10.1896

Morrow, S. A. (2013). Normative data for the Stroop color word test for a North American population. *Canadian Journal of Neurological Sciences / Le Journal Canadien Des Sciences Neurologiques, 40*(6), 842–847. http://doi.org/10.1017/S0317167100015997

Morrow, S. A., Rosehart, H., & Johnson, A. M. (2015). Diagnosis and quantification of cognitive fatigue in multiple sclerosis. *Cognitive and Behavioral Neurology, 28*(1), 27–32. https://doi.org/10.1097/WNN.0000000000000050

Niccolai, C., Portaccio, E., Goretti, B., Hakiki, B., Giannini, M., Pastò, L., . . . Amato, M. P. (2015). A comparison of the brief international cognitive assessment for multiple sclerosis and the brief repeatable battery in multiple sclerosis patients. *BMC Neurology, 15*(1). http://doi.org/10.1186/s12883-015-0460-8

Nolin, P., & Heroux, L. (2006). Relations among sociodemographic, neurologic, clinical, and neuropsychologic variables, and vocational status following mild traumatic brain injury: A follow-up study. *Journal of Head Trauma Rehabilitation, 21*(6), 514–526. http://doi.org/10.1097/00001199-200611000-00006

Obradovic, D., Petrovic, M., Antanasijevic, I., Marinkovic, J., Stojanovic, T., & Obradovic, S. (2012). The Brief Repeatable Battery: Psychometrics and normative values with age, education and gender corrections in a Serbian population. *Neurological Sciences, 33*(6), 1369–1374. http://doi.org/10.1007/s10072-012-1099-5

O'Donnell, J. P., MacGregor, L. A., Dabrowski, J. J., Oestreicher, J. M., & Romero, J. J. (1994). Construct validity of neuropsychological tests of conceptual and attentional abilities. *Journal of Clinical Psychology, 50*(4), 596–600. http://doi.org/10.1002/1097-4679(199407)50:4<596::AID-JCLP2270500416>3.0.CO;2-S

Ojile, J., Ryan, L., Betz, B., Parkslevy, J., Hilsabeck, R., Rhudy, J., & Gouvier, W. (2006). Information processing following mild head injury. *Archives of Clinical Neuropsychology, 21*(4), 293–296. https://doi.org/10.1016/j.acn.2006.03.003

Parmenter, B. A., Shucard, J. L., Benedict, R. H. B., & Shucard, D. W. (2006). Working memory deficits in multiple sclerosis: Comparison between the *n*-back task and the Paced Auditory Serial Addition Test. *Journal of the International Neuropsychological Society, 12*(5), 677–687. http://doi.org/10.1017/S1355617706060826

Portaccio, E., Goretti, B., Zipoli, V., Siracusa, G., Sorbi, S., & Amato, M. P. (2009). A short version of Rao's Brief Repeatable Battery as a screening tool for cognitive impairment in multiple sclerosis. *The Clinical Neuropsychologist, 23*(2), 268–275. http://doi.org/10.1080/13854040801992815

Rachbauer, D., Kronbichler, M., Ropele, S., Enzinger, C., & Fazekas, F. (2006). Differences in cerebral activation patterns in idiopathic inflammatory demyelination using the paced visual serial addition task: An fMRI study. *Journal of the Neurological Sciences, 244*(1–2), 11–16. http://doi.org/10.1016/j.jns.2005.11.035

Ranjeva, J.–P., Audoin, B., Van Au Duong, M., Confort-Gouny, S., Malikova, I., Viout, P., . . . Cozzone, P. J. (2006). Structural and functional surrogates of cognitive impairment at the very early stage of multiple sclerosis. *Journal of the Neurological Sciences, 245*(1–2), 161–167. http://doi.org/10.1016/j.jns.2005.09.019

Rao, S. M., Leo, G. J., Bernardin, L., Unverzagt, F. (1991). Cognitive dysfunction in multiple sclerosis: Frequency, patterns and prediction. *Neurology, 41*, 685–691, *26*(7), 583–591. http://doi.org/10.1093/arclin/acr055

Riccitelli, G. C., Pagani, E., Rodegher, M., Colombo, B., Preziosa, P., Falini, A., . . . Rocca, M. A. (2017). Imaging patterns of gray and white matter abnormalities associated with PASAT and SDMT performance in relapsing-remitting multiple sclerosis. *Multiple Sclerosis (Houndmills, Basingstoke, England)*, 1352458517743091. https://doi.org/10.1177/1352458517743091

Roman, D. D., Edwall, G. E., Buchanan, R. J., & Patton, J. H. (1991). Extended norms for the paced auditory serial addition task. *The Clinical Neuropsychologist, 5*(1), 33–40. http://doi.org/10.1080/13854049108401840

Rosti-Otajärvi, E., Hämäläinen, P., Koivisto, K., & Hokkanen, L. (2008). The reliability of the MSFC and its components. *Acta Neurologica Scandinavica, 117*(6), 421–427. http://doi.org/10.1111/j.1600-0404.2007.00972.x

Royan, J., Tombaugh, T. N., Rees, L., & Francis, M. (2004). The Adjusting-Paced Serial Addition Test (Adjusting-PSAT): Thresholds for speed of information processing as a function of stimulus modality and problem complexity. *Archives of Clinical Neuropsychology, 19*, 131–143.

Rudick, R., Antel, J., Confavreux, C., Cutter, G., Ellison, G., Fischer, J., . . . Willoughby, E. (1997). Recommendations from the National Multiple Sclerosis Society Clinical Outcomes Assessment Task Force. *Annals of Neurology, 42*, 379–382.

Sampson, H. (1956). Pacing and performance on a serial addition task. *Canadian Journal of Psychology, 10*, 219–225.

Sandry, J., Paxton, J., & Sumowski, J. F. (2016). General mathematical ability predicts PASAT performance in MS patients: Implications for clinical interpretation and cognitive reserve. *Journal of the International Neuropsychological Society, 22*(03), 375–378. http://doi.org/10.1017/S1355617715001307

Sauer, S. E., & Baer, R. A. (2012). Ruminative and mindful self-focused attention in borderline personality disorder. *Personality Disorders: Theory, Research, and Treatment, 3*(4), 433–441. http://doi.org/10.1037/a0025465

Schächinger, H., Cox, D., Linder, L., Brody, S., & Ulrich, K. (2003). Cognitive and psychomotor function in hypoglycemia: Response error patterns and retest reliability. *Pharmacology, Biochemistry and Behavior, 75*(4), 915–920. http://doi.org/10.1016/S0091-3057(03)00167-9

Schweitzer, J. B., Hanford, R. B., & Medoff, D. R. (2006). Working memory deficits in adults with ADHD: Is there evidence for subtype differences? *Behavioral and Brain Functions, 2*. http://doi.org/10.1186/1744-9081-2-43

Schweitzer, J. B., Lee, D. O., Hanford, R. B., Zink, C. F., Ely, T. D., Tagamets, M. A., . . . Kilts, C. D. (2004). Effect of methylphenidate on executive functioning in adults with attention-deficit/hyperactivity disorder: Normalization of behavior but not related brain activity. *Biological Psychiatry, 56*(8), 597–606. http://doi.org/10.1016/j.biopsych.2004.07.011

Shawaryn, M. A., Schiaffino, K. M., LaRocca, N. G., & Johnston, M. V. (2002). Determinants of health-related quality of life in multiple sclerosis: The role of illness intrusiveness. *Multiple Sclerosis, 8*, 310–318.

Sherman, E. M. S., Strauss, E., & Spellacy, F. (1997). Validity of the Paced Auditory Serial Addition Test (PASAT) in adults referred for neuropsychological assessment after head injury. *The Clinical Neuropsychologist, 11*(1), 34–45. http://doi.org/10.1080/13854049708407027

Shucard, J. L., Gaines, J. J., Ambrus, J. J., & Shucard, D. W. (2007). C-reactive protein and cognitive deficits in systemic lupus erythematosus. *Cognitive and Behavioral Neurology, 20*(1), 31–37. http://doi.org/10.1097/WNN.0b013e31802e3b9a

Shucard, J. L., Parrish, J., Shucard, D. W., McCabe, D. C., Benedict, R. H. B., & Ambrus, J. J. (2004). Working memory and processing speed deficits in systemic lupus erythematosus as measured by the paced auditory serial addition test. *Journal of the International Neuropsychological Society, 10*(1), 35–45. http://doi.org/10.1017/S1355617704101057

Sjøgren, P., Thomsen, A. B., & Olsen, A. K. (2000). Impaired neuropsychological performance in chronic nonmalignant pain patients receiving long-term oral opioid therapy. *Journal of Pain and Symptom Management, 19*(2), 100–108. http://doi.org/10.1016/S0885-3924(99)00143-8

Snyder, P. J., & Cappelleri, J. C. (2001). Information processing speed deficits may be better correlated with the extent of white matter sclerotic lesions in multiple sclerosis than previously suspected. *Brain and Cognition, 46*(1-2), 279–284. http://doi.org/10.1016/S0278-2626(01)80084-1

Snyder, P. J., Cappelleri, J. C., Archibald, C. J., & Fisk, J. D. (2001). Improved detection of differential information-processing speed deficits between two disease-course types of multiple sclerosis. *Neuropsychology, 15*(4), 617–625. http://doi.org/10.1037/0894-4105.15.4.617

Staffen, W., Mair, A., Zauner, H., Unterrainer, J., Niederhofer, H., Kutzelnigg, A., . . . Ladurner, G. (2002). Cognitive function and fMRI in patients with multiple sclerosis: Evidence for compensatory cortical activation during an attention task. *Brain: A Journal of Neurology, 125*(6), 1275–1282. http://doi.org/10.1093/brain/awf125

Strauss, E., Spellacy, F., Hunter, M., & Berry, T. (1994). Assessing believable deficits on measures of attention and information processing capacity. *Archives of Clinical Neuropsychology, 9*, 483–490.

Stuss, D. T., Stethem, L. L., Hugenholtz, H., & Richard, M. T. (1989). Traumatic brain injury: A comparison of three clinical tests, and analysis of recovery. *The Clinical Neuropsychologist, 3*(2), 145–156. http://doi.org/10.1080/13854048908403287

Stuss, D. T., Stethem, L. L., & Pelchat, G. (1988). Three tests of attention and rapid information processing: An extension. *The Clinical Neuropsychologist, 2*(3), 246–250. http://doi.org/10.1080/13854048808520107

Sumowski, J. F., Chiaravalloti, N., Wylie, G., & Deluca, J. (2009). Cognitive reserve moderates the negative effect of brain atrophy on cognitive efficiency in multiple sclerosis. *Journal of the International Neuropsychological Society, 15*(4), 606–612. http://doi.org/10.1017/S1355617709090912

Tartaglia, M. C., Narayanan, S., & Arnold, D. L. (2008). Mental fatigue alters the pattern and increases the volume of cerebral activation required for a motor task in multiple sclerosis patients with fatigue. *European Journal of Neurology, 15*(4), 413–419. http://doi.org/10.1111/j.1468-1331.2008.02090.x

Thompson, K. R., Johnson, A. M., Emerson, J. L., Dawson, J. D., Boer, E. R., & Rizzo, M. (2012). Distracted driving in elderly and middle-aged drivers. *Accident Analysis and Prevention, 45*, 711–717. http://doi.org/10.1016/j.aap.2011.09.040.

Tombaugh, T. N. (1999). *Administrative manual for the Adjusting-Paced Serial Addition Test (Adjusting-PSAT)*. Ottawa, Ontario: Carleton University Press.

Tombaugh, T. N. (2006). A comprehensive review of the Paced Auditory Serial Addition Test (PASAT). *Archives of Clinical Neuropsychology, 21*(1), 53–76. http://doi.org/10.1016/j.acn.2005.07.006

Tombaugh, T. N., Berrigan, L. I., Walker, L. A. S., & Freedman, M. S. (2010). The Computerized Test of Information Processing (CTIP) offers an alternative to the PASAT for assessing cognitive processing speed in individuals with multiple sclerosis. *Cognitive and Behavioral Neurology, 23*(3), 192–198. http://doi.org/10.1097/WNN.0b013e3181cc8bd4

Tombaugh, T. N., Rees, L., Baird, B., & Kost, J. (2004). The effects of list difficulty and modality of presentation on a computerized version of the Paced Serial Addition Test (PSAT). *Journal of Clinical and Experimental Neuropsychology, 26*(2), 257–265.

Tomporowski, P. D., Cureton, K., Armstrong, L. E., Kane, G. M., Sparling, P. B., & Millard-Stafford, M. (2005). Short-term effects of aerobic exercise on executive processes and emotional reactivity. *International Journal of Sport and Exercise Psychology, 3*(2), 131–146. http://doi.org/10.1080/1612197X.2005.9671763

Townsend, L. A., Norman, R. M. G., Malla, A. K., Rychlo, A. D., & Ahmed, R. R. (2002). Changes in cognitive functioning following comprehensive treatment for first episode patients with schizophrenia spectrum disorders. *Psychiatry Research, 113*(1-2), 69–81. http://doi.org/10.1016/S0165-1781(02)00236-6

VanderKaay, M. M., & Patterson, S. M. (2006). Nicotine and acute stress: Effects of nicotine versus nicotine withdrawal on stress-induced hemoconcentration and cardiovascular reactivity. *Biological Psychology, 71*(2), 191–201. http://doi.org/10.1016/j.biopsycho.2005.04.006

Vanderploeg, R. D., Curtiss, G., & Belanger, H. G. (2005). Long-term neuropsychological outcomes following mild traumatic brain injury. *Journal of the International Neuropsychological Society, 11*(3), 228–236. http://doi.org/10.1017/S1355617705050289

Van Gerven, P. W. M., Van Boxtel, M. P. J., Meijer, W. A., Willems, D., & Jolles, J. (2007). On the relative role of inhibition in age-related working memory decline. *Aging, Neuropsychology, and Cognition, 14*(1), 95–107. http://doi.org/10.1080/138255891007038

Vollmer, T., Huynh, L., Kelley, C., Galebach, P., Signorovitch, J., DiBernardo, A., & Sasane, R. (2016). Relationship between brain volume loss and cognitive outcomes among patients with multiple sclerosis: A systematic literature review. *Neurological Sciences, 37*(2), 165–179. http://doi.org/10.1007/s10072-015-2400-1

Walker, L. A. S., Berard, J. A., Berrigan, L. I., Rees, L. M., & Freedman, M. S. (2012). Detecting cognitive fatigue in multiple sclerosis: Method matters. *Journal of the Neurological Sciences, 316*(1–2), 86–92. http://doi.org/10.1016/j.jns.2012.01.021

Ward, T. (1997). A note of caution for clinicians using the Paced Auditory Serial Addition Task. *British Journal of Clinical Psychology, 36*(2), 303–307. https://doi.org/10.1111/j.2044-8260.1997.tb01417.x

Warlop, N. P., Achten, E., Fieremans, E., Debruyne, J., & Vingerhoets, G. (2009). Transverse diffusivity of cerebral parenchyma predicts visual tracking performance in relapsing–remitting multiple sclerosis. *Brain and Cognition, 71*(3), 410–415. http://doi.org/10.1016/j.bandc.2009.05.004

Whelan, R., Lonergan, R., Kiiski, H., Nolan, H., Kinsella, K., Hutchinson, M., . . . Reilly, R. B. (2010). Impaired information processing speed and attention allocation in multiple sclerosis patients versus controls: A high-density EEG study. *Journal of the Neurological Sciences, 293*(1–2), 45–50. http://doi.org/10.1016/j.jns.2010.03.010

White, J. N., Hutchens, T. A., & Lubar, J. F. (2005). Quantitative EEG assessment during neuropsychological task performance in adults with attention deficit hyperactivity disorder. *Journal of Adult Development, 12*(2–3), 113–121. https://doi.org/10.1007/s10804-005-7027

Wiens, A. N., Fuller, K. H., & Crossen, J. R. (1997). Paced Auditory Serial Addition Test: Adult norms and moderator variables. *Journal of Clinical and Experimental Neuropsychology, 19*(4), 473–483. http://doi.org/10.1080/01688639708403737

Wills, S., & Leathem, J. (2004). The Effects of test anxiety, age, intelligence level, and arithmetic ability on Paced Auditory Serial Addition Test performance. *Applied Neuropsychology, 11*(4), 178–185. http://doi.org/10.1207/s15324826an1104_2

Wingenfeld, S. A., Holdwick, D. J. J., Davis, J. L., & Hunter, B. B. (1999). Normative data on computerized paced auditory serial addition task performance. *The Clinical Neuropsychologist, 13*(3), 268–273. http://doi.org/10.1076/clin.13.3.268.1736

Yu, H. J., Christodoulou, C., Bhise, V., Greenblatt, D., Patel, Y., Serafin, D., . . . Wagshul, M. E. (2012). Multiple white matter tract abnormalities underlie cognitive impairment in RRMS. *NeuroImage, 59*(4), 3713–3722. http://doi.org/10.1016/j.neuroimage.2011.10.053

RUFF 2 & 7 SELECTIVE ATTENTION TEST (2 & 7 TEST)

TEST NAME	**Ruff 2 & 7 Selective Attention Test (2 & 7 Test)**
DOMAIN	Attention
AGE RANGE	16 to 90 years
ADMINISTRATION TIME	5 minutes
SCORING FORMAT	Hand scored
REFERENCE	Ruff, R. M., & Allen, C. C. (1996). *Ruff 2 & 7 Selective Attention Test Professional Manual*. Odessa, FL: Psychological Assessment Resources, Inc. www.parinc.com

DESCRIPTION

The Ruff 2 & 7 Selective Attention Test (2 & 7 Test; Ruff & Allen, 1996) is a test of sustained and selective attention. The test is based on the premise that selective attention (i.e., the ability to select relevant stimuli while ignoring irrelevant information) can be evaluated by comparing automatic and controlled processing with minimal demands on other cognitive processes such as memory (Cicerone & Azulay, 2002). The test is based on the theories of Logan et al. (Logan, 1988; Logan & Klapp, 1991; Logan & Stadler, 1991), which posit two processes through which attention is allocated: automatic processing and effortful processing.

The test is a paper-and-pencil cancellation task that consists of a set of 20 trials administered consecutively in 15-second intervals. For each trial, the examinee is asked to make a line through specific targets (always the numbers 2 and 7) while ignoring other letters or numbers (see Figure 8–5).

Two types of trials are presented: *Automatic Detection* trials, where the target numbers are presented among distractor letters, and *Controlled Search* trials, where the target numbers are presented among distractor numbers. According to the authors, target selection is automatic in the first condition because targets (numbers) differ categorically from distractors (letters). This categorical difference between letters and numbers is overlearned and is thus subject to automatic processing even in individuals with limited literacy levels (Ruff & Allen, 1996). In the second condition, because both targets and numbers belong to the same stimulus category (numbers), working memory and effortful processing of stimulus characteristics are required to effectively select targets from distractors.

ADMINISTRATION

See Source for details. There are 10 Automatic Detection trials and 10 Controlled Search trials, presented semi-randomly in the test booklet. Instructions are provided verbatim. Test items are presented on the back of the Test Booklet. Each of the 20 trials consists of a line of alphanumeric characters; the examinee is given 15 seconds to cross out as many targets as possible within the time limit, working from left to right. After 15 seconds, the examiner indicates the end of the trial by saying "Next," and the examinee must begin canceling targets on the next line.

SCORING

Several scores can be derived from the test, which are derived from the concept of errors of omission (hits) and commission (incorrect responses). A summary and description of test scores is shown in Table 8–41 (see also manual).

Scoring involves first determining the number of hits (i.e., the number of targets correctly identified among the 10 possible targets for each row); this is called the Speed score. The Accuracy score is based on hits as well as the

```
2 G O X C 7 M J 7 H Z R N G A S 2 Y W Q 2 L H B Z G J N V 7 E T 2 P R V M J
H S T Q 2 C 7 K L W C 7 X M T 7 K T R 2 A V P I W O C 2 G J 7 L S 2 B N V W
7 T O X R 2 P H 7 F D A B M 2 W H K A S T 2 O P H W E D 2 T R N E Q X 2 P K

3 1 0 7 8 9 4 4 7 0 5 3 7 6 3 8 1 5 2 3 6 5 6 9 7 0 8 9 1 5 7 8 4 3 6 2 8 6
3 2 8 6 1 5 4 2 8 0 7 1 2 9 1 8 9 2 8 1 3 7 6 4 5 3 7 8 0 4 6 7 9 6 2 9 1 2
8 3 9 1 8 3 7 8 9 4 6 5 9 1 4 7 0 8 6 7 1 3 0 3 9 7 0 2 3 3 8 9 4 1 2 6 5 5
```

Figure 8–5 *Sample item from the Ruff 2 & 7 Test.*

SOURCE: Ruff et al. (1992); see manual for instructions.

TABLE 8–41 Summary and Description of Ruff 2 & 7 Scores

CONSTRUCT	2 & 7 TEST VARIABLE	COMPUTATION OF VARIABLES
Sustained Attention	Total Speed	Sum of Automatic Detection Speed T score and Controlled Search Speed T score
	Total Accuracy	Sum of Automatic Detection Accuracy T score and Controlled Search Accuracy T score
Selective Attention	Automatic Detection Speed (ADS)	Total number of targets correctly identified on the 10 Letter trials
	Automatic Detection Accuracy (ADA)	Total number of targets correctly identified on the 10 Letter trials, divided by the number of targets plus errors on the Letter trials, multiplied by 100
	Controlled Search Speed (CSS)	Total number of targets correctly identified on the 10 Digit trials
	Controlled Search Accuracy (CSA)	Total number of targets correctly identified on the 10 Digit trials, divided by the number of targets plus errors on the Digit trials, multiplied by 100
Discrepancy Analysis	Speed Difference	Automatic Detection Speed T score minus Controlled Search Speed T score
	Accuracy Difference	Automatic Detection Accuracy T score minus Controlled Search Accuracy T score
	Total Difference	Total Speed T score minus Total Accuracy T score

SOURCE: From Ruff and Allen (1996). Reproduced by special permission of the Publisher, Psychological Assessment Resources, Inc. (PAR), 16204 North Florida Avenue, Lutz, Florida 33549, from the Ruff 2&7 Test by Ronald Ruff, PhD, Copyright 1986, 1996 by PAR. Further reproduction is prohibited without permission of PAR.

Error score. The latter includes errors of omission (i.e., missed targets, which are only counted for those characters prior to the examinee's last correct response) and errors of commission (incorrectly identified targets or false alarms). Sustained attention is measured primarily by the Total Speed and Total Accuracy scores, and selective attention is measured by the Automatic Detection and Controlled Search scores.

DEMOGRAPHIC EFFECTS

AGE

Age is moderately correlated with Automatic Detection Speed and Controlled Search Speed scores (r = –.41 and –.38, respectively; see manual, also Knight et al., 2010). Age is correlated with speed in normative studies (Caban-Holt et al., 2012; Messinis et al., 2007). Note that "speed" in this context refers to number of targets rather than response time per se. Age effects on accuracy measures are reported less often (although see Knight et al., 2010).

GENDER

No significant gender differences are found (see Source; Knight et al., 2010; Messinis et al., 2007).

EDUCATION AND IQ

There are education effects on performance; these are relatively small for Automatic Detection Speed and Controlled Search Speed scores, as reported in the manual (rs = .19 to .24). Speed scores also show relationships with education in more recent studies (Caban-Holt et al., 2012; Messinis et al., 2007). Education may contribute to higher test-retest gains (see the section "Practice Effects"). Relations between education and accuracy are reported less often, but were found between education and Automatic Detection Accuracy by Messinis et al. (2007) and Caban-Holt et al. (2012).

Correlations with Full-Scale IQ (FSIQ) are negligible (Ruff & Allen, 1996). However, when demographically corrected scores are considered, modest correlations with performance IQ are found in healthy controls (rs = .22 to .25). No significant correlations between the National Adult Reading Test and the Ruff 2 & 7 were obtained in a sample of healthy, older, well-educated adults (Knight et al., 2010).

ETHNICITY, NATIONALITY, AND LINGUISTIC EFFECTS

Caban-Holt et al. (2012) reported some group differences on Automatic Detection Accuracy (i.e., Caucasian men performed better than African-American men), estimated at a relatively small magnitude of approximately 2% in raw score metrics.

NORMATIVE DATA

STANDARDIZATION SAMPLE

The standardization sample is described in Table 8–42. Because gender does not affect test scores, norms are presented by age and education in the manual. Limited information is presented in the manual regarding ethnicity composition and data collection procedures. Norms were developed by using demographically corrected T scores in a method similar to that used by Heaton, Grant, and Matthews (1991) for the Halstead-Reitan Battery. No demographic corrections were made for the Accuracy scores due to the lack of significant age or education effects on this variable.

OTHER NORMATIVE DATASETS

Caban-Holt et al. (2012) provide age- and education-adjusted normative data for the Ruff 2 & 7 in older men. The mean age was 69.5 (+/–5.7 years; Table 8–43). Age midpoints for normative data of 65, 70, 75, and 82.5

TABLE 8–42 Characteristics of the Ruff 2 & 7 Test Normative Sample

Sample size	360
Age	16 to 70 years[b]
Geographic location	65% California 30% Michigan 5% Eastern Seaboard
Sample Type	Recruited as part of larger standardization study[a]
Education	7 to 22 years[c]
Socioeconomic status	Not reported
Gender	50% Men
Men	50% Women
Ethnicity	Details not reported[d]
Screening	Exclusion based on reported history of psychiatric disorder, substance abuse, or neurological disorder

[a]San Diego Neuropsychological Test Battery (Baser & Ruff, 1987; Ruff & Crouch, 1991).

[b]Four age groups (16 to 24, 25 to 39, 40 to 54, and 55 to 70 years).

[c]Three educational bands (≤ 12 years, 13 to 15 years, ≥ 16 years); proportions within each age band are not reported.

[d]Sample "roughly approximated the 1980 US census proportions with regards to race" (manual, p. 13).

were used. There were only six participants older than 85. Accuracy and Speed scores, adjusted for age and education, are listed in Tables 8–44 through 8–47. Importantly, the authors report that using the normative data from the original standardization sample provided in the manual resulted in a much higher classification of adults older than 70 years as impaired compared to use of their data. The difference in classification of impairment (T score ≤39) is most pronounced for Controlled Search Speed, where nearly 32% of the sample was classified as impaired using original norms versus approximately 13% using their expanded norms.

Messinis et al. (2007) present normative data for 218 Greek adults. Sample characteristics are summarized in Table 8–48, with normative data in Table 8–49. Norms were stratified by age and education, with three age groups identified (17–39, 40–59, and 60–80 years of age) and levels of education stratified to reflect school system structure in Greece (1–9, 10–12 [high school], and ≥13 years; e.g., technological and other university-level education).

Knight et al. (2010) present normative data for older adults. Sample characteristics are in Table 8–50 with normative data in Table 8–51. The sample was of high IQ on average (NART-predicted WAIS-R score mean 113.23, *SD* = 8.63).

TABLE 8–43 Characteristics of the Caban-Holt et al. (2012) Ruff 2 & 7 Normative Sample

Sample size	415
Age	60 to 90 years
Geographic location	United States (medical centers in Mid-Atlantic, Southeast, Midwest, West)
Sample Type	Recruited as part of other studies[a]
Education	19% High school 27% College 54% College or more
Gender	100% Men 0% Women
Ethnicity	68% Caucasian 25% African American 4% Other
Screening	Exclusion based on study criteria (e.g., absence of prostate cancer, stroke, hypertension, dementia, memory impairment, and neurologic conditions; on stable medications)

[a]PREADVISE trial; vitamin E and selenium trial for Alzheimer's disease.

EVIDENCE FOR RELIABILITY

EVIDENCE FOR INTERNAL RELIABILITY

Internal reliability for the standardization sample is high (all coefficients ≥.80; see manual). Coefficients for Controlled Search and Automatic Detection Speed scores are especially strong (i.e., >.95). Standard errors of measurement (*SEMs*) based on alpha coefficients for Accuracy scores are relatively small (approximately 4 points; see manual). *SEMs* for each age group for the Speed scores range from 1 to 2 T score points. When generalizability coefficients are used as the basis of calculation, *SEM* estimates are lower (i.e., 1–3 points).

EVIDENCE FOR TEST-RETEST RELIABILITY, MEASURING CHANGE, AND PRACTICE EFFECTS

Most variables have adequate to high reliability. Overall, test-retest reliability is higher for Speed compared to Accuracy scores (Ruff & Allen, 1996). Stability estimates are based on 120 individuals from the normative sample with a retest interval of six months (i.e., five participants from each of the 24 subgroups defined by age, education, and gender). Speed scores are associated with very high stability coefficients ($r \geq .90$), Controlled Search Accuracy with high estimates (*rs* = .80 to .89), and Automatic Detection Accuracy with adequate coefficients (*rs* = .70 to .79). When generalizability coefficients are examined, most scores are associated with very high reliability (e.g., ≥ .90), with Automatic Detection Accuracy associated with high reliability (.80 to .89).

Over repeated sessions, reliability is excellent for some scores but not others, at least in older adults. Lemay, Bedard, Rouleau, and Tremblay (2004) administered the test three times to older adults, with intersession intervals of 14 days. Correlation coefficients exceeded .85 for Speed scores (ICC >.81), with low estimates for Accuracy scores (*rs* = .34 to .86; *ICCs* .50 to .68). The authors therefore suggested that use of Accuracy scores for repeat assessments should be avoided.

TABLE 8-44 Normative Data for Ruff 2 & 7 Automatic Detection Speed (ADS)

		AGE RANGES				
		60 TO 70	65 TO 75	70 TO 80	75 TO 90	T-SCORE
EDUCATION LEVEL	CLINICAL INTERPRETATION	65	70	75	82.5	RANGE
High School or Less	Above Average	142–300	130–300	127–300	124–300	≥55
	Average	112–141	100–129	97–126	94–123	45–54
	Below Average	97–111	86–99	83–96	80–93	40–44
	Mildly Impaired	83–96	71–85	68–82	65–79	35–39
	Mildly-to-Moderately Impaired	68–82	56–70	53–67	50–64	30–34
	Moderately Impaired	53–67	41–55	38–52	35–49	25–29
	Moderately-to-Severely Impaired	38–52	26–40	23–37	20–34	20–24
	Severely Impaired	0–37	0–25	0–22	0–19	≤19
Some College	Above Average	151–300	145–300	130–300	124–300	≥55
	Average	121–150	115–144	100–129	94–123	45–54
	Below Average	106–120	100–114	86–99	80–93	40–44
	Mildly Impaired	91–105	86–99	71–85	65–79	35–39
	Mildly-to-Moderately Impaired	77–90	71–85	56–70	50–64	30–34
	Moderately Impaired	62–76	56–70	41–55	35–49	25–29
	Moderately-to-Severely Impaired	47–61	41–55	26–40	20–34	20–24
	Severely Impaired	0–46	0–40	0–25	0–19	≤19
College or More	Above Average	160–300	151–300	139–300	124–300	≥55
	Average	130–159	118–150	109–138	94–123	45–54
	Below Average	115–129	103–117	94–108	80–93	40–44
	Mildly Impaired	100–114	88–102	80–93	65–79	35–39
	Mildly-to-Moderately Impaired	86–99	74–87	65–79	50–64	30–34
	Moderately Impaired	71–85	59–73	50–64	35–49	25–29
	Moderately-to-Severely Impaired	56–70	44–58	35–49	20–34	20–24
	Severely Impaired	0–55	0–43	0–34	0–19	≤19

SOURCE: From Caban-Holt et al. (2012).

TABLE 8-45 Normative Data for Ruff 2 & 7 Controlled Search Speed (CSS)

		AGE RANGES				
		60 TO 70	65 TO 75	70 TO 80	75 TO 90	T-SCORE
EDUCATION LEVEL	CLINICAL INTERPRETATION	65	70	75	82.5	RANGE
High School or Less	Above Average	122–300	115–300	113–300	113–300	≥55
	Average	99–121	93–114	90–112	90–112	45–54
	Below Average	88–98	81–92	79–89	79–89	40–44
	Mildly Impaired	77–87	70–80	67–78	67–78	35–39
	Mildly-to-Moderately Impaired	65–76	58–69	56–66	56–66	30–34
	Moderately Impaired	54–64	47–57	45–55	45–55	25–29
	Moderately-to-Severely Impaired	42–53	35–46	33–44	33–44	20–24
	Severely Impaired	0–41	0–34	0–32	0–32	≤19
Some College	Above Average	129–300	125–300	118–300	113–300	≥55
	Average	106–128	102–124	95–117	90–112	45–54
	Below Average	95–105	90–101	83–94	79–89	40–44
	Mildly Impaired	83–94	79–89	72–82	67–78	35–39
	Mildly-to-Moderately Impaired	72–82	67–78	61–71	56–66	30–34
	Moderately Impaired	61–71	56–66	49–60	45–55	25–29
	Moderately-to-Severely Impaired	49–60	45–55	38–48	33–44	20–24
	Severely Impaired	0–48	0–44	0–37	0–32	≤19
College or More	Above Average	134–300	127–300	118–300	113–300	≥55
	Average	111–133	104–126	95–117	90–112	45–54
	Below Average	99–110	93–103	83–94	79–89	40–44
	Mildly Impaired	88–98	81–92	72–82	67–78	35–39
	Mildly-to-Moderately Impaired	77–87	70–80	61–71	56–66	30–34
	Moderately Impaired	65–76	58–69	49–60	45–55	25–29
	Moderately-to-Severely Impaired	54–64	47–57	38–48	33–44	20–24
	Severely Impaired	0–53	0–46	0–37	0–32	≤19

SOURCE: From Caban-Holt et al. (2012).

TABLE 8–46 Normative Data for Ruff 2 & 7 Automatic Detection Accuracy (ADA)

EDUCATION LEVEL	CLINICAL INTERPRETATION	RAW SCORES	T-SCORE RANGE
High School or Less	Above Average	97.34–100.00	≥55
	Average	93.89–97.33	45–54
	Below Average	92.16–93.88	40–44
	Mildly Impaired	90.44–92.15	35–39
	Mildly-to-Moderately Impaired	88.71–90.43	30–34
	Moderately Impaired	96.99–88.70	25–29
	Moderately-to-Severely Impaired	85.26–86.98	20–24
	Severely Impaired	0.00–85.25	≤19
Some College	Above Average	98.37–100.00	≥55
	Average	94.92–98.36	45–54
	Below Average	93.20–94.91	40–44
	Mildly Impaired	91.47–93.19	35–39
	Mildly-to-Moderately Impaired	89.75–91.46	30–34
	Moderately Impaired	88.02–89.74	25–29
	Moderately-to-Severely Impaired	86.30–88.01	20–24
	Severely Impaired	0.00–86.29	≤19
College or More	Above Average	98.37–100.00	≥55
	Average	94.92–98.36	45–44
	Below Average	93.20–94.91	40–44
	Mildly Impaired	91.47–93.19	35–39
	Mildly-to-Moderately Impaired	89.75–91.46	30–34
	Moderately Impaired	88.02–89.74	25–29
	Moderately-to-Severely Impaired	86.30–88.01	20–24
	Severely Impaired	0.00–86.29	≤19

SOURCE: From Caban-Holt et al. (2012).

Messinis et al. (2007) reported similar results. Test-retest reliability was very high for Speed scores (e.g., $r \geq .94$). Accuracy scores were more variable, with Automatic Detection Accuracy showing high reliability in 20- to 39-year-olds ($n = 16$; $r = .89$) and adequate reliability in older age groups (40- to 59-year-olds, $r = .73$; 60- to 71-year-olds, $r = .78$). Controlled Search Accuracy was high in the younger age groups (20- to 39-year-olds, $r = .87$; 40- to 59-year-olds, $r = .80$), and adequate for oldest age group (60- to 71-year-olds, $r = .76$). Of note, cell sizes were small ($n = 11$ to 16).

TABLE 8–47 Normative Data for Ruff 2 & 7 Controlled Search Accuracy (CSA)

CLINICAL INTERPRETATION	RAW SCORES	T-SCORE RANGE
Above Average	95.73–100.00	≥55
Average	90.71–95.72	45–54
Below Average	88.20–90.70	40–44
Mildly Impaired	85.69–88.19	35–39
Mildly-to-Moderately Impaired	83.18–85.68	30–34
Moderately Impaired	80.67–83.17	25–29
Moderately-to-Severely Impaired	78.16–80.66	20–24
Severely Impaired	0.00–78.15	≤19

SOURCE: From Caban-Holt et al. (2012).

TABLE 8–48 Characteristics of the Ruff 2 & 7 Messinis et al. (2007) Greek Normative Sample

Sample size	218[a]
Age	17 to 80 years old ($M = 45.07$, $SD = 17.45$)
Geographic location	Greece[b]
Sample type	Sample of convenience
Education	2 to 21 years of formal education ($M = 13.01$, $SD = 4.20$)
Gender	44% Men 56% Women
Ethnicity	Not reported
Screening	Exclusion based on history of psychiatric, neurological, substance abuse/dependence, physical (e.g., cardiovascular disease, uncorrected visual impairment), non-native Greek speaker, Mini-Mental State Examination (MMSE) cutoff score.

[a] For purposes of investigating discriminative validity, two clinical groups (26 people who had completed detoxification for opioid use disorders and 23 persons with human immunodeficiency virus, HIV) were also included separately.

[b] Two large urban centers.

In their large sample ($n = 234$) of healthy older adults, Knight et al. (2010) reported high test-retest reliability for Speed scores ($r \geq .83$). Accuracy scores were associated with marginal reliability coefficients ($r = .63$ Controlled Search, $r = .64$ Automatic Detection). The authors suggest that poor reliability of Accuracy scores may have been related to ceiling effects, as few participants in their sample made errors.

Ruff et al. (1986) reported preliminary data showing that practice effects are approximately 10 raw score points in magnitude. In their large sample of healthy older adults, Knight et al. (2010) reported lower but large practice effects nonetheless, only for speeded conditions (6.1 for Automatic Detection; 3.4 for Controlled Search). Messinis et al. (2007) provided test-retest data on a subsample of 40 healthy Greek adults (47% female, 20 to 71 years old; M education = 15.1 years, $SD = 2.9$ years), with a test-retest interval of 12 to 14 weeks. Speed scores showed a practice effect, with Accuracy scores showing practice effects only in the 20- to 39-year-old age group. Of note, Lemay et al. (2004) report that test-retest gains drop considerably after the second test session. In terms of demographic influences on practice effects, education is positively correlated with greater test-retest gains across testing sessions for Speed scores ($r = .37$; Lemay et al., 2004). However, this may be due to age (52 to 80 years) and sample size restrictions.

Knight et al. (2010) presented reliable change indices based on a large sample ($n = 234$) of healthy adults older than 65 years, at a test-retest interval of approximately one year (Table 8–52). To interpret significance of a change score in an older adult, first calculate the individuals change score, and compare this change to the data provided. For

TABLE 8-49 Ruff 2 & 7 Normative Data for Greek Adults

	AGE								
	17 TO 39 YEARS			40 TO 59 YEARS			60+ YEARS		
	EDUCATION (YEARS)			EDUCATION (YEARS)			EDUCATION (YEARS)		
	1–9	10–12	13+	1–9	10–12	13+	1–9	10–12	13+
	–	*N* = 17	*N* = 70	*N* = 16	*N* = 19	*N* = 33	*N* = 31	*N* = 16	*N* = 16
Automatic Detection Speed									
Percentile 5th	–	120.0	127.0	82.0	78.0	111.0	60.0	103.0	94.0
25th	–	155.0	166.0	100.0	141.0	142.0	84.0	115.0	115.5
50th	–	175.0	186.0	144.5	156.0	163.0	96.0	127.0	147.5
75th	–	194.0	208.0	167.0	172.0	177.0	115.0	131.0	154.0
95th	–	220.0	229.0	184.0	187.0	207.0	147.0	192.0	194.0
M	–	170.9	185.1	135.7	154.2	158.8	98.3	127.7	141.6
SD	–	30.5	31.7	34.3	27.5	28.3	26.6	20.7	31.3
Automatic Detection Accuracy									
Percentile 5th	–	82.1	90.3	47.1	78.5	90.2	80.6	88.4	89.2
25th	–	96.4	97.3	93.5	88.6	93.4	83.0	96.2	94.9
50th	–	97.6	98.5	97.3	94.8	96.7	92.3	97.3	96.3
75th	–	98.9	99.3	99.1	97.1	98.2	96.7	98.1	96.9
95th	–	100.0	100.0	100.0	99.4	99.3	99.2	100.0	100.0
M	–	96.7	97.3	93.1	92.9	95.0	90.1	96.7	95.8
SD	–	4.2	3.4	12.8	5.4	6.5	7.5	2.6	2.3
Controlled Search Speed									
Percentile 5th	–	97.0	107.0	70.0	68.0	97.0	51.0	86.0	88.0
25th	–	116.0	134.0	98.5	116.0	121.0	72.0	102.0	97.5
50th	–	140.0	148.5	117.0	129.0	136.0	82.0	110.5	119.5
75th	–	157.0	166.0	125.5	140.0	154.0	111.0	120.0	150.0
95th	–	193.0	187.0	142.0	147.0	167.0	116.0	151.0	155.0
M	–	139.9	150.4	112.2	124.8	135.3	86.5	111.1	121.2
SD	–	29.5	26.2	19.8	20.3	22.2	22.4	15.7	25.8
Controlled Search Accuracy									
Percentile 5th	–	73.2	84.6	57.1	66.5	79.9	81.2	89.8	82.8
25th	–	90.9	90.7	89.3	83.5	87.5	85.5	91.3	88.5
50th	–	93.5	93.8	91.2	91.0	93.7	90.7	95.6	93.1
75th	–	95.1	97.3	97.2	95.2	96.0	93.0	97.8	94.4
95th	–	97.5	99.2	100.0	99.3	98.8	97.5	99.2	96.4
M	–	91.6	92.9	90.0	88.1	91.2	89.6	94.9	
SD	–	5.9	6.0	10.2	9.4	8.2	4.9	3.5	4.4

SOURCE: From Messinis et al. (2007).

TABLE 8-50 Characteristics of Knight et al. (2010) Ruff 2 & 7 Normative Sample of Older Adults

Sample size	234
Age	66 to 93 (M = 74.66, *SD* = 5.75)
Geographic location	New Zealand
Sample type	Participating in a study investigating the effect of lowering homocysteine via dietary supplementation in New Zealand
Education	38% Vocational Diploma 14% University
Gender	45% Men 55% Women
Ethnicity	99% self-identified as "European"
Screening	Exclusion based on neurologic conditions, medications known to interfere with folate metabolism, Center for Epidemiologic Studies-Depression (CES-D) cutoff score, psychiatric conditions, major medical condition (e.g., renal disease, diabetes, cancer), MMSE cutoff score.

example (as provided by Knight et al., 2010), if an examinee shows Automatic Detection change from 126 to 102, this represents a decline of 24. According to the table, the decline of 24 can be interpreted as a larger decline than 98% of the sample.

EVIDENCE FOR VALIDITY

FACTOR-ANALYTIC STUDIES AND RELATIONSHIPS WITH OTHER TESTS

Studies generally support relationships between the Ruff 2 & 7 and processing speed and attention; relationships with memory, executive function, intelligence, and general cognition are overall not as strong. Ruff and Allen (1996) report that three main factors are found in healthy adults: speed of processing (Speed scores), controlled processing (Speed Difference, Accuracy Difference, Controlled Search Accuracy), and automatic processing (Automatic Detection Accuracy, Accuracy Difference).

TABLE 8–51 Ruff 2 & 7 Normative Data for Older Adults

AGE RANGE	65 TO 69 (N = 59) *M*	*SD*	70 TO 74 (N = 87) *M*	*SD*	75 TO 79 (N = 59) *M*	*SD*	80+ (N = 46) *M*	*SD*
Automatic Detection								
Speed	112.6	24.9	106.3	20.2	101.1	19.6	85.3	23.7
Accuracy	4.8	7.3	3.8	3.8	4.7	3.7	4.9	4.7
Accuracy (%)	96.2	4.1	96.6	3.2	95.5	3.5	94.4	5.9
Controlled Search								
Speed	102.8	19.3	98.2	16.4	94.0	15.6	81.9	19.8
Accuracy	6.6	6.3	6.8	6.4	8.2	5.3	7.8	5.7
Accuracy (%)	94.2	4.4	93.7	5.1	91.9	5.0	91.5	5.8
Speed Difference	9.85	11.85	8.14	8.05	7.05	8.10	3.46	6.91

NOTE: Speed Difference Controlled Search Speed — Automatic Detection Speed.
SOURCE: From Knight et al. (2010).

Processing speed is an important contributor to performance. When demographically corrected scores are considered, the Ruff 2 & 7 is most highly correlated with Digit Symbol in healthy controls (*r* = .35 to .40). Smaller correlations are found with block span tests (*r* = .18 to .24) and with trail learning tests (Baser & Ruff, 1987).

The test is also related to attention. For example, the Ruff 2 & 7 appears to correlate highly with other selective attention tests from the Test of Everyday Attention (TEA) in patients with TBI (*r* = .62 and –.69, for Map Search and Telephone Search, respectively; Bate et al., 2001). Significant correlations with TEA subtests measuring different attentional components such as attentional switching, divided attention, and sustained attention, although not as large, are also substantial (*rs* = .30 to –.57). PCA of the Ruff 2 & 7 and other tests of attention indicates that the test loads on a visual selective attention factor, along with measures such as the Stroop, SDMT, and selective attention tests from the TEA (i.e., Map Search and Telephone Search; Bate et al., 2001). In a mixed group of patients with schizophrenia and TBI, Controlled Search Speed loaded on an attention factor, and the Speed Difference score loaded on a planning and flexibility factor (Baser & Ruff, 1987).

Small correlations are reported between the Ruff 2 & 7 and other domains. Small correlations with word fluency are reported (*r* = .17 to .22), but not with other executive functioning tests such as the Wisconsin Card Sorting Test (WCST). Correlations with motor speed and conventional memory tests, both visual and auditory, are negligible (Ruff & Allen, 1996). However, when present, motor slowing may contribute to lower Speed scores (Ruff, 1994; Ruff & Allen, 1996). Although correlations with the MMSE have been reported (i.e., with Speed scores, *r* = .36, .35; with Accuracy scores *r* = –.18, –.22), the test appears to correlate minimally with IQ overall (see "Demographic Effects").

CLINICAL STUDIES

Accuracy is reportedly lower in the Controlled versus Automatic Detection conditions in individuals with lesions in the frontal lobes compared to those with posterior lesions (*n* = 30; Ruff & Allen, 1996; Ruff et al., 1992). The test also appears sensitive to injury severity in adults with TBI (Allen & Ruff, 1990; Bate et al., 2001), who show selective deficits in Controlled compared to Automatic conditions (although note Dymowski et al., 2015, who found that patients with TBI crossed out fewer targets than controls

TABLE 8–52 Ruff 2 & 7 Reliable Change Indices

	SEM	SE *DIFF*	90% CI DETERIORATE (P = .05)	90% CI IMPROVE (P = .05)	95% CI DETERIORATE (P = .025)	98% CI DETERIORATE (P = .01)
Automatic Detection						
Speed	7.93	11.22	−12.3	24.5	−15.9	−20.0
Accuracy	3.00	4.24	−6.7	7.6	−8.0	−9.6
Accuracy (%)	2.45	3.47	−5.7	5.5	−6.8	−8.1
Controlled Search						
Speed	7.46	10.55	−13.9	20.7	−17.3	−21.2
Accuracy	3.65	5.16	−8.3	8.7	−9.9	−11.8
Accuracy (%)	3.21	4.54	−7.8	7.2	−9.2	−10.9
Speed Difference	5.53	7.82	−10.1	15.6	−12.6	−15.5

NOTE: *SEM*, Standard Error of Measurement; SE *diff*, Standard Error of the Difference; CI, Confidence Interval; Speed Difference – Controlled Search Speed – Automatic Detection Speed.
SOURCE: From Knight et al. (2010).

in both Controlled and Automatic Detection conditions). The Ruff 2 & 7 was found to be a good predictor of return to school or employment after TBI (Ruff et al., 1993). The test has also been used to index cognitive fatigue in patients with TBI (Möller et al., 2014).

Diagnostic accuracy has been examined by Cicerone and Azulay (2002) in a group of patients with PCS and matched controls screened for performance validity. Scores were associated with low sensitivity (Speed 10%, Accuracy 13%), but high specificity (Speed, 100%, Accuracy, 83%). Findings indicate scores have limited utility in ruling in PCS, but high specificity in ruling out PCS (i.e., persons without PCS were unlikely to have impaired scores). PPP of the Speed score was strong (100% vs. 44% for Accuracy scores), indicating the diagnostic utility of impaired scores on the test. NPP was poor (Speed 50%, Accuracy 46%).

The Ruff 2 & 7 has also been used in patients with HIV (Messinis et al., 2007) and AIDS (Schmitt et al., 1988), substance use disorders (Messinis et al., 2007), toxic exposure (Tröster et al., 1991), postural tachycardia syndrome (Arnold et al., 2015), psychiatric conditions (Baser & Ruff, 1987; Judd & Ruff, 1993; Ruff, 1994; Weiss, 1996), evaluation of the effects of working memory training post-stroke (Westerberg et al., 2007), and in incarcerated men (LaDuke et al., 2017).

Null findings have also been reported. No group differences were reported between women with postpartum depression and those without (Messinis et al., 2010), the test was reportedly not related to pain variables in a veteran sample (Legarreta et al., 2016), and performance did not differ between people who meditated compared to those who did not (Lykins et al., 2012).

Of note, the test has shown promise in clinical trials where a rapid assessment protocol that maximizes the likelihood of compliance is needed. This has been demonstrated in the case of an outcome trial for patients with brain metastases, where the test shows an excellent pretreatment compliance rate (≥90%) and adequate posttreatment compliance rate (≥70%) after whole-brain radiation (Regine et al., 2004).

NEUROANATOMICAL CORRELATES AND IMAGING STUDIES

No information is available.

PERFORMANCE VALIDITY

No information is available.

COMMENT

The Ruff 2 & 7 is a brief and portable paper-and-pencil cancellation task that is likely to be understandable by most examinees. Although scores generated are labeled according to "Speed" and "Accuracy" parameters, this is a misnomer to some extent, as Speed scores actually reflect percentage of accurate responses rather than response time per se.

Speed scores are generally affected by age and education, with age and education reportedly exerting less effect on Accuracy scores. Gender differences are not found. Information on the effects of ethnicity and other sociodemographic variables is limited. Normative studies have been published that provide valuable data, especially for older adults (e.g., see Caban-Holt et al., 2012; Knight et al., 2010).

The test is associated with strong internal reliability, especially for Speed scores. Test-retest reliability is also strong for Speed scores. Accuracy scores are typically associated with more variable estimates. Practice effects are reported, especially on Speed scores. Reliable change indices are available, as calculated in a sample of older adults (Knight et al., 2010).

Some factor-analytic and correlational studies provide evidence of convergent and divergent validity, specifically that the Ruff 2 & 7 is associated with processing speed and attention more so than other cognitive domains. The manual also includes a discussion of base rates of impairment in clinical groups, such as persons with cerebral lesions. The test demonstrates decrements in performance in a number of clinical conditions, as may be expected given that many conditions are associated with attentional impairment. However, there is at present not a large and coherent body of literature on this test in any one clinical group.

There are also limitations associated with this test. Normative data provided in the manual are over 20 years old, although more normative data are available, especially for older adults. Accuracy scores are vulnerable to ceiling effects (e.g., 11% of individuals in the normative sample had scores at ceiling on the Automatic Detection and Controlled Search conditions; see also Knight et al., 2010; Lemay et al., 2004). Clinically, errors of omission and errors of commission may provide distinct information, and it may be informative if these were normed separately. Limited information is available on neuroanatomical correlates and performance validity.

REFERENCES

Allen, C. C., & Ruff, R. M. (1990). Self-rating versus neuropsychological performance in moderate versus severe head injury patients. *Brain Injury, 4*, 7–17.

Arnold, A. C., Haman, K., Garland, E. M., Raj, V., Dupont, W. D., Biaggioni, I., . . . Raj, S. R. (2015). Cognitive dysfunction in postural tachycardia syndrome. *Clinical Science, 128*(1), 39–45. https://doi.org/10.1042/CS20140251

Baser, C. A., & Ruff, R. R. (1987). Construct validity of the San Diego Neuropsychological Test Battery. *Archives of Clinical Neuropsychology, 2*, 13–32.

Bate, A. J., Mathias, J. L., & Crawford, J. R. (2001). Performance on the Test of Everyday Attention and standard tests of attention following severe traumatic brain injury. *The Clinical Neuropsychologist, 15*(3), 405–422.

Caban-Holt, A., Abner, E., Kryscio, R. J., Crowley, J. J., & Schmitt, F. A. (2012). Age-expanded normative data for the Ruff 2&7 Selective Attention Test: Evaluating cognition in older males. *The Clinical Neuropsychologist, 26*(5), 751–768. http://doi.org/10.1080/13854046.2012.690451

Cicerone, K. D., & Azulay, J. (2002). Diagnostic utility of attention measures in postconcussion syndrome. *The Clinical Neuropsychologist, 16*(3), 280–289.

Dymowski, A. R., Owens, J. A., Ponsford, J. L., & Willmott, C. (2015). Speed of processing and strategic control of attention after traumatic brain injury. *Journal of Clinical and Experimental Neuropsychology, 37*(10), 1024–1035. https://doi.org/10.1080/13803395.2015.1074663

Heaton, R. K., Grant, I., & Matthews, C. G. (1991). *Comprehensive Norms for an Expanded Halstead-Reitan Battery: Demographic corrections, research findings, and clinical applications*. Odessa, FL: Psychological Assessment Resources.

Judd, P. H., & Ruff, R. M. (1993). Neuropsychological dysfunction in patients with borderline personality disorder. *Journal of Personality Disorders, 7*, 275–284.

Knight, R. G., McMahon, J., Skeaff, C. M., & Green, T. J. (2010). Reliable change indices for the Ruff 2 and 7 Selective Attention Test in older adults. *Applied Neuropsychology, 17*(4), 239–245. http://doi.org/10.1080/09084282.2010.499796

LaDuke, C., DeMatteo, D., Heilbrun, K., Gallo, J., & Swirsky-Sacchetti, T. (2017). The neuropsychological assessment of justice-involved men: Descriptive analysis, preliminary data, and a case for group-specific norms. *Archives of Clinical Neuropsychology, 32*(8), 929–942. https://doi.org/10.1093/arclin/acx042

Legarreta, M., Bueler, E., DiMuzio, J. M., McGlade, E., & Yurgelun-Todd, D. (2016). Pain catastrophizing, perceived pain disability, and pain descriptors in veterans: The association with neuropsychological performance. *Professional Psychology: Research and Practice, 47*(6), 418–426. https://doi.org/10.1037/pro0000104

Lemay, S., Bedard, M.–A., Rouleau, I., & Tremblay, P.–L. G. (2004). Practice effect and test-retest reliability of attentional and executive tests in middle-aged to elderly subjects. *The Clinical Neuropsychologist, 18*(2), 284–302.

Logan, G. D. (1988). Toward an instance theory of automatization. *Psychological Review, 95*, 492–527.

Logan, G. D., & Klapp, S. T. (1991). Automatizing alphabet arithmetic: Is extended practice necessary to produce automaticity? *Journal of Experimental Psychology: Learning, Memory and Cognition, 17*, 179–195.

Logan, G. D., & Stadler, M. A. (1991). Mechanism of performance improvement and consistent mapping memory search: Automaticity or strategy search? *Journal of Experimental Psychology: Learning, Memory, and Cognition, 17*, 478–496.

Lykins, E. L. B., Baer, R. A., & Gottlob, L. R. (2012). Performance-based tests of attention and memory in long-term mindfulness meditators and demographically matched nonmeditators. *Cognitive Therapy and Research, 36*(1), 103–114. https://doi.org/10.1007/s10608-010-9318-y

Messinis, L., Kosmidis, M., Tsakona, I., Georgiou, V., Aretouli, E., & Papathanasopoulos, P. (2007). Ruff 2 and 7 Selective Attention Test: Normative data, discriminant validity and test–retest reliability in Greek adults. *Archives of Clinical Neuropsychology, 22*(6), 773–785. http://doi.org/10.1016/j.acn.2007.06.005

Messinis, L., Vlahou, C. H., Tsapanos, V., Tsapanos, A., Spilioti, D., & Papathanasopoulos, P. (2010). Neuropsychological functioning in postpartum depressed versus nondepressed females and nonpostpartum controls. *Journal of Clinical and Experimental Neuropsychology, 32*(6), 661–666. http://doi.org/10.1080/13803390903468863

Möller, M. C., Nygren de Boussard, C., Oldenburg, C., & Bartfai, A. (2014). An investigation of attention, executive, and psychomotor aspects of cognitive fatigability. *Journal of Clinical and Experimental Neuropsychology, 36*(7), 716–729. https://doi.org/10.1080/13803395.2014.933779

Regine, W. F., Schmitt, F. A., Scott, C. B., Dearth, C., Patchell, R. A., Nichols, R. C., . . . Mehta, M. P. (2004). Feasibility of neurocognitive outcome evaluations in patients with brain metastases in a multi-institutional cooperative group setting: Results of radiation therapy oncology group trial BR-0018. *International Journal of Radiation Oncology and Biology and Physiology 58*(5), 1346–1352.

Ruff, R. M. (1994). What role does depression play on the performance of the Ruff 2 & 7 Selective Attention Test? *Perceptual and Motor Skills, 78*(1), 63–66.

Ruff, R. M., & Allen, C. C. (1996). *Ruff 2 & 7 Selective Attention Test Professional Manual.* Odessa, FL: Psychological Assessment Resources, Inc.

Ruff, R. M., Evans, R. W., & Light, R. H. (1986). Automatic Detection vs Controlled Search: A Paper-and-Pencil Approach. *Perceptual and Motor Skills, 62*(2), 407–416. https://doi.org/10.2466/pms.1986.62.2.407

Ruff, R. M., & Crouch, J. A. (1991). Neuropsychological test instruments in clinical trials. In E. Mohr & P. Brouwers (Eds.), *Handbook of clinical trials: The neurobehavioral approach* (pp. 89–119). Lisse, The Netherlands: Swets & Zeitlinger.

Ruff, R. M., Marshall, L. F., Crouch, J. A., Klauber, M. R., Levin, H. S., Barth, J. T., . . . Marmarou, A. (1993). Predictors of outcome following severe head injury: Follow-up data from the TCDB. *Brain Injury, 7*, 101–111.

Ruff, R. M., Neimann, H., Allen, C. C., Farrow, C. E., & Wylie, T. (1992). The Ruff 2 & 7 Selective Attention Test: A neuropsychological application. *Perceptual and Motor Skills, 75*(3, Pt 2), 1311–1319.

Schmitt, F. A., Bigley, J. W., McKinnis, R., Logue, P. E., Evans, R. W., Drucker, J. L., & the AZT Collaborative Working Group. (1988). Neuropsychological outcome of Zidovudine (AZT) treatment of patients with AIDS and AIDS-related complex. *New England Journal of Medicine, 319*, 1573–1578.

Tröster, A. I., Ruff, R. M., & Watson, D. P. (1991). Dementia as a neuropsychological consequence of chronic occupational exposure to polychlorinated biphenyls (PCBs). *Archives of Clinical Neuropsychology, 6*, 301–318.

Weiss, K. M. (1996). A simple clinical assessment of attention in schizophrenia. *Psychiatry Research, 60*, 147–154.

Westerberg, H., Jacobaeus, H., Hirvikoski, T., Clevberger, P., Östensson, M.–L., Bartfai, A., & Klingberg, T. (2007). Computerized working memory training after stroke–A pilot study. *Brain Injury, 21*(1), 21–29. http://doi.org/10.1080/02699050601148726

SYMBOL DIGIT MODALITIES TEST (SDMT)

TEST NAME	**Symbol Digit Modalities Test (SDMT)**
DOMAIN	Attention
AGE RANGE	In adults, to 91 years
ADMINISTRATION TIME	5 minutes
SCORING FORMAT	Hand scored
REFERENCE	Smith, A. (1991). *Symbol Digit Modalities Test*. Los Angeles, CA: Western Psychological Services. www.wpspublish.com

DESCRIPTION

The Symbol Digit Modalities Test (SDMT; Smith, 1991) has been used as a test of divided attention (Ponsford & Kinsella, 1992) but also requires complex visual scanning and tracking (Shum et al., 1990), perceptual speed, motor speed, and memory (Laux & Lane, 1985). The test was originally published in 1973 as a screening measure for cerebral dysfunction. The original task can be found in the Army Beta Test and originated even earlier, in 1915 (Tulsky et al., 2003). A coding key is presented consisting of nine abstract symbols, each paired with a number, and the examinee is asked to scan the key and write down the number corresponding to each symbol as quickly as possible. The test can be administered either in written or oral form. Group administration of the written form is also possible.

Wechsler reversed the task requirements to create the Digit Symbol or Coding subtest (i.e., the examinee must write down the symbol rather than the digit). Because SDMT responses consist of overlearned numbers, the written response is simpler than that required by Digit Symbol/Coding. However, from an attentional perspective, Digit Symbol may be somewhat easier than the SDMT (Glosser et al., 1977). On Digit Symbol/Coding, cues to spatial location are contained in the key since stimulus items (numbers) are arranged in arithmetic progression across the page. In the case of the SDMT, the sequence of symbols is random, with no cues to spatial location in the key (Glosser et al., 1977).

Alternate forms have been developed (e.g., Royer, 1971; Royer et al., 1981; Tung et al., 2016; Uchiyama et al., 1994). Uchiyama et al. (1994) also provide an incidental learning version, whereby a line of 15 symbols is provided after standard administration, and the examinee is asked to fill in the number associated with the symbols from memory. The SDMT has also been adapted for computer use (e.g., Feinstein et al., 1994), including versions adapted as part of computerized assessment packages (e.g., CNS Vital Signs) and those aimed at evaluating sports-related concussion such as the Immediate Post-Concussion Assessment and Cognitive Testing (ImPACT; Maroon et al., 2000) and the Concussion Resolution Index (CRI; Erlanger et al., 2003). Tung et al. (2016) provide a tablet-based version, which has shown promise in patients with stroke and schizophrenia (see the section "Evidence for Reliability").

ADMINISTRATION

Administration instructions are provided in the manual. When administering both oral and written forms of the test, the recommended procedure is to give the written version first. Importantly, dysarthria has been shown to partially, but not fully, account for variance in performance on the oral SDMT in patients with MS (approximately 33% performance reduction; Smith & Arnett, 2007), suggesting that oral motor speed may partially confound performance in some patients. A significant relationship between visual acuity and performance in MS patients with reportedly adequate vision has been reported ($r = .37$; Bruce et al., 2007), suggesting that mild visual acuity deficits may negatively impact performance. People with MS perform more slowly on the paper-based than computer-based version (Hughes et al., 2013). The oral administration of the test has been positively reviewed as a measure for use in persons with upper limb dysfunction (see Jaywant et al., 2016).

SCORING

The number of correct responses within the 90-second interval is recorded. The maximum score is 110 on each form (i.e., written and oral). SDMT scores 1 to 1.5 *SD* below the mean are considered suggestive of impairment according to the manual (Smith, 1991).

DEMOGRAPHIC EFFECTS

AGE

SDMT scores decline with advancing age on written and oral forms in healthy and clinical populations Bosworth (range of *rs* = −.26 to −.55; see manual; Ayotte et al., 2009; Berrigan et al., 2014; Clark et al., 2004; Gonzalez et al., 2007; Goretti et al., 2014; Hsieh & Tori, 2007; Kochunov et al., 2010; Lam et al., 2013; Manly et al., 2011; Motl et al., 2013; Selnes et al., 1991; Smith & Arnett, 2007; Spedo et al., 2015; Spitz et al., 2013; Uchiyama et al., 1994; Vogel, Stokholm, & Jørgensen, 2013). In one normative study, age explained approximately 23% of the variance in SDMT performance (Pena-Casanova et al., 2009b).

In a large-scale Australian study (Kiely et al., 2014), scores on the SDMT were stable until age 35, after which decline was noted, with most prominent decline after age 55. A similar pattern was noted by Sheridan et al. (2006) in their review of normative studies. Age-related decline may reflect changes in speed of motor response and speed of information processing, including symbol encoding, visual search (Gilmore et al., 1983), and memory (Joy et al., 2004).

GENDER

Many studies report that women perform better than men (Manual; Gonzalez et al., 2007; Hsieh & Tory, 2007; Laux & Lane, 1985; Spitz et al., 2013; Yeudall et al., 1986). In a large community-based study (*n* > 7,000), women generally outperformed men on the SDMT, which remained after sociodemographic and health variables were accounted for (Jorm et al., 2004). Note, however, that gender differences have not always been found (Gilmore et al., 1983; Pena-Casanova et al., 2009).

EDUCATION AND IQ

Education is related to better performance in healthy and clinical groups (*rs* = .24 to .78; Ayotte et al. 2009; Berrigan et al., 2014; Chan et al., 2004; Gonzalez et al., 2007; Harris et al., 2007; Hsieh & Tori, 2007; Lam et al., 2013; Manly et al., 2011; Sheridan et al., 2006; Spedo et al., 2015; Vogel et al., 2013).

In normative studies, the effects of education on SDMT performance are often prominent. For example, Pena-Casanova et al. (2009b) reported that education explained 44% of the variance in test scores. In their sample of older women, Clark et al. (2004) reported that education was the greatest demographic predictor of performance, accounting for nearly 5% of SDMT scores. Education accounted for 29% of the variance in SDMT scores in a group of patients with hepatitis C (O'Bryant et al., 2007).

Examinees with higher levels of education (≥13 years of school) have higher scores than individuals with lower levels of education (≤12 years of school; see manual; Clark et al., 2004; Pena-Casanova et al., 2009; Selnes et al., 1991; Uchiyama et al., 1994). In patients with MS tested five years apart, SDMT performance did not show significant change in patients with greater than 14 years of education, but declined in patients with 14 years of education or less (Benedict et al., 2010). The manual presents means and standard deviations by age and educational level (≤12 years vs. ≥13 years).

Performance also improves with increasing IQ (Nielsen et al., 1989; Uchiyama et al., 1994; Yeudall et al., 1986). Reading ability is also correlated with performance (*r* = .32, .38; Manly et al., 2011; Vogel et al., 2012). However, note that the correlations between the SDMT and the NAART and education were small in an MS sample (*r* = .10, .13; Benedict et al., 2010).

ETHNICITY, NATIONALITY, AND LINGUISTIC EFFECTS

The SDMT has been used in clinical and normative populations internationally (including as a component of MS test batteries), including but not limited to Saudi Arabia (Al-Zahrani & Elsayed, 2009), Brazil (Azambuja et al., 2012), France (Baudic et al., 2013), Greece (Polychroniadou et al., 2016), Hong Kong (Chan et al., 2004), and Japan (Hashimoto et al., 2008; Niino et al., 2017). As part of the test's international use, the SDMT has also been translated into many other languages (e.g., Dusankova et al., 2012; Eshaghi et al., 2012).

Effects of ethnicity have been reported, although in some studies findings may be confounded by secondary variables such as socioeconomic status, education, and language proficiency. African-American participants have been reported to score lower on the test (Ayotte et al., 2009; Manly et al., 2011). Level of acculturation for African-American individuals is related to SDMT performance, but seemingly less so for the oral version (Kennepohl et al., 2004). Caribbean Black Americans were found to perform worse than African-Americans and Non-Latino white participants on a modified SDMT (Gonzalez et al., 2007). In this study, influence of age and gender were found to be similar across ethnic groups. Ethnicity was found to account for 2 to 3% of the variance in SDMT scores in both an ethnically diverse sample of college students and hepatitis C patients (O'Bryant et al., 2007). In another study, Aboriginal and Torres Strait Islanders attained lower scores than non-indigenous Australians (Kiely et al., 2014). Cores et al. (2015) reported differences on the SDMT even after participants were matched on demographic characteristics between participants in the United States and Argentina.

Agranovich, Panter, Puente, and Touradji (2011) examined effects of cultural differences in time attitudes on timed cognitive test performance, including the SDMT, in healthy Russians and Americans. US participants performed better than Russian participants, with an effect that was medium in magnitude (Cohen's d = .47). Less familiarity with standardized testing was related to poorer performance ($r = -.32$). These results suggest that attitudes toward time and familiarity with timed testing procedures, which may vary culturally, can impact scores on the SDMT.

Linguistic variables may also play a role. Scores are lower among respondents from non–English-speaking backgrounds born outside of Australia compared with native English speakers (Kiely et al., 2014). Harris et al. (2007) reported that when dominant Spanish-speaking participants were divided into high and low education groups, the lower-educated groups achieved lower scores compared to the other groups (English-speaking non-Hispanic and Hispanic bilingual).

NORMATIVE DATA

STANDARDIZATION SAMPLE

Smith (1982, manual) provides data based on a sample of 1,307 healthy adults, 18 to 78 years of age, presented by age and education (≤12 years or ≥13 years). See Table 8–53 for sample characteristics. Exclusion criteria included apparent disability or reported neurological involvement, or performance on a double simultaneous stimulation screening test.

Note that the data for the oral version are based on administration shortly after the written form. More importantly, users should note that the norms shown in the manual are, as of this writing, over 40 years old. These norms appear to be collected via a convenience sample in a nonsystematic, nonstandardized manner, including data collected for a 1975 dissertation and by psychologists participating in a neuropsychology workshop. Other normative sources are therefore preferable; a large number of alternative normative sources are available.

Dickinson and Hiscock (2011) reported a probable Flynn effect for the oral version of the SDMT. Comparison of SDMT norms based on two normative studies, including the standardization sample (Smith, 1982; norm collection reportedly 1973 to 1975) and Yeudall et al. (1986), yielded an effect corresponding to .12 to .78 standard deviations, approximately 6 points per decade. The authors provide an example to illustrate the impact of this effect on test scores in an individual examinee. If a 40-year-old examinee obtains a raw score of approximately 60 on the SDMT, the corresponding percentile according to Smith norms is the 50th percentile versus the 26th percentile according to Yeudall et al. norms. Note that due to age differences in the normative samples compared, the authors used extrapolated data for part of their analysis. Nonetheless, these data emphasize the importance of using relatively current norms to evaluate performance.

TABLE 8–53 Symbol Digit Modalities Test (SDMT) Standardization Sample Normative Data

Sample size	1,307[a]
Age	18 to 78 years[b]
Geographic location	New Jersey and Michigan, US
Education	≤12 years (*n* = 477) ≥13 years (*n* = 830)
Gender	Reportedly evenly distributed
Ethnicity	Not reported

[a] From two sources: adult volunteers for a 1975 doctoral dissertation (*n* = 420), and healthy volunteers obtained by psychologists in private practice who participated in a workshop on clinical neuropsychology in Ann Arbor, Michigan; each psychologist contributed 20 participants (*n* = 887).

[b] Age groupings: 18 to 24, 25 to 34, 35 to 44, 45 to 54, 55 to 64, and ≥65.

SOURCE: Adapted from Smith (1982).

NORMATIVE STUDIES

ORAL SDMT, AUSTRALIAN SAMPLE (JORM ET AL., 2004)

Jorm et al. (2004) provide data for the oral version based on a large, community-based sample of more than 7,000 individuals from Australia selected from the electoral roll of the region, with relatively high education levels (about 14 years). Data for women and men are presented separately in Table 8–54; three age cohorts are provided (20 to 24, 40 to 44, and 60 to 64). These data were collected between 1999 and 2001.

WRITTEN SDMT, AUSTRALIAN NORMS (KIELY ET AL., 2014)

Kiely et al. (2014) provide data for perhaps the largest normative sample to date for the written SDMT, with sample characteristics summarized in Table 8–55 and normative data in Tables 8–56 to 8–58. Participant data were collected as part of a larger longitudinal study, and participants were excluded if they had physical or neurologic conditions impacting performance (e.g., sight problems, loss of consciousness, learning difficulties, brain injury, stroke).

Exclusion criteria were tested empirically, examining physical and neurologic conditions that independently predicted lower SDMT scores after consideration of sociodemographic factors. Common disorders were included in the sample to enhance representativeness (e.g., speech problems; emotional condition or mental illness; hearing difficulty; breathing difficulty or pain), even though many of these conditions were related to poorer SDMT performance. Those with a psychiatric disorder would be expected, based on Kiely et al. data, to show three-symbol digit pairing decrement in performance (.25 *SD* to .33 *SD*, depending on normative group). Interestingly, speech problems predicted the largest decrement in performance, at approximately .5 *SD*.

Although the SDMT is reportedly generally well-tolerated by examinees, Kiely et al. reported that those participants with missing data were more likely to be older, male, less educated, from a non–English-speaking background, be an Aboriginal or Torres Strait Islander, or have a long-term health condition (odds ratio [OR] = 1.78).

TABLE 8–54 Normative Data for the Oral Symbol Digit Modalities Test (SDMT) for a Large, Community-Based Australian Sample by Gender (N = 7,485)

	WOMEN			MEN		
AGE	*N*	EDUCATION	MEAN (SD)	*N*	EDUCATION	MEAN (*SD*)
20–24	1,241	14.7	64.90 (9.89)	1,163	14.5	62.82 (10.19)
40–44	1,338	14.5	60.71 (9.42)	1,192	14.8	58.98 (9.09)
60–64	1,232	13.3	49.95 (10.0)	1,319	14.2	49.39 (9.52)

SOURCE: From Jorm et al. (2004).

MODIFIED SDMT VERSION, US SAMPLE (GONZALEZ ET AL., 2007)

Gonzalez et al. (2007) provide norms for a modified version of the SDMT based on a sample of African Americans, Caribbean Black Americans, and non-Latino white participants. The SDMT was modified to have two parts (Part A and B), each lasting 45 seconds with 50 cells per part. A subgroup of participants in the National Survey of American Life was included in this study, with characteristics detailed in Table 8–59, and normative data in Tables 8–60 to 8–62. Exclusionary criteria included psychiatric conditions (as determined via structured diagnostic interview) and incompletion of the SDMT. Detailed information regarding sampling procedures and recruitment is found in Gonzalez et al. (2007).

SPANISH SDMT NORMATIVE SAMPLE (PENA-CASANOVA ET AL., 2009A, B)

Pena-Casanova et al. (2009a, b) provide normative data for 354 Spanish adults 50–90 years of age as part of the Spanish Multicenter Normative Studies (NEURONORMA project), a large project that presented co-normed data for neuropsychological tests. The study was performed across nine different Spanish regions. All participants were Caucasian and living in Spain, educated in Spanish, and enrolled between 2004 and 2007. Participants were excluded if they were not independent or presented with cognitive impairment on the MMSE, neurologic disorder, Modified Ischemia Scale score, alcohol or psychotropic substance abuse, unmanaged medical condition that could interfere with cognition (e.g., diabetes mellitus, hypothyroidism, B_{12} deficiency), psychiatric diseases, or sensory impairment. Table 8–63 presents characteristics of the normative sample; Table 8–64 presents age-adjusted normative data, with education adjustments described in Table 8–65.

TABLE 8–55 Characteristics of the Kiely et al. (2014) Written Symbol Digit Modalities Test (SDMT) Version Normative Sample

Sample size	14,456
Age	15 to 100
Geographic location	Australia
Education	25% Tertiary qualification 30% Technical qualification (diploma or trade certificate) 16% Completed Year 12 (final year of high school) 29% Completed Year 11 or below
Gender	47% Men 53% Women
Ethnicity	Generally English-speaking background 10% males non–English-speaking background <1% males Aboriginal and Torres Strait Islander 11% females non–English-speaking background <1% females Aboriginal and Torres Strait Islander

DANISH SDMT NORMATIVE DATA (VOGEL ET AL., 2013)

Vogel et al. (2013) provide norms for 100 Danish older adults (M = 70.9 years, SD = 6.4 years). Exclusion criteria included the presence of medical or psychiatric conditions and alcohol abuse, and MMSE and Addenbrooke's Cognitive Examination performance. Characteristics of the sample are described in Table 8–66. Norms are presented in Table 8–67. The mean Danish Adult Reading Test (DART; Danish equivalent of the NART) score was 32.1 (SD = 7.9, range 11–46).

OTHER NORMATIVE STUDIES

There are a number of other SDMT normative studies. Berrigan et al. (2014) provide regression-based normative data for the oral SDMT, with application to MS, using both a healthy control sample and samples with MS. Normative information used significantly affected the classification of impairment reported; for example, in the representative clinical sample of patients with MS, 33% were classified as impaired using cross validated T scores, 47% using original T scores, and 23% using the discrete norms.

Goretti et al. (2014) provide regression-based norms for an Italian sample as part of the Brief International Cognitive Assessment System for MS (BICAMS). The sample was approximately 66% female, ranging in age from 18 to 65 years, with a mean age of 38.9 years (SD = 13). Education levels ranged from 5 to 21 years (M = 14.9 years, SD = 3.1). Spedo et al. (2015) provide normative data for 58 healthy controls as part of a Brazilian-Portuguese adaptation of the BICAMS. Others have provided cutoff scores. For example

TABLE 8–56 Australian Normative Data for the Written SDMT (Males, Age- and Education-Adjusted)

AGE GROUP	TERTIARY			POSTSECONDARY, NONTERTIARY			COMPLETED HIGH SCHOOL			YEAR 11 OR BELOW		
	N	MEAN	(SD)	*N*	MEAN	(*SD*)	*N*	MEAN	(*SD*)	*N*	MEAN	(*SD*)
15 to 19							196	57.28	(13.35)	444	52.76	(12.05)
20 to 24	65	59.54	(9.38)	182	51.87	(12.10)	296	56.86	(9.52)	145	46.13	(11.80)
25 to 29	170	55.76	(7.74)	227	53.59	(11.91)	162	53.18	(9.72)	100	49.37	(11.55)
30 to 34	186	56.17	(9.62)	214	51.49	(9.82)	76	56.16	(9.49)	70	49.93	(10.82)
35 to 39	191	56.07	(8.04)	238	50.93	(9.71)	82	50.67	(9.85)	62	45.62	(11.97)
40 to 44	180	55.63	(9.86)	255	49.37	(9.67)	57	51.31	(10.25)	93	44.08	(10.76)
45 to 49	162	52.79	(8.69)	251	46.14	(9.83)	42	50.57	(7.22)	134	45.19	(10.28)
50 to 54	148	48.91	(9.92)	271	45.89	(8.81)	47	46.27	(8.77)	115	41.68	(10.56)
55 to 59	153	47.60	(9.28)	195	46.15	(10.48)	42	43.53	(11.45)	99	39.80	(9.66)
60 to 64	101	47.60	(7.90)	170	42.59	(9.25)	38	40.35	(9.54)	106	39.14	(10.60)
65 to 69	87	45.13	(8.57)	143	39.00	(10.20)	29	40.19	(10.50)	104	35.15	(10.74)
70 to 74	49	41.13	(9.26)	114	34.60	(10.43)	25	37.85	(10.60)	84	31.10	(10.51)
75 to 79							129	31.70	(10.69)	71	26.21	(10.02)
80 to 84							65	30.85	(11.23)	57	23.07	(9.59)
85+							46	26.54	(8.52)	25	25.86	(8.78)

NOTE: Due to small cell sizes, tertiary and postsecondary education levels were collapsed to "completed high school" for age groups 15 to 19, 75 to 79, 80 to 84, and 85+. Data exclude people reporting sight problems not corrected by lenses, blackouts, "fits" and loss of consciousness, learning difficulties, and brain injury or stroke.

SOURCE: From Kiely et al. (2014).

a cutoff score of 44 or less was identified as maximizing sensitivity and specificity and represented function 1.5 *SD* below the mean; a cutoff score of 38 or less represented function 2 *SD* or more below the mean (Beier et al., 2017).

Hsieh and Tori (2007) provide normative data based on a large sample of young (n = 26, M age = 35.77 years), middle-age (n = 57, M age = 52.65), and older (n = 111, M age = 69.27) Mandarin-speaking adults in Beijing. Written SDMT for the young adult group was a mean of 48.06 (*SD* = 12.56), with oral SDMT at a mean of 55.74 (*SD* = 13.95). For the middle adult group, the written SDMT had a mean of 35.09 (*SD* = 11.54) with a mean for the oral SDMT of 43.72 (*SD* = 12.39). The older group (n = 111) had a written SDMT mean of 30.29 (*SD* = 13.16) for men and 23.56 (*SD* = 16.75) for women, with an oral SDMT mean of 38.13 (*SD* = 15.21) for men and 29.81 (*SD* = 19.51) for women.

Norms for specific groups are available. For example, Manly et al. (2011) provide normative data for a large sample (n = 1,653) of women living with HIV as well as a group of women identified as high risk without HIV. Clark et al. (2004) provide norms for 257 Australian women aged 56 to 67. Sheridan et al. (2006) provide normative data for 238 participants (aged 20 to 39 years; 69% female) who

TABLE 8–57 Australian Normative Data for the Written SDMT (Females, Age- and Education-Adjusted)

AGE GROUP	TERTIARY			POSTSECONDARY, NONTERTIARY			COMPLETED HIGH SCHOOL			YEAR 11 OR BELOW		
	N	MEAN	(SD)	*N*	MEAN	(*SD*)	*N*	MEAN	(*SD*)	*N*	MEAN	(*SD*)
15 to 19							262	59.48	(11.27)	422	55.45	(10.56)
20 to 24	128	61.34	(9.71)	189	57.96	(11.45)	326	59.04	(10.01)	119	52.57	(10.54)
25 to 29	253	58.47	(9.18)	221	55.47	(10.84)	138	56.85	(9.98)	90	53.97	(10.68)
30 to 34	264	57.73	(9.63)	182	57.51	(11.04)	87	55.75	(11.30)	63	49.57	(10.83)
35 to 39	261	56.87	(9.14)	196	54.60	(11.03)	87	54.32	(10.44)	99	50.20	(11.04)
40 to 44	242	57.06	(9.03)	204	53.28	(10.44)	97	52.26	(9.86)	153	50.69	(10.36)
45 to 49	198	53.60	(10.81)	198	50.67	(10.14)	85	51.13	(11.10)	173	45.90	(11.63)
50 to 54	198	51.93	(7.74)	201	50.83	(9.08)	65	50.92	(13.00)	184	47.49	(11.78)
55 to 59	154	51.19	(9.66)	167	48.70	(9.53)	59	46.22	(10.09)	195	45.60	(10.58)
60 to 64	113	48.23	(10.89)	126	43.49	(9.62)	37	45.85	(12.39)	213	42.58	(12.25)
65 to 69	79	43.53	(10.98)	91	42.92	(10.01)	35	42.26	(8.14)	219	38.97	(10.59)
70 to 74	40	40.56	(8.22)	63	38.00	(10.18)	20	39.80	(11.36)	188	35.07	(11.59)
75 to 79							64	37.97	(9.65)	129	32.00	(10.89)
80 to 84							57	32.34	(11.53)	108	28.31	(10.09)
85 +							24	27.37	(6.62)	88	22.62	(8.84)

NOTE: Due to small cell sizes, tertiary and postsecondary education levels were collapsed to "completed high school" for age groups 15 to 19, 75 to 79, 80 to 84, and 85+. Data exclude people reporting sight problems not corrected by lenses, blackouts, "fits" and loss of consciousness, learning difficulties, and brain injury or stroke.

SOURCE: From Kiely et al. (2014).

TABLE 8–58 Australian Normative Data for the Written SDMT (Males and Females, Age-Adjusted)

	MALES						FEMALES					
AGE GROUP	MEAN	(SD)	20TH PERCENTILE	40TH PERCENTILE	60TH PERCENTILE	80TH PERCENTILE	MEAN	(SD)	20TH PERCENTILE	40TH PERCENTILE	60TH PERCENTILE	80TH PERCENTILE
15–19	54.09	(12.31)	45	50	56	63	56.91	(11.25)	49	54	58	65
20–24	53.98	(11.27)	46	51	57	63	58.21	(10.97)	50	56	61	67
25–29	53.74	(9.79)	46	50	56	62	56.87	(10.36)	49	54	60	65
30–34	53.87	(10.00)	46	50	57	63	56.63	(10.91)	48	55	59	66
35–39	52.29	(9.66)	44	50	55	60	54.66	(10.79)	47	52	58	63
40–44	50.71	(10.44)	43	48	53	60	53.80	(10.45)	46	52	57	62
45–49	48.23	(9.76)	40	46	51	57	50.16	(11.61)	41	48	53	60
50–54	45.92	(9.56)	38	44	49	53	50.20	(10.41)	43	49	53	59
55–59	44.92	(10.30)	36	43	49	53	47.91	(10.59)	39	47	50	57
60–64	42.58	(9.68)	34	41	46	51	44.22	(11.97)	35	43	48	53
65–69	39.14	(10.58)	31	37	42	49	40.95	(10.76)	33	40	45	49
70–74	34.79	(10.65)	26	32	38	44	36.65	(11.40)	28	35	40	46
75–79	29.76	(10.54)	20	28	32	39	33.97	(11.13)	24	31	36	44
80–84	27.08	(10.87)	18	23	29	38	29.53	(10.92)	19	28	32	39
85 +	26.29	(8.42)	19	23	29	34	23.55	(8.77)	15	18	25	32

NOTE: Data exclude people reporting sight problems not corrected by lenses, blackouts, fits and loss of consciousness, learning difficulties, and brain injury or stroke.
SOURCE: From Kiely et al. (2014).

were part of a longitudinal study of families who were determined to be at elevated risk for alcohol use disorder.

There are also a number of older studies for specific subgroups (see Hinton-Bayre and colleagues; Nielsen et al., 1989; Uchiyama et al., 1994; Yeudall et al., 1986). See also Levine, Miller, Beckham, Selnes, and Cohen (2004) for test-retest norms and reliable change information. As noted previously, older norms are more likely to yield inflated estimates of ability; current norms are preferred.

EVIDENCE FOR RELIABILITY

EVIDENCE FOR INTERNAL RELIABILITY

Internal reliability information is not reported, likely because the SDMT is a timed task.

EVIDENCE FOR TEST-RETEST RELIABILITY, MEASURING CHANGE, AND PRACTICE EFFECTS

Test-retest reliability at relatively short retest intervals (e.g., days to weeks) is generally adequate to high overall in healthy and clinical groups (e.g., range *r*s = .70 to .91, ICCs >.85; Eshaghi et al., 2012; Goretti et al., 2014; Hinton-Bayre et al., 1999; Koh et al., 2011; Lee et al., 2011; Pereira et al., 2015; Smith, 1991; Spedo et al., 2015; Tang et al., 2017). Note, however, that Pereira, Costa, and Cerquier (2015) reported only adequate (r = .70) reliability over a 150-minute test-retest interval in high school students.

Retest stability over longer intervals is also relatively good. In a large study involving men (n > 1,000), Uchiyama et al. (1994) found adequate test-retest coefficients at six months (r = .79). Retest coefficients for longer test intervals, based on smaller numbers of participants, were also adequate (r = .72 at one year and two years; n = 39).

Test-retest reliability of the incidental learning trial developed by Uchiyama et al. (1994) is variable (r = .46, .52, and .71, for six-month, one-year, and two-year retest intervals, respectively). Hinton-Bayre et al. (1997) found that use of a derived index score for accuracy (i.e., percentage correct) yielded lower reliabilities than the number correct score (Hinton-Bayre et al., 1997).

The manual reports gains of about 4 points at retest (Smith, 1991). Hinton-Bayre et al. (1997), using alternate forms, found a 2% increase in the number correct over repeat assessment. Koh et al. (2011) reported a small practice effect (Cohen's d = .26) in patients with stroke tested over a one-week interval for the oral SDMT. Lee et al. (2011) reported a significant but small practice effect (5% improvement) in individuals with schizophrenia tested one week apart. In contrast, persons with mild cognitive impairment (MCI) tend to show minimal practice effects on the test (Duff et al., 2017).

Uchiyama et al. (1994) reported no significant practice effects when the written version was given at yearly intervals

TABLE 8–59 Characteristics of the Gonzalez et al. (2007) US Normative Sample for the Modified SDMT

Sample size	*N* = 2,651 African American	*N* = 1,291 Caribbean Black	*N* = 570 Non-Latino white
Age	42 (.58 *SE*)	40 (.84 *SE*)	45 (1.06 *SE*)
Geographic location	Regions in the US		
Education	13 (.09 *SE*)	13 (.17 *SE*)	13 (.32 *SE*)
Gender	46% Men 54% Women	50% Men 50% Women	49% Men 51% Women
Ethnicity	See sample size, above		

TABLE 8–60 US Normative Data for Part A of the Modified SDMT by Age, Education, Gender, and Ethnicity

	TOTAL SAMPLE				MALES				FEMALES			
	TOTAL M (*SD*); *N*	AFRICAN AMERICANS M (*SD*); *N*	CARIBBEAN BLACKS M (*SD*); *N*	NON–LATINO WHITES M (*SD*); *N*	TOTAL M (*SD*); *N*	AFRICAN AMERICANS M (*SD*); *N*	CARIBBEAN BLACKS M (*SD*); *N*	NON–LATINO WHITES M (*SD*); *N*	TOTAL M (*SD*); *N*	AFRICAN AMERICANS M (*SD*); *N*	CARIBBEAN BLACKS M (*SD*); *N*	NON–LATINO WHITES M (*SD*); *N*
Total sample	21.61 (9.74); 4537	21.49 (8.58); 2670	19.95 (3.41); 1297	21.89 (19.58); 570	21.00 (10.76); 1772	20.80 (9.27); 984	19.34 (3.61); 543	21.38 (21.54); 245	22.16 (9.00); 2765	22.08 (8.12); 1686	20.57 (3.24); 754	22.39 (17.96); 325
Education ≤ 12	20.22 (9.24); 2589	20.08 (8.66); 1673	18.56 (3.32); 631	20.59 (17.64); 285	19.40 (10.18); 1024	19.58 (9.58); 625	17.40 (3.40); 275	19.32 (19.19); 124	20.98 (8.53); 1565	20.51 (8.05); 1048	19.66 (3.22); 356	21.89 (16.15); 161
Education > 12	23.35 (10.12); 1923	23.94 (7.92); 978	21.37 (3.42); 660	23.03 (21.15); 285	23.05 (11.16); 738	22.99 (8.19); 351	21.10 (3.69); 266	23.27 (23.17); 121	23.62 (9.41); 1185	24.72 (7.71); 627	21.67 (3.23); 394	22.81 (19.59); 164
Age 18 to 34												
All	25.11 (9.44); 1589	25.01 (8.48); 957	23.28 (3.47); 487	25.47 (21.53); 145	24.35 (9.67); 600	24.48 (9.48); 332	22.16 (4.01); 211	24.49 (20.15); 57	25.70 (9.27); 989	25.46 (7.88); 625	24.57 (2.96); 276	26.10 (22.40); 88
Education ≤ 12	24.09 (8.51); 886	24.23 (8.27); 600	22.15 (3.14); 220	24.03 (17.91); 66	23.20 (8.88); 334	23.76 (9.66); 214	20.36 (3.22); 100	21.90 (16.38); 20	24.73 (8.24); 552	24.64 (7.39); 386	24.32 (2.94); 120	24.91 (18.47); 46
Education > 12	26.33 (10.39); 695	26.49 (8.62); 333	24.27 (3.68); 263	26.43 (24.04); 79	25.61 (10.42); 263	26.00 (8.87); 116	23.48 (4.55); 110	25.59 (21.74); 37	26.91 (10.36); 432	26.85 (8.50); 237	25.19 (2.88); 153	27.13 (26.08); 42
Age 35 to 50												
All	22.07 (8.93); 1607	21.67 (7.66); 941	19.70 (3.11); 488	22.82 (19.54); 178	21.82 (10.47); 638	20.26 (8.11); 361	18.72 (3.12); 186	23.73 (21.58); 91	22.36 (7.76); 969	23.01 (7.20); 580	20.50 (3.08); 302	21.54 (17.04); 87
Education ≤ 12	20.86 (8.26); 836	20.27 (7.93); 537	19.09 (3.27); 219	22.03 (16.04); 80	20.46 (9.04); 356	19.06 (8.46); 222	17.15 (3.73); 86	22.54 (15.11); 48	21.39 (7.62); 480	21.60 (7.41); 315	20.62 (2.85); 133	21.05 (17.47); 32
Education > 12	23.41 (9.45); 763	23.65 (6.83); 397	20.33 (2.97); 268	23.44 (22.00); 98	23.62 (11.78); 277	22.37 (6.92); 134	20.24 (2.38); 100	24.92 (27.04); 43	23.22 (7.83); 486	24.64 (6.67); 263	20.40 (3.27); 168	21.82 (16.93); 55
Age 51 to 65												
All	18.91 (9.40); 821	18.77 (7.69); 466	15.83 (2.90); 216	19.24 (17.62); 139	17.44 (10.79); 345	18.13 (8.48); 188	15.49 (2.98); 99	17.02 (21.17); 58	20.30 (8.06); 476	19.33 (7.10); 278	16.23 (2.84); 117	21.52 (13.84); 81
Education ≤ 12	17.65 (9.18); 500	16.99 (7.45); 300	15.57 (2.77); 124	18.49 (17.98); 76	15.27 (10.45); 201	15.73 (8.26); 113	13.35 (2.57); 55	15.00 (20.75); 33	19.82 (7.78); 299	17.91 (6.85); 187	17.02 (2.82); 69	22.64 (13.38); 43
Education > 12	20.53 (9.52); 317	21.61 (7.47); 162	16.13 (3.08); 92	20.05 (17.20); 63	20.13 (10.60); 143	21.19 (7.89); 74	16.89 (3.30); 44	19.58 (21.16); 25	20.94 (8.54); 174	22.10 (7.12); 88	14.37 (2.84); 48	20.46 (14.30); 38
Age 66+												
All	14.86 (8.90); 520	12.79 (7.22); 306	12.85 (2.63); 106	16.59 (14.54); 108	15.30 (10.25); 189	12.95 (7.78); 103	15.07 (2.84); 47	16.80 (18.07); 39	14.51 (8.03); 331	12.69 (6.93); 203	10.49 (2.18); 59	16.40 (12.25); 69
Education ≤ 12	13.68 (8.92); 367	11.13 (6.63); 236	11.97 (2.86); 68	16.34 (16.04); 63	14.29 (11.16); 133	11.23 (7.61); 76	14.23 (3.09); 34	16.51 (22.15); 23	13.21 (7.35); 234	11.07 (6.14); 160	9.11 (2.23); 34	16.16 (11.49); 40
Education > 12	17.29 (8.28); 148	18.14 (7.03); 66	15.67 (1.96); 37	16.94 (12.30); 45	17.23 (7.28); 55	17.05 (6.88); 27	19.41 (1.62); 12	17.26 (10.32); 16	17.34 (8.85); 93	19.05 (7.13); 39	13.54 (1.86); 25	16.69 (13.43); 29

SOURCE: From Gonzalez et al. (2007).

TABLE 8–61 US Normative Data for Part B of the Modified SDMT by Age, Education, Gender, and Ethnicity

	TOTAL SAMPLE				MALES				FEMALES			
	TOTAL M (*SD*); *N*	AFRICAN AMERICANS M (*SD*); *N*	CARIBBEAN BLACKS M (*SD*); *N*	NON–LATINO WHITES M (*SD*); *N*	TOTAL M (*SD*); *N*	AFRICAN AMERICANS M (*SD*); *N*	CARIBBEAN BLACKS M (*SD*); *N*	NON–LATINO WHITES M (*SD*); *N*	TOTAL M (*SD*); *N*	AFRICAN AMERICANS M (*SD*); *N*	CARIBBEAN BLACKS M (*SD*); *N*	NON–LATINO WHITES M (*SD*); *N*
Total sample	23.19 (9.87); 4522	22.85 (8.86); 2664	21.80 (3.55); 1294	23.71 (19.51); 564	22.69 (10.99); 1767	22.41 (9.57); 982	21.47 (3.86); 543	23.11 (21.83); 242	23.64 (9.07); 2755	23.23 (8.40); 1682	22.14 (3.31); 751	24.29 (17.55); 322
Education ≤ 12	21.62 (9.34); 2581	21.48 (9.04); 1670	20.03 (3.34); 630	21.97 (17.04); 281	20.95 (10.19); 1021	21.11 (9.95); 624	19.24 (3.32); 275	20.88 (18.43); 122	22.24 (8.71); 1560	21.81 (8.45); 1046	20.78 (3.34); 355	23.10 (15.74); 159
Education > 12	25.16 (10.22); 1916	25.25 (8.02); 975	23.60 (3.65); 658	25.22 (21.33); 283	24.92 (11.57); 736	24.77 (8.28); 350	23.51 (4.20); 266	25.16 (24.21); 120	25.38 (9.27); 1180	25.65 (7.86); 625	23.71 (3.23); 392	25.27 (19.02); 163
Age 18 to 34												
All	26.37 (9.86); 1587	25.94 (8.85); 957	25.37 (3.55); 486	27.10 (22.54); 144	25.95 (10.46); 600	25.59 (9.84); 332	24.96 (4.35); 211	26.70 (22.87); 57	26.69 (9.47); 987	26.22 (8.28); 625	25.85 (2.78); 275	27.36 (22.44); 87
Education ≤ 12	25.02 (8.79); 885	25.22 (8.76); 600	23.62 (3.24); 220	24.75 (17.68); 65	24.26 (9.35); 334	24.87 (10.20); 214	21.90 (3036); 100	22.66 (17.00); 20	25.58 (8.41); 551	25.53 (7.85); 386	25.70 (3.02); 120	25.64 (17.91); 45
Education > 12	27.96 (10.87); 694	27.31 (8.82); 353	26.80 (3.70); 262	28.64 (25.48); 79	27.82 (11.38); 263	27.18 (8.82); 116	27.20 (4.89); 110	28.42 (24.87); 37	28.06 (10.57); 431	27.41 (8.85); 237	26.33 (2.52); 152	28.82 (26.29); 42
Age 35 to 50												
All	23.96 (8.82); 1601	23.52 (7.80); 939	21.81 (3.12); 486	24.72 (18.80); 176	23.77 (10.11); 636	22.65 (8.37); 361	20.90 (2.82); 186	25.22 (20.47); 89	24.16 (7.85); 965	24.36 (7.37); 578	22.56 (3.28); 300	24.04 (16.96); 87
Education ≤ 12	22.55 (8.13); 833	22.40 (8.12); 536	20.48 (3.08); 218	23.03 (14.96); 79	22.23 (8.54); 355	21.59 (8.71); 222	19.39 (3.01); 86	23.29 (13.13); 47	22.98 (7.80); 478	23.30 (7.62); 314	21.35 (3.10); 132	22.52 (17.51); 32
Education > 12	25.51 (9.28); 760	25.16 (7.01); 396	23.15 (3.11); 267	26.07 (21.18); 97	25.84 (11.44); 276	24.61 (7.23); 134	22.36 (2.55); 100	27.15 (26.00); 42	25.21 (7.79); 484	25.59 (6.89); 262	23.83 (3.39); 167	24.90 (16.62); 55
Age 51 to 65												
All	20.32 (9.47); 818	20.27 (7.92); 464	16.31 (3.31); 216	20.64 (17.39); 138	18.83 (10.84); 343	19.66 (8.47); 186	15.71 (3.41); 99	18.38 (21.14); 58	21.75 (8.15); 475	20.79 (7.52); 278	17.00 (3.23); 117	23.02 (13.27); 80
Education ≤ 12	19.06 (9.33); 499	18.26 (7.93); 299	16.21 (3.06); 124	20.11 (17.50); 76	17.03 (10.50); 200	16.65 (8.11); 112	14.41 (2.92); 55	17.47 (21.00); 33	20.91 (8.14); 299	19.41 (7.70); 187	17.39 (3.12); 69	23.25 (13.07); 43
Education > 12	21.97 (9.48); 315	23.49 (7.02); 161	16.43 (3.64); 92	21.23 (17.35); 62	21.07 (10.86); 142	23.50 (7.45); 73	16.56 (3.93); 44	19.53 (21.56); 25	22.90 (8.12); 173	23.47 (6.68); 88	16.11 (3.39); 48	22.79 (13.66); 37
Age 66+												
All	16.68 (9.40); 516	13.76 (8.00); 304	15.24 (2.82); 106	19.07 (14.39); 106	16.80 (10.77); 188	13.40 (8.57); 103	17.53 (3.17); 47	18.93 (18.12); 38	16.60 (8.53); 328	13.99 (7.72); 201	12.81 (2.25); 59	19.20 (11.97); 68
Education ≤ 12	15.42 (9.62); 364	12.05 (7.32); 235	14.72 (3.04); 68	18.88 (16.63); 61	15.98 (11.76); 132	11.63 (8.08); 76	16.74 (3.48); 34	19.13 (22.72); 22	14.98 (8.16); 232	12.30 (6.94); 159	12.16 (2.22); 34	18.63 (12.30); 39
Education > 12	19.28 (8.17); 147	19.31 (8.28); 65	16.94 (2.37); 37	19.33 (10.81); 45	18.35 (7.81); 55	17.64 (8.63); 27	21.66 (1.77); 12	18.61 (9.29); 16	20.03 (8.34); 92	20.74 (7.91); 38	14.25 (2.28); 25	19.90 (11.64); 29

SOURCE: From Gonzalez et al. (2007).

TABLE 8–62 US Normative Data for Parts A and B of the Modified SDMT by Age, Education, Gender, and Ethnicity

	TOTAL SAMPLE				MALES				FEMALES			
	TOTAL M (*SD*); N	AFRICAN AMERICANS M (*SD*); N	CARIBBEAN BLACKS M (*SD*); N	NON-LATINO WHITES M (*SD*); N	TOTAL M (*SD*); N	AFRICAN AMERICANS M (*SD*); N	CARIBBEAN BLACKS M (*SD*); N	NON-LATINO WHITES M (*SD*); N	TOTAL M (*SD*); N	AFRICAN AMERICANS M (*SD*); N	CARIBBEAN BLACKS M (*SD*); N	NON-LATINO WHITES M (*SD*); N
Total sample	44.89 (18.83); 4522	44.39 (16.72); 2664	41.77 (6.46); 1294	45.77 (37.73); 564	43.76 (20.94); 1767	43.23 (18.17); 982	40.81 (6.88); 543	44.61 (41.90); 242	45.92(17.30); 2755	45.37 (15.77); 1682	42.75 (6.13); 751	46.89 (34.22); 322
Education ≤ 12	41.92 (17.92); 2581	41.59 (17.08); 1670	38.59 (6.36); 630	42.75 (33.53); 281	40.41 (19.62); 1021	40.70 (18.85); 624	36.64 (6.37); 275	40.33 (36.31); 122	43.33 (16.63); 1560	42.35 (15.91); 1046	40.44 (6.29); 355	45.24 (30.83); 159
Education >12	48.63 (19.38); 1916	49.26 (14.98); 975	45.01 (6.38); 658	48.40 (40.93); 283	48.05 (21.80); 736	47.81 (15.79); 350	44.61 (7.05); 266	48.57 (45.71); 120	49.13 (17.69); 1180	50.46 (14.45); 625	45.46 (5.89); 392	48.25 (37.16); 163
Age 18 to 34												
All	51.53 (18.45); 1587	50.95 (16.41); 957	48.67 (6.21); 486	52.69 (42.84); 144	50.30 (19.30); 600	50.07 (18.59); 332	47.12 (7.35); 211	51.19 (41.58); 57	52.47 (17.88); 987	51.68 (15.11); 625	50.45 (5.11); 275	53.66 (43.77); 87
Education ≤ 12	49.19 (16.55); 885	49.45 (16.23); 600	45.76 (6.02); 220	49.05 (34.45); 65	47.46 (17.56); 334	48.63 (19.03); 214	42.27 (6.15); 100	44.56 (32.86); 20	50.45 (15.83); 551	50.18 (14.45); 386	50.03 (5.62); 120	50.94 (34.90); 45
Education > 12	54.29 (20.30); 694	53.80 (16.28); 353	51.10 (6.19); 262	55.06 (48.26); 79	53.44 (20.78); 263	53.18 (17.13); 116	50.68 (7.99); 110	54.01 (44.79); 37	54.97 (20.00); 431	54.26 (15.87); 237	51.59 (4.49); 152	55.95 (51.59); 42
Age 35 to 50												
All	46.12 (16.83); 1601	45.24 (16.64); 939	41.56 (5.81); 486	47.71 (36.45); 176	45.72 (19.58); 636	42.91 (15.73); 361	39.62 (5.57); 186	49.25 (39.97); 89	46.58 (14.74); 965	47.47 (13.68); 578	43.14 (5.91); 300	45.59 (32.36); 87
Education ≤ 12	43.48 (15.63); 833	42.69 (15.32); 536	39.58 (5.97); 218	45.20 (29.62); 79	42.78 (16.62); 355	40.65 (16.39); 222	36.54 (6.28); 86	46.06 (26.30); 47	44.40 (14.83); 478	44.94 (14.33); 314	42.00 (5.65); 132	43.57 (34.20); 32
Education > 12	49.06 (17.60); 760	48.89 (12.79); 396	43.56 (5.63); 267	49.69 (40.99); 97	49.65 (22.10); 276	46.98 (13.38); 134	42.60 (4.69); 100	52.45 (50.70); 42	48.52 (14.44); 484	50.38 (12.36); 262	44.37 (6.12); 167	46.72 (31.40); 55
Age 51 to 65												
All	39.34 (18.19); 818	39.10 (15.07); 464	32.14 (6.00); 216	40.06 (33.73); 138	36.33 (20.93); 343	37.91 (16.25); 186	31.20 (6.15); 99	35.40 (41.12); 58	42.24 (15.50); 475	40.12 (14.20); 278	33.23 (5.87); 117	44.95 (25.34); 80
Education ≤ 12	36.73 (17.91); 499	35.28 (14.84); 299	31.77 (5.69); 124	38.61 (34.36); 76	32.33 (20.13); 200	32.44 (15.69); 112	27.77 (5.41); 55	32.47 (40.15); 33	40.73 (15.49); 299	37.33 (14.12); 187	34.41 (5.76); 69	45.89 (25.78); 43
Education > 12	42.77 (18.12); 315	45.22 (13.84); 161	32.56 (6.41); 92	41.68 (32.99); 62	41.30 (20.89); 142	44.92 (14.44); 73	33.45 (6.84); 44	39.11 (42.14); 25	44.31 (15.41); 173	45.56 (13.41); 88	30.48 (6.02); 48	44.03 (25.09); 37
Age 66+												
All	31.67 (17.74); 516	26.61 (14.86); 304	28.08 (5.18); 106	35.86 (27.88); 106	32.16 (20.41); 188	26.35 (15.97); 103	32.61 (5.76); 47	35.85 (35.10); 38	31.28 (16.04); 328	26.77 (14.29); 201	23.30 (4.11); 59	35.86 (23.19); 68
Education ≤ 12	29.27 (17.95); 364	23.23 (13.52); 235	26.70 (5.59); 68	35.55 (31.54); 61	30.36 (22.33); 132	22.86 (15.35); 76	30.97 (6.28); 34	35.84 (43.90); 22	28.40 (14.91); 232	23.45 (12.61); 159	21.26 (4.04); 34	35.26 (22.48); 39
Education > 12	36.60 (15.93); 147	37.57 (15.01); 65	32.61 (4.18); 37	36.27 (22.30); 45	35.58 (14.36); 55	34.69 (15.02); 27	41.07 (3.16); 12	35.87 (18.44); 16	37.43 (16.83); 92	40.03 (14.86); 38	27.79 (3.98); 25	36.58 (24.47); 29

SOURCE: From Gonzalez et al. (2007).

TABLE 8-63 Characteristics of the Pena-Casanova et al. (2009) SDMT Normative Sample

Sample size	354
Age	50 to 90
Geographic location	Spain
Education	<12 years education 59% ≥12 years education 41% "Blue collar" 50% Administrative 17% Professional 32%
Gender	40% Men 60% Women
Ethnicity	100% Caucasian
First language (native language)	60% Castilian (Spanish) 32% Catalan 6% Galician 2% Basque

over a two-year period, suggesting relative stability over longer time intervals. Hinton-Bayre et al. (1999) found that the size of the practice effect was dependent on the retesting interval, with alternate forms not fully eliminating practice effects. They consequently recommend two baseline assessments prior to using the SDMT to assess concussion in athletes. Tang et al. (2017) found continued practice effects over five administrations, with one-week spacing between each session, in patients with schizophrenia. Others have recommended changing the key on repeat assessments to minimize practice effects (Roar et al., 2016).

RELIABLE CHANGE INDEX

Norms for assessing change can be found in Levine et al. (2004), based on a sample similar to the normative sample used by Uchiyama et al. (1994). The sports concussion literature also provides reliable change index (RCI) cutoffs for the SDMT (see Erlanger et al., 2003; Hinton-Barye & Geffen, 2005; Hinton-Bayre et al., 1997, 1999, for additional details). Performance on the four forms used was relatively comparable; however, practice effects were found at one-week test-retest intervals and use of RCI was recommended. Koh et al. (2011) provide an RCI modified for practice effects to be −5.29 at the lower bound and 10.89 at the upper bound in patients post-stroke. Tang et al. (2017) provide minimum and maximum RCIs at the 90% confidence interval (across four test administrations) for the SDMT as ranging from −7.2 to 12.4, with smaller values for the tablet-based version (−6.3, 9.7).

EVIDENCE FOR RELIABILITY OF ALTERNATE, SHORT, OR COMPUTER FORMS

Hinton-Bayre et al. (1997) developed three new written forms, including the three mirrored pairs of symbols appearing in the original, with high ICCs reported (.87 to .98; Hinton-Barye & Geffen, 2005). Comparison of the standard form and the alternate form (Form 2) developed by Uchiyama et al. (1994) suggests these forms were not equivalent in their level of difficulty. Although the two forms are related ($r = .74$), Form 2 is more difficult than the original SDMT. However, use of form-specific normative data, which the authors provide, alleviates this discrepancy to some extent. Form 2 may also be less reliable in longer term follow-ups (i.e., two years). Royer et al.'s alternate

TABLE 8-64 Spanish Symbol Digit Modalities Test (SDMT) Normative Data (Age-Adjusted)

		SDMT									
SCALED SCORE	PERCENTILE RANGE	AGE 50 TO 60	AGE 57 TO 59	AGE 60 TO 62	AGE 63 TO 65	AGE 66 TO 68	AGE 69 TO 71	AGE 72 TO 74	AGE 75 TO 77	AGE 78 TO 80	AGE 81 TO 90
2	<1	≤5	≤5	≤5	≤6	≤8	≤8	≤8	≤8	<7	≤9
3	1	6	6	6	–	–	–	–	–	8	–
4	2	7–12	7–11	7–11	7–11	9	–	–	–	–	10
5	3–5	13–17	12–16	12–15	12–14	10–12	9–11	9	9–10	9–10	11
6	6–10	18–21	17–19	16–18	15–16	13–15	12–14	10–13	11–12	11	12
7	11–18	22–27	20–24	19–21	17–20	16–19	15–19	14–17	13–15	12–14	13–15
8	19–28	28–33	25–30	22–28	21–24	20–24	20–22	18–21	16–19	15–19	16–18
9	29–40	34–36	31–34	29–33	25–30	25–27	23–26	22–24	20–22	20–21	19–20
10	41–59	37–48	35–44	34–37	31–36	28–34	27–31	25–30	23–28	22–26	21–24
11	60–71	49–52	45–49	38–46	37–40	35–39	32–35	31–33	29–31	27–29	25–27
12	72–81	53–54	50–52	47–49	41–46	40–44	36–40	34–38	32–34	30–33	28–30
13	82–89	55–56	53–55	50–53	47–50	45–48	41–47	39–42	35–41	34–35	31–33
14	90–94	57–59	56–57	54–56	51–54	49–50	48–50	46–50	42–49	36–40	34–40
15	95–97	60–63	58–59	57–58	55	51–56	51–55	51–55	50–55	41–42	41–42
16	98	64–67	60–63	59	56	57	–	–	–	43–46	–
17	99	68–69	64–67	60–63	57	58	56–58	56–58	58	–	–
18	>99	≥70	≥68	≥64	≥58	≥59	≥59	≥59	≥59	≥47	≥43
Sample Size		137	132	123	106	121	126	117	101	68	

SOURCE: From Pena-Casanova et al. (2009).

TABLE 8-65 Spanish Symbol Digit Modalities Test (SDMT) Normative Data Education Adjustment

	EDUCATION (YEARS)																				
NSS_A	0	1	2	3	4	5	6	7	8	9	10	11	12	13	14	15	16	17	18	19	20
2	5	5	5	4	4	4	3	3	3	2	2	2	2	1	1	1	0	0	0	–1	–1
3	6	6	6	5	5	5	4	4	4	3	3	3	3	2	2	2	1	1	1	0	0
4	7	7	7	6	6	6	5	5	5	4	4	4	4	3	3	3	2	2	2	1	1
5	8	8	8	7	7	7	6	6	6	5	5	5	5	4	4	4	3	3	3	2	2
6	9	9	9	8	8	8	7	7	7	6	6	6	6	5	5	5	4	4	4	3	3
7	10	10	10	9	9	9	8	8	8	7	7	7	7	6	6	6	5	5	5	4	4
8	11	11	11	10	10	10	9	9	9	8	8	8	8	7	7	7	6	6	6	5	5
9	12	12	12	11	11	11	10	10	10	9	9	9	9	8	8	8	7	7	7	6	6
10	13	13	13	12	12	12	11	11	11	10	10	10	10	9	9	9	8	8	8	7	7
11	14	14	14	13	13	13	12	12	12	11	11	11	11	10	10	10	9	9	9	8	8
12	15	15	15	14	14	14	13	13	13	12	12	12	12	11	11	11	10	10	10	9	9
13	16	16	16	15	15	15	14	14	14	13	13	13	13	12	12	12	11	11	11	10	10
14	17	17	17	16	16	16	15	15	15	14	14	14	14	13	13	13	12	12	12	11	11
15	18	18	18	17	17	17	16	16	16	15	15	15	15	14	14	14	13	13	13	12	12
16	19	19	19	18	18	18	17	17	17	16	16	16	16	15	15	15	14	14	14	13	13
17	20	20	20	19	19	19	18	18	18	17	17	17	17	16	16	16	15	15	15	14	14
18	21	21	21	20	20	20	19	19	19	18	18	18	18	17	17	17	16	16	16	15	15

NOTE: Education adjustment applying the following formula: $NSS_{A\&E} = NSS_A - (\beta * (Education_{(years)} - 12))$, where $\beta = 0.32136$.

To use the table, select the appropriate column corresponding to the patient's years of education, find the patient's NSS_A, and subsequently refer to the corresponding $NSS_{A\&E}$.

SOURCE: From Pena-Casanova et al. (2009).

forms (1981) vary in difficulty from the standard form; these cannot therefore be used in serial evaluations.

A tablet-based form of the SDMT has high correlations with the conventional SDMT at two testing points ($r > .90$) and smaller practice effects compared to the conventional SDMT in patients with stroke (4.7% vs. 5.6%; Tung et al., 2016). Similarly, in patients with schizophrenia, excellent test-retest reliability was reported for both the conventional and tablet versions of the test (ICCs > .89; Tang et al., 2017).

EVIDENCE FOR VALIDITY

WRITTEN VERSUS ORAL ADMINISTRATION

In healthy adults, the correlation between written and oral forms is greater than .78 (Smith, 1991), and is also high in patients with TBI ($r = .88$; Ponsford & Kinsella, 1992) and MS ($r = .89$; Sandroff et al., 2013). However, despite relatively high correlations between versions, mean scores on the two forms may differ. Sheridan et al. (2006) reviewed SDMT normative studies, which overall yielded higher mean scores on the oral rather than the written administration of the test (about 6 to 12 points, depending on age group).

FACTOR-ANALYTIC STUDIES AND RELATIONSHIPS WITH OTHER TESTS

Wechsler Digit Symbol. As discussed (see "Description"), the SDMT is very similar in format to the Wechsler Digit Symbol/Coding subtest. Accordingly, correlations between the two tests are large across studies (e.g., *rs* = .62 to .91; Bowler et al., 1992; Harris et al., 2007; Hinton-Barye et al., 1997; Hinton-Barye & Geffen, 2005; Morgan & Wheelock, 1992). Digit Symbol generally yields higher scores than the SDMT (Hinton-Barye & Geffen, 2005; Harris et al., 2007; see also "Description").

Attention and Executive Function Tests. The SDMT primarily assesses the scanning and tracking aspects of attention, similar to abilities required in Letter Cancellation, the TMT, Digit Symbol, and choice reaction-time tests (McCaffrey et al., 1988; Ponsford & Kinsella, 1992; Royan et al., 2004; Shum et al., 1990). For example, the SDMT correlates moderately with the TMT in normative and

TABLE 8-66 Characteristics of the Vogel et al. (2013) Symbol Digit Modalities Test (SDMT) Normative Sample

Sample size	100
Age	60 to 87 (M = 72 years, *SD* = 6.4)
Geographic location	Denmark
Education	23 years (*SD* = 2.6)
Gender	44% Men 56% Women
Ethnicity	Not available

TABLE 8-67 Symbol Digit Modalities Test (SDMT) Danish Normative Data (by Age)

AGE	N	SDMT	5TH PERCENTILE	10TH PERCENTILE
60 to 67	34	45.5 (7.1)	27	36
68 to 74	39	39.7 (7.5)[a]	26	29
75 to 87	27[a]	33.4 (8.6)[b]	19	23

NOTE: Data shown as mean (SD) and percentiles.

[a]Significant difference from age group 60 to 67.

[b]Significant difference from age group 60 to 67 and age group 68 to 74.

SOURCE: From Vogel et al. (2013).

clinical populations, with correlations between the SDMT and the TMT A ranging from −.49 to −.47 and with the TMT B ranging from −.51 to −.62 (e.g., Berrigan et al., 2014; Clark et al., 2004, Manly et al., 2011; Ryan et al., 2011). Correlations between Color Trails and the SDMT are of similar magnitude in a sample of older adults (*rs* = −.58, −.64; Vogel et al., 2012). Smaller correlations are reported between the SDMT and TMT errors (*r* = .38, Manly et al., 2011).

The SDMT also correlates with the Stroop (*rs* = .51, .54; Morrow, 2013; Vogel et al., 2012), Letter-Number Sequencing (*r* = −.36, Clark et al., 2004), and Digits Backward (*r* = .23, Ryan et al., 2011). The test has also been found to measure aspects of selective attention. For example, it loads highly on a factor described as Visual Selective Attention along with measures such as Stroop, TEA Map Search, TEA Telephone Search, and the Ruff 2 & 7 (Bate et al., 2001; Chan, 2000). Smaller correlations have been reported for the SDMT and Tower tests (not significant to *r* = .19; Clark et al., 2004; Nigg et al., 2001; Ryan et al., 2011) and fluency tasks (*r* = .25; Tam & Schmitter-Edgecombe, 2013).

Processing Speed. In addition to the relationships between the SDMT and attention and executive function tests, the SDMT relates to processing speed and reaction time (e.g., correlations between the SDMT and reaction time measures in patients with MS range from *r* = .29 to .44; Berrigan et al., 2014; Hughes et al., 2011).

In athletes, the SDMT appears to load with other processing speed tasks (Erlanger et al., 2003). The SDMT correlated with scores from the ImPACT test in a sample of athletes with concussion (range −.60 to .70), with ImPACT processing speed and reaction time demonstrating the highest correlations (Iverson et al., 2005). A PCA of five ImPACT composite scores and the SDMT yielded three components that accounted for approximately 82% of the variance; the SDMT and reaction time and processing speed factors of the ImPACT represented the first factor (Iverson et al., 2005).

Similarly, Kochunov et al. (2010) reported that the factor analysis of select neuropsychological tests (Category Fluency, Grooved Pegboard, Coding) yielded two factors that accounted for approximately 80% of the variance in scores. The SDMT loaded on the first factor along with Pegboard and Coding, labeled by the authors as psychomotor cognitive processing speed due to the common motor component.

PASAT and the SDMT. Most research using both the SDMT and the PASAT has been completed in MS studies. See also the PASAT review elsewhere in this chapter for additional discussion. Overall, moderate correlations have been reported between the SDMT and the PASAT (*rs* = .33 to .59; Berrigan et al., 2014; Benedict et al., 2010; Morrow, 2013; Royan et al., 2004; Sandroff et al., 2013). The SDMT and the Wechsler Digits Backward subtest accounted for nearly 50% of the variance in PASAT performance in healthy controls and patients with MS (Forn, Belenguer, Parcet-Ibars, & Ávila, 2008).

Memory. The SDMT is related to memory. For example, Tam and Schmitter-Edgecombe (2013) reported that after controlling for age and visuoconstructional ability, the SDMT uniquely predicted Brief Visuospatial Memory Test (BVMT-R) learning and memory performance. The SDMT correlates with measures of memory, including the BVMT-R (*r* = .46 to .39; Tam & Schmitter-Edgecombe, 2013) and the CVLT-II (*rs* = .50 to .69; Spedo et al., 2015).

CLINICAL STUDIES

The SDMT is one of the most commonly used tests across clinical populations, including TBI, MS, HD, concussion, epilepsy, stroke, PD, schizophrenia, HIV infection, and substance use disorders.

TBI. Large group differences are found on the SDMT between individuals with TBI and controls (Willmott et al., 2009). Ponsford and Kinsella (1992) found that the oral version of the SDMT was the single best indicator of information processing impairments in TBI compared with other tasks such as reaction time, Stroop, and the PASAT.

The task differentiates between individuals who are early versus late in the recovery process post-TBI (Bate et al., 2001). Draper and Ponsford (2008) reported that TBI patients performed worse than controls on the SDMT 10 years post-injury, with the SDMT identified as one of the strongest differentiators between the groups (Cohen's *d* = .61). Spitz et al. (2013) reported that increased time post-injury was related to better SDMT performance. Duration of posttraumatic amnesia also correlates with SDMT performance (Spearman rho = −.42, Draper & Ponsford, 2008; Spitz et al., 2013). Harmful or hazardous alcohol use pre-injury was associated with poorer performance on the SDMT and CVLT in a sample of individuals who sustained moderate to severe TBI (Ponsford et al., 2013).

The test is sensitive to the cognitive effects of diffuse axonal injury (DAI) in patients with severe TBI (Felmingham et al., 2004), and is related to ventricular enlargement (a marker of DAI) in individuals with TBI (Johnson et al., 1994). The test predicts change in level of daily functioning five years after TBI (Hammond et al., 2004).

The SDMT is sensitive to the effects of concussion in athletes (e.g., Erlanger et al., 2003; Hinton-Bayre et al., 1997, 1999; Zillmer, 2003), including change over time (Hinton-Bayre et al., 1999) and rate of recovery for injuries differing in severity (e.g., Mrazik et al., 2000). It is part of standard batteries for use in sports in determining return-to-play (Erlanger et al., 2003; Lovell & Collins, 1998; Maroon et al., 2000; see "Description").

MS. The SDMT has repeatedly been identified as one of the most sensitive tests to cognitive impairment in MS (e.g., Benedict et al., 2017; Dusankova et al., 2012; Einarsson et al., 2003; Esaghi et al., 2012; Henry & Beatty, 2006;

Possa, 2010). The SDMT is part of standardized batteries for MS (e.g., Beatty et al., 1995; Benedict et al., 2017; Polychroniadou et al., 2016; Rao & the Cognitive Function Study Group of the National Multiple Sclerosis Society, 1990; Solari et al., 2002).

Healthy controls perform better than patients with MS on the SDMT, even when demographic factors are considered (Spedo et al., 2015). Differences between controls and MS patients are large in magnitude (Esaghi et al., 2012, Hughes et al., 2011, 2013; Lafosse et al., 2007; Niccolai et al., 2015; Rodgers et al., 2013). Of note, a 30-second version of the task has been shown to have similar diagnostic classification accuracy in patients with MS compared to a longer form version (Gromisch et al., 2016).

The SDMT shows significant deterioration over five-year follow-up in patients with early MS (Glanz, Healy, Hviid, Chitnis, & Weiner, 2012), and the test correlates with the duration of MS (*rs* = −.23, −.60; Motl et al., 2013; Warlop et al., 2013). The test has been identified as a valid and reliable outcome measure in MS treatment, with a responder definition proposed as a change of 4 points, or 10% in magnitude (Benedict et al., 2017). However, practice effects must be taken into account when using the test as an outcome measure in the context of repeated assessments (Roar et al., 2016; see "Evidence for Reliability").

The SDMT is correlated with physical disability measures that are also part of MS test batteries, including the 9-Hole Peg Test (r = −.42) and the Timed 25-Foot Walk (r = −.21; Eshaghi et al., 2012). The SDMT correlates with ambulatory measures in MS (r = −.68 to .57, Motl et al., 2013) and is related to physical activity parameters in MS patients when age and disability are covaried (Sandroff et al., 2013). A composite score comprised of the PASAT and SDMT is a significant predictor of speech and articulation rate in MS (Rodgers et al., 2013).

The SDMT is highly correlated with disability in MS patients (absolute value of *rs* = .34 to .72; Caneda & Vecino, 2016; Eshaghi et al., 2012; Hughes et al., 2011; Motl et al., 2013; Warlop et al., 2013). The SDMT was found to correlate significantly (r = −.27, −.32) with the Multiple Sclerosis Impact Scale, a questionnaire assessing psychological and physical impact of MS from the patient's perspective (Schäffler et al., 2013). The SDMT, along with the Timed 25-Foot Walk, has been identified as one of the best predictors of functional decline in MS (Benedict et al., 2016). The SDMT significantly predicted disability conversion and worsening disease state in MS (Moccia et al., 2016) and is one of the best predictors of deterioration in work performance, with an OR of 4.2 after controlling for demographic and MS characteristics (Morrow et al., 2010). The SDMT relates to income level in MS, even when physical disability and other clinical and sociodemographic variables are accounted for (Kavaliunas et al., 2017).

The SDMT has also been used to differentiate between MS subtypes (e.g., Huijbregts et al., 2004, 2006), and patients with progressive MS perform worse than patients with relapsing-remitting MS. Rodrigues, Paes, Vasconcelos, Landeira-Fernandez, and Alvarenga (2011) reported that 50% of patients with relapsing-remitting MS and 69% of patients with primary progressive MS showed impairment on the SDMT.

MCI and Dementia. The SDMT has been identified as a sensitive test to predict conversion from healthy aging to MCI (Cherbuin et al., 2010) and MCI to Alzheimer's disease (AD; Fleisher et al., 2007). Patients with non-amnestic MCI perform worse on the SDMT than patients with amnestic MCI (Wang, 2012). The test has been used as an outcome measure in exercise interventions in MCI and dementia (e.g., Baker et al., 2010; Hoffman et al., 2016).

HD. Lafosse et al. (2007) reported that patients with HD performed worse than healthy controls and patients with MS on the SDMT. The SDMT is part of standard assessment methods for HD, such as the Unified Huntington's Disease Rating Scale (UH-DRS; Huntington Study Group, 1996).

The SDMT has also been used to track disease progression and identify markers of disease severity. The rate of progression of HD is estimated to be 2 SDMT points per year (Mahant et al., 2003). Beglinger et al. (2010) reported that decline occurred in SDMT performance over a 16-month test-retest interval in a sample of patients with HD. Tabrizi et al. (2012) reported that cognitive performance declined over a 24-month period to a greater extent in an early HD group compared with controls, with the SDMT showing the largest effect size of cognitive measures used. The SDMT was recommended as an outcome measure for therapeutic trials in HD.

In patients with HD, disability is predicted by cognitive impairment as measured by the SDMT and negative motor features (Mahant et al., 2003). SDMT performance is also related to the presence of obsessive-compulsive symptoms in patients with HD (Anderson et al., 2001). The SDMT has been identified as a predictor of apathy in HD (Reedeker et al., 2011). Devos, Nieuwboer, Tant, De Weerdt, and Vandenberghe (2010) identified the SDMT as one of the most accurate tests in classifying at-risk drivers among persons with HD. Like Digit Symbol, the SDMT is one of the few tests sensitive to cognitive impairments in asymptomatic carriers of the HD gene (Lemiere, Decruyenaere, & Evers-Kiebooms, 2002) and has been identified as one of the tests able to detect cognitive change in prodromal HD (Paulsen et al., 2017). It is therefore an important tool for assessing the earliest symptoms of HD.

Psychiatric Conditions. People with schizophrenia perform worse than controls on the test (Chan et al., 2004; Elahipanah et al., 2011). In one study, people with nonparanoid schizophrenia performed worse than a paranoid subgroup on the SDMT (Chan et al., 2004). Elahipanah, Christensen, and Reingold (2011) examined eye movements during a computerized adaptation of the SDMT in people with schizophrenia and healthy controls and found that people with schizophrenia spent increased time searching for the target symbol and searched the key area more often. This pattern was interpreted to be reflective of less efficient visual search.

Older adults with depression and remitted depression perform worse than controls on the SDMT (Ayotte et al., 2009; Yuan et al., 2009). Hasselbalch, Knorr, Hasselbalch, Gade, and Kessing (2012) reported that a diagnosis of depression predicted performance on the SDMT after adjustment for demographic and clinical variables. Comorbid depression with an existing neurologic condition (e.g., MS) may result in worse performance on the test (Patel et al., 2016). Hashimoto et al. (2008) reported that people with obsessive-compulsive disorder performed worse than demographically matched controls.

Other Populations. Rivastigmine is associated with improved SDMT performance in individuals with PD dementia (Schmitt et al., 2010). The SDMT has been associated with driving performance in driver simulator studies in PD (Ranchet et al., 2012).

The SDMT has also been used to investigate attention in a number of other conditions, including hepatitis C (Crystal et al., 2011; O'Bryant et al., 2007), epilepsy (Meador et al., 2003), effects of neurotoxic substances (Coxon, 2002), substance abuse (Al-Zahrani & Elsayed, 2009; Cuyàs et al., 2011), brain tumors (Torres et al., 2003), and sleep apnea (Verstraeten et al., 2004). After adjustment for age, education, ethnic classification, and reading level, the SDMT was the only measure on which group differences in performance remained between women with HIV and those without (Manly et al., 2011).

The SDMT has also been used to evaluate hormonal fluctuations in postmenopausal women (Ryan et al., 2011). In a longitudinal study of women at midlife, lower physical scores were associated with lower SDMT scores, with this association remaining after controlling for socioeconomic status, depressive symptoms, and metabolic syndrome (Ford et al., 2010). The ratio of free testosterone to estradiol is related to scores on the SDMT in postmenopausal women (Ryan et al., 2011).

Poorer SDMT performance has been associated with anticholinergic medication use in older age (Low, Anstey, & Sachdev, 2009). The SDMT has been used to study the effects of repetitive transcranial magnetic stimulation in patients with fibromyalgia, with improvement reported after treatment (Baudic et al., 2013). Dong, Simon, Rajan, and Evans (2011) found associations between SDMT performance and increased risk of elder abuse, with associations also reported between SDMT and elder self-neglect (Dong et al., 2009, 2010).

NEUROANATOMICAL CORRELATES AND IMAGING STUDIES

As may be expected for an attentional test with processing speed demands, neuroimaging research has implicated frontal-parietal networks as well as regions rich in white matter as neural substrates of this task.

The SDMT has been demonstrated to be one of the tests most strongly associated with neuroimaging indices of disease in MS, including central atrophy accounting for approximately half the shared variance in patients with mild to moderate cognitive impairment (Christodoulou et al., 2003). In a systematic review, Vollmer et al. (2016) reported that brain volume loss was related to SDMT performance in patients with MS. Decreased gray matter volume was associated with poorer SDMT performance in the thalamus, cerebellum, putamen, and occipital cortex in MS (Bisecco et al., 2017). Sumowski, Chiaravalloti, Wylie, and Deluca (2009) reported that brain atrophy predicted scores on a composite measure comprised of SDMT and PASAT scores. An interaction was reported, such that individuals with higher levels of premorbid intelligence or cognitive reserve were better able to sustain atrophy without a concomitant impact on scores. Patterns of activation during SDMT performance in patients with MS suggest reduced cognitive efficiency, with greater resources expended to perform the task (Fittipaldi-Márquez et al., 2017).

The SDMT is significantly related to transverse diffusivity (i.e., diffusion across fibers rather than along fibers), a marker for axonal loss and demyelination, as measured by DTI in patients with MS (Warlop et al., 2009). Reduction of fractional anisotropy values in the posterior thalamic radiation, sagittal stratum, and corpus callosum is related to cognitive function in individuals with relapsing-remitting MS, with the strongest correlations observed for the SDMT among the tests examined (Yu et al., 2012). In patients with MS, slower SDMT performance is related to smaller corpus callosal area (Bergendal et al., 2013).

Forn et al. (2011) reported that the PASAT and SDMT were associated with activation in the left frontal and parietal areas, with the PASAT activating more frontal regions than the SDMT; the SDMT further showed bilateral occipital activation. Forn et al. (2013) evaluated the utility of an oral fMRI-adapted version of the SDMT, incorporating three different interstimulus intervals. All conditions were associated with activation in the frontoparietal networks. Shorter intervals were related to greater activation in occipital regions and greater network activation overall, including frontal areas.

Kochunov et al. (2010) examined relationships between declines in processing speed and frontal lobe MRI/magnetic resonance spectroscopy in older adults. The SDMT and other tests were factor analyzed, with a substantial proportion of variance in cognitive factor scores related to atrophic changes in frontal white matter. SDMT performance was also correlated with decreased gray matter thickness. Gautam, Cherbuin, Sachdev, Wen, and Anstey (2011) reported relationships between lateral frontal cortical volume and thickness and SDMT performance in early old-age adults.

Hou et al. (2012) reported that in remitted geriatric depressed patients, positive correlations were observed between right hippocampal volumes and the SDMT. Segura et al. (2010) reported that DTI fractional anisotropy values correlated with SDMT scores in the anterior and posterior corpus callosum in patients with metabolic syndrome.

PERFORMANCE VALIDITY

There is limited research on whether the test can be used as a measure of performance validity. Unsurprisingly, the medicolegal context may affect performance on the SDMT. Lees-Hayley (1990) gave the test to 20 personal injury litigants with no history of brain injury and no claim for brain injury. One-half of the sample scored in the potentially impaired range (≤1.5 *SD* from the mean).

COMMENT

The SDMT has a long history in neuropsychology and is an elegant yet multifactorial task that is brief and easy to administer. Users should note that MS research has suggested that mild visual impairment and dysarthria (on the oral version) can impact performance and that the oral version of the test may be a suitable alternative in the case of upper limb dysfunction.

The SDMT is affected by demographic variables. Age effects are generally moderate, with most noted decline after 55 years of age. Although some studies report no significant gender differences, others report a female advantage. Education exerts a significant effect. Ethnicity and other sociodemographic variables may be influential on performance, although performance can be complicated by other factors. There are many published studies on the SDMT, and, given demographic influences, a Flynn effect, and other limitations of the standardization sample, users are encouraged to utilize more recent normative datasets that reflect their examinee's characteristics and take demographic factors (age, gender, education, ethnicity) into account.

Overall, the SDMT shows high test-retest reliability over days to weeks, with adequate reliability or better at longer intervals (e.g., six months, years). Reliability estimates for the total score are typically reported, with limited information regarding reliability for other variables (e.g., incidental learning, percentage correct). Most research indicates that practice effects exist, but that these are generally small in magnitude. Reliable change indices and alternate forms have been created, including a tablet administration.

Although highly correlated, oral forms are typically associated with higher scores than written versions. The Wechsler Digit Symbol/Coding test also typically yields higher scores than the SDMT. The test correlates, at least moderately, with other attention and executive function tests, such as the TMT, Stroop, Digits Backward, and the PASAT, and less so with Tower and fluency tasks. Factor-analytic and correlational studies also indicate a strong processing speed component.

The SDMT has been used in a number of clinical populations, with a particularly extensive body of research in MS. Group differences are often found between patients with various conditions and controls, many of large magnitude. Much research, especially in MS, not only suggests group differences, but also that the SDMT relates to disease staging, daily functioning (e.g., physical activity variables, disability, vocational skills), and neuroimaging in a variety of different conditions. As may be expected for an attentional test with processing speed demands, neuroimaging research implicates frontoparietal networks as well as regions rich in white matter as neural substrates of this task.

REFERENCES

Agranovich, A. V., Panter, A. T., Puente, A. E., & Touradji, P. (2011). The culture of time in neuropsychological assessment: Exploring the effects of culture-specific time attitudes on timed test performance in Russian and American samples. *Journal of the International Neuropsychological Society, 17*(04), 692–701. http://doi.org/10.1017/S1355617711000592

Al-Zahrani, M. A., & Elsayed, Y. A. (2009). The impacts of substance abuse and dependence on neuropsychological functions in a sample of patients from Saudi Arabia. *Behavioral and Brain Functions, 5*(1), 48. http://doi.org/10.1186/1744-9081-5-48

Anderson, K. E., Louis, E. D., Stern, Y., & Marder, K. S. (2001). Cognitive correlates of obsessive and compulsive symptoms in Huntington's disease. *American Journal of Psychiatry, 158*, 799–801.

Ayotte, B. J., Potter, G. G., Williams, H. T., Steffens, D. C., & Bosworth, H. B. (2009). The moderating role of personality factors in the relationship between depression and neuropsychological functioning among older adults. *International Journal of Geriatric Psychiatry, 24*(9), 1010–1019. http://doi.org/10.1002/gps.2213

Azambuja, M. J., Radanovic, M., Haddad, M. S., Adda, C. C., Barbosa, E. R., & Mansur, L. L. (2012). Language impairment in Huntington's disease. *Arquivos de Neuro-Psiquiatria, 70*(6), 410–415.

Baker, L. D., Frank, L. L., Foster-Schubert, K., Green, P. S., Wilkinson, C. W., McTiernan, A., . . . Craft, S. (2010). Effects of a controlled trial of aerobic exercise for mild cognitive impairment: A controlled trial. *Archives of Neurology, 67*(1), 71–79. https://doi.org/10.1001/archneurol.2009.307

Bate, A. J., Mathias, J. L., & Crawford, J. R. (2001). Performance on the Test of Everyday Attention and standard tests of attention following severe traumatic brain injury. *The Clinical Neuropsychologist, 15*(3), 405–422.

Baudic, S., Attal, N., Mhalla, A., Ciampi de Andrade, D., Perrot, S., & Bouhassira, D. (2013). Unilateral repetitive transcranial magnetic stimulation of the motor cortex does not affect cognition in patients with fibromyalgia. *Journal of Psychiatric Research, 47*(1), 72–77. http://doi.org/10.1016/j.jpsychires.2012.09.003

Beatty, W. W., Paul, R. H., Wilbanks, S. L., Hames, K. A., Blanco, C. R., & Goodkin, D. E. (1995). Identifying multiple sclerosis patients with mild or global cognitive impairment using the screening examination for cognitive impairment (SEFCI). *Neurology, 45*, 718–723.

Beglinger, L. J., Duff, K., Allison, J., Theriault, D., O'Rourke, J. J. F., Leserman, A., & Paulsen, J. S. (2010). Cognitive change in patients with Huntington disease on the Repeatable Battery for the Assessment of Neuropsychological Status. *Journal of Clinical and Experimental Neuropsychology, 32*(6), 573–578. http://doi.org/10.1080/13803390903313564

Beier, M., Gromisch, E. S., Hughes, A. J., Alschuler, K. N., Madathil, R., Chiaravalloti, N., & Foley, F. W. (2017). Proposed cut scores for tests of the Brief International Cognitive Assessment of Multiple Sclerosis (BICAMS). *Journal of the Neurological Sciences, 381*, 110–116. https://doi.org/10.1016/j.jns.2017.08.019

Benedict, R. H., DeLuca, J., Phillips, G., LaRocca, N., Hudson, L. D., Rudick, R., & Multiple Sclerosis Outcome Assessments Consortium. (2017). Validity of the Symbol Digit Modalities Test as a cognition performance outcome measure for multiple sclerosis. *Multiple Sclerosis (Houndmills, Basingstoke, England), 23*(5), 721–733. https://doi.org/10.1177/1352458517690821

Benedict, R. H., Drake, A. S., Irwin, L. N., Frndak, S. E., Kunker, K. A., Khan, A. L., . . . Weinstock-Guttman, B. (2016). Benchmarks of meaningful impairment on the MSFC and BICAMS. *Multiple Sclerosis (Houndmills, Basingstoke, England), 22*(14), 1874–1882. https://doi.org/10.1177/1352458516633517

Benedict, R. H. B., Morrow, S. A., Weinstock Guttman, B., Cookfair, D., & Schretlen, D. J. (2010). Cognitive reserve moderates decline in information processing speed in multiple sclerosis patients. *Journal of the International Neuropsychological Society, 16*(05), 829–835. http://doi.org/10.1017/S1355617710000688

Bergendal, G., Martola, J., Stawiarz, L., Kristoffersen-Wiberg, M., Fredrikson, S., & Almkvist, O. (2013). Callosal atrophy in multiple sclerosis is related to cognitive speed. *Acta Neurologica Scandinavica, 127*(4), 281–289. http://doi.org/10.1111/ane.12006

Berrigan, L. I., Fisk, J. D., Walker, L. A. S., Wojtowicz, M., Rees, L. M., Freedman, M. S., & Marrie, R. A. (2014). Reliability of regression-based normative data for the Oral Symbol Digit Modalities Test: An evaluation of demographic influences, construct validity, and impairment classification rates in multiple sclerosis samples. *The Clinical Neuropsychologist, 28*(2), 281–299. http://doi.org/10.1080/13854046.2013.871337

Bisecco, A., Stamenova, S., Caiazzo, G., d'Ambrosio, A., Sacco, R., Docimo, R., . . . Gallo, A. (2017). Attention and processing speed performance in multiple sclerosis is mostly related to thalamic volume. *Brain Imaging and Behavior*. https://doi.org/10.1007/s11682-016-9667-6

Bowler, R., Sudia, S., Mergler, D., Harrison, R., & Cone, J. (1992). Comparison of Digit Symbol and Symbol Digit Modalities Tests for assessing neurotoxic exposure. *The Clinical Neuropsychologist, 6*, 103–104.

Bruce, J. M., Bruce, A. S., & Arnett, P. A. (2007). Mild visual acuity disturbances are associated with performance on tests of complex visual attention in MS. *Journal of the International Neuropsychological Society, 13*(03), 544–548.

Caneda, M. A. G. de, & Vecino, M. C. A. de. (2016). The correlation between EDSS and cognitive impairment in MS patients. Assessment of a Brazilian population using a BICAMS version. *Arquivos De Neuro-Psiquiatria, 74*(12), 974–981. https://doi.org/10.1590/0004-282X20160151

Chan, M. W. C., Yip, J. T. H., & Lee, T. M. C. (2004). Differential impairment on measures of attention in patients with paranoid and nonparanoid schizophrenia. *Journal of Psychiatric Research, 38*(2), 145–152.

Chan, R. C. K. (2000). Attentional deficits in patients with closed head injury: A further study of the discriminative validity of the Test of Everyday Attention. *Brain Injury, 14*, 227–236.

Cherbuin, N., Sachdev, P., & Anstey, K. J. (2010). Neuropsychological predictors of transition from healthy cognitive aging to mild cognitive impairment: The PATH Through Life Study. *American Journal of Geriatric Psychiatry, 18*(8), 723–733. https://doi.org/10.1097/JGP.0b013e3181cdecf1

Christodoulou, C., Krupp, L. E., & Liang, Z. (2003). Cognitive performance and MR markers of cerebral injury in cognitively impaired MS patients. *Neurology, 60*(11), 1793–1798.

Clark, M. S., Dennerstein, L., Elkadi, S., Guthrie, J. R., Bowden, S. C., & Henderson, V. W. (2004). Normative data for tasks of executive function and working memory for Australian-born women aged 56-67. *Australian Psychologist, 39*(3), 244–250. http://doi.org/10.1080/00050060412331295126

Cores, E. V., Vanotti, S., Eizaguirre, B., Fiorentini, L., Garcea, O., Benedict, R. H. B., & Cáceres, F. (2015). The effect of culture on two information-processing speed tests. *Applied Neuropsychology. Adult, 22*(4), 241–245. https://doi.org/10.1080/23279095.2014.910214

Coxon, L. (2002). Neuropsychological assessment of a group of BAe 146 aircraft crew members exposed to jet engine oil emissions. *Journal of Occupational Health Safety (Austria and New Zealand), 18*(4), 313–319.

Crystal, H. A., Weedon, J., Holman, S., Manly, J., Valcour, V., Cohen, M., . . . others. (2011). Associations of cardiovascular variables and HAART with cognition in middle-aged HIV-infected and uninfected women. *Journal of Neurovirology, 17*(5), 469–476.

Cuyàs, E., Verdejo-García, A., Fagundo, A. B., Khymenets, O., Rodríguez, J., Cuenca, A., . . . de la Torre, R. (2011). The influence of genetic and environmental factors among MDMA users in cognitive performance. *PLoS ONE, 6*(11), e27206. http://doi.org/10.1371/journal.pone.0027206

Devos, H., Nieuwboer, A., Tant, M., De Weerdt, W., & Vandenberghe, W. (2012). Determinants of fitness to drive in Huntington disease. *Neurology, 79*(19), 1975–1982. https://doi.org/10.1212/WNL.0b013e3182735d11

Dickinson, M. D., & Hiscock, M. (2011). The Flynn Effect in neuropsychological assessment. *Applied Neuropsychology, 18*(2), 136–142. http://doi.org/10.1080/09084282.2010.547785

Dong, X., Simon, M., Rajan, K., & Evans, D. A. (2011). Association of cognitive function and risk for elder abuse in a community-dwelling population. *Dementia and Geriatric Cognitive Disorders, 32*(3), 209–215. http://doi.org/10.1159/000334047

Dong, X., Simon, M. A., Wilson, R. S., Mendes de Leon, C. F., Rajan, K. B., & Evans, D. A. (2010). Decline in cognitive function and risk of elder self-neglect: Finding from the Chicago Health Aging Project: Decline in cognitive function and elder self-neglect. *Journal of the American Geriatrics Society, 58*(12), 2292–2299. http://doi.org/10.1111/j.1532-5415.2010.03156.x

Dong, X., Wilson, R. S., Mendes de Leon, C. F., & Evans, D. A. (2009). Self-neglect and cognitive function among community-dwelling older persons. *International Journal of Geriatric Psychiatry, 25*(8), 798–806. http://doi.org/10.1002/gps.2420

Draper, K., & Ponsford, J. (2008). Cognitive functioning ten years following traumatic brain injury and rehabilitation. *Neuropsychology, 22*(5), 618–625. http://doi.org/10.1037/0894-4105.22.5.618

Duff, K., Atkinson, T. J., Suhrie, K. R., Dalley, B. C. A., Schaefer, S. Y., & Hammers, D. B. (2017). Short-term practice effects in mild cognitive impairment: Evaluating different methods of change. *Journal of Clinical and Experimental Neuropsychology, 39*(4), 396–407. https://doi.org/10.1080/13803395.2016.1230596

Dusankova, J. B., Kalincik, T., Havrdova, E., & Benedict, R. H. B. (2012). Cross cultural validation of the Minimal Assessment of Cognitive Function in Multiple Sclerosis (MACFIMS) and the Brief International Cognitive Assessment for Multiple Sclerosis (BICAMS). *The Clinical Neuropsychologist, 26*(7), 1186–1200. http://doi.org/10.1080/13854046.2012.725101

Einarsson, U., Gottberg, K., & Fredrikson, S. (2003). Multiple sclerosis in Stockholm county: A pilot study exploring the feasibility of assessment of impairment disability and handicap by home visits. *Clinical Rehabilitation, 17*(3), 294–303.

Elahipanah, A., Christensen, B. K., & Reingold, E. M. (2011). What can eye movements tell us about Symbol Digit substitution by patients with schizophrenia? *Schizophrenia Research, 127*(1–3), 137–143. http://doi.org/10.1016/j.schres.2010.11.018

Erlanger, D., Feldman, D., Kutner, K., Kaushik, T., Kroger, H., Festa, J., Barth, J., Freeman, J., & Broshek, D. (2003). Development and validation of a web-based neuropsychological test protocol for sports-related return-to-play decision-making. *Archives of Clinical Neuropsychology, 18*, 293–316.

Eshaghi, A., Riyahi-Alam, S., Roostaei, T., Haeri, G., Aghsaei, A., Aidi, M. R., . . . Sahraian, M. A. (2012). Validity and reliability of a Persian translation of the Minimal Assessment of Cognitive Function in Multiple Sclerosis (MACFIMS). *The Clinical Neuropsychologist, 26*(6), 975–984. http://doi.org/10.1080/13854046.2012.694912

Feinstein, A., Brown, R., & Ron, M. (1994). Effects of practice on serial tests of attention in healthy subjects. *Journal of Clinical and Experimental Neuropsychology, 16*, 436–447.

Felmingham, K. L., Baguley, I. J., & Green, A. M. (2004). Effects of diffuse axonal injury on speed of information processing following a severe traumatic brain injury. *Neuropsychology, 18*(3), 564–571.

Fittipaldi-Márquez, M. S., Cruz-Gómez, Á. J., Sanchis-Segura, C., Belenguer, A., Ávila, C., & Forn, C. (2017). Exploring neural efficiency in multiple sclerosis patients during the Symbol Digit Modalities Test: A functional magnetic resonance imaging study. *Neuro-Degenerative Diseases, 17*(4–5), 199–207. https://doi.org/10.1159/000460252

Fleisher, A. S., Sowell, B. B., Taylor, C., Gamst, A. C., Petersen, R. C., & Thal, L. J. (2007). Clinical predictors of progression to Alzheimer disease in amnestic mild cognitive impairment. *Neurology, 68*(19), 1588–1595. https://doi.org/10.1212/01.wnl.0000258542.58725.4c

Ford, K., Sowers, M., Seeman, T. E., Greendale, G. A., Sternfeld, B., & Everson-Rose, S. A. (2010). Cognitive functioning is related to physical functioning in a longitudinal study of women at midlife. *Gerontology, 56*(3), 250–258. http://doi.org/10.1159/000247132

Forn, C., Belenguer, A., Belloch, V., Sanjuan, A., Parcet, M. A., & Ávila, C. (2011). Anatomical and functional differences between the Paced Auditory Serial Addition Test and the Symbol Digit Modalities Test. *Journal of Clinical and Experimental Neuropsychology, 33*(1), 42–50. http://doi.org/10.1080/13803395.2010.481620

Forn, C., Belenguer, A., Parcet-Ibars, M. A., & Ávila, C. (2008). Information-processing speed is the primary deficit underlying the poor performance of multiple sclerosis patients in the Paced Auditory Serial Addition Test (PASAT). *Journal of Clinical and Experimental Neuropsychology, 30*(7), 789–796. https://doi.org/10.1080/13803390701779560

Forn, C., Ripollés, P., Cruz-Gómez, A. J., Belenguer, A., González-Torre, J. A., & Ávila, C. (2013). Task-load manipulation in the Symbol Digit Modalities Test: An alternative measure of information processing speed. *Brain and Cognition, 82*(2), 152–160. http://doi.org/10.1016/j.bandc.2013.04.003

Gautam, P., Cherbuin, N., Sachdev, P. S., Wen, W., & Anstey, K. J. (2011). Relationships between cognitive function and frontal gray matter volumes and thickness in middle aged and early old-aged adults: The PATH Through Life Study. *NeuroImage, 55*(3), 845–855. http://doi.org/10.1016/j.neuroimage.2011.01.015

Gilmore, G. C., Royer, F. L., & Gruhn, J. J. (1983). Age differences in symbol-digit substitution task performance. *Journal of Clinical Psychology, 39*, 114–124.

Glanz, B. I., Healy, B. C., Hviid, L. E., Chitnis, T., & Weiner, H. L. (2012). Cognitive deterioration in patients with early multiple sclerosis: a 5-year study. *Journal of Neurology, Neurosurgery & Psychiatry, 83*(1), 38–43. http://doi.org/10.1136/jnnp.2010.237834

Glosser, G., Butters, N., & Kaplan, E. (1977). Visuoperceptual processes in brain-damaged patients on the digit symbol substitution task. *International Journal of Neuroscience, 7*, 59–66.

Gonzalez, H., Whitfield, K., West, B., Williams, D., Lichtenberg, P., & Jackson, J. (2007). Modified-Symbol Digit Modalities Test for African Americans, Caribbean Black Americans, and non-Latino Whites: Nationally representative normative data from the National Survey of American Life. *Archives of Clinical Neuropsychology, 22*(5), 605–613. http://doi.org/10.1016/j.acn.2007.04.002

Goretti, B., Niccolai, C., Hakiki, B., Sturchio, A., Falautano, M., Minacapelli, E., . . . Amato, M. P. (2014). The brief international cognitive assessment for multiple sclerosis (BICAMS): Normative values with gender, age and education corrections in the Italian population. *BMC Neurology, 14*(1). http://doi.org/10.1186/s12883-014-0171-6

Gromisch, E. S., Zemon, V., Holtzer, R., Chiaravalloti, N. D., DeLuca, J., Beier, M., . . . Foley, F. W. (2016). Assessing the criterion validity of four highly abbreviated measures from the Minimal Assessment of Cognitive Function in Multiple Sclerosis (MACFIMS). *The Clinical Neuropsychologist, 30*(7), 1032–1049. https://doi.org/10.1080/13854046.2016.1189597

Hammond, F. M., Grattan, K. D., & Sasser, H. (2004). Five years after traumatic brain injury: A study of individual outcomes and predictors of change in function. *NeuroRehabilitation, 19*(1), 25–35.

Harris, J. G., Wagner, B., & Munro Cullum, C. (2007). Symbol vs. digit substitution task performance in diverse cultural and linguistic groups. *The Clinical Neuropsychologist, 21*(5), 800–810. http://doi.org/10.1080/13854040600801019

Hashimoto, T., Shimizu, E., Koike, K., Orita, Y., Suzuki, T., Kanahara, N., . . . Iyo, M. (2008). Deficits in auditory P50 inhibition in obsessive–compulsive disorder. *Progress in Neuro-Psychopharmacology and Biological Psychiatry, 32*(1), 288–296. http://doi.org/10.1016/j.pnpbp.2007.08.021

Hasselbalch, B. J., Knorr, U., Hasselbalch, S. G., Gade, A., & Kessing, L. V. (2012). Cognitive deficits in the remitted state of unipolar depressive disorder. *Neuropsychology, 26*(5), 642–651. http://doi.org/10.1037/a0029301

Henry, J. D., & Beatty, W. W. (2006). Verbal fluency deficits in multiple sclerosis. *Neuropsychologia, 44*(7), 1166–1174. http://doi.org/10.1016/j.neuropsychologia.2005.10.006

Hinton-Bayre, A., & Geffen, G. (2005). Comparability, reliability, and practice effects on alternate forms of the Digit Symbol Substitution and Symbol Digit Modalities Tests. *Psychological Assessment, 17*(2), 237–241. http://doi.org/10.1037/1040-3590.17.2.237

Hinton-Bayre, A. D., Geffen, G., Geffen, L. B., McFarland, K. A., & Friis, P. (1999). Concussion in contact sports: Reliable change indices of impairment and recovery. *Journal of Clinical and Experimental Neuropsychology, 21*(1), 70–86.

Hinton-Bayre, A. D., Geffen, G., & McFarland, K. (1997). Mild head injury and speed of information processing: A prospective study of professional rugby league players. *Journal of Clinical and Experimental Neuropsychology, 19*, 275–289.

Hoffmann, K., Sobol, N. A., Frederiksen, K. S., Beyer, N., Vogel, A., Vestergaard, K., . . . Hasselbalch, S. G. (2016). Moderate-to-high intensity physical exercise in patients with Alzheimer's disease: A randomized controlled trial. *Journal of Alzheimer's Disease: JAD, 50*(2), 443–453. https://doi.org/10.3233/JAD-150817

Hsieh, S., & Tori, C. (2007). Normative data on cross-cultural neuropsychological tests obtained from Mandarin-speaking adults across the life span. *Archives of Clinical Neuropsychology, 22*(3), 283–296. http://doi.org/10.1016/j.acn.2007.01.004

Hou, Z., Yuan, Y., Zhang, Z., Bai, F., Hou, G., & You, J. (2012). Longitudinal changes in hippocampal volumes and cognition in remitted geriatric depressive disorder. *Behavioural Brain Research, 227*(1), 30–35. http://doi.org/10.1016/j.bbr.2011.10.025

Hughes, A. J., Denney, D. R., & Lynch, S. G. (2011). Reaction time and rapid serial processing measures of information processing speed in multiple sclerosis: complexity, compounding, and augmentation. *Journal of the International Neuropsychological Society, 17*(06), 1113–1121. http://doi.org/10.1017/S1355617711001135

Hughes, A. J., Denney, D. R., Owens, E. M., & Lynch, S. G. (2013). Procedural variations in the Stroop and the Symbol Digit Modalities Test: Impact on patients with multiple sclerosis. *Archives of Clinical Neuropsychology, 28*(5), 452–462. http://doi.org/10.1093/arclin/act041

Huijbregts, S. C. J., Kalkers, N. F., de Sonneville, L. M. J., de Groot, V., & Polman, C. H. (2006). Cognitive impairment and decline in different MS subtypes. *Journal of the Neurological Sciences, 245*(1-2), 187–194. http://doi.org/10.1016/j.jns.2005.07.018

Huijbregts, S. C. J., Kalkers, N. F., de Sonneville, L. M. J., de Groot, V., Reuling, I. E. W., & Polman, C. H. (2004). Differences in cognitive impairment of relapsing, remitting, secondary, and primary progressive MS. *Neurology, 63*, 335–339.

Huntington Study Group. (1996). Unified Huntington's Disease Rating Scale: Reliability and consistency. *Movement Disorders, 11*, 136–142.

Iverson, G. L., Lovell, M. R., & Collins, M. W. (2005). Retrieved from http://www.impacttest.com/ArticlesPage_images/Articles_Docs/6ValidityofImPACT2004.doc

Jaywant, A., Barredo, J., Ahern, D. C., & Resnik, L. (2016). Neuropsychological assessment without upper limb involvement: A systematic review of oral versions of the Trail Making Test and Symbol-Digit Modalities Test. *Neuropsychological Rehabilitation*, 1–23. https://doi.org/10.1080/09602011.2016.1240699

Johnson, S. C., Bigler, E. D., Burr, R. B., & Blatter, D. D. (1994). White matter atrophy, ventricular dilation, and intellectual functioning following traumatic brain injury. *Neuropsychology, 8*, 301–315.

Jorm, A. F., Anstey, K. J., Christensen, H., & Rodgers, B. (2004). Gender differences in cognitive abilities: The mediating role of health state and health habits. *Intelligence, 32*, 7–23.

Joy, S., Kaplan, E., & Fein, D. (2004). Speed and memory in the WAIS-III Digit Symbol- Coding subtest across the adult lifespan. *Archives of Clinical Neuropsychology, 19*, 759–767.

Kavaliunas, A., Danylaite Karrenbauer, V., Gyllensten, H., Manouchehrinia, A., Glaser, A., Olsson, T., . . . Hillert, J. (2017). Cognitive function is a major determinant of income among multiple sclerosis patients in Sweden acting independently from physical disability. *Multiple Sclerosis (Houndmills, Basingstoke, England)*. https://doi.org/10.1177/1352458517740212

Kennepohl, S., Shore, D., & Nabors, N. (2004). African American acculturation and neuropsychological test performance following traumatic brain injury. *Journal of the International Neuropsychological Society, 10*(4), 566–577.

Kiely, K. M., Butterworth, P., Watson, N., & Wooden, M. (2014). The Symbol Digit Modalities Test: Normative data from a large nationally representative sample of Australians. *Archives of Clinical Neuropsychology, 29*(8), 767–775. http://doi.org/10.1093/arclin/acu055

Kochunov, P., Coyle, T., Lancaster, J., Robin, D. A., Hardies, J., Kochunov, V., . . . Fox, P. T. (2010). Processing speed is correlated with cerebral health markers in the frontal lobes as quantified by neuroimaging. *NeuroImage, 49*(2), 1190–1199. http://doi.org/10.1016/j.neuroimage.2009.09.052

Koh, C.–L., Lu, W.–S., Chen, H.–C., Hsueh, I.–P., Hsieh, J.–J., & Hsieh, C.–L. (2011). Test-Retest Reliability and Practice effect of the oral-format Symbol Digit Modalities Test in patients with stroke. *Archives of Clinical Neuropsychology, 26*(4), 356–363. http://doi.org/10.1093/arclin/acr029

Lafosse, J. M., Corboy, J. R., Leehey, M. A., Seeberger, L. C., & Filley, C. M. (2007). MS vs. HD: Can white matter and subcortical gray matter pathology be distinguished neuropsychologically? *Journal of Clinical and Experimental Neuropsychology, 29*(2), 142–154. http://doi.org/10.1080/13803390600582438

Lam, M., Eng, G. K., Rapisarda, A., Subramaniam, M., Kraus, M., Keefe, R. S. E., & Collinson, S. L. (2013). Formulation of the age–education index: Measuring age and education effects in neuropsychological performance. *Psychological Assessment, 25*(1), 61–70. http://doi.org/10.1037/a0030548

Laux, L. F., & Lane, D. M. (1985). Information processing components of substitution test performance. *Intelligence, 9*(2), 111–136.

Lee, P., Li, P.–C., Liu, C.–H., & Hsieh, C.–L. (2011). Test-Retest Reliability of Two Attention Tests in Schizophrenia. *Archives of Clinical Neuropsychology, 26*(5), 405–411. http://doi.org/10.1093/arclin/acr038

Lees-Haley, P. (1990). Contamination of neuropsychological testing by litigation. *Forensic Reports, 3*(4), 421–426.

Lemiere, J., Decruyenaere, M., Evers-Kiebooms, G., Vandenbussche, E., & Dom, R. (2002). Longitudinal study evaluating neuropsychological changes in so-called asymptomatic carriers of the Huntington's disease mutation after 1 year. *Acta Neurologica Scandinavica, 106*(3), 131–141. https://doi.org/10.1034/j.1600-0404.2002.01192.x

Levine, A. J., Miller, E. N., Becker, J. T., Selnes, O. A., & Cohen, B. A. (2004). Normative data for determining significance of test-retest differences on eight common neuropsychological instruments. *The Clinical Neuropsychologist, 18*, 373–384.

Lovell, M. R., & Collins, M. W. (1998). Neuropsychological assessment of the college football player. *Journal of Head Trauma Rehabilitation, 13*, 9–26.

Low, L.-F., Anstey, K. J., & Sachdev, P. (2009). Use of medications with anticholinergic properties and cognitive function in a young-old community sample. *International Journal of Geriatric Psychiatry, 24*(6), 578–584. https://doi.org/10.1002/gps.2157

Mahant, N., McCusker, E. A., Byth, K., & the Huntington Study Group. (2003). Huntington's disease: Clinical correlates of disability and progression. *Neurology, 61*(8), 1085-1092.

Manly, J. J., Smith, C., Crystal, H. A., Richardson, J., Golub, E. T., Greenblatt, R., . . . Young, M. (2011). Relationship of ethnicity, age, education, and reading level to speed and executive function among HIV+ and HIV– women: The Women's Interagency HIV Study (WIHS) Neurocognitive Substudy. *Journal of Clinical and Experimental Neuropsychology, 33*(8), 853–863. http://doi.org/10.1080/13803395.2010.547662

Maroon, J. C., Lovell, M. R., Norwig, J., Podell, K., Powell, J. W., & Hartl, R. (2000). Cerebral concussion in athletes: Evaluation and neuropsychological testing. *Neurosurgery, 47*, 659–672.

McCaffrey, R. J., Krahula, M. M., Heimberg, R. G., Keller, K. E., & Purcell, M. J. (1988). A comparison of the Trail Making Test, Symbol Digit Modalities Test, and the Hooper Visual Organization Test in an inpatient substance abuse population. *Archives of Clinical Neuropsychology, 3*, 181–187.

Meador, K. J., Loring, D. W., Hulihan, J. F., Kamin, M., Karim, R., & CAPSS-027 Study Group. (2003). Differential cognitive and behavioural effects of topiramate and valproate. *Neurology, 60*(9), 1483–1488.

Moccia, M., Lanzillo, R., Palladino, R., Chang, K. C.–M., Costabile, T., Russo, C., . . . Brescia Morra, V. (2016). Cognitive impairment at diagnosis predicts 10-year multiple sclerosis progression. *Multiple Sclerosis (Houndmills, Basingstoke, England), 22*(5), 659–667. https://doi.org/10.1177/1352458515599075

Morgan, S. F., & Wheelock, J. (1992). Digit Symbol and Symbol Digit Modalities Tests: Are they directly interchangeable? *Neuropsychology 4*(6), 327–330.

Morrow, S. A. (2013). Normative data for the Stroop Color Word Test for a North American population. *The Canadian Journal of Neurological Sciences/Le Journal Canadien Des Sciences Neurologiques, 40*(6), 842–847. https://doi.org/10.1017/S0317167100015997

Morrow, S. A., Drake, A., Zivadinov, R., Munschauer, F., Weinstock-Guttman, B., & Benedict, R. H. B. (2010). Predicting loss of employment over three years in multiple sclerosis: Clinically meaningful cognitive decline. *The Clinical Neuropsychologist, 24*(7), 1131–1145. http://doi.org/10.1080/13854046.2010.511272

Motl, R. W., Cadavid, D., Sandroff, B. M., Pilutti, L. A., Pula, J. H., & Benedict, R. H. B. (2013). Cognitive processing speed has minimal influence on the construct validity of Multiple Sclerosis Walking Scale-12 scores. *Journal of the Neurological Sciences, 335*(1-2), 169–173. http://doi.org/10.1016/j.jns.2013.09.024

Mrazik, M., Ferrara, M. S., & Peterson, C. L. (2000). Injury severity and neuropsychological and balance outcomes of four college athletes. *Brain Injury, 14*(10), 921–931.

Niccolai, C., Portaccio, E., Goretti, B., Hakiki, B., Giannini, M., Pastò, L., . . . Amato, M. P. (2015). A comparison of the brief international cognitive assessment for multiple sclerosis and the brief repeatable battery in multiple sclerosis patients. *BMC Neurology, 15*(1). http://doi.org/10.1186/s12883-015-0460-8

Nielsen, H., Knidsen, L., & Daugbjerg, O. (1989). Normative data for eight neuropsychological tests based on a Danish sample. *Scandinavian Journal of Psychology, 30*, 37–45.

Nigg, J. T., Glass, J. M., & Wong, M. M. (2001). Neuropsychological executive functioning in children at elevated risk for alcoholism: Findings in early adolescence. *Journal of Abnormal Psychology, 113*(2), 302–314.

Niino, M., Fukazawa, T., Kira, J.–I., Okuno, T., Mori, M., Sanjo, N., . . . Matsui, M. (2017). Validation of the Brief International Cognitive Assessment for Multiple Sclerosis in Japan. *Multiple Sclerosis Journal—Experimental, Translational and Clinical, 3*(4), 2055217317748972. https://doi.org/10.1177/2055217317748972

O'Bryant, S. E., Humphreys, J. D., Bauer, L., McCaffrey, R. J., & Hilsabeck, R. C. (2007). The influence of ethnicity on Symbol Digit Modalities Test performance: An analysis of a multi-ethnic college and hepatitis C patient sample. *Applied Neuropsychology, 14*(3), 183–188.

Patel, V. P., Walker, L. A. S., & Feinstein, A. (2017). Deconstructing the Symbol Digit Modalities Test in multiple sclerosis: The role of memory. *Multiple Sclerosis and Related Disorders, 17*, 184–189. https://doi.org/10.1016/j.msard.2017.08.006

Patel, V. P., Zambrana, A., Walker, L. A., Herrmann, N., Swartz, R. H., & Feinstein, A. (2016). Distractibility in multiple sclerosis: The role of depression. *Multiple Sclerosis Journal—Experimental, Translational and Clinical, 2*, 2055217316653150. https://doi.org/10.1177/2055217316653150

Paulsen, J. S., Miller, A. C., Hayes, T., & Shaw, E. (2017). Cognitive and behavioral changes in Huntington disease before diagnosis. *Handbook of Clinical Neurology, 144*, 69–91. https://doi.org/10.1016/B978-0-12-801893-4.00006-7

Pena-Casanova, J., Blesa, R., Aguilar, M., Gramunt-Fombuena, N., Gomez-Anson, B., Oliva, R., . . . for the NEURONORMA Study Team. (2009a). Spanish Multicenter Normative Studies (NEURONORMA Project): Methods and Sample Characteristics. *Archives of Clinical Neuropsychology, 24*(4), 307–319. http://doi.org/10.1093/arclin/acp027

Pena-Casanova, J., Quinones-Ubeda, S., Quintana-Aparicio, M., Aguilar, M., Badenes, D., Molinuevo, J. L., . . . for the NEURONORMA Study Team. (2009b). Spanish Multicenter Normative Studies (NEURONORMA Project): Norms for Verbal Span, Visuospatial Span, Letter and Number Sequencing, Trail Making Test, and Symbol Digit Modalities Test. *Archives of Clinical Neuropsychology, 24*(4), 321–341. http://doi.org/10.1093/arclin/acp038

Pereira, D. R., Costa, P., & Cerqueira, J. J. (2015). Repeated assessment and practice effects of the written Symbol Digit Modalities Test using a short inter-test interval. *Archives of Clinical Neuropsychology, 30*, 424-434.

Polychroniadou, E., Bakirtzis, C., Langdon, D., Lagoudaki, R., Kesidou, E., Theotokis, P., . . . Grigoriadis, N. (2016). Validation of the Brief International Cognitive Assessment for Multiple Sclerosis (BICAMS) in Greek population with multiple sclerosis. *Multiple Sclerosis and Related Disorders, 9*, 68–72. https://doi.org/10.1016/j.msard.2016.06.011

Ponsford, J., & Kinsella, G. (1992). Attentional deficits following closed head injury. *Journal of Clinical and Experimental Neuropsychology, 14*, 822–838.

Ponsford, J., Tweedly, L., & Taffe, J. (2013). The relationship between alcohol and cognitive functioning following traumatic brain injury. *Journal of Clinical and Experimental Neuropsychology, 35*(1), 103–112. http://doi.org/10.1080/13803395.2012.752437

Possa, M. F. (2010). Neuropsychological measures in clinical practice. *Neurological Sciences, 31*(S2), 219–222. http://doi.org/10.1007/s10072-010-0374-6

Ranchet, M., Broussolle, E., Poisson, A., & Paire-Ficout, L. (2012). Relationships between cognitive functions and driving behavior in Parkinson's disease. *European Neurology, 68*(2), 98–107.

Rao, S. M., in collaboration with the Cognitive Function Study Group of the National Multiple Sclerosis Society. (1990). *A manual for the Brief, Repeatable Battery of Neuropsychological Tests in Multiple Sclerosis.* Milwaukee, WI: Medical College of Wisconsin.

Reedeker, N., Bouwens, J. A., van Duijn, E., Giltay, E. J., Roos, R. A., & van der Mast, R. C. (2011). Incidence, course, and predictors of apathy in Huntington's disease: a two-year prospective study. *Journal of Neuropsychiatry and Clinical Neurosciences, 23*(4), 434–441.

Roar, M., Illes, Z., & Sejbaek, T. (2016). Practice effect in Symbol Digit Modalities Test in multiple sclerosis patients treated with natalizumab. *Multiple Sclerosis and Related Disorders, 10*, 116–122. https://doi.org/10.1016/j.msard.2016.09.009

Rodgers, J. D., Tjaden, K., Feenaughty, L., Weinstock-Guttman, B., & Benedict, R. H. B. (2013). Influence of cognitive function on speech and articulation rate in multiple sclerosis. *Journal of the International Neuropsychological Society, 19*(02), 173–180. http://doi.org/10.1017/S1355617712001166

Rodrigues, D.–N., Paes, R. A., Vasconcelos, C. C. F., Landeira-Fernandez, J., & Alvarenga, M. P. (2011). Different cognitive profiles of Brazilian patients with relapsing-remitting and primary progressive multiple sclerosis. *Arquivos de Neuro-Psiquiatria, 69*(4), 590–595.

Royan, J., Tombaugh, T. N., & Rees, L. (2004). The Adjusting-Paced Serial Addition Test (Adjusting-PSAT): Thresholds for speed of information processing as a function of stimulus modality and problem complexity. *Archives of Clinical Neuropsychology, 19*(1), 131–143.

Royer, F. L. (1971). Spatial orientational and figural information in free recall of visual figures. *Journal of Experimental Psychology, 91*, 326–332.

Royer, F. L., Gilmore, G. C., & Gruhn, J. J. (1981). Normative data for the symbol substitution task. *Journal of Clinical Psychology, 37*, 608–614.

Ryan, J., Stanczyk, F. Z., Dennerstein, L., Mack, W. J., Clark, M. S., Szoeke, C., & Henderson, V. W. (2011). Executive functions in recently postmenopausal women: Absence of strong association with serum gonadal steroids. *Brain Research, 1379*, 199–205. http://doi.org/10.1016/j.brainres.2010.10.093

Sandroff, B. M., Pilutti, L. A., Dlugonski, D., & Motl, R. W. (2013). Physical activity and information processing speed in persons with multiple sclerosis: A prospective study. *Mental Health and Physical Activity, 6*(3), 205–211. http://doi.org/10.1016/j.mhpa.2013.08.001

Sastre-Garriga, J., Arévalo, M. J., Renom, M., Alonso, J., González, I., Galán, I., . . . Rovira, A. (2009). Brain volumetry counterparts of cognitive impairment in patients with multiple sclerosis. *Journal of the Neurological Sciences, 282*(1–2), 120–124. http://doi.org/10.1016/j.jns.2008.12.019

Schäffler, N., Schönberg, P., Stephan, J., Stellmann, J.–P., Gold, S. M., & Heesen, C. (2013). Comparison of patient-reported outcome measures in multiple sclerosis. *Acta Neurologica Scandinavica, 128*(2), 114–121. http://doi.org/10.1111/ane.12083

Schmitt, F. A., Farlow, M. R., Meng, X., Tekin, S., & Olin, J. T. (2010). Efficacy of rivastigmine on executive function in patients with Parkinson's disease dementia: Efficacy of rivastigmine on EF in patients with PDD. *CNS Neuroscience & Therapeutics, 16*(6), 330–336. http://doi.org/10.1111/j.1755-5949.2010.00182.x

Segura, B., Jurado, M. Á., Freixenet, N., Bargalló, N., Junqué, C., & Arboix, A. (2010). White matter fractional anisotropy is related to processing speed in metabolic syndrome patients: A case-control study. *BMC Neurology, 10*(1), 1.

Selnes, O. A., Jacobson, L., Machado, A. M., Becker, J. T., Wesch, J., Miller, E. N., Visscher, B., & McArthur, J. C. (1991). Normative data for a brief neuropsychological screening battery. *Perceptual and Motor Skills, 73*, 539–550.

Sheridan, L., Fitzgerald, H., Adams, K., Nigg, J., Martel, M., Puttler, L., . . . Zucker, R. (2006). Normative Symbol Digit Modalities Test performance in a community-based sample. *Archives of Clinical Neuropsychology, 21*(1), 23–28. http://doi.org/10.1016/j.acn.2005.07.003

Shum, D. H. K., McFarland, K. A., & Bain, J. D. (1990). Construct validity of eight tests of attention: Comparison of normal and closed head injured samples. *The Clinical Neuropsychologist, 4,* 151–162.

Smith, A. (1991). *Symbol Digit Modalities Test.* Los Angeles, CA: Western Psychological Services.

Smith, M. M., & Arnett, P. A. (2007). Dysarthria predicts poorer performance on cognitive tasks requiring a speeded oral response in an MS population. *Journal of Clinical and Experimental Neuropsychology, 29*(8), 804–812. http://doi.org/10.1080/13803390601064493

Solari, A., Mancuso, L., Motta, A., Mendozzi, L., & Serrati, C. (2002). Comparison of two brief neuropsychological batteries in people with multiple sclerosis. *Multiple Sclerosis, 8,* 169–176.

Spedo, C. T., Frndak, S. E., Marques, V. D., Foss, M. P., Pereira, D. A., Carvalho, L. de F., . . . Barreira, A. A. (2015). Cross-cultural adaptation, reliability, and validity of the BICAMS in Brazil. *The Clinical Neuropsychologist, 29*(6), 836–846. http://doi.org/10.1080/13854046.2015.1093173

Spitz, G., Schönberger, M., & Ponsford, J. (2013). The relations among cognitive impairment, coping style, and emotional adjustment following traumatic brain injury. *Journal of Head Trauma Rehabilitation, 28*(2), 116–125. http://doi.org/10.1097/HTR.0b013e3182452f4f

Sumowski, J. F., Chiaravalloti, N., Wylie, G., & Deluca, J. (2009). Cognitive reserve moderates the negative effect of brain atrophy on cognitive efficiency in multiple sclerosis. *Journal of the International Neuropsychological Society, 15*(04), 606. http://doi.org/10.1017/S1355617709090912

Tabrizi, S. J., Reilmann, R., Roos, R. A., Durr, A., Leavitt, B., Owen, G., Jones, R., Johnson, H., Craufurd, D., Hicks, S. L., Kennard, C., Landwehrmeyer, B., Stout, J. C., Borowsky, B., Scahill, R. I., Frost, C., & Langbehn, D. R. (2012). Potential endpoints for clinical trials in premanifest and early Huntington's disease in the TRACK-HD study: Analysis of 24 month observational data. *The Lancet Neurology, 11*(1), 42–53. https://doi.org/10.1016/S1474-4422(11)70263-0

Tam, J. W., & Schmitter-Edgecombe, M. (2013). The role of processing speed in the Brief Visuospatial Memory Test—Revised. *The Clinical Neuropsychologist, 27*(6), 962–972. http://doi.org/10.1080/13854046.2013.797500

Tang, S.–F., Chen, I.–H., Chiang, H.–Y., Wu, C.–T., Hsueh, I.–P., Yu, W.–H., & Hsieh, C.–L. (2017). A comparison between the original and Tablet-based Symbol Digit Modalities Test in patients with schizophrenia: Test-retest agreement, random measurement error, practice effect, and ecological validity. *Psychiatry Research, 260,* 199–206. https://doi.org/10.1016/j.psychres.2017.11.066

Tung, L.–C., Yu, W.–H., Lin, G.–H., Yu, T.–Y., Wu, C.–T., Tsai, C.–Y., . . . Hsieh, C.–L. (2016). Development of a Tablet-based Symbol Digit Modalities Test for reliably assessing information processing speed in patients with stroke. *Disability and Rehabilitation, 38*(19), 1952–1960. https://doi.org/10.3109/09638288.2015.1111438

Torres, I. J., Mundt, A. J., & Sweeney, P. J. (2003). A longitudinal neuropsychological study of partial brain radiation in adults with brain tumors. *Neurology, 60*(7), 1113–1118.

Tulsky, D. S., Saklofske, D. H., & Zhu, J. (2003). Revising a standard: An evaluation of the origin and development of the WAIS-III. In D. S. Tulsky, D. H. Saklofske, R. K. Heaton, R. Bornstein, & M. F. Ledbetter (Eds.), *Clinical interpretation of the WAIS-III and WMS-III* (pp. 43–92). New York: Academic Press.

Uchiyama, C. L., D'Elia, L. F., Delinger, A. M., Selnes, O. A., Becker, J. T., Wesch, J. E., . . . Miller, E. N. (1994). Longitudinal comparison of alternate versions of the Symbol Digit Modalities Test: Issues of form comparability and moderating demographic variables. *The Clinical Neuropsychologist, 8,* 209–218.

Verstnaeten, E., Cluydts, R., Pevernagie, D., & Hoffman, G. (2004). Executive function in sleep apnea: Controlling for attentional capacity in assessing executive attention. *Sleep, 27*(4), 685–93.

Vogel, A., Stokholm, J., & Jørgensen, K. (2013). Performances on Symbol Digit Modalities Test, Color Trails Test, and modified Stroop test in a healthy, elderly Danish sample. *Aging, Neuropsychology, and Cognition, 20*(3), 370–382. http://doi.org/10.1080/13825585.2012.725126

Vollmer, T., Huynh, L., Kelley, C., Galebach, P., Signorovitch, J., DiBernardo, A., & Sasane, R. (2016). Relationship between brain volume loss and cognitive outcomes among patients with multiple sclerosis: A systematic literature review. *Neurological Sciences, 37*(2), 165–179. http://doi.org/10.1007/s10072-015-2400-1

Wang, B., Guo, Q., Zhao, Q., & Hong, Z. (2012). Memory deficits for non-amnestic mild cognitive impairment: Memory deficits. *Journal of Neuropsychology, 6*(2), 232–241. http://doi.org/10.1111/j.1748-6653.2011.02024.x

Warlop, N. P., Achten, E., Fieremans, E., Debruyne, J., & Vingerhoets, G. (2009). Transverse diffusivity of cerebral parenchyma predicts visual tracking performance in relapsing–remitting multiple sclerosis. *Brain and Cognition, 71*(3), 410–415. http://doi.org/10.1016/j.bandc.2009.05.004

Willmott, C., Ponsford, J., Hocking, C., & Schönberger, M. (2009). Factors contributing to attentional impairments after traumatic brain injury. *Neuropsychology, 23*(4), 424–432. https://doi.org/10.1037/a0015058

Yeudall, L. T., Fromm, D., Reddon, J. R., & Stefanyk, W. O. (1986). Normative data stratified by age and sex for 12 neuropsychological tests. *Journal of Clinical Psychology, 42,* 918–946.

Yu, H. J., Christodoulou, C., Bhise, V., Greenblatt, D., Patel, Y., Serafin, D., . . . Wagshul, M. E. (2012). Multiple white matter tract abnormalities underlie cognitive impairment in RRMS. *NeuroImage, 59*(4), 3713–3722. http://doi.org/10.1016/j.neuroimage.2011.10.053

Yuan, Y., Zhang, Z., Bai, F., Yu, H., You, J., Shi, Y., . . . Jiang, T. (2009). Larger regional white matter volume is associated with executive function deficit in remitted geriatric depression: An optimized voxel-based morphometry study. *Journal of Affective Disorders, 115*(1–2), 225–229. http://doi.org/10.1016/j.jad.2008.09.018

Zillmer, E. A. (2003). The Neuropsychology of Repeated 1- and 3-Meter Springboard Diving Among College Athletes. *Applied Neuropsychology, 10*(1), 23–30. https://doi.org/10.1207/S15324826AN1001_4

TEST OF EVERYDAY ATTENTION (TEA)

TEST NAME	**Test of Everyday Attention (TEA)**
DOMAIN	Attention
AGE RANGE	In adults, to 80 years
ADMINISTRATION TIME	45 to 60 minutes
SCORING FORMAT	Hand scored
REFERENCE	Robertson, I. H., Ward, T., Ridgeway, V., & Nimmo-Smith, I. (1994). *The Test of Everyday Attention*. Bury St. Edmunds, UK: Thames Valley Test Company. www.pearsonclinical.com

DESCRIPTION

The Test of Everyday Attention (TEA; Robertson et al., 1994) is a test battery designed to measure sustained, selective, and divided attention, and attentional switching. Three versions are provided for use in repeat assessments (Versions A, B, and C). In particular, the TEA is thought to provide a clinically useful measure to assist in predicting recovery of function and function in day-to-day life after brain injury (Robertson et al., 1994), but it has been used in other populations as well. The theoretical basis of the test is the attentional model of Posner and Peterson (1990), which proposes the attentional systems of *orientation*, *vigilance*, and *selection*. Vigilance and selection are models tested by the TEA, using familiar materials designed to approximate day-to-day activities. For example, TEA subtests are presented in the context of a mock trip to Philadelphia, where specific activities are required (i.e., using a map in Map Search, finding information in a telephone directory in Telephone Search, attending to elevator floors in Elevator subtests, listening for lottery numbers in Lottery). The TEA is comprised of eight subtests, with task demands, scores, and modalities summarized in Table 8–68.

ADMINISTRATION

Detailed instructions are found in the manual. The TEA is portable and does not require a computer for administration. Of the three versions provided for use in repeat assessments (Versions A, B, and C), Version A is always to be administered first. For a discussion of repeat assessment with the TEA, see the sections "Reliability" and "Comment."

After verbatim instructions are provided, the examiner may paraphrase to facilitate understanding. Note that when testing individuals with sensory impairments, some subtests may be affected by difficulties with hearing or vision. For example, Bruce, Bruce, and Arnett (2007) reported that even mild visual acuity disturbances are related to poorer performance on Visual Elevator in people with MS ($r = -.33$).

TABLE 8–68 Summary of Test of Everyday Attention (TEA) Subtests, Scores, and Modalities

FACTOR		SUBTEST	TASK	SCORES	MODALITY
Visual Selective Attention	1	Map Search	Timed visual search task (circling target objects)	Number of targets within 2 minutes (maximum 80)	Visual-Motor
	6	Telephone Search	Search target symbols next to phone numbers	Time to find all targets divided by number of hits	Visual-Motor
Attentional Switching	4	Visual Elevator	Mixed forward and backward counting following visual cues	Accuracy (correctly counted strings) and timing score	Visual
	5	Elevator Counting with Reversal	Mixed forward and backward counting following auditory cues	Correctly counted strings (maximum 10)	Auditory
Auditory-Verbal Working Memory	3	Auditory Elevator Counting with Distraction	Target tones mixed with distractor tones; count strings as in subtest 5	Correctly counted strings (maximum 10)	Auditory
Sustained Attention	8	Lottery	Listen to number-letter combinations, note letters attached to target numbers	Number of correctly identified letters attached to target numbers	Auditory/Motor
	2	Elevator Counting	Count seven strings of tones	Sum of correctly counted strings (maximum 7)	Auditory
	7	Telephone Search While Counting	Search telephone strings as in subtest 2 while counting target tones	Time-per-target score corrected by dual-task decrement	Auditory/Visual

NOTE: Numbers refer to the order of administration.
SOURCE: From Sterr (2004).

When controlling for visual acuity, MS patients and controls did not differ on Visual Elevator, and visual acuity accounted for 10% of the variance in Visual Elevator performance.

Of note, care may be needed to administer this test in specific groups. In a study of very old adults (≥80 years of age), 8–19% of the participants, depending on subtest, were unable to complete the test due to a lack of comprehension of test instructions, despite repetition and practice; however, more than 90% of participants were able to complete at least three of the four tests administered (van der Leeuw et al., 2017).

SCORING

Detailed score calculations are available in the manual. Scores are presented as scaled scores ($M = 10$, $SD = 3$) and percentiles. The range of scores is generally from 1 to 19, but some subtests have a restricted range due to floor and ceiling effects. Elevator Counting has a prominent ceiling effect (i.e., no examinees in the standardization sample made greater than one error), so raw scores are designated a qualitative label (i.e., 7 out of 7 is "Normal", 6 is "Doubtful", 4 or fewer is "Definitely Abnormal"). Subtest scores, rather than composite scores, are used. The manual provides detailed interpretations of each subtest and its relevance to day-to-day life.

Crawford, Sommerville, and Robertson (1997) developed additional tables to assist in the interpretation of scores. Table 8–69 shows the size of the difference between each subtest and an individual's mean subtest score on the TEA required for statistical significance and the magnitude of the difference between a subtest and a mean subtest score that is expected to occur in less than a given percentage of the general population. A computer program can also be downloaded to calculate the differences for any combination of TEA subtests; visit (https://homepages.abdn.ac.uk/j.crawford/pages/dept/psychom.htm).

TABLE 8–69 Difference Between Test of Everyday Attention (TEA) Subtest Score and Mean Score on All Subtests Required for Statistical Significance

TEA SUBTEST	SE_{DIFF}	CRITICAL VALUE FOR A GIVEN *P* .15	.10	.05	.01
Map Search	1.11	2.56	2.73	2.99	3.55
EC with Distraction	1.48	3.41	3.64	3.99	4.73
Visual Elevator	1.48	3.41	3.64	3.99	4.73
EC with Reversal	1.59	3.65	3.89	4.27	5.07
Telephone Search	1.11	2.56	2.73	2.99	3.55
Telephone Search While Counting	1.72	3.97	4.22	4.64	5.50
Lottery	1.35	3.10	3.30	3.63	4.30

NOTE: Size of difference (regardless of sign) between each subtest and an individual's mean subtest score on the TEA required for statistical significance at the .15, .10, .05 and .01 levels. Mean subtest performance must include the individual subtest being compared in addition to all the other subtests. For determination of significant differences using shorter TEA forms, a computer program may be used (see text). EC, Elevator Counting; SE_{diff}, standard error of the difference.

SOURCE: From Crawford et al. (1997).

TABLE 8–70 Expected Difference Between Test of Everyday Attention (TEA) Subtest Score and Mean Score on All Subtests in a Healthy Population

TEA SUBTEST	SD_{DA}	PERCENTAGE OF HEALTHY POPULATION 15	10	5	1
Map Search	2.61	3.76	4.29	5.12	6.74
EC with Distraction	2.37	3.42	3.89	4.65	6.12
Visual Elevator	2.40	3.46	3.94	4.71	6.20
EC with Reversal	2.21	3.18	3.62	4.33	5.70
Telephone Search	2.18	3.14	3.57	4.27	5.62
Telephone Search While Counting	2.56	3.68	4.20	5.02	6.60
Lottery	2.46	3.54	4.03	4.81	6.34

NOTE: Size of difference (regardless of sign) between each subtest and an individual's mean subtest score on the TEA such that it would be expected to occur in less than 15, 10, 5, and 1 percent of the healthy population; the standard deviation of the difference is also presented. Mean subtest performance must include the individual subtest being compared in addition to all the other subtests. For determination of significant differences using shorter TEA forms, a computer program may be used (see text). EC, Elevator Counting; SD_{da}, Standard deviation of the difference.

SOURCE: From Crawford, et al. (1997).

DEMOGRAPHIC EFFECTS

AGE

Age effects are present on the TEA, but are not described in detail in the manual.

GENDER

There are reportedly no gender differences on any of the subtests (Robertson et al., 1994).

EDUCATION

Information regarding the influence of education is not available.

ETHNICITY, NATIONALITY, AND LINGUISTIC EFFECTS

Chan (2002) adapted the TEA for use in Hong Kong (see "Normative Data"). The authors report reservations about the applicability of this version to individuals from mainland China and the suitability of some subtests for individuals who have never traveled abroad considering the travel theme of some of the tasks. There is also an Italian standardization (Cantagallo & Zoccolotti, 1998). Bilinguals perform better than monolinguals on auditory, but not visual, subtests (Bak et al., 2014).

NORMATIVE DATA

Norms construction is detailed in the manual; some raw score distributions were not normal. Details pertaining to the normative sample are listed in Table 8–71. Recruitment process, data collection procedure, means of screening, ethnicity, and geographic location are not provided. Note that cell sizes are modest in each of the four age bands ($n = 33$ to 39), with some age and IQ groupings comprised of small numbers of individuals (e.g., $n = 11$ adults at age 50 to 64 years with IQ <100). Version A has a much larger sample size than Versions B and C.

Van der Leeuw et al. (2017) provide data for 249 older adults (80 to 101 years of age), with a mean age of 87 years ($SD = 4$), 67% female, who were part of a longitudinal study in Boston. Exclusion criteria included unable to communicate in English, moderate to severe impairment (MMSE cutoff score), not living in Boston, unable to walk without personal assistance, presence of severe health deterioration, and residence in a nursing home facility. The majority of the sample (90%) completed three or more tests administered. Participants who did not complete all four subtests were more likely to have fewer years of education, be African American, and have fair to poor self-rated health or hearing problems. For the persons who completed all four TEA subtests administered, 78% had attained college education, and 22% had attained high school or fewer years of education. The sample of completers was 86% Caucasian, 10% African American, and 4% members of another ethnic group. The means and SDs for the subtests were Visual Elevator ($M = 4.67, SD = 1.80$), Map Search ($M = 32.25, SD = 15.58$), Telephone Search ($M = 5.54$, $SD = 3.20$), Telephone Search While Counting ($M = 7.03$; $SD = 4.97$), and Dual Task Decrement Score ($M = 4.90$, $SD = 9.54$).

Chan (2002) provide norms for 49 Chinese individuals living in Hong Kong, as described in Table 8–72, along with alternate-form reliability estimates. Education level was based on scores obtained on the NART (i.e., above or below a score of 100); however, NART scores are estimates of IQ, which may differ from actual education levels. Furthermore, NART score distributions are uneven in the sample (i.e., 65% of the sample had an estimated IQ >100), leading to an overrepresentation of individuals with high IQ in the TEA norms. Nevertheless, the authors note that this is not likely to cause a problem in score interpretation because of the low correlation between TEA scores and estimated verbal intelligence. However, TEA score equivalence between high- and low-NART scorers is needed to support this conclusion.

TABLE 8–71 Characteristics of the Test of Everyday Attention (TEA) Standardization Sample

Sample size[a]	154 (Version A) 118 (Version B) 39 (Version C)
Region	UK
Education	Based on NART score; 65% of sample had a NART score >100
Gender	45% Men 55% Women
Ethnicity	Not reported

[a]Norms are stratified into four age bands (18 to 34, 35 to 49, 50 to 64, 65 to 80), and two educational levels (NART score above vs. below 100). Note that 65% of the sample had an estimated IQ greater than 100. NART, National Adult Reading Test.

TABLE 8–72 Norms and Alternate Form Reliability for the Cantonese Version of the Test of Everyday Attention (TEA)

	VERSION A (N = 49)		VERSION B (N = 35)		
SUBTEST	MEAN	(SD)	MEAN	(SD)	CORRELATION (P < 0.01)
Map Search in 1 min	51.69	(10.89)	51.57	(9.81)	0.75
Map Search in 2 min	73.69	(6.96)	74.31	(3.97)	0.69
Elevator Counting	6.93	(0.47)	7.00	(0.00)	—[a]
Elevator Counting with Distraction	8.90	(1.42)	9.14	(1.26)	0.86
Visual Elevator (number correct)	8.69	(1.29)	8.82	(0.95)	0.46
Visual Elevator (time per switch)	3.07	(1.04)	2.99	(1.01)	0.94
Elevator Counting with Reversal	8.18	(1.81)	8.63	(1.54)	0.81
Telephone Search (time per target)	2.69	(1.40)	2.41	(0.48)	0.84
Telephone Search While Counting	0.84	(1.34)	0.83	(0.77)	0.59
Lottery	9.31	(1.62)	9.63	(0.64)	0.19

[a]Unable to calculate due to no variance in the sample.
SOURCE: From Chan (2002).

EVIDENCE FOR RELIABILITY

EVIDENCE FOR INTERNAL RELIABILITY

No information on internal reliability or standard error of measurement of TEA subtests is provided in the manual, which may be due to the speeded nature of the tasks.

EVIDENCE FOR TEST-RETEST RELIABILITY, ALTERNATE FORMS, MEASURING CHANGE, AND PRACTICE EFFECTS

Test-retest reliability information for repeat administrations of Version A is not provided in the manual. Instead, stability information for the TEA is based on Versions A and B administered sequentially, and thus estimates reflect both alternate form and test-retest reliability. Normative sample subgroups were administered Version A then Version B with a one-week test-retest interval ($n = 118$). Of this subgroup, 39 were then administered Version C after a one-week interval following Version B. Test-retest reliability was also computed for a sample of patients who had sustained a unilateral stroke ($n = 74$). Map Search evidences consistently high reliability, with variable reliability for other subtests; most range from adequate to high, although some estimates are marginal to low. Generally, reliability coefficients are higher in the stroke sample. Elevator Counting with

Distraction had adequate to high coefficients in the normative subsamples and high coefficients in the stroke sample. Visual Elevator had adequate reliability in the normative subsamples and very high coefficients in the stroke sample. Elevator Counting with Reversal had marginal reliability in the normative subsample. Telephone Search was high to very high in normative subsamples, and adequate for stroke. Telephone Search While Counting was low to marginal across groups. Elevator Counting had high reliability in the stroke sample, with adequate reliability in the stroke sample for the Lottery subtest.

In a reliability study with the Cantonese version of the TEA (Chan, 2002), test-retest reliability was adequate to high for most TEA subtests, with the exception of low reliability for Visual Elevator (number correct), Telephone Search While Counting, and Lottery ($r < .60$). In another study, 90 patients with chronic stroke (≥6 months or more) completed one of three combinations of the TEA (Version A, Version B; Version B, Version C; Version C, Version A) at a one-week retest interval (Chen et al., 2013). Subtests had good to excellent test reliability (ICCs ≥. 66), except for Telephone Search While Counting (ICCs .51 to .59) and accuracy for Visual Elevator (ICCs .36 to .49).

The Elevator and Lottery subtests have large ceiling effects in the normative sample; however, the test authors report high percentage agreement from test to retest (i.e., 96% and 82%, respectively). Of note, ceiling effects are commonly reported for Elevator Counting in both healthy and clinical populations, including on a Cantonese version of the test (Chan, 2002), a nonclinical Chinese sample (Chan et al., 2006, mean score of 6.96, $SD = .53$), individuals with learning disability (Sterr, 2004), dementia (Lincoln et al., 2006), chronic stroke (Chen et al., 2013), and Friedreich's ataxia (Klopper et al., 2011).

No practice effect information (i.e., means and *SD*s) or information pertaining to the clinical significance of Version A–Version B scaled score differences (e.g., frequencies of various difference scores in the standardization sample) is provided in healthy samples. The practice effects when Version C is administered after Version B are presented in the manual and vary across subtests. The largest practice effect was obtained for Map Search 1-minute score ($M = 4.5$ points, $SD = 8.4$) and the smallest for Visual Elevator accuracy ($M = 0$, $SD = 1.58$). Chen et al. (2013) provide information regarding reliable change estimates and practice effects in a chronic stroke sample (Table 8–73). Practice effects were generally small.

TABLE 8–73 Test-Retest Reliability, Practice Effects, and Reliable Change Estimates for the Test of Everyday Attention (TEA) in a Chronic Stroke Sample

					PRACTICE EFFECTS			
SUBTEST	FORM	M_1 (SD_1)	M_2 (SD_2)	ICC (95% CI)	M_{DIFF} (SD_{DIFF})	P VALUE	SE_{DIFF}	90% CI RCI
Map Search	AB	55.8 (15.4)	57.6 (16.4)	0.72 (0.50–0.86)	1.8 (10.7)	0.345	11.5	−17.2, 20.8
	BC	48.7 (16.9)	52.8 (17.2)	0.57 (0.26–0.77)	4.1 (16.0)	0.188	15.7	−21.7, 29.9
	CA	55.9 (16.1)	59.9 (15.4)	0.70 (0.43–0.85)	4.0 (12.3)	0.090	12.5	−16.5, 24.5
Elevator Counting	AB	6.6 (1.0)	6.8 (0.9)	nc	0.2 (0.4)	0.006	0.0	0.2
	BC	6.6 (1.0)	6.8 (0.5)	nc	0.2 (0.8)	0.184	0.6	−0.8, 1.2
	CA	6.7 (0.6)	6.8 (0.4)	nc	0.1 (0.7)	0.231	0.4	−0.5, 0.7
EC with Distraction	AB	4.9 (3.4)	5.8 (3.4)	0.77 (0.55–0.88)	0.9 (2.2)	0.034	3.4	−4.7, 6.5
	BC	5.6 (3.2)	6.4 (3.6)	0.81 (0.62–0.91)	0.8 (2.0)	0.052	3.6	−5.2, 6.8
	CA	6.5 (3.4)	6.9 (3.2)	0.81 (0.63–0.91)	0.4 (2.1)	0.367	2.0	−2.9, 3.7
Visual Elevator accuracy	AB	6.8 (2.5)	7.8 (2.1)	0.49 (0.16–0.72)	1.0 (2.3)	0.017	2.5	−3.2, 5.2
	BC	7.1 (2.3)	8.1 (2.0)	0.36 (0.03–0.63)	1.0 (2.4)	0.030	2.6	−3.3, 5.3
	CA	7.8 (2.1)	7.9 (2.2)	0.83 (0.67–0.92)	0.1 (1.3)	0.669	1.2	−1.9, 2.1
Visual Elevator time per switch	AB	5.1 (2.5)	4.6 (1.6)	0.82 (0.63–0.92)	−0.5 (1.2)	0.021	1.5	−3.0, 2.0
	BC	4.7 (1.4)	4.0 (1.1)	0.70 (0.10–0.89)	−0.7 (0.8)	<0.001	1.1	−2.5, 1.1
	CA	4.9 (2.0)	4.6 (2.0)	0.92 (0.81–0.96)	−0.3 (0.7)	0.019	0.8	−1.6, 1.0
Telephone Search	AB	5.0 (1.9)	4.4 (1.2)	0.66 (0.36–0.83)	−0.6 (1.3)	0.011	1.6	−3.2, 2.0
	BC	5.5 (2.5)	4.9 (2.2)	0.85 (0.68–0.93)	−0.6 (1.2)	0.022	1.4	−2.9, 1.7
	CA	4.9 (2.0)	4.2 (1.5)	0.82 (0.51–0.92)	−0.7 (0.9)	0.001	1.2	−2.7, 1.3
Telephone Search While Counting	AB	6.8 (10.6)	4.4 (5.8)	0.54 (0.23–0.75)	−2.4 (8.1)	0.130	10.2	−19.1, 14.3
	BC	3.6 (4.4)	2.7 (3.2)	0.59 (0.30–0.79)	−0.9 (3.4)	0.176	4.0	−7.5, 5.7
	CA	5.9 (6.5)	5.1 (7.3)	0.51 (0.19–0.74)	−0.8 (6.9)	0.514	6.4	−11.4, 9.8
Lottery	AB	8.5 (2.2)	8.9 (1.7)	0.67 (0.41–0.83)	0.4 (1.6)	0.197	1.8	−2.5, 3.3
	BC	8.8 (2.5)	8.8 (2.0)	0.85 (0.71–0.93)	0.0 (1.3)	0.769	1.4	−2.3, 2.3
	CA	8.4 (2.7)	8.0 (2.7)	0.82 (0.66–0.91)	−0.4 (1.6)	0.222	1.6	−3.2, 2.3

NOTE: EC, Elevator Counting; ICC, intra-class correlation coefficients; CI, confidence interval; M_{diff}, the group mean of the test-retest difference scores (M_2-M_1); RCI, Reliable Change Index; SD_{diff}, the standard deviation of the test-rest difference scores; SE_{diff}, standard error of difference; nc, not calculated due to little variance.

SOURCE: From Chen et al. (2013).

EVIDENCE FOR VALIDITY

WITHIN-TEST CORRELATIONS

TEA subtests relate to one another. Chan et al. (2006) reported correlations generally ranging from −.63 to .59 (Elevator Counting with Reversal with Visual Elevator Time Score Switch, Elevator Counting with Reversal with Elevator Counting with Distraction, respectively). Chan and Lai (2006) reported that correlations between subtests were generally in the moderate range, ranging from −.58 to .7 (Map Search with Telephone Search, Telephone Search with Visual Elevator Time, respectively).

FACTOR-ANALYTIC STUDIES AND RELATIONSHIPS WITH OTHER TESTS

The manual reports a four-factor solution yielded by principal components analysis with varimax rotation of TEA subtests along with other tests of attention (d2 Visual Search Task, Stroop, TMT, PASAT, WCST, Digits Backward), involving (a) visual selective attention/speed (Map Search, Telephone Search, d2 Visual Search Task, Stroop, TMT B), (b) attentional switching (Visual Elevator, WCST), (c) sustained attention (Lottery, Elevator Counting, Telephone Search While Counting), and (d) auditory-verbal working memory (Elevator Counting with Reversal, Elevator Counting with Distraction, Digits Backward, PASAT).

Subsequent research has partially replicated this factor structure; the auditory-verbal working memory factor is typically not found, however. Chan (2002) replicated the selective and sustained attention factors using the Hong Kong version, and the switching factor was partially replicated with Visual Elevator loading on this factor as well. However, the auditory-verbal working memory factor was not replicated. Chan et al. (2006) reported a three-factor model consisting of visual selection (Map Search, Telephone Search), sustained attention (Telephone Search dual task; Lottery), and switching (Elevator Counting with Distraction, Visual Elevator, Visual Elevator Switch, Elevator Counting with Reversal) best reflected the structure of the TEA in a nonclinical Chinese sample. Chan and Lai (2006) reported that the TEA yielded a three-factor model comprised of visual selection (i.e., Map Search), sustained attention (Telephone Search, Elevator Counting, Lottery Task, Visual Elevator), and switching (variables from Elevator Counting, Visual Elevator) in a sample of TBI patients with chronic postconcussive symptoms. Bate et al. (2001) replicated the visual selective attention, attentional switching, and sustained attention factor, but not the auditory-verbal working memory factor, in their mixed sample of healthy people and patients with severe TBI. When factor analyzed along with other measures of more basic components, such as alerting and orienting, the TEA subtests load on a separate factor (Stewart & Amitay, 2015).

However, the test relates to other measures of complex attention and executive function. Robertson et al. (1996) report moderate to high (r = .42 to .63) correlations between selected TEA subtests and other attention tests [Stroop, TMT-B, PASAT, WCST, Digits Backward], with the exception of Lottery, Elevator Counting, and Telephone Search While Counting. Chan et al. (2002) used the Hong Kong version of the TEA, which also showed significant correlations with a number of attention and executive functioning tests (TMT, Color Trails, Symbol Digit Modalities Test, Modified Six Elements Test, Digits Backward, Stroop, Design Fluency, Word Fluency). Van der Leeuw et al. (2017) similarly reported moderate to large correlations between TEA subtests and attention and executive functions in their sample of older adults.

Bate, Mathias, and Crawford (2001) reported that the TEA correlated with attention measures such as the Stroop, PASAT, and Ruff Selective Attention Test, with the exception of Elevator Counting and Elevator Counting with Distraction, in a combined sample of healthy controls and individuals with severe TBI. Greene, Hodges, and Baddeley (1995) reported that Telephone Search While Counting was moderately correlated with another dual-performance task involving simultaneous digit span recall and cancellation. The Behavioural Assessment of the Dysexecutive Syndrome (BADS) also correlates moderately with the TEA in people with schizophrenia (r = .31 to .44, Tyson et al., 2008).

The Elevator Counting subtest is significantly correlated with verbal fluency (r = .65) in patients with lesions of the left lateral or medial frontal lobes and is also related to the Graded Naming Test (r = .69; MacPherson et al., 2010). The manual reports that correlations between the TEA and the NART are small (i.e., <.30) for all TEA subtests except Visual Elevator, which shows moderate correlations (r = .39). In their sample of older adults, van der Leeuw et al. (2017) reported moderate correlations between TEA subtests and the MMSE as well as the Hooper Visual Learning Test.

CLINICAL STUDIES

The TEA has been used with patients with dementia, stroke, TBI, and schizophrenia, among other conditions. Overall, research suggests that the TEA is useful in differentiating patients from controls, but is less useful in differentiating between clinical conditions.

Dementia. The sensitivity and specificity of Map Search is good in terms of differentiating individuals with mild cognitive impairment or dementia from healthy matched controls, but the test does not differentiate well between the two conditions (De Jager et al., 2003). Lincoln et al. (2006)

reported that individuals with dementia performed worse than healthy controls on Elevator Counting with Distraction, Telephone Search, and Telephone Search dual task.

Greene et al. (1995) found that Telephone Search While Counting was sensitive to disease stage in early AD. Lincoln et al. (2006) reported that individuals with dementia who were assessed as unsafe to drive performed worse on the Telephone Search task than those with dementia considered to be safe to drive. Equations were generated using specific test variables that were found to correctly classify 92% of drivers with dementia as safe to drive, although TEA variables were not included in these formulas. However, Yamin, Stinchcombe, and Gagnon (2016) reported that sustained attention measures from the TEA were related to driving in people with mild AD ($r = -.65$).

Stroke. In terms of stroke, older patients with unilateral stroke perform worse on the TEA than age-matched controls, as do younger stroke patients (aged 50–64 years); exceptions are Elevator Counting, Telephone Search (time per target), and Lottery (see manual). Patients with small white matter infarcts also show impaired performance on the TEA (Van Zandvoort et al., 2003).

Map Search and Elevator Counting are moderately correlated with ADLs ($rs = .34$ to $.48$). Correlations with other TEA subtests are not presented. Other conventional measures of attention (Stroop, PASAT, Digits Backward) are not consistently correlated with functional measures. As described in the manual, moderate correlations ($rs = -.30, -.45$) are found in stroke patients between an attention questionnaire completed by a collateral and two TEA subtests (Map Search and Elevator Counting), but no consistent correlations between other attention measures (Stroop, PASAT, Digit Span Backward) and the attentional rating scale were found (see manual).

The TEA has also been used as an outcome measure in evaluating the efficacy of a visual retraining program designed to improve driving skills after stroke (Mazer et al., 2003). The TEA was identified as the most commonly endorsed measure of attention in a pre-driving assessment for people with stroke by an occupational therapy group in Ireland (Stapleton & Connelly, 2010).

TBI. The manual describes 15 patients with moderate or severe TBI (mean of 17 days posttraumatic amnesia) who completed the TEA 14 months post-injury. Compared with age- and NART-matched controls, TBI patients had worse scores on subtests measuring selective and sustained attention (i.e., Map Search, Telephone Search, Telephone Search While Counting, and Lottery). Chan (2000) also found that people with TBI performed worse on a Cantonese version of the TEA compared to matched controls (except for Elevator Counting). However, Bate et al. (2001) found that only three TEA subtests measuring primarily selective attention (Map Search, Visual Elevator, and Telephone Search) differentiated between a group of individuals with severe TBI and a matched control group. Furthermore, only the TEA Map Search test, along with the Stroop, differentiated between individuals with severe TBI and controls when shared variance was taken into account (Bate et al., 2001).

Ziino and Ponsford (2006) reported that patients with TBI had a greater mean time per target score on the Telephone Search task, without significant differences on the dual task component indexed by comparison of Telephone Search and Telephone Search While Counting. Telephone Search and Telephone Search While Counting were related to subjective fatigue ratings ($rs = .29$ to $.37$). Anxiety did not correlate, but a depression rating correlated with Telephone Search misses ($r = .30$). Wiseman-Hakes et al. (2013) reported significant improvement on TEA scores measuring auditory selective working memory and selective visual attention after treatment for sleep disturbances in TBI; however, differences were no longer significant following correction for multiple comparisons.

Psychiatric Conditions. Tyson et al. (2008) administered Elevator Counting, Elevator Counting with Distraction, and Telephone Search While Counting to a group of people with schizophrenia and healthy controls. Controls performed better on each subtest (Cohen's $d = .59$ to 1.1). Using the fifth percentile as a cutoff for impairment, the majority of patients were impaired on Elevator Counting with Distraction and Telephone Search While Counting, while most patients performed within typical limits on Elevator Counting. No relationship was found between TEA subtests and disease parameters (i.e., symptom ratings, medication, or length of illness), although correlations were found between social functioning and the TEA ($r = .34$ to $.45$).

Individuals with obsessive compulsive disorder perform worse on the majority of selective attention subtests compared to people with panic disorder and controls (Clayton et al., 1999). University students classified as high in obsessionality perform worse on select TEA subtests than those with low obsessionality, most notably on the Visual Elevator subtest (Pleva & Wade, 2002).

Other Conditions. MacPherson et al. (2010) reported that patients with medial and left lateral prefrontal lesions were significantly impaired on the Elevator Counting subtest compared to healthy controls; no difference was found between right lateral, orbital, and posterior groups and healthy controls. Although statistically significant differences were found, the lowest performance was a raw score of 5.80 ($SD = 1.14$; left lateral group), near the ceiling of 7 correct.

Two TEA subtests (Lottery and Elevator Counting with Distraction) best discriminate between patients with progressive supranuclear palsy and age-matched controls compared with other neuropsychological tests, as described in the manual (Esmonde et al., 1996, as cited by Robertson et al., 1996). People with PD show improvements on the TEA following a therapeutic dance program (Ventura et al., 2016). People with Wilson's disease and neurologic symptoms perform worse than patients with Wilson's disease who are neurologically asymptomatic, especially on TEA subtests that involve switching (Iwański et al., 2015). Sterr (2004) reported worse performance in individuals with learning disabilities compared to the control group on several subtests (i.e., Map Search, Telephone Search, Visual Elevator, Elevator Counting with Distraction, Lottery). Visual selective attention (defined as Map Search and Telephone Search) was consistently impaired in learning disability. Persons who stutter are found to score lower than demographically matched controls, especially on subtests demanding selective and divided attention (Doneva et al., 2017).

Klopper et al. (2011) reported that individuals with Friedreich's ataxia performed worse than age-, gender-, and IQ-matched controls on TEA subtests (Elevator Counting with Distraction; Visual Elevator; Elevator Counting with Reversal; Lottery), with the exception of Elevator Counting, for which a ceiling effect was found. Significant correlations were reported between Visual Elevator and an ataxia rating scale (Spearman rho = −.61) and Elevator Counting with Reversal and repeat length on the short allele of FXN gene (Spearman rho = −.74).

A large effect size is found for ecstasy users with a polysubstance use history on Map Search, with dosage related to impairment on other TEA subtests (Zakzanis et al., 2002). The TEA has also been used to study the effects of environmental duress in a field survival exercise, with individuals completing the exercise performing worse than controls on specific subtests, including Map Search and Lottery, at specific testing points (Leach & Ansell, 2008).

NEUROANATOMICAL CORRELATES AND IMAGING STUDIES

No information is available.

PERFORMANCE VALIDITY

No information is available.

COMMENT

The TEA is founded on a theoretical model of attention, and the authors have made efforts to make the test ecologically valid. The TEA addresses a range of attentional domains (e.g., selective, sustained, switching) in co-normed subtests, including dual-task conditions. Profile analysis is also possible using the tables developed by Crawford et al. (1997) and the related computer program, as previously discussed.

Subtests of the TEA are moderately correlated, and the test shows correlations with other attention tasks, generally in the moderate range. Although factor-analytic studies in the manual report a four-factor solution, subsequent research often yields three factors (e.g., visual selective attention, attentional switching, and sustained attention) with an auditory-verbal working memory factor typically not found. The test has been used in a number of clinical conditions, although typically select subtests, rather than the entire test, are given. Most research indicates group differences between controls and patient groups, although there is not a coherent body of research in specific clinical groups. Additional research relating to clinical and ecological correlates and neuroanatomical substrates of performance would be beneficial.

The test has some significant limitations. More information is needed with respect to demographic effects, particularly influence of age, IQ, education, and ethnicity. The standardization sample has significant weaknesses; information regarding many important aspects of norming is not available (e.g., recruitment process, means of screening, ethnicity), and cell sizes are small, especially when further subdivided by both age and education. Note that normative data for older adults (≥80 years of age) have since been published.

As different forms of the TEA were administered twice, alternate-form reliability is conflated with test-retest reliability. Map Search is associated with high test-retest reliability, but also practice effects; test-retest reliability of other subtests tends to be variable overall, with many coefficients insufficient for clinical use. Given the small size of the normative sample who completed Version C, it may have limited use. Version A has the largest normative sample and is most often used in research, so it would be the version of choice for use in most clinical practice situations.

Elevator Counting has ceiling effects in both normative and clinical samples, and thus is unlikely to provide useful information for the majority of examinees. In older individuals, floor effects are evident on a number of subtests. For example, in the oldest age range of the normative sample, the lowest score possible (i.e., a score of 0) is equivalent to a scaled score of 7 on the Elevator Counting with Reversal subtest. Floors also appears to differ depending on whether Version A or Version B is employed. Users should note that on some subtests, Version B has a slightly higher floor, which means that examinees obtaining very poor scores on Version A might obtain slightly higher scaled scores on Version B due to the restriction of range in some Version B subtests. For example, in the oldest age group, the minimum scaled score for Version A Map Search 2 is a scaled score of 1, but the minimum scaled score for Version B is 5. However, these differences do not appear to be consistent across subtests (for Map Search B, the reverse is true: in the oldest age group, the minimum score for Version A is a scaled score of 6, whereas the minimum score for Version B is 3). Although these differences may be minimal when healthy individuals are assessed, they can potentially cause interpretation problems for low-functioning individuals and when evaluating change.

REFERENCES

Bak, T. H., Vega-Mendoza, M., & Sorace, A. (2014). Never too late? Advantage on tests of auditory attention extends to late bilinguals. *Frontiers in Psychology, 5*, 485.

Bate, A. J., Mathias, J. L., & Crawford, J. R. (2001). Performance on the Test of Everyday Attention and standard tests of attention following severe traumatic brain injury. *The Clinical Neuropsychologist, 15*(3), 405–422.

Bruce, J. M., Bruce, A. S., & Arnett, P. A. (2007). Mild visual acuity disturbances are associated with performance on tests of complex visual attention in MS. *Journal of the International Neuropsychological Society, 13*(03), 544–548.

Cantagallo, A., & Zoccolotti, P. (1998). *Il Test dell'Attenzione nella vita Quotidiana (T. A. Q.): Il contributo alla standardizzazione italiana.* [A contribution on the Italian standardization of the Test of Everyday Attention.] *Rassegna di Psicologia, 15*(3), 137–147.

Chan, R., Lai, M., & Robertson, I. (2006). Latent structure of the Test of Everyday Attention in a non-clinical Chinese sample. *Archives of Clinical Neuropsychology, 21*(5), 477–485. http://doi.org/10.1016/j.acn.2006.06.007

Chan, R. C. (2000). Attentional deficits in patients with closed head injury: A further study of the discriminative validity of the Test of Everyday Attention. *Brain Injury, 14*(3), 227–236.

Chan, R. C., Hoosain, R., & Lee, T. M. (2002). Reliability and validity of the Cantonese version of the Test of Everyday Attention among normal Hong Kong Chinese: a preliminary report. *Clinical Rehabilitation, 16*(8), 900–909.

Chan, R. C. K., & Lai, M. K. (2006). Latent structure of the Test of Everyday Attention: Convergent evidence from patients with traumatic brain injury. *Brain Injury, 20*(6), 653–659. http://doi.org/10.1080/02699050600676974

Chen, H.-C., Koh, C.-L., Hsieh, C.-L., & Hsueh, I.-P. (2013). Test of Everyday Attention in patients with chronic stroke: test-retest reliability and practice effects. *Brain Injury, 27*(10), 1148–1154. https://doi.org/10.3109/02699052.2013.775483

Clayton, I. C., Richards, J. C., & Edwards, C. J. (1999). Selective attention in obsessive-compulsive disorder. *Journal of Abnormal Psychology, 108*, 171–175.

Crawford, J. R., Sommerville, J., & Robertson, I. H. (1997). Assessing the reliability and abnormality of subtest differences on the Test of Everyday Attention. *British Journal of Clinical Psychology, 36*, 609–617.

De Jager, C. A., Hogervorst, E., Combrinck, M., & Budge, M. M. (2003). Sensitivity and specificity of neuropsychological tests for mild cognitive impairment, vascular cognitive impairment and Alzheimer's disease. *Psychological Medicine, 33*, 1039–1050.

Doneva, S., Davis, S., & Cavenagh, P. (2017). Comparing the performance of people who stutter and people who do not stutter on the Test of Everyday Attention. *Journal of Clinical and Experimental Neuropsychology*, 1–15. https://doi.org/10.1080/13803395.2017.1386162

Fonseca, J., Ferreira, J. J., & Pavão Martins, I. (2017). Cognitive performance in aphasia due to stroke: a systematic review. *International Journal on Disability and Human Development, 16*(2). https://doi.org/10.1515/ijdhd-2016-0011

Greene, J. D. W., Hodges, J. R., & Baddeley, A. D. (1995). Autobiographical memory and executive function in early dementia of the Alzheimer's type. *Neuropsychologia, 33*, 1647–1670.

Iwański, S., Seniów, J., Leśniak, M., Litwin, T., & Członkowska, A. (2015). Diverse attention deficits in patients with neurologically symptomatic and asymptomatic Wilson's disease. *Neuropsychology, 29*(1), 25–30. http://doi.org/10.1037/neu0000103

Klopper, F., Delatycki, M. B., Corben, L. A., Bradshaw, J. L., Rance, G., & Georgiou-Karistianis, N. (2011). The Test of Everyday Attention reveals significant sustained volitional attention and working memory deficits in Friedreich ataxia. *Journal of the International Neuropsychological Society, 17*(01), 196–200. http://doi.org/10.1017/S1355617710001347

Leach, J., & Ansell, L. (2008). Impairment in attentional processing in a field survival environment. *Applied Cognitive Psychology, 22*(5), 643–652. http://doi.org/10.1002/acp.1385

Lincoln, N. B., Radford, K. A., Lee, E., & Reay, A. C. (2006). The assessment of fitness to drive in people with dementia. *International Journal of Geriatric Psychiatry, 21*(11), 1044–1051. http://doi.org/10.1002/gps.1604

MacPherson, S. E., Turner, M. S., Bozzali, M., Cipolotti, L., & Shallice, T. (2010). Frontal subregions mediating Elevator Counting task performance. *Neuropsychologia, 48*(12), 3679–3682. http://doi.org/10.1016/j.neuropsychologia.2010.07.033.

Mazer, B. L., Sofer, S., Korner-Bitensky, N., Gelinas, I., Hanley, J., & Wood-Dauphinee, S. (2003). Effectiveness of a visual attention retraining program on the driving performance of clients with stroke. *Archives of Physical Medicine and Rehabilitation, 84*, 541–550.

Pleva, J., & Wade, T. D. (2002). An investigation of the relationship between responsibility and attention deficits characteristic of obsessive-compulsive phenomena. *Behavioural and Cognitive Psychotherapy, 30*, 399–414.

Posner, M. I., & Peterson, S. E. (1990). The attention system of the human brain. *Annual Review of Neuroscience, 13*, 25–42.

Robertson, I. H., Ward, T., Ridgeway, V., & Nimmo-Smith, I. (1994). *The Test of Everyday Attention.* Bury St. Edmunds, UK: Thames Valley Test Company.

Robertson, I. H., Ward, T., Ridgeway, V., & Nimmo-Smith, I. (1996). The structure of human attention: The Test of Everyday Attention. *Journal of the International Neuropsychological Society, 2*, 525–534.

Stapleton, T., & Connelly, D. (2010). Occupational therapy practice in predriving assessment post stroke in the Irish context: Findings from a nominal group technique meeting. *Topics in Stroke Rehabilitation, 17*(1), 58–68. http://doi.org/10.1310/tsr1701-58

Sterr, A. M. (2004). Attention performance in young adults with learning disabilities. *Learning and Individual Differences, 14*(2), 125–133. http://doi.org/10.1016/j.lindif.2003.10.001

Stewart, H. J., & Amitay, S. (2015). Modality-specificity of selective attention networks. *Frontiers in Psychology, 6*, 1826. https://doi.org/10.3389/fpsyg.2015.01826

Tyson, P. J., Laws, K. R., Flowers, K. A., Mortimer, A. M., & Schulz, J. (2008). Attention and executive function in people with schizophrenia: Relationship with social skills and quality of life. *International Journal of Psychiatry in Clinical Practice, 12*(2), 112–119. http://doi.org/10.1080/13651500701687133

van der Leeuw, G., Leveille, S. G., Jones, R. N., Hausdorff, J. M., McLean, R., Kiely, D. K., . . . Milberg, W. P. (2017). Measuring attention in very old adults using the Test of Everyday Attention. *Neuropsychology, Development, and Cognition. Section B, Aging, Neuropsychology and Cognition, 24*(5), 543–554. https://doi.org/10.1080/13825585.2016.1226747

Van Zandvoort, M., De Haan, E., Van Gijn, J., & Kappelle, L. J. (2003). Cognitive functioning in patients with a small infarct in the brainstem. *Journal of the International Neuropsychological Society, 9*, 490–494.

Ventura, M. I., Barnes, D. E., Ross, J. M., Lanni, K. E., Sigvardt, K. A., & Disbrow, E. A. (2016). A pilot study to evaluate multidimensional effects of dance for people with Parkinson's disease. *Contemporary Clinical Trials, 51*, 50–55. https://doi.org/10.1016/j.cct.2016.10.001

Wiseman-Hakes, C., Murray, B., Moineddin, R., Rochon, E., Cullen, N., Gargaro, J., & Colantonio, A. (2013). Evaluating the impact of treatment for sleep/wake disorders on recovery of cognition and communication in adults with chronic TBI. *Brain Injury, 27*(12), 1364–1376. http://doi.org/10.3109/02699052.2013.823663

Yamin, S., Stinchcombe, A., & Gagnon, S. (2016). Deficits in attention and visual processing but not global cognition predict simulated driving errors in drivers diagnosed with mild Alzheimer's disease. *American Journal of Alzheimer's Disease and Other Dementias, 31*(4), 351–360. http://doi.org/10.1177/1533317515618898

Zakzanis, K. K., Young, D. A., & Radkhoshnoud, N. F. (2002). Attentional processes in abstinent methylenedioxymethamphetamine (Ecstasy) users. *Applied Neuropsychology, 9*(2), 84–91.

Ziino, C., & Ponsford, J. (2006). Selective attention deficits and subjective fatigue following traumatic brain injury. *Neuropsychology, 20*(3), 383–390. http://doi.org/10.1037/0894-4105.20.3.383

TEST OF VARIABLES OF ATTENTION (T.O.V.A.)

TEST NAME	**Test of Variables of Attention (T.O.V.A.)**
DOMAIN	Attention
AGE RANGE	In adults, to 80 years
ADMINISTRATION TIME	22 minutes
SCORING FORMAT	Computerized
REFERENCE	Leark, R., Dupuy, T. R., Greenberg, L. M., Kindschi, C., & Hughes, S. (2017). *T.O.V.A: Test of Variables of Attention: Professional Manual 8.2.* Los Alamitos, CA: The T.O.V.A. Company. www.tovatest.com

DESCRIPTION

The Test of Variables of Attention (T.O.V.A.; Leark et al., 2017) is a computerized test of sustained attention. Responses are collected by USB-based timing hardware and an accurate (±1 ms) microswitch. The test is designed to measure attention and inhibitory control, in order to assist in evaluating attention problems, such as ADHD. The T.O.V.A. is comprised of a visual CPT (Visual T.O.V.A.) and an auditory CPT (Auditory T.O.V.A.), which are collectively termed the T.O.V.A. The test has a lengthy history, from beginning "life as a large rack of electronics controlling a tachistoscopic shutter and slide projector" (Leark et al., 2017, p. 1) in the 1960s to the present-day version.

There are three manuals associated with the T.O.V.A. The User's Manual (Swalwell et al., 2016) includes technical instructions for the installation, configuration, and use of T.O.V.A. software and hardware. The Clinical Manual (Greenberg et al., 2016) is focused on aiding interpretation of the computerized report. The Professional Manual (Leark et al., 2017) provides psychometric details regarding construction of the test. The authors have also published a Research User's Manual. When the term "manual" or Leark et al. (2017) is used here, the reference is to the Professional Manual. The most recent version of the T.O.V.A. does not include rating scales, but an Observation Form is included and can be found at: https://files.tovatest.com/documentation/9/Observation%20Form.pdf. Users may also find the authors' bibliography of research on the T.O.V.A. useful: https://www.tovatest.com/research-and-education/annotated_bibliography.

The T.O.V.A. employs a Go/No-Go paradigm. In the Visual T.O.V.A., the examinee is presented with stimuli consisting of a white square within a large black square. Targets are stimuli whereby the small square is at the top of the large square, and nontargets are stimuli whereby the small square is at the bottom of the large square (see Figure 8–6). Note that the stimuli are not alphanumeric and do not require left-right differentiation or color perception.

For the Auditory T.O.V.A., two distinct tones are used to differentiate the target from the nontarget. The test requires the use of a switchbox with a single button connected to a computer via a parallel port. The examinee presses the button every time a target is presented.

The test consists of four intervals. During the first two intervals, the target appears on 22.5% of the trials (stimulus-infrequent condition). During the second two intervals, the target appears on 77.5% of the trials (stimulus-frequent condition). In the latter intervals, the ISI is reduced, which means that the examinee must respond more quickly in addition to responding more frequently. Thus, the first half of the test is designed to maximize demands on sustained attention (and elicit errors of omission), whereas the second half demands inhibitory control (and elicits errors of commission).

ADMINISTRATION

Detailed administration instructions are found in the manuals. The examiner should be present for the administration, without prompting the examinee. Computer system requirements are described at this

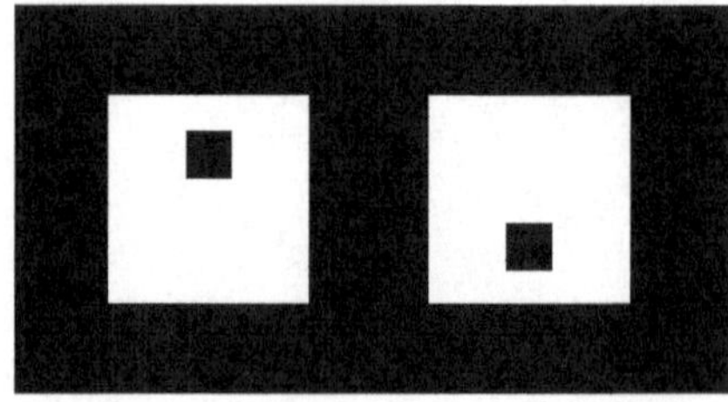

Figure 8–6 *Test of Variables of Attention (T.O.V.A.) visual stimuli.*

link: https://www.tovatest.com/system-requirements. According to the test developers, it is no longer recommended that the T.O.V.A. be administered in the morning only. However, when multiple T.O.V.A. sessions are planned, testing at the same time of day is recommended for consistency. Additionally, the authors recommend that the test be the first administered in a test battery in order to prevent artifacts due to fatigue.

Other research has examined the effects of administration time on performance. Hunt, Bienstock, and Qiang (2012) found no significant differences between morning and afternoon administration of the T.O.V.A. in young adults with ADHD. In healthy young adults, participants responded faster and made more commission errors in the afternoon compared to the morning, with no significant effects on the ADHD score (Hunt, Momjian, & Wong, 2011). Hunt et al. also reported that caffeine consumption was related to faster response times in healthy young adults who typically consumed little caffeine, suggesting caffeine consumption can impact T.O.V.A. performance, as it likely does most CPTs.

The switchbox device optimizes accurate timing (i.e., ±1 ms variance), unlike response devices used in other CPTs (mouse, spacebar, or keyboard) that may introduce additional variability (Leark et al., 2017). This device also minimizes the motor component of the task. As well, because the keyboard can be moved out of reach of the examinee, use of a microswitch prevents impulsive examinees from inadvertently pressing other computer keys and disrupting the test session, as can occur with CPTs that use the space bar or the mouse.

SCORING

Scores reflect variability (consistency), response time (speed), commissions (impulsivity), and omissions (focus and vigilance). Raw scores are converted to standard scores ($M = 100, SD = 15$) based on age and gender, with variables presented for quarters, halves, and the entire test. After the test is completed, a report is generated that compares the examinee's score with age- and gender-corrected scores. T.O.V.A. scores are summarized in Table 8–74. Of note, the ADHD score is based on a combination of scores that have strong predictive validity in detecting ADHD based on ROC analyses, and both omission and commission error scores reflect ratio scores rather than raw scores of the number of missed (omission) or incorrectly identified (commission) stimuli.

Performance is determined to be invalid if any of the following criteria are met: variability or response time is equal to zero, the test is interrupted, there are excessive anticipatory responses, or there are errors for every response (across any quarter, half, or total). Detailed interpretive steps can be found in the Professional and Clinical Manuals.

TABLE 8–74 Summary of Test of Variables of Attention (T.O.V.A.) Scores

T.O.V.A. SCORE	DESCRIPTION
Omission Errors	Measures inattention; reflects missed targets; calculated as the ratio of correctly identified targets to the actual number of targets, minus anticipatory responses toward targets, presented as a percentage.
Commission Errors	Measures impulsivity and disinhibition; reflects responses to non-targets; calculated as the ratio of incorrect responses (to non-targets) to the actual number of non-targets, minus anticipatory responses to non-targets, presented as a percentage.
Response Time	Provides the mean time taken to respond correctly to targets, in milliseconds, reported for each quarter, half, and total.
Response Time Variability	Measures consistency of response time; consists of the *SD* of the mean correct response times, for each quarter, half, and total.
D Prime	Measures response sensitivity, with regard to the ratio of the hit rate to false alarm rate; measures performance decrement according to signal detection theory, accuracy of signal-to-noise discrimination.
Attention Comparison Score[a]	Compares the examinee's performance to that of an Attention-Deficit/Hyperactivity Disorder (ADHD) sample.
Post-Commission Response Time	Mean time taken to respond to targets immediately after a commission error, in milliseconds.
Anticipatory Responses	Responses occurring when the subject responds within 150 ms after stimulus presentation; these are not included in omissions, commissions, response times, or response variability; calculated as a percentage of the total stimuli.
Multiple Responses	Occurs when the microswitch is pressed more than once per stimulus presentation; calculated as the sum of multiple responses, regardless of whether the response was to a target or non-target.

[a] Note that in early versions of T.O.V.A., the Attention Comparison Score was termed the Attention Performance Index. In earlier versions, this variable was labeled the ADHD Score. If the Attention Comparison Score is greater than 0, this indicates the examinee's performance resembles the normative sample; if less than 0, the examinee's performance is more similar to an independently diagnosed ADHD sample. See Leark et al. (2017) for more details.

The T.O.V.A. also includes an internal validity measure, termed Performance Validity (PV), which was termed Symptom Exaggeration Index (SEI) in earlier versions. The PV applies to individuals 17 years of age or older when performance is not within normal limits. PV reflects unusual patterns of performance that are not seen in samples with ADHD. It is important to note that this pattern of performance may be reflective of malingering, but also of severe disability or poor test adherence. Thus, the PV does not attribute an underlying cause to suspect performance, which must be interpreted by the clinician in the context of the assessment. PV criteria are outlined in the manual. See also the section "Performance Validity," in this review, for additional information on use of the T.O.V.A. variables as indices of noncredible performance.

DEMOGRAPHIC EFFECTS

AGE

T.O.V.A. performance follows a curvilinear progression with age. Commission errors, response time, and response time variability decrease with age, particularly in the second half of the test (see Leark et al., 2017). The test may be particularly sensitive at detecting attentional impairment in ADHD adults, compared to youth with ADHD (Ben-Sheetrit et al., 2017).

GENDER

Gender differences are discussed in the manual (Leark et al., 2017). In summary, males tend to commit more omission and commission errors, and women tend toward slower response times. These interact somewhat with age and time point in the test (e.g., more pronounced later in the test). Hunt et al. (2011) reported a main effect on the T.O.V.A. for order of presentation for women only, specifically that women who completed the WAIS-IV first performed significantly better on the T.O.V.A. However, not all research has found gender differences; for example, no gender differences were found on the T.O.V.A. in chronic pain patients (Byas-Smith et al., 2005).

EDUCATION

Information on the effects of education is limited. The T.O.V.A. was not related to education in a chronic pain sample (Byas-Smith et al., 2005).

ETHNICITY, NATIONALITY, AND LINGUISTIC EFFECTS

The effects of ethnicity have apparently not been studied directly, but the T.O.V.A. has been used cross-culturally (e.g., Anckarsater et al., 2012; Grane et al., 2014; Shen et al., 2013; Thompson et al., 2015). Test instructions are available in eight languages (i.e., English, Spanish, Hebrew, Korean, French, German, Danish, and Swedish).

NORMATIVE DATA

The adult normative sample for the Visual T.O.V.A. consists of 250 undergraduate students and participants in college communities in Minnesota. The sample was predominantly Caucasian (99%) and female (69%). Exclusion criteria were current use of psychoactive medication or a history of neurologic disorder or injury. Normative data are age- and gender-corrected and are provided in 10-year age bands, ranging from 20 to 29 as the first age band to 80+ as the last age band.

In terms of the Auditory T.O.V.A., norms are preliminary at this time according to the authors, pending release of normative data (see Leark et al., 2017). Norms will extend to age 29 ($n = 129$, 58% female) and will be corrected for age and gender. It should be noted that there is an extensive normative database for children and adolescents.

EVIDENCE FOR RELIABILITY

EVIDENCE FOR INTERNAL RELIABILITY

Internal reliability estimates derive mainly from child samples. Internal reliability was calculated as the degree of association between the first and second halves of the test. Overall, internal reliability is highest for reaction time and lowest for commissions and d' (i.e., $rs > .80$, $rs \leq .60$, respectively; see manual for more details; see also Llorente et al., 2001, 2008; Wu et al., 2007).

EVIDENCE FOR TEST-RETEST RELIABILITY, MEASURING CHANGE, AND PRACTICE EFFECTS

As with internal reliability, test-retest reliability is primarily derived from child samples. *SEM*s are provided as raw scores in the manual. *SEM*s, in standard score format, are found in Leark, Wallace, and Fitzgerald (2004). *SEM*s are quite large; use of test-retest data, rather than internal reliability estimates, may have inflated *SEM* values. Test-retest reliability based on a subset of the normative sample is in the adequate to high range ($r = .74$ for commissions to $r = .87$ for response time variability). See also Leark et al. (2004) and Llorente et al. (2001).

EVIDENCE FOR VALIDITY

FACTOR-ANALYTIC STUDIES AND RELATIONSHIPS WITH OTHER TESTS

A factor analysis completed with the standardization sample for the Visual T.O.V.A. yielded three factors: response time (response time, variability, and d'), commissions, and omissions (Leark et al., 2017). A factor analysis of the Auditory T.O.V.A. yielded a five-factor solution, including a response time factor (comprised of response time and variability), but with further subdivision of omissions and commissions based on stimulus-frequent and stimulus-infrequent conditions.

The different factor solutions yielded from each version of the T.O.V.A. suggest that test modality affects the underlying constructs being measured (Riccio et al., 2001). Comparison of the Visual and Auditory T.O.V.A. in the standardization sample indicates that about twice as many omissions are made on the auditory version but that more commissions are made on the visual test. Response times are also faster on the visual test, but variability is greater on the auditory version. Auditory and Visual T.O.V.A. error score counterparts were correlated in a sample of young adults with ADHD (omission errors, $r = .48$; commission errors, $r = .59$; Weyandt et al., 2005).

The T.O.V.A. appears to relate to rating scales of ADHD symptoms. In one study, symptoms of inattention on a self-report questionnaire (Barkley and Murphy Current Symptoms Scale) were moderately correlated with the T.O.V.A. ADHD score, response time variability, and omission errors (rs = −.31 to −.42) in a young adult ADHD sample (Hunt et al., 2011). The T.O.V.A. is also related to a self-reported questionnaire on mindfulness (Keith et al., 2017).

Negligible effects regarding the relationships between IQ and T.O.V.A. have been reported in young adults (with and without ADHD; Weyandt et al., 2002). The T.O.V.A. showed minimal correlations with the Montreal Cognitive Assessment (MoCA) following subarachnoid hemorrhage (Wallmark, Lundstrom, Wikstrom, & Ronne-Engstrom, 2015). Grane et al. (2014) reported generally small to no associations between the T.O.V.A. and the Behavior Rating Inventory of Executive Function-Adult Version (BRIEF-A) with some minor exceptions. Depression and anxiety ratings on the Achenbach System of Empirically Based Assessment (ASEBA) were not related to T.O.V.A. performance scores (Grane et al., 2014). In addition to these studies with adults, there are also studies on relationships between the T.O.V.A. and other measures in children.

CLINICAL STUDIES

Most clinical studies have been done in child populations. Some studies have been conducted in adults with ADHD. Group studies indicate impairments on specific T.O.V.A. variables in young adults with ADHD compared with controls (i.e., omission errors, Weyandt et al., 2002; see also Weyandt et al., 1998). Grane et al. (2014) reported that ADHD treatment-naïve adults performed worse than controls on multiple variables (e.g., delayed response time, increased reaction time variability, and higher omission errors). Some support for the T.O.V.A.'s sensitivity and specificity in ADHD diagnosis is provided in the manual (Leark et al., 2017). Manor, Rozen, Zemishlani, Weizman, and Zalsman (2011) reported that the T.O.V.A. was sensitive to methylphenidate response in older adults (≥55 years) with ADHD, with improvements across all variables except commissions.

The T.O.V.A. has been used in a number of other populations, including depression. Oral et al. (2012) reported that individuals with major depressive disorder performed worse on the T.O.V.A. (response time, omissions, d', but not commissions), but contrary to expectations there were not significant correlations between brain-derived neurotrophic factor (BDNF) and most neurocognitive tests, including the T.O.V.A. Shen et al. (2013) reported that individuals with major depressive disorder made more omissions and demonstrated greater variability and longer response times on the T.O.V.A. compared with healthy controls, with no significant effects for commission errors.

The T.O.V.A. has been used to examine the effects of substances. For example, Byas-Smith et al. (2005) found no group differences on the T.O.V.A. between chronic pain patients managed with opioid analgesics compared to healthy controls. Severtson and Latimer (2008) reported that T.O.V.A. commissions moderated the association between cocaine use and incarceration in intravenous drug use. Other studies have reported decreased T.O.V.A. performance following subarachnoid hemorrhage (Wallmark et al., 2015) and in people with mucopolysaccharidoses (i.e., rare genetic lysosomal disorders; Ahmed et al., 2016).

The T.O.V.A. has been used to examine the effects of different interventions. In a mixed clinical sample, Putnam, Othmer, Othmer, and Pollock (2005) reported statistically significant improvements in some T.O.V.A. variables (i.e., omissions, commissions, variability, but not response time) following neurofeedback, as have others (Surmeli et al., 2017). Null results have also been reported on the T.O.V.A. following neurofeedback (Cowley et al., 2016). Scott, Kaiser, Othmer, and Sideroff (2005) reported significant improvements on the T.O.V.A. following an electroencephalogram (EEG) biofeedback protocol in a mixed clinical sample of inpatients with substance use disorders. In addition, the T.O.V.A. was found to be sensitive to the effect of glucose on attentional performance in healthy adults (Flint & Turek, 2003).

NEUROANATOMICAL CORRELATES AND IMAGING STUDIES

Caudate asymmetry (larger right relative to left volumes) was correlated with T.O.V.A. performance in adults with ADHD in one study (Dang et al., 2016).

PERFORMANCE VALIDITY

Henry (2005) reported that in a sample predominantly comprised of patients with mild TBI involved in personal injury litigation, half the sample (n = 26) was classified as probable malingerers based on performance below established cutoff scores on a performance validity measure (e.g., Test of Memory Malingering, Word Memory Test, Computerized Assessment of Response Bias) and meeting Slick, Sherman, and Iverson's (1999) criteria of definite malingered neurocognitive dysfunction (MND). The malingering group performed significantly worse across all T.O.V.A. variables examined (e.g., omission, response time, variability), with the exception of commissions. Effect sizes were large overall. Omissions were found to be particularly useful in terms of consistently emerging as a strong predictor of group membership in regression analyses. Sensitivity and specificity were good, although cutoffs need to be adjusted to reduce false-positive errors in nonmalingerers (i.e., nearly 89% of the malingering group and nearly 81% of the not malingering group were correctly identified).

The T.O.V.A. has been identified as showing utility in persons referred for ADHD assessment, with T.O.V.A. omission errors associated with 63% sensitivity at a 90% specificity rate (Marshall et al., 2010). Persons evaluated for ADHD assessment and designated as noncredible made more commission errors and omission errors and showed greater reaction time variability than those who were deemed credible (Marshall, Hoelzle, Heyerdahl, & Nelson, 2016). Although a high proportion of patients overall showed impaired performance on the T.O.V.A., 80% of noncredible patients could be identified as such using the T.O.V.A. cutoff scores for noncredible performance, as suggested by Marshall et al. (2010; i.e., total response time variability exceeding 180 ms, ≥26 omission errors, and ≥31 commission errors).

COMMENT

The T.O.V.A. incorporates visual and auditory sustained attention measures in a computerized format, and has a relatively long history of use. The test presents with many strengths, including requiring responses on a precise microswitch that is reportedly accurate within 1 ms. In addition, the test offers a rich amount of data typical of Go/No-Go paradigms that pertain to error and response time parameters collected under differing levels of target frequency. The manuals are highly detailed, and the T.O.V.A. is updated frequently.

In terms of demographic effects, test performance generally follows a curvilinear progression with age, and, overall, there is some evidence for gender differences. Age- and gender-adjusted normative data are provided. There is little information on the influence of education. Although the test has been translated into many languages and used cross-culturally, the effect of ethnicity is unclear. As well, the adult subsample comprising the normative sample is relatively small ($n = 250$ for the Visual T.O.V.A.) and not representative of the general population (e.g., predominantly college students, 99% Caucasian, 69% female), although well-suited for some groups (e.g., ADHD screening in young adults). Auditory T.O.V.A. norms are reportedly forthcoming.

Reliability estimates are derived mainly from child samples, with lack of data in adult samples a weakness of the test. Practice effects and reliable change estimates for adults are lacking. Factor-analytic studies suggest a three-factor solution for the Visual T.O.V.A. and a five-factor solution for the Auditory T.O.V.A. In adults, more information on the relationship between cognitive measures and the T.O.V.A. is needed. Some research suggests the T.O.V.A. shows at least a moderate relation with ADHD rating scales, with other research indicating no significant relationship exists between the T.O.V.A. and executive function rating scales.

Studies of adults with ADHD indicate that there are group differences on most T.O.V.A. variables and that the T.O.V.A. is sensitive to medication effects in ADHD and the effects of neurostimulation in other populations. The T.O.V.A. has also been used in other adult clinical populations, for example showing group differences between people diagnosed with depression and controls. Other research suggests promise for omissions as an indicator of performance validity, especially in ADHD groups, but further research is needed. In addition, the test's utility in populations with attentional difficulty other than ADHD (e.g., TBI) remains to be determined.

In light of these limitations and because CPTs can miss correctly identifying examinees with ADHD, the test, if used, should only be one component of an ADHD assessment. Other elements of an assessment focused on ADHD must include a history, physical screening examination, evaluation of classroom/work environment, structured interview, and behavioral ratings, with additional elements incorporated as indicated.

REFERENCES

Ahmed, A., Shapiro, E., Rudser, K., Kunin-Batson, A., King, K., & Whitley, C. B. (2016). Association of somatic burden of disease with age and neuropsychological measures in attenuated mucopolysaccharidosis types I, II and VI. *Molecular Genetics and Metabolism Reports, 7*, 27–31. https://doi.org/10.1016/j.ymgmr.2016.03.006

Anckarsäter, H., Hofvander, B., Billstedt, E., Gillberg, I. C., Gillberg, C., Wentz, E., & Råstam, M. (2012). The sociocommunicative deficit subgroup in anorexia nervosa: autism spectrum disorders and neurocognition in a community-based, longitudinal study. *Psychological Medicine, 42*(9), 1957–1967. https://doi.org/10.1017/S0033291711002881

Ben-Sheetrit, J., Tasker, H., Avnat, L., Golubchik, P., Weizman, A., & Manor, I. (2017). Possible age-related progression of attentional impairment in ADHD and its attenuation by past diagnosis and treatment. *Journal of Attention Disorders*, 1087054717743328.

Byas-Smith, M. G., Chapman, S. L., Reed, B., & Cotsonis, G. (2005). The effect of opioids on driving and psychomotor performance in patients with chronic pain. *Clinical Journal of Pain, 21*(4), 345–352.

Cowley, B., Holmström, É., Juurmaa, K., Kovarskis, L., & Krause, C. M. (2016). Computer enabled neuroplasticity treatment: A clinical trial of a novel design for neurofeedback therapy in adult ADHD. *Frontiers in Human Neuroscience, 10*. https://doi.org/10.3389/fnhum.2016.00205

Dang, L. C., Samanez-Larkin, G. R., Young, J. S., Cowan, R. L., Kessler, R. M., & Zald, D. H. (2016). Caudate asymmetry is related to attentional impulsivity and an objective measure of ADHD-like attentional problems in healthy adults. *Brain Structure and Function, 221*(1), 277–286. https://doi.org/10.1007/s00429-014-0906-6

Flint, R. W., & Turek, C. (2003). Glucose effects on a continuous performance test of attention in adults. *Behavioural Brain Research, 142*, 217–228.

Grane, V. A., Endestad, T., Pinto, A. F., & Solbakk, A.–K. (2014). Attentional control and subjective executive function in treatment-naive adults with attention deficit hyperactivity disorder. *PloS One, 9*(12), e115227.

Greenberg, L., Kindschi, C., Dupuy, T., & Hughes, S. (2016). *T.O.V.A: Test of Variables of Attention: Clinical Manual*. Los Alamitos, CA: The TOVA Company.

Henry, G. K. (2005). Probable malingering and performance on the Test of Variables of Attention. *The Clinical Neuropsychologist, 19*(1), 121–129. https://doi.org/10.1080/13854040490516604

Hunt, M. G., Momjian, A. J., & Wong, K. (2011). Effects of diurnal variation and caffeine consumption on Test of Variables of Attention (T.O.V.A.) performance in healthy young adults. *Psychological Assessment, 23*(1), 226.

Keith, J. R., Blackwood, M. E., Mathew, R. T., & Lecci, L. B. (2017). Self-reported mindful attention and awareness, go/no-go response-time variability, and attention-deficit hyperactivity disorder. *Mindfulness, 8*(3), 765–774. https://doi.org/10.1007/s12671-016-0655-0

Leark, R., Dupuy, T., Greenberg, L., Kindschi, C., & Hughes, S. (2017). *T.O.V.A: Test of Variables of Attention: Professional Manual 8.2.* Los Alamitos, CA: The TOVA Company.

Leark, R. A., Wallace, D. R., & Fitzgerald, R. (2004). Test-retest reliability and standard error of measurement for the Test of Variables of Attention (T.O.V.A.) with healthy school-age children. *Assessment, 11*(4), 285–289.

Llorente, A. M., Amado, A. J., Voigt, R. G., Berretta, M. C., Fraley, J. K., Jensen, C. L., & Heird, W. C. (2001). Internal consistency, temporal stability, and reproducibility of individual index scores of the Test of Variables of Attention in children with attention-deficit/hyperactivity disorder. *Archives of Clinical Neuropsychology, 16*, 535–546.

Llorente, A. M., Voigt, R., Jensen, C. L., Fraley, J. K., Heird, W. C., & Rennie, K. M. (2008). The Test of Variables of Attention (T.O.V.A.): Internal consistency (Q_1 vs. Q_2 and Q_3 vs. Q_4) in children with attention deficit/hyperactivity disorder (ADHD). *Child Neuropsychology, 14*(4), 314–322. https://doi.org/10.1080/09297040701563578

Manor, I., Rozen, S., Zemishlani, Z., Weizman, A., & Zalsman, G. (2011). When does it end? Attention-deficit/hyperactivity disorder in the middle aged and older populations: *Clinical Neuropharmacology, 34*(4), 148–154. https://doi.org/10.1097/WNF.0b013e3182206dc1

Marshall, P., Schroeder, R., O'Brien, J., Fischer, R., Ries, A., Blesi, B., & Barker, J. (2010). Effectiveness of symptom validity measures in identifying cognitive and behavioral symptom exaggeration in adult attention deficit hyperactivity disorder. *The Clinical Neuropsychologist, 24*(7), 1204–1237. https://doi.org/10.1080/13854046.2010.514290

Marshall, P. S., Hoelzle, J. B., Heyerdahl, D., & Nelson, N. W. (2016). The impact of failing to identify suspect effort in patients undergoing adult attention-deficit/hyperactivity disorder (ADHD) assessment. *Psychological Assessment, 28*(10), 1290.

Oral, E., Canpolat, S., Yildirim, S., Gulec, M., Aliyev, E., & Aydin, N. (2012). Cognitive functions and serum levels of brain-derived neurotrophic factor in patients with major depressive disorder. *Brain Research Bulletin, 88*(5), 454–459. https://doi.org/10.1016/j.brainresbull.2012.03.005

Putnam, J. A., Othmer, S. F., Othmer, S., & Pollock, V. E. (2005). TOVA results following inter-hemispheric bipolar EEG training. *Journal of Neurotherapy, 9*(1), 37–52. https://doi.org/10.1300/J184v09n01_04

Riccio, C. A., Reynolds, C. R., & Lowe, P. A. (2001). *Clinical applications of continuous performance tests: Measuring attention and impulsive responding in children and adults.* New York: John Wiley & Sons.

Scott, W. C., Kaiser, D., Othmer, S., & Sideroff, S. I. (2005). Effects of an EEG biofeedback protocol on a mixed substance abusing population. *American Journal of Drug and Alcohol Abuse, 31*(3), 455–469. https://doi.org/10.1081/ADA-200056807

Severtson, S. G., & Latimer, W. W. (2008). Factors related to correctional facility incarceration among active injection drug users in Baltimore, MD. *Drug and Alcohol Dependence, 94*(1–3), 73–81. https://doi.org/10.1016/j.drugalcdep.2007.10.007

Shen, T.–W., Liu, F.–C., Chen, S.–J., & Chen, S.–T. (2013). Changes in heart rate variability during T.O.V.A. testing in patients with major depressive disorder: HRV and depression. *Psychiatry and Clinical Neurosciences, 67*(1), 35–40. https://doi.org/10.1111/j.1440-1819.2012.02404.x

Slick, D. J., Sherman, E. M., & Iverson, G. L. (1999). Diagnostic criteria for malingered neurocognitive dysfunction: Proposed standards for clinical practice and research. *The Clinical Neuropsychologist, 13,* 545–561. http://dx.doi.org/10.1076/1385-4046(199911)13:04;1-Y;FT545

Surmeli, T., Eralp, E., Mustafazade, I., Kos, I. H., Özer, G. E., & Surmeli, O. H. (2017). Quantitative EEG neurometric analysis–guided neurofeedback treatment in postconcussion syndrome (PCS): Forty cases. How is neurometric analysis important for the treatment of PCS and as a biomarker? *Clinical EEG and Neuroscience, 48*(3), 217–230.

Swalwell, S., Greenberg, A., & Dupuy, T. (2016). *TOVA 8 User's Manual.* Los Alamitos, CA: The TOVA Company.

Thompson, M., Thompson, L., & Reid-Chung, A. (2015). Treating postconcussion syndrome with Loreta z-score neurofeedback and heart rate variability biofeedback: Neuroanatomical/neurophysiological rationale, methods, and case examples. *Biofeedback,* 43(1) 15.

Weyandt, L. L., Mitzlaff, L., & Thomas, L. (2002). The relationship between intelligence and performance on the Test of Variables of Attention (T.O.V.A.). *Journal of Learning Disabilities, 35*(2), 114–120.

Weyandt, L. L., Rice, J. A., Linterman, H. I., Mitzlaff, L., & Emert, E. (1998). Neuropsychological performance of a sample of adults with ADHD, developmental reading disorder, and controls. *Developmental Neuropsychology, 14*, 643–656.

Weyandt, L., Hays, B., & Schepman, S. (2005). The construct validity of the Internal Restlessness Scale. *Assessment for Effective Intervention, 30*(3), 53–63.

Wu, Y.–Y., Huang, Y.–S., Chen, Y.–Y., Chen, C.–K., Chang, T.–C., & Chao, C.–C. (2007). Psychometric study of the test of variables of attention: Preliminary findings on Taiwanese children with attention-deficit/hyperactivity disorder. *Psychiatry and Clinical Neurosciences, 61*(3), 211–218. https://doi.org/10.1111/j.1440-1819.2007.01658.x

9 | EXECUTIVE FUNCTIONING

BEHAVIOR RATING INVENTORY OF EXECUTIVE FUNCTION—ADULT VERSION (BRIEF-A)

TEST NAME	**Behavior Rating Inventory of Executive Function—Adult Version (BRIEF-A)**
DOMAIN	Executive functioning
AGE RANGE	18 to 90 years
ADMINISTRATION TIME	10 minutes
SCORING FORMAT	Computerized or hand scored
REFERENCE	Roth, R. M., Isquith, P. K., & Gioia, G. A. (2005). *Behavioral Rating Inventory of Executive Function—Adult Version.* Lutz, FL: Psychological Assessment Resources, Inc. www.parinc.com

DESCRIPTION

Measuring executive functions through standard performance-based tests is more challenging than measuring other domain-specific functions such as language, memory and visual-spatial skills (Gioia et al., 2000). Because tests are administered in a structured, novel, quiet, one-on-one testing environment, performance-based tests of executive functioning do not always allow executive deficits to emerge during test administration. As well, many executive functioning tests are designed to measure specific subcomponent parts of executive function rather than the integrated, complex, multidimensional executive functions seen in everyday life (Roth et al., 2005). In addition, although performance-based measures may inform on ability level, they do not provide information on whether those abilities are actually deployed in real life. Last, some executive tests were developed with the explicit goal of facilitating neuroanatomical localization before the advent of modern imaging, and so these tests may not be as sensitive to executive deficits in daily life (Bulzacka et al., 2013).

The Behaviour Rating Inventory of Executive Function-Adult Version (BRIEF-A; Roth et al., 2005) is a 75-item questionnaire designed to measure executive functioning in the everyday environment. Like its predecessor for children, the Behavior Rating Inventory of Executive Function (BRIEF; Gioia et al., 2000), the BRIEF-A is intended as one component of a comprehensive evaluation of executive functioning, suitable for developmental, psychiatric and neurological conditions (Roth et al., 2005).

The BRIEF-A yields an overall composite, the Global Executive Composite (GEC), along with two broad indexes: the Behavioral Regulation Index (BRI) and the Metacognition Index (MI; Table 9–1). These are comprised of nine theoretically and empirically derived Clinical Scales, each of which reflects a specific aspect of executive functioning (Inhibit, Shift, Emotional Control, Self-Monitor, Initiate, Working Memory, Plan/Organize, Task Monitor, and Organization of Materials; Table 9–2).

In addition, the BRIEF-A includes three scales designed to assess validity (Negativity, Infrequency, and Inconsistency). The manual presents a brief yet instructive review of the ways in which disruptions and diseases affect frontal brain systems to cause executive dysfunction in the

TABLE 9–1 Clinical Scales and Composites of the BRIEF-A

GLOBAL EXECUTIVE COMPOSITE (GEC)	
BEHAVIORAL REGULATION INDEX (BRI)	METACOGNITION INDEX (MI)
Inhibit	Initiate
Shift	Working Memory
Emotional Control	Plan/Organize
Self-Monitor	Task Monitor Organization of Materials

SOURCE: Reproduced by special permission of the Publisher, Psychological Assessment Resources, Inc. (PAR), 16204 North Florida Avenue, Lutz, Florida 33549, from the Behavior Rating Inventory of Executive Function-Adult Version by Robert M. Roth, PhD, Peter K. Isquith, PhD and Gerard A. Gioia, PhD, Copyright 1996, 1998, 2001, 2003, 2004, 2005 by PAR. Further reproduction is prohibited without permission from PAR.

context of common brain disorders and developmental factors, including normal aging.

The BRIEF-A has two kinds of rating forms: the Self-Report form and the Informant Report, completed by an informant who knows the examinee well. Both provide a multidimensional estimate of the nature and severity of executive deficits. Ideally, both forms are completed for an examinee, but the Informant Report can be used alone in cases where the target patient is unable to complete the Self-Report due to illness, lack of cooperation, incapacity, or low reading skills. Comparisons between forms may yield clinically relevant information, including self-awareness of executive dysfunction compared to that of the informant. Large discrepancies between the Self-Report and Informant Report may point to unawareness, denial of deficits, or limitations in self-understanding that may be informative in terms of diagnostic evaluation and treatment planning (Roth et al., 2005), although the sensitivity of the Informant Report to executive deficits may vary by clinical condition (see the section "Validity").

TABLE 9–2 Description of BRIEF-A Clinical Scales

CLINICAL SCALE	DESCRIPTION
Inhibit	Impulse control; stopping/modulating behavior
Shift	Ability to shift from one activity, situation or problem to another or solve problems flexibly
Emotional Control	The ability to modulate emotional responses
Self-Monitor	Monitoring of own behavior in relation to others', especially in social situations
Initiate	The ability to start an activity or generate ideas
Working Memory	The process of holding information in mind for the purposes of completing a task; staying with an activity
Plan/Organize	The ability to anticipate future events, set goals and develop steps ahead of time to complete tasks
Task Monitor	Monitoring of one's work and performance in relation to a goal
Organization of Materials	The ability to maintain order in one's workspace, home and possessions.

SOURCE: Adapted from Roth et al. (2005). Reproduced by special permission of the Publisher, Psychological Assessment Resources, Inc. (PAR), 16204 North Florida Avenue, Lutz, Florida 33549, from the Behavior Rating Inventory of Executive Function-Adult Version by Robert M. Roth, PhD, Peter K. Isquith, PhD and Gerard A. Gioia, PhD, Copyright 1996, 1998, 2001, 2003, 2004, 2005 by PAR. Further reproduction is prohibited without permission from PAR.

ADMINISTRATION

The BRIEF-A consists of the Professional Manual, the BRIEF-A Self-Report, the BRIEF-A Informant Report, and scoring sheets for both forms. The Informant Report can be given to a spouse, parent, adult child, caregiver, or professional (nurse, mental health worker). The test authors recommend that the informant have at minimum a twice-per-week face-to-face interaction with the person being rated (Roth et al., 2005). Instructions for respondents are printed on the forms. The self and informant forms should be given in one sitting, but separately, to prevent the examinee and informant from influencing each other's responses on the scales.

Respondents are asked to rate the behavior described in each item on a three-point scale ("Never," "Sometimes" and "Often") in terms of how often, in the last month, the particular behavior has been a problem. The manual includes additional detailed instructions that may be used as a guide for instructing raters (Roth et al., 2005, p. 8).

Respondents with reading skills below a fifth-grade level or limited English proficiency should not complete the BRIEF-A. In our experience, it is not uncommon for some raters to inadvertently omit responses on the rating form. It is therefore important to check the form for missed items at the end of the administration and have the rater fill in missing responses if need be. This is also indicated in the manual.

SCORING

SCORES

T scores and percentiles can be derived for all the Clinical Scales and composite scores grouped according to seven age ranges for the two forms. As well, 90% confidence intervals can be calculated for scales and indexes. A T score 1.5 standard deviations (*SD*s) above the mean (T ≥65) is the recommended cutoff for abnormal elevation and potential clinical significance.

BRIEF-A data from the normative group are positively skewed, with the majority of cases at the lower end of the distribution (i.e., with few executive deficits). Consequently, conversions from T scores to percentiles are not uniform across all subscales because not all normative raw score distributions were normally distributed. This means that different scales may yield slightly different percentile values for the same T score, reflecting the shape of the underlying raw score distribution for that particular scale. T scores derive from smoothed linear or polynomial transformations of the clinical scale raw scores (Roth et al., 2005).

Validity scales (Negativity, Infrequency, and Inconsistency) are scored with regard to specific cutoffs indicated on the scoring form (Table 9–5).

INDEX DISCREPANCIES AND GEC INTERPRETATION

The GEC is best interpreted when the BRI and MI are at the same general level. To assess whether this is the case, a table of cumulative percentages of index T-score differences is shown in the manual on p. 23. Overall, T-score differences of greater than 12 (Self-Report) or greater than 11 (Informant Report) were found in less than 10% of the normative sample (Roth et al., 2005); these cutoffs can therefore serve as benchmarks for determining whether the GEC should be interpreted. Thus, if the BRI and MI are too discrepant, interpretation of the GEC would probably not provide the best estimate of the examinee's level of function. No guidelines are provided for determining whether the BRI or MI themselves are interpretable, with regard to discrepancies among Clinical Scales. Users are urged to use clinical judgment in making this determination and to not interpret BRI and MI scales if their respective Clinical Scales appear very discrepant.

SELF-REPORT VERSUS INFORMANT REPORT DISCREPANCIES

To determine whether Self-Informant differences are clinically significant, Self-Informant discrepancy base rates can be examined based on data from a mixed clinical/healthy sample (N = 180; Table 9–3), along with some possible discrepancy interpretations based on those provided in the manual (Table 9–4). See "Validity" for further discussion of discrepancies.

TABLE 9–3 BRIEF-A Self-Informant Discrepancies: Frequencies for Differences Larger Than 20 T Score Points

	SELF < INFORMANT (20 POINTS OR MORE; %)	SELF > INFORMANT (20 POINTS OR MORE; %)
Inhibit	2.8	4.5
Shift	6.7	6.7
Emotional Control	2.8	6.7
Self-Monitor	4.5	6.7
Initiate	5.6	5.0
Working Memory	4.5	10.6
Plan/Organize	6.1	10.1
Task Monitor	6.1	6.7
Organization of Materials	3.9	1.7
BRI	4.5	8.4
MI	5.0	8.9
GEC	5.6	6.7

NOTE: Percentages reflect the Mixed Clinical/Healthy Adult Sample (N = 180) described in the manual.

GEC, Global Executive Composite (GEC); BRI, Behavioral Regulation Index; MI.

SOURCE: Adapted from Roth et al. (2005). Reproduced by special permission of the Publisher, Psychological Assessment Resources, Inc. (PAR), 16204 North Florida Avenue, Lutz, Florida 33549, from the Behavior Rating Inventory of Executive Function-Adult Version by Robert M. Roth, PhD, Peter K. Isquith, PhD and Gerard A. Gioia, PhD, Copyright 1996, 1998, 2001, 2003, 2004, 2005 by PAR. Further reproduction is prohibited without permission from PAR.

NEGATIVITY SCALE

The Negativity Scale reflects the extent of negative bias on the part of the rater compared to raters in the BRIEF-A normative and clinical samples. A high Negativity score indicates that the respondent endorsed "Often" for the majority of items on the Negativity scale and that this tendency was higher than 99% of the normative and clinical samples. Negativity scores of 6 or higher are considered "Elevated"; this corresponds to higher than the 99th percentile in the normative/clinical sample. The authors recommend that protocols should only be deemed invalid after a careful review of items in the context of other test scores, history, and observations because severe executive dysfunction can be associated with elevated Negativity, since items making up the Negativity scale also appear on the Clinical Scales.

INFREQUENCY SCALE

This scale includes items that are generally answered in only one direction by most respondents. The scale is made up of five items, and thus scores range from 0 to 5. Scores of 3 or more are considered "Infrequent," a level consistent with higher than the 99th percentile in the combined sample. Protocols with scores in this range should be examined for (1) random responding or (2) purposeful bias toward endorsing extreme symptoms. The test authors note that the Infrequency scale is not designed to prove or disprove malingering, which necessitates a thorough evaluation of test performance, behavior, and clinical findings (Roth et al., 2005). Its value in detecting malingered neurocognitive dysfunction is also questionable because of the item content; a high Infrequency rating reflects both endorsement of extreme/implausible symptoms suggestive of cognitive impairment (e.g., items similar to "I forget who I am"), but also an attempt to show oneself in an implausibly positive light, through the denial of common complaints (e.g., items similar to "I am never fatigued"). Unlike the other validity scales, items from the Infrequency scale do not contribute to the Clinical Scales.

INCONSISTENCY SCALE

The Inconsistency scale consists of 10 item pairs that are similar but not identical in content, with possible scores ranging from 0 to 20. High scores on this scale indicate that the rater responded in an inconsistent manner within item pairs compared to the normative sample and a mixed clinical/healthy sample. The manual notes that the calculation of the Inconsistency scale must be made carefully because it is somewhat complex. For each pair, the absolute value of the difference between items is calculated. The Inconsistency scale is the sum of the absolute differences for each item pair. Based on this total, protocols are rated as "Acceptable" or "Inconsistent." Acceptable protocols are those with scores up to and including 7; scores of 8 or more are considered "Inconsistent," corresponding to higher than

TABLE 9–4 Possible Interpretive Significance of Self-Informant Discrepancies on the BRIEF-A

SHAPE OF PROFILE (SELF VS. INFORMANT)	SCALE ELEVATIONS (SELF VS. INFORMANT)	POSSIBLE INTERPRETATION
Same	Self = Informant	• Both parties agree on areas of difficulties • Both parties agree on severity of issues • Executive profile is likely reliable across situations
Same	Self < Informant	• Both parties agree about strengths and weaknesses, but informant sees a greater impact of the problem • Examinee has mild self-awareness problem
Different	Self < Informant	• Examinee has poor self-awareness • Informant has excessively negative view of the examinee • Informant is exaggerating severity of deficits
Different	Self > Informant	• Informant is unaware of examinee's deficits • Informant has overly positive view of the examinee • Examinee has a high level of distress • Examinee is overly critical of self • Examinee is exaggerating severity of deficits

SOURCE: Adapted from Roth et al. (2005). Reproduced by special permission of the Publisher, Psychological Assessment Resources, Inc. (PAR), 16204 North Florida Avenue, Lutz, Florida 33549, from the Behavior Rating Inventory of Executive Function-Adult Version by Robert M. Roth, PhD, Peter K. Isquith, PhD and Gerard A. Gioia, PhD, Copyright 1996, 1998, 2001, 2003, 2004, 2005 by PAR. Further reproduction is prohibited without permission from PAR.

the 99th percentile (i.e., an extremely rare score). The test authors note that inconsistent profiles should be examined for the possibility that there is a logical reason for the inconsistent ratings but note that this is likely to occur in only rare circumstances.

DEMOGRAPHIC EFFECTS

AGE

There are age effects on the BRIEF-A. Younger adults (18–39) have higher scores than older adults on almost all the clinical scales (40–90 years; Roth et al., 2005). However, in clinical studies, age effects are typically minimal to nonexistent (e.g., Rabin et al., 2006).

GENDER

There are few gender effects on the BRIEF-A. On the Self-Report, women tend to report higher elevations on Emotional Control and men higher elevations on the Initiate scale. However, gender accounts for only about 2% of the variance in ratings. On the Informant Report, men have higher elevations on Organization of Materials. Again, this accounts for less than 1% of the variance in scores. Consequently, gender-specific norms for the BRIEF-A are not provided. In clinical studies, gender effects are typically minimal to non-existent (e.g., Rabin et al., 2006).

TABLE 9–5 BRIEF-A Validity Scales

VALIDITY SCALES	DESCRIPTION
Negativity	Extent to which respondent responded to selected items in a negative manner
Infrequency	Extent to which respondent responds in an atypical or infrequent manner
Inconsistency	Extent of inconsistency of respondent on selected similar items

SOURCE: Adapted from Roth et al. (2005). Reproduced by special permission of the Publisher, Psychological Assessment Resources, Inc. (PAR), 16204 North Florida Avenue, Lutz, Florida 33549, from the Behavior Rating Inventory of Executive Function-Adult Version by Robert M. Roth, PhD, Peter K. Isquith, PhD and Gerard A. Gioia, PhD, Copyright 1996, 1998, 2001, 2003, 2004, 2005 by PAR. Further reproduction is prohibited without permission from PAR.

EDUCATION AND SES

The manual indicates that there is a low, negative correlation between education and BRIEF-A Self-Report ratings, evident on Emotional Control (r = .14) and Self Monitor scales (r = –.10). On the Informant Report, education is inversely related to Inhibit, Self Monitor, Initiate, Working Memory, and Plan/Organize (r = –.07 to –.12), but the largest of these correlations accounts for only 2% of the variance in scores (Roth et al., 2005). In clinical studies, education effects are typically minimal to non-existent (e.g., Rabin et al., 2006). In clinical studies, the BRIEF-A is not usually associated with IQ (Rabin et al., 2006; Løvstad et al., 2012; Matheson, 2010).

ETHNICITY, NATIONALITY, AND LINGUISTIC EFFECTS

Ethnicity is not related to Self-Report BRIEF-A scores in the standardization sample apart from a slight difference between African-American and Hispanic respondents on the Organization of Materials scale, with the former reporting slightly higher scores. This is interpreted as a negligible difference accounting for only 1% of the variance (Roth et al., 2005). On the Informant Report, individuals self-identifying as "Other" in terms of ethnicity report higher Task Monitor scores. Again, this difference is seen as negligible, accounting for about 1% of the variance in scores (Roth et al., 2005).

There may be differences in scores for healthy individuals in other countries, as suggested by data presented by Løvstad et. al. (2016), with healthy Norwegians having BRIEF A T scores 0.5 to .75 SDs below the US normative mean.

NORMATIVE DATA

STANDARDIZATION SAMPLE

The BRIEF-A normative sample was obtained via Internet sampling methodology. Specifically, "individuals were invited to participate anonymously in the normative data collection if they met initial demographic selection criteria" (Roth et al., 2005, p. 51). Those who completed surveys "were compensated with an entry into a survey sampling company's nationwide monthly drawing for over 100 cash prizes worth $10,000." Informed consent was obtained via the Internet. The manual does not describe how individuals were selected for contact, how they were contacted, how many potential participants declined participation, how respondents selected informants for the Informant Report, and whether identities were confirmed. Exclusion criteria for the sample are listed in Table 9–6. Whether exclusion criteria were applied to informants is not reported in the manual.

TABLE 9–6 Characteristics of the BRIEF-A Normative Sample

	SELF-REPORT	INFORMANT REPORT
Sample size	1,050	1,200
Age	18 to 90	18 to 90
Geographic Location	20% Northeast 22% Midwest 35% South 23% West	19% Northeast 27% Midwest 35% South 19% West
Sample Type	Collected via Internet	Collected via Internet
Education	15% ≤11 years 31% 12 years 28% 13–15 years 26% ≥16 years	11% ≤11 years 38% 12 years 25% 13–15 years 26% ≥16 years
Gender	50% Men 50% Women	45% Men 55% Women
Race/Ethnicity	73% Caucasian 12% Hispanic 9% African American 6% Other	72% Caucasian 13% African American 9% Hispanic 7% Other
Screening	Excluded if: 1) diagnosis or history of treatment of psychiatric illness, LD, neurological disorder or serious medical illness (e.g., cancer, heart or kidney surgery), 2) history of psychotropic medication usage	Not reported

NOTE: Norms are organized according to seven age groupings and are based on US Census bureau information for 2002. Percents rounded to the nearest decimal.

SOURCE: Adapted from Roth et al. (2005). Reproduced by special permission of the Publisher, Psychological Assessment Resources, Inc. (PAR), 16204 North Florida Avenue, Lutz, Florida 33549, from the Behavior Rating Inventory of Executive Function-Adult Version by Robert M. Roth, PhD, Peter K. Isquith, PhD and Gerard A. Gioia, PhD, Copyright 1996, 1998, 2001, 2003, 2004, 2005 by PAR. Further reproduction is prohibited without permission from PAR.

NORMATIVE CELL SIZES

Overall, the age- and sex-based cell sizes are relatively uniform (see pp. 55–60 in the manual). For the Self-Report ratings, cell sizes range from 120 to 170. Informant Report cell sizes range from 68 to 227. The smallest cell sizes for the Informant Report are found for 80- to 90-year-olds, the oldest cell size in the normative sample (N = 30 men and 38 women).

EVIDENCE FOR RELIABILITY

EVIDENCE FOR INTERNAL RELIABILITY

Cronbach's alpha for the BRIEF-A GEC, BRI and MI are high to very high (r = .93 to .98, Roth et al., 2005). Reliabilities for clinical scales range from adequate to high, with most reliabilities in the .80 to .90 range; this applies in both the normative group and a mixed clinical/healthy sample described in the manual, and for both the Self-Report and Informant Report (see manual for details). The lowest reliabilities are found for Inhibit (.73 to .85) and Task Monitor (.74 to .89), but even these are adequate to high. High reliabilities have also been reported in clinical groups including traumatic brain injury (TBI) (Waid-Ebbs et al., 2012), eating disorders (Ciszewski et al., 2014; Rouel et al., 2016), and hearing-impaired students with and without Attention-Deficit/Hyperactivity Disorder (ADHD) (Hauser et al., 2013). The Informant report also shows high reliability in moderate to severe TBI (Waid-Ebbs et al., 2012).

EVIDENCE FOR TEST-RETEST RELIABILITY, MEASURING CHANGE, AND PRACTICE EFFECTS

Test-retest reliability coefficients are high to very high, with rs ranging from .82 to .94, and .91 to .96, for the Self-Report and Informant Report. These estimates are based on Ns for healthy adults of 50 (Self-Report) and 44 (Informant Report) aged between 19 and 72 years who were readministered the form after an average interval of four weeks. Test-retest correlations for the GEC, BRI, and MI are especially high (Self-Report: rs = .94, .93, .93, respectively, and r = .96 for all three Informant index scores; Roth et al., 2005).

The test authors examined the magnitude of T-score changes over time for the test-retest groups to see whether ratings increase or decrease after readministration. For the Self- and Informant Reports, T-score changes were minimal, on average (i.e., three points or less for the Self-Report, two points or less for the Informant Report). On the Self-Report, scales showing the largest changes included the Initiate, Plan/Organize, and Task Monitor scales (3.26, 2.94, and 2.94, respectively). On the Informant Report, the Self-Monitor and Task Monitor scales showed the largest change (2.18 and 1.95 points). Overall, these results indicate that the BRIEF has minimal practice effects on repeat assessments.

EVIDENCE FOR INTERRATER RELIABILITY

Interrater reliability is not provided in the manual; this would be useful for estimating the degree of agreement between different family members or caregivers for the same examinee.

EVIDENCE FOR VALIDITY

The BRIEF-A content was derived from the original BRIEF and its related scales, as well as from literature review of executive functioning across the lifespan (Roth et al., 2005). Items were rewritten for adults, and additional items were developed based on reviews of clinical interview notes from the three authors' clinical work. In particular, two broad kinds of items were included: items reflecting concrete instances of particular behavioral domains along with general descriptions of the same domains. Common behavior rating scales were also reviewed to minimize redundancy with other general scales. From an initial pool of 160 items, 75 items were retained after eliminating redundancies and after item tryouts with a mixed clinical–healthy sample, followed by item-total analyses and principal factor analyses. For further details on item content, see Roth et al. (2005).

FACTOR-ANALYTIC STUDIES

The manual describes results from principal factor analysis with oblique rotation (Promax) on the normative sample. For the Self-Report, a one-factor solution was rejected in favor of a two-factor solution based on theoretical grounds. The two-factor solution accounted for 73% of the variance, and yielded factors consistent with BRI and MI and their respective subscales. The two factors are noted to be strongly related ($r = .78$; Roth et al., 2005). The results were replicated in a mixed clinical/healthy sample, with again, highly intercorrelated factors ($r = .80$, Roth et al., 2005). Two factors were also found in younger and older adults, and in men and women. Similar results were replicated for the Informant Report (see manual for details). Of note, the high interrelation of factors in the two-factor solution may raise questions about interpreting these as separate components of executive function, although clinical studies do show different patterns for the factors (see the section "Clinical Studies").

In other studies, confirmatory factor analysis indicates three main factors in healthy young adults (Roth et al., 2013) and mild TBI (Donders & Strong, 2016), with both solutions reflecting factors of Metacognition, Behavioral Regulation, and Emotional Regulation. The three-factor solution (particularly Behavioral Regulation) has higher validation in ADHD than the original two-factor solution in the BRIEF-A manual, providing clinical support for a three-factor model. Similarly, confirmatory factor analysis of the Informant Report completed by mental health practitioners of patients with schizophrenia shows a three-factor solution, although it differs in content (Emotional Regulation, Problem-Solving, and Orderliness; Power et al., 2012). Nevertheless, cross-validation samples seem to indicate that three-factor solutions may reflect the emotional/volitional and metacognitive dimensions of executive functioning more adequately than the original factor solution.

SELF VERSUS INFORMANT RATING CONCORDANCE

Self-Report and Informant ratings are moderately to highly correlated, indicating that both measure a similar dimension of behavior. The correlation between Self-Report and Informant ratings presented in the manual for a mixed clinical/healthy sample was .63 for the GEC, with clinical scale intercorrelations ranging between .44 to .68 ($N = 180$, Roth et al., 2005). The highest agreement is found for Emotional Control ($r = .68$), and the lowest for Shift ($r = .44$). Interestingly, the magnitude of these correlations far exceeds those found for parent–teacher and parent–caregiver agreement for BRIEF scales intended for younger patients (Strauss et al., 2006). Nevertheless, as evidenced by the intercorrelations of .68 for Emotional Control, equivalent to a maximum of 46% of common variance, each rater brings unique elements to the assessment of executive function with the BRIEF-A. Thus, Self-Report and Informant ratings are not interchangeable; judicious review of each rater's viewpoint is essential in making inferences about patients' level of executive function.

Clinical studies indicate substantial correlations between Self-Report and Informant ratings in a variety of conditions, including Alzheimer's disease (AD), mild cognitive impairment (MCI), and healthy people with cognitive complaints, with the most substantial correlations occurring between the scales comprising the Metacognition Index ($rs. = .41–.57$; Rabin et al., 2006), as well as high intercorrelations for the Emotional Control scale ($r = .61$; Rabin et al., 2006). There are also strong self-informant correlations in mild TBI (Donders et al., 2015).

Importantly, high correlations do not necessarily mean equivalence of T-score levels or similar sensitivity to clinical deficits (i.e., there may be high concordance in terms of correlation, but poor agreement in terms of severity of scores). Discrepancies between Self-Report and Informant T scores, while useful in terms of shedding light on the different viewpoints of the examinee and the informant, may have particular utility in assessing for awareness of deficit as lack of insight is associated with some neurological conditions such as dementia, brain injury, and ADHD. These discrepancies may also inform on degree of caregiver burden. Consequently, low Self-Report T scores in the context of high Informant Reports may have clinical potential, but confirmation that this is a clinically useful metric is still needed.

According to the manual, Self-Informant discrepancies are relatively rare, particularly those involving low Self-Reports and high Informant ratings. For instance, in the Mixed Clinical/Healthy sample in the manual, only about 7% of individuals had lower Self-Report GEC compared to Informant Report of a magnitude exceeding a 10-point difference. Differences in the opposite direction, that is, with examinees rating themselves as having more difficulty than did their informant, appear more frequently. Fully 29% of persons in this sample rated themselves as having worse GEC than their informant (i.e., GEC 10 points higher than the GEC on the Informant Report).

The literature appears to indicate that the rate of clinically significant BRIEF-A Self-Informant discrepancies differs across clinical conditions. For example, whereas more than 55% of persons with MCI report clinically elevated problems with working memory, only 10% of informants report elevations on this score (Rabin et al., 2006), raising questions about the clinical sensitivity of informant ratings of executive dysfunction in the early stages of cognitive decline. Similarly, individuals with mild AD report elevations on the BRIEF-A, particularly on the Working Memory scale, but informants report lesser severity of symptoms (Fogarty et al., 2017). In addition, informant ratings are of limited utility in tracking changes attributable to stimulant medication in adults with ADHD (De Bruyckere et al., 2016), and no differences are found on informant ratings of patients with different kinds of frontal lesions despite differences on the self-report (Løvstad et al., 2012). Self-ratings are also higher than informant ratings after mild TBI compared to controls (Donders et al., 2015), which runs counter to the notion that brain injury is associated with insight difficulties. Some research on schizophrenia indicates lower self-report ratings than informant ratings (Kumbhani et al., 2010), possibly consistent with the low insight associated with this condition.

CORRELATIONS WITH EXECUTIVE FUNCTIONING TESTS

Most studies indicate no significant association with performance-based executive tests. This includes most of the well-known executive tests such as Wisconsin Card Sorting Test (WCST), Trail Making Test (TMT), Delis-Kaplan Executive Function System (D-KEFS), and Stroop, and involves a variety of populations, including AD, MCI, older adults with cognitive complaints, psychiatric conditions, TBI, focal frontal lobe damage, learning disability, and schizophrenia (e.g., Løvstad et al., 2016; Donders et al., 2015; Garcia-Molina et al., 2012; Meltzer et al., 2017; Rabin et al., 2006). BRIEF-A scores are especially sensitive to ADHD and are commonly elevated in the majority of adults with ADHD compared to a much lower rate of deficits on performance-based measures of executive functioning (Biederman et al., 2011). In other groups, the BRIEF-A is better than performance-based measures like the Stroop, Iowa Gambling Task, or TMT at differentiating clinical cases from controls (e.g., Hagen et al., 2016).

Some exceptions do exist. In particular, in ADHD, BRIEF-A scores are moderately correlated with scores from the Test of Variables of Attention (TOVA), a sustained attention task with both attentional and inhibition demands (Grane et al., 2014), and this is true for both Self-Report and Informant ratings. In schizophrenia, an association between BRIEF-A Initiation and Working Memory and Digit Span Backward has been reported (Bulzacka et al., 2013), but not always in the expected direction (Garlinghouse et al., 2010). Conversely, some clinical groups have deficits on performance-based executive functioning tests but show no elevations on BRIEF-A scores (Sakamoto et al., 2013; Sølsnes et al., 2014), suggesting reduced sensitivity to executive functioning deficits compared to performance-based tests. In other clinical groups, neurological disability indicators predict performance-based executive functioning tests but not BRIEF-A scores (e.g., Hanssen et al., 2014; Pham et al., 2015). Because of this, some researchers have concluded that sole reliance on the BRIEF-A for screening for executive deficits in populations at risk is insufficient (Liemburg et al., 2014). Other authors propose that rating scales such as the BRIEF-A may be particularly suited to detect deficits related to orbital frontal functions affecting the behavioral aspects of executive functioning, whereas performance-based tests are more sensitive to dorsolateral deficits affecting the cognitive aspects of executive functioning (e.g., Løvstad et al., 2012), which is an appealing explanation but may not fully account for the conflicting studies on concordance.

CORRELATIONS WITH EXECUTIVE FUNCTIONING RATING SCALES

According to data presented in the manual, BRIEF-A ratings appear moderately correlated with other rating scales tapping executive function such as the Frontal Systems Behavior Scale (FrSBe) and Dysexecutive Questionnaire (DEX) (reviewed elsewhere in this chapter), although the issue deserves further study due to small *N*s in these studies. First, in a small sample of adults with mixed diagnoses ($N = 18$), the BRIEF-A GEC demonstrated high correlation with the FrSBe Executive Dysfunction and Apathy scales ($r = .67, .57$) and moderate correlation with the Disinhibition scale ($r = .44$; Roth et al., 2005). In an even smaller group ($N = 9$), the concordance of BRIEF-A Informant Report and FrSBe Family Rating Form was assessed. Correlations were extremely high, particularly between the GEC and FrsBe Disinhibition, and GEC and FrsBe Executive Dysfunction (*rs* = .82 and .74; Roth et al., 2005); small *N* limits generalizability of these findings. With regard to the DEX, strong correlations were observed in a mixed sample ($N = 40$), with DEX total score highly related to BRIEF-A Self-Report BRI, MI and GEC (*rs* = .84, .73 and .84, respectively; Roth et al., 2005). Similar findings were reported for Informant Report concordance in 32 informants (*rs* = .82, .78, and .87 for the BRI, MI, and GEC, respectively, with DEX total score). Apart from these data, there are very few independent studies on concordance with other executive questionnaires. Of note, in one study, the BRIEF-A was predictive of self-reported scores on a time management questionnaire in young adults with dyslexia (Sharfi & Rosenblum, 2016).

CORRELATIONS WITH DEPRESSION AND ANXIETY SCALES

Several studies indicate an association between emotional functioning and BRIEF-A scores and recommend that interpretation of BRIEF-A scores take into account mood and personality. For example, in a large same of community-dwelling older adults, BRIEF-A scores were related to worry, oversensitivity, anxiety, fear of aging, lower conscientiousness, neuroticism, and depression (Meltzer et al., 2016). There are also moderate correlations with the Geriatric Depression Scale (GDS) in persons with MCI or cognitive complaints (*rs* = .36 to 37; Rabin et al., 2006) and associations between the BRIEF-A Emotional Control scale and mood and emotional distress, in particular (e.g., Løvstad et al., 2012). The manual describes correlational analyses involving the BRIEF-A and depression rating scales, with all scales yielding moderate to high correlations with the BRIEF-A, including the Beck Depression Inventory (BDI-II; *rs* = .49, .56, and .59 for the BRI, MI, and GEC) and the GDS (*r* = .49, .46, and .50 for the BRI, MI, and GEC, respectively). Associations between mood and BRIEF-A ratings are also reported in ADHD and multiple sclerosis (MS), with the recommendation that these be taken into account when interpreting ratings (Grane et al., 2014; Hanssen et al., 2014).

Executive dysfunction is frequently found in mood disorders, as discussed in the manual, so associations between mood scales and the BRIEF-A are not unexpected. For example, BRIEF-A scores improve after stimulant treatment in partially or fully remitted major depression with persisting executive dysfunction (Madhoo et al., 2014), suggesting that the BRIEF-A may be a useful tracking tool in depression. While some attribute the sizable correlations between BRIEF-A and depression scales to common elements of executive dysfunction in depression, more research is needed on the relationship between BRIEF-A ratings and depression. This could include clarifying whether the BRIEF-A should be interpreted differently in individuals with depression, or whether there are items that are specifically affected by depressive disorders (e.g., apathy, avolition).

CLINICAL STUDIES

There is extensive support for the clinical utility and sensitivity of the test to different manifestations of executive dysfunction in the context of identified clinical disorders across a wide variety of studies spanning a number of clinical conditions.

AD, MCI, and Parkinson's Disease (PD). The BRIEF-A is sensitive to executive dysfunction in AD, MCI, and in healthy people with cognitive complaints that may be precursors to MCI (Rabin et al., 2006), with potential to use as a tool to identify at-risk individuals as executive dysfunction is thought to be an early sign of cognitive decline (see also Fogarty et al., 2016). Although improvements in BRIEF-A scores occur after subthalamic deep brain stimulation in PD, these are not related to improvements in motor function, with preoperative depressed mood appearing to predict improvement in executive function (Pham et al., 2015).

MS. Moderate to severe depression predicts BRIEF-A scores in persons with MS, whereas neurological disability predicts performance-based executive functioning tests (Hanssen et al., 2014). Although stimulant medication improves measures of memory and processing speed in people with MS (i.e., California Verbal Learning Test [CVLT-II] and Symbol Digit Modalities Test [SDMT]), BRIEF-A scores are unchanged by treatment (Morrow et al., 2013).

TBI. In mild TBI, BRIEF-A scores appear to be mostly driven by pre-injury factors such as prior psychiatric treatment and lower levels of education (Donders et al., 2015; Donders & Strong, 2016). In moderate and severe brain injury, BRIEF-A Self-Report scores are elevated, and Informant scores are related to head injury severity, with the most frequent elevations on Working Memory (Matheson, 2010; Olsen et al., 2015). BRIEF-A Self-Report scores are also correlated with number of lifetime concussions and are elevated in healthy individuals with a prior history of concussion (Vynorius et al., 2016), with the Working Memory scale most sensitive to the number of prior concussions. In line with these findings, elite college and professional football players in general have elevated BRIEF-A scores, with players 40 and older having more elevations across scales than younger football players (Seichepine et al., 2013) and with number of years playing football correlated with the Working Memory scale in particular (*r* = .29 to .37). Notably, in this sample, the average number of concussions ranged from 22 in younger players to more than 500 in the older players, and so these findings do not apply to the typical concussion case seen in community settings. In TBI, BRIEF-A ratings are not related to traditional executive functioning tests but are related to functional competencies in everyday life (Garcia-Molina et al., 2012). Of note, the BRIEF-A has also been used with some success in outcome studies on heart rate variability training in TBI using biofeedback to help train emotional control (Waid-Ebbs et al., 2012). BRIEF-A Informant items can also be ranked according to difficulty and used to develop behavioral hierarchies for rehabilitation goals for patients with moderate to severe brain injury (see Waid-Ebbs et al., 2012).

Schizophrenia. The BRIEF-A is sensitive to executive deficits in schizophrenia, with some studies showing that the highest elevations are found on the Initiation scale (Bulzacka et al., 2013), although other elevations are also reported. The Informant scale has been used by mental health practitioners to rate chronic schizophrenia patients in a rehabilitation setting; used in this way, the scale shows good association with measures of overall functioning and of behavioral adjustment (Power et al., 2012), indicating that the Informant Report is a useful tool when self-ratings are unavailable, or in populations with limited cooperation or capacity to complete self-ratings.

ADHD. BRIEF-A scores are elevated in ADHD, particularly on the Working Memory scale, but with both BRI and MI showing clinical elevations and with Self-Reports showing larger differences than Informant ratings, which tend to be in the average range (Grane et al., 2014). Studies provide considerable support for the use of the BRIEF-A in the assessment and treatment of adult ADHD. For example, compared to 40% of people with ADHD with deficits on performance-based measures of executive functioning, more than 90% of adults with ADHD have two or more scale elevations on the BRIEF-A (Biederman et al., 2011).

The test has also been used to track response to ADHD medications such as stimulants; studies indicate that BRIEF-A executive deficits may not clearly modulate or predict response to methylphenidate. With atomoxetine treatment, improvements in Self-Report but not Informant Report are found, with some correlation between BRIEF-A and ADHD symptoms (De Bruyckere et al., 2016). Similar results have been reported with lisdexamfetamine in ADHD (e.g., Adler et al., 2013). In college students, the BRIEF-A Metacognition appears useful for predicting academic adjustment over and above subthreshold ADHD symptoms (Sheeban & Iarocci et al., 2015). This may relate to its association with learning disability (see later discussion). The BRIEF-A also has good predictive validity in terms of its ability to classify hearing-impaired students with and without ADHD (Hauser et al., 2012).

Learning Disability. Adults with reading disability show significantly poorer BRIEF-A scores than matched controls (Sharfi & Rosenblum, 2016), particularly on the Metacognition scales, consistent with the view that deficits in reading disability are not restricted to phonological processing (Smith-Spark et al., 2016). Although both group have clinically elevated scores on the BRIEF-A, young adults with combined ADHD and reading disability tend to have more impaired scores on Working Memory and Metacognition compared to young adults with only ADHD, consistent with the idea that effective reading depends on working memory capacity (Miranda et al., 2017; see also Sharfi & Rosenblum, 2016). BRIEF-A scores are also inversely correlated with measures of quality of life in young adults with learning disabilities (Sharfi & Rosenblum, 2016).

Other Clinical Groups. The scale has been used in a variety of clinical conditions associated with executive dysfunction, including pathological gambling (Reid et al., 2012), intoxicated aggression (where the BRI is particularly predictive; Giancola et al., 2012), distracted driving (Pope et al., 2017), nicotine and ecstasy consumption (Hadjiefthyvoulou et al., 2012), hypersexual behavior (Reid et al., 2010), and binge-eating disorder (Rouel et al., 2016).

In polysubstance use disorders, one-year sobriety is associated with improvements on the BRIEF-A compared to both those who relapse and controls (Hagen et al., 2017), showing responsiveness of the scale to real change in function. The BRIEF-A is better at predicting correlates of substance use status and social adjustment than performance-based executive tests (Hagen et al., 2016), with recommendations that it be an integral measure for screening in substance abusers.

The scale has also been used in identifying deficits associated with breast cancer chemotherapy (see "Neuroanatomical Correlates") and shows responsivity to treatment, with scores improving after an online cognitive training program for breast cancer survivors aimed at improving executive function (Kesler et al., 2013).

Patients with chronic pain also demonstrate elevated BRIEF-A scores, particularly in terms of Working Memory and Emotional Control, with BRIEF-A scores predicted in part by medication, negative emotional state, and pain interference (Baker et al., 2016). BRIEF-A scores also improve in patients with chronic fatigue after treatment with stimulant medication (Young et al., 2013). In fibromyalgia, BRIEF-A scores are elevated but are largely accounted for by depression and anxiety except for elevations on the Working Memory scale (Gelonch et al., 2016). On the other hand, the scale has not demonstrated sensitivity to improved cognitive flexibility after aortic valve replacement surgery despite improvements on other measures of executive functioning (Liimatainen et al., 2016).

NEUROANATOMICAL CORRELATES AND IMAGING STUDIES

There are a small number of studies on neuroanatomical correlates, with more studies expected to emerge in the coming years given how many studies use the BRIEF-A as an outcome measure. For example, Working Memory deficits on the BRIEF-A are associated with smaller right and left frontal lobe gray matter volumes in schizophrenia (Garlinghouse et al., 2010). Similarly, adult survivors of acute lymphoblastic leukemia demonstrate smaller surface area in the prefrontal regions, including the superior frontal gyri and left anterior cingulate, and this is associated with elevations on BRIEF-A Emotional Control and Self-Monitoring (Tamnes et al., 2015). One study with a relatively small sample of patients with lateral prefrontal and orbital prefrontal injuries suggested that orbital prefrontal injuries in particular are related to BRIEF-A scores, whereas lateral prefrontal lesions are related to performance-based neuropsychological tests of executive function (Løvstad et al., 2012). Notably, Informant reports showed no group differences, and BRIEF-A scores correlated highly with emotional distress.

Increased brain activation in individuals with TBI is inversely related to BRIEF-A scores (Olsen et al., 2015) and is thought to possibly reflect successful compensatory mechanisms. Reduced lateral prefrontal cortex activation has been associated with elevations in BRIEF-A scores in chemotherapy-treated women with breast cancer (Kesler et al., 2011). Similarly, decreased frontal gray matter density after breast cancer chemotherapy is associated with reductions in BRIEF-A scores over time compared to baseline levels, with most changes detected on the Initiation scale (McDonald et al., 2013).

PERFORMANCE VALIDITY

Very little information is available on this topic to our knowledge. In one study, 5% of self-ratings and 5% of informant ratings in a mixed group of primarily mild TBI patients involved in workers' compensation or litigation had invalid scores on one or more of the BRIEF-A validity scales (Matheson, 2010). This is quite low for this kind of sample and raises questions about the BRIEF-A validity scale sensitivities to symptom exaggeration and overreporting.

Of note, the BRIEF-A Infrequency scale may be useful in identifying invalid profiles, but its value in detecting malingered neurocognitive dysfunction in particular (i.e., feigned or exaggerated impairment) is questionable because of the item content; a high Infrequency rating reflects both endorsement of extreme/implausible symptoms suggestive of cognitive impairment (e.g., items similar to "I forget who I am"), but also an attempt to show oneself in an implausibly positive light through the denial of common complaints (e.g., items similar to "I am never fatigued"). Anecdotal experience with the BRIEF-A from our own practice suggests that this scale is less sensitive than performance validity tests and symptom validity tests designed expressly for detecting exaggeration and feigning, but research studies are needed to support or disconfirm this impression.

COMMENT

Although the field is rapidly expanding, there exist few psychometrically robust and validated scales for assessing executive dysfunction in everyday life in adults. The BRIEF-A stands alone in having impressive psychometrics (internal and test-retest reliabilities), a large normative dataset, a comprehensive and well-written manual, and a large amount of validity data, with a virtual explosion of studies since its publication date in 2005. It has been featured in numerous studies on clinical groups, including AD, MCI, TBI, MS, schizophrenia, ADHD, learning disability, substance abuse, cancer, and multiple conditions involving executive dysfunction and impulse control disorders.

Some limitations of the BRIEF-A deserve mention, although some of these are relatively minor. First, BRIEF-A scores tend to be elevated in anxiety and depression, and this needs to be taken into account in interpretation. Second, although the normative data are substantial, norms were gathered via Internet, and the scales were completed electronically, also via Internet, a methodology that is subject to bias in that it may limit participation of economically or culturally disadvantaged groups and where veracity of participant identity is difficult to establish conclusively. On the other hand, electronic norms and administration are ideally suited for some applications and will become increasingly relevant as online data capture overtakes paper-and-pencil administration for questionnaires as the field moves forward. Third, Self–Informant discrepancies hold promise in measuring self-awareness and insight, but more research is needed on the sensitivity of the Informant scale in different conditions including caregiver burden. Studies show that individuals with conditions associated with reduced insight do not necessarily show the expected Self–Informant discrepancies reflective of reduced self-reporting of executive deficits (e.g., AD, MCI, brain injury). Fourth, research on exaggeration, feigning, and malingering is required, especially given its use in adult ADHD, a population with an elevated rate of malingering related to accessing controlled substances, accommodations for standardized testing, and workplace accommodations. More research on the validity scales is needed as there is virtually no information on their associations with other validity indictors such as performance validity or symptom validity tests. Last, the BRIEF-A's 75-item format is somewhat long for most clinical settings, and a short form would be useful.

Importantly, the authors emphasize that the BRIEF-A is not intended as a tool for independently diagnosing specific disorders and note that many adults with identified conditions have normal-range scores on the BRIEF-A. More information on sensitivity, specificity, and other classification accuracy statistics across conditions are needed, but existing studies demonstrate the scale's responsiveness to change associated with treatment or to progression of neurological conditions with prominence of executive dysfunction, such as dementia. The BRIEF-A may also have potential in identifying individuals at risk of transitioning to MCI and should be considered for inclusion in evaluations of people with memory complaints.

Overall, the BRIEF-A appears to be very useful component of the neuropsychological assessment of adults that serves to confirm clinical inferences derived from executive functioning tests, provide an ecologically valid index of executive dysfunction, and yield a multidimensional, cost-effective, and user-friendly measure of executive functioning suitable for most clinical settings.

REFERENCES

Adler, L. A., Dirks, B., Deas, P., Raychaudhuri, A., Dauphin, M., Saylor, K., & Weisler, R. (2013). Self-Reported quality of life in adults with attention-deficit/hyperactivity disorder and executive function impairment treated with lisdexamfetamine dimesylate: A randomized, double-blind, multicenter, placebo-controlled, parallel-group study. *BMC Psychiatry, 13*, 253. https://doi.org/10.1186/1471-244X-13-253

Baker, K. S., Gibson, S., Georgiou-Karistianis, N., Roth, R. M., & Giummarra, M. J. (2016). Everyday executive functioning in chronic pain: specific deficits in working memory and emotion control, predicted by mood, medications, and pain interference. *Clinical Journal of Pain, 32*(8), 673–680. https://doi.org/10.1097/AJP.0000000000000313

Biederman, J., Mick, E., Fried, R., Wilner, N., Spencer, T. J., & Faraone, S. V. (2011). Are stimulants effective in the treatment of executive function deficits? Results from a randomized double blind study of OROS-methylphenidate in adults with ADHD. *European Neuropsychopharmacology, 21*(7), 508–515. https://doi.org/10.1016/j.euroneuro.2010.11.005

Bulzacka, E., Vilain, J., Schürhoff, F., Méary, A., Leboyer, M., & Szöke, A. (2013). A self-administered executive functions ecological questionnaire (the Behavior Rating Inventory of Executive Function—Adult Version) shows impaired scores in a sample of patients with schizophrenia. *Mental Illness, 5*(1), e4. https://doi.org/10.4081/mi.2013.e4

Ciszewski, S., Francis, K., Mendella, P., Bissada, H., & Tasca, G. A. (2014). Validity and reliability of the Behavior Rating Inventory of Executive Function—Adult Version in a clinical sample with eating disorders. *Eating Behaviors, 15*(2), 175–181. https://doi.org/10.1016/j.eatbeh.2014.01.004

De Bruyckere, K., Bushe, C., Bartel, C., Berggren, L., Kan, C. C., & Dittmann, R. W. (2016). Relationships between functional outcomes and symptomatic improvement in atomoxetine-treated adult patients with Attention-Deficit/Hyperactivity Disorder: Post hoc analysis of an integrated database. *CNS Drugs, 30*(6), 541–558. https://doi.org/10.1007/s40263-016-0346-3

Donders, J., Oh, Y. I., & Gable, J. (2015). Self- and informant ratings of executive functioning after mild traumatic brain injury. *Journal of Head Trauma Rehabilitation, 30*(6), E30-39. https://doi.org/10.1097/HTR.0000000000000120

Donders, J., & Strong, C.-A. H. (2016). Latent structure of the Behavior Rating Inventory of Executive Function-Adult Version (BRIEF-A) after mild traumatic brain injury. *Archives of Clinical Neuropsychology, 31*(1), 29–36. https://doi.org/10.1093/arclin/acv048

Fogarty, J., Almklov, E., Borrie, M., Wells, J., & Roth, R. M. (2017). Subjective rating of executive functions in mild Alzheimer's disease. *Aging & Mental Health, 21*(11), 1184–1191. https://doi.org/10.1080/13607863.2016.1207750

García-Molina, A., Tormos, J. M., Bernabeu, M., Junqué, C., & Roig-Rovira, T. (2012). Do traditional executive measures tell us anything about daily life functioning after traumatic brain injury in Spanish-speaking individuals? *Brain Injury, 26*(6), 864–874. https://doi.org/10.3109/02699052.2012.655362

Garlinghouse, M. A., Roth, R. M., Isquith, P. K., Flashman, L. A., & Saykin, A. J. (2010). Subjective rating of working memory is associated with frontal lobe volume in schizophrenia. *Schizophrenia Research, 120*(1–3), 71–75. https://doi.org/10.1016/j.schres.2010.02.1067

Gelonch, O., Garolera, M., Valls, J., Rosselló, L., & Pifarré, J. (2016). Executive function in fibromyalgia: Comparing subjective and objective measures. *Comprehensive Psychiatry, 66*, 113–122. https://doi.org/10.1016/j.comppsych.2016.01.002

Giancola, P. R., Godlaski, A. J., & Roth, R. M. (2012). Identifying component-processes of executive functioning that serve as risk factors for the alcohol-aggression relation. *Psychology of Addictive Behaviors, 26*(2), 201–211. https://doi.org/10.1037/a0025207

Gioia, G. A., Isquith, P. K., Guy, S. C., & Kenworthy, L. (2000). *Behavior Rating Inventory of Executive Function*. Odessa, FL: Psychological Assessment Resources, Inc.

Grane, V. A., Endestad, T., Pinto, A. F., & Solbakk, A.-K. (2014). Attentional control and subjective executive function in treatment-naive adults with attention deficit hyperactivity disorder. *PloS One, 9*(12), e115227. https://doi.org/10.1371/journal.pone.0115227

Hadjiefthyvoulou, F., Fisk, J. E., Montgomery, C., & Bridges, N. (2012). Self-reports of executive dysfunction in current ecstasy/polydrug Users. *Cognitive and Behavioral Neurology, 25*(3), 128–138. https://doi.org/10.1097/WNN.0b013e318261459c

Hagen, E., Erga, A. H., Hagen, K. P., Nesvåg, S. M., McKay, J. R., Lundervold, A. J., & Walderhaug, E. (2016). Assessment of executive function in patients with substance use disorder: A comparison of inventory- and performance-based assessment. *Journal of Substance Abuse Treatment, 66*, 1–8. https://doi.org/10.1016/j.jsat.2016.02.010

Hagen, E., Erga, A. H., Hagen, K. P., Nesvåg, S. M., McKay, J. R., Lundervold, A. J., & Walderhaug, E. (2017). One-year sobriety improves satisfaction with life, executive functions and psychological distress among patients with polysubstance use disorder. *Journal of Substance Abuse Treatment, 76*, 81–87. https://doi.org/10.1016/j.jsat.2017.01.016

Hanssen, K. T., Beiske, A. G., Landrø, N. I., & Hessen, E. (2014). Predictors of executive complaints and executive deficits in multiple sclerosis. *Acta Neurologica Scandinavica, 129*(4), 234–242. https://doi.org/10.1111/ane.12177

Hauser, P. C., Lukomski, J., & Samar, V. (2013). Reliability and validity of the BRIEF-A for assessing deaf college students' executive function. *Journal of Psychoeducational Assessment, 31*(4), 363–374. https://doi.org/10.1177/0734282912464466

Kesler, S., Hadi Hosseini, S. M., Heckler, C., Janelsins, M., Palesh, O., Mustian, K., & Morrow, G. (2013). Cognitive training for improving executive function in chemotherapy-treated breast cancer survivors. *Clinical Breast Cancer, 13*(4), 299–306. https://doi.org/10.1016/j.clbc.2013.02.004

Kesler, S. R., Kent, J. S., & O'Hara, R. (2011). Prefrontal cortex and executive function impairments in primary breast cancer. *Archives of Neurology, 68*(11), 1447–1453. https://doi.org/10.1001/archneurol.2011.245

Kumbhani, S. R., Roth, R. M., Kruck, C. L., Flashman, L. A., & McAllister, T. W. (2010). Nonclinical obsessive-compulsive symptoms and executive functions in schizophrenia. *Journal of Neuropsychiatry and Clinical Neurosciences, 22*(3), 304–312. https://doi.org/10.1176/jnp.2010.22.3.304

Liimatainen, J., Peräkylä, J., Järvelä, K., Sisto, T., Yli-Hankala, A., & Hartikainen, K. M. (2016). Improved cognitive flexibility after aortic valve replacement surgery. *Interactive Cardiovascular and Thoracic Surgery, 23*(4), 630–636. https://doi.org/10.1093/icvts/ivw170

Løvstad, M., Funderud, I., Endestad, T., Due-Tønnessen, P., Meling, T. R., Lindgren, M., . . . Solbakk, A. K. (2012). Executive functions after orbital or lateral prefrontal lesions: neuropsychological profiles and self-reported executive functions in everyday living. *Brain Injury, 26*(13–14), 1586–1598. https://doi.org/10.3109/02699052.2012.698787

Løvstad, M., Sigurdardottir, S., Andersson, S., Grane, V. A., Moberget, T., Stubberud, J., & Solbakk, A. K. (2016). Behavior Rating Inventory of Executive Function-Adult Version in patients with neurological and neuropsychiatric conditions: Symptom levels and relationship to emotional distress. *Journal of the International Neuropsychological Society, 22*(6), 682–694. https://doi.org/10.1017/S135561771600031X

Matheson, L. (2010). Executive dysfunction, severity of traumatic brain injury, and IQ in workers with disabilities. *Work (Reading, Mass.), 36*(4), 413–422. https://doi.org/10.3233/WOR-2010-1043

McDonald, B. C., Conroy, S. K., Smith, D. J., West, J. D., & Saykin, A. J. (2013). Frontal gray matter reduction after breast cancer chemotherapy and association with executive symptoms: A replication and extension study. *Brain, Behavior, and Immunity, 30 Suppl*, S117–125. https://doi.org/10.1016/j.bbi.2012.05.007

Miranda, A., Mercader, J., Fernández, M. I., & Colomer, C. (2017). Reading performance of young adults with ADHD diagnosed in childhood. *Journal of Attention Disorders, 21*(4), 294–304. https://doi.org/10.1177/1087054713507977

Morrow, S. A., Smerbeck, A., Patrick, K., Cookfair, D., Weinstock-Guttman, B., & Benedict, R. H. B. (2013). Lisdexamfetamine dimesylate improves processing speed and memory in cognitively impaired MS patients: A phase II study. *Journal of Neurology, 260*(2), 489–497. https://doi.org/10.1007/s00415-012-6663-7

Olsen, A., Brunner, J. F., Indredavik Evensen, K. A., Finnanger, T. G., Vik, A., Skandsen, T., . . . Håberg, A. K. (2015). Altered cognitive control activations after moderate-to-severe traumatic brain injury and their relationship to injury severity and everyday-life function. *Cerebral Cortex (New York, N. Y.: 1991), 25*(8), 2170–2180. https://doi.org/10.1093/cercor/bhu023

Pham, U. H. G., Andersson, S., Toft, M., Pripp, A. H., Konglund, A. E., Dietrichs, E., . . . Solbakk, A.-K. (2015). Self-reported executive functioning in everyday life in Parkinson's disease after three months of subthalamic deep brain stimulation. *Parkinson's Disease, 2015*, 461453. https://doi.org/10.1155/2015/461453

Pope, C. N., Bell, T. R., & Stavrinos, D. (2017). Mechanisms behind distracted driving behavior: The role of age and executive function in the engagement of distracted driving. *Accident; Analysis and Prevention, 98*, 123–129. https://doi.org/10.1016/j.aap.2016.09.030

Power, B. D., Dragović, M., & Rock, D. (2012). Brief screening for executive dysfunction in schizophrenia in a rehabilitation hospital. *Journal of Neuropsychiatry and Clinical Neurosciences, 24*(2), 215–222. https://doi.org/10.1176/appi.neuropsych.11060145

Rabin, L. A., Roth, R. M., Isquith, P. K., Wishart, H. A., Nutter-Upham, K. E., Pare, N., . . . Saykin, A. J. (2006). Self- and informant reports of executive function on the BRIEF-A in MCI and older adults with cognitive complaints. *Archives of Clinical Neuropsychology, 21*(7), 721–732. https://doi.org/10.1016/j.acn.2006.08.004

Reid, R. C., Karim, R., McCrory, E., & Carpenter, B. N. (2010). Self-reported differences on measures of executive function and hypersexual behavior in a patient and community sample of men. *International Journal of Neuroscience, 120*(2), 120–127. https://doi.org/10.3109/00207450903165577

Reid, R. C., McKittrick, H. L., Davtian, M., & Fong, T. W. (2012). Self-reported differences on measures of executive function in a patient sample of pathological gamblers. *International Journal of Neuroscience, 122*(9), 500–505. https://doi.org/10.3109/00207454.2012.673516

Roth, R. M., Isquith, P. K., & Gioia, G. A. (2005). *Behavioural Rating Inventory of Executive Function—Adult Version.* Lutz, FL: Psychological Assessment Resources, Inc.

Roth, R. M., Lance, C. E., Isquith, P. K., Fischer, A. S., & Giancola, P. R. (2013). Confirmatory factor analysis of the Behavior Rating Inventory of Executive Function-Adult Version in healthy adults and application to attention-deficit/hyperactivity disorder. *Archives of Clinical Neuropsychology, 28*(5), 425–434. https://doi.org/10.1093/arclin/act031

Rouel, M., Raman, J., Hay, P., & Smith, E. (2016). Validation of the Behaviour Rating Inventory of Executive Function—Adult Version (BRIEF-A) in the obese with and without binge eating disorder. *Eating Behaviors, 23*, 58–65. https://doi.org/10.1016/j.eatbeh.2016.07.010

Sakamoto, M., Woods, S. P., Kolessar, M., Kriz, D., Anderson, J. R., Olavarria, H., . . . Huckans, M. (2013). Protective effects of higher cognitive reserve for neuropsychological and daily functioning among individuals infected with hepatitis C. *Journal of Neurovirology, 19*(5), 442–451. https://doi.org/10.1007/s13365-013-0196-4

Seichepine, D. R., Stamm, J. M., Daneshvar, D. H., Riley, D. O., Baugh, C. M., Gavett, B. E., . . . Stern, R. A. (2013). Profile of self-reported problems with executive functioning in college and professional football players. *Journal of Neurotrauma, 30*(14), 1299–1304. https://doi.org/10.1089/neu.2012.2690

Sharfi, K., & Rosenblum, S. (2016). Executive functions, time organization and quality of life among adults with learning disabilities. *PloS One, 11*(12), e0166939. https://doi.org/10.1371/journal.pone.0166939

Sheehan, W. A., & Iarocci, G. (2015). Executive functioning predicts academic but not social adjustment to university. *Journal of Attention Disorders*. https://doi.org/10.1177/1087054715612258

Smith-Spark, J. H., Henry, L. A., Messer, D. J., Edvardsdottir, E., & Zięcik, A. P. (2016). Executive functions in adults with developmental dyslexia. *Research in Developmental Disabilities, 53–54*, 323–341. https://doi.org/10.1016/j.ridd.2016.03.001

Sølsnes, A. E., Skranes, J., Brubakk, A.-M., & Løhaugen, G. C. C. (2014). Executive functions in very-low-birth-weight young adults: A comparison between self-report and neuropsychological test results. *Journal of the International Neuropsychological Society, 20*(5), 506–515. https://doi.org/10.1017/S1355617714000332

Strauss, E., Sherman, E. M. S., & Spreen, O. (2006). *A compendium of neuropsychological tests: Administration, norms, and commentary* (3rd ed.). Oxford University Press.

Tamnes, C. K., Zeller, B., Amlien, I. K., Kanellopoulos, A., Andersson, S., Due-Tønnessen, P., . . . Fjell, A. M. (2015). Cortical surface area and thickness in adult survivors of pediatric acute lymphoblastic leukemia. *Pediatric Blood & Cancer, 62*(6), 1027–1034. https://doi.org/10.1002/pbc.25386

Vynorius, K. C., Paquin, A. M., & Seichepine, D. R. (2016). Lifetime multiple mild traumatic brain injuries are associated with cognitive and mood symptoms in young healthy college students. *Frontiers in Neurology, 7*, 188. https://doi.org/10.3389/fneur.2016.00188

Waid-Ebbs, J. K., Wen, P.-S., Heaton, S. C., Donovan, N. J., & Velozo, C. (2012). The item level psychometrics of the Behavior Rating Inventory of Executive Function—Adult (BRIEF-A) in a TBI sample. *Brain Injury, 26*(13–14), 1646–1657. https://doi.org/10.3109/02699052.2012.700087

Young, J. L. (2013). Use of lisdexamfetamine dimesylate in treatment of executive functioning deficits and chronic fatigue syndrome: a double blind, placebo-controlled study. *Psychiatry Research, 207* (1–2), 127–133. https://doi.org/10.1016/j.psychres.2012.09.007

BEHAVIOURAL ASSESSMENT OF THE DYSEXECUTIVE SYNDROME (BADS)

TEST NAME	**Behavioural Assessment of the Dysexecutive Syndrome (BADS)**
DOMAIN	Executive functioning
AGE RANGE	16 to 87
ADMINISTRATION TIME	40 minutes
SCORING FORMAT	Hand scored
REFERENCE	Wilson, B. A., Alderman, N., Burgess, P. W., Emslie, H., & Evans, J. J. (1996). *Behavioural Assessment of the Dysexecutive Syndrome*. Bury St. Edmunds, UK: Thames Valley Test Company. www.pearsonclinical.com

DESCRIPTION

The purpose of this battery is to predict everyday problems arising from executive dysfunction. The authors (Wilson et al., 1996) note that most neuropsychological tests consist of an explicit task to solve, a short trial, examiner-prompted task initiation, and task success that is clearly defined. Rarely are examinees required to organize or plan their behavior over longer time periods or set priorities when faced with two or more competing tasks despite the fact that these types of executive abilities are a major component of everyday activities.

The Behavioural Assessment of the Dysexecutive Syndrome (BADS) is comprised of a collection of six tests that are thought to be similar to everyday activities that could pose challenging for patients with difficulties with executive function. Table 9–7 lists specific task requirements and scoring variables. The demands involved in the BADS subtests are as follows:

1. The *Rule Shift Cards Test* uses non-picture playing cards and examines the individual's ability to respond correctly to a rule and to shift from one rule to another. It measures rule-shifting ability and working memory.
2. The *Action Program Test* was adapted from a task originally described by Klosowaska (1976) and requires the examinee to solve a novel problem by developing a five-step plan of action.
3. In the *Key Search Test*, examinees are presented with the task of finding something that has been lost. The efficiency of the search strategy is evaluated.
4. The *Temporal Judgment Test* comprises four short questions concerning commonplace events. The task evaluates the examinee's ability to make reasonable guesses or estimates.
5. The *Zoo Map Test* requires examinees to show how they would visit a series of designated locations on a map of a zoo, following certain rules. Planning ability is evaluated.
6. The *Modified Six Elements Test* is modeled after a task (Shallice & Burgess, 1991) that requires examinees to organize their activities to carry out six tasks in a limited time period and without breaking certain rules.

The BADS also includes a questionnaire (the DEX) that can be administered to both the patient and a rater. This questionnaire is not normed and intended to supplement the BADS via qualitative information (Malloy & Grace, 2005). The DEX is not technically part of the BADS in the sense that it is not formally used in the calculation of the Profile score for the battery and is reviewed separately in this volume.

SCORING

Scoring guidelines are found in the manual. See also Table 9–7. The method of scoring was devised so that a score, ranging from 0 to 4, is calculated for each test, with an overall Profile score that ranges from 0 to 24. Standardized scores are not calculated for each subtest. Although it is recommended that all six tests of the BADS be administered to obtain the Profile score, it is possible to prorate on the basis of five tests. The Profile score can be converted into a standardized score with a mean (*M*) of 100 and an *SD* of 15. The score is further classified categorically as impaired, borderline, low average, average, high average, or superior. The Profile score is referenced to three age groups (40 or younger, 41–65, 65–87).

ADMINISTRATION

Detailed administration instructions are provided in the manual.

TABLE 9–7 Description of Behavioural Assessment of the Dysexecutive Syndrome (BADS) Tasks

TASK	DESCRIPTION	SCORING
Rule Shift Cards	Uses 21 spiral-bound non-picture playing cards. In the first part of the test, the examinee is asked to say "Yes" to a red card and "No" to a black card. This rule, typed on a card, is left in full view to reduce memory constraints. In the second part, the examinee must "forget" the first rule and concentrate on applying a new rule. The examinee is asked to respond "Yes" if the card that has just been turned over is the same color as the previously turned card and "No" if it is a different color. This new, typed rule is left in full view.	The measures are time taken and number of errors on the second trial.
Action Program	Requires five steps to its solution. The examinee is presented with a rectangular stand; in one end is set a large transparent beaker with a removable lid that has a small central hole in it. The beaker is two-thirds full of water. A thin transparent tube is set at the other end, at the bottom of which is a small piece of cork. To the left of the stand is placed an L-shaped metal rod, which is not long enough to reach the cork, and a small screw-top container, with its lid unscrewed and lying beside it. Examinees are asked to get the cork out of the tube using any of the objects in front of them without lifting up the stand, the tube, or the beaker, and without touching the beaker lid with their fingers. There is no time limit.	A score is obtained according to the number of stages completed.
Key Search	Examinees are presented with a piece of paper with a square in the middle and a small black dot below. They are told to imagine that the square is a large field and that they have lost their keys. They are asked to draw a line, starting at the black dot, to show where they would walk to search the field to make absolutely certain that they would find their keys.	The time required and efficiency of the search plan are evaluated.
Temporal Judgment	The task comprises four short questions concerning commonplace events that take a few seconds (e.g., how long does it take to blow up a party balloon?) to several years (how long do most dogs live?).	Each of the four questions is scored 0 or 1.
Zoo Map	Examinees show how they would visit a series of designated locations on a map of a zoo, following certain rules. The first trial consists of a high-demand version of the task in which the planning abilities of the examinee are rigorously tested. In the second, low-demand trial, the examinee is simply required to follow the instructions to produce an error-free performance.	The score reflects the sequence produced, the number of errors made, and the time to task completion.
Modified Six Elements	The examinee is given instructions to do three tasks (dictating or describing an event, arithmetic, and picture naming), each of which is divided into two parts, A and B. The examinee is required to attempt at least something from each of the six subtasks within a 10-minute period. In addition, the examinee is told that there is one rule that must not be broken: do not do two parts of the same task consecutively.	The score is based on the number of tasks completed, the number of tasks where rule breaks were made, and the time spent on any one task.

SOURCE: Adapted from Wilson et al. (1996).

DEMOGRAPHIC EFFECTS

AGE

Age affects task performance, with poorer overall scores for people 65 years and older (Wilson et al., 1996). Older participants score marginally worse than younger adults on the Temporal Judgment task (Gillespie et al., 2002). Age, along with positive symptoms, predicts the Profile score (younger perform better) in a sample of individuals with bipolar disorder (Amann et al., 2012).

GENDER

Limited information is available on gender effects. Males reportedly outperform females on Key Search, and women outperform men on Six Elements (Proctor & Zhang, 2008). There are no sex differences on the Temporal Judgment task (Gillespie et al., 2002).

EDUCATION

No information is available regarding the effect of education on performance.

ETHNICITY, NATIONALITY, AND LINGUISTIC EFFECTS

Proctor and Zhang (2008) reported that European Americans outperformed other ethnic groups on the Zoo Map test in a sample of college students. When classification categories were compared, more African-American students were classified as "borderline" or "impaired" on the BADS (15%) compared with Latino Americans (9%) and European Americans (2%). Of note, the test has been translated into Spanish (Vargas et al., 2009).

NORMATIVE DATA

Description of the standardization sample is sparse (Table 9–8). Wilson et al. (1996) normed the test on a group of 216 healthy individuals (age, $M = 46.6$, $SD = 19.8$) in each of three ability bands (below average, average, above average according to the National Adult Reading Test [NART]; mean NART Full-Scale IQ [FSIQ] = 102.7; $SD = 16.2$; range 69–129) and balanced to have approximately equal numbers of men and women in each of the bands from

TABLE 9–8 Characteristics of the Behavioural Assessment of the Dysexecutive Syndrome (BADS) Normative Sample

Sample size	216
Age	16 to 87 years
Geographic location	England
Sample type	Volunteers selected to comprise approximately equal numbers in each of three NART IQ-based ability bands: below average (≤89), average (90–109), and above average (110+), Mean NART FSIQ = 102.7 (*SD* = 16.2, range 69–129)
Education	Not reported
Gender	Balanced to have approximately equal numbers of men and women in each of the IQ bands from each of four age groups: 16 to 31, 32 to 47, 48 to 63, and 64+
Race/ethnicity	Not reported
Screening	Reported to be neurologically healthy but the screening method was not provided

NOTE: FSIQ, Full-Scale IQ; NART, National Adult Reading Test.

SOURCE: Adapted from Wilson et al. (1996).

each of four age groups (16–31, 32–47, 48–63, and 64+; age, *M* = 58.93, *SD* = 15.35; education, *M* = 13.83 years, *SD* = 2.70). Although the Profile score is evaluated with reference to age, no age-based norms are provided for the individual subtests.

Examination of Table 9–9 suggests that performance was at ceiling for some tasks (especially Action Program, Six Elements, and Rule Shift). Gillespie et al. (2002) examined a group of 101 community-dwelling older adults who were negative for neurological disorders by self-report (age, *M* = 71.2 years; range 56 to 89 years) on the Temporal Judgment task. The median score was two, a value similar to that reported by Wilson et al. (1996). Younger (*M* = 38.20, *SD* = 3.44; range 31 to 46) and older (*M* = 59.60, *SD* = 4.27; range 53 to 64) healthy adults on a variant of the Six Elements task showed no midlife declines in task performance (Garden et al., 2001).

TABLE 9–9 Behavioural Assessment of the Dysexecutive Syndrome (BADS) Subtest Means and Standard Deviations for Healthy Controls (*n* = 216)

	MEAN (*SD*)
Profile score	18.05 (3.05)
Action Program	3.77 (0.52)
Key Search	2.60 (1.32)
Modified Six Elements	3.52 (0.80)
Rule Shift Cards	3.56 (0.87)
Zoo Map	2.44 (1.13)
Temporal Judgment	2.15 (0.91)

SOURCE: Adapted from Wilson et al. (1998).

EVIDENCE FOR RELIABILITY

EVIDENCE FOR INTERNAL RELIABILITY

Internal reliability is relatively low for the Profile score (Cronbach alpha .60 to .73; Bennett et al., 2005; Gillespie et al., 2002; Vargas et al., 2009).

EVIDENCE FOR TEST-RETEST RELIABILITY, MEASURING CHANGE, AND PRACTICE EFFECTS

Wilson et al. (1996) report that 29 healthy people were retested on the battery along with three other executive tasks (Modified Card Sorting Test, Cognitive Estimation, and FAS Letter Fluency) after an interval of 6–12 months. Test-retest correlations for the BADS tests ranged from –.08 (Rule Shift Cards) to .71 (Key Search), with most below acceptable levels. Test-retest reliability for the Profile score was not reported. Ceiling effects in conjunction with small sample sizes likely adversely affected the correlation coefficients. Percentage agreement of the same scores also tended to be low. On only two tasks (Action Program and Rule Shift Cards) did more than 70% the sample obtain the same score at both testing points. Similar results were obtained with shorter retest intervals in a sample of 22 psychiatric patients (Jelicic et al., 2001). On repeat administration, patients obtained higher scores (about one point) on one test (Action Program) and on the Profile score (about two points).

EVIDENCE FOR INTERRATER RELIABILITY

Wilson et al. (1996) report that high interrater reliability (≥.88) was obtained when 25 healthy individuals were tested with a second tester present.

EVIDENCE FOR VALIDITY

FACTOR-ANALYTIC STUDIES AND RELATIONSHIPS WITH OTHER TESTS

In a study of the BADS in people with schizophrenia, Vargas et al. (2009) reported that a principal components analysis yielded a sole factor accounting for approximately 43% of the variance in performance. In terms of factor structure when other tests are also considered, factor-analytic studies have generally suggested that BADS subtests load with other executive tests. Bennett et al. (2005) reported that four factors were extracted from the BADS and other executive tests in a brain injury sample. On the first factor, Zoo Map loaded with Porteus Mazes and the TMT; the second factor consisted of the Modified Six Elements and the WCST; the third factor was comprised of Action Program, TMT, and the Cognitive Estimation Test (CET); and the fourth factor included Rule Shift, Key Search, and the Tinker Toy test. Wood and Liossi (2006) performed a principal components analysis with the Hayling and Brixton, BADS

Zoo Map and Key Search, TMT-B and the Controlled Oral Word Association (COWA), in a study of severe brain injury, finding that Zoo Map and Key Search loaded on a second factor with other executive function tests.

Executive Function and Attention Tests. The BADS generally shows small to moderate correlations with other measures of executive function in a variety of populations. Norris and Tate (2000) examined healthy individuals and a mixed group of neurological patients and found moderate correlations between the BADS and other measures of executive function (e.g., WCST, TMT-B, Porteus Mazes, Rey-Osterreith Complex Figure Copy strategy, CET, and COWA). In particular, the Profile score and the Action and Rule Shift subtests showed small to moderate correlations (*rs* = .20 to .54) with each executive task. Although the Zoo Map and Key Search tasks showed a statistically significant relationship with another measure of planning (i.e., Porteus Mazes, *rs* = .41, .28, respectively), the Temporal Judgment task had low and nonsignificant correlations with the executive tasks. In a mixed clinical sample, planning, rather than measures of other aspects of cognition (e.g., memory, inhibition) was the strongest predictor of the total score on the Zoo Map test, with overall time to complete the task related to processing speed (Oosterman et al., 2013). Thus, there appears to be converging support for the Zoo Map test as a measure of planning ability.

Vargas et al. (2009) reported that, after controlling for IQ, correlations between the BADS and other executive tests were small to moderate, as follows: Wechsler Working Memory Index (WMI; r = .18), Stroop (r = .31), TMT (r = –.42), and WCST (r = –.38, .50, depending on variable). In a sample of patients with schizophrenia, moderate correlations were found between the BADS Profile score and the Test of Everyday Attention (TEA) sustained and divided attention tests (Elevator Counting r = .44, TEA Telephone Search While Counting r = .33; Tyson et al., 2008).

In a sample of people who sustained a severe brain injury, after controlling for IQ, correlations between Zoo Map and other executive functioning tests such as the Hayling and TMT-B were significant (*rs* = .18 to .27; Wood & Liossi, 2007). Key Search was also similarly correlated with the Hayling, Brixton, and TMT-B (*rs* = .23 to .47). The BADS was not correlated with the TMT, but was correlated with other executive function tests, such as the WCST and the Tower of London (TOL; *rs* = .43 to .51; Perfetti et al., 2010). In a college sample, Rule Shift correlated with WCST variables (*rs* = –.21 to –.27; Proctor & Zhang, 2008).

IQ Tests. The BADS is significantly correlated with IQ, generally in the moderate to large range. Vargas et al. (2009) reported that correlations between the BADS and Wechsler IQ were approximately .50. High correlations were reported between the BADS and IQ in a sample of adults with Prader-Willi syndrome, especially for Rule Shift, Zoo Map, Modified Six Elements, and Key Search (*rs* = .43 to .78), with Action Program unrelated to IQ (Chevalère et al., 2013). In their sample of people who had sustained a severe TBI, Woods and Liossi (2007) reported moderate correlations between the Wechsler Adult Intelligence Scale (WAIS-III) IQ and Zoo Map and Key Search (*rs* = .35, .41, respectively). IQ scores correlated with the BADS Profile score, Temporal Judgment, and Zoo Map subtests (*rs* = 0.45 to .58) in a sample of persons with schizophrenia (Jovanovski et al., 2007). Null findings have also been reported (e.g., Gillespie et al., 2002).

BADS and the DEX. The relationship between the BADS subtests and the DEX has been examined, with mixed results reported (see also DEX review elsewhere in this chapter). Some research has reported low correlations overall between various BADS subtests and the DEX, with the exception of Rule Shift (Boelen et al., 2009). Similarly, no significant relationships between the BADS and DEX have been reported in a sample of patients who sustained a severe TBI (Wood & Liossi, 2006) or patients with neurologic conditions (Norris & Tate, 2000). As many as 29% of patients with MS showed discrepant impairment between BADS performance and DEX ratings (van der Hiele et al., 2012).

However, Wilson et al. (1996) reported that there were moderate negative correlations between the DEX ratings made by others and performance on the six individual tests; that is, poor awareness of deficit was correlated with poor executive functioning on each BADS test. A moderate association was reported between various BADS subtests (particularly Action Program, Modified Six Elements) and DEX ratings by clinicians in a TBI sample (Bennett et al., 2005).

The identity of the rater may impact whether relationships are found or not (see also DEX review in this chapter and Wilson et al., 1996); for example, in a study of patients with brain injury due to various etiologies, the DEX-Other as completed by therapists significantly correlated with BADS subtests, whereas the DEX-Self did not (Emmanouel et al., 2014).

Other Tests. Correlations between BADS Profile score and Cognistat subtests were not significant overall in a sample of patients with schizophrenia in the chronic illness stage, with the exception of construction and naming subtests (Katz et al., 2007). There appears to be little relationship between performance on the BADS tests and memory test scores (Evans et al., 1997). In a sample of people with schizophrenia, the BDI-II moderately correlated with Temporal Judgment (Jovanovski et al., 2007).

CLINICAL STUDIES

MCI and Dementia. In one study, BADS performance differed among people with AD, MCI, and healthy controls (da Costa Armentano et al., 2013). For example, Zoo Map effectively differentiated between controls and patients with MCI, with every one-point increase associated with a reduced risk of classification of MCI of 46%. Differentiation between MCI and early onset AD was best achieved by Rule Shift and Modified Six Elements, with a one-point increase associated with 87% and 69% risk reductions in diagnosis, respectively. Regression analyses suggested that early- and late-onset AD were differentiated via Modified Six Elements, Action Program, and Key Search subtests.

Other research has indicated that AD patients perform worse on the BADS than MCI patients, who in turn perform better than controls (Espinosa et al., 2009). Rule Shift and Action Program appear best at discriminating MCI and controls; Zoo Map and Modified Six Elements best at differentiating between MCI and AD; and Action Program, Zoo Map, and Modified Six Elements appear to be the best differentiator between AD and controls. BADS performance was not related to irritability in patients with Huntington's disease (HD; Nimmagadda et al., 2011).

TBI and Mixed Neurologic Samples. Wilson et al. (1996, 1998) reported that the Profile score differentiated the performance of healthy controls from a group of 76 patients with neurological disorders, mostly comprised of patients with TBI. In addition, the performance of neurological patients was poorer than that of controls on all six of the individual tests making up the BADS. In Boelen et al.'s (2009) study of patients with brain injury referred for outpatient rehabilitation who both complained of executive function problems and were observed to exhibit such problems, Key Search, Modified Six Elements, and Zoo Map emerged as significant predictors of group membership. Along with other variables (Verbal Fluency, Everyday Descriptions Task, 20 Questions), nearly 88% of patients were correctly classified.

The BADS appears comparable to standard executive tasks in discriminating between neurological (TBI, MS) and non-neurological groups (Norris & Tate, 2000). Significant group differences are observed on three subtests (Action Program, Zoo Map, and Six Elements), along with the Profile score and other measures (Porteus Mazes, COWA). Correct classification of individuals without brain injury is high (84%), but classification accuracy for the neurologically impaired individuals (patients with TBI or MS) is poorer (64%). The overall classification rate is 74%. Similar results were obtained for other executive tasks (e.g., Porteus Mazes, COWA).

There is mixed evidence with respect to congruence between BADS performance and loci of damage. Shallice and Burgess (1991) described several atypical behaviors (e.g., spending a disproportionately long time on one subtask, misinterpreting task instructions) in patients with frontal lobe damage performing the Six Elements task. However, Garden et al. (2001) reported that unusual behaviors may be seen in healthy as well as patient populations. Left frontal lobe patients, but not right frontal lobe patients, were impaired on an adapted version of the Modified Six Elements Test, along with other conventional measures of executive function (Gouveia et al., 2007). Deficits were primarily related to disordered planning, including more rule violations.

There is mixed evidence regarding congruence between the BADS and functional and clinical correlates. A mixed sample of TBI patients performed worse than controls on the BADS except for Temporal Judgment and Action Program, with the Modified Six Elements task related to behavioral changes (externalizing) as rated by relatives (Rochat et al., 2009). BADS subtests were not significantly related to posttraumatic amnesia or time since trauma. Norris and Tate (2000) reported that performance on the Action Program, Zoo Map, and Six Elements tests predicted clinicians' ratings of everyday role functioning in neurological patients. Standard measures (COWA, errors on the Progressive Matrices) failed to predict role functioning. See also "Factor-Analytic Studies and Relationships with Other Tests" for information regarding relationships between BADS and DEX ratings in brain injury samples.

PD. The BADS has some promise in the assessment of PD. Perfetti et al. (2010) reported that the Profile score was sensitive in discriminating between PD patients without dementia and demographically matched controls, with the Six Elements task the best predictor at the subtest level. Group differences were noted on BADS subtests except Action Program and Temporal Judgment. A regression model with predictors including the Profile score and the TOL yielded a group classification accuracy rate of nearly 86%, with a model comprised of the BADS Six Elements task and the TOL yielding an accuracy rate of nearly 90%. Low plasmic uric acid level was related to decreased performance on the Rule Shift subtest (Annanmaki et al., 2008). The test is related to physical parameters in persons with PD, such as measurements related to gait (Teramoto et al., 2014) and posture (Ninomiya et al., 2015). The BADS has also been used to assess response to dopaminergic treatment in people with PD (Murakami et al., 2017).

Psychiatric Conditions. Impaired performance has been reported in people with schizophrenia (Evans et al., 1997; Ihara et al., 2000; Jovanovski et al., 2007; Peters et al., 2007). Tyson et al. (2008) reported that a large effect size discrepancy for the Profile score in favor of healthy controls. Vargas et al. (2009) report nearly 47% of a sample of persons with schizophrenia were impaired relative to controls (in which 3% of the sample were classified as impaired), with high diagnostic accuracy reported (88% sensitivity and 77% specificity). Jovanovski et al. (2007) report similar figures, with approximately 57% of their sample performing in the impaired range. Zoo Map was the most impaired, and Temporal Judgment evidenced near-ceiling performance levels.

Tyson, Laws, Flowers, Mortimer, and Schulz (2008) reported that controls performed better than people with schizophrenia on the Rule Shift subtest and the Profile score, in the magnitude of medium to large effect sizes, respectively (Amann et al., 2012). People with schizophrenia, bipolar disorder, and schizoaffective disorder also perform worse than controls on the BADS, without differences between clinical groups (Amann et al., 2012). In the bipolar group, a rating of symptom severity, along with age, was a significant predictor of BADS performance.

In addition to group differences and relatively high classification accuracy, correlates between the BADS and clinical and real-world outcomes have been reported in patients with schizophrenia. Chronic patients perform worse than acute patients; controls outperform both patient groups (Katz et al., 2007). Within the chronic group, BADS score is a predictor of activities of daily living (ADLs) and communication on a measure of functional outcome. The BADS is related to greater symptoms, poorer function, poorer social adjustment, greater clinical severity, and length of illness (Vargas et al., 2009) and emerges as a significant predictor of social function and quality of life in schizophrenia (Tyson et al., 2008). Duration of illness predicts BADS performance (Amann et al., 2012).

Jovanovski et al. (2007) reported the degree of insight into the illness correlated with most BADS subtests, except Rule Shift, with attenuated correlations overall when intelligence was controlled for. The Profile score and WCST errors predict memory efficiency in patients with schizophrenia (Peters et al., 2007). A relationship is reported between restrained eating behavior, disinhibition in eating situations, and worse BADS performance in individuals with schizophrenia (Knolle-Veentjer et al., 2008).

Null findings have also been reported. No post-treatment effects in BADS performance in individuals with schizophrenia randomized to individualized therapy or cognitive remediation therapy have been reported (Franck et al., 2013), with absence of significant change also reported following an intervention based on virtual reality (Amado et al., 2016). In patients diagnosed with psychotic disorder, stress sensitivity is related to performance on the TMT and the Stroop, but not on the BADS (Morrens et al., 2007). Coping with psychosis was not related to performance on Zoo Map and other cognitive measures (Bak et al., 2008).

Euthymic patients with a diagnosis of major depressive disorder perform worse than demographically matched controls on the BADS, with greater executive function difficulty in patients classified into severe versus mild depression groups (Paelecke-Habermann et al., 2005). A planning composite generated the largest discrepancy in favor of controls, with a smaller but medium sized effect between patient groups. Patients with anorexia nervosa are also found to be impaired on Zoo Map, with eating and depressive symptoms significantly related to performance (Carral-Fernández et al., 2016).

Korsakoff's Syndrome and Substance Use Disorders. The BADS is sensitive to cognitive deficits related to substance use disorders (Moriyama et al., 2002), particularly Korsakoff's syndrome. Patients with Korsakoff's syndrome perform significantly worse than patients with chronic alcoholism on the BADS, with 87% of a Korsakoff sample showing impairment compared with 13% of a chronic alcoholism sample (Maharasingam et al., 2013). Eighty percent of a sample of patients with Korsakoff's syndrome evidenced impairment on at least one BADS subtest, with the Six Elements test associated with the highest frequency of impairment, and Temporal Judgment with the lowest (55% impaired vs. 5% impaired; Van Oort & Kessels, 2009).

In another study, a sample of people with polysubstance use disorders performed worse than controls on the BADS, with the exception of Action Program; effect sizes ranged from .53 to 1.3 (Verdejo-García & Pérez-García, 2007); 3,4-methylenedioxymethamphetamine (MDMA) and alcohol use was inversely related to the Profile score ($rs = -.24$ to $-.39$). The BADS predicted problems in day-to-day life on the FrsBE in the areas of apathy, disinhibition, and executive dysfunction. No relationship was found between binge drinking in college students and Zoo Map and Key Search performance (Parada et al., 2012).

Other Populations. Performance on the BADS is impaired in a variety of other conditions thought to adversely impact executive functioning, such as Prader-Willi syndrome (Chevalere et al., 2013). Lower Profile scores are reported for patients with epilepsy who had been seizure-free for less than three months compared to controls, and patients with epilepsy who were seizure-free for three months performed worse than controls on the Zoo Map test (Treitz et al., 2009). Correlations between duration of the seizure-free period and BADS performance were significant ($r = -.24$).

NEUROANATOMICAL CORRELATES AND IMAGING STUDIES

In patients with AD, Rule Shift was related to cortical thickness of the right middle frontal gyrus (Vasconcelos et al., 2014).

PERFORMANCE VALIDITY

No information is available.

COMMENT

The BADS is a task designed to be similar to everyday activities that involve executive functioning, which renders this task appealing despite drawbacks as discussed later. The test shows small to moderate correlations with other executive function and complex attention tasks, while also loading with executive tasks in factor-analytic studies. The test is moderately correlated with IQ. The test has been used in multiple clinical samples, including TBI, MCI, dementia, and PD, among others, and has shown group differences in these populations. Clinical research in schizophrenia using this measure is compelling, with large group differences reported as well also associations with performance and clinical variables and daily function. Associations with its companion rating scale, the DEX, have yielded mixed results in brain injury samples, with some studies reporting significant relationships and others not finding significant associations (see also DEX review elsewhere in this chapter).

By emphasizing ecological validity, the BADS differs from many conventional executive tasks that place relative emphasis on compartmentalization of executive skills according to theoretical models. The emphasis on ecological validity is conceptually appealing but also renders the tasks complex and the underlying processes somewhat unclear. For example, the BADS subtests appear to involve inhibition, working memory, planning, and reasoning, although the relative salience of each of these component processes required for each task is not apparent. This notion is further supported by the finding that the BADS subtests tend to correlate with a variety of executive measures to a small to moderate degree.

Age appears to affect performance, particularly over the age of 65 years. However, there is little information available regarding the influence of other demographic variables. The normative sample is relatively small but includes three ability levels based on NART performance, and age bands are reportedly balanced for gender. Although the overall score is evaluated with reference to age, no age-based norms are provided for the individual subtests. Information regarding education and screening methodology is not provided. Note that there appear to be ceiling effects, particularly on Action Program, Six Elements, and Rule Shift.

Interrater reliability is strong; however, internal reliability and test-retest reliability appear relatively weak overall. It may be most prudent to administer the entire battery as the Profile score can be compared to normative standards and is associated with somewhat better psychometric properties than individual subtests. However, generally speaking, the test should not be used for high-stakes clinical decision making due to significant normative and psychometric limitations, although it has been used fairly extensively in some research populations. There is little information regarding neuroanatomical substrates of performance or performance validity.

REFERENCES

Amado, I., Brénugat-Herné, L., Orriols, E., Desombre, C., Dos Santos, M., Prost, Z., . . . Piolino, P. (2016). A serious game to improve cognitive functions in schizophrenia: A pilot study. *Frontiers in Psychiatry, 7*. https://doi.org/10.3389/fpsyt.2016.00064

Amann, B., Gomar, J. J., Ortiz-Gil, J., McKenna, P., Sans-Sansa, B., Sarró, S., . . . Pomarol-Clotet, E. (2012). Executive dysfunction and memory impairment in schizoaffective disorder: A comparison with bipolar disorder, schizophrenia and healthy controls. *Psychological Medicine, 42*(10), 2127–2135. https://doi.org/10.1017/S0033291712000104

Annanmaki, T., Pessala-Driver, A., Hokkanen, L., & Murros, K. (2008). Uric acid associates with cognition in Parkinson's disease. *Parkinsonism & Related Disorders, 14*(7), 576–578. https://doi.org/10.1016/j.parkreldis.2007.11.001

Bak, M., Krabbendam, L., Delespaul, P., Huistra, K., Walraven, W., & van Os, J. (2008). Executive function does not predict coping with symptoms in stable patients with a diagnosis of schizophrenia. *BMC Psychiatry, 8*(1). https://doi.org/10.1186/1471-244X-8-39

Bennett, P. C., Ong, B., & Ponsford, J. (2005). Measuring executive dysfunction in an acute rehabilitation setting: Using the dysexecutive questionnaire (DEX). *Journal of the International Neuropsychological Society, 11*(04), 376. https://doi.org/10.1017/S1355617705050423

Boelen, D. H. E., Spikman, J. M., Rietveld, A. C. M., & Fasotti, L. (2009). Executive dysfunction in chronic brain-injured patients: Assessment in outpatient rehabilitation. *Neuropsychological Rehabilitation, 19*(5), 625–644. https://doi.org/10.1080/09602010802613853

Carral-Fernández, L., González-Blanch, C., Goddard, E., González-Gómez, J., Benito-González, P., Bustamante-Cruz, E., & Gómez del Barrio, A. (2016). Planning abilities in patients with anorexia nervosa compared with healthy controls. *The Clinical Neuropsychologist, 30*(2), 228–242. https://doi.org/10.1080/13854046.2016.1147603

Chevalère, J., Postal, V., Jauregui, J., Copet, P., Laurier, V., & Thuilleaux, D. (2013). Assessment of executive functions in Prader–Willi syndrome and relationship with intellectual level. *Journal of Applied Research in Intellectual Disabilities, 26*(4), 309–318. https://doi.org/10.1111/jar.12044

da Costa Armentano, C. G., Porto, C. S., Nitrini, R., & Brucki, S. M. D. (2013). Ecological evaluation of executive functions in mild cognitive impairment and Alzheimer disease. *Alzheimer Disease & Associated Disorders, 27*(2), 95–101.

Emmanouel, A., Mouza, E., Kessels, R. P. C., & Fasotti, L. (2014). Validity of the Dysexecutive Questionnaire (DEX). Ratings by patients with brain injury and their therapists. *Brain Injury, 28*(12), 1581–1589. https://doi.org/10.3109/02699052.2014.942371

Espinosa, A., Alegret, M., Boada, M., Vinyes, G., Valero, S., MartíNez-Lage, P., . . . TáRraga, L. (2009). Ecological assessment of executive functions in mild cognitive impairment and mild Alzheimer's disease. *Journal of the International Neuropsychological Society, 15*(05), 751. https://doi.org/10.1017/S135561770999035X

Evans, J. J., Chua, S. E., McKenna, P. J., & Wilson, B. A. (1997). Assessment of the dysexecutive syndrome in schizophrenia. *Psychological Medicine, 27*(3), 635–646.

Franck, N., Duboc, C., Sundby, C., Amado, I., Wykes, T., Demily, C., . . . Vianin, P. (2013). Specific vs general cognitive remediation for executive functioning in schizophrenia: A multicenter randomized trial. *Schizophrenia Research, 147*(1), 68–74. https://doi.org/10.1016/j.schres.2013.03.009

Garden, S. E., Phillips, L. H., & MacPherson, S. E. (2001). Midlife aging, open-ended planning, and laboratory measures of executive function. *Neuropsychology, 15*(4), 472–482. https://doi.org/10.1037/0894-4105.15.4.472

Gillespie, D. C., Evans, R. I., Gardener, E. A., & Bowen, A. (2002). Performance of older adults on tests of cognitive estimation. *Journal of Clinical and Experimental Neuropsychology (Neuropsychology, Development and Cognition: Section A), 24*(3), 286–293. https://doi.org/10.1076/jcen.24.3.286.988

Gouveia, P. A. R., Brucki, S. M. D., Malheiros, S. M. F., & Bueno, O. F. A. (2007). Disorders in planning and strategy application in frontal lobe lesion patients. *Brain and Cognition, 63*(3), 240–246. https://doi.org/10.1016/j.bandc.2006.09.001

Ihara, H., Berrios, G. E., & McKenna, P. J. (2000). Dysexecutive syndrome in schizophrenia: A cross-cultural comparison between Japanese and British patients. *Behavioural Neurology, 12*(4), 209–220. https://doi.org/10.1155/2000/825727

Jelicic, M., Henquet, C. E. C., Derix, M. M. A., & Jolles, J. (2001). Test-retest stability of the Behavioural Assessment of the Dysexecutive Syndrome in a sample of psychiatric patients. *International Journal of Neuroscience, 110*(1–2), 73–78. https://doi.org/10.3109/00207450108994222

Jovanovski, D., Zakzanis, K. K., Young, D. A., & Campbell, Z. (2007). Assessing the relationship between insight and everyday executive deficits in schizophrenia: A pilot study. *Psychiatry Research, 151* (1–2), 47–54. https://doi.org/10.1016/j.psychres.2006.09.012

Katz, N., Tadmor, I., Felzen, B., & Hartman-Maeir, A. (2007). The Behavioural Assessment of the Dysexecutive Syndrome (BADS) in schizophrenia and its relation to functional outcomes. *Neuropsychological Rehabilitation, 17*(2), 192–205. https://doi.org/10.1080/09602010600685053

Klosowaska, D. (1976). Relation between ability to program actions and location of brain damage. *Polish Psychological Bulletin, 7*, 245–255.

Knolle-Veentjer, S., Huth, V., Ferstl, R., Aldenhoff, J. B., & Hinze-Selch, D. (2008). Delay of gratification and executive performance in individuals with schizophrenia: Putative role for eating behavior and body weight regulation. *Journal of Psychiatric Research, 42*(2), 98–105. https://doi.org/10.1016/j.jpsychires.2006.10.003

Maharasingam, M., Macniven, J. A. B., & Mason, O. J. (2013). Executive functioning in chronic alcoholism and Korsakoff syndrome. *Journal of Clinical and Experimental Neuropsychology, 35*(5), 501–508. https://doi.org/10.1080/13803395.2013.795527

Malloy, P., & Grace, J. (2005). A review of rating scales for measuring behavior change due to frontal systems damage. *Cognitive and Behavioral Neurology, 18*(1), 18–27.

Moriyama, Y., Mimura, M., Kato, M., Yoshino, A., Hara, T., Kashima, H., . . . Watanabe, A. (2002). Executive dysfunction and clinical outcome in chronic alcoholics. *Alcoholism: Clinical and Experimental Research, 26*(8), 1239–1244. https://doi.org/10.1097/00000374-200208000-00016

Morrens, M., Krabbendam, L., Bak, M., Delespaul, P., Mengelers, R., Sabbe, B., . . . Myin-Germeys, I. (2007). The relationship between cognitive dysfunction and stress sensitivity in schizophrenia: A replication study. *Social Psychiatry and Psychiatric Epidemiology, 42*(4), 284–287. https://doi.org/10.1007/s00127-007-0170-7

Murakami, H., Nohara, T., Shozawa, H., Owan, Y., Kuroda, T., Yano, S., . . . Ono, K. (2017). Effects of dopaminergic drug adjustment on executive function in different clinical stages of Parkinson's disease. *Neuropsychiatric Disease and Treatment, 13*, 2719–2726. https://doi.org/10.2147/NDT.S145916

Nimmagadda, S. R., Agrawal, N., Worrall-Davies, A., Markova, I., & Rickards, H. (2011). Determinants of irritability in Huntington's disease. *Acta Neuropsychiatrica, 23*(06), 309–314. https://doi.org/10.1111/j.1601-5215.2011.00563.x

Ninomiya, S., Morita, A., Teramoto, H., Akimoto, T., Shiota, H., & Kamei, S. (2015). Relationship between postural deformities and frontal function in Parkinson's disease. *Parkinson's Disease, 2015*, 1–5. https://doi.org/10.1155/2015/462143

Norris, G., & Tate, R. L. (2000). The Behavioural Assessment of the Dysexecutive Syndrome (BADS): Ecological, concurrent and construct validity. *Neuropsychological Rehabilitation, 10*(1), 33–45. https://doi.org/10.1080/096020100389282

Oosterman, J. M., Wijers, M., & Kessels, R. P. C. (2013). Planning or something else? Examining neuropsychological predictors of Zoo Map performance. *Applied Neuropsychology, 20*(2), 103–109. https://doi.org/10.1080/09084282.2012.670150

Paelecke-Habermann, Y., Pohl, J., & Leplow, B. (2005). Attention and executive functions in remitted major depression patients. *Journal of Affective Disorders, 89*(1–3), 125–135. https://doi.org/10.1016/j.jad.2005.09.006

Parada, M., Corral, M., Mota, N., Crego, A., Rodríguez Holguín, S., & Cadaveira, F. (2012). Executive functioning and alcohol binge drinking in university students. *Addictive Behaviors, 37*(2), 167–172. https://doi.org/10.1016/j.addbeh.2011.09.015

Perfetti, B., Varanese, S., Mercuri, P., Mancino, E., Saggino, A., & Onofrj, M. (2010). Behavioural Assessment of the Dysexecutive Syndrome in Parkinson's disease without dementia: A comparison with other clinical executive tasks. *Parkinsonism & Related Disorders, 16*(1), 46–50. https://doi.org/10.1016/j.parkreldis.2009.07.011

Peters, M. J. V., Cima, M. J., Smeets, T., de Vos, M., Jelicic, M., & Merckelbach, H. (2007). Did I say that word or did you? Executive dysfunctions in schizophrenic patients affect memory efficiency, but not source attributions. *Cognitive Neuropsychiatry, 12*(5), 391–411. https://doi.org/10.1080/13546800701470145

Proctor, A., & Zhang, J. (2008). Performance of three racial/ethnic groups on two tests of executive function: Clinical implications for traumatic brain injury (TBI). *NeuroRehabilitation, 23*(6), 529–536.

Rochat, L., Ammann, J., Mayer, E., Annoni, J.-M., & Linden, M. (2009). Executive disorders and perceived socio-emotional changes after traumatic brain injury. *Journal of Neuropsychology, 3*(2), 213–227. https://doi.org/10.1348/174866408X397656

Shallice, T., & Burgess, P. W. (1991). Deficits in strategy application following frontal lobe damage in man. *Brain, 114 (Pt 2)*, 727–741.

Teramoto, H., Morita, A., Ninomiya, S., Shiota, H., & Kamei, S. (2014). Relation between freezing of gait and frontal function in Parkinson's disease. *Parkinsonism & Related Disorders, 20*(10), 1046–1049. https://doi.org/10.1016/j.parkreldis.2014.06.022

Treitz, F. H., Daum, I., Faustmann, P. M., & Haase, C. G. (2009). Executive deficits in generalized and extrafrontal partial epilepsy: Long versus short seizure-free periods. *Epilepsy & Behavior, 14*(1), 66–70. https://doi.org/10.1016/j.yebeh.2008.08.005

Tyson, P. J., Laws, K. R., Flowers, K. A., Mortimer, A. M., & Schulz, J. (2008). Attention and executive function in people with schizophrenia: Relationship with social skills and quality of life. *International Journal of Psychiatry in Clinical Practice, 12*(2), 112–119. https://doi.org/10.1080/13651500701687133

van der Hiele, K., Spliethoff-Kamminga, N. G. A., Ruimschotel, R. P., Middelkoop, H. A. M., & Visser, L. H. (2012). The relationship between self-reported executive performance and psychological characteristics in multiple sclerosis. *European Journal of Neurology, 19*(4), 562–569. https://doi.org/10.1111/j.1468-1331.2011.03538.x

Van Oort, R., & Kessels, R. P. C. (2009). Executive dysfunction in Korsakoff's syndrome: Time to revise the DSM criteria for alcohol-induced persisting amnestic disorder? *International Journal of Psychiatry in Clinical Practice, 13*(1), 78–81. https://doi.org/10.1080/13651500802308290

Vargas, M. L., Sanz, J. C., & Marín, J. J. (2009). Behavioural Assessment of the Dysexecutive Syndrome battery (BADS) in schizophrenia: A pilot study in the Spanish population. *Cognitive and Behavioral Neurology, 22*(2), 95–100.

Vasconcelos, L., Jackowski, A., Oliveira, M., Ribeiro Flor, Y., Souza, A., Bueno, O., & Brucki, S. (2014). The thickness of posterior cortical areas is related to executive dysfunction in Alzheimer's disease. *Clinics, 69*(01), 28–37. https://doi.org/10.6061/clinics/2014(01)05

Verdejo-García, A., & Pérez-García, M. (2007). Profile of executive deficits in cocaine and heroin polysubstance users: Common and differential effects on separate executive components. *Psychopharmacology, 190*(4), 517–530. https://doi.org/10.1007/s00213-006-0632-8

Wilson, B. A., Alderman, N., Burgess, P. W., Emslie, H., & Evans, J. J. (1996). *Behavioural Assessment of the Dysexecutive Syndrome.* Bury St. Edmunds, UK: Thames Valley Test Company.

Wilson, B. A., Evans, J. J., Emslie, H., Alderman, N., & Burgess, P. (1998). The Development of an Ecologically Valid Test for Assessing Patients with a Dysexecutive Syndrome. *Neuropsychological Rehabilitation, 8*(3), 213–228. https://doi.org/10.1080/713755570

Wood, R., & Liossi, C. (2006). The ecological validity of executive tests in a severely brain injured sample. *Archives of Clinical Neuropsychology, 21*(5), 429–437. https://doi.org/10.1016/j.acn.2005.06.014

Wood, R. L., & Liossi, C. (2007). The relationship between general intellectual ability and performance on ecologically valid executive tests in a severe brain injury sample. *Journal of the International Neuropsychological Society, 13*(1), 90–98.

CATEGORY TEST (CAT)

TEST NAME	**Category Test (CAT)**
DOMAIN	Executive functioning
AGE RANGE	15 to 80
ADMINISTRATION TIME	30 to 60 minutes
SCORING FORMAT	Hand scored (computerized version available)
REFERENCES	DeFilippis, N. A., & McCampbell, E. (1979, 1991, 1997). *Manual for the Booklet Category Test.* Odessa, FL: Psychological Assessment Resources. Reitan, R. M., & Davison, L. A. (1974). *Clinical neuropsychology: Current status and applications.* Oxford: V. H. Winston & Sons. www.parinc.com

DESCRIPTION

The Category Test (CAT) was developed by Halstead (1947) and is part of the Reitan test battery (Halstead-Reitan Category Test, HRCT; Reitan & Davison, 1974). This test measures abstraction, concept formation, cognitive flexibility, and an ability to learn from experience. Items are presented in sets, and each set is organized on the basis of a different principle (e.g., number of objects, spatial position of a specific stimulus). For example, Roman numerals from I to IV are presented in the first set of stimuli, and the examinee is asked to indicate the number (one to four) on the response key suggested by the design (see Figure 9–1). Examinees are provided with feedback regarding accuracy of responses and are expected to infer the underlying principle behind the subtest. No clues are given as to what the principle might be. Therefore, the test requires the deduction of a classification principle by means of response-contingent feedback, the use of the principle while it remains effective, and the ability to abandon the principle when it is no longer effective.

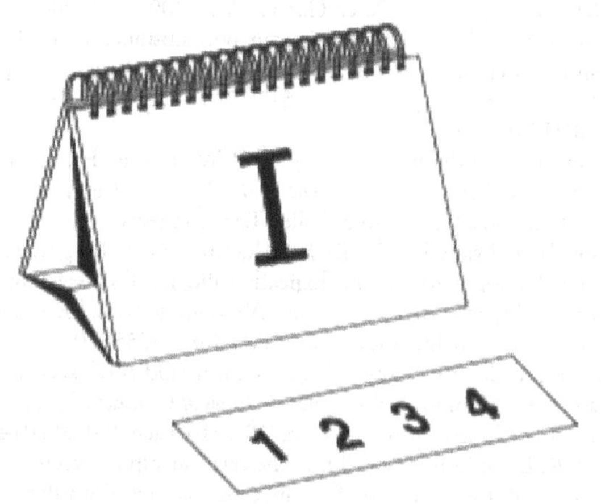

Figure 9–1 Example of an item from the Category Test.

Different types of category tests have been published, which use different materials. The original Halstead-Reitan version requires a projection box, an examiner's control panel, and a projector. Other versions include the Booklet Version that uses paper-based stimuli (available via Psychological Assessment Resources; DeFilippis & McCampbell, 1997) and computer versions, including a computerized version of the original Halstead-Reitan version (developed by Choca, Laatsch, Garside, Gupta, and Fenstermacher and available via Multi-Health Systems). Of note, evidence suggests that paper-based and computer-based forms of the test yield results similar to the original Halstead slide version (Choca & Morris, 1992; DeFilippis & McCampbell, 1997; Holz et al., 1996; Mercer et al., 1997; Nici & Hom, 2013; Silk-Eglit et al., 2014). The majority of recent research uses paper or computer versions of the test.

The test can take an exceptionally long time to complete (i.e., up to two hours), especially in people with significant impairment. Short forms of the test have been developed (e.g., Boyle, 1986; Caslyn et al., 1980; Charter et al., 1997; Gregory et al., 1979; Russell & Levy, 1987; Wetzel & Boll, 1987). The Short Category Test, Booklet Format (SCT) consists of 100 items (Wetzel & Boll, 1987). The SCT appears to function similarly to the Halstead-Retian version in terms of psychometric properties, discriminative ability, and relationship with other neuropsychological tests (Gelowitz & Paniak, 1992; Gontkovsky & Souheaver, 2002).

ADMINISTRATION

See Source for details.

SCORING

The total number of errors are recorded. Raw error scores must be converted initially to scaled scores and then to demographically corrected T scores for use with the Heaton et al. (2004) norms (see the section "Normative Data"). Other scores are also available. For example, Webster and Lopez (2006) devised novel scores for the fifth and sixth subtests of the Halstead-Reitan version, which were selected because they are sensitive to interference effects from previous subtests. Patients with TBI performed worse on these measures, with moderate to high classification accuracy reported. The description and calculation of these novel scores are detailed in the authors' paper for the interested reader. McNally, Dsurney, McGovern, DeFilippis, and Chan (2015) demonstrated concurrent validity for 13 subscales derived for the Booklet Category Test, with derived scores reflecting concept formation, learning, construction, and perseveration (see their paper for details).

DEMOGRAPHIC EFFECTS

AGE

Error scores increase with age (e.g., Golden et al., 1998; Heaton et al., 2004; Kamat et al., 2012; Leckliter & Matarazzo, 1989; Mitrushina et al., 2005; Sherrill-Pattison et al., 2000; Sweeney & Johnson, 2001). Heaton et al. (2004) report that in adults 20 to 85 years of age, age accounts for the largest amount of the variance in test scores among demographic variables examined (29% in Caucasians, 42% in African Americans).

GENDER

Gender has little impact on test scores (Heaton et al., 2004; Kamat et al., 2012; Sherrill-Pattison et al., 2000). Heaton reported that gender contributed to 1% of the variance in scores in Caucasian participants, and 2% in African-American participants.

EDUCATION AND IQ

Scores are inversely related to education (e.g., Golden et al., 1998; Greiffenstein & Baker, 2003; Kamat et al., 2012; Leckliter & Matarazzo, 1989; Pavol et al., 2006; but see Mitrushina et al., 2005). Education impacts performance even after accounting for neurological variables (e.g., severity of brain injury; Sherrill-Pattison et al., 2000). Heaton reported education accounted for 13% of the variance in scores in Caucasian participants and 4% in African-American participants. See "Construct Validity" for relationships with IQ.

ETHNICITY, NATIONALITY, AND LINGUISTIC EFFECTS

Level of acculturation is inversely related to performance (Arnold et al., 1994; Manly et al., 1998). Kamat et al. (2012) reported that bilingualism (Marathi and Hindi) did not relate to performance.

NORMATIVE DATA

Reitan and Wolfson (1985, see Table 9–10) provide reference standards for impairment, although the normative sample on which these are based is unclear.

Russell and Starkey (1993) developed the Halstead-Russell Neuropsychological Evaluation System (HRNES), which includes the Halstead-Reitan Category Test. The HRNES computer scoring system evaluates an individual's performance relative to a sample that consists of 576 people with neurologic conditions and a comparison group of 200 individuals (i.e., with negative neurologic exams). The data are further partitioned into seven age groups and four levels of education/IQ. Mitrushina et al. (2005) provide age-based metanorms, based on 1,579 participants, 16 to 79 years of age. The sample size is large, but the data are not subdivided by variables (e.g., education/IQ) that have been shown to impact performance. Note that the data derive from 11 studies dating largely from the 1970s to the 1980s, and the inclusion of old normative data may introduce the potential for considerable score inflation (i.e., Flynn effect; Flynn, 1984).

Heaton et al. (2004) provide normative data based on 1,212 healthy adults between 20 and 85 years of age. Their data are preferable as they are subdivided by age, gender, education, and ethnicity (see Table 9–11). Note, however, that participants were tested over a period of about 25 years, and it is not known to what extent the normative set includes dated norms.

Because intellectual level correlates with performance, IQ scores can be used to predict expected error scores and to determine if obtained scores are as expected. Titus et al. (2002) developed regression equations to predict error scores from WAIS-III Verbal Intelligence Quotient (VIQ), Performance Intelligence Quotient (PIQ), and FSIQ scores. The equations for predicting Halstead-Reitan Category Test scores and predictor tables for VIQ, PIQ, and FSIQ are shown in Table 9–12. Cutoff scores were calculated by averaging the standard deviations of Category Test scores in their study with standard deviations observed in prior studies using healthy individuals. Doubling and rounding the average standard deviation (*SD* = 15) created cutoff scores that were two standard deviations above

TABLE 9–10 Severity Ranges for the Standard Form of the Category Test

	PERFECTLY NORMAL	NORMAL	MILDLY IMPAIRED	SEVERELY IMPAIRED
Errors	0–25	26–45	46–65	65+

SOURCE: From Reitan and Wolfson (1985).

TABLE 9–11 Characteristics of the Category Test Normative Sample Provided by Heaton et al. (2004)

Sample size	1,212
Age	20 to 85
Geographic location	Various states in United States and Manitoba, Canada
Sample type	Individuals recruited as part of multicenter studies
Education	0 to 20 years
Gender	57% Men 43% Women
Race/Ethnicity	52% Caucasian 48% African American
Screening	Participants completed structured interviews and reported no history of learning disability, neurological disorder, serious psychiatric disorder, or alcohol or drug abuse.

NOTE: Age: 20 to 34, 35 to 39, 40 to 44, 45 to 49, 50 to 54, 55 to 59, 60 to 64, 65 to 69, 70 to 74, 75 to 79, 80 to 89. Education: 7 to 8, 9 to 11, 12, 13 to 15, 16 to 17, 18 to 20 years.

SOURCE: Reproduced by special permission of the Publisher, Psychological Assessment Resources, Inc. (PAR), 16204 North Florida Avenue, Lutz, FL 33549, from *Revised Comprehensive Norms for an Expanded Halstead-Reitan Battery Professional Manual*, Copyright 1991, 1992, 2004 by Psychological Assessment Resources, Inc. All rights reserved.

the projected means for each IQ level. Note that the equations were developed using a sample of 51 Caucasian university students (mean age = 19.51, range 17–34 years). Accordingly, it is difficult to generalize these findings to individuals with differing sociodemographic characteristics that affect performance (e.g., age).

For the SCT (Wetzel & Boll, 1987), normative data are based on a relatively small number of healthy individuals (n = 120). The manual provides tables broken down by age (45 years and younger; 46 years and older). A raw score cutoff of 41 is recommended for people 45 years of age and younger, while a cutoff score of 46 is suggested for people 46 years of age or older. Gontkovsky and Souheaver (2002) suggest that these cutoffs may require downward adjustment to increase sensitivity.

EVIDENCE FOR RELIABILITY

EVIDENCE FOR INTERNAL RELIABILITY

The odd-even split-half method and coefficient alpha have been used to calculate internal reliability estimates. Very high reliability coefficients (>.95) are found for the total score in healthy and clinical samples (Charter et al., 1987; Lopez et al., 2000; Moses, 1985; Shaw, 1966). However, some individual subtest reliability estimates are poor (i.e., Subtest I r = .46 and Subtest II r = .65). Split-half reliability coefficients are high for the total score for the booklet versions (.81 on the SCT). Some research suggests that the first and second subtests are too easy (evaluated according to the number of individuals passing an item) and show

TABLE 9–12 Predicted Category Test Error Scores

	VIQ		PIQ		FSIQ	
OBSERVED IQ	PREDICTED CAT	CUTOFF	PREDICTED CAT	CUTOFF	PREDICTED CAT	CUTOFF
150	10	40	9	39	6	36
145	12	42	11	41	9	39
140	14	44	14	44	11	41
135	16	46	16	46	14	44
130	18	48	19	49	17	47
125	20	50	21	51	19	49
120	22	52	23	53	22	52
115	24	54	26	56	25	55
110	27	57	28	58	27	57
105	29	59	31	61	30	60
100	31	61	33	63	33	63
95	33	63	36	66	35	65
90	35	65	38	68	38	68
85	37	67	40	70	41	71
80	39	69	43	73	43	73
75	42	72	45	75	46	76
70	44	74	48	78	49	79
65	46	76	50	80	51	81
60	48	78	53	83	54	84
55	50	80	55	85	57	87
50	52	82	57	87	59	89

NOTE: Regression equations are as follows:

(1) CAT = –.427 (WAIS-III VIQ) + 73.552, R^2 = .084, SE = 16.86

(2) CAT = –.486 (WAIS-III PIQ) + 81.77, R^2 = .112, SE = 16.60

(3) CAT = –.534 (WAIS-III FSIQ) + 86.00, R^2 = .129, SE = 16.51

PIQ, performance IQ; VIQ, verbal IQ; WAIS, Wechsler Adult Intelligence Scale.

SOURCE: Adapted from Titus et al. (2002).

poor discrimination (low correlation between test item and total score; Lopez et al., 2000).

EVIDENCE FOR TEST-RETEST RELIABILITY, MEASURING CHANGE, AND PRACTICE EFFECTS

Test-retest reliability in healthy samples is marginal to high over relatively short or long intervals (e.g., three weeks vs. up to 1 year; *rs* = .60 to .85; Bornstein et al., 1987; Dikmen et al., 1999; Matarazzo et al., 1974). Low values may be related to a restriction in the range of scores and a learning effect (Russell, 1992). According to some studies, patients with severe neurologic impairment show very high test-retest reliability, greater than .90, even after intervals of two years (Goldstein & Watson, 1989; Matarazzo et al., 1974).

Practice effects have been reported in moderately impaired neurological patients (DeFilippis & McCampbell, 1997; Dodrill & Troupin, 1975). In light of this finding, the absence of improvement (practice effects) has been considered an indicator of abnormal performance. In healthy adults (mean age = 32.3 years, *SD* = 10.3; VIQ, *M* = 105, *SD* = 10.8; PIQ, *M* = 105.0, *SD* = 10.5), following short retest intervals (about three weeks), an average raw score change of 23.5 (*SD* = 18.5) points has been reported (Bornstein et al., 1987). The average percentage of change in relation to initial performance was reportedly 46% in this sample. Dikmen et al. (1999) report an average decline in errors of about 10 points in a sample of 384 healthy or neurologically stable individuals (aged 15–83 years, *M* = 34.2, *SD* = 16.7) who were retested about 9 months after initial testing.

Table 9–13 provides information to determine if there has been substantial change in performance after accounting for practice effects. To use this information, first subtract the mean T2-T1 change (column 3) from the difference between the two testing points for the individual and then compare it to 1.64 times the standard deviation of the difference. The figure of 1.64 comes from the normal distribution and is exceeded in the positive or negative direction only 10% of the time if there is no actual change in clinical condition.

There are a number of factors other than clinical variables that can influence practice effects (Dikmen et al., 1999). For example, young age, higher education, higher initial competency, and short retest interval associated with larger score increase on retest. Regression to the mean also occurs, with a large positive change for people initially scoring poorly and a much smaller improvement or even deterioration for those initially scoring well.

TABLE 9–13 Test-Retest Data for the Category Test Based on a Sample of Healthy or Neurologically Stable Adults

TIME 1		TIME 2		T2 - T1		
MEAN	*SD*	*MEAN*	*SD*	*MEAN*	*SD*	*R*
40.97	26.07	30.42	25.01	−10.54	14.13	.85

NOTE: N = 384; interval of about 9 months; ages 15 to 83 (M = 34.2, *SD* = 16.7).
SOURCE: Adapted from Dikmen et al. (1999).

EVIDENCE FOR VALIDITY

FACTOR-ANALYTIC STUDIES

There is general agreement that the Category Test is a complex measure, loading on a number of different factors. The multifaceted nature of the test may be obscured by the fact that typically a single composite score is interpreted (Donders & Nesbitt-Greene, 2004). For example, in McNally et al.'s (2016) study of patients with TBI, a novel decomposition of the Booklet Category Test into 13 subcomponents suggested different abilities were involved in different subparts of the task (as evidenced by patterns of moderate and minimal correlations with subscales and conventional measures of memory, executive function, and conceptual reasoning). Similar findings have also been reported in a mixed clinical sample, showing convergence of Booklet Category Test subscales that measure learning, set loss, and memory with conventional measures, with somewhat weaker divergent validity (Roye et al., 2016).

Several studies using a variety of different clinical and healthy samples have suggested that the Category Test measures at least two factors, identified as spatial position reasoning (Subtests III, IV, and VII), and proportional reasoning (Subtests V and VI and sometimes VII; Allen et al., 1999, 2007a, b; Donders, 2001; Johnstone et al., 1997). In one study, these factors, in addition to a counting/symbol recognition factor (Subtests I and II), accounted for nearly 78% of the variance in performance (Allen et al., 2007a). The subtests loading on the spatial positioning factor are affected by age, whereas performance on the subtests loading on the proportional reasoning factor is affected more by education and appears sensitive to the severity of brain injury (Donders, 2001). Donders (2001) also noted that Subtest III does not show any relationship to injury variables.

CORRELATIONS WITH EXECUTIVE FUNCTION TESTS

The relationship between executive function tests and the Category Test is mixed. In a sample of individuals with schizophrenia, the Short Category Test correlated with the WCST perseverative errors score (*r* = 0.37, Josman & Katz, 2006). In a sample of adults with neurofibromatosis, COWA was minimally correlated with the Category Test (Spearman rho = −.23; Pavol et al., 2006). Verdejo-Garcia and Perez-Garcia (2007) reported that in a factor analysis of executive function tests in polysubstance users, a computerized version of the Category Test loaded with Go/No-Go and WCST variables on a third factor labeled "shifting." Letter-Number Sequencing is also moderately related to performance (Dugbarty et al., 1999; Titus et al., 2002).

CORRELATIONS WITH IQ

Scores are related to IQ (e.g., Golden et al., 1998; Leckliter & Matarazzo, 1989; Mitrushina et al., 2005; Titus et al., 2002). The total score shows moderate relations with the Wechsler FSIQ, especially the perceptual reasoning subtests (Berger, 1998; Dugbarty et al., 1999; Golden et al., 1998; Lansdell & Donnelly, 1977; Titus et al., 2002) and the proportional reasoning factor score (as described earlier; $r = -.47$; Allen et al., 2007a). Despite moderate relationships between visual reasoning and the Category Test, others have reported only a modest amount of shared variance between Wechsler PIQ and total score (11% to 13%; Titus et al., 2002).

CORRELATIONS WITH OTHER TESTS

There is a modest association between the Category Test and measures of learning and memory (Bertram et al., 1990; Fischer & Dean, 1990), consistent with the test's purported utility as a measure of learning ability. Consistent with the test's relationship with visual reasoning, Pavol et al. (2006) reported that the Booklet Category Test was moderately to highly correlated with a number of other visuospatial and fine motor tests in a sample of adults with neurofibromatosis (e.g., Developmental Test of Visual-Motor Integration, Judgment of Line Orientation [JLO]; *rs* = –.43 to –.66). In support of divergent validity, Halstead-Reitan Category Test factor scores are weakly related to Grip Strength (Allen et al., 2007a).

CLINICAL STUDIES

Neurologic Impairment. The Category Test is sensitive to a variety of neurologic conditions (see Choca et al., 1997, for a review) and is almost as sensitive as the full Halstead-Reitan battery in determining the presence or absence of neurological impairment (Adams & Trenton, 1981). Similarly, Allen, Caron, Duke, and Goldstein (2007) reported that the spatial positional factor of the Halstead-Reitan version for detection of neurologic impairment is comparable to the total error score of the test (i.e., sensitivity of 78%, specificity of 83%).

Impairment on the Category Test does not appear to consistently relate to specific location or laterality of neurologic impairment (Allen et al., 2007a; Anderson et al., 1995; Bornstein, 1986; Demakis, 2004; Donders, 2001; Lansdell & Donnelly, 1977; Pendleton & Heaton, 1982; Reitan & Wolfson, 1995). Combining subtests into a single summary score may also limit sensitivity of the test (see Donders & Nesbitt-Greene, 2004; McNally et al., 2016; Roye et al., 2016). The test has been used to index neurocognitive decline, in contrast to "hold" measures believed to be less prone to decline, such as IQ measures (Sweeney & Johnson, 2017).

Other Populations. Diminished performance is not specific to neurologic groups and also occurs in depressed individuals (Savard et al., 1980; but see Ruttan & Heinrichs, 2003), persons with posttraumatic stress disorder (PTSD) (Brenner et al., 2009), and people with schizophrenia (Goldstein et al., 1996; Steindl & Boyle, 1995). Group differences have also been reported in polysubstance users (Verdejo-Garcia & Perez-Garcia, 2007) and persons with human immunodeficiency virus (HIV; Spies et al., 2012). Osmon, Smerz, Braun, and Plambeck (2006) reported that the Category Test, along with JLO and a fluid reasoning subtest from the Woodcock-Johnson, Revised, predicted 16% of the variance in math skills in college adults referred for learning concerns, after controlling for intelligence. State variables, such as caffeine withdrawal after sleep deprivation, also apparently decrease performance (Killgore et al., 2007). Null findings have also been reported. For example, the Halstead-Reitan version did not differ between recently detoxified alcohol-dependent patients and controls (Alhassoon et al., 2012) or adults with neurofibromatosis and healthy controls (Pavol et al., 2006).

The test shows some evidence of predictive validity. For example, Barreca et al. (1999) found that patients who sustained a stroke and made few errors on the Category Test subsequently showed the greatest improvement in arm and hand function. Josman and Katz (2006) examined associations between the SCT and day-to-day tasks involving sorting skills (e.g., sorting laundry, organizing invoices, etc.) in individuals with schizophrenia, patients post-stroke, and healthy controls. The SCT was low to moderately (Spearman rho = –.36 to –.51) correlated with daily categorization tests in the schizophrenia group.

NEUROANATOMICAL CORRELATES AND IMAGING STUDIES

See "Clinical Studies" for lesion and laterality studies. Alhasoon et al. (2012) reported no significant relationship between diffusion tensor imaging values of the corpus callosum and Halstead-Reitan Category Test performance. Event-related potential correlates of error processing on the Halstead-Reitan version have been reported (Santos et al., 2016).

PERFORMANCE VALIDITY

Various cutoff scores have shown promise in the evaluation of performance validity, although findings are limited due to confounding with actual neurologic impairment and educational attainment. Performance validity cutoffs are mostly based on the fact that very few healthy individuals make errors on Subtests I and II (see Forrest et al., 2004; Simmel & Counts, 1957; Sweet & King, 2002). Tenhula and Sweet (1996) reported that an excessive number of errors on Subtests I, II, and VII might also raise the suspicion of compromised performance validity and that a cutoff of three infrequently missed items was quite effective

TABLE 9–14 Booklet Category Test False-Positive Error Rates and Sensitivity for Malingered Neurocognitive Dysfunction

		ALL TBI		MILD TBI		MODERATE TO SEVERE TBI	
	CUTOFF	FALSE POSITIVES	SENSITIVITY (%)	FALSE POSITIVES (%)	SENSITIVITY (%)	FALSE POSITIVES (%)	SENSITIVITY (%)
Total errors	>87	10.4	47.5	9.3	44.2	11.8	56.3
Subtest I and II	>1	3.9	15.3	4.7	16.3	23.5	13.5
Subtest VII	>5	32.7	52.5	30.2	51.2	29.4	56.3
Bolter items	>3	2.6	5.1	2.3	7.0	2.9	0.0
"Easy" items	>2	7.8	28.8	9.3	37.2	5.9	6.3

NOTE: TBI, traumatic brain injury.

SOURCE: Greve et al. (2007).

in differentiating patients with brain injury from healthy participants who were instructed to malinger (84% hit rate, 51% sensitivity, 98% specificity; see also DiCarlo et al., 2000). Forrest et al. (2004) recommend a liberal cutoff of two or more errors to reduce the likelihood of false positives (see also Williamson et al., 2003). Performance inconsistency can also suggest compromised validity, specifically with respect to a lack of performance improvement or even significant worsening of performance on retest (see Reitan & Wolfson, 1996; see also "Evidence for Test-Retest Reliability, Measuring Change, and Practice Effects").

Greve, Bianchini, and Roberson (2007) provide Booklet Category Test cutoffs for TBI patients validated against malingered neurocognitive dysfunction criteria based on Slick, Sherman, and Iverson (1999). Total raw error scores on the Booklet Category Test were associated with the highest accuracy rates, and this metric was also associated with an acceptable 10% false-positive rate in both mild and moderate to severe TBI. They also evaluated other indices of malingering from the Category Test used previously, with associated cutoffs (see Table 9–14). Overall, false-positive rates were variable depending on the score examined (see also Williamson et al., 2003).

Misialek, Fazio, Denney, and Myers (2013) classified incarcerated men into malingering and nonmalingering groups based on Slick et al. (1999) malingering criteria. Of the validity indicators examined, errors on Booklet Category Test Subtests I and II had the best classification accuracy (71%) with a specificity of 95% and a sensitivity of 49%, with an odds ratio of 27.

COMMENT

The Category Test was devised in 1947 and, at one time, was a very commonly used test. The original Halstead slide version is no longer being used as frequently, and the booklet, computerized, and short-form versions of the task have largely taken its place. Overall, research suggests that alternate versions approximate the original test in a number of ways. Note however, that the normative data for the short version are based on a relatively small sample and collected a number of years ago. When administering the test to individuals with significant cognitive impairment, users should note that the test may require a lengthy time to complete.

The Category Test is multifaceted and comprised of at least two factors, with some research suggesting multiple subparts can be meaningfully identified. It is not a unitary measure of executive functioning, and the test correlates with IQ in addition to other cognitive domains such as visuospatial function, suggesting that there are large reasoning and spatial components to the task. Modest relations are also reported between the test and measures of academic performance, memory, and fine motor function. Evidence regarding the relationship between the test and measures of executive function is mixed.

There are demographic effects on this test. Available research indicates that the Category Test is affected by age, education, IQ, and ethnicity. Gender is typically reported to have little effect. Most of the normative data were collected a number of years ago, with Heaton et al. (2004) providing the most comprehensive normative set that considers a number of sociodemographic factors and is not based on cutoff scores, unlike much of the other normative data available. In terms of reliability, internal reliability is generally strong (note that low coefficients have been reported for Subtests I and II), test-retest reliability is variable, and there are significant practice effects.

The test is reportedly sensitive to neurologic impairment and shows group differences between patients and healthy controls in some populations, but its ability to discriminate between conditions and its clinical and functional correlates are less clear. Despite the fact that the Category Test is comprised of multiple subtests, clinical interpretations and most studies tend to rely on a single composite score, which some have suggested limits the sensitivity of the test. Further definition of subscales within the test may be of benefit. There is some compelling data regarding evaluation of performance validity using the Category Test. As is the case for several PVTs, due to modest sensitivity and confounds of actual neurologic impairment, the test should not be used in isolation for the purpose of performance validity assessment.

REFERENCES

Adams, R. L., & Trenton, S. L. (1981). Development of a paper-and-pen form of the Halstead Category Test. *Journal of Consulting and Clinical Psychology, 49*, 298–299.

Alhassoon, O. M., Sorg, S. F., Taylor, M. J., Stephan, R. A., Schweinsburg, B. C., Stricker, N. H., Gongvatana, A., & Grant, I. (2012). Callosal White Matter Microstructural Recovery in Abstinent Alcoholics: A Longitudinal Diffusion Tensor Imaging Study. *Alcoholism: Clinical and Experimental Research, 36*(11), 1922–1931. https://doi.org/10.1111/j.1530-0277.2012.01808.x

Allen, D. N., Caron, J. E., Duke, L. A., & Goldstein, G. (2007a). Sensitivity of the Halstead Category Test factor scores to brain damage. *The Clinical Neuropsychologist, 21*(4), 638–652. http://doi.org/10.1080/13854040600744821

Allen, D. N., Goldstein, G., & Mariano, E. (1999). Is the Halstead Category Test a multidimensional instrument? *Journal of Clinical and Experimental Neuropsychology, 21*, 237–244.

Allen, D. N., Strauss, G. P., Kemtes, K. A., & Goldstein, G. (2007b). Hemispheric contributions to nonverbal abstract reasoning and problem-solving. *Neuropsychology, 21*(6), 713–720. http://doi.org/10.1037/0894-4105.21.6.713

Anderson, C. V., Bigler, E. D., & Blatter, D. D. (1995). Frontal lobe lesions, diffuse damage, and neuropsychological functioning of traumatic brain-injured patients. *Journal of Clinical and Experimental Neuropsychology, 17*, 900–908.

Arnold, B. R., Montgomery, G. T., Castaneda, I., & Longoria, R. (1994). Acculturation and performance of Hispanics on selected Halstead-Reitan neuropsychological tests. *Assessment, 1*, 239–248.

Barreca, S. R., Finlayson, A. J., Gowland, C. A., & Basmajian, J. V. (1999). Use of the Halstead Category Test as a cognitive predictor of functional recovery in the hemiplegic upper limb: A cross-validation study. *The Clinical Neuropsychologist, 13*, 171–181.

Berger, S. (1998). The WAIS-R factors: Usefulness and construct validity in neuropsychological assessments. *Applied Neuropsychology, 5*, 37–42.

Bertram, K. W., Abeles, N., & Snyder, P. J. (1990). The role of learning in performance on Halstead's Category Test. *The Clinical Neuropsychologist, 4*, 244–252.

Brenner, L. A., Ladley-O'Brien, S. E., Harwood, J. E., Filley, C. M., Kelly, J. P., Homaifar, B. Y., & Adler, L. E. (2009). An exploratory study of neuroimaging, neurologic, and neuropsychological findings in veterans with traumatic brain injury and/or posttraumatic stress disorder. *Military Medicine, 174*(4), 347–352.

Bornstein, R. A. (1986). Contribution of various neuropsychological measures to detection of frontal lobe impairment. *International Journal of Clinical Neuropsychology, 8*, 18–22.

Bornstein, R. A., Baker, R. B., & Douglass, A. B. (1987). Short-term retest reliability of the Halstead-Reitan battery in a normal sample. *The Journal of Nervous and Mental Disease, 175*, 229–232.

Boyle, G. L. (1986). Clinical neuropsychological assessment: Abbreviating the Halstead Category Test of brain dysfunction. *Journal of Clinical Psychology, 42*, 615–625.

Caslyn, D. A., O'Leary, M. R., & Chaney, E. F. (1980). Shortening the Category Test. *Journal of Consulting and Clinical Psychology, 48*, 788–789.

Charter, R. A., Adkins, T. G., Alekoumbides, A., & Seacat, G. F. (1987). Reliability of the WAIS, WMS, and Reitan Battery: Raw scores and standardization scores corrected for age and education. *The International Journal of Clinical Neuropsychology, 9*, 28–32.

Charter, R. A., Swift, K. M., & Blusewicz, M. J. (1997). Age- and education-corrected, standardized short form of the Category Test. *The Clinical Neuropsychologist, 11*, 142–145.

Choca, J., & Morris, J. (1992). Administering the Category Test by computer: Equivalence of results. *The Clinical Neuropsychologist, 6*, 9–15.

Choca, J. P., Laatsch, L., Wetzel, L., & Agresti, A. (1997). The Halstead Category Test: A fifty year perspective. *Neuropsychology Review, 7*, 61–75.

DeFilippis, N. A., & McCampbell, E. (1979, 1991, 1997). *Manual for the Booklet Category Test.* Odessa, FL: Psychological Assessment Resources.

Demakis, G. J. (2004). Frontal lobe damage and tests of executive processing: A meta-analysis of the Category Test, Stroop Test, and Trail-Making Test. *Journal of Clinical and Experimental Neuropsychology, 26*, 441–450.

DiCarlo, M. A., Gfeller, J. D., & Oliveri, M. V. (2000). Effects of coaching on detecting feigned cognitive impairment with the Category Test. *Archives of Clinical Neuropsychology, 15*, 399–413.

Dikmen, S. S., Heaton, R. K., Grant, I., & Temkin, N. R. (1999). Test-retest reliability and practice effects of expanded Halstead-Reitan neuropsychological test battery. *Journal of the International Neuropsychological Society, 5*, 346–356.

Dodrill, C. B., & Troupin, A. S. (1975). Effects of repeated administrations of a comprehensive neuropsychological battery among chronic epileptics. *Journal of Nervous and Mental Disease, 161*, 185–190.

Donders, J. (2001). Clinical utility of the Category Test as a multidimensional instrument. *Psychological Assessment, 13*, 592–594.

Donders, J., & Nesbitt-Greene, K. (2004). Predictors of neuropsychological test performance after pediatric traumatic brain injury. *Assessment, 11*, 275–284.

Dugbarty, A. T., Sanchez, P. N., Rosenbaum, J. G., Mahurin, R. K., Davis, M., & Townes, B. (1999). WAIS-III Matrix Reasoning test performance in a mixed clinical sample. *The Clinical Neuropsychologist, 13*, 396–404.

Fischer, W. E., & Dean, R. S. (1990). Factor structure of the Halstead Category Test by age and gender. *International Journal of Clinical Neuropsychology, 12*, 180–183.

Forrest, T. J., Allen, D. N., & Goldstein, G. (2004). Malingering indexes for the Halstead Category Test. *The Clinical Neuropsychologist, 18*, 334–347.

Flynn, J. R. (1984). The mean IQ of Americans: Massive gains 1932–1978. *Psychological Bulletin, 95*, 29–51.

Gelowitz, D. L., & Paniak, C. E. (1992). Cross-validation of the Short Category Test-Booklet Format. *Neuropsychology, 6*, 287–292.

Golden, C. J., Kushner, T., Lee, B., & McMorrow, M. A. (1998). Searching for the meaning of the Category Test: A comparative analysis. *International Journal of Neuroscience, 93*, 141–150.

Goldstein, G., & Watson, J. R. (1989). Test-retest reliability of the Halstead-Reitan Battery and the WAIS in a neuropsychiatric population. *The Clinical Neuropsychologist, 3*, 265–273.

Goldstein, G., Beers, S. R., & Shemansky, W. J. (1996). Neuropsychological differences between schizophrenic patients with heterogeneous Wisconsin Card Sorting Test performance. *Schizophrenia Research, 21*(1), 13–18. https://doi.org/10.1016/0920-9964(96)00019-9

Gontkovsky, S. T., & Souheaver, G. T. (2002). T-score and raw-score comparisons in detecting brain dysfunction using the Booklet Category Test and the Short Category Test. *Perceptual and Motor Skills, 94*, 319–322.

Gregory, R. J., Paul, J. J., & Morrison, M. W. (1979). A short form of the Category Test for adults. *Journal of Clinical Psychology, 35*, 795–798.

Greve, K. W., Bianchini, K. J., & Roberson, T. (2007). The Booklet Category Test and malingering in traumatic brain injury: Classification accuracy in known groups. *The Clinical Neuropsychologist, 21*(2), 318–337. http://doi.org/10.1080/13854040500488552

Greiffenstein, M. F., & Baker, W. J. (2003). Premorbid clues? Preinjury scholastic performance and present neuropsychological functioning in late postconcussion syndrome. *The Clinical Neuropsychologist, 17*, 561–573.

Halstead, W. C. (1947). *Brain and intelligence.* Chicago: University of Chicago Press.

Heaton, R. K., Miller, S. W., Taylor, M. J., & Grant, I. (1991, 1992, 2004). *Revised comprehensive norms for an expanded Halstead-Reitan Battery: Demographically adjusted neuropsychological norms for African American and Caucasian adults.* Lutz, FL: PAR.

Holz, J. L., Gearhart, L. P., & Watson, C. G. (1996). Comparability of scores on projector- and booklet-administration of the Category Test in brain-impaired veterans and controls. *Neuropsychology, 10*, 194–196.

Johnstone, B., Holland, D., & Hewett, J. E. (1997). The construct validity of the Category Test: Is it a measure of reasoning or intelligence? *Psychological Assessment, 9*, 28–33.

Josman, N., & Katz, N. (2006). Relationships of categorization on tests and daily tasks in patients with schizophrenia, post-stroke patients and healthy controls. *Psychiatry Research, 141*(1), 15–28. http://doi.org/10.1016/j.psychres.2004.03.015

Kamat, R., Ghate, M., Gollan, T. H., Meyer, R., Vaida, F., Heaton, R. K., . . . the HIV Neurobehavioral Research Program (HNRP) group. (2012). Effects of Marathi-Hindi bilingualism on neuropsychological performance. *Journal of the International Neuropsychological Society, 18*(02), 305–313. http://doi.org/10.1017/S1355617711001731

Killgore, W. D., Kahn-Greene, E. T., Killgore, D. B., Kamimori, G. H., & Balkin, T. J. (2007). Effects of acute caffeine withdrawal on Short Category Test performance in sleep-deprived individuals. *Perceptual and Motor Skills, 105*(3 suppl), 1265–1274.

Lansdell, H., & Donnelly, E. F. (1977). Factor analysis of the Wechsler Adult Intelligence Scale and the Halstead-Reitan Category and Tapping Tests. *Journal of Consulting and Clinical Psychology, 3*, 412–416.

Leckliter, I. N., & Matarazzo, J. D. (1989). The influence of age, education, IQ, gender, and alcohol abuse on Halstead-Reitan neuropsychological test battery performance. *Journal of Clinical Psychology, 45*, 484–512.

Lopez, M. N., Charter, R. A., & Newman, J. R. (2000). Psychometric properties of the Halstead Category Test. *The Clinical Neuropsychologist, 14*, 157–161.

Manly, J. J., Miller, S. W., Heaton, R. K., Byrd, D., Reilly, J., Velasquez, R. J., Saccuzzo, D. P., Grant, I., & the HIV Neurobehavioral Research Center (HNRC) group. (1998). The effect of African American acculturation on neuropsychological test performance in normal and HIV-positive individuals. *Journal of the International Neuropsychological Society, 4*, 291–302.

Matarazzo, J. D., Wiens, A. N., Matarazzo, R. G., & Goldstein, S. G. (1974). Psychometric and test-retest reliability of the Halstead impairment index in a sample of healthy, young, normal men. *Journal of Nervous and Mental Disease, 158*, 37–49.

McNally, S., Dsurney, J., McGovern, J., DeFilippis, N., & Chan, L. (2015). Concurrent validity of new subscale scores for the Booklet Category Test. *Assessment*, 1073191115588783.

Mercer, W. N., Harrell, E. H., Miller, D. C., Childs, H. W., & Rockers, D. M. (1997). Performance of brain-injured versus healthy adults on three versions of the Category Test. *The Clinical Neuropsychologist, 11*, 174–179.

Misialek, L., Fazio, R. L., Denney, R. L., & Myers, W. G. (2013). Limited predictive accuracy of the Booklet Category Test in a criminal forensic sample. *Applied Neuropsychology, 20*(2), 77–82. http://doi.org/10.1080/09084282.2012.670162

Mitrushina, M. N., Boone, K. B., Razani, J., & D'Elia, L. F. (2005). *Handbook of normative data for neuropsychological assessment* (2nd ed.). New York: Oxford University Press.

Moses, J. A. (1985). Internal consistency of standard and short forms of three itemized Halstead-Reitan neuropsychological battery tests. *International Journal of Clinical Neuropsychology, 3*, 164–166.

Nici, J., & Hom, J. (2013). Comparability of the computerized Halstead Category Test with the original version. *Archives of Clinical Neuropsychology, 28*(8), 824–828. http://doi.org/10.1093/arclin/act075

Osmon, D. C., Smerz, J. M., Braun, M. M., & Plambeck, E. (2006). Processing abilities associated with math skills in adult learning disability. *Journal of Clinical and Experimental Neuropsychology, 28*(1), 84–95. http://doi.org/10.1080/13803390490918129

Pavol, M., Hiscock, M., Massman, P., Moore, B., Foorman, B., & Meyers, C. (2006). Neuropsychological function in adults with von Recklinghausen's neurofibromatosis. *Developmental Neuropsychology, 29*(3), 509–526.

Pendleton, M. G., & Heaton, R. K. (1982). A comparison of the Wisconsin Card Sorting Test and the Category Test. *Journal of Clinical Psychology, 38*, 392–396.

Reitan, R. M., & Davison, L. A. (1974). *Clinical neuropsychology: Current status and applications.* Oxford: V. H. Winston & Sons.

Reitan, R. M., & Wolfson, D. (1985). *The Halstead-Reitan Neuropsychological Test Battery: Theory and clinical interpretation.* Tucson, AZ: Neuropsychology Press.

Reitan, R. M., & Wolfson, D. (1995). Category Test and Trail Making Test as measures of frontal lobe functions. *The Clinical Neuropsychologist, 9*, 50–56.

Reitan, R. M., & Wolfson, D. (1996). The question of validity of neuropsychological test scores among head-injured litigants: Development of a dissimulation index. *Archives of Clinical Neuropsychology, 11*, 573–580.

Roye, S., Calamia, M., Greve, K., Bianchini, K., Aguerrevere, L., & Curtis, K. (2016). Further validation of booklet category test subscales for learning, set loss, and memory in a mixed clinical sample. *Applied Neuropsychology. Adult*, 1–8. https://doi.org/10.1080/23279095.2016.1230120

Russell, E. W. (1992). Reliability of the Halstead Impairment Index: A simulation and reanalysis of Matarazzo et al. (1974). *Neuropsychology, 6*, 251–259.

Russell, E. W., & Levy, M. (1987). Revision of the Halstead Category Test. *Journal of Consulting and Clinical Psychology, 55*, 898–901.

Russell, E. W., & Starkey, R. I. (1993). *Halstead Russell Neuropsychological Evaluation System (HRNES).* Los Angeles: Western Psychological Services.

Ruttan, L. A., & Heinrichs, R. W. (2003). Depression and neurocognitive functioning mild traumatic brain injury patients referred for assessment. *Journal of Clinical and Experimental Neuropsychology, 25*, 407–419.

Santos, I. M., Teixeira, A. R., Tomé, A. M., Pereira, A. T., Rodrigues, P., Vagos, P., . . . Silva, C. F. (2016). ERP correlates of error processing during performance on the Halstead Category Test. *International Journal of Psychophysiology, 106*, 97–105. https://doi.org/10.1016/j.ijpsycho.2016.06.010

Savard, R. J., Rey, A. C., & Post, R. M. (1980). Halstead-Reitan Category Test in bipolar and unipolar affective disorders: Relationship to age and phase in illness. *Journal of Nervous and Mental Disease, 168*, 297–304.

Shaw, D. J. (1966). The reliability and validity of the Halstead Category Test. *Journal of Clinical Psychology, 37*, 847–848.

Sherrill-Pattison, S., Donders, J., & Thompson, E. (2000). Influence of demographic variables on neuropsychological test performance after traumatic brain injury. *The Clinical Neuropsychologist, 14*, 496–503.

Silk-Eglit, G. M., Gunner, J. H., Miele, A. S., Lynch, J. K., & McCaffrey, R. J. (2014). A comparison of the standard category test with a new computer version. *Applied Neuropsychology. Adult, 21*(1), 9–13. https://doi.org/10.1080/09084282.2012.716802

Simmel, M. S., & Counts, S. (1957). Some stable determinants of perception, thinking, and learning: A study based on the analysis of a single test. *Genetic Psychology Monographs, 56*, 3–157.

Slick, D. J., Sherman, E. M., & Iverson, G. L. (1999). Diagnostic criteria for malingered neurocognitive dysfunction: Proposed standards for clinical practice and research. *The Clinical Neuropsychologist, 13*(4), 545–561. https://doi.org/10.1076/1385-4046(199911)13:04;1-Y;FT545

Spies, G., Fennema-Notestine, C., Archibald, S. L., Cherner, M., & Seedat, S. (2012). Neurocognitive deficits in HIV-infected women and victims of childhood trauma. *AIDS Care, 24*(9), 1126–1135. http://doi.org/10.1080/09540121.2012.687813

Steindl, S. R., & Boyle, G. J. (1995). Use of the Booklet Category Test to assess abstract concept formation in schizophrenic disorders. *Archives of Clinical Neuropsychology, 10*, 205–210.

Sweeney, J. E., & Johnson, A. M. (2001). Age and neuropsychological status following exposure to violent nonimpact acceleration forces in MVAs. *Journal of Forensic Neuropsychology, 2,* 31–40.

Sweeney, J. E., & Johnson, A. M. (2017). An index of decline or recovery following nonimpact and impact mTBI. *Applied Neuropsychology. Adult,* 1–5. https://doi.org/10.1080/23279095.2017.1392304

Sweet, J. J., & King, J. H. (2002). Category Test validity indicators: Overview and practice recommendations. *Journal of Forensic Neuropsychology, 3,* 241–274.

Tenhula, W. N., & Sweet, J. J. (1996). Double cross-validation of the Booklet Category Test in detecting malingered traumatic brain injury. *The Clinical Neuropsychologist, 10,* 104–116.

Titus, J. B., Retzlaff, P. D., & Dean, R. S. (2002). Predicting scores of the Halstead Category Test with the WAIS-III. *International Journal of Neuroscience, 112,* 1099–1114.

Verdejo-García, A., & Pérez-García, M. (2007). Profile of executive deficits in cocaine and heroin polysubstance users: Common and differential effects on separate executive components. *Psychopharmacology, 190*(4), 517–530. http://doi.org/10.1007/s00213-006-0632-8

Webster, J. S., & Lopez, M. N. (2006). New scores for the Category Test: Measures of interference for subtests 5 and 6. *The Clinical Neuropsychologist, 20*(4), 678–694. http://doi.org/10.1080/138540491005848

Wetzel, L., & Boll, T. J. (1987). *Short Category Test, booklet format.* Los Angeles: Western Psychological Services.

Williamson, D. J. G., Green, P., Allen, L., & Rohling, M. L. (2003). Evaluating effort with the Word Memory Test and Category Test—or not: Inconsistencies in a compensation-seeking sample. *Journal of Forensic Neuropsychology, 3,* 19–44.

CLOCK DRAWING TEST (CDT)

TEST NAME	**Clock Drawing Test (CDT)**
DOMAIN	Dementia screening
AGE RANGE	17 to 98 years
ADMINISTRATION TIME	5 minutes
SCORING FORMAT	Hand scored
REFERENCES	Tuokko, H., Hadjistavropoulos, T., Miller, J. A., Horton, A., & Beattie, B. L. (1995). *The Clock Test: Administration and scoring manual.* Toronto, Ont.: Multi-Health Systems. Royall, D. R., Cordes, J. A., & Polk, M. (1998). CLOX: An executive clock drawing task. *Journal of Neurology, Neurosurgery, and Psychiatry, 64*(5), 588–594. Freedman, M., Kaplan, E., Delis, D., & Morris, R. (1994). *Clock Drawing: A neuropsychological analysis.* New York: Oxford University Press. www.mhs.com

DESCRIPTION

The Clock Drawing Test (CDT) is a dementia screener and executive function test with visual-spatial, constructional, and executive demands. The simple freehand drawing of a clock face is a long-standing component of the brief mental status examination in neurology and has a long history of use as a screening instrument, dating to 1915 (see review by Hazan, Frankenburg, Brenkel, & Shulman, 2018). The test is one of the most commonly used dementia screeners (Maruta et al., 2011; Strauss et al., 2012) and is also commonly used to assess executive function (de Assis Faria et al., 2015). In contrast to the primarily verbal content of most dementia scales, the Clock Drawing Test relies on visual-spatial, constructional, and higher order cognitive abilities.

Many different versions of the test have been published (see Table 9–15). More than 2,000 publications exist on the CDT (Hazan et al., 2018), and it has been subject to many reviews, including by Hazan et al. (2018), Lezak (2012), Pinto and Peters (2009), Shulman (2000), Smedslund, Siqveland, and Leiknes (2015), Spenciere, Alves, and Charchat-Fichman (2017), and Tuokko and O'Connell (2006). No specific test material is required. A commercial version is offered (e.g., Tuokko et al., 1995) via Multi-Health Systems (www.mhs.com), and the test is incorporated into a number of batteries (e.g., 7 Minute Screen [Solomon et al., 1998]; CAMCOG [Roth et al., 1986]; Spatial-Quantitative Battery in the Boston Diagnostic Aphasia Examination [Goodglass & Kaplan, 1983, 2001]; the Montreal Cognitive Assessment [Nasreddine et al., 2005], and the Kaplan Baycrest Neurocognitive Assessment [Leach et al., 2000]).

Versions of the test vary. One major distinguishing feature between them is the requirement to free-draw a clock versus complete a predrawn circle with the numbers and hands set toward a specific time. An advantage of versions involving predrawn circles are that they emphasize number and hand placement, thereby limiting confounds as a poorly drawn circle confounds the remainder of the clock drawing (Tuokko, 2000). Several authors (Libon et al., 1993, 1996; Rouleau et al., 1992; Royall et al., 1998) also include copying conditions to improve understanding of performance.

Another differentiating feature is the time setting. A commonly used time setting is "10 after 11" (or "10 past 11"); this time setting may enhance the inhibitory demands of the task, given the proximity of the 10 and 11 on the clock (Freedman et al., 1994; Manos & Wu, 1994). This time setting also requires both visual fields, which can facilitate identification of hemilateral neglect or hemianopia.

The versions in Table 9–15 have been used in various populations. Each version has been used in cognitively healthy older adults and people with AD. Most others have also been used in other dementia subtypes, including mixed dementia (Manos & Wu, 1994; Mendez et al., 1992; Rouleau et al., 1992; Tuokko et al., 1992), vascular dementia (Freedman et al., 1994; Manos & Wu, 1994; Rouleau et al., 1992), frontotemporal dementia (FTD; Manos & Wu, 1994), HD, dementia with Lewy bodies (Rouleau et al., 1992), and PD (Freedman et al., 1994; Rouleau et al., 1992). Versions have also been used following stroke (Freedman et al., 1994; Mendez et al., 1992; Rouleau et al., 1992), in mood and anxiety disorders (Freedman et al., 1994; Mendez et al., 1992; Rouleau et al., 1992; Shulman, 2000), schizophrenia (Freedman et al., 1994; Mendez et al., 1992), and young- to middle-age adults (Freedman et al., 1994).

TABLE 9–15 Summary of Select Clock Drawing Test Versions

AUTHOR	CIRCLE	TIME SETTING	TOTAL SCORE	CUTOFF
Mendez et al. (1992; Clock Drawing Interpretation Score, CDIS)	Free-drawn	11:10	20	<18
Royall et al. (1998; CLOX)	CLOX1 (Free-drawn) CLOX2 (Copying)	1:45	15	CLOX1 (<10) CLOX2 (<12)
Rouleau et al. (1992)	Free-drawn	11:10	Quantitative (out of 10) Qualitative (errors)	NA
Freedman et al. (1994)	Free-drawn Predrawn	6:45 6:05	15 13	NA
Sunderland et al. (1989)	Predrawn	2:45	10	<6
Lin et al. (2003)	Predrawn	10:10	16	<23
Wolf-Klein et al. (1989)	Predrawn		10	<7
Manos & Wu (1994)	Predrawn	11:10	10	<8
Tuokko et al. (1992)	Predrawn	11:10	Error tally	>2 errors
Shulman et al. (1986), Shulman (2000)	Predrawn	11:10	5	<4

SOURCE: Adapted from Tuokko and O'Connell (2006).

Of note, a digital CDT has also been introduced, which uses a digitizing pen that functions both as a regular pen and also records position with a high level of spatial and temporal accuracy, which is then analyzed by software designed for this purpose (Souillard-Mandar et al., 2016). A digitized version of the CDT has shown promise in delineating age-related decline in performance on the CDT (Piers et al., 2017) and in the diagnosis of dementia (Müller, Preische, Heymann, Elbing, & Laske, 2017).

ADMINISTRATION

There are a number of ways the test can be administered. A review of methods (Pinto & Peters, 2009) suggests that the most common instructions are: "Please draw a clock face, placing all the numbers on it. Now set the time to 10 past 11." Other instructions are more detailed. For example, in the free-drawn version (e.g., Goodglass and Kaplan, 1983; Libon et al., 1993; Rouleau et al., 1992), the examiner is instructed to place upright a standard, unlined letter-size sheet of paper and a pencil in front of the examinee and say: "I want you to draw the face of a clock with all the numbers on it. Make it large." After completion of the clock face, the instructions are as follows: "Now, please set the time to 10 after 11 (or 20 to 4)." Instructions may be repeated or rephrased if the examinee does not understand but no other assistance should be given. The time taken to complete the task may be noted.

If using a predrawn circle, provide a sheet with a circle about 4 inches (10 cm) in diameter (Shulman, 2000) and say: "This circle represents a clock face. Please put in the numbers so that it looks like a clock and then set the time to 10 minutes past 11." Shulman (2000) recommended that the examiner should not use the word "hands" in the instructions.

Sensory impairments, such as hemianopia and visual neglect, affect test performance and can be manifest as unilateral errors (see Ogden, 1985). Chokron, Colliot, and Bartolomeo (2004) found that patients with left neglect performed better on the CDT when their eyes were closed, which may relate to deficits in visual scanning (i.e., disengaging attention from right-sided visual stimuli). Subtle alterations in administration may also affect results. For example, Chan, Remington, Paskavitz, and Shea (2008) reported that individuals younger than 60 years of age showed similar performance with a digital prompt (e.g., 12:45) and analog prompt (e.g., quarter to 1), whereas people older than 70 years performed better with an analog prompt.

SCORING

Scoring systems range from a three-point system (Goodglass & Kaplan, 1983, 2001) to more complex systems (e.g., a 20-point scale by Mendez et al., 1992). A number of authors (e.g., Cosentino et al., 2004; Libon et al., 1996; Rouleau et al., 1992; Suhr et al., 1998; Tuokko et al., 1992) have developed qualitative scoring systems that include evaluation of clock size, omissions, graphic difficulties (e.g., numbers hard to read, distortions in the hands), stimulus-bound errors (e.g., setting the hands on 10 and 11), conceptual errors (e.g., writing the time on the clock rather than setting the hands, lack of numbers on the clock), perseverations (e.g., more than two hands, writing numbers beyond "12"), and spatial/planning errors (e.g., neglect, gaps in number spacing, numbers outside clock face or counterclockwise). Some of the most common scoring systems are provided in Tables 9–16 to 9–20. Normative data for several of these versions are presented in the section "Normative Data." Scoring methods tend to be highly correlated ($r \geq .67$; e.g., Kozora & Cullum, 1994; Lourenço et al., 2008; Santana et al., 2013; Tuokko, 2000).

TABLE 9–16 Freedman (1994) Scoring Criteria for the Clock Drawing Test

SUBTEST	CRITICAL ITEMS	POINTS
Numbers	1) Numbers 1–12 only without additions or omissions	1
	2) Arabic characters	1
	3) Written in correct order	1
	4) No rotations of paper while drawing numbers	1
	5) Correct position of numbers	1
	6) All numbers included inside circle	1
		Subtotal /6
Hands	7) Clock has two hands or marks	1
	8) Hour target indicated	1
	9) Minute target indicated	1
	10) Hands in correct proportion	1
	11) No superfluous marking	1
	12) Hands joined or within ½′ of joining	1
		Subtotal /6
Center of Clock	13) Clock has a center—either drawn or inferred	1
		Subtotal /1 Predrawn Total /13
Clock Circle	14) Acceptable circle drawn	1
	15) Circle is not too small or big, nor reproduced repeatedly	1
		Subtotal /2 Free-Drawn Total /15

SOURCE: Adapted from Freedman (1994).

Ricci et al. (2016) also presented a scoring system for the CDT based on factors extracted from a principal components analysis that included an omissions cluster (omission of numbers and hands), a code cluster (coding of numbers and hands), and a position cluster (incorrect positioning of hands, numbers in reverse order and incorrect position).

DEMOGRAPHIC EFFECTS

AGE

Age affects clock drawing (e.g., Freedman et al., 1994; Hubbard et al., 2008; Menon et al., 2012; Nyborn et al., 2013; Piers et al., 2017; Pinto & Peters, 2009; Santana et al., 2013; Sugawara et al., 2010), with performance declining particularly after 60 or 70 years of age, depending on the study (Bozikas et al., 2008; Caffarra et al., 2011; Kozora & Cullum, 1994; Marcopulos et al., 1997) and others suggesting the most dramatic decline after 75 years of age (Hubbard et al., 2008).

GENDER

Gender differences are reported to be small or not significant (Bozikas et al., 2008; Caffarra et al., 2011; Crowe et al., 2010; Hubbard et al., 2008; Kim & Chey, 2010). In their large

TABLE 9–17 Rouleau (1992) Quantitative Scoring Criteria for the Clock Drawing Test

QUALITATIVE FEATURE	RATING
Integrity of Clock Faces	2 points—if it is present without major distortion 1 point—if it is incomplete or with some distortion 0 points—if it is absent or totally inappropriate
Numbers	4 points—all present, in right order, with minimal error in spatial arrangement 3 points—all present, but errors in spatial arrangement 2 points—missing or added numbers, but no gross distortion of remaining numbers, or—numbers placed in counterclockwise direction, or—numbers all present, but gross distortions in spatial layout (e.g., hemi-neglect, numbers outside the clock) 1 point—missing or added numbers and gross spatial distortion 0 points—absence or poor representation of numbers
Hands	4 points—hands are in correct position and the appropriate size difference is represented 3 points—slight errors in the placement of the hands, or no representation of size difference 2 points—major errors in the placement of the hands 1 point—only one hand or poor representation of both hands 0 points—no hands or perseveration on hands

SOURCE: Adapted from Rouleau (1992).

TABLE 9–18 Rouleau (1992) Qualitative Scoring Criteria for the Clock Drawing Test

QUALITATIVE ERROR	HOW DEFINED
Size	Size of clock was small if less than 1.5″ or large if more than 5″
Graphic Difficulty	Mild—some distortions present in the lines of the clock face and/or hands and/or numbers, but overall performance is adequate. Moderate—distortions are evident, but overall performance is interpretable. Severe—distortions are evident and in some cases make it very difficult to interpret the overall performance
Stimulus Bound	A—hands are set to 10 to 11 instead of 10 after 11 (in free-drawn condition) B—time is written in letters or numbers, hands are either absent, hands are present but pointed between the numbers 10 and 11
Conceptual Deficit	A—misrepresentation of the clock itself B—misrepresentation of the time set on the clock or time is written on the clock.
Spatial/ Planning	A—neglect on left side of clock B—deficit in planning—with gap before 12, 3, 6, or 9 C—deficit in spatial layout of numbers without any pattern D—numbers written outside clock circle E—numbers written counterclockwise
Perseveration	A—perseveration of hands (more than 2 hands) B—perseveration of numbers or writing numbers beyond 1–12

SOURCE: Adapted from Rouleau (1992).

TABLE 9–19 Shulman (2000) Scoring Criteria for the Clock Drawing Test

5	Perfect clock
4	Minor visual-spatial errors
3	Inaccurate representation of "10 after 11" when the visual-spatial organization is well done
2	Moderate visual-spatial disorganization of numbers such that accurate denotation of "10 after 11" is impossible
1	Severe level of visual-spatial disorganization
0	Inability to make any reasonable representation of a clock

SOURCE: Adapted from Shulman (2000).

sample, Nyborn et al. (2013) reported minimal gender effects overall but noted on error analysis that women make more centering errors whereas men make more time setting/outline errors. Although men outperformed women across three scoring systems in one study, effects were small and did not require incorporation into normative data (Santana et al., 2013). Menon et al. (2012) found gender differences only for non-Hispanic white participants and only on CLOX 1 and not on CLOX 2. Sugawara et al. (2010) reported that CDT scores were higher for women in free and predrawn conditions.

EDUCATION

Education impacts performance (Bozikas et al., 2008; Cecato et al., 2012; Crowe et al., 2010; Kim & Chey, 2010; Nyborn et al., 2013; Pinto & Peters, 2009; Santana et al., 2013; Siciliano et al., 2016; Sugawara et al., 2010; von Gunten et al., 2008), with reading ability also related to performance (Hubbard et al., 2008; Kim & Chey, 2010; Nielsen & Jørgensen, 2013). In a review by Pinto and Peters (2009), effects of education were mixed; the authors concluded that the CDT may be overly simplistic for individuals with high education, and, at the same time, low literacy levels can impact performance. Thus, the CDT may be most suitable for use in groups with moderate levels of education. See "Evidence for Validity" for relationships between the CDT and IQ.

TABLE 9–20 Sunderland et al. (1989) and Libon et al. (1993) Scoring Criteria for the Clock Drawing Test

10	Normal drawing, numbers and hands in approximately correct positions, hour hand distinctly different from minute hand and approaching 4 o'clock.
9	Slight errors in placement of hands—not exactly on 8 and 4 (or 10 and 11), but not on one of the adjoining numbers—or one missing number on clock face.
8	More noticeable errors in placement of hour and minute hand (off by one number); number spacing shows a gap.
7	Placement of hands significantly off course (more than one number); very inappropriate spacing of numbers (e.g., all on one side).
6	Inappropriate use of clock hands (use of digital display or circling of numbers despite repeated instructions); crowding of numbers at one end of the clock or reversal of numbers.
5	Perseverative or otherwise inappropriate arrangement of numbers (e.g., numbers indicated by dots). Hands may be represented but do not clearly point at a number.
4	Numbers absent, written outside of clock, or in distorted sequence. Integrity of clock face missing. Hands not clearly represented or drawn outside of clock face.
3	Numbers and clock face no longer connected in the drawing. Hands not recognizably present.
2	Drawing reveals some evidence of instructions received, but representation of clock is only vague; inappropriate spatial arrangement of numbers.
1	Irrelevant, uninterpretable figure or no attempt.

NOTE: Roman numerals and embellishments of the clock (clock feet, bells) are acceptable.
SOURCE: Adapted from Sunderland et al. (1989) and Libon et al. (1993).

Interpretation of CDT performance should be done cautiously in people with limited levels of education (Kim & Chey, 2010; Lourenço et al., 2008). In one study of the impact of education on CDT performance, education accounted for nearly 22% of the variance, with literacy accounting for an additional 17% of the variance (Kim & Chey, 2010). Furthermore, qualitative errors made by individuals with low levels of formal education (<6 years) were similar to those made by patients with AD, indicating the importance of avoiding false positives in populations with low education levels. Specificity is improved in people with limited literacy when the CDT is combined with other instruments (Aprahamian et al., 2010).

ETHNICITY, NATIONALITY, AND LINGUISTIC EFFECTS

The CDT is commonly used internationally (e.g., Maruta et al., 2011, see also "Normative Data"). However, data regarding the influence of ethnicity and language on this test are limited. Some have reported no effect (e.g., Marcopulos et al., 1997), and others have reported that ethnicity effects are attenuated when education or reading level is accounted for (Crowe et al., 2010; Hubbard et al., 2008). La Rue et al. (1999) reported that participants who spoke only English scored higher than patients who spoke only Spanish. Some interaction effects have been reported, such that on CLOX 1, age, education, and gender affected performance only in non-Hispanic white participants, with age the only influential variable for Hispanic participants (Menon et al., 2012).

NORMATIVE DATA

Unlike many neuropsychological tests, the CDT is often interpreted according to cutoff values rather than normative reference standards (see Table 9–15). However, a number of normative studies have been published, as summarized in Table 9–21. Descriptions of administration/scoring referenced in Table 9–21 can be found under "Scoring" in this review.

Data from the majority of normative studies that corrected for age and education are presented in this section. The studies varied in screening criteria and sociodemographic characteristics of samples, with details described here.

Bozikas et al. (2008) normative data are based on Greek community-dwelling adults (45% female) with mean age of 45.99 (SD = 18.82) years. Screening was completed via interview (exclusion included history of

TABLE 9–21 Summary of Clock Drawing Test Normative Studies

REFERENCE	COUNTRY	SAMPLE SIZE	ADMINISTRATION/SCORING SYSTEM	AGE RANGE	NORM ADJUSTMENT: AGE	NORM ADJUSTMENT: GENDER	NORM ADJUSTMENT: EDUCATION OR WRAT-3 SCORE
Bozikas et al. (2008)	Greece	223	Freedman et al. (1994)	17 to 80	✓		✓
Caffara et al. (2011)[a]	Italy	248	Freedman et al. (1994)	20 to 89	✓		
Sugawara et al. (2010)	Japan	873	Freedman et al. (1994)	30 to 79	✓		✓
Kim & Chey (2010)	Korea	240	Todd et al. (1995) Rouleau et al. (1992)	55 to 84			✓
Santana et al. (2013)	Portugal	630	Rouleau et al. (1992) Cahn et al. (1996) Babins et al. (2008)	25 to 91	✓		✓
Von Guten et al. (2008)	Switzerland	242	Montani et al. (1997) Rouleau et al. (1992)[d]	60 to 90	✓		✓
Crowe et al. (2010)	USA	375	Royall (CLOX)	65 to 89	✓		✓
Hubbard et al. (2008)[a]	USA	207	Mendez et al. (1992) Cahn et al. (1996) Freund et al. (2005)	55 to 98	✓		✓
Menon et al. (2011)[b]	USA	278 and 168	Royall (CLOX)	40 to 93	✓		✓
Nyborn et al. (2013)[c]	USA	1476	Nyborn et al. (2013)[e] (KMFHSClock Drawing Test)	43 to 91	✓	✓	✓

NOTE: Administration/Scoring System shown under the section "Scoring" in this chapter.

[a]Crowe et al. (2010) and Hubbard et al. (2008) provide normative data based on Wide Range Achievement Test, Third Edition (WRAT-3) score, rather than education.

[b]Menon et al. (2011) present normative data for sub-samples of Caucasian and Hispanic individuals.

[c]Nyborn et al. (2013) present normative data simultaneously corrected for age and education, with gender specific normative data presented separately.

[d]Modification of Montani and Rouleau scoring systems.

[e]KMFHSClock Drawing Test = Kaplan Modified Framingham Heart Study Clock Drawing Test.

neurological disease, head injury, psychiatric disorder, subjective memory problems, or substance abuse). See Table 9–22.

Caffara et al. (2011) provided Italian norms which included younger participants via university student and employee populations and older individuals via senior citizen centers and parish communities. Participants were screened for substance abuse, psychiatric disorders, TBI, stroke, transient ischemic attacks, seizures, dementia, or memory complaints. Participants had a Mini-Mental State Examination (MMSE) score of at least 24. Highly educated participants were somewhat underrepresented in older age groups. See Tables 9–23 and 9–24.

US NORMATIVE SAMPLES

Crowe et al. (2010) recruited their normative sample of American community-dwelling older adults as part of a longitudinal study of aging (see Allman, Sawyer, & Roseman, 2006). Exclusion was based on an MMSE cutoff or a dementia diagnosis. Average age was 72.8 years

TABLE 9–22 Normative Data for the Clock Drawing Test in a Greek Sample, by Age and Education

		MEAN CLOCK DRAWING SCORES OF THE GROUPS BASED ON AGE AND EDUCATIONAL LEVEL											
		AGE 17 TO 59 YEARS (N = 146)						AGE 60 TO 80 YEARS (N = 77)					
		EDUC. 1–9 YEARS (*N* = 31)		EDUC. 10–12 YEARS (*N* = 43)		EDUC. 13 YEARS (*N* = 72)		EDUC. 1–9 YEARS (*N* = 24)		EDUC. 10–12 YEARS (*N* = 24)		EDUC. 13+ YEARS (*N* = 29)	
CLOCK		MEAN	*SD*	MEAN	*SD*	MEAN	*SD*	MEAN	*SD*	MEAN	*SD*	MEAN	*SD*
A	(6:45)	14.35	0.80	14.56	0.63	14.67	0.58	12.92	2.04	14.17	1.10	14.38	1.08
B	(6:05)	12.45	0.72	12.63	0.66	12.85	0.40	10.96	1.94	12.13	1.33	12.59	1.18
C	(11:10)	10.68	0.60	10.74	0.49	10.90	0.34	9.63	1.90	10.25	1.42	10.79	0.49
D	(8:20)	10.26	0.82	10.26	0.62	10.60	0.57	8.88	1.78	10.63	0.68	10.76	0.51
E	(3:00)	10.58	0.67	10.53	0.80	10.94	0.23	9.29	2.22	10.54	1.25	10.88	0.44

NOTE: Clock A = free-drawn and 6:45; Clock B = predrawn and 6:05; Clock C = clock face and numbers provided by examiner and examinee sets hands for 11:10; Clock D = clock face and numbers provided by examiner and examinee sets hands for 8:20, Clock E = clock face and numbers provided by examiner and examinee sets hands for 3:00.

SOURCE: Adapted from Bozikas et al. (2008).

TABLE 9–23 Clock Drawing Test Normative Data for an Italian Sample for Free-Drawn, Predrawn, and Examiner-Drawn Conditions

	AGE GROUP (IN YEARS)						
CONDITION	20 TO 29	30 TO 39	40 TO 49	50 TO 59	60 TO 69	70 TO 79	80 TO 89
Free-Drawn	12.25 (2.55)	13.37 (1.58)	13.13 (1.69)	12.14 (2.43)	12.31 (2.19)	11.91 (2.49)	11.83 (2.82)
Predrawn	10.77 (1.95)	10.87 (2.05)	11.59 (1.75)	10.76 (1.79)	10.74 (2.05)	10.72 (2.31)	10.73 (2.48)
Examiner-Drawn	31.82 (1.93)	30.87 (2.35)	31.37 (1.53)	30.89 (1.48)	30.78 (3.13)	30.06 (4.58)	30.26 (4.75)
Total	53.09 (4.33)	54.26 (4.01)	55.86 (3.45)	53.91 (4.17)	54.10 (5.69)	53.18 (8.30)	53.47 (7.88)

NOTE: Standard deviations in parentheses.

SOURCE: Adapted from Caffara et al. (2011).

(*SD* = 5.3 years). The sample was 53% female, 47% African American, and 48% rural-dwelling. The majority of the sample had 13 or more years of education (40% of the sample), with 30% with 12 years of education, and 24% with seven to 11 years. Participants were from three rural and two urban counties in central Alabama and stratified by ethnicity (African American/Caucasian), gender, and county (rural/urban). The normative sample for the CLOX in this study was comprised of people who completed cognitive testing at baseline and at four-year follow-up. See Tables 9–25 and 9–26.

Hubbard et al. (2008) recruited participants from a US patient control registry; participants were at least 55 years of age, evaluated annually with physical and neurological examinations, informant interviews, and neuropsychological tests. Inclusion criteria were: received a consensus diagnosis of "non-case" status, nonimpaired performance (i.e., ≤1.5 *SD*s) on neuropsychological tests, above cutoffs on the Clinical Dementia Rating Scale (CDR), the MMSE, and the GDS. Participants were a mean age of 71.3 (8.4 *SD*), and the sample was approximately 65% female, 84% Caucasian, and 15% African American, with a mean education of 16.6 years (*SD* = 2.7).

Menon et al. (2012) provide US normative data from a sample of English- and Spanish-speaking Hispanic and non-Hispanic white participants who were part of a study of health among people from rural areas, with participants from regions along the Texass–New Mexico border. Half of the Hispanic sample self-identified as being of Mexican origin and had greater mastery of Spanish than English, and tests were administered in Spanish for these participants.

Participants were recruited in the community. Participants underwent medical examination, laboratory investigations, neuropsychological testing, and participant and informant interviews. Cutoff scores from the MMSE and CDR, as well as executive function and visuospatial tests, were used to exclude participants from CLOX 1 and CLOX 2, respectively. For the CLOX 1 subsample, the mean age was 58.6 (*SD* = 11.4); this subsample was 81% female, 38% Hispanic, and had a mean education level of 12.2 years (*SD* = 3.8). For the CLOX 2 subsample, the mean age was 58.5 (*SD* = 11.2), with sample composition as 73% female, 39% Hispanic, and with a mean education level of 12.1 years (*SD* = 4.1). See Tables 9–27 and 9–28.

Nyborn et al. (2013) provide US normative data from volunteers in the Framingham Heart Study (FHS) Offspring Cohort, which included offspring and spouses of participants involved in the Framingham heart study to identify risk factors for cardiovascular and cerebrovascular diseases. Examinations occurred every four years (medical history, physical examinations, and laboratory tests). People who had sustained stroke, dementia, or other neurological diseases were excluded. The mean age of participants was 67.46 (*SD* = 8.93); the sample was 54% female, Caucasian, with approximately 40% of the sample having a college education (57% had college or high school; 3% had less than high school).

TABLE 9–24 Clock Drawing Test Cutoff Scores for an Italian Sample for Free-Drawn, Predrawn, and Examiner-Drawn Conditions

EQUIVALENT SCORE	FREE-DRAWN	PREDRAWN	EXAMINER-DRAWN	TOTAL
0	≤7.56	≤6.54	≤24.49	≤42.16
1	7.57–9.37	6.55–8.18	24.50–26.81	42.17–46.34
2	9.38–11.18	8.19–9.82	26.82–29.13	46.35–50.52
3	1.19–12.99	9.83–11.46	29.14–31.46	50.53–54.69
4	≥13.00	≥11.47	≥31.47	≥54.70

SOURCE: Adapted from Caffara et al. (2011).

TABLE 9–25 US Normative Data for the Clock Drawing Test, CLOX 1, by Reading Ability and Age Group

	AGE GROUP					
	AGE 65 TO 69		AGE 70 TO 74		75+	
WRAT 3 SCORE	N	MEAN (SD)	N	MEAN (SD)	N	MEAN (SD)
≤38	31	11.23 (2.33)	50	11.06 (1.79)	45	10.36 (2.36)
39–46	51	11.75 (2.31)	40	11.50 (2.44)	33	12.18 (2.34)
≥47	38	12.63 (2.05)	45	12.51 (1.63)	42	11.31 (2.89)

NOTE: *SD*, standard deviation; CLOX, Executive Clock Drawing Test; WRAT 3, Wide Range Achievement Test, 3rd edition.

SOURCE: Adapted from Crowe et al. (2010).

TABLE 9–26 US Normative Data for the Clock Drawing Test, CLOX 2, by Reading Ability and Age Group

WRAT 3 SCORE	AGE GROUP					
	AGE 65 TO 69		AGE 70 TO 74		75+	
	N	MEAN (*SD*)	*N*	MEAN (*SD*)	*N*	MEAN (*SD*)
≤38	31	13.16 (1.32)	50	12.90 (1.44)	45	12.47 (1.44)
39–46	51	13.76 (0.86)	40	13.58 (0.90)	33	13.72 (0.91)
≥47	38	13.86 (0.91)	45	14.02 (0.83)	42	13.54 (1.21)

NOTES: *SD;* standard deviation; CLOX, Executive Clock Drawing Test; WRAT-3, Wide Range Achievement Test, 3rd edition.

SOURCE: Adapted from Crowe et al. (2010).

KOREAN NORMATIVE SAMPLE

Kim and Chey (2010) recruited older participants from community centers, workplaces, senior citizen pavilions, and churches in Korea. The mean age was 69.13 years (*SD* = 8.11), with a mean education level of 7.48 years (*SD* = 5.06). Inclusion criteria were absence of cognitive disorders leading to functional impairments in everyday life, living independently, absence of dementia, psychiatric, and neurologic conditions, absence of physical conditions with impact on cognition, thyroid disease, and no loss of consciousness for more than 1 hour. Some participants were further evaluated on the basis of a neuropsychological interview (see the paper for details).

PORTUGUESE NORMATIVE SAMPLE

Santana et al. (2013) recruited a Portuguese community-based sample. Inclusion criteria included being a native speaker of Portuguese; absence of motor, visual, or auditory deficits, independent ADLs, and absence of substance abuse, psychiatric, neurologic disorders, chronic systemic diseases, significant depressive symptoms, or medication that can impact cognition. The normative sample had a mean age of approximately 56 years (*SD* = 15.3) and was approximately 64% female, with a mean of 8.08 years of education (*SD* = 4.58). See Tables 9–29 and 9–30.

JAPANESE NORMATIVE SAMPLE

Sugawara et al. (2010) reported Japanese normative data for a 63% female sample, with a mean age of 57.5 years (*SD* = 11.9) and a mean education of 11.3 years (*SD* = 2.1)

TABLE 9–27 US Hispanic Normative Data for the Clock Drawing Test, CLOX 1, by Age Group

AGE GROUP			
40 TO 51 YEARS		52 OR MORE YEARS	
N	MEAN (*SD*)	*N*	MEAN (*SD*)
57	12.7 (1.6)	47	12.4 (1.8)

NOTE: *SD*, standard deviation; CLOX, Executive Clock Drawing Test.

SOURCE: Adapted from Menon et al. (2011).

participating in a broader study. Inclusion/exclusion criteria were not detailed. The Freedman et al. (1994) scoring method was used to generate the norms. The data are presented in Tables 9–31 to 9–34.

SWISS NORMATIVE SAMPLE

Von Gunten et al. (2008) recruited 242 participants (72% female) from a French-speaking area of the Swiss cantons. The inclusion criteria were independent, home-dwelling, first language French, eyesight sufficiently adequate to read, hearing sufficiently adequate to repeat a sentence, and an MMSE cutoff. Exclusion criteria were subjective memory impairment that interfered with ADLs, neurologic or psychiatric disorder, substance abuse, MMSE and GDS cutoffs, and performance on additional cognitive tests (details not provided). The mean age was 73.4 years (*SD* = 8.4), with 26% of the sample with low levels of education, 36% with intermediate levels, and 38% with high levels of education. The overall mean MMSE score was 27.66. A modification of Montani and Rouleau scoring systems was used. Interested readers should refer to the source for the full description of the modified scoring and norms.

EVIDENCE FOR RELIABILITY

EVIDENCE FOR INTERNAL RELIABILITY

Santana et al. (2013) reported that in a Portuguese population, the Rouleau et al. (1992) and Cahn et al. (1996) scoring systems showed weak internal reliability (.49 and .49), and the Babins system was associated with good internal reliability (.88).

EVIDENCE FOR TEST-RETEST RELIABILITY, MEASURING CHANGE, AND PRACTICE EFFECTS

Retest reliability for clock drawing after 12 weeks is adequate ($r = .78$) for patients with AD (Mendez et al., 1992; see also Jørgensen et al., 2015; Lezak, 2012; Nair et al., 2010; Royall et al., 1998; Suhr et al., 1998; Tene et al., 2016; Tuokko, 2000; Tuokko et al., 1995).

EVIDENCE FOR INTERRATER RELIABILITY

Overall, interrater and/or intrarater reliability is high to very high ($r > .80$) for most methods that have been examined (Jørgensen et al., 2015; Mazancova, Nikolai, Stepankova, Kopecek, & Bezdicek, 2017; Lezak, 2012; Nair et al., 2010; Nyborn et al., 2013; Royall et al., 1998; Suhr et al., 1998; Tene et al., 2016; Tuokko, 2000).

EVIDENCE FOR VALIDITY

RELATIONSHIPS WITH OTHER TESTS

Given its integrative nature, it is perhaps unsurprising that the CDT relates to a number of abilities. It shows moderate correlations with measures of temporal orientation

TABLE 9–28 US Non-Hispanic Whites Normative Data for the Clock Drawing Test, CLOX 1, by Age, Education, and Gender Groups

	AGE GROUP			
	40 TO 61 YEARS		62 OR MORE YEARS	
EDUCATION	FEMALES	MALES	FEMALES	MALES
8 to 13 years	*N* = 32, Mean = 12.9, *SD* = 1.6	*N* = 6, Mean = 12.8, *SD* = 1.5	*N* = 35, Mean = 12.7, *SD* = 1.6	*N* = 17, Mean = 11.5, *SD* = 2.3
14+ years	*N* = 29, Mean = 13.8, *SD* = 1.1	*N* = 16, Mean = 12.5, *SD* = 2.1	*N* = 24, Mean = 13.1, *SD* = 2.0	*N* = 13, Mean = 12.7, *SD* = 1.3

NOTE: *SD*, standard deviation; CLOX, Executive Clock Drawing Test.
SOURCE: Adapted from Menon et al. (2011).

(Suhr et al., 1998), visual-spatial/visual-constructional skill (Libon et al., 1993, 1996; Suhr et al., 1998), and executive functioning and attention (Libon et al., 1993; Parsey & Schmitter-Edgecombe, 2011; Suhr et al., 1998; Terwindt et al., 2016). Semantic and verbal memory is also implicated (Ahmed et al., 2016; Libon et al., 1996; Parsey & Schmitter-Edgecombe, 2011). The CDT also provides an indication of general cognitive functioning, correlating moderately to highly with global measures such as the MMSE, dementia screeners, and other global measures (Aprahamian et al., 2010; Fuzikawa et al., 2007; Mendez et al., 1992; Royall et al., 1998; Santana et al., 2013; Shulman, 2000; Smedslund et al., 2015; Terwindt et al., 2016).

It has also been suggested that different clock drawing conditions show differential relationships with cognitive skills. For example, Royall and colleagues (Royall & Espino, 2002; Royall et al., 1998, 2004) argue that the CLOX 1 (free-drawn) is sensitive to executive functioning, correlating highly with measures of executive function, whereas CLOX 2 (copying) is more dependent on visual-constructional skills. Evidence for this is mixed (see Cosentio et al., 2004; Libon et al., 1993, 1996; Royall & Espino, 2002; Royall et al., 1992; Royall et al., 2004).

CLINICAL STUDIES

Dementia. With respect to diagnostic accuracy in dementia, sensitivity tends to be relatively high, with specificity typically variable (e.g., sensitivity from 59% to 98%, specificity from 38% to 95%; see Chen et al., 2018; Smedslund et al., 2015; Tuokko, 2000). The Shulman method (see "Scoring") frequently yields among the highest sensitivity and specificity estimates (Brodaty & Moore, 1997; Ehreke et al., 2011; Schramm et al., 2002; Storey et al., 2002). A comparison of five clock drawing methods in 462 consecutive memory clinic patients (Berger et al., 2008) suggested that all methods that involved time setting were associated with higher sensitivities (81 to 93%) and negative predictive values. Specificity was relatively higher for methods that did not require time setting (64%, 81%). Inadequate sensitivity (approximately 41 to 56%) and specificity (approximately 71 to 85%) of the CDT was reported using other scoring systems (Lee et al., 2008). A modified Rouleau method based on qualitative errors was found to have greater sensitivity than a standard version (Parsey & Schmitter-Edgecombe, 2011). Importantly, scoring systems need not be long to be accurate. Existing scoring systems have been modified to include six or fewer scoring dimensions that simplify scoring while also retaining diagnostic accuracy (Jørgensen et al., 2015; Jouk & Tuokko, 2012; Ricci et al., 2016).

The CDT has utility in differentiating healthy controls from persons with dementia (e.g., Manos, 1999; Royall et al., 1998; Tuokko et al., 1992; Freedman et al., 1994; Rouleau et al., 1992). The CDT also appears useful in documenting severity of cognitive impairment (Manos & Wu, 1994;

TABLE 9–29 Portuguese Normative Data for the Clock Drawing Test, Using Rouleau et al. (1992) Scoring System, by Age and Education

	AGE					
EDUCATION	25 TO 49	50 TO 64	≥65	65 TO 74	≥75	ALL AGES
N	25	89	–	87	49	250
1 to 4 years	8.44 (1.94)	8.06 (1.93)	–	7.15 (2.52)	6.49 (2.41)	7.47 (2.33)
N	63	58	44	–	–	165
5 to 9 years	9.02 (1.59)	8.37 (1.55)	8.23 (1.99)			8.72 (1.71)
N	55	33	18	–	–	106
10 to 12 years	9.35 (1.14)	9.30 (1.02)	9.11 (1.23)			9.29 (1.11)
N	60	31	18	–	–	109
>12 years	9.65 (0.76)	9.45 (1.12)	9.33 (0.77)			9.54 (0.88)
N	203	211	216	–	–	630
All education	9.22 (1.37)	8.65 (1.69)	7.56 (2.38)	–	–	8.46 (1.99)

SOURCE: Adapted from Santana et al. (2013).

TABLE 9-30 Portuguese Normative Data for the Clock Drawing Test, Using Babins et al. (2008) Scoring System, by Age and Education

	AGE					
EDUCATION	25 TO 49	50 TO 64	≥65	65 TO 74	≥75	ALL AGES
N	25	89	–	87	49	250
1 to 4 years	14.88 (3.37)	13.57 (3.57)		12.10 (4.59)	11.32 (4.40)	12.71 (4.24)
N	63	58	44	–	–	165
5 to 9 years	15.92 (2.84)	15.41 (2.47)	14.48 (3.55)			15.36 (2.97)
N	55	33	18	–	–	106
10 to 12 years	16.91 (1.44)	16.33 (1.85)	16.11 (2.35)			16.59 (1.77)
N	60	31	18	–	–	109
>12 years	17.22 (1.20)	16.84 (1.70)	16.72 (0.96)			17.03 (1.33)
N	203	211	216	–	–	630
All education	16.44 (2.33)	14.99 (3.10)	13.08 (4.39)			14.80 (3.67)

SOURCE: Adapted from Santana et al. (2013).

Petrova et al., 2016; Royall et al., 1998; Sunderland et al., 1989; Tuokko, 2000). In their systematic review of the CDT as a cognitive screener, Pinto and Peters (2009) reported that it had low sensitivity and variable specificity in patients with mild dementia, with improved diagnostic accuracy in moderate and severe dementia.

The utility of the CDT in differential diagnosis between dementia subtypes is less clear. Some authors have reported that the CDT has some value in differentiating AD from vascular dementia (Heinik et al., 2002; Kitabayashi et al., 2001). Others, however, have not found evidence for the test's utility in this regard (Barr et al., 1992; Cosentino et al., 2004; Libon et al., 1993, 1996; Tan et al., 2015; Wolf-Klein et al., 1989).

In one study, errors were not found to discriminate between dementia subtypes (Lee et al., 2011). However, spatial and planning errors were found to be most common in moderate dementia and conceptual deficits more common in severe dementia. A four-point scoring system was able to differentiate between healthy controls and patients with AD, but sensitivity and specificity was very poor for differentiation of vascular dementia from AD (55 to 69% sensitivity vs. 22 to 33% specificity; Tan et al., 2015).

Research suggests that qualitative data may be more effective than the overall score at differentiating between dementia subtypes (Tan et al., 2015; see also Libon et al., 1993, 1996; Rouleau et al., 1992). Although total CDT score did not differentiate early-onset AD from FTD, qualitative analysis, specifically hand placement, effectively discriminated between groups, with early-onset AD performing worse than FTD (Barrows et al., 2015).

TABLE 9-31 Japanese CDT Norms for Males as a Function of Age Groups

	30–39 YEARS	40–49 YEARS	50–59 YEARS	60–69 YEARS	70–79 YEARS
N	32	63	77	74	60
Free-drawn	13.19 (1.55)	13.25 (1.40)	11.94 (3.07)	12.49 (2.54)	11.27 (3.95)
Predrawn	12.44 (0.67)	12.59 (0.61)	12.01 (1.81)	11.91 (1.84)	11.52 (2.63)
Examiner 1	10.75 (0.51)	10.81 (0.50)	10.68 (0.64)	10.70 (0.64)	10.03 (2.25)
Examiner 2	10.31 (0.64)	10.57 (0.61)	10.38 (0.63)	10.24 (0.74)	9.67 (2.24)
Examiner 3	10.94 (0.25)	10.95 (0.21)	10.91 (0.49)	10.70 (0.64)	10.20 (2.33)

NOTE: Mean (*SD*).

Free-drawn = 6:45. Predrawn = 6:05, Examiner 1 = clock face and numbers provided by examiner and examinee sets hands for 11:10; Examiner 2 = clock face and numbers provided by examiner and examinee sets hands for 8:20; Examiner 3 = clock face and numbers provided by examiner and examinee sets hands for 3:00.

SOURCE: Sugawara et al. (2010).

TABLE 9-32 Japanese CDT Norms for Females as a Function of Age Groups

	30–39 YEARS	40–49 YEARS	50–59 YEARS	60–69 YEARS	70–79 YEARS
N	43	81	162	155	93
Free-drawn	13.51 (1.24)	13.57 (1.38)	13.06 (2.17)	12.62 (2.99)	11.94 (4.03)
Predrawn	12.70 (0.67)	12.54 (0.84)	12.30 (1.54)	12.30 (1.50)	11.88 (2.11)
Examiner 1	10.70 (0.51)	10.78 (0.45)	10.78 (0.49)	10.60 (0.84)	10.05 (2.07)
Examiner 2	10.19 (0.82)	10.42 (0.61)	10.38 (0.68)	10.18 (0.76)	9.61 (2.02)
Examiner 3	10.95 (0.30)	10.90 (0.30)	10.90 (0.49)	10.79 (0.63)	10.26 (1.80)

NOTE: Mean (*SD*).

Free-drawn = 6:45, Predrawn = 6:05, Examiner 1 = clock face and numbers provided by examiners and examinees set hands for 11:10, Examiner 2 = clock face and numbers provided by examiners and examinees set hands for 8:20, Examiner 3 = clock face and numbers provided by examiners and examinees set hands for 3:00.

SOURCE: Sugawara et al. (2010).

TABLE 9-33 Japanese CDT Norms for Males as a Function of Age and Education

	AGE 30 TO 59 YEARS (*N* = 172)			AGE 60 TO 79 YEARS (*N* = 134)		
	EDUCATION			EDUCATION		
	1–9 YEARS	10–12 YEARS	13+ YEARS	1–9 YEARS	10–12 YEARS	13+ YEARS
N	16	125	31	64	58	12
Free-drawn	12.19 (2.66)	12.69 (2.50)	12.74 (1.81)	11.19 (3.89)	12.71 (2.49)	12.25 (2.45)
Predrawn	11.94 (2.72)	12.35 (1.14)	12.29 (0.90)	11.58 (2.38)	11.91 (2.05)	11.67 (2.27)
Examiner 1	10.81 (0.40)	10.72 (0.62)	10.77 (0.43)	10.34 (1.36)	10.57 (1.49)	9.92 (2.94)
Examiner 2	10.31 (0.60)	10.42 (0.65)	10.58 (0.56)	9.91 (1.42)	10.12 (1.51)	9.75 (2.80)
Examiner 3	10.75 (1.00)	10.94 (0.23)	10.97 (0.18)	10.47 (1.45)	10.59 (1.52)	10.00 (2.86)

NOTE: Mean (*SD*).

Free-drawn = 6:45, Predrawn = 6:05, Examiner 1 = clock face and numbers provided by examiners and examinees set hands for 11:10, Examiner 2 = clock face and numbers provided by examiners and examinees set hands for 8:20, Examiner 3 = clock face and numbers provided by examiners and examinees set hands for 3:00.

SOURCE: Sugawara et al. (2010).

Diagnostic accuracy of the CDT is improved in differentiating between dementia and nondementia groups (e.g., healthy controls, MCI, depression) when combined with other methods, such as the MMSE (Aprahamian et al., 2010; Cacho et al., 2010; Heinik & Shaikewitz, 2009; Milian et al., 2013; Zhou & Jia, 2008). Similarly, the CDT has been described to have improved utility when combined with an enhanced cued recall measure, accurately classifying 70% of a sample comprised of persons with dementia and MCI subtypes (Saka & Elibol, 2009).

The CDT appears less effective at differentiating MCI from healthy controls compared to differentiating persons with dementia from healthy controls. For example, Nair et al. (2010) randomly assigned clocks from predetermined groups diagnosed via consensus (cognitive control, MCI, and AD). Dichotomous ratings yielded high sensitivity and specificity rates (75%, 81%) in differentiating between AD and healthy controls. However, decreased sensitivity estimates were associated with differentiation between patients with MCI and controls (sensitivity 47%; specificity 81%).

Diagnostic accuracy may relate to the nature of the scoring systems used. For example more complex scoring systems have been found to be better at identifying MCI than simple scoring systems (Rubínová et al., 2014). However, although sensitivity was high, specificity was poor for all methods (see also Donnelly et al., 2008). In a systematic review, variable sensitivity (range 50 to 80%) and specificity (range 65 to 90%) of the CDT in detecting MCI was reported (Ehreke et al., 2010). However, not all research has reported this pattern of findings, for example, finding high specificity but weaker sensitivity (Forti et al., 2010).

Similar to differentiation of dementia subtypes, examination of qualitative errors, as opposed to total scores, may be of benefit. For example, Parsey and Schmitter-Edgecombe (2011) reported that conceptual and graphic errors were more common in MCI, with more errors across categories in persons with AD. Using an 18-item scoring system (modification of Freedman et al., 1994), Babins et al. (2008) reported individual features of the clock (e.g., two hands, hour hand toward the correct number) differentiated those who progressed to dementia from those who did not.

Clock drawing is useful for predicting cognitive decline. In one study, the CDT and episodic memory measures were

TABLE 9-34 Japanese CDT Norms for Females as a Function of Age and Education

	AGE 30 TO 59 YEARS (*N* = 286)			AGE 60 TO 79 YEARS (*N* = 248)		
	EDUCATION			EDUCATION		
	1–9 YEARS	10–12 YEARS	13+ YEARS	1–9 YEARS	10–12 YEARS	13+ YEARS
N	32	181	73	147	80	21
Free-drawn	12.72 (2.49)	13.25 (1.84)	13.58 (1.54)	11.94 (3.67)	13.01 (2.87)*	12.86 (3.28)
Predrawn	11.94 (2.44)	12.45 (1.01)	12.60 (1.10)	11.97 (2.03)	12.49 (0.83)	12.05 (2.22)
Examiner 1	10.75 (0.51)	10.78 (0.47)	10.74 (0.50)	10.22 (1.73)	10.73 (0.53)	10.38 (1.53)
Examiner 2	10.09 (1.03)	10.38 (0.60)	10.44 (0.69)	9.78 (1.65)	10.30 (0.58)	10.05 (1.53)
Examiner 3	10.81 (0.47)	10.94 (0.26)	10.86 (0.65)	10.44 (1.47)	10.88 (0.33)	10.57 (1.43)

NOTE: Mean (*SD*). *$p < 0.05$ by Mann-Whitney test with Bonferroni correction.

Free-drawn = 6:45, Predrawn = 6:05, Examiner 1 = clock face and numbers provided by examiners and examinees set hands for 11:10, Examiner 2 = clock face and numbers provided by examiners and examinees set hands for 8:20, Examiner 3 = clock face and numbers provided by examiners and examinees set hands for 3:00.

SOURCE: Sugawara et al. (2010).

the best predictors of conversion from MCI to AD over four-year follow-up, even when other variables were considered, including demographic variables, APOE genotype, and biomarkers (Gomar et al., 2014). The CDT, when combined with the MMSE and biomarkers, yielded the highest diagnostic accuracy (85%) for predicting subsequent development of dementia among individuals with MCI compared to cognitive tests or biomarkers alone (Palmqvist et al., 2012).

In a systematic review of studies involving longitudinal analysis of the CDT, conceptual clock drawing errors were the most influential variable for prediction of decline (Amodeo et al., 2015). The CDT was able to differentiate cognitively intact older adults from those who would progress to dementia up to two years after baseline assessment. Additionally, the CDT differentiated between people with MCI and those who subsequently developed dementia up to six years post-baseline.

Clock drawing was moderately correlated with ADLs in AD according to a meta-analysis (Martyr & Clare, 2012). The CDT was also part of a predictive model found to accurately predict driving in patients with dementia (Carr et al., 2011); see also the section "Driving and Daily Functioning."

In dementia populations, the CDT has been used primarily as a diagnostic tool or screener. However, the CDT has also been used in studies aimed to evaluate treatment outcomes in patients with dementia, including memantine (Paskavitz et al., 2007), donepezil (Fukui et al., 2006), rivastigmine (Seibert et al., 2012), dual-task physical activity training (Pedroso et al., 2012), exercise (Stevens & Killeen, 2006), vitamin E treatment (Lloret et al., 2009), and Ginkgo biloba (Napryeyenko et al., 2009; Yancheva et al., 2009).

Stroke. The CDT appears to have less utility in stroke compared to dementia, although data are limited. Nøkleby et al. (2008) reported that clock drawing has relatively poor sensitivity and specificity in screening for cognitive impairment after stroke when compared with other cognitive screens, such as Cognistat and the Screening Instrument for Neuropsychological Impairments in Stroke (Nokleby et al., 2008). Rasch analysis of the CLOX 1 and 2 in stroke patients suggested that CLOX 1 met Rasch model expectations, with CLOX 2 having two items with misfit, as well as a ceiling effect, leading the authors to suggest omission of CLOX 2 (Zuverza-Chavarria & Tsanadis, 2011).

However, some research has reported that the CDT, particularly qualitative features of clock drawing, is more accurate than quantitative features at differentiating stroke subgroups by location (Suhr et al., 1998). Other research has noted relationships between the CDT and neurologic deficits post-stroke (Pustokhanova & Morozova, 2013) and improvements on the CDT following cognitive rehabilitation (Prokopenko et al., 2013).

PD. Patients with PD have been found to perform poorly on the CDT (Stella et al., 2007). In one study, sensitivity and specificity of diagnosing dementia in PD patients was reported to be 71% and 69%; diagnostic accuracy was poorer in patients with comorbid depression (specificity of 56% vs. 71% in non-depressed patients; Riedel et al., 2013).

Patients with left-sided onset of PD as well as non-tremor subtypes perform worse on the CDT than controls, with the Rouleau method identified as the most accurate scoring system for differentiating among groups in one study (Seichepine et al., 2015).

The CDT predicts pedestrian safety errors in patients with PD (Lin et al., 2013) and has been used to assess outcome in patients with PD with dementia treated with memantine (Litvinenko et al., 2010) or galantamine (Litvinenko et al., 2008).

Psychiatric Conditions. The CDT appears to have promise in schizophrenia. Patients with schizophrenia perform significantly worse than matched healthy controls on the CDT (Kaneda et al., 2013), even when matched on the MMSE (Bozikas et al., 2004; Herrmann et al., 1999; Tene et al., 2016). In patients with psychotic disorders, the CDT is inversely related to severity of psychosis and improves from admission to discharge (Tene et al., 2016). The CDT is related to symptom severity and length of current hospitalization, as well as to life skills in patients with chronic schizophrenia (Okamura et al., 2012).

The effect of depression on CDT performance is mixed. For example, in one study, depressive symptoms were negatively correlated with CDT scores (Santana et al., 2013). In contrast, Herrmann et al. (1998) found that, although patients with AD were impaired on the test, patients with major affective disorder did not differ from age-matched controls (Bodner et al., 2004). Others have also reported little impact of depression on performance (Bodner et al., 2004; Brodaty & Moore, 1997; Manos, 1997).

Other Conditions. The CDT has been identified as a useful screener in evaluating cognitive impairment in primary care (Janssen et al., 2017), older adults with heart failure (Piotrowicz, Fedyk-Łukasik, Skalska, & Grodzicki, 2018), HD (Terwindt et al., 2016), and TBI (Hazan, Zhang, Brenkel, Shulman, & Feinstein, 2017) among other groups. For example, people with moderate to severe TBI performed worse on the CDT than did mild TBI patients, and the CDT and the TMT-B in combination were associated with a sensitivity of 65% and a specificity of 82% in an acute rehabilitation setting (de Guise et al., 2011). In carriers of the HD gene mutation, mean sensitivity across scoring methods examined was 82% and mean specificity was 79% (Terwindt et al., 2016). CDT performance is worse in patients with fibromyalgia compared to controls and correlated with pain intensity (Can & Gencay-Can, 2012). The CDT was associated with a sensitivity of 92% and specificity of 73% in a hospice population (Henderson et al., 2007). Metabolic syndrome also predicts decline on the CDT (Viscogliosi et al., 2016).

Driving and Daily Functioning. The CDT appears to relate to driving safety. The CDT was found to be a predictor of pedal errors in healthy older adult drivers, and unsafe drivers performed worse on the CDT than did safe and restricted drivers (Freund & Colgrove, 2008). A specificity of 85% and a sensitivity of 80% for a battery that included the CDT was reported for predicting on-road driving performance, with the CDT identified as the third best predictor in the battery after the TMT-A and age (De Raedt & Ponjaert-Kristoffersen, 2001).

In addition to driving, the CDT relates to a number of other functional outcomes, including functional outcome of hip fracture (Adunsky et al., 2002) and functional impairment in community-dwelling older adults (Royall & Espino, 2002; Royall et al., 2000, 2004). Clock drawing is related to knowledge of medication regime in older adults (Sela-Katz et al., 2010) and history of falls (Yamada et al., 2013). Age, CLOX 1, and executive measures independently contributed to prediction of the level of care required in an older retiree sample, with a classification accuracy rate exceeding 60% (Royall et al., 2005).

NEUROANATOMICAL CORRELATES AND IMAGING STUDIES

Most of the research relating to neuroanatomical correlates of clock drawing has been conducted via lesion studies and in dementia populations. Consistent with its multifaceted nature, performance on the CDT has been associated with frontal, temporal, and parietal regions (de Guise et al., 2010; Shoyama et al., 2011).

There is some research to suggest that areas in the right hemisphere are relatively more involved in construction, whereas left regions are relatively more involved in processing detailed elements on the test (Trojano et al., 2002). There also may be differences in performance related to the location of the lesion. Based on case studies, Freedman et al. (1994) suggested that major spatial disorganization (sometimes with retention of the essential elements of the clock) can be expected in patients with focal right parietal lesions; those with frontal lesions show difficulty integrating the multiple task demands of clock drawing (e.g., number sequence and spatial layout); patients with left posterior lesions may show difficulty with numbers and time settings because of receptive aphasia; and similar problems may occur with left anterior lesions (e.g., setting the clock after instead of before). Similarly, impairments on the CDT are associated with damage to right parietal regions (supramarginal gyrus) and left inferior frontoparietal regions; visuospatial errors are more common following right-sided damage, and time setting errors are more common following left hemisphere damage (Tranel et al., 2008).

Research with patients with AD using a number of neuroimaging methods indicates that a broad range of brain regions and networks are involved in the CDT, including frontal, temporal, and parietal regions (Brugnolo et al., 2010; Hirjak, Sambataro et al., 2019; Hirjak, Wolf et al., 2017; Kim et al., 2009; Matsuoka et al., 2013; Nakashima et al., 2016; Takahashi et al., 2008; Thomann et al., 2008; Ueda et al., 2002).

Error type has been linked to specific neuroanatomical regions in AD studies. For example, patients with AD who show reversed clock drawing exhibit greater frontotemporal dysfunction in the right hemisphere compared to patients with AD who demonstrate typical errors and show left posterior temporoparietal hypoperfusion (Brugnolo et al., 2010). Nakashima et al. (2016) reported that error type was correlated with regional cerebral blood flow in specific neuroanatomical regions (e.g., missing numbers with right parietal lobe, deviated clock center with left frontal lobe, etc.).

Studies of patients with dementia with Lewy bodies have implicated a left-hemispheric posterofrontal network involving temporoparietal and dorsal premotor cortices (Perneczky et al., 2010) and a frontal-subcortical network involving frontal and supplementary eye fields and the thalamus (Nagahama et al., 2008).

PERFORMANCE VALIDITY

No information is available.

COMMENT

The CDT has a long history of use in neuropsychology, used primarily as a dementia screener. Although seemingly quite simple in nature, the construction of a clock on request relies on a number of higher-order cognitive skills, including visuospatial, constructional, and executive cognitive abilities. The multifactorial nature of the test is supported by its pattern of relationships with other tests, including moderate to large correlations with tests of visuospatial ability, executive function, semantic and verbal memory, and general cognitive function, as well as neuroanatomical substrates involving frontal, temporal, and parietal regions. This renders the task quite effective as a general screener, but at the same time renders identification of specific processes underlying poor performance difficult. Clinically, inclusion of various conditions (e.g., copying, clock reading) and examination of the nature of qualitative errors is desirable. Certainly, poor performance on this test simply indicates that further inquiry is required, rather than that a diagnosis can be made with certainty.

There are a number of versions of the CDT, which vary significantly in terms of specific task parameters (e.g., free-drawn or predrawn clocks, time setting) and scoring. Research suggests that scoring methods are highly correlated. A gold standard measure has not yet emerged, with choice of method likely guided in practical terms by the amount of clinical time available for scoring and the depth of information desired. Longer scoring systems provide rich information but may require more time to score and interpret than is available. Additionally, the quality of available normative data may guide the selection of which CDT is to be used. In dementia research, the Shulman method is often associated with relatively high sensitivity and specificity estimates when compared to other versions.

The CDT is affected by demographic factors, with well-established effects of age (especially after 60–70 years), education, and reading level. Gender is generally found not to be influential. Some research has reported effects of ethnicity, although these appear to be attenuated to some degree by consideration of sociodemographic factors. When possible, these sociodemographic influences should be considered in the selection of normative data. Fortunately, many normative studies using popular scoring systems have been published, and most are corrected for age and education. The Nyborn et al. (2013) normative data are particularly impressive but are based on a fairly lengthy scoring protocol. Menon et al. (2012) also provide separate data for Hispanic and Caucasian participants.

Using normative data, rather than cutoffs, may be quite important in capturing the range of normal performance. For example, in the Hubbard et al. (2008) study, only one participant obtained a perfect clock drawing score. Using conventional scoring cutoffs, the scores of a number of participants would be considered abnormal. The authors suggest that previous cutoffs are overly stringent, noting that commonplace guidelines would result in a substantial proportion of healthy participants in their sample being referred for driving evaluation. Additionally, the well-established effects of age and education on this test further highlights the importance of normative data adjusted for these influences.

The CDT is effective at differentiating between controls and patients with dementia, and diagnostic accuracy statistics are enhanced when the test is combined with other measures such as the MMSE. The evidence is mixed with respect to differential diagnosis of dementia subtypes, with performance often found to be worse with increasing dementia severity. The CDT also has predictive validity in terms of identifying progression to dementia. Research in other clinical populations is emerging, and the CDT has particular promise in predicting driving ability and other variables relating to functional abilities. Psychometrically, the test has strong test-retest reliability and inter- and intrarater reliability coefficients for the majority of versions examined. There are limited data regarding internal reliability of various versions, and information regarding practice effects and measurement of reliable change is scant.

REFERENCES

Adunsky, A., Fleissig, Y., Levenkrohn, S., Arad, M., & Noy, S. (2002). A comparative study of Mini-Mental Test, Clock Drawing Task and Cognitive-FIM in evaluating functional outcome of elderly hip fracture patients. *Clinical Rehabilitation, 16*(4), 414–419. https://doi.org/10.1191/0269215502cr514oa

Ahmed, S., Brennan, L., Eppig, J., Price, C. C., Lamar, M., Delano-Wood, L., . . . Libon, D. J. (2016). Visuoconstructional impairment in subtypes of mild cognitive impairment. *Applied Neuropsychology: Adult, 23*(1), 43–52. https://doi.org/10.1080/23279095.2014.1003067

Allman, R. M., Sawyer, P., & Roseman, J. M. (2006). The UAB Study of Aging: background and insights into life-space mobility among older Americans in rural and urban settings. In H. Goodglass & E. Kaplan (ed., 1972). *The assessment of aphasia and related disorders.* Lea & Febiger.

Amodeo, S., Mainland, B. J., Herrmann, N., & Shulman, K. I. (2015). The times they are a-changin': Clock drawing and prediction of dementia. *Journal of Geriatric Psychiatry and Neurology, 28*(2), 145–155. https://doi.org/10.1177/0891988714554709

Aprahamian, I., Martinelli, J. E., Neri, A. L., & Yassuda, M. S. (2010). The accuracy of the Clock Drawing Test compared to that of standard screening tests for Alzheimer's disease: Results from a study of Brazilian elderly with heterogeneous educational backgrounds. *International Psychogeriatrics, 22*(01), 64. https://doi.org/10.1017/S1041610209991141

Babins, L., Slater, M. E., Whitehead, V., & Chertkow, H. (2008). Can an 18-point clock-drawing scoring system predict dementia in elderly individuals with mild cognitive impairment?. *Journal of Clinical and Experimental Neuropsychology, 30*(2), 173–186.

Barrows, R. J., Barsuglia, J., Paholpak, P., Eknoyan, D., Sabodash, V., Lee, G. J., & Mendez, M. F. (2015). Executive abilities as reflected by clock hand placement: Frontotemporal dementia versus early onset Alzheimer disease. *Journal of Geriatric Psychiatry and Neurology, 28*(4), 239–248. https://doi.org/10.1177/0891988715598228

Berger, G., Frölich, L., Weber, B., & Pantel, J. (2008). Diagnostic accuracy of the Clock Drawing Test: The relevance of "time setting" in screening for dementia. *Journal of Geriatric Psychiatry and Neurology, 21*(4), 250–260.

Bodner, T., Delazer, M., Kemmler, G., Gurka, P., Marksteiner, J., & Fleischhacker, W. W. (2004). Clock drawing, clock reading, clock setting, and judgment of clock faces in elderly people with dementia and depression: clock tasks in dementia. *Journal of the American Geriatrics Society, 52*(7), 1146–1150. https://doi.org/10.1111/j.1532-5415.2004.52313.x

Bozikas, V. P., Giazkoulidou, A., Hatzigeorgiadou, M., Karavatos, A., & Kosmidis, M. H. (2008). Do age and education contribute to performance on the clock drawing test? Normative data for the Greek population. *Journal of Clinical and Experimental Neuropsychology, 30*(2), 199–203. https://doi.org/10.1080/13803390701346113

Bozikas, V. P., Kosmidis, M. H., Gamvrula, K., Hatzigeorgiadou, M., Kourtis, A., & Karavatos, A. (2004). Clock Drawing Test in patients with schizophrenia. *Psychiatry Research, 121*(3), 229–238.

Brodaty, H., & Moore, C. M. (1997). The Clock Drawing Test for dementia of the Alzheimer's type: A comparison of three scoring methods in a memory disorders clinic. *International Journal of Geriatric Psychiatry, 12*(6), 619–627.

Brugnolo, A., Morbelli, S., Dessi, B., Girtler, N., Mazzei, D., Famà, F., . . . Nobili, F. (2010). The reversed Clock Drawing Test phenomenon in Alzheimer's disease: A perfusion SPECT study. *Dementia and Geriatric Cognitive Disorders, 29*(1), 1–10. https://doi.org/10.1159/000270898

Cacho, J., Benito-León, J., García-García, R., Fernández-Calvo, B., Vicente-Villardón, J. L., & Mitchell, A. J. (2010). Does the combination of the MMSE and clock drawing test (mini-clock) improve the detection of mild Alzheimer's disease and mild cognitive impairment? *Journal of Alzheimer's Disease, 22*(3), 889–896.

Caffarra, P., Gardini, S., Zonato, F., Concari, L., Dieci, F., Copelli, S., . . . Venneri, A. (2011). Italian norms for the Freedman version of the Clock Drawing Test. *Journal of Clinical and Experimental Neuropsychology, 33*(9), 982–988. https://doi.org/10.1080/13803395.2011.589373

Cahn, D. A., Salmon, D. P., Monsch, A. U., Butters, N., Wiederholt, W. C., & Corey-Bloom, J. (1996). Screening for dementia of Alzheimer type in the community: The utility of the Clock Drawing Test. *Archives of Clinical Neuropsychology, 2,* 529–539.

Can, S. S., & Gencay-Can, & A. (2012). Assessment of cognitive function in patients with fibromyalgia using the Clock Drawing Test. *Journal of Musculoskeletal Pain, 20*(3), 177–182. https://doi.org/10.3109/10582452.2012.704145

Carr, D. B., Barco, P. P., Wallendorf, M. J., Snellgrove, C. A., & Ott, B. R. (2011). Predicting road test performance in drivers with dementia. *Journal of the American Geriatrics Society, 59*(11), 2112–2117. https://doi.org/10.1111/j.1532-5415.2011.03657.x

Cecato, J. F., Fiorese, B., Montiel, J. M., Bartholomeu, D., & Martinelli, J. E. (2012). Clock Drawing Test in elderly individuals with different education levels: Correlation with Clinical Dementia Rating. *American Journal of Alzheimer's Disease and Other Dementias, 27*(8), 620–624. https://doi.org/10.1177/1533317512463954

Chan, A., Remington, R., Paskavitz, J., & Shea, T. B. (2008). The Clock-Drawing Test: Time for a change? *American Journal of Alzheimer's Disease and Other Dementias, 23*(4), 377–381. https://doi.org/10.1177/1533317508316680

Chen, L., Xu, S., Jin, X., Lu, X., Liu, L., Lou, Y., Wang, Y., Li, Y., & Jin, Y. (2018). A comparison of six clock-drawing test scoring methods in a nursing home. *Aging Clinical and Experimental Research, 30*(7), 775–781. https://doi.org/10.1007/s40520-017-0843-3

Chokron, S., Colliot, P., & Bartolomeo, P. (2004). The role of vision in spatial representation. *Cortex, 40*(2), 281–290. https://doi.org/10.1016/S0010-9452(08)70123-0

Cosentino, S., Jefferson, A., Chute, D. L., Kaplan, E., & Libon, D. J. (2004). Clock drawing errors in dementia: Neuropsychological and neuroanatomical considerations. *Cognitive and Behavioral Neurology, 17*(2), 74–84.

Crowe, M., Allman, R. M., Triebel, K., Sawyer, P., & Martin, R. C. (2010). Normative Performance on an executive Clock Drawing Task (CLOX) in a community-dwelling sample of older adults. *Archives of Clinical Neuropsychology, 25*(7), 610–617. https://doi.org/10.1093/arclin/acq047

de Assis Faria, C., Dias Alves, H. V., & Charchat-Fichman, H. (2015). The most frequently used tests for assessing executive functions in aging. *Dementia & Neuropsychologia, 9*(2), 149–155. https://doi.org/10.1590/1980-57642015DN92000009

de Guise, E., Gosselin, N., LeBlanc, J., Champoux, M.-C., Couturier, C., Lamoureux, J., . . . Feyz, M. (2011). Clock Drawing and Mini-Mental State Examination in patients with traumatic brain injury. *Applied Neuropsychology, 18*(3), 179–190. https://doi.org/10.1080/09084282.2011.595444

de Guise, E., LeBlanc, J., Gosselin, N., Marcoux, J., Champoux, M.-C., Couturier, C., . . . Feyz, M. (2010). Neuroanatomical correlates of the clock drawing test in patients with traumatic brain injury. *Brain Injury, 24*(13–14), 1568–1574. https://doi.org/10.3109/02699052.2010.523052

De Raedt, R., & Ponjaert-Kristoffersen, I. (2001). Short cognitive/neuropsychological test battery for first-tier fitness-to-drive assessment of older adults. *The Clinical Neuropsychologist, 15*(3), 329–336. https://doi.org/10.1076/clin.15.3.329.10277

Donnelly, K., Donnelly, J. P., & Cory, E. (2008). Primary care screening for cognitive impairment in elderly veterans. *American Journal of Alzheimer's Disease and Other Dementias, 23*(3), 218–226. https://doi.org/10.1177/1533317508315932

Ehreke, L., Luppa, M., König, H.-H., & Riedel-Heller, S. G. (2010). Is the Clock Drawing Test a screening tool for the diagnosis of mild cognitive impairment? A systematic review. *International Psychogeriatrics, 22*(01), 56. https://doi.org/10.1017/S1041610209990676

Ehreke, L., Luppa, M., König, H.-H., Villringer, A., & Riedel-Heller, S. G. (2011). Does the Clock Drawing Test predict dementia results of the Leipzig Longitudinal Study of the Aged (LEILA 75+). *Dementia and Geriatric Cognitive Disorders, 31*(2), 89–97. https://doi.org/10.1159/000323317

Freedman, M., Kaplan, E., Delis, D., & Morris, R. (1994). *Clock Drawing: A neuropsychological analysis.* New York: Oxford University Press.

Forti, P., Olivelli, V., Rietti, E., Maltoni, B., & Ravaglia, G. (2010). Diagnostic performance of an executive Clock Drawing Task (CLOX) as a screening test for mild cognitive impairment in elderly persons with cognitive complaints. *Dementia and Geriatric Cognitive Disorders, 30*(1), 20–27. https://doi.org/10.1159/000315515

Freund, B., & Colgrove, L. A. A. (2008). Error specific restrictions for older drivers: Promoting continued independence and public safety. *Accident Analysis & Prevention, 40*(1), 97–103. https://doi.org/10.1016/j.aap.2007.04.010

Freund, B., Gravenstein, S., Ferris, R., Burke, B. L., & Shaheen, E. (2005). Drawing clocks and driving cars: Use of brief tests of cognition to screen driving competency in older adults. *Journal of General Internal Medicine, 20,* 240–244.

Fukui, T., Hieda, S., & Bocti, C. (2006). Do Lesions involving the cortical cholinergic pathways help or hinder efficacy of donepezil in patients with Alzheimer's disease? *Dementia and Geriatric Cognitive Disorders, 22*(5–6), 421–431. https://doi.org/10.1159/000095801

Fuzikawa, C., Lima-Costa, M. F., Uchôa, E., & Shulman, K. (2007). Correlation and agreement between the Mini-Mental State Examination and the Clock Drawing Test in older adults with low levels of schooling: The Bambuí Health Aging Study (BHAS). *International Psychogeriatrics, 19*(04), 657. https://doi.org/10.1017/S1041610207005467

Gomar, J. J., Conejero-Goldberg, C., Davies, P., & Goldberg, T. E. (2014). Extension and refinement of the predictive value of different classes of markers in ADNI: Four-year follow-up data. *Alzheimer's & Dementia, 10*(6), 704–712. https://doi.org/10.1016/j.jalz.2013.11.009

Hazan, E., Frankenburg, F., Brenkel, M., & Shulman, K. (2018). The test of time: A history of clock drawing: History of clock drawing. *International Journal of Geriatric Psychiatry, 33*(1), e22–e30. https://doi.org/10.1002/gps.4731

Hazan, E., Zhang, J., Brenkel, M., Shulman, K., & Feinstein, A. (2017). Getting clocked: screening for TBI-related cognitive impairment with the clock drawing test. *Brain Injury, 31*(11), 1501–1506.

Heinik, J., & Shaikewitz, D. (2009). The Clock Drawing Test: Modified and integrated approach (Clock Drawing Test-MIA) as an instrument for detecting mild cognitive impairment in a specialized outpatient setting. *Journal of Geriatric Psychiatry and Neurology, 22*(3), 171–180. https://doi.org/10.1177/0891988709332940

Heinik, J., Solomesh, I., Shein, V., & Becker, D. (2002). Clock Drawing Test in mild and moderate dementia of the Alzheimer's type: A comparative and correlation study. *International Journal of Geriatric Psychiatry, 17*(5), 480–485. https://doi.org/10.1002/gps.616

Henderson, M., Scott, S., & Hotopf, M. (2007). Use of the Clock-Drawing Test in a hospice population. *Palliative Medicine, 21*(7), 559–565. https://doi.org/10.1177/0269216307081936

Herrmann, N., Kidron, D., Shulman, K. I., Kaplan, E., Binns, M., Leach, L., & Freedman, M. (1998). Clock tests in depression, Alzheimer's disease, and elderly controls. *International Journal of Psychiatry in Medicine, 28,* 437–447.

Herrmann, N., Kidron, D., Shulman, K. I., Kaplan, E., Binns, M., Soni, J., Leach, L., & Freedman, M. (1999). The use of clock tests in schizophrenia. *General Hospital Psychiatry, 21,* 70–73.

Hirjak, D., Sambataro, F., Remmele, B., Kubera, K. M., Schröder, J., Seidl, U., . . . Thomann, P. A. (2019). The relevance of hippocampal subfield integrity and clock drawing test performance for the diagnosis of Alzheimer's disease and mild cognitive impairment. *The World Journal of Biological Psychiatry, 20*(3), 197–208.

Hirjak, D., Wolf, R. C., Pfeifer, B., Kubera, K. M., Thomann, A. K., Seidl, U., . . . Thomann, P. A. (2017). Cortical signature of clock drawing performance in Alzheimer' disease and mild cognitive impairment. *Journal of Psychiatric Research, 90*, 133–142.

Hubbard, E., Santini, V., Blankevoort, C., Volkers, K., Barrup, M., Byerly, L., . . . Green, R. (2008). Clock drawing performance in cognitively normal elderly. *Archives of Clinical Neuropsychology, 23*(3), 295–327. https://doi.org/10.1016/j.acn.2007.12.003

Janssen, J., Koekkoek, P. S., van Charante, E. P. M., Kappelle, L. J., Biessels, G. J., & Rutten, G. E. (2017). How to choose the most appropriate cognitive test to evaluate cognitive complaints in primary care. *BMC Family Practice, 18*(1), 101.

Jørgensen, K., Kristensen, M. K., Waldemar, G., & Vogel, A. (2015). The six-item Clock Drawing Test—reliability and validity in mild Alzheimer's disease. *Neuropsychology, Development, and Cognition. Section B, Aging, Neuropsychology and Cognition, 22*(3), 301–311. https://doi.org/10.1080/13825585.2014.932325

Jouk, A., & Tuokko, H. (2012). A reduced scoring system for the Clock Drawing Test using a population-based sample. *International Psychogeriatrics, 24*(11), 1738–1748. https://doi.org/10.1017/S1041610212000804

Kaneda, Y., Ohmori, T., Okahisa, Y., Sumiyoshi, T., Pu, S., Ueoka, Y., . . . Sora, I. (2013). Measurement and treatment research to improve cognition in Schizophrenia Consensus Cognitive Battery: Validation of the Japanese version. *Psychiatry and Clinical Neurosciences, 67*(3), 182–188. https://doi.org/10.1111/pcn.12029

Kim, H., & Chey, J. (2010). Effects of education, literacy, and dementia on the Clock Drawing Test performance. *Journal of the International Neuropsychological Society, 16*(06), 1138–1146. https://doi.org/10.1017/S1355617710000731

Kim, Y.-S., Lee, K.-M., Choi, B. H., Sohn, E.-H., & Lee, A. Y. (2009). Relation between the clock drawing test (Clock Drawing Test) and structural changes of brain in dementia. *Archives of Gerontology and Geriatrics, 48*(2), 218–221. https://doi.org/10.1016/j.archger.2008.01.010

Kitabayashi, Y., Ueda, H., Narumoto, J., Nakamura, K., Kita, H., & Fukui, K. (2001). Qualitative analyses of clock drawings in Alzheimer's disease and vascular dementia. *Psychiatry and Clinical Neurosciences, 55*(5), 485–491. https://doi.org/10.1046/j.1440-1819.2001.00894.x

Kozora, E., & Cullum, C. M. (1994). Qualitative features of clock drawings in normal aging and Alzheimer's disease. *Assessment, 1*(2), 179–187. https://doi.org/10.1177/107319119400100200８

LaRue, A., Romero, L. J., Ortiz, I. E., Chi Lang, H., & Lindeman, R. D. (1999). Neuropsychological performance of Hispanic and non-Hispanic older adults: An epidemiologic survey. *The Clinical Neuropsychologist, 13*(4), 474–486.

Leach, L., Kaplan, E., Rewilak, D., Richards, B., & Proulx, B-B. (2000). *Kaplan Baycrest Neurocognitive Assessment*. San Antonio, TX: The Psychological Corporation.

Lee, K. S., Kim, E. A., Hong, C. H., Lee, D.-W., Oh, B. H., & Cheong, H.-K. (2008). Clock Drawing Test in mild cognitive impairment: Quantitative analysis of four scoring methods and qualitative analysis. *Dementia and Geriatric Cognitive Disorders, 26*(6), 483–489. https://doi.org/10.1159/000167879

Lezak, M. D. (Ed.). (2012). *Neuropsychological Assessment* (5th ed.). Oxford, New York: Oxford University Press.

Libon, D., Swenson, R., Barnoski, E., & Sands, L. (1993). Clock drawing as an assessment tool for dementia. *Archives of Clinical Neuropsychology, 8*(5), 405–415. https://doi.org/10.1016/0887-6177(93)90004-K

Libon, D. J., Malamut, B. L., Swenson, R., Sands, L. P., & Cloud, B. S. (1996). Further analyses of clock drawings among demented and nondemented older subjects. *Archives of Clinical Neuropsychology, 11*(3), 193–205.

Litvinenko, I. V., Odinak, M. M., Mogil'naya, V. I., & Emelin, A. Y. (2008). Efficacy and safety of galantamine (reminyl) for dementia in patients with Parkinson's disease (an open controlled trial). *Neuroscience and Behavioral Physiology, 38*(9), 937–945. https://doi.org/10.1007/s11055-008-9077-3

Litvinenko, I. V., Odinak, M. M., Mogil'naya, V. I., & Perstnev, S. V. (2010). Use of memantine (akatinol) for the correction of cognitive impairments in Parkinson's disease complicated by dementia. *Neuroscience and Behavioral Physiology, 40*(2), 149–155.

Lloret, A., Badía, M.-C., Mora, N. J., Pallardó, F. V., Alonso, M.-D., & Viña, J. (2009). Vitamin E paradox in Alzheimer's disease: It does not prevent loss of cognition and may even be detrimental. *Journal of Alzheimer's Disease, 17*(1), 143–149.

Lourenço, R. A., Ribeiro-Filho, S. T., Moreira, I. de F. H., Paradela, E. M. P., & Miranda, A. S. de. (2008). The Clock Drawing Test: Performance among elderly with low educational level. *Revista Brasileira de Psiquiatria, 30*(4), 309–315.

Manos, P. J. (1997). The utility of the 10-point clock test as a screen for cognitive impairment in general hospital patients. *General Hospital Psychiatry, 19*, 439–444.

Manos, P. J. (1999). Ten-point clock test sensitivity for Alzheimer's disease in patients with MMSE scores greater than 23. *International Journal of Geriatric Psychiatry, 14*(6), 454–458.

Manos, P. J., & Wu, R. (1994). The ten point clock test: A quick screen and grading method for cognitive impairment in medical and surgical patients. *International Journal of Psychiatry in Medicine, 24*(3), 229–244. https://doi.org/10.2190/5A0F-936P-VG8N-0F5R

Marcopulos, B. A., McLain, C. A., & Giuliano, A. J. (1997). Cognitive impairment or inadequate norms? A study of healthy, rural, older adults with limited education. *The Clinical Neuropsychologist, 11*(2), 111–131. https://doi.org/10.1080/13854049708407040

Martyr, A., & Clare, L. (2012). Executive function and activities of daily living in Alzheimer's disease: A correlational meta-analysis. *Dementia and Geriatric Cognitive Disorders, 33*(2–3), 189–203.

Maruta, C., Guerreiro, M., de Mendonça, A., Hort, J., & Scheltens, P. (2011). The use of neuropsychological tests across Europe: The need for a consensus in the use of assessment tools for dementia: The use of neuropsychological tests across Europe. *European Journal of Neurology, 18*(2), 279–285. https://doi.org/10.1111/j.1468-1331.2010.03134.x

Matsuoka, T., Narumoto, J., Okamura, A., Taniguchi, S., Kato, Y., Shibata, K., . . . Fukui, K. (2013). Neural correlates of the components of the clock drawing test. *International Psychogeriatrics, 25*(08), 1317–1323. https://doi.org/10.1017/S1041610213000690

Mazancova, A. F., Nikolai, T., Stepankova, H., Kopecek, M., & Bezdicek, O. (2017). The reliability of clock drawing test scoring systems modeled on the normative data in healthy aging and nonamnestic mild cognitive impairment. *Assessment, 24*(7), 945–957.

Mendez, M. F., Ala, T., & Underwood, K. L. (1992). Development of scoring criteria for the clock drawing task in Alzheimer's disease. *Journal of the American Geriatrics Society, 40*(11), 1095–1099.

Menon, C., Hall, J., Hobson, V., Johnson, L., & O'Bryant, S. E. (2012). Normative performance on the executive clock drawing task in a multi-ethnic bilingual cohort: a project FRONTIER study: An executive clock drawing task: normative performance. *International Journal of Geriatric Psychiatry, 27*(9), 959–966. https://doi.org/10.1002/gps.2810

Milian, M., Leiherr, A.-M., Straten, G., Müller, S., Leyhe, T., & Eschweiler, G. W. (2013). The Mini-Cog, Clock Drawing Test, and the Mini-Mental State Examination in a German Memory Clinic: Specificity of separation dementia from depression. *International Psychogeriatrics, 25*(01), 96–104. https://doi.org/10.1017/S104161021200141X

Montani, C., Bouati, N., Pelissier, C., Couturier, P., Jasso-Mosqueda, G., Hugonot, R., & Franco, A. (1997). Cotation et validation du test du cadran de l'horloge en psychométrie chez le sujet âgé. *Encéphale, 23*, 194–199.

Müller, S., Preische, O., Heymann, P., Elbing, U., & Laske, C. (2017). Increased diagnostic accuracy of digital vs. conventional clock drawing test for discrimination of patients in the early course of Alzheimer's disease from cognitively healthy individuals. *Frontiers in Aging Neuroscience, 9*, 101.

Nagahama, Y., Okina, T., Suzuki, N., & Matsuda, M. (2008). Cerebral substrates related to impaired performance in the Clock-Drawing Test in dementia with Lewy bodies. *Dementia and Geriatric Cognitive Disorders, 25*(6), 524–530. https://doi.org/10.1159/000131665

Nair, A. K., Gavett, B. E., Damman, M., Dekker, W., Green, R. C., Mandel, A., . . . others. (2010). Clock Drawing Test ratings by dementia specialists: Interrater reliability and diagnostic accuracy. *Journal of Neuropsychiatry and Clinical Neurosciences, 22*(1), 85–92.

Nakashima, H., Umegaki, H., Makino, T., Kato, K., Abe, S., Suzuki, Y., & Kuzuya, M. (2016). Neuroanatomical correlates of error types on the Clock Drawing Test in Alzheimer's disease patients. *Geriatrics & Gerontology International, 16*(7), 777–784.

Napryeyenko, O., Sonnik, G., & Tartakovsky, I. (2009). Efficacy and tolerability of Ginkgo biloba extract EGb 761® by type of dementia: Analyses of a randomised controlled trial. *Journal of the Neurological Sciences, 283*(1–2), 224–229. https://doi.org/10.1016/j.jns.2009.02.353

Nasreddine, Z. S., Phillips, N. A., Bedirian, V., Charbonneau, S., Whitehead, V., Collin, I., et al. (2005). The Montreal Cognitive Assessment, MoCA: A brief screening tool for mild cognitive impairment. *Journal of the American Geriatric Society, 53* (4), 695-699.

Nielsen, T. R., & Jørgensen, K. (2013). Visuoconstructional abilities in cognitively healthy illiterate Turkish immigrants: A quantitative and qualitative investigation. *The Clinical Neuropsychologist, 27*(4), 681–692. https://doi.org/10.1080/13854046.2013.767379

Nokleby, K., Boland, E., Bergersen, H., Schanke, A.-K., Farner, L., Wagle, J., & Wyller, T. B. (2008). Screening for cognitive deficits after stroke: a comparison of three screening tools. *Clinical Rehabilitation, 22*(12), 1095–1104. https://doi.org/10.1177/0269215508094711

Nyborn, J. A., Himali, J. J., Beiser, A. S., Devine, S. A., Du, Y., Kaplan, E., . . . Au, R. (2013). The Framingham Heart Study clock drawing performance: Normative data from the offspring cohort. *Experimental Aging Research, 39*(1), 80–108. https://doi.org/10.1080/0361073X.2013.741996

Ogden, J. A. (1985). Anterior-posterior interhemispheric differences in the loci of lesions producing visual hemineglect. *Brain and Cognition, 4*(1), 59–75.

Okamura, A., Kitabayashi, Y., Kohigashi, M., Shibata, K., Ishida, T., Narumoto, J., . . . Fukui, K. (2012). Neuropsychological and functional correlates of clock-drawing test in elderly institutionalized patients with schizophrenia: Clock-Drawing Test in schizophrenia. *Psychogeriatrics, 12*(4), 242–247. https://doi.org/10.1111/j.1479-8301.2012.00425.x

Palmqvist, S., Hertze, J., Minthon, L., Wattmo, C., Zetterberg, H., Blennow, K., . . . Hansson, O. (2012). Comparison of brief cognitive tests and CSF biomarkers in predicting Alzheimer's disease in mild cognitive impairment: Six-year follow-up study. *PloS One, 7*(6), e38639. https://doi.org/10.1371/journal.pone.0038639

Parsey, C. M., & Schmitter-Edgecombe, M. (2011). Quantitative and qualitative analyses of the Clock Drawing Test in mild cognitive impairment and Alzheimer disease: Evaluation of a modified scoring system. *Journal of Geriatric Psychiatry and Neurology, 24*(2), 108–118. https://doi.org/10.1177/0891988711402349

Paskavitz, J. F., Gunstad, J. J., & Samuel, J. E. (2007). Clock drawing and frontal lobe behavioral effects of memantine in Alzheimer's disease: A rater-blinded study. *American Journal of Alzheimer's Disease and Other Dementias, 21*(6), 454–459. https://doi.org/10.1177/1533317506294474

Pedroso, R. V., Coelho, F. G. de M., Santos-Galduróz, R. F., Costa, J. L. R., Gobbi, S., & Stella, F. (2012). Balance, executive functions and falls in elderly with Alzheimer's disease (AD): A longitudinal study. *Archives of Gerontology and Geriatrics, 54*(2), 348–351. https://doi.org/10.1016/j.archger.2011.05.029

Perneczky, R., Drzezga, A., Boecker, H., Ceballos-Baumann, A. O., Valet, M., Feurer, R., . . . Häussermann, P. (2010). Metabolic alterations associated with impaired clock drawing in Lewy body dementia. *Psychiatry Research: Neuroimaging, 181*(2), 85–89. https://doi.org/10.1016/j.pscychresns.2009.08.001

Petrova, M., Pavlova, R., Zhelev, Y., Mehrabian, S., Raycheva, M., & Traykov, L. (2016). Investigation of neuropsychological characteristics of very mild and mild dementia with Lewy bodies. *Journal of Clinical and Experimental Neuropsychology, 38*(3), 354–360. https://doi.org/10.1080/13803395.2015.1117058

Piers, R. J., Devlin, K. N., Ning, B., Liu, Y., Wasserman, B., Massaro, J. M., . . . Penney, D. L. (2017). Age and graphomotor decision making assessed with the digital clock drawing test: the Framingham Heart Study. *Journal of Alzheimer's Disease, 60*(4), 1611–1620.

Pinto, E., & Peters, R. (2009). Literature review of the Clock Drawing Test as a tool for cognitive screening. *Dementia and Geriatric Cognitive Disorders, 27*(3), 201–213. https://doi.org/10.1159/000203344

Piotrowicz, K., Fedyk-Łukasik, M., Skalska, A., & Grodzicki, T. (2018). Is the Clock Drawing Test useful in the screening assessment of aged patients with chronic heart failure?. *Advances in Medical Sciences, 63*(1), 199–204.

Prokopenko, S. V., Mozheyko, E. Y., Petrova, M. M., Koryagina, T. D., Kaskaeva, D. S., Chernykh, T. V., . . . Bezdenezhnih, A. F. (2013). Correction of post-stroke cognitive impairments using computer programs. *Journal of the Neurological Sciences, 325*(1–2), 148–153. https://doi.org/10.1016/j.jns.2012.12.024

Pustokhanova, L., & Morozova, E. (2013). Cognitive impairment and hypothymia in post stroke patients. *Journal of the Neurological Sciences, 325*(1–2), 43–45. https://doi.org/10.1016/j.jns.2012.11.013

Ricci, M., Pigliautile, M., D'Ambrosio, V., Ercolani, S., Bianchini, C., Ruggiero, C., . . . Mecocci, P. (2016). The Clock Drawing Test as a screening tool in mild cognitive impairment and very mild dementia: A new brief method of scoring and normative data in the elderly. *Neurological Sciences, 37*(6), 867–873. https://doi.org/10.1007/s10072-016-2480-6

Riedel, O., Klotsche, J., Forstl, H., Wittchen, H.-U., & for the GEPAD Study Group. (2013). Clock Drawing Test: Is it useful for dementia screening in patients having Parkinson disease with and without depression? *Journal of Geriatric Psychiatry and Neurology, 26*(3), 151–157. https://doi.org/10.1177/0891988713490994

Roth, M., Huppert, F. A., Tym, E., & Mountjoy, C. Q. (1988). *CAMDEX: The Cambridge Exomination for Mental Disorders of the Elderb*. Cambridge: Cambridge University Press.

Roth, M., Tym, E., Mountjoy, C. Q., Huppert, F. A., Hendrie, H., Verma, S., & Goddard, R. (1986). CAMDEX: A standardised instrument for the diagnosis of mental disorder in the elderly with special reference to the early detection of dementia. *British Journal of Pychiatry, 149*, 698–709.

Rouleau, I., Salmon, D. P., Butters, N., Kennedy, C., & McGuire, K. (1992). Quantitative and qualitative analyses of clock drawings in Alzheimer's and Huntington's disease. *Brain and Cognition, 18*(1), 70–87.

Royall, D. R., Chiodo, L. K., & Polk, M. J. (2005). An empiric approach to level of care determinations: The importance of executive measures. *The Journals of Gerontology Series A: Biological Sciences and Medical Sciences, 60*(8), 1059–1064.

Royall, D. R., Cordes, J. A., & Polk, M. (1998). CLOX: an executive clock drawing task. *Journal of Neurology, Neurosurgery, and Psychiatry, 64*(5), 588–594.

Royall, D. R., & Espino, D. V. (2002). Not all clock-drawing tasks are the same. *Journal of the American Geriatric Society, 30,* 1166–1167.

Royall, D. R., Mahurin, R. K., & Gray, K. F. (1992). Bedside assessment of executive cognitive impairment: the Executive Interview (EXIT). *Journal of American Geriatric Society, 40,* 1221–1226.

Royall, D. R., Mulroy, A. R., Chiodo, L. K., & Polk, M. J. (2000). Clock drawing is sensitive to executive control: A comparison of six methods. *Journal of Gerontology: Psychological Sciences, 54B,* P328–P333.

Rubínová, E., Nikolai, T., Marková, H., Siffelová, K., Laczó, J., Hort, J., & Vyhnálek, M. (2014). Clock Drawing Test and the diagnosis of amnestic mild cognitive impairment: can more detailed scoring systems do the work? *Journal of Clinical and Experimental Neuropsychology, 36*(10), 1076–1083. https://doi.org/10.1080/13803395.2014.977233

Saka, E., & Elibol, B. (2009). Enhanced cued recall and clock drawing test performances differ in Parkinson's and Alzheimer's disease-related cognitive dysfunction. *Parkinsonism & Related Disorders, 15*(9), 688–691. https://doi.org/10.1016/j.parkreldis.2009.04.008

Santana, I., Duro, D., Freitas, S., Alves, L., & Simoes, M. R. (2013). The Clock Drawing Test: Portuguese norms, by age and education, for three different scoring systems. *Archives of Clinical Neuropsychology, 28*(4), 375–387. https://doi.org/10.1093/arclin/act016

Schramm, U., Berger, G., Müller, R., Kratzsch, T., Peters, J., & Frölich, L. (2002). Psychometric properties of Clock Drawing Test and MMSE or Short Performance Test (SKT) in dementia screening in a memory clinic population. *International Journal of Geriatric Psychiatry, 17*(3), 254–260. https://doi.org/10.1002/gps.585

Seibert, J., Tracik, F., Articus, K., & Spittler, S. (2012). Effectiveness and tolerability of transdermal rivastigmine in the treatment of Alzheimer's disease in daily practice. *Neuropsychiatric Disease and Treatment, 8*, 141–147. https://doi.org/10.2147/NDT.S29116

Seichepine, D. R., Neargarder, S., Davidsdottir, S., Reynolds, G. O., & Cronin-Golomb, A. (2015). Side and type of initial motor symptom influences visuospatial functioning in Parkinson's disease. *Journal of Parkinson's Disease, 5*(1), 75–83.

Sela-Katz, P., Rabinowitz, I., Shugaev, I., & Shigorina, G. (2010). Basic knowledge of the medication regimen correlates with performance on cognitive function tests and diagnosis of dementia in elderly patients referred to a geriatric assessment unit. *Gerontology, 56*(5), 491–495. https://doi.org/10.1159/000304738

Shoyama, M., Nishioka, T., Okumura, M., Kose, A., Tsuji, T., Ukai, S., & Shinosaki, K. (2011). Brain activity during the Clock-Drawing Test: Multichannel near-infrared spectroscopy study. *Applied Neuropsychology, 18*(4), 243–251. https://doi.org/10.1080/09084282.2011.595450

Shulman, K. I., Shedletzky, R., & Silver, I. L. (1986). The challenge of time: Clock drawing and cognitive function in the elderly. *International Journal of Geriatric Psychiatry, 1*, 135–140.

Shulman, K. I. (2000). Clock-drawing: Is it the ideal cognitive screening test? *International Journal of Geriatric Psychiatry, 15*(6), 548–561.

Siciliano, M., Santangelo, G., D'Iorio, A., Basile, G., Piscopo, F., Grossi, D., & Trojano, L. (2016). Rouleau version of the Clock Drawing Test: age-and education-adjusted normative data from a wide Italian sample. *The Clinical Neuropsychologist, 30*(sup1), 1501–1516.

Smedslund, G., Siqveland, J., & Leiknes, K. A. (2015). *Psychometric Assessment of the Clock Drawing Test*. Knowledge Centre for the Health Services at The Norwegian Institute of Public Health (NIPH). http://www.ncbi.nlm.nih.gov/books/NBK390574/

Solomon, P. R., Hirschoff, A., Kelly, B., Relin, M., Brush, M., DeVeaux, R. D., & Pendlebury, W. W. (1998). A 7 minute neurocognitive screening battery highly sensitive to Alzheimer's disease. *Archives of Neurology, 55*(3), 349–355.

Souillard-Mandar, W., Davis, R., Rudin, C., Au, R., Libon, D. J., Swenson, R., . . . Penney, D. L. (2016). Learning classification models of cognitive conditions from subtle behaviors in the Digital Clock Drawing Test. *Machine Learning, 102*(3), 393–441. https://doi.org/10.1007/s10994-015-5529-5

Spenciere, B., Alves, H., & Charchat-Fichman, H. (2017). Scoring systems for the Clock Drawing Test: A historical review. *Dementia & Neuropsychologia, 11*(1), 6–14. https://doi.org/10.1590/1980-57642016dn11-010003

Stella, F., Gobbi, L. T., Gobbi, S., Oliani, M. M., Tanaka, K., & Pieruccini-Faria, F. (2007). Early impairment of cognitive functions in Parkinson's disease. *Arquivos de Neuro-Psiquiatria, 65*(2B), 406–410.

Stevens, J., & Killeen, M. (2006). A randomised controlled trial testing the impact of exercise on cognitive symptoms and disability of residents with dementia. *Contemporary Nurse, 21*(1), 32–40. https://doi.org/10.5555/conu.2006.21.1.32

Storey, J. E., Rowland, J. T., Basic, D., & Conforti, D. A. (2002). Accuracy of the clock drawing test for detecting dementia in a multicultural sample of elderly Australian patients. *International Psychogeriatrics, 14*(3), 259–271.

Strauss, H.-M., Leathem, J., Humphries, S., & Podd, J. (2012). The use of brief screening instruments for age-related cognitive impairment in New Zealand. *New Zealand Journal of Psychology, 41*(2), 11–20.

Sugawara, N., Yasui-Furukori, N., Umeda, T., Sato, Y., Kaneda, A., Tsuchimine, S., . . . Kaneko, S. (2010). Clock drawing performance in a community-dwelling population: Normative data for Japanese subjects. *Aging & Mental Health, 14*(5), 587–592. https://doi.org/10.1080/13607860903586086

Suhr, J., Grace, J., Allen, J., Nadler, J., & McKenna, M. (1998). Quantitative and qualitative performance of stroke versus normal elderly on six clock drawing systems. *Archives of Clinical Neuropsychology, 13*(6), 495–502.

Sunderland, T., Hill, J. L., Mellow, A. M., Lawlor, B. A., Gundersheimer, J., Newhouse, P. A., & Grafman, J. H. (1989). Clock drawing in Alzheimer's disease: A novel measure of dementia severity. *Journal of the American Geriatric Association, 37*, 725–729.

Takahashi, M., Sato, A., Nakajima, K., Inoue, A., Oishi, S., Ishii, T., & Miyaoka, H. (2008). Poor performance in Clock-Drawing Test associated with visual memory deficit and reduced bilateral hippocampal and left temporoparietal regional blood flows in Alzheimer's disease patients. *Psychiatry and Clinical Neurosciences, 62*(2), 167–173. https://doi.org/10.1111/j.1440-1819.2008.01750.x

Tan, L. P. L., Herrmann, N., Mainland, B. J., & Shulman, K. (2015). Can clock drawing differentiate Alzheimer's disease from other dementias? *International Psychogeriatrics, 27*(10), 1649–1660. https://doi.org/10.1017/S1041610215000939

Tene, O., Sigler, M., Shiloh, R., Weizman, A., & Aizenberg, D. (2016). The Clock-Drawing Test as a possible indicator of acute psychosis. *International Clinical Psychopharmacology, 31*(3), 155–158. https://doi.org/10.1097/YIC.0000000000000118

Terwindt, P. W., Hubers, A. A., Giltay, E. J., van der Mast, R. C., & van Duijn, E. (2016). Screening for cognitive dysfunction in Huntington's disease with the clock drawing test. *International Journal of Geriatric Psychiatry, 31*(9), 1013–1020.

Thomann, P. A., Toro, P., Santos, V. D., Essig, M., & Schröder, J. (2008). Clock drawing performance and brain morphology in mild cognitive impairment and Alzheimer's disease. *Brain and Cognition, 67*(1), 88–93. https://doi.org/10.1016/j.bandc.2007.11.008

Todd, M. E., Dammers, P. M., Adams, S. G., Jr, Todd, H. M., & Morrison, M. (1995). An examination of a proposed scoring procedure for clock drawing test: Reliability and predictive validity of the clock scoring system (CSS). *American Journal of Alzheimer's Disease and Other Dementias, 10*, 22–26.

Tranel, D., Rudrauf, D., Vianna, E. P. M., & Damasio, H. (2008). Does the Clock Drawing Test have focal neuroanatomical correlates? *Neuropsychology, 22*(5), 553–562. https://doi.org/10.1037/0894-4105.22.5.553

Trojano, L., Grossi, D., Linden, D. E. J., Formisano, E., Goebel, R., Cirillo, S., . . . Di Salle, F. (2002). Coordinate and categorical judgements in spatial imagery. An fMRI study. *Neuropsychologia, 40*(10), 1666–1674.

Tuokko, H. (2000). A Comparison of alternative approaches to the scoring of clock drawing. *Archives of Clinical Neuropsychology, 15*(2), 137–148. https://doi.org/10.1016/S0887-6177(99)00003-7

Tuokko, H., Hadjistavropoulos, T., Miller, J. A., & Beattie, B. L. (1992). The Clock Test: a sensitive measure to differentiate normal elderly from those with Alzheimer disease. *Journal of the American Geriatrics Society, 40*(6), 579–584.

Tuokko, H., Hadjistavropoulos, T., Miller, J. A., Horton, A., & Beattie, B. L. (1995). *The Clock Test: Administration and scoring manual.* Toronto, Ont.: Multi-Health Systems.

Tuokko, H., & O'Connell, M. (2006). A review of quantified approaches to the qualitative assessment of clock drawing. In A. Poreh (Ed.), *Quantified process approach*. Lisse: Swetts & Zeitlinger.

Ueda, H., Kitabayashi, Y., Narumoto, J., Nakamura, K., Kita, H., Kishikawa, Y., & Fukui, K. (2002). Relationship between clock drawing test performance and regional cerebral blood flow in

Alzheimer's disease: A single photon emission computed tomography study. *Psychiatry and Clinical Neurosciences*, *56*(1), 25–29. https://doi.org/10.1046/j.1440-1819.2002.00940.x

Viscogliosi, G., Chiriac, I. M., Andreozzi, P., & Ettorre, E. (2016). The metabolic syndrome predicts longitudinal changes in Clock Drawing Test performance in older nondemented hypertensive individuals. *American Journal of Geriatric Psychiatry*, *24*(5), 359–363. https://doi.org/10.1016/j.jagp.2015.09.001

von Gunten, A., Ostos-Wiechetek, M., Brull, J., Vaudaux-Pisquem, I., Cattin, S., & Duc, R. (2008). Clock-Drawing Test performance in the normal elderly and its dependence on age and education. *European Neurology*, *60*(2), 73–78. https://doi.org/10.1159/000131895

Wolf-Klein, G. P., Silverstone, F. A., Levy, A. P., Brod, M. S., & Breuer, J. (1989). Screening for Alzheimer's disease by clock drawing. *Journal of the American Geriatric Association, 37,* 730–734.

Yamada, M., Takechi, H., Mori, S., Aoyama, T., & Arai, H. (2013). Global brain atrophy is associated with physical performance and the risk of falls in older adults with cognitive impairment: Global brain atrophy and falls. *Geriatrics & Gerontology International*, *13*(2), 437–442. https://doi.org/10.1111/j.1447-0594.2012.00927.x

Yancheva, S., Ihl, R., Nikolova, G., Panayotov, P., Schlaefke, S., Hoerr, R., & for the GINDON Study Group. (2009). *Ginkgo biloba* extract EGb 761®, donepezil or both combined in the treatment of Alzheimer's disease with neuropsychiatric features: A randomised, double-blind, exploratory trial. *Aging & Mental Health*, *13*(2), 183–190. https://doi.org/10.1080/13607860902749057

Zhou, A., & Jia, J. (2008). The value of the Clock Drawing Test and the Mini-Mental State Examination for identifying vascular cognitive impairment no dementia. *International Journal of Geriatric Psychiatry*, *23*(4), 422–426. https://doi.org/10.1002/gps.1897

Zuverza-Chavarria, V., & Tsanadis, J. (2011). Measurement properties of the CLOX Executive Clock Drawing Task in an inpatient stroke rehabilitation setting. *Rehabilitation Psychology*, *56*(2), 138–144. https://doi.org/10.1037/a0023465

COGNITIVE ESTIMATION TEST (CET)

TEST NAME	**Cognitive Estimation Test (CET)**
DOMAIN	Executive functioning
AGE RANGE	17 to 91
ADMINISTRATION TIME	5 minutes
SCORING FORMAT	Hand scored
REFERENCE	Shallice, T., & Evans, M. E. (1978). The involvement of the frontal lobes in cognitive estimation. *Cortex, 14*, 292–303.

DESCRIPTION

The Cognitive Estimation Test (CET) is used to evaluate the ability to generate effective problem-solving strategies. There is no commercial source. Shallice and Evans (1978) designed the CET so that the task requires examinees to respond to questions that do not have readily apparent answers. For example, answering questions such as "What is the average length of a man's spine?" requires selecting an appropriate estimate and checking the plausibility of the estimate, but does not require performing any complex computation. Preliminary normative data were provided based on a sample of 25 British neurologically healthy individuals (Shallice & Evans, 1978).

The task has subsequently been revised. For example, in 1994, Axelrod and Millis adapted the task for use with North-American populations, eliminated items that required non-numerative responses, and provided an empirically-based, standardized scoring method and preliminary normative data. The test consists of 10 items, shown in Figure 9–2. The task has been modified further (Levinoff et al., 2006). Two parallel nine-item versions of the CET for use have also been created (MacPherson et al., 2014) and adopted for use with Italian speakers (Scarpina et al., 2015). A seven-item version (CET-R-7) has also been created (Gansler et al., 2014).

Please answer the following questions in the space provided. Although you may not know the exact answer, make a best guess. Be sure to complete all items.

1. How tall is the Empire State Building? feet
2. How fast do race horses gallop? miles per hour
3. How long is the average necktie? feet, inches
4. What is the average length of a man's spine? feet, inches
5. How tall is the average woman? feet, inches
6. How heavy is a full-grown elephant? pounds
7. How much does one quart of milk weigh? pound(s)
8. How fast does a commercial jet fly? miles per hour
9. On average, how many TV programs are there on any one channel between the hours of 6 PM and 11 PM?
10. What is the average temperature in Anchorage, Alaska, on Christmas Day? degrees F.

Total Deviation score =

Figure 9–2 Cognitive Estimation Test (CET).
SOURCE: From Axelrod and Millis (1994).

The Biber Cognitive Estimation Test, or Biber CET (Bullard et al., 2004) represents an attempt to establish quantitative rather than subjective judgments of normality for items in several content areas. Thus, it consists of 20 items, five in each category of time/duration, quantity, weight, and distance/length. The items are shown in Figure 9–3. To define the range of acceptable responses, items were given to healthy volunteers, and the responses that fell within the 5th to 95th percentile were considered normal; those that fell outside those percentiles were considered abnormal.

ADMINISTRATION

For the CET, the examiner provides a response sheet with the test questions and requests that the examinee complete the questions with "best guesses" in the spaces provided. There is no time limit. The instructions for the Biber CET are provided in Figure 9–3.

SCORING

In terms of scoring the CET, each response is compared with answers provided on the Deviation Scoring Sheet (see Axelrod & Millis version, Figure 9–4). The deviation scores for each CET item were developed from percentiles based on the mean performance of the standardization sample (e.g., deviation score of 0 for responses between the 16th and 84th percentiles; deviation score of 1 for responses between the 2nd and 16th as well as 84th to 98th percentiles; deviation score of 2 for responses less than the 2nd and greater than the 98th percentiles). The total deviation score is computed by summing item deviation scores for all 10 CET items. Thus, higher deviation scores imply more impaired (bizarre) performance. O'Carroll et al. (1994) use a somewhat different scoring system, with each response scored from 0 (good estimate) to 3 (bizarre).

1. How many seeds are there in a watermelon?
2. How much does a telephone weigh?
3. How many sticks of spaghetti are there in a one-pound package?
4. What is the distance an adult can walk in an afternoon?
5. How high off a trampoline can a person jump?
6. How long does it take a builder to construct an average-sized house?
7. How much do a dozen medium-sized apples weigh?
8. How far could a horse pull a farm cart in one hour?
9. How many brushings can someone get from a large tube of toothpaste?
10. How many potato chips are there in a small, one-ounce bag?
11. How long would it take an adult to hand-write a one-page letter?
12. What is the age of the oldest living person in the United States?
13. How long is a tablespoon?
14. How much does a bridge (folding) chair weigh?
15. How long does it take to iron a shirt?
16. How long is a giraffe's neck?
17. How many slices are there in a one-pound loaf?
18. How much does a pair of men's shoes weigh?
19. How much does the fattest man in the United States weigh?
20. How long does it take for fresh milk to go sour in the refrigerator?

It is unlikely that anyone would know the exact answer to any of the above questions, so please give your best guess. Provide only a single guess to each, not a range. For example, do not write "between 10 and 20," or "about 50." In addition to the number, be sure to indicate how many "what." In other words, do not just write "30." Write "30 miles" or "30s" or 30 pounds," etc. Please answer every question no matter how unsure you are or how unusual the question seems.

Figure 9–3 *Biber Cognitive Estimation Test (CET) Items and Instructions.*
SOURCE: From Bullard et al. (2004).

In terms of the Biber CET, Table 9–35 shows the item number, category, units of measurement, and percentile ranges. Responses that fall within the 5th to 95th percentile are considered normal; those that fall outside of those percentiles are considered abnormal. The number of items within the normal range is the total score.

DEMOGRAPHIC EFFECTS

AGE

In some studies, age has a negligible effect on performance on the CET (Axelrod & Millis, 1994; Gansler et al., 2014; Gillespie et al., 2002; Roth et al., 2012; Scarpina et al., 2015) and the Biber CET (Bullard et al., 2004). However, others have reported significant age effects (Fortune & Richards, 2017; MacPherson et al., 2014; Parente et al., 2013).

GENDER

On the CET, some research has suggested than men perform better than women (O'Carroll, Egan, & Mackenzie, 1994; Spencer & Johnson-Greene, 2009), whereas others have noted no relationship between gender and estimation ability (Gillespie et al., 2002). In a regression model, a revised version of the CET was related to gender (Gansler et al., 2014; MacPherson et al., 2014), and Scarpina et al. (2015) reported that men outperformed women on items with a stereotypically male bias.

On the Biber CET, gender effects are typically not found in healthy individuals; however, in patients with dementia, women performed slightly better in the time domain than their male counterparts (Bullard et al., 2004). In one study, performance on the Biber CET was compared in men and women following sleep deprivation, with women receiving placebo or caffeine performing worse than men (Killgore et al., 2008).

EDUCATION

On the CET, level of education impacts performance (Axelrod & Millis, 1994; Gansler et al., 2014; MacPherson et al., 2014; Parente et al., 2013; Spencer & Johnson-Greene, 2009; however, see Scarpina et al., 2015), with deviation scores lower for individuals with more education. Education effects on the Biber CET have been reported in some studies (Fortune & Richards, 2017) but not others (Bullard et al., 2004).

ETHNICITY, NATIONALITY, AND LINGUISTIC EFFECTS

Spencer and Johnson-Greene (2009) reported that Caucasian participants performed better than African-American participants on the test. College students who spoke English as a native language performed better than non-native English-speaking college students (Kisser et al., 2012). When ethnicity was covaried, differences on the CET remained, suggesting that language, rather than ethnicity, was related to the difference in performance.

NORMATIVE DATA

CET

Axelrod and Millis (1994) reported that the average deviation score for a sample of 164 adults (age, M = 39.0, SD = 16.1; education, M = 16.2 years, SD = 2.8; 74% female, 26% male; 75% Caucasian, 23% African American, 2% other) was 4.4 (SD = 2.2). Factually correct responses for each item on the CET result in a total deviation score of 3, which falls within one standard deviation of the sample mean. In general, deviation scores were lower for individuals with more education (Table 9–36).

Schretlen, Testa, and Pearlson (2010) provide norms for 312 adults as part of the Calibrated Neuropsychological Normative System (CNNS) available through Psychological Assessment Resources (PAR; www.parinc.com). These provide T scores and discrepancies based on a large sample of older adults from the northeastern United States. A major advantage of these norms is the option to correct for demographic variables such as age, sex, education, and ethnicity.

Response	Deviation	Response	Deviation
Empire State Building (ft)		Elephant Weight (lbs)	
<78	2	<500	2
78–499	1	500–1000	1
500–3555	0	1001–4999	0
3556–66,900	1	5000–20,880	1
>66,900	2	>20,880	2
Race Horse (mph)		Quart of Milk Weight (lbs)	
<5	2	<0.3	2
5–20	1	0.3–0.99	1
21–49	0	1.0–2.2	0
50–100	1	2.3–5.0	1
>100	2	>5.0	2
Necktie Length (inches)		Speed of Commercial Jet (mph)	
<10.5	2	<83	2
10.5–18	1	83–250	1
19–47	0	251–787	0
48–70	1	788–6720	1
>70	2	>6720	2
Spine Length (inches)		Number of TV Shows	
<12	2	<1.3	2
12–24	1	1.3–5.0	1
25–42	0	5. 1–9.9	0
43–64	I	10–88	1
>64	2	>88	2
Height of Woman (inches)		Temperature in Anchorage (°F)	
<60.5	2	<-37	2
60.5–64.0	1	-37 to -10	1
64.1–65.9	0	-9 to +32	0
66.0–68.0	1	+33 to +59	1
>68	2	>59	2

Figure 9–4 *Cognitive Estimation Test (CET) Deviation Scoring Sheet.*
SOURCE: From Axelrod and Millis (1994).

Several other commonly used neuropsychological tests are co-normed using this sample, which facilitates cross-test comparisons.

O'Carroll et al. (1994) provide normative data for a 10-item British version of the CET. The data are based on a sample of 150 healthy individuals, aged 17 to 91 years (education, M = 11.6 [SD = 2.9] years), living in the United Kingdom. The mean CET score for the entire sample was 5.3 (SD = 3.6).

Levinoff et al. (2006) modified the CET to include 23 questions from the original CET as well as new items generated by the authors. Items were administered to 69 older adults in Montreal, Canada. The mean age of the sample was 52 years (SD = 23 years), with a mean education level of 15.5 years (SD = 4.0 years), recruited from employees of a research institute and people from a research cohort who underwent routine neuropsychological testing. Eight questions were discarded due to deviation from normality, resulting in retention of five items from the original version and 10 new items. This version is available at http://dx.doi.org/10.1037/0894-4105.20.1.123.supp. Normative data are shown in Table 9–37. Of note, the authors also administered the test to another group of healthy older controls, individuals with MCI, and people with AD; see "Clinical Studies."

Two novel parallel forms of the CET have been introduced (MacPherson et al., 2014). They were administered to 184 participants in Britain (18 to 79 years of age, M = 48.07 years, SD = 17.51 years; M = 14.33 years, SD = 2.92, nine to 22 years of education; 56% female). Exclusion criteria were history of brain injury or stroke, neurologic or psychiatric condition, and substance abuse. Participants were grouped into six age bands (18–29, 30–39, 40–49, 50–59, 60–69, and 70–79 years) and three education bands (9–11 years [O-level or standard grade examinations], 12–15 years [A-level or higher grades examinations, as well as college-level higher education] and 16 plus years [university level education]). All participants spoke English as their first language. Normative data are provided in Tables 9–38 and 9–39. The versions were also administered to a

TABLE 9–35 Biber Cognitive Estimation Test (CET) Item Statistics

ITEM	CATEGORY	UNITS	5TH PERCENTILE	95TH PERCENTILE
1	Quantity	Seeds	30	1,000
2	Weight	Pounds	0.5	10
3	Quantity	Sticks	50	500
4	Distance/length	Miles	2.7	25
5	Distance/length	Feet	3	20
6	Time/age	Months	0.4	8
7	Weight	Pounds	1.5	9.3
8	Distance/length	Miles	1	15
9	Quantity	Brushings	34.2	250
10	Quantity	Chips	10	93
11	Time/age	Minutes	5	33
12	Time/age	Years	102	122.9
13	Distance/length	Inches	1.5	10
14	Weight	Pounds	0.90	15.9
15	Time/age	Minutes	2	20
16	Distance/length	Feet	2.5	15
17	Quantity	Slices	12	30.6
18	Weight	Pounds	0.7	5
19	Weight	Pounds	350	1200
20	Distance/length	Days	4	21

SOURCE: From Bullard et al. (2004).

sample of patients with frontal lesions and demographically matched controlled (see "Clinical Studies").

Scarpina et al. (2015) present normative data for 217 participants on two parallel modified nine-item versions of the CET (see MacPherson et al., 2014). Participants were Italian speaking, and reportedly did not have a history of neurologic or psychiatric conditions or alcohol abuse. The sample was 56% women, aged 19 to 91 years (M = 47.37 years, SD 17.13 years), with education levels between five and 24 years (M = 14.95 years, SD 4.35 years). Normative data are provided in Table 9–40.

BIBER CET

In the initial development of the Biber CET with 113 healthy individuals (age, M = 37.3, SD = 16.1, range 17–85; education, M = 16.5, SD = 2.6; 42% male, 95% Caucasian), the authors reported a mean score of 18.9 (SD = 1.1) and a range of 16 to 20. Cross-validation in a second sample of 49 healthy individuals (age, M = 40.3, SD = 14, range 17–78; education, M = 13.7, SD = 3.1; 39% male, 90% Caucasian) suggested a revised cutoff score of three standard deviations below the mean (i.e., below 15.6).

TABLE 9–36 Mean Deviation Score for Cognitive Estimation Test Performance across Education Groups

EDUCATION LEVEL	N	MEAN DEVIATION SCORE	SD
≤12	16	5.9	2.3
13–15	32	4.8	2.1
16	32	4.2	2.4
17–18	37	3.8	1.9
≥19	25	4.2	2.0

SOURCE: From Axelrod and Millis (1994).

EVIDENCE FOR RELIABILITY

EVIDENCE FOR INTERNAL RELIABILITY

The broad content represented in the CET appears to be multidimensional, and internal reliability estimates have suggested poor reliability across studies and versions examined (e.g., Cronbach's alpha .23 to .62; Gansler et al., 2014; MacPherson et al., 2014; Scarpina et al., 2015; Silverberg et al., 2007; Spencer & Johnson-Greene, 2009).

For the Biber CET, Bullard et al. (2004) reported that in patients with dementia, values are marginally acceptable, revealing a Cronbach's alpha of .62 and a Guttman split-half reliability coefficient of .74. In a sample of patients with acquired brain injury (Fortune & Richards, 2017), however, internal reliability was reportedly strong for the entire scale (Cronbach's alpha = .86), although subscale scores were comparatively weaker (Cronbach's alpha = .57 to .73).

EVIDENCE FOR TEST-RETEST RELIABILITY, MEASURING CHANGE, AND PRACTICE EFFECTS

Test-retest reliability information is not available.

EVIDENCE FOR RELIABILITY OF ALTERNATE FORMS

Two parallel nine-item CETs (MacPherson et al., 2014) were moderately correlated, and yielded similar descriptive values (Version A: M = 5.02, SD = 3.51, range = 0–24; Version B: M = 5.42, SD = 3.89, range = 0–22).

EVIDENCE FOR INTERRATER RELIABILITY

O'Carroll et al. (1994) reported that the interrater reliability coefficient was high (r = .91) for a group of 50 healthy subjects given the British version of the CET in which responses were scored from 0 (good estimate) to 3 (bizarre estimate).

EVIDENCE FOR VALIDITY

FACTOR-ANALYTIC STUDIES

Multiple factors have been extracted from the CET. For example Gansler et al. (2014) reported that 10 items yielded four factors; subsequently two factors were extracted that jointly accounted for 32% of the variance. Factors were labeled Length (Items 1, 2, 4, 5) and Speed and Time (Items, 8, 9, and 2). Three items were excluded (7, 10, 6). For the Biber CET, a factor analysis in an acquired brain injury sample suggested a four-factor structure that did not conform to the purported dimensions of quantity, weight, time, and distance (Fortune & Richards, 2017).

TABLE 9–37 Normative Data for a Modified Version of the Cognitive Estimation Test (CET)

QUESTION (UNIT OF MEASUREMENT)	<2ND PERCENTILE	2ND–16TH PERCENTILE	16TH–84TH PERCENTILE	84TH–98TH PERCENTILE	>98TH PERCENTILE
Race horses (km/hr)	<17	18–27	28–70	71–98	>99
Spine length (inches)	<55	56–63	64–100	101–134	>135
Oldest age (years)	<104.0	105–110	111–121	122–126.0	>127
Height woman (inches)	<58	59–63	64–66	67–68	>69
Necktie length (inches)	<20	20–26	26.0–48.0	48.1-59.7	>59.7
Weight elephant (lbs)	<489	490–1,000	1,001–5,000	5,001–30,480	>30,480
Jet speed (km/hr)	<240	241–480	481–1,082	1,083–2,160	>2,161
Temperature, Paris (°C)	< –14	–14 to –3	–2 to 10	11–19	>20
TV programs	<4	4–4.9	5–8.4	8.5–18.1	>18.1
Marathon time (hrs)	<2	2.1–2.9	3.0–8.0	8.1–15.0	>15.0
Weight hammer (lbs)	<0.75	0.76–1.5	1.5–5.1	5.2–12.8	>12.9
Shower water (L)	<6	7–11.3	12–100	100–349	>350
Height giraffe (feet)	<8	8–10	11–20	21–30	>31
Liquid consumption (L)	<0.4	0.4–0.9	1.0–3.9	3.9–7.0	>7.1
Pyramid age (years)	<500	501–1,999	2,000–5,000	5,001–6,660	>6,660

NOTE: An answer that fell within the 16th–84th percentile was assigned a score of 0, an answer that fell within the 84th–98th percentiles was assigned a score of 1, and an answer that was given above the 98th percentile and below the 2nd percentile was assigned a score of 2.

SOURCE: From Levinoff et al. (2006).

CORRELATIONS WITH OTHER TESTS

Executive Function. Correlations between the CET and other executive function tests tend to be variable; some studies report modest correlations, whereas others report no significant correlations. Overall, a pattern of moderate correlations is reported between the CET and executive function and/or complex attention tests (e.g., Brief Test of Attention, Digit Span, TOL, TMT, WCST, letter and semantic fluency, depending on the study) in patient populations (Brand et al., 2003; Canellopoulou & Richardson, 1998; D'Aniello et al., 2015; Kopelman, 1991; Roth et al., 2012; Scarpina et al., 2017).

The CET has been found to be unrelated to one measure of estimation (the Temporal Judgment Test of the Behavioural Assessment of the Dysexecutive Syndrome; Gillespie et al., 2002) and moderately related (r = .47) to others (Brand et al., 2003). In a mixed group of adult neurological patients, the CET was one of the few putative measures of executive function that failed to correlate significantly with everyday executive problems (Burgess et al., 1998).

In patients 1 to 15 years post-TBI, the Biber CET demonstrates moderate correlations with other executive function tests (e.g., Letter-Number Sequencing, TMT, Stroop), with correlations attenuated significantly after Information was partialled out (Silverberg et al., 2007). Similarly, modest to moderate correlations were reported overall between the Biber CET and executive measures, such as the Modified Six Elements Test, phonemic fluency, and the TMT (Fortune & Richards, 2017).

TABLE 9–38 Normative Data by Age, Education, and Gender for the CET A

		AGE					
EDUCATION	GENDER	18–29	30–39	40–49	50–59	60–69	70–79
9–11 years	M	6.00 (1.41)	6.67 (4.04)	7.20 (1.30)	3.00 (4.36)	2.50 (1.76)	8.00 (8.49)
	F	7.80 (3.42)	– –	5.00 (4.58)	4.33 (4.16)	6.83 (2.14)	9.80 (8.29)
12–15 years	M	3.89 (1.76)	6.25 (2.63)	6.33 (3.51)	3.33 (1.75)	3.67 (4.72)	5.00 (2.58)
	F	6.60 (3.05)	7.75 (2.06)	5.43 (3.46)	7.00 (4.00)	3.80 (2.95)	3.20 (2.49)
16–22 years	M	3.14 (1.95)	4.40 (4.28)	3.60 (2.30)	1.20 (1.30)	5.67 (4.04)	2.67 (3.79)
	F	5.88 (3.40)	5.64 (2.58)	6.00 (3.22)	4.33 (2.90)	2.67 (2.07)	5.20 (4.09)

SOURCE: From MacPherson et al. (2014).

TABLE 9–39 Normative Data by Age, Education, and Gender for the CET B

		AGE					
EDUCATION	GENDER	18–29	30–39	40–49	50–59	60–69	70–79
9–11 years	M	8.50	5.33	3.20	4.67	3.67	5.00
		(3.54)	(3.79)	(2.28)	(1.53)	(3.33)	(5.66)
	F	9.00	–	7.67	10.33	7.33	10.60
		(5.29)	–	(6.43)	(4.93)	(4.50)	(7.77)
12–15 years	M	5.89	5.25	4.67	1.67	4.67	1.50
		(3.22)	(3.86)	(4.51)	(1.75)	(1.86)	(1.29)
	F	9.60	9.25	5.57	7.57	5.80	5.80
		(3.85)	(6.55)	(2.44)	(2.57)	(2.17)	(4.55)
16–22 years	M	5.71	2.80	3.20	3.20	6.33	1.33
		(1.50)	(2.39)	(2.59)	(2.49)	(4.73)	(0.58)
	F	5.25	5.36	4.83	4.67	4.67	3.20
		(4.23)	(3.23)	(2.14)	(3.89)	(1.21)	(1.92)

SOURCE: From MacPherson et al. (2014).

Intelligence. Level of intelligence and general knowledge contributes significantly to CET performance (Brand et al., 2003; Gillespie et al., 2002; Kopelman, 1991; MacPherson et al., 2014; Scarpina et al., 2017). Most research has found moderate to large correlations between the CET and measures of general intelligence, such as Wechsler scales and indices and the NART (absolute value of *rs* = .30 to .63; Diaz-Asper, Schretlen, & Pearlson, 2004; Gillespie et al., 2002; Kopelman, 1991; Levinoff et al., 2006; O'Carroll et al., 1994; Spencer & Johnson-Greene, 2009). General cognitive status measured via MMSE is also reportedly related to performance on the Biber CET, although other measures (e.g., fund of general information, abstract reasoning) are not (Bullard et al., 2004). In an acquired brain injury sample, composites from the Repeatable Battery for the Assessment of Neuropsychological Status (RBANS) were modestly to moderately related to the Biber CET (Fortune & Richards, 2017).

Other Tests. Aspects of memory appear to be involved in cognitive estimation, generally with correlations in the moderate range in neurologic populations (*rs* = .32 to .67; Kopelman, 1991, Mendez, Doss, & Cherrier, 1998; Roth et al., 2012; Spencer & Johnson-Greene, 2009; however see Gansler et al., 2014) and healthy controls (Levinoff et al., 2006). The bulk of evidence also suggests that naming ability and word retrieval are related to performance (Levinoff et al., 2006; MacPherson et al., 2014; Spencer & Johnson-Greene, 2009). In patients 1 to 15 years post-TBI, the Biber CET moderately correlates with nonexecutive measures (absolute values of *rs* = .35 to .36; i.e., JLO, Grooved Pegboard; Silverberg et al., 2007).

Numerical ability and the capacity to construct and make appropriate use of mental images may also be important (Canellopoulou & Richardson, 1998; MacPherson et al., 2014; Mendez et al., 1998; Scarpina et al., 2017; but see Goldstein et al., 1996, and Shallice & Evans, 1978, who failed to find a relationship with arithmetic ability). In sum, research suggests that the CET may measure several other cognitive domains in addition to executive function, depending on the population studied (see also Spencer & Johnson-Greene, 2009).

CLINICAL STUDIES

Dementia. Impaired performance on the CET has been noted in patients with AD (Brand et al., 2003; Goldstein et al., 1996; Kopelman, 1991; Mendez et al., 1998). Mendez et al. (1998) gave the CET to patients with FTD and AD. Both groups gave more extreme answers than controls, and, contrary to expectation, AD patients gave more extreme estimates than the patients with FTD. Although people with AD perform worse on the CET than healthy controls, no differences between individuals with MCI and healthy controls are reported (Levinoff et al., 2006). Similar findings are reported in patients with FTD and corticobasal syndrome or posterior cortical atrophy who perform worse than controls on the Biber CET; no differences are found between MCI and controls (Bisbing et al., 2015).

Impaired performance has been reported in patients with Korsakoff's syndrome (Brand, Fujiwara et al., 2003; Brand, Kalbe et al., 2003; Kopelman, 1991; Shoqueirat et al., 1990; Taylor & O'Carroll, 1995; but see Leng & Parkin, 1988). Brand, Kalbe, et al. (2003) constructed their own CET version and found that in AD patients, the dimensions of size and weight were the most affected, while patients with Korsakoff's syndrome had the most difficulties in estimating time questions.

Impairments on the Biber CET have also been reported in patients with PD (Bullard et al., 2004). Mild impairments were found in patients with PD without dementia, particularly on length-related items (Scarpina et al., 2017).

Lesion Studies. Mixed evidence has been found in lesion studies, with Shallice and Evans (1978) reporting

TABLE 9–40 Normative Data for a Modified Version of the Cognitive Estimation Test (CET)

		CET A						CET B					
		AGE						AGE					
EDUCATION	GENDER	19–29	30–39	40–49	50–59	60–69	70–91	19–29	30–39	40–49	50–59	60–69	70–91
3–5 years	M	–	–	–	–	–	3.00	–	–	–	–	–	4.00
	F	–	–	–	5.00	4.00	13.33 (4.04)	–	–	–	6.00	8.00	9.67 (5.51)
6–8 years	M	–	1.00	–	4.00 (2.00)	7.40 (5.50)	–	–	5.00	–	4.50 (4.12)	4.40 (2.70)	–
	F	–	7.00	4.00 (1.41)	4.40 (2.07)	7.00 (5.94)	9.50 (4.95)	–	9.00	3.50 (3.54)	6.20 (2.17)	8.75 (2.22)	6.50 (0.71)
9–13 years	M	6.67 (3.20)	5.83 (2.99)	4.33 (3.21)	3.88 (2.30)	5.78 (2.64)	4.00 (4.00)	5.83 (4.31)	4.50 (2.17)	3.33 (3.06)	5.63 (3.29)	2.89 (2.32)	4.33 (1.53)
	F	7.60 (4.62)	5.50 (2.12)	5.83 (2.48)	5.25 (2.21)	7.80 (3.96)	9.50 (4.68)	9.40 (1.95)	2.50 (0.71)	6.17 (2.99)	5.94 (2.64)	5.20 (2.49)	8.83 (5.42)
>13 years	M	6.15 (3.26)	4.17 (2.57)	4.17 (2.40)	4.24 (3.46)	6.50 (3.00)	5.00 (7.07)	5.08 (2.75)	4.78 (3.17)	4.67 (3.88)	4.41 (2.40)	3.50 (3.00)	5.50 (3.54)
	F	5.96 (3.27)	4.86 (3.72)	5.22 (3.19)	5.50 (3.21)	7.50 (2.38)	11.50 (4.95)	5.17 (3.08)	6.00 (4.61)	4.33 (3.24)	5.60 (3.50)	4.00 (3.74)	8.50 (3.54)

NOTE: Values represent means and standard deviations.

SOURCE: Scarpina et al. (2015).

that patients with anterior lesions performed significantly worse than patients with posterior lesions, whereas Taylor and O'Carroll (1995) did not find differential evidence of anterior vs. posterior lesion location. Frontal lobe damage was associated with impaired performance on a modified version of the CET compared to controls and those with posterior lesions, with extreme and very extreme incorrect responses more common in people with frontal lesions (Cipolotti et al., 2017). Similarly, persons with frontal lesions perform worse on the CET than demographically matched controls (MacPherson et al., 2014).

TBI. Axelrod and Millis (1994) reported that patients with severe brain injuries were impaired on the CET relative to a sample of medical outpatients. However, TBI patients had significantly less education than controls, raising the possibility that the test may be more sensitive to education than to brain injury. Silverberg et al. (2007) reported that Biber CET scores did not predict functional status in patients after brain injury. However, Fortune and Richards (2017) reported that the Biber CET accounted for significant variance in community integration in an acquired brain injury sample even after severity of disability, executive function and general neuropsychological status were considered.

Epilepsy. Patients with epilepsy with various seizure-free periods do not differ from controls on CET performance (Treitz et al., 2009) but patients with intractable temporal lobe epilepsy performed worse than controls on the CET (Parente et al., 2013). In one study, patients with right temporal lobe epilepsy performed significantly worse, although also had earlier age of seizure onset than individuals with left temporal lobe epilepsy and fewer years of education than controls. Seizure onset prior to 12 years of age was related with worse CET performance. Age of seizure onset and semantic fluency predicted CET total and bizarreness scores, and bizarreness scores related to age, education, and visual attention.

Psychiatric Conditions. Roth et al. (2012) reported that patients with schizophrenia performed worse than demographically matched controls on the CET. Impairments on the Biber CET have also been reported in schizophrenia (Jackson et al., 2001).

Measures of anxiety and depression appear unrelated to cognitive estimation (Roth et al., 2012), but manic and euthymic patients perform worse than other groups (Buoli et al., 2014). Longer duration of psychiatric illness is predictive of bizarreness on the CET.

Other Populations. Impairments in CET performance have been found in detoxified chronic alcohol abuse (Steinmetz & Federspiel, 2012), postencephalitic amnesia (Kopelman, 1991), following prenatal alcohol exposure (Kopera-Frye et al., 1996), and in anterior communicating artery aneurysm (Leng & Parkin, 1988). No differences between patients with subcortical ischemic vascular disease and healthy controls on the CET have been reported (Margraf et al., 2009).

NEUROANATOMICAL CORRELATES AND IMAGING STUDIES

Magnetic resonance imaging (MRI) analyses of performance in patient with FTD, corticobasal syndrome, and posterior cortical atrophy implicated a frontal-parietal network in cognitive estimation. Specifically, gray matter atrophy in the right lateral prefrontal and orbital frontal cortices appears related to Biber CET performance in patients with FTD, and atrophy in the right inferior parietal cortex, right insula, and fusiform cortices was related to performance in patients with corticobasal syndrome or posterior cortical atrophy (Bisbing et al., 2015).

PERFORMANCE VALIDITY

No information is available.

COMMENT

The CET is a brief test that requires few materials. The specific abilities underlying performance on the CET are not clear, and there are a number of findings that suggest that performance may be a reflection of a rather diverse set of abilities, including intelligence, general fund of knowledge and semantic stores, and retrieval of information. Specifically, the CET appears to correlate more with intelligence (moderate to large correlations overall) than measures of executive function and attention. The test appears to also be related to other cognitive abilities, including naming, word retrieval, and memory, among others. Factor-analytic studies suggest that this test, despite being comprised of relatively few items, yields multiple factors.

In terms of demographic influences, unlike many tests, significant age effects are generally not reported. The effect of gender is mixed. Overall, the CET is related to education, with less prominent effects reported for the Biber CET. Effects of ethnicity and language ability have also been reported. Certainly, many items on this test appear to rely at least in part on experience, much of which may be culturally based. Most normative datasets are unsophisticated and inadequate for use in most clinical applications, and in some cases are quite dated. Sample sizes and cell sizes are small, and the effect of education or IQ is generally not considered in normative data, although note Schretlen et al. (2010), MacPherson et al. (2014), and Scarpina et al. (2015) who provide up-to-date normative information adjusted for demographic factors.

Internal reliability is poor overall and information on test-retest reliability is lacking, although the test appears to have high interrater reliability. In clinical populations, evidence for the ability of the CET to discriminate between patients with anterior versus posterior lesions is mixed.

Impaired performance has been reported in patients with dementia, which perhaps relates to the degradation of semantic knowledge involved in the disease, which could manifest as poor performance on the CET. Other research has suggested some group differences between patients and controls (see "Clinical Studies"). Limited information is available regarding neuroanatomical correlates. Overall, given the lack of precision of abilities measured, the poor reliability, limited validity, and limited normative data, this test should be used with caution in clinical settings but might have utility for research purposes.

REFERENCES

Axelrod, B. N., & Millis, S. R. (1994). Preliminary standardization of the Cognitive Estimation Test. *Assessment, 1*(3), 269–274. https://doi.org/10.1177/107319119400100307

Bisbing, T. A., Olm, C. A., McMillan, C. T., Rascovsky, K., Baehr, L., Ternes, K., . . . Grossman, M. (2015). Estimating frontal and parietal involvement in cognitive estimation: a study of focal neurodegenerative diseases. *Frontiers in Human Neuroscience, 9*. https://doi.org/10.3389/fnhum.2015.00317

Brand, M., Kalbe, E., Fujiwara, E., Huber, M., & Markowitsch, H. J. (2003). Cognitive estimation in patients with probable Alzheimer's disease and alcoholic Korsakoff patients. *Neuropsychologia, 41*(5), 575–584. https://doi.org/10.1016/S0028-3932(02)00183-5

Bullard, S. E., Fein, D., Gleeson, M. K., Tischer, N., Mapou, R. L., & Kaplan, E. (2004). The Biber Cognitive Estimation Test. *Archives of Clinical Neuropsychology, 19*(6), 835–846. https://doi.org/10.1016/j.acn.2003.12.002

Buoli, M., Caldiroli, A., Caletti, E., Zugno, E., & Altamura, A. C. (2014). The impact of mood episodes and duration of illness on cognition in bipolar disorder. *Comprehensive Psychiatry, 55*(7), 1561–1566. https://doi.org/10.1016/j.comppsych.2014.06.001

Burgess, P. W., Alderman, N., Evans, J., Emslie, H., & Wilson, B. A. (1998). The ecological validity of tests of executive function. *Journal of the International Neuropsychological Society, 4*(6), 547–558.

Canellopoulou, M., & Richardson, J. T. (1998). The role of executive function in imagery mnemonics: evidence from multiple sclerosis. *Neuropsychologia, 36*(11), 1181–1188. https://doi.org/10.1016/S0028-3932(97)00173-5

Cipolotti, L., MacPherson, S. E., Gharooni, S., van-Harskamp, N., Shallice, T., Chan, E., & Nachev, P. (2017). Cognitive estimation: Performance of patients with focal frontal and posterior lesions. *Neuropsychologia*. https://doi.org/10.1016/j.neuropsychologia.2017.08.017

D'Aniello, G. E., Scarpina, F., Albani, G., Castelnuovo, G., & Mauro, A. (2015). Disentangling the relationship between cognitive estimation abilities and executive functions: A study on patients with Parkinson's disease. *Neurological Sciences, 36*(8), 1425–1429. https://doi.org/10.1007/s10072-015-2158-5

Diaz-Asper, C. M., Schretlen, D. J., & Pearlson, G. D. (2004). How well does IQ predict neuropsychological test performance in normal adults? *Journal of the International Neuropsychological Society, 10*(1), 82–90. https://doi.org/10.1017/S1355617704101100

Fortune, D. G., & Richards, H. L. (2017). Assessing cognitive estimation and its effects on community integration in people with acquired brain injury undergoing rehabilitation. *BioMed Research International, 2017*, 1–13. https://doi.org/10.1155/2017/2874819

Gansler, D. A., Varvaris, M., Swenson, L., & Schretlen, D. J. (2014). Cognitive estimation and its assessment. *Journal of Clinical and Experimental Neuropsychology, 36*(6), 559–568. https://doi.org/10.1080/13803395.2014.915933

Gillespie, D. C., Evans, R. I., Gardener, E. A., & Bowen, A. (2002). Performance of older adults on tests of cognitive estimation. *Journal of Clinical and Experimental Neuropsychology (Neuropsychology, Development and Cognition: Section A), 24*(3), 286–293. https://doi.org/10.1076/jcen.24.3.286.988

Goldstein, F. C., Green, J., Presley, R. M., O'Jile, J., Freeman, A., Watts, R., & Green, R. C. (1996). Cognitive estimation in patients with Alzheimer's disease. *Neuropsychiatry, Neuropsychology, and Behavioural Neurology, 9*, 35–42.

Jackson, C. T., Fein, D., Essock, S. M., & Mueser, K. T. (2001). The effects of cognitive impairment and substance abuse on psychiatric hospitalizations. *Community Mental Health Journal, 37*(4), 303–312. https://doi.org/10.1023/A:1017593423538

Killgore, W. D. S., Muckle, A. E., Grugle, N. L., Killgore, D. B., & Balkin, T. J. (2008). Sex differences in cognitive estimation during sleep deprivation: Effects of stimulant countermeasures. *International Journal of Neuroscience, 118*(11), 1547–1557. https://doi.org/10.1080/00207450802323970

Kisser, J. E., Wendell, C. R., Spencer, R. J., & Waldstein, S. R. (2012). Neuropsychological performance of native versus non-native English speakers. *Archives of Clinical Neuropsychology, 27*(7), 749–755. https://doi.org/10.1093/arclin/acs082

Kopelman, M. D. (1991). Frontal dysfunction and memory deficits in the alcoholic Korsakoff syndrome and Alzheimer-type dementia. *Brain: A Journal of Neurology, 114 (Pt 1A)*, 117–137.

Kopera-Frye, K., Dehaene, S., & Streissguth, A. P. (1996). Impairments of number processing induced by prenatal alcohol exposure. *Neuropsychologia, 34*(12), 1187–1196. https://doi.org/10.1016/0028-3932(96)00043-7

Leng, N. R. C., & Parkin, A. J. (1988). Double dissociation of frontal dysfunction in organic amnesia. *British Journal of Clinical Psychology, 27*(4), 359–362. https://doi.org/10.1111/j.2044-8260.1988.tb00800.x

Levinoff, E. J., Phillips, N. A., Verret, L., Babins, L., Kelner, N., Akerib, V., & Chertkow, H. (2006). Cognitive estimation impairment in Alzheimer disease and mild cognitive impairment. *Neuropsychology, 20*(1), 123–132. https://doi.org/10.1037/0894-4105.20.1.123

MacPherson, S. E., Wagner, G. P., Murphy, P., Bozzali, M., Cipolotti, L., & Shallice, T. (2014). Bringing the Cognitive Estimation Task into the 21st century: Normative data on two new parallel forms. *PloS One, 9*(3), e92554. https://doi.org/10.1371/journal.pone.0092554

Margraf, N., Bachmann, T., Schwandner, W., Gottschalk, S., & Seidel, G. (2009). Bedside screening for executive dysfunction in patients with subcortical ischemic vascular disease. *International Journal of Geriatric Psychiatry, 24*(9), 1002–1009. https://doi.org/10.1002/gps.2212

Mendez, M. F., Doss, R. C., & Cherrier, M. M. (1998). Use of the cognitive estimations test to discriminate frontotemporal dementia from Alzheimer's disease. *Journal of Geriatric Psychiatry and Neurology, 11*(1), 2–6. https://doi.org/10.1177/089198879801100102

O'Carroll, R., Egan, V., & MacKenzie, D. M. (1994). Assessing cognitive estimation. *British Journal of Clinical Psychology, 33*(2), 193–197.

Parente, A., Manfredi, V., Villani, F., Franceschetti, S., & Giovagnoli, A. R. (2013). Investigating higher-order cognitive functions in temporal lobe epilepsy: Cognitive estimation. *Epilepsy & Behavior, 29*(2), 330–336. https://doi.org/10.1016/j.yebeh.2013.07.031

Roth, R. M., Pixley, H. S., Kruck, C. L., Garlinghouse, M. A., Giancola, P. R., & Flashman, L. A. (2012). Performance on the Cognitive Estimation Test in Schizophrenia. *Applied Neuropsychology, 19*(2), 141–146. https://doi.org/10.1080/09084282.2011.595461

Scarpina, F., D'Aniello, G. E., Mauro, A., Castelnuovo, G., & MacPherson, S. E. (2015). How many segments are there in an orange: normative data for the new Cognitive Estimation Task in an Italian population. *Neurological Sciences, 36*(10), 1889–1895. https://doi.org/10.1007/s10072-015-2276-0

Scarpina, F., Mauro, A., D'Aniello, G. E., Albani, G., Castelnuovo, G., Ambiel, E., & MacPherson, S. E. (2017). Cognitive estimation in non-demented Parkinson's disease. *Archives of Clinical Neuropsychology, 32*(4), 381–390. https://doi.org/10.1093/arclin/acx019

Shallice, T., & Evans, M. E. (1978). The involvement of the frontal lobes in cognitive estimation. *Cortex, 14*(2), 294–303.

Schretlen, D. J., Testa, S. M., & Pearlson, G. D. (2010). *Calibrated Neuropsychological Normative System*. Lutz, FL: PAR.

Silverberg, N. D., Hanks, R. A., & Mckay, C. (2007). Cognitive estimation in traumatic brain injury. *Journal of the International Neuropsychological Society, 13*(05), 898–902.

Spencer, R. J., & Johnson-Greene, D. (2009). The Cognitive Estimation Test (CET): Psychometric limitations in neurorehabilitation populations. *Journal of Clinical and Experimental Neuropsychology, 31*(3), 373–377. https://doi.org/10.1080/13803390802206398

Steinmetz, J.-P., & Federspiel, C. (2012). Alcohol-Related cognitive and affective impairments in a sample of long-term care residents. *GeroPsych, 25*(2), 83–95. https://doi.org/10.1024/1662-9647/a000057

Taylor, R. J., & O'Carroll, R. (1995). Cognitive estimation in neurological disorders. *British Journal of Clinical Psychology, 34,* 223–228.

Treitz, F. H., Daum, I., Faustmann, P. M., & Haase, C. G. (2009). Executive deficits in generalized and extrafrontal partial epilepsy: Long versus short seizure-free periods. *Epilepsy & Behavior, 14*(1), 66–70. https://doi.org/10.1016/j.yebeh.2008.08.005

DELIS-KAPLAN EXECUTIVE FUNCTION SYSTEM (D-KEFS)

TEST NAME	**Delis-Kaplan Executive Function System (D-KEFS)**
DOMAIN	Executive functioning
AGE RANGE	In adults, to 89 years
ADMINISTRATION TIME	90 minutes
SCORING FORMAT	Computerized or hand scored
REFERENCE	Delis, D. C., Kaplan, E., & Kramer, J. H. (2001). *Delis-Kaplan Executive Function System*. San Antonio, TX: The Psychological Corporation. www.pearsonclinical.com

DESCRIPTION

The Delis-Kaplan Executive Function System (D-KEFS; Delis et al., 2001) battery includes tests to evaluate component processes of executive functioning. The D-KEFS includes nine tests that derive from existing experimental and clinical measures. The tests, descriptions, and intended function assessed are listed in Table 9–41. The tests embrace a process-oriented approach, specifically that each task provides multiple scores to delineate the source of any difficulties. For example, the D-KEFS Sorting Test yields five primary measures and more than 20 optional measures of different components of problem-solving skills. In this way, the examiner can isolate the fundamental components resulting in impaired performance and can assess the fundamental skill itself.

A number of features are incorporated in the D-KEFS that are designed to increase the sensitivity of the tests to mild neurologic dysfunction. For example, a number of switching conditions are included in the tasks. In addition to traditional Stroop procedures of naming color patches, reading color words in black ink, and naming the ink color in which a color word is written (an interference condition), a fourth condition involves switching between naming the dissonant ink color and reading the actual word.

Because patients with frontal lobe damage may have difficulty disengaging their attention from salient aspects of the physical environment, the authors added "capture" stimuli to several of the test materials, compelling more automatic, effortless responding. For example, on the switching condition of the TMT where the examinee must alternate connecting numbers and letters in sequence, two pairs of capture stimuli were placed strategically in each quadrant of the stimulus page. For instance, a 4 is printed immediately adjacent to the 3 along the same path as the B-to-3 connection. Furthermore, to maximize detection of subtle executive deficits, processing demands of tasks were increased. For example, the D-KEFS Sorting Test requires the examinee to identify a maximum of 16 different conceptual rules for sorting the card sets.

The D-KEFS was designed to be used in a flexible manner. Thus, the tests can be used singly or in combination with other D-KEFS tests. Test conditions may also be omitted. An alternate form is provided for three of the tests that are most susceptible to practice effects: Sorting, Twenty Questions, and Verbal Fluency.

ADMINISTRATION

Detailed administration instructions are found in the manual.

SCORING

Scoring guidelines for each test are found in the Examiner's Manual and the Record Form. For most of the measures, raw scores are converted to age-scaled scores (M = 10, SD = 3). Some process measure raw scores (e.g., error or ratio measures) have limited ranges in healthy populations. Thus, the raw scores are converted to cumulative percentile ranks corrected for each of the 16 age groups. A few measures have limited raw score ranges and show minimal age effects across the normative sample (e.g., set-loss errors on Verbal Fluency). In those cases, raw scores are converted to cumulative percentile ranks corrected for the entire normative sample.

The D-KEFS includes contrast measures that quantify relative performance on (a) a baseline task and a higher level task (e.g., Trail Making Contrast = Number-Letter Switching minus Motor Speed) or (b) two higher level tasks (e.g., Verbal Fluency Contrast = Letter Fluency minus Category Fluency). Scaled score differences are treated like raw scores and are converted to a new scaled score (M = 10, SD = 3). In addition, some measures are combined into new scaled scores so that tasks that are thought to measure similar cognitive functions can be evaluated (e.g., Design Fluency

TABLE 9–41 Delis-Kaplan Executive Function System (D-KEFS) Tests and Their Functions

D-KEFS TESTS	DESCRIPTION	KEY FUNCTIONS ASSESSED
Trail Making Test	The examinee is to scan letters and numbers and mark the number 3 (Condition 1), connect the number in ascending order (Condition 2), connect just the letters in alphabetical order (Condition 3), switch between connecting numbers and letters (Condition 4), and draw a line over a dotted line as quickly as possible (Condition 5).	Assesses visual scanning, number sequencing, letter sequencing, number-letter switching, and motor speed
Verbal Fluency Test	The examinee is asked to say words that begin with a specified letter (Letter Fluency), say words that belong to a designated semantic category (Category Fluency) and alternate between saying words from two different semantic categories (Category Switching).	Fluent productivity in the verbal domain
Design Fluency Test	The examinee is presented with rows of boxes containing an array of dots and must make as many designs as possible in one minute by connecting filled dots (Condition 1), connecting unfilled dots only (Condition 2), and alternating connections between filled and unfilled dots (Condition 3).	Fluent productivity in the nonverbal domain
Color-Word Interference Test	A variant of the Stroop procedure in which the examinee names color patches (Condition 1), reads words that denote colors printed in black ink (Condition 2), names the ink color in which color words are printed (Condition 3), and switches back and forth between naming the dissonant ink colors and reading the conflicting words (Condition 4).	Inhibition of an overlearned response and flexibility
Sorting Test	In Condition 1 (Free Sorting), the examinee is asked to sort six cards into two groups, according to as many rules as possible. In Condition 2 (Sort Recognition), the examinee is to identify and describe the correct rules the examiner used to generate the sort.	Problem solving, verbal and nonverbal concept formation, and flexibility of thinking on a conceptual task
Twenty Questions Test	The examinee is presented with a stimulus page containing 30 common objects and has to ask the fewest number of yes/no questions to identify the target.	Categorical processing and ability to use feedback to guide problem solving
Word Context Test	The examinee is to discover the meaning of made-up words based on cues given in sentences.	Deductive reasoning, verbal abstract thinking, and hypothesis testing
Tower Test	The examinee's task is to move five disks across three pegs to build a target tower in the fewest number of moves possible.	Planning, rule learning, and inhibition
Proverb Test	The examinee is to interpret proverbs orally (Free Inquiry) and select the best interpretation from four alternatives (Multiple Choice).	Metaphorical thinking and generating versus comprehending abstract thought

SOURCE: Adapted from Delis et al. (2001).

Composite = Condition 1 Filled Dots plus Condition 2 Empty Dots). The D-KEFS distinguishes between "primary" and "optional" measures. Primary measures either provide a global overall characterization of performance on the task or they provide process scores for key components of the task.

DEMOGRAPHIC EFFECTS

AGE

Age affects performance on the D-KEFS (Wecker et al., 2000). Performance on measures that are highly dependent on processing speed tend to peak in the adolescent and young adult groups, whereas performance on tests of verbal conceptual reasoning tends to peak in the adult age groups.

Older age is associated with fewer correct sorts on the Sorting Test (manual, Mattioli et al., 2014), which may be due in part to diminished working memory for previous sorts. Age differences are reduced when cues related to verbal descriptions of previous sorts are provided to examinees, which assists them in monitoring and organizing information necessary for decision making (Hartman et al., 2004). Age also accounts for a significant portion of variance on the Color-Word Interference condition and switching conditions of the Trail Making, Design Fluency, and Verbal Fluency tasks, a relationship that remains even when component process are accounted for (Wecker et al., 2000; Wecker et al., 2005).

GENDER

Overall, gender effects are minimal (Clark et al., 2010; Davis et al., 2011; Mattioli et al., 2014; Mitchell & Miller, 2008), although some have reported effects (Kalkut et al., 2009).

EDUCATION AND IQ

The manual does not provide information regarding the effects of education on performance; however, subsequent research has suggested a relationship. There is a significant effect of education level and vocabulary on the TMT (Fine et al., 2011; see also the section "Normative Data"). A factor score reflecting inhibition on the D-KEFS relates to education in patients with schizophrenia (Clark et al., 2010).

Moderate correlations between the Sorting Test and education in patients with MS have been reported (Parmenter et al., 2007). See "Evidence for Validity" for information on IQ effects.

ETHNICITY, NATIONALITY, AND LINGUISTIC EFFECTS

The impact of these sociodemographic variables has not been reported. Of note, the D-KEFS has been translated into other languages, including Hebrew (Heled et al., 2012).

NORMATIVE DATA

The D-KEFS was normed on a sample of 1,750 individuals aged 8 to 89 years selected to match the US population in terms of age, gender, ethnicity, education, and geographic region. The characteristics of adults in the standardization sample are shown in Table 9–42.

For the alternate forms, a normative equating study was conducted with a sample of 286 individuals (105 males, 181 females; aged 16–89 years, $M = 47.5$, $SD = 23.5$; 84% Caucasian; 89% with ≥12 years of education) who were administered both the standard and alternate forms in counterbalanced order. Norms for each alternate form were derived from linear transformations of the standard form normative values for each age group; however, use of the norms may be problematic given the low correlations between forms for many of the key variables (see "Evidence for Reliability").

Fine et al. (2011) provide education-adjusted norms for the adult standardization sample on the D-KEFS, derived via inferential norming. Their study involved 875 participants. The average age of the sample was 51.5 years ($SD = 20.7$ years). The sample was 52% female, predominantly Caucasian (80% Caucasian, 11% African American, 7% Hispanic American). Most of the sample had at least 12 years of education (81%; see paper for additional details).

Vocabulary-adjusted normative data were also provided for 1,191 individuals who completed the Wechsler Abbreviated Scale of Intelligence (WASI) Vocabulary subtest, including both children and adults. The mean age was 35.9 years ($SD = 25$). The sample was 54% female and predominantly Caucasian (83% Caucasian, 9% African American, 6% Hispanic American). Most of the sample had a Grade 12 education or higher (87%; see paper for details). The average IQ of the sample was 102.3 ($SD = 13.8$). Normative data are provided in Tables 9–43 to 9–50.

Mattioli et al. (2014) provide Italian normative data for 195 participants 20 to 69 years of age for the Sorting Test, standard and alternate forms. The sample was 54% female, with an average age of 43.76 years ($SD = 13.85$) and a mean education of 12.44 years ($SD = 4.39$). Exclusion criteria included neurologic or psychiatric condition, learning disability, substance abuse, subjective complaint of cognitive impairment, MMSE cutoff score, major medical condition, and inadequate (or uncorrected) vision and hearing. Normative data are provided in the online version of their article.

TABLE 9–42 Characteristics of the D-KEFS Normative Sample

Sample size	1,750
Age	8 to 89
Geographic location	From geographic regions in proportions consistent with 2000 US Census data
Sample type	Based on a representative sample of the US population stratified on the basis of age, gender, ethnicity, education level, and geographic region
Education	<8 to >16 years and consistent with US Census proportions; for examinees ≤19 years of age, parental education was used
Gender	Roughly an equal number of males and females in each age group with the exception that the older age groups included more women than men, in proportions consistent with 2000 US Census data
Ethnicity	The proportions of Caucasians, African Americans, Hispanics and other ethnic groups were based on ethnic proportions within each age band according to 2000 US Census data
Screening	Screened via self-report for sensory, substance abuse, medical, psychiatric, or motor condition that could affect performance

NOTE: *The adult* sample was divided into the following age groups: 16 to 19, 20 to 29, 30 to 39, 40 to 49, 50 to 59, 60 to 69, 70 to 79, 80 to 89 years. The *n* in each age band ranged from 70 to 175, depending on the age group.

SOURCE: Adapted from Delis et al. (2001).

TABLE 9–43 Education-Adjusted Normative Data for the Delis-Kaplan Executive Function System (D-KEFS) Trail Making Number Sequencing Condition

	EDUCATION				
TRAIL MAKING NUMBER SEQUENCING AGE-SCALED SCORE	≤8 YEARS	9–11 YEARS	12 YEARS	13–15 YEARS	≥16 YEARS
1	2	1	1	1	1
2	3	1	1	1	1
3	4	2	2	2	2
4	5	3	3	3	3
5	6	4	4	4	4
6	7	5	5	5	5
7	8	6	6	6	6
8	8	7	7	7	6
9	9	8	8	8	7
10	10	10	9	9	8
11	10	10	10	10	9
12	11	11	11	11	10
13	12	12	12	12	11
14	13	13	13	13	12
15	14	14	14	14	14
16	15	15	15	15	15
17	16	16	16	16	16
18	17	17	17	17	17
19	19	18	18	18	18

SOURCE: Fine et al. (2011).

TABLE 9–44 Delis-Kaplan Executive Function System (D-KEFS) Trail Making Letter Sequencing Education-Adjusted Normative Data

TRAIL MAKING LETTER SEQUENCING AGE-SCALED SCORE	EDUCATION				
	≤8 YEARS	9–11 YEARS	12 YEARS	13–15 YEARS	≥16 YEARS
1	2	1	1	1	1
2	3	1	1	1	1
3	4	2	1	1	1
4	5	3	2	2	1
5	6	4	3	3	2
6	7	5	4	4	3
7	8	7	6	5	4
8	9	8	7	6	5
9	10	9	9	8	6
10	10	10	10	9	7
11	11	11	10	10	9
12	12	12	11	11	10
13	13	13	12	12	11
14	13	13	13	13	13
15	14	14	14	14	14
16	15	15	15	15	15
17	16	16	16	16	16
18	17	17	17	17	17
19	19	18	18	18	18

SOURCE: Fine et al. (2011).

Methods have been provided for calculating supplemental D-KEFS scores from data presented in the Technical Manual (Crawford et al., 2011), including base rate data (i.e., the number of abnormally low scores in comparison with normative estimates of the number of low scores) and a composite executive function index score and confidence intervals. A computerized program is provided, which is recommended rather than manual calculations. The program is found at https://homepages.abdn.ac.uk/j.crawford/pages/dept/psychom.htm. Base rate data were generated using a Monte Carlo method. The reliabilities of

TABLE 9–45 Education-Adjusted Normative Data for the Delis-Kaplan Executive Function System (D-KEFS) Trail Making Number-Letter Switching Condition

TRAIL MAKING NUMBER-LETTER SWITCHING AGE-SCALED SCORE	EDUCATION				
	≤8 YEARS	9–11 YEARS	12 YEARS	13–15 YEARS	≥16 YEARS
1	2	2	1	1	1
2	3	3	2	1	1
3	4	4	3	1	1
4	5	5	4	2	1
5	6	5	5	3	2
6	7	6	5	4	3
7	8	7	6	5	4
8	9	8	7	6	5
9	10	9	8	8	7
10	10	10	9	9	8
11	11	10	10	10	9
12	11	11	11	11	10
13	12	12	12	12	11
14	13	13	13	13	13
15	14	14	14	14	14
16	15	15	15	15	15
17	16	16	16	16	16
18	17	17	17	17	17
19	19	18	18	18	18

SOURCE: Fine et al. (2011).

TABLE 9–46 Education-Adjusted Normative Data for the Delis-Kaplan Executive Function System (D-KEFS) Trail Making Motor Speed Condition

TRAIL MAKING MOTOR SPEED AGE-SCALED SCORE	EDUCATION				
	≤ 8 YEARS	9–11 YEARS	12 YEARS	13–15 YEARS	≥16 YEARS
1	1	1	1	1	1
2	1	1	1	1	1
3	2	2	2	2	1
4	3	3	3	3	1
5	4	4	4	4	2
6	6	5	5	5	3
7	8	6	6	6	5
8	9	7	7	7	6
9	10	9	8	8	8
10	10	10	9	9	9
11	11	11	10	10	10
12	12	12	11	11	11
13	13	12	12	12	11
14	13	13	13	13	12
15	14	14	14	13	13
16	15	15	15	14	14
17	16	16	16	15	15
18	17	17	17	16	16
19	19	18	18	17	17

SOURCE: Fine et al. (2011).

TABLE 9–47 Vocabulary-Adjusted Normative Data for the Delis-Kaplan Executive Function System (D-KEFS) Trail Making Number Sequencing Condition

TRAIL MAKING NUMBER SEQUENCING AGE-SCALED SCORE	VOCABULARY SCALED SCORE						
	1–3	4–5	6–7	8–9	10–11	12–13	>13
1	4	3	2	1	1	1	1
2	5	4	3	2	1	1	1
3	6	5	4	3	2	2	2
4	6	5	4	4	3	3	3
5	7	6	5	5	4	4	4
6	8	7	6	6	5	5	5
7	9	8	7	7	6	6	6
8	10	9	9	8	7	7	7
9	11	10	10	9	8	8	8
10	12	11	11	10	10	9	9
11	14	12	12	11	11	10	10
12	15	14	13	12	12	11	11
13	16	15	14	13	13	12	12
14	17	16	15	15	14	14	13
15	18	17	16	16	15	15	15
16	19	18	18	18	17	17	17
17	19	19	19	19	18	18	18
18	19	19	19	19	19	19	19
19	19	19	19	19	19	19	19

NOTE: Vocabulary scaled scores are from the Wechsler Abbreviated Scale of Intelligence (WASI).

SOURCE: Fine et al. (2011).

TABLE 9-48 Vocabulary-Adjusted Normative Data for the Delis-Kaplan Executive Function System (D-KEFS) Trail Making Letter Sequencing Condition

TRAIL MAKING LETTER SEQUENCING AGE-SCALED SCORE	VOCABULARY SCALED SCORE						
	1–3	4–5	6–7	8–9	10–11	12–13	>13
1	4	3	2	1	1	1	1
2	5	4	3	2	1	1	1
3	6	5	4	3	2	2	1
4	7	6	5	4	3	3	2
5	8	7	6	5	4	4	3
6	9	8	7	6	5	5	4
7	10	9	8	7	6	6	5
8	11	10	9	8	7	7	7
9	12	11	10	9	8	8	8
10	13	12	11	10	10	9	9
11	14	13	12	11	11	10	10
12	15	14	13	12	12	12	11
13	16	15	14	13	13	13	12
14	17	16	15	15	14	14	14
15	18	17	16	16	16	16	15
16	19	18	17	17	17	17	17
17	19	19	18	18	18	18	18
18	19	19	19	19	19	19	19
19	19	19	19	19	19	19	19

NOTE: Vocabulary scaled scores are from the Wechsler Abbreviated Scale of Intelligence (WASI).

SOURCE: Fine et al. (2011).

TABLE 9-49 Vocabulary-Adjusted Normative Data for the Delis-Kaplan Executive Function System (D-KEFS) Trail Making Number-Letter Switching Condition

TRAIL MAKING NUMBER-LETTER SWITCHING AGE-SCALED SCORE	VOCABULARY SCALED SCORE						
	1–3	4–5	6–7	8–9	10–11	12–13	>13
1	5	4	2	1	1	1	1
2	6	5	3	2	1	1	1
3	7	6	4	3	2	1	1
4	8	7	5	4	3	2	2
5	9	8	6	5	4	3	3
6	10	9	7	6	5	4	4
7	10	9	8	7	6	5	5
8	11	10	9	9	8	7	7
9	12	11	10	10	9	8	8
10	13	12	11	11	10	9	9
11	14	13	12	12	11	10	10
12	14	14	13	13	12	11	11
13	15	15	14	13	13	13	12
14	16	16	15	14	14	14	13
15	17	17	16	15	15	15	14
16	18	18	17	16	16	16	15
17	19	19	18	17	17	17	16
18	19	19	19	18	18	18	17
19	19	19	19	19	19	19	19

NOTE: Vocabulary scaled scores arc from the Wechsler Abbreviated Scale of Intelligence (WASI).

SOURCE: Fine et al. (2011).

TABLE 9-50 Vocabulary-Adjusted Normative Data for the Delis-Kaplan Executive Function System (D-KEFS) Trail Making Motor Speed Condition

TRAIL MAKING MOTOR SPEED AGE-SCALED SCORE	VOCABULARY SCALED SCORE						
	1–3	4–5	6–7	8–9	10–11	12–13	>13
1	3	2	2	1	1	1	1
2	4	3	3	2	2	2	1
3	5	4	4	3	3	3	2
4	6	5	5	4	4	4	3
5	7	6	6	5	5	4	4
6	8	7	7	6	6	5	5
7	10	9	8	7	7	6	6
8	11	10	9	8	8	7	7
9	12	11	10	9	9	8	8
10	13	12	11	10	10	9	9
11	14	13	12	11	11	10	10
12	15	14	13	12	12	11	11
13	16	15	14	14	13	13	13
14	17	16	15	15	15	14	14
15	18	17	16	16	16	16	16
16	19	18	17	17	17	17	17
17	19	19	19	19	19	19	19

NOTE: Vocabulary scaled scores are from the Wechsler Abbreviated Scale of Intelligence (WASI).

SOURCE: Fine et al. (2011).

the Executive Index were calculated to be very high, ranging from .90 to .92 for three age bands. To calculate the Composite Executive Index, the formula in Figure 9–5 is used. Tables 9–51 and 9–52 depict base rate data. As the authors discuss, as shown in Table 9–51, if an abnormally low score is defined as a score of 5 or less, then nearly half of the normative population between the ages of 20 to 49 are expected to exhibit at least one low score of this magnitude. Using the cutoff of 5 or less, 25% of the population is expected to exhibit two or more low scores (Crawford et al., 2011).

Karr, Garcia-Barrera, Holdnack, and Iverson (2017) provide base rate data of low scores for 1,050 adult participants from the D-KEFS standardization sample. Test scores from the TMT, the Color-Word Interference Test, and the Verbal Fluency Test were analyzed, and are presented in Tables 9–53 and 9–54. Low test scores were common, with 36%

To form a composite executive index, the available achievement scores for an individual are simply summed and entered into the following formula to convert this sum to an index score having a mean of 100 and standard deviation of 15.

$$\text{Executive Index score} = \frac{15}{S_{sum}}(X_{sum} - \bar{X}) + 100, \qquad (2)$$

where X_{sum} is the sum of an individual's achievement score, S_{sum} is the population standard deviation of the sum of the achievement scores, and $\bar{X}$ is the population mean of the sum of the achievement scores (Crawford, 2004).

Figure 9–5 *Formula for the calculation of the Composite Executive Index.*

SOURCE: Crawford et al. (2011)

TABLE 9–51 Base Rate Data for Delis-Kaplan Executive Function System (D-KEFS) Low Scores for Ages 20–49 Years

	NUMBER OF LOW SCORES															
CRITERION	1	2	3	4	5	6	7	8	9	10	11	12	13	14	15	16
<7 (PR = 15.9)	84.98	66.25	50.48	37.75	27.67	19.82	13.81	9.30	6.02	3.71	2.14	1.21	0 52	0.19	0.05	0.00
<6 (PR = 9.12)	69.09	44.83	29.52	19.38	12.52	7.95	4.94	2.97	1.72	0.95	0.48	0.22	0.08	0.03	0.00	0.00
<5 (PR = 4.78)	**49.36**	**25.60**	**14.15**	**8.00**	**4.51**	**2.51**	**1.37**	**0.73**	**0.37**	**0.18**	**0.08**	**0.03**	**0.01**	**0.00**	**0.00**	**0.00**
<4 (PR = 2.27)	30.56	12.24	5.56	2.62	1.29	0.63	0.30	0.14	0.06	0.03	0.01	0.00	0.00	0.00	0.00	0.00
<3 (PR = 0.98)	16.34	4.91	1.80	0.71	0.29	0.12	0.05	0.02	0.01	0.00	0.00	0.00	0.00	0.00	0.00	0.00

NOTE: Increasingly stringent criteria for an abnormally low score are applied, ranging from a score of 7 or lower (PR = 15.9) to a score of 3 or lower (PR = .98). The figures in this table assume that all 16 scores were obtained. A score of 5 or lower is the preferred criterion for an abnormally low score. Therefore, the percentages for this criterion appear in bold. PR, percentile rank.

SOURCE: Crawford et al. (2011).

of the sample with one or more scores at or lower than the 5th percentile. The prevalence of low scores increased with lower levels of intelligence as measured by the WASI and fewer years of education.

EVIDENCE FOR RELIABILITY

EVIDENCE FOR INTERNAL RELIABILITY

Internal reliability is provided in the Technical Manual for primary measures in the normative sample. Coefficients range from inadequate (e.g., Verbal Fluency Category Switching Total Correct) to adequate or higher (e.g., Twenty Questions Initial Abstraction), depending on the particular measure and the age group. Low reliability coefficients of contrast measures obtained from the D-KEFS have been reported, with none exceeding .70, and a median reliability of .30 (Crawford et al., 2008).

EVIDENCE FOR TEST-RETEST RELIABILITY, MEASURING CHANGE, AND PRACTICE EFFECTS

Test-retest reliability provided in the manual was based on a sample of 101 participants, distributed across age groups. The time between administrations ranged from nine to 74 days, with an average retest interval of 25 days. Test-retest correlations ranged from low (e.g., Trail Making, Design Fluency) to adequate/high (e.g., Letter and Category Fluency Total Correct; see Table 9–55). Practice effects are evident for most of the tasks, with gains of about one to two scaled-score points on each task.

EVIDENCE FOR RELIABILITY OF ALTERNATE, SHORT, OR COMPUTER FORMS

The D-KEFS provides alternate forms for the Sorting, Verbal Fluency, and Twenty Questions tests. The two forms were given in counterbalanced order to 286 people, ranging in age from 16 to 89 years ($M = 47.5$, $SD = 23.5$). The Technical Manual provides means, standard deviations, and correlations for the key variables of the standard and alternate forms. As shown in Table 9–56, correlations between forms for key variables range from low (e.g., Twenty Questions) to high (e.g., Letter Fluency Total Correct).

EVIDENCE FOR INTERRATER RELIABILITY

No information is available. Interrater reliability estimates would be informative for tasks that require examiner judgment (e.g., Proverbs, Twenty Questions, Word Context).

EVIDENCE FOR VALIDITY

WITHIN-TEST RELATIONSHIPS

A number of within- and between-task correlational analyses subdivided by specified age bands in the normative sample are presented in the manual. The magnitude of the

TABLE 9–52 Base Rate Data for Delis-Kaplan Executive Function System (D-KEFS) Low Scores for Ages 50–89 Years

	NUMBER OF LOW SCORES															
CRITERION	1	2	3	4	5	6	7	8	9	10	11	12	13	14	15	16
<7 (PR = 15.9)	84.90	64.67	49.05	36.85	27.41	20.09	14.46	10.07	6.78	4.36	2.64	1.45	0.69	0.27	0.07	0.00
<6 (PR = 9.12)	68.52	43.35	28.65	19.18	12.83	8.52	5.54	3.49	2.12	1.24	0.67	0.32	0.13	0.04	0.01	0.00
<5 (PR = 4.78)	**48.51**	**24.70**	**14.00**	**8.23**	**4.91**	**2.91**	**1.70**	**0.98**	**0.53**	**0.27**	**0.13**	**0.06**	**0.02**	**0.00**	**0.00**	**0.00**
<4 (PR = 2.27)	29.85	11.90	5.67	2.89	1.52	0.81	0.42	0.22	0.10	0.05	0.02	0.01	0.00	0.00	0.00	0.00
<3 (PR = 0.98)	15.95	4.86	1.92	0.85	0.39	0.18	0.08	0.04	0.01	0.01	0.00	0.00	0.00	0.00	0.00	0.00

NOTE: Increasingly stringent criteria for an abnormally low score are applied ranging from a score of 7 or lower (PR = 15.9) to a score of 3 or lower (PR = .98). The figures in this table assume that all 16 scores were obtained. A score of 5 or lower is the preferred criterion for an abnormally low score. Therefore, the percentages for this criterion appear in bold. PR, percentile rank.

SOURCE: Crawford et al. (2011).

TABLE 9–53 Delis-Kaplan Executive Function System (D-KEFS) Base Rates of Low Scores According to Percentile Cutoffs for Ages 16–89 Years by IQ and Education

NUMBER OF LOW SCORES	TOTAL SAMPLE	WASI FSIQ				EDUCATION				
		≤89	90–99	100–109	110+	≤8	9–11	12	13–15	16+
Sample size	1,028	160	163	243	241	57	125	351	275	220
≤25th percentile										
7 low scores	0.3	1.3	–	–	–	3.5	–	–	0.4	–
6 or more	2.9	7.5	1.8	1.2	0.4	10.5	5.6	3.4	0.7	1.4
5 or more	8.4	22.5	6.1	5.3	0.8	21.1	17.6	8.5	4.7	4.1
4 or more	18.2	44.4	18.4	11.9	2.9	33.3	36.8	19.9	12.4	8.2
3 or more	32.3	63.8	33.7	25.9	10.8	52.6	50.4	35.6	25.5	20.0
2 or more	50.9	83.1	58.3	42.0	27.8	77.2	70.4	57.8	42.2	32.7
1 or more	76.6	95.0	85.9	71.2	60.2	96.5	92.0	81.8	70.5	61.8
No low scores	23.4	5.0	14.1	28.8	39.8	3.5	8.0	18.2	29.5	38.2
≤16th percentile										
7 low scores	0.2	1.3	–	–	–	3.5	–	–	–	–
6 or more	1.5	4.4	1.2	0.4	–	7.0	4.8	1.1	–	0.5
5 or more	2.8	9.4	1.2	1.6	0.4	12.3	5.6	2.6	1.1	1.4
4 or more	8.9	23.1	8.6	4.1	0.4	22.8	18.4	11.1	4.7	1.8
3 or more	18.7	44.4	17.8	9.9	2.9	36.8	37.6	20.5	12.7	7.7
2 or more	35.8	67.5	37.4	28.0	14.9	57.9	54.4	38.7	30.2	21.8
1 or more	62.8	88.1	67.5	58.4	38.6	87.7	78.4	70.1	54.9	45.9
No low scores	37.2	11.9	32.5	41.6	61.4	12.3	21.6	29.9	45.1	54.1
≤9th percentile										
7 low scores	–	–	–	–	–	–	–	–	–	–
6 or more	0.5	1.3	–	–	–	5.3	1.6	–	–	–
5 or more	1.6	5.6	0.6	0.8	–	7.0	3.2	1.4	0.4	0.9
4 or more	5.2	15.0	4.9	2.1	–	15.8	9.6	6.6	2.2	1.4
3 or more	11.4	28.8	12.3	5.3	1.2	26.3	24.0	13.1	6.9	3.2
2 or more	24.4	51.9	25.2	18.5	6.6	49.1	42.4	24.8	19.6	13.2
1 or more	48.1	78.1	51.5	41.6	23.7	77.2	64.8	51.0	41.1	35.0
No low scores	51.9	21.9	48.5	58.4	76.3	22.8	35.2	49.0	58.9	65.0
≤5th percentile										
7 low scores	–	–	–	–	–	–	–	–	–	–
6 or more	0.1	–	–	–	–	–	0.8	–	–	–
5 or more	0.3	–	–	–	–	1.8	1.6	–	–	–
4 or more	1.9	6.3	1.2	0.8	–	5.3	4.8	2.6	0.4	0.5
3 or more	6.0	16.3	7.4	2.5	–	17.5	14.4	6.6	2.5	1.8
2 or more	14.0	33.8	13.5	7.8	2.5	33.3	28.0	13.7	9.5	7.3
1 of more	36.1	66.9	41.1	25.5	16.2	59.6	53.6	39.9	29.5	22.3
No low scores	63.9	33.1	58.9	74.5	83.8	40.4	46.4	60.1	70.5	77.7
≤2nd percentile										
7 low scores	–	–	–	–	–	–	–	–	–	–
6 or more	–	–	–	–	–	–	–	–	–	–
5 or more	0.1	–	–	–	–	–	0.8	–	–	–
4 or more	0.5	1.3	–	0.4	–	–	2.4	0.6	–	–
3 or more	2.6	6.9	4.3	0.4	–	10.5	5.6	3.7	0.4	–
2 or more	8.9	23.1	10.4	3.7	1.2	19.3	16.0	10.3	4.7	5.0
1 or more	26.8	50.6	33.1	16.5	9.1	42.1	43.2	30.2	21.1	15.5
No low scores	73.2	49.4	66.9	83.5	90.9	57.9	56.8	69.8	78.9	84.5

NOTE: WASI, Wechsler Abbreviated Scale of Intelligence. Subtests and scores included were Trail Making Test Condition 4: Number-Letter Switching, Verbal Fluency Test Condition 1: Letter Fluency, Condition 2: Category Fluency, Condition 3: Category Switching Total Correct Responses, and Condition 4: Category Switching Total Switching Accuracy, and Color-Word Interference Test Condition 3: Inhibition, and Condition 4: Inhibition/Switching. All values represent cumulative percentages except for the rows labeled "No low scores" which provide the percentage of the sample with no scores under the low score cutoffs.

SOURCE: Karr et al. (2017).

correlations of scores within tasks varies significantly by the task, measure, and age group. In general, primary measures derived from the same test correlate more highly than scores across tests. Correlations between tasks tend to be modest. For example, median correlations between summary scores for Sorting, Tower, Letter Fluency, and Figural Fluency tasks were $r = .25$ for 20- to 49-year-olds and $r = .33$ for 50-89-year-olds. These relatively modest values suggest that the tasks may measure different aspects of executive function (Delis et al., 2001). However, modest values may also suggest weak convergent validity of the executive functioning construct (Salthouse et al., 2003).

The D-KEFS provides many process variables, including several measures reflecting initiation of problem-solving behavior (e.g., the number of attempted sorts on the Sorting Test and the number of total responses generated on Verbal

TABLE 9–54 Base Rate Data for Delis-Kaplan Executive Function System (D-KEFS) Low Scores for Ages 16–89 Years by IQ and Education (Qualitative Descriptor)

		WASI FSIQ				EDUCATION				
	TOTAL SAMPLE	≤89	90–99	100–109	110+	≤8	9–11	12	13–15	16+
	N = 1,028	N = 160	N = 163	N = 243	N = 241	N = 57	N = 125	N = 351	N = 275	N = 220
Number of scores ≤25th percentile										
Above average	0	0–1	0	–	–	0–1	0–1	0	–	–
Average	1–3	2–4	1–3	0–3	0–2	2–4	2–4	1–3	0–3	0–2
Below average	4	5	4	4	3	5–6	5	4	4	3
Unusually low	5	6	5	5	–	7	6	5–6	5	4–5
Extremely low	6–7	7	6–7	6–7	4–7	–	7	7	6–7	6–7
Number of scores ≤16th percentile										
Above average	–	0	–	–	–	0	0	–	–	–
Average	0–2	1–3	0–2	0–2	0–1	1–3	1–3	1–2	1–2	0–1
Below average	3	4	3	–	2	4–5	4	3–4	3	2
Unusually low	4	5–6	4	3–4	–	6–7	5–6	4	4	3
Extremely low	5–7	7	5–7	5–7	3–7	–	7	5–7	5–7	4–7
Number of scores ≤9th percentile										
Above average	–	0	–	–	–	0	–	–	–	–
Average	0–1	1–3	0–2	0–1	0	1–3	0–2	0–1	0–1	0–1
Below average	2–3	4	3	2	1	4	3	2–3	2	2
Unusually low	4	5	4	3	2	5–6	4–5	4	3	3
Extremely low	5–7	6–7	5–7	4–7	3–7	7	6–7	5–7	4–7	4–7
Number of scores <5th percentile										
Above average	–	–	–	–	–	–	–	–	–	–
Average	0–1	0–2	0–1	0–1	0	0–2	0–2	0–1	0–1	0
Below average	2	3	2	–	1	3	3	2	–	1
Unusually low	3	4	3	2	–	4	4	3	2	2
Extremely low	4–7	5–7	4–7	3–7	2–7	5–7	5–7	4–7	3–7	3–7
Number of scores <2nd percentile										
Above average	–	–	–	–	–	–	–	–	–	–
Average	0–1	0–1	0–1	0	0	0–1	0–1	0–1	0	0
Below averse	–	2	2	1	–	2–3	2	2	1	1
Unusually low	2	3	3	2	1	–	3	3	2	2
Extremely low	3–7	4–7	4–7	3–7	2–7	4–7	4–7	4–7	3–7	3–7

NOTE: WASI, Wechsler Abbreviated Scale of Intelligence. Subtests and scores included were Trail Making Test Condition 4: Number-Letter Switching; Verbal Fluency Test Condition 1: Letter Fluency, Condition 2: Category Fluency. Condition 3: Category Switching Total Correct Responses, and Condition 4: Category Switching Total Switching Accuracy: and Color-Word Interference Test Condition 3: Inhibition, and Condition 4: Inhibition/Switching. The normative classification ranges in the first column were as follows: Above Average: >75th percentile, fewer than 25% score in this range; Average: 25th to 75th percentile ranks in the cumulative frequency distribution; Below Average: 10th to 24th percentile ranks in the cumulative frequency distribution; Unusually Low: 3rd to 9th percentile; and Extremely Low: <3rd percentile.

To use this table for your client, comparison with the IQ score or education level may be used to determine if the number of scores within each score band obtained is considered above average or extremely low relative to others who obtained the same IQ score or education level.

SOURCE: Karr et al. (2017).

Fluency). The correlations among these measures are unexpectedly modest (rs = .10–.30), given that they are purported to measure a similar underlying construct. Indicators of speed of processing also tend to be low across tasks (typically r < .20). Correlations between error scores (e.g., repetition, set-loss) across tasks are also low. These low correlations raise concerns regarding the meaning of the various scores and the possibility that measures with the same classification (e.g., repetition, set-loss errors) may actually measure different constructs.

FACTOR-ANALYTIC STUDIES AND RELATIONSHIPS WITH OTHER TESTS

Factor-analytic studies generally yield two to three factors. Factors include a cognitive flexibility factor and an inhibition factor (Clark et al., 2010; Latzman & Markon, 2010; manual) or have identified a cognitive flexibility and abstraction factor (Savla et al., 2010). A third factor, termed monitoring (switching from fluency measures) has also been identified (see manual). The inhibition factor typically reflects variables from Color-Word Interference, Trail Making, and fluency measures, with the flexibility factor reflecting Sorting Test variables and/or other measures.

Research typically suggests moderate correlations between the D-KEFS and other executive function measures, such as the WCST (absolute value of rs = .27 to .59; manual; Parmenter et al., 2007) and verbal fluency (McKinlay et al., 2009).

Studies comparing the D-KEFS Tower Test to other tower tests suggest that some distinct abilities are measured.

TABLE 9–55 Magnitude of Reliability Coefficients for the Delis-Kaplan Executive Function System (D-KEFS)

	INTERNAL RELIABILITY	TEST-RETEST
Very high (.90+)		
High (.80 to .89)	**Verbal Fluency**: Condition 1 Letter Fluency Total Correct **Twenty Questions**: Initial Abstraction **Proverb Test**: Total Achievement	**Verbal Fluency**: Condition 1 Letter Fluency Total Correct
Adequate (.70 to .79)	**Trail Making**: Combined Number and Letter Sequencing Composite **Color Word**: Combined Color Naming and Word Reading Composite **Sorting**: Condition 1 Free Sorting Confirmed, Condition 2 Free Sorting Description, Condition 3 Sorting Recognition Total	**Trail Making**: Condition 5 Motor Speed Seconds to Complete **Verbal Fluency**: Condition 2 Category Fluency Total Correct **Color-Word**: Condition 1 Color Naming Seconds to Complete, Condition 3 Inhibition Seconds to Complete **Word Context**: Total First Trial Consistency Correct **Proverb Test**: Total Achievement
Marginal (.60 to .69)	**Verbal Fluency**: Condition 2 Category Fluency, Condition 3 Category Switching Total Switching **Word Context**: Total Consecutively Correct **Tower Test**: Total Achievement	**Color-Word**: Condition 2 Word Reading Seconds to Complete, Condition 4 Inhibition/Switching Seconds to Complete Trail Making: Combined Number and Letter Sequencing
Low (≤.59)	**Trail Making**: Conditions 1–4 Verbal Fluency: Category Switching Total Correct **Twenty Questions**: Total Weighted Achievement	**Design Fluency** **Sorting Test** **Twenty Questions** **Tower Test**: Total Achievement **Verbal Fluency**: Condition 3 Category Switching Total Correct and Total Switching Accuracy

SOURCE: Adapted from Delis et al. (2001).

Although the D-KEFS Tower Test is moderately correlated with the TOL (r = .47), there are no order effects, thus suggesting no beneficial effect of practice from one task to the next, and the tasks are found to share a small amount of variance (Larochette et al., 2009). In addition, the D-KEFS Tower takes longer to complete overall, although earlier items on the D-KEFS are completed faster and with fewer moves than counterparts on the TOL. Similarly, other research indicates that the Cambridge Neuropsychological Test Automated Battery (CANTAB) Tower and D-KEFS are not interchangeable. McKinlay et al. (2009) reported that patients with PD performed worse than controls on CANTAB Tower, but not on the D-KEFS Tower Test. The tests only shared between 7% and 24% of variance, and inhibition and spatial working memory were related to the CANTAB Tower, whereas only spatial working memory was related to the D-KEFS Tower Test. The D-KEFS Design Fluency task has also been examined. Suchy, Kraybill, and Larson (2010) reported that the generation of novel designs relied on motor planning, the capacity to generate novel designs, and motor speed.

TABLE 9–56 Correlations Between Standard and Alternate Forms of the Delis-Kaplan Executive Function System (D-KEFS) Verbal Fluency, Sorting Test, and Twenty Questions Test

SUBTEST	R
Verbal Fluency	Ranges from .44 (Condition 3 Category Switching Total Switching Accuracy) to .83 (Condition 1 Letter Fluency Total Correct)
Sorting Test	Ranges from .39 (Condition 1 Free Sorting Description Total Score) to .72 (Condition 2 Sort Recognition Total Description Score)
Twenty Questions Test	Ranges from .25 (Total Questions Asked) to .61 (Total Abstraction Score)

SOURCE: Adapted from Delis et al. (2001).

Research suggests there is a large amount of shared variance between the D-KEFS and the WAIS-III (e.g., 54%; Davis et al., 2011), with group effects on the D-KEFS attenuated to nonsignificance after controlling for intelligence (Barbey et al., 2012; Keifer & Tranel, 2013; see also "Clinical Studies"). The Sorting Test, in particular, appears to be strongly related to IQ (Davis et al., 2011; Kalkut et al., 2009; although see Fulford, Feldman, Tabak, McGillicuddy, & Johnson, 2013). A measure of word reading in college students was only weakly related to D-KEFS Verbal Fluency (Davis et al., 2016).

The D-KEFS is moderately related to the CVLT-II (Yochim et al., 2013). Complex action planning was found to relate to a composite measure of D-KEFS performance in community-dwelling older adults (Niermeyer et al., 2017).

CLINICAL STUDIES

Dementia. Group differences between patients with dementia and controls have been described, as well as differentiation between dementia subtypes. For example, patients with FTD and AD perform worse than healthy controls on the D-KEFS, with patients with FTD making more rule violations on the Tower Test (Carey et al., 2008) and more errors on Design Fluency than other dementia groups (Possin et al., 2012). Twenty Questions is the best differentiator between patients with FTD and corticobasal syndrome (Huey et al., 2009). In addition, the Color-Word Interference Test is associated with high classification accuracy, sensitivity, and specificity (73%, 80%, 71%, respectively) in the identification of cognitive decline, even after performance on memory measures is accounted for (Clark et al., 2012).

Lesion Studies. Patients with frontal lobe lesions perform worse than healthy controls on D-KEFS tests (Ghawami et al., 2017), including fluency tests (Baldo et al., 2001), the Twenty Questions Test, the Sorting Test (Baldo et al., 2004), the TMT (Yochim et al., 2007), and the Tower Test (Yochim et al., 2009). Of note, rule violations on the Tower Test have been associated with high sensitivity (83%) and specificity (100%) in differentiating patients with prefrontal lesions from those without (Yochim et al., 2009).

Laterality effects have also been noted, with patients with left frontal lesions showing relatively greater impairment on the Verbal Fluency Test (Baldo et al., 2001) and the Word Context Test (Keil et al., 2005). In addition to laterality effects, the specific site of frontal lesions appears to impact performance, although this may be secondary to processing speed. For example, Keifer and Tranel (2013) reported that patients with dorsolateral prefrontal cortex lesions obtained lower scores on multiple D-KEFS tests when compared to patients with ventromedial prefrontal or nonfrontal lesions. However, between-group differences were no longer significant after intelligence was accounted for, with subsequent analyses suggesting that processing speed was the primary variable accounting for differences. Similar findings have been reported in a sample of veterans with focal brain injury (Barbey et al., 2012).

TBI. The D-KEFS has utility in TBI. Amongst a number of executive function measures, the D-KEFS Sorting Test was identified as one of the best predictors in differentiating between severe TBI and healthy controls (Heled et al., 2012), with attempted sorts associated with a sensitivity of 88% and a specificity of 65%. Verbal Fluency (letter and category switching) is also able to differentiate groups (Strong et al., 2011), with a sensitivity of 66% and a specificity of 65%. Coma length is related to Verbal Fluency, with partial mediation by processing speed; after controlling for sociodemographic and clinical factors, length of coma predicts performance on the Color–Word Inhibition/Switching subtest, and the presence of diffuse lesions is related to Verbal Fluency Category Switching in persons with mild to severe TBI (Anderson et al., 2017). Additionally, persons with moderate to severe TBI perform worse on Category Switching and Color-Word Inhibition/Switching compared to persons with mild uncomplicated TBI and healthy controls, with a classification accuracy for Color-Word and Verbal Fluency of 66%.

PD. Some research suggests that individuals with PD show impairment on D-KEFS tests, including the TMT and Twenty Questions (Kudlicka et al., 2013). The D-KEFS TMT is highly correlated (*rs* = .59 to .86) with ADLs in patients with PD without dementia (Higginson et al., 2013). Performance improvement has also been noted following treatment with rivastigmine (Schmitt et al., 2010).

MS. After controlling for depression, MS patients can be differentiated from controls using the D-KEFS Sorting Test, which also predicts vocational status (Parmenter et al., 2007). The Sorting Test has been used as an outcome measurement in MS pharmacologic (Comi et al., 2017) and nonpharmacologic multimodal interventions (Lee et al., 2017). The test has also been truncated in length to Free Card Sort 1 without significantly compromising diagnostic accuracy in MS batteries (Gromisch et al., 2016).

Psychiatric Conditions. Persons with schizophrenia obtain lower scores than controls on the D-KEFS TMT and Color-Word Interference Test (Neill & Rossell, 2013). Group differences are attenuated after accounting for processing speed and basic components of the tasks (Neill & Rossell, 2013; Savla et al., 2011). In schizophrenia, D-KEFS factor scores are also associated with clinical variables, such as negative symptomatology and cognitive symptoms (Clark et al., 2010), psychopathology, illness duration (Savla et al., 2011), and patient illness awareness (Lysaker et al., 2006). Of note, oververbalization has been associated with improved performance on the switching condition of the D-KEFS TMT, with worsened performance on basic component tasks (Harvey, Gallety, Field, & Proeve, 2009).

People with depression reportedly show relatively poor performance on the D-KEFS, including the Color-Word Interference Test, the Verbal Fluency Test (Hammar et al., 2011; Schmid et al., 2011; Yochim et al., 2013), and the TMT (Yochim et al., 2013). Self-reported depressive symptomatology correlates with the D-KEFS TMT in patients with PD (e.g., GDS; *rs* = .37 to .67; Higginson et al., 2013). Poor performance may be amplified in people with neurologic conditions with comorbid depression, such as those with temporal lobe epilepsy and a comorbid mood disorder. Some research has suggested that the D-KEFS does not relate to clinical outcomes, such as measures of mood, general function, number of hospitalizations, or duration of time in hospital (Hammar et al., 2011). However, other research has suggested clinical correlates, such as depression relapse, are associated with worse performance on Inhibition/Switching conditions of the Color-Word Interference Test (Schmid & Hammar, 2013).

Relationships between D-KEFS tests and anxiety have also been reported. For example, in patients with panic disorder, the inhibition condition of the Color-Word Interference Test is related to heart rate variability, duration of illness, panic-related distress (Hovland et al., 2012), and sleep disturbance (Hovland et al., 2013). In community-dwelling older adults, anxiety and depression are related to decreased performance on switching conditions of the D-KEFS TMT, with anxiety predictive of D-KEFS Twenty

Questions Test and depression predictive of performance on Verbal Fluency (Yochim et al., 2013).

Other Populations. Weaknesses in D-KEFS performance have also been reported in other groups, including adults with ADHD (set shifting of the Color-Word Interference Test; Halleland et al., 2012), frontal lobe epilepsy (switching condition of the TMT; McDonald et al., 2005), persons with HIV (Willen et al., 2017), agenesis of the corpus callosum (Color-Word Interference Test, TMT; Marco et al., 2012), subcortical ischemic vascular disease (Kramer, 2002), persisting pain (TMT; Karp et al., 2006), and PTSD (Color-Word Interference Test; Aupperle et al., 2012). Self-reported impulsivity in university undergraduates has been associated with Tower performance (Lyvers et al., 2015).

The D-KEFS has relationships with clinical and functional outcomes. A subgroup of adults with ADHD who showed executive deficits on select D-KEFS tests also showed higher rates of unemployment, more reading and writing problems, lower IQ scores, and more self-reported childhood ADHD symptoms compared to a subgroup of adults with ADHD without executive deficits on the D-KEFS (Halleland et al., 2015). In one study, D-KEFS tests (TMT, Tower Test, Verbal and Design Fluency) accounted for 26% of the variance in day-to-day functional ability of older adults after controlling for education and depressive symptoms (Mitchell & Miller, 2008). A composite D-KEFS score (switching conditions of the D-KEFS TMT, Tower, Verbal Fluency, Design Fluency) entirely mediated the relationship between cognitive reserve and functional ability in community-dwelling older adults (Puente et al., 2015). Interestingly, a prominent role of heritability on TMT performance has been reported in twin studies (Vasilopoulos et al., 2012).

NEUROANATOMICAL CORRELATES AND IMAGING STUDIES

The neuroanatomical correlates of D-KEFS tasks vary depending on the specific test examined. Generally, frontal regions are implicated, along with other regions depending on other processes involved in the task. For example, the Tower Test also involves parietal regions, whereas verbal tasks such as Proverbs involve left temporal regions. For example, in patients with neurodegenerative conditions as well as healthy controls, set Shifting conditions of Design Fluency, TMT, and Color-Word Interference correlate with focal regions in prefrontal and posterior parietal cortex, and bilateral prefrontal and right posterior parietal lobe regions (Pa et al., 2010). Reduced fractional anisotropy across broad networks is associated with poor performance on both Color-Word Interference and the TMT in MS (Genova et al., 2013). When processing speed is controlled for, however, these correlations are attenuated or not significant. Neuronal density in the left and right inferior frontostriatal tract is related to worse performance on Switching measures (Category Switching of Verbal Fluency, Color-Word Interference) in patients with temporal lobe epilepsy (Reyes et al., 2018). Increased dorsolateral prefrontal activation is associated with Color-Word Interference performance in women with PTSD (Aupperle et al., 2012). The middle frontal gyrus plays a prominent role in performing complex conditions of the Color-Word Interference Test (Adólfsdóttir et al., 2014).

Older age is related to slower performance on the Number and Letter Sequencing conditions of the TMT and fractional anisotropy values in the right uncinate fasciculus and the left hippocampal portion of the cingulum for patients with euthymic bipolar disorder but not healthy controls (Dev et al., 2017).

Design Fluency is related to right and left frontal lobe volumes, especially in patients with FTD as opposed to AD, semantic dementia, and healthy controls (Kramer et al., 2007). Relationships remain after MMSE and basic task component performance are accounted for. The Design Fluency Test is also correlated with cerebral volumes in the orbitofrontal cortex, the right inferior frontal gyrus, and the right striatum (Possin et al., 2012).

The Sorting Test is related to brain atrophy on MRI in patients with MS (Parmenter et al., 2007). Enlarged Virchow-Robin spaces in MS are also related to performance on the Sorting Test (Favaretto et al., 2017). Relationships are found between diffusion tensor imaging measurements of the lateral mediodorsal thalamus and the Sorting Test (Jakab et al., 2012). Relationships between left prefrontal performance and the Sorting Test have also been found. Left frontal lobe volumes significantly predicted Free Description scores on the D-KEFS Sorting Test in a mixed clinical sample (Fine et al., 2009). The left dorsolateral prefrontal cortex is implicated in patients with FTD (Huey et al., 2009). Decreased gray matter volume of the left lateral ventral prefrontal cortex is associated with poor performance on the Sorting Test and Twenty Questions tests in patients with FTD and corticobasal syndrome (Huey et al., 2015). Sorting Test performance is related to reduced left prefrontal and left parietal cortical thickness in people with amyotrophic lateral sclerosis as measured by MRI (Libon et al., 2012).

Tower performance is related to smaller brain volumes in bilateral frontal and parietal regions, and increased rule violations are related to decreased frontal volume bilaterally in patients with dementia (Carey et al., 2008). Patients with FTD show decreased performance on the Proverb Test compared to people with AD, with tensor-based morphometry indices indicating correlations between performance and the left anterior temporal region, especially on the left side (Kaiser et al., 2013).

PERFORMANCE VALIDITY

No information is available as of this writing.

COMMENT

The D-KEFS is an executive battery that offers a process-oriented approach to task analysis and co-norming of many conventional executive function tasks. These features provide a within-subjects design that reduces variability inherent in comparing an individual's performance across different sets of normative data. Demographic effects exist on the D-KEFS, with age affecting performance on the majority of tests, following the expected trajectory (i.e., tasks with prominent processing speed components peak earlier in adulthood than tasks emphasizing verbal reasoning). Overall, gender appears to not exert a significant effect (though see Kalkut et al., 2009), and more information overall would be beneficial regarding the effect of gender, education, and other sociodemographic factors on D-KEFS tests. For example, significant effect of education and verbal abilities have been identified on the D-KEFS TMT, and Fine et al. (2011) provide normative data for education- and vocabulary-adjusted scores for this test. Similar normative adjustments, particularly for other tests in the battery that emphasize processing speed, would be a welcome addition to the clinician's toolbox.

The standardization sample has many strengths: it is large in number, spans a wide range of ages, and is Census-stratified in terms of geographic region, age, gender, ethnicity, and educational level. Users should note that alternate-form data are based on a substantially smaller group of individuals and were derived from linear transformations of the standard form norms. For this reason, in addition to the low reliability coefficients between the standard form and alternate forms for some variables, the alternate forms should not be viewed as precise equivalents of the standard forms.

In addition to the high quality of normative data, recent extensions have increased utility, including Fine et al.'s (2011) adjustment for education and vocabulary on the D-KEFS TMT, and Crawford et al.'s (2011) and Karr et al.'s (2017) base rate data. Examination of tables presented in this review by these authors suggests that the effect of education and consideration of base rates of low scores in normative samples is important in interpreting D-KEFS scores. For example, Fine et al.'s data suggest that individuals with high education levels would be expected to perform relatively better than individuals with low education on the D-KEFS TMT. Base rate data suggest that the presence of some low scores on the D-KEFS is relatively common in healthy people (note that base rates of low scores vary depending on cutoff used) and interact with IQ and education.

The reliability of many tests on the D-KEFS is a relative weakness. Adequate to high reliability has been reported for various scores on Verbal Fluency, Twenty Questions, Proverbs, Sorting, Trail Making, and Color-Word Interference, with contrast scores faring poorly according to Crawford et al.'s (2008) data. Thus, a limited number of process scores have sufficient reliability for clinical use.

Additionally, although the D-KEFS adopts a process approach in that each task provides multiple conditions to delineate the specific source of poor performance, it is not always clear that these subscores capture more basic processes. For example, in patients seeking outpatient neuropsychological evaluation, approximately 57% performed better on less complex conditions of the Color-Word Interference Test than more complex conditions, suggesting that more complex tasks on the D-KEFS may not always be associated with poorer performance than less complex tasks (Lippa & Davis, 2010). Others have reported that people showing this pattern are more likely to perform better than persons showing the expected pattern on tests of memory and semantic fluency (Berg et al., 2016).

Research indicates that the D-KEFS may reflect a set of disparate abilities. Within-task correlations are in the low to moderate range overall, including primary scores as well as process variables such as errors. Factor-analytic studies generally yield two to three factors, with inhibition and cognitive flexibility typically identified. Correlations between D-KEFS variables and nonexecutive measures such as memory are of similar magnitude as correlations between D-KEFS variables and executive tests. IQ also plays a significant role in performance for many tests. Overall, it is perhaps inaccurate to consider the D-KEFS as a measure of a single construct, but rather reflective of diverse subcomponents.

The D-KEFS has been used in many clinical populations, including brain injury, dementia, PD, schizophrenia, mood and anxiety disorders, and a range of other populations. Most research has reported group differences, but some utility with respect to differential diagnosis, clinical correlates, and relationships with daily function has also been reported. Neuroanatomical correlates of D-KEFS performance are generally as expected, showing frontal and prefrontal activation as well as recruitment of additional brain regions depending on test-specific processes. Information on assessing performance validity using the D-KEFS would be of utility, although this is not common among most executive functioning measures.

REFERENCES

Adólfsdóttir, S., Haász, J., Wehling, E., Ystad, M., Lundervold, A., & Lundervold, A. J. (2014). Salient measures of inhibition and switching are associated with frontal lobe gray matter volume in healthy middle-aged and older adults. *Neuropsychology*, *28*(6), 859–869. https://doi.org/10.1037/neu0000082

Anderson, L. B., Jaroh, R., Smith, H., Strong, C.-A. H., & Donders, J. (2017). Criterion validity of the D-KEFS color-word and verbal fluency switching paradigms following traumatic brain injury. *Journal of Clinical and Experimental Neuropsychology*, *39*(9), 890–899. https://doi.org/10.1080/13803395.2016.1277513

Aupperle, R. L., Allard, C. B., Grimes, E. M., Simmons, A. N., Flagan, T., Behrooznia, M., . . . others. (2012). Dorsolateral prefrontal cortex activation during emotional anticipation and neuropsychological performance in posttraumatic stress disorder. *Archives of General Psychiatry, 69*(4), 360–371.

Baldo, J. V., Shimamura, A. P., Delis, D. C., Kramer, J., & Kaplan, E. (2001). Verbal and design fluency in patients with frontal lobe lesions. *Journal of the International Neuropsychological Society, 7*(5), 586–596.

Baldo, Juliana V., Delis, D. C., Wilkins, D. P., & Shimamura, A. P. (2004). Is it bigger than a breadbox? Performance of patients with prefrontal lesions on a new executive function test. *Archives of Clinical Neuropsychology, 19*(3), 407–419. https://doi.org/10.1016/S0887-6177(03)00074-X

Barbey, A. K., Colom, R., Solomon, J., Krueger, F., Forbes, C., & Grafman, J. (2012). An integrative architecture for general intelligence and executive function revealed by lesion mapping. *Brain, 135*(4), 1154–1164. https://doi.org/10.1093/brain/aws021

Berg, J.-L., Swan, N. M., Banks, S. J., & Miller, J. B. (2016). Atypical performance patterns on Delis-Kaplan Executive Functioning System Color-Word Interference Test: Cognitive switching and learning ability in older adults. *Journal of Clinical and Experimental Neuropsychology, 38*(7), 745–751. https://doi.org/10.1080/13803395.2016.1161734

Carey, C. L., Woods, S. P., Damon, J., Halabi, C., Dean, D., Delis, D. C., . . . Kramer, J. H. (2008). Discriminant validity and neuroanatomical correlates of rule monitoring in frontotemporal dementia and Alzheimer's disease. *Neuropsychologia, 46*(4), 1081–1087. https://doi.org/10.1016/j.neuropsychologia.2007.11.001

Clark, L. R., Schiehser, D. M., Weissberger, G. H., Salmon, D. P., Delis, D. C., & Bondi, M. W. (2012). Specific measures of executive function predict cognitive decline in older adults. *Journal of the International Neuropsychological Society: JINS, 18*(1), 118–127. https://doi.org/10.1017/S1355617711001524

Clark, L. K., Warman, D., & Lysaker, P. H. (2010). The relationships between schizophrenia symptom dimensions and executive functioning components. *Schizophrenia Research, 124*(1–3), 169–175. https://doi.org/10.1016/j.schres.2010.08.004

Comi, G., Patti, F., Rocca, M. A., Mattioli, F. C., Amato, M. P., . . . For the Golden Study Group. (2017). Efficacy of fingolimod and interferon beta-1b on cognitive, MRI, and clinical outcomes in relapsing–remitting multiple sclerosis: An 18-month, open-label, rater-blinded, randomised, multicenter study (the GOLDEN study). *Journal of Neurology, 264*(12), 2436–2449. https://doi.org/10.1007/s00415-017-8642-5

Crawford, J. R., Garthwaite, P. H., Sutherland, D., & Borland, N. (2011). Some supplementary methods for the analysis of the Delis–Kaplan Executive Function System. *Psychological Assessment, 23*(4), 888–898. https://doi.org/10.1037/a0023712

Crawford, J. R., Sutherland, D., & Garthwaite, P. H. (2008). On the reliability and standard errors of measurement of contrast measures from the D-KEFS. *Journal of the International Neuropsychological Society, 14*(06), 1069–1073.

Davis, A. S., Finch, W. H., Drapeau, C., Nogin, M., E Moss, L., & Moore, B. (2016). Predicting verbal fluency using Word Reading: Implications for premorbid functioning. *Applied Neuropsychology. Adult, 23*(6), 403–410. https://doi.org/10.1080/23279095.2016.1163262

Davis, A. S., Pierson, E. E., & Finch, W. H. (2011). A Canonical correlation analysis of intelligence and executive functioning. *Applied Neuropsychology, 18*(1), 61–68. https://doi.org/10.1080/09084282.2010.523392

Delis, D. C., Kaplan, E., & Kramer, J. H. (2001). *Delis-Kaplan Executive Function System.* San Antonio, TX: The Psychological Corporation.

Dev, S. I., Nguyen, T. T., McKenna, B. S., Sutherland, A. N., Bartsch, H., Theilmann, R. J., & Eyler, L. T. (2017). Steeper slope of age-related changes in white matter microstructure and processing speed in bipolar disorder. *American Journal of Geriatric Psychiatry, 25*(7), 744–752. https://doi.org/10.1016/j.jagp.2017.02.014

Favaretto, A., Lazzarotto, A., Riccardi, A., Pravato, S., Margoni, M., Causin, F., . . . Gallo, P. (2017). Enlarged Virchow Robin spaces associate with cognitive decline in multiple sclerosis. *PloS One, 12*(10), e0185626. https://doi.org/10.1371/journal.pone.0185626

Fine, E. M., Delis, D. C., Dean, D., Beckman, V., Miller, B. L., Rosen, H. J., & Kramer, J. H. (2009). Left frontal lobe contributions to concept formation: A quantitative MRI study of performance on the Delis–Kaplan Executive Function System Sorting Test. *Journal of Clinical and Experimental Neuropsychology, 31*(5), 624–631. https://doi.org/10.1080/13803390802419017

Fine, E. M., Delis, D. C., & Holdnack, J. (2011). Normative adjustments to the D-KEFS Trail Making Test: Corrections for education and vocabulary level. *The Clinical Neuropsychologist, 25*(8), 1331–1344. https://doi.org/10.1080/13854046.2011.609838

Fulford, D., Feldman, G., Tabak, B. A., McGillicuddy, M., & Johnson, S. L. (2013). Positive Affect Enhances the Association of Hypomanic Personality and Cognitive Flexibility. *International Journal of Cognitive Therapy, 6*(1), 1–16.

Genova, H. M., DeLuca, J., Chiaravalloti, N., & Wylie, G. (2013). The relationship between executive functioning, processing speed, and white matter integrity in multiple sclerosis. *Journal of Clinical and Experimental Neuropsychology, 35*(6), 631–641. https://doi.org/10.1080/13803395.2013.806649

Ghawami, H., Sadeghi, S., Raghibi, M., & Rahimi-Movaghar, V. (2017). Executive functioning of complicated-mild to moderate traumatic brain injury patients with frontal contusions. *Applied Neuropsychology. Adult, 24*(4), 299–307. https://doi.org/10.1080/23279095.2016.1157078

Gromisch, E. S., Zemon, V., Holtzer, R., Chiaravalloti, N. D., DeLuca, J., Beier, M., . . . Foley, F. W. (2016). Assessing the criterion validity of four highly abbreviated measures from the Minimal Assessment of Cognitive Function in Multiple Sclerosis (MACFIMS). *The Clinical Neuropsychologist, 30*(7), 1032–1049. https://doi.org/10.1080/13854046.2016.1189597

Halleland, H. B., Haavik, J., & Lundervold, A. J. (2012). Set-shifting in adults with ADHD. *Journal of the International Neuropsychological Society, 18*(04), 728–737. https://doi.org/10.1017/S1355617712000355

Halleland, H. B., Sørensen, L., Posserud, M.-B., Haavik, J., & Lundervold, A. J. (2015). Occupational status is compromised in adults with ADHD and psychometrically defined executive function deficits. *Journal of Attention Disorders.* https://doi.org/10.1177/1087054714564622

Hammar, Å., Strand, M., Årdal, G., Schmid, M., Lund, A., & Elliott, R. (2011). Testing the cognitive effort hypothesis of cognitive impairment in major depression. *Nordic Journal of Psychiatry, 65*(1), 74–80. https://doi.org/10.3109/08039488.2010.494311

Hartman, M., Nielsen, C., & Stratton, B. (2004). The contributions of attention and working memory to age differences in concept identification. *Journal of Clinical and Experimental Neuropsychology, 26*(2), 227–245. https://doi.org/10.1076/jcen.26.2.227.28083

Harvey, K. E., Galletly, C. A., Field, C., & Proeve, M. (2009). The effects of verbalisation on cognitive performance in schizophrenia: A pilot study using tasks from the Delis Kaplan Executive Function System. *Neuropsychological Rehabilitation, 19*(5), 733–741. https://doi.org/10.1080/09602010902732892

Heled, E., Hoofien, D., Margalit, D., Natovich, R., & Agranov, E. (2012). The Delis–Kaplan Executive Function System Sorting Test as an evaluative tool for executive functions after severe traumatic brain injury: A comparative study. *Journal of Clinical and Experimental Neuropsychology, 34*(2), 151–159. https://doi.org/10.1080/13803395.2011.625351

Higginson, C. I., Lanni, K., Sigvardt, K. A., & Disbrow, E. A. (2013). The contribution of trail making to the prediction of performance-based instrumental activities of daily living in Parkinson's disease without dementia. *Journal of Clinical and Experimental Neuropsychology, 35*(5), 530–539. https://doi.org/10.1080/13803395.2013.798397

Hovland, A., Pallesen, S., Hammar, Å., Hansen, A. L., Thayer, J. F., Sivertsen, B., . . . Nordhus, I. H. (2013). Subjective sleep quality in relation to inhibition and heart rate variability in patients with panic disorder. *Journal of Affective Disorders, 150*(1), 152–155. https://doi.org/10.1016/j.jad.2012.12.017

Hovland, A., Pallesen, S., Hammar, Å., Hansen, A. L., Thayer, J. F., Tarvainen, M. P., & Nordhus, I. H. (2012). The relationships among heart rate variability, executive functions, and clinical variables in patients with panic disorder. *International Journal of Psychophysiology, 86*(3), 269–275. https://doi.org/10.1016/j.ijpsycho.2012.10.004

Huey, E. D., Goveia, E. N., Paviol, S., Pardini, M., Krueger, F., Zamboni, G., . . . Grafman, J. (2009). Executive dysfunction in frontotemporal dementia and corticobasal syndrome. *Neurology, 72*(5), 453–459. https://doi.org/10.1212/01.wnl.0000341781.39164.26

Huey, E. D., Lee, S., Brickman, A. M., Manoochehri, M., Griffith, E., Devanand, D. P., . . . Grafman, J. (2015). Neuropsychiatric effects of neurodegeneration of the medial versus lateral ventral prefrontal cortex in humans. *Cortex, 73*, 1–9. https://doi.org/10.1016/j.cortex.2015.08.002

Jakab, A., Blanc, R., & Berényi, E. L. (2012). Mapping changes of in vivo connectivity patterns in the human mediodorsal thalamus: Correlations with higher cognitive and executive functions. *Brain Imaging and Behavior, 6*(3), 472–483. https://doi.org/10.1007/s11682-012-9172-5

Kaiser, N. C., Lee, G. J., Lu, P. H., Mather, M. J., Shapira, J., Jimenez, E., . . . Mendez, M. F. (2013). What dementia reveals about proverb interpretation and its neuroanatomical correlates. *Neuropsychologia, 51*(9), 1726–1733. https://doi.org/10.1016/j.neuropsychologia.2013.05.021

Kalkut, E. L., Han, S. D., Lansing, A. E., Holdnack, J. A., & Delis, D. C. (2009). Development of set-shifting ability from late childhood through early adulthood. *Archives of Clinical Neuropsychology, 24*(6), 565–574. https://doi.org/10.1093/arclin/acp048

Karp, J. F., Reynolds, C. F., Butters, M. A., Dew, M. A., Mazumdar, S., Begley, A. E., . . . Weiner, D. K. (2006). The relationship between pain and mental flexibility in older adult pain clinic patients. *Pain Medicine, 7*(5), 444–452.

Karr, J. E., Garcia-Barrera, M. A., Holdnack, J. A., & Iverson, G. L. (2017). Using multivariate base rates to interpret low scores on an abbreviated battery of the Delis-Kaplan Executive Function System. *Archives of Clinical Neuropsychology, 32*(3), 297–305. https://doi.org/10.1093/arclin/acw105

Keifer, E., & Tranel, D. (2013). A neuropsychological investigation of the Delis-Kaplan Executive Function System. *Journal of Clinical and Experimental Neuropsychology, 35*(10), 1048–1059. https://doi.org/10.1080/13803395.2013.854319

Keil, K., Baldo, J., Kaplan, E., Kramer, J., & Delis, D. C. (2005). Role of frontal cortex in inferential reasoning: Evidence from the word context test. *Journal of the International Neuropsychological Society, 11*(4), 426–433.

Kramer, J. H. (2002). Executive dysfunction in subcortical ischaemic vascular disease. *Journal of Neurology, Neurosurgery & Psychiatry, 72*(2), 217–220. https://doi.org/10.1136/jnnp.72.2.217

Kramer, J. H., Quitania, L., Dean, D., Neuhaus, J., Rosen, H. J., Halabi, C., . . . others. (2007). Magnetic resonance imaging correlates of set shifting. *Journal of the International Neuropsychological Society, 13*(3), 386–392.

Kudlicka, A., Clare, L., & Hindle, J. V. (2013). Pattern of executive impairment in mild to moderate Parkinson's disease. *Dementia and Geriatric Cognitive Disorders, 36*(1–2), 50–66. https://doi.org/10.1159/000348355

Larochette, A.-C., Benn, K., & Harrison, A. G. (2009). Executive Functioning: A Comparison of the Tower of London [DX] and the D-KEFS Tower Test. *Applied Neuropsychology, 16*(4), 275–280. https://doi.org/10.1080/09084280903098695

Latzman, R. D., & Markon, K. E. (2010). The factor structure and age-related factorial invariance of the Delis-Kaplan Executive Function System (D-KEFS). *Assessment, 17*(2), 172–184. https://doi.org/10.1177/1073191109356254

Libon, D. J., McMillan, C., Avants, B., Boller, A., Morgan, B., Burkholder, L., . . . Grossman, M. (2012). Deficits in concept formation in amyotrophic lateral sclerosis. *Neuropsychology, 26*(4), 422–429. https://doi.org/10.1037/a0028668

Lippa, S. M., & Davis, R. N. (2010). Inhibition/switching is not necessarily harder than inhibition: An analysis of the D-KEFS Color-Word Interference Test. *Archives of Clinical Neuropsychology, 25*(2), 146–152. https://doi.org/10.1093/arclin/acq001

Lysaker, P. H., Whitney, K. A., & Davis, L. W. (2006). Awareness of illness in schizophrenia: Associations with multiple assessments of executive function. *Journal of Neuropsychiatry and Clinical Neurosciences, 18*(4), 516–520. https://doi.org/10.1176/appi.neuropsych.18.4.516

Lyvers, M., Basch, V., Duff, H., & Edwards, M. S. (2015). Trait impulsivity predicts D-KEFS Tower Test performance in university students. *Applied Neuropsychology. Adult, 22*(2), 88–93. https://doi.org/10.1080/23279095.2013.850693

Marco, E. J., Harrell, K. M., Brown, W. S., Hill, S. S., Jeremy, R. J., Kramer, J. H., . . . Paul, L. K. (2012). Processing speed delays contribute to executive function deficits in individuals with agenesis of the corpus callosum. *Journal of the International Neuropsychological Society, 18*(03), 521–529. https://doi.org/10.1017/S1355617712000045

Mattioli, F., Stampatori, C., Bellomi, F., Scarpazza, C., Galli, P., Guarneri, C., . . . Capra, R. (2014). Assessing executive function with the D-KEFS Sorting Test: Normative data for a sample of the Italian adult population. *Neurological Sciences, 35*(12), 1895–1902. https://doi.org/10.1007/s10072-014-1857-7

McDonald, C. R., Delis, D. C., Norman, M. A., Tecoma, E. S., & Iragui-Madozi, V. I. (2005). Is impairment in set-shifting specific to frontal-lobe dysfunction? Evidence from patients with frontal-lobe or temporal-lobe epilepsy. *Journal of the International Neuropsychological Society, 11*(4), 477–481.

McKinlay, A., Grace, R. C., Kaller, C. P., Dalrymple-Alford, J. C., Anderson, T. J., Fink, J., & Roger, D. (2009). Assessing cognitive impairment in Parkinson's disease: A comparison of two tower tasks. *Applied Neuropsychology, 16*(3), 177–185. https://doi.org/10.1080/09084280903098661

Mitchell, M., & Miller, L. S. (2008). Prediction of functional status in older adults: The ecological validity of four Delis–Kaplan Executive Function System tests. *Journal of Clinical and Experimental Neuropsychology, 30*(6), 683–690. https://doi.org/10.1080/13803390701679893

Neill, E., & Rossell, S. L. (2013). Executive functioning in schizophrenia: The result of impairments in lower order cognitive skills? *Schizophrenia Research, 150*(1), 76–80. https://doi.org/10.1016/j.schres.2013.07.034

Niermeyer, M. A., Suchy, Y., & Ziemnik, R. E. (2017). Motor sequencing in older adulthood: relationships with executive functioning and effects of complexity. *The Clinical Neuropsychologist, 31*(3), 598–618. https://doi.org/10.1080/13854046.2016.1257071

Pa, J., Possin, K. L., Wilson, S. M., Quitania, L. C., Kramer, J. H., Boxer, A. L., . . . Johnson, J. K. (2010). Gray matter correlates of set-shifting among neurodegenerative disease, mild cognitive impairment, and healthy older adults. *Journal of the International Neuropsychological Society, 16*(04), 640–650. https://doi.org/10.1017/S1355617710000408

Parmenter, B. A., Zivadinov, R., Kerenyi, L., Gavett, R., Weinstock-Guttman, B., Dwyer, M. G., . . . Benedict, R. H. B. (2007). Validity of the Wisconsin Card Sorting and Delis–Kaplan Executive Function System (D-KEFS) Sorting Tests in multiple sclerosis. *Journal of Clinical and Experimental Neuropsychology, 29*(2), 215–223. https://doi.org/10.1080/13803390600672163

Possin, K. L., Chester, S. K., Laluz, V., Bostrom, A., Rosen, H. J., Miller, B. L., & Kramer, J. H. (2012). The frontal-anatomic specificity of design fluency repetitions and their diagnostic relevance for behavioral variant frontotemporal dementia. *Journal of the International Neuropsychological Society, 18*(5), 834–844. https://doi.org/10.1017/S1355617712000604

Puente, A. N., Lindbergh, C. A., & Miller, L. S. (2015). The relationship between cognitive reserve and functional ability is mediated by executive functioning in older adults. *The Clinical Neuropsychologist, 29*(1), 67–81. https://doi.org/10.1080/13854046.2015.1005676

Reyes, A., Uttarwar, V. S., Chang, Y.-H. A., Balachandra, A. R., Pung, C. J., Hagler, D. J., . . . McDonald, C. R. (2018). Decreased neurite density within frontostriatal networks is associated with executive dysfunction in temporal lobe epilepsy. *Epilepsy & Behavior, 78*, 187–193. https://doi.org/10.1016/j.yebeh.2017.09.012

Salthouse, T. A., Atkinson, T. M., & Berish, D. E. (2003). Executive functioning as a potential mediator of age-related cognitive decline in normal adults. *Journal of Experimental Psychology. General, 132*(4), 566–594. https://doi.org/10.1037/0096-3445.132.4.566

Savla, G. N., Twamley, E. W., Delis, D. C., Roesch, S. C., Jeste, D. V., & Palmer, B. W. (2010). Dimensions of executive functioning in schizophrenia and their relationship with processing speed. *Schizophrenia Bulletin*, sbq149.

Savla, G. N., Twamley, E. W., Thompson, W. K., Delis, D. C., Jeste, D. V., & Palmer, B. W. (2011). Evaluation of specific executive functioning skills and the processes underlying executive control in schizophrenia. *Journal of the International Neuropsychological Society, 17*(01), 14–23. https://doi.org/10.1017/S1355617710001177

Schmid, M., & Hammar, A. (2013). A follow-up study of first episode major depressive disorder. Impairment in inhibition and semantic fluency-potential predictors for relapse? *Frontiers in Psychology, 4*, 633. https://doi.org/10.3389/fpsyg.2013.00633

Schmid, M., Strand, M., Ardal, G., Lund, A., & Hammar, A. (2011). Prolonged impairment in inhibition and semantic fluency in a follow-up study of recurrent major depression. *Archives of Clinical Neuropsychology, 26*(7), 677–686. https://doi.org/10.1093/arclin/acr048

Schmitt, F. A., Farlow, M. R., Meng, X., Tekin, S., & Olin, J. T. (2010). Efficacy of rivastigmine on executive function in patients with Parkinson's disease dementia: Efficacy of rivastigmine on EF in patients with PDD. *CNS Neuroscience & Therapeutics, 16*(6), 330–336. https://doi.org/10.1111/j.1755-5949.2010.00182.x

Strong, C.-A. H., Tiesma, D., & Donders, J. (2011). Criterion Validity of the Delis-Kaplan Executive Function System (D-KEFS) fluency subtests after traumatic brain injury. *Journal of the International Neuropsychological Society, 17*(02), 230–237. https://doi.org/10.1017/S1355617710001451

Suchy, Y., Kraybill, M. L., & Gidley Larson, J. C. (2010). Understanding design fluency: Motor and executive contributions. *Journal of the International Neuropsychological Society, 16*(1), 26–37. https://doi.org/10.1017/S1355617709990804

Vasilopoulos, T., Franz, C. E., Panizzon, M. S., Xian, H., Grant, M. D., Lyons, M. J., . . . Kremen, W. S. (2012). Genetic architecture of the Delis-Kaplan executive function system Trail Making Test: Evidence for distinct genetic influences on executive function. *Neuropsychology, 26*(2), 238–250. https://doi.org/10.1037/a0026768

Wecker, N. S., Kramer, J. H., Hallam, B. J., & Delis, D. C. (2005). Mental flexibility: age effects on switching. *Neuropsychology, 19*(3), 345–352. https://doi.org/10.1037/0894-4105.19.3.345

Wecker, N. S., Kramer, J. H., Wisniewski, A., Delis, D. C., & Kaplan, E. (2000). Age effects on executive ability. *Neuropsychology, 14*(3), 409–414.

Willen, E. J., Cuadra, A., Arheart, K. L., Post, M. J. D., & Govind, V. (2017). Young adults perinatally infected with HIV perform more poorly on measures of executive functioning and motor speed than ethnically matched healthy controls. *AIDS Care, 29*(3), 387–393. https://doi.org/10.1080/09540121.2016.1234677

Yochim, B., Baldo, J., Nelson, A., & Delis, D. C. (2007). D-KEFS Trail Making Test performance in patients with lateral prefrontal cortex lesions. *Journal of the International Neuropsychological Society, 13*(04), 704–709.

Yochim, B. P., Baldo, J. V., Kane, K. D., & Delis, D. C. (2009). D-KEFS Tower Test performance in patients with lateral prefrontal cortex lesions: The importance of error monitoring. *Journal of Clinical and Experimental Neuropsychology, 31*(6), 658–663. https://doi.org/10.1080/13803390802448669

Yochim, B. P., Mueller, A. E., & Segal, D. L. (2013). Late life anxiety is associated with decreased memory and executive functioning in community dwelling older adults. *Journal of Anxiety Disorders, 27*(6), 567–575. https://doi.org/10.1016/j.janxdis.2012.10.010

DESIGN FLUENCY TEST

TEST NAME	**Design Fluency Test**
DOMAIN	Executive functioning
AGE RANGE	In adults, to 72 years
ADMINISTRATION TIME	15 minutes
SCORING FORMAT	Hand scored
REFERENCES	Jones-Gotman, M. (1991). Localization of lesions by neuropsychological testing. *Epilepsia, 32,* S41–S52. Jones-Gotman, M., & Milner, B. (1977). Design Fluency: The invention of nonsense drawings after focal cortical lesions. *Neuropsychologia, 15,* 653–674.

DESCRIPTION

The Design Fluency Test (Jones-Gotman, 1991; Jones-Gotman & Milner, 1977) was developed as a nonverbal analog to word fluency tasks. The task requires the examinee to generate as many different abstract designs as possible. The test is comprised of a free-response condition, lasting five minutes, in which few restrictions are imposed on design generation, and a fixed-response condition, lasting four minutes, in which the examinee must produce designs that contain exactly four lines or components. Other stand-alone Design Fluency tests are the Ruff Figural Fluency Test (RFFT; Ruff, 1996, 1998) and the Five-Point Test (Regard et al., 1982), also reviewed elsewhere in this chapter. Variants of Design Fluency are part of larger test batteries, including the D-KEFS (Delis et al., 2001), reviewed elsewhere in this chapter. A modification of the fixed-response condition is also part of the HRNES (Russell & Starkey, 1993, 2001).

ADMINISTRATION

Detailed instructions are provided in Figure 9–6 (from M. Jones-Gotman, personal communication with previous authors, April 1995).

As per Jones-Gotman and Milner (1977), Kingery et al. (2006) implemented instructions as per Figure 9–7, administering only the fixed-response condition.

SCORING

There is one basic score for each condition: a *novel output score,* which is defined as the total output (total number of drawings) minus the sum of all perseverative responses, nameable drawings, and drawings with the wrong number of lines. To score the Design Fluency Test, first determine the perseverative responses. These include rotations or mirror-image versions of previous drawings, variations on a theme, complicated drawings that differ from previous ones by small details, and scribbles. The perseverative responses must be scored strictly and then subtracted from the total number drawn; the remaining drawings should be quite different from one another. Occasionally, the examinee might reproduce the drawing made by the examiner. This is not counted as a perseverative error.

For nameable drawings, the examiner will have asked "What is this?" for at least one drawing at the end of each condition. Most often examinees will deny knowing what the drawing represents, but they sometimes answer with the name of a concrete object or a letter that has been elaborated, and so on. The examiner must also use his or her own judgment when something looks nameable.

Jones-Gotman (1991) noted that it is not uncommon for examinees to produce some drawings that are too similar to others, although healthy individuals produce relatively few perseverations (see "Normative Data"). Furthermore, the greater the total number of drawings produced, the higher the likelihood that some will be repeated. The drawings of an individual may also have a certain resemblance reflecting the individual's style; however, Jones-Gotman suggests that this is distinct from the repetitiveness or perseveration that is often seen in the productions made by patients with right frontal dysfunction.

Of note, Harter, Hart, and Harter (1999) have developed an expanded scoring system to improve the reliability of scoring the number of novel designs, complexity of designs, variations in designs, and concrete, perseverative, and scribbled responses. Likewise, Kingery et al. (2006) describe an approach to administering and scoring the fixed-response condition of the Design Fluency Test that was modified from the Jones-Gotman and Milner (1997) version and was intended to more clearly delineate procedural ambiguities. Participants included individuals from a

Use a stopwatch and have the patient comfortably seated before giving the instructions. If more than one page is used per condition, provide new blank paper and place the old one so that the patient can always see what he or she has already drawn. Always use a ballpoint pen to avoid erasures. Use a separate page for examples provided during the instructions, and hide that page after giving the directions. Draw the examples one under the other to illustrate what is expected from the patient.

A. Free Condition (five minutes)

I want you to do some drawing for me. This test is different from others that you have done, because in this test you must make up the drawings in your head. Do not make drawings that represent something. Do not draw anything you have ever seen before. Do not make drawings that anybody could name; if you draw something that can be named I won't count it. Instead, what you must do is to make up designs out of your head. For example, you could draw something like this:

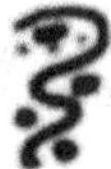

It's nothing, I just made it up. Or you could draw something like this: 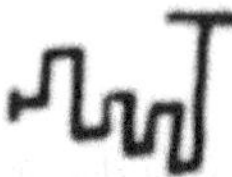

It's also nothing and I made it up. But if you were to draw, for example, something like this:  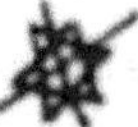

I would call it a star and I would not count it. The only other thing that is not accepted is scribbling. If you draw

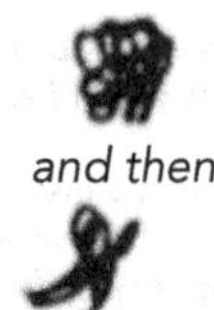

each might be slightly different from the other, but they do not require much effort from you and they are too much alike, so they are also not accepted and wouldn't count in your score. All of your drawings must be very different from each other.

Do you have any questions? When I say go, begin drawing. Make as many different drawings as you can in five minutes. You can start here, and draw them in columns like I have done. Go.

Remove the examiner's drawings from the patient's view. It is important to watch while the patient draws, so that warnings can be given at the appropriate moment. One warning only is given for each of the following: Scribbling *(That is a scribble. Remember scribbling is not allowed.)*; Nameable Drawing *(I can name that. It's a ______. Do not make drawings that represent something.)*; Too Similar to a Previous Drawing *(That is too much like … indicate which one … remember, all of your drawings must be very different from each other.)*; Too Elaborate *(Remember, you must make as many different drawings as you can.)* At the end, always question at least one design to probe for nameable drawings (What is this?).

B. Four-Line Condition (four minutes)

Give the patient a separate sheet of paper and write "4 lines" at the top. Use your instruction page to draw examples. Count the lines aloud while drawing the examples in this condition.

There is a second part to this test. It is like the first one because again you have to make up designs that you invent yourself, but this time each design must be made with exactly four lines. I will show you what I mean by 'a line' for the purposes of this test.

Figure 9–6 *Instructions for administration of the Design Fluency Test.*

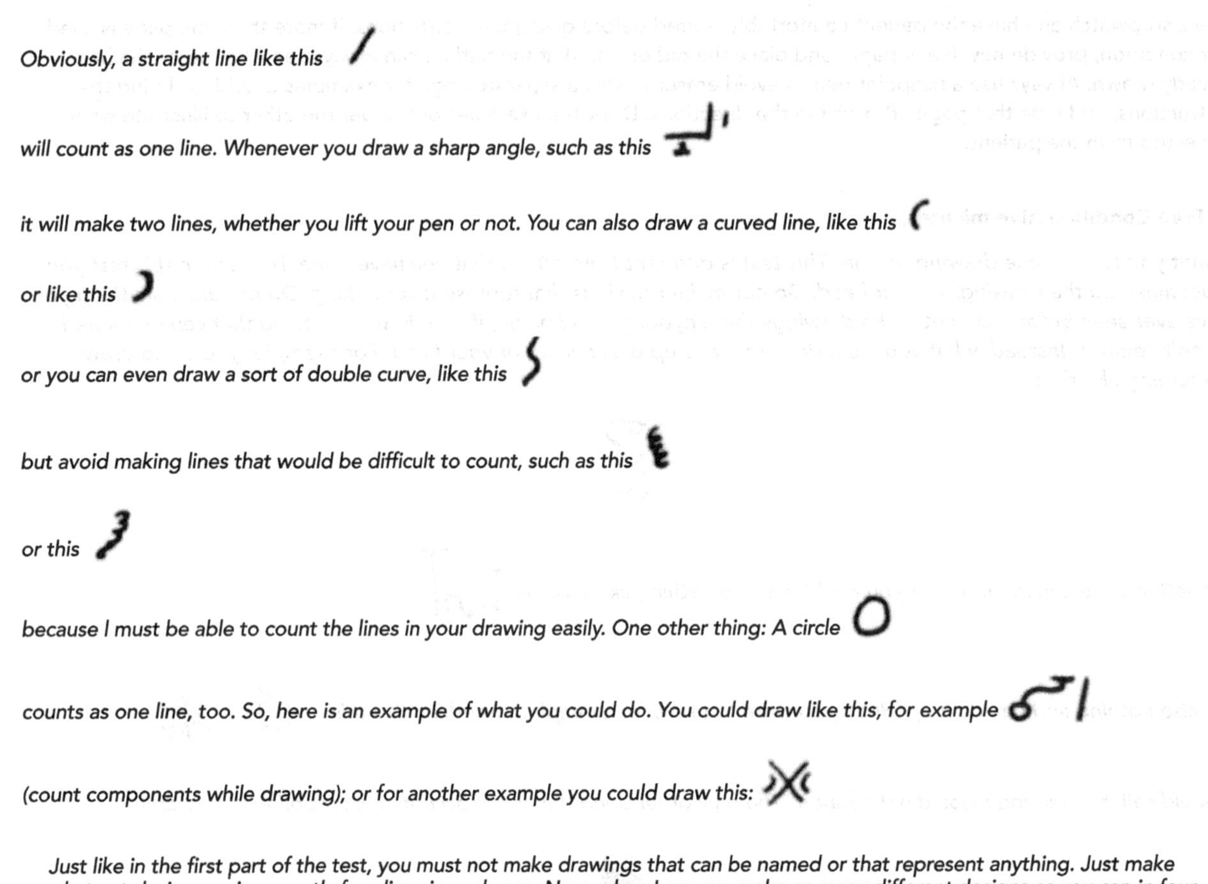

Obviously, a straight line like this

will count as one line. Whenever you draw a sharp angle, such as this

it will make two lines, whether you lift your pen or not. You can also draw a curved line, like this

or like this

or you can even draw a sort of double curve, like this

but avoid making lines that would be difficult to count, such as this

or this

because I must be able to count the lines in your drawing easily. One other thing: A circle

counts as one line, too. So, here is an example of what you could do. You could draw like this, for example

(count components while drawing); or for another example you could draw this:

Just like in the first part of the test, you must not make drawings that can be named or that represent anything. Just make up abstract designs, using exactly four lines in each one. Now, when I say go, make as many different designs as you can in four minutes. Go.

As before, remove the examiner's drawings from the patient's view. Watch the patient so that warnings can be given at the appropriate moment. One warning only is given for each of the following: Too similar to a Previous Drawing *(That is too much like... indicate which one... remember, all of your drawings must be very different from each other);* Nameable Drawings (often a letter or a square in this condition); Wrong Number of Lines (count the lines aloud and remind patient to use exactly four lines). Question at least one drawing at the end to probe for nameable designs that you may not recognize as such *(What is this?).*

Figure 9-6 *Continued*

SOURCE: From M. Jones-Gotman, personal communication with previous authors, April 1995.

longitudinal study of healthy aging, with additional participant details provided in "Evidence for Reliability."

In Kingery et al.'s (2006) scoring scheme, the total number of designs is the sum of all designs drawn within the four-minute time period. Rule-break errors are drawings that include line violations (i.e., too few or too many elements, scribbles) and nameable designs (i.e., those readily identified as an object or symbol). Perseverative responses include exact copies or rotations (identical or rotated versions) or minimal variations (designs that differ by just one element) of previous designs. The novel design total is the number of complete drawings minus the sum of unacceptable designs. A ratio of the total number of errors to total number of designs can also be calculated.

Now I want to see how many different designs you can think of in four minutes. I do have some rules, however. Each design must have four and only four parts. A "part" can be either: a straight line, a curved line (or arc), or a circle. Let me show you an example [show examples]. See how this figure has four parts: one, two, three, four [point to each part] and it includes a curved line, a circle and two straight lines. This design [point to second design] also has four parts: one, two, three, four [point to each part], but it includes two straight lines and two circles. A drawing does not have to include all three kinds of parts, but it must include a total of four parts. Do you understand? Remember, I want to see how many original designs you can think of, so do not copy the examples and do not make your designs too similar to each other. Also, do not draw a figure that is namable; for example, if you drew this [draw a square], I could point to it and say "That is a square." Does that make sense? When I say "begin," draw as many different designs with four parts each as you can. Ready? Begin!

Figure 9–7 *Instructions for administration of the Design Fluency Test, Fixed-Response Condition.*

SOURCE: Kingery et al. (2006).

DEMOGRAPHIC EFFECTS

AGE

In adulthood, performance decreases with advancing age (Jones-Gotman, 1990; Mittenberg et al., 1989, although see Turner, 1999; Varney et al., 1996). Daigneault, Braun, and Whitaker (1992) reported a higher incidence of perseverative errors in older adults (aged 45 to 65) without any reduction in the number of correct designs. In contrast, Kingery et al. (2006) reported that older age predicted rule breaks and line violations but not perseverative errors; age also predicted novel designs and unacceptable designs on repeat testing. Regression formulas are provided in their paper that incorporate relevant demographic influences of age and education, when applicable, to predict performance on the Design Fluency Test.

GENDER

Most studies report no significant gender differences (Demakis & Harrison, 1997; Varney et al., 1996; Kingery et al., 2006).

EDUCATION AND IQ

In general, performance appears to be related to education or IQ (e.g., Diaz-Asper et al., 2004, Kingery et al., 2006; however, see Harter et al., 1999; Turner, 1999; Varney et al., 1996). Crane, Pring, Ryder, and Hermelin (2011) reported that the overall number of designs as well as the number of novel designs produced was highly correlated with both verbal and performance IQ in individuals with learning difficulties (*rs* = .69 to .84). Similarly, IQ as measured by Raven's Progressive Matrices, was related to performance on both free-response and fixed-response conditions in patients with frontal lesions (*rs* = .34, .60, respectively; Robinson et al., 2012).

ETHNICITY, NATIONALITY, AND LINGUISTIC EFFECTS

Ethnicity is not found to predict change in scores over time (Kingery et al., 2006).

NORMATIVE DATA

Normative data are summarized in Table 9–57. Jones-Gotman (personal communication with previous authors, June 1995) has collected normative data for adults on both the free (five-minute) and fixed or four-line (four-minute) condition. Data are available for persons aged 14 to 55 years (*n* = 45) as well as a very small sample of people aged 58 to 72 (*n* = 10). Carter, Shore, Harnadek, and Kubu (1998) obtained similar data for a slightly larger sample of adults 19 to 56 years of age (*n* = 66; age, *M* = 25.06 years, *SD* = 7.83, range 19–56; education, *M* = 15.21, *SD* = 1.60; WAIS-R FSIQ = 100.85, *SD* = 11.07) using the revised scoring criteria described previously. Data are also available for errors on the free-response condition (mean perseverative errors = 7.1, *SD* = 7.8) and the fixed-response condition (mean perseverative errors = 6.4, *SD* = 5.5). Data from other sources suggest similar values (*n* = 33, mean age 33.8 years, Nelson et al., 2012; *n* = 35, mean age = 47.8 years, Robinson et al., 2012). Data are also available for combined samples of children and adults (Daigneault et al., 1992; Levin et al., 1991; Varney et al., 1996; Woodward et al., 1992).

Schretlen, Testa, and Pearlson (2010) also provide norms for 319 adults on the fixed condition as part of the CNNS available through Psychological Assessment Resources (PAR; www.parinc.com). These provide T scores and discrepancies based on a large sample of older adults from the northeastern United States. A major advantage of these norms is the option to correct for demographic variables such as age, sex, education, and ethnicity. Several other commonly used neuropsychological tests are co-normed using this sample, which facilitates cross-test comparisons.

Healthy people make one or no nameable errors (Carter et al., 1998; Kingery et al., 2006; Varney et al., 1996) and produce very few designs (less than three) with an incorrect number of lines on the fixed-response condition (Carter et al., 1998). In one study, errors were most likely to be designs that minimally varied from others or were perseverative in nature (Kingery et al., 2006).

TABLE 9–57 Summary of Normative Data for the Design Fluency Test

AUTHOR	FREE-RESPONSE CONDITION, MEAN (*SD*)	FIXED-RESPONSE CONDITION, MEAN (*SD*)
Jones-Gotman (1995)	15.5 (6.1), age 14–55 11.8 (4.4), age 58–72	18.9 (5.6), age 14–55 12.6 (4.3), age 58–72
Carter et al. (1998)	13.9 (6.3)	16.7 (6.1)
Nelson et al. (2012)	20.8 (7.8)	20.4 (7.8)
Robinson et al. (2012)	17.9 (8.3)	21.3 (8.7)
Kingery et al. (2006)	*n/a*	21.44 (9.36)

EVIDENCE FOR RELIABILITY

EVIDENCE FOR INTERNAL RELIABILITY

No information is available.

EVIDENCE FOR TEST-RETEST RELIABILITY, MEASURING CHANGE, AND PRACTICE EFFECTS

Test-retest reliability is variable. For example, Harter et al. (1999) found marginal test-retest reliability for the number of novel designs in the free-response condition (*r* = .69) but higher reliability for concreteness and complexity of the protocol (*r* = .91, .77, respectively). Goebel, Fischer, Ferstl, and Mehdorn (2009) reported strong test-retest reliability for a sample of healthy individuals aged 18 to 61 years of age, with a test-retest interval of 26 to 34 days (intraclass correlation coefficients [ICCs] for total designs and perseverations from .74 to .89), with the exception of repetition errors (ICCs of .36, .44).

TABLE 9–58 Test-Retest Reliability of the Design Fluency Test, Fixed Condition

DESIGN FLUENCY SCORE	TIME 1 MEAN	TIME 1 *SD*	TIME 2 MEAN	TIME 2 *SD*	MEAN DIFFERENCE	*r*	ICC
Total Designs	21.44	9.36	19.85	9.18	− 1.59	.79	.78
Nameable Designs	0.14	0.38	0.13	0.37	− 0.01	.12	.13
Line Violations	1.79	2.80	1.26	2.40	− 0.48	.06	.06
Sum Rule Breaks	1.93	2.81	1.39	2.45	− 0.49	.06	.06
Exact Copy/Rotation	0.43	0.94	0.72	1.30	0.27	.26	.24
Minimal Variations	3.56	3.46	4.64	4.52	0.93	.47	.45
Sum Perseverative Designs	3.99	3.99	5.37	5.34	1.20	.46	.43
Sum Unacceptable Designs	5.92	4.40	6.76	5.59	0.70	.39	.37
Novel Designs	15.52	7.48	13.09	6.87	− 2.79	.71	.67

NOTE: *SD*, standard deviation; r, Pearson correlation coefficient; ICC, intraclass correlation coefficient; Sum Rule Breaks = nameable designs + line violations; Sum Perseverative Designs = exact copy/rotation + minimal variations; Sum Unacceptable Designs = sum rule breaks ± sum perseverative designs.

SOURCE: From Kingery et al. (2006).

Kingery et al. (2006) provide follow-up testing data for approximately 87 healthy adults for the fixed-response condition (some were excluded due to severe health problems or poor MMSE score), an average of 5.5 years after initial testing. Participants ranged in age from 20 to 88 years (M = 55.6 years, SD = 16.5), with a mean education level of approximately 14 years (M = 13.9 years, SD = 3.1 years). Women and men were approximately equally represented (56% female), with non-Hispanic Caucasians predominant (88%; 12% African American).

As shown in Table 9–58, test-retest reliability of the Design Fluency Test was low overall and adequate only for total and novel designs. ICCs followed a similar pattern. Although total designs decrease from time 1 to time 2, as do novel designs (Kingery et al., 2006), other research has reported that previous exposure to the task results in an increase in design production, both in terms of total and novel designs (Harter et al., 1999), as well as an increase in test-taking efficiency, marked by a relative decrease in the proportion of perseverative responses. Reliable change indices, as calculated by Kingery et al. (2006) at the 90% confidence interval (CI) for the fixed-response condition, are large (see Table 9–59). This suggests that a large change would be required to reflect actual change in test performance.

TABLE 9–59 Reliable Change Indices for the Design Fluency Test, Fixed Condition

VARIABLE	MAGNITUDE OF CHANGE REQUIRED (90% CI)
Total Designs	+/-9.86
Nameable Designs	+/-.82
Line Violations	+/-5.87
Sum of Rule Breaks	+/-5.93
Exact Copy/Rotations	+/-2.26
Minimal Variations	+/-6.8
Sum of Perseverative Errors	+/-8.04
Sum Unacceptable Designs	+/-9.11
Novel Designs	+/-8.97

NOTE: CI, confidence interval; Sum Rule Breaks, nameable designs + line violations; Sum Perseverative Designs, exact copy/rotation + minimal variations; Sum Unacceptable Designs, sum rule breaks ± sum perseverative designs.

SOURCE: From Kingery et al. (2006).

EVIDENCE FOR INTERRATER RELIABILITY

When the original scoring criteria described in Jones-Gotman and Milner (1977) are used, there is marginal to adequate interrater agreement and consistency for the majority of scoring parameters in both conditions (e.g., r = .64 for novel output in the free-response condition and r = .71 in the fixed-response condition; Woodward et al., 1992). Other research has found high agreement between raters (e.g., 90% agreement for novel designs in the free-response condition; Varney et al., 1996).

Expanded scoring criteria (see "Scoring") enhance the reliability of most scores. Jones-Gotman (1991) assessed scoring reliability in a study of 324 children and 50 adults, with reliability coefficients at or exceeding .74 across three raters. Carter et al. (1998) reported good to excellent reliability for novel output scores and perseverative errors across three raters (ICCs ranging from .73–.99). However, nameable errors and designs with the incorrect number of lines yielded lower reliability coefficients.

Kingery et al. (2006) randomly selected 50 protocols for independent scoring by five raters. Average ICCs across five raters were excellent overall, ranging from .67 (copy rotation) to .99 (total designs), with most exceeding .82. Interrater reliability was high for total designs and novel designs (r = .79, .71, respectively) and substantially lower for minimal variations, perseverative designs, unacceptable designs, and exact copy/rotation (rs = .26 to .47). Goebel et al. (2009) similarly reported strong interrater reliabilities for free-response and fixed-response conditions (ICCs >.89).

EVIDENCE FOR VALIDITY

WITHIN-TEST CORRELATIONS AND RELATIONSHIPS WITH OTHER TESTS

Creating novel designs is a complex task and likely involves several cognitive processes, including creativity, constructional abilities, working memory, shifting set from one design to the next, and inhibiting repetition of a design (Foldi et al., 2003). Moderately strong correlations have been reported between the free-response and fixed-response conditions in healthy individuals (rs = .55 to .78; Demakis & Harrison, 1997). Scores on the Design Fluency Test and a similar task, the RFFT, are modestly correlated (Demakis & Harrison, 1997), with correlations between the fixed-response condition and the RFFT somewhat larger than correlations between the free-response condition (r = .38 vs. r = .25). The degree of association with word fluency varies, with most studies reporting at least modest overlap between the Design Fluency Test and verbal fluency (moderate to large correlations, Robinson et al., 2012; Turner, 1999; Varney et al., 1996; modest correlations, Demakis & Harrison, 1997).

The free-response condition shows strong relationships with visual constructional and memory tasks such as the copy and recall of the Rey-Osterreith Complex Figure Test and the Recognition Memory Test (range of r = .23 to .65; Mickanin et al., 1994). The Hayling Test, a measure of executive functioning, is correlated with both the free- and fixed-response conditions (rs = .30, .55, respectively; Robinson et al., 2012).

CLINICAL STUDIES

Dementia. The test has shown some utility in detecting FTD (Neary et al., 1990), particularly in those with right-sided FTD (Boone et al., 1999). Impairment in Design Fluency has also been found in patients with AD (Bigler et al., 1988; Harter et al., 1999; Mickanin et al., 1994); however, in one study, only 3% of patients with mild AD were found to be impaired on Design Fluency despite impairment on TMT-B and the Stroop in more than 40% of patients (Stokholm et al., 2006).

Lesion Studies. Jones-Gotman (1991) and Jones-Gotman and Milner (1977) reported that patients with right frontal or central damage show the greatest impairment on the task, although patients with lesions in other brain regions (e.g., right temporal, left frontal) also generate fewer novel designs than healthy people. Newer studies indicate that people with right frontal or central damage create few new designs and/or tend to make numerous perseverative errors. Robinson et al. (2012) examined verbal, design, gestural, and ideational fluency tests in a sample of patients with focal frontal and posterior lesions, as well as in demographically matched controls. Consistent with previous research, all participants with frontal lesions were impaired on each fluency task, with right-sided lesions associated with greater Design Fluency deficits than left-sided lesions.

Psychiatric Conditions. Some studies report group differences in favor of controls and relationships with the Design Fluency Test and interpersonal function (e.g., Zanello et al., 2006), whereas others have reported no relationships between the Design Fluency Test and social function in individuals with schizophrenia (Xiang et al., 2010).

Nelson et al. (2012) reported that individuals with comorbid anxiety and depression performed worse than depressed and control patients on this test. Obsessionality has been associated with reduced Design Fluency Test performance (Mataix-Cols et al., 1999). Delorme et al. (2007) reported no differences between relatives of people with autism and obsessive-compulsive disorder (OCD) and healthy controls on this test.

Other Populations. Impaired performance has been reported in people with MS (Tong et al., 2002), amyotrophic lateral sclerosis (Abrahams et al., 2000; for number of rule violations only), and autism (Turner, 1999), and in pain sufferers following bilateral anterior cingulotomy (Cohen et al., 1999). Savants with autism spectrum disorder and a group of people with learning difficulties produced more responses and more novel responses on the Design Fluency Test than a group with autism spectrum disorder (Crane et al., 2011). Higher levels of free thyroglobulin antibodies appear to be related to errors on the Design Fluency test and other executive function measures in healthy, euthyroid women (Grigorova & Sherwin, 2012).

NEUROANATOMICAL CORRELATES AND NEUROIMAGING STUDIES

Regional cerebral blood flow augmentation is seen in both frontal lobes during Design Fluency performance compared with baseline (Elfgren & Risberg, 1998). This is particularly evident when a visuospatial strategy is used to generate designs; however, when participants thought about a nameable object while also using a visuospatial strategy, the left frontal lobe was engaged. Design fluency scores are predicted by brain-derived neurotrophic factor and left temporal fractional anisotropy in patients with epilepsy (Chen et al., 2016).

PERFORMANCE VALIDITY

No information is available.

COMMENT

The Design Fluency test is a relatively brief task that requires little equipment. The Jones-Gotman (1977, 1991) version involves both a free-response condition that incorporates relatively few restrictions and a fixed-response condition, where production is relatively more constrained. As may be anticipated with a task requiring free-form production by an examinee, rigorous scoring is needed, with several modifications since inception of the original task that assist in delineating scoring procedures. The primary score is a novel output score, reflecting the total sum of designs minus errors.

Demographic influences on performance are not well-defined. Some research suggests worse performance with age, whereas others do not. Gender differences are generally not found. Research on the effects of education and IQ is mixed, with moderate correlations reported overall between Design Fluency and IQ. Limited information is available on the effects of ethnicity and other sociodemographic variables.

Normative data are sparse and lack precision, with small sample sizes and a lack of age bands, and are generally not of sufficient rigor for clinical decision making, at least for the original test. Kingery et al. (2006) and Schretlen et al. (2010) offer the most recent normative data for the fixed-response condition only, and so this may be the most appropriate version of the test to use. Of note, strong interrater reliability estimates are found when rigorous scoring criteria are used.

The processes underlying design fluency performance are not well-defined. In general, the test appears to moderately correlate with a range of tests, including other fluency measures, psychomotor speed, memory, and some executive function tests. In clinical populations, the test has shown sensitivity to frontal lesions, particularly right-sided lesions. Data are relatively sparse for other populations, and neuroanatomical correlates are limited, as is the utility of the test as a performance validity estimate.

REFERENCES

Abrahams, S., Leigh, P. N., Harvey, A., Vythelingum, G. N., Grise, D., & Goldstein, L. H. (2000). Verbal fluency and executive dysfunction in amyotrophic lateral sclerosis (ALS). *Neuropsychologia, 38*, 734–747.

Bigler, E. D., Schultz, R., Grant, M., Knight, G., Lucas, J., Roman, M., Hall, S., & Sullivan, M. (1988). Design Fluency in dementia of the Alzheimer's type: Preliminary findings. *Neuropsychology, 2*, 127–133.

Boone, K. B., Miller, B. L., Lee, A., Berman, N., Sherman, D., & Stuss, D. T. (1999). Neuropsychological patterns in right versus left frontotemporal dementia. *Journal of the International Neuropsychological Society, 5*, 612–622.

Carter, S. L., Shore, D., Harnadek, M. S., & Kubu, C. S. (1998). Normative data and interrater reliability of the Design Fluency Test. *The Clinical Neuropsychologist, 12*, 531–534.

Chen, N.-C., Chuang, Y.-C., Huang, C.-W., Lui, C.-C., Lee, C.-C., Hsu, S.-W., . . . Chang, C.-C. (2016). Interictal serum brain-derived neurotrophic factor level reflects white matter integrity, epilepsy severity, and cognitive dysfunction in chronic temporal lobe epilepsy. *Epilepsy & Behavior, 59*, 147–154. https://doi.org/10.1016/j.yebeh.2016.02.029

Cohen, R. A., Kaplan, R. F., Zuffante, P., Moser, D. J., Jenkines, M. A., Salloway, S., & Wilkinson, H. (1999). Alteration of intention and self-initiated action associated with bilateral anterior cingulotomy. *Journal of Neuropsychiatry and Clinical Neuroscience, 11*, 444–453.

Crane, L., Pring, L., Ryder, N., & Hermelin, B. (2011). Executive functions in savant artists with autism. *Research in Autism Spectrum Disorders, 5*(2), 790–797. http://doi.org/10.1016/j.rasd.2010.09.007

Daigneault, S., Braun, C. M. J., & Whitaker, H. A. (1992). Early effects of normal aging on perseverative and nonperseverative prefrontal measures. *Developmental Neuropsychology, 8*, 99–114.

Delis, D. C., Kaplan, E., & Kramer, J. H. (2001). *Delis-Kaplan Executive Function System.* San Antonio, TX: The Psychological Corporation.

Delorme, R., Goussé, V., Roy, I., Trandafir, A., Mathieu, F., Mouren-Siméoni, M.-C., . . . Leboyer, M. (2007). Shared executive dysfunctions in unaffected relatives of patients with autism and obsessive-compulsive disorder. *European Psychiatry, 22*(1), 32–38. http://doi.org/10.1016/j.eurpsy.2006.05.002

Demakis, G. J., & Harrison, D. W. (1997). Relationships between verbal and nonverbal fluency measures: Implications for assessment of executive functioning. *Psychological Reports, 81*, 443–448.

Diaz-Asper, C., Schretlen, D. J., & Pearlson, G. D. (2004). How well does IQ predict neuropsychological test performance in normal adults. *Journal of the International Neuropsychological Society, 10*, 82–90.

Elfgren, C. I., & Risberg, J. (1998). Lateralized frontal blood flow increases during fluency tasks: Influence of cognitive strategy. *Neuropsychologia, 36*, 505–512.

Foldi, N. S., Helm-Estabrooks, N., Redfield, J., & Nickel, D. G. (2003). Perseveration in normal aging: A comparison of perseveration rates on Design Fluency and verbal generative tasks. *Aging, Neuropsychology and Cognition, 10*, 268–280.

Goebel, S., Fischer, R., Ferstl, R., & Mehdorn, H. M. (2009). Normative data and psychometric properties for qualitative and quantitative scoring criteria of the Five-point Test. *The Clinical Neuropsychologist, 23*(4), 675–690. http://doi.org/10.1080/13854040802389185

Grigorova, M., & Sherwin, B. B. (2012). Thyroid hormones and cognitive functioning in healthy, euthyroid women: A correlational study. *Hormones and Behavior, 61*(4), 617–622. http://doi.org/10.1016/j.yhbeh.2012.02.014

Harter, S. L., Hart, C. C., & Harter, G. W. (1999). Expanded scoring criteria for the Design Fluency Test: Reliability and validity in neuropsychological and college samples. *Archives of Clinical Psychology, 14*, 419–432.

Jones-Gotman, M. (1991). Localization of lesions by neuropsychological testing. *Epilepsia, 32*, S41–S52.

Jones-Gotman, M., & Milner, B. (1977). Design Fluency: The invention of nonsense drawings after focal cortical lesions. *Neuropsychologia, 15*, 653–674.

Kingery, L. R., Schretlen, D. J., Sateri, S., Langley, L. K., Marano, N. C., & Meyer, S. M. (2006). Interrater and test–retest reliability of a fixed condition Design Fluency Test. *The Clinical Neuropsychologist, 20*(4), 729–740. http://doi.org/10.1080/13854040500350992

Levin, H. S., Culhane, K. A., Hartmann, J., Harword, H., Ringholtz, G., Ewing-Cobbs, L., & Fletcher, J. M. (1991). Developmental changes in performance on tests of purported frontal lobe functioning. *Developmental Neuropsychology, 7*, 377–395.

Mataix-Cols, D., Barrios, M., Sanchez-Turet, M., & Vallejo, J. (1999). Reduced Design Fluency in subclinical obsessive-compulsive subjects. *Journal of Neuropsychiatry & Clinical Neurosciences, 11*, 395–397.

Mickanin, J., Grossman, M., Onishi, K., Auriacombe, S., & Clark, C. (1994). Verbal and nonverbal fluency in patients with probable Alzheimer's disease. *Neuropsychology, 8*, 385–394.

Mittenberg, W., Seidenberg, M., O'Leary, D. S., & DiGiulio, D. V. (1989). Changes in cerebral functioning associated with normal aging. *Journal of Clinical and Experimental Neuropsychology, 11*, 918–932.

Neary, D., Snowden, J. S., Mann, D. M. A., Northen, B., Goulding, P. J., & Macdermott, N. (1990). Frontal lobe dementia and motor neuron disease. *Journal of Neurology, Neurosurgery, and Psychiatry, 53*, 23–32.

Nelson, B. D., Sarapas, C., Robison-Andrew, E. J., Altman, S. E., Campbell, M. L., & Shankman, S. A. (2012). Frontal brain asymmetry in depression with comorbid anxiety: A neuropsychological investigation. *Journal of Abnormal Psychology, 121*(3), 579–591. http://doi.org/10.1037/a0027587

Regard, M., Strauss, E., & Knapp, P. (1982). Children's production of verbal and nonverbal fluency tasks. *Perceptual and Motor Skills, 55*, 839–844.

Robinson, G., Shallice, T., Bozzali, M., & Cipolotti, L. (2012). The differing roles of the frontal cortex in fluency tests. *Brain, 135*(7), 2202–2214. http://doi.org/10.1093/brain/aws142

Ruff, R. (1996, 1998). *Ruff Figural Fluency Test.* Odessa, FL: PAR.

Russell, E. W., & Starkey, R. I. (1993, 2001). *Halstead Russell Neuropsychological Evaluation System (HRNES-R).* Los Angeles: Western Psychological Services.

Schretlen, D. J., Testa, S. M., & Pearlson, G. D. (2010). *Calibrated Neuropsychological Normative System*. Lutz, FL: PAR.

Stokholm, J., Vogel, A., Gade, A., & Waldemar, G. (2006). Heterogeneity in executive impairment in patients with very mild Alzheimer's disease. *Dementia and Geriatric Cognitive Disorders, 22*(1), 54–59. http://doi.org/10.1159/000093262

Tong, B. S., Yip, J. T. H., Lee, T. M. C., & Li, L. S. W. (2002). Frontal fluency and memory functioning among multiple sclerosis patients in Hong Kong. *Brain Injury, 16*, 987–995.

Turner, M. A. (1999). Generating novel ideas: Fluency performance in high-functioning and learning disabled individuals with autism. *Journal of Child Psychology and Psychiatry, 40*, 189–201.

Varney, N. R., Roberts, R. J., Struchen, M. A., Hanson, T. V., Franzen, K. M., & Connell, S. K. (1996). Design Fluency among normals and patients with closed head injury. *Archives of Clinical Neuropsychology, 11*, 345–353.

Woodward, J. L., Axelrod, B. N., & Henry, R. R. (1992). Interrater reliability of scoring parameters for the Design Fluency Test. *Neuropsychology, 6*, 173–178.

Xiang, Y.-T., Shum, D., Chiu, H. F., Tang, W.-K., & Ungvari, G. S. (2010). Association of demographic characteristics, symptomatology, retrospective and prospective memory, executive functioning and intelligence with social functioning in schizophrenia. *Australian and New Zealand Journal of Psychiatry, 44*(12), 1112–1117.

Zanello, A., Perrig, L., & Huguelet, P. (2006). Cognitive functions related to interpersonal problem-solving skills in schizophrenic patients compared with healthy subjects. *Psychiatry Research, 142*(1), 67–78. http://doi.org/10.1016/j.psychres.2003.07.009

DYSEXECUTIVE QUESTIONNAIRE (DEX)

TEST NAME	**Dysexecutive Questionnaire (DEX)**
DOMAIN	Executive functioning
AGE RANGE	16 to 87
ADMINISTRATION TIME	15 minutes
SCORING FORMAT	Hand scored
REFERENCE	Wilson, B. A., Alderman, N., Burgess, P. W., Emslie, H., & Evans, J. J. (1996). *Behavioural Assessment of the Dysexecutive Syndrome.* Bury St. Edmunds, UK: Thames Valley Test Company. www.pearsonclinical.com

DESCRIPTION

The Dysexecutive Questionnaire (DEX; Wilson et al., 1996) is a questionnaire that is included with the BADS battery (Wilson et al., 1996). The BADS is reviewed elsewhere in this chapter. The DEX is not technically part of the BADS in the sense that it is not included in the calculation of the Profile score for the BADS. It is not normed, and it is intended to supplement information from the BADS via qualitative data provided by self-report and informant ratings.

The DEX purports to assess a number of characteristics including difficulty with abstract thinking, impulsivity, confabulation, perseveration, planning problems, euphoria, lack of insight, apathy, disinhibition, distractibility, knowledge-response dissociation, and lack of concern for social rules. The DEX includes 20 items that can be subdivided into four broad areas: emotional or personality changes, motivational changes, behavioral changes, and cognitive changes. Items include statements such as: "I act without thinking, doing the first thing that comes to mind" or "I have difficulty thinking ahead and planning for the future."

The questionnaire compares responses in two versions, one of which is designed to be completed by the patient (DEX-Self) and another by a relative or a caregiver who has close, preferably daily, contact with the patient (DEX-Other). Of note, on the basis of factor analysis, a 15-item revised version of the DEX has also been introduced (Shaw et al., 2015).

ADMINISTRATION

See the manual.

SCORING

The DEX is intended to be used to provide qualitative information and supplement information obtained from the BADS. Each of the 20 items is scored on a five-point (0–4) Likert scale, ranging from "Never" to "Very Often." The DEX yields a maximum raw score of 80 points, with higher scores indicating greater impairment.

DEMOGRAPHIC EFFECTS

AGE

No relationships with age are found in severe TBI samples (Azouvi et al., 2015; Jourdan et al., 2013) or people with learning disabilities (Masson et al., 2010).

GENDER

No relationships with gender are reported in TBI samples (Azouvi et al., 2015; Bodenburg & Dopslaff, 2008; Jourdan et al., 2013) or a learning disability sample (Masson et al., 2010). However, women were found to perform better than men in a healthy sample (Takeuchi et al., 2013).

EDUCATION AND IQ

The DEX is negatively related to education in severe TBI, indicating that higher education levels are related to lower levels of impairment (Azouvi et al., 2015; Jourdan et al., 2013); similar findings have been reported in older adults with diabetes (Munshi et al., 2012). See the section "Evidence for Validity" for information on IQ effects.

ETHNICITY, NATIONALITY, AND LINGUISTIC EFFECTS

The DEX has been used in a number of countries, but information specifically concerning the impact of sociodemographic variables on performance is not available.

NORMATIVE DATA

No normative data are provided for the DEX in the manual. Evans, Chua, McKenna, and Wilson (1997) examined a small group of healthy controls (n = 26; age, M = 39.1,

TABLE 9–60 Dysexecutive Questionnaire (DEX) DEX-Self and DEX-Other Scores in a Healthy Hong Kong Sample

ITEMS	DEX-SELF MEAN	(SD)	RANGE	DEX-OTHER MEAN	(SD)	RANGE
1. Abstract thinking problems	1.28	(0.85)	0–4	1.08	(0.81)	0–3
2. Impulsivity	1.04	(0.79)	0–3	0.94	(0.88)	0–4
3. Confabulation	0.61	(0.77)	0–3	0.75	(0.88)	0–3
4. Planning problems	1.52	(0.79)	0–4	1.34	(1.03)	0–4
5. Euphoria	1.27	(0.86)	0–4	1.25	(0.95)	0–4
6. Temporal sequencing problems	1.24	(0.72)	0–3	0.91	(0.78)	0–3
7. Lack of insight and social awareness	0.90	(0.81)	0–4	0.79	(0.77)	0–3
8. Apathy and lack of drive	1.37	(0.89)	0–4	1.30	(0.96)	0–3
9. Disinhibition	0.70	(0.62)	0–2	0.60	(0.67)	0–3
10. Variable motivation	0.78	(0.77)	0–4	0.83	(0.92)	0–3
11. Shallowing of affective responses	1.29	(0.82)	0–4	1.14	(1.06)	0–3
12. Aggression	0.94	(0.83)	0–4	1.18	(0.95)	0–3
13. Lack of concern	0.98	(0.76)	0–2	0.83	(0.81)	0–4
14. Perseveration	1.10	(0.85)	0–3	0.96	(0.88)	0–4
15. Restlessness-hyperkinesis	0.75	(0.90)	0–3	0.68	(0.76)	0–3
16. Inability to inhibit response	1.10	(0.73)	0–4	1.13	(0.88)	0–4
17. Knowing-doing dissociation	0.97	(0.78)	0–4	0.85	(0.86)	0–3
18. Distractibility	1.61	(0.94)	0–4	1.11	(0.91)	0–4
19. Poor decision-making ability	1.38	(0.82)	0–4	1.18	(0.94)	0–4
20. No concern for social rules	1.31	(1.00)	0–4	1.20	(1.04)	0–4

NOTE: Range of total score is 0–80.

SOURCE: From Chan (2001).

SD = 19.02; mean estimated NART IQ = 110.3, *SD* = 8.95) and reported DEX-Self ratings (*M* = 21.81, *SD* = 8.16) and DEX-Other ratings (*M* = 11.25, *SD* = 6.71). The relationship of the collateral raters to the controls was not reported.

Chan (2001) recruited a sample of 93 healthy Hong Kong Chinese participants (29 males, 64 females) between the ages of 18 and 50 years (*M* = 34.7, *SD* = 10.39) and their relatives. The reported DEX values (self and relatives) are summarized in Table 9–60. The values are reported to be similar to those obtained in the United Kingdom (Chan & Manly, 2002).

Quartile distributions are provided for the DEX-Self (see Table 9–61) for a sample of 191 patients (73 women, 118 men) with an average age of 42.5 years. This was an unselected clinical sample with acquired brain injury seen via outpatient neuropsychological practice in Germany (Bodenburg & Dopslaff, 2008). The time since brain injury ranged from one to 39 months (*M* = 6.9 months; *SD* = 8.4 months). The components in Table 9–61 refer to those yielded by the authors' factor analysis of the structure of the DEX (see "Evidence for Validity").

EVIDENCE FOR RELIABILITY

EVIDENCE FOR INTERNAL RELIABILITY

Internal reliability is high (>.85; Azouvi et al., 2015; Bennett et al., 2005; Bodenburg & Dopslaff, 2008; Hellebrekers et al., 2017; McGuire et al., 2014; Moreno & McKerral, 2018; Takeuchi et al., 2013). A 15-item revised DEX questionnaire has been introduced based on factor analysis, which had high internal reliability, exceeding .85 (Shaw et al., 2015).

EVIDENCE FOR TEST-RETEST RELIABILITY, MEASURING CHANGE, AND PRACTICE EFFECTS

Test-retest reliability for the DEX-Self is strong (r = .88) but weaker for the DEX-Other (r = .60), as reported in a

TABLE 9–61 Quartile Distributions for DEX-Self Ratings in People with Acquired Brain Injury

QUARTILE	COMPONENT: INITIATE, SUSTAIN	IMPULSE CONTROL, SEQUENCING	EXCITABILITY	REGARD FOR SOCIAL STANDARDS	OVERALL TEST
25% (mild)	8	5	3	2	20
50% (moderate)	12	7	5	4	28
75% (strong)	17	10	7	5	36

NOTE: The totals for the four scales are based on summing item responses. Factor 1 (Initiate, Sustain): items 2, 4, 8, 10, 17, 18, 19; Factor 2 (Impulse Control, Sequencing): items 1, 6, 12. 14, 16; Factor 3 (Excitability): items 5, 7, 15; and Factor 4 (Regard for Social Standard): items 9, 13, 20; Overall Test: sum of all scale scores.

SOURCE: Adapted from Bodenburg and Dopslaff (2008).

study of patients with acquired brain injury (Hellebrekers et al., 2017).

EVIDENCE FOR INTERRATER RELIABILITY

No information is available.

EVIDENCE FOR VALIDITY

FACTOR-ANALYTIC STUDIES

The number of factors underlying DEX performance may range from one to five (for discussion, see Pedrero-Pérez et al., 2015; Shaw et al., 2015). Similarly, Rasch analysis of items in an acquired brain injury sample has suggested that both the DEX-Self and the DEX-Other are multifaceted and reflect a number of latent traits (Simblett et al., 2012; Simblett & Bateman, 2011).

Factor analysis of informant ratings on the DEX has suggested that the questionnaire measures change in at least three (Hellebrekers et al., 2017; Shaw et al., 2015; Wilson et al., 1996), four (Bodenburg & Dopslaff, 2008) or five (Burgess et al., 1998; Chan, 2001) factors (note that some authors have reported a one-factor solution; McGuire et al., 2014; Pedrero-Pérez et al., 2015). Four factors, accounting for nearly 50% of the variance in scores, reflected initiating and sustaining actions, impulse control and sequencing, psychophysical and mental excitability, and social conventions in one study (Bodenburg & Dopslaff, 2008). Of note, principal components analysis of the DEX-Self in an acquired brain injury sample generally suggested fewer factors than for the DEX-Other, including a one-factor (McGuire et al., 2014) or two-factor structure (Hellebrekers et al., 2017).

WITHIN-TEST RELATIONSHIPS

DEX-Self and DEX-Other. The DEX-Self and DEX-Other may yield different results (see also Alderman et al., 2001; Burgess et al., 1998; Wilson et al., 1996). When agreement is compared via ICC in an acquired brain injury sample (McGuire et al., 2014), agreement is fair between DEX ratings provided by self and significant others (average ICC = .41) and inadequate between DEX ratings provided by self, significant others, and clinicians (average ICCs ≤. 31). The DEX-Other completed by therapists revealed significant group differences between patients with anterior compared to posterior lesions, whereas differences on the DEX-Self were reported only between patient groups and healthy controls (Emmanouel et al., 2014). In addition, the DEX-Other indicated greater severity of executive difficulty in patients with anterior compared to posterior lesions. However, note that some studies have reported that DEX-Self ratings may be higher or equivalent to DEX-Other ratings, such as in mild TBI (Erez et al., 2009) or patients with PD (Koerts et al., 2012).

SHORT FORMS

The shortened 15-item version of the DEX introduced by Shaw et al. (2015; see "Description") accurately classified 69% of cases overall into community, psychiatric, and neurologic groups; however, note that only one-quarter of the psychiatric sample was correctly classified. Also note that although there were some differences between neurologic, psychiatric, and community-dwelling groups in DEX ratings, the community-dwelling and neurologically impaired groups did not differ on the revised DEX score. Overall, receiver operating characteristic (ROC) analysis suggested optimal differentiation at a revised DEX score cutoff of 37.5, which was associated with relatively high sensitivity (90%) and specificity (70%).

RELATIONSHIPS WITH THE BADS

BADS and DEX. The relationship between the BADS subtests and the DEX has been examined, with mixed results reported. Some research has found low correlations overall between various BADS subtests and the DEX, with the exception of Rule Shift (Boelen et al., 2009). Similarly, no significant relationships between the BADS and DEX have been reported in severe TBI (Wood & Liossi, 2006) or patients with neurologic conditions (Norris & Tate, 2000). As many as 29% of patients with MS show discrepant impairment between BADS performance and DEX ratings (van der Hiele et al., 2012).

However, Wilson et al. (1996) reported that there were moderate negative correlations between the DEX ratings made by others and performance on the six individual BADS tests; that is, poor awareness of deficit was correlated with poor executive functioning on each BADS test. A moderate association was reported between various BADS subtests (particularly Action Program, Modified Six Elements) and DEX ratings by clinicians in a TBI sample (Bennett et al., 2005).

The identity of the rater may impact whether relationships are found or not (see also previous discussion and also Wilson et al., 1996); for example, in a study of patients with brain injury due to various etiologies, the DEX-Other as completed by therapists significantly correlated with BADS subtests, whereas the DEX-Self did not (Emmanouel et al., 2014).

CORRELATIONS WITH OTHER TESTS AND SCALES

The DEX appears to correlate with broad measures of cognition, generally in the moderate to large range of magnitude, including an adapted version of the Montreal Cognitive Assessment (MoCA) in persons with learning disability (Edge et al., 2015). In a severe TBI sample, the DEX-Self correlated with cognitive status as measured by the Neurobehavioral Rating Scale–Revised (Azouvi et al., 2015). In a sample of patients with MS, the DEX was moderately correlated with Wechsler Similarities (Cerezo García et al., 2015). See also Wilson et al. (1996) who reported moderate correlations between the WAIS-R and the DEX.

In terms of executive function, mixed results have been reported. In a sample of patients with AD, the DEX-Self was moderately related to CLOX 1, the Luria Test, and Rule Shift Cards (Canali et al., 2011). In people with intellectual disability, the DEX-Other was related to TOL performance (Masson et al., 2010). However, note that other studies have found no significant correlations between the DEX and performance-based measures of executive function such as the TMT and Verbal Fluency (Munshi et al., 2012).

Evidence consistently suggests relationships between the DEX and measures of mood. In a series of studies in non-clinical samples, DEX ratings were found to correlate with neuroticism and low levels of conscientiousness (medium to large effect sizes) but not with performance-based measures of executive function such as the TMT, Verbal Fluency, or Digit Span (Buchanan, 2016). Similarly, in patients with MS, the DEX was significantly related to depressive and anxiety symptoms (Cerezo García et al., 2015), with similar findings reported in TBI (Moreno & McKerral, 2018; Azouvi et al., 2015) and psychiatric outpatients (Oei et al., 2016). Similarly, patients with PD and comorbid depression showed higher DEX-Self and DEX-Other ratings indicating greater difficulty than PD patients without depression (Koerts et al., 2012). Depressive symptoms and diabetes-related distress were also significantly related to DEX ratings in a sample of older adults with diabetes (Munshi et al., 2012). Patients with MS who rated themselves poorly on the DEX compared to performance-based measures tended to have more depression, anxiety, and stress symptoms than persons whose ratings aligned with BADS scores (van der Hiele et al., 2012).

CLINICAL STUDIES

The DEX-Other has been found to be useful in the prediction of progression in MCI (Aretouli et al., 2013). For example, the DEX-Self was found to differentiate patients with AD from controls with a sensitivity of 49% and a specificity of 71% at a cutoff of 18 (Canali et al., 2011). In another study, however, the DEX-Self ratings were lower (i.e., indicating less impairment) when completed by persons with MCI who declined compared to persons with MCI who were stable, potentially indicating decreased awareness in the declining group (Johnson et al., 2010). No differences were found in the DEX-Other ratings between the groups. Patients with MCI characterized by greater executive than amnestic disturbance obtain worse scores on the DEX (Pa et al., 2009).

The DEX (Self and Other) is sensitive to the presence of mild to moderate TBI (Chan, 2001). DEX ratings made by professionals are also linked to severity of injury (Bennett et al., 2005). In patients with severe TBI, distractibility and shallowing of affective responses are most commonly reported (>40% of patients), as well as abstract thinking problems, impulsivity, planning problems, apathy, aggression, restlessness-hyperkinesis and poor decision making in more than 30% of the sample (Azouvi et al., 2015).

The DEX has been used in other clinical populations, including in people with PD (Koerts et al., 2012; Vlagsma et al., 2017), subarachnoid hemorrhage (Buunk et al., 2016), and persons with acromegaly (Shan et al., 2017), and the DEX has been shown to be impaired in a large proportion of adults with ADHD (Fuermaier et al., 2015).

The DEX has functional and clinical correlates in a number of populations. Although the DEX-Self does not relate to injury severity (Glasgow Coma Scale, post-traumatic amnesia), the scale is significantly related to disability, ADLs, and return to work in severe TBI at four-year follow-up (Azouvi et al., 2015). DEX ratings are also related to risky sexual behavior in persons with TBI (Moreno & McKerral, 2018) and to coping (Rakers et al., 2017). In an MS sample, caregiver burden was correlated with DEX scores (Bayen et al., 2016). Although the DEX was not related to indices of glycemic control in older adults with diabetes, ratings were related to a number of other clinical variables, including number of falls, fear of falling, and fewer medications (Munshi et al., 2012).

The DEX has also been used as a treatment outcome measure following rehabilitation after acquired brain injury (Goodwin et al., 2016), following cognitive rehabilitation in patients with spina bifida (Stubberud et al., 2015), following treatment for persons with AD after galantamine therapy (Oka et al., 2016), and following chemotherapy in breast cancer (Kitahata et al., 2017).

NEUROANATOMICAL CORRELATES AND IMAGING STUDIES

A factor score from the DEX was correlated with an index of cerebral blood flow in a study of patients with moyamoya disease (Fang et al., 2016). Single-photon emission computed tomography (SPECT) findings indicate that lower baseline regional cerebral blood values in frontal areas are associated with improved DEX scores following galantamine therapy in patients with AD (Oka et al., 2016). DEX ratings are also related to orbitofrontal cortex activation and bilateral white matter areas near the temporal regions (Takeuchi et al., 2013).

PERFORMANCE VALIDITY

No information is available.

COMMENT

The DEX provides useful qualitative information regarding executive function, both from the perspective of the patient (DEX-Self) and a collateral informant (DEX-Other). It is relatively brief and easy to administer and may be particularly useful when a more comprehensive assessment of executive function is not available.

In terms of demographic effects, the questionnaire is generally found not to be significantly related to age or gender; however, relationships with education are reported. There is insufficient information relating to the influence of other sociodemographic variables, such as ethnicity, nationality, or language. The DEX is not normed, but cutoff scores and rudimentary normative data have been provided in some studies.

Internal reliability is strong and test-retest reliability appears strong for the DEX-Self. An alternative 15-item version of the DEX has been introduced, which appears to have some promise. Research suggests there is different information obtained by the self- and other-ratings, with poor agreement between raters. Although a lack of insight on the part of the patient has been identified as a potential reason for the discrepancy between raters, there is also evidence that third-party raters differ from one another (e.g., therapists, family members). Discrepancies between ratings, when found, may provide valuable clinical information in terms of designing rehabilitation or other interventions to accommodate for the stages of change the patient and family may be at regarding treatment readiness. Mixed results have been reported in terms of correlations between the BADS and the DEX, which may be related in part to whether the ratings have been completed by self or other. However, generally speaking, correlations between executive functioning ratings and tests of executive functioning are moderate at best and often fairly low depending on the test, the informant, and the dimension of executive functioning measured.

The evidence is mixed with respect to the number of factors underlying DEX performance, with anywhere from one to five factors identified, suggesting that the DEX is unlikely to be a unitary measure of executive function. The test correlates with global measures of cognition, such as mental status, other screeners, and IQ, with mixed evidence for correlation with other tests of executive function. The DEX is highly correlated with measures of mood, and consideration of depression and anxiety must be factored in when interpreting results. There is research in a number of clinical populations, including TBI, MCI, dementia, and others. Functional and clinical correlates have been reported. There is some evidence to suggest DEX ratings are related to areas in the frontal cortex, although research is limited. Information on performance validity is not available. Of note, this test has relatively weak normative data and no validity scale, which is an important omission compared to other normed scales such as the BRIEF-A.

REFERENCES

Alderman, N., Dawson, K., Rutterford, N. A., & Reynolds, P. J. (2001). A comparison of the validity of self-report measures amongst people with acquired brain injury: A preliminary study of the usefulness of EuroQol-5D. *Neuropsychological Rehabilitation, 11*, 529–537.

Aretouli, E., Tsilidis, K. K., & Brandt, J. (2013). Four-year outcome of mild cognitive impairment: The contribution of executive dysfunction. *Neuropsychology, 27*(1), 95–106. https://doi.org/10.1037/a0030481

Azouvi, P., Vallat-Azouvi, C., Millox, V., Darnoux, E., Ghout, I., Azerad, S., . . . Jourdan, C. (2015). Ecological validity of the Dysexecutive Questionnaire: Results from the PariS-TBI study. *Neuropsychological Rehabilitation, 25*(6), 864–878. https://doi.org/10.1080/09602011.2014.990907

Bayen, E., Jourdan, C., Ghout, I., Darnoux, E., Azerad, S., Vallat-Azouvi, C., . . . Azouvi, P. (2016). Objective and subjective burden of informal caregivers 4 years after a severe traumatic brain injury: Results from the Paris-TBI study. *The Journal of Head Trauma Rehabilitation, 31*(5), E59–E67. https://doi.org/10.1097/HTR.0000000000000079

Bennett, P. C., Ong, B., & Ponsford, J. (2005). Measuring executive dysfunction in an acute rehabilitation setting: Using the dysexecutive questionnaire (DEX). *Journal of the International Neuropsychological Society, 11*(04), 376. https://doi.org/10.1017/S1355617705050423

Bodenburg, S., & Dopslaff, N. (2008). The Dysexecutive Questionnaire advanced: Item and test score characteristics, 4-factor solution, and severity classification. *Journal of Nervous and Mental Disease, 196*(1), 75–78. https://doi.org/10.1097/NMD.0b013e31815faa2b

Boelen, D. H. E., Spikman, J. M., Rietveld, A. C. M., & Fasotti, L. (2009). Executive dysfunction in chronic brain-injured patients: Assessment in outpatient rehabilitation. *Neuropsychological Rehabilitation, 19*(5), 625–644. https://doi.org/10.1080/09602010802613853

Buchanan, T. (2016). Self-report measures of executive function problems correlate with personality, not performance-based executive function measures, in nonclinical samples. *Psychological Assessment, 28*(4), 372–385. https://doi.org/10.1037/pas0000192

Burgess, P. W., Alderman, N., Evans, J., Emslie, H., & Wilson, B. A. (1998). The ecological validity of tests of executive function. *Journal of the International Neuropsychological Society, 4*, 547–558.

Buunk, A. M., Groen, R. J. M., Veenstra, W. S., Metzemaekers, J. D. M., van der Hoeven, J. H., van Dijk, J. M. C., & Spikman, J. M. (2016). Cognitive deficits after aneurysmal and angiographically negative subarachnoid hemorrhage: Memory, attention, executive functioning, and emotion recognition. *Neuropsychology, 30*(8), 961–969. https://doi.org/10.1037/neu0000296

Canali, F., Brucki, S. M. D., Bertolucci, P. H. F., & Bueno, O. F. A. (2011). Reliability study of the Behavioral Assessment of the Dysexecutive Syndrome adapted for a Brazilian sample of older-adult controls and probable early Alzheimer's disease patients. *Revista Brasileira de Psiquiatria, 33*(4), 1–8. https://doi.org/10.1590/S1516-44462011005000015

Cerezo García, M., Martín Plasencia, P., & Aladro Benito, Y. (2015). Alteration profile of executive functions in multiple sclerosis. *Acta Neurologica Scandinavica, 131*(5), 313–320. https://doi.org/10.1111/ane.12345

Chan, R. K. C. (2001). Dysexecutive symptoms among a non-clinical sample: A study with the use of the dysexecutive questionnaire. *British Journal of Psychology, 92*, 551–565.

Chan, R. C., & Manly, T. (2002). The application of "dysexecutive syndrome" measures across cultures: Performance and checklist assessment in neurologically healthy and traumatically brain-injured Hong Kong Chinese volunteers. *Journal of the International Neuropsychological Society, 8*(6), 771–780.

Edge, D., Oyefeso, A., Evans, C., & Evans, A. (2015). The utility of the Montreal Cognitive Assessment as a mental capacity assessment tool for patients with a learning disability. *British Journal of Learning Disabilities*. https://doi.org/10.1111/bld.12157

Emmanouel, A., Mouza, E., Kessels, R. P. C., & Fasotti, L. (2014). Validity of the Dysexecutive Questionnaire (DEX). Ratings by patients with brain injury and their therapists. *Brain Injury, 28*(12), 1581–1589. https://doi.org/10.3109/02699052.2014.942371

Erez, A. B.-H., Rothschild, E., Katz, N., Tuchner, M., & Hartman-Maeir, A. (2009). Executive functioning, awareness, and participation in daily life after mild traumatic brain injury: A preliminary study. *American Journal of Occupational Therapy, 63*(5), 634–640. https://doi.org/10.5014/ajot.63.5.634

Evans, J. J., Chua, S. E., McKenna, P. J., & Wilson, B. A. (1997). Assessment of the dysexecutive syndrome in schizophrenia. *Psychological Medicine, 27*(3), 635–646. https://doi.org/10.1017/s0033291797004790

Fang, L., Huang, J., Zhang, Q., Chan, R. C. K., Wang, R., & Wan, W. (2016). Different aspects of dysexecutive syndrome in patients with moyamoya disease and its clinical subtypes. *Journal of Neurosurgery, 125*(2), 299–307. https://doi.org/10.3171/2015.7.JNS142666

Fuermaier, A. B. M., Tucha, L., Koerts, J., Aschenbrenner, S., Kaunzinger, I., Hauser, J., . . . Tucha, O. (2015). Cognitive impairment in adult ADHD: Perspective matters! *Neuropsychology, 29*(1), 45–58. https://doi.org/10.1037/neu0000108

Goodwin, R. A., Lincoln, N. B., & Bateman, A. (2016). Dysexecutive symptoms and carer strain following acquired brain injury: Changes measured before and after holistic neuropsychological rehabilitation. *NeuroRehabilitation, 39*(1), 53–64. https://doi.org/10.3233/NRE-161338

Hellebrekers, D., Winkens, I., Kruiper, S., & Van Heugten, C. (2017). Psychometric properties of the awareness questionnaire, patient competency rating scale and Dysexecutive Questionnaire in patients with acquired brain injury. *Brain Injury, 31*(11), 1469–1478. https://doi.org/10.1080/02699052.2017.1377350

Johnson, J. K., Pa, J., Boxer, A. L., Kramer, J. H., Freeman, K., & Yaffe, K. (2010). Baseline predictors of clinical progression among patients with dysexecutive mild cognitive impairment. *Dementia and Geriatric Cognitive Disorders, 30*(4), 344–351. https://doi.org/10.1159/000318836

Jourdan, C., Bosserelle, V., Azerad, S., Ghout, I., Bayen, E., Aegerter, P., . . . Azouvi, P. (2013). Predictive factors for 1-year outcome of a cohort of patients with severe traumatic brain injury (TBI): Results from the PariS-TBI study. *Brain Injury, 27*(9), 1000–1007. https://doi.org/10.3109/02699052.2013.794971

Kitahata, R., Nakajima, S., Uchida, H., Hayashida, T., Takahashi, M., Nio, S., . . . Mimura, M. (2017). Self-rated cognitive functions following chemotherapy in patients with breast cancer: a 6-month prospective study. *Neuropsychiatric Disease and Treatment, Volume 13*, 2489–2496. https://doi.org/10.2147/NDT.S141408

Koerts, J., van Beilen, M., Leenders, K. L., Brouwer, W. H., Tucha, L., & Tucha, O. (2012). Complaints about impairments in executive functions in Parkinson's disease: The association with neuropsychological assessment. *Parkinsonism & Related Disorders, 18*(2), 194–197. https://doi.org/10.1016/j.parkreldis.2011.10.002

Masson, J. D., Dagnan, D., & Evans, J. (2010). Adaptation and validation of the Tower of London test of planning and problem-solving in people with intellectual disabilities. *Journal of Intellectual Disability Research, 54*(5), 457–467. https://doi.org/10.1111/j.1365-2788.2010.01280.x

McGuire, B. E., Morrison, T. G., Barker, L. A., Morton, N., McBrinn, J., Caldwell, S., . . . Walsh, J. (2014). Impaired self-awareness after traumatic brain injury: Inter-rater reliability and factor structure of the Dysexecutive Questionnaire (DEX) in patients, significant others and clinicians. *Frontiers in Behavioral Neuroscience, 8*, 352.

Moreno, J. A., & McKerral, M. (2018). Relationships between risky sexual behaviour, dysexecutive problems, and mental health in the years following interdisciplinary TBI rehabilitation. *Neuropsychological Rehabilitation, 28*(1), 34–56. https://doi.org/10.1080/09602011.2015.1136222

Munshi, M. N., Hayes, M., Iwata, I., Lee, Y., & Weinger, K. (2012). Which aspects of executive dysfunction influence ability to manage diabetes in older adults? *Diabetic Medicine, 29*(9), 1171–1177. https://doi.org/10.1111/j.1464-5491.2012.03606.x

Norris, G., & Tate, R. L. (2000). The Behavioural Assessment of the Dysexecutive Syndrome (BADS): Ecological, concurrent and construct validity. *Neuropsychological Rehabilitation, 10*(1), 33–45. https://doi.org/10.1080/096020100389282

Oei, T. P. S., Shaw, S., & Healy, K. L. (2016). Executive function deficits in psychiatric outpatients in Australia. *International Journal of Mental Health and Addiction, 14*(3), 337–349. https://doi.org/10.1007/s11469-016-9634-x

Oka, M., Nakaaki, S., Negi, A., Miyata, J., Nakagawa, A., Hirono, N., & Mimura, M. (2016). Predicting the neural effect of switching from donepezil to galantamine based on single-photon emission computed tomography findings in patients with Alzheimer's disease. *Psychogeriatrics, 16*(2), 121–134. https://doi.org/10.1111/psyg.12132

Pa, J., Boxer, A., Chao, L. L., Gazzaley, A., Freeman, K., Kramer, J., . . . Johnson, J. K. (2009). Clinical-neuroimaging characteristics of dysexecutive mild cognitive impairment. *Annals of Neurology, 65*(4), 414–423. https://doi.org/10.1002/ana.21591

Pedrero-Pérez, E. J., Ruiz-Sánchez-de-León, J. M., & Winpenny-Tejedor, C. (2015). Dysexecutive Questionnaire (DEX): Unrestricted structural analysis in large clinical and non-clinical samples. *Neuropsychological Rehabilitation, 25*(6), 879–894. https://doi.org/10.1080/09602011.2014.993659

Rakers, S. E., Scheenen, M. E., Westerhof-Evers, H. J., de Koning, M. E., van der Horn, H. J., van der Naalt, J., & Spikman, J. M. (2017). Executive functioning in relation to coping in mild versus moderate-severe traumatic brain injury. *Neuropsychology*. https://doi.org/10.1037/neu0000399

Shan, S., Fang, L., Huang, J., Chan, R. C. K., Jia, G., & Wan, W. (2017). Evidence of dysexecutive syndrome in patients with acromegaly. *Pituitary, 20*(6), 661–667. https://doi.org/10.1007/s11102-017-0831-9

Shaw, S., Oei, T. P. S., & Sawang, S. (2015). Psychometric validation of the Dysexecutive Questionnaire (DEX). *Psychological Assessment, 27*(1), 138–147. https://doi.org/10.1037/a0038195

Simblett, S. K., Badham, R., Greening, K., Adlam, A., Ring, H., & Bateman, A. (2012). Validating independent ratings of executive functioning following acquired brain injury using Rasch analysis. *Neuropsychological Rehabilitation, 22*(6), 874–889. https://doi.org/10.1080/09602011.2012.703956

Simblett, S. K., & Bateman, A. (2011). Dimensions of the Dysexecutive Questionnaire (DEX) examined using Rasch analysis. *Neuropsychological Rehabilitation, 21*(1), 1–25. https://doi.org/10.1080/09602011.2010.531216

Stubberud, J., Langenbahn, D., Levine, B., Stanghelle, J., & Schanke, A.-K. (2015). Emotional health and coping in spina bifida after goal management training: A randomized controlled trial. *Rehabilitation Psychology, 60*(1), 1–16. https://doi.org/10.1037/rep0000018

Takeuchi, H., Taki, Y., Sassa, Y., Hashizume, H., Sekiguchi, A., Fukushima, A., & Kawashima, R. (2013). Brain structures associated with executive functions during everyday events in a non-clinical sample. *Brain Structure & Function, 218*(4), 1017–1032. https://doi.org/10.1007/s00429-012-0444-z

van der Hiele, K., Spliethoff-Kamminga, N. G. A., Ruimschotel, R. P., Middelkoop, H. A. M., & Visser, L. H. (2012). The relationship between self-reported executive performance and psychological characteristics in multiple sclerosis. *European Journal of Neurology, 19*(4), 562–569. https://doi.org/10.1111/j.1468-1331.2011.03538.x

Vlagsma, T. T., Koerts, J., Tucha, O., Dijkstra, H. T., Duits, A. A., van Laar, T., & Spikman, J. M. (2017). Objective versus subjective measures of executive functions: Predictors of participation and quality of life in Parkinson disease? *Archives of Physical Medicine and Rehabilitation, 98*(11), 2181–2187. https://doi.org/10.1016/j.apmr.2017.03.016

Wilson, B. A., Alderman, N., Burgess, P. W., Emslie, H., & Evans, J. J. (1996). *Behavioral Assessment of the Dysexecutive Syndrome.* Bury St. Edmunds, UK: Thames Valley Test Company.

Wilson, B. A., Evans, J. J., Emslie, H., Alderman, N., & Burgess, P. (1998). The development of an ecologically valid test for assessing patients with a dysexecutive syndrome. *Neuropsychological Rehabilitation, 8*, 213–228.

Wood, R., & Liossi, C. (2006). The ecological validity of executive tests in a severely brain injured sample. *Archives of Clinical Neuropsychology, 21*(5), 429–437. https://doi.org/10.1016/j.acn.2005.06.014

FIVE-POINT TEST

TEST NAME	**Five-Point Test**
DOMAIN	Executive functioning
AGE RANGE	In adults, to 80 years
ADMINISTRATION TIME	5 to 7 minutes
SCORING FORMAT	Hand scored
REFERENCE	Regard, M., Strauss, E., & Knapp, P. (1982). Children's production of verbal and nonverbal fluency tasks. *Perceptual and Motor Skills, 55*, 839–844.

DESCRIPTION

The Five-Point Test (Regard et al., 1982) requires production of novel designs under time constraints. There are a number of adaptations of the Five-Point Test, including the RFFT (Ruff, 1988; Ruff et al., 1987) and the D-KEFS Design Fluency Test (Delis et al., 2001) described elsewhere in this chapter. A computer variant of design fluency has also been developed (Woods et al., 2016).

Figural fluency tests have been developed as nonverbal analogs to word fluency tasks. One of the first figural fluency tasks, Jones-Gotman and Milner's Design Fluency Test (1977; see review elsewhere in this volume), presents with challenges that restrict its widespread use. These include inadequate normative data and difficulty interpreting the performance of patients with visuoconstructive and/or motor challenges. In addition, patients with cognitive impairment may have difficulty understanding the task demands.

In an attempt to overcome some of these limitations, Regard et al. (1982) provided the Five-Point Test as an alternative figural fluency task. This task consists of a sheet of paper with 40 dot matrices arranged in eight rows and five columns. The matrices are identical to the five-dot arrangement on dice (see Figure 9–8). Examinees are asked to produce as many different figures as possible by connecting the dots within each rectangle.

ADMINISTRATION

Regard et al. (1982) provided five minutes to perform the test. Using the Regard et al. stimuli, Lee, Loring, Newell, and McCloskey (1994) adapted the task for use within a three-minute time limit to make it more comparable to the time limits used for the COWA test. Given its brevity and high correlations with the five-minute version, the three-minute version may be preferable (Lee et al., 1997). Note also that the most recent normative data provided are based on shortened versions of the task (see the section "Normative Data").

To administer the Five-Point Test, the examiner places a protocol sheet in front of the examinee and indicates that the aim of the task is to produce as many different figures or designs as possible in three minutes by connecting the dots in each rectangle. The examinee is told that only straight lines are to be used, that all lines must connect dots, that no figures are to be repeated, and that only single lines are to be used. One caution is provided on the first (and only the first) violation of each of these rules. The rules are not repeated on any subsequent rule violation.

At the start of the test, two sample solutions are drawn by the examiner. The first sample design is drawn using all dots and the second is drawn using just two dots in order to demonstrate to the examinee that it is possible to make either simple or complex designs using some or all of the dots. The examinee is permitted to copy the sample designs drawn by the examiner. When an examinee exhausts a page, the examiner smoothly and quickly gives the examinee a second page while repositioning the first page so that the examinee can easily see it. Examinees may ask whether a seemingly trivial variation of a design constitutes a unique production. The examiner should reassure the examinee that the second design counts. Another frequent question is whether all dots need to be used. The examiner should repeat that the examinee need not use all dots.

SCORING

A number of scores can be calculated, including the total number of Unique Designs and the number of repeated, or Perseverative Designs (also termed Perseverations). Examinees who are more productive have a greater opportunity to make more Perseverations, so to adjust for this, the Percentage of Perseverations ((Perseverative Designs/Total Unique Designs) × 100) can be calculated (also called Flexibility in the scoring scheme provided later).

Goebel, Fischer, Ferstl, and Mehdorn (2009) have extended the scores available from the Five-Point Test to include other scores:

Name ______________ Date ______________ Tested by ______________

Total Designs ________ Total Unique Designs ________ % Correct ________ Repetitions ________

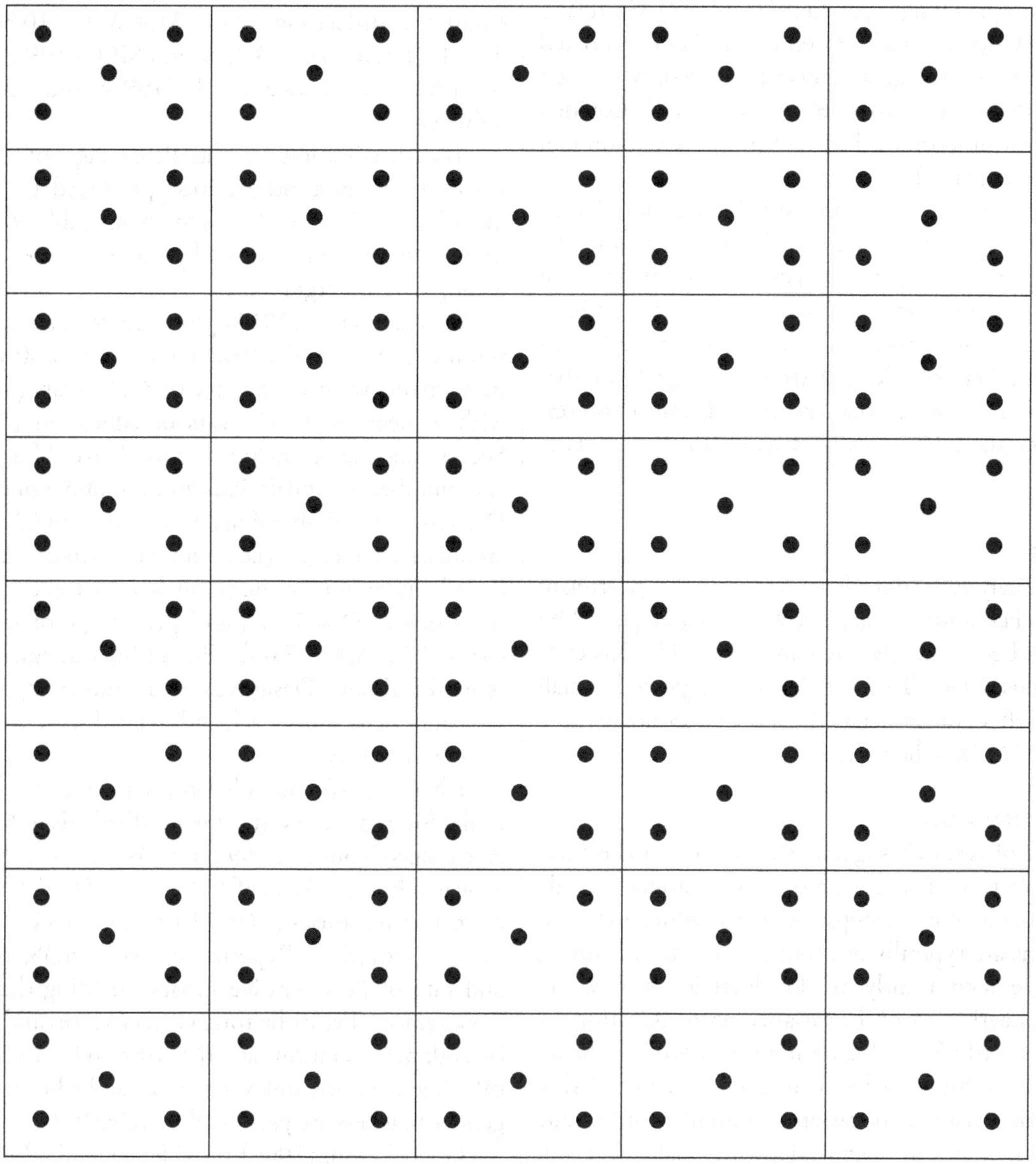

Figure 9–8 Five-Point Test stimuli.
SOURCE: Regard et al. (1982).

a. *Productivity*: the number of Unique Designs. Total produced designs minus Perseverative Designs and Rule Breaking Errors.

b. *Flexibility*: Percentage of Perseverations. The number of Perseverative Designs is divided by the number of Unique Designs and multiplied by 100.

c. *Strategy Score*: A strategic item is one whereby the examinee rotates and/or mirrors an item, so that it becomes different from the item directly before it. The number of strategic items is divided by the number of Unique Designs and multiplied by 100 to yield the Strategy Score. Note that if the rotated or mirrored item is an error, the strategy point is not given.

d. *Rule Breaking*: Non-Perseverative Errors (e.g., connecting dots from different squares, drawing curled lines or lines not connecting dots). Rule-breaking is rare. The authors present a cutoff value valid for all participants (see "Normative Data").

DEMOGRAPHIC EFFECTS

AGE

Overall, age appears to affect performance, but this has not been found in all studies or for each variable. For example, age accounted for nearly 19% of the variance in Productivity scores, nearly 11% of the variance in Strategy Score, and 9% of the variance in Perseverations (Goebel et al., 2009). Fernandez, Moroni, Carranza, Fabbro, and Lebowitz (2009) also reported that age was related to the number of Unique Designs produced ($r = -.53$). Cattelani, Dal Sasso, Corsini, and Posteraro (2011) reported relationships between age and Five-Point scores in their sample of Italian adults 16 to 60 years old and provided age- and education-corrected scores for variables examined (see "Normative Data").

Although Tucha, Aschenbrenner, Koerts, and Lange (2012) reported a large correlation between age and the number of Unique Designs, a relatively smaller, but still significant correlation was reported between age and Rule Violations (i.e., failure to connect dots), and no relationship was found between Perseverations and age. Note that some research has reported that age has little impact on test scores (Lee et al., 1997; Rinaldi et al., 2014; Santa Maria et al., 2001).

GENDER

Gender generally does not affect performance (Cattelani et al., 2011; Fernandez et al., 2009; Goebel et al., 2009; Khalil, 2010; Lee et al., 1997; Regard et al., 1982; Risser & Andrikopoulos, 1996). Tucha et al. (2012) reported a small to negligible effect of gender, with women producing more Perseverative Designs than men.

EDUCATION AND IQ

The majority of research suggests that scores on the Five-Point Test are related to education (e.g., Cattelani et al., 2011), although relationships between education and Perseverations are typically not found. Education is found to contribute significantly to Productivity scores, accounting for nearly 27% of the variance, with education accounting for nearly 20% of the variance in Strategy Score (Goebel et al., 2009). Tucha et al. (2012) reported that the correlation between education and number of Unique Designs was medium in magnitude, with smaller but still significant correlations between education and the number of Rule Violations. No relationship was found between education and Perseverations. Ferandez et al. (2009) similarly reported that education correlated with number of Unique Designs ($r = .55$), but not with Perseverative Errors. Note that some research has reported limited influence of education on performance (Glosser & Goodglass, 1990; Lee et al., 1997; Rinaldi et al., 2014; Santa Maria et al., 2001). IQ appears correlated with the number of Unique Designs produced ($r = .64$; Lee et al., 1997). Goebel et al. (2009) similarly reported significant correlations between the Strategy Score and IQ ($r = .47$).

ETHNICITY, NATIONALITY, AND LINGUISTIC EFFECTS

No information is available, although normative data have been provided from a number of countries.

NORMATIVE DATA

Normative data based on a sample of 62 adults with psychiatric disorders (age, $M = 35.4$, $SD = 10.3$; education, $M = 13.4$ years, $SD = 3.4$; mean FSIQ = 109.1, $SD = 11.9$) are provided by Lee et al. (1997) and are shown in Table 9–62.

The distribution of the Percentage of Perseverative Errors (with percentile ranks) produced by participants described in Lee et al. is shown in Table 9–63. Similar findings have been reported by Santa Maria et al. (2001) in a sample of undergraduates.

Cattelani et al. (2011) provided normative data (three-minute limit) for 332 Italian adults 16 to 60 years of age; participants were a mean age of 37.24 years ($SD = 12.72$), with a mean of 13.11 years of education ($SD = 3.41$). Scores calculated included cumulative Unique Designs (i.e., number of total designs minus number of Perseverative Designs and Rule-Breaking errors; $M = 34.03$, $SD = 8.72$), cumulative strategies (i.e., number of Unique Designs produced under one strategy, such as a rotational strategy; $M = 6.98$, $SD = 7.21$), and percentage of failed designs ($M = 7.59$, $SD = 7.06$). The authors designated a cutoff score for Unique Designs as 23.83, indicating unusual performance below this level, and a cutoff score for cumulative strategies of 1.89.

Khalil (2010) provided normative data (three-minute limit) for 215 Arabic-speaking individuals in Saudi Arabia. Age ranged from 17 to 59 years ($M = 27.4$, $SD = 6.2$), with a mean education level of 11.9 years ($SD = 5.4$). In addition to correct responses ($M = 32.14$, $SD = 6.84$), Perseverative Errors (scored as Repetitions; $M = 4.38$, $SD = 2.41$) and rate of Perseverative Errors (dividing the number of Perseverative Errors by total correct scores and multiplying by 100; perseveration rate $M = 10.4$, $SD = 13.58$) were also calculated. Means and *SD*s for age and education as well as gender brackets are presented in Table 9–64.

Goebel et al. (2009) provide age and education stratified normative data for 280 German 18- to 80-year-olds (three-minute time limit). Exclusion criteria were based on self-report, with participants with neurologic or psychiatric conditions and people 60 years of age or older scoring below an MMSE cutoff excluded. The normative sample consisted of 280 adults, split between males and females (approximately 53% female), with a mean age of 44.85 ($SD = 17.90$). Participants were classified into lower (1 to 13 years) or higher (≥13 years) education groups.

TABLE 9–62 Five-Point Test (Three-Minute Time Limit): Mean Unique Designs and Perseverations in Adults with Psychiatric Disorders

N	UNIQUE DESIGNS	PERSEVERATIONS	% PERSEVERATIONS
62	31.95 (8.4)	1.39 (1.8)	4.82 (6.6)

SOURCE: Adapted from Lee et al. (1997).

TABLE 9–63 Five-Point Test (Three-Minute Time Limit): Percentile Ranks Associated with the Percentage of Perseverative Errors in a Psychiatric Sample

PERCENT OF PERSEVERATIONS	CUMULATIVE PERCENTILE
0	100
1	56
2	56
3	48
4	39
5	32
6	31
7	27
8	27
9	21
10	21
11	16
12	15
13	11
14	6
15 (cutoff score)	6
16	5
17	0

NOTE: $N = 62$.

SOURCE: Adapted from Lee et al. (1997).

Data on the portion of participants working inside/outside the home and retired were also provided. Cell sizes varied from $n = 21$ to $n = 86$ (60- to 80-year-olds, 13 or more years of education; and 18- to 39-year-olds, 13 or more years of education, respectively). Simultaneous age and education stratified norms are as depicted in Tables 9–65 to 9–67. Given the rarity of rule-breaking errors in their sample (approximately 4% of participants) Goebel et al. (2009) recommended use of cutoff scores to evaluate level of performance (two errors = <1st percentile, "impaired"; one error = 4th percentile, "borderline"; zero errors = 5th to 100th percentile, "unimpaired").

Tucha et al. (2012) provided normative data for 608 healthy participants in Germany. Participants were provided

TABLE 9–64 Normative Data for the Five-Point Test by Age, Education, and Gender in a Saudi-Arabian Sample

CATEGORY	N	DESIGN FLUENCY *M*	*SD*
Age (years)			
17–29	98	30.81	7.14
30–39	70	32.91	4.00
40–59	47	32.45	4.65
Education (years)			
0–9	80	31.01	8.37
10–12	95	32.11	5.22
13+	40	33.40	5.98
Gender			
Male	125	32.19	6.00
Female	90	32.08	7.52
Total	215	32.14	6.84

SOURCE: From Khalil (2010).

TABLE 9–65 Normative Data for the Five-Point Test (Number of Unique Designs) by Age and Education in a German Sample

	PRODUCTIVITY (NUMBER OF UNIQUE DESIGNS)					
	AGE 19 TO 39		AGE 40 TO 59		AGE 60 TO 80	
PERCENTILE	EDUC 1–13	EDUC 13+	EDUC 1–13	EDUC 13+	EDUC 1–13	EDUC 13+
2	11	23	11	16	10	20
5	16	25	14	18	12	22
10	18	29	22	24	15	
16	20	32	24	26	16	23
20	22	33	25	27	17	24
25	23	34	26	29	19	26
30	24	35	27	31	20	27
40	25	37	28	35	23	28
50	28	41	31	36	24	29
60	29	44	32	37	26	31
70	31	47	33	40	30	32
75	33	49	35	42	31	35
80	35	51	37	45	32	42
84	37	52	38	47	33	46
90	39	57	40	49	34	48
95	46	58	42	55	37	51
98	47	60	44	56	41	53

NOTE: Educ, years of education.

SOURCE: Goebel et al. (2009).

with a 1- and 2-minute time limit to complete the test. Exclusion criteria included self-reported history of neurologic or psychiatric condition and medications affecting central nervous system function, as well as MMSE performance. Of the 608 participants (55% female), the mean age was 41.8 years ($SD = 15.4$), with an educational level mean

TABLE 9–66 Normative Data for the Five-Point Test (Percent of Perseverations) by Age and Education in a German Sample

	FLEXIBILITY (PERCENTAGE OF PERSEVERATIONS)					
	AGE 19 TO 39		AGE 40 TO 59		AGE 60 TO 80	
PERCENTILE	EDUC 1–13 (%)	EDUC 13+ (%)	EDUC 1–13 (%)	EDUC 13+ (%)	EDUC 1–13 (%)	EDUC 13+ (%)
2	21.5	19.9	28.6	35.3	44.5	22.2
5	20.2	16.7	23.0	28.9	41.9	17.8
10	18.8	11.9	17.9	17.6	32.0	14.2
16	13.2	7.7	7.7	17.1	22.9	13.4
20	12.1	7.0	11.2	14.8	22.0	12.4
25	11.4	6.4	9.0	13.6	19.9	11.9
30	7.0	6.0	8.4	11.5	16.7	10.9
40	5.2	4.0	6.3	8.1	12.3	8.4
50	4.0	2.7	4.1	7.4	9.3	6.7
60	0.0	2.0	3.3	5.2	8.0	5.6
70		0.0	2.9	4.2	5.2	4.2
75			2.5	3.1	4.1	3.8
80			0.0	2.8	2.8	3.1
84				2.5	0.0	1.9
90				0.0	0.0	0.0

NOTE: Educ, years of education.

SOURCE: From Goebel et al. (2009).

TABLE 9–67 Normative Data for the Five-Point Test (Strategy Score) by Age and Education in a German Sample

	STRATEGY SCORE (PERCENTAGE OF ROTATED AND/OR MIRRORED ITEMS)					
	AGE 19 TO 39		AGE 40 TO 59		AGE 60 TO 80	
PERCENTILES	EDUC 1–13 (%)	EDUC 13+ (%)	EDUC 1–13 (%)	EDUC 13+ (%)	EDUC 1–13 (%)	EDUC 13+ (%)
2		6.0		12.0		
5	0	12.0	0	14.5	0	0
10	4.5	24.0	10.1	18.5	2.7	11.6
16	6.5	31.5	14.9	26.0	5.1	14.5
20	12.0	35.5	17.3	29.4	5.8	23.5
25	16.7	39.4	25.6	32.4	7.0	29.5
30	20.5	40.0	27.9	34.3	8.3	34.9
40	23.1	43.0	32.1	37.0	14.3	39.2
50	30.4	48.1	35.4	47.5	17.8	40.3
60	35.9	53.2	38.5	49.0	20.2	41.9
70	39.2	59.2	46.2	55.1	28.0	46.5
75	42.4	61.3	48.1	56.8	30.7	49.3
80	45.1	63.3	51.5	59.3	36.0	54.3
84	45.8	65.8	55.2	61.6	37.1	55.4
90	48.1	67.6	60.9	67.1	47.7	59.4
95	54.1	70.6	62.3	68.9	53.1	64.7
98	59.5	71.3	63.5	70.9	61.5	65.4

NOTE: Educ, years of education.
SOURCE: Goebel et al. (2009).

of 11.8 years (*SD* = 3.2). Nearly 88% of participants were right-handed. Norm groupings were based on six age categories. Tucha et al. also provide a correction for education (<10 years, 10 to 12 years, >12 years). Normative data are provided in Tables 9–68 to 9–69.

Fernandez et al. (2009) provided data from 212 healthy participants (65% female; age *M* = 47.79, *SD* = 21.76; education *M* = 13.10, *SD* = 4.55; 86% right-handed) in Argentina. Exclusion criteria was a history of neurologic or psychiatric conditions, substance abuse, diabetes, thyroid disease, Chagas disease (an infectious disease resulting in heart dysfunction), heart disease, unmanaged blood pressure, and other physical health conditions. Participants produced a mean number of Unique Designs of 26.63 (*SD* = 9.71) and a mean Percentage of Perseverative Errors of 9 (*SD* = 9.35).

Of note, Woods et al. (2016) compared normative data from various sources for the Five-Point Test, noting relatively large discrepancies across samples in terms of Unique Designs completed per minute and percent of repetitions (Table 9–70). The reasons for the discrepancy are unclear and may reflect cultural differences or variability in test instruction, administration, and scoring procedures followed.

EVIDENCE FOR RELIABILITY

EVIDENCE FOR INTERNAL RELIABILITY

Fernandez et al. (2009) reported split-half reliability in a group of healthy individuals to be strong for Unique Designs (.80) and limited for Perseverations (.48).

EVIDENCE FOR TEST-RETEST RELIABILITY, MEASURING CHANGE, AND PRACTICE EFFECTS

Most research suggests that test-retest reliability is generally adequate to high for Unique Designs and variable for Perseverations. There are significant practice effects, particularly for the number of Unique Designs across sessions.

Fernandez et al. (2009) provide data on a subset of 142 individuals who completed the Five-Point Test with a 38-day test-retest interval, with coefficients of .78 for Unique Designs and .51 for Perseverative Errors. Goebel et al. (2009) reported reliability data from 34 participants who were retested after a four-week interval. Participants in the reliability study ranged from 19 to 67 years (*M* = 29.4, *SD* = 11.1), with the majority (84%) attaining more than 13 years of education. ICCs were calculated as .84 (Unique Designs), .35 (percentage Perseverations), and .72 (% percentage Strategy). Similar values were obtained for Unique Designs in healthy older adults, with ICCs of .71 or greater (Donath et al., 2017). Goebel, Atanassov, Köhnken, Mehdorn, and Leplow (2013) reported retest reliability for the test in a group of healthy participants aged 18 to 61 tested within a month (*M* = 30.33 days) as ICCs of .85 (Productivity), .95 (Perseverations), .45 (Repetitions), and .82 (Strategy Score). Test-retest reliability as reported by Tucha et al. (2012) was r = .65 for Unique Designs in one minute, and r = .77 for Unique Designs in two minutes.

In terms of practice effects, Goebel et al. (2009) reported that although Unique Designs improved from Time 1 to Time 2 (mean of 5 points), as did percent Perseverations (decrease of approximately 2%), the Strategy Score did not differ. However, other research has suggested improved strategy use over short retest intervals (Peter et al., 2016). Tucha et al. (2012) reported significant improvements across testing sessions (medium effect size; three-week test-retest interval) approximating an improvement of four designs, indicating substantial practice effects. Perseverative Errors and Rule Violations, however, did not change across sessions. Fernandez et al. (2009) report that the standard error of prediction was 6.25 for Unique Designs, and 5.08 for Percentage of Perseverative Errors; 90% CIs were +/− 10 for Unique Designs and +/−8 for Perseverative Errors. Thus, changes exceeding these values are needed to demonstrate actual change.

EVIDENCE FOR RELIABILITY OF ALTERNATE FORMS

No information is available.

EVIDENCE FOR INTERRATER RELIABILITY

Interrater reliability is strong, with correlation coefficients and ICCs exceeding .97 for variables examined (Goebel et al., 2009, 2013; Tucha et al., 2012).

TABLE 9–68 Normative Data for the Five-Point Test by Age in a German Sample (One- and Two-Minute Time Limit)

RAW SCORE	ONE-MINUTE TIME LIMIT 20–29 YEARS	30–39 YEARS	40–49 YEARS	50–59 YEARS	60–69 YEARS	OVER 69 YEARS	TWO-MINUTE TIME LIMIT 20–29 YEARS	30–39 YEARS	40–49 YEARS	50–59 YEARS	60–69 YEARS	OVER 69 YEARS	RAW SCORE
3				1		6						3	3
4				3	2	19							4
5	1			5	7	42						10	5
6	2			6	12	52				1		13	6
7			2	7		71						16	7
8	3	1	4	10		84				3		26	8
9	3		5	12	20	90				5	5	39	9
10	4	3	8	16	35	94				6	12	48	10
11	6	4	9	23	42			1	1	7	15	55	11
12	9	6	14	27	57	97					17	61	12
13		8	17	35	65	99			2	8		71	13
14	10	10	23	41					3		20	81	14
15	13	14	36	51	70		1			12	25	84	15
16	16	19	45	62	78		2		4	13	35	90	16
17	19	24	52	69	85					15	40	97	17
18	24	32	61	71	90				7	21	45		18
19	33	41	70	80	95		5		11	22	50		19
20	39	53	78	83			6	2	14	27	55		20
21	48	61	82	88			7	6	16	31	57		21
22	56	70	85	89			8	8	18	33	60		22
23	64	72	90	92				13	23	41	62	99	23
24	74	78	92	94			9	15	32	50	68		24
25	81	85	96	98			11	16	38	56	72		25
26	84	89	98	99	98		13	23	46	60	82		26
27	88	93	99		99		15	30	49	60			27
28	90	94					18	32	51	62	85		28
29	92						20	38	57	68	87		29
30	94	96					25	43	62	74	90		30
31	95	98					26	48	70	76			31
32	98	99					30	54	75	81			32
33	99						40	61	78	86	95		33
34							46	63	81	88			34
35							58	70	87	91			35
36							65	76	88	95	98		36
37							70	81		96			37
38							72	83	92	97			38
39							79	86	93	98			39
40								89	95				40
41							82		96				41
42							83	92	98				42
43							85	94	99	99			43
44							89	96					44
45							90						45
46							95	98					46
47							97						47
48													48
49													49
50								99					50
51							98						51
52							99						52

SOURCE: Tucha et al. (2012).

TABLE 9–69 Correction of Raw Scores for Education Level for the Five-Point Test in a German Sample (One- and Two-Minute Time Limit)

YEARS OF EDUCATION	ONE-MINUTE TIME LIMIT 20–29 YEARS	30–39 YEARS	40–49 YEARS	50–59 YEARS	60–69 YEARS	OVER 69 YEARS	TWO-MINUTE TIME LIMIT 20–29 YEARS	30–39 YEARS	40–49 YEARS	50–59 YEARS	60–69 YEARS	OVER 69 YEARS	YEARS OF EDUCATION
Under 10	+5	+3	+2	+2	+1	0	+4	+5	+4	+3	+2	0	Under 10
10–12	+2	+1	0	0	−2	0	+3	+2	0	0	−3	0	10–12
Over 12	−1	−2	−2	−2	−2	−1	−1	−2	−3	−3	−3	−3	Over 12

SOURCE: Tucha et al. (2012).

TABLE 9-70 Comparison of Five-Point Test Normative Data

	N	AGE	EDUCATION	UNIQUE PATTERNS	SD	COEFFICIENT OF VARIATION	TIME LIMIT	UNIQUE PATTERNS/ MIN	REPEATED PATTERNS	% REPEATED PATTERNS
Santa Maria et al. (2001)	80	23.96	15.50	74.22			10	7.42	11.73	13.65%
Femandez et al. (2009)	212	47.80	13.10	26.63	9.71	36.46%	3	8.88	2.40	9.00%
Goebel et al. (2009)	280	44.90	13.30	32.81			3	10.94		8.39%
Cattelani el al. (2011)	332	37.20	13.11	34.03	8.72	25.62%	3	11.34	2.58	7.59%
Tucha el al. (2012)	608	41.80	11.80	28.91	9.34	32.32%	2	14.45	1.63	5.34%
Khali (2010)	215	27.40	11.90	32.14	6.84	21.28%	3	10.71	4.38	11.99%

NOTE: *SD*, standard deviation.
SOURCE: Woods et al. (2016).

EVIDENCE FOR VALIDITY

FACTOR-ANALYTIC STUDIES AND RELATIONSHIPS WITH OTHER TESTS

Factor-analytic studies suggest that speed and executive/inhibition are involved in task demands associated with the Five-Point Test. Factor analysis of the Five-Point Test and other tests was completed by Goebel et al. (2009), with four factors accounting for approximately 57% of the variance in scores. The first factor was reflective of productivity and speed (TMT-B, TMT-A, Productivity), the second factor of verbal working memory (Digit Span Forward and Backward), the third factor of executive function (Strategy, Perseverations), and the fourth factor of verbal abilities (verbal IQ, verbal fluency). Factor-analytic findings in patients with seizure disorders suggests that the number correct loaded together with other tasks involving attention and speed (e.g., mazes time, letter cancellation, word fluency) while errors loaded on a response inhibition factor (e.g., mazes errors, Stroop Interference; Helmstaedter et al., 1996). The Paced Auditory Serial Addition Test (PASAT) loaded on the same factor as the Five-Point Test in patients with MS (Hansen et al., 2017); substitution of the Five-Point Test in place of the PASAT did not significantly alter the proportion of patients classified as impaired.

In terms of relationships with other fluency tests, Goebel et al. (2013) reported that Productivity was highly correlated between different figural fluency tasks (Five-Point, Design Fluency, RFFT; r = .74 to .86). The test is moderately correlated with measures of verbal fluency (Regard et al., 1982; Risser & Andrikopoulos, 1996). In their sample of Arabic-speaking individuals in Saudi Arabia, Khalil (2010) reported moderate correlations between verbal fluency tasks and the Five-Point Test (r = .29 to .31), with Tucha et al. (2012) reporting large correlations between Unique Designs and verbal fluency.

Overall, design fluency involves a number of abilities, including motor speed, visuoperceptual and visuospatial function, and executive function. For example, Goebel et al. (2013) reported moderate to large correlations with motor speed (TMT-A), construction (Rey-Osterreith Complex Figure Copy), and visuoperceptual skills (rs = .36 to .74). Goebel et al. (2009) reported significant correlations between the Strategy Score and the TMT-B (r = –.41) and inverse scores with Perseverations and Digit Span Backward (r = –.52). Similarly, Tucha et al. (2012) reported large correlations between Unique Designs and both TMT-A and TMT-B.

The number of Unique Designs is also correlated with visual short-term memory and working memory (Visual Memory Span), problem-solving (TOL), and inhibition (Stroop). The Frontal Assessment Battery score is significantly correlated with the number of Unique Designs produced by patients with schizophrenia (Rinaldi et al., 2014). The Five-Point Test and its variant (an untimed version by Glosser & Goodglass, 1990) are also moderately to highly (r = .40 to .70) correlated with visual-spatial and visual-constructive measures (e.g., Wechsler Picture Completion, Block Design) and measures of executive control (e.g., WCST) but not with linguistic function (Glosser & Goodglass, 1990). In contrast, a study of neurosurgical patients with right-side lesions reported minimal correlations between Unique Designs and the TMT and Digit Symbol, among other measures (Hansen et al., 2017).

CLINICAL STUDIES

Lesion Studies and Neurologic Populations. There is mixed evidence regarding whether patients with frontal lobe involvement perform worse on the Five-Point Test compared to those with nonfrontal neurologic involvement, as well as whether left- versus right-hemispheric involvement is meaningfully associated with performance (e.g., Glosser & Goodglass, 1990; Helmstaedter et al., 1996; Lee et al., 1997; Tucha et al., 1999). In one study (Marin et al., 2017), just over 20% of neurosurgical patients with right-sided lesions were impaired on the Five-Point Test, which was apparently related to a lack of a strategic approach employed (i.e., absence of a rotational strategy). Analysis of lesion location implicated a broad right frontoparietal network in performance.

PD. Tucha et al. (2012) reported that patients with PD produce fewer Unique Designs than healthy participants (large effect size), without differences in Perseverations or Rule Violations. In a study involving comparison of figural fluency tasks, individuals with PD demonstrated impaired performance on the Five-Point Test, Design Fluency Test, and the RFFT (Goebel et al., 2013). However, the Five-Point Test and the RFFT were better able to differentiate PD from healthy controls than Design Fluency.

Qualitative variables from the Five-Point Test (e.g., perseverative, repetitive, or strategic behavior) were identified as particularly beneficial in the assessment of PD patients, as deficits remain following control for visuomotor speed (TMT-A) and visuoconstruction (RCFT Copy; Goebel et al., 2013). Patients with PD are impaired relative to healthy controls on the test, with effect sizes ranging from .63 (Repetitions) to 1.36 (Productivity). However, note that the overall percentage of patients who are classified as impaired can be quite low, ranging from 18% to 50%, depending on the variable (Goebel et al., 2013).

Other Populations. Performance is compromised relative to controls in persons with MCI (Ávila-Villanueva et al., 2016), both in terms of accuracy and strategy use (Peter et al., 2016). Performance improves following cognitive rehabilitation in MCI (Barekatain et al., 2016). Margraf, Bachmann, Schwandner, Gottschalk, and Seidel (2009) reported that the Five-Point Test evidenced poor to fair accuracy in differentiating between those with subcortical ischemic vascular disease and demographically matched healthy controls (75% sensitivity, 50% specificity). Individuals who have sustained a stroke performed worse on the Five-Point Test, which along with the Tinker Toy test, differentiates between employed and unemployed groups (Ownsworth & Shum, 2008). Persons with anorexia show impairment relative to controls (Heled et al., 2016).

Patients with schizophrenia produce fewer designs than healthy controls, and negative symptoms are correlated with Perseverations (Rinaldi et al., 2014). Psychiatric patients produce significantly more Unique Designs and a lower Percentage of Perseverative Errors than patients with neurological disorders (Lee et al., 1997). Reduced performance has been documented in patients with OCD, a condition that is thought to involve frontostriatal dysfunction (Schmidtke et al., 1998).

NEUROANATOMICAL CORRELATES AND IMAGING STUDIES

Superior frontal gyrus volume predicts Five-Point Test performance and strategy use in healthy controls and persons with MCI (Peter et al., 2016). A frontoparietal network has been implicated in lesion studies (see Marin et al., 2017).

PERFORMANCE VALIDITY

No information is available.

COMMENT

The Five-Point Test is a brief task that requires little equipment, requiring the examinee to produce as many different figures as possible by connecting the dots within each provided rectangle, within specific task constraints. The most common scores calculated are the number of Unique Designs produced as well as Perseverations. Goebel et al. (2009) have also provided additional scores with apparent clinical utility (see "Scoring").

In terms of demographic effects, overall, age and education are influential, particularly for the Unique Designs score. Most research suggests that gender has negligible effects on performance. In recent years a number of normative datasets have been published, most of which use the three-minute time limit (though note Tucha et al., 2012, with a one- and two-minute limit). The norms provided by Goebel et al. (2009) and Tucha et al. (2012) are specifically recommended as these are larger in size and enable adjustment for both age and education for a number of variables. Normative data vary across dataset examined. Note that few normative data are available for individuals older than 60, so caution is recommended in use of this test with older adults.

Test-retest reliability and internal reliability are high for Unique Designs and low for Perseverations, suggesting caution in interpreting Perseverations, particularly across repeat assessments. There are significant practice effects, which should be considered when interpreting repeat assessments. Interrater reliability is uniformly high across variables. The Five-Point Test is correlated moderately with other measures, including fluency tests, motor speed, visuoperceptual and constructional tasks, inhibition/executive tasks, and speeded tests, suggesting that performance involves a number of abilities.

There is limited information overall in clinical samples and limited information on the effects of ethnicity, other sociodemographic variables, and neuroanatomical correlates and performance validity. Overall, however, this task has a number of compelling features, especially when compared to other stand-alone fluency tasks, including ease of instruction, minimal administration time, high reliability of specific scores, and availability of age- and education-adjusted normative data.

REFERENCES

Ávila-Villanueva, M., Rebollo-Vázquez, A., Ruiz-Sánchez de León, J. M., Valentí, M., Medina, M., & Fernández-Blázquez, M. A. (2016). Clinical relevance of specific cognitive complaints in determining mild cognitive impairment from cognitively normal states in a study of healthy elderly controls. *Frontiers in Aging Neuroscience, 8*. https://doi.org/10.3389/fnagi.2016.00233

Barekatain, M., Alavirad, M., Tavakoli, M., Emsaki, G., & Maracy, M. (2016). Cognitive rehabilitation in patients with nonamnestic mild cognitive impairment. *Journal of Research in Medical Sciences, 21*(1), 101. https://doi.org/10.4103/1735-1995.193173

Cattelani, R., Dal Sasso, F., Corsini, D., & Posteraro, L. (2011). The Modified Five-Point Test: Normative data for a sample of Italian healthy adults aged 16–60. *Neurological Sciences, 32*(4), 595–601. http://doi.org/10.1007/s10072-011-0489-4

Delis, D. C., Kaplan, E., & Kramer, J. H. (2001). *Delis-Kaplan Executive Function System.* San Antonio, TX: The Psychological Corporation.

Donath, L., Ludyga, S., Hammes, D., Rossmeissl, A., Andergassen, N., Zahner, L., & Faude, O. (2017). Absolute and relative reliability of acute effects of aerobic exercise on executive function in seniors. *BMC Geriatrics, 17*(1). https://doi.org/10.1186/s12877-017-0634-x

Fernandez, A. L., Moroni, M. A., Carranza, J. M., Fabbro, N., & Lebowitz, B. K. (2009). Reliability of the Five-Point Test. *The Clinical Neuropsychologist, 23*(3), 501–509. http://doi.org/10.1080/13854040802279675

Glosser, G., & Goodglass, H. (1990). Disorders in executive control functions among aphasic and other brain-damaged patients. *Journal of Clinical and Experimental Neuropsychology, 12,* 485–501.

Goebel, S., Atanassov, L., Köhnken, G., Mehdorn, H. M., & Leplow, B. (2013). Understanding quantitative and qualitative figural fluency in patients with Parkinson's disease. *Neurological Sciences, 34*(8), 1383–1390. http://doi.org/10.1007/s10072-012-1245-0

Goebel, S., Fischer, R., Ferstl, R., & Mehdorn, H. M. (2009). Normative data and psychometric properties for qualitative and quantitative scoring criteria of the Five-point Test. *The Clinical Neuropsychologist, 23*(4), 675–690. http://doi.org/10.1080/13854040802389185

Hansen, S., Muenssinger, J., Kronhofmann, S., Lautenbacher, S., Oschmann, P., & Keune, P. M. (2017). Cognitive screening in multiple sclerosis: The Five-Point Test as a substitute for the PASAT in measuring executive function. *The Clinical Neuropsychologist, 31*(1), 179–192. https://doi.org/10.1080/13854046.2016.1241894

Heled, E., Hoofien, D., Bachar, E., & Ebstein, R. P. (2016). Verbal versus figural fluency tests in currently ill and weight restored anorexia nervosa patients: Fluency tests in anorexia nervosa. *European Eating Disorders Review, 24*(3), 206–213. https://doi.org/10.1002/erv.2387

Helmstaedter, C., Kemper, B., & Elger, C. E. (1996) Neuropsychological aspects of frontal lobe epilepsy. *Neuropsychologia, 34,* 399–406.

Jones-Gotman, M., & Milner, B. (1977). Design fluency: The invention of nonsense drawings after focal cortical lesions. *Neuropsychologia, 15,* 653–674.

Khalil, M. S. (2010). Preliminary Arabic normative data of neuropsychological tests: The verbal and design fluency. *Journal of Clinical and Experimental Neuropsychology, 32*(9), 1028–1035. http://doi.org/10.1080/13803391003672305

Lee, G. P., Loring, D. W., Newell, J., & McCloskey, L. (1994). Figural fluency on the Five-Point Test: Preliminary normative and validity data. *International Neuropsychological Society Program and Abstracts, 1,* 51.

Lee, G. P., Strauss, E., Loring, D. W., McCloskey, L., & Haworth, J. M. (1997). Sensitivity of figural fluency on the Five-Point Test to focal neurological disease. *The Clinical Neuropsychologist, 11,* 59–68.

Margraf, N., Bachmann, T., Schwandner, W., Gottschalk, S., & Seidel, G. (2009). Bedside screening for executive dysfunction in patients with subcortical ischemic vascular disease. *International Journal of Geriatric Psychiatry, 24*(9), 1002–1009. http://doi.org/10.1002/gps.2212

Marin, D., Madotto, E., Fabbro, F., Skrap, M., & Tomasino, B. (2017). Design fluency and neuroanatomical correlates in 54 neurosurgical patients with lesions to the right hemisphere. *Journal of Neuro-Oncology, 135*(1), 141–150. https://doi.org/10.1007/s11060-017-2560-3

Ownsworth, T., & Shum, D. (2008). Relationship between executive functions and productivity outcomes following stroke. *Disability and Rehabilitation, 30*(7), 531–540. http://doi.org/10.1080/09638280701355694

Peter, J., Kaiser, J., Landerer, V., Köstering, L., Kaller, C. P., Heimbach, B., . . . Klöppel, S. (2016). Category and design fluency in mild cognitive impairment: Performance, strategy use, and neural correlates. *Neuropsychologia, 93,* 21–29. https://doi.org/10.1016/j.neuropsychologia.2016.09.024

Regard, M., Strauss, E., & Knapp, P. (1982). Children's production of verbal and nonverbal fluency tasks. *Perceptual and Motor Skills, 55,* 839–844.

Rinaldi, R., Trappeniers, J., & Lefebvre, L. (2014). Shall we use nonverbal fluency in schizophrenia? A pilot study. *Psychiatry Research, 216*(3), 314–319. http://doi.org/10.1016/j.psychres.2014.01.029

Risser, A. H., & Andrikopoulos, J. (1996). *Regard's Five-Point Test: Adolescent cohort stability.* Paper presented to the International Neuropsychological Society, Chicago.

Ruff, R. (1988). *Ruff Figural Fluency Test.* San Diego, CA: Neuropsychological Resources.

Ruff, R. M., Light, R., & Evans, R. (1987). The Ruff Figural Fluency Test: A normative study with adults. *Developmental Neuropsychology, 3,* 37–51.

Santa Maria, M. P., Martin, J. A., Morrow, C. M., & Gouvier, W. D. (2001). On the duration of spatial fluency measures. *International Journal of Neuroscience, 7,* 586–596.

Schmidtke, K., Schorb, A., Winkelmann, G., & Hohagen, F. (1998). Cognitive frontal lobe dysfunction in obsessive-compulsive disorder. *Society of Biological Psychiatry, 43,* 666–673.

Tucha, L., Aschenbrenner, S., Koerts, J., & Lange, K. W. (2012). The Five-Point Test: Reliability, validity and normative data for children and adults. *PloS One, 7*(9), e46080. http://doi.org/10.1371/journal.pone.0046080

Tucha, O., Smely, C., & Lange, K. W. (1999). Verbal and figural fluency in patients with mass lesions of the left or right frontal lobes. *Journal of Clinical and Experimental Neuropsychology, 21,* 229–236.

Woods, D. L., Wyma, J. M., Herron, T. J., & Yund, E. W. (2016). A computerized test of design fluency. *PloS One, 11*(5), e0153952.

FRONTAL SYSTEMS BEHAVIOR SCALE (FRSBE)

TEST NAME	**Frontal Systems Behavior Scale (FrSBe)**
DOMAIN	Executive Functioning
AGE RANGE	18 to 95 years
ADMINISTRATION TIME	10 minutes
SCORING FORMAT	Online scoring available, but can be hand scored
REFERENCE	Grace, J., & Malloy, P. (2001). *Frontal Systems Behavior Scale.* Lutz, FL: PAR. www.parinc.com

DESCRIPTION

The Frontal Systems Behavior Scale (FrSBe) is a 46-item rating scale designed to measure behaviors associated with damage to the frontal lobes and to the frontal systems of the brain (Grace & Malloy, 2001; Table 9–71). It measures both pre- and post-injury behaviors and is specifically designed to detect three main frontal behavioral syndromes: apathy, disinhibition, and executive dysfunction. The FrSBe was formerly known as the Frontal Lobe Personality Scale (FloPS; Grace et al., 1999). The FrSBe provides both self-rated and informant questionnaires—the Self-Rating Form and Family Rating Form—and has been translated into over a dozen languages (www.parinc.com), including a Spanish version validated in both healthy and patient groups (Caracuel et al., 2008, 2012; Verdejo-García & Pérez-García, 2008).

The FrSBe is intended as an assessment tool for a variety of populations, but the authors mention specifically its utility in focal lesion patients (tumor, stroke), dementia, head injury, and psychiatric disorders with frontal dysfunction such as depression, schizophrenia, and adult ADHD. It is designed to be more sensitive than neuropsychological tests of executive function because persons with frontal lobe dysfunction may perform well on neuropsychological tests yet display problem behaviors in their daily lives that lead to significant occupational and social dysfunction. According to the authors, an important feature of the FrSBe is the ability to track behavior over time.

TABLE 9–71 Frontal Systems Behavior Scale (FrSBe) Subscale Descriptions

SUBSCALE	MEANING OF SUBSCALE ELEVATIONS
Apathy	Reduced initiation, psychomotor retardation, aspontaneity, reduced drive, lack of persistence, low energy, loss of interest, reduced self-care, and blunted affective expression
Disinhibition	Impulsive behavior, hyperactivity, socially inappropriate behavior, reduced ability to conform to social conventions, poor emotional control (i.e., lability, irritability, explosiveness)
Executive Dysfunction	Problems with sustained attention, working memory, organization, planning, future orientation, sequencing, problem-solving, insight, mental flexibility, self-monitoring, and modulation of behavior in response to feedback

SOURCE: Adapted from Grace and Malloy (2001). Reproduced by special permission of the Publisher, Psychological Assessment Resources, Inc. (PAR), 16204 North Florida Avenue, Lutz, Florida 33549, from the Frontal Systems Behavior Scale by Janet Grace, PhD and Paul F. Malloy, PhD, Copyright 1992, 2000, 2001 by PAR. Further reproduction is prohibited without permission of PAR.

ADMINISTRATION

Administration instructions are printed on the record form and further detailed in the manual; the scale can also be administered via computer. The examinee is instructed to provide ratings on a series of behaviors in terms of how severe these are according to a five-point Likert scale, and in terms of severity (1) "before illness or injury" and (2) "at the present time." A sixth-grade reading level is required.

SCORING

The scale contains both negative and positive behaviors, the latter of which are reverse scored. Scoring is very straightforward and typically takes about 10 minutes, less if scored via computer. Scores are converted to T scores, with scores 65 or higher defined as falling in the clinical range. T scores between 60 and 64 are interpreted as reflecting borderline impairment.

Although this is not mentioned as a problem in the manual, the reverse-coding of some items may be confusing for some examinees, at least based on one study involving preclinical HD patients and controls (Duff et al., 2010). Therefore, it might be useful for the examiner to check that these items have been completed correctly by the examinee.

TABLE 9–72 Frontal Systems Behavior Scale (FrSBe) Self-Rating Form Standardization Sample Characteristics

Age	18 to 95 Mean = 48.1 (18.0)
Sample size	436
Sample type	Community and volunteer organizations
Geographic location	New England states, Indiana, Iowa, and New Jersey
Gender	57% Women 43% Men
Ethnicity	100% Caucasian
Education	14.2 (2.4) years; range: 10 years to doctoral level
Exclusion criteria	History of neurological illness, major psychiatric disorder, substance abuse, current psychotropic medications

SOURCE: Adapted from Grace and Malloy (2001). Reproduced by special permission of the Publisher, Psychological Assessment Resources, Inc. (PAR), 16204 North Florida Avenue, Lutz, Florida 33549, from the Frontal Systems Behavior Scale by Janet Grace, PhD and Paul F. Malloy, PhD, Copyright 1992, 2000, 2001 by PAR. Further reproduction is prohibited without permission of PAR.

NORMATIVE DATA

Characteristics of the normative sample ($N = 436$) for the Self-Rating Form are shown in Table 9–72 . Participants were Caucasian, community-dwelling individuals in the northern US, with about 14 years of education. Norms are provided according to education, gender, and three age groupings ($N = 147$, ages 18 to 39; $N = 165$, ages 40 to 59, and $N = 124$ in those older than 59 years). Informants who completed the Family Rating Form were either spouses or significant others having daily contact with the individual.

Although the Spanish version is intended to be used with the existing US norms, there are minor differences between groups, with lower raw scores in healthy Spanish examinees compared to norms from the US standardization sample. Norms and standard deviations for a small Spanish sample of primarily male, healthy volunteers in Spain (Caracuel et al., 2008) are shown in Table 9–73.

DEMOGRAPHIC EFFECTS

For the Self-Rating Form, demographic effects of age, gender, and education account for 11% of the variance in scores; for the Family Rating Form, these account for 18% of the variance (Grace & Malloy, 2001).

TABLE 9–73 Raw Score Means and Standard Deviations for the Self-Report Spanish Version of the Frontal Systems Behavior Scale (FrSBe) in Healthy Controls

	MEAN	*SD*
Apathy	25.17	5.80
Disinhibition	27.40	6.55
Executive Dysfunction	32.91	6.65
Total	85.49	16.60

NOTE: $N = 37$ (35 men, 2 women); mean age = 33.1 ($SD = 7.7$), range 18–50 years, mean years of education = 10.7 ($SD = 2.4$), range 6–17 years.

SOURCE: Adapted from Caracuel et al. (2008).

AGE

Age is inversely related to FrSBe scores (Spinella & Lyke, 2004); accordingly, scores are presented based on three age groupings (Grace & Malloy, 2001).

GENDER

Gender is also related to scores, with men scoring higher than women (Spinella & Lyke, 2004), although this is not found in all studies (Caracuel et al., 2008).

EDUCATION AND IQ

Education is inversely related to FrSBe scores (Spinella & Lyke, 2004), with separate norms provided for those with less than or equal to 12 years of education and those with 12 years or more of education (Grace & Malloy, 2001). IQ effects are not reported.

ETHNICITY, NATIONALITY, AND LINGUISTIC EFFECTS

Although the test has been translated in several languages by the publisher, the FrSBe normative sample is US Caucasian. Comparison of the Spanish and original US version suggest differences attributed to culture, with the Spanish version yielding lower scores overall in healthy people but not clinical samples, of moderate size, and of likely minimal clinical significance (Caracuel et al., 2008).

EVIDENCE FOR RELIABILITY

EVIDENCE FOR INTERNAL RELIABILITY

The internal reliabilities for post-injury scores for the standardization sample are high to very high for the Total FrSBe score, with adequate to high reliabilities for Apathy, Disinhibition, and Executive Dysfunction subscales (r = .72 to .87). No internal reliability data are provided for pre-injury subscale scores. In a mixed clinical group, internal consistency estimates for the pre-injury scales are strong for the Family Rating Form, as are post-injury ratings for a mixed clinical-healthy group (r = .95 for both scores, $N = 39$ and $N = 87$, respectively; Grace et al., 1999, as cited in the manual). In TBI and schizophrenia, the FrSBe demonstrates good internal reliability (r = .89 to .92; Niemeier et al., 2013; Velligan et al., 2002).

The Spanish version also demonstrates adequate to high internal reliabilities (Total r = .91, and .76 to .82 for subscales; Caracuel et al., 2008). However, Rasch analysis of the Spanish version indicates that the test is not a unidimensional instrument (Caracuel et al., 2012), with support for use of the three subscales, but not for the Total score. Overall, the Family Rating Form had more validity evidence than the Self-Rating Form, but some items have questionable relevance for non-neurological populations with minimal deficits (e.g., items relating to incontinence).

EVIDENCE FOR TEST-RETEST RELIABILITY, MEASURING CHANGE, AND PRACTICE EFFECTS

Test-retest reliability is not reported in the manual, nor are practice effects or techniques for measuring change. This is surprising, given that the authors specifically indicate that the FrSBe is useful for tracking change. As well, although the test provides post-injury and pre-injury ratings, there is no statistical technique for determining whether scores are psychometrically different from each other.

A test-retest reliability of .78 has been reported in schizophrenia (Velligan et al., 2002). Neimeier et al. (2013) reported adequate test-retest reliability for the Total Family Rating Form score in an acute TBI sample (r = .72), with some marginal to adequate Family Rating Form subscale test-retest reliabilities (r = .68 to .74). Self-rated Total and subscale scores were marginal to low (r = .42 to .57), suggesting caution in using self-ratings clinically in this group (Niemeier et al., 2013).

EVIDENCE FOR INTERRATER RELIABILITY

Not reported.

EVIDENCE FOR VALIDITY

CONTENT-RELATED VALIDITY

Items were selected based on theoretical grounds, according to review of the literature on frontal lobe or frontal systems damage, followed by review by neuropsychologists (see manual).

FACTOR-ANALYTIC STUDIES

In the manual, the authors cite a factor-analytic study of the Family Rating Form on a large sample of neurological patients that supported a three-factor solution that had been initially based on theoretical grounds. A later confirmatory factor analysis of the Family Rating Form by the authors indicated that a better fit would be obtained by eliminating eight items (Carvalho et al., 2013, 2016). In contrast, a study on a TBI sample found that the three-factor solution did not fit the data well, nor did a one-factor solution, concluding that the scale likely would benefit from elimination of problematic items as many items did not correlate significantly with their own scales. Reanalysis of the original version with eight problematic items removed showed that this reduced version had good validity, as shown by associations with basic and instrumental ADLs (Carvalho et al., 2016).

In a large sample of patients with behavioral variant FTD, primary progressive aphasia, and corticobasal syndrome, informant FrSBe ratings and D-KEFS executive functioning tasks (Verbal Fluency, Tower Test, and Sorting Test) were reported to reflect distinct but related constructs using latent variable factor analysis (r = –.48; Gansler et al., 2017).

SCALE INTERCORRELATIONS

Self-ratings and family ratings are only modestly related for Apathy (r = .26), but the Disinhibition and Executive Dysfunction scales are moderately correlated (r = .46 to .48; Barrett et al., 2013). The subscales show high associations in some patient groups, demonstrating that the two subscales have significant overlap (r = .44 to .71; Zamboni et al., 2008).

CORRELATIONS WITH OTHER NEUROPSYCHOLOGICAL TESTS

Evidence for associations between FrSBe scores and standard tests of executive functioning are generally positive, although some evidence is mixed; there are differences in associations with standard executive functioning tests depending on the rater (self vs. informant), the population, and the severity and disease stage. There does appear to be incremental validity of using the FrSBe over standard neuropsychological tests in some cases.

In neurological patients, informant FrSBe scores are related to National Institutes of Health (NIH) EXAMINER scores, a computerized battery of executive functioning tests (Possin et al., 2014), and to Stroop and TMT-B scores. The self-rating Disinhibition score also correlates modestly with verbal reasoning as measured by Wechsler Similarities (r = .30, Pluck et al., 2012).

In vascular dementia, the Family Rating Form demonstrates modest to moderate correlations with the DRS, with the largest associations found for FrSBe Apathy (Zawacki et al., 2002 but see Zamboni et al., 2008). In nondemented individuals with PD, those with high Apathy perform more poorly on D-KEFS category and letter fluency tasks and on the DRS conceptualization subtest (Zgaljardic et al., 2007). However, in other studies on PD, correlations with executive tests are mixed, with only modest correlations with TMT (r = .29) and negligible correlations with verbal fluency and Tower tests (Puente et al., 2016).

There appears to be incremental utility in the conjoint use of the FrSBe and neuropsychological tests of executive functioning; at low but not high levels of dysexecutive behavior, the FrSBe was the more robust modality for assessing executive deficits compared to the D-KEFS, particularly in discriminating between frontal variant FTD and corticobasal syndrome (Gansler et al., 2017). In MS, FrSBe informant ratings and self-ratings both correlate with measures of information processing, working memory, and executive control (Chiaravalloti & DeLuca, 2003). In presymptomatic individuals with HD, self-ratings are not related to neuropsychological tests of executive function, but family ratings are related to Symbol Digit and Stroop performance (Duff et al., 2010).

In patients with TBI, Executive Dysfunction self-ratings are highly related to neuropsychological measures of executive dysfunction ($r = -.50$) and moderately related to measures of working memory ($r = -.39$), whereas family ratings show no associations with neuropsychological tests of similar constructs; self-reported Apathy appears to be modestly related to working memory ($r = -.28$; Barrett et al., 2013). In other studies in patients with TBI, self-reported FrSBe ratings are related to measures of attention and processing speed, but not to executive functioning or memory tests (Schiehser et al., 2011). In moderate to severe TBI, self-ratings are moderately related to attention tasks such as Digit Span, but only Disinhibition is related to verbal fluency; self-ratings are not related to memory measures (CVLT-II), switching tasks (TMT, WCST, D-KEFS Color-Word), or planning tasks such as the D-KEFS Tower Test. Similarly, family ratings are unrelated to neuropsychological executive functioning tasks except for a moderate relationship between Disinhibition and verbal fluency and WCST (Lengenfelder et al., 2015). Negligible associations were found between family FrSBe ratings and Thurstone Word Fluency and Rey Auditory Verbal Learning Test (RAVLT) in a TBI sample (Lane-Brown & Tate, 2009). One study found an association between FrSBe scores and performance on a virtual reality executive functioning test requiring acquired brain injury participants to multitask to complete everyday errands in a virtual city, but few associations with standard measures of executive functioning were found (Jovanovski et al., 2012). Last, FrSBe ratings predict community integration following TBI, whereas conventional neuropsychological tests fail to add predictive value (Reid-Arndt et al., 2007). Compared to D-KEFS scores, FrSBe scores are stronger predictors of substance use in healthy college students (Meil et al., 2016), a behavior associated with executive dysfunction.

CORRELATIONS WITH OTHER SCALES AND QUESTIONNAIRES

Correlations between the FrSBe and scales designed to measure impulsivity are very high, mostly due to high correlations with the Executive Functioning subscale, not with the Disinhibition scale (Spinella, 2007). FrSBe scores are, however, moderately correlated with disinhibition on eating behavior inventories, but only modestly with measures of cognitive restraint, supporting a role for frontal circuits in the regulation of eating-related behaviors (Spinella & Lyke, 2004).

In stroke patients, FrSBe scores are inversely related to emotional intelligence (EI), with self-report scores correlating more highly with EI than informant-rated scores ($r = -.60$ vs. $-.39$; Hoffmann et al., 2010).

In TBI, the scale demonstrates moderate correlations with scales that measure self-awareness; the FrSBe Apathy subscale also correlates highly with the Apathy Evaluation Scale in TBI patients ($r = .71$; Lane-Brown & Tate, 2009). In TBI, some studies indicate that FrSBe self-ratings are highly related to depressive symptoms as measured by the BDI (Schiehser et al., 2011), whereas others find only modest correlations and conclude that the FrSBe is able to discriminate between apathy and depression (Lane-Brown & Tate, 2009).

CLINICAL STUDIES

Overall, there is an impressive body of literature supporting the clinical validity of the FrSBe in a variety of clinical populations with executive deficits, dementia, TBI, various neurological conditions, substance abuse, and psychiatric conditions, with the exception of adult ADHD, where studies are scant.

Dementia. FrSBe scores are able to detect early changes in apathy and executive dysfunction in very early and MCI, before functional decline occurs (Ready et al., 2003). In AD, FrSBe scores are elevated by approximately two standard deviations, whereas in amnestic MCI, scores are elevated by only one standard deviation. Within amnestic MCI patients, those with the APOE E4 allele have higher Executive Dysfunction scores than noncarriers and have overall scores that are 1.5 *SD* higher than the mean, midway between noncarrier MCI patients and AD patients (Mikos et al., 2013). These results suggest that the FrSBe may be a useful tool to detect early frontal neurobehavioral dysfunction in MCI patients prior to decline on neuropsychological tests and prior to functional decline. In AD, clinical elevations on the FrSBe are present regardless of stage of dementia, whereas those with dementia with Lewy bodies show problems only in later stages of the disease, indicating that frontal system neuropathology is an early occurring feature in AD but a late occurring feature in dementia with Lewy bodies (Peavy et al., 2013).

In mild to moderate AD, discrepancies between pre-injury and post-injury scores on the Family Rating Form predict deficits in basic and instrumental ADLs over and above general estimates of cognition such as the DRS, with Apathy particularly useful in combination with DRS Initiation/Perseveration to predict deficits (Boyle et al., 2003). FrSBe Apathy is also highly related to instrumental ADLs as measured by the Lawton scale ($r = -.63$; Boyle et al., 2003), demonstrating an independent effect of frontally dependent behaviors on daily functioning, over and above general cognition. In younger general neurology referrals, the addition of the informant FrSBe increases prediction of instrumental ADLs by 50% over neuropsychological tests of executive functioning, adding more predictive ability than intelligence tests, and with Executive Dysfunction providing higher prediction than the other two FrSBe scales (Karzmark et al., 2012). Overall, Apathy may be a more important predictor of instrumental ADLs in older patients and Executive Dysfunction a more important predictor in younger patients.

In FTD, those with behavioral variant FTD are more impaired on FrSBe Disinibition than those with aphasic FTD, but both have clinically elevated scores on the Total,

Apathy, and Executive Dysfunction subscales (Zamboni et al., 2008). Patients with behavioral variant FTD also have more impaired scores than primary progressive aphasia or corticobasal syndrome patients (Gansler et al., 2017). The FrSBe is felt by some authors to be superior to other rating scales such as the Neuropsychiatric Inventory (NPI) in capturing the specific subtypes of apathetic and disinhibited behaviors in FTD (Zamboni et al., 2008).

In mild to moderate dementia, the FrSBe Family Rating Form is also much more predictive of caregiver burden compared to length of diagnosis and hours of daily care, and this is particularly true for the Executive Dysfunction and Disinhibition subscales, but not Apathy (Davis & Tremont, 2007). These results suggest that active behaviors related to executive dysfunction (but not passive behaviors related to apathy) are more difficult for caregivers to manage in dementia. In contrast, both FrSBe Apathy and Disinhibition scores predict caregiver burden in FTD and corticobasal syndrome; caregivers of patients with elevated FrSBe scores had 10 times the odds of caregiver burden compared to those without; almost all patients had elevated Executive Dysfunction in this clinical group (Armstrong et al., 2013). In vascular dementia, Apathy and Executive Dysfunction are at least 2.5 standard deviations from the mean, but with Disinhibition within normal limits; however, only Apathy predicts ADLs (Zawacki et al., 2002).

In PD, 40% to more than 50% of patients have elevations on the Apathy scale (Schiehser et al., 2013; Zgaljardic et al., 2007). PD patients with high Apathy scores tend to have worse performance on neuropsychological tests and more depression symptoms and behavioral disturbance (Zgaljardic et al., 2007). The FrSBe is also a strong predictor of instrumental ADLs in PD, demonstrating significantly higher correlations than standard executive functioning tests. Self-ratings and caregiver ratings are moderately correlated in PD and show the highest agreement for Apathy, but discrepancies between raters on prediagnosis and postdiagnosis ratings are present in some cases and can be influenced by caregiver burden, caregiver depression, and medication status (Schiehser et al., 2013).

In HD, asymptomatic genetic carriers (individuals with trinucleotide repeat expansion for HD but insufficient motor symptoms for diagnosis) have higher scores than individuals who are gene-negative for HD, with both self-rated and family FrSBe ratings related to HD markers. Individuals closest in time to clinical diagnosis show the greatest discrepancies between self-ratings and family ratings, suggesting that insight problems occur in the 10 years prior to HD diagnosis (Duff et al., 2010), supporting the sensitivity of the FrSBe to disorders involving dysfunction in the frontal circuitry causing loss of self-awareness. In HD patients, only informant reports are related to disease severity, suggesting that self-ratings become less accurate as the disease progresses, likely due to reduced self-awareness (Hergert et al., 2015).

TBI. The FrSBe is recommended as one of several common data elements to measure neurobehavioral deficits in TBI (Wilde et al., 2010). Studies on TBI generally indicate elevations on FrSBe scales, although there is variability in terms of which scales are elevated depending on the study (e.g., Reid-Arndt et al., 2007), possibly related to recovery stage (acute vs. subacute vs. chronic), but less clearly related to injury severity. Some studies indicate that moderate to severe TBI is associated with clinically significant elevations on FrSBe Executive Dysfunction, whereas mild TBI is associated with elevations on the Disinhibition scale and borderline scores on Apathy (Barrett et al., 2013). Others find no elevations in mild TBI and suggest that some elevations in TBI research may relate to exaggeration of deficits (Schiehser et al., 2011).

Self-family discrepancies in FrSBe ratings are larger in men than women with TBI, indicating better self-awareness in women after TBI, possibly attributable to hormonal neuroprotection (Niemeier et al., 2014). At discharge, women's average discrepancy score was 7.3 versus 11.1 for men.

The sensitivity of self- versus family ratings may depend on time since injury. For example, in the acute setting, family ratings are more reliable and demonstrate more clinical elevations than do self-ratings (Niemeier et al., 2013); one year or more after injury, self- and informant ratings are fairly similar in terms of severity of deficits (Lengenfelder et al., 2015). In adults who sustained traumatic brain injuries in childhood, self-ratings indicate more problems than do family ratings, and these correlate more highly with neuropsychological tests of executive functioning, suggesting that self-ratings have predictive utility in adults with TBI compared to family ratings (Barrett et al., 2013).

The FrSBe appears to be sensitive to treatment effects in TBI according to a small number of studies. In a randomized control trial of the efficacy of intensive metacognitive skill training for problem solving and emotional regulation in a mixed TBI group, self-rated FrSBe Executive Dysfunction improved after treatment compared to a waitlist control group, whereas standard neuropsychological tests and measures of mood and wellbeing were not affected by treatment (Cantor et al., 2014). Similarly, FrSBe scores improved after videogame-based group therapy designed to improve self-awareness in a primarily severe, chronic TBI group (Llorens et al., 2015). Self- and family ratings in moderate to severe TBI indicate that substance use disorder is associated with more negative family ratings but not self-ratings, suggesting worse self-awareness and executive deficits in TBI patients with a history of substance use disorder (Niemeier et al., 2016).

Other Neurological Conditions. In ALS, some studies report elevations on self- and family ratings of Apathy (Terada et al., 2011; Witgert et al., 2010), with FrSBe scores correlating highly with scales designed to measure behavioral changes specific to ALS (Elamin et al., 2017), and that the self-report predicts disease severity (Terada et al., 2011). Others have found elevations on all FrSBe scales (Strutt et al., 2012) or only in cognitively impaired patients (Witgert et al., 2010). However, significantly more respiratory-impaired patients are rated by caregivers as having elevations on the Executive Functioning scale before ALS and on the Disinhibition scales after ALS, with different patterns depending on whether bulbar-onset or limb-onset type (Strutt et al., 2012). ALS patients without dementia have normal insight as defined as minimal self-informant discrepancies on the FrSBe, compared to patients with ALS-FTD (Woolley et al., 2010).

In MS, the Apathy and Executive Dysfunction scales are elevated; however, physical disease progression correlates with FrSBe family ratings, not FrSBe self-ratings (Chiaravalloti et al., 2003). At the same time, self-ratings have been shown to be potent indicators of cognitive and functional impairment in MS (Basso et al., 2008).

Psychiatric Conditions and Healthy Populations. FrSBe scores are related to measures of negative emotional states, such as the Profile of Mood States (POMS), and to measures of depression and anxiety, with FrSBe Total score and overall scores on anxiety and depression scales tending to be moderately to highly correlated (r = .46 to .53; Spinella, 2007). FrSBe scores also differentiate between patients with refractory OCD and healthy controls, demonstrating utility in psychiatric conditions. Older adults with depression with elevated self-reported FrSBe scores have a slower response to escitalopram treatment than those without (Manning et al., 2015), raising the possibility of using the FrSBe to determine treatment responsiveness in late-life depression. In a small sample of eight patients, FrSBe scores improved after mindfulness-based cognitive therapy for bipolar disorder (Stange et al., 2011).

In chronic schizophrenia, discrepancy scores between patients and psychologists have been used to estimate insight, with more than half of patients showing positive discrepancies (i.e., rating themselves as less cognitively impaired), but overestimation of executive deficits occurred in more than 30%. Furthermore, correlations between insight into executive deficits and insight into illness are only modest, indicating that self-awareness is a multidimensional concept (González-Suárez et al., 2011). All three FrSBe subscales correlate with adaptive functioning in schizophrenia (Velligan et al., 2002).

FrSBe scores are related to risk of substance abuse. In healthy college students, the FrSBe Disinhibition scale is predictive of alcohol, tobacco, and marijuana use, consistent with the view that addiction is related to frontal dysfunction (Meil et al., 2016). Discrepancies between self-ratings of substance users and informant ratings increase during periods of substance abuse, but decrease during abstinence, indicating sensitivity of the FrSBe to self-awareness deficits and denial of problems during active substance abuse. During periods of drug and alcohol abuse, FrSBe scores are more than two standard deviations above the mean and decrease to only a mild increase during abstinence (Verdejo-García & Pérez-García, 2008).

In opiate users, the Apathy scores and the Total scores are both elevated, supporting the view of frontal lobe dysfunction in this group (Pluck et al., 2012). Furthermore, in community samples of substance users, including those using tobacco, cannabis, major stimulants such as cocaine, and dissociative hallucinogens such as ketamine, there are modest associations between drug use and FrSBe scores, particularly with the Disinhibition scale (Spinella, 2003; see also Winhusen, Somoza, et al., 2013, for similar results in stimulant users), supporting the association between prefrontal lobe function and addiction. The FrSBe has been used in a variety of studies on addiction, including measuring oxidative damage in stimulant abusers (Winhusen, Walker, et al., 2013) and showing preexisting deficits in self-rated executive functioning in stimulant-dependent patients (Winhusen, Somoza, et al., 2013), and it has been shown to be superior in identifying those at risk of cocaine dependence and identifying trait impulsivity compared to personality questionnaires such as the NEO Personality Inventory (LoBue et al., 2014).

The FrSBe has also been used in the field of neuroeconomics, with higher scores associated with specific attitudes toward money (e.g., seeing money as a means to impress) and to reduced concern about long-term financial security, with scores inversely related to income in healthy people (Spinella et al., 2008). FrSBe Executive Dysfunction but not Apathy or Disinhibition scales are related to credit card debt (Spinella et al., 2004). Last, FrSBe scores are inversely related to scales measuring empathy, particularly emotional empathy and perspective taking in community samples (Spinella, 2005).

NEUROANATOMICAL CORRELATES AND IMAGING STUDIES

In FTD, FrSBe Family Rating Form subscale scores are associated with imaging findings of the prefrontal cortex, medial temporal structures, and basal ganglia, with Apathy correlating with degree of atrophy in the right dorsolateral prefrontal cortex and Disinhibition with atrophy in the right nucleus accubens, right superior temporal sulcus, and right mediotemporal limbic structures (Zamboni et al., 2008). In dementia, FrSBe family ratings are also uniquely associated with cortical thickness of the cingulate gyrus bilaterally, right subcallosal, and right anterior frontal cortex, while both FrSBe and standard neuropsychological tests of executive functioning are related to rostral aspects of the prefrontal cortex bilaterally (Gansler et al., 2017). In presymptomatic individuals with HD, there is a small but significant association between family ratings of Apathy and Disinhibition and striatal volume; similarly, Apathy self-ratings are associated with reduced striatal volumes (Duff et al., 2010). In ALS, FrSBe Apathy scores correlate with atrophy of the prefrontal cortex, including the orbitofrontal, dorsolateral, and right frontal gyrus (Tsujimoto et al., 2011); the FrSBe also correlates with white matter abnormalities in the corpus callosum and the left superior longitudinal fasciculus (Trojsi et al., 2013). In moderate to severe TBI with evidence of diffuse axonal injury, disrupted structural connectivity and reduced brain network efficiency were associated with lower informant-reported FrSBe scores (Kim et al., 2014). In a small study, FrSBe self-informant rating discrepancies were reliably associated with decreased awareness of deficits as measured by event-related potentials (Larson & Perlstein, 2009). Finally, in schizophrenia, FrSBe Executive Dysfunction scores are correlated with volume reduction in the bilateral dorsolateral prefrontal cortex (Kawada et al., 2009).

PERFORMANCE VALIDITY

The FrSBe does not contain any scales to assess symptom validity. One study in mild to moderate TBI indicated that those examinees who fell below the cutoffs on at least one of two embedded performance validity measures on neuropsychological tests (i.e., Reliable Digit Span and the forced-choice recognition trial of the CVLT-II) had greater FrSBe Executive Dysfunction and Apathy scores than those who passed embedded validity indicators (Schiehser et al., 2011), indicating that the scale is vulnerable to exaggeration of deficits.

COMMENT

The FrSBe is a brief, clinically useful scale for use in many clinical populations where executive functioning deficits are prominent. It has a vast number of clinical studies supporting its use across populations, including various dementia syndromes, TBI, and substance abuse, although studies are needed on its use in adult ADHD. Imaging studies on FrSBe correlates are also impressive. Like other rating scales of executive function, the FrSBe may be an especially useful addition to neuropsychological batteries because it increases incremental validity over standard neuropsychological tests of executive functioning while avoiding redundancy (Karzmark et al., 2012). Unlike some other executive functioning scales, this incremental validity has been demonstrated in a number of clinical populations. Notably, there are few standardized scales for measuring apathy in the clinical setting, and the FrSBe seems to be a valid and reliable tool for this purpose, particularly in dementia, where it is a strong predictor of capacity for ADLs. The Disinhibition scale seems to have particular sensitivity to potential for substance abuse. FrSBe scores are also useful in TBI, where deficits predict community integration.

The self-report questionnaire format is an asset when executive testing itself is not an option, and the availability of an informant form is very helpful when self-ratings cannot be completed due to severe cognitive deficit or lack of insight, as in dementia. Importantly, however, users should not assume that informant ratings on the FrSBe are more accurate than self-ratings as there is research showing this is not the case for specific populations where self-ratings are likely to provide more accurate information.

The normative data are substantial but restricted to the northern US states and completely Caucasian. There are a number of translations, but no information on the influence of ethnicity apart from one Spanish study. There are questions about its factor structure and about inclusion of a small number of lesser quality items. On the plus side, the sample is stratified by gender and education, and the scale has been used with success in an impressive variety of clinical samples, showing that the inclusion of a small number of problematic items does not interfere with its clinical sensitivity to executive dysfunction. The questionnaire form is divided into columns for before and after injury or illness and so is ideally suited to examinees having experienced specific clinical events (e.g., stroke, head injury), but it is less suited for examinees with more general conditions or developmental conditions with no clear onset (e.g., psychiatric conditions)—although several studies have used the scale in these groups by simply omitting the pre-injury ratings.

More data on test-retest reliability are needed as this is not reported in the manual, nor are practice effects or techniques for measuring change. This is surprising, given that the authors specifically indicate that the FrSBe is useful for tracking change. As well, although the test provides pre-injury and post-injury ratings, normative data on discrepancies for determining whether scores are psychometrically different from each other, other than visual inspection of the profile sheet, would be useful. Last, there are no validity scales in this questionnaire for confirming the accuracy of self- or informant reports, so the addition of additional scales to measure symptom validity is recommended when assessing examinees with the FrSBe.

REFERENCES

Armstrong, N., Schupf, N., Grafman, J., & Huey, E. D. (2013). Caregiver burden in frontotemporal degeneration and corticobasal syndrome. *Dementia and Geriatric Cognitive Disorders, 36*(5–6), 310–318. https://doi.org/10.1159/000351670

Barrett, R. D., McLellan, T. L., & McKinlay, A. (2013). Self versus family ratings of the Frontal Systems Behaviour Scale and measured executive functions: Adult outcomes following childhood traumatic brain injury. *PloS One, 8*(10), e76916. https://doi.org/10.1371/journal.pone.0076916

Basso, M. R., Shields, I. S., Lowery, N., Ghormley, C., Combs, D., Arnett, P. A., & Johnson, J. (2008). Self-reported executive dysfunction, neuropsychological impairment, and functional outcomes in multiple sclerosis. *Journal of Clinical and Experimental Neuropsychology, 30*(8), 920–930. https://doi.org/10.1080/13803390801888733

Boyle, P. A., Malloy, P. F., Salloway, S., Cahn-Weiner, D. A., Cohen, R., & Cummings, J. L. (2003). Executive dysfunction and apathy predict functional impairment in Alzheimer disease. *American Journal of Geriatric Psychiatry, 11*(2), 214–221.

Cantor, J., Ashman, T., Dams-O'Connor, K., Dijkers, M. P., Gordon, W., Spielman, L., . . . Oswald, J. (2014). Evaluation of the short-term executive plus intervention for executive dysfunction after traumatic brain injury: A randomized controlled trial with minimization. *Archives of Physical Medicine and Rehabilitation, 95*(1), 1–9.e3. https://doi.org/10.1016/j.apmr.2013.08.005

Caracuel, A., Verdejo-García, A., Fernández-Serrano, M. J., Moreno-López, L., Santago-Ramajo, S., Salinas-Sánchez, I., & Pérez-García, M. (2012). Preliminary validation of the Spanish version of the Frontal Systems Behavior Scale (FrSBe) using Rasch analysis. *Brain Injury, 26*(6), 844–852. https://doi.org/10.3109/02699052.2012.655365

Caracuel, A., Verdejo-García, A., Vilar-Lopez, R., Perez-Garcia, M., Salinas, I., Cuberos, G., . . . Puente, A. E. (2008). Frontal behavioral and emotional symptoms in Spanish individuals with acquired brain injury and substance use disorders. *Archives of Clinical Neuropsychology, 23*(4), 447–454. https://doi.org/10.1016/j.acn.2008.03.004

Carvalho, J. O., Buelow, M. T., Ready, R. E., & Grace, J. (2016). Associations between original and a reduced Frontal Systems Behavior Scale (FrSBe), cognition, and activities of daily living in a large neurologic sample. *Applied Neuropsychology. Adult, 23*(2), 125–132. https://doi.org/10.1080/23279095.2015.1012759

Carvalho, J. O., Ready, R. E., Malloy, P., & Grace, J. (2013). Confirmatory factor analysis of the Frontal Systems Behavior Scale (FrSBe). *Assessment, 20*(5), 632–641. https://doi.org/10.1177/1073191113492845

Chiaravalloti, N. D., & DeLuca, J. (2003). Assessing the behavioral consequences of multiple sclerosis: An application of the Frontal Systems Behavior Scale (FrSBe). *Cognitive and Behavioral Neurology, 16*(1), 54–67.

Davis, J. D., & Tremont, G. (2007). Impact of frontal systems behavioral functioning in dementia on caregiver burden. *Journal of Neuropsychiatry and Clinical Neurosciences, 19*(1), 43–49. https://doi.org/10.1176/jnp.2007.19.1.43

Duff, K., Paulsen, J. S., Beglinger, L. J., Langbehn, D. R., Wang, C., Stout, J. C., . . . Predict-HD Investigators of the Huntington Study Group. (2010). "Frontal" behaviors before the diagnosis of Huntington's disease and their relationship to markers of disease progression: evidence of early lack of awareness. *Journal of Neuropsychiatry and Clinical Neurosciences, 22*(2), 196–207. https://doi.org/10.1176/jnp.2010.22.2.196

Elamin, M., Pinto-Grau, M., Burke, T., Bede, P., Rooney, J., O'Sullivan, M., . . . Hardiman, O. (2017). Identifying behavioural changes in ALS: Validation of the Beaumont Behavioural Inventory (BBI). *Amyotrophic Lateral Sclerosis & Frontotemporal Degeneration, 18*(1–2), 68–73. https://doi.org/10.1080/21678421.2016.1248976

Gansler, D. A., Huey, E. D., Pan, J. J., Wasserman, E., & Grafman, J. H. (2017). Assessing the dysexecutive syndrome in dementia. *Journal of Neurology, Neurosurgery, and Psychiatry, 88*(3), 254–261. https://doi.org/10.1136/jnnp-2016-313576

Grace, J., & Malloy, P. (2001). *Frontal Systems Behavior Scale*. Lutz, FL: PAR.

Grace, J., Stout, J. C., & Malloy, P. F. (1999). Assessing frontal lobe behavioral syndromes with the Frontal Lobe Personality Scale. *Assessment, 6*, 269-284.

González-Suárez, B., Gomar, J. J., Pousa, E., Ortiz-Gil, J., García, A., Salvador, R., . . . McKenna, P. J. (2011). Awareness of cognitive impairment in schizophrenia and its relationship to insight into illness. *Schizophrenia Research, 133*(1–3), 187–192. https://doi.org/10.1016/j.schres.2011.08.023

Hergert, D. C. B., Sanchez-Ramos, J., & Cimino, C. R. (2015). Examining Huntington's disease patient and informant concordance on frontally mediated behaviors. *Journal of Clinical and Experimental Neuropsychology, 37*(9), 981–987. https://doi.org/10.1080/13803395.2015.1073226

Hoffmann, M., Cases, L. B., Hoffmann, B., & Chen, R. (2010). The impact of stroke on emotional intelligence. *BMC Neurology, 10*, 103. https://doi.org/10.1186/1471-2377-10-103

Jovanovski, D., Zakzanis, K., Ruttan, L., Campbell, Z., Erb, S., & Nussbaum, D. (2012). Ecologically valid assessment of executive dysfunction using a novel virtual reality task in patients with acquired brain injury. *Applied Neuropsychology. Adult, 19*(3), 207–220. https://doi.org/10.1080/09084282.2011.643956

Karzmark, P., Llanes, S., Tan, S., Deutsch, G., & Zeifert, P. (2012). Comparison of the Frontal Systems Behavior Scale and neuropsychological tests of executive functioning in predicting instrumental activities of daily living. *Applied Neuropsychology. Adult, 19*(2), 81–85. https://doi.org/10.1080/09084282.2011.643942

Kawada, R., Yoshizumi, M., Hirao, K., Fujiwara, H., Miyata, J., Shimizu, M., . . . Murai, T. (2009). Brain volume and dysexecutive behavior in schizophrenia. *Progress in Neuro-Psychopharmacology & Biological Psychiatry, 33*(7), 1255–1260. https://doi.org/10.1016/j.pnpbp.2009.07.014

Kim, J., Parker, D., Whyte, J., Hart, T., Pluta, J., Ingalhalikar, M., . . . Verma, R. (2014). Disrupted structural connectome is associated with both psychometric and real-world neuropsychological impairment in diffuse traumatic brain injury. *Journal of the International Neuropsychological Society, 20*(9), 887–896. https://doi.org/10.1017/S1355617714000812

Lane-Brown, A. T., & Tate, R. L. (2009). Measuring apathy after traumatic brain injury: Psychometric properties of the Apathy Evaluation Scale and the Frontal Systems Behavior Scale. *Brain Injury, 23*(13–14), 999–1007. https://doi.org/10.3109/02699050903379347

Larson, M. J., & Perlstein, W. M. (2009). Awareness of deficits and error processing after traumatic brain injury. *Neuroreport, 20*(16), 1486–1490. https://doi.org/10.1097/WNR.0b013e32833283fe

Lengenfelder, J., Arjunan, A., Chiaravalloti, N., Smith, A., & DeLuca, J. (2015). Assessing frontal behavioral syndromes and cognitive functions in traumatic brain injury. *Applied Neuropsychology. Adult, 22*(1), 7–15. https://doi.org/10.1080/23279095.2013.816703

Llorens, R., Noé, E., Ferri, J., & Alcañiz, M. (2015). Videogame-based group therapy to improve self-awareness and social skills after traumatic brain injury. *Journal of Neuroengineering and Rehabilitation, 12*, 37. https://doi.org/10.1186/s12984-015-0029-1

LoBue, C., Cullum, C. M., Braud, J., Walker, R., Winhusen, T., Suderajan, P., & Adinoff, B. (2014). Optimal neurocognitive, personality and behavioral measures for assessing impulsivity in cocaine dependence. *American Journal of Drug and Alcohol Abuse, 40*(6), 455–462. https://doi.org/10.3109/00952990.2014.939752

Manning, K. J., Alexopoulos, G. S., Banerjee, S., Morimoto, S. S., Seirup, J. K., Klimstra, S. A., . . . Gunning-Dixon, F. (2015). Executive functioning complaints and escitalopram treatment response in late-life depression. *American Journal of Geriatric Psychiatry, 23*(5), 440–445. https://doi.org/10.1016/j.jagp.2013.11.005

Meil, W. M., LaPorte, D. J., Mills, J. A., Sesti, A., Collins, S. M., & Stiver, A. G. (2016). Sensation seeking and executive deficits in relation to alcohol, tobacco, and marijuana use frequency among university students: Value of ecologically based measures. *Addictive Behaviors, 62*, 135–144. https://doi.org/10.1016/j.addbeh.2016.06.014

Mikos, A. E., Piryatinsky, I., Tremont, G., & Malloy, P. F. (2013). The APOE ε4 allele is associated with increased frontally mediated neurobehavioral symptoms in amnestic MCI. *Alzheimer Disease and Associated Disorders, 27*(2), 109–115. https://doi.org/10.1097/WAD.0b013e318266c6c3

Niemeier, J. P., Leininger, S. L., Whitney, M. P., Newman, M. A., Hirsch, M. A., Evans, S. L., . . . Perrin, P. B. (2016). Does history of substance use disorder predict acute traumatic brain injury rehabilitation outcomes? *NeuroRehabilitation, 38*(4), 371–383. https://doi.org/10.3233/NRE-161328

Niemeier, J. P., Perrin, P. B., Holcomb, M. G., Nersessova, K. S., & Rolston, C. D. (2013). Factor structure, reliability, and validity of the Frontal Systems Behavior Scale (FrSBe) in an acute traumatic brain injury population. *Rehabilitation Psychology, 58*(1), 51–63. https://doi.org/10.1037/a0031612

Niemeier, J. P., Perrin, P. B., Holcomb, M. G., Rolston, C. D., Artman, L. K., Lu, J., & Nersessova, K. S. (2014). Gender differences in awareness and outcomes during acute traumatic brain injury recovery. *Journal of Women's Health (2002), 23*(7), 573–580. https://doi.org/10.1089/jwh.2013.4535

Peavy, G. M., Salmon, D. P., Edland, S. D., Tam, S., Hansen, L. A., Masliah, E., . . . Hamilton, J. M. (2013). Neuropsychiatric features of frontal lobe dysfunction in autopsy-confirmed patients with Lewy bodies and "pure" Alzheimer disease. *American Journal of Geriatric Psychiatry, 21*(6), 509–519. https://doi.org/10.1016/j.jagp.2012.10.022

Pluck, G., Lee, K.-H., Rele, R., Spence, S. A., Sarkar, S., Lagundoye, O., & Parks, R. W. (2012). Premorbid and current neuropsychological function in opiate abusers receiving treatment. *Drug and Alcohol Dependence, 124*(1–2), 181–184. https://doi.org/10.1016/j.drugalcdep.2012.01.001

Possin, K. L., LaMarre, A. K., Wood, K. A., Mungas, D. M., & Kramer, J. H. (2014). Ecological validity and neuroanatomical correlates of the NIH EXAMINER executive composite score. *Journal of the International Neuropsychological Society, 20*(1), 20–28. https://doi.org/10.1017/S1355617713000611

Puente, A. N., Cohen, M. L., Aita, S., & Brandt, J. (2016). Behavioral ratings of executive functioning explain instrumental activities of daily living beyond test scores in Parkinson's disease. *The Clinical Neuropsychologist, 30*(1), 95–106. https://doi.org/10.1080/13854046.2015.1133847

Ready, R. E., Ott, B. R., Grace, J., & Cahn-Weiner, D. A. (2003). Apathy and executive dysfunction in mild cognitive impairment and Alzheimer disease. *American Journal of Geriatric Psychiatry, 11*(2), 222–228.

Reid-Arndt, S. A., Nehl, C., & Hinkebein, J. (2007). The Frontal Systems Behaviour Scale (FrSBe) as a predictor of community integration following a traumatic brain injury. *Brain Injury, 21*(13–14), 1361–1369. https://doi.org/10.1080/02699050701785062

Schiehser, D. M., Delis, D. C., Filoteo, J. V., Delano-Wood, L., Han, S. D., Jak, A. J., . . . Bondi, M. W. (2011). Are self-reported symptoms of executive dysfunction associated with objective executive function performance following mild to moderate traumatic brain injury? *Journal of Clinical and Experimental Neuropsychology, 33*(6), 704–714. https://doi.org/10.1080/13803395.2011.553587

Schiehser, D. M., Liu, L., Lessig, S. L., Song, D. D., Obtera, K. M., Burke Iii, M. M., . . . Vincent Filoteo, J. (2013). Predictors of discrepancies in Parkinson's disease patient and caregiver ratings of apathy, disinhibition, and executive dysfunction before and after diagnosis. *Journal of the International Neuropsychological Society, 19*(3), 295–304. https://doi.org/10.1017/S1355617712001385

Spinella, M. (2003). Relationship between drug use and prefrontal-associated traits. *Addiction Biology, 8*(1), 67–74. https://doi.org/10.1080/1355621031000069909

Spinella, M. (2005). Prefrontal substrates of empathy: Psychometric evidence in a community sample. *Biological Psychology, 70*(3), 175–181. https://doi.org/10.1016/j.biopsycho.2004.01.005

Spinella, M. (2007). Measuring the executive regulation of emotion with self-rating scales in a nonclinical population. *Journal of General Psychology, 134*(1), 101–111. https://doi.org/10.3200/GENP.134.1.101-111

Spinella, M., & Lyke, J. (2004). Executive personality traits and eating behavior. *International Journal of Neuroscience, 114*(1), 83–93. https://doi.org/10.1080/00207450490249356

Spinella, M., Yang, B., & Lester, D. (2004). Prefrontal system dysfunction and credit card debt. *International Journal of Neuroscience, 114*(10), 1323–1332. https://doi.org/10.1080/00207450490476011

Spinella, M., Yang, B., Lester, D. (2008). Prefrontal cortex dysfunction and attitudes toward money: A study in neuroeconomics. *Journal of Socio-Economics, 37,* 1785-1788.

Stange, J. P., Eisner, L. R., Hölzel, B. K., Peckham, A. D., Dougherty, D. D., Rauch, S. L., . . . Deckersbach, T. (2011). Mindfulness-based cognitive therapy for bipolar disorder: Effects on cognitive functioning. *Journal of Psychiatric Practice, 17*(6), 410–419. https://doi.org/10.1097/01.pra.0000407964.34604.03

Strutt, A. M., Palcic, J., Wager, J. G., Titus, C., Macadam, C., Brown, J., . . . York, M. K. (2012). Cognition, behavior, and respiratory function in amyotrophic lateral sclerosis. *ISRN Neurology, 2012,* 912123. https://doi.org/10.5402/2012/912123

Terada, T., Obi, T., Yoshizumi, M., Murai, T., Miyajima, H., & Mizoguchi, K. (2011). Frontal lobe-mediated behavioral changes in amyotrophic lateral sclerosis: Are they independent of physical disabilities? *Journal of the Neurological Sciences, 309*(1–2), 136–140. https://doi.org/10.1016/j.jns.2011.06.049

Trojsi, F., Corbo, D., Caiazzo, G., Piccirillo, G., Monsurrò, M. R., Cirillo, S., . . . Tedeschi, G. (2013). Motor and extramotor neurodegeneration in amyotrophic lateral sclerosis: a 3T high angular resolution diffusion imaging (HARDI) study. *Amyotrophic Lateral Sclerosis & Frontotemporal Degeneration, 14*(7–8), 553–561. https://doi.org/10.3109/21678421.2013.785569

Tsujimoto, M., Senda, J., Ishihara, T., Niimi, Y., Kawai, Y., Atsuta, N., . . . Sobue, G. (2011). Behavioral changes in early ALS correlate with voxel-based morphometry and diffusion tensor imaging. *Journal of the Neurological Sciences, 307*(1–2), 34–40. https://doi.org/10.1016/j.jns.2011.05.025

Velligan, D. I., Ritch, J. L., Sui, D., DiCocco, M., & Huntzinger, C. D. (2002). Frontal Systems Behavior Scale in schizophrenia: relationships with psychiatric symptomatology, cognition and adaptive function. *Psychiatry Research, 113*(3), 227–236.

Verdejo-García, A., & Pérez-García, M. (2008). Substance abusers' self-awareness of the neurobehavioral consequences of addiction. *Psychiatry Research, 158*(2), 172–180. https://doi.org/10.1016/j.psychres.2006.08.001

Wilde, E. A., Whiteneck, G. G., Bogner, J., Bushnik, T., Cifu, D. X., Dikmen, S., . . . von Steinbuechel, N. (2010). Recommendations for the use of common outcome measures in traumatic brain injury research. *Archives of Physical Medicine and Rehabilitation, 91*(11), 1650–1660.e17. https://doi.org/10.1016/j.apmr.2010.06.033

Winhusen, T. M., Somoza, E. C., Lewis, D. F., Kropp, F. B., Horigian, V. E., & Adinoff, B. (2013). Frontal systems deficits in stimulant-dependent patients: Evidence of pre-illness dysfunction and relationship to treatment response. *Drug and Alcohol Dependence, 127*(1–3), 94–100. https://doi.org/10.1016/j.drugalcdep.2012.06.017

Winhusen, T., Walker, J., Brigham, G., Lewis, D., Somoza, E., Theobald, J., & Somoza, V. (2013). Preliminary evaluation of a model of stimulant use, oxidative damage and executive dysfunction. *American Journal of Drug and Alcohol Abuse, 39*(4), 227–234. https://doi.org/10.3109/00952990.2013.798663

Witgert, M., Salamone, A. R., Strutt, A. M., Jawaid, A., Massman, P. J., Bradshaw, M., . . . Schulz, P. E. (2010). Frontal-lobe mediated behavioral dysfunction in amyotrophic lateral sclerosis. *European Journal of Neurology, 17*(1), 103–110. https://doi.org/10.1111/j.1468-1331.2009.02801.x

Woolley, S. C., Moore, D. H., & Katz, J. S. (2010). Insight in ALS: awareness of behavioral change in patients with and without FTD. *Amyotrophic Lateral Sclerosis, 11*(1–2), 52–56. https://doi.org/10.3109/17482960903171110

Zamboni, G., Huey, E. D., Krueger, F., Nichelli, P. F., & Grafman, J. (2008). Apathy and disinhibition in frontotemporal dementia: Insights into their neural correlates. *Neurology, 71*(10), 736–742. https://doi.org/10.1212/01.wnl.0000324920.96835.95

Zawacki, T. M., Grace, J., Paul, R., Moser, D. J., Ott, B. R., Gordon, N., & Cohen, R. A. (2002). Behavioral problems as predictors of functional abilities of vascular dementia patients. *Journal of Neuropsychiatry and Clinical Neurosciences, 14*(3), 296–302. https://doi.org/10.1176/jnp.14.3.296

Zgaljardic, D. J., Borod, J. C., Foldi, N. S., Rocco, M., Mattis, P. J., Gordon, M. F., . . . Eidelberg, D. (2007). Relationship between self-reported apathy and executive dysfunction in nondemented patients with Parkinson disease. *Cognitive and Behavioral Neurology, 20*(3), 184–192. https://doi.org/10.1097/WNN.0b013e318145a6f6

HAYLING AND BRIXTON TESTS

TEST NAME	**Hayling and Brixton Tests**
DOMAIN	Executive functioning
AGE RANGE	To 90 years or older
ADMINISTRATION TIME	15 minutes
SCORING FORMAT	Hand scored
REFERENCE	Burgess, P. W., & Shallice, T. (1997). *The Hayling and Brixton tests.* Thurston, UK: Thames Valley Test Company. www.pearsonclinical.co.uk

DESCRIPTION

The Hayling and Brixton Tests (HBT; Burgess & Shallice, 1997) are comprised of the Hayling Sentence Completion Test (Hayling) and the Brixton Spatial Anticipation Test (Brixton). The Hayling consists of two sets of 15 sentences, each with the last word missing. The Brixton is a rule attainment task that yields three different measures of executive function. These two tests are thought to assess behavioral regulation. These can be considered separately or combined into an overall score. The Hayling tends to be used more often than the Brixton, and in clinical research these tasks are often used separately.

ADMINISTRATION

Administration instructions are detailed in the manual. The Hayling consists of two sets of 15 sentences, each with the last word missing. In the first part, Section 1, the examiner reads each sentence aloud and the examinee is to complete the sentence as quickly as possible. This section yields a simple measure of response speed, with some authors terming this initiation. In Section 2, the examinee is faced with the more novel task of completing the sentence with a word that is unconnected to the sentence. Therefore, the examinee has to inhibit a strongly activated (automatic) response before generating a new response. This section yields two scores, an error score and a measure of response speed, with many researchers associating this with suppression. The Hayling thus yields three measures (response latencies from Sections 1 and 2 and error score from Section 2) which can be combined into an overall score.

The Brixton consists of a 56-page Stimulus Booklet, each page showing an array of 10 numbered circles in two rows, with one blue circle. The position of the circle changes from one page to the next; the change in position is governed by rules that vary without warning. The examinee's task is to provide a response (orally or by pointing) indicating where the blue circle will be, based on what the examinee has deduced from previous pages. Total errors are recorded. The scoring sheet prompts the examiner regarding scoring procedures. The Hayling requires an oral response, whereas the Brixton requires an oral or nonverbal (pointing) response.

SCORING

Scoring is detailed in the manual. The Hayling yields response latencies (whole second units, no rounding; Section 1 and Section 2) and error scores (Section 2). Section 1 is the sum of all the individual item latencies converted to a scaled score (range: 1 = Impaired to 7 = High Average). Section 2 time is similarly scored and converted to a scaled score (range: 1 = Impaired to 8 = Good). Responses on Section 2 are scored according to three categories: 0 points (word unconnected to sentence), Category B error (word somewhat connected), or Category A error (plausible). Scores from Category A and B are converted according to tables on the scoring sheet, then error scores and response latency scores are summed and transformed to an overall scaled score. Time scores compared to error scores perform differently and yield unique information (Baryard et al., 2017a; Martyr et al., 2017). Some authors have elaborated the Hayling scoring system (e.g., Robinson et al., 2015). For the Brixton, the total number of errors is converted to a scaled score (range: 1 = Impaired to 10 = Very Superior), with the answer to the first item disregarded.

DEMOGRAPHIC EFFECTS

AGE

Overall, age impacts performance (Andres & Van der Linden, 2000; Bayard et al., 2017a; Bielak et al., 2006; Burgess & Shallice, 1997; de Frias et al., 2006; Lin et al., 2007) with older adults showing slower responding and more errors (see Andres & van der Linden, 2000; Bielak et al., 2006; de Frias et al., 2006). The age effect persists with mild attenuation after accounting for processing speed (Andres & Van der Linden, 2000) and fluid intelligence (Bielak et al., 2006). A meta-analysis suggested large effects of age on response latencies for both Hayling sections and moderate effect of age on Section 2 errors (Cervera-Crespo & González-Alvarez, 2017).

GENDER

Overall, gender does not significantly impact Hayling scores (Bielak et al., 2006; Burgess & Shallice, 1997; deFrias et al., 2006; van den Berg et al., 2009). Bielak et al. (2006) reported that although female gender was associated with more errors on the Brixton, the effect was small compared with age (i.e., 1% vs. 11%, respectively).

EDUCATION AND IQ

Education appears to be minimally related to Hayling and Brixton scores (although see Bayard et al., 2017a). For example, Bielak et al. (2006) reported that education accounted for only approximately 1% of the variance in Hayling scores and approximately 2% of the variance in Brixton scores. Van den Berg et al. (2009) reported that the Brixton was minimally correlated with education and NART performance (r = −.18 and −.22, respectively). However, Burgess and Shallice recommend that the tests be used with caution in individuals with relatively low educational achievement or whose estimated premorbid IQ would be within the lower 15% of the population distribution on measures of general intelligence (i.e., IQ ≤85). Higher IQ is linked to fewer errors (Bielak et al., 2006; Burgess & Shallice, 1997; Clark et al., 2000) and reduced time required on the second part of the Hayling (Clark et al., 2000).

ETHNICITY, NATIONALITY, AND LINGUISTIC EFFECTS

No information is available.

NORMATIVE DATA

Burgess and Shallice (1997) normed the Hayling on a group of 118 healthy individuals, aged 18–80 (M = 45.3, SD = 18.1) living in the United Kingdom. The NART estimated IQ for a subsample (n = 71) of these individuals was in the above-average range (M = 110.9, SD = 6.7). Characteristics of the sample are shown in Table 9–74. Note that participants with low NART scores were excluded. Therefore, a scaled score of 6 is the average for all three measures yielded by the Hayling.

The Brixton was normed on a sample of 121 healthy people, aged 18 to 80 (M = 45.6, SD = 17.8). The NART estimated IQ of a subsample was in the upper end of the average range (M = 109.9, SD = 7.1, n = 73). Characteristics of the sample are shown in Table 9–75. As with the Hayling, participants with low NART scores were excluded. For each test, age, IQ, and age- and IQ-related 5% cutoff scores are provided in the manual.

TABLE 9–74 Characteristics of the Hayling Normative Sample

Sample size	118
Age	18 to 80 years[a]
Geographic location	England
Sample type	A mix of patient relatives, volunteers for research studies, people from a job-employment program, and non-academic staff at a university; mean NART estimated IQ of 71 participants = 110.9 (SD = 6.7)
Education	Not reported
Gender	52% Women 48% Men
Ethnicity	Not reported
Screening	Reported to have no history of neurologic or psychiatric conditions or substance use disorders. However, the method used to screen was not reported. Participants were excluded based on low NART scores.

[a]Age distributions as follows: 18 to 45, n = 48; 46 to 65, n = 51; 66 to 80, n = 19.
SOURCE: Adapted from Burgess and Shallice (1997).

Bielak et al. (2006) provided additional normative data for a sample of 457 healthy older community-dwelling adults in Victoria, British Columbia, Canada. The sample ranged in age from 53 to 90 years, was well-educated (M = 15.23; SD = 2.86), predominantly female (70%), and Caucasian (98%). Most participants were native English speakers (90%), and had 12 years of education or more (92%). Exclusion criteria were an MMSE cutoff score, moderate/severe visual or auditory impairment despite corrective aids, and a history of significant neurological or psychiatric disorders. The data for the Hayling

TABLE 9–75 Characteristics of the Brixton Normative Sample

Number	121
Age	18 to 80 years[a]
Geographic location	England
Sample type	A mix of patient relatives, volunteers for research studies, people from a job-employment program, and non-academic staff at a university; mean NART estimated IQ of a subsample of 73 participants = 109.9 (SD = 7.1)
Education	Not reported
Socioeconomic status	Not reported
Gender	
Females	55%
Males	45%
Ethnicity	Not reported
Screening	Reported to have no history of neurologic or psychiatric conditions or substance use disorders. However, the method used to screen was not reported. Participants were excluded based on low NART scores.

[a]Age distributions as follows: 18 to 45, n = 58; 46 to 65, n = 45; 66 to 80, n = 18.
SOURCE: Adapted from Burgess and Shallice (1997).

TABLE 9–76 Hayling: Response Latencies and Error Scores by Age Midpoints

VARIABLE	MIDPOINT AGE 57	MIDPOINT AGE 60	MIDPOINT AGE 65	MIDPOINT AGE 70	MIDPOINT AGE 75	MIDPOINT AGE 80	MIDPOINT AGE 85
Age range	53–60	55–65	60–70	60–75	70–80	75–85	80–90
M	57.34	60.19	64.80	69.93	75.11	79.47	82.69
n	88	167	161	141	128	105	55
Time to Section 1							
M	4.49	5.24	5.25	4.57	6.56	8.62	9.13
(SD)	(5.21)	(6.65)	(6.30)	(4.34)	(7.77)	(8.64)	(6.41)
Time to Section 2							
M	19.93	20.83	24.80	34.38	40.41	43.65	51.38
(SD)	(16.43)	(19.24)	(21.43)	(33.23)	(40.45)	(41.48)	(41.89)
Category A errors							
M	0.83	0.82	0.76	0.87	1.03	1.05	1.11
(SD)	(1.04)	(0.98)	(0.91)	(0.01)	(1.18)	(1.28)	(1.41)
Category B errors							
M	2.43	2.23	2.52	3.33	3.36	3.30	3.64
(SD)	(2.25)	(2.15)	(2.27)	(2.63)	(2.53)	(2.34)	(2.67)

NOTE: Age is calculated to the exact date of the participant's first testing session. Times are rounded down to nearest second and out of 15 trials.
SOURCE: Bielak et al. (2006).

are presented in Table 9–76, based on overlapping midpoint age ranges. The values for the Hayling time scores are somewhat lower than those reported by Burgess and Shallice (1997). Table 9–77 provides data for the Brixton Test based on the same sample. The scores are generally consistent with those reported by others (Andres & Van der Linden, 2000; Burgess & Shallice, 1997).

Spitoni et al. (2017) adapted an Italian version of the Hayling and Brixton with normative data provided for 240 Italian participants collected between 2014 and 2016. Participants were between 16 and 94 years of age (*M* = 45.80 years, *SD* = 18.83 years), 55% female, with an education range of three to 18 years (*M* = 12.29 years, *SD* = 4.05 years). Inclusion criteria were 16 to 99 years of age, absence of cognitive or functional impairment, native language of Italian, or corrected or intact vision and hearing. Exclusion criteria were neurologic or psychiatric conditions, use of psychotropic medications, substance use disorders, subjective cognitive complaints, MMSE cutoff score, or major medical condition. Because the response time and errors for Hayling Section 1 was typically 0, a constant of 1 was added to all scores for both times and errors. Normative data are provided in Tables 9–78 to 9–80.

Bayard et al. (2017a) provide regression-based normative data for the Hayling for 426 community-dwelling adults in France between 20 and 87 years of age (*M* = 56.5 years; *SD* = 17.9), 58% female, with an education level ranging from five to 22 years (*M* = 12.4 years; *SD* = 3.4). Exclusion criteria were a history of neurologic or psychiatric conditions and a score below cutoff on the MMSE (for participants > 50 years of age). Error scores on Section 1 were rare; 98% of participants made fewer than two errors. On Section 2, errors ranged from 0 to 18. In terms of time scores, Section 1 was also completed easily by most participants, with nearly all (99.5%) latencies of two seconds or less. Time latencies in the second condition of the Hayling were more variable (range 0–24).

Based on relationships between Hayling scores and age and education, regression-based models were created taking these variables into account. Raw scores are converted into standardized residuals through the following steps. First, predicted scores of the examinee are calculated. Second, residuals are calculated. Finally, residuals are standardized. The authors provide the following example: a 73-year-old man with 12 years of education took 11 seconds to complete Section 2, and his error score was 10. To determine whether or not this examinee obtained a response time score within the typical range, a predicted score was calculated using the equation: $0.592 + (0.002 \times 73) - (0.008 \times 12) = 0.642$. The residual was -0.437 [$= 0.642 - \log_{10}(11 + 1)$] and the standardized

TABLE 9–77 Brixton: Total Number of Errors by Age Midpoints

VARIABLE	MIDPOINT AGE 57	MIDPOINT AGE 60	MIDPOINT AGE 65	MIDPOINT AGE 70	MIDPOINT AGE 75	MIDPOINT AGE 80	MIDPOINT AGE 85
Age range	53–60	55–65	60–70	65–75	70–80	75–85	80–90
M	57.30	60.19	64.72	69.98	75.17	79.36	82.72
n	89	172	165	143	134	107	53
Errors score							
M	16.1	17.23	17.93	18.71	21.19	22.92	24.08
(SD)	(5.32)	(6.86)	(7.37)	(6.93)	(8.08)	(8.53)	(7.37)

NOTE: Age is calculated to the exact date of the participant's first testing session.
SOURCE: Bielak et al. (2006).

TABLE 9–78 Descriptive Statistics and Percentiles for the Hayling and Brixton by Age

VARIABLE	AGE RANGE 16–29 YEARS (N = 50)	30–39 YEARS (N = 62)	40–49 YEARS (N = 70)	50–59 YEARS (N = 75)	60–69 YEARS (N = 65)	70–90 YEARS (N = 41)
Hayling test						
Time to Section 1 (S1)						
M ± *SD*	2.80 ± 2.78	2.21 ± 2.21	6.56 ± 6.81	9.04 ± 6.82	11.26 ± 6.54	14.83 ± 5.80
Percentiles						
5	7	6	20	18	19	24
25	5	4	15	15	16	17
50	2	2	4	8	15	15
75	0	0	0	3	5	12
95	0	0	0	0	0	5
Time to Section 2 (S2)						
M ± *SD*	15.22 ± 14.37	16.35 ± 13.46	22.73 ± 17.60	26.91 ± 14.74	34.86 ± 20.20	47.56 ± 29.07
Percentiles						
5	44	46	62	60	80	109
25	25	26	30	36	45	58
50	10	12	21	24	31	39
75	3	5	9	16	21	27
95	0	0	1	6	11	14
Category A errors						
M ± *SD*	0.90 ± 1.42	0.73 ± 1.16	1.59 ± 2.07	2.23 ± 2.65	2.83 ± 3.09	4.29 ± 4.18
Percentiles						
5	4	3	6	7	9	11
25	2	1	3	4	5	7
50	0	0	1	1	1	3
75	0	0	0	0	0	1
95	0	0	0	0	0	0
Category B errors						
M ± *SD*	3.00 ± 2.56	3.69 ± 2.92	4.56 ± 3.39	4.23 ± 3.21	4.35 ± 3.20	4.20 ± 2.68
Percentiles						
5	8	9	10	9	9	9
25	5	5	7	7	7	6
50	3	3	4	4	4	4
75	1	1	2	2	2	3
95	0	0	0	0	0	0
Brixton test						
Error score						
M ± *SD*	15.68 ± 4.34	15.32 ± 6.8	16.06 ± 6.42	16.36 ± 6.19	18.11 ± 8.44	21.24 ± 9.14
Percentiles						
5	40	24	29	27	38	37
25	17	17	19	19	20	23
50	14	14	15	15	15	19
75	12	11	11	12	13	14
95	8	7	8	9	9	11
Age midpoint	22.5	34.5	44.5	54.5	64.5	82.5

SOURCE: Spitoni et al. (2017).

residual was −2.30 [= −0.437/0.19], which is an atypical score. The predicted score for the number of errors was computed as follows: 0.782 + (0.003 × 73) − (0.02 × 12) = 0.761. The residual was −0.28 [= 0.761 − $\log_{10}(10 + 1)$] and the standardized residual was −1.168 [= −0.28/0.24], which is a borderline score.

Pérez-Pérez et al. (2016) developed a Spanish version of the Hayling (see supplementary material at https://academic.oup.com/acn/article/31/5/411/2364792#supplementary-data) and provide normative data for 185 healthy controls between 18 and 99 years of age (*M* = 57.73, *SD* = 16.28), 58% female, with a mean education of 12.07 years (*SD* = 5.10 years). Participants were healthy volunteers who met the following inclusion criteria: between 18 and 99 years of age, absence of cognitive and functional impairment (based on MMSE and Clinical Dementia Rating Scale cutoffs), and Spanish as their native language. Exclusion criteria were neurologic condition, systemic disease that could be associated with cognitive impairment, psychiatric condition, substance use disorder, or auditory impairment. Information on major medical conditions is also provided ranging from less than 1% of participants with heart disease to 10% of participants with hypertension.

TABLE 9–79 Age-Adjusted Scores for the Hayling (Section 2 + 1)/(Section 1 + 1) Time Scores by Age

			AGE RANGE					
CLASSIFICATION[a]	SCALED SCORE	PERCENTILE RANK	16–29 YEARS (N = 50)	30–39 YEARS (N = 62)	40–49 YEARS (N = 70)	50–59 YEARS (N =75)	60–69 YEARS (N = 65)	70–90 YEARS (N = 41)
Impaired	1	<1	>23	>20	>18	>16	>14	>10
	2	<1	22–23	19–20	17–18	16	14	10
Abnormal	3	1	20–21	18	16	14–15	13	–
	4	2	18–19	16–17	14–15	–13	11–12	9
Poor	5	5	16–17	14–15	13	11–12	10	8
Low average	6	9	14–15	12–13	11–12	10	9	7
	7	16	12–13	10–11	10	9	8	6
Moderate average	8	25	10–11	9	8–9	7–8	6–7	5
	9	37	8–9	7–8	6–7	6	5	4
Average	10	50	6–7	5–6	5	4–5	4	3
	11	63	4–5	3–4	3–4	3	3	2
High average	12	75	2–3	2	2	2	2	–
	13	84	1	1	1	1	1	1
Good	14	91	–	–	–	–	–	–
Superior	15	95	–	–	–	–	–	–
	16	98	–	–	–	–	–	–
Highly superior	17	99	–	–	–	–	–	–
	18	>99	–	–	–	–	–	–
	19	>99	<1	<1	<1	<1	<1	<1
	Age midpoint		22.5	34.5	44.5	54.5	64.5	82.5

[a]Classification based on scaled score convention used for Hayling and Brixton tests.

SOURCE: Spitoni et al. (2017).

An overlapping interval strategy was used, yielding 13 intervals. The following formula was used to estimate scaled scores adjusted by age and education: SSAE = SSA − (b × [Education − 12]), where SSAE was the scaled score adjusted by Age and Education, SSA was the scaled score adjusted only by Age, and b was the regression coefficient for education. The scores presented were the ratio between Section 2 and Section 1; because the final score in Section 1 would be zero in many examinees, normative data were created by adding a constant of 10 points to each score. Normative data are provided in Tables 9–78 to 9–84. An example of how to use these data is provided by the authors

TABLE 9–80 Age-Adjusted Scores for the Hayling (Errors Section 2 + 1)/(Errors Section 1 + 1) Error Scores by Age

			AGE RANGE					
CLASSIFICATION[a]	SCALED SCORE	PERCENTILE RANK	16–29 YEARS (N = 50)	30–39 YEARS (N = 62)	40–49 YEARS (N = 70)	50–59 YEARS (N = 75)	60–69 YEARS (N = 65)	70–90 YEARS (N = 41)
Impaired	1	<1	>15	>15	>15	>15	>15	>15
	2	<1	14–15	–	–	–	–	–
Abnormal	3	1	13	15	–	–	–	–
	4	2	12	14	15	–	–	–
Poor	5	5	11	12–13	14	15	–	–
Low average	6	9	10	11	12–13	13–14	15	–
	7	16	8–9	10	11	12	13–14	15
Moderate average	8	25	7	8–9	9–10	10–11	11–12	13–14
	9	37	6	7	8	9	10	11–12
Average	10	50	5	6	6–7	7–8	8–9	9–10
	11	63	4	4–5	5	6	6–7	7–8
High average	12	75	2–3	3	3–4	4–5	4–5	5–6
	13	84	1	2	2	2–3	3	3–4
Good	14	91	–	1	1	1	1–2	2
Superior	15	95	–	–	–	–	–	1
	16	98	–	–	–	–	–	–
Highly superior	17	99	–	–	–	–	–	–
	18	>99	–	–	–	–	–	–
	19	>99	<1	<1	<1	<1	<1	
	Age midpoint		22.5	34.5	44.5	54.5	64.5	82.5

[a]Classification based on scaled score convention used for Hayling and Brixton tests.

SOURCE: Spitoni et al. (2017).

TABLE 9–81 Age-Adjusted Scores for the Hayling (Time; Section 2/Section 1)

SCALED SCORE	PERCENTILE RANGE	AGE RANGE 20–27	28–32	33–37	38–42	43–47	48–52	53–57	58–62	63–67	68–72	73–77	78–82	83–90
2	<1	>11.0	>8.86	>6.03	>9.37	>12.29	>26.91	>29.18	>29.52	>13.02	>11.06	>11.51	>11.29	>9.79
3	1	–	–	–	–	–	–	–	–	–	–	–	–	–
4	2	–	–	–	–	–	–	–	–	–	–	–	–	–
5	3–5	–	–	–	–	–	12.50–26.91	19.00–29.18	20.00–29.52	10.20–13.02	9.50–11.06	11.30–11.51	–	–
6	6–10	9.5–11.0	6.90–8.86	–	–	8.00–12.29	7.30–12.49	8.00–18–99	8.00–19.99	7.30–10.19	8.75–9.49	9.43–11.29	9.60–11.29	–
7	11–18	6.9–9.4	6.17–6.89	5.86–6.03	6.60–9.37	6.45–7.99	6.40–739	6.52–7.99	5.50–7.99	6.70–7.29	7.20–8.74	7.68–9.42	7.98–9.59	7.67–9.79
8	19–28	5.90–6.89	5.74–6.16	5.67–5.85	6.02–6.59	5.94–6.44	5.25–639	4.86–6.51	4.68–5.49	4.87–6.69	6.00–7.19	6.34–7.67	6.26–7.97	6.92–7.66
9	29–40	4.4–5.85	4.80–5.73	5.27–5.66	4.80–6.01	4.73–5.93	4.66–5.24	4.20–4.85	4.20–4.67	4.30–4.86	5.24–5.99	5.60–6.33	5.44–6.25	6.16–6.91
10	41–59	3.48–4.39	3.33–4.79	4.01–5.26	3.10–4.79	3.67–4.72	3.72–4.65	3.44–4.19	3.58–4.19	3.64–4.29	4.20–5.23	4.64–5.59	4.63–5.43	4.58–6.15
11	60–71	3.11–3.47	2.73–3.32	2.84–4.00	2.40–3.09	3.10–3.66	3.11–3.71	2.89–3.43	3.16–3.57	3.27–3.63	3.72–4.19	4.06–4.63	4.05–4.62	3.94–4.57
12	72–81	2.36–3.10	2.42–2.72	2.48–2.83	2.25–2.39	2.30–3.09	2.43–3.10	2.31–2.88	2.67–3.15	2.69–336	3.37–3.71	3.73–4.05	3.60–4.04	2.80–3.93
13	82–89	2.15–2.35	2.22–2.41	2.38–2.47	1.40–2.24	1.43–2.29	1.85–2.42	2.00–2.30	2.25–2.66	2.19–2.68	2.70–3.36	3.09–3.72	2.98–3.59	1.93–2.79
14	90–94	<2.03–2.14	2.06–2.21	2.29–2.37	1.28–1.39	1.27–1.42	1.42–1.84	1.58–1–99	1.83–2.24	1,83–2.18	2.32–2.69	2.36–3.08	1.80–2.97	1.82–1.92
15	95–97	–	2.02–2.05	–	–	1.20–1.26	1.25–1.41	1.47–1.57	157–1.82	1.57–1.82	2.14–2.31	1.68–2.35	1.48–1.79	–
16	98	–	–	–	–	–	1.20–134	1.42–1.46	154–1.56	1.54–156	2.12–2.14	1.48–1.68	–	–
17	99	–	–	–	–	–	–	–	–	–	–	–	–	–
18	>99	<2.02	<2.02	<2.29	<1.28	<1.20	<1.20	<1.42	<1.54	<1.54	<2.12	<1.48	<1.48	<1.82
Age range		*18–30*	*25–35*	*30–40*	*35–45*	*40–50*	*45–55*	*50–60*	*55–65*	*60–70*	*65–75*	*70–80*	*75–85*	*80–90*
Age midpoint		*25*	*30*	*35*	*40*	*45*	*50*	*55*	*60*	*65*	*70*	*75*	*80*	*85*
Sample size		*16*	*20*	*14*	*15*	*32*	*41*	*46*	*44*	*44*	*40*	*43*	*28*	*14*

SOURCE: Pérez-Pérez et al. (2016).

TABLE 9–82 Education Adjustment for the Hayling (Time; Section 2/Section 1)

SCALED SCORE	EDUCATION (YEARS) 0	1	2	3	4	5	6	7	8	9	10	11	12	13	14	15	16	17	18
2	4	4	4	3	3	3	3	3	2	2	2	2	2	1	1	1	1	0	0
3	5	5	5	4	4	4	4	4	3	3	3	3	3	2	2	2	2	1	1
4	6	6	6	5	5	5	5	5	4	4	4	4	4	3	3	3	3	2	2
5	7	7	7	6	6	6	6	6	5	5	5	5	5	4	4	4	4	3	3
6	8	8	8	7	7	7	7	7	6	6	6	6	6	5	5	5	5	4	4
7	9	9	9	8	8	8	8	8	7	7	7	7	7	6	6	6	6	5	5
8	10	10	10	9	9	9	9	9	8	8	8	8	8	7	7	7	7	6	6
9	11	11	11	10	10	10	10	10	9	9	9	9	9	8	8	8	8	7	7
10	12	12	12	11	11	11	11	11	10	10	10	10	10	9	9	9	9	8	8
11	13	13	13	12	12	12	12	12	11	11	11	11	11	10	10	10	10	9	9
12	14	14	14	13	13	13	13	13	12	12	12	12	12	11	11	11	11	10	10
13	15	15	15	14	14	14	14	14	13	13	13	13	13	12	12	12	12	11	11
14	16	16	16	15	15	15	15	15	14	14	14	14	14	13	13	13	13	12	12
15	17	17	17	16	16	16	16	16	15	15	15	15	15	14	14	14	14	13	13
16	18	18	18	17	17	17	17	17	16	16	16	16	16	15	15	15	15	14	14
17	19	19	19	18	18	18	18	18	17	17	17	17	17	16	16	16	16	15	15
18	20	20	20	19	19	19	19	19	18	18	18	18	18	17	17	17	17	16	16

SOURCE: Pérez-Pérez et al. (2016).

as follows: a 69-year-old participant with a Hayling score (Section 2 + 10)/(Section 1 + 10) of 2.22 corresponds to an age-adjusted scaled score of 7. If the participant has six years of formal education, the age- and education-adjusted score would be 8, and if the participant has 18 years of education, the scaled score would be 5.

Van den Berg et al. (2009) provide normative data for the Brixton based on 283 healthy participants. Participants ranged in age from 55 to 92 years (M = 67.4, SD = 8.5 years). Cell sizes varied from 23 to 108 participants (>80 years old and 60–69 years old, respectively). Data for clinical groups were also included, such as patients with stroke (n = 106), diabetes (n = 376), MCI or early dementia (n = 70), psychiatric conditions (n = 63), and Korsakoff's syndrome (n = 41). All participants were Caucasian and spoke Dutch. The mean education level was 10.7 years (SD = 3.4). Exclusion criteria included uncorrected visual impairment, neglect, a fasting blood glucose cutoff suggestive of diabetes, history of alcohol abuse, psychiatric condition, or neurological disease.

Of note, patients with Korsakoff's syndrome, stroke, and psychiatric conditions performed worse on the Brixton than healthy controls (see also the section "Clinical Studies" for group differences). The following equation was derived via linear regression analyses for the expected error total score on the Brixton: Expected Total score = 6.12 + (0.23 × Age) – (0.24 × Education in years). A residual score is then calculated by subtracting the expected score from the observed score. The frequency distribution for the residual score was converted into a percentile distribution, as provided in Table 9–85. A score below the 5th percentile is interpreted as indicative of impairment.

EVIDENCE FOR RELIABILITY

EVIDENCE FOR INTERNAL RELIABILITY

For the Hayling, Burgess and Shallice (1997) report that split-half reliability coefficients were variable for healthy adults but adequate to very high for patients with anterior lesions (range of rs = .35 to .83 and rs = .72 to .93, respectively). For the Brixton, split-half reliability in healthy individuals is modest (r = .62; Burgess & Shallice, 1997).

EVIDENCE FOR TEST-RETEST RELIABILITY, MEASURING CHANGE, AND PRACTICE EFFECTS

Test-retest reliability was assessed in a group of 31 healthy adults retested between two days and four weeks after the first assessment (Burgess & Shallice, 1997). Reliabilities were adequate for the overall score (.76) and for Section 2 of the Hayling (r = .76, .78, respectively), but modest for the other scores (rs = .52, .62). Practice effects were not reported.

For the Brixton, test-retest reliability was assessed in a group of 31 healthy people retested either two days or four weeks after the first assessment (Burgess & Shallice, 1997). Reliability was adequate (r = .71). van den Berg et al. (2009) reported somewhat lower scores in a subsample of 83 healthy older tested within intervals ranging from six to 48 months (r = .61). There does not appear to be a significant practice effect on the Brixton, at least over relatively lengthy retest intervals (Burke et al., 2014; van den Berg et al., 2009).

EVIDENCE FOR INTERRATER RELIABILITY

Significant judgment is required in terms of assigning responses to particular categories. Unfortunately, no information is provided in the manual regarding interrater reliability. One study (Andres & Van der Linden,

TABLE 9–83 Age-Adjusted Scores for the Hayling (Section 2+10)/(Section 1+10) Scoring

SCALED SCORE	PERCENTILE RANGE	AGE RANGE												
		20–27	28–32	33–37	38–42	43–47	48–52	53–57	58–62	63–67	68–72	73–77	78–82	83–90
2	<1	≥2.50	≥2.49	≥2.15	≥2.30	≥2.34	≥2.38	≥2.36	≥2.30	≥2.74	≥2.82	≥2.78	≥2.72	≥2.8
3	1	–	–	–	–	–	–	–	–	–	–	–	–	–
4	2	–	–	–	–	–	–	–	–	–	–	–	–	–
5	3–5	–	2.45–2.48	–	–	–	2.26–2.37	2.30–2.35	–	2.36–2.73	2.48–2.81	2.51–2.77	–	–
6	6–10	2.33–2.49	2.25–2.45	2.05–2.14	2.25–2.29	2.21–2.33	2.00–2.25	2.21–2.29	2.23–2.29	2.30–2.35	2.36–2.47	2.42–2.50	2.45–2.71	–
7	11–18	2.19–2.32	2.02–2.24	2.00–2.04	2.01–2.24	1.71–2.20	1.80–1.99	2.00–2.20	2.10–2.22	2.21–2.29	2.21–2.35	2.21–2.41	2.33–2.44	2.53–2.79
8	19–28	1.87–2.18	1.80–2.01	1.58–1.99	1.80–2.00	1.56–1.70	1.61–1.79	1.80–1.99	1.81–2.09	1.93–2.20	2.11–2.20	2.11–2.20	2.17–2.32	2.41–252
9	29–40	1.56–1.82	1.50–1.79	1.50–1.57	1.60–1.79	1.47–1.55	1.60–1.51	1.63–1.79	1.61–1.80	1.61–1.92	2.00–2.10	2.00–2.10	2.11–2.16	2.30–2.40
10	41–59	1.50–1.55	1.36–1.49	1.42–1.49	1.30–1.59	1.31–1.46	1.40–1.50	1.40–1.62	1.35–1.60	1.31–1.60	1.87–1.99	1.91–1.99	1.99–2.10	2.11–2.29
11	60–71	1.30–1.49	1.21–1.35	1.31–1.41	1.16–1.29	1.21–1.30	1.29–1.39	1.30–1.39	1.21–1.34	1.26–1.30	1.61–1.86	1.71–1.90	1.91–1.98	2.03–2.10
12	72–81	1.12–1.29	1.10–1.20	1.28–1.30	1.09–1.15	1.11–1.20	1.20–1.28	1.11–1.29	1.11–1.20	1.11–1.25	1.45–1.60	1.51–1.70	1.64–1.90	1.88–2.02
13	82–89	1.10–1.11	–	1.16–1.27	1.00–1.08	1.00–1.10	1.00–1.19	1.00–1.10	1.00–1.10	1.00–1.10	1.22–1.44	1.36–1.50	1.40–1.63	1.60–1.87
14	90–94	–	–	1.10–1.15	–	–	–	–	0.95–0.99	0.95–0.99	1.10–1.21	1.15–1.35	1.13–1.39	1.20–1.59
15	95–97	–	–	–	–	–	–	–	0.92–0.94	0.92–0.94	–	1.10–1.14	1.00–1.12	–
16	98	–	–	–	–	–	–	–	–	–	–	–	–	–
17	99	–	–	–	–	–	–	–	–	–	–	–	–	–
18	>99	<1.10	<1.10	<1.10	<1.00	<1.00	<1.00	<1.00	<0.92	<0.92	<1.10	<1.10	<1.00	<1.20
Age range		*18–30*	*25–35*	*30–40*	*35–45*	*40–50*	*45–55*	*50–60*	*55–65*	*60–70*	*65–75*	*70–80*	*75–85*	*80–90*
Age midpoint		*25*	*30*	*35*	*40*	*45*	*50*	*55*	*60*	*65*	*70*	*75*	*80*	*85*
Sample size		*16*	*20*	*14*	*15*	*32*	*41*	*46*	*44*	*44*	*40*	*43*	*28*	*14*

SOURCE: Pérez-Pérez et al. (2016).

TABLE 9–84 Education Adjustment for the Hayling (Section 2 + 10)/(Section 1 + 10) Scoring

SEALED SCORE	EDUCATION (YEARS)																		
	0	1	2	3	4	5	6	7	8	9	10	11	12	13	14	15	16	17	18
2	4	4	4	4	3	3	3	3	2	2	2	2	2	1	1	1	1	0	0
3	5	5	5	5	4	4	4	4	3	3	3	3	3	2	2	2	2	1	1
4	6	6	6	6	5	5	5	5	4	4	4	4	4	3	3	3	3	2	2
5	7	7	7	7	6	6	6	6	5	5	5	5	5	4	4	4	4	3	3
6	8	8	8	8	7	7	7	7	6	6	6	6	6	5	5	5	5	4	4
7	9	9	9	9	8	8	8	8	7	7	7	7	7	6	6	6	6	5	5
8	10	10	10	10	9	9	9	9	8	8	8	8	8	7	7	7	7	6	6
9	11	11	11	11	10	10	10	10	9	9	9	9	9	8	8	8	8	7	7
10	12	12	12	12	11	11	11	11	10	10	10	10	10	9	9	9	9	8	8
11	13	13	13	13	12	12	12	12	11	11	11	11	11	10	10	10	10	9	9
12	14	14	14	14	13	13	13	13	12	12	12	12	12	11	11	11	11	10	10
13	15	15	15	15	14	14	14	14	13	13	13	13	13	12	12	12	12	11	11
14	16	16	16	16	15	15	15	15	14	14	14	14	14	13	13	13	13	12	12
15	17	17	17	17	16	16	16	16	15	15	15	15	15	14	14	14	14	13	13
16	18	18	18	18	17	17	17	17	16	16	16	16	16	15	15	15	15	14	14
17	19	19	19	19	18	18	18	18	17	17	17	17	17	16	16	16	16	15	15
18	20	20	20	20	19	19	19	19	18	18	18	18	18	17	17	17	17	16	16

SOURCE: Pérez-Pérez et al. (2016).

2000) noted that two raters agreed on only 77% of 1,425 responses. In another study, however, an independently scored sample of 20 randomly selected Hayling tests yielded high-average interrater agreement (96%; Bielak et al., 2006).

EVIDENCE FOR VALIDITY

RELATIONSHIPS BETWEEN HAYLING AND BRIXTON TESTS

Research regarding the degree of relationships between Hayling and Brixton tests is mixed. Correlations between the tasks tend to be low in community-dwelling older adults (r = .12 or less; Bielak et al., 2006; de Frias et al., 2006), with others reporting a variable pattern of correlations (Wood & Liossi, 2006; see also Marczewski et al., 2001). Similarly, a factor analysis involving the Hayling and Brixton and other executive measures suggested a distinct pattern of loadings, suggesting the tasks reflect different aspects of executive function (Kahokehr et al., 2004).

However, de Frias et al. (2006) noted that these tests share some common variance at the latent construct level, even though they appear quite disparate based on zero-order correlations. Burgess and Shallice (1997) reported that in healthy individuals, correlations between the Hayling and Brixton tests are reduced significantly after controlling for age and IQ (see also Andres & Van der Linden, 2000).

TABLE 9–85 Brixton Percentile Distribution of Residual Scores

PERCENTILE	RESIDUAL SCORE
2	18.93
5	13.24
10	8.00
15	5.73
20	4.34
30	2.44
40	0.47
50	-1.09
60	-2.83
70	-4.37
80	-5.97
85	-6.71
90	-7.79
95	-9.55

SOURCE: Van den Berg et al. (2009).

RELATIONSHIPS WITH OTHER TESTS

Overall, the tests generally correlate moderately with other measures of executive function (e.g., COWA Test, Digit Span Backward; Kahokehr et al., 2004) and minimally to moderately with the DEX in patient populations (Kahokehr et al., 2004; Odhuba et al., 2005; Woods & Liossi, 2006). The Hayling shows moderate correlations (rs = .40 to .65) with the Six Elements Test (Clark et al., 2000), the TOL (Andres & Van der Linden, 2000; Marczewski et al., 2001), and the TMT-B (Rohling et al., 2009). However, minimal correlations between the Hayling and executive tests have also been reported (see de Frias et al., 2006; Wood & Liossi, 2006).

The Brixton is moderately related to other measures of executive function (e.g., TOL; r = .58, Marczewski et al., 2001). However, minimal correlations between the test and executive function have also been reported (e.g., Color Trails Part 2, Stroop; de Frias et al., 2006).

The task loads with the TMT in community-dwelling older adults (van den Berg et al., 2009). Scores from the Hayling and Brixton generally show larger correlations with fluid than crystallized intelligence (e.g., Bielak et al., 2006; de Frias et al., 2006). See also "Demographic Effects." Kahokehr et al. (2004) reported that the Hayling correlated with the GDS and the MMSE in older rehabilitation inpatients.

CLINICAL STUDIES

TBI. Utility of the test in brain injury is mixed. Some research has suggested low rates of impairment on the test after severe brain injury (Wood & Liossi, 2006), whereas Draper and Ponsford (2008) reported that errors on the Hayling were effective at differentiating controls from patients with TBI at 10-year follow-up. The test also appears to minimally to moderately correlate with disability in patients with acquired brain injury of diverse etiologies (Odhuba et al., 2005).

PD. Research in patients with PD is mixed. Group differences have been reported between patients with moderate PD on versus off medication (Lord et al., 2011), whereas others have not reported group differences between patients with PD and controls (Rochester et al., 2005). Bayard et al. (2017b) reported that errors were rare on the Hayling Section 1 in people with PD; however, 46% of patients with PD showed impaired performance on error scores on Section 2, and 25% had poor performance on Section 2 time scores. The test shows small relationships with measures of depression and fatigue in patients with PD (Rochester et al., 2005). The Brixton, physical fatigue, and depression variables account for up to 39% of the variation in walking speed in patients with PD (Rochester et al., 2004).

Psychiatric Conditions. Impaired performance has been reported in patients with schizophrenia on the Hayling (Marczewski et al., 2001; Martin et al., 2016) relative to demographically matched healthy controls, with differences remaining after fluid intelligence is controlled for (Martin et al., 2015). The Hayling has been used extensively in patients with schizophrenia, with a meta-analysis suggesting medium to large effect sizes on the test (Wang et al., 2013) and impairments also found in first-episode psychosis (Chan et al., 2012). Bayard et al. (2017b) reported that errors were rare on the Hayling Section 1 in people with schizophrenia; however, 61% showed poor performance on Section 2 errors, and 23% showed impaired time scores on Section 2.

A meta-analysis has suggested that patients with schizophrenia and bipolar disorders show similar levels of impairment on the Hayling (Wang et al., 2013), with other studies reporting that patients with schizophrenia perform worse than patients with bipolar disorder (Joshua et al., 2009). Strategy use on the Hayling also relates to symptoms of formal thought disorder (Martin et al., 2016). In patients with schizophrenia, social impulsivity symptoms are moderately linked to performance on the Hayling (Chan et al., 2004). See also "Neuroanatomical Correlates and Imaging Studies." Group differences have also been reported on the Brixton (Marczweski et al., 2001).

Major depressive disorder impacts performance on the Hayling (Gohier et al., 2009; Richard-Devantoy et al., 2013), with differences not reported on the Brixton in one study (Gohier et al., 2009). The Hayling and Brixton appear to relate to lifetime occurrence of psychotic symptoms, prior number of episodes, and previous hospitalizations in patients with bipolar disorder (Rocca et al., 2008).

Other Populations. Performance is impaired on the Hayling in a variety of conditions thought to disrupt executive functioning, including AD (Collette et al., 2000, 2002; Martyr et al., 2017; Nash et al., 2007), alcohol use disorders (Noel et al., 2001), Klinefelter's syndrome (Temple & Sanfilippo, 2003), and ADHD (Baylis & Roodenrys, 2000; Clark et al., 2000). Hornberger, Piquet, Kipps, and Hodges (2008) reported that 86% of patients could be classified on the basis of Hayling and Digit Span scores as progressive versus nonprogressive FTD.

In terms of the Brixton, impaired performance has been reported in disorders thought to adversely impact executive processes such as eating disorders, with patients with anorexia performing worse than patients with bulimia, and inpatients with anorexia performing worse than outpatients (Tchanturia et al., 2004). Although the test differentiated stroke patients from healthy controls, relatively modest sensitivity and specificity was reported (56% and 58%, respectively, van den Berg et al., 2009). Korsakoff's syndrome was associated with strong sensitivity (81%) but relatively modest specificity (62%; van den Berg et al., 2009). The Brixton was found to relate to a measure of functional independence in stroke patients, even after considering performance on the RBANS (Vordenberg et al., 2014).

Null effects have also been reported. No group differences were found on the Hayling and Brixton between patients with seizure disorders and healthy controls (Treitz et al., 2009). However, the test was related to the length of seizure-free period. On follow-up years after organic solvent exposure, no effects on performance were found (Wood & Liossi, 2005).

NEUROANATOMICAL CORRELATES AND IMAGING STUDIES

Neural correlates of the Hayling have been analyzed according to response process involved, including initiation and suppression, with research reporting slightly different networks involved in each. Positron emission tomography research with the Hayling suggests that, in healthy individuals, activation of the left prefrontal regions (frontal operculum, inferior frontal gyrus) and right anterior cingulate is associated with response suppression and selection on Section 2 (Nathaniel-James et al., 1997). During response initiation (Section 1), activation is in left prefrontal, left middle temporal, and right anterior cingulate gyri. Allen et al. (2008) reported that, in healthy participants, response suppression was related to activation in left middle and orbitofrontal gyrus and bilateral precuneus compared to response initiation, with subsequent analyses implicating that the connection from the left middle temporal gyrus was related to increased activation in suppression versus initiation.

Patients with lesions involving the frontal lobe appear to perform worse on both the Hayling and Brixton than people with posterior lesions and healthy controls (Hayling; Burgess & Shallice, 1997; although see Andres & Van der Linden, 2001). Research has combined lesion and imaging approaches, finding impairment in all lesion groups on this test, but impairments in certain scores (e.g., suppression errors as in Robinson et al., 2015) are more likely to be obtained in patients with frontal lesions. For example, Volle et al. (2012) reported that Brodmann's Area 10 (medial rostral prefrontal cortex) was implicated in the initiation condition, and posterior inferolateral lesions were related to both initiation and suppression scores. Orbitoventral lesions were related to errors in suppression. Robinson et al. (2015) used a similar combined lesion and neuroimaging approach to investigate people with focal frontal lesions versus posterior lesions versus demographically matched controls. Frontal patients were found to show poorer performance than healthy controls on all scores examined (e.g., overall score, initiation time, suppression time, suppression errors), whereas overall score and suppression errors were more likely to be impaired in frontal patients compared to posterior patients. All frontal patients produced clear suppression errors, with the right lateral group showing more subtle errors. Right frontal patients produced fewer correct responses that implied strategy use, whereas right lateral lesions were associated with verbal suppression and strategy generation and use.

Neuroimaging data of individuals at risk for schizophrenia suggest increased recruitment of temporal regions compared to controls. Whalley et al (2009) compared individuals who were at high genetic risk for schizophrenia who became symptomatic versus those who were at high risk but remained asymptomatic over an 18-month interval. Participants who became symptomatic showed more activation in the left medial temporal gyrus on functional MRI (fMRI) during the Hayling than those who were asymptomatic. Whalley et al. (2008) also compared those at high risk for schizophrenia with depression versus those at high risk without depression versus controls; analyses according to fMRI suggested that people who were at high risk with depressive symptoms showed increased left superior temporal gyrus activation and decreased right middle and superior frontal gyrus activation compared to other groups. Whalley and colleagues also investigated comparisons between relatives of individuals with bipolar disorder versus healthy controls. Relatives of bipolar patients showed increased amygdala activation; across all groups, depression was correlated with ventral striatum activation during Hayling performance and cyclothymia with ventral prefrontal activation.

McIntosh et al. (2008) compared patients with bipolar disorder with patients with schizophrenia and healthy controls. Patients with bipolar disorder showed different patterns of activation compared to those with schizophrenia, particularly in the insula and dorsolateral prefrontal cortex. In addition, orbitofrontal and ventral striatal activation was increased in patients with bipolar disorder compared to controls. Noel et al. (2001) reported a relationship between Hayling performance and regional cerebral blood flow measures in the bilateral inferior and medial frontal gyrus in patients with alcohol use disorder.

In terms of the Brixton, there is evidence indicating that brain regions in addition to the frontal lobe contribute to task performance. Collette et al. (2002) found that patients with AD with hypometabolism restricted to posterior cerebral areas and those with hypometabolism in both posterior and anterior regions obtained similar scores. Andres and Van der Linden (2001) compared patients with discrete lesions in the frontal lobes who were in the post-acute phase with controls. The number of errors made did not differ between groups, despite a longer response latency in the frontal group. That is, patients with frontal lesions could inhibit a prepotent response, but it took them longer. Crescentini et al. (2011) reported that rule acquisition (responses provided up to rule deduction) and rule following (correct responses after rule acquisition) were associated with different activation according to fMRI imaging of healthy young adults; rule acquisition was associated with dorsolateral prefrontal cortex, and rule following with a broader network of temporal, motor, and medial and anterior prefrontal cortex. Frontopolar activation was found in both phases.

PERFORMANCE VALIDITY

No information is available.

COMMENT

Although they are available together as one test, the Hayling and Brixton reflect different executive abilities. Specifically, the Hayling appears to be more reflective of inhibition and the Brixton more reflective of planning. The tasks tend to be weakly correlated, are associated with different patterns of neural activation, and place different demands on examinees (e.g., verbal vs. nonverbal responses).

Demographic effects exist. Age is influential, both in terms of slower responding and increased errors, which appear to remain after processing speed and intelligence are controlled for. Gender is generally found to have no significant effect on performance. Education affects performance, although overall less so than age. Information on other sociodemographic factors, such as culture and ethnicity, is limited. The standardization sample is quite small, based on a relatively high IQ group, and over 20 years old, although some high-quality normative data have been published since.

In terms of reliability, internal reliability is variable for the Hayling and relatively modest for the Brixton. Test-retest reliability fares a bit better, generally in the adequate range. No significant practice effects are reported on the Hayling or Brixton. The degree of interrater agreement is somewhat mixed, which is an important consideration given that the test requires a degree of subjective judgment to score.

Overall, the Hayling and Brixton correlate moderately with other executive tests, including objective tasks and rating scales (e.g., DEX). In general, both tests overall show stronger relationships with fluid than crystallized intelligence. The test has been used in a variety of clinical populations, including TBI and PD. The Hayling has been used fairly extensively in schizophrenia, showing not only group differences but clinical and functional correlates. There is also a relatively large body of research on the neuroanatomical substrates involved in the test in patients with lesions, schizophrenia, and healthy controls. Although the networks are still being elucidated, frontal areas are consistently found to play a role, with recruitment of other regions apparently relatively more commonly observed in clinical groups. There is limited information on performance validity.

REFERENCES

Allen, P., Mechelli, A., Stephan, K. E., Day, F., Dalton, J., Williams, S., & McGuire, P. K. (2008). Fronto-temporal interactions during overt verbal initiation and suppression. *Journal of Cognitive Neuroscience, 20*(9), 1656–1669. http://doi.org/10.1162/jocn.2008.20107

Andres, P., & Van der Linden, M. (2000). Age-related differences in supervisory attentional system functions. *Journal of Gerontology: Psychological Sciences, 55B*, P373–P380.

Andres, P., & Van der Linden, M. (2001). Supervisory attentional system in patients with focal frontal lesions. *Journal of Clinical and Experimental Neuropsychology, 23*, 225–239.

Bayard, S., Gély Nargeot, M.-C., Raffard, S., Guerdoux-Ninot, E., Kamara, E., Gros-Balthazard, F., . . . Collège des Psychologues Cliniciens spécialisés en Neuropsychologie du Languedoc Roussillon (CPCN-Languedoc Roussillon). (2017a). French version of the Hayling Sentence Completion Test, Part I: Normative data and guidelines for error scoring. *Archives of Clinical Neuropsychology, 32*(5), 585–591. https://doi.org/10.1093/arclin/acx010

Bayard, S., Moroni, C., Gély Nargeot, M.-C., Rossignol-Arifi, A., Kamara, E., Raffard, S., & Collège des Psychologues Cliniciens spécialisés en Neuropsychologie du Languedoc Roussillon (CPCN-Languedoc Roussillon). (2017b). French Version of the Hayling Sentence Completion Test, Part II: Clinical utility in schizophrenia and Parkinson's disease. *Archives of Clinical Neuropsychology, 32*(5), 592–597. https://doi.org/10.1093/arclin/acx011

Baylis, D. M., & Roodenrys, S. (2000). Executive processing and attention deficit disorder: An application of the supervisory attentional system. *Developmental Neuropsychology, 17*, 161–180.

Bielak, A., Mansueti, L., Strauss, E., & Dixon, R. (2006). Performance on the Hayling and Brixton tests in older adults: Norms and correlates. *Archives of Clinical Neuropsychology, 21*(2), 141–149. http://doi.org/10.1016/j.acn.2005.08.006

Burgess, P. W., & Shallice, T. (1997). *The Hayling and Brixton tests.* Thurston, Suffolk: Thames Valley Test Company.

Burke, T., Wynne, B., O'Brien, C., Elamin, M., Bede, P., Hardiman, O., & Pender, N. (2014). Retrospective investigations of practice effects on repeated neuropsychological measures of executive functioning. *Irish Journal of Psychology, 35*(4), 178–187. http://doi.org/10.1080/03033910.2015.1044554

Cervera-Crespo, T., & González-Alvarez, J. (2017). Age and semantic inhibition measured by the Hayling Task: A meta-analysis. *Archives of Clinical Neuropsychology, 32*(2), 198–214. https://doi.org/10.1093/arclin/acw088

Chan, K. K. S., Xu, J. Q., Liu, K. C. M., Hui, C. L. M., Wong, G. H. Y., & Chen, E. Y. H. (2012). Executive function in first-episode schizophrenia: A three-year prospective study of the Hayling Sentence Completion Test. *Schizophrenia Research, 135*(1–3), 62–67. http://doi.org/10.1016/j.schres.2011.12.022

Chan, R. C. K., Chen, E. Y. H., Cheung, E. F. C., & Cheung, H. K. (2004). Executive dysfunctions in schizophrenia: Relationships to clinical manifestation. *European Archives of Psychiatry and Clinical Neuroscience, 254*, 256–262.

Clark, C., Prior, M., & Kinsella, G. J. (2000). Do executive function deficits differentiate between adolescents with ADHD and oppositional/defiant/conduct disorder? A neuropsychological study using the Six Elements Test and Hayling Sentence Completion Test. *Journal of Abnormal Child Psychology, 28*, 403–414.

Collette, F., Van der Linden, M., Delrue, G., & Salmon, E. (2002). Frontal hypometabolism does not explain inhibitory dysfunction in Alzheimer disease. *Alzheimer Disease & Related Disorders, 16*, 228–238.

Collette, F., Van der Linden, M., & Salmon, E. (2000). Relationships between cognitive performance and cerebral metabolism in Alzheimer's disease. *Current Psychology Letters, 1*, 55–69.

Crescentini, C., Seyed-Allaei, S., De Pisapia, N., Jovicich, J., Amati, D., & Shallice, T. (2011). Mechanisms of rule acquisition and rule following in inductive reasoning. *Journal of Neuroscience, 31*(21), 7763–7774. http://doi.org/10.1523/JNEUROSCI.4579-10.2011

de Frias, C. M., Dixon, R. A., & Strauss, E. (2006). Structure of four executive functioning tests in healthy older adults. *Neuropsychology, 20*(2), 206–214. http://doi.org/10.1037/0894-4105.20.2.206

Draper, K., & Ponsford, J. (2008). Cognitive functioning ten years following traumatic brain injury and rehabilitation. *Neuropsychology, 22*(5), 618–625. http://doi.org/10.1037/0894-4105.22.5.618

Gohier, B., Ferracci, L., Surguladze, S. A., Lawrence, E., El Hage, W., Kefi, M. Z., . . . Le Gall, D. (2009). Cognitive inhibition and working memory in unipolar depression. *Journal of Affective Disorders, 116*(1-2), 100–105. http://doi.org/10.1016/j.jad.2008.10.028

Hornberger, M., Piguet, O., Kipps, C., & Hodges, J. R. (2008). Executive function in progressive and nonprogressive behavioral variant frontotemporal dementia. *Neurology, 71*(19), 1481–1488. http://doi.org/10.1212/01.wnl.0000334299.72023.c8

Joshua, N., Gogos, A., & Rossell, S. (2009). Executive functioning in schizophrenia: A thorough examination of performance on the Hayling Sentence Completion Test compared to psychiatric and non-psychiatric controls. *Schizophrenia Research, 114*(1–3), 84–90. http://doi.org/10.1016/j.schres.2009.05.029

Kahokehr, A., Siegert, R. J., & Weatherall, M. (2004). The frequency of executive cognitive impairment in elderly rehabilitation inpatients. *Journal of Geriatric Psychiatry and Neurology, 17*, 68-72.

Lin, H., Chan, R. C. K., Zheng, L., Yang, T., & Wang, Y. (2007). Executive functioning in healthy elderly Chinese people. *Archives of Clinical Neuropsychology, 22*(4), 501–511. http://doi.org/10.1016/j.acn.2007.01.028

Lord, S., Baker, K., Nieuwboer, A., Burn, D., & Rochester, L. (2011). Gait variability in Parkinson's disease: An indicator of non-dopaminergic contributors to gait dysfunction? *Journal of Neurology, 258*(4), 566–572. http://doi.org/10.1007/s00415-010-5789-8

Marczewski, P., Van der Linden, M., & Laroi, F. (2001). Further investigation of the supervisory attentional system in schizophrenia: Planning, inhibition, and rule abstraction. *Cognitive Neuropsychiatry, 6*, 175–192.

Martin, A. K., Gibson, E. C., Mowry, B., & Robinson, G. A. (2016). Verbal initiation, suppression, and strategy use and the relationship with clinical symptoms in schizophrenia. *Journal of the International Neuropsychological Society, 22*(7), 735–743. http://doi.org/10.1017/S1355617716000552

Martin, A. K., Mowry, B., Reutens, D., & Robinson, G. A. (2015). Executive functioning in schizophrenia: Unique and shared variance with measures of fluid intelligence. *Brain and Cognition, 99*, 57–67. http://doi.org/10.1016/j.bandc.2015.07.009

Martyr, A., Boycheva, E., & Kudlicka, A. (2017). Assessing inhibitory control in early stage Alzheimer's and Parkinson's disease using the Hayling Sentence Completion Test. *Journal of Neuropsychology*. https://doi.org/10.1111/jnp.12129

McIntosh, A. M., Whalley, H. C., McKirdy, J., Hall, J., Sussmann, J. E. D., Shankar, P., . . . Lawrie, S. M. (2008). Prefrontal function and activation in bipolar disorder and schizophrenia. *American Journal of Psychiatry, 165*(3), 378–384. http://doi.org/10.1176/appi.ajp.2007.07020365

Nash, S., Henry, J. D., McDonald, S., Martin, I., Brodaty, H., & Peek-O'Leary, M.-A. (2007). Cognitive disinhibition and socioemotional functioning in Alzheimer's disease. *Journal of the International Neuropsychological Society, 13*(6), 1060–1064. http://doi.org/10.1017/S1355617707071184

Nathaniel-James, D. A., Fletcher, P., & Frith, C. D. (1997). The functional anatomy of verbal initiation and suppression using the Hayling Test. *Neuropsychologia, 35*, 559–566.

Noel, X., Paternot, J., Van der Linden, M., Sferrazza, R., Verhas, M., Hanak, C., Kornreich, C., Martin, P., De Mol, J., Pelc, I., & Verbanck, P. (2001). Correlation between inhibition, working memory and delimited frontal area blood flow measured by –super (99m)-Tc-Bicisate Spect in alcohol-dependent patients. *Alcohol & Alcoholism, 36*, 556–563.

Odhuba, R. A., Broek, M. D., & Johns, L. C. (2005). Ecological validity of measures of executive functioning. *British Journal of Clinical Psychology, 44*(2), 269–278. http://doi.org/10.1348/014466505X29431

Pérez-Pérez, A., Matias-Guiu, J. A., Cáceres-Guillén, I., Rognoni, T., Valles-Salgado, M., Fernández-Matarrubia, M., . . . Matías-Guiu, J. (2016). The Hayling Test: Development and normalization of the Spanish version. *Archives of Clinical Neuropsychology, 31*(5), 411–419. https://doi.org/10.1093/arclin/acw027

Richard-Devantoy, S., Deguigne, F., Annweiler, C., Letourneau, G., & Beauchet, O. (2013). Influence of gender and age on cognitive inhibition in late-onset depression: A case-control study. *International Journal of Geriatric Psychiatry, 28*(11), 1125–1130.

Robinson, G. A., Cipolotti, L., Walker, D. G., Biggs, V., Bozzali, M., & Shallice, T. (2015). Verbal suppression and strategy use: A role for the right lateral prefrontal cortex? *Brain, 138*(4), 1084–1096. http://doi.org/10.1093/brain/awv003

Rocca, C., Macedo-Soares, M., Gorenstein, C., Tamada, R., Isller, C., Dias, R., et al. (2008). Verbal fluency dysfunction in euthymic bipolar patients: A controlled study. *Journal of Affective Disorders, 107*, 187–192.

Rochester, L., Hetherington, V., Jones, D., Nieuwboer, A., Willems, A.-M., Kwakkel, G., et al. (2004) Attending to the task: Interference effects of functional tasks on walking in Parkinson's Disease and the roles of cognition, depression, fatigue, and balance. *Archives of Physical Medicine and Rehabilitation, 85*, 1578–1585.

Rochester, L., Hetherington, V., Jones, D., Nieubower, A., Willems, A.-M., Kwakkel, G., et al. (2005). The effect of external rhythmic cues (auditory and visual) on walking during a functional task in homes of people with Parkinson's disease. *Archives of Physical Medicine and Rehabilitation, 86*, 999–1006.

Rohling, M. L., Faust, M. E., Beverly, B., & Demakis, G. (2009). Effectiveness of cognitive rehabilitation following acquired brain injury: A meta-analytic re-examination of Cicerone et al.'s (2000, 2005) systematic reviews. *Neuropsychology, 23*(1), 20–39. https://doi.org/10.1037/a0013659.

Spitoni, G. F., Bevacqua, S., Cerini, C., Ciurli, P., Piccardi, L., Guariglia, P., . . . Antonucci, G. (2017). Normative data for the Hayling and Brixton Tests in an Italian population. *Archives of Clinical Neuropsychology*, 1–11. https://doi.org/10.1093/arclin/acx072

Tchanturia, K., Anderluh, M. B., Morris, R. G., Rabe-Hesketh, S., Collier, D. A., Sanchex, P., & Treaure, J. L. (2004). Cognitive flexibility in anorexia nervosa and bulimia nervosa. *Journal of the International Neuropsychological Society, 10*, 513–520.

Temple, C. M., & Sanfilippo, P. M. (2003). Executive skills in Klinefelter's syndrome. *Neuropsychologia, 41*, 1547–1559.

Treitz, F. H., Daum, I., Faustmann, P. M., & Haase, C. G. (2009). Executive deficits in generalized and extrafrontal partial epilepsy: Long versus short seizure-free periods. *Epilepsy & Behavior, 14*, 66-70.

van den Berg, E., Nys, G. M. S., Brands, A. M. A., Ruis, C., Van Zandvoort, M. J. E., & Kessels, R. P. C. (2009). The Brixton Spatial Anticipation Test as a test for executive function: Validity in patient groups and norms for older adults. *Journal of the International Neuropsychological Society, 15*(05), 695. http://doi.org/10.1017/S1355617709990269

Volle, E., de Lacy Costello, A., Coates, L. M., McGuire, C., Towgood, K., Gilbert, S., . . . Burgess, P. W. (2012). Dissociation between verbal response initiation and suppression after prefrontal lesions. *Cerebral Cortex, 22*(10), 2428–2440. http://doi.org/10.1093/cercor/bhr322

Vordenberg, J. A., Barrett, J. J., Doninger, N. A., Contardo, C. P., & Ozoude, K. A. (2014). Application of the Brixton Spatial Anticipation Test in stroke: Ecological validity and performance characteristics *The Clinical Neuropsychologist, 28*(2), 300–316. http://doi.org/10.1080/13854046.2014.881555

Wang, K., Song, L.-L., Cheung, E. F. C., Lui, S. S. Y., Shum, D. H. K., & Chan, R. C. K. (2013). Bipolar disorder and schizophrenia share a similar deficit in semantic inhibition: A meta-analysis based on Hayling Sentence Completion Test performance. *Progress in Neuro-Psychopharmacology & Biological Psychiatry, 46*, 153–160. http://doi.org/10.1016/j.pnpbp.2013.07.012

Whalley, H. C., Gountouna, V.-E., Hall, J., McIntosh, A. M., Simonotto, E., Job, D. E., . . . Lawrie, S. M. (2009). fMRI changes over time and reproducibility in unmedicated subjects at high genetic risk of schizophrenia. *Psychological Medicine, 39*(7), 1189–1199. http://doi.org/10.1017/S0033291708004923

Whalley, H. C., Mowatt, L., Stanfield, A. C., Hall, J., Johnstone, E. C., Lawrie, S. M., & McIntosh, A. M. (2008). Hypofrontality in subjects at high genetic risk of schizophrenia with depressive symptoms. *Journal of Affective Disorders, 109*(1–2), 99–106. http://doi.org/10.1016/j.jad.2007.11.009

Wood, R. L. I., & Liossi, C. (2005). Long-term neuropsychological impact of brief occupational exposure to organic solvents. *Archives of Clinical Neuropsychology, 20,* 655–665.

Wood, R., & Liossi, C. (2006). The ecological validity of executive tests in a severely brain injured sample. *Archives of Clinical Neuropsychology, 21*(5), 429–437. http://doi.org/10.1016/j.acn.2005.06.014

RUFF FIGURAL FLUENCY TEST (RFFT)

TEST NAME	**Ruff Figural Fluency Test (RFFT)**
DOMAIN	Executive functioning
AGE RANGE	16 to 70 years
ADMINISTRATION TIME	7 minutes
SCORING FORMAT	Hand scored; computer scoring software available
REFERENCE	Ruff, R. (1996, 1998). *Ruff Figural Fluency Test*. Odessa, FL: PAR. www.parinc.com

DESCRIPTION

The Ruff Figural Fluency Test (RFFT; Ruff, 1996, 1998) measures the production of novel designs under time constraints and was developed to assess divergent thinking, cognitive flexibility, and planning. Figural fluency tests have been developed as nonverbal analogs to word fluency tasks. Other stand-alone design fluency tests include a variant presented by Jones-Gotman (1991; Jones-Gotman & Milner, 1977) and the Five-Point Test (Regard et al., 1982), reviewed elsewhere in this chapter. Variants of design fluency are also part of larger test batteries, including the D-KEFS (Delis et al., 2001), reviewed elsewhere in this chapter. A modification of the fixed-response condition is also part of the HRNES (Russell & Starkey, 1993, 2001).

Ruff (1996, 1998) developed a variant of the Five-Point Test that consists of five parts. The test is made up of five pages (parts), each consisting of 35 five-dot matrices, arranged in seven rows and five columns on a sheet of paper. Each part consists of a different stimulus pattern of dots (see Figure 9–9). Parts 2 and 3 contain the dot pattern of Part 1 with various distractors (Part 2: triangles, Part 3: lines); Parts 4 and 5 contain variations of the original dot pattern without distracting elements.

Each stimulus sheet is preceded by a page containing three samples of the specific stimulus to provide the examinee with an opportunity to practice. The task in each part is to draw as many Unique Designs as possible in a one-minute interval by connecting the dots in the different patterns. If the same design is repeated, then the design is scored as a Perseverative Error (also called a Perseveration).

ADMINISTRATION

Administration details are provided in the manual.

SCORING

The number of Unique Designs and Perseverative Errors (also termed Perseverations) appears to be fairly consistent across the five parts of the test, suggesting no significant practice or learning effects. Accordingly, only total test scores summed across conditions are evaluated. Standard RFFT indices include:

- The total number of Unique Designs;
- The total number of Perseverative Errors across the five parts of the test; and
- An Error Ratio calculated by dividing the total number of Perseverative Errors by the total number of Unique Designs. The Error Ratio represents an index of planning efficiency (Ruff, 1996, 1998).

The total number of Unique Designs and Error Ratio scores are converted to T scores and descriptive ranges ("Impaired" to "Very Superior") based on age. Corrections for education are available for each of the age groups,

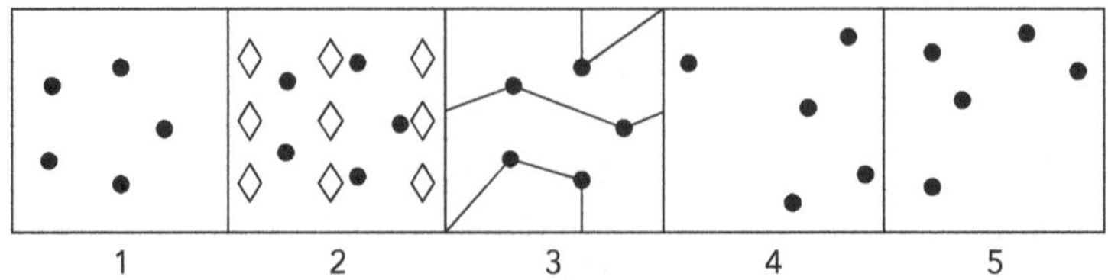

Figure 9–9 *Examples of Dot Patterns in Parts 1 to 5 of the Ruff Figural Fluency Test (RFFT).*

SOURCE: Ruff (1998). Reproduced by special permission of the Publisher, Psychological Assessment Resources, Inc. (PAR), 16204 North Florida Avenue, Lutz, Florida 33549, from the Ruff Figural Fluency Test by Ronald M. Ruff, PhD Copyright 1988, 1996, by PAR. Further reproduction is prohibited without permission of PAR.

and these corrections are listed in the manual for Unique Designs and Error Ratios. Of note, a novel computer scoring software program has been developed, which shows high reliability between computer and human raters (Elderson et al., 2016).

Qualitative scores to evaluate strategy have been developed (Ross et al., 2003) involving three or more consecutive designs for which the examinee has employed a systematic process to generate designs. These "strategic clusters" are categorized as two types. The first is a rotational strategy that involves simply rotating a drawing systematically clockwise or counterclockwise within the array of dots to make it appear differently in each square. The second is a quantitative strategy whereby examinees alter a design by systematically adding or removing one line. Two other indices of strategy were developed: mean cluster size (reflecting the extent to which an examinee applied a single strategy across consecutive designs) and percentage of designs used in strategies (the number of designs incorporated into production strategies divided by the number of designs overall, including Perseverative Errors). In healthy college students, the most common spontaneously generated strategy used was rotational (Gardner et al., 2013). Strategy use was generally related to the production of more Unique Designs.

DEMOGRAPHIC EFFECTS

AGE

Age affects performance (Fama et al., 1998; Izaks et al., 2011b; Ruff et al., 1987; Salthouse et al., 2003). There is also evidence that age interacts with practice effects (see the section "Evidence for Reliability").

GENDER

Gender has little impact on performance (Demakis & Harrison, 1997; Kraybill & Suchy, 2008; Ross, 2014).

EDUCATION AND IQ

Education and IQ impact performance (Izaks et al., 2011b; Ruff et al., 1987).

ETHNICITY, NATIONALITY, AND LINGUISTIC EFFECTS

In a study of the effect of cultural attitudes toward time on neuropsychological test performance, Agranovich, Panter, Puente, and Touradji (2011) reported that Russian and American volunteers did not differ in performance on the RFFT, with an earlier study reporting, however, that Americans scored higher than Russians (Agranovich & Puente, 2007). The difference in performance between the groups approximated a mean difference of approximately 11 Unique Designs. Bilingual adults with stronger language abilities perform better on the test (Festman et al., 2010).

NORMATIVE DATA

Normative data provided in the manual are based on a sample of 358 healthy individuals ranging in age from 16 to 70 years. Test scores (Unique Designs, Error Ratio) are provided according to four age and three educational groupings, as shown in Table 9–86.

Izaks et al. (2011b) provide data for 1,651 adults (35 to 82 years), predominantly of Western-European descent living in the Netherlands. Demographic characteristics are summarized in Table 9–87. Data were collected from a sample of the general population as part of a larger medical study, and no exclusion criteria were applied. Normative data are presented based on age and education. The number of Unique Designs was lower than the US standardization sample. Normative data are presented in Tables 9–88 to 9–91.

A large study based in the Netherlands (van Eersel et al., 2015) provided longitudinal data separated by age and education for 2,515 participants at three time points (see Tables 9–90 and 9–91). Participants were part of a larger renal and cardiovascular study in the general population, and thus the study included a broad range of participants who were 28 to 75 years of age, selected based on their urinary albumin excretion. Participants were a mean age of 53 years ($SD = 10$), 47% female, and 96% were of Western-European descent. Second or third measurements were more likely to be obtained from younger participants with higher education levels.

TABLE 9–86 Characteristics of the Ruff Figural Fluency Test (RFFT) Standardization Sample

Number	358
Age	
16–24	22%
25–39	28%
40–54	26%
55–70	23%
Geographic location	65% California; 30% Michigan; 5% Eastern United States
Sample type	Volunteers
Education	32% ≤12 years 36% 13–15 years 32% ≥16 years
Gender	45% Male 55% Female
Race/ethnicity	Not reported
Screening	Examinees excluded with a positive history of psychiatric hospitalization, chronic polysubstance abuse, or neurological disorder.

SOURCE: Adapted from Ruff (1996). Reproduced by special permission of the Publisher, Psychological Assessment Resources, Inc. (PAR), 16204 North Florida Avenue, Lutz, Florida 33549, from the Ruff Figural Fluency Test by Ronald M. Ruff, PhD Copyright 1988, 1996, by PAR. Further reproduction is prohibited without permission of PAR.

TABLE 9–87 Characteristics of Izaks et al. (2011b) Ruff Figural Fluency Test (RFFT) Normative Sample

Sample size	1,651
Age	35 to 82 years (mean = 54)
Female	53%
Ethnicity	96% Western-European descent
Education	37% ≤ Grade 12 63% > Grade 12

Woods, Wyma, Herron, and Yund (2016) compared normative data from various sources for the RFFT, noting some discrepancies across samples in terms of Unique Designs completed per minute and percent of repetitions (see Table 9–92). The reasons for the discrepancy are unclear and may reflect cultural differences or variability in test instruction, administration, and scoring procedures followed. Of note, the characteristics of the samples were quite different across groups which may have also contributed to variability.

EVIDENCE FOR RELIABILITY

EVIDENCE FOR TEST-RETEST RELIABILITY, MEASURING CHANGE, AND PRACTICE EFFECTS

Test-retest reliability is relatively strong for number of Unique Designs, and lower for other scores. In healthy individuals, the test-retest reliability coefficient for the total number of Unique Designs is adequate to high over intervals of three weeks to 12 months (*rs* = .71 to .88; Basso et al., 1999; Demakis, 1999; Ross et al., 2003; Ross, 2014; Ruff et al., 1987). The reliability coefficients for the number of Perseverative Errors and Ratio Score, however, are modest (*rs* = .36 to .64; Basso et al., 1999; Ross, 2014; Ross et al., 2003; Ruff et al., 1987). Strategy scores have acceptable reliability coefficients ($r \geq .70$), with the exception of the mean cluster size ($r = .51$; Ross et al., 2003).

There are significant practice effects on the test. With relatively short intervals (about three weeks), university students show a gain of about 17 designs (Demakis, 1999). Following retest intervals of one to six months, healthy individuals tend to increase the number of Unique Designs by about eight designs, although there tends to be no commensurate increase in Perseverations (Ross et al., 2003; Ruff et al., 1987). Similarly, over longer retest intervals (12 months), healthy adults produce more Unique Designs (approximately seven more designs; Basso et al., 1999).

Van Eersel et al. (2015) report that in a large sample (n = 2,515) of individuals aged 35 to 82 years tested three times over a span of six years, the number of Unique Designs showed improvements of six points from first to second session and four points from second to third sessions. Perseverations also increased, but to a smaller degree (e.g., only one point across the time period). The increase in Unique Designs and Perseverations interacted with age, such that the mean difference in number of Unique Designs from the initial to third measurement point was 16 in 35- to 39-year-olds, with a decrease of one design on average in persons 75 years and older. See also "Normative Data."

Basso et al. (1999) used reliable change methodology to estimate the range of change in T scores that might be expected while accounting for measurement error and practice effects. Table 9–93 shows the mean estimated true scores at 12 months together with the standard error of prediction (SE_p) and resulting 90% CI. Note the large range of retest scores that may fall within the 90% CI. An examinee could increase or decrease performance by as much as 10 T-score units without displaying meaningful changes in performance. In this sample of community-dwelling healthy men, no individual obtained a score that reflected significant improvement or decline. To use the CIs, the 90%

TABLE 9–88 Normative Data for the Ruff Figural Fluency Test (RFFT) by Age and Education (≤12 Years of Education)

	AGE (YEARS)								
PERCENTILE	35–39 N = 12	40–44 N = 48	45–49 N = 71	50–54 N = 95	55–59 N = 95	60–64 N = 75	65–69 N = 85	70–74 N = 75	≥75 N = 53
10	–[a]	40	41	34	33	29	25	24	23
20	–	49	47	43	42	32	30	30	29
30	–	52	53	51	45	39	35	39	33
40	–	55	60	57	51	42	40	43	36
50	–	65	65	62	54	46	43	45	40
60	–	74	76	67	59	50	45	48	45
70	–	81	84	71	65	54	49	52	52
80	–	88	90	78	72	67	56	57	53
90	–	101	102	88	80	75	70	66	68

[a]Not calculated because of the small number of persons.

SOURCE: Izaks et al. (2011b).

TABLE 9-89 Normative Data for the Ruff Figural Fluency Test (RFFT) by Age and Education (>12 Years of Education)

	AGE (YEARS)								
PERCENTILE	35–39 N = 144	40–44 N = 161	45–49 N = 180	50–54 N = 191	55–59 N = 164	60–64 N = 74	65–69 N = 46	70–74 N = 44	≥75 N = 38
10	57	50	57	52	47	42	44	36	25
20	71	67	66	62	52	49	48	43	38
30	82	76	73	69	60	62	52	45	43
40	86	82	78	75	65	66	57	52	47
50	93	86	83	82	72	70	59	57	52
60	98	91	88	88	79	75	63	65	57
70	104	96	94	95	85	81	65	71	59
80	111	104	102	102	90	85	80	76	63
90	121	114	111	110	102	94	93	83	79

SOURCE: Izaks et al. (2011b).

confidence band should be summed with an individual's estimated true score

$$(Y_{TRUE} = M + r[Y_{OBS} - M])$$

where M is the sample mean of the test and Y_{OBS} is the actual score obtained by the individual.

Significant changes reflect the frequency of obtained scores that fall above or below the CI.

EVIDENCE FOR INTERRATER RELIABILITY

Interrater reliability is generally strong. For example, in a sample of 102 healthy undergraduates, Ross (2014) reported ICCs ranging from .84 (Error Ratio) to .98 (Unique Designs), with most coefficients exceeding .90. In another university sample, Ross et al. (1996, 2003) reported high interrater reliability for quantitative (*rs* = .80 to .98) and qualitative scores (*rs* = .79 to .95). However, despite reporting excellent interrater reliability for Unique Designs (*r* = .93), Berning, Weed, and Aloia (1998) reported only adequate coefficients for Perseverative Errors (*r* = .74) and modest estimates for Error Ratio scores (*r* = .66). Similarly, strong inter- and intrarater agreement has been reported for Unique Designs (≥95%), with somewhat lower, but still high, coefficients (≥85%) for qualitative variables (Murray, 2017). A novel computer scoring software program has been developed, which shows high reliability between computer and human raters (Elderson et al., 2016).

TABLE 9-90 Normative Data for the Ruff Figural Fluency Test (RFFT) by Age

PERFORMANCE ON THE RFFT	CONSECUTIVE MEASUREMENT (PERIOD) 1 (2003–2006)	2 (2006–2008)	3 (2008–2012)
Number of Unique Designs, mean (*SD*)			
35–39 years	91 (23)	102 (23)	107 (24)
40–44 years	83 (25)	92 (24)	98 (25)
45–49 years	80 (24)	86 (24)	93 (24)
50–54 years	75 (24)	79 (23)	84 (24)
55–59 years	68 (23)	74 (23)	77 (24)
60–64 years	63 (22)	66 (20)	67 (22)
65–69 years	55 (19)	57 (21)	57 (19)
70–74 years	50 (18)	52 (18)	52 (18)
≥75 years	50 (17)	53 (19)	49 (21)
All	73 (26)	79 (27)	83 (28)
Number of Perseverative Errors, median (interquartile range)			
35–39 years	6 (3–11)	8 (4–12)	9 (4–15)
40–44 years	7 (4–14)	9 (5–14)	10 (5–17)
45–49 years	7 (4–12)	8 (4–16)	8 (4–16)
50–54 years	7 (4–15)	7 (4–15)	9 (4–16)
55–59 years	7 (3–15)	7 (3–14)	7 (4–14)
60–64 years	7 (3–13)	8 (4–14)	9 (3–17)
65–69 years	7 (3–15)	7 (3–16)	7 (4–14)
70–74 years	6 (3–11)	7 (3–16)	5 (3–11)
≥75 years	8 (5–15)	6 (3–10)	7 (2–10)
All	7 (3–13)	7 (4–14)	8 (4–15)

SOURCE: van Eersel et al. (2015).

EVIDENCE FOR VALIDITY

WITHIN-TEST RELATIONSHIPS

Perseverative Errors and Error Ratio scores are highly correlated (*r* = .89); however, the number of Unique Designs shows only small correlations with the Error Ratio score (*r* = .24) and no relationship with the number of

TABLE 9-91 Normative Data for the Ruff Figural Fluency Test (RFFT) by Education

PERFORMANCE ON THE RFFT	CONSECUTIVE MEASUREMENT (PERIOD) 1 (2003–2006)	2 (2006–2008)	3 (2008–2012)
Number of Unique Designs, mean (*SD*)			
Primary school	51 (20)	56 (23)	56 (24)
Lower secondary education	61 (22)	66 (23)	70 (25)
Higher secondary education	73 (24)	79 (24)	83 (26)
University	85 (23)	92 (24)	96 (25)
Number of Perseverative Errors, median (interquartile range)			
Primary school	7 (3–15)	7 (3–15)	7 (3–15)
Lower secondary education	7 (3–15)	8 (4–16)	8 (4–17)
Higher secondary education	7 (4–14)	7 (4–14)	8 (4–15)
University	7 (4–12)	7 (4–14)	8 (4–15)

SOURCE: van Eersel et al. (2015).

TABLE 9–92 Comparison of Ruff Figural Fluency Test (RFFT) Normative Data

REFERENCE	*N*	MEAN AGE	YEARS OF EDUCATION	UNIQUE PATTERNS (UP)	*SD*	COEFFICIENT OF VARIATION	DURATION OF TEST (MINUTES)	UP/MIN	REPEATED PATTERNS (RPS)	% RPS
Ruff et al. 1978	358	44.30	14.40	93.67			5	18.73	9.01	8.77%
Izaks et al. 2011	1,651	54.00	13.00	70.00	26	37.14%	5	14.00	7.7	9.91%
Ross, 2014	102	21.70	14.00	93.72	21.62	23.07%	5	18.74	5.67	5.70%
van Eersel et al. 2015	2,515	53.00	14.00	73.00	26	34.93%	5	14.60	7	8.75%

NOTE: *SD*, standard deviation; UP/min, average unique patterns per minute; % RPs, percentage of total patterns that were repeated.

Perseverative Errors ($r = .06$; Ross et al., 2003; see also Ross, 2014, who found moderate correlations between Unique Designs and other variables but minimal correlations with Unique Designs and Error Ratio scores).

FACTOR-ANALYTIC STUDIES AND RELATIONSHIPS WITH OTHER TESTS

Factor-analytic studies suggest that the test involves a number of abilities, including motor planning, executive function, and intelligence. For example, Unique Designs loads on two factors: general intelligence (WAIS-R) and attention/speed (Ruff 2 & 7, Finger Tapping; Ruff, 1996, 1998). The Error Ratio loads on a planning factor (e.g., Rey-Osterrieth Complex Figure Test-Copy, Grooved Pegboard, WCST) and error scores load on a complex intelligence factor (WAIS-R) and a planning factor (Ruff-Light Trail Learning Test, Ruff 2 & 7). Kraybill and Suchy (2008) found that executive function tests (e.g., TMT-B, Push-Turn-Tap Task, and a motor sequencing fluency task) significantly contributed to performance.

The various figural fluency tasks are not interchangeable. Scores on the RFFT are modestly correlated with those of other figural fluency tasks (Demakis & Harrison, 1997). Performance on the RFFT is less consistently related to phonemic fluency (COWA Test; Demakis & Harrison, 1997; Fama et al., 1998; Ruff et al., 1987) than semantic fluency (Fama et al., 1998), although even with the latter task, the coefficients tend to vary in size (*rs* = .28 to .67; Fama et al., 1998). In summary, the RFFT and verbal fluency tasks measure both similar and unique components. For example, structural equation analyses indicate that phonemic fluency is more closely related to speed and vocabulary abilities, whereas the RFFT is more closely related to fluid intelligence and speed abilities (Salthouse et al., 2003).

Unique Designs is moderately related to a number of executive function measures, including Stroop, TMT, Tower of Hanoi, the WCST (*rs* = .20 to .41, Ross, 2014), and the D-KEFS Tower Test ($r = .30$, Gardner et al., 2013). Strategy scores are similarly moderately related to the D-KEFS Tower Test (Gardner et al., 2013) and the Self-Ordered Pointing Test (Ross et al., 2007). In a sample of individuals with cardiovascular disease, the RFFT correlated moderately with other attention and executive function tests ($r = .34$ to .46, Jefferson et al., 2006). Similarly, moderate to large correlations were found between RFFT variables and attention and executive measures in patients with right or left hemisphere lesions, although the magnitude and pattern of correlations differed somewhat between groups (see Murray, 2017).

RFFT scores are moderately correlated with measures of general cognitive status (*rs* = .38 to .57) such as the Performance IQ of the WAIS-R (Ruff et al., 1987), Block Design (Ross, 2014), the WAIS-III Similarities (Woo et al., 2010), the MMSE (Fama et al., 1998, 2000; Woo et al., 2010), the Dementia Rating Scale (DRS; Woo et al., 2010), and the NART (Fama et al., 1998). The RFFT was modestly to moderately correlated with tasks from the Cogstate battery (Kuiper et al., 2017).

Reduced motor speed contributes to lower scores on the RFFT; however, it does not fully account for impaired performance (Fama et al., 1998; Milders et al., 2003; Ruff et al., 1987). Memory for temporal order also appears to

TABLE 9–93 Descriptive Statistics and Confidence Intervals for Ruff Figural Fluency Test (RFFT) Estimated True Scores at 12-Month Follow-Up

	M	R_{Y1Y2}	SE_P	90% CI	SIGNIFICANT INCREASES	SIGNIFICANT DECREASES
Unique Designs	58.66	.71	6.22	±10	0	0
Ratio Score	49.20	.39	7.64	±13	0	0

NOTE: Based on a sample of 50 community-dwelling healthy males, predominantly Caucasian, ranging in age from 20 to 59 (*M* = 32.5, *SD* = 9.27), with a mean education of 14.98 years (*SD* = 1.93).

SOURCE: From Basso et al. (1999).

be moderately associated with performance (Parkin et al., 1995). Correlations with language have also been reported (Murray, 2017).

CLINICAL STUDIES

The RFFT has been used in a number of studies with diverse clinical populations, with impairments noted in AD (Fama et al., 1998, 2000), PD (Fama et al., 1998), HIV (Basso & Bornstein, 2003), and substance use disorders (Fernández-Serrano, Pérez-García, Perales, & Verdejo-García, 2010; Oscar-Berman et al., 2009). Patients with moderate to severe TBI tend to produce fewer designs than controls but do not seem more likely to break the rules (Milders et al., 2003). Major depression has also been found to negatively impact test scores (Lugtenburg et al., 2017).

The RFFT has also been used in genetic studies. Izaks et al. (2011a) reported homozygous APOE E4 carriers performed worse than heterozygous carriers and noncarriers. *CETP* I405V valine homozygosity (associated with lower risk of cognitive decline) was related to better performance (Izaks et al., 2012). Data regarding relationships between the RFFT and clinical and functional correlates are limited, but test performance shows no significant correlation with ADLs in patients with cardiovascular disease (Jefferson et al., 2006).

Associations of performance on the RFFT with hemispheric laterality are not clear. Ruff et al. (1994) reported that the test accurately classified 60% of right-frontal cases and 96% of non–right frontal cases. Foster, Williamson, and Harrison (2005) reported that healthy university students who perform poorly exhibit heightened right frontal delta magnitude compared with those who perform well. Unfortunately, left-sided activity was not measured in this study nor was activity at other brain sites (e.g., posterior). Jaywant, Musto, Neargarder, Gilbert, and Cronin-Golomb (2014) reported that patients with PD with left-sided onset of tremor generated more Unique Designs than patients with tremor of right-sided onset.

Some research has reported that fluency performance tends to be affected more by anterior than posterior cerebral involvement (Ruff et al., 1994; Suchy et al., 2003). However, classification accuracy is relatively modest (67% hit rate in patients with frontal compared to temporal seizure foci). Persons with aphasia and those with right-hemisphere lesions perform worse than controls, with qualitative differences in approach noted between persons with right-hemisphere lesions and controls (Murray, 2017). Patients with mesial temporal lobe epilepsy are impaired relative to patients with lateral temporal lobe epilepsy, potentially suggesting a role for the hippocampus and medial temporal lobe structures in performance (Zalonis et al., 2017). See also "Neuroanatomical Correlates and Imaging Studies."

NEUROANATOMICAL CORRELATES AND IMAGING STUDIES

Neuroimaging studies have generally implicated right frontal regions in performance. In a study of patients with AD, Woo et al. (2010) reported that low metabolic rate in right temporal and right parietal lobes was related to performance. Heightened right frontal delta magnitude (an index of abnormality) was found in a group of individuals who performed more poorly compared to a group who performed well (Foster et al., 2005). Repetitive transcranial magnetic stimulation over the right dorsolateral prefrontal cortex does not affect performance on the RFFT or other executive measures (Schaller et al., 2013).

Others, however, have reported no association between laterality and performance (Fama et al., 2000; Suchy et al., 2003). For example, in patients with AD, fluency was selectively associated with bilateral frontal gray matter volumes, suggesting that both regions contribute to the generation of nonverbal exemplars (Fama et al., 2000). Similarly, Suchy et al. (2003) reported that the RFFT was sensitive to both left and right frontal impairment in patients with epilepsy.

PERFORMANCE VALIDITY

There are few studies on this question. Unsurprisingly, individuals instructed to simulate symptoms of TBI tend to depress their performance on the test (Demakis, 1999).

COMMENT

The RFFT includes five conditions designed to vary in level of difficulty (e.g., through the use of different levels of interfering stimuli). The basic scores calculated are the number of Unique Designs, Perseverative Errors, and an Error Ratio derived from Perseverative Errors and Unique Designs. A number of qualitative scores have also been devised (see "Scoring"). Although there are five different conditions, the total score alone is typically interpreted.

Demographically, age and education appear influential. Gender effects are not found. There may be ethnicity and linguistic effects, although more research is needed in this regard. Although original standardization data are based on a relatively large sample and stratified by age and education, the data are more than 20 years old. Izaks et al. (2011b) have presented age- and education-based normative data on a sample of more than 1,600 healthy participants. The strengths of this dataset are its recency, large size, and stratification by relevant demographic variables. Users should note, however, that stringent participant exclusion criteria are absent and that the number of Unique Designs was overall lower than in the US standardization sample.

Like other figural fluency tests (e.g., the Five-Point Test, see review elsewhere in this chapter), Unique Designs tends to be associated with stronger reliability than other scores.

Interrater reliability is generally high for most variables. Large practice effects are reported on this test, especially for young adults, and use of reliable change calculations may be of value on repeat assessments. Note, however, that the sample these are based on is predominantly Caucasian, male, young, and relatively well-educated. Therefore, these data may not be generalizable to dissimilar groups (e.g., older, low education levels).

Like other figural fluency tasks, the RFFT is related to a number of abilities. The RFFT is moderately correlated with other fluency tasks, executive tasks, and general cognition and IQ. There does not appear to be a coherent body of clinical research involving the RFFT. Neuroimaging and clinical studies, however, provide some evidence to suggest that right frontal regions are important for performance on the test (although note mixed findings). There are limited data regarding performance validity.

REFERENCES

Agranovich, A., & Puente, A. (2007). Do Russian and American normal adults perform similarly on neuropsychological tests? Preliminary findings on the relationship between culture and test performance. *Archives of Clinical Neuropsychology, 22*(3), 273–282. http://doi.org/10.1016/j.acn.2007.01.003

Agranovich, A. V., Panter, A. T., Puente, A. E., & Touradji, P. (2011). The culture of time in neuropsychological assessment: Exploring the effects of culture-specific time attitudes on timed test performance in Russian and American samples. *Journal of the International Neuropsychological Society, 17*(04), 692–701. http://doi.org/10.1017/S1355617711000592

Basso, M. R., & Bornstein, R. A. (2003). Effects of past noninjection drug abuse upon executive function and working memory in HIV infection. *Journal of Clinical and Experimental Neuropsychology, 25*, 893–903.

Basso, M. R., Bornstein, R. A., & Lang, J. M. (1999). Practice effects on commonly used measures of executive function across twelve months. *The Clinical Neuropsychologist, 13*, 283–292.

Berning, L. C., Weed, N. C., & Aloia, M. S. (1998). Interrater reliability of the Ruff Figural Fluency Test. *Assessment, 5*, 181–186.

Delis, D. C., Kaplan, E., & Kramer, J. H. (2001). *Delis-Kaplan Executive Function System.* San Antonio, TX: The Psychological Corporation.

Demakis, G. J. (1999). Serial malingering on verbal and nonverbal fluency and memory measures: An analog investigation. *Archives of Clinical Neuropsychology, 14*, 401–410.

Demakis, G. J., & Harrison, D. W. (1997). Relationships between verbal and nonverbal fluency measures: Implications for assessment of executive functioning. *Psychological Reports, 81*, 443–448.

Elderson, M. F., Pham, S., van Eersel, M. E. A., LifeLines Cohort Study, Wolffenbuttel, B. H. R., Kok, J., . . . Izaks, G. J. (2016). Agreement between computerized and human assessment of performance on the Ruff Figural Fluency Test. *PLOS ONE, 11*(9), e0163286. https://doi.org/10.1371/journal.pone.0163286

Fama, R., Sullivan, E. V., Shear, P. K., Cahn-Weiner, D. A., Marsh, L., Lim, K. O., Yesavage, J. A., & Tinklenberg, J. R. (2000). Structural brain correlates of verbal and nonverbal fluency measures in Alzheimer's disease. *Neuropsychology, 14*, 29–40.

Fama, R., Sullivan, E. V., Shear, P. K., Cahn-Weiner, D. A., Yesavage, J. A., Tinklenberg, J. R, & Pfefferbaum, A. (1998). Fluency performance patterns in Alzheimer's disease and Parkinson's disease. *The Clinical Neuropsychologist, 12*, 487–499.

Fernández-Serrano, M. J., Pérez-García, M., Perales, J. C., & Verdejo-García, A. (2010). Prevalence of executive dysfunction in cocaine, heroin and alcohol users enrolled in therapeutic communities. *European Journal of Pharmacology, 626*(1), 104–112. http://doi.org/10.1016/j.ejphar.2009.10.019

Festman, J., Rodriguez-Fornells, A., & Münte, T. F. (2010). Individual differences in control of language interference in late bilinguals are mainly related to general executive abilities. *Behavioral and Brain Functions, 6*(1), 1.

Foster, P. S., Williamson, J. B., & Harrison, D. W. (2005). The Ruff Figural Fluency Test: Heightened right frontal lobe delta activity as a function of performance. *Archives of Clinical Neuropsychology, 20*, 427–434.

Gardner, E., Vik, P., & Dasher, N. (2013). Strategy use on the Ruff Figural Fluency Test. *The Clinical Neuropsychologist, 27*(3), 470–484. http://doi.org/10.1080/13854046.2013.771216

Izaks, G. J., Gansevoort, R. T., van der Knaap, A. M., Navis, G., Dullaart, R. P. F., & Slaets, J. P. J. (2011a). The association of APOE genotype with cognitive function in persons aged 35 years or older. *PloS One, 6*(11), e27415. http://doi.org/10.1371/journal.pone.0027415

Izaks, G. J., Joosten, H., Koerts, J., Gansevoort, R. T., & Slaets, J. P. (2011b). Reference data for the Ruff Figural Fluency Test stratified by age and educational level. *PloS One, 6*(2), e17045. http://doi.org/10.1371/journal.pone.0017045

Izaks, G. J., van der Knaap, A. M., Gansevoort, R. T., Navis, G., Slaets, J. P. J., & Dullaart, R. P. F. (2012). Cholesteryl Ester Transfer Protein (CETP) genotype and cognitive function in persons aged 35 years or older. *Neurobiology of Aging, 33*(8), 1851.e7–1851.e16. http://doi.org/10.1016/j.neurobiolaging.2012.02.022

Jaywant, A., Musto, G., Neargarder, S., Stavitsky Gilbert, K., & Cronin-Golomb, A. (2014). The effect of Parkinson's disease subgroups on verbal and nonverbal fluency. *Journal of Clinical and Experimental Neuropsychology, 36*(3), 278–289. http://doi.org/10.1080/13803395.2014.889089

Jefferson, A., Paul, R., Ozonoff, A., & Cohen, R. (2006). Evaluating elements of executive functioning as predictors of instrumental activities of daily living (IADLs). *Archives of Clinical Neuropsychology, 21*(4), 311–320. http://doi.org/10.1016/j.acn.2006.03.007

Jones-Gotman, M. (1991). Localization of lesions by neuropsychological testing. *Epilepsia, 32*, S41–S52.

Jones-Gotman, M., & Milner, B. (1977). Design fluency: The invention of nonsense drawings after focal cortical lesions. *Neuropsychologia, 15*, 653–674.

Kraybill, M. L., & Suchy, Y. (2008). Evaluating the role of motor regulation in figural fluency: Partialing variance in the Ruff Figural Fluency Test. *Journal of Clinical and Experimental Neuropsychology, 30*(8), 903–912. http://doi.org/10.1080/13803390701874361

Kuiper, J. S., Oude Voshaar, R. C., Verhoeven, F. E. A., Zuidema, S. U., & Smidt, N. (2017). Comparison of cognitive functioning as measured by the Ruff Figural Fluency Test and the CogState computerized battery within the LifeLines Cohort Study. *BMC Psychology, 5*(1). https://doi.org/10.1186/s40359-017-0185-0

Lugtenburg, A., Oude Voshaar, R. C., Van Zelst, W., Schoevers, R. A., Enriquez-Geppert, S., & Zuidersma, M. (2017). The relationship between depression and executive function and the impact of vascular disease burden in younger and older adults. *Age and Ageing, 46*(4), 697–701. https://doi.org/10.1093/ageing/afx043

Milders, M., Fuchs, S., & Crawford, J. R. (2003). Neuropsychological impairments and changes in emotional and social behavior following severe traumatic brain injury. *Journal of Clinical and Experimental Neuropsychology, 25*, 157–172.

Murray, L. L. (2017). Design fluency subsequent to onset of aphasia: A distinct pattern of executive function difficulties? *Aphasiology, 31*(7), 793–818. https://doi.org/10.1080/02687038.2016.1261248

Oscar-Berman, M., Valmas, M. M., Sawyer, K. S., et al. (2009). Frontal brain dysfunction in alcoholism with and without antisocial personality disorder. *Neuropsychiatr Dis Treat, 5,* 309–326. doi:10.2147/ndt.s4882

Parkin, A. J., Walter, B. M., & Hunkin, N. M. (1995). Relationship between normal aging, frontal lobe function, and memory for temporal and spatial information. *Neuropsychology, 9,* 304–312.

Regard, M., Strauss, E., & Knapp, P. (1982). Children's production of verbal and nonverbal fluency tasks. *Perceptual and Motor Skills, 55,* 839–844.

Ross, T., Hanouskova, E., Giarla, K., Calhoun, E., & Tucker, M. (2007). The reliability and validity of the self-ordered pointing task. *Archives of Clinical Neuropsychology, 22*(4), 449–458. http://doi.org/10.1016/j.acn.2007.01.023

Ross, T. P. (2014). The reliability and convergent and divergent validity of the Ruff Figural Fluency Test in healthy young adults. *Archives of Clinical Neuropsychology, 29*(8), 806–817. http://doi.org/10.1093/arclin/acu052

Ross, T. P., Foard, E. L., Hiott, F. B., & Vincent, A. (2003). The reliability of production strategy scores for the Ruff Figural Fluency Test. *Archives of Clinical Neuropsychology, 18,* 879–891.

Ruff, R. (1996, 1998). *Ruff Figural Fluency Test.* Odessa, FL: PAR.

Ruff, R. M., Allen, C. C., Farrow, C. E., Niemann, H., & Wylie, T. (1994). Figural fluency: Differential impairment in patients with left versus right frontal lobe lesions. *Archives of Clinical Neuropsychology, 9,* 41–45.

Ruff, R. M., Light, R., & Evans, R. (1987). The Ruff Figural Fluency Test: A normative study with adults. *Developmental Neuropsychology, 3,* 37–51.

Russell, E. W., & Starkey, R. I. (1993, 2001). *Halstead Russell Neuropsychological Evaluation System (HRNES-R).* Los Angeles: Western Psychological Services.

Salthouse, T. A., Atkinson, T. M., & Berish, D. E. (2003). Executive functioning as a potential mediator of age-related cognitive decline in normal adults. *Journal of Experimental Psychology: General, 132,* 566–594.

Schaller, G., Lenz, B., Friedrich, K., Dygon, D., Richter-Schmidinger, T., Sperling, W., & Kornhuber, J. (2013). No evidence for effects of a high-frequency repetitive transcranial magnetic stimulation series on verbal and figural fluency and tap task performance in healthy male volunteers. *Neuropsychobiology, 67*(2), 69–73. https://doi.org/10.1159/000343502

Suchy, Y., Sands, K., & Chelune, G. J. (2003). Verbal and nonverbal fluency performance before and after surgery. *Journal of Clinical and Experimental Neuropsychology, 25,* 190–200.

van Eersel, M. E., Joosten, H., Koerts, J., Gansevoort, R. T., Slaets, J. P., & Izaks, G. J. (2015). Longitudinal study of performance on the Ruff Figural Fluency Test in persons aged 35 years or older. *PloS One, 10*(3), e0121411.

Woo, B. K. P., Harwood, D. G., Melrose, R. J., Mandelkern, M. A., Campa, O. M., Walston, A., & Sultzer, D. L. (2010). Executive deficits and regional brain metabolism in Alzheimer's disease. *International Journal of Geriatric Psychiatry, 25*(11), 1150–1158. http://doi.org/10.1002/gps.2452

Woods, D. L., Wyma, J. M., Herron, T. J., & Yund, E. W. (2016). A computerized test of design fluency. *PloS One, 11*(5), e0153952.

Zalonis, I., Christidi, F., Artemiadis, A., Psarros, C., Papadopoulos, G., Tsivgoulis, G., . . . Karavasilis, E. (2017). Verbal and figural fluency in temporal lobe epilepsy: Does hippocampal sclerosis affect performance? *Cognitive and Behavioral Neurology, 30*(2), 48–56.

STROOP TEST (STROOP)

TEST NAME	**Stroop Test (Stroop)**
DOMAIN	Executive functioning
AGE RANGE	Up to 96 years
ADMINISTRATION TIME	5 to 15 minutes, depending on version
SCORING FORMAT	Hand scored or computerized
REFERENCES	Comalli Jr., P. E., Wapner, S., & Werner, H. (1962). Interference effects of Stroop Color-Word Test in childhood, adulthood and aging. *Journal of Genetic Psychology, 100*, 47–53. Delis, D. C., Kaplan, E., & Kramer, J. H. (2001). *Delis-Kaplan Executive Function System*. San Antonio, TX: The Psychological Corporation. Golden, C. J. (1976). Identification of brain disorders by the Stroop Color and Word Test. *Journal of Clinical Psychology, 32*, 654–658. Golden, C. J. (1978). *Stroop Color and Word Test: A manual for clinical and experimental uses*. Chicago, IL: Stoelting Co. Golden, C. J., & Freshwater, S. M. (2002). *Stroop Color and Word Test: Revised examiner's manual*. Wood Dale, IL: Stoelting Co. Spreen, O., & Strauss, E. (1998). *A compendium of neuropsychological tests: Administration, norms, and commentary*. Oxford University Press. Stroop, J. R. (1935). Studies of interference in serial verbal reaction. *Journal of Experimental Psychology, 18*, 643–662.

DESCRIPTION

The Stroop is an executive functioning test with inhibitory demands that assesses the ease with which an examinee can maintain a goal in mind and suppress a habitual response in favor of a less familiar one. This measure of selective attention and cognitive flexibility was originally developed by Stroop (1935), although the paradigm dates back to the work of Cattell in the late 1800s (Mitrushina et al., 2005).

Stroop's original version consists of three white cards, each containing 10 rows of five items. There are four parts to the test. In Part 1, the examinee reads randomized color names (blue, green, red, brown, purple) printed in black type. In Part 2, the examinee reads the color names (blue, green, red, brown, purple) printed in colored ink (blue, green, red, yellow), ignoring the color of the print (the print color never corresponds to the color name). In Part 3, the examinee names the color of squares (blue, green, red, brown, purple). In Part 4, the examinee is given the card used in Part 2, but this time, the task is to name the color in which the color names are printed and disregard their word content.

The primary variable of interest is performance when presented with colored words printed in nonmatching colored ink (i.e., the interference trial). Stroop reported that healthy people can read color words printed in colored ink as quickly as when the words are presented in black ink (Part 2 vs. Part 1). However, the time to complete the task increases significantly when the examinee is asked to name the color of the ink rather than read the word (Part 4 vs. Part 3). This decrease in color naming speed is called the "color-word interference effect."

A number of versions of the Stroop have been developed or are incorporated into multiple computerized assessment batteries, such as the CNS Vital Signs (see review elsewhere in this volume). Tests differ along various dimensions, including the number of conditions (e.g., see D-KEFS version, Delis et al., 2001; Graf et al., 1995; Trenerry et al., 1989), use of stimuli (e.g., colored patches/dots vs. colored X's, see Comalli version, Comalli et al., 1962; Victoria version, Regard, 1981; D-KEFS version, Delis et al., 2001; compared to Golden, 1978 and Graf et al., 1995 versions), the number of items in each condition (e.g., 24 per card on the Victoria version, 50 items on the D-KEFS version, Delis et al., 2001; 100 items on the Golden and Comalli versions), and the number of colors used (e.g., three in the versions by Comalli, Delis et al., Golden, and Graf et al.; four in the Victoria version; and five in the original form used by Stroop).

STROOP COLOR AND WORD TEST (GOLDEN)

The Golden version (Golden, 1978; Golden & Freshwater, 2002) is frequently used. It consists of a Word Page with 100 color words (red, green, blue) printed in black ink, a Color Page with 100 Xs printed in either red, green, or blue ink, and a Color-Word Page with 100 words from the first page (red, green, blue) printed in colors from the second page (the color and the word do not match). The examinee looks at each sheet and moves down the columns, reading words or naming the ink color as quickly as possible within a time limit (45 seconds). The test yields three scores based on the number of items completed on each of the three stimulus sheets. An interference score can also be calculated.

VICTORIA STROOP TEST (VST)

The Victoria version (Regard, 1981) has several advantages (Troyer et al., 2006). First, in contrast to other versions, which have a large number of items (i.e., ≥60) on each condition, the Victoria Stroop Test (VST) has only 24 items on each of three tasks (naming the color of dots, neutral words, and color words printed in contrasting colors). Thus, The VST may be beneficial in capturing difficulties with response inhibition because the examinee does not get extended practice with the task (see Klein et al., 1997). Second, scores that are relatively independent of cognitive speed can be evaluated, including an error score and an interference (ratio) score that corrects for generalized slowing. Third, a reasonable normative database is available (see later discussion). Finally, the VST is in the public domain, and users may make their own stimuli.

The VST consists of three cards, each containing six rows of four items. In Part D (Dots), the examinee is asked to name, as quickly as possible, the color of 24 dots printed in blue, green, red, or yellow. Each color is used six times, and the four colors are arranged in a pseudorandom order within the array, each color appearing once in each row. Unlike the original Stroop, Part W (Words) is similar to Part D, except that the dots are replaced by common words ("when," "hard," and "over"), printed in lowercase letters. The examinee is required to name the colors in which the stimuli are printed and to disregard their verbal content. Part C (Colors) is similar to Parts D and W, but in this condition the colored stimuli are the color names "blue, green, red, and yellow" printed in lowercase so that the print color never corresponds to the color name (e.g., "red" is written in blue ink). This latter task thus requires the examinee to inhibit an automatic reading response and to produce a more effortful color-naming response. The interference effect is determined by calculating the extra time required to name colors in the interference task in comparison to the time required to name colors in the control task.

COMALLI AND COMALLI-KAPLAN VERSION

This version (Comalli et al., 1962) consists of three cards, each containing 100 items (10 × 10). The first card contains the words red, blue, and green printed in black ink, randomly selected and arranged in 10 rows of 10 items each. The second card contains patches of the colors red, blue, and green randomly selected and presented in a 10 × 10 array. The third card contains color names printed in a discrepant ink color. Time to completion on each of the three conditions is used as the dependent variable. The Comalli-Kaplan modification requires that the color naming card be presented first and that errors be recorded. The rationale underlying this modification is that (a) individuals who are color blind can be quickly identified and (b) the procedure maximizes the interference effect by presenting the word-reading condition just prior to the interference task. Normative data are provided in Mitrushina et al. (2005).

DELIS-KAPLAN EXECUTIVE FUNCTION SYSTEM (D-KEFS) VERSION

The D-KEFS version (Delis et al., 2001) incorporates the Comalli-Kaplan modification; the D-KEFS is reviewed elsewhere in this chapter.

COMPUTERIZED VERSIONS

Although Stroop paradigms are commonly included in many computerized batteries (e.g., CNS Vital Signs, reviewed elsewhere in this volume), formats vary considerably across tests and validation of each version is not always available.

ADMINISTRATION

STROOP COLOR AND WORD TEST (GOLDEN)

See Source for administration instructions. For all trials, examinees are asked to complete the trials as quickly as possible. Errors are indicated by the examiner, cueing the examinee to correct the error and continue. After 45 seconds, the item last named on each stimulus sheet (trial) is noted. Errors are not counted.

VICTORIA STROOP TEST (VST)

In this version, the three cards are always presented as follows: Dots (Part D), Words (Part W), and Colors (Part C). The examinee is instructed to read or call out the color name as quickly as possible. The examiner starts the timer immediately after providing instructions (see Figure 9–10 for administration instructions).

The errors in color naming on each part are corrected by the examiner immediately and the examinee is then asked to continue as quickly as possible. The examiner notes the number of errors and time taken for each section.

Part D. "*Name the colors of the dots as quickly as you can. Begin here and go across the rows from left to right.*" Direct the examinee's eyes across the rows from left to right.

Part W. "*This time, name the colors of the words as quickly as you can. Begin here and go across the rows from left to right.*" Clarify, if necessary: "*Name the colors in which the words are printed.*"

Part C. "*Again, name the colors in which the words are printed as quickly as you can.*" Clarify if necessary: "*Don't read the word, tell me the color in which the word is printed.*"

Figure 9–10 Administration instructions for the Victoria Stroop Test.

INFLUENCES ON PERFORMANCE

A number of factors affect performance. For example, the medium of presentation may be influential. Patients with MS perform better on the paper-based version of the Golden compared with a computer-based version (Hughes et al., 2013). Time of testing (i.e., level of circadian arousal) may also impact the magnitude of the Stroop interference effect, particularly for older adults (see May & Hasher, 1998). In older adults, results may be confounded by age-related declines in visual acuity or color vision (see Anstey et al., 2000, 2002; Van Boxtel et al., 2001).

The degree of interference also depends on the examinee's familiarity with the stimuli and the semantic relatedness of the material (e.g., pictures vs. words; Graf et al., 1995). The degree of automaticity of the reading response is also a critical factor. Cox et al. (1997) recommend that interpretation of the interference score as a measure of response inhibition be restricted to those whose single-word reading skills are at least equal to their FSIQs. Average reading skills thus appear to be a minimal requirement for this test.

SCORING

STROOP COLOR AND WORD TEST (GOLDEN)

This version yields three scores: the Word reading (W) score consists of the number of items completed in 45 seconds on the first condition; the Color naming (C) score is made up of the number of items completed in 45 seconds on the second condition; and the Color-Word (CW) score is made up of the number of items completed on the third condition. An interference score is also calculated.

The scoring system for adults incorporates adjusted scores derived from the prediction of intact performance based on an examinee's age and years of education. Thus, predicted Word (W), Color (C), and Color-Word scores (CW) are determined from tables provided in the test manual. The age-/education-adjusted scores are then subtracted from the raw scores to yield a residual score for each measure. These residual scores are translated into T scores (M = 50, SD = 10) using another table. A derived score, the Color-Word minus predicted Color-Word score, is used as the measure of interference (interference T score). For the three basic scores, higher T scores reflect better performance. For the interference score, lower scores (a T score of ≤40) are generally indicative of problems.

Some conceptual challenges in the use of this version have been identified. Franzen (2000) cautions that there is insufficient information about the appropriateness or the size of the samples used in the derivation of these standardized scores (see also "Normative Data"). In addition, Chafetz and Matthews (2004) have questioned the theoretical model underlying Golden's interference score. They note that the interference score is based on the assumption that the brain *adds* word-reading to color-naming processes to produce the results on the CW card (i.e., the time to read a CW item is an additive function of the time to read a word plus the time to name a color). However, discussion of the Stroop effects in neuropsychology has not focused on addition, but rather on inhibition or suppression. Consistent with this notion, they propose a different interference score based on the notion that the time to read a CW item reflects the time to *suppress* the reading of a word plus the time to name a color.

VICTORIA STROOP TEST (VST)

For each part, the examiner records both the time to complete the task and the number of errors. Spontaneous corrections are scored as correct. Figure 9–11 shows a sample scoring sheet. Researchers have typically relied on a difference score, defined as the difference in the amount of time required for the interference card (e.g., Part C) versus the Color card (e.g., Part D; MacLeod, 1991). Graf et al. (1995) contend that a difference score is not independent of age-related slowing and recommend the use of a ratio index of interference (e.g., Part C/ Part D). Errors are found to be rare in control conditions compared with the interference condition (Bayard et al., 2011).

DEMOGRAPHIC EFFECTS

AGE

An age effect on the Stroop is consistently reported across samples internationally and across age groups (e.g., Andrews et al., 2012; Bayard et al., 2011; Bezdicek et al., 2015; Campanhalo et al., 2014; Kang et al., 2013; Llinas-Regla et al., 2013; Lubrini et al., 2014; Morrow, 2013; Oosthuizen & Phipps, 2012; Pavao Martins et al., 2013; Pena-Casanova et al., 2009; Seo et al., 2008; Troyer et al., 2006; van der Elst,

Name________________________________ Date ____________________

Age______________

Dots:

G	B	Y	R
Y	R	G	B
B	G	Y	R
B	Y	R	G
R	G	B	Y
Y	G	B	R

Colors:

G	B	Y	R
Y	R	G	B
B	G	Y	R
B	Y	R	G
R	G	B	Y
Y	G	B	R

Words:

G	B	Y	R
Y	R	G	B
B	G	Y	R
B	Y	R	G
R	G	B	Y
Y	G	B	R

	Time	*Errors*
Dots		
Colors		
Words		

Figure 9–11 *Sample score sheet for the Victoria Stroop Test.*

2006; Vogel et al., 2013; Zalonis et al., 2009; Zimmerman et al., 2015). Age accounts for 10 to 33% of the variance in performance on the interference score, and age and interference are moderately correlated (generally *rs* = –.40 to –.47; Bayard et al., 2011; Lubrini et al., 2014; Mitrushina et al., 2005; Morrow, 2013; Pena-Casanova et al., 2009; Troyer et al., 2006; van der Elst et al., 2006).

However, there is mixed evidence with respect to whether age-related decrements on the Stroop are specific to interference effects or are accounted for by underlying processes. Studies of aging and Stroop interference have been somewhat mixed (Troyer et al., 2006), with some suggesting processing speed is influential in age-related performance decline (e.g., Graf et al., 1995; Uttl & Graf, 1997) and others implicating color vision as the primary variable underlying age-related decline (e.g., Antsey et al., 2002). However, other research has suggested that age-related increases in the interference effect persist even after generalized slowing is considered (e.g., Troyer et al., 2006). Of note, increased errors also occur with age (Delis et al., 2001; Troyer et al., 2006), suggesting that age-related decrements on the Stroop task are related to cognitive processes (e.g., response inhibition) other than, or perhaps in addition to, generalized slowing.

GENDER

Gender differences on interference tend to be insignificant (Anstey et al., 2000; Campanholo et al., 2014; Golden & Freshwater, 2002; Morrow, 2013; Pavao Martins et al., 2013; Pena-Casanova et al., 2009; Troyer et al., 2006) or minimal (Lucas et al., 2005). However, note that a female advantage has also been reported in some research (Llinas-Regla et al.,

2013; Norman et al., 2011; Seo et al., 2008; van der Elst et al., 2006).

EDUCATION AND IQ

Education affects performance (e.g., Bayard et al., 2011; Bezdicek et al., 2015; Campanhalo et al., 2014; Foss et al., 2009; Kang et al., 2015; Llinas et al., 2013; Lubrini et al., 2014; Morrow, 2013; Pavao Martins et al., 2013; Pena-Casanova et al., 2009; Seo et al., 2008; Troyer et al., 2006; van der Elst et al., 2006; Vogel et al., 2013; Zalonis et al., 2009; Zimmerman et al., 2015). For example, Pena-Casanova et al. (2009) reported that education and the Stroop are moderately correlated (r = .42), with age accounting for 17 to 27% of variance, and Campanholo et al. (2014) also reported moderate correlations between education and Stroop conditions (rs = −.44 to −.53).

Of note, although education effects are generally found, other research has suggested a modest relation between Stroop interference and education (<.30; Anstey et al., 2000; Razani et al., 2007; Steinberg et al., 2005; Troyer et al., 2006; but see Mitrushina et al., 2005).

Effects of education on performance may interact with ethnicity (see also "Ethnicity, Nationality, and Linguistic Effects"). In African Americans, Moering, Schinka, Mortimer, and Graves (2004) found that education had the strongest effect on Stroop scores, accounting for 8 to 26% of the variance, followed by gender (<1% to 6%) and age (1 to 2%). However, Lucas et al. (2005) reported that in African-American participants both age and education each accounted for about 8 to 9% of the variance in performance on the interference trial. Reading ability, but not education, was significantly related to Golden Stroop performance in older African Americans (Schneider & Lichtenberg, 2011). When participants in the study were dichotomized into high versus low reading groups based on Wide Range Achievement Test (WRAT-3) performance, effect sizes were large.

Other interaction effects have been reported. In addition to those with higher education exhibiting better Stroop performance, Avila et al. (2009) reported that education and depression interacted, such that low level of education and high levels of depression exerted a negative influence of Stroop performance. Research suggests that age effects are particularly pronounced in low education groups (van der Elst et al., 2006).

Some research has reported that IQ shows a stronger relationship to test scores than education (Steinberg et al., 2005). Although correlations with years of education decrease as task complexity increases (reading color names versus naming incongruent ink colors), correlations with intelligence increase across these conditions (Steinberg et al., 2005). In general, the higher an individual's intelligence (particularly fluid intelligence) scores are, the less interference they are likely to experience (Shilling et al., 2002).

ETHNICITY, NATIONALITY, AND LINGUISTIC EFFECTS

The Stroop is used internationally and has been translated into Spanish, Cantonese (e.g., Artiola I Fortuny et al., 1999; Lee, 2003), and a number of other languages (see "Normative Data"). The test is frequently used in Europe (Maruta et al., 2011).

Research has suggested that African Americans obtain lower scores than Caucasians even when education is taken into account (Moering et al., 2004). See also "Education and IQ." Furthermore, Norman et al. (2011) reported that the effects of demographic factors, particularly age, were more pronounced for African-American participants compared to Caucasian participants. Age and education were related to interference in Caucasian participants, but age, education, and gender were related to most variables for African-American participants. The authors note that use of normative data that do not take into account the differential effect of sociodemographic factors on performance may overestimate impairment in African-American individuals.

Razani et al. (2007) reported that a sample of English-speaking Anglo Americans performed better on the Stroop than an ethnically diverse (Hispanic, Asian, Middle-Eastern descent) sample; the authors further reported that acculturation variables (e.g., scores on an acculturation scale, time educated outside of the United States, and degree of English language growing up) correlated moderately with Stroop performance.

Performance tends to be slower in bilinguals (Spanish-English) than in monolinguals, particularly on the Color Naming condition (Rosselli et al., 2002). Gasquoine, Croyle, Cavazos-Gonzalez, and Sandoval (2007) reported that significant effects of language on Stroop performance for English-dominant bilingual Hispanic Texans are found, with significantly better performance in the English version compared with the Spanish version. Buré-Reyes et al. (2013) reported no significant differences in performance on the Stroop test between Spanish-speaking individuals from four different countries.

NORMATIVE DATA

There are a number of normative datasets available (see Table 9–94). Most of the normative data presented in Table 9–94 are age- and education-adjusted, with many also adjusted for gender (e.g., Bezdicek et al., 2015; Llinas-Regla et al., 2013, Seo et al., 2008; van der Elst, 2006). Details are discussed later in this section.

In addition to the norms described in Table 9–94, other norms for specific groups are available. Andrews, Shuttleworth-Edwards, and Radloff (2012) provide norms for a sample of 33 Xhosa-speaking unskilled workers in South Africa with an educational level of Grade 11 or 12. Oosthuizen and Phipps (2011) provide normative data

TABLE 9–94 Summary of Stroop Normative Studies

REFERENCE	COUNTRY	SAMPLE SIZE	ADMINISTRATION/SCORING SYSTEM	AGE RANGE
Norman et al. (2011)	USA	143 Caucasian 103 African American	Golden	Caucasian 20–66 African American 20–69
Schneider (2011)	USA	86	Golden	56–91
Morrow (2013)	Canada	146	Golden	18–56
Llinas-Regla et al. (2013)	Spain	2,151	Golden	55–82
Lubrini et al. (2014)	Spain	258	Golden	15–80
Pena-Casanova et al. (2009)	Spain	344	Golden	50–90
Seo et al. (2008)	Korea	564	Golden	60–90
Campanholo et al. (2014)	Brazil	1,025	Victoria	18+
Bayard et al. (2011)	France	244	Victoria	50–94
Troyer et al. (2006)	Canada	272	Victoria	18–94
Martins et al. (2013)	Portugal	479	Stroop 1935 cited[a]	50–95
Zimmerman et al. (2015)	Brazil	158	Stroop 1935 with modification[b]	19–75
Van der elst et al. (2006)	Netherlands	1,788	Hammes 1973[c]	24–81
Kang et al. (2013)	USA	153	Kaplan	50–89
Vogel et al. (2013)	Denmark	100	Klein et al., 1997[d]	60–87
Bezdicek et al. (2015)	Czech Republic	539	Prague[e]	60–96
Zalonis et al. (2009)	Greece	605	Trennery	18–84

NOTE: References provided in alphabetical order by author.
[a]Version used was similar to Golden.
[b]Version used was similar to Golden.
[c]Version used was similar to Comalli.
[d]Version used was similar to Comalli (however, 40 items per trial).
[e]Modification of Victoria Stroop.

for a computerized Stroop (Bohnen et al. version) for 102 Setswana-speaking university students.

STROOP COLOR AND WORD TEST (GOLDEN)

North-American Normative Samples

Normative data from the standardization sample are based on a sample of individuals ranging from 15 to 90 years. However, the characteristics of the sample (e.g., sample size, gender distribution, and age groupings) are not clearly provided in the manual (see Table 9–95 for sample characteristics). Mitrushina et al. (2005) note that the norms presented in the 1978 manual were derived from data from Golden's own studies as well as from normative data provided by other sources (e.g., Stroop, 1935, Comalli et al., 1962). However, the procedures and formats used by others differed from Golden's (e.g., examinees completed the entire stimulus card rather than stopping at 45 seconds, used colored rectangles rather than colored Xs, used a wall chart presentation rather than a standard page presented in front of the examinee).

TABLE 9–95 Characteristics of the Stroop Adult Normative Sample Provided by Golden and Freshwater (2002)

Number	≥300
Age	15 to 90 years
Geographic location	Not reported
Sample type	Not reported
Education	2 to 20 years
Gender	Not reported
Ethnicity	Not reported
Screening	Not reported

Ivnik, Malek, Smith, and Tangalos (1996) provide normative data for the three conditions based on a sample of 356 Caucasian individuals of average IQ (MayoFSIQ = 106.2, *SD* = 14.0), 56 to 94 years of age as part of the Mayo's Older Americans Normative Studies (MOANS). Participants were independently functioning, community-dwelling persons who had been recently examined by a physician and who had no active neurological or psychiatric disorder with potential to affect cognition. Data are stratified by age using the midpoint interval technique. The data are shown in Tables 9–96 to 9–106. Education contributes minimally to test performance in this dataset (correlations <.30 between age and the three test trials). Nonetheless, a computational formula is also provided (Table 9–107) to derive age- and education-corrected scaled scores.

Some research has suggested that IQ is more strongly related to performance than education (see "Demographic Effects"). Steinberg et al. (2005) reanalyzed data from the MOANS and provided age- (≥55 years) and IQ-adjusted percentile equivalents of age-adjusted Stroop scores. All FSIQs are Mayo age-adjusted scores which are based on the WAIS-R, not the WAIS-III. Given the upward shift in scores with the passage of time (Flynn effect), use of the WAIS-R FSIQ rather than the WAIS-III might result in a given Stroop score appearing less favorable. The interested reader is referred to their article for the relevant tables.

TABLE 9–96 Stroop Golden Version: MOANS Scaled Scores for Persons Whose Ages Range from 56 to 62 Years

SCALED SCORES	RAW SCORES EARNED STROOP WORD	COLOR	COLOR-WORD	PERCENTILE RANGES
2	<60	<41	<17	<1
3	60–63	41–42	17–18	1
4	64–65	43–44	19–20	2
5	66–72	45–50	21–23	3–5
6	73–77	51–54	24–25	6–10
7	78–82	55–59	26–28	11–18
8	83–88	60–64	29–30	19–28
9	89–93	65–66	31–34	29–40
10	94–101	67–71	35–38	41–59
11	102–107	72–75	39–40	60–71
12	108–111	76–81	41–43	72–81
13	112–116	82–85	44–47	82–89
14	117–122	86–88	48–49	90–94
15	123–125	89–91	50–55	95–97
16	126–129	92–93	56–57	98
17	130–139	94–104	58–62	99
18	>139	>104	>62	>99
Type of score for each test	Correct Count	Correct Count	Correct Count	
Age range (years) used for each test's norms	56–66	56–66	56–66	
Normative sample size (*n*) for each test	160	160	160	

SOURCE: From Ivnik et al. (1996).

TABLE 9–97 Stroop Golden Version: MOANS Scaled Scores for Persons Whose Ages Range from 63 to 65 Years

SCALED SCORES	RAW SCORES EARNED STROOP WORD	COLOR	COLOR-WORD	PERCENTILE RANGES
2	<58	<39	<16	<1
3	58	39–40	16	1
4	59	41–43	17	2
5	60–68	44–48	18–21	3–5
6	69–76	49–53	22–23	6–10
7	77–81	54–58	24–26	11–18
8	82–86	59–61	27–29	19–28
9	87–91	62–64	30–32	29–40
10	92–98	65–70	33–36	41–59
11	99–103	71–73	37–39	60–71
12	104–109	74–80	40–42	72–81
13	110–115	81–82	43–45	82–89
14	116–122	83–86	46–48	90–94
15	123–125	87–89	49–51	95–97
16	126–127	90–92	52–54	98
17	128–132	93–104	55–62	99
18	>132	>104	>62	>99
Type of score for each test	Correct Count	Correct Count	Correct Count	
Age range (years) used for each test's norms	59–69	59–69	59–69	
Normative sample size (*n*) for each test	206	206	206	

SOURCE: From Ivnik et al. (1996).

Mitrushina et al. (2005) compiled six datasets comprising 490 adults, aged 25 to 74 years. Data for the word-reading and color-naming conditions were sparse and therefore were not analyzed. Metanorms are provided for the interference condition only.

Normative data for older African Americans are provided by Moering et al. (2004) and Lucas et al. (2005). The data by Lucas et al. (2005) are shown here given the somewhat larger normative sample (303 vs. 236), a somewhat wider age range (56 to 94 years vs. 60 to 84 years), and the availability of co-normed tests. Their data for Stroop raw scores are shown in Tables 9–108 and 9–109 and are based on a sample of 303 African-American community-dwelling participants from the Mayo Older African American Normative Studies (MOAANS) project in Jacksonville, Florida. Participants were predominantly female (75%), ranged in age from 56 to 94 years (M = 69.6, SD = 6.87), with education levels varying from 0 to 20 years (M = 12.2, SD = 3.48). Exclusion criteria included active neurological, psychiatric, or other conditions that might reasonably be expected to affect cognition. Table 9–108 presents the age-scaled scores and Table 9–109 provides the computational formula used to calculate age- and education-adjusted MOAANS scaled scores. The authors urge that their data be used with caution since the number of very old adults is somewhat small and they used a sample of convenience.

Norman et al. (2011) recruited 243 healthy individuals who were controls without HIV infection as part of a longitudinal HIV study in San Diego, California; distribution of ethnic groups matched the 2000 US Census and was used to generate normative data. Participants were excluded if they presented with a history of neurologic conditions, substance abuse, psychiatric disorders, or major medical conditions. A sample of Caucasian (n = 143) and African-American (n = 103) individuals was included. Caucasian participants were an average age of 37.6 years (SD = 12.3), 31% female, with an average education of 14.1 (SD = 2.4) years. African-American participants were an average age of 40.6 years (SD = 12.3), 50% female, with an average education of 13.8 (SD = 2.1) years. See Table 9–110 for normative data.

Morrow (2013) provides data for a sample of 146 community-dwelling Canadian adults. Participants completed the Golden Stroop and were excluded if they

TABLE 9–98 Stroop Golden Version: MOANS Scaled Scores for Persons Whose Ages Range from 66 to 68 Years

SCALED SCORES	RAW SCORES EARNED: STROOP WORD	COLOR	COLOR-WORD	PERCENTILE RANGES
2	<58	<32	<16	<1
3	58	32–40	16	1
4	59	41–42	17	2
5	60–68	43–47	18–21	3–5
6	69–74	48–51	22	6–10
7	75–80	52–57	23–26	11–18
8	81–85	58–59	27–29	19–28
9	86–91	60–63	30–31	29–40
10	92–97	64–69	32–35	41–59
11	98–103	70–72	36–38	60–71
12	104–109	73–78	39–42	72–81
13	110–115	79–81	43–44	82–89
14	116–122	82–85	45–47	90–94
15	123–125	86–87	48–50	95–97
16	126–127	88–90	51–52	98
17	128–131	91–104	53–60	99
18	>131	>104	>60	>99
Type of score for each test	Correct Count	Correct Count	Correct Count	
Age range (years) used for each test's norms	62–72	62–72	62–72	
Normative sample size (*N*) for each test	152	152	152	

SOURCE: From Ivnik et al. (1996).

TABLE 9–99 Stroop Golden Version: MOANS Scaled Scores for Persons Whose Ages Range from 69 to 71 Years

SCALED SCORES	RAW SCORES EARNED: STROOP WORD	COLOR	COLOR-WORD	PERCENTILE RANGES
2	<44	<24	<16	<1
3	44–46	24–30	16	1
4	47–50	31–41	17	2
5	51–59	42–45	18–19	3–5
6	60–71	46–48	20–21	6–10
7	72–79	49–52	22–24	11–18
8	80–83	53–57	25–27	19–28
9	84–87	58–60	28–29	29–40
10	88–94	61–65	30–32	41–59
11	95–98	66–71	33–35	60–71
12	99–103	72–76	36–39	72–81
13	104–111	77–81	40–44	82–89
14	112–120	82–85	45	90–94
15	121–125	86–87	46–50	95–97
16	126–127	88–90	51–52	98
17	128–131	91–104	53–60	99
18	>131	>104	>60	>99
Type of score for each test	Correct Count	Correct Count	Correct Count	
Age range (years) used for each test's norms	65–75	65–75	65–75	
Normative sample size (*N*) for each test	134	134	134	

SOURCE: From Ivnik et al. (1996).

presented with a history of neurologic conditions, psychiatric disorders, substance abuse, visual or auditory impairment, or major medical conditions. Participants were an average of 37.5 years old (*SD* = 10.9), 69% female, predominantly Caucasian (90%) with a mean education level of 14.3 (*SD* = 2.1), with a North American Adult Reading Test (NAART) score of 107.8 (*SD* = 7.4). The mean Stroop score was 45.4 ± 10.4 with a range of 21 to 85.

Spanish Normative Samples

Llinas-Regla et al. (2013) provide data for 2151 Catalan adults in Spain for the Golden Stroop. Participants were recruited through an ongoing study and excluded if they presented with visual, auditory, or motor disorders that could affect performance. The average age in the sample was 67.4 (*SD* = 8.2), 53% were female, with just over half presenting with low levels of education (56%; eight years or less), a quarter average levels (eight to 12 years), and the remainder above-average education levels. Approximately 73% of the sample spoke Catalan as their first language. Descriptive norms (by age and education) are provided in Table 9–111, with regression-based norms provided in their paper.

Lubrini et al. (2014) provide norms for the Golden Stroop for 258 Spanish adults, including a sample of healthy controls, people with schizophrenia, and people who had sustained a TBI. Healthy participants were an average age of 39.1 (*SD* = 18.4) years, 60% female, with a mean education level of 12.6 (*SD* = 3.7). Healthy controls were recruited from university classes, university staff, social organizations, hospitals, and healthcare centers. Exclusion criteria were the presence of medical complications, psychiatric conditions, substance abuse, or neurologic disease. The interested reader is referred to their study for additional details regarding demographic characteristic of the clinical sample. Normative data are provided in Table 9–112.

Pena-Casanova et al. (2009) provide normative data for 344 Spanish adults 50–90 years of age as part of the Spanish Multicenter Normative Studies (NEURONORMA project), a large project that presents co-normed data for neuropsychological tests. All participants were Caucasian and living in Spain, educated in Spanish, and enrolled between 2004 and 2007. Informants were also interviewed.

Participants were excluded if they were out of the age range of the study, did not live or function independently,

TABLE 9–100 Stroop Golden Version: MOANS Scaled Scores for Persons Whose Ages Range from 72 to 74 Years

	RAW SCORES EARNED			
	STROOP			
SCALED SCORES	WORD	COLOR	COLOR-WORD	PERCENTILE RANGES
2	<42	<24	<4	<1
3	42–45	24–30	4–6	1
4	46–48	31–39	7–15	2
5	49–56	40–41	16–17	3–5
6	57–63	42–44	18–20	6–10
7	64–76	45–49	21–22	11–18
8	77–81	50–53	23–26	19–28
9	82–85	54–58	27–28	29–40
10	86–93	59–63	29–31	41–59
11	94–96	64–67	32–33	60–71
12	97–100	68–71	34–36	72–81
13	101–105	72–74	37–40	82–89
14	106–111	75–80	41–44	90–94
15	112–115	81	45	95–97
16	116–122	82–84	46–49	98
17	123–130	85–90	50–52	99
18	>130	>90	>52	>99
Type of score for each test	Correct Count	Correct Count	Correct Count	
Age range (years) used for each test's norms	68–78	68–78	68–78	
Normative sample size (*n*) for each test	124	124	124	

SOURCE: Ivnik et al. (1996).

TABLE 9–101 Stroop Golden Version: MOANS Scaled Scores for Persons Whose Ages Range from 75 to 77 Years

	RAW SCORES EARNED			
	STROOP			
SCALED SCORES	WORD	COLOR	COLOR-WORD	PERCENTILE RANGES
2	<42	<23	<4	<1
3	42–45	23	4–6	1
4	46–48	24–26	7–13	2
5	49–54	27–39	14–15	3–5
6	55–63	40–43	16–17	6–10
7	64–72	44–48	18–21	11–18
8	73–80	49–51	22–25	19–28
9	81–84	52–55	26–27	29–40
10	85–91	56–60	28–30	41–59
11	92–96	61–65	31–32	60–71
12	97–98	66–70	33–34	72–81
13	99–105	71–73	35–38	82–89
14	106–110	74–80	39–42	90–94
15	111–115	81	43–45	95–97
16	116–122	82–84	—	98
17	123–130	85–90	46	99
18	>130	>90	>46	>99
Type of score for each test	Correct Count	Correct Count	Correct Count	
Age range (years) used for each test's norms	71–81	71–81	71–81	
Normative sample size (*n*) for each test	111	111	111	

SOURCE: Ivnik et al. (1996).

scored below a cutoff on the MMSE, had a neurologic disorder, scored below a cutoff on the Modified Ischemia Scale, presented with substance abuse, or had an unmanaged medical condition that could interfere with cognition (e.g., diabetes mellitus, hypothyroidism, B_{12} deficiency), a psychiatric condition, or sensory impairment. The sample was approximately 61% female; 21% of participants had 16 years or more of education, 20% had 12 to 15 years of education, and the remainder had fewer than 12 years of education. Age-adjusted data are shown in Tables 9–113 to 9–122. To calculate the education-adjusted score, find the appropriate column in Tables 9–123 to 9–125 that corresponds to the examinee's years of education, find the NSS_A, and refer to the corresponding $NSS_{A\&E}$.

KOREAN NORMATIVE SAMPLE

Seo et al. (2008) recruited 564 participants in Korea from a sample of older individuals participating in a community service program aimed at dementia diagnosis and care who completed the Golden Stroop. Inclusion criteria included: independent living, Consortium to Establish a Registry for Alzheimer's Disease (CERAD) cutoff score, and corroboration of cognitive and functional status by an informant. Exclusion criteria included the presence of a neurologic or neurodegenerative disorder, psychiatric condition, serious medical condition, or hearing or visual impairment. Participants were an average age of 70.7 years (*SD* = 6.1), 63% female, with a mean of 7.5 years education (*SD* = 44.9). Data are shown in Tables 9–126 to 9–128.

VICTORIA STROOP TEST

NORTH-AMERICAN NORMATIVE SAMPLES

Normative data using overlapping age groups are based on 272 healthy, community-dwelling adults aged 18 to 94 years of age living in Victoria, British Columbia, or Toronto, Ontario, Canada (64% females; mean education 13 years; Troyer et al., 2006). They were recruited from a university-based older adult participant pool, senior centers, and advertisements posted in the community and at the university. Participants were interviewed to screen for neurological disorders and psychiatric disorders that could affect cognitive functioning. All participants were fluent in English. Scaled scores and percentiles for time and error scores are shown in Tables 9–129 to 9–133.

TABLE 9–102 Stroop Golden Version: MOANS Scaled Scores for Persons Whose Ages Range from 78 to 80 Years

	RAW SCORES EARNED			
	STROOP			
SCALED SCORES	WORD	COLOR	COLOR-WORD	PERCENTILE RANGES
2	<41	<23	<4	<1
3	41–44	23	4–6	1
4	45–48	24–26	7–13	2
5	49–52	27–39	14	3–5
6	53–63	40–41	15	6–10
7	64–70	42–45	16–20	11–18
8	71–76	46–48	21–22	19–28
9	77–82	49–51	23–25	29–40
10	83–88	52–57	26–28	41–59
11	89–93	58–60	29	60–71
12	94–96	61–65	30–32	72–81
13	97–98	66–71	33–36	82–89
14	99–104	72–75	37–39	90–94
15	105	76–80	40–43	95–97
16	106–109	81	44	98
17	110–114	82	45	99
18	>114	>82	>45	>99
Type of score for each test	Correct Count	Correct Count	Correct Count	
Age range (years) used for each test's norms	74–84	74–84	74–84	
Normative sample size (*n*) for each test	88	88	88	

SOURCE: Ivnik et al. (1996).

TABLE 9–103 Stroop Golden Version: MOANS Scaled Scores for Persons Whose Ages Range from 81 to 83 Years

	RAW SCORES EARNED			
	STROOP			
SCALED SCORES	WORD	COLOR	COLOR-WORD	PERCENTILE RANGES
2	<41	<23	<4	<1
3	41–44	23	4	1
4	45–47	24–25	5–6	2
5	48–52	26–30	7–10	3–5
6	53–63	31–39	11–15	6–10
7	64–69	40–42	16	11–18
8	70–74	43–45	17–19	19–28
9	75–80	46–49	20–22	29–40
10	81–86	50–53	23–25	41–59
11	87–91	54–56	26–28	60–71
12	92–96	57–59	29–30	72–81
13	97–98	60–64	31–32	82–89
14	99–104	65–71	33–38	90–94
15	105	72–78	39–40	95–97
16	106–109	79–80	41–43	98
17	110–114	81	44	99
18	>114	>81	>44	>99
Type of score for each test	Correct Count	Correct Count	Correct Count	
Age range (years) used for each test's norms	>76	>76	>76	
Normative sample size (*n*) for each test	79	79	79	

SOURCE: Ivnik et al. (1996).

French Normative Sample

Regression-based norms are also available. Bayard et al. (2011) provide data for the Victoria Stroop based on a sample of 244 community-dwelling adults recruited from a participants pool and senior citizen associations in France. Participants were screened for neurological and psychiatric disorders, all had normal or corrected hearing and vision, and all had an MMSE score above the 10th percentile. The sample had a mean age of 65.83 (*SD* = 10.71), was 51% female, and all participants were native French speakers.

Brazilian Portuguese Normative Sample

Campanholo et al. (2014) adapted the Victoria version for use in Brazilian, Portuguese-speaking community-dwelling adults recruited via community associations, adult schools, senior care centers, and other sources. Participants were excluded if they presented with a history of neurologic or psychiatric disorders, psychotropic drug use, sensory or motor disorders, IQ lower than 80, MMSE scores below education-based cutoffs, or anxiety and depression cutoffs on a questionnaire. The sample was 67% female and had an average age of 41 (*SD* = 16.4), with 11.9 (*SD* = 5.6) years of education; average IQ was 103.2 (*SD* = 12.0). See Table 9–134.

Other Versions

Versions Similar to the Golden Version. Pavão Martins, Maruta, Freitas, and Mares (2013) provide norms for older Portuguese-speaking adults with low levels of education. The version of the Stroop used was similar in structure to the Golden. Participants were part of a longitudinal study regarding aging and cognition. The average age of the sample was 66.4 years, with a median education of seven years; 64% of the sample was female. Inclusion criteria were the absence of neurologic and neurodegenerative disease, psychiatric disorders, uncontrolled medical diseases, independent ADLs, and an MMSE cutoff.

Zimmerman et al. (2015) recruited community-dwelling Brazilian Portuguese speakers. The version used was similar to the Golden. Participants were excluded if they did not comprehend test instructions; presented with a history of neurologic conditions,

TABLE 9–104 Stroop Golden Version MOANS Scaled Scores for Persons Whose Ages Range from 84 to 86 Years

SCALED SCORES	RAW SCORES EARNED: STROOP WORD	COLOR	COLOR-WORD	PERCENTILE RANGES
2	<41	<23	<4	<1
3	41–44	23	4	1
4	45–47	24–25	5–6	2
5	48–52	26–30	7–10	3–5
6	53–63	31–39	11–15	6–10
7	64–69	40–42	16	11–18
8	70–74	43–45	17–19	19–28
9	75–80	46–49	20–22	29–40
10	81–86	50–53	23–25	41–59
11	87–91	54–56	26–28	60–71
12	92–96	57–59	29–30	72–81
13	97–98	60–64	31–32	82–89
14	99–104	65–71	33–38	90–94
15	105	72–78	39–40	95–97
16	106–109	79–80	41–43	98
17	110–114	81	44	99
18	>114	>81	>44	>99
Type of score for each test	Correct Count	Correct Count	Correct Count	
Age range (years) used for each test's norms	>76	>76	>76	
Normative sample size (*N*) for each test	79	79	79	

SOURCE: Ivnik et al. (1996).

TABLE 9–105 Stroop Golden Version MOANS Scaled Scores for Persons Whose Ages Range from 87 to 89 Years

SCALED SCORES	RAW SCORES EARNED: STROOP WORD	COLOR	COLOR-WORD	PERCENTILE RANGES
2	<41	<23	<4	<1
3	41–44	23	4	1
4	45–47	24–25	5–6	2
5	48–52	26–30	7–10	3–5
6	53–63	31–39	11–15	6–10
7	64–69	40–42	16	11–18
8	70–74	43–45	17–19	19–28
9	75–80	46–49	20–22	29–40
10	81–86	50–53	23–25	41–59
11	87–91	54–56	26–28	60–71
12	92–96	57–59	29–30	72–81
13	97–98	60–64	31–32	82–89
14	99–104	65–71	33–38	90–94
15	105	72–78	39–40	95–97
16	106–109	79–80	41–43	98
17	110–114	81	44	99
18	>114	>81	>44	>99
Type of score for each test	Correct Count	Correct Count	Correct Count	
Age range (years) used for each test's norms	>76	>76	>76	
Normative sample size (*n*) for each test	79	79	79	

SOURCE: Ivnik et al. (1996).

psychiatric disorders, or substance abuse; scored below an MMSE cutoff; or had difficulty with vision or hearing. Participants ranged in age from 19 to 75 years. Education level varied per age group, and there was an overall predominance of female participants. Normative data are provided in the paper.

Prague Stroop. Bezdicek et al. (2015) provide data for the Prague Stroop, a modification of the Victoria Stroop, for 539 Czech adults. Participants were community-dwelling older adults participating in an ongoing longitudinal project. Nonrandom quota sampling was used, with participants in each demographic category described in five-year age intervals and balanced for gender ratios and education levels. Participants were excluded if they presented with neurodegenerative or neurologic conditions, a history of substance abuse or psychiatric conditions, unstable medical disorders, uncorrected visual difficulties, or hearing difficulties. Participants were further excluded if they performed two standard deviations or lower within normative expectations on cognitive tests. A sample of participants with PD (see "Clinical Studies") was also included. Supplemental tables outlining normative data are available at (http://dx.doi.org/10.1080/13803395.2015.1057106) or from the author.

Kaplan Version. Kang et al. (2013) provide data for 153 older adults who were part of an ongoing longitudinal study in California. Participants were recruited from a Memory Disorders Clinic or the community. Exclusion criteria included scores of 1.5 standard deviations or lower on a neuropsychological test battery, MCI or dementia, neurologic condition, psychiatric disorder, systemic illness, or unstable medical condition with potential to impact cognition. Participants were a mean age of 70.2 years (SD = 8), and the sample was 42% female and predominantly Caucasian (92%), with a mean education level of 16.8 years (SD = 2.6). Age-adjusted data for the entire test and data for the first and second half of the test are presented in their paper.

Hammes Version. Van der Elst (2006) included Danish participants for the Hammes version of the Stroop who were participating in a longitudinal study regarding cognitive aging in the Netherlands. The version was similar to the Comalli. Participants were recruited after being seen by physicians in primary care. Individuals were excluded

TABLE 9-106 Stroop Golden Version MOANS Scaled Scores for Persons Whose Ages Range from 90 to 97 Years

	RAW SCORES EARNED			
	STROOP			
SCALED SCORES	WORD	COLOR	COLOR-WORD	PERCENTILE RANGES
2	<41	<23	<4	<1
3	41–44	23	4	1
4	45–47	24–25	5–6	2
5	48–52	26–30	7–10	3–5
6	53–63	31–39	11–15	6–10
7	64–69	40–42	16	11–18
8	70–74	43–45	17–19	19–28
9	75–80	46–49	20–22	29–40
10	81–86	50–53	23–25	41–59
11	87–91	54–56	26–28	60–71
12	92–96	57–59	29–30	72–81
13	97–98	60–64	31–32	82–89
14	99–104	65–71	33–38	90–94
15	105	72–78	39–40	95–97
16	106–109	79–80	41–43	98
17	110–114	81	44	99
18	>114	>81	>44	>99
Type of score for each test	Correct Count	Correct Count	Correct Count	
Age range (years) used for each test's norms	>76	>76	>76	
Normative sample size (*n*) for each test	79	79	79	

SOURCE: Ivnik et al. (1996).

who presented with neurologic or neurodegenerative conditions, medical conditions that could impact cognition, significant psychiatric conditions, substance abuse, MMSE cutoff, or greater than 20 errors on the third Stroop condition. Participants were a mean age of 51.41 years (*SD* = 16.37), 50% female, Caucasian and native Dutch speakers, with 36% with a low education level, 41% with average education levels (junior vocational), and 23% with high levels of education (senior or academic). Normative data are presented in their paper.

TABLE 9-107 Computational Formula for Age- and Education-Corrected Stroop Golden Version MOANS Scaled Scores

Age- and education-corrected MOANS scaled score = k (constant) + (W_1 × Age-MOANS Scaled Score) - (W_2 × number of years of formal schooling).
The specific values are:

STROOP	K	W_1	W_2
Word	3.47	1.10	0.34
Color	1.88	1.10	0.23
Color-Word	1.38	1.09	0.19

SOURCE: From Ivnik et al. (1996).

Klein et al. (1997) Version. Vogel et al. (2012) provide norms for 100 Danish older adults. The version was similar to the Comalli version, but it used 40 items per trial. Newspaper advertisements were the method of recruitment. Inclusion criteria were medical or psychiatric conditions, alcohol abuse, and MMSE and Addenbrooke's Cognitive Examination performance. Participants were average age of 71 years (*SD* = 6.4), were 56% female, and presented with an average of 11.9 (*SD* = 2.6) years of education. Normative data are presented in their paper.

Trenerry Version. Zalonis et al. (2009) provide normative data for the Trenerry version for 605 adults in Greece. Participants were excluded if they presented with a history of neurologic conditions, psychiatric conditions, substance abuse, major medical condition or treatment impacting cognition, and sensory limitations (e.g., visual disturbance, effortful verbal response, color blindness). In addition, an MMSE cutoff and TMT cutoff were used. Participants presented with a mean age of 53.72 years (*SD* = 16.27), a mean education of 11.69 years (*SD* = 3.64), and were 44% female. Normative data are provided in their paper.

EVIDENCE FOR RELIABILITY

EVIDENCE FOR INTERNAL RELIABILITY

Kang et al. (2013) reported strong split-half reliability (all conditions ≥.80). Oosthuizen and Phipps (2012) similarly reported strong reliability, with Cronbach's alpha exceeding .77 in each condition.

EVIDENCE FOR TEST-RETEST RELIABILITY, MEASURING CHANGE, AND PRACTICE EFFECTS

Across multiple versions, test-retest reliability coefficients are generally high, and practice effects are found (e.g., Delis et al., 2001; Dikmen et al., 1999; Graf et al., 1995; Trenerry et al., 1989). Reliabilities for the interference trial tend to be somewhat lower, in the adequate range.

Golden (1975) reported adequate to high test-retest reliabilities of *r* = .86 (Word), *r* = .82 (Color), and *r* = .73 (Color-Word). Similar correlations were reported at a two-week retest interval (Franzen et al., 1987) and a four-week retest interval (Seo et al., 2008), with values for the Word condition exceeding .83, the Color condition exceeding .74, and the Color-Word condition exceeding .67. Franzen et al. (1987) reported significant increases in scores, with gains approximating five points on the Word and Color trials and four points on the Color-Word trial.

RELIABILITY OF ALTERNATE FORMS

Due to the presence of significant practice effects, examiners interested in documenting change by repeat measurement

TABLE 9–108 MOAANS Age-Based Golden Stroop Norms in African-American Adults

AGES	56–62			63–65			66–68			
SCALED SCORE	WORD	COLOR	COLOR-WORD	WORD	COLOR	COLOR-WORD	WORD	COLOR	COLOR-WORD	PERCENTILE RANGES
2	0–45	0–32	0–3	0–45	0–32	0–3	0–37	0–23	0–3	<1
3	46–48	—	4–5	46–48	—	4	38–44	24–32	4	1
4	49–51	33	6–8	49–51	33	—	45–46	33	—	2
5	52–62	34–38	9–12	52–62	34–38	5–8	47–50	34–36	5–8	3–5
6	63–67	39–44	13–14	63–66	39–44	9–12	52–64	37–41	9–10	6–10
7	68–73	45–49	15–16	67–71	45–48	13–15	65–69	42–47	11–14	11–18
8	74–79	50–52	17–20	72–76	49–52	16–18	70–74	48–50	15–16	19–28
9	80–83	53–57	21–23	77–82	53–57	19–21	75–79	51–55	17–20	29–40
10	84–90	58–62	24–28	83–88	58–62	22–26	80–87	56–61	21–25	41–59
11	91–96	63–69	29–31	89–95	63–67	27–29	88–92	62–64	26–28	60–71
12	97–101	70–73	32–36	96–99	68–72	30–34	93–97	65–71	29–32	72–81
13	102–107	74–76	37–38	100–106	73–76	35–37	98–105	72–76	33–37	82–89
14	108–112	77–80	39–40	107–109	77–79	38–40	106–107	77–79	38–39	90–94
15	113–123	81–82	41–42	110–121	80–82	41–42	108–110	80–82	40–42	95–97
16	124–125	83–85	43–44	122–125	83–84	43–44	111–112	83	43–44	98
17	126–130	86–89	—	126–130	85–88	—	113–121	84–87	—	99
18	131+	90+	45+	131+	89+	45+	122+	88+	45+	>99
N	106	106	106	128	128	128	165	165	165	

AGES	69–71			72–74			75–77			
SCALED SCORE	WORD	COLOR	COLOR-WORD	WORD	COLOR	COLOR-WORD	WORD	COLOR	COLOR-WORD	PERCENTILE RANGES
2	0–34	0–20	0–3	0–34	0–20	0–3	0–34	0–20	0–3	<1
3	35–44	21–30	4	35–37	21–25	4	35–37	21–25	4	1
4	45–46	31	—	38–46	26–29	—	38–42	26–27	—	2
5	47–49	32–34	5–8	47–48	30–33	5–8	43–47	28–32	5–8	3–5
6	50–63	35–40	9–10	49–60	34–37	9–10	48–58	33–36	9–10	6–10
7	64–67	41–44	11–13	61–66	38–43	11–13	59–64	37–41	11–13	11–18
8	68–73	45–49	14–16	67–70	44–47	14–16	65–70	42–46	14–16	19–28
9	74–78	50–54	17–19	71–76	48–51	17–19	71–76	47–50	17–18	29–40
10	79–87	55–60	20–24	77–87	52–59	20–24	77–87	51–59	19–23	41–59
11	88–92	61–62	25–27	88–92	60–62	25–26	88–92	60–61	24–26	60–71
12	93–97	63–68	28–31	93–97	63–67	27–29	93–96	62–64	27–29	72–81
13	98–101	69–73	32–36	98–101	68–73	30–32	97–101	65–73	30–32	2–89
14	102–106	74–78	37–38	102–106	74–78	33–37	102–105	74–78	33–36	90–94
15	107–109	79–82	39–42	107–109	79–82	38–39	106–109	79–82	37–38	95–97
16	110	83	43	110	83	40–42	110	83	—	98
17	111–112	84–87	44	111–112	84–87	43	111–112	84–87	39–43	99
18	113+	88+	45+	113+	88+	44+	113+	88+	44+	>99
N	182	182	182	156	156	156	119	119	119	

AGES	78+			
SCALED SCORE	WORD	COLOR	COLOR-WORD	PERCENTILE RANGES
2	0–30	0–20	0–3	<1
3	31–37	21–23	4	1
4	38–42	—	—	2
5	43–47	24–26	5–8	3–5
6	48–57	27–33	9–10	6–10
7	58–61	33–39	11–12	11–18
8	62–69	40–42	13–15	19–28
9	70–74	43–48	16–17	29–40
10	75–83	49–55	18–20	41–59
11	84–90	56–59	21–24	60–71
12	91–95	60–64	25–27	72–81

TABLE 9–108 Continued

AGES	78+			
SCALED SCORE	WORD	COLOR	COLOR-WORD	PERCENTILE RANGES
13	96–99	65–70	28–29	82–89
14	100–103	71–76	30–31	90–94
15	104–107	77–79	32–34	95–97
16	108–109	80–81	35–36	98
17	—	82–83	37–38	99
18	110+	84+	39+	>99
N	78	78	78	

SOURCE: Lucas et al. (2005).

on the same or alternate forms should ensure that examinees have sufficient practice with the test, at least more than one practice trial (Franzen et al., 1987; Sachs et al., 1991). Connor, Franzen, and Sharp (1988) report that gains plateau after three administrations.

EVIDENCE FOR VALIDITY

WITHIN-TEST CORRELATIONS

Correlations among test trials are moderate to high (Chafetz & Matthew, 2004; Pineda & Merchan, 2003).

CORRELATIONS WITH OTHER EXECUTIVE FUNCTION AND ATTENTION TESTS

The Stroop is moderately correlated with a number of attention and executive tasks, including the TMT (absolute value of *r*s = .34 to .55; Pavao Martins et al., 2013; Sánchez-Cubillo et al., 2009), Color Trails (Vogel et al., 2013), Wechsler Digit Symbol (*r*s = .23 to .48; Pavao Martins et al., 2013; Sánchez-Cubillo et al., 2009), the SDMT (*r* = .51; Morrow, 2013), the PASAT (*r* = .40; Morrow, 2013), and the Stop-Signal task (absolute value *r*s = .33 to .56; May & Hasher, 1998; also see Friedman & Miyake, 2004). Pavao Martins et al. reported that Stroop interference correlated modestly with verbal fluency (*r* = .23 to .29). Kane and Engle (2003) reported that individual differences in working memory capacity predict performance on the Stroop task.

TABLE 9–109 Computational Formula for Age- and Education-Corrected Golden Stroop MOAANS Scaled Scores

	K	W_1	W_2
Word Reading	2.49	1.10	0.29
Color Naming	2.82	1.09	0.31
Stroop Interference	2.77	1.08	0.28

Age- and education-corrected MOAANS Scaled Scores ($MSS_{A\&E}$) can be calculated for Stroop scores by using aged-corrected MOAANS scaled scores (MSS_A) and education (expressed in years completed) in the following formula: $MSS_{A\&E} = K + (W_1 \times MSS_A) - (W_2 \times EDUC)$

SOURCE: From Lucas et al. (2005).

CORRELATIONS WITH GENERAL COGNITION AND SPEED OF PROCESSING

Conceptual ability and speed of processing are related to performance (e.g., Anstey et al., 2002; Graf et al., 1995). Stroop interference should be interpreted within the context of processing speed. For instance, in healthy older adults, 85% of age-related variance in the Stroop interference trial is due to overall processing speed (Salthouse & Meinz, 1995). Furthermore, in clinical samples, Stroop interference loads on factors that appear to represent speed of processing (e.g., Digit Symbol, TMT-A, phonemic fluency) to a greater extent than executive function (Bondi et al., 2002; Boone et al., 1998). See "Age" for an additional discussion of processing speed on performance.

The Stroop relates to measures of conceptual ability. For example, Anstey et al. (2002) found that, in healthy older adults, Stroop interference loads on the same factor as a measure of fluid intelligence (the Raven's Progressive Matrices). Similarly, Graf et al. (1995) reported that, in healthy older adults,

TABLE 9–110 US Normative Data for the Golden Stroop

	RAW		
	STROOP COLOR AND WORD TEST		
SCALED	WORD READING	COLOR NAMING	COLOR-WORD
18	≥145	≥107	
17	134–144	100–106	≥65
16	128–133	97–99	63–64
15	123–127	93–96	59–62
14	118–122	89–92	56–58
13	114–117	85–88	53–55
12	109–113	80–84	49–52
11	106–108	76–79	46–48
10	101–105	74–75	42–45
9	97–100	70–73	39–41
8	89–96	66–69	36–38
7	83–88	62–65	32–35
6	77–82	58–61	29–31
5	71–76	49–57	25–28
4	67–70	43–48	22–24
3	66	40–42	0–21
2	<66	0–39	

SOURCE: Norman et al. (2011).

TABLE 9–111 Catalan Spanish Normative Data for Golden Stroop Adjusted for Age, Gender, and Education Level

MEASURE	SEX	EDUCATION	55–61	62–64	65–67	68–70	71–73	74–76	77–79	80–82	82+
Word											
Mean (*SD*)	M and F	L	82.1 (17.1)	79.5 (17.6)	77.4 (18.3)	74.0 (18.6)	71.2 (18.8)	68.9 (19.4)	66.0 (19.2)	65.9 (19.0)	64.9 (18.8)
PC 5/50/95			55/83/110	50/80/108	48/78/106	41/75/102	38/73/100	34/71/99	31/67/97	31/66/96	30/66/95
n			476	513	521	515	469	444	401	300	185
Mean (*SD*)		A	94.9 (15.3)	94.4 (15.8)	92.6 (15.9)	89.5 (16.1)	85.3 (16.8)	81.0 (16.0)	79.7 (17.0)	77.0 (15.0)	75.5 (16.3)
PC 5/50/95			69/95/123	69/95/123	67/94/123	63/90/119	59/86/110	56/82/103	55/79/100	52/77/100	52/75/98
n			334	300	249	193	139	115	100	71	46
Mean (*SD*)		H	98.8 (14.7)	98.2 (14.5)	97.5 (15.2)	96.0	92.3 (15.4)	87.4 (15.1)	84.9 (14.4)	83.5 (15.4)	81.0 (14.6)
PC 5/50/95			74/98/123	74/98/123	73/97/123	73/96/123	70/92/122	63/88/113	62/85/106	54/84/106	54/81/105
n			227	202	176	137	109	91	85	59	31
Color											
Mean (*SD*)	M	L	56.6 (12.1)	54.5 (12.5)	52.7 (13.0)	51.1 (13.1)	50.2 (12.1)	48.6 (12.2)	47.8 (12.2)	46.2 (12.4)	43.4 (11.8)
PC 5/50/95			35/56/77	34/54/75	30/53/74	30/50/73	30/50/69	29/48/68	25/48/68	25/47/66	23/44/64
n			207	216	222	217	188	189	183	146	92
Mean (*SD*)		A	63.9 (11.1)	63.4 (11.3)	62.5 (10.8)	60.6 (11.2)	58.5 (12.8)	53.4 (12.3)	53.2 (12.2)	51.4 (10.1)	50.1 (10.4)
PC 5/50/95			42/63/83	42/62/82	42/62/80	40/61/80	38/58/80	34/52/78	34/52/77	34/52/72	29/52/71
n			141	134	108	76	61	51	46	34	21
Mean (*SD*)		H	64.6 (12.0)	64.0 (11.7)	62.8 (12.1)	62.2 (12.9)	59.2 (12.3)	54.7 (11.6)	54.4 (11.7)	53.0 (11.9)	53.1 (11.2)
PC 5/50/95			46/65/83	45/65/83	42/63/83	41/61/82	39/59/82	37/55/77	37/54/75	33/51/72	33/51/72
n			124	123	111	94	75	63	58	39	23
Mean (*SD*)	F	L	58.9 (11.9)	57.5 (11.8)	56.8 (11.9)	54.8 (11.7)	53.1 (11.6)	51.9 (11.3)	49.6 (10.7)	48.0 (10.9)	47.2 (11.4)
PC 5/50/95			39/60/79	38/59/78	37/57/78	37/55/75	36/53/75	33/52/73	32/49/68	30/48/65	26/46/65
n			269	297	299	298	281	255	218	154	93
Mean (*SD*)		A	65.4 (11.0)	64.7 (10.8)	63.2 (10.7)	62.0 (11.5)	58.6 (11.3)	55.8 (9.9)	54.7 (10.0)	53.0 (10.6)	51.6 (11.0)
PC 5/50/95			48/63/85	48/63/87	44/63/82	42/61/82	40/59/81	40/57/75	34/57/68	33/57/66	29/57/66
n			193	166	141	117	78	64	54	37	25
Mean (*SD*)		H	66.4 (11.5)	65.0 (11.4)	63.6 (10.5)	61.9 (12.1)	61.3 (13.5)	59.1 (11.8)	57.5 (11.1)	56.9 (11.5)	54.0 (10.5)
PC 5/50/95			49/66/90	47/65/84	46/65/83	40/61/83	40/60/82	39/60/81	38/59/79	37/59/79	37/59/62
n			103	79	65	43	34	28	27	20	8
Word–Color											
Mean (*SD*)	M and F	L	31.6 (9.2)	30.9 (9.3)	30.4 (9.9)	28.9 (10.1)	28.3 (10.5)	26.7 (9.3)	25.3 (9.1)	24.7 (9.1)	23.1 (7.9)
PC 5/50/95			17/31/47	16/30/46	15/29/46	14/28/46	14/27/45	14/26/42	12/24/42	12/24/41	10/23/37
n			476	513	521	515	469	444	401	300	185
Mean (*SD*)		A	37.9 (9.5)	37.2 (9.4)	35.9 (9.5)	33.9 (9.3)	32.2 (9.2)	29.8 (8.8)	29.1 (8.8)	27.0 (8.3)	25.7 (8.7)
PC 5/50/95			22/38/55	22/37/35	20/35/54	19/33/50	18/31/48	17/30/46	15/30/44	14/26/44	13/24/44
n			334	300	249	193	139	115	100	71	46
Mean (*SD*)		H	40.3 (9.1)	39.7 (8.9)	38.2 (9.7)	36.0 (11.1)	33.0 (10.6)	30.8 (11.6)	29.6 (10.7)	29.2 (11.0)	29.3 (12.6)
PC 5/50/35			26/43/55	25/40/54	23/38/53	16/36/53	14/33/50	13/29/50	13/28/48	13/28/48	13/27/58
n			227	202	176	137	109	91	85	59	31

TABLE 9–111 Continued

MEASURE	SEX	EDUCATION	55–61	62–64	65–67	68–70	71–73	74–76	77–79	80–82	82+
Interference 1											
Mean (*SD*)	M	L	−1.7 (7.9)	−1.1 (7.7)	−1.1 (9.2)	−1.4 (9.1)	−0.5 (9.9)	−1.5 (8.5)	−1.0 (8.9)	−0.5 (9.1)	−1.0 (8.7)
PC 5/50/95			−14/−2/12	−13/−1/12	−14/−2/13	−14/ −2/12	−14/−1/17	−14/−2/14	−12/−2/12	−13/−2/12	−12/−2/9
n			207	216	222	217	188	189	183	146	92
Mean (*SD*)		A	−0.5 (7.1)	−0.5 (7.4)	−0.8 (7.7)	−0.8 (7.6)	−0.4 (7.3)	−0.7 (6.2)	−2.1 (6.5)	−3.9 (6.2)	−4.9 (6.9)
PC 5/50/95			−14/0/11	−13/0/12	−13/−1/12	−13/−2/12	−13/−1/11	−13/−1/9	−15/−2/9	−17/−3/7	−18/−3/9
n			141	134	108	76	61	51	46	34	21
Mean (*SD*)		H	1.5 (8.3)	1.2 (7.5)	0.5 (8.4)	−1.4 (8.4)	−3.0 (7.6)	−2.6 (10.7)	−3.1 (10.5)	−1.8 (7.5)	−2.2 (13.7)
PC 5/50/95			−10/1/13	−10/1/12	−14/1/14	−15/−1/9	−16/−2/9	−17/−2/15	−20/−3/9	−19/−2/10	−20/−3/12
n			124	123	111	94	75	63	58	39	23
Mean (*SD*)	F	L	−2.2 (8.3)	−2.1 (8.9)	−1.5 (8.9)	−1.7 (8.8)	−1.8 (9.7)	−2.2 (8.9)	−3.3 (8.8)	−3.6 (8.6)	−4.5 (7.3)
PC 5/50/95			−16/−3/12	−15/−3/13	−15/−2/15	−15/−3/13	−16/−3/13	−16/−3/12	−17/−4/10	−17/−4/9	−17/−5/6
n			269	297	299	298	281	255	218	154	93
Mean (*SD*)		A	−0.3 (7.7)	−1.0 (7.7)	−1.6 (8.0)	−3.2 (7.5)	−3.5 (7.4)	−4.0 (8.2)	−3.5 (8.6)	−3.9 (9.7)	−4.5 (7.3)
PC 5/50/95			−13/−1/12	−14/−1/12	−15/−2/10	−16/−3/9	−16/−3/7	−16/−3/12	−16/−3/14	−17/−6/14	−17/−7/13
n			193	166	141	117	78	64	54	37	25
Mean (*SD*)		H	1.6 (7.9)	0.5 (7.5)	−0.5 (7.7)	−1.7 (8.9)	−3.2 (8.9)	−4.0 (7.8)	−4.5 (7.3)	−2.7 (7.5)	−2.8 (8.1)
PC 5/50/95			−12/2/13	−11/0/13	−12/0/15	−16/−1/18	−21/−3/15	−22/−3/11	−22/−3/8	−21/−3/9	−12/−5/10
n			103	79	65	43	34	28	27	20	8
Interference 2											
Mean (*SD*)	M	L	−7.2 (7.7)	−7.1 (7.6)	−7.2 (8.8)	−7.9 (8.9)	−7.7 (8.8)	−9.1 (7.1)	−9.3 (7.1)	−8.8 (6.9)	−9.0 (6.8)
PC 5/50/95			−20/−7/7	−19/−7/5	−19/−7/5	−21/−9/5	−21/−9/5	−21/−10/3	−21/−10/3	−21/−10/3	−21/−10/1
n			207	216	222	217	188	189	183	146	92
Mean (*SD*)		A	−3.3 (7.7)	−3.5 (7.9)	−4.2 (8.2)	−5.1 (8.0)	−4.8 (8.6)	−5.8 (7.9)	−7.7 (8.3)	−10.7 (6.1)	−12.1 (6.8)
PC 5/50/95			−17/−2/10	−17/−3/10	−18/−3/10	−18/−5/10	−18/−5/9	−18/−6/7	−19/−8/6	−23/−10/4	−25/−12/1
n			141	134	108	76	61	51	46	34	21
Mean (*SD*)		H	−0.7 (8.3)	−1.0 (7.6)	−1.6 (8.6)	−3.6 (9.1)	−6.4 (7.9)	−6.7 (11.2)	−8.0 (11.2)	−7.1 (12.5)	−7.9 (14.1)
PC 5/50/95			−15/−1/13	−14/−2/12	−15/−2/12	−17/−3/8	−20/−6/7	−22/−8/8	−22/−9/7	−22/−8/7	−22/−10/6
n			124	123	111	94	75	63	58	39	23
Mean (*SD*)	F	L	−8.6 (7.7)	−8.8 (8.5)	−8.8 (8.3)	−9.6 (8.3)	−9.9 (9.3)	−10.7 (8.2)	−11.8 (8.3)	−12.8 (8.2)	−13.0 (6.7)
PC 5/50/95			−21/−9/5	−21/−9/5	−21/−9/4	−21/−10/4	−22/−11/4	−23/−11/3	−25/−12/0	−25/−12/0	−25/−12/−2
n			269	297	299	298	281	255	218	154	93
Mean (*SD*)		A	−3.7 (8.4)	−4.5 (8.3)	−5.6 (8.2)	−7.7 (7.7)	−9.4 (7.4)	−10.6 (7.8)	−9.9 (8.6)	−9.9 (9.3)	−9.8 (10.2)
PC 5/50/95			−18/−4/10	−19/−5/10	−21/−5/9	−21/−7/5	−23/−9/4	−23/−11/4	−23/−10/4	−23/−10/4	−24/−10/4
n			193	166	141	117	78	64	54	37	25
Mean (*SD*)		H	−1.0 (7.9)	−1.9 (7.9)	−2.9 (8.5)	−4.6 (10.3)	−6.5 (10.5)	−9.0 (8.7)	−10.0 (6.8)	−8.7 (6.4)	−13.0 (6.7)
PC 5/50/95			−16/−1/13	−17/−1/13	−17/−2/13	−20/−5/13	−22/−6/12	−24/−9/11	−24/−10/8	−24/−10/2	−25/−12/−2
n			103	79	65	43	34	28	27	20	8

NOTES: M, men; F, women; L, low; A, average; H, high; PC, percentile.

SOURCE: Llinas-Regla et al. (2013).

TABLE 9-112 Spanish Normative Data for the Golden Stroop by Age, Gender, and Education

Young group *N* = 149; male = 66; female = 83		
	M	*SD*
Age	23.8	4
Edu	13.1	3.3
WR	108.8	15.2
CN	81.1	13.6
CW	55.2	11.6
IS	9	8.9
Middle-age group; Low Education = 0–11 years; *N* = 69; male = 17; female = 52		
	M	*SD*
Age	58.2	10.8
Edu	8.6	1.5
WR	95.6	17
CN	66.2	12
CW	37.6	9.7
IS	−1.2	8.5
Middle-age group; High Education = 12+ years; *N* = 67; male = 32; female = 35		
	M	*SD*
Age	53.3	13.5
Edu	15.6	2.6
WR	103.7	16.6
CN	70.5	14.6
CW	42.5	11.6
IS	0.7	9

NOTE: Edu, Education in years; WR, Word Reading; CN, Color Naming; CW, Color Word; IS, Interference Score.

SOURCE: Lubrini et al. (2014).

TABLE 9-113 NEURONORMA Spanish Normative Data for the Golden Stroop Age 50–56

SCALED SCORE	PERCENTILE RANGE	WORD SCORE	COLOR SCORE	WORD-COLOR SCORE
2	<1	≤24	≤21	≤6
3	1	25–43	22–32	7
4	2	44–55	33–42	8–11
5	3–5	56–60	43–46	12–19
6	6–10	61–71	47–48	20–21
7	11–18	72–79	49–55	22–25
8	19–28	80–88	56–58	26–31
9	29–40	89–96	59–61	32–33
10	41–59	97–100	62–69	34–39
11	60–71	101–107	70–74	40–41
12	72–81	108–112	75–78	42–46
13	82–89	113–119	79–81	47–50
14	90–94	120–123	82–86	51–54
15	95–97	124–126	87–93	55–56
16	98	127–130	94–98	57–66
17	99	–	99–100	67–72
18	>99	≥131	≥101	≥73
Sample size		136	136	136

SOURCE: Pena-Casanova et al. (2009).

TABLE 9-114 NEURONORMA Spanish Normative Data for the Golden Stroop Age 57–59

SCALED SCORE	PERCENTILE RANGE	WORD SCORE	COLOR SCORE	WORD-COLOR SCORE
2	<1	≤43	≤32	≤6
3	1	–	33–36	7
4	2	44–46	–	8–11
5	3–5	47–64	37–45	12–18
6	6–10	65–68	46–48	19–20
7	11–18	69–79	49–51	21–25
8	19–28	80–86	52–57	26–29
9	29–40	87–93	58–60	30–32
10	41–59	94–99	61–67	33–38
11	60–71	100–105	68–74	39–41
12	72–81	106–110	75–78	42–44
13	82–89	111–119	79	45–49
14	90–94	120–123	80–85	50–54
15	95–97	124–126	86–90	55–56
16	98	127–130	91–93	57–66
17	99	–	94–98	67–72
18	>99	≥131	≥99	≥73
Sample size		133	133	133

SOURCE: Pena-Casanova et al. (2009).

Stroop interference loads on the same factor as several WAIS subtests that involve speed of processing and conceptual abilities (Digit Symbol, Block Design, Similarities; see also "Other Executive Function and Attention Tests"). Pavao Martins et al. (2013) reported that Stroop interference correlated with Matrix Reasoning (r = .33) after controlling for education. See also "Education and IQ."

TABLE 9-115 NEURONORMA Spanish Normative Data for the Golden Stroop Age 60–62

SCALED SCORE	PERCENTILE RANGE	WORD SCORE	COLOR SCORE	WORD-COLOR SCORE
2	<1	≤42	≤20	≤6
3	1	43	21–32	7
4	2	–	33–36	8–9
5	3–5	44–55	37–40	10–18
6	6–10	56–66	41–46	19–20
7	11–18	67–73	47–49	21–24
8	19–28	74–80	50–54	25–26
9	29–40	81–90	55–58	27–30
10	41–59	91–99	59–65	31–36
11	60–71	100–104	66–70	37–41
12	72–81	105–110	71–76	42–43
13	82–89	111–119	77–79	44–47
14	90–94	120–123	80–82	48–50
15	95–97	124–126	83–86	51–55
16	98	127–130	87–89	–
17	99	–	90	56
18	>99	≥131	≥91	≥57
Sample size		123	123	123

SOURCE: Pena-Casanova et al. (2009).

TABLE 9-116 NEURONORMA Spanish Normative Data for the Golden Stroop Age 63–65

SCALED SCORE	PERCENTILE RANGE	WORD SCORE	COLOR SCORE	WORD-COLOR SCORE
2	<1	≤42	≤20	≤6
3	1	43	21–32	7
4	2	44–45	33–36	8–9
5	3–5	46–53	37–40	10–13
6	6–10	54–60	41–42	14–15
7	11–18	61–70	43–47	16–21
8	19–28	71–76	48–49	22–24
9	29–40	77–84	50–56	25–28
10	41–59	85–97	57–62	29–34
11	60–71	98–99	63–68	35–38
12	72–81	100–103	69–74	39–41
13	82–89	104–114	75–78	42–45
14	90–94	115–120	79	46–49
15	95–97	121–124	80–82	50–53
16	98	125–130	83–84	54
17	99	–	85–90	55
18	>99	≥131	≥91	≥56
Sample size		106	106	106

SOURCE: Pena-Casanova et al. (2009).

TABLE 9-118 NEURONORMA Spanish Normative Data for the Golden Stroop Age 69–71

SCALED SCORE	PERCENTILE RANGE	WORD SCORE	COLOR SCORE	WORD-COLOR SCORE
2	<1	≤23	≤21	≤5
3	1	24–30	–	–
4	2	31–32	21–23	6–9
5	3–5	33–53	24–32	10–11
6	6–10	54–59	33–38	12–14
7	11–18	60–70	39–43	15–19
8	19–28	71–73	44–47	20–23
9	29–40	74–79	48–50	24–25
10	41–59	80–90	51–56	26–29
11	60–71	91–96	57–60	30–33
12	72–81	97–98	61–63	34–36
13	82–89	99–106	64–70	37–42
14	90–94	107–112	71–74	43–44
15	95–97	113–115	75–76	45–46
16	98	116–120	77	47–50
17	99	121–130	78–82	51
18	>99	≥131	≥83	≥52
Sample size		124	124	124

SOURCE: Pena-Casanova et al. (2009).

CORRELATIONS WITH OTHER TESTS

The interference trial also involves the semantic system and perhaps aspects of planning. Bondi et al. (2002) noted that in healthy individuals, the interference trial loaded on a factor representing semantic knowledge (verbal fluency, Boston Naming Test, Vocabulary) and attention (Digit Span). Hanes, Andrewes, Smith, and Pantelis (1996) found that in patients with schizophrenia, PD, and HD, Stroop interference showed strong relations with performance on a semantic fluency task ($r = .58$) and the number of trials to completion on the TOL ($r = .65$), but only modest or little relations with other tasks, such as delayed recall of the Rey-Osterrieth Complex Figure Test ($r = .31$) and the Purdue Pegboard ($r = .12$). Pavao Martins et al. (2013) reported that Stroop interference correlated with CVLT-II recall ($r = .22$) and WMS-III Faces ($r = .21$), but not CVLT-II recognition ($r = .06$), after controlling for education.

TABLE 9-117 NEURONORMA Spanish Normative Data for the Golden Stroop Age 66–68

SCALED SCORE	PERCENTILE RANGE	WORD SCORE	COLOR SCORE	WORD-COLOR SCORE
2	<1	≤30	≤20	≤5
3	1	31–42	21–23	–
4	2	43–45	24–26	6–9
5	3–5	46–57	27–38	10–13
6	6–10	58–65	39–40	14–17
7	11–18	66–71	41–45	18–21
8	19–28	72–77	46–49	22–24
9	29–40	78–82	50–53	25–26
10	41–59	83–91	54–59	27–30
11	60–71	92–98	60–62	31–35
12	72–81	99–108	63–67	36–39
13	82–89	109–115	68–73	40–43
14	90–94	116–120	74–76	44–47
15	95–97	121–124	77–79	48–50
16	98	125–130	80–82	51
17	99	–	83–84	52–54
18	>99	≥131	≥85	≥55
Sample size		119	119	119

SOURCE: Pena-Casanova et al. (2009).

TABLE 9-119 NEURONORMA Spanish Normative Data for the Golden Stroop Age 72–74

SCALED SCORE	PERCENTILE RANGE	WORD SCORE	COLOR SCORE	WORD-COLOR SCORE
2	<1	≤23	≤21	≤5
3	1	24–30	–	6–8
4	2	31–32	22–23	–
5	3–5	33–47	24–29	9–10
6	6–10	48–59	30–36	11–13
7	11–18	60–67	37–40	14–17
8	19–28	68–75	41–45	18–20
9	29–40	76–81	46–49	21–24
10	41–59	82–89	50–55	25–27
11	60–71	90–95	56–60	28–30
12	72–81	96–98	61–62	31–36
13	82–89	99–104	63–67	37–40
14	90–94	105–111	68–71	41–44
15	95–97	112–114	72–76	45–46
16	98	115–120	77	–
17	99	121–123	78–82	47–50
18	>99	≥124	≥83	≥51
Sample size		124	124	124

SOURCE: Pena-Casanova et al. (2009).

TABLE 9-120 NEURONORMA Spanish Normative Data for the Golden Stroop Age 75–77

SCALED SCORE	PERCENTILE RANGE	WORD SCORE	COLOR SCORE	WORD-COLOR SCORE
2	<1	≤22	≤20	≤4
3	1	23	-	5
4	2	24–30	21	6–8
5	3–5	31–41	22–27	9
6	6–10	42–54	28–32	10–11
7	11–18	55–61	33–39	12–15
8	19–28	62–70	40–45	16–18
9	29–40	71–77	46–48	19–21
10	41–59	78–85	49–54	22–26
11	60–71	86–91	55–57	27–28
12	72–81	92–96	58–60	29–34
13	82–89	97–100	61–66	35–38
14	90–94	101–109	67–69	39–43
15	95–97	110–114	70–73	44
16	98	115–119	74	45
17	99	120	75–77	–
18	>99	≥121	≥78	≥46
Sample size		98	98	98

SOURCE: Pena-Casanova et al. (2009).

TABLE 9-122 NEURONORMA Spanish Normative Data for the Golden Stroop Age 81–90

SCALED SCORE	PERCENTILE RANGE	WORD SCORE	COLOR SCORE	WORD-COLOR SCORE
2	<1	≤20	≤17	≤7
3	1	–	–	–
4	2	21	18	8
5	3–5	22–41	19–21	9
6	6–10	42–50	22–32	10
7	11–18	51–54	33–35	11–14
8	19–28	55–65	36–40	15–16
9	29–40	66–75	41–46	17–18
10	41–59	76–83	47–49	19–22
11	60–71	84–88	50–54	23–25
12	72–81	89–95	55–58	26–27
13	82–89	96–99	59–60	28–34
14	90–94	100–104	61–66	35–36
15	95–97	105–114	67–68	37
16	98	115–119	69–71	38–40
17	99	–	–	–
18	>99	≥120	≥72	≥41
Sample size		41	41	41

SOURCE: Pena-Casanova et al. (2009).

CLINICAL STUDIES

TBI. Overall, slowed processing accounts for difficulties on the Stroop in patients with TBI rather than inhibition difficulty per se. In their meta-analysis of Stroop performance after TBI, Ben-David, Nguyen, and van Lieshout (2011) reported a larger interference effect for persons with TBI compared to controls. However, the authors note that analysis of data suggests that this effect may be secondary to slowed processing speed and sensory factors (e.g., latency difference between reading and naming font color of a color neutral word) rather than selective attention per se. Similarly, persons with TBI are typically slower to respond on all conditions of the Stroop, rather than showing disproportionate difficulty on the interference condition (e.g., Felmingham et al., 2004; Lubrini et al., 2014; Ponsford & Kinsella, 1992; Rios et al., 2004). In patients with postconcussion syndrome (PCS) screened for performance validity, the Stroop showed limited sensitivity and high specificity (Cicerone & Azulay, 2002).

TABLE 9-121 NEURONORMA Spanish Normative Data for the Golden Stroop Age 78–80

SCALED SCORE	PERCENTILE RANGE	WORD SCORE	COLOR SCORE	WORD-COLOR SCORE
2	<1	≤31	≤20	≤7
3	1	32	21	8
4	2	–	–	–
5	3–5	33–41	22–27	9
6	6–10	42–50	28–32	10–11
7	11–18	51–55	33–35	12–14
8	19–28	56–67	36–40	15–17
9	29–40	68–75	41–46	18–19
10	41–59	76–83	47–51	20–23
11	60–71	84–89	52–54	24–26
12	72–81	90–97	55–60	27–31
13	82–89	98–100	61–64	32–36
14	90–94	101–104	65–68	37–38
15	95–97	105–114	69	39–40
16	98	115–119	70–71	41–42
17	99	–	–	–
18	>99	≥120	≥72	≥43
Sample size		65	65	65

SOURCE: Pena-Casanova et al. (2009).

ADHD. People with ADHD with high IQ perform worse than high-IQ adults without ADHD. In one study, the Stroop was predictive, along with other executive function tasks, of functional outcomes, including arrest history and traffic violations (Antshel et al., 2010). Lower performance was noted particularly in persons with ADHD with comorbid anxiety or bipolar disorder (Silva et al., 2013).

Dementia. Increased Stroop interference has been reported in patients with dementia (e.g., Bondi et al., 2002; Nathan et al., 2001). The breakdown in inhibitory processes appears to occur early in the course of AD, and the magnitude of the interference effect is moderately related to the severity of dementia (Bondi et al., 2002). With regard to predictive validity, better performance on the Stroop at baseline is related to longer survival in patients with AD (Zhou et al., 2010).

The Stroop has some utility in other dementia subtypes, including HD (Hanes et al., 1996; Snowden et al., 2001). Johns et al. (2009) reported that the Stroop (particularly errors) was the most useful among executive function tasks examined at differentiating Lewy body dementia from

FTD. Sudo, Amado, Alves, Laks, and Engelhardt (2017) reported that Stroop performance was impaired in vascular MCI. Baseline interference scores on the Golden version are predictive of functional status at one-year follow-up in patients with vascular dementia (Boyle et al., 2004). The Stroop was identified as one of the most useful tests in detecting cognitive change in prodromal HD (Paulsen et al., 2017).

PD. Increased interference has been found in patients with PD (Hanes et al., 1996). Bezdicek et al. (2015) used a variation of the Victoria Stroop and reported that the interference score was associated with a sensitivity of 82% and a specificity of 53% in differentiating controls from patients with PD.

MS. Patients with MS show difficulties on the Stroop, particularly in terms of greater response times and slowed processing speed (Bodling et al., 2012; Denney & Lynch, 2009; Hughes et al., 2013; Lynch et al., 2010). Relationships between processing speed on the Stroop and disability status have also been reported (Lynch et al., 2010).

Psychiatric Conditions. An interference effect has been demonstrated in patients with schizophrenia (Hanes et al., 1996; Moritz et al., 2002). Lubrini et al. (2014) reported that people with schizophrenia showed greater interference than people with TBI and healthy controls. Stroop performance improved in people with schizophrenia following treatment (Szöke et al., 2008). Relatives of individuals with schizophrenia performed worse on the Stroop than healthy controls (Hou et al., 2016; Szöke et al., 2005).

Diminished performance on the Stroop has also been documented in depressed patients (Moritz et al., 2002; Nathan et al., 2001; Videbach et al., 2004). In their meta-analysis of executive function deficit in major depressive disorder, Wagner, Doering, Helmreich, Lieb, and Tadić (2012) reported greater Stroop interference in patients with major depressive disorder compared with controls, with improved performance following antidepressant treatment.

The Stroop test has been identified as an important instrument in the assessment of cognitive impairment in people with bipolar disorder (Yatham et al., 2010). Twins with bipolar disorder and healthy co-twins both perform worse on the Stroop than healthy controls (Juselius et al., 2009). Processing speed on the Stroop is slower among euthymic patients than healthy controls, with a medium effect size reported (Pattanayak et al., 2012).

Impaired Stroop performance is reported in patients with OCD (Gruner & Pittenger, 2017). Patients with treatment refractory OCD showed improved Stroop scores after treatment via anterior capsulotomy (Csigó et al., 2010). D'alcante et al. (2012) reported that errors on the Stroop, along with measures of verbal intellectual function and memory, were found to predict treatment response after cognitive behavioral therapy or fluoxetine in patients with OCD. In a mixed psychiatric sample of older adults treated at a community mental health center, the Stroop yielded a sensitivity rate of 89% and a specificity rate of 37% (Mackin et al., 2010).

Other Populations. Increased interference has been found in a variety of patient groups thought to have executive disturbance, such as Friedreich's ataxia (White et al., 2000), alcohol use disorders (Dao-Castellana et al., 1998), and HIV infection (Castellon et al., 2000). Improved Stroop performance was reported following physical exercise and rehabilitation post-stroke (Rand et al., 2010).

NEUROANATOMICAL CORRELATES AND IMAGING STUDIES

Evidence suggests that prefrontal regions are implicated in Stroop performance, with recruitment of a broader based network of association areas. Lesion studies have suggested that patients with focal frontal lesions tend to show greater than typical levels of interference on Stroop tests (Regard, 1981; Stuss et al., 2001), with left lateral superior and middle frontal gyri implicated in performance in people with prefrontal lesions (Cipolotti et al., 2016). In a meta-analysis, Demakis (2004) compared patients with frontal lobe damage with those with damage to posterior brain regions. Significant differences between groups were found for all trials of the Stroop (weighted effect sizes of −.33 for Word, −.36 for Color, −.45 for Color-Word). However, use of Stroop performance alone was not sufficient to differentiate between frontal and nonfrontal groups. In fact, the amount of overlap between the distributions of these two groups was 70 to 79%, indicating little separation of groups and relatively poor sensitivity (true positives) and specificity (true negatives).

Although neuroimaging studies suggest that frontal systems are critical for performance (Kerns et al., 2004; Ravnkilde et al., 2002; Stuss et al., 2001), Stroop performance is mediated by a more broadly based system, which has been found in both healthy and clinical samples. fMRI activation obtained in healthy adults during performance of the Stroop includes not only frontal regions but also inferior temporal and parietal cortices, as well as the caudate nuclei (Peterson et al., 2002). In healthy adults, the volume of thalamofrontal projections is related to Stroop performance (Hughes et al., 2012). Stroop performance is associated with AD pathology in the hippocampus and a number of cortical regions, including posterior cerebral areas (Bondi et al., 2002; Collette et al., 2002).

White matter abnormalities are related to performance. In healthy older adults, Söderlund et al. (2006) reported that periventricular white matter hyperintensities predicted worse Stroop (time) performance, and subcortical atrophy predicted Stroop (errors) after adjustment for demographic variables. In patients with age-related white matter hypertensities, atrophy of the corpus callosum was associated with poorer Stroop performance (Jokinen et al., 2007). Increased interference has also been reported in nondemented

TABLE 9–123 NEURONORMA Spanish Education Adjustment for the Golden Stroop Part A

	EDUCATION (YEARS)																				
NSS_A	0	1	2	3	4	5	6	7	8	9	10	11	12	13	14	15	16	17	18	19	20
2	5	4	4	4	4	3	3	3	3	2	2	2	2	1	1	1	0	0	0	0	-1
3	6	5	5	5	5	4	4	4	4	3	3	3	3	2	2	2	1	1	1	1	0
4	7	6	6	6	6	5	5	5	5	4	4	4	4	3	3	3	2	2	2	2	1
5	8	7	7	7	7	6	6	6	6	5	5	5	5	4	4	4	3	3	3	3	2
6	9	8	8	8	8	7	7	7	7	6	6	6	6	5	5	5	4	4	4	4	3
7	10	9	9	9	9	8	8	8	8	7	7	7	7	6	6	6	5	5	5	5	4
8	11	10	10	10	10	9	9	9	9	8	8	8	8	7	7	7	6	6	6	6	5
9	12	11	11	11	11	10	10	10	10	9	9	9	9	8	8	8	7	7	7	7	6
10	13	12	12	12	12	11	11	11	11	10	10	10	10	9	9	9	8	8	8	8	7
11	14	13	13	13	13	12	12	12	12	11	11	11	11	10	10	10	9	9	9	9	8
12	15	14	14	14	14	13	13	13	13	12	12	12	12	11	11	11	10	10	10	10	9
13	16	15	15	15	15	14	14	14	14	13	13	13	13	12	12	12	11	11	11	11	10
14	17	16	16	16	16	15	15	15	15	14	14	14	14	13	13	13	12	12	12	12	11
15	18	17	17	17	17	16	16	16	16	15	15	15	15	14	14	14	13	13	13	13	12
16	19	18	18	18	18	17	17	17	17	16	16	16	16	15	15	15	14	14	14	14	13
17	20	19	19	19	19	18	18	18	18	17	17	17	17	16	16	16	15	15	15	15	14
18	21	20	20	20	20	19	19	19	19	18	18	18	18	17	17	17	16	16	16	16	15

NOTE: Education adjustment applying the following formula: $NSS_{A\&E} = NSS_A - (\beta \times [Education_{(years)} - 12])$, where $\beta = 0.25663$.

SOURCE: Pena-Casanova et al. (2009).

patients with subcortical lacunar infarcts, with the extent of white matter signal hyperintensity correlated with Stroop performance (Kramer et al., 2002). Melrose et al. (2017) reported that hypometabolism of the inferior parietal lobe was associated with poorer Stroop performance in patients with dementia, with interference related to metabolism in the medial prefrontal cortex and insula. Hoshi et al. (2010) reported that interference on a modified Stroop was related to serum inflammatory marker levels and white matter lesions on MRI in patients with atherosclerotic risk factors. Videbech et al. (2004) reported that Stroop performance was correlated with the number of white matter lesions in the frontal lobes, insula, and a region adjacent to the basal ganglia in patients with depression.

Patients with OCD show less activation in the anterior cingulate gyrus and cerebellum than controls on MRI during the Stroop. After symptom improvement following behavioral therapy, the cerebellum and parietal lobe demonstrate increased activation, and decreased activation was reported in the orbitofrontal cortex, middle frontal gyrus, and temporal regions (Nabeyama et al., 2008).

TABLE 9–124 NEURONORMA Spanish Education Adjustment for the Golden Stroop Part B

	EDUCATION (YEARS)																				
NSS_A	0	1	2	3	4	5	6	7	8	9	10	11	12	13	14	15	16	17	18	19	20
2	4	4	4	3	3	3	3	3	2	2	2	2	2	1	1	1	1	0	0	0	0
3	5	5	5	4	4	4	4	4	3	3	3	3	3	2	2	2	2	1	1	1	1
4	6	6	6	5	5	5	5	5	4	4	4	4	4	3	3	3	3	2	2	2	2
5	7	7	7	6	6	6	6	6	5	5	5	5	5	4	4	4	4	3	3	3	3
6	8	8	8	7	7	7	7	7	6	6	6	6	6	5	5	5	5	4	4	4	4
7	9	9	9	8	8	8	8	8	7	7	7	7	7	6	6	6	6	5	5	5	5
8	10	10	10	9	9	9	9	9	8	8	8	8	8	7	7	7	7	6	6	6	6
9	11	11	11	10	10	10	10	10	9	9	9	9	9	8	8	8	8	7	7	7	7
10	12	12	12	11	11	11	11	11	10	10	10	10	10	9	9	9	9	8	8	8	8
11	13	13	13	12	12	12	12	12	11	11	11	11	11	10	10	10	10	9	9	9	9
12	14	14	14	13	13	13	13	13	12	12	12	12	12	11	11	11	11	10	10	10	10
13	15	15	15	14	14	14	14	14	13	13	13	13	13	12	12	12	12	11	11	11	11
14	16	16	16	15	15	15	15	15	14	14	14	14	14	13	13	13	13	12	12	12	12
15	17	17	17	16	16	16	16	16	15	15	15	15	15	14	14	14	14	13	13	13	13
16	18	18	18	17	17	17	17	17	16	16	16	16	16	15	15	15	15	14	14	14	14
17	19	19	19	18	18	18	18	18	17	17	17	17	17	16	16	16	16	15	15	15	15
18	20	20	20	19	19	19	19	19	18	18	18	18	18	17	17	17	17	16	16	16	16

NOTE: Education adjustment applying the following formula: $NSS_{A\&E} = NSS_A - (\beta \times [Education_{(years)} - 12])$, where $\beta = 0.2099$.

SOURCE: Pena-Casanova et al. (2009).

TABLE 9–125 NEURONORMA Spanish Education Adjustment for the Golden Stroop Part C

	EDUCATION (YEARS)																				
NSS_A	0	1	2	3	4	5	6	7	8	9	10	11	12	13	14	15	16	17	18	19	20
2	4	3	3	3	3	3	3	2	2	2	2	2	2	1	1	1	1	1	0	0	0
3	5	4	4	4	4	4	4	3	3	3	3	3	3	2	2	2	2	2	1	1	1
4	6	5	5	5	5	5	5	4	4	4	4	4	4	3	3	3	3	3	2	2	2
5	7	6	6	6	6	6	6	5	5	5	5	5	5	4	4	4	4	4	3	3	3
6	8	7	7	7	7	7	7	6	6	6	6	6	6	5	5	5	5	5	4	4	4
7	9	8	8	8	8	8	8	7	7	7	7	7	7	6	6	6	6	6	5	5	5
8	10	9	9	9	9	9	9	8	8	8	8	8	8	7	7	7	7	7	6	6	6
9	11	10	10	10	10	10	10	9	9	9	9	9	9	8	8	8	8	8	7	7	7
10	12	11	11	11	11	11	11	10	10	10	10	10	10	9	9	9	9	9	8	8	8
11	13	12	12	12	12	12	12	11	11	11	11	11	11	10	10	10	10	10	9	9	9
12	14	13	13	13	13	13	13	12	12	12	12	12	12	11	11	11	11	11	10	10	10
13	15	14	14	14	14	14	14	13	13	13	13	13	13	12	12	12	12	12	11	11	11
14	16	15	15	15	15	15	15	14	14	14	14	14	14	13	13	13	13	13	12	12	12
15	17	16	16	16	16	16	16	15	15	15	15	15	15	14	14	14	14	14	13	13	13
16	18	17	17	17	17	17	17	16	16	16	16	16	16	15	15	15	15	15	14	14	14
17	19	18	18	18	18	18	18	17	17	17	17	17	17	16	16	16	16	16	15	15	15
18	20	19	19	19	19	19	19	18	18	18	18	18	18	17	17	17	17	17	16	16	16

NOTE: Education adjustment applying the following formula: $NSS_{A\&E} = NSS_A - (\beta \times [Education_{(years)} - 12])$, where $\beta = 0.17826$.

SOURCE: Pena-Casanova et al. (2009).

PERFORMANCE VALIDITY

Although it is not usually thought of in this way, the Stroop shows promise as a performance validity test. Van Gorp et al. (1999) reported that probable malingerers take significantly more time to complete the Color and Color-Word trials than nonmalingerers, although the task does not reliably identify those who are malingering. Lu, Boone, Jimenez, and Razami (2004) noted that the Stroop test may be particularly useful in patients complaining of complete illiteracy. They describe six patients who claimed that they were unable to perform the Word trial, but on the Color-Word trial, they all

TABLE 9–126 Korean Normative Data for the Golden Stroop Word Condition by Age, Gender, and Education

		MEN			WOMEN		
EDUCATION (YEARS)		0–3	4–9	≥10	0–3	4–9	≥10
Age 60–69	*n*	12	45	85	68	128	65
	Mean	51.25	60.38	71.71	50.38	65.33	79.68
	SD	11.01	11.84	15.27	12.87	14.56	13.54
	5th percentile	40.00	42.30	38.00	27.00	41.45	54.00
	Median	48.50	59.00	54.00	51.00	66.00	80.00
	95th percentile	72.00	84.20	72.70	71.65	93.00	100.70
70–74	*n*	15	60	85	78	126	51
	Mean	50.47	59.90	69.79	46.60	61.49	75.10
	SD	8.52	10.41	14.96	13.70	15.07	11.94
	5th percentile	40.00	43.00	44.60	23.95	35.05	52.00
	Median	51.00	59.00	70.00	47.50	60.50	76.00
	95th percentile	67.00	77.00	95.70	70.15	88.65	97.60
75–79	*n*	13	53	54	65	86	29
	Mean	47.77	57.92	66.50	44.54	57.45	71.83
	SD	7.70	10.81	12.86	12.95	14.09	11.55
	5th percentile	40.00	40.00	43.75	23.30	33.35	48.50
	Median	45.00	58.00	67.00	43.00	57.50	75.00
	95th percentile	62.00	77.90	89.00	71.20	79.65	91.00
80–90	*n*	8	35	23	39	45	11
	Mean	46.25	56.43	66.13	42.18	56.58	71.18
	SD	9.68	12.29	15.21	12.65	13.75	13.36
	5th percentile	30.00	30.60	40.20	21.00	30.90	48.00
	Median	46.00	58.00	67.00	42.00	57.00	73.00
	95th percentile	60.00	77.60	97.40	67.00	84.70	96.00

NOTE: The normative data were established by using overlapping strata of the ages 60 74, 65 79, 70 84, and 75 90.

SOURCE: Seo et al. (2008).

TABLE 9-127 Korean Normative Data for the Golden Stroop Color Condition by Age, Gender, and Education

		MEN			WOMEN		
EDUCATION (YEARS)		0–3	4–9	≥10	0–3	4–9	≥10
Age 60–69	*n*	12	45	85	68	128	65
	Mean	47.17	51.44	54.18	50.34	57.56	65.23
	SD	9.28	10.21	11.01	10.59	10.73	10.88
	5th percentile	30.00	33.60	38.00	31.45	39.50	47.30
	Median	48.50	49.00	54.00	50.50	58.50	66.00
	95th percentile	72.00	68.70	72.70	70.55	77.00	83.00
70–74	*n*	15	60	85	78	126	51
	Mean	47.87	50.78	54.14	47.73	56.31	62.63
	SD	8.36	9.09	11.31	10.29	11.05	9.78
	5th percentile	30.00	35.05	36.60	31.00	37.00	43.60
	Median	48.00	49.50	54.00	48.00	56.50	62.00
	95th percentile	68.00	67.00	73.00	70.00	77.00	78.40
75–79	*n*	13	53	54	65	86	29
	Mean	44.39	48.74	53.22	47.03	54.51	59.76
	SD	7.10	8.33	9.55	9.49	11.17	9.28
	5th percentile	30.00	35.70	39.00	31.30	34.35	41.00
	Median	46.00	48.00	53.50	46.00	55.00	60.00
	95th percentile	55.00	64.90	72.25	63.10	74.60	74.00
80–90	*n*	8	35	23	39	45	11
	Mean	43.38	47.74	53.35	45.72	53.58	58.55
	SD	8.02	8.63	10.84	8.73	11.11	8.98
	5th percentile	32.00	33.00	36.80	35.00	33.30	39.00
	Median	46.00	46.00	52.00	45.00	53.00	59.00
	95th percentile	55.00	67.00	73.80	61.00	75.70	72.00

NOTE: The normative data were established by using overlapping strata of the ages 60–74, 65–79, 70–84, and 75–90.

SOURCE: Seo et al. (2008).

TABLE 9-128 Korean Normative Data for the Golden Stroop Color-Word Condition by Age, Gender, and Education

		MEN			WOMEN		
EDUCATION (YEARS)		0–3	4–9	≥10	0–3	4–9	≥10
Age 60–69	*n*	12	45	85	68	128	65
	Mean	30.58	32.13	35.19	34.87	34.56	40.31
	SD	9.08	10.02	10.19	10.97	11.50	11.47
	5th percentile	19.00	14.80	18.60	14.00	17.00	22.60
	Median	30.50	32.00	35.00	34.00	35.00	39.00
	95th percentile	48.00	48.40	55.00	56.10	50.55	59.70
70–74	*n*	15	60	85	78	126	51
	Mean	29.60	32.70	35.37	33.18	34.21	38.77
	SD	8.64	9.87	10.51	10.99	11.96	10.64
	5th percentile	18.00	18.05	17.90	11.95	16.35	20.80
	Median	29.00	31.50	35.00	33.00	34.00	39.00
	95th percentile	48.00	48.90	55.70	52.15	53.95	54.40
75–79	*n*	13	53	54	65	86	29
	Mean	26.31	29.79	35.89	32.86	33.14	37.90
	SD	7.09	10.18	10.79	10.71	11.60	9.60
	5th percentile	17.00	12.40	16.75	11.30	15.10	21.00
	Median	26.00	29.00	35.50	33.00	34.00	38.00
	95th percentile	37.00	46.90	56.25	51.70	53.95	54.00
80–90	*n*	8	35	23	39	45	11
	Mean	25.50	29.91	35.57	30.97	32.18	38.82
	SD	8.05	10.52	12.07	10.40	10.78	10.21
	5th percentile	16.00	9.80	7.20	11.00	15.40	23.00
	Median	26.00	29.00	36.00	32.00	29.00	42.00
	95th percentile	37.00	46.40	56.60	48.00	52.70	54.00

[a]The normative data were established by using overlapping strata of the ages 60–74, 65–79, 70–84, and 75–90.

SOURCE: Seo et al. (2008).

TABLE 9–129 Scaled Score Equivalents for Victoria Stroop Dot Time Scores (in Seconds), by Age Group

AGE N	18–39 (29)	30–49 (40)	40–59 (50)	50–64 (57)	60–69 (65)	65–74 (70)	70–79 (75)	75–84 (80)	80–94 (87)
MEAN	11.0	11.1	12.3	12.0	12.1	13.3	14.2	15.1	15.1
SD	2.5	1.9	2.4	2.3	2.3	3.6	3.9	3.8	3.8
SS									
17	<7					<9	<9	<9	<9
16	7	<8	<8	<8	8	9	9	9	9
15	8	8	8	8	9	10	10	10	10
14			9	9	10			11	11
13	9	9	10	10		11	11	12	12
12		10			11		12	13	13
11	10		11	11		12	13	14	14
10		11	12	12	12	13	14	15	15–16
9	11	12	13	13	13	14	15	16	17
8	12	13	14	14	14	15	16–17	17	18–19
7	13	14	15	15	15	16–17	18–19	18–20	20–21
6	14–15	15–16	16	16	16–17	18–20	20–21	21–22	22–23
5	16–17	17	17	17	18–19	21–27	22–27	23–27	24–29
4	18	18	18	18	20	28–29	28–29	28–29	>29
3	19	19	19	19	21	30	>29	>29	
2	>19	>19	>19	>19	>21	>30			

NOTE: Midpoint ages are shown in parentheses. Overlapping age groups were used. Total *n* = 272. Education information was not recorded for the youngest age groups. Mean education was as follows: Ages 40–59: 13.2 (*SD* = 3.0); 50–64: 13.2 (2.4); 60–69: 13.6 (2.5); 65–74: 13.6 (2.9); 70–79: 12.9 (2.8); 75–84: 12.1 (2.7); 80–94: 11.5 (3.1).

SOURCE: From Troyer et al. (2006).

committed errors by reading the written words. Five of the six patients also performed substantially slower on the Color-Word trial relative to the Color trial, indicating that they were in fact inhibiting a reading response. Authors note that in the rare presentation of a report of total reading disability, failure to suppress the Stroop effect may be a valuable diagnostic tool to evaluate the veracity of this symptom presentation.

Mixed result have been reported in the identification of verified malingerers. Arentsen et al. (2013) examined

TABLE 9–130 Scaled Score Equivalents for Victoria Stroop Test Neutral Word Time Scores (in Seconds), by Age Group

AGE N	18–39 (29)	30–49 (40)	40–59 (50)	50–64 (57)	60–69 (65)	65–74 (70)	70–79 (75)	75–84 (80)	80–94 (87)
MEAN	13.0	13.9	15.2	15.4	15.9	16.9	18.6	20.7	22.1
SD	2.9	2.6	2.9	3.2	5.1	5.1	5.4	6.7	6.0
SS									
17			<10	<10	<10	<11	<11		
16	<9	<10	10	10	10	11	11–12	<14	<14
15	9	10	11	11	11	12	13	14	14
14	10	11		12	12	13	14	15	15
13	11		12	13	13		15	16	16
12		12	13			14	16	17	17–18
11	12	13	14	14	14	15	17	18	19–20
10	13	14	15	15	15	16	18	19	21–22
9	14	15	16	16	16	17	19	20–22	23–24
8	15	16	17	17	17	18–19	20–21	23–25	25–26
7	16–17	17	18	18	18	20–21	22–23	26–29	27–29
6	18–19	18–19	19	19–20	19–24	22–24	24–29	30–33	30–33
5	20	20	20	21–26	25–41	25–41	30–41	34–45	34–45
4	21	21	21–24	27–28	42–45	42–45	42–46	>45	>45
3	22	>21	>24	>28	>45	>45	>46		
2	>22								

NOTE: Midpoint ages are shown in parentheses.

SOURCE: From Troyer et al. (2006).

TABLE 9–131 Scaled Score Equivalents for Victoria Stroop Test Color Word Time Scores (in Seconds), by Age Group

AGE	18–39	30–49	40–59	50–64	60–69	65–74	70–79	75–84	80–94
N	(29)	(40)	(50)	(57)	(65)	(70)	(75)	(80)	(87)
MEAN	22.1	25.7	27.8	28.5	29.4	32.6	37.1	43.3	50.4
SD	7.2	9.0	8.2	9.5	9.0	9.6	11.9	17.7	23.9
SS									
17	<11	<15	<15	<15	<15	<19	<19	<22	<22
16	11	15	15–17	15–17	15–17	19–20	19–21	22	22–25
15	12–13	16	18	18	18–19	21	22–23	23–24	26–28
14	14–15	17	19	19	20	22	24	25–26	29–30
13	16	18	20–21	20–21	21–22	23–25	25–28	27–29	31–32
12	17–18	19–20	22–23	22–23	23–24	26–28	29–31	30–32	33–36
11	19	21–22	24–25	24–25	25–26	29–31	32–34	33–36	37–44
10	20–22	23–24	26–27	26–28	27–29	32–33	35–39	37–44	45–53
9	23–24	25–28	28–30	29–30	30–33	34–36	40–42	45–52	54–59
8	25–28	29–33	31–34	31–37	34–37	37–41	43–47	53–63	60–68
7	29–30	34–38	35–39	38–42	38–42	42–44	48–55	64–66	69–83
6	31–35	39–48	40–48	43–51	43–56	45–57	56–65	67–74	84–112
5	36–48	49–50	49–51	52–57	57–58	58–68	66–69	75–109	113–137
4	>48	>50	>51	58–59	>58	69–70	70–71	110–112	>137
3				>59		>70	>71	>112	
2									

NOTE: Midpoint ages are shown in parentheses.

SOURCE: From Troyer et al. (2006).

the utility of the Stroop (Comalli version) in detection of noncredible performance in a group meeting Slick et al.'s (1999) criteria for probable malingered neurocognitive dysfunction compared with credible neuropsychology clinic patients. The credible group outperformed the malingering group on all Stroop trials, with Word and Color particularly effective at differentiation. The following cutoff scores and sensitivity rates were reportedly associated with a specificity of 90%: Word (≥66, 54% sensitivity), Color (≥93, 49% sensitivity), with Color-Word comparatively less sensitive (≥191, 29% sensitivity). A higher risk of false positives was associated with certain clinical conditions (e.g., learning disabilities, severe TBI, psychosis, depression), age older than 80, and lower IQ.

TABLE 9–132 Scaled Score Equivalents for Victoria Stroop Test Interference Scores, by Age Group

AGE	18–39	30–49	40–59	50–64	60–69	65–74	70–79	75–84	80–94
N	(29)	(40)	(50)	(57)	(65)	(70)	(75)	(80)	(87)
MEAN	2.0	2.3	2.3	2.4	2.5	2.6	2.7	2.9	3.2
SD	0.6	0.8	0.7	0.8	0.8	0.9	1.0	1.0	1.6
SS									
18							<1.2	<1.2	<1.5
17		<1.1	<1.2	<1.2	<1.3	<1.4	1.2–1.3	1.2–1.3	1.5
16	<1.1	1.1–1.2	1.2	1.2	1.3–1.4	1.4	1.4–1.5	1.4–1.5	1.6–1.7
15	1.1–1.2	1.3	1.3–1.4	1.3–1.4	1.5–1.6	1.5–1.6	1.6	1.6–1.8	1.8
14	1.3	1.4–1.5	1.5	1.5–1.6	1.7–1.8	1.7–1.8	1.7–1.9	1.9–2.0	1.9–2.0
13	1.4–1.5	1.6–1.7	1.6–1.7	1.7–1.8	1.9	1.9	2.0	2.1	2.1–2.2
12	1.6–1.7	1.8–1.9	1.8–1.9	1.9–2.0	2.0	2.0–2.1	2.1	2.2	2.3
11	1.8–1.9	2.0–2.1	2.0–2.1	2.1	2.1	2.2	2.2–2.4	2.3–2.4	2.4–2.7
10	2.0–2.1	2.2–2.3	2.2–2.4	2.2–2.4	2.2–2.4	2.3–2.5	2.5–2.6	2.5–2.8	2.8–3.4
9	2.2–2.3	2.4–2.5	2.5–2.6	2.5–2.7	2.5–2.7	2.6–2.8	2.7–3.0	2.9–3.3	3.5–3.6
8	2.4–2.5	2.6–2.8	2.7–2.8	2.8–3.2	2.8–3.2	2.9–3.2	3.1–3.5	3.4–3.9	3.7–3.9
7	2.6–2.8	2.9–3.7	2.9–3.7	3.3–3.7	3.3–3.7	3.3–4.0	3.6–4.1	4.0–5.0	4.0–5.1
6	2.9–3.5	3.8–3.9	3.8–3.9	3.8–4.0	3.8–4.1	4.1–5.0	4.2–5.0	5.1–5.5	5.2–5.5
5	3.6–4.0	4.0–4.5	4.0–4.5	4.1–4.7	4.2–4.7	5.1–6.0	5.1–6.0	5.6–6.1	5.6–10.0
4	4.1–4.2	4.6	4.6	4.8–4.9	4.8–4.9	6.1–6.3	6.1–6.4	6.2–6.5	>10.0
3	>4.2	>4.6	>4.6	>4.9	>4.9	>6.3	>6.4	>6.5	
2									

NOTE: Midpoint ages are shown in parentheses. Interference scores were calculated as the number of seconds required to complete the Color-Word task divided by the number of seconds required to complete the Dot task.

SOURCE: From Troyer et al. (2006).

TABLE 9–133 Means and Cumulative Percentages Associated with Raw Error Scores on Victoria Stroop Test Color-Word Task, by Age Group

AGE *N*	18–39 (29)	30–49 (40)	40–59 (50)	50–64 (57)	60–69 (65)	65–74 (70)	70–79 (75)	75–84 (80)	80–94 (87)
MEAN	0.8	0.8	0.7	0.6	0.5	0.6	1.1	1.7	2.1
SD	1.0	1.0	1.0	1.0	0.9	1.2	1.6	1.8	2.0
Errors									
0	100	100	100	100	100	100	100	100	100
1	47	50	43	35	27	33	47	64	79
2	19	24	22	19	14	17	29	45	50
3	9	9	4	5	4	5	18	28	32
4	3		2	3	2	2	6	11	16
5						2	5	8	10
6						2	3	6	8
7						2	2	4	8
8									3

NOTE: Midpoint ages are shown in parentheses.

SOURCE: From Troyer et al. (2006).

Guise, Thompson, Greve, Bianchini, and West (2014) used the Golden Stroop to assess performance validity in 77 patients with a reported history of mild TBI, as well as 42 patients with moderate to severe TBI and 75 people with other clinical diagnoses. Slick et al.'s (1999) criteria for malingered neurocognitive dysfunction was used as the reference standard. Unfortunately, sensitivities were low when an optimal false-positive rate was set at 5% (i.e., 12 to 32% for Word Reading, 12 to 24% for Color Reading, and 0 to 24% for Color-Word).

COMMENT

The Stroop tests has a long history of use in neuropsychology, and various versions exist, most notably the Golden, Victoria, Comalli, and D-KEFS versions, among others. Versions vary in a number of ways including specific conditions, order of condition presentation, and number of stimuli included, but all incorporate control conditions that parse out the basic processes of word reading and color naming from the inhibitory condition of incongruent color-word naming. All versions yield response time as the primary dependent variable, with the Victoria version and D-KEFS version also allowing for tabulation of errors, which can be of qualitative value. The Golden version appears to be the most frequently used. It is not clear whether computer versions are equivalent to paper-based versions.

The test involves attention, processing speed, and conceptual abilities. There is some evidence that decrements

TABLE 9–134 Brazilian Portuguese Age- and Education-Adjusted Norms for the Victoria Stroop Test

		EDUCATION (YEARS)											
	AGE GROUP (YEARS)	0–4			5–8			9–12			≥13		
		N	*M*	*SD*	*N*	*M*	*SD*	*N*	*M*	*SD*	*N*	*M*	*SD*
STA	18–29	40	16.95	6.2	49	16.16	5.3	61	13.11	2.7	170	12.93	2.4
	30–39	23	20.70	6.7	36	15.53	4.1	60	14.34	3.7	129	13.35	2.9
	40–49	13	22.48	5.3	34	19.12	6.3	52	14.14	2.7	69	14.77	3.6
	50–59	10	22.60	6.2	19	18.25	6.4	41	15.55	5.5	48	15.23	3.5
	60–69	31	21.03	6.5	23	18.05	5.9	25	16.74	4.6	29	15.91	3.1
	>70	35	22.66	5.9	16	21.50	7.8	11	20.69	5.1	8	17.70	5.0
STB	18–29	40	19.68	7.6	49	19.69	5.9	61	15.89	4.0	171	14.19	2.5
	30–39	23	25.60	6.6	36	18.78	4.2	60	17.91	5.7	129	14.76	3.1
	40–49	13	28.54	8.8	34	22.63	5.1	52	15.94	3.5	69	17.05	3.9
	50–59	10	30.40	4.8	19	23.40	7.3	41	19.54	7.4	48	18.10	3.8
	60–69	31	26.77	6.5	23	25.48	7.6	25	21.59	4.4	29	18.86	2.7
	>70	35	30.09	8.3	16	28.50	9.6	11	28.18	7.1	8	22.08	7.0
STC	18–29	40	27.61	9.8	49	32.06	11.9	61	22.02	6.1	171	20.40	4.7
	30–39	23	36.13	10.8	36	32.56	11.5	60	27.68	8.7	129	21.90	5.5
	40–49	13	37.62	12.4	34	34.06	8.4	52	25.67	5.2	69	25.99	7.3
	50–59	10	45.40	7.7	19	34.46	9.3	41	31.76	11.1	48	27.54	7.5
	60–69	31	40.16	13.0	23	39.93	10.3	25	37.71	9.9	29	31.12	8.2
	>70	35	53.43	19.6	16	49.21	21.7	11	44.27	13.8	8	39.37	15.4

NOTE: STA, Stroop A; STB, Stroop B; STC, Stroop C.

SOURCE: Campanholo et al. (2014).

in performance are related to processing speed in some conditions such as TBI, whereas increased difficulty with interference underlies poor performance in other conditions such as schizophrenia and dementia. Neuroanatomical correlates of performance implicate frontal areas and also suggest that the task requires recruitment of a broad-based network involving white matter tracts and temporal regions. Users should note there are also a number of other influences on performance. For example, in older adults, time of testing and visual ability including visual acuity and color vision are impactful. Degree of automaticity of word reading must also be considered when interpreting results.

Demographically, age has well-established effects on performance. However, the research is somewhat mixed with respect to whether aging has specific effects on interference versus whether age-related decrements in performance are instead reflective of changes in underlying processes such as visual abilities and processing speed. In clinical practice, examination of performance on various subcomponents of the task can assist in elucidating whether the specific cause of poor performance is due to a deficiency in basic processes. Additionally, examination of other tasks within the battery administered can also help elucidate the nature of poor performance.

Gender differences are sometimes found in favor of women, although evidence is mixed overall. Education effects are often found to be nearly as influential as age; reading ability and IQ also impact performance. There appear to be effects of language and ethnicity. These demographic variables should be considered when selecting normative datasets. Fortunately, there are a large number of normative datasets, most of which adjust for age and education. Most normative data are based on the Golden version, with a few others using the Victoria version. Of note, there are weaknesses with the normative data provided in the manual for the Golden version, and thus other datasets are preferred. The choice of data will depend on the population of interest as there are many norms for specific countries, languages, and age ranges. Reliability is strong overall. Test-retest reliability coefficients are somewhat lower for the interference trials, although still in the acceptable range. Practice effects have been reported, with minimal gains after approximately three administrations.

The test has been used successfully in many diverse clinical populations, including TBI, dementia, ADHD, PD, schizophrenia, and other psychiatric conditions involving mood and anxiety. Last, although the test has some promise in performance validity assessment, research has reported variable sensitivity to feigning, suggesting that it should not be used in isolation to establish the presence of noncredible performance.

REFERENCES

Andrews, K., Shuttleworth-Edwards, A., & Radloff, S. (2012). Normative indications for Xhosa speaking unskilled workers on the Trail Making and Stroop Tests. *Journal of Psychology in Africa, 22*(3), 333–341.

Antsey, K. J., Dain, S., Andrews, S., & Drobny, J. (2002). Visual abilities in older adults explain age-differences in Stroop and fluid intelligence but not face recognition: Implications for the vision-cognition connection. *Aging, Neuropsychology, & Cognition, 9*, 253–265.

Anstey, K. J., Matters, B., Brown, A. K., & Lord, S. R. (2000). Normative data on neuropsychological tests for very old adults living in retirement villages and hostels. *The Clinical Neuropsychologist, 14*, 309–317.

Antshel, K. M., Faraone, S. V., Maglione, K., Doyle, A. E., Fried, R., Seidman, L. J., & Biederman, J. (2010). Executive functioning in high-IQ adults with ADHD. *Psychological Medicine, 40*(11), 1909–1918. http://doi.org/10.1017/S0033291709992273

Arentsen, T. J., Boone, K. B., Lo, T. T. Y., Goldberg, H. E., Cottingham, M. E., Victor, T. L., . . . Zeller, M. A. (2013). Effectiveness of the Comalli Stroop Test as a measure of negative response bias. *The Clinical Neuropsychologist, 27*(6), 1060–1076. http://doi.org/10.1080/13854046.2013.803603

Artiola I Fortuny, L., Romo, D. H., Heaton, R. K., & Pardee III, R. E. (1999). *Manual de Normas y Procedimemientos para la Bateria Neuropsicologia en Espanol.* The Netherlands: Swets & Zeitlinger.

Avila, R., Moscoso, M. A. A., Ribeiz, S., Arrais, J., Jaluul, O., & Bottino, C. M. C. (2009). Influence of education and depressive symptoms on cognitive function in the elderly. *International Psychogeriatrics, 21*(03), 560. http://doi.org/10.1017/S1041610209008928

Bayard, S., Erkes, J., Moroni, C., & the College des Psychologues Cliniciens specialises en Neuropsychologie du Languedoc Roussillon (CPCN Languedoc Roussillon). (2011). Victoria Stroop Test: Normative data in a sample group of older people and the study of their clinical applications in the assessment of inhibition in Alzheimer's disease. *Archives of Clinical Neuropsychology, 26*(7), 653–661. http://doi.org/10.1093/arclin/acr053

Ben-David, B. M., Nguyen, L. L. T., & van Lieshout, P. H. H. M. (2011). Stroop effects in persons with traumatic brain injury: Selective attention, speed of processing, or color-naming? A meta-analysis. *Journal of the International Neuropsychological Society, 17*(02), 354–363. http://doi.org/10.1017/S135561771000175X

Bezdicek, O., Lukavsky, J., Stepankova, H., Nikolai, T., Axelrod, B. N., Michalec, J., . . . Kopecek, M. (2015). The Prague Stroop Test: Normative standards in older Czech adults and discriminative validity for mild cognitive impairment in Parkinson's disease. *Journal of Clinical and Experimental Neuropsychology, 37*(8), 794–807. http://doi.org/10.1080/13803395.2015.1057106

Bodling, A. M., Denney, D. R., & Lynch, S. G. (2012). Individual variability in speed of information processing: An index of cognitive impairment in multiple sclerosis. *Neuropsychology, 26*(3), 357–367. http://doi.org/10.1037/a0027972

Bondi, M. W., Serody, A. B., Chan, A. S., Eberson-Schumate, S. C., Delis, D. C., Hansen, L. A., & Salmon, D. P. (2002). Cognitive and neuropathologic correlates of Stroop Color-Word Test performance in Alzheimer's disease. *Neuropsychology*, 16, 335–343.

Boone, K. B., Ponton, M. O., Gorsuch, R. L., Gonzalez, J. J., & Miller, B. L. (1998). Factor analysis of four measures of pre-frontal lobe functioning. *Archives of Clinical Neuropsychology, 13*, 585–595.

Boyle, P. A., Paul, R. H., Moser, D. J., & Cohen, R. A. (2004). Executive impairments predict functional declines in vascular dementia. *The Clinical Neuropsychologist, 18*, 75–82.

Buré-Reyes, A., Hidalgo-Ruzzante, N., Vilar-López, R., Gontier, J., Sánchez, L., Pérez-García, M., & Puente, A. E. (2013). Neuropsychological test performance of Spanish speakers: Is performance different across different Spanish-speaking subgroups? *Journal of Clinical and Experimental Neuropsychology, 35*(4), 404–412. http://doi.org/10.1080/13803395.2013.778232

Campanholo, K. R., Romão, M. A., Machado, M. de A. R., Serrao, V. T., Coutinho, D. G. C., Benute, G. R. G., & Lucia, M. C. S. de. (2014). Performance of an adult Brazilian sample on the Trail Making Test and Stroop Test. *Dementia & Neuropsychologia, 8*(1), 26–31.

Castellon, S. A., Hinkin, C. H., & Myers, H. F. (2000). Neuropsychiatric disturbance is associated with executive dysfunction in HIV-1 infection. *Journal of the International Neuropsychological Society, 6*, 336–347.

Chafetz, M. D., & Matthews, L. H. (2004). A new interference score for the Stroop test. *Archives of Clinical Neuropsychology, 19*, 555–567.

Cicerone, K. D., & Azulay, J. (2002). Diagnostic utility of attention measures in postconcussion syndrome. *The Clinical Neuropsychologist, 16*, 280–289.

Cipolotti, L., Spanò, B., Healy, C., Tudor-Sfetea, C., Chan, E., White, M., . . . Bozzali, M. (2016). Inhibition processes are dissociable and lateralized in human prefrontal cortex. *Neuropsychologia, 93*(Pt A), 1–12. https://doi.org/10.1016/j.neuropsychologia.2016.09.018

Collette, F., Van der Linden, M., Delrue, G., & Salmon, E. (2002). Frontal hypometabolism does not explain inhibitory dysfunction in Alzheimer disease. *Alzheimer Disease & Associated Disorders, 16*, 228–238.

Comalli Jr., P. E., Wapner, S., & Werner, H. (1962). Interference effects of Stroop Color-Word Test in childhood, adulthood and aging. *Journal of Genetic Psychology, 100*, 47–53.

Connor, A., Franzen, M., & Sharp, B. (1988). Effects of practice and differential instructions on Stroop performance. *International Journal of Clinical Neuropsychology, 10*, 1–4.

Cox, C. S., Chee, E., Chase, G. A., Baumgardner, T. L., Schuerholz, L. J., Reader, M. J., Mohr, J., & Denkla, M. B. (1997). Reading proficiency affects the construct validity of the Stroop Test Interference Score. *The Clinical Neuropsychologist, 11*, 105–110.

Csigó, K., Harsányi, A., Demeter, G., Rajkai, C., Németh, A., & Racsmány, M. (2010). Long-term follow-up of patients with obsessive–compulsive disorder treated by anterior capsulotomy: A neuropsychological study. *Journal of Affective Disorders, 126*(1-2), 198–205. http://doi.org/10.1016/j.jad.2010.02.127

D'Alcante, C. C., Diniz, J. B., Fossaluza, V., Batistuzzo, M. C., Lopes, A. C., Shavitt, R. G., . . . Hoexter, M. Q. (2012). Neuropsychological predictors of response to randomized treatment in obsessive–compulsive disorder. *Progress in Neuro-Psychopharmacology and Biological Psychiatry, 39*(2), 310–317. http://doi.org/10.1016/j.pnpbp.2012.07.002

Dao-Castellana, M. H., Samson, Y., Legaugt, F., Martinot, J. L., Aubin, H. J., Crouzel, C., . . . Syrota, A. (1998). Frontal dysfunction in neurologically normal chronic alcoholic subjects: Metabolic and neuropsychological findings. *Psychological Medicine, 28*, 1039–1048.

Delis, D. C., Kaplan, E., & Kramer, J. H. (2001). *Delis-Kaplan Executive Function System.* San Antonio, TX: The Psychological Corporation.

Demakis, G. J. (2004). Frontal lobe damage and tests of executive processing: A meta-analysis of the Category Test, Stroop Test, and Trail-Making Test. *Journal of Clinical and Experimental Neuropsychology, 26*, 441–450.

Denney, D. R., & Lynch, S. G. (2009). The impact of multiple sclerosis on patients' performance on the Stroop Test: Processing speed versus interference. *Journal of the International Neuropsychological Society, 15*(03), 451. http://doi.org/10.1017/S1355617709090730

Dikmen, S. S., Heaton, R. K., Grant, I., & Temkin, N. R. (1999). Test-retest reliability and practice effects of expanded Halstead-Reitan Neuropsychological Test Battery. *Journal of the International Neuropsychological Society, 5*, 346–356.

Felmingham, K. L., Baguley, I. J., & Green, A. M. (2004). Effects of diffuse axonal injury on speed of information processing following severe traumatic brain injury. *Neuropsychology, 18*, 564–571.

Foss, M. P., Formigheri, P., & Speciali, J. G. (2009). Heterogeneity of cognitive aging in Brazilian normal elderly. *Dementia & Neuropsychologia, 3*(4), 344–351. https://doi.org/10.1590/S1980-57642009DN30400014

Franzen, M. D. (2000). *Reliability and Validity in Neuropsychological Assessment* (2nd ed.). New York: Kluwer Academic/Plenum Publishers.

Franzen, M. D., Tishelman, A. C., Sharp, B. H., & Friedman, A. G. (1987). An investigation of the test-retest reliability of the Stroop Color-Word Test across two intervals. *Archives of Clinical Neuropsychology, 2*, 265–272.

Friedman, N. P., & Miyake, A. (2004). The relations among inhibition and interference control functions: A latent variable analysis. *JEP: General.*

Gasquoine, P., Croyle, K., Cavazosgonzalez, C., & Sandoval, O. (2007). Language of administration and neuropsychological test performance in neurologically intact Hispanic American bilingual adults. *Archives of Clinical Neuropsychology, 22*(8), 991–1001. http://doi.org/10.1016/j.acn.2007.08.003

Golden, C. J. (1975). A group version of the Stroop Color and Word Test. *Journal of Personality Assessment, 39*, 502–506.

Golden, C. J. (1976). Identification of brain disorders by the Stroop Color and Word Test. *Journal of Clinical Psychology, 32*, 654–658.

Golden, C. J. (1978). *Stroop Color and Word Test: A manual for clinical and experimental uses.* Chicago, IL: Stoelting Co.

Golden, C. J., & Freshwater, S. M. (2002). *Stroop Color and Word Test: Revised examiner's manual.* Wood Dale, IL: Stoelting Co.

Graf, P., Uttl, B., & Tuokko, H. (1995). Color- and picture-word Stroop tests: Performance changes in old age. *Journal of Clinical and Experimental Neuropsychology, 17*, 390–415.

Gruner, P., & Pittenger, C. (2017). Cognitive inflexibility in Obsessive-Compulsive Disorder. *Neuroscience, 345*, 243–255. https://doi.org/10.1016/j.neuroscience.2016.07.030

Guise, B. J., Thompson, M. D., Greve, K. W., Bianchini, K. J., & West, L. (2014). Assessment of performance validity in the Stroop Color and Word Test in mild traumatic brain injury patients: a criterion-groups validation design. *Journal of Neuropsychology, 8*(1), 20–33. https://doi.org/10.1111/jnp.12002

Hanes, K. R., Andrewes, D. G., Smith, D. J., & Pantelis, C. (1996). A brief assessment of executive control dysfunction: Discriminant validity and homogeneity of planning, set shift, and fluency measures. *Archives of Clinical Neuropsychology, 11*, 185–191.

Hoshi, T., Yamagami, H., Furukado, S., Miwa, K., Tanaka, M., Sakaguchi, M., . . . Kitagawa, K. (2010). Serum inflammatory proteins and frontal lobe dysfunction in patients with cardiovascular risk factors: Serum hsCRP and frontal lobe dysfunction. *European Journal of Neurology, 17*(9), 1134–1140. http://doi.org/10.1111/j.1468-1331.2010.02990.x

Hou, C.-L., Xiang, Y.-T., Wang, Z.-L., Everall, I., Tang, Y., Yang, C., . . . Jia, F.-J. (2016). Cognitive functioning in individuals at ultra-high risk for psychosis, first-degree relatives of patients with psychosis and patients with first-episode schizophrenia. *Schizophrenia Research, 174*(1–3), 71–76. https://doi.org/10.1016/j.schres.2016.04.034

Hughes, A. J., Denney, D. R., Owens, E. M., & Lynch, S. G. (2013). Procedural variations in the Stroop and the Symbol Digit Modalities Test: Impact on patients with multiple sclerosis. *Archives of Clinical Neuropsychology, 28*(5), 452–462. http://doi.org/10.1093/arclin/act041

Hughes, E. J., Bond, J., Svrckova, P., Makropoulos, A., Ball, G., Sharp, D. J., . . . Counsell, S. J. (2012). Regional changes in thalamic shape and volume with increasing age. *NeuroImage, 63*(3), 1134–1142. http://doi.org/10.1016/j.neuroimage.2012.07.043

Ivnik, R. J., Malec, J. F., Smith, G. E., & Tangalos, E. G. (1996). Neuropsychological test norms above age 55: COWAT, BNT, MAE token, WRAT-R reading, AMNART, Stroop, TMT, and JLO. *The Clinical Neuropsychologist, 10*, 262–278.

Johns, E. K., Phillips, N. A., Belleville, S., Goupil, D., Babins, L., Kelner, N., . . . Chertkow, H. (2009). Executive functions in frontotemporal dementia and Lewy body dementia. *Neuropsychology, 23*(6), 765–777. http://doi.org/10.1037/a0016792

Jokinen, H., Ryberg, C., Kalska, H., Ylikoski, R., Rostrup, E., Stegmann, M. B., . . . LADIS group. (2007). Corpus callosum atrophy is associated with mental slowing and executive deficits in subjects with age-related white matter hyperintensities: the LADIS Study. *Journal of Neurology, Neurosurgery, and Psychiatry, 78*(5), 491–496. https://doi.org/10.1136/jnnp.2006.096792

Juselius, S., Kieseppa, T., Kaprio, J., Lonnqvist, J., & Tuulio-Henriksson, A. (2009). Executive functioning in twins with bipolar i disorder and healthy co-twins. *Archives of Clinical Neuropsychology, 24*(6), 599–606. http://doi.org/10.1093/arclin/acp047

Kane, M. J., & Engle, R. W. (2003). Working-memory capacity and the control of attention: The contributions of goal neglect, response competition, and task set to Stroop interference. *Journal of Experimental Psychology: General, 132*, 47–70.

Kang, C., Lee, G. J., Yi, D., McPherson, S., Rogers, S., Tingus, K., & Lu, P. H. (2013). Normative data for healthy older adults and an abbreviated version of the Stroop test. *The Clinical Neuropsychologist, 27*(2), 276–289. http://doi.org/10.1080/13854046.2012.742930

Kerns, J. G., Cohen, J. D., MacDonald, A. W., Cho, R. Y., Stenger, V. A., & Carter, C. S. (2004). Anterior cingulate conflict monitoring and adjustments in control. *Science, 303*, 102–123.

Klein, M., Ponds, R. W. H. M., Houx, P. J., & Jolles, J. (1997). Effect of test duration on age-related differences in Stroop interference. *Journal of Clinical and Experimental Neuropsychology, 19*, 77–82.

Kramer, J. H., Reed, B. R., Mungas, D., Weiner, M. W., & Chui, H. C. (2002). Executive dysfunction in subcortical ischaemic vascular disease. *Journal of Neurology, Neurosurgery and Psychiatry, 72*, 217–220.

Lee, T. M. (2003). *Normative data: Neuropsychological measures for Hong Kong Chinese.* The University of Hong Kong Neuropsychology Laboratory.

Llinas-Regla, J., Vilalta-Franch, J., Lopez-Pousa, S., Calvo-Perxas, L., & Garre-Olmo, J. (2013). Demographically adjusted norms for Catalan older adults on the Stroop Color and Word Test. *Archives of Clinical Neuropsychology, 28*(3), 282–296. http://doi.org/10.1093/arclin/act003

Lu, P. H., Boone, K. B., Jiminez, N., & Razami, J. (2004). Failure to inhibit the reading response on the Stroop test: A pathognomic indicator of suspect effort. *Journal of Clinical and Experimental Neuropsychology, 26*, 180–189.

Lubrini, G., Periañez, J. A., Rios-Lago, M., Viejo-Sobera, R., Ayesa-Arriola, R., Sanchez-Cubillo, I., . . . Rodriguez-Sanchez, J. M. (2014). Clinical Spanish norms of the Stroop Test for traumatic brain injury and schizophrenia. *Spanish Journal of Psychology, 17*. http://doi.org/10.1017/sjp.2014.90

Lucas, J. A., Ivnik, R. J., Smith, G. E., Ferman, T. J., Willis, F. B., Petersen, R. C., & Graff-Radford, N. R. (2005). Mayo's Older African Americans Normative Studies: Norms for Boston naming test, Controlled Oral Word Association, Category Fluency, Animal Naming, Token Test, WRAT-3 Reading, Trail Making Test, Stroop Test, and Judgement of Line Orientation. *The Clinical Neuropsychologist, 19*, 243–269.

Lynch, S. G., Dickerson, K. J., & Denney, D. R. (2010). Evaluating processing speed in multiple sclerosis: A comparison of two rapid serial processing measures. *The Clinical Neuropsychologist, 24*(6), 963–976. http://doi.org/10.1080/13854046.2010.502128

Mackin, R. S., Ayalon, L., Feliciano, L., & Arean, P. A. (2010). The sensitivity and specificity of cognitive screening instruments to detect cognitive impairment in older adults with severe psychiatric illness. *Journal of Geriatric Psychiatry and Neurology, 23*(2), 94–99. http://doi.org/10.1177/0891988709358589

MacLeod, C. M. (1991). Half a century of research on the Stroop effect: An integrative review. *Psychological Bulletin, 109*, 163–203.

Maruta, C., Guerreiro, M., de Mendonça, A., Hort, J., & Scheltens, P. (2011). The use of neuropsychological tests across Europe: The need for a consensus in the use of assessment tools for dementia: The use of neuropsychological tests across Europe. *European Journal of Neurology, 18*(2), 279–285. http://doi.org/10.1111/j.1468-1331.2010.03134.x

May, C. P., & Hasher, L. (1998). Synchrony effects in inhibitory control over thought and action. *Journal of Experimental Psychology: Human Perception and Performance, 24*, 363–379.

Mead, L. A., Mayer, A. R., Bobholz, J. A., Woodley, S. J., Cunningham, J. M., Hammeke, T. A., & Rao, S. M. (2002). Neural basis of the Stroop interference task: Response competition or selective attention. *Journal of the International Neuropsychological Society, 8*, 735–742.

Melrose, R. J., Young, S., Weissberger, G. H., Natta, L., Harwood, D., Mandelkern, M., & Sultzer, D. L. (2017). Cerebral metabolic correlates of attention networks in Alzheimer's disease: A study of the Stroop. *Neuropsychologia, 106*, 383–389. https://doi.org/10.1016/j.neuropsychologia.2017.10.020

Mitrushina, M. M., Boone, K. B., Razani, J., & D'Elia, L. F. (2005). *Handbook of normative data for neuropsychological assessment* (2nd ed.). New York: Oxford University Press.

Moering, R. G., Schinka, J. A., Mortimer, J. A., & Graves, A. B. (2004). Normative data for elderly African Americans for the Stroop Color and Word Test. *Archives of Clinical Neuropsychology, 19*, 61–71.

Moritz, S., Birkner, C., & Kloss, M. (2002). Executive functioning in obsessive-compulsive disorder, unipolar depression, and schizophrenia. *Archives of Clinical Neuropsychology, 17*, 477–483.

Morrow, S. A. (2013). Normative data for the Stroop color word test for a North American population. *Canadian Journal of Neurological Sciences. Le Journal Canadien Des Sciences Neurologiques, 40*(6), 842–847.

Nabeyama, M., Nakagawa, A., Yoshiura, T., Nakao, T., Nakatani, E., Togao, O., . . . Kanba, S. (2008). Functional MRI study of brain activation alterations in patients with obsessive-compulsive disorder after symptom improvement. *Psychiatry Research: Neuroimaging, 163*(3), 236–247. http://doi.org/10.1016/j.pscychresns.2007.11.001

Nathan, J., Wilkinson, D., Stammers, S., & Low, J. L. (2001). The role of tests of frontal executive functioning in the detection of mild dementia. *International Journal of Geriatric Psychiatry, 16*, 18–26.

Norman, M. A., Moore, D. J., Taylor, M., Franklin, D., Cysique, L., Ake, C., . . . the HNRC Group. (2011). Demographically corrected norms for African Americans and Caucasians on the Hopkins Verbal Learning Test–Revised, Brief Visuospatial Memory Test–Revised, Stroop Color and Word Test, and Wisconsin Card Sorting Test 64-Card Version. *Journal of Clinical and Experimental Neuropsychology, 33*(7), 793–804. http://doi.org/10.1080/13803395.2011.559157

Oosthuizen, M. D., & Phipps, W. D. (2012). A preliminary standardisation of the Bohnen et al. version of the Stroop Color-Word Test for Setswana-speaking university students. *South African Journal of Psychology, 42*(3), 411–422.

Pattanayak, R. D., Sagar, R., & Mehta, M. (2012). Neuropsychological performance in euthymic Indian patients with bipolar disorder type I: Correlation between quality of life and global functioning: Neuropsychological performance and QoL. *Psychiatry and Clinical Neurosciences, 66*(7), 553–563. http://doi.org/10.1111/j.1440-1819.2012.02400.x

Paulsen, J. S., Miller, A. C., Hayes, T., & Shaw, E. (2017). Cognitive and behavioral changes in Huntington disease before diagnosis. *Handbook of Clinical Neurology, 144*, 69–91. https://doi.org/10.1016/B978-0-12-801893-4.00006-7

Pavão Martins, I., Maruta, C., Freitas, V., & Mares, I. (2013). Executive performance in older Portuguese adults with low education. *The Clinical Neuropsychologist, 27*(3), 410–425. http://doi.org/10.1080/13854046.2012.748094

Pena-Casanova, J., Quinones-Ubeda, S., Gramunt-Fombuena, N., Quintana, M., Aguilar, M., Molinuevo, J. L., . . . for the NEURONORMA Study Team. (2009). Spanish Multicenter Normative Studies (NEURONORMA Project): Norms for the Stroop Color-Word Interference Test and the Tower of London-Drexel. *Archives of Clinical Neuropsychology, 24*(4), 413–429. http://doi.org/10.1093/arclin/acp043

Perret, E. (1974). The left frontal lobe of man and the suppression of habitual responses in verbal categorical behavior. *Neuropsychologia, 12*, 323–330.

Peterson, B. S., Kane, M. J., Alexander, G. M., Lacadie, C., Skudlarski, P., Leung, H-C., May, J., & Gore, J. C. (2002). An event-related fMRI study interference effects in the Simon and Stroop tasks. *Cognitive Brain Research, 13*, 427–440.

Pineda, D. A., & Merchan, V. (2003). Executive function in young Colombian adults. *International Journal of Neuroscience, 113*, 397–410.

Ponsford, J., & Kinsella, G. (1992). Attentional deficits following closed head injury. *Journal of Clinical and Experimental Neuropsychology, 14*, 822–828.

Rand, D., Eng, J. J., Liu-Ambrose, T., & Tawashy, A. E. (2010). Feasibility of a 6-month exercise and recreation program to improve executive functioning and memory in individuals with chronic stroke. *Neurorehabilitation and Neural Repair, 24*(8), 722–729. http://doi.org/10.1177/1545968310368684

Ravnkilde, B., Videbech, P., Rosenberg, R., Gjedde, A., & Gade, A. (2002). Putative tests of frontal lobe function: A PET-study of brain activation during Stroop's test and verbal fluency. *Journal of Clinical and Experimental Neuropsychology, 24*, 534–547.

Razani, J., Burciaga, J., Madore, M., & Wong, J. (2007). Effects of acculturation on tests of attention and information processing in an ethnically diverse group. *Archives of Clinical Neuropsychology, 22*(3), 333–341. http://doi.org/10.1016/j.acn.2007.01.008

Regard, M. (1981). *Cognitive rigidity and flexibility: A neuropsychological study.* Unpublished PhD dissertation, University of Victoria.

Rios, M., Perianez, J. A., & Munoz-Cespedes, J. M. (2004). Attentional control and slowness of information processing after severe traumatic brain injury. *Brain Injury, 18*, 257–272.

Rosselli, M., Ardila, A., Santisi, M. N., Arecco, A. D. R., Salvatierra, J., Conde, A., & Lenis, B. (2002). Stroop effect in Spanish-English bilinguals. *Journal of the International Neuropsychological Society, 8*, 819–827.

Sachs, T. L., Clark, C. R., Pols, R. G., & Geffen, L. B. (1991). Comparability and stability of performance of six alternate forms of the Dodrill-Stroop Color-Word Test. *The Clinical Neuropsychologist, 5*, 220–225.

Salthouse, T. A., & Meinz, E. J. (1995). Aging, inhibition, working memory, and speed. *Journal of Gerontology, 50*, 297–306.

Sánchez-Cubillo, I., Periáñez, J. A., Adrover-Roig, D., Rodríguez-Sánchez, J. M., Ríos-Lago, M., Tirapu, J., & Barceló, F. (2009). Construct validity of the Trail Making Test: Role of task-switching, working memory, inhibition/interference control, and visuomotor abilities. *Journal of the International Neuropsychological Society, 15*(03), 438. http://doi.org/10.1017/S1355617709090626

Schneider, B. C., & Lichtenberg, P. A. (2011). Influence of reading ability on neuropsychological performance in African American elders. *Archives of Clinical Neuropsychology, 26*(7), 624–631. http://doi.org/10.1093/arclin/acr062

Seo, E. H., Lee, D. Y., Choo, Il H., Kim, S. G., Kim, K. W., Youn, J. C., . . . Woo, J. I. (2008). Normative study of the Stroop Color and Word Test in an educationally diverse elderly population. *International Journal of Geriatric Psychiatry, 23*(10), 1020–1027. http://doi.org/10.1002/gps.2027

Shilling, V. M., Chetwynd, A., & Rabbitt, P. M. A. (2002). Individual inconsistency across measures of inhibition: An investigation of the construct validity of inhibition in older adults. *Neuropsychologia, 40*, 605–619.

Silva, K. L., Guimaraes-da-Silva, P. O., Grevet, E. H., Victor, M. M., Salgado, C. A. I., Vitola, E. S., . . . Bau, C. H. D. (2013). Cognitive deficits in adults with ADHD go beyond comorbidity effects. *Journal of Attention Disorders, 17*(6), 483–488. http://doi.org/10.1177/1087054711434155

Slick, D. J., Sherman, E. M. S., & Iverson, G. L. (1999). Diagnostic Criteria for Malingered Neurocognitive Dysfunction: Proposed Standards for Clinical Practice and Research. *The Clinical Neuropsychologist, 13*(4), 545–561. https://doi.org/10.1076/1385-4046(199911)13:04;1-Y;FT545

Snowden, J., Craufurd, D., Griffiths, H., Thompson, J., & Neary, D. (2001). Longitudinal evaluation of cognitive disorder in Huntington's disease. *Journal of the International Neuropsychological Society, 7*, 33–44.

Steinberg, B. A., Bieliauskas, L. A., Smith, G. E., & Ivnik, R. J. (2005). Mayo's Older Americans Normative Studies: Age- and IQ-adjusted norms for the Trail-Making Test, the Stroop Test, and MAE Controlled Oral Word Association Test. *The Clinical Neuropsychologist, 19*, 329–377.

Stroop, J. R. (1935). Studies of interference in serial verbal reaction. *Journal of Experimental Psychology, 18*, 643–662.

Stuss, D. T., Floden, D., Alexander, M. P., Levine, B., & Katz, D. (2001). Stroop performance in focal lesion patients: Dissociation of processes and frontal lobe lesion location. *Neuropsychologia, 39*, 771–786.

Sudo, F. K., Amado, P., Alves, G. S., Laks, J., & Engelhardt, E. (2017). A continuum of executive function deficits in early subcortical vascular cognitive impairment: A systematic review and meta-analysis. *Dementia & Neuropsychologia, 11*(4), 371–380. https://doi.org/10.1590/1980-57642016dn11-040006

Szöke, A., Schürhoff, F., Mathieu, F., Meary, A., Ionescu, S., & Leboyer, M. (2005). Tests of executive functions in first-degree relatives of schizophrenic patients: A meta-analysis. *Psychological Medicine, 35*(6), 771–782. http://doi.org/10.1017/S0033291704003460

Szöke, A., Trandafir, A., Dupont, M.-E., Meary, A., Schürhoff, F., & Leboyer, M. (2008). Longitudinal studies of cognition in schizophrenia: Meta-analysis. *British Journal of Psychiatry, 192*(4), 248–257. http://doi.org/10.1192/bjp.bp.106.029009

Trenerry, M. R., Crosson, B., DeBoe, J., & Leber, W. R. (1989). *Stroop Neurological Screening Test.* Odessa, FL: Psychological Assessment Resources.

Troyer, A. K., Leach, L., & Strauss, E. (2006). Aging and response inhibition: Normative data for the Victoria Stroop Test. *Aging, Neuropsychology, and Cognition, 13*(1), 20–35. http://doi.org/10.1080/138255890968187

Uttl, B., & Graf, P. (1997). Color Word Stroop Test performance across the adult life span. *Journal of Clinical and Experimental Neuropsychology, 19*, 405–420.

Van Boxtel, M. P. J., ten Tusscher, M. P. M., Metsemakers, J. F. M., Willems, B., & Jolles, J. (2001). Visual determinants of reduced performance on the Stroop Color-Word Test in normal aging adults. *Journal of Clinical and Experimental Neuropsychology, 23*, 620–627.

Van der Elst, W. (2006). The Stroop Color-Word Test: Influence of age, sex, and education; and normative data for a large sample across the adult age range. *Assessment, 13*(1), 62–79. http://doi.org/10.1177/1073191105283427

Van Gorp, W. G., Humphrey, L. A., Kalechstein, A., Brumm, V. L., McMullen, W. J., Stoddard, M., & Pachana, N. A. (1999). How well do standard clinical neuropsychological tests identify malingering? A preliminary analysis. *Journal of Clinical and Experimental Neuropsychology, 21*, 245–250.

Videbech, P., Ravnkilde, B., Gammelgaard, L., Egander, A., Clemmensen, K., Rasmussen, N. A., . . . Rosenberg, R. (2004). The Danish PET/depression project: Performance on Stroop's test linked to white matter lesions in the brain. *Psychiatry Research: Neuroimaging, 130*(2), 117–130. http://doi.org/10.1016/j.pscychresns.2003.10.002

Vogel, A., Stokholm, J., & Jørgensen, K. (2013). Performances on Symbol Digit Modalities Test, Color Trails Test, and modified Stroop test in a healthy, elderly Danish sample. *Aging, Neuropsychology, and Cognition, 20*(3), 370–382. http://doi.org/10.1080/13825585.2012.725126

Wagner, S., Doering, B., Helmreich, I., Lieb, K., & Tadić, A. (2012). A meta-analysis of executive dysfunctions in unipolar major depressive disorder without psychotic symptoms and their changes during antidepressant treatment: Executive dysfunctions in unipolar MDD. *Acta Psychiatrica Scandinavica, 125*(4), 281–292. http://doi.org/10.1111/j.1600-0447.2011.01762.x

White, M., Lalonde, R., & Botez-Marquard, T. (2000). Neuropsychologic and neuropsychiatric characteristics of patients with Friedreich's ataxia. *Acta Neurologica Scandinavica 102*, 222–226.

Yatham, L. N., Torres, I. J., Malhi, G. S., Frangou, S., Glahn, D. C., Bearden, C. E., . . . Chengappa, K. N. R. (2010). The International Society for Bipolar Disorders-Battery for Assessment of Neurocognition (ISBD-BANC): ISBD-BANC. *Bipolar Disorders, 12*(4), 351–363. http://doi.org/10.1111/j.1399-5618.2010.00830.x

Zalonis, I., Christidi, F., Bonakis, A., Kararizou, E., Triantafyllou, N. I., Paraskevas, G., . . . Vasilopoulos, D. (2009). The Stroop Effect in Greek healthy population: Normative data for the Stroop neuropsychological screening test. *Archives of Clinical Neuropsychology, 24*(1), 81–88. http://doi.org/10.1093/arclin/acp011

Zhou, B., Zhao, Q., Teramukai, S., Ding, D., Guo, Q., Fukushima, M., & Hong, Z. (2010). Executive function predicts survival in Alzheimer disease: a study in Shanghai. *Journal of Alzheimer's Disease, 22*(2), 673–682.

Zimmermann, N., Cardoso, C. de O., Trentini, C. M., Grassi-Oliveira, R., & Fonseca, R. P. (2015). Brazilian preliminary norms and investigation of age and education effects on the Modified Wisconsin Card Sorting Test, Stroop Color and Word test and Digit Span test in adults. *Dementia & Neuropsychologia, 9*(2), 120–127. http://doi.org/10.1590/1980-57642015DN92000006

TRAIL MAKING TEST (TMT)

TEST NAME	**Trail Making Test (TMT)**
DOMAIN	Executive functioning
AGE RANGE	Up to 90+ years
ADMINISTRATION TIME	10 minutes
SCORING FORMAT	Hand scored
REFERENCE	Varies (see "Description")

DESCRIPTION

The Trail Making Test (TMT) is a measure of attention, speed, and mental flexibility. The test was originally constructed in 1938 as "Partington's Pathways" or the "Divided Attention Test" (Partington & Leiter, 1949). It was adapted by Reitan (1955) and added to the Halstead Battery. It requires the examinee to connect, by making pencil lines, 25 encircled numbers randomly arranged on a page in proper order (Part A or TMT-A) and 25 encircled numbers and letters in alternating order (Part B or TMT-B).

Variants of the TMT are included in other batteries, such as the D-KEFS (see review elsewhere in this chapter). Others variants have been developed (e.g., Drapeau et al., 2007; Franzen et al., 1996; Lewis & Rennick, 1979; Reynolds, 2002; Stanczak et al., 1998). An oral version is also available, for individuals with significant motor or visual impairments (e.g., Ricker & Axelrod, 1994; Ricker et al., 1996). A computerized version that enables a broader range of scores to be collected has also shown promise (Woods et al., 2015).

ADMINISTRATION

Administration guidelines for the TMT are provided in Figures 9–12 and 9–13 (standard and oral versions, respectively). A number of authors (e.g., Heaton et al., 2004; Lucas et al., 2005) include a time limit of five minutes (300 seconds) on the TMT-B to reduce testing time and examinee frustration. Examinees who cannot complete the TMT-B within five minutes are assigned a time of 300 or 301 seconds. Practice exercises are included. Thompson et al. (1999) provide tables related to the practice component of the task to assist the clinician in deciding whether to administer the remainder of the TMT or to discontinue, as may be done in the case of examinees with severe impairment. A 20-second TMT-A practice time cutoff resulted in optimal prediction of successful completion of the TMT-A (<180 seconds); a TMT-B practice time cutoff of 30 seconds proved optimal in predicting successful completion of the TMT-B (<300 seconds). Of note, circadian rhythm is related to TMT performance, with older adults but not younger adults tested at nonoptimal times (i.e., evening) showing compromised performance (May & Hasher, 1998).

SCORING

Scoring is expressed in terms of the time in seconds required for completion of each of the two parts of the test. Because of the difference in cognitive test demands between the TMT-A and the TMT-B, some examiners also calculate derived scores, including the TMT-B/TMT-A ratio score and a TMT-B minus TMT-A difference score. The ratio and difference scores are attempts to elucidate the added task requirements of TMT-B (i.e., divided attention, complex alternating sequencing). Normative data are available for derived scores (see "Normative Data").

In the oral version, TMT-B scores are transformed to written equivalents by multiplying them by 2.44 (written equivalent = Oral TMT-B × 2.44; Ricker et al., 1996). Mrazik, Millis, and Drane (2010) reported that in their sample, calculations of the written TMT-B to Oral TMT-B ratio suggested a ratio of 2.1 for the sample overall, ranging from 1.7 (20- to 39-year-olds) to 2.3 (59- to 79-year-olds). Their scores are provided in Table 9–135.

DEMOGRAPHIC EFFECTS

Demographic effects on the TMT are substantial, with findings generally suggesting that age is the most influential, followed by education, and gender contributing little. However, other studies have reported comparable effects of age and education (Lucas et al., 2005; Mitrushina et al., 2005), with findings from the Spanish Multicenter Normative Studies (NEURONORMA) project suggesting that education exerts comparatively more influence than age on performance (Pena-Casanova et al., 2009). Similarly, in a comparison of normative data from 10 countries, Fernández and Marcopulos (2008) reported most pervasive effects of both age and education. Of note, a number of studies have examined the relative

Part A

Sample A. When ready to begin the test, place the Part A test sheet in front of the subject, give the subject a pencil, and say: *On this page* (point) *are some numbers. Begin at number 1* (point to "1") *and draw a line from 1 to 2,* (point to "2"), *2 to 3* (point to "3"), *3 to 4* (point to "4"), *and so on, in order, until you reach the end* (pointing to the circle marked "END"). *Draw the lines as fast as you can. Do not lift the pencil from the paper. Ready! Begin!*

If the subject makes a mistake on Sample A, point it out and explain it. The following explanations of mistakes are acceptable:

1. *You started with the wrong circle. This is where you start* (point to "1").
2. *You skipped this circle* (point to the one omitted). *You should go from number 1* (point) *to 2* (point), *2 to 3* (point), *and so on, until you reach the circle marked "END"* (point).
3. *Please keep the pencil on the paper, and continue right on to the next circle.*

After the mistake has been explained, the examiner marks out the wrong part and says: *Go on from here* (point to the last circle completed correctly in the sequence).

If the subject still cannot complete Sample A, take the subject's hand and guide the pencil (eraser end down) through the trail. Then say: *Now you try it. Put your pencil, point down. Remember, begin at number 1* (point), *and draw a line from 1 to 2* (point to "2"), *2 to 3* (point to "3"), *3 to 4* (point to "4"), *and so on, in order until you reach the circle marked "END"* (point). *Do not skip around but go from one number to the next in the proper order. If you make a mistake, mark it out. Remember, work as fast as you can. Ready! Begin!*

If the subject succeeds this time, go on to Part A of the test. If not, repeat the procedure until the subject does succeed or it becomes evident that the subject cannot do it.

If the subject completes the sample item correctly, and in a manner which shows that the subject knows what to do, say: *Good! Let's try the next one.* Turn the page and give Part A of the test.

Say, On this page are numbers from 1 to 25. Do this the same way. Begin at number 1 (point) *and draw a line from 1 to 2* (point to "2"), *2 to 3* (point to "3"), *3 to 4* (point to "4"), *and so on, in order until you reach the end* (point). *Remember, work as fast as you can. Ready! Begin!*

Start timing. If the subject makes an error, call it to their attention immediately, and have the subject proceed from the point where the mistake occurred. Do not stop timing.

If the examinee completes Part A without error, remove the test sheet. Record the time in seconds. Errors count only in the increased time of perfomance. Then say: *"That's fine. Now we'll try another one."* Proceed immediately to Part B, sample.

Part B

Sample B. Place the test sheet for Part B, sample side up, flat on the table in front of the examinee, in the same position as the sheet for Part A was placed. Point with the right hand to the sample and say: *On this page are some numbers and letters. Begin at number 1* (point) *and draw a line from 1 to A,* (point to "A"), *A to 2* (point to "2"), *2 to B* (point to "B"), *B to 3* (point to "3"), *3 to C* (point to "C"), *and so on, in order, until you reach the end* (pointing to the circle marked "END"). *Remember, first you have a number* (point to "1"), *then a letter* (point to "A"), *then a number* (point to "2"), *then a letter* (point to "B"), *and so on. Draw the lines as fast as you can. Do not lift the pencil from the paper. Ready! Begin!*

If the subject makes a mistake on Sample B, point it out and explain it. The following explanations of mistakes are acceptable:

1. *You started with the wrong circle. This is where you start* (point to "1").
2. *You skipped this circle* (point to the one omitted). *You should go from 1* (point) *to A* (point), *A to 2* (point), *2 to B* (point), *B to 3* (point), *and so on, until you reach the circle marked "END"* (point). If it is clear that the subject intended to touch the circle but missed it, do not count it as an omission, but caution them to touch the circle.
3. *You only went as far as this circle* (point). *You should have gone to the circle marked "END"* (point).
4. *"Please keep the pencil on the paper and go right on to the next circle."*

After the mistake has been explained, the examiner marks out the wrong part and says: *Go on from here* (point to the last circle completed correctly in the sequence).

If the subject still cannot complete Sample B, take the subject's hand and guide the pencil (eraser end down) through the trail. Then say: *Now you try it. Put your pencil, point down. Remember, begin at number 1* (point), *and draw a line from 1 to A* (point to "A"), *A to 2* (point to "2"), *2 to B* (point to "B"), *B to 3* (point to "3"), *and so on until you reach the circle marked "END"* (point). *Ready! Begin!*

If the subject succeeds this time, go on to Part B of the test. If not, repeat the procedure until the subject does succeed or it becomes evident that they cannot do it.

If the subject completes the sample item correctly, say: *Good! Let's try the next one.* Turn the page over and proceed immediately to Part B, and say: *On this page are both numbers and letters. Do this the same way. Begin at number 1* (point) *and draw a line from 1 to A* (point to "A"), *A to 2* (point to "2"), *2 to B* (point to "B"), *B to 3* (point to "3"), *3 to C* (point to "C"), *and so on, in order until you reach the end* (point to circle marked "END"). *Remember, first you have a number* (point to "1"), *then a letter* (point to "B"), *and so on. Do not skip around, but go from one circle to the next in the proper order. Draw the lines as fast as you can. Ready! Begin!*

Start timing. If the subject makes an error, call it to their attention and have the subject proceed from the point at which the mistake occurred. Do not stop timing.

If the subject completes Part B without error, remove the test sheet. Record the time in seconds. Errors count only in the increased time of perfomance.

Figure 9–12 Instructions for the Trail Making Test (TMT).

Trails A
I would like you to count from 1 to 25 as quickly as you can. 1, 2, 3, 4, and so on. Ready? Begin.

Trails B
Now, I would like you to count again, but this time you are to switch between numbers and letters when you count. 1, A, 2, B, 3, C, and so on until you reach number 13. Ready? Begin.

If the patient makes an error on either task, direct them back to the last correct item and to start from there. Time to completion is the score for both the forms A and B.

Figure 9–13 *Instructions for the Oral Trail Making Test (TMT).*
SOURCE: Adapted from Abraham et al. (1996).

impact of demographic variables on performance in clinical samples, with many studies reporting lesser impact of demographic variables compared to studies with nonclinical populations (e.g., Horton & Roberts, 2003; Sherrill-Pattison et al., 2000; although see Manly et al., 2011, later discussion).

AGE

Performance on the TMT is affected by age, with performance declining with advancing age (Backman et al., 2004; Cangoz et al., 2009; Hankee et al., 2013; Lucas et al., 2005; Mitrushina et al., 2005; Seo et al., 2006; Tombaugh, 2004). Results across studies tend to be fairly consistent, finding that age accounts for 16 to 31% of the variance in TMT-A performance and a similar proportion (25 to 35%) of variance in TMT-B performance (Bezdicek et al., 2012; Heaton et al., 2004; Tombaugh, 2004). Most normative studies report moderate correlations between age and performance, generally in the range of r = .40 for both parts of the test (Bezdicek et al., 2012; Campanholo et al., 2014; Knight et al., 2006; Pena-Casanova et al., 2009). Bezdicek et al. (2012) noted most pronounced change after 55 years of age, whereas Hamdan, Amer, Hamdan, and Eli Mara (2009) noted performance decrements after age 50. Hashimoto et al. (2006) reported that in their sample of 70- to 85-year-olds and older, most pronounced age effects were seen after 85 years of age. In their study of older adults, Schneider et al. (2015) described a decrease in TMT-B performance of approximately 0.5 *SD* each decade. Longitudinal examination also reveals declines with advancing age and increased variability between individuals as age increases (Ratcliff et al., 2003). Age effects are typically related to processing speed (Backman et al., 2004; Salthouse & Fristoe, 1995; Salthouse et al., 2000).

TABLE 9–135 Written TMT-B to Oral TMT-B Ratio Scores

	AGE GROUPS (YEARS) (MIDPOINT)					
	20–39 (29)	29–49 (39)	39–59 (49)	49–69 (59)	59–79 (69)	69–90 (79)
WTMT-B/ OTMT-B ratio[a]	1.7	1.8	1.9	2.2	2.3	2.3
Mean Est. WTMT-B scores[b]	47.2	53.9	58.2	77.6	97.2	107.6
Estimated WTMT-B T scores	54	54	53	48	48	49

NOTE: WTMT-B, Written Trail Making Test, Part B; OTMT-B, Oral Trail Making Test, Part B. Not all Participants received the WTMT (20–39 years: n = 24, 29–49 years: n = 29, 39–59 years: n = 25, 49–69 years: n = 21, 59–79 years: n = 22, 69–90 years: n = 18).

[a]The correlation between age and ratio scores approached statistical significance (r = .22, p = .06).

[b]Mean estimated WTMT-B scores derived from calculating the OTMT-B mean from within a collapsed age group and multiplying the mean by the WTMT-B/OTMT-B ratio.

SOURCE: Mrazik et al. (2010).

GENDER

Gender generally has little impact on performance (Fernández & Marcopulos, 2008; Heaton et al., 2004; Knight et al., 2006; Lucas et al., 2005; Mitrushina et al., 2005; Pena-Casanova et al., 2009; Tombaugh, 2004; however, see Campanholo et al., 2014; Cangoz et al., 2009; Cavaco et al., 2013).

EDUCATION, IQ, AND READING ABILITY

Education is related to performance (Bezdicek et al., 2012; Cangoz et al., 2009; Campanholo et al., 2014; Cavaco et al., 2013; Clark et al., 2004; Hankee et al., 2013; Hester et al., 2005; Lucas et al., 2005; Manly et al., 2011; Mitrushina et al., 2005; Pena-Casanova et al., 2009; Perianez et al., 2007; Seo et al., 2006; Tombaugh, 2004; but see Backman et al., 2004). Research typically suggests that less influence on performance is exerted by education compared to age (e.g., 3 to 10% for the TMT-A, 7% to 16% for the TMT-B; Bezideck et al., 2012; Heaton et al., 2004; Pena-Casanova et al., 2009; Tombaugh, 2004). Some authors have reported weak correlations (Bezdicek et al., 2012; Manly et al., 2011), whereas others have reported moderate correlations between education and the TMT (Campanholo et al., 2014; Pena-Casanova et al., 2009).

In a sample of Korean elders, Seo et al. (2006) reported that education accounted for nearly 21% of the variance of scores in the TMT-A and nearly 14% in the TMT-B. Hashimoto et al. (2006) noted that education effects are most pronounced at six years of education or less in a sample of older Japanese adults. Bezdicek et al. (2012) noted the most pronounced difference in performance between those with fewer compared to more than 13 years of education. Continuation rates are highly related to education, particularly for the TMT-B. For example, Cavaco et al. (2013) reported that 84% of the people in their sample who discontinued the TMT-B had the lowest levels of education in their sample (four years), and just over 20% of people with four years of education discontinued the TMT-B.

IQ shows a moderate relationship with test performance, and lower IQ has been associated with poorer test scores (Diaz-Asper et al., 2004; Knight et al., 2006). Associations tend to become stronger as IQ increases (Steinberg et al., 2005). The effect of IQ appears slightly more pronounced on the TMT-B. For example, Steinberg et al. (2005) reported correlations with FSIQ of $r = .37$ for the TMT-A and $r = .50$ for the TMT-B. The NART was modestly related to the TMT-A ($r = .12$) but more so with the TMT-B ($r = .26$) in one study of older adults (Knight et al., 2006). General cognition and TMT performance were found to be genetically linked in a large-scale heritability study (Hagenaars et al., 2017).

Correlations between the WRAT-3 reading and the TMT have also been reported (TMT-A $r = -.22$, TMT-B $r = -.41$; Manly et al., 2011). In their large study of women with HIV infection and without, Manly et al. (2011) reported that age accounted for nearly 14% of the variance in scores (TMT and the SDMT), education 4%, and the WRAT-3 nearly 12%. Johnson, Flicker, and Lichetnberg (2006) reported that reading ability mediated performance in their sample to a larger degree than education; the relative importance of reading ability over education was also reported by Schneider and Lichtenberg (2011). Schneider and Lichtenberg (2011) reported that when high and low reading groups (split according to a WRAT-3 score of 42) were compared, there were large differences between groups on the TMT-A and the TMT-B (Cohen's $d = .77$ and 1.06, respectively).

ETHNICITY, NATIONALITY, AND LINGUISTIC EFFECTS

The TMT has been used in many countries, with translated versions available. The bulk of data suggests that cultural/linguistic variables affect test scores. Fernández and Marcopulous (2008) compared normative data from 10 countries, finding large differences between datasets even when other factors, such as age and education, were comparable. The authors concluded that sample variability and administration differences may account for differences.

Lee, Cheung, Chan, and Chan (2000) found that English monolinguals performed the TMT-A faster than Chinese-English bilinguals, suggesting that language background may exert some effect on task performance. Razani, Burciaga, Madore, and Wong (2007) reported that a monolingual English speaking Anglo-American group outperformed a fluent English-speaking ethnically diverse group (Hispanic, Asian, Middle Eastern descent) on the TMT-B. Buré-Reyes et al. (2013) reported no differences in TMT performance between Spanish speakers from different countries (e.g., Chile, Dominican Republic, Puerto Rico, Spain). Cherner et al. (2008) compared two alternate Spanish forms of the TMT (one including the sound "Ch" between letters "C" and "D," and another omitting the sound "Ch"), reporting comparability in performance on the alternate forms.

In healthy Arabic- and English-speaking college students, the Arabic TMT was associated with poorer performance than the English TMT. Acculturation variables (e.g., years of education outside of the United States, degree of English spoken growing up) were correlated with TMT performance, indicating that increased acculturation was associated with better performance. Hayden et al. (2014) reported a large difference in raw scores between Russian and American samples on the TMT-B, in favor of American participants. Manly et al. (1998) reported that acculturation variables among African Americans were associated with poor performance on the TMT-B.

Manly et al. (2011) reported that after age, education, and WRAT-3 reading score were entered, ethnicity still accounted for 3% of the variance in a composite cognitive score that included the TMT. The authors reported that African Americans were three times as likely to make errors on the TMT-B and Hispanic women were approximately 2.5 times more likely to make errors than Caucasian participants, even after adjustment for age, years of school, and WRAT-3 performance. Overall, the authors note that relative contributions of demographic variables accounted for more variance than HIV status on the TMT.

DEMOGRAPHIC EFFECTS ON THE ORAL TMT

Increasing age is associated with poorer performance on the Oral TMT-B ($r = .21$; Ruchinskas, 2003; $r = .40$; Mrazik et al., 2010). Ruchinskas (2003) reported moderate to strong correlations with education (TMT-A, $r = -.27$; TMT-B, $r = -.55$) and with general cognitive status as indexed by the MMSE (TMT-A, $r = -.21$; TMT-B, $r = -.66$). However, Mrazik et al. reported that only age was related to TMT-B performance, without associations with other demographic variables (i.e., education and gender). The TMT-A was not significantly related to any demographic variable, including age.

NORMATIVE DATA

Normative data are generally favored over the use of cutoff scores designating "organic impairment" (e.g., Reitan & Wolfson, 1985, 1988). A large number of normative datasets have been published for the TMT. The data presented here include metanorms from a large number of published studies and norms from various regions and linguistic groups (e.g., North America, New Zealand, Spain, Brazil, Portugal, and Turkey). Data based on other scoring methods such as difference and ratio scoring as well as the Oral TMT are also presented here.

METANORMS

Mitrushina et al. (2005) collected data from 28 studies for TMT-A and 29 studies for TMT-B, reflecting data points for each part based on a total of 6,317 participants aged 16–89 years of age for the TMT-A and 6,360 for the TMT-B.

TABLE 9–136A Trail Making Test (TMT) Metanorms for 35-Year-Olds and Older Adjusted by Education

	<12 YR. EDUCATION						12–14 YR. EDUCATION					
SAMPLES	11						104					
N	368						4,966					
IQ	94.6						101.6					
					95% CI						95% CI	
MEASURE	*N*	*M*	*SD*	*SE*	LOWER BOUND	UPPER BOUND	*N*	*M*	*SD*	*SE*	LOWER BOUND	UPPER BOUND
Trails A	251	25.42	8.43	1.04	24.38	26.46	3,480	25.21	9.29	0.31	24.90	25.52
Trails B	283	61.09	23.34	2.72	58.37	63.81	3,725	57.93	24.69	0.79	57.14	58.72
	>15 YR. EDUCATION						ALL LEVELS OF EDUCATION					
SAMPLES	23						138					
N	656						5,990					
IQ	109.2						102.9					
					95% CI						95% CI	
MEASURE	*N*	*M*	*SD*	*SE*	LOWER BOUND	UPPER BOUND	*N*	*M*	*SD*	*SE*	LOWER BOUND	UPPER BOUND
Trails A	286	23.00	7.04	0.82	22.18	23.82	4,017	25.06	9.10	0.28	24.78	25.34
Trails B	500	49.36	17.11	1.50	47.86	50.86	4,508	57.18	23.88	0.70	56.48	57.88

SOURCE: Greer et al. (2010).

Greer, Brewer, Cannici, and Pennett (2010) provide pooled normative data amalgamated across 96 studies and 153 samples (n = 9,489) for the TMT. Data for other Halstead-Reitan tests were also included. Of note, the studies were published from 1950 to 2003. The studies varied in the amount of demographic data reported. Occupation was rarely reported, and ethnicity was reported in only 30 studies, with an overall proportion of Caucasian participants (85%) and a male majority of 58%. Normative data for TMT, by education and age grouping, are provided in Tables 9–136a to 9–136c.

TABLE 9–136B Trail Making Test (TMT) Metanorms for 35- to 64-Year-Olds Adjusted by Education

	<12 YR. EDUCATION						12–14 YR. EDUCATION					
SAMPLES	33						60					
N	1,684						3,177					
IQ	102.5						110.6					
					95% CI						95% CI	
MEASURE	*N*	*M*	*SD*	SE	LOWER BOUND	UPPER BOUND	*N*	*M*	*SD*	SE	LOWER BOUND	UPPER BOUND
Trails A	1,072	44.19	17.42	1.04	43.15	45.23	1,171	37.72	13.87	0.79	36.93	38.51
Trails B	1,238	106.77	51.89	2.89	103.88	109.66	2,030	76.67	35.70	1.55	75.12	78.22
	>15 YR. EDUCATION						ALL LEVELS OF EDUCATION					
SAMPLES	18						111					
N	1,596						6,457					
IQ	112.7						108.8					
					95% CI						95% CI	
MEASURE	*N*	*M*	*SD*	SE	LOWER BOUND	UPPER BOUND	*N*	*M*	*SD*	SE	LOWER BOUND	UPPER BOUND
Trails A	1,509	27.41	11.28	0.57	26.84	27.98	3,752	33.86	14.07	0.45	33.41	34.31
Trails B	1,550	64.76	29.47	1.47	63.29	66.23	4,818	80.57	38.84	1.10	79.47	81.67

SOURCE: Greer et al. (2010).

TABLE 9–136C Trail Making Test (TMT) Metanorms for 65-Year-Olds and Older Adjusted by Education

	<12 YR. EDUCATION						12–14 YR. EDUCATION					
SAMPLES	20						33					
N	2,783						2,188					
IQ	99.8						109.0					
					95% CI						95% CI	
MEASURE	*N*	*M*	*SD*	*SE*	LOWER BOUND	UPPER BOUND	*N*	*M*	*SD*	SE	LOWER BOUND	UPPER BOUND
Trails A	1,316	61.86	28.92	1.56	60.30	63.42	1,454	46.10	25.85	1.33	44.77	47.43
Trails B	2,357	137.74	71.89	2.90	134.84	140.64	2,046	120.62	62.77	2.72	117.90	123.34

	>15 YR. EDUCATION						ALL LEVELS OF EDUCATION					
SAMPLES	9						62					
N	562						5,533					
IQ	108.5						102.3					
					95% CI						95% CI	
MEASURE	*N*	*M*	*SD*	SE	LOWER BOUND	UPPER BOUND	*N*	*M*	*SD*	SE	LOWER BOUND	UPPER BOUND
Trails A	562	43.25	15.76	1.30	41.95	44.55	3,332	51.88	25.77	0.88	51.00	52.76
Trails B	562	112.37	50.19	4.15	108.22	116.52	4,965	127.82	66.05	1.84	125.98	129.66

SOURCE: Greer et al. (2010).

NORTH-AMERICAN NORMS

Heaton et al. (2004) provide norms separately for Caucasians and African Americans organized by age, gender, and education. The samples are large and cover a wide range in terms of age and education, and exclusion criteria are specified (see Table 9–137). Users should note, however, that these data derive from several separate studies, some of which were conducted many years ago. Note also that individuals "generally" were given a maximum of 300 seconds to complete the TMT-B. If the TMT-B was discontinued before completion, the time score (in seconds) was prorated by dividing 300 seconds by the number of circles completed and then multiplying the resulting "time per circle" figure by 25. T scores less than 40 were classed as impaired.

Given that IQ is more strongly related to performance than education in some studies, Steinberg et al. (2005) reanalyzed data from the MOANS and provided age- (>55 years) and IQ-adjusted percentile equivalents of MOANS age-adjusted scores. Readers should note that all FSIQs are age-adjusted scores, which are based on the WAIS-R, not the WAIS-IV. Given the upward shift in scores (Flynn effect) with the passage of time, use of the WAIS-R FSIQ rather than the WAIS-IV may result in a given TMT score appearing less favorable. The interested reader is referred to their article for the relevant tables.

Lucas et al. (2005) provide age- and education-adjusted normative data based on 303 African-American community-dwelling participants from the MOAANS project in Jacksonville, Florida. Participants were predominantly female (75%), ranged in age from 56 to 94 years ($M = 69.6$,

TABLE 9–137 Characteristics of the Trail Making Test (TMT) Normative Sample

Number	1,212
Age (years)	20 to 85[a]
Geographic location	Various states in United States, and Manitoba, Canada.
Sample type	Individuals recruited as part of multicenter studies.
Education (years)	0–20[b]
Gender	
Male	57%
Female	43%
Ethnicity	
Caucasian	52%
African American	48%
Screening	No reported history of learning disability, neurological disorder, serious psychiatric disorder, or substance abuse.

[a]Age bands: 20 to 34, 35 to 39, 40 to 44, 45 to 49, 50 to 54, 55 to 59, 60 to 64, 65 to 69, 70 to 74, 75 to 79, and 80 to 89 years.

[b]Education groups: 7 to 8, 9 to 11, 12, 13 to 15, 16 to 17, and 18 to 20 years.

SOURCE: From Heaton et al. (2004). Reproduced by special permission of the Publisher, Psychological Assessment Resources, Inc. (PAR), 16204 North Florida Avenue, Lutz, FL 33549, from Revised Comprehensive Norms for an Expanded Halstead-Reitan Battery Professional Manual, Copyright 1991, 1992, 2004 by Psychological Assessment Resources, Inc. All rights reserved.

SD = 6.87), and education levels ranged from 0 to 20 years (*M* = 12.2, *SD* = 3.48). Participants were screened to exclude those with active neurological, psychiatric, or other conditions that might affect cognition. A time limit of 300 seconds was used for the TMT-B. Participants who required additional time were assigned a time of 301 seconds. Table 9–138a presents their data, and Table 9–138b provides the computational formula used to calculate age- and education-adjusted MOAANS scaled scores.

Lucas et al. (2005) reported that about 15% of their sample performed above the discontinuation cutoff on the TMT-B. Consequently, they also provide frequency distributions of error scores on the TMT-A and TMT-B. About 36% of their sample made two or more errors on the TMT-B, whereas it was much less common for that number of errors to be made on the TMT-A (3% of the normative sample). Less than 10% of their sample made four or more errors on the TMT-B. Examination of MOAANS normative estimates for the TMT-B reveal a substantial floor effect, likely because of the truncation of higher scores (i.e., longer completion times) resulting from the use of an a priori time limit. Overall, the relatively large number of study participants who discontinued the TMT-B suggests that poor performance on this measure may not be a reliable indicator of cognitive dysfunction in older African Americans (Lucas et al., 2005). The reasons for this poor performance are uncertain. Due to small sample sizes and a sample of convenience, data should be interpreted cautiously (Lucas et al., 2005).

Schneider et al. (2015) provide age, ethnicity, and education regression-based norms for a large sample (*n* = 320 African American, *n* = 392 Caucasian) of participants recruited as part of a study on atherosclerotic risk. Participants were excluded if they presented with neurologic or neurodegenerative diseases and cognitive complaints. For the African-American sample, the average age was 71 years (*SD* = 4.1), and approximately 70% of the sample was female. In terms of education, 27% had less than high school, 24% had high school, General Education Diploma (GED), or vocational training, and 50% had college or university education. For the Caucasian sample, the average age was 72.4 years (*SD* = 4.3). The sample was 57% female. In terms of education, 8% had less than high school; 45% had high school, GED, or vocational training; and 46% had college or university education. MMSE and depression scale rankings are provided in the paper.

Hankee et al. (2013) provide TMT data based on 1,907 participants who were offspring of the original cohort in the Framingham study of cardiovascular risk factors, with data collected from 2005 to 2008. Exclusion criteria included neurologic or neurodegenerative disease. Proportions of participants in each age group were as follows: 7% age 55 years or younger, 35% age 55 to 64 years, 34% age 65 to 74 years, and 24% older than 75 years. Education levels were as follows: 3% less than high school, 57% high school, and 40% college or graduate school. The sample was 54% female. TMT completion time, errors, and pen lifts are depicted separately by age and education in Tables 9–139a to 9–139c.

Tombaugh (2004) provide normative data based on a large sample (*n* = 858) of healthy, community-dwelling individuals aged 20 to 89 years of age living in Canada. The education level varied from five to 25 years (*M* = 12.6, *SD* = 2.7). All participants scored higher than 23 (*M* = 28.6, *SD* = 1.5) on the MMSE and lower than 14 (*M* = 4.1, *SD* = 3.4) on the GDS. The data, stratified by age and education, are shown in Table 9–140.

A series of regression analyses revealed that education accounts for virtually none of the variance in the 25- to 54-year-old age range. However, for the TMT-B, education becomes progressively more important with increasing age. These observations, as well as the fact that most of the participants in the 25 to 54 age range were relatively well-educated, prompted division of only the older age groups into two education levels (0 to 12 and >12 years). Some caution should be exercised in interpreting scores from the oldest age group (aged 85 to 89) because of the restricted sample size. It should also be noted that all members of the youngest group (aged 18 to 24) were university students. The normative values reported by Tombaugh (2004) are more stringent than those provided by Mitrushina et al. (2005) but appear broadly similar to those provided by Heaton et al. (2004).

NEW ZEALAND NORMS

Knight et al. (2006) provide regression-based data for 272 community-dwelling older adults 65–90 years of age (*M* = 73.67, *SD* = 5.75). The sample was 55% female. In terms of education, 9% of individuals had less than a high school education, 27% had less than three years of high school, 12% had more than three years of high school, 38% had a vocational qualification, and 14% were university-educated. The NART score was equated to a predicted FSIQ of 113. Participants were recruited as part of a baseline phase of a larger study in New Zealand. Participants were excluded if they presented with renal disease, diabetes, cancer, neurologic or neurodegenerative disease, or psychiatric conditions. The program for calculation of scores can be found at https://homepages.abdn.ac.uk/j.crawford/pages/dept/psychom.htm. This page can also be located through the home page of Professor John Crawford of the Department of Psychology, University of Aberdeen. Applying regression data using an example is in the program labeled CLREGMUL.EXE.

TABLE 9–138A MOAANS Trail Making Test (TMT) Norms in African Americans, By Age Group

SCALED SCORE	56–62 YEARS		63–65 YEARS		66–68 YEARS		69–71 YEARS		72–74 YEARS		75–77 YEARS		78+ YEARS		
TMT PART	A	B	A	B	A	B	A	B	A	B	A	B	A	B	PERCENTILE RANGES
2	120+	–	121+	–	121+	–	121+	–	125+	–	202+	–	227+	–	<1
3	112–119	–	117–120	–	117–120	–	117–120	–	118–124	–	184–201	–	202–226	–	1
4	93–111	–	101–116	–	107–116	–	113–116	–	–	–	–	–	183–201	–	2
5	88–92	301+	90–100	301+	95–106	301+	102–112	301+	112–117	301+	122–183	–	154–182	–	3–5
6	76–87	247–300	80–89	260–300	86–94	270–300	89–101	285–300	97–111	285–299	113–121	301+	121–153	301+	6–10
7	67–75	239–246	74–79	246–259	76–85	255–271	79–88	268–284	81–96	267–284	87–112	295–300	114–120	–	11–18
8	58–66	189–238	62–73	196–245	67–75	218–254	72–78	239–267	73–80	239–266	75–86	257–294	82–113	288–300	19–28
9	48–57	150–188	53–61	169–195	57–66	183–217	60–71	191–238	62–72	202–238	65–74	221–256	71–81	259–287	29–40
10	41–47	109–149	44–52	121–168	48–56	135–182	49–59	147–190	51–61	155–201	51–64	156–220	53–70	194–258	41–59
11	38–40	97–108	39–43	103–120	43–47	111–134	43–48	115–146	45–50	121–154	45–50	126–155	46–52	155–193	60–71
12	34–37	82–96	36–38	86–102	38–42	100–110	39–42	104–114	41–44	111–120	41–44	112–125	41–45	123–154	72–81
13	31–33	70–81	31–35	72–85	33–37	79–99	33–38	95–103	34–40	101–110	34–40	102–111	34–40	111–122	82–89
14	28–30	56–69	28–30	60–71	30–32	71–78	30–32	73–94	30–33	88–100	30–33	88–101	30–33	98–110	90–94
15	25–27	52–58	26–27	52–59	27–29	54–70	27–29	69–72	28–29	73–87	28–29	73–87	28–29	91–97	95–97
16	–	50–51	25	50–51	25–26	52–53	25–26	54–68	25–27	69–72	25–27	69–72	24–27	88–90	98
17	22–24	46–49	23–24	46–49	23–24	50–51	23–24	50–53	23–24	59–68	23–24	59–68	23	87–71	99
18	<22	<46	<23	<46	<23	<50	<23	<50	<23	<59	<23	<59	<23	<71	>99
N	107	107	129	129	165	165	181	181	155	155	118	118	77	77	

SOURCE: Adapted from Lucas et al. (2005).

TABLE 9–138B Computational Formula for Age- and Education-Corrected MOAANS Scaled Scores

	K	W_1	W_2
TMT-A	2.93	1.12	0.35
TMT-B	3.10	1.19	0.40

NOTE: Age- and education-corrected MOAANS Scaled Scores ($MSS_{A\&E}$) can be calculated for TMT scores by using age-corrected MOAANS Scaled Scores (MSS_A) and education (expressed in years completed) in the following formula: $MSS_{A\&E} = K + (W_1 \times MSS_A) - (W_2 \times EDUC)$.
SOURCE: Adapted from Lucas et al. (2005).

SPANISH NORMS

Pena-Casanova et al. (2009) present data as part of the Spanish NEURONORMA project, a large project that presented co-normed data for neuropsychological tests. The study was performed across nine different Spanish regions. All participants were Caucasian, living in Spain, educated in Spanish, and enrolled between 2004 and 2007. Informants were also interviewed. Participants were excluded if they were out of the age range of the study; did not live/function independently; performed below a cutoff on the MMSE; presented with a neurologic disorder; scored above a cutoff on the Modified Ischemia Scale; or presented with alcohol or psychotropic substance abuse, an unmanaged medical condition that could interfere with cognition (e.g., diabetes mellitus, hypothyroidism, B_{12} deficiency), psychiatric conditions, or sensory impairment. The sample sizes of persons who completed the TMT-A and TMT-B were 350 and 327, respectively.

The sample was 58% female and the following education levels were represented: 17% with five years of education or fewer, 7% with six to seven years of education, 19% with eight to nine years of education, 12% with 10 to 11 years of education, 11% with 12 to 13 years of education, 10% with 14 to 15 years of education, and 23% with 16 years of education or more. Tables 9–141a and 9–141b are presented for education adjustment. To calculate the education-adjusted score, find the appropriate column in Tables 9–141a to 9–141b that corresponds to the examinee's years of education, find the NSS_A, and refer to the corresponding $NSS_{A\&E}$.

TABLE 9–139A TMT-A Normative Data Adjusted Separately by Age and Education

TEST PARAMETER	AGE, YEARS (*N*)			
	<55 (134)	55–64 (659)	65–74 (639)	≥75 (422)
Errors	0.1 (0.3)	0.1 (0.4)	0.1 (0.4)	0.2 (0.4)
Pen lifts	0.5 (0.7)	0.7 (1.0)	1.0 (1.6)	1.6 (2.2)
Early start	0.1 (0.3)	0.1 (0.3)	0.2 (0.4)	0.2 (0.4)
	EDUCATION (*N*)			
	<HIGH SCHOOL (62)	HIGH SCHOOL (1,043)	COLLEGE (398)	≥GRADUATE (351)
Errors	0.1 (0.4)	0.2 (0.4)	0.1 (0.4)	0.1 (0.4)
Pen lifts	1.4 (1.5)	1.1 (1.6)	0.9 (1.9)	0.8 (1.2)
Early start	0.3 (0.5)	0.2 (0.4)	0.1 (0.4)	0.1 (0.4)

SOURCE: Hankee et al. (2013).

TABLE 9–139B TMT-B Normative Data Adjusted by Age

TEST PARAMETER	AGE (YEARS)				
	<55	55–64	65–74	≥75	TOTAL
Completion time	66.7 (25.0)	74.2 (34.8)	95.0 (48.5)	124.4 (57.3)	91.8 (49.1)
Total errors	0.4 (0.7)	0.4 (0.8)	0.7 (1.0)	0.9 (1.3)	0.6 (1.0)
Pen lifts	0.7 (0.9)	1.0 (1.5)	1.5 (2.3)	2.3 (2.9)	1.4 (2.2)
	n = 130	*n* = 652	*n* = 616	*n* = 393	*n* = 1791

SOURCE: Hankee et al. (2013).

PORTUGUESE NORMS

Campanholo et al. (2014) administered the TMT to 1,025 Brazilian, Portuguese-speaking, community-dwelling adults. Participants were excluded if they presented with a history of neurologic or psychiatric disorders, psychotropic drugs, sensory or motor disorders, IQ lower than 80, MMSE scores below education-based cutoffs, or anxiety and depression scores above cutoffs on questionnaires. The sample was 67% female, with an average age of 41 years (SD = 16.4) and an average education level of 11.9 years (SD = 5.6). The average IQ of the sample was 103.2 (SD = 12). Age- and education-adjusted normative data are depicted in Table 9–142.

Cavaco et al. (2013) provide data for 1,038 Portuguese community-dwelling individuals, ranging in age from 18 to 93 years with three to 22 years of education. Inclusion criteria were Portuguese as a native language, living in Portugal for the previous five years, three or more years of education, over half of formal schooling in Portugal, and absence of significant sensory or motor deficits. "Cognitive normalcy" of participants was corroborated via an informant. Participants were excluded if they presented with a history of neurologic, developmental, or psychiatric conditions, or substance abuse. The sample was 69% female, and thus women were overrepresented. However, age and education were representative of the Portuguese population when compared to that country's 2011 Census. Participants were a mean age of 52.2 years (SD = 17.5) with a mean education of 10.2 years (SD = 4.7).

The authors calculated conventional scores (time to complete the TMT-A and the TMT-B and errors), as well as a number of derived scores, including a difference score (TMT-B – TMT-A), a ratio score (TMT-B/TMT-A), a sum score (TMT-A + TMT-B), and a multiplication score (TMT-A × TMT-B/100).

The example provided by the authors regarding application of their data is as follows: A 43-year-old male client (9 years of education) completes the TMT-A in 60 seconds and the TMT-B in 160 seconds. The adjusted scores are thus 21.7 for TMT-A and 21.8 for TMT-B, which correspond to a percentile range of 3 to 5 (i.e., 3 to 5% of the

TABLE 9–139C TMT-B Normative Data Adjusted by Education

	EDUCATION (DEGREE)				
TEST PARAMETER	<HIGH SCHOOL	HIGH SCHOOL	COLLEGE	≥GRADUATE	TOTAL
Completion time	147.8 (68.1)	98.8 (52.2)	82.7 (41.8)	74.4 (31.3)	91.8 (49.1)
Total errors	1.5 (1.7)	0.7 (1.1)	0.5 (0.9)	0.4 (0.7)	0.6 (1.0)
Pen lifts	2.1 (2.3)	1.6 (2.4)	1.2 (2.1)	1.0 (1.5)	1.4 (2.2)
	n = 47	*n* = 1005	*n* = 395	*n* = 344	*n* = 1791

SOURCE: Hankee et al. (2013).

healthy male Portuguese population with similar age and education level require ≥60 seconds to complete the TMT-A and ≥160 seconds to complete the TMT-B).

TURKISH NORMS

Cangoz et al. (2009) provide normative data for 484 Turkish community-dwelling adults 50 years and older. The sample was 49% female. Approximately 31% of participants presented with an elementary school education, 33% with a high school education, and the remainder were university-educated. Participants presenting with neurologic or neurodegenerative disease, psychiatric conditions, substance abuse, or significant medical disorders (e.g., chronic lung or renal disease, cerebrovascular disease) were excluded. Cutoff scores on the MMSE, GDS, Clinical Dementia Rating Scale-Long Form (CDR), and Functional Activities Questionnaire (FAQ) also acted as exclusion criteria. Age-, education-, and gender-adjusted norms (for the TMT-A, TMT-B, and a difference score) are presented in Table 9–143a to 9–143c.

DIFFERENCE AND RATIO SCORING

In addition to conventional scores (e.g., time to complete the TMT-A and the TMT-B, errors), some authors have also reported derived scores, such as difference scores (TMT-B − TMT-A) or ratio scores (TMT-B/TMT-A; for information regarding derived scores see Cangoz et al., 2009; Cavaco et al., 2013; Hester et al., 2005).

Demographic variables can affect supplemental TMT indices (Drane et al., 2002), although the impact of age and education may be reduced if ratio scores are considered (Hester et al., 2005). Therefore, scores that take into account demographic variables are likely to result in less erroneous interpretation than simple fixed cutoffs. Tom Tombaugh (personal communication with previous authors, July 20, 2003) has provided ratio (percentage; TMT-B/TMT-A × 100) and difference score (TMT-B − TMT-A) data based on a large sample ($N = 858$) of healthy, community-dwelling individuals aged 20–89 years (described earlier). The data are shown in Tables 9–144a and 9–144b. As is evident in the tables, derived scores tend to increase, particularly after age 70 years. In addition, derived scores tend to be smaller for people with more years of education (but see Drane et al., 2002).

ADDITIONAL NORMATIVE DATA

A number of contemporary normative studies on the TMT are available for specific groups, as noted in Table 9–145.

ORAL TMT NORMS

The oral version is performed considerably more quickly than the written version (Ricker & Axelrod, 1994). One way to evaluate the TMT-B score is to transform it to a written equivalent (see "Scoring") and then evaluate it using the demographically based norms described earlier. Alternatively, some normative data were provided by Ricker and Axelrod (1994) based on small samples of healthy individuals (mean education not reported; see Table 9–146). Ricker and Axelrod (Abraham et al., 1996; Ricker & Axelrod, 1994; Ricker et al., 1996) administered both the oral and written versions in counterbalanced order to individuals in three age groups (see Table 9–146). They converted raw scores to T scores demographically corrected for age, education, and gender and found a consistent relationship between the oral and written versions across age groups. In addition, correlations between versions (oral, written) for each form were strong ($r = -.68$ for the TMT-A; $r = -.72$ for the TMT-B).

Somewhat faster times were reported by Ruchinksas (2003) for a sample of 27 healthy older adults aged 60 years and older ($M = 70.3$, $SD = 6.4$) with a mean education of 12.5 years ($SD = 2.9$). The means and *SD*s were as follows: TMT-A, $M = 7.0$ seconds, $SD = 1.7$; TMT-B, $M = 35.1$ seconds, $SD = 14.4$.

Mrazik et al. (2010) provide data for 81 community-dwelling adults 20–90 years old ($M = 49.62$, $SD = 19.56$), nearly 73% female, with a mean education level of 14.2 years ($SD = 2.15$ years). Participants were recruited as part of a neuropsychological normative project. Participants were excluded if they presented with neurologic or psychiatric disorders or substance abuse. All participants additionally performed within typical ranges on a screening measure (Cognistat) and the BDI. Table 9–147a provides the normative data, and Table 9–147b depicts the cumulative

TABLE 9–140 Canadian TMT Normative Data by Age and Education

	EDUCATION 0–12 YEARS		EDUCATION >12 YEARS		TOTAL	
PERCENTILE	TMT-A	TMT-B	TMT-A	TMT-B	TMT-A	TMT-B
Age group 18–24 (university students; *n*)					155	
90					16	35
80					17	38
70					19	41
60					20	44
50					22	47
40					23	49
30					25	54
20					27	61
10					31	66
Age group 25–34 (*n*)					33	
90					14	33
80					17	38
70					19	45
60					21	48
50					23	50
40					25	53
30					27	58
20					33	63
10					40	67
Age group 35–44 (*n*)					39	
90					16	40
80					20	45
70					23	50
60					24	53
50					26	58
40					28	60
30					32	62
20					36	70
10					46	87
Age group 45–54 (*n*)					41	
90					19	42
80					23	50
70					27	59
60					29	62
50					31	64
40					33	68
30					34	72
20					38	75
10					50	84
Age group 55–59 (*n*)	58		37		95	
90	25	56	22	42	23	56
80	27	64	24	56	25	58
70	29	66	25	57	27	64
60	31	71	26	61	30	66
50	32	74	30	65	32	73
40	34	81	32	71	33	74
30	38	87	33	74	35	83
20	40	98	37	81	40	90
10	50	105	53	102	53	104
Age Group 60–64 (*n*)	55		31		86	
90	21	56	22	45	22	48
80	24	58	25	48	24	56
70	26	62	26	53	26	59
60	30	67	27	59	29	62

TABLE 9–140 Continued

PERCENTILE	EDUCATION 0–12 YEARS		EDUCATION >12 YEARS		TOTAL	
	TMT-A	TMT-B	TMT-A	TMT-B	TMT-A	TMT-B
50	33	72	31	60	32	68
40	37	75	33	66	34	72
30	40	79	35	71	37	77
20	43	92	37	77	42	84
10	45	96	43	87	45	96
Age Group 65–69 (*n*)	65		32		95	
90	24	60	26	52	25	56
80	30	71	28	57	29	62
70	32	74	30	63	31	70
60	36	81	31	67	32	73
50	39	86	32	68	37	76
40	40	93	34	71	39	83
30	44	103	39	73	42	91
20	47	110	40	75	45	104
10	56	137	45	77	53	121
Age Group 70–74 (*n*)	76		30		106	
90	25	70	26	59	26	64
80	30	79	29	63	30	76
70	35	74	31	68	34	81
60	37	83	33	80	36	85
50	38	95	36	84	38	97
40	42	101	41	85	41	105
30	46	112	42	103	45	112
20	52	146	46	109	49	138
10	57	172	71	112	61	159
Age Group 75–79 (*n*)	74		34		108	
90	30	78	22	57	27	65
80	37	92	27	59	34	79
70	39	96	34	66	38	88
60	45	107	37	73	40	98
50	50	120	40	87	46	115
40	53	140	43	105	50	128
30	56	156	46	126	54	148
20	61	167	58	141	58	163
10	72	189	66	178	70	185
Age Group 80–84 (*n*)	84		34		118	
90	31	72	37	89	31	84
80	39	101	38	100	39	101
70	43	112	41	111	42	111
60	49	119	46	113	47	116
50	53	140	48	128	52	133
40	59	154	56	131	58	144
30	66	176	58	139	63	159
20	78	204	64	151	75	193
10	90	259	101	227	93	241
Age Group 85–89 (*n*)	16		13		29	
90	37	89	35	70	36	81
80	39	95	42	81	39	87
70	43	112	49	87	47	95
60	47	132	52	90	51	121
50	55	143	53	121	54	138
40	56	188	60	143	56	150
30	63	194	67	156	65	194
20	72	214	78	212	68	199
10	94	317	125	290	120	296

SOURCE: From Tombaugh (2004).

TABLE 9–141A Education Adjustment for the Spanish TMT-A

	EDUCATION (YEARS)																				
NSS_A	0	1	2	3	4	5	6	7	8	9	10	11	12	13	14	15	16	17	18	19	20
2	3	3	3	3	2	2	2	2	2	1	1	1	1	0	0	0	0	0	−1	−1	−1
3	4	4	4	4	3	3	3	3	3	2	2	2	2	1	1	1	1	1	0	0	0
4	5	5	5	5	4	4	4	4	4	3	3	3	3	2	2	2	2	2	1	1	1
5	6	6	6	6	5	5	5	5	5	4	4	4	4	3	3	3	3	3	2	2	2
6	7	7	7	7	6	6	6	6	6	5	5	5	5	4	4	4	4	4	3	3	3
7	8	8	8	8	7	7	7	7	7	6	6	6	6	5	5	5	5	5	4	4	4
8	9	9	9	9	8	8	8	8	8	7	7	7	7	6	6	6	6	6	5	5	5
9	10	10	10	10	9	9	9	9	9	8	8	8	8	7	7	7	7	7	6	6	6
10	11	11	11	11	10	10	10	10	10	9	9	9	9	8	8	8	8	8	7	7	7
11	12	12	12	12	11	11	11	11	11	10	10	10	10	9	9	9	9	9	8	8	8
12	13	13	13	13	12	12	12	12	12	11	11	11	11	10	10	10	10	10	9	9	9
13	14	14	14	14	13	13	13	13	13	12	12	12	12	11	11	11	11	11	10	10	10
14	15	15	15	15	14	14	14	14	14	13	13	13	13	12	12	12	12	12	11	11	11
15	16	16	16	16	15	15	15	15	15	14	14	14	14	13	13	13	13	13	12	12	12
16	17	17	17	17	16	16	16	16	16	15	15	15	15	14	14	14	14	14	13	13	13
17	18	18	18	18	17	17	17	17	17	16	16	16	16	15	15	15	15	15	14	14	14
18	19	19	19	19	18	18	18	18	18	17	17	17	17	16	16	16	16	16	15	15	15

NOTE: Education adjustment applying the following formula: $NSS_{A\&E} = NSS_A - (\beta * [Education_{(years)} - 12])$, where $\beta = 0.21832$.

SOURCE: Pena-Casanova et al. (2009).

percentages of written to Oral TMT ratio scores (see also "Scoring").

EVIDENCE FOR RELIABILITY

EVIDENCE FOR TEST-RETEST RELIABILITY, MEASURING CHANGE, AND PRACTICE EFFECTS

Test-retest variability varies significantly, generally from low to adequate for the TMT-A and low to high for the TMT-B. For example, Bornstein, Baker, and Douglas (1987) reported low coefficients for the TMT-A (r = .55) but adequate reliability coefficients for the TMT-B (r = .75) in a young adult sample tested over a three-week interval. Matarazzo, Wiens, Matarazzo, and Goldstein (1974) reported poor coefficients at a 12-week test-retest interval (rs = .46 and .44 for the TMT-A and the TMT-B, respectively). At 1-year intervals, several authors have similarly reported low TMT-A reliability and adequate TMT-B reliability (e.g., rs = .53 to .64 and rs = .67 to .72, respectively; Mitrushina & Satz, 1991; Snow et al., 1988).

TABLE 9–141B Education Adjustment for the Spanish TMT-B

	EDUCATION (YEARS)																				
NSS_A	0	1	2	3	4	5	6	7	8	9	10	11	12	13	14	15	16	17	18	19	20
2	4	3	3	3	3	2	2	2	2	1	1	1	0	0	0	0	−1	−1	−1	−2	−2
3	5	4	4	4	4	3	3	3	3	2	2	2	1	1	1	1	0	0	0	−1	−1
4	6	5	5	5	5	4	4	4	4	3	3	3	2	2	2	2	1	1	1	0	0
5	7	6	6	6	6	5	5	5	5	4	4	4	3	3	3	3	2	2	2	1	1
6	8	7	7	7	7	6	6	6	6	5	5	5	4	4	4	4	3	3	3	2	2
7	9	8	8	8	8	7	7	7	7	6	6	6	5	5	5	5	4	4	4	3	3
8	10	9	9	9	9	8	8	8	8	7	7	7	6	6	6	6	5	5	5	4	4
9	11	10	10	10	10	9	9	9	9	8	8	8	7	7	7	7	6	6	6	5	5
10	12	11	11	11	11	10	10	10	10	9	9	9	8	8	8	8	7	7	7	6	6
11	13	12	12	12	12	11	11	11	11	10	10	10	9	9	9	9	8	8	8	7	7
12	14	13	13	13	13	12	12	12	12	11	11	11	10	10	10	10	9	9	9	8	8
13	15	14	14	14	14	13	13	13	13	12	12	12	11	11	11	11	10	10	10	9	9
14	16	15	15	15	15	14	14	14	14	13	13	13	12	12	12	12	11	11	11	10	10
15	17	16	16	16	16	15	15	15	15	14	14	14	13	13	13	13	12	12	12	11	11
16	18	17	17	17	17	16	16	16	16	15	15	15	14	14	14	14	13	13	13	12	12
17	19	18	18	18	18	17	17	17	17	16	16	16	15	15	15	15	14	14	14	13	13
18	20	19	19	19	19	18	18	18	18	17	17	17	16	16	16	16	15	15	15	14	14

NOTE: Education adjustment applying the following formula: $NSS_{A\&E} = NSS_A - (\beta * [Education_{(years)} - 12])$, where $\beta = 0.27320$.

SOURCE: Pena-Casanova et al. (2009).

TABLE 9-142 Trail Making Test (TMT) Normative Data Adjusted by Age and Education, Based on a Brazilian, Portuguese-Speaking Sample

	AGE GROUP (YEARS)	EDUCATION (YEARS) 0–4 *N*	*M*	*SD*	5–8 *N*	*M*	*SD*	9–12 *N*	*M*	*SD*	>13 *N*	*M*	*SD*
TMT-A	18–29	40	38.06	20.9	49	37.73	15.2	61	34.57	9.1	170	29.63	9.1
	30–39	22	49.96	12.0	36	40.25	16.1	60	35.36	10.7	129	30.92	11.6
	40–49	11	62.65	20.4	33	54.16	23.9	52	34.71	11.8	69	30.81	9.6
	50–59	10	52.40	36.8	19	43.54	19.0	41	37.00	10.1	48	37.46	11.0
	60–69	31	63.42	26.9	22	54.84	16.1	25	44.20	13.9	29	40.59	11.8
	>70	35	75.66	30.9	18	55.78	9.2	11	59.09	16.8	8	44.75	12.8
TMT-B	18–29	40	98.06	50.8	48	83.44	39.3	58	70.90	27.5	170	56.97	20.8
	30–39	19	125.68	45.9	35	113.57	37.3	59	69.58	26.3	127	55.49	18.1
	40–49	10	149.30	66.2	29	105.48	52.3	51	73.76	32.5	67	64.42	21.6
	50–59	9	88.67	48.4	18	86.35	34.9	41	79.69	26.2	48	76.58	24.0
	60–69	31	173.03	67.3	21	138.14	51.2	25	100.84	43.7	29	91.14	30.0
	>70	34	191.65	57.0	17	143.18	53.0	10	130.30	41.3	8	94.50	18.1

SOURCE: Campanhalo et al. (2014).

Others have reported adequate to high reliabilities in healthy and neurologically stable adults at 11-month test-retest interval (*rs* = .79, .89 for the TMT-A and the TMT-B; Dikmen et al., 1999; see also Levine et al., 2004, with coefficients exceeding *r* = .70). Cangoz et al. (2009) and Seo et al. (2006) reported similarly adequate to high reliabilities in older adults (*rs* = .78, .79 and *rs* = .73, .82, for the TMT-A and the TMT-B).

Some research suggests reliability coefficients in healthy samples tend to be higher than in clinical groups, including schizophrenia (*rs* = .36 for the TMT-A, .63 for the TMT-B; Goldstein & Watson, 1989) and persons with HIV infection (*rs* = .40 to .50 for TMT-A; *rs* = .54 to .62 for TMT-B; Bardi et al., 1995). Others have reported coefficients similar to those found in healthy controls for mixed neurologic samples (Goldstein & Watson, 1989), patients with cerebrovascular disease (Matarazzo et al., 1974), and people with epilepsy (although a range of reliability coefficients were noted across repeat administrations; see Dodrill & Troupin, 1975). Overall, these studies suggest that the TMT may not be uniformly reliable across populations and time intervals.

Over short retest intervals, practice effects emerge; however, these appear to diminish after several administrations. For example, Bornstein et al. (1987) retested a sample of healthy adults after a three-week interval and noted significant improvement (about three seconds) for the TMT-A only. However, Dye (1979), Stuss, Stethem, and Poirier (1987) and Stuss, Stehem, and Pelchat (1988) reported significant practice effects after a 1-week interval for both

TABLE 9-143A TMT-A Normative Data Adjusted by Age, Education, and Gender for a Turkish Sample

N = 484		50–54 YEARS	55–59 YEARS	60–64 YEARS	65–69 YEARS	70–74 YEARS	75–79 YEARS	80 YEARS AND OVER
Primary school	F	69.67	72.77	82.23	100.00	110.20	158.20	238.30
(0–5 years)		(21.59)	(21.41)	(29.80)	(33.33)	(34.29)	(57.48)	(89.47)
		n = 12	*n* = 13	*n* = 13	*n* = 11	*n* = 10	*n* = 10	*n* = 10
	M	88.00	69.70	78.90	97.40	89.20	121.40	286.40
		(21.90)	(7.67)	(27.02)	(38.74)	(35.39)	(30.89)	(28.23)
		n = 12	*n* = 10	*n* = 10	*n* = 10	*n* = 10	*n* = 10	*n* = 10
High school	F	60.31	61.69	77.00	63.70	93.83	110.50	195.90
(6–11 years)		(13.24)	(24.55)	(22.57)	(13.66)	(47.53)	(44.24)	(74.72)
		n = 13	*n* = 13	*n* = 10	*n* = 10	*n* = 12	*n* = 10	*n* = 10
University	F	53.53	53.14	58.00	78.60	107.60	132.00	183.10
(12 years and over)		(10.81)	(13.60)	(20.01)	(31.54)	(43.50)	(23.88)	(13.43)
		n = 17	*n* = 14	*n* = 10	*n* = 10	*n* = 10	*n* = 10	*n* = 10
	M	52.38	51.16	71.60	54.27	83.40	91.10	128.90
		(16.23)	(7.54)	(39.18)	(14.95)	(28.70)	(43.29)	(41.25)
		n = 16	*n* = 19	*n* = 15	*n* = 11	*n* = 10	*n* = 10	*n* = 10

NOTE: Scores were calculated in seconds.

SOURCE: Cangoz et al. (2009).

TABLE 9–143B TMT-B Normative Data Adjusted by Age, Education, and Gender for a Turkish Sample

N = 484		50–54 YEARS	55–59 YEARS	60–64 YEARS	65–69 YEARS	70–74 YEARS	75–79 YEARS	80 YEARS AND OVER
Primary school (0–5 years)	F	108.83 (15.22) *n* = 12	127.85 (26.90) *n* = 13	141.62 (49.28) *n* = 13	168.91 (66.00) *n* = 11	235.30 (27.84) *n* = 10	236.10 (55.33) *n* = 10	301.10 (78.71) *n* = 10
	M	126.17 (27.61) *n* = 12	122.90 (15.65) *n* = 10	121.40 (20.50) *n* = 10	161.10 (37.86) *n* = 10	219.20 (61.58) *n* = 10	228.50 (43.22) *n* = 10	351.70 (26.05) *n* = 10
High school (6–11 years)	F	94.92 (16.91) *n* = 13	122.15 (27.12) *n* = 13	140.10 (30.45) *n* = 10	105.70 (28.14) *n* = 10	226.50 (105.29) *n* = 12	234.50 (50.34) *n* = 10	309.50 (22.07) *n* = 10
	M	89.47 (16.69) *n* = 17	123.91 (31.00) *n* = 11	117.08 (32.79) *n* = 12	130.15 (38.78) *n* = 13	206.80 (63.31) *n* = 10	167.60 (49.80) *n* = 10	2542.50 (51.58) *n* = 10
University (12 years and over)	F	89.71 (18.03) *n* = 17	109.07 (41.46) *n* = 14	110.70 (32.51) *n* = 10	122.00 (30.34) *n* = 10	229.80 (43.04) *n* = 10	186.60 (43.74) *n* = 10	252.00 (46.54) *n* = 10
	M	86.25 (23.02) *n* = 16	109.07 (41.46) *n* = 19	125.40 (56.23) *n* = 15	108.55 (31.40) *n* = 11	193.90 (71.35) *n* = 10	185.50 (51.07) *n* = 10	226.10 (53.64) *n* = 10

NOTE: Scores were calculated in seconds.
SOURCE: Cangoz et al. (2009).

parts (see Table 9–148), and Durvasula et al. (1996) found continuing improvement for both parts during repeat testing at six-month intervals, which plateaued after five administrations. McCaffrey, Ortega, and Haase (1993) reported steady improvement across three sessions followed by a sudden decrement on the fourth session.

TABLE 9–143C Trail Making Test (TMT) Difference Scores (TMT-B minus TMT-A) Normative Data Adjusted by Age, Education, and Gender for a Turkish Sample

AGE GROUP	SCORE B–A
50–54 years	36.12 (17.93) *n* = 87
55–59 years	61.08 (26.32) *n* = 80
60–64 years	54.57 (26.86) *n* = 70
65–69 years	55.94 (26.86) *n* = 65
70–74 years	122.60 (74.46) *n* = 62
75–79 years	74.46 (64.05) *n* = 60
80 years and over	84.00 (60.04) *n* = 60

NOTE: Score B-A values were calculated in seconds.
SOURCE: Cangoz et al. (2009).

After longer intervals, TMT scores show little or only modest change, at least in healthy adults. For example, Basso, Bornstein, and Lang (1999) retested a group of 50 healthy men after a 12-month interval and found that retesting had no effect on performance. The presence and magnitude of practice effects were similar between individuals of average and above average IQ. The authors also calculated reliable change indices (RCIs) using the standard error of prediction to estimate the range of change in scores that might be expected while accounting for measurement error and practice effects. They noted that a wide range of retest scores could fall within the 90% CI and still reflect measurement error rather than meaningful change. An individual could increase or decrease performance by as much as 24 seconds on the TMT-B without displaying meaningful change in performance.

Similar findings were reported by Levine et al. (2004). Drawing from a database of 605 well-educated, mostly

TABLE 9–144A Total Scores (Mean and Standard Deviation [*SD*]) for Two Derived Measures on the TMT-A and TMT-B

AGE GROUP (YEARS)	RATIO % (B/A%)	DIFFERENCE SCORE (B – A)
18–24	224.79 (71.40)	26.03 (12.08)
25–54	218.22 (65.48)	29.60 (12.95)
55–59	234.06 (73.05)	41.20 (1942)
60–64	223.93 (54.50)	38.41 (16.45)
65–69	230.47 (68.51)	42.07 (20.82)
70–74	261.68 (90.80)	61.43 (30.72)
75–79	263.33 (96.56)	73.23 (39.64)
80–84	263.20 (72.17)	89.44 (45.42)
85–89	261.93 (90.47)	95.31 (62.17)

SOURCE: Tom Tombaugh, personal communication with previous authors (July 20, 2003).

TABLE 9–144B TMT Derived Scores

	EDUCATION 0–12 YEARS		EDUCATION 12+ YEARS		TOTAL	
PERCENTILE	B/A%	B–A	B/A%	B–A	B/A%	B–A
Age Group 18–24 (University Students)						
90					150	13
80					172	15
70					182	18
60					196	21
50					206	23
40					222	26
30					245	30
20					271	35
10					313	43
Age Group 25–54						
90					135	13
80					164	18
70					188	22
60					203	26
50					210	29
40					222	32
30					238	37
20					256	41
10					309	46
Age Group 55–59						
90	153	23	152	12	153	22
80	167	27	167	25	168	26
70	200	31	178	26	187	30
60	214	34	194	30	212	32
50	225	39	221	33	223	36
40	235	43	232	37	233	41
30	261	50	243	46	258	48
20	303	59	292	51	292	54
10	335	75	336	61	333	68
Age Group 60–64						
90	168	24	154	16	160	21
80	175	28	163	20	173	25
70	191	34	167	25	180	28
60	213	35	189	28	208	33
50	230	36	213	31	214	35
40	246	40	222	33	240	39
30	261	49	232	36	255	45
20	280	51	244	44	264	50
10	312	60	259	51	285	56
Age Group 65–69						
90	147	23	151	21	151	23
80	177	34	157	24	177	26
70	185	38	179	26	185	34
60	221	41	190	27	197	38
50	231	46	196	31	221	41
40	249	53	197	36	235	46
30	275	60	217	38	266	51
20	297	65	262	46	284	60
10	351	94	274	48	344	81
Age Group 70–74						
90	172	34	151	28	165	32
80	198	41	182	29	193	38
70	206	45	191	34	205	41
60	224	49	201	38	211	45
50	244	55	210	41	230	50
40	287	72	216	44	260	57
30	320	81	231	49	295	76

TABLE 9–144B Continued

	EDUCATION 0–12 YEARS		EDUCATION 12+ YEARS		TOTAL	
PERCENTILE	B/A%	B–A	B/A%	B–A	B/A%	B–A
20	382	104	275	68	334	83
10	429	121	343	77	406	117
Age Group 75–79						
90	176	36	165	26	173	31
80	190	43	176	27	184	37
70	211	50	189	35	201	43
60	222	64	224	38	223	52
50	238	71	249	43	247	66
40	251	82	260	63	259	76
30	296	91	268	77	287	83
20	346	119	293	83	329	105
10	405	131	349	112	376	128
Age Group 80–84						
90	196	43	172	45	190	44
80	214	54	194	47	213	52
70	226	65	215	55	222	56
60	242	69	223	55	232	67
50	262	83	228	70	249	73
40	269	103	244	73	265	91
30	281	111	275	91	281	106
20	305	126	297	104	302	124
10	364	168	382	130	365	164
Age Group 85–89						
90	197	47	128	15	152	28
80	208	51	152	28	187	48
70	219	71	180	43	213	52
60	249	77	200	52	223	71
50	274	96	223	54	248	83
40	294	108	244	85	267	100
30	337	125	248	109	285	124
20	350	136	286	135	338	134
10	470	253	337	164	359	181

NOTE: B/A% = ratio of scores on Trails A and Trails B expressed as a percentage. B - A = difference score. Readers can convert B - A scores into a percent difference change score (B - A/A × 100) by subtracting 100 from the B/A% score.

SOURCE: Tom Tombaugh, personal communication with previous authors (July 22, 2003).

Caucasian men (education M = 16.4 years, SD = 2.3; age M = 39.5 years, SD = 8.7), they used the regression approach to derive estimates of change. The retest interval ranged from four to 24 months. Table 9–149 shows the regression formulas used to estimate Time 2 scores. The residual SDs for the regression formulas are also shown and can be used to establish the typically expected range for retest scores. For example, a 90% CI can be created around the scores by multiplying the residual SD by 1.645, which allows for 5% of people to fall outside of both the upper and lower extremes. Individuals whose scores exceed the extremes are considered to show significant change. The length of the retest interval did not contribute significantly to the regression equation.

Dikmen et al. (1999) retested a sample of 384 healthy or neurologically stable adults (age M = 34.1, SD = 16.7;

TABLE 9–145 Additional Normative Studies for Specific Groups

REFERENCE	SAMPLE SIZE	SAMPLE CHARACTERISTICS
Andrews et al. (2012)	33	Xhosa-speaking unskilled workers in South Africa
Carrion-Baralt et al. (2009)	81	Spanish-speaking Puerto Rican nonagenarians
Hashimoto et al. (2006)	155	Japanese older adults (70 to over 85 years)
Lovell & Solomon (2011)	513	Professional football athletes (National Football League, US)
Manly et al. (2011)	1,653; 511	Women with human immunodeficiency virus (HIV), women without HIV (US)
Martins et al. (2013)	479	Portuguese-speaking older adults 50 years and older with low levels of education
Perianez et al. (2007)	90; 127; 223	Traumatic brain injury (TBI), schizophrenia, healthy controls (Spain)
Bezdicek et al. (2014)	421	Czech adults, including two clinical groups [mild cognitive impairment (MCI) and Alzheimer's disease (AD)]
Seo et al. (2006)	997	60- to 89-year-old Korean elders

education M = 12.1, SD = 2.6; 66% male) after retest intervals of about nine months (range, about two to 16 months) and also noted that mean difference scores were small. However, some individuals did show large differences, as reflected in the large SD of the difference score (see Table 9–150). This table also provides information needed to determine whether there has been substantial change (RCI) taking practice effects into account. One first subtracts the mean score change for all examinees (T2 – T1) from the difference between the two testing sessions for the individual and then compares the resulting value to 1.64 times the standard deviation of the difference. The 1.64 is derived from the normal distribution and is exceeded in the positive or negative direction only 10% of the time if there is no actual change in clinical condition.

EVIDENCE FOR RELIABILITY OF ALTERNATE FORMS

Alternate forms have been created, with generally high reliabilities ($rs \geq .78$; Charter et al., 1987; des Rosiers & Kavanaugh, 1987; Franzen, 1996; Franzen et al., 1996). Of note, using linear growth modeling, Buck, Atkinson, and Ryan (2008) reported improved performance across three serial administrations of variants of the TMT across one-week intervals. Other studies suggest invariance of latent factors across test administrations, leading authors to advocate for use of alternate forms of the TMT rather than serial administrations of the same form (e.g., Atkinson et al., 2010, 2011).

TABLE 9–146 Raw Scores (Mean and Standard Deviation [*SD*]) on the Oral Trail Making Test in Three Age Groups

	YOUNG ADULTS	MIDDLE-AGED ADULTS	OLDER ADULTS
Age (years)	18.9 (1.1)	31.9 (8.9)	83.5 (6.6)
N	20	18	20
TMT-A	6.4 (0.9)	6.4 (1.0)	10.6 (0.8)
TMT-B	24.1 (10.6)	22.8 (10.6)	40.2 (5.6)

SOURCE: Adapted from Ricker and Axelrod (1994).

EVIDENCE FOR INTERRATER RELIABILITY

Interrater reliability is excellent (i.e., $rs \geq .94$ for the TMT-A and $rs \geq .90$ for the TMT-B; Cangoz et al., 2009).

EVIDENCE FOR RELIABILITY FOR THE ORAL TMT

Information regarding reliability and practice effects for the oral version is not available.

EVIDENCE FOR VALIDITY

WITHIN-TEST CORRELATIONS

The TMT-A and the TMT-B are moderately correlated ($rs \geq .31$; Pineda & Merchan, 2003; Royan et al., 2004). There are additional structural differences between the TMT-A and the TMT-B beyond increased switching demands in the TMT-B. In the TMT-B, the actual distances between circles are longer compared to the TMT-A (i.e., the TMT-B incorporates 57 cm more line length). The TMT-B also includes more visual interference: there are 11 items within a 3-cm distance from the lines to be drawn in the TMT-A, compared to 28 items in the TMT-B. Hence, the TMT-B places greater demands on visual search and motor speed than the TMT-A (Gaudino et al., 1995; Woodruff et al., 1995). Therefore, a low score on the TMT-B relative to the TMT-A does not necessarily indicate reduced cognitive efficiency, but may reflect the increased demands on motor speed and visuoperceptual processes.

ALTERNATE VERSIONS OF THE TMT

Variants of the TMT correlate moderately overall with the conventional TMT, although departures from the format (e.g., oral or computerized vs. written) may decrease task concordance. For example, Drapeau et al. (2007) found a larger difference between the TMT-A and the TMT-B in the conventional, paper version compared to a computer version, with versions failing to show high correlations. Atkinson and Ryan (2007) reported that variants of tests involving trail making (including the D-KEFS and Connections Test) were moderately correlated (r = –.45 to r = .33). According to a confirmatory factor analysis, the best fitting model for trail making tests was reflected in two factors, sequencing and shifting. Mrazik et al. (2010) reported comparable correlations between the TMT-A and the TMT-B of the oral and written versions of the tests (r = .54, r = .62, respectively); however, the Oral TMT-A

TABLE 9–147A Means, Standard Deviations (SDs), and Percentiles for the Oral Trail Making Test

AGE GROUPS (YEARS) (MIDPOINT)	20–39 (29)	29–49 (39)	39–59 (49)	49–69 (59)	59–79 (69)	69–90 (79)
Group size	31	31	31	27	23	18
OTMT-A	6.25 (1.3)	6.56 (1.4)	7.02 (2.0)	7.16 (2.3)	6.98 (2.3)	7.48 (2.1)
9th percentile	8.0	8.0	9.6	9.6	9.1	9.1
25th percentile	7.4	7.3	7.6	8.2	8.9	8.4
50th percentile	6.0	6.0	6.4	6.4	7.1	8.0
75th percentile	5.0	5.3	5.7	5.5	5.3	5.9
OTMT-B	27.77 (14.8)	29.97 (15.2)	30.65 (14.1)	35.27 (16.2)	42.25 (19.1)	46.78 (20.6)
2nd percentile	55.0	58.0	58.0	60.0	73.0	82.3
9th percentile	44.0	53.0	53.0	56.0	69.7	73.0
25th percentile	33.0	34.1	34.0	42.0	52.9	52.9
50th percentile	22.0	22.9	24.2	30.1	32.1	36.1
75th percentile	16.0	17.2	20.0	23.6	25.0	31.4

NOTE: 9th percentile score distribution as a cutoff point for possible impairment. Of note, however, cutpoints may vary on the basis of the screening context.

SOURCE: Mrazik et al. (2010).

was not correlated to either of the written conditions. See also "Scoring" and "Evidence for Reliability."

FACTOR-ANALYTIC STUDIES

Factor-analytic studies have suggested that processing speed and visual scanning and search are also important components of test performance. For example, González-Blanch et al. (2011) report on the factor structure of a neuropsychological battery in healthy older controls, completed as part of the MOANS project. A five-factor model was found to best fit the data, with the TMT and Digit Symbol loading on a factor termed motor speed. Similarly, Greenaway, Smith, Tangalos, Geda, and Ivnik (2009) subjected the expanded MOANS cognitive battery to a factor analysis, finding that that the TMT loaded on a motor speed factor with WAIS-III Processing Speed subtests in a five-factor solution. See also "Age." Processing speed and TMT performance were found to be genetically linked in a large-scale heritability study (Hagenaars et al., 2017).

TABLE 9–147B Cumulative Percentage of Written to Oral TMT-B Ratio Scores (Mrazik et al., 2010)

	AGE GROUP (YEARS)						
RATIOS	20–39	29–49	39–59	49–69	59–79	69–90	TOTAL
6.70	–	–	–	4.8	9.5	–	1.5
5.50	5.0	3.6	–	–	–	–	3.1
4.40	–	–	–	9.5	14.3	5.6	5.4
4.20	–	–	–	–	–	11.1	6.2
4.00	–	–	–	–	–	16.7	6.9
3.40	–	7.1	5.0	14.3	23.8	–	10.0
3.30	10.0	10.7	–	–	–	22.2	13.1
3.20	–	14.3	–	19.0	33.3	–	15.4
3.10	15.0	–	–	–	–	27.8	17.7
3.00	–	–	–	23.8	42.9	–	19.2
2.90	–	17.9	15.0	28.6	–	–	22.3
2.80	–	21.4	20.0	33.3	–	–	24.6
2.70	–	28.6	35.0	42.9	52.4	–	30.8
2.60	–	–	–	47.6	61.9	44.4	35.4
2.50	–	32.1	40.0	–	–	50	38.5
2.40	–	35.7	–	52.4	–	–	40.0
2.30	–	39.3	–	–	–	–	40.8
2.20	20.0	46.4	50.0	57.1	–	61.1	47.7
2.10	25.0	50.0	55.0	61.9	71.4	72.2	54.6
2.00	30.0	53.6	60.0	–	–	–	56.9
1.90	40.0	60.7	65.0	71.4	81.0	–	63.1
1.80	55.0	67.9	70.0	76.2	–	77.8	70.0
1.70	65.0	71.4	–	81.0	90.5	83.3	74.6
1.60	75.0	75.0	75.0	85.7	100	88.9	81.5
1.50	80.0	78.6	–	–	–	–	83.1
1.40	–	–	–	–	–	100	86.2
1.30	–	–	–	–	–	–	–
1.20	85.0	85.7	85.0	90.5	–	–	90.8
1.10	–	92.9	95.0	95.2	–	–	95.4
1.00	–	–	100	100.0	–	–	96.9
0.90	95.0	96.4	–	–	–	–	98.5
0.70	100.0	100.0	–	100.0	–	–	100.0

SOURCE: Mrazik et al. (2010).

Other factor-analytic research has suggested that the TMT derived scores may be more reflective of executive control than the conventional scores. Oosterman et al. (2010) reported that neuropsychological variables examined in their study (e.g., select CANTAB subtests, Wechsler Digit Span, Stockings of Cambridge, Stroop, Auditory Verbal Learning Test) predicted TMT-B performance, but only executive function predicted the ratio score of TMT-B/TMT-A. The authors note the multiplicity of cognitive functions involved in TMT performance and recommend use of the TMT ratio score in interpretation of the TMT as a test of executive ability.

CORRELATIONS WITH ATTENTION, EXECUTIVE FUNCTION, PROCESSING SPEED, AND VISUAL SEARCH

Executive control plays a role in performance, with correlations between the TMT and executive tests involving working memory, inhibition, and fluency in the moderate range overall. Research suggests that visual search, visual-spatial sequencing, scanning abilities, and speed are also important components. In contrast, memory tests (CVLT, Wechsler Memory Scale Faces) have been reported to show weak or nonsignificant correlations with the TMT-B (Pavao Martins et al., 2013), as do language tests

TABLE 9–148 Completion Time in Seconds (Means and SDs) for the TMT-A and the TMT-B by Age, Based on Two Test Sessions Spaced One Week Apart

N	AGE	EDUCATION (YEARS)	TMT-A TEST 1	TMT-A TEST 2	TMT-B TEST 1	TMT-B TEST 2
30	16–29	14.1	21.48 (6.44)	19.68 (7.32)	48.77 (18.66)	42.18 (15.54)
30	30–49	14.9	27.58 (9.43)	22.95 (6.23)	61.30 (17.88)	61.52 (22.79)
30	50–69	13.2	36.73 (13.68)	29.30 (14.73)	76.97 (30.52)	67.10 (28.37)

SOURCE: Adapted from Stuss et al. (1988).

(Token Test, Peabody Picture Vocabulary Test, and Picture Naming; Ehrenstein et al., 1982).

A number of authors have reported that the TMT is moderately correlated with executive and attention measures (i.e., absolute value of correlations from r = .23 to r = .63), including Wechsler Digit Span (Pavao Martins et al., 2013; Sánchez-Cubillo et al., 2009), the SDMT (Manly et al., 2011; Royan et al., 2004), the Stroop (Pavao Martins et al., 2013; Sánchez-Cubillo et al., 2009), the PASAT (Royan et al., 2004), the CANTAB (Smith et al., 2013), phonemic fluency (Pavao Martins et al., 2013), and the Category Test (Pavao Martins et al., 2013). Overall, slightly higher correlations are reported between the TMT-B and executive and attention measures compared to the TMT-A, which is consistent with the greater executive demands made by the TMT-B. Regression analyses have also suggested that the TMT-B is more sensitive to cognitive flexibility (see Kortte et al., 2002). In terms of the Oral TMT, Ricker et al. (1996) reported moderate correlations between the Oral TMT and the WCST percent perseverative errors (r = .35), but not with verbal fluency (r = .17).

Sánchez-Cubillo et al. (2009) examined relative contributions of working memory, inhibition, interference control, task switching, and visuomotor speed to TMT performance in 41 healthy older participants. Multiple regression analyses of TMT-A performance suggested that 45% of the variance could be explained by Digit Symbol performance, whereas multiple regression analyses of the TMT-B suggested that Digit Backward and a novel task switching measure accounted for 48% of the variance. Multiple regression analyses of the TMT-B – TMT-A difference scores suggested that 30% of the variance could be accounted for by the novel task switching paradigm. The authors interpreted their findings to suggest that that the TMT-A involves predominantly visuoperceptual abilities, the TMT-B involves working memory and task switching, and the TMT-B – TMT-A difference score reflects a relatively pure indicator of executive control.

TABLE 9–149 Trail Making Test (TMT) Regression Equations for Estimating Retest (Time 2) Scores

MEASURE	REGRESSION EQUATION	RESIDUAL *SD*
TMT-A	9.55 + (.545 × Time 1 score)	5.35
TMT-B	21 + (.553 × Time 1 score)	11.61

SOURCE: Adapted from Levine et al. (2004).

CORRELATIONS WITH IQ

See "Demographic Effects."

CORRELATIONS WITH SENSORY AND MOTOR SKILLS

In a mixed neuropsychiatric sample, visual acuity showed a modest correlation (r = –.27) with the TMT-B, whereas motor speed and dexterity were moderately correlated with the task (rs = –.42, –.46; Schear & Sato, 1989; see also Skeel et al., 2003). In addition, only the motor tests were significant predictors of TMT performance in a regression analysis. See also "Age" and "Administration."

CLINICAL STUDIES

Dementia. The TMT-B has been identified as an important test in the diagnosis of dementia (Steenland et al., 2010), and is sensitive to AD (Cahn et al., 1995; Chen et al., 2000; Lafleche & Albert, 1995). In a mixed sample of patients referred for dementia evaluation, Schmitt et al. (2010) investigated the diagnostic utility of scoring the TMT-B based on the ability to complete or not complete the test. The authors reported that TMT-B completion was associated with a sensitivity of 69% and specificity of 100% in differentiating dementia versus nondementia.

TABLE 9–150 Trail Making Test (TMT) Test-Retest Data (Means and Standard Deviations [SDs]) Based on a Sample (N = 384) of Healthy or Neurologically Stable Adults, Aged 15–83 Years

TRAIL MAKING TEST	TIME 1	TIME 2	T2 – T1	SD_{DIFF}	*R*
TMT-A	26.52 (11.66)	25.56 (11.66)	–.96	7.54	.79
TMT-B	72.05 (45.22)	68.19 (46.13)	–3.86	21.64	.89

M = 34.2, *SD* = 16.7.

NOTE: In order to reduce testing time and patient fatigue, time limits were imposed on the TMT-A (100 seconds) and the TMT-B (300 seconds). The mean test-retest interval was about nine months. One first subtracts the mean change (T1 score – T2 score) from the difference between the two testing sessions for the examinee and then compares this value to 1.64 times the standard deviation of the difference. The 1.64 is derived from the normal distribution and is exceeded in the positive or negative direction only 10% of the time if there is no actual change in clinical condition.

SOURCE: Adapted from Dikmen et al. (1999).

The test has demonstrated some utility in differentiating between dementia subtypes (although see Barr et al., 1992). Patients with dementia with Lewy bodies (DLB) performed worse than patients with AD on the TMT-B (Kraybill et al., 2005). The TMT has been identified as part of a battery that effectively differentiates DLB from healthy aging and AD (Ferman et al., 2006). With the inclusion of the TMT-A, the Benton Visual Form Discrimination, and the RAVLT, sensitivity was nearly 89% and specificity was approximately 96% in differentiating DLB from healthy controls. In terms of differentiating DLB from AD, the TMT-A, Boston Naming Test, RAVLT, and the copy condition of the Rey-Osterrieth Complex Figure were associated with a sensitivity of 83% and specificity of 91%.

The TMT has shown utility in MCI, including in identifying MCI in patients with PD (Biundo et al., 2013) and predicting progression rates from MCI to dementia, especially when the test is used in conjunction with other variables (e.g., Zhou et al., 2012). Blacker et al. (2007) reported that the TMT and the CVLT significantly predicted time to progress from MCI to AD. The TMT-A, as part of a battery that included semantic fluency and memory tests, significantly predicted development of dementia in a group of patients with amnesia (53% accuracy at two-year follow-up; Molinuevo et al., 2011). The TMT-B was identified as a significant predictor, along with the Alzheimer's Disease Assessment Scale-Cognitive and independent ADLs, of conversion from amnestic MCI to dementia at one-year follow-up (Rozzini et al., 2007). See also "Driving" and "Activities of Daily Living."

TBI. Heled, Hoofien, Margalit, Natovich, and Agranov (2012) reported that the TMT-B was able to effectively differentiate severe TBI from healthy controls, with the TMT-B associated with a sensitivity of 90% and a specificity of 82%. TMT completion times increase with increasing severity of injury (Dikmen et al., 1995; Iverson et al., 2002; Martin et al., 2003). Felmingham, Baguley, and Green (2004) noted that diffuse axonal injury is associated with slowed performance on the TMT in patients with severe TBI.

In terms of long-term outcome, longitudinal studies reveal that there is marked heterogeneity of TMT outcome after moderate to severe injury. Five years after injury, a substantial proportion of individuals with moderate to severe TBI show TMT performance within typical limits, although a significant number continue to show deficits on the test. Millis et al. (2001) found that about 43% of individuals who show impairment show poor performance on the TMT-A, compared to 33% of patients who demonstrate deficits on the TMT-B. Outcome may interact with individual characteristics. For example, Millis et al. (2001) reported that older age at the time of injury was an important risk factor for neuropsychological outcome. In addition, patients carrying the APOE-Ɛ4 allele performed worse on the TMT-B after moderate and severe TBI than did noncarriers (Ariza et al., 2006).

The TMT is generally less affected by mild TBI and postconcussive effects than more severe forms of TBI. Cicerone and Azulay (2002) administered the TMT to a group of patients with PCS and matched controls, screened for performance validity. Sensitivity was poor for the TMT-A (31%) and the TMT-B (14%), with excellent specificity (100% for each condition). Iverson, Lange, and Franzen (2005) also noted that patients with acute, uncomplicated mild TBI could not be reliably differentiated by the TMT from patients with substance abuse problems.

Some authors have reported that derived scores are more sensitive to the effects of TBI than are conventional scores. For example, Felmingham et al. (2004) recommended the use of a ratio score because slower performance on the TMT-A appears to underlie deficits in the TMT-B. That is, slowing of information processing speed may account for difficulties on more complex cognitive tasks. Although Iverson et al. (2002) reported that the TMT ratio scores (but not errors) increased with injury severity, Martin et al. (2003) reported that the TMT ratio score did not demonstrate sensitivity to injury severity.

The TMT is related to functional outcomes in TBI. A subset of veterans who sustained a mild TBI were found to perform poorly on the TMT, which subsequently predicted performance on several other cognitive measures (Thaler et al., 2013). The TMT is also related to a measure of everyday competence in patients who sustained a moderate to severe TBI (Garcia Molina et al., 2012). TMT performance is associated with vocational outcome in adulthood after childhood TBI. Similar findings were reported for injury incurred in adulthood (Atchison et al., 2004). People with TBI working full-time tend to perform faster on the TMT-B (Nybo et al., 2004). In addition, psychosocial outcome after TBI can be predicted by the TMT-A and the TMT-B (Acker & Davis, 1989; Colantonio et al., 2000; Millis et al., 1994; Ross et al., 1997). See also "Driving."

HIV. The TMT has shown to be useful in identifying cognitive impairment in HIV infection (de Almeida et al., 2017). In a Thai sample of patients with HIV infection, the TMT-A improved the sensitivity of the International HIV Dementia Scale in identification of HIV-associated neurocognitive disorder (HAND), with a sensitivity of 86% and specificity of 79% (Chalermchai et al., 2013). Muñoz-Moreno et al. (2013) reported that a screening battery for detecting HIV-related cognitive impairment involving the TMT and verbal fluency was associated with a sensitivity of nearly 75% and specificity of nearly 82%. In a randomized, double-blind, placebo-controlled, crossover study of the efficacy and safety of rivastigmine in patients with HAND, improvements in the TMT-A were noted following treatment (Simioni et al., 2013).

Demographic variables are an important consideration. Manly et al. (2011) reported that once demographic variables were considered, there was no significant difference in performance on the TMT between women in their sample with HIV and those without. Levine et al. (2007) evaluated the generalizability of data derived from a healthy sample in detecting change among two groups: persons with HIV who were demographically similar to the healthy sample and persons with HIV who were demographically dissimilar to the healthy sample. The authors reported greater generalizability of simple regression-based methods when demographic features were consistent.

Psychiatric Conditions. Patients with schizophrenia tend to show deficits on the TMT (Moritz et al., 2002; Nielsen et al., 2013; Woelwer, 2002; Zalla et al., 2004), with the TMT relating to the severity of negative symptoms, general psychopathology, employment readiness (Hanuszkiewicz et al., 2009), and improvements after antipsychotic use (Crespo-Facorro et al., 2009; Harvey et al., 2008). The test also relates to the duration of psychosis (Allott et al., 2017). In one study, the TMT-B differentiated between patients with and without later clinical deterioration at the level of group analyses (Wölwer et al., 2008). However, relatively low sensitivity and specificity were reported (72%, 51%, respectively), with improved prediction when psychopathological variables were also considered.

Major depression also affects performance negatively, with many authors reporting that the TMT-B is particularly sensitive (Elderkin-Thompson et al., 2003; Messinis et al., 2010; Naismith et al., 2003). However, a meta-analysis suggested that the TMT-A is one of the most effective measures differentiating depressed from nondepressed controls, with the TMT-B not found to be effective (Lim et al., 2013). Persons with remitted depression may also show worse performance on the TMT (King et al., 1995), even after adjustment for demographic variables (Hasselbalch et al., 2012).

Other research suggests that it is important to consider a number of factors. Jungwirth et al. (2011) reported that after accounting for neurologic comorbidity (e.g., stroke, PD), gender, education, and antidepressant and benzodiazepine use, only a minor slowing effect of depression on TMT-A and TMT-B performance was found. The effect of neurologic comorbidity and education, in contrast, strongly influenced TMT performance.

The TMT-B has been identified as one of the most robust measures differentiating controls from patients with bipolar disorder, with an overall effect size of .63 across reanalysis of primary datasets (Bourne et al., 2013). In a meta-analytic review, patients with bipolar disorder and psychosis showed greater impairment on the TMT than patients without psychosis (Cohen's d = .30; Bora et al., 2010). Juselius, Kieseppa, Kaprio, Lonnqvist, and Tuulio-Henriksson (2009) reported that the duration of illness and number of hospitalizations were correlated with TMT performance in patients with bipolar disorder. The TMT-B was found to predict psychological and social aspects of quality of life in patients with bipolar disorder (Pattanayak et al., 2012), psychosocial outcome (Soni et al., 2017), and functional outcome when combined with depressive symptomatology (Solé et al., 2011).

Other Populations. Larrabee, Millis, and Meyers (2008) reported that the TMT-B was associated with a large effect size (Cohen's d = .89) in differentiating patients with neurologic conditions from controls, and it has been suggested that the TMT is useful as a general indicator of neurologic function (Reitan & Wolfson, 1995, 2004). The TMT has been found to be sensitive to a variety of conditions, including Joseph-Machado disease (Braga-Neto et al., 2012), fragile X syndrome (Moore et al., 2004), MS (Papathanasiou et al., 2017), prodromal HD (Park et al., 2017), toxic exposure (Stewart et al., 1999; Summers et al., 2011), iron deficiency (Lukowski et al., 2010), vitamin D deficiency (meta-analysis; Annweiler et al., 2013), essential tremor (Benito-León, Louis, & Bermejo-Pareja, 2006), anorexia nervosa (effect size estimates of .49; Stedal et al., 2012), history of critical illness (Pandharipande et al., 2013), long-term use of anticholinergic medications (Bottiggi et al., 2006), and as a screening test for cognitive impairment in unhoused adults (Hurstak et al., 2017).

The test is sensitive to substance use disorders (e.g., Grant et al., 1984, 1987; McCaffrey et al., 1988). The TMT-A accurately classified 59% of older adults with alcohol use disorders with minor neurocognitive disorder (Kaufmann et al., 2017). Improvements on the TMT have been noted following inpatient treatment for substance use (Schrimsher & Parker, 2008).

Driving. Studies have suggested that the TMT effectively predicts driving ability and differentiates levels of driving ability in older adults (Mathias & Lucas, 2009; Niewoehner et al., 2012; Ott et al., 2013), as well as in patients who have sustained a TBI (Aslaksen et al., 2013; Cullen et al., 2014; Demery et al., 2010; Hargrave et al., 2012). In combination with a test of visual acuity, the MMSE, and the CDT, the TMT-A showed 85% specificity and 80% sensitivity in predicting real-world road test performance in older adults (De Raedt, 2001). However, no significant differences were reported between older drivers with a crash history compared to those without (Woolnough et al., 2013).

In terms of dementia, the TMT-A was identified as part of a screening battery that predicted performance on an on-road driving test (Carr et al., 2011). The TMT-A was related to safety errors in drivers with AD (Dawson et al., 2009). In patients with PD, TMT performance is correlated with performance in driving simulator studies and an on-road evaluation (Ranchet et al., 2012). The TMT was one of the most effective cognitive tests in classifying fitness to drive in HD (Devos et al., 2012).

Marshall et al. (2007) identified the TMT as one of the best cognitive predictors of on-road driving assessment in patients following stroke. In a systematic review and meta-analysis of fitness to drive after stroke, Devos et al. (2011)

found that the TMT-B identified unsafe drivers with 80% accuracy.

Activities of Daily Living. The TMT also appears useful for predicting instrumental ADLs in community-dwelling older adults (Cahn-Weiner et al., 2002; Bell-McGinty et al., 2002), in cognitively impaired older adults (Baum et al., 1996; Boyle et al., 2004; Tierney et al., 2001), and in patients with stroke (Park et al., 2017). For example, Tierney et al. (2001) reported that the TMT-B was significantly related to self-care deficits, use of emergency services, experiencing harm, and loss of property as judged by independent raters and primary care physicians in patients with cognitive impairment who lived alone. The TMT-B predicted change in ADLs in patients one year after cardiac surgery (Benvenuti et al., 2013). Hirota et al. (2010) reported that the mean difference between performance on the TMT-A and TMT-B was related to variables pertaining to walking performance in older Japanese adults. See also previous sections in "Clinical Studies" for relationships between the TMT and functional outcomes in specific groups.

NEUROANATOMICAL CORRELATES AND IMAGING STUDIES

Lesion Studies. In a meta-analysis, Demakis (2004) compared patients with frontal damage to those with damage to posterior brain regions. Significant differences between groups were found for the TMT-A but not for the TMT-B (weighted effect size = –.23 and –.16, respectively). However, use of the TMT-A alone was not sufficient to discriminate between those with frontal versus nonfrontal brain injury. The degree of overlap between the distributions of these two groups at this effect size was about 85%, indicating little separation of groups and thus relatively poor sensitivity and specificity.

The TMT-B may be sensitive to damage to specific frontal subregions, but specificity is not detected due to data aggregation in meta-analytic research. Stuss et al. (2001) found notable slowing of TMT in patients with frontal lobe injury but found that error analysis was more informative than time-based scores. All patients who made more than one error on the TMT-B had frontal lesions, with the greatest impairment in patients with dorsolateral frontal cortex involvement and the least impairment in persons with lesions affecting the inferior (ventromedial/orbitofrontal) region.

Neuroimaging. Research beyond lesion studies has implicated frontal regions in TMT performance, in both healthy and clinical populations. Other regions have also been identified as important, including temporal regions and white matter tracts.

Healthy Samples. In healthy populations, a functional near-infrared spectroscopy (fNIRS) study of healthy older people (50 to 75 years of age; Hagen et al., 2014) reported that frontal activation was noted in the dorsolateral prefrontal cortex, the frontopolar area, and Broca's area during performance of the TMT, along with activation in the left motor, somatosensory, and somatosensory association cortices. Participants older than 58 years of age showed less focused prefrontal activation. Lu et al. (2013) reported that age-related slowing on the TMT is mediated by myelin breakdown in late myelinating regions, such as the prefrontal cortex and genu of the corpus callosum in healthy older adults. See also "Age." Kubo et al. (2008) reported increased blood flow in the prefrontal cortex during performance of the TMT, as measured by near-infrared spectroscopy (NIRS). In addition to prefrontal activation, more global measures may also be related to TMT performance; Hankee et al. (2013) reported that the TMT was related to total cerebral brain volume in addition to frontal lobe volume via MRI.

Consistent with their disparate task demands, the TMT-A and the TMT-B have been shown to be associated with different patterns of activation. Jacobson, Blanchard, Connolly, Cannon, and Garavan (2011) reported greater activation in right inferior/middle frontal cortices, right precentral gyrus, left angular gyrus, and left middle temporal gyrus on a computer modification of the TMT-B relative to the TMT-A in healthy participants. Zakzanis, Mraz, and Graham (2005) report left-sided dorsolateral and medial frontal activity in a modified TMT-B relative to the TMT-A in healthy young adults using fMRI, also noting additional activation in left middle and superior temporal gyrus regions.

Schizophrenia and Psychosis. Patients with schizophrenia show relationships between TMT performance and the frontal cortex, as well as the temporal lobe and cerebellar regions, among other areas. Performance on the TMT-B was related to decreased Brodmann's Area 9 (part of the dorsolateral and medial prefrontal cortex) gray matter volume in people with schizophrenia (Bonilha et al., 2008). Reduced gray matter volume in the left cerebellum as measured by a cerebellum-optimized voxel-based morphometry procedure was correlated with TMT performance in patients with schizophrenia (Kuhn et al., 2012).

Oosterman et al. (2010) reported that medial temporal lobe atrophy was the strongest predictor of TMT-B performance relative to other neuroanatomical variables (e.g., periventricular hyperintensities, deep white matter hyperintensities) and neuropsychological variables (e.g., memory, executive function, processing speed, attention). Patients with first-episode psychosis demonstrated correlations between TMT performance and reduced fractional anisotropy in the right and left anterior thalamic radiation, inferior frontal-occipital fasciculus, forceps minor, and left superior and inferior longitudinal fasciculi (Pérez-Iglesias et al., 2010). People defined clinically as at risk for psychosis showed correlations between the TMT-B and the ventromedial prefrontal cortex, cerebellum, and frontocallosal white matter (Koutsouleris et al., 2010).

Dementia and MCI. In terms of dementia and MCI, Terada et al. (2013) compared amnestic MCI and AD patients dichotomized as either showing better or worse scores on the TMT-B. Patients with poorer scores on the TMT-B demonstrated significant hypoperfusion in the bilateral anterior cingulate extending to the posterior region on the right, bilateral caudate nucleus and putamen, and thalamus bilaterally. Blood flow in the right cingulate cortex was related to TMT-B scores. Sudo et al. (2013) reported that the TMT was related to an index of white matter hyperintensities in patients with vascular MCI. Impairments in ADLs were related to worse TMT-A scores and smaller hippocampal volumes in patients with amnestic MCI or AD (Brown et al., 2011). The TMT-B and the TMT difference score were related to gray matter volume of the inferior frontal gyrus, precuneus, and superior temporal cortex in patients with neurocognitive disorder (Lu et al., 2017).

PERFORMANCE VALIDITY

A number of authors have reported suppressed performance in simulator groups and persons suspected of performing noncredibly compared to persons with verifiable injury (Binder et al., 2003; Egeland et al., 2007; Powell et al., 2011; Ruffolo et al., 2000; Youngjohn et al., 1995). Sensitivity and specificity vary across studies.

Iverson et al. (2002) examined a group of 571 patients with acute TBI and developed cutoff scores that could be used to indicate inadequate performance validity (see Table 9–151). Using cutoff scores at the 5th percentile, Iverson et al. (2002) noted that the group with compromised performance validity performed more poorly than controls on both conditions of the TMT. Although the TMT-A and the TMT-B time-to-completion scores appeared to be reasonable indicators of inadequate performance validity at the group level, this was only the case with very mild injury. At the level of individual classification, the scores were unlikely to detect malingerers; sensitivity varied between 7% and 19%, and there was a low degree of confidence in the classification of nonmalingerers, with a negative predictive value ranging from 66% to 78%. There was also little benefit in the use of the ratio scores to identify compromised performance validity (see also Martin et al., 2003).

The authors concluded that scores that fall in the range of possible biased responding can be considered "red flags" for the clinician because they do not make biological or psychometric sense. However, the sensitivity of the TMT to deliberate exaggeration is very low, so clinicians who rely on this test to identify invalid performance will fail to identify the vast majority of cases. Similar findings have been reported by others (e.g., Van Gorp et al., 1999; O'Bryant et al., 2003). Stand-alone performance validity tests intended for this purpose tend to perform better (Merten et al., 2004).

Other studies show some utility, but specificity rates vary, at times indicating unacceptable false-positive rates. For example, Busse and Whiteside (2012) report on the comparative value of various neuropsychological tests (TMT, Brief Test of Attention, Continuous Performance Test, the Test of Memory Malingering [TOMM]) in performance validity assessment in a mixed clinical sample of 413 clients assessed in private practice. TBI was the most common diagnosis. Participants were further classified as exhibiting biased responding or unbiased responding according to TOMM performance. The TMT-A was found to have unacceptably poor classification accuracy. The TMT-B was found to yield a sensitivity of 61% and specificity of 85% at a cutoff of 120 seconds. When the TMT-A and the TMT-B time scores were combined, a cutoff score of 170 seconds yielded a sensitivity of 48% and specificity of 85%.

Similarly, Powell et al. (2011) grouped 76 patients evaluated for treatment in a brain injury rehabilitation program based on TOMM Trial 2 performance, resulting in a group with compromised performance validity and an adequate performance validity group. The adequate performance validity group completed the TMT-A faster than the TMT-B. The TMT-A yielded a 72% sensitivity rate and an 80% specificity rate, with the TMT-B yielding rates of 50% sensitivity and 80% specificity.

Egeland et al. (2007) reported data from clients seeking financial compensation classified as possibly malingering or nonmalingering based on performance on the Victoria Symptom Validity Test. The participants deemed as nonmalingering were further classified into impaired/unimpaired. Possible malingerers performed worse on the TMT-A compared to both impaired and nonimpaired clients. A TMT ratio score of less than 2.5 yielded sensitivity

TABLE 9–151 Trail Making Test (TMT) Performance Validity Cutoff Values for Time-to-Completion Scores

	TMT-A TIME (PERCENTILE)			TMT-B TIME (PERCENTILE)			TMT-B/TMT-A RATIO (PERCENTILE)		
	10TH	5TH	1ST	10TH	5TH	1ST	10TH	5TH	1ST
Total Clinical Sample (n = 571)	52	63	86	155	200	288	1.66	1.49	1.25

NOTE: Age M = 34.7, SD = 15; Education M = 11.8, SD = 1.8.

SOURCE: Adapted from Iverson et al. (2002).

rates of 68% and specificity of 57%, the latter indicating an unacceptable false-positive rate at this cutoff.

Errors may be helpful in the detection of performance validity, primarily because they tend to be infrequent (Hankee et al., 2013). For example, in their normative sample, Cavaco et al. (2013) reported that the majority of their sample did not make errors on the TMT-A or the TMT-B. More than one error on the TMT-A and two errors or more on the TMT-B were obtained by less than 5% of the sample. Errors are relatively few even in patients with severe TBI (Iverson et al., 2002; Ruffulo et al., 2000). Iverson et al. (2002) reported that it was unusual for individuals with moderate to severe TBI to demonstrate two or more errors on the TMT-A, and four or more errors on TMT-B; fewer than about 5% of the clinical sample obtained a similar score. Therefore, a large number of errors may alert the examiner to noncredible performance, at least in TBI. However, more research is needed in populations with known cognitive impairments to better delineate appropriate cutoffs that do not overidentify impaired examinees as noncredible, including examinees with neurological compromise, suspected dementia, or low IQ.

COMMENT

The TMT has a long history of use in neuropsychology and a correspondingly well-characterized body of literature. Demographic effects are well-established, including a prominent age effect, especially after 50 years and later in older adulthood. Research suggests age-related effects may relate to decrements in processing speed. Education, reading ability, and IQ effects are significant, particularly in examinees with low levels of education. Gender is generally not influential. There is evidence that ethnicity and other sociodemographic variables influence performance.

Given these influences, normative data should be chosen that incorporate adjustments for demographic effects. Fortunately, more than 70 normative studies have been published on the TMT, many of which have been published relatively recently and offer high-quality and comprehensive data. Cangoz et al. (2009) and Cavaco et al. (2013) provide normative data on derived measures, which may confer additional advantages over conventional measures alone (see "Normative Data"). In addition to conventional measures, Hankee et al. (2013) provide qualitative data for a large number of participants on error rates and pen lifts. Pena-Casanova et al. (2009) offer age- and education-adjusted data in narrow age increments for older adults as part of the NEURONORMA project, which is a dataset that also has the advantage of being co-normed with many other neuropsychological tests. Schneider et al. (2015) provide TMT data separately based on ethnicity.

Strong interrater and alternate form reliability have been reported, whereas test-rest reliability is variable across ages and populations, overall ranging from low to adequate for the TMT-A and low to high for the TMT-B. Practice effects are generally reported, which tend to plateau after repeated administrations. Reliable change data are provided and are recommended for evaluating results from repeated assessments.

Relationships with other tests suggest that the TMT involves a number of abilities, not only attention and executive function, but also visual scanning, visual search, and processing speed. Limited associations with memory and language tests provide support for divergent validity. Neuroimaging studies in clinical and healthy populations have similarly implicated not only frontal regions, but also broad-based networks, including white matter tracts likely related to processing speed and temporal regions, among others. There is evidence that the derived scores may be a relatively purer measure of executive ability than completion-time scores and may also show relatively greater sensitivity in some clinical populations such as TBI. However, less is known about the psychometric properties of derived scores, including their reliability. The TMT-A and the TMT-B share some common components, although evidence suggests that the TMT-B involves greater executive demands.

Clinically, the TMT has shown sensitivity to a wide range of both neurologic and neuropsychiatric conditions, including TBI, dementia, HIV, schizophrenia, mood disorders, and anxiety, among others. The test also shows impressive relationships with clinical correlates and functional activities in both healthy controls and clinical samples, particularly regarding driving.

In terms of performance validity, diagnostic accuracy is somewhat variable and not generally impressive, and the test would benefit from research in cognitively compromised groups to better delineate cutoffs that do not unduly raise false-positive rates.

In participants who may have visual or motor impairments precluding administration of the conventional written TMT, the Oral TMT is an alternative option. However, note that the Oral TMT is not equivalent to the written version. For example, when compared with the written TMT, the oral version is performed much more quickly, shows a discrepant pattern of demographic influence, has less rigorous normative data, has limited information regarding reliability, and has been the subject of less research overall. Although data are provided to convert an oral score to a written score, given the discrepancies between these two tasks, use of the Oral TMT norms may provide more precision than score conversion.

REFERENCES

Abraham, E., Axelrod, B. N., & Ricker, J. H. (1996). Application of the oral Trail Making Test to a mixed clinical sample. *Archives of Clinical Neuropsychology, 11*, 697–701.

Acker, M. B., & Davis, J. R. (1989). Psychology test scores associated with late outcome in head injury. *Neuropsychology, 3,* 1–10.

Allott, K., Fraguas, D., Bartholomeusz, C. F., Díaz-Caneja, C. M., Wannan, C., Parrish, E. M., . . . Rapado-Castro, M. (2017). Duration of untreated psychosis and neurocognitive functioning in first-episode psychosis: A systematic review and meta-analysis. *Psychological Medicine,* 1–18. https://doi.org/10.1017/S0033291717003002

Andrews, K., Shuttleworth-Edwards, A., & Radloff, S. (2012). Normative indications for Xhosa speaking unskilled workers on the Trail Making and Stroop Tests. *Journal of Psychology in Africa, 22*(3), 333–341.

Annweiler, C., Montero-Odasso, M., Llewellyn, D. J., Richard-Devantoy, S., Duque, G., & Beauchet, O. (2013). Meta-analysis of memory and executive dysfunctions in relation to vitamin D. *Journal of Alzheimer's Disease, 37*(1), 147–171. https://doi.org/10.3233/JAD-130452

Ariza, M., Pueyo, R., Matarín, M. del M., Junqué, C., Mataró, M., Clemente, I., . . . Sahuquillo, J. (2006). Influence of APOE polymorphism on cognitive and behavioural outcome in moderate and severe traumatic brain injury. *Journal of Neurology, Neurosurgery, and Psychiatry, 77*(10), 1191–1193. https://doi.org/10.1136/jnnp.2005.085167

Aslaksen, P. M., Ørbo, M., Elvestad, R., Schäfer, C., & Anke, A. (2013). Prediction of on-road driving ability after traumatic brain injury and stroke. *European Journal of Neurology, 20*(9), 1227–1233. http://doi.org/10.1111/ene.12172

Atchison, T. B., Sander, A. M., Struchen, M. A., High, W. M., Roebuck, T. M., Contant, C. F., Wefel, J. S., Novack, T. A., & Sherer, M. (2004). Relationship between neuropsychological test performance and productivity at 1-year following traumatic brain injury. *The Clinical Neuropsychologist, 18,* 249–265.

Atkinson, T. M., & Ryan, J. P. (2007). The use of variants of the Trail Making Test in serial assessment: A construct validity study. *Journal of Psychoeducational Assessment, 26*(1), 42–53. http://doi.org/10.1177/0734282907301592

Atkinson, T. M., Ryan, J. P., Kryza, M., & Charette, L. M. (2011). Using versions of the Trail Making Test as alternate forms. *The Clinical Neuropsychologist, 25*(7), 1193–1206. http://doi.org/10.1080/13854046.2011.589410

Atkinson, T. M., Ryan, J. P., Lent, A., Wallis, A., Schachter, H., & Coder, R. (2010). Three trail making tests for use in neuropsychological assessments with brief interest intervals. *Journal of Clinical and Experimental Neuropsychology, 32*(2), 151–158. http://doi.org/10.1080/13803390902881934

Backman, L., Wahlin, A., Small, B. J., Herlitz, A., Winblad, B., & Fratiglioni, L. (2004). Cognitive functioning in aging and dementia: The Kungsholmen Project. *Aging, Neuropsychology and Cognition, 11,* 212–244.

Bardi, C. A., Hamby, S. L., & Wilkins, J. W. (1995). Stability of several brief neuropsychological tests in an HIV+ longitudinal sample [Abstract]. *Archives of Clinical Neuropsychology, 10,* 295.

Barr, A., Benedict, R., Tune, L., & Brandt, J. (1992). Neuropsychological differentiation of Alzheimer's disease from vascular dementia. *International Journal of Geriatric Medicine, 7,* 621–627.

Basso, M. R., Bornstein, R. A., & Lang, J. M. (1999). Practice effects on commonly used measures of executive function across twelve months. *The Clinical Neuropsychologist, 13,* 283–292.

Baum, C., Edwards, D., Yonan, C., & Storandt, M. (1996). The relation of neuropsychological test performance to performance on functional tasks in dementia of the Alzheimer type. *Archives of Clinical Neuropsychology, 11,* 69–75.

Bell-McGinty, S., Podell, K., Baird, A., & Williams, M. J. (2002). Standard measures of executive function in predicting instrumental activities of daily living in older adults. *International Journal of Geriatric Psychiatry, 17,* 828–834.

Bezdicek, O., Motak, L., Axelrod, B. N., Preiss, M., Nikolai, T., Vyhnalek, M., . . . Ruzicka, E. (2012). Czech version of the Trail Making Test: Normative data and clinical utility. *Archives of Clinical Neuropsychology, 27*(8), 906–914. http://doi.org/10.1093/arclin/acs084

Binder, L. M., Kelly, M. P., Villanueva, M. R., & Winslow, M. W. (2003). Motivation and neuropsychological test performance following mild head injury. *Journal of Clinical and Experimental Neuropsychology, 25,* 420–430.

Biundo, R., Weis, L., Pilleri, M., Facchini, S., Formento-Dojot, P., Vallelunga, A., & Antonini, A. (2013). Diagnostic and screening power of neuropsychological testing in detecting mild cognitive impairment in Parkinson's disease. *Journal of Neural Transmission, 120*(4), 627–633. http://doi.org/10.1007/s00702-013-1004-2

Blacker, D., Lee, H., Muzikansky, A., Martin, E. C., Tanzi, R., McArdle, J. J., . . . Albert, M. (2007). Neuropsychological measures in normal individuals that predict subsequent cognitive decline. *Archives of Neurology, 64*(6), 862–871.

Bonilha, L., Molnar, C., Horner, M. D., Anderson, B., Forster, L., George, M. S., & Nahas, Z. (2008). Neurocognitive deficits and prefrontal cortical atrophy in patients with schizophrenia. *Schizophrenia Research, 101*(1-3), 142–151. http://doi.org/10.1016/j.schres.2007.11.023

Bora, E., Yücel, M., & Pantelis, C. (2010). Neurocognitive markers of psychosis in bipolar disorder: A meta-analytic study. *Journal of Affective Disorders, 127*(1-3), 1–9. http://doi.org/10.1016/j.jad.2010.02.117

Bornstein, R. A., Baker, G. B., & Douglas, A. B. (1987). Short-term retest reliability of the Halstead-Reitan Battery in a normal sample. *Journal of Nervous and Mental Disease, 175,* 229–232.

Bottiggi, K. A., Salazar, J. C., Yu, L., Caban-Holt, A. M., Ryan, M., Mendiondo, M. S., & Schmitt, F. A. (2006). Long-term cognitive impact of anticholinergic medications in older adults. *American Journal of Geriatric Psychiatry, 14*(11), 980–984. https://doi.org/10.1097/01.JGP.0000224619.87681.71

Bourne, C., Aydemir, Ö., Balanzá-Martínez, V., Bora, E., Brissos, S., Cavanagh, J. T. O., . . . Goodwin, G. M. (2013). Neuropsychological testing of cognitive impairment in euthymic bipolar disorder: An individual patient data meta-analysis. *Acta Psychiatrica Scandinavica, 128*(3), 149–162. http://doi.org/10.1111/acps.12133

Boyle, P. A., Paul, R. H., Moser, D. J., & Cohen, R. A. (2004). Executive impairments predict functional declines in vascular dementia. *The Clinical Neuropsychologist, 18,* 75–82.

Braga-Neto, P., Pedroso, J. L., Alessi, H., Dutra, L. A., Felício, A. C., Minett, T., . . . Barsottini, O. G. P. (2012). Cerebellar cognitive affective syndrome in Machado Joseph disease: Core clinical features. *Cerebellum, 11*(2), 549–556. http://doi.org/10.1007/s12311-011-0318-6

Brown, P. J., Devanand, D. P., Liu, X., & Caccappolo, E. (2011). Functional impairment in elderly patients with mild cognitive impairment and mild Alzheimer disease. *Archives of General Psychiatry, 68*(6), 617–626.

Buck, K. K., Atkinson, T. M., & Ryan, J. P. (2008). Evidence of practice effects in variants of the Trail Making Test during serial assessment. *Journal of Clinical and Experimental Neuropsychology, 30*(3), 312–318. http://doi.org/10.1080/13803390701390483

Buré-Reyes, A., Hidalgo-Ruzzante, N., Vilar-López, R., Gontier, J., Sánchez, L., Pérez-García, M., & Puente, A. E. (2013). Neuropsychological test performance of Spanish speakers: Is performance different across different Spanish-speaking subgroups? *Journal of Clinical and Experimental Neuropsychology, 35*(4), 404–412. http://doi.org/10.1080/13803395.2013.778232

Busse, M., & Whiteside, D. (2012). Detecting suboptimal cognitive effort: Classification accuracy of the Conner's Continuous Performance Test-II, Brief Test of Attention, and Trail Making Test. *The Clinical Neuropsychologist, 26*(4), 675–687. http://doi.org/10.1080/13854046.2012.679623

Cahn, D. A., Salmon, D. P., Butters, N., Wiederholt, W. C., Corey-Bloom, J., Edelstein, S. L., & Barrett-Connor, E. (1995). Detection of dementia of the Alzheimer type in a population-based sample: Neuropsychological test performance. *Journal of the International Neuropsychological Society, 1,* 252–260.

Cahn-Weiner, D. A., Boyle, P. A., & Malloy, P. F. (2002). Tests of executive function predict instrumental activities of daily living in community-dwelling older individuals. *Applied Neuropsychology, 9,* 187–191.

Campanholo, K. R., Romão, M. A., Machado, M. de A. R., Serrao, V. T., Coutinho, D. G. C., Benute, G. R. G., & Lucia, M. C. S. de. (2014). Performance of an adult Brazilian sample on the Trail Making Test and Stroop Test. *Dementia & Neuropsychologia, 8*(1), 26–31.

Cangoz, B., Karakoc, E., & Selekler, K. (2009). Trail Making Test: Normative data for Turkish elderly population by age, sex and education. *Journal of the Neurological Sciences, 283*(1–2), 73–78. http://doi.org/10.1016/j.jns.2009.02.313

Carr, D. B., Barco, P. P., Wallendorf, M. J., Snellgrove, C. A., & Ott, B. R. (2011). Predicting road test performance in drivers with dementia. *Journal of the American Geriatrics Society, 59*(11), 2112–2117. http://doi.org/10.1111/j.1532-5415.2011.03657.x

Carrión-Baralt, J. R., Meléndez-Cabrero, J., Schnaider Beeri, M., Sano, M., & Silverman, J. M. (2009). The neuropsychological performance of nondemented Puerto Rican nonagenarians. *Dementia and Geriatric Cognitive Disorders, 27*(4), 353–360. http://doi.org/10.1159/000209213

Cavaco, S., Goncalves, A., Pinto, C., Almeida, E., Gomes, F., Moreira, I., . . . Teixeira-Pinto, A. (2013). Trail Making Test: Regression-based norms for the Portuguese population. *Archives of Clinical Neuropsychology, 28*(2), 189–198. http://doi.org/10.1093/arclin/acs115

Chalermchai, T., Valcour, V., Sithinamsuwan, P., Pinyakorn, S., Clifford, D., . . . The SEARCH 007 and 011 study groups. (2013). Trail Making Test A improves performance characteristics of the International HIV Dementia Scale to identify symptomatic HAND. *Journal of NeuroVirology, 19*(2), 137–143. http://doi.org/10.1007/s13365-013-0151-4

Charter, R. A., Adkins, T. G., Alekoumbides, A., & Seacat, G. F. (1987). Reliability of the WAIS, WMS, and Reitan Battery: Raw scores and standardized scores corrected for age and education. *International Journal of Clinical Neuropsychology, 9,* 28–32.

Chen, P., Ratcliff, G., Belle, S. H., Cauley, J. A. De Kosky, S. T., Ganguli, M., & Phil, D. (2000). Cognitive tests that best discriminate between presymptomatic AD and those who remain nondemented. *Neurology, 55,* 1847–1853.

Cherner, M., Suárez, P., Posada, C., Fortuny, L. A. i, Marcotte, T., Grant, I., . . . the HNRC group. (2008). Equivalency of Spanish language versions of the Trail Making Test Part B including or excluding "CH." *The Clinical Neuropsychologist, 22*(4), 662–665. http://doi.org/10.1080/13854040701476976

Cicerone, K. D., & Azulay, J. (2002). Diagnostic utility of attention measures in postconcussion syndrome. *The Clinical Neuropsychologist, 16,* 280–289.

Clark, M. S., Dennerstein, L., Elkadi, S., Guthrie, J. R., Bowden, S. C., & Henderson, V. W. (2004). Normative data for tasks of executive function and working memory for Australian-born women aged 56–67. *Australian Psychologist, 39,* 244–250.

Colantonio, A., Ratcliff, G., Chase, S., & Escobar, M. (2000). Is cognitive performance related to level of community integration many years after traumatic brain injury? *Brain and Cognition, 44,* 19–20.

Crespo-Facorro, B., Rodríguez-Sánchez, J. M., Pérez-Iglesias, R., Mata, I., Ayesa, R., Ramirez-Bonilla, M., . . . Vázquez-Barquero, J. L. (2009). Neurocognitive effectiveness of haloperidol, risperidone, and olanzapine in first-episode psychosis: a randomized, controlled 1-year follow-up comparison. *Journal of Clinical Psychiatry, 70*(5), 717–729. https://doi.org/10.4088/JCP.08m04634

Cullen, N., Krakowski, A., & Taggart, C. (2014). Early neuropsychological tests as correlates of return to driving after traumatic brain injury. *Brain Injury, 28*(1), 38–43. http://doi.org/10.3109/02699052.2013.849005

Dawson, J. D., Anderson, S. W., Uc, E. Y., Dastrup, E., & Rizzo, M. (2009). Predictors of driving safety in early Alzheimer disease. *Neurology, 72*(6), 521–527. https://doi.org/10.1212/01.wnl.0000341931.35870.49

de Almeida, S. M., Kamat, R., Cherner, M., Umlauf, A., Ribeiro, C. E., de Pereira, A. P., . . . Ellis, R. J. (2017). Improving detection of HIV-associated cognitive impairment: Comparison of the International HIV Dementia Scale and a brief screening battery. *Journal of Acquired Immune Deficiency Syndromes (1999), 74*(3), 332–338. https://doi.org/10.1097/QAI.0000000000001224

D'Elia, L. F., Satz, P., Uchiyama, C. L., & White, T. (1996). *Color Trails Test.* Odessa, Fla.: PAR.

Demakis, G. J. (2004). Frontal lobe damage and tests of executive processing: A meta-analysis of the Category Test, Stroop Test, and Trail-Making Test. *Journal of Clinical and Experimental Neuropsychology, 26,* 441–450.

Demery, J. A., Larson, M. J., Dixit, N. K., Bauer, R. M., & Perlstein, W. M. (2010). Operating characteristics of executive functioning tests following traumatic brain injury. *The Clinical Neuropsychologist, 24*(8), 1292–1308. http://doi.org/10.1080/13854046.2010.528452

De Raedt, R. (2001). Short, cognitive neuropsychological test battery for first-tier fitness-to-drive assessment of older adults. *The Clinical Neuropsychologist, 15,* 329–336.

Des Rosiers, G., & Kavanagh, D. (1987). Cognitive assessment in closed head injury: Stability, validity and parallel forms for two neuropsychological measures of recovery. *International Journal of Clinical Neuropsychology, 9,* 162–173.

Devos, H., Akinwuntan, A. E., Nieuwboer, A., Truijen, S., Tant, M., & De Weerdt, W. (2011). Screening for fitness to drive after stroke: a systematic review and meta-analysis. *Neurology, 76*(8), 747–756. https://doi.org/10.1212/WNL.0b013e31820d6300

Devos, H., Nieuwboer, A., Tant, M., De Weerdt, W., & Vandenberghe, W. (2012). Determinants of fitness to drive in Huntington disease. *Neurology, 79*(19), 1975–1982. https://doi.org/10.1212/WNL.0b013e3182735d11

Diaz-Asper, C., Schretlen, D. J., & Pearlson, G. D. (2004). How well does IQ predict neuropsychological test performance in normal adults. *Journal of the International Neuropsychological Society, 10,* 82–90.

Dikmen, S. S., Heaton, R. K., Grant, I., & Temkin, N. R. (1999). Test-retest reliability and practice effects of expanded Halstead-Reitan Neuropsychological Test Battery. *Journal of the International Neuropsychological Society, 5,* 346–356.

Dikmen, S. S., Machamer, J. E., Winn, H. R., & Temkin, N. R. (1995). Neuropsychological outcome at 1-year post head injury. *Neuropsychology, 9,* 80–90.

Dodrill, C. B., & Troupin, A. S. (1975). Effects of repeated administration of a comprehensive neuropsychological battery among chronic epileptics. *Journal of Nervous and Mental Disease, 161,* 185–190.

Drane, D. L., Yuspeh, R. L., Huthwaite, J. S., & Klingler, L. K. (2002). Demographic characteristics and normative observations for derived Trail Making indices. *Neuropsychiatry, Neuropsychology, and Behavioral Neurology, 15,* 39–43.

Drapeau, C. E., Bastien-Toniazzo, M., Rous, C., & Carlier, M. (2007). Nonequivalence of computerized and paper-and-pencil versions of Trail Making Test. *Perceptual and Motor Skills, 104*(3), 785–791.

Durvasula, R. S., Satz, P., Hinkin, C. H., et al. (1996). Does practice make perfect? Results of a six-year longitudinal study with semiannual testing [Abstract]. *Archives of Clinical Neuropsychology, 11,* 386.

Dye, O. A. (1979). Effects of practice on Trail Making Test performance. *Perceptual and Motor Skills, 48,* 296.

Egeland, J., Langtjaeran, T., & Egeland, J. (2007). *Applied Neuropsychology, 14,* 113–119.

Ehrenstein, W. H., Heister, G., & Cohen, R. (1982). Trail Making Test and visual search. *Archiv fuer Psychiatrie und Nervenkrankheiten, 231,* 333–338.

Elderkin-Thompson, V., Kumar, A., Bilker, W. B., Dunkin, J. J., Mintz, J., Moberg, P. J., Mesholam, R. I., & Gur, R. E. (2003). Neuropsychological deficits among patients with late-onset minor and major depression. *Archives of Clinical Neuropsychology, 18,* 529–549.

Felmingham, K. L., Baguley, I. J., & Green, A. M. (2004). Effects of diffuse axonal injury on speed of information processing following severe traumatic brain injury. *Neuropsychology, 18,* 564–571.

Ferman, T. J., Smith, G. E., Boeve, B. F., Graff-Radford, N. R., Lucas, J. A., Knopman, D. S., . . . Dickson, D. W. (2006). Neuropsychological differentiation of dementia with Lewy bodies from normal aging and Alzheimer's disease. *The Clinical Neuropsychologist, 20*(4), 623–636. http://doi.org/10.1080/13854040500376831

Fernández, A. L., & Marcopulos, B. A. (2008). A comparison of normative data for the Trail Making Test from several countries: Equivalence of norms and considerations for interpretation. *Scandinavian Journal of Psychology, 49*(3), 239–246. http://doi.org/10.1111/j.1467-9450.2008.00637.x

Franzen, M. D. (1996). Cross-validation of the alternate forms reliability of the Trail Making Test [Abstract]. *Archives of Clinical Neuropsychology, 11,* 390.

Franzen, M. D., Paul, D., & Iverson, G. L. (1996). Reliability of alternate forms of the Trail Making Test. *The Clinical Neuropsychologist, 10,* 125–129.

García-Molina, A., Tormos, J. M., Bernabeu, M., Junqué, C., & Roig-Rovira, T. (2012). Do traditional executive measures tell us anything about daily life functioning after traumatic brain injury in Spanish-speaking individuals? *Brain Injury, 26*(6), 864–874. https://doi.org/10.3109/02699052.2012.655362

Gaudino, E. A., Geisler, M. W., & Squires, N. K. (1995). Construct validity in the Trail Making Test: What makes Trail B harder? *Journal of Clinical and Experimental Neuropsychology, 17,* 529–535.

Goldstein, G., & Watson, J. R. (1989). Test-retest reliability of the Halstead-Reitan battery and the WAIS in a neuropsychiatric population. *The Clinical Neuropsychologist, 3,* 265–273.

González-Blanch, C., Pérez-Iglesias, R., Rodríguez-Sánchez, J. M., Pardo-García, G., Martínez-García, O., Vázquez-Barquero, J. L., & Crespo-Facorro, B. (2011). A digit symbol coding task as a screening instrument for cognitive impairment in first-episode psychosis. *Archives of Clinical Neuropsychology, 26*(1), 48–58. https://doi.org/10.1093/arclin/acq086

Grant, I., Adams, K. M., & Reed, R. (1984). Aging, abstinence, and medical risk in the prediction of neuropsychological deficit among long-term alcoholics. *Archives of General Psychiatry, 41,* 710–716.

Grant, I., Reed, R., & Adams, K. M. (1987). Diagnosis of intermediate-duration and subacute organic mental disorders in abstinent alcoholics. *Journal of Clinical Psychiatry, 48,* 319–323.

Greenaway, M. C., Smith, G. E., Tangalos, E. G., Geda, Y. E., & Ivnik, R. J. (2009). Mayo Older Americans Normative Studies: Factor analysis of an expanded neuropsychological battery. *The Clinical Neuropsychologist, 23*(1), 7–20. http://doi.org/10.1080/13854040801891686

Greer, S. E., Brewer, K. K., Cannici, J. P., & Pennett, D. L. (2010). Level of performance accuracy for core Halstead-Reitan measures by pooling normal controls from published studies: Comparison with existing norms in a clinical sample. *Perceptual and Motor Skills, 111*(1), 3–18. http://doi.org/10.2466/03.22.27.PMS.111.4.3-18

Hagen, K., Ehlis, A.-C., Haeussinger, F. B., Heinzel, S., Dresler, T., Mueller, L. D., . . . Metzger, F. G. (2014). Activation during the Trail Making Test measured with functional near-infrared spectroscopy in healthy elderly subjects. *NeuroImage, 85,* 583–591. http://doi.org/10.1016/j.neuroimage.2013.09.014

Hagenaars, S. P., Cox, S. R., Hill, W. D., Davies, G., Liewald, D. C. M., CHARGE consortium Cognitive Working Group, . . . Deary, I. J. (2017). Genetic contributions to Trail Making Test performance in UK Biobank. *Molecular Psychiatry.* https://doi.org/10.1038/mp.2017.189

Hamdan, A. C., & Hamdan, E. M. L. R. (2009). Effects of age and education level on the Trail Making Test in a healthy Brazilian sample. *Psychology & Neuroscience, 2*(2), 199–203. https://doi.org/10.3922/j.psns.2009.2.012

Hankee, L. D., Preis, S. R., Beiser, A. S., Devine, S. A., Liu, Y., Seshadri, S., . . . Au, R. (2013). Qualitative neuropsychological measures: Normative data on executive functioning tests from the Framingham Offspring study. *Experimental Aging Research, 39*(5), 515–535. http://doi.org/10.1080/0361073X.2013.839029

Hanuszkiewicz, I., Cechnicki, A., & Kalisz, A. (2009). The relationship between cognitive deficits and the course of schizophrenia. Preliminary research on participants of a rehabilitation programme. *Archives of Psychiatry and Psychotherapy, 3,* 27–34.

Hargrave, D. D., Nupp, J. M., & Erickson, R. J. (2012). Two brief measures of executive function in the prediction of driving ability after acquired brain injury. *Neuropsychological Rehabilitation, 22*(4), 489–500. http://doi.org/10.1080/09602011.2012.662333

Harvey, P. D., Sacchetti, E., Galluzzo, A., Romeo, F., Gorini, B., Bilder, R. M., & Loebel, A. D. (2008). A randomized double-blind comparison of ziprasidone vs. clozapine for cognition in patients with schizophrenia selected for resistance or intolerance to previous treatment. *Schizophrenia Research, 105*(1–3), 138–143. http://doi.org/10.1016/j.schres.2007.11.014

Hashimoto, R., Meguro, K., Lee, E., Kasai, M., Ishii, H., & Yamaguchi, S. (2006). Effect of age and education on the Trail Making Test and determination of normative data for Japanese elderly people: The Tajiri Project. *Psychiatry and Clinical Neurosciences, 60*(4), 422–428. http://doi.org/10.1111/j.1440-1819.2006.01526.x

Hasselbalch, B. J., Knorr, U., Hasselbalch, S. G., Gade, A., & Kessing, L. V. (2012). Cognitive deficits in the remitted state of unipolar depressive disorder. *Neuropsychology, 26*(5), 642–651. http://doi.org/10.1037/a0029301

Hayden, K. M., Makeeva, O. A., Newby, L. K., Plassman, B. L., Markova, V. V., Dunham, A., . . . Roses, A. D. (2014). A comparison of neuropsychological performance between US and Russia: Preparing for a global clinical trial. *Alzheimer's & Dementia, 10*(6), 760–768.e1. http://doi.org/10.1016/j.jalz.2014.02.008

Heaton, R. K., Miller, S. W., Taylor, M. J., & Grant, I. (2004). *Revised comprehensive norms for an expanded Halstead-Reitan Battery: Demographically adjusted neuropsychological norms for African American and Caucasian adults.* Lutz, FL: PAR.

Heled, E., Hoofien, D., Margalit, D., Natovich, R., & Agranov, E. (2012). The Delis–Kaplan Executive Function System Sorting Test as an evaluative tool for executive functions after severe traumatic brain injury: A comparative study. *Journal of Clinical and Experimental Neuropsychology, 34*(2), 151–159. http://doi.org/10.1080/13803395.2011.625351

Hester, R. L., Kinsella, G. J., Ong, B., & McGregor, J. (2005). Demographic influences on baseline and derived scores from the Trail Making Test in healthy older Australian adults. *The Clinical Neuropsychologist, 19,* 45–54.

Hirota, C., Watanabe, M., Sun, W., Tanimoto, Y., Kono, R., Takasaki, K., & Kono, K. (2010). Association between the Trail Making Test and physical performance in elderly Japanese. *Geriatrics & Gerontology International, 10*(1), 40–47. http://doi.org/10.1111/j.1447-0594.2009.00557.x

Horton, A. M., & Roberts, C. (2003). Demographic effects on the Trail Making Test in a drug abuse treatment sample. *Archives of Clinical Neuropsychology, 18,* 49–56.

Hurstak, E., Johnson, J. K., Tieu, L., Guzman, D., Ponath, C., Lee, C. T., . . . Kushel, M. (2017). Factors associated with cognitive impairment in a cohort of older homeless adults: Results from the HOPE HOME study. *Drug and Alcohol Dependence, 178,* 562–570. https://doi.org/10.1016/j.drugalcdep.2017.06.002

Iverson, G. L., Lange, R. T., & Franzen, M. D. (2005). Effects of mild traumatic brain injury cannot be differentiated from substance abuse. *Brain Injury, 19,* 11–18.

Iverson, G. L., Lange, R. T., Green, P., & Franzen, M. (2002). Detecting exaggeration and malingering with the Trail Making Test. *The Clinical Neuropsychologist, 16,* 398–406.

Jacobson, S. C., Blanchard, M., Connolly, C. C., Cannon, M., & Garavan, H. (2011). An fMRI investigation of a novel analogue to the Trail-Making Test. *Brain and Cognition, 77*(1), 60–70. http://doi.org/10.1016/j.bandc.2011.06.001

Johnson, A. S., Flicker, L. J., & Lichtenberg, P. A. (2006). Reading ability mediates the relationship between education and executive function tasks. *Journal of the International Neuropsychological Society, 12*(01), 64–71.

Jungwirth, S., Zehetmayer, S., Hinterberger, M., Kudrnovsky-Moser, S., Weissgram, S., Tragl, K. H., & Fischer, P. (2011). The influence of depression on processing speed and executive function in nondemented subjects aged 75. *Journal of the International Neuropsychological Society, 17*(05), 822–831. http://doi.org/10.1017/S135561771100083X

Juselius, S., Kieseppa, T., Kaprio, J., Lonnqvist, J., & Tuulio-Henriksson, A. (2009). Executive functioning in twins with bipolar i disorder and healthy co-twins. *Archives of Clinical Neuropsychology, 24*(6), 599–606. http://doi.org/10.1093/arclin/acp047

Kaufmann, L., Huber, S., Mayer, D., Moeller, K., & Marksteiner, J. (2017). The CERAD Neuropsychological Assessment Battery is sensitive to alcohol-related cognitive deficiencies in elderly patients: A retrospective matched case-control study. *Journal of the International Neuropsychological Society*, 1–12. https://doi.org/10.1017/S1355617717001072

King, D. A., Cox, C., Lyness, J. M., & Caine, E. D. (1995). Neuropsychological effects of depression and age in an elderly sample: A confirmatory study. *Neuropsychology, 9,* 300–408.

Knight, R. G., McMahon, J., Green, T. J., & Skeaff, C. M. (2006). Regression equations for predicting scores of persons over 65 on the Rey Auditory Verbal Learning Test, the mini-mental state examination, the trail making test and semantic fluency measures. *British Journal of Clinical Psychology, 45*(3), 393–402. http://doi.org/10.1348/014466505X68032

Kortte, C. B., Horner, M. D., & Windham, W. K. (2002) The Trail Making Test, Part B: Cognitive flexibility or ability to maintain set? *Applied Neuropsychology, 9,* 106–109.

Koutsouleris, N., Patschurek-Kliche, K., Scheuerecker, J., Decker, P., Bottlender, R., Schmitt, G., . . . Meisenzahl, E. M. (2010). Neuroanatomical correlates of executive dysfunction in the at-risk mental state for psychosis. *Schizophrenia Research, 123*(2–3), 160–174. http://doi.org/10.1016/j.schres.2010.08.026

Kraybill, M. L., Larson, E. B., Tsuang, D. W., Teri, L., McCormick, W. C., Bowen, J. D., Kukull, W. A., Leverenz, J. B., & Cherrier, M. M. (2005). Cognitive differences in dementia patients with autopsy-verified AD, Lewy body pathology, or both. *Neurology, 64*(12), 2069–2073. https://doi.org/10.1212/01.WNL.0000165987.89198.65

Kubo, M., Shoshi, C., Kitawaki, T., Takemoto, R., Kinugasa, K., Yoshida, H., . . . Okamoto, M. (2008). Increase in prefrontal cortex blood flow during the Computer Version Trail Making Test. *Neuropsychobiology, 58*(3–4), 200–210. http://doi.org/10.1159/000201717

Kühn, S., Romanowski, A., Schubert, F., & Gallinat, J. (2012). Reduction of cerebellar gray matter in Crus I and II in schizophrenia. *Brain Structure and Function, 217*(2), 523–529. http://doi.org/10.1007/s00429-011-0365-2

Lafleche, G., & Albert, M. S. (1995). Executive function deficits in mild Alzheimer's disease. *Neuropsychology, 9,* 313–320.

Larrabee, G. J., Millis, S. R., & Meyers, J. E. (2008). Sensitivity to brain dysfunction of the Halstead-Reitan vs an ability-focused neuropsychological battery. *The Clinical Neuropsychologist, 22*(5), 813–825. http://doi.org/10.1080/13854040701625846

Lee, M.-S., Lee, S.-H., Moon, E.-O., Moon, Y.-J., Kim, S., Kim, S.-H., & Jung, I.-K. (2013). Neuropsychological correlates of the P300 in patients with Alzheimer's disease. *Progress in Neuro-Psychopharmacology and Biological Psychiatry, 40,* 62–69. http://doi.org/10.1016/j.pnpbp.2012.08.009

Lee, T. M. C., Cheung, C. C. Y., Chan, J., & Chan, C. C. H. (2000). Trail making across languages. *Journal of Clinical and Experimental Neuropsychology, 22,* 772–778.

Levine, A. J., Hinkin, C. H., Miller, E. N., Becker, J. T., Selnes, O. A., & Cohen, B. A. (2007). The generalizability of neurocognitive test/retest data derived from a nonclinical sample for detecting change among two HIV+ cohorts. *Journal of Clinical and Experimental Neuropsychology, 29*(6), 669–678. http://doi.org/10.1080/13803390600920471

Levine, A. J., Miller, E. N., Becker, J. T., Selnes, O. A., & Cohen, B. A. (2004). Normative data for determining significance of test-retest differences on eight common neuropsychological instruments. *The Clinical Neuropsychologist, 18,* 373–384.

Lewis, R. F., & Rennick, P. M. (1979). *Manual for the Repeatable Cognitive-Perceptual-Motor Battery.* Grosse Pointe Park, MI: Axon.

Lezak, M. D., Howieson, D. B., & Loring, D. W. (2004). *Neuropsychological assessment* (4th ed.). New York: Oxford University Press.

Lim, J., Oh, I. K., Han, C., Huh, Y. J., Jung, I.-K., Patkar, A. A., . . . Jang, B.-H. (2013). Sensitivity of cognitive tests in four cognitive domains in discriminating MDD patients from healthy controls: A meta-analysis. *International Psychogeriatrics, 25*(09), 1543–1557. http://doi.org/10.1017/S1041610213000689

Lovell, M. R., & Solomon, G. S. (2011). Psychometric Data for the NFL Neuropsychological Test Battery. *Applied Neuropsychology, 18*(3), 197–209. http://doi.org/10.1080/09084282.2011.595446

Lu, H., Chan, S. S. M., Fung, A. W. T., & Lam, L. C. W. (2017). Beyond a differential diagnosis: Cognitive and morphometric decoding of information processing speed in senior adults with DSM-5 Mild Neurocognitive Disorders. *Journal of Alzheimer's Disease, 58*(3), 927–937. https://doi.org/10.3233/JAD-161122

Lu, P. H., Lee, G. J., Tishler, T. A., Meghpara, M., Thompson, P. M., & Bartzokis, G. (2013). Myelin breakdown mediates age-related slowing in cognitive processing speed in healthy elderly men. *Brain and Cognition, 81*(1), 131–138. http://doi.org/10.1016/j.bandc.2012.09.006

Lucas, J. A., Ivnik, R. J., Smith, G. E., Ferman, T. J., Willis, F. B., Petersen, R. C., & Graff-Radford, N. R. (2005). Mayo's Older African Americans Normative Studies: Norms for Boston Naming Test, Controlled Oral Word Association, Category Fluency, Animal Naming, Token Test, WRAT-3 Reading, Trail Making Test, Stroop Test, and Judgment of Line Orientation. *The Clinical Neuropsychologist, 19,* 243–269.

Lukowski, A. F., Koss, M., Burden, M. J., Jonides, J., Nelson, C. A., Kaciroti, N., . . . Lozoff, B. (2010). Iron deficiency in infancy and neurocognitive functioning at 19 years: Evidence of long-term deficits in executive function and recognition memory. *Nutritional Neuroscience, 13*(2), 54–70. http://doi.org/10.1179/147683010X12611460763689

Manly, J. J., Smith, C., Crystal, H. A., Richardson, J., Golub, E. T., Greenblatt, R., . . . Young, M. (2011). Relationship of ethnicity, age, education, and reading level to speed and executive function among HIV+ and HIV− women: The Women's Interagency HIV Study (WIHS) Neurocognitive Substudy. *Journal of Clinical and Experimental Neuropsychology, 33*(8), 853–863. http://doi.org/10.1080/13803395.2010.547662

Manly, J. L., Miller, S. W., Heaton, R. K., Byrd, D., Reilly, J., Velasquez, R. J., Saccuzzo, D. P., Grant, I., and the HIV Neurobehavioral Research Center (HNRC) Group. (1998). The effect of African American acculturation on neuropsychological test performance in normal and HIV-positive individuals. *Journal of the International Neuropsychological Society, 4,* 291–302.

Marshall, S. C., Molnar, F., Man-Son-Hing, M., Blair, R., Brosseau, L., Finestone, H. M., . . . Wilson, K. G. (2007). Predictors of driving ability following stroke: A systematic review. *Topics in Stroke Rehabilitation, 14*(1), 98–114. http://doi.org/10.1310/tsr1401-98

Martin, T. A., Hoffman, N. M., & Donders, J. (2003). Clinical utility of the Trail Making Test ratio score. *Applied Neuropsychology, 10,* 163–169.

Martyr, A., & Clare, L. (2012). Executive function and activities of daily living in Alzheimer's disease: a correlational meta-analysis. *Dementia and Geriatric Cognitive Disorders, 33*(2-3), 189–203.

Matarazzo, J. D., Wiens, A. N., Matarazzo, R. G., & Goldstein, S. G. (1974). Psychometric and clinical test-retest reliability of the Halstead Impairment Index in a sample of healthy, young, normal men. *Journal of Nervous and Mental Disease, 158,* 37–49.

Mathias, J. L., & Lucas, L. K. (2009). Cognitive predictors of unsafe driving in older drivers: a meta-analysis. *International Psychogeriatrics, 21*(04), 637. http://doi.org/10.1017/S1041610209009119

May, C. P., & Hasher, L. (1998). Synchrony effects in inhibitory control over thought and action. *Journal of Experimental Psychology: Human Perception and Performance, 24,* 363–379.

McCaffrey, R. J., Krahula, M. M., Heimberg, R. G., Keller, K. E., et al. (1988). A comparison of the Trail Making Test, Symbol Digit Modalities Test, and the Hooper Visual Organization Test in an inpatient substance abuse population. *Archives of Clinical Neuropsychology, 3,* 181–187.

McCaffrey, R. J., Ortega, A., & Haase, R. F. (1993). Effects of repeated neuropsychological assessments. *Archives of Clinical Neuropsychology, 8,* 519–524.

Merten, T., Henry, M., & Hilsabeck, R. (2004). Symptomvalidierungstests in der neuropsycholgischen diagnostic: Eine analogstudie. *Zeitschrift fur Neuropsychologie, 15,* 81–90.

Messinis, L., Malegiannaki, A.-C., Christodoulou, T., Panagiotopoulos, V., & Papathanasopoulos, P. (2011). Color Trails Test: Normative data and criterion validity for the Greek adult population. *Archives of Clinical Neuropsychology, 26*(4), 322–330. http://doi.org/10.1093/arclin/acr027

Messinis, L., Vlahou, C. H., Tsapanos, V., Tsapanos, A., Spilioti, D., & Papathanasopoulos, P. (2010). Neuropsychological functioning in postpartum depressed versus nondepressed females and nonpostpartum controls. *Journal of Clinical and Experimental Neuropsychology, 32*(6), 661–666. http://doi.org/10.1080/13803390903468863

Millis, S. R., Rosenthal, M., & Lourie, I. F. (1994). Predicting community integration after traumatic brain injury with neuropsychological measures. *International Journal of Neuroscience, 79,* 165–167.

Millis, S. R., Rosenthal, M., Novack, T. A., Sherer, M., Nick, T. G., Kreutzer, J. S., High, W. M. Jr., & Ricker, J. H. (2001). Long-term neuropsychological outcome after traumatic brain injury. *Journal of Head Trauma Rehabilitation, 16,* 343–355.

Mitrushina, M., & Satz, P. (1991). Effect of repeated administration of a neuropsychological battery in the elderly. *Journal of Clinical Psychology, 47,* 790–801.

Mitrushina, M. N., Boone, K. B., Razani, J., & D'Elia, L. F. (2005). *Handbook of normative data for neuropsychological assessment* (2nd ed.). New York: Oxford University Press.

Molinuevo, J. L., Gómez-Anson, B., Monte, G. C., Bosch, B., Sánchez-Valle, R., & Rami, L. (2011). Neuropsychological profile of prodromal Alzheimer's disease (Prd-AD) and their radiological correlates. *Archives of Gerontology and Geriatrics, 52*(2), 190–196. http://doi.org/10.1016/j.archger.2010.03.016

Moore, C. J., Daly, E. M., Schmitz, N., Tassone, F., Tysoe, C., Hagerman, R. J., Hagerman, P. J., Morris, R. G., Murphy, K. C., & Murphy, D. G. (2004). A neuropsychological investigation of male permutation carriers of fragile X syndrome. *Neuropsychologia, 42,* 1934–1947.

Moritz, S., Birkner, C., Kloss, M., Holger, J., Hand, I., Haasen, C., & Krausz, M. (2002). Executive functioning in obsessive-compulsive disorder, unipolar depression, and schizophrenia. *Archives of Clinical Neuropsychology, 17,* 477–483.

Mrazik, M., Millis, S., & Drane, D. L. (2010). The Oral Trail Making Test: Effects of Age and Concurrent Validity. *Archives of Clinical Neuropsychology, 25*(3), 236–243. http://doi.org/10.1093/arclin/acq006

Muñoz-Moreno, J. A., Prats, A., Pérez-Álvarez, N., Fumaz, C. R., Garolera, M., Doval, E., . . . others. (2013). A brief and feasible paper-based method to screen for neurocognitive impairment in HIV-infected patients: the NEU screen. *JAIDS Journal of Acquired Immune Deficiency Syndromes, 63*(5), 585–592.

Naismith, S. L., Hickie, I. B., Turner, K., Little, C. L., Winter, V., Ward, P. B., Wilhelm. K., Mitchell, P., & Parker, G. (2003). Neuropsychological performance in patients with depression is associated with clinical, etiological and genetic risk factors. *Journal of Clinical and Experimental Neuropsychology, 25,* 866–877.

Niewoehner, P. M., Henderson, R. R., Dalchow, J., Beardsley, T. L., Stern, R. A., & Carr, D. B. (2012). Predicting road test performance in adults with cognitive or visual impairment referred to a Veterans Affairs Medical Center driving clinic. *Journal of the American Geriatrics Society.* http://doi.org/10.1111/j.1532-5415.2012.04201.x

Nybo, T., Sainio, M., & Müller, K. (2004). Stability of vocational outcome in adulthood after moderate to severe preschool brain injury. *Journal of the International Neuropsychological Society, 10*(5), 719–723. https://doi.org/10.1017/S1355617704105109

O'Bryant, S. E., Hilsabeck, R. C., Fisher, J. M., & McCaffrey, R. J. (2003). Utility of the Trail Making Test in the assessment of malingering in a sample of mild traumatic brain injury litigants. *The Clinical Neuropsychologist, 17,* 69–74.

Oosterman, J. M., Vogels, R. L. C., van Harten, B., Gouw, A. A., Poggesi, A., Scheltens, P., . . . Scherder, E. J. A. (2010). Assessing mental flexibility: Neuroanatomical and neuropsychological correlates of the trail making test in elderly people. *The Clinical Neuropsychologist, 24*(2), 203–219. http://doi.org/10.1080/13854040903482848

O'Rourke, J. J. F., Beglinger, L. J., Smith, M. M., Mills, J., Moser, D. J., Rowe, K. C., . . . the PREDICT-HD Investigators of the. (2011). The Trail Making Test in prodromal Huntington disease: Contributions of disease progression to test performance. *Journal of Clinical and Experimental Neuropsychology, 33*(5), 567–579. http://doi.org/10.1080/13803395.2010.541228

Ott, B. R., Davis, J. D., Papandonatos, G. D., Hewitt, S., Festa, E. K., Heindel, W. C., . . . Carr, D. B. (2013). Assessment of driving-related skills prediction of unsafe driving in older adults in the office setting. *Journal of the American Geriatrics Society, 61*(7), 1164–1169. http://doi.org/10.1111/jgs.12306

Pandharipande, P. P., Girard, T. D., Jackson, J. C., Morandi, A., Thompson, J. L., Pun, B. T., . . . Ely, E. W. (2013). Long-term cognitive impairment after critical illness. *New England Journal of Medicine, 369*(14), 1306–1316. http://doi.org/10.1056/NEJMoa1301372

Papathanasiou, A., Messinis, L., Zampakis, P., & Papathanasopoulos, P. (2017). Corpus callosum atrophy as a marker of clinically meaningful cognitive decline in secondary progressive multiple sclerosis. Impact on employment status. *Journal of Clinical Neuroscience, 43,* 170–175. https://doi.org/10.1016/j.jocn.2017.05.032

Park, S. H., Sohn, M. K., Jee, S., & Yang, S. S. (2017). The characteristics of cognitive impairment and their effects on functional outcome after inpatient rehabilitation in subacute stroke patients. *Annals of Rehabilitation Medicine, 41*(5), 734–742. https://doi.org/10.5535/arm.2017.41.5.734

Partington, J. E., & Leiter, R. G. (1949). Partington's Pathway Test. *Psychological Service Center Bulletin, 1,* 9–20.

Pattanayak, R. D., Sagar, R., & Mehta, M. (2012). Neuropsychological performance in euthymic Indian patients with bipolar disorder type I: Correlation between quality of life and global functioning: Neuropsychological performance and QoL. *Psychiatry and Clinical Neurosciences, 66*(7), 553–563. http://doi.org/10.1111/j.1440-1819.2012.02400.x

Paulsen, J. S., Miller, A. C., Hayes, T., & Shaw, E. (2017). Cognitive and behavioral changes in Huntington disease before diagnosis. *Handbook of Clinical Neurology, 144,* 69–91. https://doi.org/10.1016/B978-0-12-801893-4.00006-7

Pavão Martins, I., Maruta, C., Freitas, V., & Mares, I. (2013). Executive performance in older Portuguese adults with low education. *The Clinical Neuropsychologist, 27*(3), 410–425. http://doi.org/10.1080/13854046.2012.748094

Pena-Casanova, J., Quinones-Ubeda, S., Quintana-Aparicio, M., Aguilar, M., Badenes, D., Molinuevo, J. L., . . . for the NEURONORMA Study Team. (2009). Spanish Multicenter Normative Studies (NEURONORMA Project): Norms for Verbal Span, Visuospatial Span, Letter and Number Sequencing, Trail Making Test, and Symbol Digit Modalities Test. *Archives of Clinical Neuropsychology, 24*(4), 321–341. http://doi.org/10.1093/arclin/acp038

Pérez-Iglesias, R., Tordesillas-Gutiérrez, D., McGuire, P. K., Barker, G. J., Roiz-Santiañez, R., Mata, I., . . . others. (2010). White matter integrity and cognitive impairment in first-episode psychosis. *American Journal of Psychiatry*. Retrieved from http://ajp.psychiatryonline.org/doi/pdf/10.1176/appi.ajp.2009.09050716

Perianez, J., Rioslago, M., Rodriguezsanchez, J., Adroverroig, D., Sanchez-Cubillo, I., Crespofacorro, B., . . . Barcelo, F. (2007). Trail Making Test in traumatic brain injury, schizophrenia, and normal ageing: Sample comparisons and normative data. *Archives of Clinical Neuropsychology, 22*(4), 433–447. http://doi.org/10.1016/j.acn.2007.01.022

Pineda, D. A., & Merchan, V. (2003). Executive function in young Colombian adults. *International Journal of Neuroscience, 113,* 397–410.

Powell, M. R., Locke, D. E. C., Smigielski, J. S., & McCrea, M. (2011). Estimating the diagnostic value of the Trail Making Test for suboptimal effort in acquired brain injury rehabilitation patients. *The Clinical Neuropsychologist, 25*(1), 108–118. http://doi.org/10.1080/13854046.2010.532912

Ranchet, M., Broussolle, E., Poisson, A., & Paire-Ficout, L. (2012). Relationships between cognitive functions and driving behavior in Parkinson's disease. *European Neurology, 68*(2), 98–107.

Ratcliff, G., Dodge, H., Birzescu, M., & Ganguli, M. (2003). Tracking cognitive functioning over time: Ten-year longitudinal data from a community-based study. *Applied Neuropsychology, 10,* 76–88.

Razani, J., Burciaga, J., Madore, M., & Wong, J. (2007). Effects of acculturation on tests of attention and information processing in an ethnically diverse group. *Archives of Clinical Neuropsychology, 22*(3), 333–341. http://doi.org/10.1016/j.acn.2007.01.008

Razzak, R. A. (2013). A preliminary study on the Trail-Making Test in Arabic–English bilingual young adults. *Applied Neuropsychology, 20*(1), 53–60. http://doi.org/10.1080/09084282.2012.670163

Reitan, R. M. (1955). The relation of the Trail Making Test to organic brain damage. *Journal of Consulting Psychology, 19,* 393–394.

Reitan, R. M., & Wolfson, D. (1985). *The Halstead-Reitan Neuropsychological Test Battery*. Tucson, AZ: Neuropsychology Press.

Reitan, R. M., & Wolfson, D. (1988). *Traumatic brain injury. Vol. II: Recovery and rehabilitation*. Tucson, AZ.: Neuropsychology Press.

Reynolds, C. (2002). *Comprehensive Trail Making Test*. Austin, TX: Pro-Ed.

Ricker, J. H., & Axelrod, B. N. (1994). Analysis of an oral paradigm for the Trail Making Test. *Assessment, 1,* 47–51.

Ricker, J. H., Axelrod, B. N., & Houtler, B. D. (1996). Clinical validation of the oral Trail Making Test. *Neuropsychiatry, Neuropsychology, and Behavioral Neurology, 9,* 50–53.

Ross, S. R., Millis, S. R., & Rosenthal, M. (1997). Neuropsychological prediction of psychosocial outcome after traumatic brain injury. *Applied Neuropsychology, 4,* 165–170.

Royan, J., Tombaugh, T. N., Rees, L., & Francis, M. (2004). The Adjusting-Paced Serial Addition Test (Adjusting-PSAT): Thresholds for speed of information processing as a function of stimulus modality and problem complexity. *Archives of Clinical Neuropsychology, 19,* 131–143.

Rozzini, L., Chilovi, B. V., Conti, M., Bertoletti, E., Delrio, I., Trabucchi, M., & Padovani, A. (2007). Conversion of amnestic mild cognitive impairment to dementia of Alzheimer type is independent to memory deterioration. *International Journal of Geriatric Psychiatry, 22*(12), 1217–1222. http://doi.org/10.1002/gps.1816

Ruchinskas, R. A. (2003). Limitations of the oral Trail Making Test in a mixed sample of older adults. *The Clinical Neuropsychologist, 17,* 137–142.

Ruffulo, L. F., Guilmette, T. J., & Willis, W. G. (2000). Comparison of time and error analysis on the Trail Making Test among patients with head injuries, experimental malingerers, patients with suspect effort on testing, and normal controls. *The Clinical Neuropsychologist, 14,* 223–230.

Salthouse, T., Toth, J., Daniels, K., Parks, C., Pak, R., Wolbrette, M., & Hocking, K. J. (2000). Effects of aging on efficiency of task switching in a variant of the Trail Making Test. *Neuropsychology, 14,* 102–111.

Salthouse, T. A., & Fristoe, N. M. (1995). Process analysis of adult age effects on a computer-administered Trail Making Test. *Neuropsychology, 9,* 518–528.

Sánchez-Cubillo, I., Periáñez, J. A., Adrover-Roig, D., Rodríguez-Sánchez, J. M., Ríos-Lago, M., Tirapu, J., & Barceló, F. (2009). Construct validity of the Trail Making Test: Role of task-switching, working memory, inhibition/interference control, and visuomotor abilities. *Journal of the International Neuropsychological Society, 15*(03), 438. http://doi.org/10.1017/S1355617709090626

Schear, J. M., & Sato, S. D. (1989). Effects of visual acuity and visual motor speed and dexterity on cognitive test performance. *Archives of Clinical Neuropsychology, 4,* 25–33.

Schmitt, A. L., Livingston, R. B., Smernoff, E. N., Waits, B. L., Harris, J. B., & Davis, K. M. (2010). Dichotomous scoring of Trails B in patients referred for a dementia evaluation. *Perceptual and Motor Skills, 110*(2), 429–441. http://doi.org/10.2466/pms.110.2.429-441

Schneider, B. C., & Lichtenberg, P. A. (2011). Influence of reading ability on neuropsychological performance in African American elders. *Archives of Clinical Neuropsychology, 26*(7), 624–631. http://doi.org/10.1093/arclin/acr062

Schneider, A. L. C., Sharrett, A. R., Gottesman, R. F., Coresh, J., Coker, L., Wruck, L., Selnes, O. A., Deal, J., Knopman, D., & Mosley, T. H. (2015). Normative data for 8 neuropsychological tests in older blacks and whites from the atherosclerosis risk in communities (ARIC) study. *Alzheimer Disease and Associated Disorders, 29*(1), 32–44. https://doi.org/10.1097/WAD.0000000000000042

Schrimsher, G. W., & Parker, J. D. (2008). Changes in cognitive function during substance use disorder treatment. *Journal of Psychopathology and Behavioral Assessment, 30*(2), 146–153. http://doi.org/10.1007/s10862-007-9054-0

Seo, E. H., Lee, D. Y., Kim, K. W., Lee, J. H., Jhoo, J. H., Youn, J. C., . . . Woo, J. I. (2006). A normative study of the Trail Making Test in Korean elders. *International Journal of Geriatric Psychiatry, 21*(9), 844–852. http://doi.org/10.1002/gps.1570

Sherrill-Pattison, S., Donders, J., & Thompson, E. (2000). Influence of demographic variables on neuropsychological test performance after traumatic brain injury. *The Clinical Neuropsychologist, 14,* 496–503.

Simioni, S., Cavassini, M., Annoni, J.-M., Métral, M., Iglesias, K., Rimbault Abraham, A., . . . Du Pasquier, R. A. (2013). Rivastigmine for HIV-associated neurocognitive disorders: A randomized crossover pilot study. *Neurology, 80*(6), 553–560. https://doi.org/10.1212/WNL.0b013e3182815497

Skeel, R. L., Nagra, A., Van Voorst, W., & Olson, E. (2003). The relationship between performance-based visual acuity screening, self-reported visual acuity, and neuropsychological performance. *The Clinical Neuropsychologist, 17,* 129–136.

Smith, P. J., Need, A. C., Cirulli, E. T., Chiba-Falek, O., & Attix, D. K. (2013). A comparison of the Cambridge Automated Neuropsychological Test Battery (CANTAB) with "traditional" neuropsychological testing instruments. *Journal of Clinical and Experimental Neuropsychology, 35*(3), 319–328. http://doi.org/10.1080/13803395.2013.771618

Snow, W. G., Tierney, M. C., Zorzitto, M. L., Fisher, R. H., & Reid, D. W. (1988). One-year test-retest reliability of selected neuropsychological tests in older adults [Abstract]. *Journal of Clinical and Experimental Neuropsychology, 10,* 60.

Solé, B., Bonnin, C. M., Torrent, C., Balanzá-Martínez, V., Tabarés-Seisdedos, R., Popovic, D., . . . Vieta, E. (2012). Neurocognitive impairment and psychosocial functioning in bipolar II disorder: Neurocognition in bipolar II disorder. *Acta Psychiatrica Scandinavica, 125*(4), 309–317. http://doi.org/10.1111/j.1600-0447.2011.01759.x

Soni, A., Singh, P., Shah, R., & Bagotia, S. (2017). Impact of cognition and clinical factors on functional outcome in patients with bipolar disorder. *East Asian Archives of Psychiatry [Dong Ya Jing Shen Ke Xue Zhi], 27*(1), 26–34

Stanczak, D. E., Lynch, M. D., NcNeil, C. K., & Brown, B. (1998). The Expanded Trail Making Test: Rationale, development, and psychometric properties. *Archives of Clinical Neuropsychology, 13,* 473–487.

Stedal, K., Frampton, I., Landrø, N. I., & Lask, B. (2012). An examination of the Ravello Profile: A neuropsychological test battery for anorexia nervosa: Neuropsychological Test Battery. *European Eating Disorders Review, 20*(3), 175–181. http://doi.org/10.1002/erv.1160

Steenland, K., Macneil, J., Bartell, S., & Lah, J. (2010). Analyses of diagnostic patterns at 30 Alzheimer's disease centers in the US. *Neuroepidemiology, 35*(1), 19–27. http://doi.org/10.1159/000302844

Steinberg, B. A., Bieliauskas, L. A., Smith, G. E., & Ivnik, R. J. (2005). Mayo Older Americans Normative Studies: Age- and IQ-adjusted norms for the Trail-Making Test, the Stroop Test, and MAE Controlled Oral Word Association Test. *The Clinical Neuropsychologist, 19,* 329–377.

Stewart, W. F., Schwartz, B. S., Simon, D., Bola, K. I., Todd, A. C., & Links, J. (1999). Neurobehavioral function and tibial and chelatable lead levels in 543 former organolead workers. *Neurology, 52,* 1610–1617.

Stuss, D. T., Bisschop, S. M., Alexander, M. P., Levine, B., Katz, D., & Izukawa, D. (2001). The Trail Making Test: A study in focal lesion patients. *Psychological Assessment, 13,* 230–239.

Stuss, D. T., Stethem, L. L., & Pelchat, G. (1988). Three tests of attention and rapid information processing: An extension. *The Clinical Neuropsychologist, 2,* 246–250.

Stuss, D. T., Stethem, L. L., & Poirier, C. A. (1987). Comparison of three tests of attention and rapid information processing across six age groups. *The Clinical Neuropsychologist, 1,* 139–152.

Sudo, F. K., Alves, C. E. O., Alves, G. S., Ericeira-Valente, L., Tiel, C., Moreira, D. M., . . . Engelhardt, E. (2013). White matter hyperintensities, executive function and global cognitive performance in vascular mild cognitive impairment. *Arquivos de Neuro-Psiquiatria, 71*(7), 431–436. http://doi.org/10.1590/0004-282X20130057

Summers, M. J., Summers, J. J., White, T. F., & Hannan, G. J. (2011). The effect of occupational exposure to manganese dust and fume on neuropsychological functioning in Australian smelter workers. *Journal of Clinical and Experimental Neuropsychology, 33*(6), 692–703. http://doi.org/10.1080/13803395.2011.553585

Terada, S., Sato, S., Nagao, S., Ikeda, C., Shindo, A., Hayashi, S., . . . Uchitomi, Y. (2013). Trail Making Test B and brain perfusion imaging in mild cognitive impairment and mild Alzheimer's disease. *Psychiatry Research: Neuroimaging, 213*(3), 249–255. http://doi.org/10.1016/j.pscychresns.2013.03.006

Thaler, N. S., Linck, J. F., Heyanka, D. J., Pastorek, N. J., Miller, B., Romesser, J., . . . Allen, D. N. (2013). Heterogeneity in Trail Making Test performance in OEF/OIF/OND veterans with mild traumatic brain injury. *Archives of Clinical Neuropsychology, 28*(8), 798–807. http://doi.org/10.1093/arclin/act080

Thompson, M. D., Scott, J. G., Dickson, S. W., Schoenfeld, J. D., Ruwe, W. D., & Adams, R. L. (1999). Clinical utility of the Trail Making Test practice time. *The Clinical Neuropsychologist, 13,* 450–455.

Tierney, M. C., Charles, J., Jaglai, S., Snow, W. G., Szalai, J. P., Spizziri, F., & Fisher, R. H. (2001). Identification of those at greatest risk of harm among cognitively impaired people who live alone. *Aging, Neuropsychology, and Cognition, 8,* 182–191.

Tombaugh, T. N. (2004). Trail Making Test A and B: Normative data stratified by age and education. *Archives of Clinical Neuropsychology, 19,* 203–214.

Van Gorp, W. G., Humphrey, L. A., Kalechstein, A., Brumm, V. L., McMullen, W. J., Soddard, M., & Pachana, N. A. (1999). How well do standard clinical neuropsychological tests identify malingering? A preliminary analysis. *Journal of Clinical and Experimental Neuropsychology, 21,* 245–250.

Woelwer, W. (2002). Impaired Trail-Making Test-B performance in patients with acute schizophrenia is related to inefficient sequencing of planning and acting. *Journal of Psychiatric Research, 36,* 407–416.

Wölwer, W., Brinkmeyer, J., Riesbeck, M., Freimüller, L., Klimke, A., Wagner, M., . . . for the German Study Group on First Episode Schizophrenia. (2008). Neuropsychological impairments predict the clinical course in schizophrenia. *European Archives of Psychiatry and Clinical Neuroscience, 258*(S5), 28–34. http://doi.org/10.1007/s00406-008-5006-2

Woodruff, G. R., Mendoza, J. E., Dickson, A. L., Blanchard, E., & Christenberry, L. B. (1995). The effects of configural differences on the Trail Making Test [Archives]. *Archives of Clinical Neuropsychology, 10,* 408.

Woods, D. L., Wyma, J. M., Herron, T. J., & Yund, E. W. (2015). The effects of aging, malingering, and traumatic brain injury on computerized Trail-Making Test performance. *PloS One, 10*(6), e0124345. https://doi.org/10.1371/journal.pone.0124345

Woolnough, A., Salim, D., Marshall, S. C., Weegar, K., Porter, M. M., Rapoport, M. J., . . . Vrkljan, B. (2013). Determining the validity of the AMA guide: A historical cohort analysis of the Assessment of Driving Related Skills and crash rate among older drivers. *Accident Analysis & Prevention, 61,* 311–316. http://doi.org/10.1016/j.aap.2013.03.020

Youngjohn, J. R., Burrows, L., & Erdal, K. (1995). Brain damage or compensation neurosis? The controversial post-concussion syndrome. *The Clinical Neuropsychologist, 9,* 112–123.

Zakzanis, K. K., Mraz, R., & Graham, S. J. (2005). An fMRI study of the Trail Making Test. *Neuropsychologia, 43*(13), 1878–1886. http://doi.org/10.1016/j.neuropsychologia.2005.03.013

Zalla, T., Joyce, C., Szöke, A., Schürhoff, F., Pillon, B., Komano, O., . . . Leboyer, M. (2004). Executive dysfunctions as potential markers of familial vulnerability to bipolar disorder and schizophrenia. *Psychiatry Research, 121,* 207–217.

Zhou, B., Nakatani, E., Teramukai, S., Nagai, Y., Fukushima, M., & Alzheimer's Disease Neuroimaging Initiative. (2012). Risk classification in mild cognitive impairment patients for developing Alzheimer's disease. *Journal of Alzheimer's Disease: JAD, 30*(2), 367–375. https://doi.org/10.3233/JAD-2012-112117

VERBAL FLUENCY TEST

TEST NAME	**Verbal Fluency Test**
DOMAIN	Executive functioning
AGE RANGE	Up to 90 years
ADMINISTRATION TIME	5 minutes
SCORING FORMAT	Hand scored
REFERENCE	Varies, depending on version

DESCRIPTION

Phonemic and semantic fluency tasks have a long history of use in psychology, dating from the work of Thurstone (1938). The general paradigm has been described under various test names, including the Controlled Oral Word Association Test (COWAT), Word Fluency, Letter Fluency, FAS-Test or FAS, Category Fluency, Phonemic Fluency, Semantic Fluency, Controlled Verbal Fluency, and Thurstone Word Fluency Test. The test has been adapted for use in a number of countries and languages (see the sections "Demographic Effects" and "Normative Data").

PHONEMIC FLUENCY

The examinee is asked to orally produce as many words as possible beginning with a specified letter during a fixed period of time, usually one minute. Verbal fluency thus measures timed production of individual words under restricted search conditions (e.g., a given letter of the alphabet). "F," "A," and "S" are the most commonly used letters, although other letter combinations and single letters are also used. This task may also be called letter fluency. See "Normative Data" and "Evidence for Reliability" for examples and discussion of administration variants.

SEMANTIC FLUENCY

This fluency test is based on the restricted search condition of category, and is also called category fluency. The most common category is "animals" and the examinee is asked to produce as many animal names as possible within a one-minute interval. There are a number of other administration variants. See "Gender," "Normative Data," and "Alternate Form Reliability."

OTHER TYPES OF FLUENCY

In addition to phonemic and semantic fluency, a number of other variants exist. For example, some versions of the test require a combination of phonetic and semantic fluency (animal names that begin with "A"; Heller & Dobbs, 1993); alternating fluency (Costa et al., 2014); action fluency (verb naming, things that people do; Piatt et al., 1999; Woods et al., 2005); a switching format, which requires the individual to alternate between categories, such as fruits and furniture (e.g., Baldo et al., 2001; Delis et al., 2001); and excluded letter fluency (generation of words that do not contain a specific vowel, such as the letter "E"; Crawford et al., 1995).

Other tests that derive from conventional verbal fluency tasks can be found, including the Homophone Meaning Generation Test (providing multiple definitions for a series of homophones, such as *bear/bare*; Warrington, 2000). A written word fluency exists (Thurstone, 1938), which involves five minutes for written generation of words according to a specific letter, then generation of four-letter words with another letter for four minutes.

ADMINISTRATION

See Figure 9–14 for phonemic fluency instructions and Figure 9–15 for semantic fluency instructions. According to Thurstone's (1938) written fluency test, the examinee first writes as many words beginning with a specific letter (i.e., the letter "S") in a period of five minutes. Next, the examinee is required to write as many four-letter words as possible that begin with the letter "C" during a four-minute trial. Since the test is somewhat lengthy and dependent on basic spelling skills and intact motor ability, it is not suitable for patients with motor impairment.

Research has suggested there may be influences on performance that are related to administration parameters, such as time of day, third-party observation, time interval provided for word generation, and handedness of the examinee.

For example, in one study, more words were generated in the afternoon than in the morning (Bennett et al., 2008). Horwitz and McCaffrey (2008) reported that third-party

Use a stopwatch and have the patient comfortably seated before giving the following instructions: I will say a letter of the alphabet. Then I want you to give me as many words that begin with that letter as quickly as you can. For example, if I say "b" you might give me "bad, battle, bed…." I do not want you to use words that are proper names such as "Boston, Bob, or Buick." Also, do not use the same word with different ending such as "eat" and "eating." Any questions? (pause). Begin when I say the letter. The first letter is F. Go ahead.

Begin timing immediately.

Allow one minute for each letter (F, A, and S). Say *"Fine"* or *"Good"* after each one-minute performance. If the examinee stops before the end of the minute, encourage them to try to think of more words. If there is a silence of 15 seconds, repeat the basic instructions, and the letter.

For scoring purposes, write down the actual words in the order in which they are produced. If repetitions occur that may be acceptable if an alternate meaning was intended by the examinee ("Four" and "for," "sun" and "son"), ask what was meant by this word at the end of the one-minute period.

Administer all three letters: F, A, and S.

Figure 9–14 *Instructions for phonemic fluency.*

observation and trait anxiety were significantly related to decreased semantic fluency performance. Holtzer, Goldin, and Donovick (2009) reported improved group discrimination (control vs. cognitively impaired) and larger correlations between phonemic fluency and the Dementia Rating Scale, when two minutes, rather than one minute, were provided for letter generation.

Examinee characteristics may also be important considerations. Sontam, Christman, and Jasper (2009) reported increased switching between categories on a semantic fluency task in those with mixed handedness compared to those with strong single-hand preferences.

SCORING

PHONEMIC FLUENCY

Total correct is the sum of all admissible words for the three letters. Slang terms and foreign words that are part of standard English ("faux pas" or "lasagna") are acceptable. Inadmissible words under these instructions (e.g., proper names, wrong words, variations, repetitions) are errors.

SEMANTIC FLUENCY

Total correct is the sum of all admissible words for the semantic category. For animal category fluency, names of extinct, imaginary, or magic animals are admissible, but given names for animals like "Kingsley," "Hugo," "Bronco," and "Lexie" are not. Inadmissible words under these instructions (e.g., proper names, wrong words, variations, repetitions) are errors.

Errors. When viewed qualitatively, errors provide valuable process information that cannot be provided by the score of "total correct" alone. For example, errors may include repetitions of previous responses (recurrent or ideational perseverations), reverting back to a previous category (stuck in set), repeating the same item over and over (continuous perseveration), intrusions (of other letters or from another category), paraphasias, or spelling errors.

Strategy. Another important qualitative variable is strategy use, specifically clustering and switching, as discussed later. Based on studies of patients with AD, Chertkow and Bub (1990) suggested that effective verbal fluency performance requires both an intact semantic store for supplying a knowledge base of related words and an effective search process to access and retrieve this information. Thus, poor performance on verbal fluency tasks can result from deterioration of a stored knowledge base or from an inefficient search (e.g., failing to generate search strategies or failing to shift to new searches when previous ones are exhausted).

Say: *I am going to tell you the names of some things you can find in the kitchen: spoons, knives, forks, plates, faucet. Can you think of other things in the kitchen?*

Allow the examinee to name other things, and correct if they produce incorrect responses, explaining the task once again. Then say: *Now, tell me the names of as many animals as you can. Name them as quickly as possible.*

Allow one minute. If the examinee discontinues before the end of the period, encourage them to produce more names. If there is a pause of 15 or more seconds, repeat the instructions and give the starting word *"dog."* Start timing immediately after instructions have been given, but allow extra time in the period if instructions are repeated. Write down the actual words in the order in which they are produced.

Figure 9–15 *Instructions for semantic fluency.*

These store and search processes were operationalized by Troyer, Moscovitch, and Winocur (1997) as *clustering* and *switching*, respectively. According to Troyer et al., optimal fluency performance involves clustering or generating words within a subcategory and, when a subcategory is exhausted, switching to a new subcategory. Clustering involves phonemic analysis on phonemic fluency and semantic categorization on semantic fluency and is thought to be a relatively automatic process. Switching involves cognitive flexibility in shifting from one subcategory to another and is thought to involve a relatively effortful process.

Decreased clustering has been related to temporal lobe disturbance, while switching implicates frontal functioning, although some inconsistencies in this pattern have been noted (see "Evidence for Validity"). Scoring for cluster size and switches is provided in Troyer (2000; Troyer et al., 1997). Additional approaches to verbal fluency scoring have been presented by others (e.g., Abwender et al., 2001; Giovannetti et al., 2001; Giovannetti-Carew et al., 1997).

While most healthy examinees produce the majority of their responses at the beginning of the time allotted per trial and fewer over time (Delis et al., 2001), others may have difficulty with task initiation or maintenance; yet others may be affected by anxiety initially and produce the bulk of their responses later in the trial. This can be monitored by noting (with a line) and counting the number of words in each 15-second block. Delis et al. (2001) additionally provide normative data for each of the four 15-second blocks.

Qualitative scores have shown value not only in patients with AD, but supplemental scores such as clustering and switching, error types, and temporal-based responding variables also offer enhanced clinical and diagnostic information in patients with acquired brain injury (Thiele, Quinting, & Stenneken, 2016; see also "Evidence for Validity").

WRITTEN FLUENCY

The examinee obtains a score of one point for each word; duplicate words do not earn points. The score is the sum of scores for Part A (words beginning with "S") and Part B (words beginning with "C"). Misspelled words are counted as correct. The examiner should ask the examinee about any words not written clearly. If an examinee has written a word that does not resemble the one she or he identifies the word to be, it may be counted provided that the word the examinee meant to write meets the criteria specified in the instructions (Heaton et al., 2004).

DEMOGRAPHIC EFFECTS

AGE

Phonemic Fluency. Age is related to performance in normative studies ($rs = -.24, -.26$; Costa et a., 2014; $r = -.24$, Cavaco et al., 2013). Performance peaks at about age 30–39 and shows a mild decline in old age (Backman et al., 2004; Delis et al., 2001; Heaton et al., 2004; Kave, 2005; Khalil, 2010; Loonstra et al., 2001; Lucas et al., 2005; Mack et al., 2005; Mitrushina et al., 2005; Troyer, 2000). In a large sample of Dutch speakers, van der Elst, van Boxtel, van Breukelen, and Jolles (2006) reported a significant decline after 50 years of age in fluency tasks requiring generation of four-letter words beginning with "M" and profession naming; in contrast, animal fluency showed a linear decline. A meta-analysis of phonemic fluency suggested a decrease in performance after 40 years of age, with further decline after age 60 with increased decrements through the late 80s. An interaction with gender has been reported, such that women perform better than men after 60 years of age (Rodríguez-Aranda & Martinussen, 2006).

Semantic Fluency. Age also has a moderate impact on category fluency (Acevedo et al., 2000; Cavaco et al., 2013; Costa et a., 2014; Delis et al., 2001; Heaps et al., 2013; Knight et al., 2006; Sosa et al., 2009; Troyer, 2000). Some research has suggested that aging is more strongly related to the number of words generated on semantic fluency than phonemic fluency tasks (Brickman et al., 2005; Kozora & Cullum, 1995; Mathuranath et al., 2003; Ravdin et al., 2003; Troyer, 2000).

Written Fluency. Age accounts for approximately 9% of variance in performance (Heaton et al., 2004).

GENDER

Many authors find little evidence of gender effects on phonemic and semantic fluency (Backman et al., 2004; Brickman et al., 2005; Cavaco et al., 2013; Heaton et al., 2004; Kave, 2005; Khalil, 2010; Kozora & Cullum, 1995; Lucas et al., 1998, 2005; Mitrushina et al., 2005; Ryu et al., 2012; Sosa et al., 2009; Troyer, 2000).

However, some research has suggested that women perform better than men on phonemic fluency (e.g., Barr, 2003; Costa et al., 2014). Meta-analytic findings, based on an aggregate sample of 17,625 healthy individuals, indicate a small advantage on phonemic fluency for women ($M = 35.14$, $SD = 12.59$) in comparison with men ($M = 33.28$, $SD = 12.96$; Loonstra et al., 2001).

Although animal fluency is generally not reported to be affected by gender, other categories (e.g., fruits and vegetables) may show gender differences that reflect stereotypical gender patterns (Acevado et al., 2000; Knight et al., 2006; Pena-Casanova et al., 2009). Egeland et al. (2006) report a small advantage in favor of women on clothing fluency ($M = 23.5$ for women vs. $M = 22$ for men), as did Pena-Casanova et al. (2009) on kitchen tools. In examining four semantic fluency variants, a gender effect was found for vegetables and clothing, but not animals and fruit (Rosselli et al., 2009). In one large normative study, men outperformed women on profession naming only, with a difference of .75 words (van der Elst et al., 2006). In another study, men outperformed women only on brands of cars, with animals and fruits not showing gender effects (Zarino et al., 2014).

READING LEVEL AND EDUCATION

Education. Educational level exerts a significant influence on both phonemic and semantic fluency tasks with higher levels of education associated with better performance (e.g., Backman et al., 2004; Brickman et al., 2005; Cavaco et al., 2013; Costa et al., 2014; Egeland et al., 2006; Heaps et al., 2013; Kave, 2005; Lam et al., 2013; Loonstra et al., 2001; Lucas et al., 1998, 2005; Mitrushina et al., 2005; Moraes et al., 2013; Pena-Casanova et al., 2009; Sosa et al., 2009; Steinberg et al., 2005; Tallberg et al., 2008; Troyer, 2000). Van der Elst et al. (2006) reported that individuals with primary education generated approximately four fewer words on average than individuals with high levels of education on animal fluency.

Education may be more impactful than age (e.g., Egeland et al., 2006; Gonzalez et al., 2005; Kosmidis et al., 2004). Tombaugh, Kozak, and Rees (1999) reported that for phonemic fluency (e.g., FAS), education accounted for more variance than age (22% vs. 12%), while for semantic (e.g., animal) naming, the opposite relationship existed (education = 14%; age = 23%). Rosselli et al. (2009) noted that education affected all semantic fluency variants they examined, with fruit being the least affected by education. Education is similarly more influential than age in written fluency (i.e., accounting for approximately 14% of the variance in scores; Heaton et al., 2004).

Some research has suggested interaction effects. Ostrosky-Solis, Gutierrez, Flores, and Ardila (2007) reported that education influenced semantic fluency, with age as the strongest predictor in people with more than 10 years of education, but education the strongest predictor in those with fewer than 10 years of education. The relative importance of education compared to age is not found in all studies (e.g., age was the best predictor in phonemic and semantic tasks in Hebrew speakers; Kave, 2005).

Reading Level. Reading level shows a small correlation with semantic (animal) fluency ($r = .26$), but a moderate relationship with phonemic (FAS) fluency ($r = .47$; Johnson-Selfridge et al., 1998). Schneider and Lichtenberg (2011) reported that when high- and low-reading groups of African-American elders were compared, there were large differences between groups on the COWAT (Cohen's $d = 1.41$). The level of literacy may differentially impact performance depending on the particular semantic task chosen. Gonzalez da Silva, Petersson, Faisca, Ingvar, and Reis (2004) found that literacy had little impact on a supermarket fluency task but a significant impact on animal fluency.

ETHNICITY, NATIONALITY, AND LINGUISTIC EFFECTS

Fluency tests have been widely used in multiple countries and languages (e.g., Artiola I Fortuny et al., 1999; Kave, 2005; Kosmidis et al., 2004; Ostrosky-Solis et al., 1999; Ostrosky et al., 2007). See "Normative Data."

Linguistic differences may be influential. For example, predominance of one-syllable animal names in Vietnamese versus a predominance of multisyllable animal names in Spanish was proposed as an explanation of the finding that Vietnamese speakers produced more animal names than Spanish speakers (Kempler et al., 1998). Another study found that Spanish-English bilingual speakers generated fewer words than monolingual speakers on animal fluency but not on phonemic fluency, which may be related to interference between the two languages (see Rosselli et al., 2002, for further discussion).

Some studies have reported generally comparable results across languages and countries. Gonzalez et al. (2005) reported that demographic factors jointly accounted for about 10% of the variance in semantic fluency performance, and were more influential than language of administration for English- and Spanish-speaking older Mexican Americans. In their normative study, Heaps et al. (2013) reported that verbal fluency was the only test among a number of neuropsychological tests that did not differ between their sample of Thai and US individuals. Agranovich and Puente (2007) reported that Russian and American controls did not differ on semantic fluency performance. Ostrosky et al. (2007) reported differences among Spanish speakers in different countries, but reported that country variability may be due to variability in administration and scoring. Sosa et al. (2009) collated norms for animal fluency as part of the CERAD across multiple countries (Cuba, Dominican Republic, Peru, Venezuela, Mexico, China, India), noting that, with the exception of India where six fewer animals were generated on average, norms were similar between countries in North America, Europe, and Latin America.

When considering use of verbal fluency across languages, research suggests that letter frequency is an important consideration. For example, Oberg and Ramírez (2006) analyzed phonemic fluency data from 926 individuals across five countries (Mexico, Argentina, Denmark, US, and Israel) and four languages (Spanish, English, Danish, and Hebrew). They reported that when education and word frequency were considered (i.e., higher frequency letters produce more words), the number of words generated are similar across languages and cultures.

Geographical region may also impact performance. Fillenbaum et al. (2001) reported that older African Americans living in North Carolina produced fewer animals than a similar cohort in Indianapolis. Gupta et al. (2011) reported that while controlling for other demographic factors, urban participants outperformed rural participants in China.

NORMATIVE DATA

There are a large number of normative datasets. Most are adjusted for age and education and are diverse in terms of regional, ethnic, and linguistic groups on which they are based. A summary of normative data provided in this review is provided in Table 9–152.

PHONEMIC FLUENCY: FAS

Loonstra et al. (2001) provide metanorms for the FAS derived from 32 studies comprising a total of 17,625 English speakers. The studies were either normative studies or studies in which a control group of healthy participants were included. The authors note that in several of these studies, the criteria for defining cognitive health were vague or based only on self-report and that demographic data were incomplete in a number of cases. The data are stratified by age, level of education, and gender and are shown in Table 9–153.

The data do not allow for simultaneous consideration of various influences such as age and education. The values are somewhat lower than those reported by Mitrushina et al.'s (2005) metanorm set compiled of 18 studies. Use of the tables provided by Mitrushina et al.

TABLE 9–152 Summary of Normative Data

REFERENCE	TYPE OF FLUENCY	SAMPLE SIZE	AGE RANGE (YEARS)	ADJUSTMENT	SAMPLE CHARACTERISTICS
Cavaco et al. (2013)	Phonemic ("M," "R," "P"), Semantic (animal)	Phonemic, 821 Semantic, 950	18–98	Regression-based; age and education	Portuguese
Hankee et al. (2013)	Phonemic (FAS), Semantic (animals)	1,907	<55–75 and older	Age, education (separately)	US
Heaton et al. (2004)[a]	Phonemic, Semantic (animals)	1,148	20–85	Age, education, ethnicity (simultaneous)	Caucasian and African American (US)
Knight et al. (2006)	Semantic (animals, fruits and vegetables, transport)	272	65–90	Regression-based (age, IQ, gender)	New Zealand
Loonstra et al. (2001)	Phonemic (FAS)	17,625	<40–95	Age, education, gender (separately)	Metanorms (English-speakers)
Lucas et al. (2005)	Phonemic (CFL)	304	56–94	Age, education (simultaneous)	Caucasian and African American, Mayo's African American Normative Studies (MOAANS; US)
Mitrushina et al. (2005)[a]	Phonemic, Semantic (animal)	2,843	25–87	Age	Metanorms
Pena-Casanova et al. (2009)	Phonemic ("P," "M," "R"), Semantic (animals, fruits and vegetables, kitchen tools), excluded letters (excluding A, E, S)	346	50–94	Age, education (simultaneous), and gender for select scores	Part of Spanish Multicenter Normative Studies (NEURONORMA; Spanish)
Ryu et al. (2012)	Semantic (animals)	3,025	60–96	Age, education (simultaneous)	Korean
Steinberg et al. (2005)	Phonemic (CFL)	777	55 and older	Age, IQ (simultaneous)	Mayo's Older Americans Normative Studies (MOANS; US)
Tombaugh et al. (1999)	Phonemic (FAS), Semantic (animal)	1,298	16–95	Age, education (simultaneous)	Canadian
Van der Elst et al. (2006)	Phonemic (four-letter "M" words), Semantic (animal, profession)	1,856	24–81	Age, education (simultaneous)	Dutch speakers

NOTE: Studies listed alphabetically by first author.

[a]Normative data available from reference cited; not provided in this review.

TABLE 9–153 Metanorms for FAS

CATEGORY	N	M	SD
Gender			
Males	7,310	33.28	12.96
Females	9,172	35.14	12.59
Age			
<40	634	43.51	9.44
40–59	9,202	34.24	12.48
60–79	5,294	32.31	12.70
80–95	433	29.37	13.05
Education			
0–12	1,357	30.07	13.09
>12	588	41.14	12.37
Overall	17,625	34.78	12.82

NOTE: Norms derived from 32 studies comprising 17,625 English speakers.

SOURCE: From Loonstra et al. (2001).

(2005) allows evaluation of scores with respect to both age and education.

PHONEMIC FLUENCY: CFL

Steinberg et al. (2005) reanalyzed data from the MOANS and provided age and IQ-adjusted percentile equivalents of MOANS age-adjusted CFL scores for persons 55 years of age and older. Readers should note that all FSIQ scores are Mayo age-adjusted scores which are based on the WAIS-R. Given the upward shift in scores (Flynn effect) with the passage of time, use of the WAIS-R rather than the WAIS-IV might result in a given fluency score appearing less favorable. The interested reader is referred to their article for the relevant tables.

SEMANTIC FLUENCY: ANIMALS, FOODS, AND TRANSPORT

Knight et al. (2006) provide regression-based norms for semantic fluency (animals, fruits and vegetables, transport) in a sample of community-dwelling older participants aged 65 to 90 years of age (M = 73.67, SD = 5.75). The sample was 55% female. Participants' education levels were as follows: 9% with less than high school education, 27% with less than three years of high school, 12% with more than three years high school, 38% with a vocational qualification, and 14% with university education. The NART score was equated to a predicted FSIQ of 113.

Participants were recruited as part of a baseline phase of a larger study assessing the impact of lowering homocysteine concentration by vitamin supplementation in New Zealand. Participants were excluded if they presented with renal disease, diabetes, cancer, neurologic or neurodegenerative disease, or psychiatric conditions. The program for calculation can be found through the home page of Professor John Crawford of the Department of Psychology, University of Aberdeen (https://homepages.abdn.ac.uk/j.crawford/pages/dept/psychom.htm). Applying regression data using an example is in the program labeled CLREGMUL.EXE.

Ryu et al. (2012) provide normative data for animal fluency for 3,025 Korean older adults 60 to 96 years of age (M age = 71.7, SD = 6.7 years). The sample was 53% female, with an average of 7.4 years (SD = 5.2) of education. Participants were community-dwelling and participating in ongoing longitudinal studies in Korea. Participants completed clinical and diagnostic interviews. Exclusion criteria were dementia, psychiatric disorders, major medical conditions impacting cognition, neurologic disorders, uncorrected hearing or vision, and GDS cutoff score. Normative data are presented in Table 9–154.

SELECT CO-NORMED PHONEMIC AND CATEGORY FLUENCY TASKS

Heaton et al. (2004) provide data for 1,148 healthy Caucasians and African Americans for animal fluency and phonemic fluency. Use of their data allows simultaneous adjustment of age, education, and ethnicity. Mitrushina et al. (2005) compiled 11 studies for animal fluency and phonemic fluency consisting of 2,843 participants, aged 25 to 87 years. Data are corrected for age only, because education did not account for a significant amount of variance.

Tombaugh et al. (1999) provide normative data for animal fluency and FAS based on a sample of 1,298 community-dwelling healthy individuals in Canada, ranging in age from 16 to 95 years, with no evidence of cognitive impairment. English was the first language for all participants. The normative data allow for simultaneous consideration of both age and level of education and are shown in Tables 9–155 and 9–156. The values are broadly consistent with data provided in other normative studies (e.g., Gladsjo et al., 1999; Heaton et al., 2004; Kozora & Cullum, 1995, Loonstra et al., 2001; Mitrushina et al., 2005).

The lack of sociodemographic diversity of the participants in the Tombaugh et al. (1999) study (i.e., mainly Caucasians living in economically advantaged regions of North America) limits the use of these norms in individuals with dissimilar sociodemographic backgrounds. Lucas et al. (2005) provide age- and education-adjusted category fluency normative data based on 304 African-American community-dwelling participants from the MOAANS project in Jacksonville, Florida. Participants were predominantly female (75%), ranged in age from 56 to 94 years (M = 69.6, SD = 6.87) and education levels ranged from 0 to 20 years (M = 12.2, SD = 3.48). They were screened to exclude participants with active neurologic, psychiatric, or other conditions that may affect cognition. Their data are shown in Table 9–157a. The

TABLE 9–154 Age- and Education-Adjusted Normative Data for Animal Fluency

	EDUCATION (YEARS)				
	0	1–6	7–9	10–12	≥13
Age 60–69[a]					
Number	300	812	352	3.85	360
Mean ± *SD*	11.21 ± 3.82	12.66 ± 3.69	13.84 ± 4.08	14.79 ± 4.44	15.78 ± 4.10
Median	11.00	13.00	14.00	14.00	15.00
5–95 percentile	5.00–17.00	7.00–19.00	8.00–21.00	9.00–22.70	9.00–23.00
70–74[b]					
Number	381	845	353	385	373
Mean ± *SD*	10.87 ± 3.92	12.41 ± 3.64	13.42 ± 3.80	14.59 ± 4.42	15.35 ± 3.96
Median	11.00	12.00	13.00	14.00	15.00
5–95 percentile	5.00–17.00	7.00–18.70	7.00–21.00	8.00–22.70	9.00–23.00
75–79[c]					
Number	298	517	224	237	213
Mean ± *SD*	10.20 ± 3.86	11.92 ± 3.63	13.09 ± 3.99	14.42 ± 4.30	14.67 ± 3.66
Median	10.00	12.00	13.00	14.00	14.00
5–95 percentile	4.00–17.00	6.00–18.00	7.00–20.00	7.90–22.00	9.00–21.30
80–84[d]					
Number	212	253	107	99	97
Mean ± *SD*	9.65 ± 4.08	11.61 ± 3.33	12.74 ± 3.56	13.96 ± 4.53	14.07 ± 3.37
Median	10.00	12.00	13.00	14.00	14.00
5–95 percentile	2.00–17.00	6.00–17.00	7.00–19.00	7.00–22.00	9.00–20.00
≥85[e]					
Number	136	112	39	49	39
Mean ± *SD*	9.22 ± 4.18	11.16 ± 3.54	12.23 ± 3.63	13.39 ± 3.66	13.95 ± 3.47
Median	10.00	11.00	12.00	13.00	14.00
5–95 percentile	2.00–16.15	5.65–17.00	7.00–19.00	7.00–19.00	9.00–20.00

[a] Normative data from age group 60–74 years.
[b] Normative data from age group 65–79 years.
[c] Normative data from age group 70–84 years.
[d] Normative data from age group 75–89 years.
[e] Normative data from age group 80–95 years.
SOURCE: Ryu et al. (2012).

computational formula for age- and education-corrected MOAANS scaled scores is shown in Table 9–157b. The authors suggest caution in the use of their norms since there was limited representation of the oldest participants and they used a regional convenience sample of volunteers. Two sets of age-adjusted normative data are shown in Table 9–158a: one set is presented for the combined total number of words produced across all three categories (animals, fruits, and vegetables), and the second set provides norms for animal naming alone. Table 9–158b shows the computational formula used to calculate age- and education-corrected scaled scores.

Hankee et al. (2013) report on verbal fluency (FAS and animals) data from 1,907 participants who were offspring of the original cohort in the Framingham study, with data collected from 2005 to 2008. Exclusion criteria included the presence of neurologic or neurodegenerative disease. Proportions of participants in each age group were as follows: 7% were 55 years or younger, 35% were 55 to 64 years, 34% were 65 to 74 years, and 24% were older than 75 years. Education levels were as follows: 3% with less than high school, 57% with high school, and 40% with postsecondary education. The sample was 54% female. Verbal fluency total responses, perseverative errors, and errors are depicted separately by age and education in Table 9–159a and 9–159b, respectively.

Pena-Casanova et al. (2009) present data as part of the Spanish Multicenter Normative Studies (NEURONORMA project), a large project that presents co-normed data for neuropsychological tests. Participants completed three semantic fluency tasks (animals, fruit and vegetables, and kitchen tools), three phonetic fluency tasks (words beginning with "P," "M," and "R"), and three excluded letter fluency tasks (excluded "A," "E," and "S"). The study was performed across nine different Spanish regions. Informants were also interviewed.

Participants were excluded if they were out of age range, did not live/function independently, presented with

TABLE 9–155 Age- and Education-Adjusted Norms for the FAS

	AGE 16–59 YEARS			AGE 60–79 YEARS			AGE 80–95 YEARS		
	EDUCATION (YEARS)			EDUCATION (YEARS)			EDUCATION (YEARS)		
PERCENTILE SCORE	0–8 (*N* = 12)	9–12 (*N* = 268)	13–21 (*N* = 242)	0–8 (*N* = 76)	9–12 (*N* = 292)	13–21 (*N* = 185)	0–8 (*N* = 75)	9–12 (*N* = 102)	13–21 (*N* = 46)
90	48	56	61	39	54	59	33	42	56
80	45	50	55	36	47	53	29	38	47
70	42	47	51	31	43	49	26	34	43
60	39	43	49	27	39	45	24	31	39
50	36	40	45	25	35	41	22	29	36
40	35	38	42	22	32	38	21	27	33
30	34	35	38	20	28	36	19	24	30
20	30	32	35	17	24	34	17	22	28
10	27	28	30	13	21	27	13	18	23
M	38.5	40.5	44.7	25.3	35.6	42.0	22.4	29.8	37.0
(SD)	(12.0)	(10.7)	(11.2)	(11.1)	(12.5)	(12.1)	(8.2)	(11.4)	(11.2)

SOURCE: From Tombaugh et al. (1999).

cognitive impairment on the MMSE, presented with neurologic disorder, scored above a cutoff on a Modified Ischemia Scale, or presented with alcohol or psychotropic substance abuse, an unmanaged medical condition that could interfere with cognition (e.g., diabetes mellitus, hypothyroidism, B_{12} deficiency), psychiatric condition, or sensory impairment. Pena-Casanova et al. (2009) provide data for 50- to 94-year-olds, with a sample size of 346 people. The sample was approximately 60% female. The sample had the following approximate education levels: five years or fewer (21%), six to 11 years (37%), 12 to 15 years (20%), and more than 16 years (22%). All participants were Caucasian and Spanish speakers.

Age-adjusted data are shown in Tables 9–160a to 9–160j. Tables 9–160k to 9–160n are presented for education adjustment. Gender-adjusted scores for relevant measures are in Tables 9–160o and 9–160p. To calculate the education-adjusted score, find the appropriate column in Tables 9–160k to 9–160n that corresponds to the examinee's years of education, find the NSS_A, and refer to the corresponding $NSS_{A\&E}$.

Cavaco et al. (2013) provide regression-based normative data for 950 Portuguese-speaking adults 18 to 98 years of age (M = 57.8 years, SD = 19). The sample was 66% female, with an average education of 8.8 years (SD = 5.2). "M," "R," "P" and animal fluency were used. Note that the phonemic fluency test was administered to 821 participants (64% women, age M = 55.8, SD = 18.7; education M = 9.8, SD = 4.8). Inclusion criteria were native language of Portuguese, lived in Portugal in the past five years, completed the majority of schooling in Portugal, absence of uncorrected auditory problems, developmental disorders, neurologic conditions, psychiatric conditions, and substance abuse. Persons with fewer than four years of education did not complete phonemic fluency. Formulas for adjusted scores are presented in Table 9–161a, with data in Table 9–161b.

TABLE 9–156 Age- and Education-Adjusted Norms for Animal Fluency

	AGE 16–59 YEARS			AGE 60–79 YEARS			AGE 80–95 YEARS		
	EDUCATION (YEARS)			EDUCATION (YEARS)			EDUCATION (YEARS)		
PERCENTILE SCORE	0–8 (*N* = 4)	9–12 (*N* = 109)	13–21 (*N* = 78)	0–8 (*N* = 61)	9–12 (*N* = 165)	13–21 (*N* = 94)	0–8 (*N* = 75)	9–12 (*N* = 103)	13–21 (*N* = 46)
90		26	30	20	22	25	18	19	24
75		23	25	17	19	22	16	17	20
50		20	23	14	17	19	13	14	16
25		17	18	12	14	16	11	12	14
10		15	16	11	12	13	9	11	12
M		19.8	21.9	14.4	16.4	18.2	13.1	13.9	16.3
(SD)		(4.2)	(5.4)	(3.4)	(4.3)	(4.2)	(3.8)	(3.4)	(4.3)

SOURCE: From Tombaugh et al. (1999).

TABLE 9–157A MOAANS Age-Based Norms for C, F, and L in African-American Adults

SCALED SCORE	56–62	63–65	66–68	69–71	72–74	75–77	78+	PERCENTILE RANGES
2	0–7	0–7	0–6	0–6	0–5	0–5	0–5	<1
3	8–10	8–10	7–10	7–10	6–10	6–10	6–7	1
4	11–12	11–12	11	–	–	–	8–10	2
5	13–14	13–14	12–14	11–13	11–12	11–12	11–12	3–5
6	15–16	15–16	15–16	14–16	13–15	13–15	13–15	6–10
7	17–21	17–20	17–20	17–20	16–19	16–19	16–17	11–18
8	22–23	21–22	21–22	21–22	20–22	20–22	18–21	19–28
9	24–27	23–26	23–26	23–26	23–25	23–25	22–23	29–40
10	28–33	27–31	27–31	27–31	26–31	26–30	24–28	41–59
11	34–36	32–36	32–36	32–36	32–36	31–36	29–32	60–71
12	37–41	37–41	37–40	37–40	37–40	37–40	33–37	72–81
13	42–47	42–45	41–44	41–44	41–44	41–44	38–41	82–89
14	48–53	46–52	45–50	45–50	45–50	45–50	42–49	90–94
15	54–56	53–56	51–55	51–55	51–55	51–53	50–51	95–97
16	57–61	57–60	56–60	56–60	56–60	54–55	52	98
17	62+	61–62	61–62	61–62	61	56–58	53	99
18	–	63+	63+	63+	62+	59+	54+	>99
N	108	130	167	183	159	120	80	

SOURCE: Adapted from Lucas et al. (2005).

Van der Elst et al. (2006) provide normative data for 1,856 Dutch speakers 24 to 81 years of age in the Netherlands. Animal, profession, and letter "M" (four-letter words) were used. Participants were recruited from a larger study on the determinants of cognitive aging. Exclusion criteria were neurodegenerative, neurologic, or significant developmental disorders, psychiatric conditions, substance abuse, cutoff score on the MMSE, and more than five errors or repetitions on at least one verbal fluency test. The sample was approximately 50% female and all participants were Caucasian and native Dutch speakers. Participants were grouped into low education (primary school or less; 37%), average education (junior vocational; 41%), and high education (vocational or academic; 23%). Normative data is presented in Table 9–162.

OTHER NORMATIVE DATA

In addition to the aforementioned normative datasets, additional datasets are available for specific groups (see Table 9–163). A number of older normative datasets are also available (e.g., Acevedo et al., 2000; Gladsjo et al., 1999a, b; Ivnik et al., 1996; Lucas et al., 1998; Ravdin et al., 2003; Stricks et al., 1998). Select normative studies are described in more detail later.

TABLE 9–157B Computational Formula for Age- and Education-Corrected MOAANS Scaled Scores

	K	W_1	W_2
CFL	2.97	1.19	0.41

Age- and education-corrected MOAANS scaled scores ($MSS_{A\&E}$) can be calculated for CFL scores by using aged-corrected MOAANS scaled scores (MSS_A) and education (expressed in years completed) in the following formula: $MSS_{A\&E} = K + (W_1 \times MSS_A) - (W_2 \times EDUC)$

SOURCE: Adapted from Lucas et al. (2005).

DISCREPANCIES BETWEEN PHONEMIC (FAS) AND SEMANTIC (ANIMAL) FLUENCY

Discrepancies between phonemic (FAS) and category (animal) fluency may be of diagnostic value (see "Construct Validity"). Accordingly, Gladsjo et al. (1999a) and Gladsjo, Schuman, Miller, and Heaton (1999b) provide the frequency of FAS minus animal fluency T-score discrepancies of different magnitudes. Relatively large differences between phonemic (Letter) and semantic (Category) fluency were not uncommon: 10% of the total sample had a Letter > Category T-score difference of 18 or more, or had a Letter < Category T-score difference of 19 or greater. Letter-category fluency discrepancy score was not significantly related to participant's age, education, gender, or ethnicity. The D-KEFS also allows the examiner to contrast phonemic and category fluency conditions, and offers a large normative database (see review in this chapter).

CLUSTERING AND SWITCHING

Normative data for clustering and switching are provided by Troyer (2000) for tests of phonemic fluency (FAS or CFL) and semantic fluency (animals and supermarket) based on a sample of 411 healthy adults between the ages of 18 and 91 years. Percentiles for individual raw scores can be obtained by adding relevant corrections and looking up

TABLE 9–158A MOAANS Age-Based Category (Animals, Fruits, and Vegetables) and Animal Fluency Norms in African-American Adults

SCALED	56–62		63–65		66–68		69–71		72–74		75–77		78+		PERCENTILE
SCORE	C	A	C	A	C	A	C	A	C	A	C	A	C	A	RANGES
2	0–19	0–6	0–19	0–1	0–19	0–1	0–19	0–1	0–17	0–1	0–17	0–1	0–16	0–1	<1
3	20–22	–	20–22	2–6	20–21	2–6	20–21	2–6	18–19	2–6	18–19	2–6	17–19	2–4	1
4	23	7	23	–	22–23	–	22	–	20–21	–	20	–	20	5–6	2
5	24	–	24	7	24	7	23–24	7	22–24	7	21–24	7	21–23	7	3–5
6	25–29	8–9	25–28	8	25–28	8	25–27	8	25–27	8	25–26	8	24	8	6–10
7	30	10	29–30	9–10	29–30	9–10	28–29	9–10	28–29	9–10	27–29	9	25–27	9	11–18
8	31–33	11	31–33	11	31–33	11	30–32	11	30–32	11	30–32	10–11	28–29	–	19–28
9	34–37	12–14	34–36	12	34–36	12	33–35	12	33–34	12	33–34	12	30–33	10	29–40
10	38–42	15–16	37–40	13–15	37–39	13–14	36–39	13–14	35–38	13	35–38	13	34–35	11–12	41–59
11	43–45	17	41–43	16	40–42	15	40–41	15	39–41	14–15	39–41	14–15	36–39	13–14	60–71
12	46–48	18–19	44–46	17–18	43–44	16–17	42–44	16–17	42–43	16	42–43	16	40	15	72–81
13	49–53	20–21	47–49	19–20	45–47	18–19	45–47	18	44–46	17–18	44–46	17–18	41–42	16	82–89
14	54–57	22–23	50–53	21	48–51	20	48–51	19–20	47–49	19	47	19	43–46	17–18	90–94
15	58–60	24	54–58	22–24	52–54	21–22	52–54	21–22	50–54	20–21	48–54	20–21	47–51	19	95–97
16	–	25	59–60	25	55–57	23–24	55–57	23–24	55–57	22–24	55–56	22–24	52–54	20–23	98
17	61–60	26–28	61–64	26–28	58–63	25–27	58–63	25–27	58–59	–	57	–	55–57	24	99
18	29+	65+	65+	29+	64+	28+	64+	28+	60+	25+	58+	25+	58+	25+	>99
N	107	107	129	129	165	165	181	181	155	155	118	118	79	79	

SOURCE: Adapted from Lucas et al. (2005).

the corresponding corrected score in Table 9–164. For example, consider a 50-year-old woman with 13 years of education. If she produced a cluster size of 0.35 on FAS, her adjusted score would be calculated as 0.35 + 50(–.001) + 13(–0.015) + 0.094 = 0.20. This places her score at about the 50th percentile.

Written Fluency. Heaton et al. (2004) provide norms separately for two ethnicity groups (Caucasians, African Americans) organized by age, gender, and education. The samples are large (295 Caucasians, 409 African Americans), cover a wide range in terms of age (20–85 years) and education (0–20 years), and exclusion criteria are specified. T scores less than 40 are classed as impaired.

EVIDENCE FOR RELIABILITY

EVIDENCE FOR INTERNAL RELIABILITY

Internal reliability is high ($r \geq .83$, Cavaco et al., 2013; Tombaugh et al., 1999; Ruff et al., 1996).

TABLE 9–158B Computational Formula for Age- and Education-Corrected MOAANS Scaled Scores

	K	W_1	W_2
Category fluency	2.00	1.11	0.23
Animal fluency	1.84	1.11	0.24

Age- and education-corrected MOAANS scaled scores ($MSS_{A\&E}$) can be calculated for fluency scores by using aged-corrected MOAANS scaled scores (MSS_A) and education (expressed in years completed) in the following formula: $MSS_{A\&E} = K + (W_1 \times MSS_A) - (W_2 \times EDUC)$

SOURCE: Adapted from Lucas et al. (2005).

EVIDENCE FOR TEST-RETEST RELIABILITY, MEASURING CHANGE, AND PRACTICE EFFECTS

In healthy adults, test-retest correlations are adequate to high, typically greater than $r = .70$, for both phonemic and semantic fluency, at both short (e.g., one-week) and long (e.g., five-year) intervals (Basso et al., 1999; Dikmen et al., 1999; Harrison et al., 2000; Levine et al., 2004; Ross, 2003). For example, Tombaugh et al. (1999) found a test-retest reliability coefficient of $r = .74$ for FAS after an interval of more than five years in older individuals.

As might be expected, gains are more notable following short retest intervals. Wilson, Watson, Baddeley, Emslie, and Evans (2000) reported that fluency for the same letter or category shows a small but consistent increase across 20 successive administrations over a four-week period in healthy controls as well as those with severe TBI, and Basso et al. (1999) noted no gains among 50 healthy males retested with the FAS following a 12-month interval. Levine et al. (2004) reported gains of about three words for 145 healthy men retested with the FAS across a wide time interval, ranging from four to 24 months (interval $M = 191$ days, $SD = 38$). Table 9–164a shows the change score, standard deviation of the change score, and test-retest reliability coefficient for use in RCI formulas. Table 9–164b shows a regression formula that can be used to estimate Time 2 scores.

Based on this data, neither the length of retest interval nor age contributed significantly to the regression equation. The impact of educational level, while significant, only contributed an additional 2%. The residual standard deviation for the regression formula shown in Table 9–164b can be used to establish the range for retest scores that can be

TABLE 9–159A Norms for FAS Stratified by Age

TEST PARAMETER	AGE (YEARS) <55	55–64	65–74	≥75	TOTAL
FAS					
Total responses	41.6 (12.6)	41.8 (12.3)	36.3 (11.9)	33.4 (11.2)	38.0 (12.4)
%Psv errors	2.2 (3.5)	3.6 (4.2)	3.8 (4.7)	5.0 (6.3)	3.9 (4.9)
%Total errors	4.3 (5.7)	5.7 (6.2)	6.3 (6.9)	8.3 (9.8)	6.4 (7.5)
Animals					
Total responses	20.2 (4.1)	20.2 (4.9)	17.7 (4.7)	14.8 (4.5)	18.1 (5.1)
%Psv errors	2.7 (4.8)	2.7 (7.5)	3.3 (5.7)	4.1 (8.4)	3.2 (7.0)
%Total errors	2.7 (4.8)	2.9 (7.8)	3.6 (6.1)	4.6 (9.0)	3.5 (7.4)
	n = 132	*n* = 659	*n* = 635	*n* = 429	*n* = 1,855

NOTE: %Psv errors = perseverations/total responses; %Total errors = total errors/total responses.

SOURCE: Hankee et al. (2013).

TABLE 9–159B Norms for FAS Stratified by Education

TEST PARAMETER	EDUCATION (DEGREE) <HIGH SCHOOL	HIGH SCHOOL	COLLEGE	≥GRADUATE	TOTAL
FAS					
Total responses	27.6 (13.3)	35.4 (11.5)	40.7 (12.0)	44.2 (11.8)	38.0 (12.4)
%Psv errors	3.8 (4.9)	4.2 (5.4)	3.3 (4.1)	3.6 (4.4)	3.9 (4.9)
%Total errors	9.6 (9.9)	7.1 (8.2)	5.2 (5.8)	5.4 (5.9)	6.4 (7.5)
Animals					
Total responses	14.3 (5.2)	17.1 (4.7)	19.0 (5.0)	20.6 (5.2)	18.1 (5.1)
%Psv errors	3.6 (5.3)	3.7 (7.7)	2.4 (5.0)	2.7 (6.8)	3.2 (7.0)
%Total errors	3.6 (5.3)	4.0 (8.1)	2.6 (5.6)	3.0 (7.2)	3.5 (7.4)
	n = 58	*n* = 1,046	*n* = 398	*n* = 353	*n* = 1855

NOTE: %Psv errors = perseverations/total responses; %Total errors = total erros/total responses.

SOURCE: Hankee et al. (2013).

TABLE 9–160A Normative Data for Spanish Verbal Fluency for Age 50–56

		SEMANTIC			PHONOLOGICAL INITIAL LETTER			EXCLUDED LETTER		
SCALED SCORE	PERCENTILE RANGE	ANIMALS	FRUITS AND VEGETABLES	KITCHEN TOOLS	P	M	R	A	E	S
2	<1	0–10	0–9	0–7	0–4	0–1	0–1	0	0–1	0–1
3	1	–	–	–	5–6	–	–	–	–	2
4	2	11–12	10–11	–	7	2–4	–	–	2	3–4
5	3–5	13	–	8	8	5	2–4	1–2	3–4	5–6
6	6–10	14	12–13	–	–	6	5	3	–	7
7	11–18	15	14	9–10	9–10	7–8	6–7	4	5–6	8–9
8	19–28	16–17	15–16	11	11–12	9	8	5–6	8	10–11
9	29–40	18–19	17	12–13	13	10–11	9–10	7	9	12
10	41–59	20–21	18–19	14	14–17	12–13	11–13	8–9	10–11	13–15
11	60–71	22–23	20	15–16	18	14	14–15	10	12–13	16–18
12	72–81	24–26	21–22	–	19–20	15–16	16–17	11–12	14	19–20
13	82–89	27–29	23–24	17–18	21–22	17	18	13–14	15–16	21–23
14	90–94	30–31	25–26	19	23	18–20	19–22	15–16	17	24
15	95–97	32	27–28	20–21	24–27	21–22	23	17	18–20	25–26
16	98	–	29	22–24	28–29	23–24	24–25	18–19	21	27
17	99	33	–	–	30	–	26–28	20	22	28–29
18	>99	≥34	≥30	≥25	≥31	≥25	≥29	≥21	≥23	≥30
Sample size		135	135	135	135	135	135	135	135	135

SOURCE: Pena-Casanova et al. (2009).

TABLE 9-160B Normative Data for Spanish Verbal Fluency for Age 57–59

					PHONOLOGICAL					
		SEMANTIC			INITIAL LETTER			EXCLUDED LETTER		
SCALED SCORE	PERCENTILE RANGE	ANIMALS	FRUITS AND VEGETABLES	KITCHEN TOOLS	P	M	R	A	E	S
2	<1	0–7	0–9	0–6	0–3	0–1	0–1	0	0–1	0
3	1	–	–	–	4	–	–	–	–	1
4	2	8–10	10–11	–	–	2–3	–	–	–	–
5	3–5	11–12	–	7–8	5–7	4	2–4	–	2–3	2–4
6	6–10	13–14	12–13	9	8	5	5	1–2	4–5	5–6
7	11–18	15	14–15	10	9–10	6–7	6	3–4	6	7–8
8	19–28	16–17	16	11	11–12	8–9	7–8	5	7	9–10
9	29–40	18	17	12	13	10	9–10	6	8	11–12
10	41–59	19–21	18–19	13–14	14–16	11–12	11–13	7–8	9–11	13–14
11	60–71	22–23	20	15	17–19	13–14	14–15	9–10	12	15–17
12	72–81	24–26	21	16	20	15	16–17	11–12	13–15	18–20
13	82–89	27–29	22–23	17–18	21	16–17	18	13–14	16–17	21
14	90–94	30–32	24–26	19	22–23	18–20	19–21	15–16	18–20	22–23
15	95–97	–	27–28	20–21	24–25	21–22	22–23	17–19	21	24–25
16	98	33	29	22	26	23	–	–	22	26–27
17	99	34	30	23–24	27–28	24	24	20	–	28–29
18	>99	≥35	≥31	≥25	≥29	≥25	≥25	≥21	≥23	≥30
Sample size		132	132	132	132	132	132	128	132	132

SOURCE: Pena-Casanova et al. (2009).

typically expected. For example, a 90% CI can be created around the scores by multiplying the residual standard deviation by 1.645, which allows for 5% of people to fall outside of both the upper and lower extremes. Individuals whose scores exceed the extremes are considered to show significant changes.

Although test-retest reliabilities are generally reasonable for phonemic fluency, these findings suggest that relatively large changes in performance are required to conclude that a real decline or improvement has occurred as opposed to being due to the effects of practice and random measurement error (see also Basso et al., 1999).

Similar findings are reported for semantic fluency. Bird, Papadopoulou, Ricciardelli, Rossor, and Cipolotti (2004) evaluated animal fluency in 99 healthy adults drawn from a larger sample of 188 healthy volunteers retested following a

TABLE 9-160C Normative Data for Spanish Verbal Fluency for Age 60–62

					PHONOLOGICAL					
		SEMANTIC			INITIAL LETTER			EXCLUDED LETTER		
SCALED SCORE	PERCENTILE RANGE	ANIMALS	FRUITS AND VEGETABLES	KITCHEN TOOLS	P	M	R	A	E	S
2	<1	0–7	0–7	0–6	0–3	0–1	0–1	0	0–1	0
3	1	–	8	7	4	2–3	–	–	–	1
4	2	8–10	–	–	5	–	2–4	–	–	–
5	3–5	11	9–11	8	6	4	–	–	2–3	2–4
6	6–10	12–13	12	9	7–8	5	5	1–2	4	5
7	11–18	14	13–14	10	9	6	6	3	5	6–7
8	19–28	15–16	15–16	11	10	7–8	7	4	6	8–9
9	29–40	17–18	17	12	11–12	9	8–9	5–6	7–8	10–11
10	41 -59	19–20	18–19	13–14	13–14	10–11	10–13	7–8	9–10	12–14
11	60–71	21–23	20	15	15–17	12–14	14	9	11–12	15–16
12	72–81	24–26	21	16	18–19	15	15–17	10	13–15	17–19
13	82–89	27–29	22–23	17	20–21	16	18	11–13	–	20
14	90–94	30–32	24–25	18	22	17–18	19–20	14–15	16–17	21–23
15	95–97	–	26–28	19	23	19–20	21–22	16–18	18	24–25
16	98	33	29	20	–	21–22	23	19	–	26–27
17	99	34	30	21–22	24	23–24	24	20	19–21	28
18	>99	≥35	≥31	≥23	≥25	≥25	≥25	≥21	≥22	≥29
Sample size		123	123	123	123	123	123	119	123	123

SOURCE: Pena-Casanova et al. (2009).

TABLE 9–160D Normative Data for Spanish Verbal Fluency for Age 63–65

					PHONOLOGICAL					
		SEMANTIC			INITIAL LETTER			EXCLUDED LETTER		
SCALED SCORE	PERCENTILE RANGE	ANIMALS	FRUITS AND VEGETABLES	KITCHEN TOOLS	P	M	R	A	E	S
2	<1	0–7	0–7	0–6	0–4	0–3	0–2	0	0–1	0–1
3	1	8–10	8	–	5	–	–	–	–	–
4	2	–	–	7	–	4	3	–	–	2–4
5	3–5	11	9–11	8	6	5	–	–	2–3	–
6	6–10	12	12	–	7	–	4	1	–	5
7	11–18	13–14	13	9–10	8–9	6	5–6	2–3	4–5	6–7
8	19–28	15–16	14–15	11	10	7–8	7	4	6	8
9	29–40	17	16–17	12	11–12	9	8	5	7–8	9–10
10	41–59	18–20	18–19	13–14	13–15	10–12	9–11	6–8	9–10	11–14
11	60–71	21–22	20	15	16–17	13–14	12–14	9	11–12	15–16
12	72–81	23–24	21	–	18–19	15	15–16	10	13–15	17–19
11	82–89	25–26	22–23	16–17	20–21	16–17	17–18	11–13	16	20
14	90–94	27–30	24–25	18	–	18–19	19–21	14	17	21–23
15	95–97	–	26–27	19	22	20	22	15–16	18	24–26
16	98	31–33	28	20	23	–	23	17	–	27
17	99	34	30	21	24	21–22	24	18–19	19–21	28
18	>99	≥35	≥31	≥22	≥25	≥23	≥25	≥20	≥22	≥29
Sample size		107	107	107	107	107	107	103	107	107

SOURCE: Pena-Casanova et al. (2009).

one-month interval. As Table 9–166 shows, small but reliable practice effects were seen. Reliable change indices were calculated as the standard deviation of the difference scores, multiplied by 1.645, and adding the mean change in score from Time 1 to Time 2. Therefore, 10% of the sample had a change in score that fell outside of the RCI corrected for practice. Note that the RCI is large, due to the considerable variability in performance that can be expected between assessments. Neither NART IQ nor age was related to the practice effect.

As an example, suppose an examinee obtains a baseline raw score of 20 on animal fluency. Repeat testing one month later following cognitive therapy reveals a score of 26. Examination of Table 9–166 indicates that a gain of six points does not exceed the upper limits (+10.5) of the 90% CI. Of note, information regarding generalizability of RCI estimates in persons with HIV is provided for the interested reader in Levine et al. (2007).

In contrast to the total score, the supplemental fluency scores (e.g., clustering and switching) are generally

TABLE 9–160E Normative Data for Spanish Verbal Fluency for Age 66–68

					PHONOLOGICAL					
		SEMANTIC			INITIAL LETTER			EXCLUDED LETTER		
SCALED SCORE	PERCENTILE RANGE	ANIMALS	FRUITS AND VEGETABLES	KITCHEN TOOLS	P	M	R	A	E	S
2	<1	0–7	0–6	0–6	0–3	0–3	0	0	0	0–1
3	1	8	7	–	–	–	–	–	–	2–4
4	2	–	–	–	4	–	–	–	–	–
5	3–5	9–11	8–9	7	5	4	1–3	1	1–3	5
4	6–10	12	10–11	8	6	5	4	2	4	6
7	11–18	13	12–13	9	7	6	5	3	–	7
8	19–28	14–15	14	10	8–9	7–8	6–7	4	5–6	8
9	29–40	16	15	11	10–11	9	8	5	7	9–10
10	41–59	17–19	16–18	12–13	12–14	10–12	9–11	6–7	8–9	11–12
11	60–71	20–21	19	14	15–16	13–14	12–14	8–9	10–11	13–14
12	72–81	22–23	20–21	15	17	15	15	10	12–13	15–17
13	82–89	24	22	16	18–19	16–17	16	11–12	14–15	18–20
14	90–94	25–27	23	17–18	20	18–19	17–18	13	16–17	–
15	95–97	28–29	24–25	19–20	21–22	20–21	19–21	14	18	21–24
16	98	–	26	–	23	–	–	15	19–20	25
17	99	30–33	27	21	24–25	22	22	16	21	26
18	>99	≥34	≥28	≥22	≥26	≥23	≥23	≥17	≥22	≥27
Sample size		121	121	121	121	121	121	118	121	121

SOURCE: Pena-Casanova et al. (2009).

TABLE 9–160F Normative Data for Spanish Verbal Fluency for Age 69–71

					PHONOLOGICAL					
		SEMANTIC			INITIAL LETTER			EXCLUDED LETTER		
SCALED SCORE	PERCENTILE RANGE	ANIMALS	FRUITS AND VEGETABLES	KITCHEN TOOLS	P	M	R	A	E	S
2	<1	0–7	0–6	0–6	0–3	0–2	0	0	0	0
3	1	8	–	–	4	–	–	–	1	1–4
4	2	–	7–8	–	–	3	–	–	–	–
5	3–5	9–10	9	7	5	–	–	–	–	5
4	6–10	11	10	8	6	4	1–3	1	2–3	6
7	11–18	12–13	11–12	9	7	5–6	4–5	2	4	7
8	19–28	14	13	10	8–9	7	6	3	5–6	8
9	29–40	15–16	14–15	11	10	8–9	7–8	4	7	9
10	41–59	17–18	16	12	11–13	10–11	9–11	5–6	8–9	10–12
11	60–71	19–21	17–18	13–14	14–16	12–14	12–13	7–8	10	13–14
12	72–81	22–23	19–20	15	17	15	14–15	9–10	11–13	15–17
13	82–89	24	21	16	18–19	16–17	16	11	14–15	18–20
14	90–94	25–26	22–23	17–18	20–21	18	17–18	12–13	16	21
15	95–97	27–29	24–25	19–20	22–23	19–20	19–21	14	17–18	22–24
16	98	30	26	–	24	21	–	15	19	25
17	99	31–33	27	21	25	22	22	16	–	26
18	>99	≥34	≥28	≥22	≥26	≥23	≥23	≥17	≥20	≥27
Sample size		125	125	125	125	125	125	125	125	125

SOURCE: Pena-Casanova et al. (2009).

associated with weaker reliability coefficients. Ross (2003) examined the stability of phonemic fluency scores in a sample of 55 healthy college students who were retested over an average interval of six to seven weeks. He found that test-retest reliability for clustering and switching was poor (r_{icc} = .47 and .58, respectively), suggesting that any search process (strategic or otherwise) can vary considerably with each test administration.

Ross et al. (2007) reported that test-retest reliability for the qualitative scores were modest to poor (r_{icc} = .60 to .40 range), despite high test-retest reliability for the total word score (r_{icc} = .84) in 108 healthy adults on phonemic fluency. Specifically, the authors reported a test-retest coefficient of r_{icc} of .85 (range of .64 to 94) for novel words produced on the CFL, similar to PRW coefficients of .80 (range .64 to .89). Cluster scores were comparatively poorer, including .49 (range .32 to .63) for the CFL, .54 (range .13 to .75) for the PRW, as were switching scores (.50 [range .34 to .64] for the CFL and .48 [range .21 to .68]) for the PRW. Ross et al. (2005) found that informing

TABLE 9–160G Normative Data for Spanish Verbal Fluency for Age 72–74

					PHONOLOGICAL					
		SEMANTIC			INITIAL LETTER			EXCLUDED LETTER		
SCALED SCORE	PERCENTILE RANGE	ANIMALS	FRUITS AND VEGETABLES	KITCHEN TOOLS	P	M	R	A	E	S
2	<1	0–6	0–5	0–5	0–3	0–2	0	0	0	0
3	1	7	6	–	4	–	–	–	1	1–4
4	2	8	7	6	–	3	–	–	–	–
5	3–5	9–10	8	–	5	–	–	–	–	5
4	6–10	11	9	7–8	6	4	1–3	1	2–3	6
7	11–18	12–13	10–12	9	7	5	4–5	2	4	7
8	19–28	14	13	10	8–9	6–7	6	3	5–6	–
9	29–40	15–16	14	–	10	8	7–8	4	–	8
10	41–59	17–18	15–16	11–12	11–13	9–10	9–10	5–6	7–8	9–11
11	60–71	19–20	17	13	14–16	11–12	11–12	7	9–10	12
12	72–81	21–23	18	14	17	13–15	13–15	8–9	11–12	13–15
13	82–89	24	19–20	15–16	18–19	16–17	–	10	13–14	16–18
14	90–94	25–26	21	17–18	20–21	–	16	11–12	15	19–20
15	95–97	27–28	22–25	19–20	22–23	18–20	17–19	13–14	16–18	21–23
16	98	29	–	–	24	–	–	15	19	24
17	99	30	26	21	25	21	22	16	–	25
18	>99	≥31	≥27	≥22	≥26	≥22	≥23	≥17	≥20	≥26
Sample size		125	125	125	125	125	125	123	125	125

SOURCE: Pena-Casanova et al. (2009).

TABLE 9–160H Normative Data for Spanish Verbal Fluency for Age 75–77

		SEMANTIC			PHONOLOGICAL					
					INITIAL LETTER			EXCLUDED LETTER		
SCALED SCORE	PERCENTILE RANGE	ANIMALS	FRUITS AND VEGETABLES	KITCHEN TOOLS	P	M	R	A	E	S
2	<1	0–6	0–5	0–5	0–2	0–2	0	0	0	0
3	1	–	–	–	3	–	–	–	–	–
4	2	7	6	–	–	3	–	–	1	1–12
5	3–5	8–9	7	6	4	–	1–2	–	–	3–4
4	6–10	10	8–9	7	5–6	4	3	1	2	5
7	11–18	11–12	10	8	7	–	4	2	3	6
8	19–28	13	11–12	9	–	5–6	5	–	4	7
9	29–40	14–15	13	10	8–9	7	6–7	3–4	5–6	8
10	41–59	16–18	14–15	11	10–12	8–9	8–10	5	7	9–10
11	60–71	19	16–17	12	13	10–11	11–12	6	8	11
12	72–81	20–21	18	13	14–16	12–13	13–14	7–8	9–11	12–13
13	82–89	22–24	19	14–15	17–18	14–16	15	9–10	12–13	14–16
14	90–94	25–26	20–21	16–17	19	17	–	–	14–15	17–20
15	95–97	27	22–23	18–19	20	18–19	16	11–12	16–17	21–22
16	98	28	–	20	21	20	17	13–15	18	23
17	99	29	24–25	21	22–23	–	18–19	16	19	24
18	>99	≥30	≥26	≥22	≥24	≥21	≥20	≥17	≥20	≥25
Sample size		100	100	100	100	100	100	99	100	100

SOURCE: Pena-Casanova et al. (2009).

individuals of clustering strategies did not significantly improve stability coefficients for total words produced and cluster size, although stability of cluster and switch scores were improved (r_{icc} = .76 vs. .49).

In terms of written fluency, Cohen and Stanczak (2000) reported a six-week retest reliability of .79 for 70 adult students (age, $M = 20.62$, $SD = 4.36$). There was a notable practice effect of an average eight-word gain on the second administration.

EVIDENCE FOR RELIABILITY OF ALTERNATE, SHORT, OR COMPUTER FORMS

Ruff et al. (1996) administered alternate versions of phonemic fluency (CFL in the first test session, PRW in the second test session) to 120 participants with an interval of six months. A correlation of $r = .74$ was reported, with an average gain of three words on the second administration. Wilson et al. (2000) suggested that practice effects can be reduced by changing the letter or category on each test

TABLE 9–160I Normative Data for Spanish Verbal Fluency for Age 78–80

		SEMANTIC			PHONOLOGICAL					
					INITIAL LETTER			EXCLUDED LETTER		
SCALED SCORE	PERCENTILE RANGE	ANIMALS	FRUITS AND VEGETABLES	KITCHEN TOOLS	P	M	R	A	E	S
2	<1	0–6	0–5	0–5	0–3	0–2	0	0	0	0
3	1	–	6	–	4	3	–	–	–	1–2
4	2	–	–	–	–	–	–	–	–	–
5	3–5	7–8	7	6	–	–	2	–	–	3–4
4	6–10	9–11	8–9	7	5–6	4	3	1	1–2	5
7	11–18	–	10	8	–	5	4	2	3–4	–
8	19–28	12–13	11–12	9	7	–	5–6	3	–	6–7
9	29–40	14	–	–	8	6	7	–	5–6	8
10	41–59	15–17	13–14	10	9–10	7–8	8–9	4	7	9
11	60–71	18	15	11	11–13	9–10	10–11	5	8	10–11
12	72–81	19–20	16–17	12	14	11	12	6–7	9	12
13	82–89	21	–	13	15–18	12–14	13	8	10–11	13–14
14	90–94	22–25	18	14–15	19	–	14–15	9–10	12–13	15–17
15	95–97	26–27	–	16	20	15–17	16	11–12	14–16	18–21
16	98	–	19	17–18	–	18	17	13	17	22
17	99	–	–	–	–	–	–	–	–	–
18	>99	≥28	≥20	≥19	≥21	≥19	≥18	≥14	≥18	≥23
Sample size		65	65	65	65	65	65	63	65	65

SOURCE: Pena-Casanova et al. (2009).

TABLE 9–160J Normative Data for Spanish Verbal Fluency for Age 81–90

					PHONOLOGICAL					
		SEMANTIC			INITIAL LETTER			EXCLUDED LETTER		
SCALED SCORE	PERCENTILE RANGE	ANIMALS	FRUITS AND VEGETABLES	KITCHEN TOOLS	P	M	R	A	E	S
2	<1	0–7	0–6	0–4	0–3	0–2	0	0	0	0
3	1	–	–	–	–	–	–	–	–	–
4	2	8	–	5	4	3	–	–	–	1–2
5	3–5	9	7	6	5	4	2	–	–	3–4
4	6–10	10–12	8	7	6	–	3	1	2	–
7	11–18	–	9	–	–	–	–	2	3	5
8	19–28	12–13	10–11	8	7	5	4–6	–	4	6
9	29–40	14	12	9	8	6	7	3–4	5	7
10	41–59	15–16	13	10	9	7–8	8–9	5	6	8–9
11	60–71	17–18	14–15	11	10–12	9–10	10	6	7	10
12	72–81	–	16	–	13–14	11	11	7–8	8	11–12
13	82–89	19	17	12	15	12	12–13	9–10	9	13
14	90–94	20	18	–	17–18	13	–	–	10	14
15	95–97	–	–	13	–	14	–	11–12	11–12	–
16	98	21–22	19	14	–	15–16	14	13–15	–	15–16
17	99	–	–	–	–	–	–	16	–	–
18	>99	≥23	≥20	≥15	≥19	≥17	≥15	≥17	≥13	≥17
Sample size		42	42	42	42	42	42	40	42	42

SOURCE: Pena-Casanova et al. (2009).

occasion. Consistent with this proposal, Dikmen et al. (1999) found that the reliability of alternate forms of phonemic fluency (FAS, BDT) was adequate ($r = .72$) at a retest interval of about 11 months, and only small practice effects were noted. Table 9–167 provides information to assess change, taking practice into account. Using values in Table 9–167, one first subtracts the mean T2-T1 change (column 3) from the difference between the two testing sessions for the individual and then compares it to 1.64 times the *SD* of the difference (column 4). The 1.64 is from the normal distribution and is exceeded in the positive or negative direction only 10% of the time if indeed there is no real change in clinical condition.

Ross, Furr, Carter, and Weinberg (2006) examined form equivalence of novel words and qualitative scores (switching and clustering) of the CFL and PRW in healthy college students. Using a within-subjects design, no mean differences or differences in *SD* were found, with the exception of *SD* for mean cluster size. In a between-subjects design, normative data did not differ between versions, and correlations were similar between scores, suggesting comparability of forms. See also "Evidence for Validity."

TABLE 9–160K Education Adjustment for Spanish Animals Verbal Fluency

	EDUCATION (YEARS)																				
NSS_A	0	1	2	3	4	5	6	7	8	9	10	11	12	13	14	15	16	17	18	19	20
2	4	4	4	3	3	3	3	3	2	2	2	2	2	1	1	1	1	0	0	0	0
3	5	5	5	4	4	4	4	4	3	3	3	3	3	2	2	2	2	1	1	1	1
4	6	6	6	5	5	5	5	5	4	4	4	4	4	3	3	3	3	2	2	2	2
3	7	7	7	6	6	6	6	6	5	5	5	5	5	4	4	4	4	3	3	3	3
6	8	8	8	7	7	7	7	7	6	6	6	6	6	5	5	5	5	4	4	4	4
2	9	9	9	8	8	8	8	8	7	7	7	7	7	6	6	6	6	5	5	5	5
8	10	10	10	9	9	9	9	9	8	8	8	8	8	7	7	7	7	6	6	6	6
9	11	11	11	10	10	10	10	10	9	9	9	9	9	8	8	8	8	7	7	7	7
10	12	12	12	11	11	11	11	11	10	10	10	10	10	9	9	9	9	8	8	8	8
11	13	13	13	12	12	12	12	12	11	11	11	11	11	10	10	10	10	9	9	9	9
12	14	14	14	13	13	13	13	13	12	12	12	12	12	11	11	11	11	10	10	10	10
13	15	15	15	14	14	14	14	14	13	13	13	13	13	12	12	12	12	11	11	11	11
14	16	16	16	15	15	15	15	15	14	14	14	14	14	13	13	13	13	12	12	12	12
15	17	17	17	16	16	16	16	16	15	15	15	15	15	14	14	14	14	13	13	13	13
16	18	18	18	17	17	17	17	17	16	16	16	16	16	16	15	15	15	14	14	14	14
17	19	19	19	18	18	18	18	18	17	17	17	17	17	16	16	16	16	15	15	15	15
18	20	20	20	19	19	19	19	19	18	18	18	18	18	17	17	17	17	16	16	16	16

NOTE: Animals. Education adjustment applying the following formula: $NSS_{A\&E} = NSS_A - (\beta \times [Education_{(years)} - 12])$, where $\beta = 0.20588$.

SOURCE: Pena-Casanova et al. (2009).

TABLE 9–160L Education Adjustment for Letter "P" Spanish Verbal Fluency

	EDUCATION (YEARS)																				
NSS_A	0	1	2	3	4	5	6	7	8	9	10	11	12	13	14	15	16	17	18	19	20
2	4	4	4	3	3	3	3	3	2	2	2	2	2	1	1	1	1	0	0	0	0
3	5	5	5	4	4	4	4	4	3	3	3	3	3	2	2	2	2	1	1	1	1
4	6	6	6	5	5	5	5	5	4	4	4	4	4	3	3	3	3	2	2	2	2
3	7	7	7	6	6	6	6	6	5	5	5	5	5	4	4	4	4	3	3	3	3
6	8	8	8	7	7	7	7	7	6	6	6	6	6	5	5	5	5	4	4	4	4
2	9	9	9	8	8	8	8	8	7	7	7	7	7	6	6	6	6	5	5	5	5
8	10	10	10	9	9	9	9	9	8	8	8	8	8	7	7	7	7	6	6	6	6
9	11	11	11	10	10	10	10	10	9	9	9	9	9	8	8	8	8	7	7	7	7
10	12	12	12	11	11	11	11	11	10	10	10	10	10	9	9	9	9	8	8	8	8
11	13	13	13	12	12	12	12	12	11	11	11	11	11	10	10	10	10	9	9	9	9
12	14	14	14	13	13	13	13	13	12	12	12	12	12	11	11	11	11	10	10	10	10
13	15	15	15	14	14	14	14	14	13	13	13	13	13	12	12	12	12	11	11	11	11
14	16	16	16	15	15	15	15	15	14	14	14	14	14	13	13	13	13	12	12	12	12
15	17	17	17	16	16	16	16	16	15	15	15	15	15	14	14	14	14	13	13	13	13
16	18	18	18	17	17	17	17	17	16	16	16	16	16	16	15	15	15	14	14	14	14
17	19	19	19	18	18	18	18	18	17	17	17	17	17	16	16	16	16	15	15	15	15
18	20	20	20	19	19	19	19	19	18	18	18	18	18	17	17	17	17	16	16	16	16

NOTE: Initial letter P. Education adjustment applying the following formula: $NSS_{A\&E} = NSS_A - (\beta \times [Education_{(years)} - 12])$, where $\beta = 0.22078$.

SOURCE: Pena-Casanova et al. (2009).

EVIDENCE FOR INTERRATER RELIABILITY

Interrater reliability is excellent for various scores ($r \geq .90$). For example, studies have examined CFL ($r = .99$; Ross, 2003; $r = .99$ Rosselli et al., 2009); clustering and switching ($r > .95$ Ross, 2003; Rosselli et al., 2009); letters M, R, and P; and animals ($r > .98$; Cavaco et al., 2013). When a variety of scoring systems were examined, all indices yielded r_{icc} coefficients of .90 or greater (Ross et al., 2007). See also Abwender et al. (2001), and Troyer et al. (1997). In terms of written fluency, an interrater reliability of .98 was observed in university students (Cohen & Stanczak, 2000).

EVIDENCE FOR VALIDITY

CORRELATIONS AMONG FLUENCY TESTS

Correlations between phonemic fluency tasks (e.g., FAS, CFL) are high across studies of different clinical groups (e.g., *rs* ≥ .85; Cohen & Stanczak, 2000; Troyer, 2000). Other letter sets also appear highly correlated (e.g., FAS and BHR, $r = .83$; Delis et al., 2001; CFL and PRW, $r = .82$; Benton et al., 1994), as are written word fluency and phonemic fluency (FAS and CFL/PRW; $r = .72$ and .81, respectively; Cohen & Stanczak, 2000).

TABLE 9–160M Education Adjustment for Letter "M" Spanish Verbal Fluency

	EDUCATION (YEARS)																				
NSS_A	0	1	2	3	4	5	6	7	8	9	10	11	12	13	14	15	16	17	18	19	20
2	4	4	4	4	3	3	3	3	2	2	2	2	2	1	1	1	1	0	0	0	0
3	5	5	5	5	4	4	4	4	3	3	3	3	3	2	2	2	2	1	1	1	1
4	6	6	6	6	5	5	5	5	4	4	4	4	4	3	3	3	3	2	2	2	2
5	7	7	7	7	6	6	6	6	5	5	5	5	5	4	4	4	4	3	3	3	3
6	8	8	8	8	7	7	7	7	6	6	6	6	6	5	5	5	5	4	4	4	4
7	9	9	9	9	8	8	8	8	7	7	7	7	7	6	6	6	6	5	5	5	5
8	10	10	10	10	9	9	9	9	8	8	8	8	8	7	7	7	7	6	6	6	6
9	11	11	11	11	10	10	10	10	9	9	9	9	9	8	8	8	8	7	7	7	7
10	12	12	12	12	11	11	11	11	10	10	10	10	10	9	9	9	9	8	8	8	8
11	13	13	13	13	12	12	12	12	11	11	11	11	11	10	10	10	10	9	9	9	9
12	14	14	14	14	13	13	13	13	12	12	12	12	12	11	11	11	11	10	10	10	10
13	15	15	15	15	14	14	14	14	13	13	13	13	13	12	12	12	12	11	11	11	11
14	16	16	16	16	15	15	15	15	14	14	14	14	14	13	13	13	13	12	12	12	12
15	17	17	17	17	16	16	16	16	15	15	15	15	15	14	14	14	14	13	13	13	13
16	18	18	18	18	17	17	17	17	16	16	16	16	16	15	15	15	15	14	14	14	14
17	19	19	19	19	18	18	18	18	17	17	17	17	17	16	16	16	16	15	15	15	15
18	20	20	20	20	19	19	19	19	18	18	18	18	18	17	17	17	17	16	16	16	16

NOTE: Initial letter M. Education adjustment applying the following formula: $NSS_{A\&E} = NSS_A - (\beta \times [Education_{(years)} - 12])$, where $\beta = 0.24352$.

SOURCE: Pena-Casanova et al. (2009).

TABLE 9–160N Education Adjustment for Letter "R" Spanish Verbal Fluency

	EDUCATION (YEARS)																				
NSS_A	0	1	2	3	4	5	6	7	8	9	10	11	12	13	14	15	16	17	18	19	20
2	4	4	4	4	3	3	3	3	2	2	2	2	2	1	1	1	1	0	0	0	0
3	5	5	5	5	4	4	4	4	3	3	3	3	3	2	2	2	2	1	1	1	1
4	6	6	6	6	5	5	5	5	4	4	4	4	4	3	3	3	3	2	2	2	2
5	7	7	7	7	6	6	6	6	5	5	5	5	5	4	4	4	4	3	3	3	3
6	8	8	8	8	7	7	7	7	6	6	6	6	6	5	5	5	5	4	4	4	4
7	9	9	9	9	8	8	8	8	7	7	7	7	7	6	6	6	6	5	5	5	5
8	10	10	10	10	9	9	9	9	8	8	8	8	8	7	7	7	7	6	6	6	6
9	11	11	11	11	10	10	10	10	9	9	9	9	9	8	8	8	8	7	7	7	7
10	12	12	12	12	11	11	11	11	10	10	10	10	10	9	9	9	9	8	8	8	8
11	13	13	13	13	12	12	12	12	11	11	11	11	11	10	10	10	10	9	9	9	9
12	14	14	14	14	13	13	13	13	12	12	12	12	12	11	11	11	11	10	10	10	10
13	15	15	15	15	14	14	14	14	13	13	13	13	13	12	12	12	12	11	11	11	11
14	16	16	16	16	15	15	15	15	14	14	14	14	14	13	13	13	13	12	12	12	12
15	17	17	17	17	16	16	16	16	15	15	15	15	15	14	14	14	14	13	13	13	13
16	18	18	18	18	17	17	17	17	16	16	16	16	16	15	15	15	15	14	14	14	14
17	19	19	19	19	18	18	18	18	17	17	17	17	17	16	16	16	16	15	15	15	15
18	20	20	20	20	19	19	19	19	18	18	18	18	18	17	17	17	17	16	16	16	16

NOTE: Initial letter R. Education adjustment applying the following formula: $NSS_{A\&E} = NSS_A - (\beta \times [Education_{(years)} - 12])$, where $\beta = 0.24088$.

SOURCE: Pena-Casanova et al. (2009).

Similarly, normative data suggest that differences between the letter sets appear to be small (see Ross et al., 2006; Troyer, 2000; see "Normative Data"). However, in their meta-analysis, Barry, Bates, and Labouvie (2008) compared FAS and CFL forms of verbal fluency. The CFL form resulted in worse performance than FAS (small effect size) and was affected by age, education (large effect size), and sample characteristics (stricter exclusion criteria resulted in more words recalled; medium effect size). Performance on the FAS form was more variable, with age and study year (less variability in older studies) related to performance.

Correlations between forms using different semantic categories (e.g., animals and clothing, animals and foods) are moderately high (Delis et al., 2001). However, the values are not sufficiently high to establish equivalency among forms. Note, too, that demographic influences may differentially impact various categories (e.g., see "Demographic Effects"). Correlations within phonemic and semantic fluency tasks show higher indices of association than those between these

TABLE 9–160O Gender Adjustment for Kitchen Tools Spanish Verbal Fluency

	$NSS_{A\&E}$	
NSS_A	MEN	WOMEN
2	2	0
3	3	1
4	4	2
5	5	3
6	6	4
7	7	5
8	8	6
9	9	7
10	10	8
11	11	9
12	12	10
13	13	11
14	14	12
15	15	13
16	16	14
17	17	15
18	18	16

NOTE: Kitchen tools: sex adjustments formula: $NSS_{A\&E} = NSS_A - (\gamma \times sex)$, where $\gamma = 1.74961$, men = 0, and women = 1.

SOURCE: Pena-Casanova et al. (2009).

TABLE 9–160P Gender Adjustment for Fruits and Vegetables Spanish Verbal Fluency

	$NSS_{A\&E}$	
NSS_A	MEN	WOMEN
2	2	0
3	3	1
4	4	2
5	5	3
6	6	4
7	7	5
8	8	6
9	9	7
10	10	8
11	11	9
12	12	10
13	13	11
14	14	12
15	15	13
16	16	14
17	17	15
18	18	16

NOTE: Fruits and Vegetables: sex adjustments formula: $NSS_{A\&E} = NSS_A - (\gamma \times sex)$, where $\gamma = 1.24574$, men = 0, and women = 1.

SOURCE: Pena-Casanova et al. (2009).

TABLE 9–161A Algorithms for Age and Education Adjustments of Raw Scores for Portuguese Verbal Fluency

Semantic fluency	(raw score – 11.3984 – (age * 0.0795) + (age² * 0.0014) – (education * 0.8008) + (education² * 0.0165))/4.1399
Phonemic fluency	
M	(raw score – 2.5878 – (age × 0.0858) + (age² × 0.0009) – (education × 0.7495) + (education² × 0.0133))/3.6498
R	(raw score – 2.0379 – (age × 0.0817) + (age² × 0.0007) – (education × 0.7555) + (education² × 0.0150))/3.6089
P	(raw score – 2.2708 – (age × 0.0409) + (age² × 0.0002) – (education × 1.0408) + (education² × 0.0275))/3.9190
Total score	(raw score – 6.8965 – (age × 0.2084) + (age² × 0.0019) – (education × 2.5458) + (education² × 0.0558))/9.7035

SOURCE: Cavaco et al. (2013).

two types of tests. Phonemic fluency (e.g., FAS) scores correlate moderately ($rs = .34$ to $.64$) with semantic fluency (e.g., animals, foods; Kave, 2005; Kosmidis et al., 2004; Johnson-Selfridge et al., 1998; Tombaugh et al., 1999).

FACTOR-ANALYTIC STUDIES

Factor analyses suggest that attentional control and working memory play an important role in performance. Consistent with these findings, individuals who score high on a measure of working memory capacity generate more animal names than individuals who score low on the same measure (Rosen & Engle, 1997). Egeland et al. (2006) reported that a factor analysis of a number of neuropsychological tests with a mixed clinical sample yielded a three-factor solution accounting for nearly 62% of the variance. Phonemic fluency loaded with the PASAT, Stroop Interference, Dichotic Listening (Forced Left), and Similarities. The second factor representing processing speed explained nearly 24% of the variance, with highest loadings of semantic word fluency, Stroop Word Reading, and a simple reaction time measure.

Processing speed is also important for performance. A factor analysis of FAS and other tests in psychiatric patients and controls (Boone et al., 1998) suggested that FAS loaded on a speeded processing factor along with the Stroop and the Wechsler Digit Symbol subtest (see also Egeland et al., 2006). Greenaway et al. (2009) subjected the expanded MOANS cognitive battery to a factor analysis, finding that phonemic and semantic fluency loaded on a processing speed factor along with the WAIS-III Symbol Search subtest in a five-factor solution. Individual differences in speed of processing are related to fluency performance, with lower scores on fluency tasks associated with slower processing speed. Notably, aging-related effects in fluency performance appear to not be mediated entirely by declines in speed (Ratcliff et al., 2003; Sliwinski & Buschke, 1999).

Verbal Ability and IQ. Verbal fluency measures have a substantial verbal component. In fact, phonemic fluency was initially developed as a measure of VIQ (Thurstone, 1938). Not surprisingly, correlations between $r = .44$ and $r = .87$ have been reported between phonemic fluency and the VIQ (see Henry & Crawford, 2004a, for a review; although see Tomabaugh et al., 1999, who reported modest correlations). Phonemic fluency shows a somewhat stronger relationship to VIQ than PIQ (Steinberg et al., 2005). A closer relationship exists between naming

TABLE 9–161B Percentile Ranks for Age and Education Adjusted Scores for Portuguese Verbal Fluency

		ADJUSTED SCORES				
			PHONEMIC FLUENCY			
PERCENTILE RANKS	SCALED SCORES	SEMANTIC FLUENCY: ANIMALS	M	R	P	TOTAL SCORE
1	3	−1.9	−2.2	−2.2	−2.2	−2.2
2	4	−1.8	−2.0	−1.9	−2.0	−1.9
3–5	5	−1.6 to −1.5	−1.8 to 1.5	−1.8 to −1.6	−1.8 to −1.6	−1.7 to −1.6
6–10	6	−1.4 to −1.3	−1.5 to −1.2	−1.6 to −1.3	−1.5 to −1.3	−1.5 to −1.2
11–18	7	−1.2 to −0.9	−1.2 to −0.9	−1.2 to −1.0	−1.2 to −1.0	−1.2 to −0.9
19–28	8	−0.9 to −0.6	−0.9 to −0.6	−0.9 to −0.6	−1.0 to −0.6	−0.9 to −0.6
29–40	9	−0.6 to −0.3	−0.6 to −0.3	−0.6 to −0.3	−0.6 to −0.3	−0.6 to −0.3
41–59	10	−0.2 to 0.2	−0.3 to 0.1	−0.3 to 0.2	−0.3 to 0.2	−0.3 to −0.2
60–71	11	0.2–0.5	0.3–0.5	0.2–0.5	0.2–0.5	−0.2–0.6
72–81	12	0.6–0.8	0.5–0.9	0.6–0.9	0.5–0.9	0.6–0.9
82–89	13	0.9–1.2	1.0–1.3	0.9–1.2	0.9–1.3	0.9–1.3
90–94	14	1.3–1.7	1.3–1.6	1.3–1.5	1.3–1.6	1.3–1.6
95–97	15	1.8–2.0	1.7–2.0	1.6–1.9	1.7–1.9	1.7–1.9
98	16	2.3	2.1	2.1	2.1	2.2
99	17	2.8	2.4	2.4	2.4	2.3
Minimum		−2.3	−2.9	−2.7	−2.7	−2.9
Maximum		4.2	3.5	3.1	3.1	3.8

SOURCE: Cavaco et al. (2013).

TABLE 9–162 Normative Data for Dutch Semantic Fluency (Animals) by Age and Education

			MALE & FEMALE											
			AGE IN YEARS											
	Z VALUE	CUM. PROB.	25	30	35	40	45	50	55	60	65	70	75	80
LE low	1.64	.95	33.9	33.4	32.9	32.5	32.0	31.5	31.0	30.5	30.0	29.6	29.1	28.6
	1.28	.90	31.8	31.3	30.9	30.4	29.9	29.4	28.9	28.4	28.0	27.5	27.0	26.5
	0.84	.80	29.3	28.8	28.3	27.8	27.3	26.9	26.4	25.9	25.4	24.9	24.4	23.9
	0	.50	24.4	23.9	23.4	23.0	22.5	22.0	21.5	21.0	20.5	20.0	19.6	19.1
	−0.84	.20	19.5	19.1	18.6	18.1	17.6	17.1	16.6	16.1	15.7	15.2	14.7	14.2
	−1.28	.10	17.0	16.5	16.0	15.5	15.1	14.6	14.1	13.6	13.1	12.6	12.1	11.7
	−1.64	.05	14.9	14.4	13.9	13.4	13.0	12.5	12.0	11.5	11.0	10.5	10.1	9.6
LE average	1.64	.95	36.7	36.2	35.7	35.3	34.8	34.3	33.8	33.3	32.8	32.3	31.9	31.4
	1.28	.90	34.6	34.1	33.7	33.2	32.7	32.2	31.7	31.2	30.7	30.3	29.8	29.3
	0.84	.80	32.1	31.6	31.1	30.6	30.1	29.6	29.2	28.7	28.2	27.7	27.2	26.7
	0	.50	27.2	26.7	26.2	25.7	25.3	24.8	24.3	23.8	23.3	22.8	22.4	21.9
	−0.84	.20	22.3	21.8	21.4	20.9	20.4	19.9	19.4	18.9	18.5	18.0	17.5	17.0
	−1.28	.10	19.8	19.3	18.8	18.3	17.8	17.4	16.9	16.4	15.9	15.4	14.9	14.4
	−1.64	.05	17.7	17.2	16.7	16.2	15.8	15.3	14.8	14.3	13.8	13.3	12.8	12.4
LE high	1.64	.95	38.3	37.8	37.3	36.8	36.4	35.9	35.4	34.9	34.4	33.9	33.4	33.0
	1.28	.90	36.2	35.7	35.2	34.8	34.3	33.8	33.3	32.8	32.3	31.8	31.4	30.9
	0.84	.80	33.7	33.2	32.7	32.2	31.7	31.2	30.7	30.3	29.8	29.3	28.8	28.3
	0	.50	28.8	28.3	27.8	27.3	26.8	26.4	25.9	25.4	24.9	24.4	23.9	23.5
	−0.84	.20	23.9	23.4	22.9	22.5	22.0	21.5	21.0	20.5	20.0	19.6	19.1	18.6
	−1.28	.10	21.4	20.9	20.4	19.9	19.4	18.9	18.5	18.0	17.5	17.0	16.5	16.0
	−1.64	.05	19.3	18.8	18.3	17.8	17.3	16.9	16.4	15.9	15 4	14.9	14.4	13.9

NOTE: LE, Level of education; Cum. prob., cumulative probability.
SOURCE: Van der Elst et al. (2006).

(Boston Naming Test) and semantic fluency than between naming and phonemic fluency (Henry et al., 2004).

Intellectual function is related to both phonemic and semantic fluency (Diaz-Asper et al., 2004). The magnitude of the relationship tends to be moderate to large using Wechsler IQ tests (Harrison et al., 2000; Wood & Liossi, 2007). Some research has suggested that IQ shows a stronger relationship to phonemic fluency than does education, and the association becomes stronger as IQ increases (Steinberg et al., 2005). Correlations between the NART

TABLE 9–163 Summary of Additional Normative Studies

REFERENCE	TYPE OF FLUENCY TEST	SAMPLE SIZE	SAMPLE CHARACTERISTICS
Costa et al. (2014)	Phonemic (FAS), Semantic (colors, animals, fruit), novel alternating fluency task	335	20- to 90-year-olds (Italian)
Egeland et al. (2006)	Phonemic (FAS), Semantic (clothes, animals)	156	16- to 77-year-olds (Norwegian)
Elkadi et al. (2006)	Semantic (animals)	257	65- to 67-year-old women (Australian)
Fine et al. (2012)	Phonemic ('F'), Semantic (vegetables)	680	85- to 95-year-old women
Gonzalez et al. (2005)	Semantic (animals with four legs)	1276	English- and Spanish-speaking Mexican Americans 50 years old and older
Heaps et al. (2013)	Semantic (animals, first names)	477, 236	Thai, US
Khalil (2010)	Phonemic (three Arabic letters), Semantic (animals)	215	18- to 59-year-old Arabic speakers
Lovell and Solomon (2011)	Phonemic	513	Professional football athletes (US)
Roselli et al. (2009)	Semantic (animals, fruit, vegetables, clothing)	105	Hispanic-speakers 55 to 98 years old
Zarino et al. (2014)	Semantic (animals, fruit, vehicles)	290	18- to 98-year-olds (Italian)
Zimmerman et al. (2014)	Phonemic ('P'), Semantic (clothing), unconstrained fluency	300	19- to 75-year-olds (Brazilian)

TABLE 9–164 Corrections, Demographically Corrected Descriptive Data, and Percentiles for Fluency Scores

	PHONEMIC (FAS OR CFL)			ANIMALS		
	CLUSTER	SWITCHES	TOTAL	CLUSTER	SWITCHES	TOTAL
Age (years)	–0.001	+0.05	+0.04	–0.002	+0.05	+0.09
Ed (years)	–0.015	–0.38	–1.06	–0.023	–0.17	–0.51
Form (FAS)	+0.094	–2.67	–2.18	NA	NA	NA
Mean	0.24	23.9	28.6	0.75	9.8	18.1
SD	0.23	8.2	11.1	0.57	2.7	4.6
1st percentile	–0.16	6.6	4.3	–0.24	3.9	8.3
5th percentile	–0.06	10.2	11.4	0.01	5.8	10.9
16th percentile	0.01	15.6	17.0	0.23	7.3	13.5
25th percentile	0.08	18.7	20.6	0.40	7.9	14.9
50th percentile	0.19	23.3	28.7	0.64	9.6	17.9
75th percentile	0.35	29.7	36.6	1.12	11.6	21.2
84th percentile	0.44	32.3	39.3	1.39	12.4	22.8
95th percentile	0.73	37.6	47.6	1.89	14.7	26.7
99th percentile	0.97	43.2	57.4	2.43	16.7	29.3

NOTE: Based on a sample 411 healthy community-dwelling adults, aged 18 to 91 years (M = 59.8, SD = 20.7), and level of education ranging from 5 to 21 years (M = 13.9, SD = 2.9).

SOURCE: Troyer (2000).

and both types of fluency have also been reported and are generally moderate to large in magnitude (e.g., Bird et al., 2004; Crawford et al., 1992; Knight et al.; 2006; Ross, 2003). Crawford et al. (1992) suggested that expected scores in phonemic fluency could be predicted on the basis of NART scores (see Figure 9–16).

Crawford et al. (1992) compared a healthy group of participants with a neurologic group, demonstrating accurate differentiation when expected fluency scores were used. Information to convert NART errors to predicted FAS scores is presented in their paper. Users should keep in mind that the data are based on a study with the British NART and healthy British participants.

Other research has also been completed to predict fluency performance on the basis of general measures of cognition. Tallberg et al. (2008) reported that intellectual level was a significant predictor of FAS, animal fluency, and verb fluency. Formulas are provided in their paper that use an estimate of premorbid intelligence based on Swedish tests of premorbid intelligence, analogous to the NAART, as well as a lexical decision test.

CORRELATIONS WITH OTHER NEUROPSYCHOLOGICAL DOMAINS

Verbal fluency scores need to be interpreted within the context of processing speed (see also Salthouse et al., 2003) but memory contributes to performance. In a sample of people who sustained a stroke and were in the acute stage in an inpatient rehabilitation unit, phonemic fluency showed large correlations with the Language-Verbal Memory factor of the RBANS (r = .65), as well as moderate correlations with a memory factor (r = .30; Wilde, 2006). The COWAT also shows some moderate correlations with memory subtests from the CANTAB (Smith et al., 2013). However, there are reports of patients with dense amnesia who can perform at average or above-average levels on verbal fluency (Dall'Ora et al., 1989), indicating that such tests can be performed adequately despite the presence of severe episodic memory deficits.

CLINICAL STUDIES

Dementia. There is evidence that semantic fluency in particular is useful in the detection of dementia. The inclusion of verbal fluency measures has been recommended to increase the sensitivity of tests such as the MMSE (see MMSE review elsewhere in this volume). Biological correlates of fluency performance in AD have also been reported. For example, the degree of amyloid beta deposition was correlated with semantic fluency and performance on other cognitive tests in the oldest-old (average age 85 years; Snitz et al., 2013). Cosentino, Scarmeas, Albert, and Stern (2006) reported that higher verbal fluency (semantic and phonemic) at diagnosis of AD was associated with lower risk of mortality.

TABLE 9–165A FAS Change Scores, Standard Deviations (*SD*), and Reliability Coefficients

MEASURE	T1 MEAN	*SD*	T2 MEAN	*SD*	T2–T1	*SD*	R	P	COHEN'S D
FAS	45.0	11.89	48.1	11.43	3.08	7.94	.77	.001	.26

NOTE: Based on a sample of 145 well-educated men (education, M = 16.4, SD = 2.3), mostly Caucasian (age, M = 38.8, SD = 7.9), mean retest interval of 191 days.

SOURCE: Adapted from Levine et al. (2004).

TABLE 9–165B Regression Equations for Estimating Retest Scores

MEASURE	REGRESSION EQUATION	RESIDUAL *SD*
FAS	14.84 + (.739 × Time 1 score)	7.31

SOURCE: Adapted from Levine et al. (2004).

Semantic fluency has specifically been identified as a useful tool to screen for AD in patients, even those with lower literacy levels. Caramelli, Carthery-Goulart, Porto, Charchat-Fichman, and Nitrini (2007) identify semantic fluency (animals/minute) as an effective screening tool for AD across a range of education levels (illiterate to ≥8 years). Based on optimal sensitivity and specificity values, cutoff points were identified for each group, with high sensitivity and specificity values (83 to 95% and 80 to 100%, respectively) at different cutoffs for differing literacy levels. Similarly, semantic fluency was recommended as an instrument to routinely screen older individuals with low levels of education in primary care in Brazil, showing good specificity when used along with a functional activities questionnaire (Jacinto et al., 2014).

A number of studies have reported that discrepancies between phonemic and semantic fluency may be useful for the early detection of dementia and for distinguishing between cortical and subcortical dementias. In patients with AD, a common finding is that semantic fluency tends to be more affected than phonemic fluency (Henry & Crawford, 2004c; Henry et al., 2004; Monsch et al., 1994), reflecting disorganization or degradation in semantic knowledge. Some research indicates that semantic fluency is 20 times more likely to be impaired in AD than in healthy people (sensitivity 88%, specificity 96%; Cahn et al., 2004). Semantic fluency was noted to improve following addition of memantine to a rivastigmine regimen in patients with mild to moderate AD (Riepe et al., 2007).

However, some research has suggested that discrepancies between semantic and phonemic fluency have limited diagnostic utility (e.g., Sherman & Massman, 1999). In a meta-analysis, the effect sizes of semantic and phonemic discrepancies did not differ between persons with AD and controls in approximately 35% of the included studies (Laws et al., 2010). Effect sizes were large, specifically for semantic fluency (Cohen's $d = 2.10$), but also for phonemic fluency (Cohen's $d = 1.46$).

TABLE 9–166 Animal Fluency Test-Retest Reliability, Practice Effects, and Reliable Change Indices Corrected for Practice

TEST	N	R	MEAN T1 (*SD*)	MEAN T2 (*SD*)	LOWER RCI	UPPER RCI
Animals	99	.56	23.4 (5.1)	24.7 (6.3)	−7.6	+10.5

NOTE: Based on a sample of 99 healthy people, aged 39–75 years (*M* = 57.0 years, *SD* = 8.3) and 13.1 years of education (*SD* = 3.7). Retest interval was one month. RCIs are based on a 90% confidence interval.

SOURCE: Adapted from Bird et al. (2004).

The role of verbal fluency in differentiation of dementia subtypes has also been examined, with mixed results. In comparison of autopsy-confirmed cases of FTD and AD, people with AD performed worse than patients with FTD (Liscic et al., 2007). People with semantic dementia had worse scores on semantic fluency compared to phonemic fluency than in other dementias (Rogers et al., 2006). Phonemic fluency differentiated vascular dementia from AD with poor sensitivity and high specificity (sensitivity 44%, specificity 90%; Canning et al., 2004). Higher phonemic fluency scores were associated with somewhat increased odds of developing AD rather than vascular dementia in a Canadian longitudinal study (odds ratio [OR] = 1.21; Brewster et al., 2012).

Fine-grained analyses of task structure of verbal fluency have been conducted in AD. Behforuzi, Burtis, Williamson, Stamps, and Heilman (2013) reported that people with AD produced fewer words beginning with "A" than "F" and "S." The authors propose that this finding may reflect the initial vulnerability of the weakest semantic representational networks in AD (i.e., words beginning with "A," which are less frequent than words beginning with "F" or "S"). This proposal is supported by additional research. Foster et al. (2012) reported that patients with AD produced words with a higher average word frequency on semantic fluency compared to phonemic fluency. Furthermore, patients treated via acetylcholinesterase inhibitors had higher word frequency than people not taking the medication (Foster et al., 2012). Pakhomov, Hemmy, and Lim (2012) presented a means of computationally quantifying the degree of semantic similarity between words on a semantic fluency measure. The authors reported significant differences between semantically adjacent words at differing levels of severity (i.e., probable and possible AD, MCI).

MCI. In addition to findings suggesting differences between MCI and controls (Economou et al., 2007; Nutter-Upham et al., 2008), verbal fluency measures, especially semantic fluency, have also shown utility in predicting progression from MCI to dementia (Molinuevo et al., 2011). Silva et al. (2013) reported that semantic fluency was one of the measures that best differentiated persons who progressed to AD at five-year follow-up. Gallagher et al. (2010) reported that semantic fluency, combined with a delayed recall test, was associated with a diagnostic accuracy rate of 83% in predicting conversion from MCI to AD. A majority of people who converted from MCI to AD were identified from a combination of atrophy in the left temporal cortex and impaired scores on semantic fluency and a paired associates test. Phonemic fluency (number of errors) was one of the measures that best differentiated healthy controls from individuals who progressed to AD (Schmid et al., 2013).

TABLE 9–167 Verbal Fluency Test-Retest Effects in 81 Healthy Individuals Assessed Following Intervals of About 11 Months for FAS and BDT

	TIME 1 (1)		TIME 2 (2)		(3)	T2–T1 (4)	(5)	(6)	T1, T2 (7)
MEASURE	M	(*SD*)	M	(*SD*)	M	(*SD*)	P	|T2–T1|/*SD*(T1)	R
Letter Fluency	43.25	10.75	44.47	10.36	1.22	7.85	.165	.11	.72

NOTE: Tests administered in a counterbalanced order. The mean age of the sample was about 29 years, the mean education of the sample was about 12 years.
SOURCE: Adapted from Dikmen et al. (1999).

PD. Elgh et al. (2009) reported semantic fluency deficits in patients with PD, and semantic fluency has been identified as one of the most powerful predictors of cognitive decline in patients with PD (Williams-Gray et al., 2007). Meta-analytic findings suggest that patients with PD have comparatively poorer performance on semantic relative to phonemic fluency, although in patients with AD, the relative deficit in semantic fluency appears more pronounced (Henry & Crawford, 2004c; Henry et al., 2004). Functional ability is also associated with fluency in patients with PD (Sabbagh et al., 2007).

HD. Patients with HD appear to experience comparable deficits in semantic and phonemic fluency (Henry et al., 2005), and Arango-Lasprilla et al. (2006) reported that verbal fluency (letter and animal) was the only measure in a neuropsychological battery that differentiated patients with HD from patients with AD.

TBI. A meta-analysis of patients with TBI (Henry & Crawford, 2004b) reported that TBI patients were comparably impaired on tests of phonemic and semantic fluency. The phonemic fluency deficit could not be accounted for by patients' level of premorbid or current level of VIQ and was also in excess of deficits on a measure of psychomotor speed (TMT-A). Phonemic fluency was also significantly more sensitive to the presence of TBI than was the WCST. Phonemic fluency is also sensitive to the severity of TBI (Iverson et al., 1999).

Zakzanis, McDonald, and Troyer (2013) reported that cluster and switching scores for semantic fluency yielded large effect sizes differentiating between severe TBI and control groups (Cohen's $d = 1.32, 1.53$). Total words produced yielded the largest effect size for phonemic fluency (Cohen's $d = .62$). Large effect sizes were obtained for the number of switches and cluster size on semantic fluency.

Epilepsy. Buckley, Fitzgerald, Hoerold, Davey, and Doherty (2010) reported that patients with epilepsy taking topiramate performed worse than patients taking lamotrigine in a double-blind, randomized, prospective study, with others reporting that patients taking lamotrigine had better performance on phonemic fluency than patients taking carbamazepine (Lee et al., 2011). Drug withdrawal in epilepsy is also related to improved fluency performance (Hessen et al., 2007, 2009). A high presurgical verbal fluency score, language dominant hemisphere surgery, and poor seizure outcome are factors that increase the risk of verbal fluency decline following frontal lobe resection for epilepsy (Sarkis et al., 2013).

HIV and AIDS. Verbal fluency is affected by AIDS dementia complex according to a meta-analytic study, with a large effect size reported (Cysique et al., 2006). A small effect size has been reported in HIV infection, without significant discrepancy between phonemic and semantic fluency (Iudicello et al., 2007). Verbal fluency was identified as one of two measures (along with the TMT) that showed the highest sensitivity (nearly 75%) and specificity (nearly 82%) in detecting neurocognitive impairment in HIV (Muñoz-Moreno et al., 2013). Iudicello et al. (2008) reported that HIV-related deficits in semantic fluency are related to an impairment in switching.

Psychiatric Conditions. Overall, relatively greater impairment is reported in semantic fluency compared to phonemic fluency in schizophrenia. In their meta-analysis of longitudinal studies in schizophrenia, Szöke et al. (2008) identified semantic fluency as the best candidate cognitive endophenotype for schizophrenia, due to stability over time and degree of impairment noted. Impairment in semantic fluency may be related to degradation in semantic retrieval or semantic stores, although the exact mechanism is unclear.

A meta-analysis of studies comparing the performance of people with schizophrenia and healthy controls on tests of fluency suggested that patients with schizophrenia were

Predicted WF = 57.5 – 0.76 × NART errors, SE_E = 9.09; also see https://homepages.abdn.ac.uk/j.crawford/pages/dept/psychom.htm

Figure 9–16 National Adult Reading Test (NART)-predicted FAS score.
SOURCE: Crawford et al. (1992).

significantly more impaired on semantic relative to phonemic fluency (Henry & Crawford, 2005b). Neither phonemic or semantic fluency deficits constituted differential deficits relative to intelligence or psychomotor speed, and Henry and Crawford (2005b) concluded that deficits on tests of verbal fluency reflect a more generalized intellectual impairment and not particular deficits in executive control processes. Furthermore, they suggested that the larger deficit for semantic relative to phonemic fluency suggests that, in addition to general retrieval difficulties, schizophrenia is associated with compromises to the semantic store. This explanation is not reflected uniformly in research in the area (e.g., Doughty & Done, 2009), with some suggesting the impairment in schizophrenia reflects an underlying deficit of automatic activation of semantic information (Sung et al., 2012).

Several other meta-analyses have been conducted showing impaired verbal fluency in schizophrenia (e.g., Bora, Binnur Akdede, & Alptekin, 2017). In their meta-analysis focused on the relationship between cognition and age of onset of schizophrenia, Rajji, Ismail, and Mulsant (2009) compared cognition in youth-onset, late-onset, and adults with first-episode schizophrenia. All groups showed large effect sizes on fluency measures (Cohen's *d* from .83 to 1.53); those with late-onset schizophrenia demonstrated relatively larger deficits on fluency than other groups. In their meta-analysis, Bora, Yücel, and Pantelis (2010) reported deficits in semantic fluency (large effect size) in patients with affective psychoses, which included studies of people with depression and bipolar disorder. The authors also reported relatively greater impairment in individuals with bipolar disorder with psychosis compared to those without (Bora, Yücel, Pantelis, 2009). Neill, Gurvich, and Rossell (2014) found that semantic memory was a relatively larger contributor to semantic fluency deficits in schizophrenia than executive deficits.

Verbal fluency may have utility in informing progression to psychosis in at-risk populations. In their meta-analysis, Fusar-Poli et al. (2012) reported that people at high risk for psychosis were impaired on verbal fluency, with subsequent development of psychosis related to deficits in verbal fluency. Not only does decreased semantic fluency predict development of psychosis in high-risk patients (Becker et al., 2010), but Meijer et al. (2011) reported a correlation between semantic fluency scores and decreased gray matter density in the right superior and middle temporal gyrus, the right insula, and the left anterior cingulate cortex in a group who converted to psychosis.

In their meta-analysis of cognitive deficits in unaffected relatives of people with schizophrenia, Snitz, MacDonald, and Carter (2006) reported that category fluency yielded an effect size that was almost large in magnitude (Cohen's $d = .68$). The magnitude of this effect was attenuated when studies with age and psychiatric exclusion confounds (e.g., lack of matching) were excluded. In their meta-analysis of cognitive deficits in first-degree relatives of people with schizophrenia, Szöke et al. (2005) described medium to large effect sizes for fluency tests (0.65 for phonological and 0.87 for semantic).

Meta-analyses have been conducted on the effects of treatment in schizophrenia on verbal fluency. In their meta-analysis of cognitive effects of treatment in schizophrenia (i.e., clozapine, olanzapine, quetiapine, and risperidone), Woodward, Purdon, Meltzer and Zald (2007) reported that after excluding uncontrolled studies, quetiapine was associated with more improvement than risperidone and olanzapine, with effect sizes attenuated when random assignment or double-blind studies were considered. In their meta-analysis of treatment with haloperidol, Woodward, Purdon, Meltzer, and Zald (2007) reported that haloperidol was not associated with changes in verbal fluency.

Finally, fluency may have value as a brief screening measure. Hurford, Marder, Keefe, Reise, and Bilder (2011) reported that a composite score comprised of the TMT-B, semantic fluency, and Digit Symbol demonstrated strong correlations ($r = .86$) with a larger battery of tests in schizophrenia.

Depression has an impact on fluency, with lower levels of distress associated with higher fluency scores. A meta-analysis (Lim et al., 2013) reported that fluency was significantly worse among those with depression compared to healthy controls, with deficits persisting at remission after a first episode of depression (Ahern & Semkovska, 2017).

Another meta-analysis of 42 studies that included 2,206 participants (Henry & Crawford, 2005a) concluded that both phonemic and semantic fluency are broadly equivalent in sensitivity to depression and that neither qualified as a differential deficit relative to psychomotor speed. Thus, for patients with depression, low scores on these fluency tasks may not reflect executive dysfunction or a degraded semantic store, but a more generalized impairment, such as cognitive slowing. Similarly, patients with depression who did not respond to fluoxetine had worse fluency scores, thought to be secondary to psychomotor slowing (Taylor et al., 2006). Verbal fluency is also more impaired in depressed individuals treated with electroconvulsive therapy (ECT) compared to transcranial magnetic stimulation (TMS; Ren et al., 2014). However, note that in a normative study of women in midlife, no relationship was found between a rating scale of depression and semantic fluency (Elkadi et al., 2006).

Several meta-analyses have been conducted regarding verbal fluency in bipolar disorder, finding moderate (Raucher-Chéné, Achim, Kaladjian, & Besche-Richard, 2017) to large effect sizes (Arts et al., 2008; Robinson et al., 2006), with smaller effect sizes for unaffected first-degree relatives. A meta-analysis suggested that people with bipolar disorder I performed worse than people with bipolar disorder II on semantic fluency (Cohen's $d = .35$; Bora, Yücel, Pantelis, & Berk, 2011). In a meta-analytic review,

Kertz and Gerraty (2009) reported that bipolar patients in a depressed state demonstrated relatively greater difficulty with fluency (large effect size) than those in other phases (moderate to large effect sizes overall).

In their meta-analysis of cognitive function in OCD, Shin, Lee, Kim, and Kwon (2014) reported that verbal fluency impairments were small to medium in effect size. Henry's (2006) meta-analysis concluded that fluency deficits in OCD may be related to generalized cognitive impairment. Hwang et al. (2007) reported that late-onset OCD patients (onset age ≥21 years) had worse phonemic and semantic fluency than early-onset OCD patients and controls.

Other Populations. Verbal fluency has been included in research on cognitive function in a number of populations, including aphasia (Sarno et al., 2005), chronic hepatitis (Lieb et al., 2006), and hepatic encephalopathy (Malaguarnera et al., 2011). Impairments have also been reported in substance use disorder, including alcohol use disorders (Stavro et al., 2013) and chronic opioid use (Baldacchino et al., 2012).

In terms of research in MS, verbal fluency, when combined with verbal memory measures, has a sensitivity of 81% and a specificity of 97% in differentiating patients with MS (relapsing-remitting subtype) from demographically matched controls (Negreiros et al., 2008). Among vocational rehabilitation patients with MS, verbal fluency emerges as the only significant predictor of vocational stability (Fraser et al., 2009).

Strategy scores have also shown utility in clinical samples. Lepow et al. (2010) reported that amyotrophic lateral sclerosis patients without cognitive impairment generated fewer clusters and more switches on a phonemic fluency test, with lower clustering on semantic fluency related to increased temporal involvement. Tucha et al. (2005) reported that adults with ADHD produced fewer words than controls and produced fewer switching responses, but did not differ in terms of repetitions or rule violations.

Diagnostic Utility of Clustering/Switching Scores and Error Scores. Traditionally, the number of acceptable responses within the allotted time is used as the main dependent variable on verbal fluency tests. However, fluency measures yield considerable qualitative information as well (e.g., clustering and switching), and examination of the qualitative aspects of the output may help to clarify the nature of poor performance. As discussed in "Scoring," Troyer et al. (1997) proposed that clustering (i.e., contiguous words from the same subcategory) is related to temporal lobe processes such as retrieval from verbal memory, whereas switching (the ability to shift between clusters) implicates frontal processes involving mental flexibility and mental search processes.

Evidence supportive of this proposal includes impaired clustering following temporal lobectomy versus impaired switching in people with left dorsolateral and superior medial frontal lobe lesions (Troyer et al., 1998a) and that switching decreases with advancing age (Kosmidis et al., 2004; Troyer et al., 1997) and conditions that demand divided attention (Troyer et al., 1997). Decreased switching has been observed in a number of clinical groups who have purported involvement of frontal areas as part of the neuropathology of their conditions, including PD (perhaps restricted to those with dementia; Troester et al., 1998; Troyer et al., 1998b), pallidotomy patients (Troester et al., 2002; York et al., 2003), HD (Ho et al., 2002; Rich et al., 1999), MS (Troester et al., 1998), AIDS (Millikin et al., 2004), and schizophrenia (Robert et al., 1998; Zakzanis et al., 2000). See also the sections discussing "TBI," "HIV and AIDS," and "Other Populations."

Despite these findings, the expected relationship between qualitative scores and neuropathological site is not always found (see Epker et al., 1999; Troyer et al., 1998b). It has also been suggested that qualitative fluency variables are of greater utility in individuals with relatively mild cognitive difficulty and in patients with focal lesions, rather than in patients with severe or widespread neuropathology or cognitive impairment. Finally, the precise interpretation of clustering and switching scores remains unresolved, and it has been suggested that switching may be secondary to deficits in general cognitive function or processing speed (Mayr, 2002).

In terms of errors, recurrent perseverations are the most commonly observed type of perseverative error, with greater frequency among individuals with a variety of neurological conditions (see Baldo & Shimamura, 1998, Ho et al., 2002, Suhr & Jones, 1998). Errors are relatively rare in healthy adults (see Azuma, 2004, for a review), and repetitions are the most common type of errors in healthy populations (see Hankee et al., 2013 in "Normative Data").

Written Fluency. Early studies of written word fluency were designed for individuals with frontal lobe disease (e.g., Milner's [1964] examination of the performance of patients with left and right frontal and temporal lobectomies in which she reported the test's sensitivity to left frontal lobe involvement). Patients with frontal lesions perform worse on written fluency than those with nonfrontal lesions, but the test does not differentiate between focal and diffuse lesions (Pendleton et al., 1982). Cohen and Stanczak (2000) reported that a mixed neurologic sample was differentiated from healthy controls with a sensitivity of 97% and specificity of 38%, without accurate delineation of side or site (e.g., anterior, posterior) of damage.

NEUROANATOMICAL CORRELATES AND IMAGING STUDIES

Left frontal lesions often reportedly impair performance on phonemic fluency tasks (e.g., Baldo et al., 2001). Stuss et al. (1998) found that, as a group, left frontal lesions impair phonemic fluency, but not all patients with left frontal pathology are impaired. Stuss et al. examined both phonemic (FAS) and semantic (animals) fluency performance in a sample of 74 adults with restricted brain lesions, finding that patients with lesions of the dorsolateral and/or striatal areas of the left frontal lobe were the most impaired. Superior medial frontal lobe regions of either hemisphere had a moderate impact on performance. Nonfrontal left hemisphere regions also have a role in phonemic fluency, as evidenced by the finding that left parietal lobe lesions were also associated with performance deficits.

Meta-analytic findings suggest that both phonemic and semantic fluency make comparable demands on frontal structures, but semantic fluency is also relatively more dependent on temporal structures (Henry & Crawford, 2004a; Henry et al., 2004). Henry and Crawford (2004a) also note that for frontal, but not nonfrontal patients, phonemic fluency deficits are disproportionately impaired when considered in the context of IQ and psychomotor speed. Thus, the integrity of the semantic system and generalized slowing should also be considered in evaluating fluency performance.

The lesion data are supported by imaging studies in healthy individuals, implicating frontal regions (especially inferior frontal gyrus) and temporal areas. COWAT scores were correlated with gray matter volume in 221 cognitively healthy adults in the left lateral inferior and middle frontal gyri (Newman et al., 2007), and Hirshorn and Thompson-Schill (2006) reported that switching during semantic fluency was associated with activation in the left inferior frontal gyrus. Consistent with fMRI, near-infrared spectroscopy showed that phonemic fluency was associated with prefrontal activation, and semantic fluency with temporal regions (Hatta et al., 2008). In a large normative study, Hankee et al. (2013) reported that total cerebral volume measured via MRI was related to FAS total responses.

Gender may interact with patterns of activation. For example, a differential relationship was found for men compared to women, with phonemic fluency performance related to different regions within the superior longitudinal fasciculus (i.e., fractional anisotropy of temporal regions related to better performance for men and parietal regions related to worse performance in women; Madhavan et al., 2014).

Neuroimaging studies have also been conducted in clinical populations. These studies similarly find associations between semantic fluency and the temporal cortex, and phonemic fluency and the frontal cortex. These studies include voxel-based lesion symptom mapping in left hemisphere stroke (Baldo et al., 2006), relationships between semantic fluency deficits and atrophy of the medial temporal lobe in AD (Venneri et al., 2011), and relationships between phonemic fluency and the left prefrontal cortex in patients with epilepsy (Keller et al., 2009). Relationships have also been found between verbal fluency and broader patterns of activation. For example, relationships are reported between verbal fluency and the parietal lobe in left hemisphere stroke (Baldo et al., 2006), the right ventral striatum and phonemic fluency via diffusion tensor imaging in severe TBI (Shah et al., 2012), white matter tracts in lacunar infarction and white matter hyperintensities (Croall et al., 2017), and the left hippocampus via MRI in patients with epilepsy (Keller et al., 2009). See also "Clinical Studies."

PERFORMANCE VALIDITY

The test shows promise as a performance validity indicator. Johnson, Silverberg, Millis, and Hanks (2012) employed Bayesian model averaging to determine the set of predictors that differentiated between mild TBI patients presenting with and without malingered neurocognitive dysfunction. Use of an equation incorporating the COWAT total score and a measure reflecting change in output over time yielded a 78% correct classification rate, a sensitivity of 67%, and a specificity of 88%. Although other models had similar diagnostic accuracy, they required more time, making the weighted combination more practicable. Others have also found that some response patterns, such as reduced trial difficulty effect, more stable word generation over time, and decreased phonemic clustering, show promise, with an 80% classification rate (Silverberg et al., 2008).

Curtis, Thompson, Greve, and Bianchini (2008) also evaluated the classification accuracy of verbal fluency in detecting malingered neurocognitive dysfunction in TBI. They reported that an education-adjusted FAS total correct T score of less than 32 was associated with a sensitivity of 27% at a 5% false-positive error rate, while an FAS total correct T score of less than 34 was associated with a sensitivity of 36% at a 10% false-positive error rate. Although FAS total correct differentiated between malingered neurocognitive dysfunction and the credible performance group in mild TBI, it did not differentiate between levels of performance validity in moderate to severe brain injury.

Sugarman and Axelrod (2015) reported that semantic fluency was able to differentiate between credible and noncredible performance groups in a veteran sample with 90% specificity and 40% or greater sensitivity, with poorer sensitivity for phonemic fluency. Combining both types of fluency into a regression model yielded 90% specificity and greater than 44% sensitivity. The best performing variable was the Animals raw score cutoff of less than 13, which was associated with 90% specificity and 50% sensitivity.

COMMENT

Verbal fluency has a long history in neuropsychology and remains widely used. Likely due its history, popularity, utility in many clinical populations, and ease of administration, the corresponding body of clinically relevant research is legion. The clinician therefore stands to benefit from the high degree of information available for this test, including underlying processes, reliability data, a wide range of normative studies, and highly relevant studies in a range of clinical populations.

Performance on verbal fluency is related to a number of abilities other than attention and executive function, including processing speed, verbal ability, IQ, and memory. Research suggests that both a semantic store that supplies the knowledge base of words and an efficient search process are important cognitive processes operating during the task. Neuroanatomical correlates generally suggest that the frontal cortex plays a dominant role, especially regions of the inferior frontal gyrus, with temporal activation also implicated in semantic fluency.

There are many variants of fluency measures. The most commonly used phonemic fluency test is FAS, although other letters are also used, especially in other countries and languages. Letters used for phonemic fluency tend to be adapted for the specific language in which normative data are intended. The most common semantic fluency task is animal fluency, which also has a vast body of normative data across many different countries and languages and generally does not show a gender effect.

The demographic effects on this test are well-established. Age affects fluency performance, as does education. Many studies suggest that education may be relatively more influential than age. Reading level is also influential, particularly for phonemic fluency, although less research exists on this relationship. Gender generally does not affect performance, and, when differences are found, they tend to favor females and are small in magnitude. Note, however, that certain category prompts can be affected by gender. Verbal fluency measures have been subject to more cross-cultural and international comparisons than many other neuropsychological tests. The bulk of evidence suggests effects of ethnicity, language, and geographic region. However, some studies have not found differences once other important variables are considered, such as demographic variables, letter frequency, scoring, and administration procedures. Fortunately, there are a number of high-quality, relatively recent normative studies relevant for specific cultural and linguistic groups, many of which are co-normed for both phonemic and semantic fluency.

Phonemic and semantic fluency both require generation of words according to specific constraints, but differ in important ways. Semantic fluency tends to be somewhat easier than phonemic fluency. The tests have different patterns of neuroanatomical activation and differ in clinical populations.

Most research supports the reliability of this test. Phonemic fluency is internally reliable (high range). Test-retest reliabilities of verbal fluency total scores tend to be strong after both short and long intervals, with comparatively poorer test-retest reliability for qualitative scores such as clustering and switching. Practice effects are usually found, and reliable change calculations are recommended when interpreting repeat assessments. Alternate form reliability appears adequate overall. Interrater reliability is excellent for all scores examined, including total correct and strategy scores.

In addition to total correct, which is the conventional measure, examination of errors and strategy variables such as clustering and switching, as well as words generated initially compared to those generated later in the task, provide additional qualitative information that can assist in informing processes involved in task execution. Notably, although these scores have demonstrated some utility in clinical populations, they tend to have relatively low test-retest reliability, and the evidence base is insufficient at present to use these scores diagnostically.

The test has been used in a number of clinical populations, including dementia, TBI, epilepsy, HIV, schizophrenia, mood and anxiety disorders, and a host of other conditions. Although impairments are often noted in both phonemic and semantic fluency, relatively poorer semantic fluency has been reported in some conditions such as dementia and schizophrenia. This may reflect impairments in semantic systems associated with these conditions. Other conditions do not show relatively more impairment in one type of fluency or another, such as TBI and depression. The clinical research is impressive, showing not only group differences, but also examination of differential diagnosis, diagnostic accuracy statistics, staging of clinical severity, treatment effects, and correlates with daily function. Several meta-analyses have also been conducted. Last, the task has promise in performance validity assessment, although more studies are needed in clinical groups before it can be considered an established performance validity test.

REFERENCES

Abwender, D. A., Swan, J. G., Bowerman, J. T., & Connolly, S. W. (2001). Qualitative analysis of verbal fluency output: Review and comparison of several scoring methods. *Assessment, 8,* 323–336.

Acevedo, A., Loewenstein, D. A., Barker, W. B., Harwood, D. G., Luis, C., Bravo, M., . . . Duara, R. (2000). Category fluency test: Normative data for English- and Spanish-speaking elderly. *Journal of the International Neuropsychological Society, 6,* 760–769.

Agranovich, A., & Puente, A. (2007). Do Russian and American normal adults perform similarly on neuropsychological tests? Preliminary findings on the relationship between culture and test performance. *Archives of Clinical Neuropsychology, 22*(3), 273–282. https://doi.org/10.1016/j.acn.2007.01.003

Ahern, E., & Semkovska, M. (2017). Cognitive functioning in the first-episode of major depressive disorder: A systematic review and meta-analysis. *Neuropsychology, 31*(1), 52–72. https://doi.org/10.1037/neu0000319

Arango-Lasprilla, J. C., Rogers, H., Lengenfelder, J., Deluca, J., Moreno, S., & Lopera, F. (2006). Cortical and subcortical diseases: do true neuropsychological differences exist? *Archives of Clinical Neuropsychology, 21*(1), 29–40. https://doi.org/10.1016/j.acn.2005.07.004

Artiola I Fortuny, L., Romo, D. H., Heaton, R. K., & Pardee III, R. E. (1999). *Manual de Normas y Procedimemientos para la Bateria Neuropsicologia en Espanol.* The Netherlands: Swets & Zeitlinger.

Arts, B., Jabben, N., Krabbendam, L., & van Os, J. (2008). Meta-analyses of cognitive functioning in euthymic bipolar patients and their first-degree relatives. *Psychological Medicine, 38*(6), 771–785. https://doi.org/10.1017/S0033291707001675

Azuma, T. (2004). Working memory and perseveration in verbal fluency. *Neuropsychology, 18,* 69–77.

Backman, L., Wahlin, A., Small, B. J., Herlitz, A., Winblad, B., & Fratiglioni, L. (2004). Cognitive functioning in aging and dementia: The Kugsholmen project. *Aging Neuropsychology & Cognition, 11,* 212–244.

Baldacchino, A., Balfour, D. J. K., Passetti, F., Humphris, G., & Matthews, K. (2012). Neuropsychological consequences of chronic opioid use: A quantitative review and meta-analysis. *Neuroscience and Biobehavioral Reviews, 36*(9), 2056–2068. http://doi.org/10.1016/j.neubiorev.2012.06.006

Baldo, J. V., Schwartz, S., Wilkins, D., & Dronkers, N. F. (2006). Role of frontal versus temporal cortex in verbal fluency as revealed by voxel-based lesion symptom mapping. *Journal of the International Neuropsychological Society, 12*(6), 896–900. http://doi.org/10.1017/S1355617706061078

Baldo, J. V., & Shimamura, A. P. (1998). Letter and category fluency in patients with frontal lobe lesions. *Neuropsychology, 12,* 259–267.

Baldo, J. V., Shimamura, A., Delis, D. C., Kramer, J., & Kaplan, E. (2001). Verbal and design fluency in patients with frontal lobe lesions. *Journal of the International Neuropsychological Society, 7,* 586–596.

Barr, W. (2003). Neuropsychological testing of high school athletes Preliminary norms and test–retest indices. *Archives of Clinical Neuropsychology, 18*(1), 91–101. https://doi.org/10.1016/S0887-6177(01)00185-8

Barry, D., Bates, M. E., & Labouvie, E. (2008). FAS and CFL forms of verbal fluency differ in difficulty: A meta-analytic study. *Applied Neuropsychology, 15*(2), 97–106. http://doi.org/10.1080/09084280802083863

Basso, M. R., Bornstein, R. A., & Lang, J. M. (1999). Practice effects on commonly used measures of executive function across twelve months. *The Clinical Neuropsychologist, 13,* 283–292.

Becker, H. E., Nieman, D. H., Dingemans, P. M., van de Fliert, J. R., De Haan, L., & Linszen, D. H. (2010). Verbal fluency as a possible predictor for psychosis. *European Psychiatry, 25*(2), 105–110. https://doi.org/10.1016/j.eurpsy.2009.08.003

Behforuzi, H., Burtis, D. B., Williamson, J. B., Stamps, J. J., & Heilman, K. M. (2013). Impaired initial vowel versus consonant letter-word fluency in dementia of the Alzheimer type. *Cognitive Neuroscience, 4*(3–4), 163–170. https://doi.org/10.1080/17588928.2013.854200

Bennett, C. L., Petros, T. V., Johnson, M., & Ferraro, F. R. (2008). Individual Differences in the influence of time of day on executive functions. *American Journal of Psychology, 121*(3), 349. http://doi.org/10.2307/20445471

Benton, A. L., deS, K., & Sivan, A. B. (1994). *Multilingual aphasia examination.* AJA associates.

Bird, C. M., Papadopoulou, K., Ricciardelli, P., Rossor, M. N., & Cipolotti, L. (2004). Monitoring cognitive changes: Psychometric properties of six cognitive tests. *British Journal of Clinical Psychology, 43,* 197–210.

Boone, K. B., Ponton, M. O., Gorsuch, R. L., Gonzales, J. J., & Miller, B. L. (1998). Factor analysis of four measures of prefrontal lobe functioning. *Archives of Clinical Neuropsychology, 13,* 585–595.

Bora, E., Binnur Akdede, B., & Alptekin, K. (2017). Neurocognitive impairment in deficit and non-deficit schizophrenia: A meta-analysis. *Psychological Medicine, 47*(14), 2401–2413. https://doi.org/10.1017/S0033291717000952

Bora, E., Yücel, M., & Pantelis, C. (2009). Cognitive endophenotypes of bipolar disorder: A meta-analysis of neuropsychological deficits in euthymic patients and their first-degree relatives. *Journal of Affective Disorders, 113*(1–2), 1–20. http://doi.org/10.1016/j.jad.2008.06.009

Bora, E., Yücel, M., & Pantelis, C. (2010). Cognitive impairment in affective psychoses: A meta-analysis. *Schizophrenia Bulletin, 36*(1), 112–125. http://doi.org/10.1093/schbul/sbp093

Bora, E., Yücel, M., Pantelis, C., & Berk, M. (2011). Meta-analytic review of neurocognition in bipolar II disorder: Cognition and BD II. *Acta Psychiatrica Scandinavica, 123*(3), 165–174. https://doi.org/10.1111/j.1600-0447.2010.01638.x

Brewster, P. W. H., McDowell, I., Moineddin, R., & Tierney, M. C. (2012). Differential prediction of vascular dementia and Alzheimer's disease in nondemented older adults within 5 years of initial testing. *Alzheimer's & Dementia, 8*(6), 528–535. http://doi.org/10.1016/j.jalz.2011.09.233

Brickman, A. M., Paul, R. H., Cohen, R. A., Williams, L. M., MacGregor, K. L., Jefferson, A. L., Tate, D. F., Gunstad, J., & Gordon, E. (2005). Category and letter verbal fluency across the adult lifespan: Relationship to EEG theta power. *Archives of Clinical Neuropsychology, 20,* 561–573.

Buckley, A., Fitzgerald, M., Hoerold, D., Davey, G. P., & Doherty, C. (2010). Effects of the anticonvulsant topiramate on language abilities in people with epilepsy: A cross-sectional study. *Irish Journal of Psychological Medicine, 27*(04), 179–183. https://doi.org/10.1017/S0790966700001488

Canning, S. J. D., Leach, L., Stuss, D., Ngo, L., & Black, S. E. (2004). Diagnostic utility of abbreviated fluency measures in Alzheimer disease and vascular dementia. *Neurology, 62*(4), 556–562. https://doi.org/10.1212/WNL.62.4.556

Caramelli, P., Carthery-Goulart, M. T., Porto, C. S., Charchat-Fichman, H., & Nitrini, R. (2007). Category fluency as a screening test for Alzheimer disease in illiterate and literate patients. *Alzheimer Disease and Associated Disorders, 21*(1), 65–67. http://doi.org/10.1097/WAD.0b013e31802f244f

Cavaco, S., Goncalves, A., Pinto, C., Almeida, E., Gomes, F., Moreira, I., . . . Teixeira-Pinto, A. (2013). Semantic fluency and phonemic fluency: Regression-based norms for the Portuguese population. *Archives of Clinical Neuropsychology, 28*(3), 262–271. http://doi.org/10.1093/arclin/act001

Chertkow, H., & Bub, D. (1990). Semantic memory loss in dementia of the Alzheimer's type. *Brain, 113,* 397–417.

Cohen, M. J., & Stanczak, D. E. (2000). On the reliability, validity, and cognitive structure of the Thurstone Word Fluency Test. *Archives of Clinical Neuropsychology, 15,* 267–279.

Cosentino, S., Scarmeas, N., Albert, S. M., & Stern, Y. (2006). Verbal fluency predicts mortality in Alzheimer disease. *Cognitive and Behavioral Neurology, 19*(3), 123–129. https://doi.org/10.1097/01.wnn.0000213912.87642.3d

Costa, A., Bagoj, E., Monaco, M., Zabberoni, S., De Rosa, S., Papantonio, A. M., . . . Carlesimo, G. A. (2014). Standardization and normative data obtained in the Italian population for a new verbal fluency instrument, the phonemic/semantic alternate fluency test. *Neurological Sciences, 35*(3), 365–372. http://doi.org/10.1007/s10072-013-1520-8

Crawford, J. R., Moore, J. W., & Cameron, I. M. (1992). Verbal fluency: A NART-based equation for estimation of premorbid performance. *British Journal of Clinical Psychology, 31,* 327–329.

Crawford, J. R., Wright, R., & Bate, A. (1995). Verbal, figural and ideational fluency in CHI. *Journal of the International Neuropsychological Society, 1,* 321.

Croall, I. D., Lohner, V., Moynihan, B., Khan, U., Hassan, A., O'Brien, J. T., Morris, R. G., Tozer, D. J., Cambridge, V. C., Harkness, K., Werring, D. J., Blamire, A. M., Ford, G. A., Barrick, T. R., & Markus, H. S. (2017). Using DTI to assess white matter microstructure in cerebral small vessel disease (SVD) in multicentre studies. *Clinical Science, 131*(12), 1361–1373. https://doi.org/10.1042/CS20170146

Curtis, K. L., Thompson, L. K., Greve, K. W., & Bianchini, K. J. (2008). Verbal Fluency Indicators of Malingering in Traumatic Brain Injury: Classification Accuracy in Known Groups. *The Clinical Neuropsychologist, 22*(5), 930–945. https://doi.org/10.1080/13854040701563591

Cysique, L. A. J., Maruff, P., & Brew, B. J. (2006). The neuropsychological profile of symptomatic AIDS and ADC patients in the pre-HAART era: A meta-analysis. *Journal of the International Neuropsychological Society, 12*(3), 368–382. http://doi.org/10.1017/S1355617706060401

Dall'Ora, P., Della Sala, S., & Spinnler, H. (1989). Autobiographical memory. Its impairments in amnesic syndromes. *Cortex, 25,* 197–217.

Delis, D. C., Kaplan, E., & Kramer, J. H. (2001). *Delis-Kaplan Executive Function System*. San Antonio, TX: Psychological Corporation.

Diaz-Asper, C., Schretlen, D. J., & Pearlson, G. D. (2004). How well does IQ predict neuropsychological test performance in normal adults. *Journal of the International Neuropsychological Society, 10,* 82–90.

Dikmen, S. S., Heaton, R. K., Grant, I., & Temkin, N. R. (1999). Test-retest reliability and practice effects of expanded Halstead-Reitan neuropsychological test battery. *Journal of the International Neuropsychological Society, 5,* 346–356.

Doughty, O. J., & Done, D. J. (2009). Is semantic memory impaired in schizophrenia? A systematic review and meta-analysis of 91 studies. *Cognitive Neuropsychiatry, 14*(6), 473–509. http://doi.org/10.1080/13546800903073291

Economou, A., Papageorgiou, S. G., Karageorgiou, C., & Vassilopoulos, D. (2007). Nonepisodic memory deficits in amnestic MCI. *Cognitive and Behavioral Neurology, 20*(2), 99–106. https://doi.org/10.1097/WNN.0b013e31804c6fe7

Egeland, J., Landrø, N. I., Tjemsland, E., & Walbækken, K. (2006). Norwegian norms and factor-structure of phonemic and semantic word list generation. *The Clinical Neuropsychologist, 20*(4), 716–728. http://doi.org/10.1080/13854040500351008

Elgh, E., Domellöf, M., Linder, J., Edström, M., Stenlund, H., & Forsgren, L. (2009). Cognitive function in early Parkinson's disease: A population-based study. *European Journal of Neurology, 16*(12), 1278–1284. https://doi.org/10.1111/j.1468-1331.2009.02707.x

Elkadi, S., Clark, M. S., Dennerstein, L., Guthrie, J. R., Bowden, S. C., & Henderson, V. W. (2006). Normative data for Australian midlife women on category fluency and a short form of the Boston Naming Test. *Australian Psychologist, 41*(1), 37–42. http://doi.org/10.1080/00050060500421634

Epker, M. O., Lacritz, L. H., & Cullum, M. C. (1999). Comparative analysis of qualitative verbal fluency performance in normal elderly and demented populations. *Journal of Clinical and Experimental Neuropsychology, 21,* 425–434.

Fillenbaum, G. G., Heyman, A., Huber, M. S., Gangull, M., & Unverzagt, F. W. (2001). Performance of elderly African American and white community residents on the CERAD neuropsychological battery. *Journal of the International Neuropsychological Society, 7,* 502–509.

Fine, E. M., Kramer, J. H., Lui, L.-Y., Yaffe, K., & the Study of Osteoporotic Fractures. (2012). Normative data in women aged 85 and older: Verbal Fluency, Digit Span, and the CVLT-II Short Form. *The Clinical Neuropsychologist, 26*(1), 18–30. http://doi.org/10.1080/13854046.2011.639310

Foster, P. S., Branch, K. K., Witt, J. C., Giovannetti, T., Libon, D., Heilman, K. M., & Drago, V. (2012). Acetylcholinesterase inhibitors reduce spreading activation in dementia. *Neuropsychologia, 50*(8), 2093–2099. https://doi.org/10.1016/j.neuropsychologia.2012.05.010

Foster, P. S., Drago, V., Yung, R. C., Pearson, J., Stringer, K., Giovannetti, T., Libon, D., & Heilman, K. M. (2013). Differential Lexical and Semantic Spreading Activation in Alzheimer's Disease. *American Journal of Alzheimer's Disease & Other Dementiasr, 28*(5), 501–507. https://doi.org/10.1177/1533317513494445

Fraser, R. T., Clemmons, D., Gibbons, L., Koepnick, D., Getter, A., & Johnson, E. (2009). Predictors of vocational stability in multiple sclerosis. *Journal of Vocational Rehabilitation, 31*(2), 129–135. https://doi.org/10.3233/JVR-2009-481

Fusar-Poli, P., Deste, G., Smieskova, R., Barlati, S., Yung, A. R., Howes, O., . . . Borgwardt, S. (2012). Cognitive functioning in prodromal psychosis: A meta-analysis. *JAMA Psychiatry, 69*(6), 562–571.

Gallagher, D., Mhaolain, A. N., Coen, R., Walsh, C., Kilroy, D., Belinski, K., . . . Lawlor, B. A. (2010). Detecting prodromal Alzheimer's disease in mild cognitive impairment: Utility of the CAMCOG and other neuropsychological predictors. *International Journal of Geriatric Psychiatry, 25*(12), 1280–1287. https://doi.org/10.1002/gps.2480

Giovanetti, T., Lamar, M., Cloud, B. S., Swenson, R., Fein, D., Kaplan, E., & Libon, D. J. (2001). Different underlying mechanisms for deficits in concept formation in dementia. *Archives of Clinical Neuropsychology, 16,* 547–560.

Giovanetti-Carew, T. G., Lamar, M., Cloud, B. S., Grossman, M., & Libon, D. J. (1997). Impairment in category fluency in ischaemic vascular dementia. *Neuropsychology, 11,* 400–412.

Gladsjo, J. A., Schuman, C. C. Evans, J. D., Peavy, G. M., Miller, S. W., & Heaton, R. K. (1999a). Norms for letter and category fluency: Demographic corrections for age, education, and ethnicity. *Assessment, 6,* 147–178.

Gladsjo, J. A., Schuman, C. C. Miller, S. W., & Heaton, R. K. (1999b). *Norms for letter and category fluency: Demographic corrections for age, education, and ethnicity*. Odessa, FL: PAR.

Gonzalez, H. M., Mungas, D., & Haan, M. N. (2005). A semantic verbal fluency test for English- and Spanish-speaking older Mexican Americans. *Archives of Clinical Neuropsychology, 20,* 199–208.

Gonzalez da Silva, C., Petersson, K. M., Faisca, L., Ingvar, M., & Reis, A. (2004). The effects of literacy and education on the quantitative and qualitative aspects of semantic verbal fluency. *Journal of Clinical and Experimental Neuropsychology, 26,* 266–277.

Greenaway, M. C., Smith, G. E., Tangalos, E. G., Geda, Y. E., & Ivnik, R. J. (2009). Mayo Older Americans Normative Studies: Factor analysis of an expanded neuropsychological battery. *The Clinical Neuropsychologist, 23*(1), 7–20. http://doi.org/10.1080/13854040801891686

Gruner, P., & Pittenger, C. (2017). Cognitive inflexibility in obsessive-compulsive disorder. *Neuroscience, 345,* 243–255. https://doi.org/10.1016/j.neuroscience.2016.07.030

Guise, B. J., Thompson, M. D., Greve, K. W., Bianchini, K. J., & West, L. (2014). Assessment of performance validity in the Stroop Color and Word Test in mild traumatic brain injury patients: A criterion-groups validation design. *Journal of Neuropsychology, 8*(1), 20–33. https://doi.org/10.1111/jnp.12002

Gupta, S., Vaida, F., Riggs, K., Jin, H., Grant, I., Cysique, L., . . . The HIV Neurobehavioral Research Center (HNRC) Group. (2011). Neuropsychological performance in mainland China: The effect of urban/rural residence and self-reported daily academic skill use. *Journal of the International Neuropsychological Society, 17*(01), 163–173. http://doi.org/10.1017/S1355617710001384

Hankee, L. D., Preis, S. R., Beiser, A. S., Devine, S. A., Liu, Y., Seshadri, S., . . . Au, R. (2013). Qualitative neuropsychological measures: Normative data on executive functioning tests from the Framingham Offspring Study. *Experimental Aging Research, 39*(5), 515–535. http://doi.org/10.1080/0361073X.2013.839029

Harrison, J. E., Buxton, P., Husain, M., & Wise, R. (2000). Short test of semantic and phonological fluency: Normal performance, validity and test-retest reliability. *British Journal of Clinical Psychology, 39,* 181–191.

Hatta, T., Kanari, A., Mase, M., Kabasawa, H., Ogawa, T., Shirataki, T., . . . Yamada, K. (2008). Brain mechanisms in Japanese Verbal Fluency Test: Evidence from examination by NIRS (near-infrared spectroscopy). *Asia Pacific Journal of Speech, Language and Hearing, 11*(2), 103–110. https://doi.org/10.1179/136132808805297250

Heaps, J., Valcour, V., Chalermchai, T., Paul, R., Rattanamanee, S., Siangphoe, U., . . . Ananworanich, J. (2013). Development of normative neuropsychological performance in Thailand for the assessment of HIV-associated neurocognitive disorders. *Journal of Clinical and Experimental Neuropsychology, 35*(1), 1–8. http://doi.org/10.1080/13803395.2012.733682

Heaton, R. K., Miller, S. W., Taylor, M. J., & Grant, I. (2004). *Revised comprehensive norms for an expanded Halstead-Reitan Battery: Demographically adjusted neuropsychological norms for African American and Caucasian adults.* Lutz, FL: PAR.

Heller, R. B., & Dobbs, A. R. (1993) Age differences in word finding in discourse and nondiscourse situations. *Psychology and Aging, 8*, 443–450.

Henry, J. (2006). A meta-analytic review of Wisconsin Card Sorting Test and verbal fluency performance in obsessive-compulsive disorder. *Cognitive Neuropsychiatry, 11*(2), 156–176. https://doi.org/10.1080/13546800444000227

Henry, J. D., & Crawford, J. R. (2004a). A meta-analytic review of verbal fluency performance following focal cortical lesions. *Neuropsychology, 18*, 284–295.

Henry, J. D., & Crawford, J. R. (2004b). A meta-analytic review of verbal fluency performance in patients with traumatic brain injury. *Neuropsychology, 18*, 621–628.

Henry, J. D., & Crawford, J. R. (2004c). Verbal fluency deficits in Parkinson's disease: A meta-analysis. *Journal of the International Neuropsychological Society, 10*, 608–622.

Henry, J. D., & Crawford, J. R. (2005a). A meta-analytic review of verbal fluency deficits in depression. *Journal of Clinical and Experimental Neuropsychology, 27*, 78–101.

Henry, J. D., & Crawford, J. R. (2005b). A meta-analytic review of verbal fluency deficits in schizophrenia relative to other neurocognitive deficits. *Cognitive Neuropsychiatry, 10*, 1–33.

Henry, J. D., Crawford, J. R., & Phillips, L. H. (2004). Verbal fluency performance in dementia of the Alzheimer's type: A meta-analysis. *Neuropsychologia, 42*, 1212–1222.

Henry, J. D., Crawford, J. R., & Phillips, L. H. (2005). A meta-analytic review of verbal fluency deficits in Huntington's disease. *Neuropsychology, 19*, 243–252.

Hessen, E., Lossius, M. I., & Gjerstad, L. (2009). Antiepileptic monotherapy significantly impairs normative scores on common tests of executive functions. *Acta Neurologica Scandinavica, 119*(3), 194–198. https://doi.org/10.1111/j.1600-0404.2008.01109.x

Hessen, E., Lossius, M. I., Reinvang, I., & Gjerstad, L. (2007). Influence of major antiepileptic drugs on neuropsychological function: Results from a randomized, double-blind, placebo-controlled withdrawal study of seizure-free epilepsy patients on monotherapy. *Journal of the International Neuropsychological Society, 13*(3), 393–400. https://doi.org/10.1017/S1355617707070555

Hirshorn, E. A., & Thompson-Schill, S. L. (2006). Role of the left inferior frontal gyrus in covert word retrieval: Neural correlates of switching during verbal fluency. *Neuropsychologia, 44*(12), 2547–2557. https://doi.org/10.1016/j.neuropsychologia.2006.03.035

Ho, A. K., Sahakian, B. J., Robbins, T. W., Barker, R. A., Rosser, A. E., & Hodges, J. R. (2002). Verbal fluency in Huntington's disease: A longitudinal analysis of phonemic and semantic clustering and switching. *Neuropsychologia, 40*, 1277–1284.

Holtzer, R., Goldin, Y., & Donovick, P. (2009). Extending the administration time of the Letter Fluency Test increases sensitivity to cognitive status in aging. *Experimental Aging Research, 35*(3), 317–326. https://doi.org/10.1080/03610730902922119

Horwitz, J., & Mccaffrey, R. (2008). Effects of a third party observer and anxiety on tests of executive function. *Archives of Clinical Neuropsychology, 23*(4), 409–417. https://doi.org/10.1016/j.acn.2008.02.002

Hurford, I. M., Marder, S. R., Keefe, R. S. E., Reise, S. P., & Bilder, R. M. (2011). A brief cognitive assessment tool for schizophrenia: Construction of a tool for clinicians. *Schizophrenia Bulletin, 37*(3), 538–545. http://doi.org/10.1093/schbul/sbp095

Hwang, S. H., Kwon, J. S., Shin, Y.-W., Lee, K. J., Kim, Y. Y., & Kim, M.-S. (2007). Neuropsychological profiles of patients with obsessive-compulsive disorder: Early onset versus late onset. *Journal of the International Neuropsychological Society: JINS, 13*(1), 30–37. https://doi.org/10.1017/S1355617707070063

Iudicello, J. E., Woods, S. P., Parsons, T. D., Moran, L. M., Carey, C. L., & Grant, I. (2007). Verbal fluency in HIV infection: A meta-analytic review. *Journal of the International Neuropsychological Society, 13*(1), 183–189. http://doi.org/10.1017/S1355617707070221

Iverson, G. L., Franzen, M. D., & Lovell, M. R. (1999). Normative comparisons for the Controlled Oral Word Association Test following acute traumatic brain injury. *The Clinical Neuropsychologist, 13*, 437–441.

Ivnik, R., Malec, J. F., Smith, G. F., Tangelos, E. G., & Petersen, R. C. (1996). Neuropsychological tests' norms above age 55: COWAT, BNT, MAE token, WRAT-R reading, AMNART, Stroop, TMT, and JLO. *The Clinical Neuropsychologist, 10*, 262–278.

Jacinto, A. F., Brucki, S. M. D., Porto, C. S., Martins, M. de A., Citero, V. de A., & Nitrini, R. (2014). Suggested instruments for general practitioners in countries with low schooling to screen for cognitive impairment in the elderly. *International Psychogeriatrics, 26*(07), 1121–1125. http://doi.org/10.1017/S1041610214000325

Jacobs, D. M., Sano, M., Albert, S., Schofield, P., Dooneief, G., & Stern, Y. (1997). Cross-cultural neuropsychological assessment: A comparison of randomly selected, demographically matched cohorts of English- and Spanish-speaking older adults. *Journal of Clinical and Experimental Neuropsychology, 19*, 331–339.

Johnson, S. C., Silverberg, N. D., Millis, S. R., & Hanks, R. A. (2012). Symptom validity indicators embedded in the Controlled Oral Word Association Test. *The Clinical Neuropsychologist, 26*(7), 1230–1241. http://doi.org/10.1080/13854046.2012.709886

Johnson-Selfridge, M. T., Zalewski, C., & Aboudarham, J-F. (1998). The relationship between ethnicity and word fluency. *Archives of Clinical Neuropsychology, 13*, 319–325.

Kave, G. (2005). Phonemic fluency, semantic fluency, and difference scores: Normative data for adult Hebrew speakers. *Journal of Clinical and Experimental Neuropsychology, 27*, 690–699.

Keller, S. S., Baker, G., Downes, J. J., & Roberts, N. (2009). Quantitative MRI of the prefrontal cortex and executive function in patients with temporal lobe epilepsy. *Epilepsy & Behavior, 15*(2), 186–195. http://doi.org/10.1016/j.yebeh.2009.03.005

Kempler, D., Teng, E. L., Dick, M., Taussig, I. M., & Davis, D. S. (1998). The effects of age, education, and ethnicity on verbal fluency. *Journal of the International Neuropsychological Society, 4*, 531–538.

Khalil, M. S. (2010). Preliminary Arabic normative data of neuropsychological tests: The verbal and design fluency. *Journal of Clinical and Experimental Neuropsychology, 32*(9), 1028–1035. http://doi.org/10.1080/13803391003672305

Knight, R. G., McMahon, J., Green, T. J., & Skeaff, C. M. (2006). Regression equations for predicting scores of persons over 65 on the Rey Auditory Verbal Learning Test, the Mini-Mental State Examination, the Trail Making Test and semantic fluency measures. *British Journal of Clinical Psychology, 45*(3), 393–402. http://doi.org/10.1348/014466505X68032

Kosmidis, M. H., Vlahou, C. H., Panagiotaki, P., & Kiosseoglou, G. (2004). The verbal fluency task in the Greek population: Normative data, and clustering and switching strategies. *Journal of the International Neuropsychological Society, 10*, 164–172.

Kozora, E., & Cullum, C. M. (1995). Generative naming in normal aging: Total output and qualitative changes using phonetic and semantic constraints. *The Clinical Neuropsychologist, 9*, 313–325.

Kurtz, M. M., & Gerraty, R. T. (2009). A meta-analytic investigation of neurocognitive deficits in bipolar illness: Profile and effects of clinical state. *Neuropsychology, 23*(5), 551–562. https://doi.org/10.1037/a0016277

La Rue, A., Romero, L. J., Ortiz, I. E., Liang, H. C., & Kindeman, R. D. (1999). Neuropsychological performance of Hispanic and non-Hispanic older adults: An epidemiologic survey. *The Clinical Neuropsychologist, 13*, 474–486.

Lam, M., Eng, G. K., Rapisarda, A., Subramaniam, M., Kraus, M., Keefe, R. S. E., & Collinson, S. L. (2013). Formulation of the age-education index: measuring age and education effects in neuropsychological performance. *Psychological Assessment, 25*(1), 61–70. https://doi.org/10.1037/a0030548

Laws, K. R., Duncan, A., & Gale, T. M. (2010). "Normal" semantic–phonemic fluency discrepancy in Alzheimer's disease?

A meta-analytic study. *Cortex, 46*(5), 595–601. http://doi.org/10.1016/j.cortex.2009.04.009

Lee, S.-A., Lee, H.-W., Heo, K., Shin, D.-J., Song, H.-K., Kim, O.-J., . . . Lee, B.-I. (2011). Cognitive and behavioral effects of lamotrigine and carbamazepine monotherapy in patients with newly diagnosed or untreated partial epilepsy. *Seizure, 20*(1), 49–54. https://doi.org/10.1016/j.seizure.2010.10.006

Lepow, L., Van Sweringen, J., Strutt, A. M., Jawaid, A., MacAdam, C., Harati, Y., . . . York, M. K. (2010). Frontal and temporal lobe involvement on verbal fluency measures in amyotrophic lateral sclerosis. *Journal of Clinical and Experimental Neuropsychology, 32*(9), 913–922. https://doi.org/10.1080/13803391003596439

Levine, A. J., Miller, E. N., Becker, J. T., Selnes, O. A., & Cohen, B. A. (2004). Normative data for determining significance of test-retest differences on eight common neuropsychological instruments. *The Clinical Neuropsychologist, 18,* 373–384.

Levine, A. J., Hinkin, C. H., Miller, E. N., Becker, J. T., Selnes, O. A., & Cohen, B. A. (2007). The generalizability of neurocognitive test/retest data derived from a nonclinical sample for detecting change among two HIV+ cohorts. *Journal of Clinical and Experimental Neuropsychology, 29*(6), 669–678. http://doi.org/10.1080/13803390600920471

Lieb, K., Engelbrecht, M. A., Gut, O., Fiebich, B. L., Bauer, J., Janssen, G., & Schaefer, M. (2006). Cognitive impairment in patients with chronic hepatitis treated with interferon alpha (IFNalpha): Results from a prospective study. *European Psychiatry, 21*(3), 204–210. https://doi.org/10.1016/j.eurpsy.2004.09.030

Lim, J., Oh, I. K., Han, C., Huh, Y. J., Jung, I.-K., Patkar, A. A., . . . Jang, B.-H. (2013). Sensitivity of cognitive tests in four cognitive domains in discriminating MDD patients from healthy controls: A meta-analysis. *International Psychogeriatrics, 25*(9), 1543–1557. http://doi.org/10.1017/S1041610213000689

Liscic, R. M., Storandt, M., Cairns, N. J., & Morris, J. C. (2007). Clinical and psychometric distinction of frontotemporal and Alzheimer dementias. *Archives of Neurology, 64*(4), 535–540.

Loewenstein, D. A., Duara, R., Arguelles, T., & Arguelles, S. (1995). Use of the Fuld Object Memory Evaluation in the detection of mild dementia among Spanish-speaking and English-speaking groups. *American Journal of Geriatric Psychiatry, 3,* 448–454.

Loonstra, A. S., Tarlow, A. R., & Sellers, A. H. (2001). COWAT metanorms across age, education, and gender. *Applied Neuropsychology, 8,* 161–166.

Lovell, M. R., & Solomon, G. S. (2011). Psychometric data for the NFL Neuropsychological Test Battery. *Applied Neuropsychology, 18*(3), 197–209. http://doi.org/10.1080/09084282.2011.595446

Lucas, J. A., Ivnik, R. J., Smith, G. E., Bohac, D. L., Tangalos, E. G., Graff-Radford, N. R., & Peterson, R. C. (1998). Mayo's Older Americans Normative Study: Category fluency norms. *Journal of Clinical and Experimental Neuropsychology, 20,* 194–200.

Lucas, J. A., Ivnik, R. J., Smith, G. E., Ferman, T. J., Willis, F. B., Petersen, R. C., & Graff-Radford, N. R. (2005). Mayo's Older African Americans Normative Studies: Norms for Boston Naming Test, Controlled Oral Word Association, Category Fluency, Animal Naming, Token Test, WRAT-3 Reading, Trail Making Test, Stroop Test, and Judgement of Line Orientation. *The Clinical Neuropsychologist, 19,* 243–269.

Mack, W. J., Teng, E., Zheng, L., Paz, S., Chui, H., & Varma, R. (2005). Category fluency in a Latino sample: Associations with age, education, gender, and language. *Journal of Clinical and Experimental Neuropsychology, 27,* 591–598.

Madhavan, K. M., McQueeny, T., Howe, S. R., Shear, P., & Szaflarski, J. (2014). Superior longitudinal fasciculus and language functioning in healthy aging. *Brain Research, 1562,* 11–22. https://doi.org/10.1016/j.brainres.2014.03.012

Malaguarnera, M., Vacante, M., Motta, M., Giordano, M., Malaguarnera, G., Bella, R., . . . Pennisi, G. (2011). Acetyl-L-carnitine improves cognitive functions in severe hepatic encephalopathy: A randomized and controlled clinical trial. *Metabolic Brain Disease, 26*(4), 281–289. https://doi.org/10.1007/s11011-011-9260-z

Martins, I. P., Maruta, C., Freitas, V., & Mares, I. (2013). Executive performance in older Portuguese adults with low education. *The Clinical Neuropsychologist, 27*(3), 410–425. http://doi.org/10.1080/13854046.2012.748094

Mathuranath, P. S., George, A., Cherian, P. J., Alexander, A., Sarma, S. G., & Sarma, P. S. (2003). Effects of age, education and gender on verbal fluency. *Journal of Clinical and Experimental Neuropsychology, 25,* 1057–1064.

Mayr, U. (2002). On the dissociation between clustering and switching in verbal fluency: Comment on Troyer, Moscovitch, Winocur, Alexander and Stuss. *Neuropsychologia, 40*(5), 562–566. https://doi.org/10.1016/s0028-3932(01)00132-4

Meijer, J. H., Schmitz, N., Nieman, D. H., Becker, H. E., van Amelsvoort, T. A. M. J., Dingemans, P. M., . . . de Haan, L. (2011). Semantic fluency deficits and reduced gray matter before transition to psychosis: A voxelwise correlational analysis. *Psychiatry Research, 194*(1), 1–6.

Melrose, R. J., Young, S., Weissberger, G. H., Natta, L., Harwood, D., Mandelkern, M., & Sultzer, D. L. (2017). Cerebral metabolic correlates of attention networks in Alzheimer's Disease: A study of the Stroop. *Neuropsychologia, 106,* 383–389. https://doi.org/10.1016/j.neuropsychologia.2017.10.020

Millikin, C. P., Trepanier, L. L., & Rourke, S. B. (2004). Verbal fluency component analysis in adults with HIV/AIDS. *Journal of Clinical and Experimental Neuropsychology, 26,* 933–942.

Mitrushina, M. M., Boone, K. B., Razani, J., & D'Elia, L. F. (2005). *Handbook of normative data for neuropsychological assessment* (2nd ed.). New York: Oxford University Press.

Molinuevo, J. L., Gómez-Anson, B., Monte, G. C., Bosch, B., Sánchez-Valle, R., & Rami, L. (2011). Neuropsychological profile of prodromal Alzheimer's disease (Prd-AD) and their radiological correlates. *Archives of Gerontology and Geriatrics, 52*(2), 190–196. https://doi.org/10.1016/j.archger.2010.03.016

Monsch, A. U., Bondi, M. W., Butters, N., Paulsen, J. S., Salmon, D. P., Brugger, P., & Swenson, M. R. (1994). A comparison of category and letter fluency in Alzheimer's disease and Huntington's disease. *Neuropsychology, 8,* 25–30.

Moraes, A. L., Guimarães, L. S. P., Joanette, Y., Parente, M. A. de M. P., Fonseca, R. P., & Almeida, R. M. M. de. (2013). Effect of aging, education, reading and writing, semantic processing and depression symptoms on verbal fluency. *Psicologia: Reflexão e Crítica, 26*(4), 680–690. https://doi.org/10.1590/S0102-79722013000400008

Muñoz-Moreno, J. A., Prats, A., Pérez-Álvarez, N., Fumaz, C. R., Garolera, M., Doval, E., Negredo, E., Ferrer, M. J., & Clotet, B. (2013). A Brief and Feasible Paper-Based Method to Screen for Neurocognitive Impairment in HIV-Infected Patients: The NEU Screen. *JAIDS Journal of Acquired Immune Deficiency Syndromes, 63*(5), 585–592. https://doi.org/10.1097/QAI.0b013e31829e1408

Neill, E., Gurvich, C., & Rossell, S. L. (2014). Category fluency in schizophrenia research: Is it an executive or semantic measure? *Cognitive Neuropsychiatry, 19*(1), 81–95. https://doi.org/10.1080/13546805.2013.807233

Negreiros, M. A., Mattos, P., Landeira-Fernandez, J., Paes, R. A., & Alvarenga, R. P. (2008). A brief neuropsychological screening test battery for cognitive dysfunction in Brazilian multiple sclerosis patients. *Brain Injury, 22*(5), 419–426. http://doi.org/10.1080/02699050801998243

Newman, L. M., Trivedi, M. A., Bendlin, B. B., Ries, M. L., & Johnson, S. C. (2007). The relationship between gray matter morphometry and neuropsychological performance in a large sample of cognitively healthy adults. *Brain Imaging and Behavior, 1*(1-2), 3–10. http://doi.org/10.1007/s11682-007-9000-5

Nutter-Upham, K. E., Saykin, A. J., Rabin, L. A., Roth, R. M., Wishart, H. A., Pare, N., & Flashman, L. A. (2008). Verbal fluency performance in amnestic MCI and older adults with cognitive complaints. *Archives of Clinical Neuropsychology, 23*(3), 229–241. https://doi.org/10.1016/j.acn.2008.01.005

Oberg, G., & Ramírez, M. (2006). Cross-linguistic meta-analysis of phonological fluency: Normal performance across cultures. *International Journal of Psychology, 41*(5), 342–347. http://doi.org/10.1080/00207590500345872

Ostrosky-Solis, F., Ardila, A., & Roselli, M. (1999). NEUROPSI: A brief neuropsychological test battery in Spanish with norms by age and educational level. *Journal of the International Neuropsychological Society, 5,* 413–433.

Ostrosky-Solis, F., Gutierrez, A., Flores, M., & Ardila, A. (2007). Same or different? Semantic verbal fluency across Spanish-speakers from different countries. *Archives of Clinical Neuropsychology, 22*(3), 367–377. http://doi.org/10.1016/j.acn.2007.01.011

Paulsen, J. S., Miller, A. C., Hayes, T., & Shaw, E. (2017). Cognitive and behavioral changes in Huntington disease before diagnosis. *Handbook of Clinical Neurology, 144,* 69–91. https://doi.org/10.1016/B978-0-12-801893-4.00006-7

Pena-Casanova, J., Quinones-Ubeda, S., Gramunt-Fombuena, N., Quintana-Aparicio, M., Aguilar, M., Badenes, D., . . . for the NEURONORMA Study Team. (2009). Spanish Multicenter Normative Studies (NEURONORMA Project): Norms for Verbal Fluency Tests. *Archives of Clinical Neuropsychology, 24*(4), 395–411. http://doi.org/10.1093/arclin/acp042

Pendleton, M. G., Heaton, R. K., Lehman, R. A. W., & Hulihan, D. (1982). Diagnostic utility of the Thurstone Word Fluency Test in neuropsychological evaluations. *Journal of Clinical Neuropsychology, 4,* 307–317.

Piatt, A. L., Fields, J. A., Paolo, A. M., & Troester, A. I. (1999). Action (verb naming) fluency as a unique executive function measure: Convergent and divergent evidence of validity. *Neuropsychologia, 37,* 1499–1503.

Rajji, T. K., Ismail, Z., & Mulsant, B. H. (2009). Age at onset and cognition in schizophrenia: Meta-analysis. *British Journal of Psychiatry, 195*(4), 286–293. https://doi.org/10.1192/bjp.bp.108.060723

Ratcliff, G., Dodge, H., Birzescu, M., & Ganguli, M. (2003). Tracking cognitive functioning over time: Ten-year longitudinal data from a community-based study. *Applied Neuropsychology, 10, 76–88.*

Raucher-Chéné, D., Achim, A. M., Kaladjian, A., & Besche-Richard, C. (2017). Verbal fluency in bipolar disorders: A systematic review and meta-analysis. *Journal of Affective Disorders, 207,* 359–366. https://doi.org/10.1016/j.jad.2016.09.039

Ravdin, L. D., Katzen, H. L., Agrawal, P., & Relkin, N. R. (2003). Letter and semantic fluency in older adults: Effects of mild depressive symptoms and age-stratified normative data. *The Clinical Neuropsychologist, 17,* 195–202.

Ren, J., Li, H., Palaniyappan, L., Liu, H., Wang, J., Li, C., & Rossini, P. M. (2014). Repetitive transcranial magnetic stimulation versus electroconvulsive therapy for major depression: A systematic review and meta-analysis. *Progress in Neuro-Psychopharmacology and Biological Psychiatry, 51,* 181–189. https://doi.org/10.1016/j.pnpbp.2014.02.004

Rich, J. B., Troyer, A. K., Blysma, F. W., & Brandt, J. (1999). Longitudinal analysis of phonemic clustering and switching during word list generation in Huntington's disease. *Neuropsychology, 13,* 525–531.

Riepe, M. W., Adler, G., Ibach, B., Weinkauf, B., Tracik, F., & Gunay, I. (2007). Domain-specific improvement of cognition on memantine in patients with Alzheimer's disease treated with rivastigmine. *Dementia and Geriatric Cognitive Disorders, 23*(5), 301–306. https://doi.org/10.1159/000100875

Robert, P. H., Lafont, V., Medecin, I., Berthet, L., Thauby, S., Baudu, C., & Darcourt, G. (1998). Clustering and switching strategies in verbal fluency tasks: Comparison between schizophrenic and healthy subjects. *Journal of the International Neuropsychological Society, 4,* 539–546.

Robinson, H., Calamia, M., Gäscher, J., Bruss, J., & Tranel, D. (2014). Neuroanatomical correlates of executive functions: A neuropsychological approach using the EXAMINER Battery. *Journal of the International Neuropsychological Society, 20*(1), 52–63. http://doi.org/10.1017/S135561771300060X

Robinson, L. J., Thompson, J. M., Gallagher, P., Goswami, U., Young, A. H., Ferrier, I. N., & Moore, P. B. (2006). A meta-analysis of cognitive deficits in euthymic patients with bipolar disorder. *Journal of Affective Disorders, 93*(1-3), 105–115. http://doi.org/10.1016/j.jad.2006.02.016

Rodríguez-Aranda, C., & Sundet, K. (2006). The frontal hypothesis of cognitive aging: factor structure and age effects on four frontal tests among healthy individuals. *Journal of Genetic Psychology, 167*(3), 269–287.

Rogers, T. T., Ivanoiu, A., Patterson, K., & Hodges, J. R. (2006). Semantic memory in Alzheimer's disease and the frontotemporal dementias: A longitudinal study of 236 patients. *Neuropsychology, 20*(3), 319–335. https://doi.org/10.1037/0894-4105.20.3.319

Rosen, V. M., & Engle, R. W. (1997). The role of working memory capacity in retrieval. *Journal of Experimental Psychology: General, 126,* 211–227.

Ross, T. P. (2003). The reliability of cluster and switch scores for the Controlled Oral Word Association Test. *Archives of Clinical Neuropsychology, 18,* 153–164.

Ross, T. P., Calhoun, E., Cox, T., Wenner, C., Kono, W., & Pleasant, M. (2007). The reliability and validity of qualitative scores for the Controlled Oral Word Association Test. *Archives of Clinical Neuropsychology, 22*(4), 475–488. https://doi.org/10.1016/j.acn.2007.01.026

Ross, T. P., Furr, A. E., Carter, S. E., & Weinberg, M. (2006). The psychometric equivalence of two alternate forms of the Controlled Oral Word Association Test. *The Clinical Neuropsychologist, 20*(3), 414–431. https://doi.org/10.1080/13854040590967153

Ross, T. P., Weinberg, M., Furr, A. E., Carter, S. E., Evans-Blake, L., & Parham, S. (2005). The temporal stability of cluster and switch scores using a modified COWAT procedure. *Archives of Clinical Neuropsychology, 20*(8), 983–996. https://doi.org/10.1016/j.acn.2005.05.002

Rosselli, M., Ardila, A., Salvatierra, J., Marquez, M., Matos, L., & Weekes, V. A. (2002). A cross-linguistic comparison of verbal fluency tests. *International Journal of Neuroscience, 112,* 759–776.

Rosselli, M., Tappen, R., Williams, C., Salvatierra, J., & Zoller, Y. (2009). Level of education and Category Fluency task among Spanish speaking elders: Number of words, clustering, and switching strategies. *Aging, Neuropsychology, and Cognition, 16*(6), 721–744. http://doi.org/10.1080/13825580902912739

Ruff, R. M., Light, R. H., Parker, S. B., & Levin, H. S. (1996). Benton Controlled Oral Word Association Test: Reliability and updated norms. *Archives of Clinical Neuropsychology, 11,* 329–338.

Ryu, S.-H., Kim, K. W., Kim, S., Park, J. H., Kim, T. H., Jeong, H.-G., . . . Cho, M. J. (2012). Normative study of the category fluency test (CFT) from nationwide data on community-dwelling elderly in Korea. *Archives of Gerontology and Geriatrics, 54*(2), 305–309. http://doi.org/10.1016/j.archger.2011.05.010

Sabbagh, M. N., Lahti, T., Connor, D. J., Caviness, J. N., Shill, H., Vedders, L., Mahant, P., Samanta, J., Burns, R. S., Evidente, V. G. H., Driver-Dunckley, E., Reisberg, B., Bircea, S., & Adler, C. H. (2007). Functional Ability Correlates with Cognitive Impairment in Parkinson's Disease and Alzheimer's Disease. *Dementia and Geriatric Cognitive Disorders, 24*(5), 327–334. https://doi.org/10.1159/000108340

Sarkis, R. A., Busch, R. M., Floden, D., Chapin, J. S., Kalman Kenney, C., Jehi, L., . . . Najm, I. (2013). Predictors of decline in verbal fluency after frontal lobe epilepsy surgery. *Epilepsy & Behavior: E&B, 27*(2), 326–329. https://doi.org/10.1016/j.yebeh.2013.02.015

Salthouse, T. A., Atkinson, T. M., & Berish, D. E. (2003). Executive functioning as a potential mediator of age-related cognitive decline in normal adults. *Journal of Experimental Psychology: General, 132,* 566–594.

Sarno, M. T., Postman, W. A., Cho, Y. S., & Norman, R. (2005). Evolution of phonemic word fluency performance in post-stroke aphasia. *Journal of Communication Disorders, 38,* 83–107.

Schmid, N. S., Taylor, K. I., Foldi, N. S., Berres, M., & Monsch, A. U. (2013). Neuropsychological signs of Alzheimer's disease 8 years prior to diagnosis. *Journal of Alzheimer's Disease, 34*(2), 537–546. https://doi.org/10.3233/JAD-121234

Schneider, B. C., & Lichtenberg, P. A. (2011). Influence of Reading Ability on Neuropsychological Performance in African American Elders. *Archives of Clinical Neuropsychology, 26*(7), 624–631. http://doi.org/10.1093/arclin/acr062

Shah, S., Yallampalli, R., Merkley, T. L., McCauley, S. R., Bigler, E. D., MacLeod, M., . . . Wilde, E. A. (2012). Diffusion tensor imaging and volumetric analysis of the ventral striatum in adults with traumatic brain injury. *Brain Injury, 26*(3), 201–210. http://doi.org/10.3109/02699052.2012.654591

Sherman, A. M., & Massman, P. J. (1999). Prevalence and correlates of category versus letter fluency discrepancies in Alzheimer's disease. *Archives of Clinical Neuropsychology: The Official Journal of the National Academy of Neuropsychologists, 14*(5), 411–418.

Shin, N. Y., Lee, T. Y., Kim, E., & Kwon, J. S. (2014). Cognitive functioning in obsessive-compulsive disorder: A meta-analysis. *Psychological Medicine, 44*(6), 1121–1130. http://doi.org/10.1017/S0033291713001803

Silva, D., Guerreiro, M., Santana, I., Rodrigues, A., Cardoso, S., Maroco, J., & de Mendonça, A. (2013). Prediction of long-term (5 years) conversion to dementia using neuropsychological tests in a memory clinic setting. *Journal of Alzheimer's Disease: JAD, 34*(3), 681–689. https://doi.org/10.3233/JAD-122098

Silverberg, N. D., Hanks, R. A., Buchanan, L., Fichtenberg, N., & Millis, S. R. (2008). Detecting response bias with performance patterns on an expanded version of the Controlled Oral Word Association Test. *The Clinical Neuropsychologist, 22*(1), 140–157. http://doi.org/10.1080/13854040601160597

Sliwinski, M., & Buschke, H. (1999). Cross-sectional and longitudinal relationships among age, cognition, and processing speed. *Psychology and Aging, 14*, 18–33.

Smith, P. J., Need, A. C., Cirulli, E. T., Chiba-Falek, O., & Attix, D. K. (2013). A comparison of the Cambridge Automated Neuropsychological Test Battery (CANTAB) with "traditional" neuropsychological testing instruments. *Journal of Clinical and Experimental Neuropsychology, 35*(3), 319–328. http://doi.org/10.1080/13803395.2013.771618

Snitz, B. E., Macdonald, A. W., & Carter, C. S. (2006). Cognitive deficits in unaffected first-degree relatives of schizophrenia patients: A meta-analytic review of putative endophenotypes. *Schizophrenia Bulletin, 32*(1), 179–194. https://doi.org/10.1093/schbul/sbi048

Snitz, B. E., Weissfeld, L. A., Lopez, O. L., Kuller, L. H., Saxton, J., Singhabahu, D. M., . . . DeKosky, S. T. (2013). Cognitive trajectories associated with -amyloid deposition in the oldest-old without dementia. *Neurology, 80*(15), 1378–1384. https://doi.org/10.1212/WNL.0b013e31828c2fc8

Sontam, V., Christman, S. D., & Jasper, J. D. (2009). Individual differences in semantic switching flexibility: Effects of handedness. *Journal of the International Neuropsychological Society, 15*(06), 1023. https://doi.org/10.1017/S1355617709990440

Sosa, A. L., Albanese, E., Prince, M., Acosta, D., Ferri, C. P., Guerra, M., . . . Stewart, R. (2009). Population normative data for the 10/66 Dementia Research Group cognitive test battery from Latin America, India and China: A cross-sectional survey. *BMC Neurology, 9*(1). http://doi.org/10.1186/1471-2377-9-48

Stavro, K., Pelletier, J., & Potvin, S. (2013). Widespread and sustained cognitive deficits in alcoholism: A meta-analysis. *Addiction Biology, 18*(2), 203–213. http://doi.org/10.1111/j.1369-1600.2011.00418.x

Steinberg, B. A., Bieliauskas, L. A., Smith, G. E., & Ivnik, R. J. (2005). Mayo's Older Americans Normative Studies: Age- and IQ-adjusted norms for the Trail-Making Test, the Stroop Test, and MAE Controlled Oral Word Association Test. *The Clinical Neuropsychologist, 19*, 329–377.

Stricks, L., Pittman, J., Jacobs, D. M., Sano, M., & Stern, Y. (1998). Normative data for a brief neuropsychological battery administered to English- and Spanish-speaking community-dwelling elders. *Journal of the International Neuropsychological Society, 4*, 311–318.

Stuss, D. T., Alexander, M. P., Hamer, L., Paumbo, C., Dempster, R., Binns, M., Levine, B., & Izukawa, D. (1998). The effects of focal anterior brain lesions on verbal fluency. *Journal of the International Neuropsychological Society, 4*, 265–278.

Sudo, F. K., Amado, P., Alves, G. S., Laks, J., & Engelhardt, E. (2017). A continuum of executive function deficits in early subcortical vascular cognitive impairment: A systematic review and meta-analysis. *Dementia & Neuropsychologia, 11*(4), 371–380. https://doi.org/10.1590/1980-57642016dn11-040006

Sugarman, M. A., & Axelrod, B. N. (2015). Embedded measures of performance validity using verbal fluency tests in a clinical sample. *Applied Neuropsychology. Adult, 22*(2), 141–146. https://doi.org/10.1080/23279095.2013.873439

Suhr, J. A., & Jones, R. D. (1998). Letter and semantic fluency in Alzheimer's, Huntington's, and Parkinson's dementias. *Archives of Clinical Neuropsychology, 13*, 447–454.

Sung, K., Gordon, B., Vannorsdall, T. D., Ledoux, K., Pickett, E. J., Pearlson, G. D., & Schretlen, D. J. (2012). Semantic clustering of category fluency in schizophrenia examined with singular value decomposition. *Journal of the International Neuropsychological Society, 18*(03), 565–575. https://doi.org/10.1017/S1355617712000136

Szöke, A., Trandafir, A., Dupont, M.-E., Méary, A., Schürhoff, F., & Leboyer, M. (2008). Longitudinal studies of cognition in schizophrenia: Meta-analysis. *British Journal of Psychiatry, 192*(4), 248–257. http://doi.org/10.1192/bjp.bp.106.029009

Tallberg, I. M., Ivachova, E., Jones Tinghag, K., & Östberg, P. (2008). Swedish norms for word fluency tests: FAS, animals and verbs. *Scandinavian Journal of Psychology, 49*(5), 479–485. http://doi.org/10.1111/j.1467-9450.2008.00653.x

Taussig, I. M., Henderson, V. W., & Mack, W. (1992). Spanish translation and evaluation of a neuropsychological battery: Performance of Spanish and English-speaking Alzheimer's disease patients and normal comparison subjects. Paper presented at the Gerontological Society of America.

Taylor, B. P., Bruder, G. E., Stewart, J. W., McGrath, P. J., Halperin, J., Ehrlichman, H., & Quitkin, F. M. (2006). Psychomotor slowing as a predictor of fluoxetine nonresponse in depressed outpatients. *American Journal of Psychiatry, 163*(1), 73-78.

Thiele, K., Quinting, J. M., & Stenneken, P. (2016). New ways to analyze word generation performance in brain injury: A systematic review and meta-analysis of additional performance measures. *Journal of Clinical and Experimental Neuropsychology, 38*(7), 764–781. https://doi.org/10.1080/13803395.2016.1163327

Thurstone, L. L. (1938). *Primary mental abilities*. Chicago: University of Chicago Press.

Tombaugh, T. N., Kozak, J., & Rees, L. (1999). Normative data stratified by age and education for two measures of verbal fluency: FAS and animal naming. *Archives of Clinical Neuropsychology, 14*, 167–177.

Troester, A. I., Fields, J. A., Testa, J. A., Paul, R. H., Blanco, C. R., Hames, K. A., Salmon, D. P., & Beatty, W. W. (1998). Cortical and subcortical influences on clustering and switching in the performance of verbal fluency tasks. *Neuropsychologia, 36*, 295–304.

Troester, A. I., Woods, S. P., Fields, J. A., Hanisch, C., & Beatty, W. W. (2002). Declines in switching underlie verbal fluency changes after unilateral pallidal surgery in Parkinson's disease. *Brain and Cognition, 50*, 207–217.

Troyer, A. K. (2000). Normative data for clustering and switching on verbal fluency tasks. *Journal of Clinical and Experimental Neuropsychology, 22*, 370–378.

Troyer, A. K., Moscovitch, M., & Winocur, G. (1997). Clustering and switching as two components of verbal fluency: Evidence from younger and healthy adults. *Neuropsychology, 11*, 138–146.

Troyer, A. K., Moscovitch, M., Winocur, G., Alexander, M. P., & Stuss, D. (1998a). Clustering and switching on verbal fluency: The effects of focal frontal- and temporal-lobe lesions. *Neuropsychologia, 36*, 449–504.

Troyer, A. K., Moscovitch, M., Winocur, G., Leach, L., & Freedman, M. (1998b). Clustering and switching on verbal fluency tests in Alzheimer's disease and Parkinson's disease. *Journal of the International Neuropsychological Society, 4*, 137–143.

Tucha, O., Mecklinger, L., Laufkötter, R., Kaunzinger, I., Paul, G. M., Klein, H. E., & Lange, K. W. (2005). Clustering and switching on verbal and figural fluency functions in adults with attention deficit hyperactivity disorder. *Cognitive Neuropsychiatry, 10*(3), 231–248. https://doi.org/10.1080/13546800444000047

Van der Elst, W., Van Boxtel, M. P., Van Breukelen, G. J., & Jolles, J. (2006). Normative data for the Animal, Profession and Letter M Naming verbal fluency tests for Dutch speaking participants and the effects of age, education, and sex. *Journal of the International Neuropsychological Society, 12*(01), 80–89.

Venneri, A., Gorgoglione, G., Toraci, C., Nocetti, L., Panzetti, P., & Nichelli, P. (2011). Combining neuropsychological and structural neuroimaging indicators of conversion to Alzheimer's disease in amnestic mild cognitive impairment. *Current Alzheimer Research, 8*(7), 789–797. http://doi.org/10.2174/156720511797633160

Warrington, E. D. (2000). Homophone meaning generation: A new test of verbal switching for the detection of frontal lobe dysfunction. *Journal of the International Neuropsychological Society, 6*, 643–648.

Wilde, M. C. (2006). The validity of the repeatable battery of neuropsychological status in acute stroke. *The Clinical Neuropsychologist, 20*(4), 702–715.

Williams-Gray, C. H., Foltynie, T., Brayne, C. E. G., Robbins, T. W., & Barker, R. A. (2007). Evolution of cognitive dysfunction in an incident Parkinson's disease cohort. *Brain: A Journal of Neurology, 130*(Pt 7), 1787–1798. https://doi.org/10.1093/brain/awm111

Wilson, B. A., Watson, P. C., Baddeley, A. D., Emslie, H., & Evans, J. J. (2000). Improvement or simply practice? The effects of twenty repeated assessments on people with and without brain injury. *Journal of the International Neuropsychological Society, 6*, 469–479.

Wood, R. L., & Liossi, C. (2007). The relationship between general intellectual ability and performance on ecologically valid executive tests in a severe brain injury sample. *Journal of the International Neuropsychological Society, 13*(1), 90–98.

Woods, S. P., Scott, J. C., Sires, D. A., Grant, I., Heaton, R. K., Troster, A. I., & the HIV Neurobehavioral Research Center (HNRC) Group. (2005). Action (verb) fluency: Test-retest reliability, normative standards, and construct validity. *Journal of the International Neuropsychological Society, 11*, 408–415.

Woodward, N. D., Purdon, S. E., Meltzer, H. Y., & Zald, D. H. (2007). A meta-analysis of cognitive change with haloperidol in clinical trials of atypical antipsychotics: Dose effects and comparison to practice effects. *Schizophrenia Research, 89*(1-3), 211–224. http://doi.org/10.1016/j.schres.2006.08.021

York, M. K., Levin, H. S., Grossman, R. G., Lai, E. C., & Krauss, J. K. (2003). Clustering and switching in phonemic fluency following pallidotomy for the treatment of Parkinson's disease. *Journal of Clinical and Experimental Neuropsychology, 25*, 110–121.

Zakzanis, K. K., McDonald, K., & Troyer, A. K. (2011). Component analysis of verbal fluency in patients with mild traumatic brain injury. *Journal of Clinical and Experimental Neuropsychology, 33*(7), 785–792. http://doi.org/10.1080/13803395.2011.558496

Zakzanis, K. K., McDonald, K., & Troyer, A. K. (2013). Component analysis of verbal fluency scores in severe traumatic brain injury. *Brain Injury, 27*(7–8), 903–908. http://doi.org/10.3109/02699052.2013.775505

Zakzanis, K. K., Troyer, A. K., Rich, J. B., & Heinrichs, W. (2000). Component analysis of verbal fluency in patients with schizophrenia. *Neuropsychiatry, Neuropsychology, & Behavioral Neurology, 13*, 239–245.

Zarino, B., Crespi, M., Launi, M., & Casarotti, A. (2014). A new standardization of semantic verbal fluency test. *Neurological Sciences, 35*(9), 1405–1411. http://doi.org/10.1007/s10072-014-1729-1

Zimmermann, N., Parente, M. A. de M. P., Joanette, Y., & Fonseca, R. P. (2014). Unconstrained, phonemic and semantic verbal fluency: Age and education effects, norms and discrepancies. *Psicologia: Reflexão E Crítica, 27*(1), 55–63.

WISCONSIN CARD SORTING TEST (WCST)

TEST NAME	**Wisconsin Card Sorting Test (WCST)**
DOMAIN	Executive functioning
AGE RANGE	Up to 89 years
ADMINISTRATION TIME	30 minutes
SCORING FORMAT	Computerized or hand scored
REFERENCE	Heaton, R. K., Chelune, G. J., Talley, J. L., Kay, G. G., & Curtis, G. (1993). *Wisconsin Card Sorting Test (WCST) manual, revised and expanded.* Odessa, FL: Psychological Assessment Resources. www.parinc.com

DESCRIPTION

The purpose of the Wisconsin Card Sorting Test (WCST; Heaton et al., 1993) is to evaluate the ability to form abstract concepts, shift and maintain set, and utilize feedback. The test requires strategic planning, organized search, the ability to use environmental feedback to shift cognitive set, goal-oriented behavior, and modulation of impulsive responding. Cognitive persistence, or the ability to overcome task difficulty in pursuit of a goal, is another important skill involved in test performance that is distinct from cognitive flexibility or set-shifting (Teubner-Rhodes et al., 2017).

This test was developed by Berg and Grant (Berg, 1948; Grant & Berg, 1948). Heaton (1981) standardized the test instructions and scoring procedures and published it as a clinical instrument. In the updated manual (Heaton et al., 1993), scoring rules were refined, the recording form was revised, and normative data were provided for individuals up to 89 years of age. Relatively recent literature has focused on identifying cognitive component processes underlying WCST performance, including sequential learning models (e.g., differential attention shifting for reward and punishment, decision consistencies across individuals, and attentional focus; see Bishara et al., 2010 for an in-depth discussion).

The test consists of four stimulus cards placed in front of the examinee, the first with a red triangle, the second with two green stars, the third with three yellow crosses, and the fourth with four blue circles (see Figure 9–17). The examinee is given two packs each containing 64 response cards, which have designs similar to those on the stimulus cards, varying in color, geometric form, and number. The examinee is asked to match each of the cards in the decks to one of the four key cards and is given feedback after each selection on whether it is right or wrong. No warning is provided that the sorting rule changes. There is no time limit for this test.

Task Variations. The abbreviated form of the standard WCST, the WCST-64 (Axelrod et al., 1992; Kongs et al., 2000), involves giving only the first deck of 64 cards. Although most use Heaton's procedure, there are also other versions of the test (e.g., Modified Card Sorting Test, Cianchetti et al., 2005; Nelson, 1976; Milwaukee Card Sorting Test, Osmon & Suchy, 1996). The Modified Wisconsin Card Sorting Test (MWCST), as originally designed by Nelson (1976), is similar in concept to the WCST and involves 48 cards. A tactile version of the WCST for use with visually impaired individuals has also been developed (Beauvais et al., 2004), as has a computer version (as discussed later). Other modifications of the WCST include the Cleveland Sorting Test (Poreh et al., 2012).

Computer administration of the WCST is also available (see Source). Some research has reported similar performance between the computerized and standard versions (Artiola i Fortuny & Heaton, 1996; Hellman et al., 1992; Wagner & Trentini, 2009). In contrast, others have not found equivalence on distributional properties

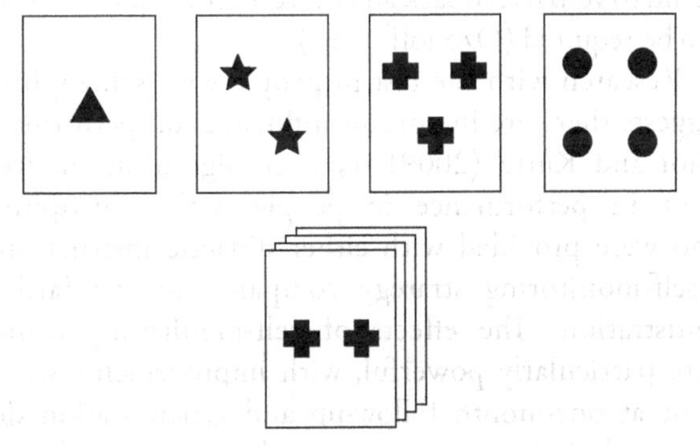

Figure 9–17 Example of Wisconsin Card Sorting Test (WCST) stimuli.
NOTE: 1 Red Triangle; 2 Green Stars; 3 Yellow Crosses; 4 Blue Circles.

Reproduced by special permission of the Publisher, Psychological Assessment Resources, Inc. (PAR), 16204 North Florida Avenue, Lutz, Florida 33549, from the Wisconsin Card Sorting Test by David A. Grant, PhD and Esta A. Berg, PhD, Copyright 1981, 1993 by PAR. Further reproduction is prohibited without permission of PAR.

(central tendency, variability, shape) of the scores between the standard and computerized versions in healthy groups (Feldstein et al., 1999). Steinmetz, Brunner, Loarer, and Houssemand (2010) similarly reported minimal psychometric equivalence (i.e., in terms of variance, alternate form reliability, temporal stability) between scores on the two versions in healthy adults. Overall, given the various discrepancies in the literature, it is unclear whether norms collected under standard administration conditions may be used with computerized administrations.

ADMINISTRATION

See Source for details. Although it is permissible to clarify the meaning of the stimulus (key) cards and the manner in which the examinee is to respond, the examiner is not to provide any indication of the sorting principles or the nature of the shift from one category to the next. Recording performance, particularly if the examinee works quickly, can be difficult (see Source for instructions).

INFLUENCES OF SITUATIONAL PARAMETERS ON PERFORMANCE

Fatigue may impact performance. Young, healthy adults who work on cognitively demanding tasks for a considerable time (e.g., two hours) discover fewer categories and are more perseverative on the WCST, in comparison to individuals who are not fatigued (van der Linden et al., 2003). Similarly, Bennett, Petros, Johnson, and Ferraro (2008) reported that participants classified as having morning-type circadian rhythms performed better on the WCST in the morning compared to later in the day.

Other influences have also been reported. High cortisol levels at the beginning of a testing session were related to more errors in women than men (McCormick et al., 2007). In contrast, Yantz and McCaffrey (2007) reported that examiner presence during computerized WCST performance did not appear to significantly alter results. Motivation to attend to verbal feedback and a level of social awareness may also be required (Ozonoff, 1995).

Research with the test in people with schizophrenia suggests there are important influences on performance. Choi and Kurtz (2009) reported significant improvement in performance in people with schizophrenia who were provided with either didactic instruction or a self-monitoring strategy compared to standard administration. The effects of self-monitoring training were particularly powerful, with improvements still evident at one-month follow-up and generalization demonstrated via improvement on other executive function tests. Kantrowitz, Revheim, Pasternak, Silipo, and Javitt (2009) reported that individuals with schizophrenia performed better on a variant of the WCST that employed faces rather than abstract stimuli.

SCORING

Scoring the WCST can be challenging, and the manual provides detailed scoring criteria and clarifications (Heaton et al., 1993). Scoring errors are common, even among experienced clinicians (Greve, 1993; Paolo et al., 1994) and are most likely to occur when response cards match a stimulus card on two attributes (Paolo et al., 1994). A computer scoring program is available and is recommended to avoid recording and scoring errors. Berry (1996) also summarizes the relevant rules for scoring perseverations in a diagrammatic format that can be used as a scoring aid.

Number of Categories Completed is often referred to as *Categories Completed*, and reflects the number of categories (i.e., each sequence of 10 consecutive correct matches to the criterion sorting category) completed during the test. Scores can range from 0 to 6, at which point the test is discontinued. When an examinee persists in responding to a stimulus characteristic that is incorrect, the response is said to match the "perseverated-to" principle and is scored as perseverative ("p"). The perseverative response may reflect an inability to relinquish the old category for the new one or the inability to see a new possibility.

The score for *Failure to Maintain Set* is the number of times the examinee makes five or more correct responses in a row and then makes an error before successfully achieving a category. It indicates the inability to continue using a strategy that has been successful. *Percent Conceptual Level Responses* is defined as consecutive correct responses occurring in runs of three or more. It is thought to reflect some insight into correct sorting principles. The number of trials administered, total number correct, and total number of errors are also recorded. *Percent Errors, Percent Perseverative Responses,* and *Percent Non-Perseverative Errors* can also be calculated to assist in research investigations. Use of these latter scores is not recommended for clinical interpretation, in part due to weaker reliability compared to basic scores.

There are a number of redundancies in the various WCST scores. For example, correlations are high between Categories Completed and Total Errors (*rs* = −.76 to −.89; e.g., Bowden et al., 1998; Iverson et al., 2000; Pineda & Merchan, 2003) and between Perseverative Errors and Perseverative Responses (*rs* = .69 to .95; Bowden et al., 1998; Iverson et al., 2000). Some scores (e.g., Total Errors) are linear combinations of other scores (Perseverative Errors and Non-Perseverative Errors).

The most common measures used to assess executive control on the WCST are Categories Completed and Perseverative Errors. The measure of Perseverative Errors is marginally more sensitive to age-related decline in comparison with Categories Completed and may be a better metric of executive function if only a single score from the WCST is to be used (Rhodes, 2004). Klein, Foerster, and Hartnegg (2007) provide equations to predict an examinee's score on the WCST; however, this was modeled on healthy participants six to 26 years of age, rather than on an exclusively adult sample.

DEMOGRAPHIC EFFECTS

AGE

Age has a significant effect on performance, accounting for about 20% of the variance in test scores (Heaton et al., 1993; Rhodes, 2004). In one normative study, age effects were medium and larger than education effects (Norman et al., 2011). Performance remains fairly stable between the second to fifth decades of life. Declines in some aspects of performance (e.g., Categories Completed, Perseverative Errors) become apparent after 60 years of age (see Rhodes [2004] for a meta-analysis).

Some have proposed that declines with age are linked to age-related declines in working memory (e.g., Hartman et al., 2001), switching (Gamboz et al., 2009), or rule inference (Lange et al., 2016). Using a qualitative approach involving participants verbalizing their response strategy during task completion, Ashendorf and McCaffrey (2008) interpreted results to suggest poor set-shifting and maintenance, suggestive of poor use of feedback utilization, as processes underlying age-associated decline in WCST performance. However, others have suggested that age differences in performance on the WCST are the result of underlying deficits in processing speed rather than executive control (see Fristoe et al., 1997; Salthouse et al., 1996).

GENDER

The influence of gender is typically found to be nonsignificant (e.g., Heaton et al., 1993; Laiacona et al., 2000; Norman et al., 2011).

EDUCATION

Education level is modestly correlated with test scores (Boone et al., 1993, 1999; Heaton et al., 1993; Heinrichs, 1990) and contributes a small but significant proportion of variance in addition to that explained by age (i.e., 4 to 7%; Heaton et al., 1993; Rhodes, 2004). Large effect sizes on a modified WCST for low versus highly educated groups have been reported (Zimmerman et al., 2015). See the section "Evidence for Validity" for information on the effects of IQ.

ETHNICITY, NATIONALITY, AND LINGUISTIC EFFECTS

Effects of culture and ethnicity are often reported. Boone, Victor, Wen, Razani, and Ponton (2007) reported that WCST performance differed in their sample of Caucasian, African-American, Hispanic, and Asian persons referred for neuropsychological evaluation. Specifically, Caucasian and Hispanic patients obtained better scores than African Americans on Categories Completed. Higher levels of acculturation in Mexican-American participants were associated with better performance using English norms, with no significant differences using Spanish norms (Coffey et al., 2005). Norman et al. (2011) reported that Caucasian participants performed better than African Americans on the computerized WCST-64, with effect sizes medium to large in magnitude, depending on the variable.

In other studies, performance appears similar among groups (Rey et al., 1999). When bilingual Hispanic Americans were subdivided into Spanish-dominant, balanced, and English-dominant bilingual speakers, the WCST did not show a language administration effect when it was alternatively administered in Spanish and English (Gasquoine et al., 2007).

NORMATIVE DATA

WCST

Norms for individuals up to 89 years of age are provided in the manual (Heaton et al., 1993). The data were derived from 899 healthy people aggregated from six samples. The characteristics of the sample are shown in Table 9–168. The educational level of this sample was somewhat higher than that of the US population in 1987. Information is not

TABLE 9–168 Description of Wisconsin Card Sorting Test (WCST) Standardization Sample

Number	899
Age	Up to 89 years, 11 months
Geographic location	United States
Sample type	Aggregate of six different samples, including child and youth samples (Sample 1 and 2) and: Sample 3: 150 subjects aged 15 to 77 from Texas and Colorado Sample 4: 50 subjects aged 58 to 84 from Colorado Sample 5: 124 pilots aged 24 to 65 from Colorado Sample 6: 73 adults aged 51 to 89 from Detroit and 384 adults age 20+ matched with 1995 projections of US population with regard to age[a]
Education	6 to 20 years[b]
Gender	
Female	42%
Ethnicity	Not reported
Screening	Not reported for adults

[a]For the adult normative sample, participants in the younger age ranges are slightly underrepresented, while participants in the older age ranges are slightly overrepresented.

[b]Mean education of this sample is about three years higher (M = 14.95, SD = 2.97) than the US population in 1987.

SOURCE: Heaton et al. (1993). Reproduced by special permission of the Publisher, Psychological Assessment Resources, Inc. (PAR), 16204 North Florida Avenue, Lutz, Florida 33549, from the Wisconsin Card Sorting Test by David A. Grant, PhD and Esta A. Berg, PhD, Copyright 1981, 1993 by PAR. Further reproduction is prohibited without permission of PAR.

provided for a number of important variables (e.g., ethnicity, screening method).

Tables are provided (see Source) based on the examinee's age or combination of age and years of education. Raw scores are converted to percentile scores. For some scores, corresponding standard scores ($M = 100$, $SD = 15$) and T scores ($M = 50$, $SD = 10$) are also recorded. Because both age and education influence performance, demographically corrected normative data are recommended, particularly for diagnostic purposes. When making inferences about a person's capacity for everyday functioning (e.g., job placement), US Census-based data for the general adult population may be preferred (see manual). Standard scores of 84 or lower or T scores of 39 or lower are considered to be in the impaired range. Base rate information is also provided (see manual). Some concerns have been raised that the norms overcorrect for age, thereby artificially enhancing performance, especially in older adults (Fastenau, 1998). However, other data suggest the norms perform adequately in older adults (Heaton et al., 1999).

In addition to normative data provided by the standardization sample, other normative data can be found. A meta-analysis of 34 studies published between 1990 and 2003 comprising about 3,000 participants examined age-related differences in young (ages 20–35, $M = 24$ years, $SD = 3$; education, $M = 14$ years; $n = 1{,}350$; 55% female) and older (≥55 years, $M = 71$ years, $SD = 7$; education, $M = 13$ years; $n = 1{,}650$; 58% female) healthy adults on the standard and the Nelson versions of the WCST (Rhodes, 2004). The study documented robust age-related changes in performance on both versions for Categories Completed and Perseverative Errors. The data are shown in Table 9–169 and appear to be more stringent than those reported by Heaton et al. (1993) for young and older adults.

Artiola i Fortuny, Romo, Heaton, and Pardee (1999) provide data for Spanish speakers. Normative data for Italians are also available (Laiacona et al., 2000) and for 93 Setswana-speaking students aged 18 to 29 years of age in South Africa (Gadd & Phipps, 2012).

TABLE 9–169 Metanorms for the Wisconsin Card Sorting Test (WCST)

VARIABLE	OLDER PARTICIPANTS (55+)	YOUNGER PARTICIPANTS (20–35)
N	1,650	1,350
Mean categories achieved	3.99	5.58
SD	1.83	1.10
Mean perseverative errors	15.85	6.92
SD	11.44	5.04

NOTE: Norms based on 34 studies comprising about 3,000 healthy adults. The standard deviation refers to the mean of the standard deviations reported across all studies examined.

SOURCE: From Rhodes (2004).

WCST-64

Use of the standard WCST Manual's norms for 128 cards to estimate normative data for the WCST-64 is not recommended (Axelrod et al., 1997). Normative data have been published for the WCST-64 (Kongs et al., 2000). Norman et al. (2011) collected normative data for the WCST-64 in 246 healthy individuals who were controls as part of a longitudinal HIV study in San Diego, California. The distribution of ethnic groups matched the 2000 US Census and was used in the generation of normative data. Participants were excluded if they presented with a history of neurologic conditions, substance abuse, psychiatric disorders, or major medical conditions. A sample of Caucasian ($n = 143$) and African-American ($n = 103$) individuals were included. Caucasian participants were an average age of 37.6 years ($SD = 12.3$), 31% female, with an average education of 14.1 years ($SD = 2.4$). African-American participants were an average age of 40.6 years ($SD = 12.3$), 50% female, with an average education of 13.8 years ($SD = 2.1$).

Raw scores are first converted to scaled scores (Table 9–170), then formulas are used to adjust for demographic effects (Table 9–171). Norman et al.'s (2011) data reinforce the importance of using demographically corrected norms. Using their derived norms, impairment rates in African Americans ranged from 10% to 15%, depending on the WCST variables examined. When using conventional norms, however, impairment rates in this group ranged from 40% to 50%. However, Caucasian participants

TABLE 9–170 Raw to Scaled Score Conversions for the WCST-64

	RAW		
SCALED	TOTAL ERRORS	PERSEVERATIVE ERRORS	CONCEPTUAL LEVEL RESPONSES
18		0–3	
17	0–6		≥58
16	7		57
15	8		56
14		4	54–55
13	9–10		53
12	11	5	51–52
11	12	6	49–50
10	13–15	7	45–48
9	16–19	8	39–44
8	20–22	9–10	34–38
7	23–28	11–13	28–33
6	29–32	14–15	20–27
5	33–35	16–18	16–19
4	36–39	19–26	13–15
3	40–48	26–41	6–12
2	≥49	≥42	≤5
1			

NOTE: WCST-64 = Wisconsin Card Sorting Test 64-Card Version.

SOURCE: Norman et al. (2011).

TABLE 9–171 Formulas for Demographic Adjustments for the WCST-64

T SCORE FORMULAS	
Caucasian	
WCST-64 Total Errors	[(Total errors scaled score – (0.3187) × (edu – 14.13) + (-0.01) × (age – 37.37) + 0.1608 × gender + 10.4049) – (-0.0017))/2.674] × 10 + 50
WCST-64 Perseverative Errors	[(Perseverative errors scaled score – (0.2357 × (edu – 14.13) + (-0.0941) × (age – 37.37) + 0.0341 × gender + 10.33) – (-0.0012))/2.5506] × 10 + 50
WCST-64 Conceptual Level Responses	[(Conceptual level responses scaled score -(0.3223) × (edu – 14.13) + (-0.0941) × (age – 37.37) + 0.0577 × gender + 10.4292) – (-0.0016))/2.568] × 10 + 50
African American	
WCST-64 Total Errors	[(Total errors scaled score – (0.3321) × (edu – 13.97) + (-0.0838) × (age – 40.7) + 0.3215 × sex + 8.1621) – (-0.0006))/2.7911] × 10 + 50
WCST-64 Perseverative Errors	[(Perseverative errors scaled score – (0.3599 × (edu – 13.97) + (-0.0776) × (age – 40.7) + (-0.1093) × sex + 8.5524) – (-0.0006))/3.0124] × 10 + 50
WCST-64 Conceptual Level Responses	[(Conceptual level responses scaled score - (0.4002) × (edu – 13.97) + (-0.0874) × (age – 40.7) + 0.2546 × gender + 8.2248) – (-0.0006))/2.5887] × 10 + 50

NOTE: Sex: male = 0, female = 1. Edu, education: years of education were determined using a previously defined and standardized procedure where education level ranges from 1 to 20 based on number of years of schooling completed (Heaton et al., 2004).

SOURCE: Norman et al. (2011).

showed roughly the same level of impairment irrespective of the normative dataset used.

Normative data from a sample of 303 patients with acute, uncomplicated, mild TBI has been provided by Iverson et al. (2000). They note that their data may be of value in interpreting test performance of individuals in the post-acute period. The interested reader is referred to their article for the norms.

MODIFIED WISCONSIN CARD SORTING TEST (MWCST)

Zimmerman et al. (2015) recruited community-dwelling Brazilian Portuguese speakers who completed a MWCST, originally designed by Nelson (1976). The test is similar in concept to the WCST and involves 48 cards. Participants were excluded if they did not comprehend test instructions, presented with a history of neurologic conditions, psychiatric disorders, or substance abuse, scored below a MMSE cutoff, or had an uncorrected vision or hearing impairment. Participants ranged in age from 19 to 75 years, with varying education levels in each of the three age groups and an overall predominance of female participants. Age- and education-adjusted normative data are provided in Table 9–172.

Schretlen, Testa, and Pearlson (2010) provide norms for 323 adults for the MWCST as part of the CNNS available through Psychological Assessment Resources (www.parinc.com). These provide T scores and discrepancies based on a large sample of older adults from the northeastern United States. A major advantage of these norms is the option to correct for demographic variables such as age, sex, education, and ethnicity. Several other commonly used neuropsychological tests are co-normed using this sample, which facilitates cross-test comparisons.

TABLE 9–172 Normative Data for the Modified Wisconsin Card Sorting Test (MWCST) Adjusted by Age and Education

AGE	19–39 YEARS OLD				40–59 YEARS OLD				60–75 YEARS OLD			
YEARS OF EDUCATION	5–8		≥ 9		5–8		≥ 9		5–8		≥ 9	
VARIABLES	MEAN	*SD*	MEAN	*SD*	MEAN	*SD*	MEAN	*SD*	MEAN	*SD*	MEAN	*SD*
	(*n* = 19)		(*n* = 24)		(*n* = 15)		(*n* = 16)		(*n* = 18)		(*n* = 31)	
Categories Completed	3.74	1.24	5.71	0.69	3.6	1.54	5.19	1.32	3.22	1.59	5.61	0.66
Perseverative Errors	12.05	5.94	2.82	2.63	13.13	5.92	4.04	3.16	13.13	6.07	4.43	4.65
Non-Perseverative Errors	5.21	2.46	2.46	3.53	4.47	2.94	1.94	2.29	4.56	3.39	2.31	2.54
Failure to Maintain Set	0.79	0.71	0.46	0.83	1.00	0.84	0.44	0.72	0.94	1.11	0.41	0.68

SOURCE: Zimmerman et al. (2015).

EVIDENCE FOR RELIABILITY

EVIDENCE FOR INTERNAL RELIABILITY

Gadd and Phipps (2012) reported strong internal reliability (Cronbach's alpha = .85).

EVIDENCE FOR TEST-RETEST RELIABILITY, MEASURING CHANGE, AND PRACTICE EFFECTS

Test-retest reliability is variable, but typically reported to be in the low range, with generally weak coefficients for Learning to Learn and higher coefficients for error scores. Practice effects are often reported to be substantial (but see Tate et al., 1998). Some authors have argued that once an examinee has figured out the category sorts and shift principle, the WCST no longer measures problem-solving ability (Lezak, 2012). This suggests that the low stability of the WCST for healthy people may reflect that, on retesting, it is no longer measuring problem-solving abilities in the same manner as on novel presentation (Paolo et al., 1996a). Procedural knowledge of test demands and test-taking strategies are likely retained, facilitating subsequent performance, rather than knowledge of the progression of rule change per se (Basso et al., 1999). Of note, however, reliability estimates are often higher in clinical than healthy samples, suggesting that the test may be more sensitive to change in clinical populations.

Paolo et al. (1996a) retested 87 healthy older adults following an interval of about one year. To ensure that each participant displayed intact cognitive function at both assessment points, each participant had to have an initial Dementia Rating Scale score greater than 130 and display no evidence of significant decline (i.e., 10 points or more). Stability coefficients were generally low, ranging from $r = .12$ for Learning to Learn to $r = .66$ for Total Errors. The majority of individuals improved on retest, with five WCST scores demonstrating significant average retest gains of 5 to 7 standard score points.

Paolo et al. (1996a) also calculated standard error of prediction, standard error of difference, and abnormal test-retest discrepancy scores to assist in detecting possible meaningful changes in WCST scores on retest. Table 9–173 presents the 90% cutoff scores for WCST standard scores, with 5% of the cases indicating gain (positive) and 5% indicating loss (negative).

To use the cutoff scores, the user must first convert the raw scores to normalized age- and education-corrected standard scores according to the manual. Next, subtract the initial score from the score obtained on retest. If the difference score is negative, it reflects a loss on retest. If it is positive, the score represents a retest gain. Next, compare the difference score to the cutoff values provided in Table 9–173. If the difference score equals or exceeds the tabled values, then the test-retest change is considered unusual because it occurred in 5% or less of the sample. Note that the magnitude of the difference required for an unusual change on retest is quite large, typically more than one standard deviation.

TABLE 9–173 Cutoff Scores at the 90% Confidence Interval Level of Abnormality for the Detection of Change on Retest in Older Adults

SCALE	LOSS	GAIN
Total Number of Errors	18	35
Perseverative Responses	12	30
Perseverative Errors	15	35
Non-Perseverative Errors	29	40
Percent Conceptual Level Response	24	35

NOTE: Mean age of individuals was 68.79 years (*SD* = 6.21). The retest interval was on average 13.55 months (*SD* = 2.19). To calculate losses and gains, see the section "Evidence for Reliability."

SOURCE: From Paolo et al. (1996a).

Basso et al. (1999) retested a group of 50 healthy men (age, $M = 32.5$ years, $SD = 9.27$) following a 12-month interval and found that retesting resulted in significant improvement on nearly all indices, especially the number of trials needed to complete the test. On average, approximately 101 cards were required at baseline, whereas only approximately 85 trials were needed 12 months later. As well, the number of Perseverative Errors and Perseverative Responses decreased by nearly half on retesting (but see Tate et al., 1998, and Ferland et al., 1998, who found somewhat smaller practice effects in healthy individuals when test-retest intervals were about 5 months in length). The presence and magnitude of practice effects was similar among individuals of average and above-average IQ.

The authors also calculated reliable change indices using the standard error of prediction to estimate the range of change in scores that might be expected while accounting for measurement error and practice effects. Table 9–174 shows the mean estimated true scores at 12 months together with the standard error of prediction (SE_P) and resulting 90% CI.

Note that a wide range of retest scores are within the 90% CI and reflect measurement error rather than meaningful change (see also Tate et al., 1998, for similar findings). To use the CIs, the 90% confidence band should be summed with an individual's estimated true score ($Y_{TRUE} = M + r[Y_{OBS} - M]$), where M is the sample mean of the test, Y_{OBS} is

TABLE 9–174 Descriptive Statistics and Confidence Intervals for Estimated True Scores at 12-Month Follow-Up

	M	R_{Y1Y2}	SE_P	90% CI
Categories Completed	5.42	.54	1.30	±2
Number of Trials	84.73	.30	17.71	±29
Errors	16.68	.50	10.29	±17
Perseverative Errors	8.43	.52	5.25	±9
Percent Conceptual Responses	76.11	.54	15.74	±26
Perseverative Responses	9.34	.50	6.65	±11
Learning to Learn	.73	.36	3.63	±6
Failure to Maintain Set	.80	–.02	1.15	±2

NOTE: Based on a sample of 50 community-dwelling healthy males, for the most part Caucasian, ranging in age from 20–59 (*M* = 32.5, *SD* = 9.27) and mean education of 14.98 years (*SD* = 1.93). For information on how to use these formulas, see the section "Evidence for Reliability."

SOURCE: From Basso et al. (1999).

the actual score obtained by the individual, and r is the reliability coefficient. Significant changes reflect the frequency of obtained scores that fall above or below the CI.

In terms of clinical populations, Ingram et al. (1999) retested patients with obstructive sleep apnea a median of 12 days apart (range 1–71 days) and reported correlations ranging from r = .34 to r = .83, with a mean of r = .64. Perseverative Errors and Non-Perseverative Errors had high correlation coefficients (rs = .83 and .80, respectively), while coefficients for Trials to Complete First Category, Failure to Maintain Set, Total Correct, and Learning to Learn were low (rs = .34 to .61).

Greve, Love, Sherwin, Mathias, Houston, and Brennan (2002) examined temporal stability in survivors of severe TBI, whose conditions were stable (tested at least one-year post-injury, with a median retest interval of 54 weeks). On average, scores improved by about 5 T-score points. Stability coefficients were generally marginal/good (r > .60) except for Non-Perseverative Errors, Categories Completed, Trials to First Category, Failure to Maintain Set, and Learning to Learn, which were low.

The authors also provide 90% CI s to determine whether the test-retest difference scores (Time 2 minus Time 1) are unusual in TBI patients. The cutoff values for improvement and decline are shown in Table 9–175. A negative difference score indicates that the WCST score at Time 2 was lower than at Time 1. Depending on the variable, this can indicate improvement (e.g., Total Errors, Perseverative Responses, Perseverative Errors, and Trials to Complete First Category) or decline (e.g., Percent Conceptual Level Responses, Categories Completed, and Learning to Learn).

TABLE 9–175 Discrepancy Cutoff Scores for Wisconsin Card Sorting Test (WCST-128 and WCST-64) Variables

	WCST-128	WCST-128	WCST-64	WCST-64
	LOWER BOUND	UPPER BOUND	LOWER BOUND	UPPER BOUND
T Scores				
TE	−16	2	−16	8
PR	−27	7	−22	10
PE	−24	5	−20	10
NPE	−13	18	−15	12
%CLR	−16	2	−15	5
Raw Scores				
TE	−6	36	−8	17
PR	−20	58	−19	32
PE	−15	33	−15	20
NPE	−21	13	−9	9
%CLR	−39	12	−23	7
CAT	−5	1	−3	1
TTF	−15	100		
FMS	−3	3	−2	2
LL	−13	4	−38	8

NOTE: Based on Time 2 minus Time 1 scores in a TBI sample. An individual difference score must be outside the 90% confidence interval—indicated by the Lower and Upper Bound—to indicate a significant change.

SOURCE: Adapted from Greve et al. (2002).

EVIDENCE FOR RELIABILITY OF ALTERNATE, SHORT OR COMPUTER FORMS

Bowden et al. (1998) created an alternate form with the order of correct sorting of cards changed. That is, participants were required to sort first to form, then color, then number. University students were administered both versions in the same test session, with the order of presentation counterbalanced. Reliability coefficients were low (r ≤ .63). Therefore, use of this type of alternate form does not appear to improve reliability over retesting in comparison with the standard form administered twice.

Greve, Love, Sherwin, Mathias, Ramzinski, and Levy (2002) noted that stability of the WCST-64 was poorer than for the standard WCST and for most of the variables (except Total Errors and Percent Conceptual Level Responses), and coefficients were thus below acceptable levels. As the authors note, in this study, the 64-card version was extracted from the standard version and these individuals had as much as double the experience with the WCST-64 after the first testing point than would be the case if only the first 64 cards were given.

EVIDENCE FOR INTERRATER RELIABILITY

Interscorer and intrascorer reliability are excellent in some studies (ICCs higher than .83; Axelrod, Goldman, & Woodard, 1992; Greve, 1993), whereas another study indicated that interscorer reliability on indices of perseveration is quite low (Flashman, 1991). The detailed criteria provided in the manual and/or the use of computer software may increase reliability, although this remains to be evaluated.

EVIDENCE FOR VALIDITY

WITHIN-TEST RELATIONSHIPS

WCST variables are intercorrelated (see "Scoring"). Numerous factor-analytic studies have also been published investigating the structure of the WCST (e.g., Bell et al., 1997; Goldman et al., 1996; Greve et al., 1993, 1998, 1999; Koren et al., 1998; Paolo et al., 1995; Salthouse et al., 1996; Salthouse et al., 2003; Sullivan et al., 1993; Wiegner & Donders, 1999) using a variety of populations (e.g., mixed psychiatric or neurologic patients, patients with schizophrenia, TBI, stroke, healthy older adults). Most have used exploratory factor analysis and have found evidence in favor of two or more factors (see also review by Polgár et al., 2010). These processes include combinations of the ability to shift set, problem solve/hypothesis test, and maintain responses (Greve et al., 2005).

For example, in their study of people with schizophrenia, Polgár et al. (2010) reported two factors accounting for 95% of the variance (general executive function, which was comprised of a number of variables, and the second factor comprised of Non-Perseverative Errors). Similar factor structure has been reported for the WCST-64 (Su et al.,

2008). Principal components analysis of WCST variables in a severe TBI sample suggested a three-factor solution, accounting for 96% of the variance, with factors anchored by Percent Conceptual Level Responses, Failure to Maintain Set, and Non-Perseverative Errors (Benge et al., 2007). Similarly, in a sample of patients who had sustained a stroke, Jodzio and Biechowska (2010) reported that a three-factor solution accounted for approximately 90% of the variance.

A large-scale confirmatory factor analysis from a mixed sample of neurologic (n = 620) and psychiatric (n = 228) patients and healthy controls (n = 373) found support for the three-factor solution reported in the exploratory factor analysis literature (Greve et al., 2005). However, the second factors were less stable than the first factor (first factor: Perseverative Responses, Percent Conceptual Level Responses, Categories Completed, and Total Correct; second factor: Percent Conceptual Level Responses, Categories Completed, Total Correct, and Non-Perseverative Errors; third factor: Total Correct and Failure to Maintain Set). Greve et al. (2005) also suggest that having dual termination criteria (i.e., completion of six categories or all 128 cards, whichever is first) has likely contributed to varied factor-analytic solutions reported in the literature, and recommend use of all 128 cards.

WCST AND WCST-64 COMPARISON IN CLINICAL STUDIES

The WCST-64 is highly correlated with corresponding scores on the long form (r > .70; Axelrod, 2002; Merrick et al., 2003; Sherer et al., 2003). However, the WCST-64 may not produce results that are consistent with the full WCST on an individual basis. For example, in a mixed clinical sample, Axelrod (2002) observed that WCST-64 demographically adjusted scores capture about 59% of the full WCST scores within a 5-point margin of error, suggesting relatively moderate congruence. Sherer et al. (2003) reported that although scores were within 10 T-score points of each other for only 72% of participants, there was relatively high agreement in classification of performance as impaired (<40 T score) or not impaired (i.e., 86% agreement). Merrick et al. (2003) found that about one-quarter of a sample of adult patients who sustained a TBI obtained WCST-64 Perseverative Response T-scores that were more than 10 points below the corresponding WCST variable. The findings appeared to covary with age, with results from tests of older people showing stronger consistency between WCST/WCST-64 scores than those of younger adults (Donders & Wildeboer, 2004).

There is some evidence that the short form is sensitive to deficits in dementia (Paolo et al., 1996b), as well as to recovery in TBI (Merrick et al., 2003). The WCST appears to be more sensitive to impairment in the post-acute phase following TBI (median time post-injury of three months) than the WCST-64, as a higher percentage of individuals produce impaired scores on the standard WCST (58% versus 32%; Sherer et al., 2003). However, the WCST-64 performs comparably to the WCST in predicting level of disability in patients with TBI at discharge from inpatient rehabilitation (Sherer et al., 2003) and in differentiating between patients with AD and controls (Sánchez et al., 2017).

FACTOR-ANALYTIC STUDIES

Factor-analytic findings in both healthy adults (e.g., Pukrop et al., 2003) and clinical groups (e.g., Greve et al., 1998, 1999) have found that WCST scores load on the same factor as tasks that require speeded processing and aspects of working memory/attention involved in the comparison of information (e.g., Digit Symbol, TMT-B, CPT). Shifting appears to contribute significantly to performance. Miyake, Friedman, Emerson, Witzki, and Howerter (2000) reported that in healthy young adults, structural equation modeling indicated that performance on the WCST was significantly predicted by "shifting" ability. Once "shifting" ability was taken into account, neither "inhibition" nor "updating" abilities contributed to performance. Fisk and Sharp (2004) reported findings consistent with those of Miyake et al.

Interestingly, when the WCST is analyzed along with other measures of executive function, the WCST tends to load on a separate factor. For example, in individuals with autism (Minshew et al., 2002), variables from the WCST (Categories Completed, Perseverative Errors) loaded on one factor, while other tasks (e.g., 20 Questions, Stanford-Binet Verbal and Pictorial Absurdities subtests, Category Test, TMT-B) loaded on separate factors. Similar findings have been reported by others (e.g., Boone et al., 1998; Fisk & Sharp, 2004; Pineda & Merchan, 2003).

The WCST appears to measure a dimension of conceptual processing similar to that of other tests of rule derivation such as the Weigl Test (Laiacona et al., 2000) and the Category Test (e.g., Golden et al., 1997; O'Donnell et al., 1994; Pendleton & Heaton, 1982; Perrine, 1993). Based on a factor analysis with the WAIS-R subtests in a mixed clinical sample, Golden et al. (1997) suggested that the Category Test reflects spatial-analytic skills (loading with the Performance subtests), while the WCST loads on factors independent of the other tasks. Perrine (1993) noted that the WCST was associated with attribute identification, which entails discrimination of relevant features (i.e., the correct answer is based on the stimulus attribute of color, form, or number). Perrine noted about 30% shared variance between the WCST and Category Test. Minshew et al. (2002) also noted that the task involves hypothesis formation.

CORRELATIONS WITH EXECUTIVE AND ATTENTION MEASURES

The WCST has generally been found to relate to other measures of attention and executive function, although with generally lower associations than may be expected (see also Boone et al., 1998; Paolo et al., 1995). Some investigators have reported that indices of perseveration on the WCST show modest correlations (*rs* = .19 to .42) with measures of attention/working memory (e.g., TMT-B, CPT, Digit Span; e.g., Koren et al., 1998; O'Donnell et al., 1994; Somerville et al., 2000; Vanderploeg et al., 1994). Steinmetz and Houssemand (2011) reported that inhibition errors on Go No-Go and Stop-Signal paradigms predicted errors, particularly Non-Perseverative Errors.

CORRELATIONS WITH MEMORY TESTS

Memory appears modestly to moderately related to performance (*rs* = .19 to .42; Koren et al., 1998; O'Donnell et al., 1994; Somerville et al., 2000; Vanderploeg et al., 1994; though note Boone et al., 1998; Paolo et al., 1995). Rempfer, Hamera, Brown, and Bothwell (2006) categorized individuals with schizophrenia, bipolar disorder, or depression into learner subgroups based on WCST performance, with learners showing better verbal and working memory than those classified as nonretainers, suggesting that learning and memory ability impact performance.

The shorter version of the WCST also appears to be related to memory. Egan et al. (2011) found that memory measures (Benton Visual Retention Test, CVLT) were significantly correlated with Perseverative Errors and Categories Completed on the WCST-64 in patients with schizophrenia spectrum disorder (Spearman's rho = –.62, .54, respectively), but not healthy controls. Similarly, Greenwood et al. (2012) reported moderate correlations between WCST-64 Perseverative Errors as well as Categories Completed with measures of immediate and delayed recall (absolute value of *rs* = .34 to .53).

CORRELATIONS WITH IQ AND GENERAL COGNITION

A number of authors have reported a modest relation between IQ and WCST scores (e.g., Ardila et al., 2000; Boone, 1999; Diaz-Asper et al., 2004; Heaton, 1981; Greve et al., 1999; Koren et al., 1998; Parkin et al., 1995; Sherman et al., 1995). In healthy adults, Total Errors appear to closely relate to fluid intelligence (Salthouse et al., 2003). Differences between patients with bipolar disorder and controls were attenuated to nonsignificance when intelligence was accounted for (Chiu et al., 2017).

CLINICAL STUDIES

TBI. Patients with TBI often perform poorly on the WCST, with severity of injury correlating moderately with WCST variables (*rs* = .28 to .49; Anderson et al., 1995; King et al., 2002). However, a meta-analysis of 30 studies comprising 1,269 TBI patients suggests that phonemic fluency is more sensitive to TBI than the WCST (Categories Completed, Perseverative Errors; Henry & Crawford, 2004b). See also "Daily Function."

Stroke. The WCST appears to have some utility in stroke. Su et al. (2008) reported via discriminant function analysis that error variables of the WCST and Total Correct were most effective at differentiating cognitively impaired patients from those who were not cognitively impaired, with a classification rate of nearly 70%; 89% of the patients with cognitive impairment were correctly classified, and 50% of the patients with no cognitive impairment were correctly classified.

Jodzio and Biechowska (2010) reported that the WCST had good negative predictive power overall in detecting executive function deficit in their sample of patients with stroke (ranging from 65% for Learning to Learn to 95% for Trials to Complete First Category), but poor positive predictive power (17% for Perseverative and Non-Perseverative Errors, and Perseverative Responses, to 34% for Percent Conceptual Level Responses and Learning to Learn), which resulted in a low classification accuracy rate (43% for Perseverative Errors to 59% for Trials to Complete First Category). WCST performance is also impaired in patients with thalamic stroke, particularly those with left medial thalamic damage (Liebermann et al., 2013). Categories and Total Correct are moderately related to ADLs in stroke (Chiu et al., 2017). Starchina et al. (2007) reported improvement on the WCST in stroke patients following antihypertensive therapy.

MS. Impaired performance has been reported in patients with MS (Arnett et al., 1994; Beatty & Aupperle, 2002; Beatty & Monson, 1996). The WCST has been used as an outcome measure in MS following drug treatment (Mattioli et al., 2011; Mattioli, Stampatori, Zanotti, Parrinello, & Capra, 2009).

PD. Impaired performance has been described in PD (Green et al., 2002; Henry & Crawford, 2004c; Monchi et al., 2004; Paolo et al., 1995). Woods and Troster (2003) monitored patients with PD over a one-year interval and found that perseveration indices on the WCST demonstrated a degree of diagnostic classification accuracy in identifying PD patients who later developed dementia from those who did not (overall predictive power of 68%).

Psychiatric Conditions. Individuals with schizophrenia demonstrate performance decrements on the WCST (e.g., Heinrichs & Zakzanis, 1998; Holmén et al., 2012; Johnson-Selfridge & Zalewski, 2001; Koren et al., 1998; Moritz et al., 2002; Van der Does & Van den Bosch, 1992) consistent with a frontal model of the condition (Ragland et al., 2007). Some evidence has suggested that patients with clinical profiles characterized by negative symptomatology show particular impairments on the WCST (Polgár et al., 2010; Vogel et al., 2013).

However, some authors report that when VIQ is taken into account, differences between patients and controls can be significantly attenuated (Pukrop et al., 2003; see also similar finding in PD; Roca et al., 2012). Thus, deficits on the WCST may be more reflective of a generalized intellectual deficit rather than specific difficulties with executive control (Henry & Crawford, 2005). Moreover, some research has suggested deficits found are not specific to schizophrenia and extend to other psychiatric conditions as well. For example, aspects of WCST performance do not differentiate between schizophrenia spectrum, depression, and bipolar disorder (Rady et al., 2011; Waford & Lewine, 2010).

WCST performance is associated with a number of functional and clinical outcomes in individuals with schizophrenia. Errors on the WCST and a modified WCST are correlated with insight (Chan et al., 2012; Kao et al., 2013). Perseverative Errors on the WCST were found to be a significant predictor of relapse in individuals with schizophrenia spectrum disorder (OR = 2.4; Chen et al., 2005). WCST performance and negative symptoms have been associated with social function (Rocca et al., 2009; Xiang et al., 2010). Tomida et al. (2010) reported that WCST performance significantly predicted aspects of quality of life in chronic schizophrenia.

The test has been used in a range of investigations in schizophrenia, including in studies of cognitive outcome following alterations in drug treatment (e.g., Chen et al., 2008; Ehrenreich et al., 2007; Gibel & Ritsner, 2008; Kim et al., 2009; Shim et al., 2012) and investigation of genetic substrates of schizophrenia (Barnett et al., 2007; Greenwood et al., 2012; Lien et al., 2010). WCST performance was also related to autonomic regulation in schizophrenia (Mathewson et al., 2012).

The WCST has been identified as a beneficial inclusion to a battery designed to study first-episode psychosis (González-Ortega et al., 2013), and Perseverative Errors have been associated with duration of untreated illness in first-episode psychosis (Allott et al., 2017). Peña, Ojeda, Segarra, Eguiluz, García, and Gutiérrez et al. (2011) reported that WCST performance was accurate in identifying individuals with first-episode psychosis who were subsequently diagnosed with schizophrenia at 2-year follow-up, with a diagnostic accuracy rate of approximately 84%, even when symptoms, depression, premorbid function, and duration of psychosis were considered. In a meta-analysis, patients with bipolar disorder and psychosis presented with greater impairment on the WCST than patients with bipolar disorder without psychosis, with Categories Completed reflecting the largest difference (Cohen's d = .55; Bora et al., 2010).

The WCST has been used in research on cognitive function in bipolar disorder (Yatham et al., 2010). In their meta-analysis of cognitive deficits in euthymic bipolar patients, Bourne et al. (2013) reported that deficits remained after controlling for age, IQ, gender, and residual mood symptoms, although effect sizes were significant reduced. The authors suggested that this may be due to heterogeneity of factors between studies. Other research has similarly suggested that poorer performance on the WCST persists in bipolar disorder even after controlling for demographic and clinical factors (O'Donnell et al., 2017). Long-term follow-up of individuals at risk for major mood disorders suggests an association between impairment on the WCST and subsequent development of bipolar disorder (Meyer et al., 2004).

In addition, the literature suggests that depression and anxiety may affect performance on the WCST. In their meta-analysis, Lim et al. (2013) reported significant differences between patients with major depressive disorder and healthy controls (standardized mean difference = –.40). Improvement, as measured via reliable change methodology, has been reported following treatment (Chang et al., 2012). Withall, Harris, and Cumming (2009) reported that Perseverative Errors on admission predicted worse outcome in depression. Impaired performance on the WCST has also been described in OCD (Aigner et al., 2007; Cavedini et al., 2010; Lacerda et al., 2003).

WCST performance has also been investigated in eating disorders (Abbatte-Daga et al., 2011; Van Autreve et al., 2013; Tchanturia et al., 2012). For example, Fagundo et al. (2012) reported that, relative to healthy controls, people with disordered eating (i.e., anorexia and obesity) made more errors and had fewer correct responses.

Substance Use. WCST performance has been investigated in substance use populations (Brokate et al., 2003; Nowakowska et al., 2008) and, according to a meta-analysis, is one of the most sensitive executive function measures to the cognitive effects of alcohol use disorders (Stephan et al., 2017). Persons with substance use disorders differ in cognitive processing aspects of WCST performance compared to healthy controls (e.g., slower attention shifting following punished trials and reduced decision consistency; Bishara et al., 2010; Woicik et al., 2011). In a sample of young adults, blood alcohol concentration was associated with Perseverative Errors (Lyvers & Tobias-Webb, 2010). Perseverative Errors have also been found to relate to treatment retention in individuals with cocaine dependency (Turner et al., 2009).

Other Populations. Impaired performance has been reported in a number of conditions purported to involve disturbances in executive control, such as ADHD (Antshel et al., 2010), autism spectrum disorder (Braden et al., 2017), and impulse control disorders such as pathological gambling (Marazziti et al., 2008) and kleptomania (Grant et al., 2007). Other research has reported limited utility of the WCST in differentiating between mild AD and controls (Huang et al., 2017). In one study, WCST performance was found to be associated with greater suicide risk in individuals with temporal lobe epilepsy (Garcia Espinosa et al., 2010).

Daily Function. The WCST has functional correlates in a number of groups (see also "Schizophrenia"). For example, Failure to Maintain Set was related to better occupational outcomes and Non-Perseverative Errors to supervision needs in a severe TBI sample one year post-injury (Benge et al., 2007). In a Spanish sample, the WCST was significantly correlated with ADLs in patients who sustained a moderate to severe TBI (García-Molina et al., 2012).

There is also some evidence that the WCST may have some value as a predictor of the capacity to manage independently outside of a hospital setting (Heinrichs, 1990), of vocational outcome (Nybo & Koskiniem, 1999), and of functional status at discharge from hospital following stroke (Greve et al., 1999).

NEUROANATOMICAL CORRELATES AND IMAGING STUDIES

Lesion Studies. In her classic study with the WCST, Milner (1963) found clear differences between patients with dorsolateral frontal excisions and those with orbitofrontal and posterior lesions. Patients with dorsolateral lesions showed an inability "to shift from one sorting principle to another, apparently due to perseverative interference from previous modes of response" (p. 99). Similarly, a meta-analysis (Demakis, 2003) comparing individuals with frontal lobe damage to those with posterior brain damage indicated significantly poorer performance for participants with frontal damage, particularly those with dorsolateral damage or acute injuries. However, Demakis noted that even though effect sizes were large for patients with dorsolateral damage, the overlap in scores between frontal and nonfrontal groups was large (about 35%) and thus scores were insufficient for classification purposes.

Others have reported normal performance in some individuals with considerable frontal pathology (e.g., Anderson, Damasio, Jones, & Tranel, 1991; Eslinger & Damasio, 1985). In addition, meta-analytic findings in patients with focal cortical excisions show that phonemic fluency is more strongly and specifically related to the presence of frontal lesions than the WCST scores (Henry & Crawford, 2004a). In their meta-analysis, Alvarez and Emory (2006) reported that the majority of lesion studies indicated that those with frontal lobe lesions performed worse than healthy controls, as well as worse than patients with nonfrontal lesions. However, some studies did not find significant differences. This suggests that the WCST may be sensitive to frontal lesions but lacking in specificity to frontal lesions.

The literature is mixed regarding laterality of dysfunction, with some suggesting greater sensitivity of the test to lesions in the left compared to the right dorsolateral prefrontal cortex (Milner, 1963) and others reporting increased perseveration with right-sided lesions (Bornstein, 1986; Drewe, 1974; Lombardi et al., 1999; Robinson et al., 1980). Meta-analytic findings suggest no significant differences between patients with right- compared to left-sided lesions (Demakis, 2003). A study of stroke patients found no effects of side or anterior or posterior location of damage on performance (Jodzio & Biechowska, 2010).

Overall, lesion studies and neuroimaging studies suggest that the WCST engages frontal cortices, and a broad neural network is also involved in performance that includes areas such as regions of the parietal lobes, temporal-parietal association areas, and visual cortices (see a review of neuroimaging studies in healthy participants by Nyhus & Barcelo, 2009, and a meta-analysis by Yuan & Raz, 2014).

In patients with schizophrenia, a number of brain regions have been implicated in performance, including gray matter in Brodmann's area 9 (BA9; part of dorsolateral prefrontal and medial prefrontal cortex; Bonihla et al., 2008), white matter in the right inferior frontooccipital fasiculus and the right external capsule (Lee et al., 2013), and white matter in the rostral middle frontal gyrus-striatal tract (Quan et al., 2013). In patients with AD and MCI, regions implicated include frontal and parietal periventricular white matter (Chen et al., 2009), bilateral precentral, callosomarginal, pericallosal, right thalamus, left central and parietal regions (Takeda et al., 2010), and bilateral orbital gyri (Terada et al., 2011).

Matsui et al. (2007) reported that poor WCST performance in patients with PD was related to decreased fractional anisotropy in the left parietal region. Guo et al. (2013) reported relations between WCST errors and medial prefrontal cortex activation in fMRI in first-episode, drug-naïve, major depressive disorder. Vasic, Walter, Höse, and Wolf (2008) reported that decreased gray matter of the right medial and inferior frontal gyrus was related to WCST performance, as was decreased gray matter hippocampal volume in patients with depression. Depressive symptomatology was also related to neuroimaging indices. Of note, much of the research on neuroimaging correlates of WCST performance has been conducted in early disease state (e.g., first-episode schizophrenia, early dementia), which further strengthens the associations found by minimizing confounds that tend to accompany disease progression (e.g., medication complications, social risk factors).

PERFORMANCE VALIDITY

Performance on the WCST may also be useful in detecting malingering. Examinees suspected of inadequate performance validity tend to perform more poorly on WCST variables than those classified as performing credibly (e.g., Greve, Bianchini, Mathias, Heaton, & Courch, 2002; King et al., 2002; Larrabee, 2003; but see Binder et al., 2002). For example, Failure to Maintain Set scores greater than 1 have been considered as potentially suggestive of compromised performance validity (Suhr & Boyer, 1999), and Larrabee (2003) noted that no patient with moderate to severe TBI had scores greater than 3 on Failure to Maintain Set.

DenBoer and Hall (2007) examined the pattern of WCST performance in coached and uncoached TBI simulators. Successful simulators performed worse on many WCST variables than controls. However, the pattern of performance was unusual in that the successful simulator group performed worse on Total Errors and Failure to Maintain Set but not on Perseverative Errors.

Ord, Greve, Bianchini, and Aguerrevere (2010) evaluated WCST performance in patients with mild TBI and patients with moderate to severe TBI compared to those with dementia and healthy controls. In the presence of adequate performance validity, mild TBI patients had no significant deficits in WCST performance, whereas moderate to severe TBI patients were impaired. When effect sizes were examined, performance validity exerted a larger effect (Cohen's $d = .42$) than injury severity.

Prediction formulas have been proposed based on the concept that individuals who malinger may suppress performance on obvious measures such as Categories Completed but less so on more subtle ones such as Perseverative Errors or may avoid too many consecutive correct responses (e.g., Bernard et al., 1996; King et al., 2002; Suhr & Boyer, 1999). The Suhr and Boyer (1999) and King et al. (2002) are the most well-known, as follows:

Suhr & Boyer (1999) formula: (−.75 × Categories Completed) + (1.01 × Failure to Maintain Set) + 3.16

King et al. (2002) formula: (−.752 × Categories Completed) + (.345 × Failure to Maintain Set Errors) − (.007% × Conceptual Level Responses) + 1.537

The equations provided by Suhr and Boyer (1999) and King et al. (2002) appear to provide reasonably good classification rates in TBI samples (Table 9–176). However, other research indicates that although specificity tends to be good with these formulas, sensitivity appears more limited (Greve et al., 2002; King et al., 2002). Greve, Heinly, Bianchini, and Love (2009) reported that Failure to Maintain Set, the Suhr and Boyer formula, and the King et al. formula detected approximately 30% of malingerers at cutoffs associated with a false-positive error rate of 11%.

In older adults, these formulas may result in a high rate of false positives and therefore may be inappropriate for use in this population (Ashendorf et al., 2003). Larrabee (2003) found that Failure to Maintain Set alone was more effective than the Suhr and Boyer discriminant score in differentiating litigants identified as malingering from patients with moderate to severe TBI.

TABLE 9–176 Wisconsin Card Sorting Test (WCST) Logistic Regression Equation to Determine Invalid Performance

KING ET AL. (2002) LOGISTIC REGRESSION SCORE	PROBABILITY OF NONCREDIBLE PERFORMANCE	SUHR & BOYER (1999) LOGISTIC REGRESSION SCORE
4.29	0.99	4.69
2.90	0.95	3.68
2.13	0.90	3.16
1.74	0.85	2.41
1.32	0.80	1.69
1.09	0.75	1.43
0.87	0.70	1.17
0.57	0.65	.91
0.34	0.60	.42
0.20	0.55	.16
0.00	0.50	0.00

NOTE: King et al. (2002) formula: (-.752 × Categories Completed) + (.345 × Failure to Maintain Set Errors) − (.007% × Conceptual Level Responses) + 1.537;
Suhr & Boyer (1999) formula: (-.75 × Categories Completed) + (1.01 × Failure to Maintain Set) + 3.16.

SOURCE: Adapted from King et al. (2002) and Suhr & Boyer (1999).

COMMENT

The WCST has a long history of use in neuropsychology. In contrast to many other executive measures that emphasize a final outcome score, the WCST provides additional quantitative information regarding aspects of problem-solving behavior beyond task failure or successful completion (e.g., Perseverative Errors, Failure to Maintain Set, Categories Completed). Research literature has further extended examination of cognitive component processes underlying performance (see Bishara et al., 2010).

The WCST is generally found to reflect two or more factors, broadly reflecting shifting, problem solving, and response maintenance. The WCST shows modest to moderate correlations with attention and executive measures, as well as memory measures and IQ. Overall, factor-analytic studies suggest that the WCST often loads separately from other measures of executive function.

The nature of the cognitive processes underlying successful performance is complex. The task requires numerous skills including basic visual processing, numerical ability, rule induction, the ability to identify the most relevant stimulus attributes, speeded processing, the ability to maintain the current sorting category in working memory, and the ability to shift mental set. In addition, the test has been reported by some to reflect conceptual processing and problem solving, rather than specific executive processes such as working memory alone. Any significant deficit in one or more of these processes may lead to impairments. Overall, lesion studies and neuroimaging studies reflect the gestalt nature of the task. Although frontal cortices are engaged in task performance, a broad neural network is also involved that includes areas such as regions of the parietal lobes, temporal-parietal association areas, white-matter tracts, and visual cortices.

There are a number of influences on performance related to administration parameters and examinee characteristics, including fatigue and circadian rhythm, cortisol levels, awareness and responsivity to social feedback, and strategy use. A number of scores are available on the WCST, some of which appear to be highly correlated. The most common measures used to assess executive control on the WCST are Categories Completed and Perseverative Errors.

There are a number of variants of the WCST, including short (WCST-64) and computer forms. There is mixed evidence regarding equivalency between the WCST and computerized versions. Although some research has suggested that groups do not differ in performance between the versions, examination of psychometric properties suggests the tasks are not equivalent; there is mixed evidence regarding their comparable utility in clinical groups.

Administration of the conventional WCST takes a fair amount of practice to master, and the scoring can be nuanced. Although hand scoring facilitates an in-depth understanding of the task, in routine clinical practice computerized scoring is likely to be optimal for minimizing clerical errors and reducing the scoring time required.

The WCST is affected by demographic factors, with most research indicating that age is the most influential demographic variable. Education also significantly affects performance, and there is evidence that other sociodemographic variables, such as ethnicity, also impact performance. Gender is generally not reported to affect task performance.

The original normative data for the WCST are large and age- and education-adjusted, yet have some limitations including that they are dated and produced by aggregation of various studies. Additionally, important information relating to characteristics of the samples is lacking. More recent normative data have been provided by Norman et al. (2011) for the computerized WCST-64. This dataset is valuable because it offers adjustments for demographic variables, which are important to consider in interpreting performance.

Reliability is a weakness of the WCST. Test-retest reliability is generally unacceptably low for most scores, with error scores yielding somewhat higher reliability estimates than other variables, such as Learning to Learn. However, all scores examined appear to be quite unstable on retest. Some authors have proposed that this is due to the nature of the test, in that once the principle underlying shifting is deduced by the examinee, the WCST no longer measures problem solving on retest. Limited research is available on internal reliability. Data on interrater reliability are mixed.

The WCST has been used in a variety of clinical populations, including TBI, stroke, schizophrenia, mood and anxiety disorders, eating disorders, substance abuse, and impulse control disorders, among others. In stroke, poor specificity and positive predictive power have been reported in classification of cognitively impaired versus not cognitively impaired patients. The test has shown utility in schizophrenia, including associations with functional outcomes and some diagnostic utility. Last, the test may have some value as an adjunct to other performance validity measures, especially Failure to Maintain Set, the Suhr and Boyer (1999) formula, and the King et al. (2002) formula, although users should note some of these variables are associated with less-than-optimal classification rates in some studies and deserve further validation.

REFERENCES

Abbate-Daga, G., Buzzichelli, S., Amianto, F., Rocca, G., Marzola, E., McClintock, S. M., & Fassino, S. (2011). Cognitive flexibility in verbal and nonverbal domains and decision making in anorexia nervosa patients: A pilot study. *BMC Psychiatry, 11*(1), 1.

Aigner, M., Sachs, G., Bruckmüller, E., Winklbaur, B., Zitterl, W., Kryspin-Exner, I., . . . Katschnig, H. (2007). Cognitive and emotion recognition deficits in obsessive–compulsive disorder. *Psychiatry Research, 149*(1-3), 121–128. http://doi.org/10.1016/j.psychres.2005.12.006

Allott, K., Fraguas, D., Bartholomeusz, C. F., Díaz-Caneja, C. M., Wannan, C., Parrish, E. M., . . . Rapado-Castro, M. (2017). Duration of untreated psychosis and neurocognitive functioning in first-episode psychosis: A systematic review and meta-analysis. *Psychological Medicine*, 1–18. https://doi.org/10.1017/S0033291717003002

Alvarez, J. A., & Emory, E. (2006). Executive function and the frontal lobes: A meta-analytic review. *Neuropsychology Review, 16*(1), 17–42. https://doi.org/10.1007/s11065-006-9002-x

Anderson, S. W., Damasio, H., Jones, R. D., & Tranel, D. (1991). Wisconsin Card Sorting Test Performance as a Measure of Frontal Lobe Damage. *Journal of Clinical and Experimental Neuropsychology, 13*(6), 909–922. https://doi.org/10.1080/01688639108405107

Anderson, C. V., Bigler, E. D., & Blatter, D. D. (1995). Frontal lobe lesions, diffuse damage, and neuropsychological functioning in traumatic brain-injured patients. *Journal of Clinical and Experimental Neuropsychology, 17*, 900–908.

Antshel, K. M., Faraone, S. V., Maglione, K., Doyle, A. E., Fried, R., Seidman, L. J., & Biederman, J. (2010). Executive functioning in high-IQ adults with ADHD. *Psychological Medicine, 40*(11), 1909–1918. http://doi.org/10.1017/S0033291709992273

Ardila, A., Pineda, D., & Rosseli, M. (2000). Correlation between intelligence test scores and executive function measures. *Archives of Clinical Neuropsychology, 15*, 31–36.

Arnett, P. A., Rao, S. M., Bernardin, L., Grafman, J., Yetkin, F. Z., & Lobeck, L. (1994). Relationship between frontal lobe lesions and Wisconsin Card Sorting Test performance in patients with multiple sclerosis. *Neurology, 44*, 420–425.

Artiola i Fortuny, L. A., & Heaton, R. K. (1996). Standard versus computerized administration of the Wisconsin Card Sorting Test. *The Clinical Neuropsychologist, 10*, 419–424.

Ashendorf, L., & McCaffrey, R. J. (2008). Exploring age-related decline on the Wisconsin Card Sorting Test. *The Clinical Neuropsychologist, 22*(2), 262–272. http://doi.org/10.1080/13854040701218436

Ashendorf, L., O'Bryant, S. E., & McCaffrey, R. J. (2003). Specificity of malingering detection strategies in older adults using the CVLT and WCST. *The Clinical Neuropsychologist, 17*, 255–262.

Axelrod, B. N. (2002). Are normative data from the 64-card version of the WCST comparable to the full WCST? *The Clinical Neuropsychologist, 16*, 7–11.

Axelrod, B. N., Goldman, R. S., & Woodard, J. L. (1992). Interrater reliability in scoring the Wisconsin Card Sorting Test. *The Clinical Neuropsychologist, 6*, 143–155.

Axelrod, B. N., Paolo, A. M., & Abraham, E. (1997). Do normative data from the full WCST extend to the abbreviated WCST? *Assessment, 4*, 41–46.

Axelrod, B. N., Woodard, J. L., & Henry, R. R. (1992). Analysis of an abbreviated form of the Wisconsin Card Sorting Test. *The Clinical Neuropsychologist, 6*, 27–31.

Barnett, J. H., Jones, P. B., Robbins, T. W., & Müller, U. (2007). Effects of the catechol-O-methyltransferase Val158Met polymorphism on executive function: A meta-analysis of the Wisconsin Card Sort Test in schizophrenia and healthy controls. *Molecular Psychiatry, 12*(5), 502–509.

Basso, M. R., Bornstein, R. A., & Lang, J. M. (1999). Practice effects on commonly used measures of executive function across twelve months. *The Clinical Neuropsychologist, 13*, 283–292.

Beatty, W. W., & Aupperle, R. L. (2002). Sex differences in cognitive impairment in multiple sclerosis. *The Clinical Neuropsychologist, 16,* 472–480.

Beatty, W. W., & Monson, N. (1996). Problem solving by patients with multiple sclerosis: Comparison of performance on the Wisconsin and California Card Sorting Tests. *Journal of the International Neuropsychological Society, 2,* 134–140.

Beauvais, J. E., Woods, S. P., Delaney, R. C., & Fein, D. (2004). Development of a tactile Wisconsin Card Sorting Test. *Rehabilitation Psychology, 49,* 282–287.

Bell, M. D., Greig, T. C., Kaplan, E., & Bryson, G. (1997). Wisconsin Card Sorting Test dimensions in schizophrenia: Factorial, predictive, and divergent validity. *Journal of Clinical and Experimental Neuropsychology, 19,* 933–941.

Benge, J. F., Caroselli, J. S., & Temple, R. O. (2007). Wisconsin Card Sorting Test: Factor structure and relationship to productivity and supervision needs following severe traumatic brain injury. *Brain Injury, 21*(4), 395–400. http://doi.org/10.1080/02699050701311091

Bennett, C. L., Petros, T. V., Johnson, M., & Ferraro, F. R. (2008). Individual differences in the influence of time of day on executive functions. *American Journal of Psychology, 121*(3), 349. http://doi.org/10.2307/20445471

Berg, E. A. (1948). A simple objective technique for measuring flexibility in thinking. *Journal of General Psychology, 39,* 15–22.

Bernard, L. C., McGrath, M. J., & Houston, W. (1996). The differential effects of simulating malingering, closed head injury, and other CNS pathology on the Wisconsin Card Sorting Test: Support for the "pattern of performance" hypothesis. *Archives of Clinical Neuropsychology, 11,* 231–245.

Berry, S. (1996). Diagrammatic procedure for scoring the Wisconsin Card Sorting Test. *The Clinical Neuropsychologist, 10,* 117–121.

Bishara, A. J., Kruschke, J. K., Stout, J. C., Bechara, A., McCabe, D. P., & Busemeyer, J. R. (2010). Sequential learning models for the Wisconsin card sort task: Assessing processes in substance dependent individuals. *Journal of Mathematical Psychology, 54*(1), 5–13. http://doi.org/10.1016/j.jmp.2008.10.002

Bonilha, L., Molnar, C., Horner, M. D., Anderson, B., Forster, L., George, M. S., & Nahas, Z. (2008). Neurocognitive deficits and prefrontal cortical atrophy in patients with schizophrenia. *Schizophrenia Research, 101*(1-3), 142–151. http://doi.org/10.1016/j.schres.2007.11.02

Boone, K. B. (1999). Neuropsychological assessment of executive functions: Impact of age, education, gender, intellectual level, and vascular status on executive test scores. In B. Miller & J. L. Cummings (Eds.), *The human frontal lobes: Functions and disorders* (pp. 247–260). New York: Guilford Press.

Boone, K., Victor, T., Wen, J., Razani, J., & Ponton, M. (2007). The association between neuropsychological scores and ethnicity, language, and acculturation variables in a large patient population. *Archives of Clinical Neuropsychology, 22*(3), 355–365. http://doi.org/10.1016/j.acn.2007.01.010

Boone, K. B., Gharffarian, S., Lesser, I. M., Hill-Gutierrez, E., & Berman, N. G. (1993). Wisconsin Card Sorting Test performance in healthy, older adults: Relationship to age, sex, education, and IQ. *Journal of Clinical Psychology, 49,* 54–60.

Boone, K. B., Ponton, M. O., Gorsuch, R. L., Gonzalez, J. J., & Miller, B. L. (1998). Factor analysis of four measures of pre-frontal lobe functioning. *Archives of Clinical Neuropsychology, 13,* 585–595.

Bora, E., Yücel, M., & Pantelis, C. (2010). Neurocognitive markers of psychosis in bipolar disorder: A meta-analytic study. *Journal of Affective Disorders, 127*(1-3), 1–9. http://doi.org/10.1016/j.jad.2010.02.117

Bornstein, R. A. (1986). Contribution of various neuropsychological measures to detection of frontal lobe impairment. *International Journal of Clinical Neuropsychology, 8,* 18–22.

Bourne, C., Aydemir, Ö., Balanzá-Martínez, V., Bora, E., Brissos, S., Cavanagh, J. T. O., . . . Goodwin, G. M. (2013). Neuropsychological testing of cognitive impairment in euthymic bipolar disorder: An individual patient data meta-analysis. *Acta Psychiatrica Scandinavica, 128*(3), 149–162. http://doi.org/10.1111/acps.1213

Bowden, S. C., Fowler, K. S., Bell, R. C., Whelan, G., Clifford, C., Ritter, A. J., & Long, C. M. (1998). The reliability and internal validity of the Wisconsin Card Sorting Test. *Neuropsychological Rehabilitation, 8,* 243–254.

Braden, B. B., Smith, C. J., Thompson, A., Glaspy, T. K., Wood, E., Vatsa, D., . . . Baxter, L. C. (2017). Executive function and functional and structural brain differences in middle-age adults with autism spectrum disorder. *Autism Research, 10*(12), 1945–1959. https://doi.org/10.1002/aur.1842

Brokate, B., Hildebrandt, H., Eling, P., Fichtner, H., Rnge, K., & Timm, C. (2003). Frontal lobe dysfunction in Korsakoff 's syndrome and chronic alcoholism: Continuity or discontinuity? *Neuropsychology, 17,* 420–428.

Cavedini, P., Zorzi, C., Piccinni, M., Cavallini, M. C., & Bellodi, L. (2010). Executive dysfunctions in obsessive-compulsive patients and unaffected relatives: Searching for a new intermediate phenotype. *Biological Psychiatry, 67*(12), 1178–1184. http://doi.org/10.1016/j.biopsych.2010.02.012

Chan, S. K. W., Chan, K. K. S., Lam, M. M. L., Chiu, C. P. Y., Hui, C. L. M., Wong, G. H. Y., . . . Chen, E. Y. H. (2012). Clinical and cognitive correlates of insight in first-episode schizophrenia. *Schizophrenia Research, 135*(1-3), 40–45. http://doi.org/10.1016/j.schres.2011.12.013

Chang, H. H., Lee, I. H., Gean, P. W., Lee, S.-Y., Chi, M. H., Yang, Y. K., . . . Chen, P. S. (2012). Treatment response and cognitive impairment in major depression: Association with C-reactive protein. *Brain, Behavior, and Immunity, 26*(1), 90–95. http://doi.org/10.1016/j.bbi.2011.07.239

Chen, E. Y.-H., Hui, C. L.-M., Dunn, E. L.-W., Miao, M. Y.-K., Yeung, W.-S., Wong, C.-K., . . . Tang, W.-N. (2005). A prospective 3-year longitudinal study of cognitive predictors of relapse in first-episode schizophrenic patients. *Schizophrenia Research, 77*(1), 99–104. http://doi.org/10.1016/j.schres.2005.02.020

Chen, T.-F., Chen, Y.-F., Cheng, T.-W., Hua, M.-S., Liu, H.-M., & Chiu, M.-J. (2009). Executive dysfunction and periventricular diffusion tensor changes in amnesic mild cognitive impairment and early Alzheimer's disease. *Human Brain Mapping, 30*(11), 3826–3836. http://doi.org/10.1002/hbm.20810

Chen, Z., Wang, G., Wang, X., Chen, R., Wang, H., Yang, M., . . . Mei, H. (2008). Effects of warm-supplementing kidney yang (WSKY) capsule added on risperidone on cognition in chronic schizophrenic patients: A randomized, double-blind, placebo-controlled, multi-center clinical trial. *Human Psychopharmacology: Clinical and Experimental, 23*(6), 465–470. http://doi.org/10.1002/hup.958

Chiu, E.-C., Wu, W.-C., Hung, J.-W., & Tseng, Y.-H. (2017). Validity of the Wisconsin Card Sorting Test in patients with stroke. *Disability and Rehabilitation,* 1–5. https://doi.org/10.1080/09638288.2017.1323020

Cianchetti, C., Corona, S., Foscoliano, M., Scalas, F., & Sanniofancello, G. (2005). Modified Wisconsin Card Sorting Test: Proposal of a supplementary scoring method. *Archives of Clinical Neuropsychology, 20*(4), 555–558. http://doi.org/10.1016/j.acn.2004.12.002

Coelho, L. F., do Rosário, M. C., Mastrorosa, R. S., Miranda, M. C., & Amodeo Bueno, O. F. (2012). Performance of a Brazilian sample on the computerized Wisconsin Card Sorting Test. *Psychology & Neuroscience,* 5(2), 147–156. http://doi.org/10.3922/j.psns.2012.2.04

Coffey, D., Marmol, L., Schock, L., & Adams, W. (2005). The influence of acculturation on the Wisconsin Card Sorting Test by Mexican Americans. *Archives of Clinical Neuropsychology, 20*(6), 795–803. http://doi.org/10.1016/j.acn.2005.04.009

Demakis, G. J. (2003). A meta-analytic review of the sensitivity of the Wisconsin Card Sorting Test to frontal and lateralized frontal brain damage. *Neuropsychology, 17,* 255–264.

DenBoer, J. W., & Hall, S. (2007). Neuropsychological test performance of successful brain injury simulators. *The Clinical Neuropsychologist, 21*(6), 943–955. http://doi.org/10.1080/13854040601020783

Diaz-Asper, C., Schretlen, D. J., & Pearlson, G. D. (2004). How well does IQ predict neuropsychological test performance in normal adults. *Journal of the International Neuropsychological Society, 10*, 82–90.

Donders, J., & Wildeboer, M. A. (2004). Validity of the WCST-64 after traumatic brain injury in children. *The Clinical Neuropsychologist, 18*(4), 521–527. https://doi.org/10.1080/13854040490524l1

Drewe, E. A. (1974). The effect of type and area of brain lesion on Wisconsin Card Sorting Test performance. *Cortex, 10*, 159–170.

Egan, G. J., Hasenkamp, W., Wilcox, L., Green, A., Hsu, N., Boshoven, W., . . . Duncan, E. (2011). Declarative memory and WCST-64 performance in subjects with schizophrenia and healthy controls. *Psychiatry Research, 188*(2), 191–196. http://doi.org/10.1016/j.psychres.2011.02.026

Ehrenreich, H., Hinze-Selch, D., Stawicki, S., Aust, C., Knolle-Veentjer, S., Wilms, S., . . . others. (2007). Improvement of cognitive functions in chronic schizophrenic patients by recombinant human erythropoietin. *Molecular Psychiatry, 12*(2), 206–220.

Eslinger, P. J., & Damasio, A. R. (1985). Severe disturbance of higher cortical function after frontal lobe ablation. *Neurology, 35*, 421–429.

Fagundo, A. B., de la Torre, R., Jiménez-Murcia, S., Agüera, Z., Granero, R., Tárrega, S., . . . Fernández-Aranda, F. (2012). Executive functions profile in extreme eating/weight conditions: From anorexia nervosa to obesity. *PloS One, 7*(8), e43382. http://doi.org/10.1371/journal.pone.0043382

Fastenau, P. S. (1998). Validity of regression-based norms: An empirical test of the comprehensive norms with older adults. *Journal of Clinical and Experimental Neuropsychology, 20*, 906–916.

Feldstein, S. N., Keller, F. R., Portman, R. E., Durham, R. L., Klebe, K. J., & Davis, H. P. (1999). A comparison of computerized and standard versions of the Wisconsin Card Sorting Test. *The Clinical Neuropsychologist, 13*, 303–313.

Ferland, M. B., Ramsay, J., Engeland, C., & O'Hara, P. (1998). Comparison of the performance of normal individuals and survivors of traumatic brain injury on repeat administrations of the Wisconsin Card Sorting Test. *Journal of Clinical and Experimental Neuropsychology, 20*, 473–482.

Fisk, J. E., & Sharp, C. A. (2004). Age-related impairment in executive functioning: Updating, inhibition, shifting, and access. *Journal of Clinical and Experimental Neuropsychology, 26*, 874–890.

Flashman, L. A., Horner, M. D., & Freides, D. (1991). Note on scoring perseveration on the Wisconsin Card Sorting Test. *The Clinical Neuropsychologist, 5*, 190–194.

Flavia, M., Stampatori, C., Zanotti, D., Parrinello, G., & Capra, R. (2010). Efficacy and specificity of intensive cognitive rehabilitation of attention and executive functions in multiple sclerosis. *Journal of the Neurological Sciences, 288*(1-2), 101–105. http://doi.org/10.1016/j.jns.2009.09.024

Fristoe, N. M., Salthouse, T. A., & Woodard, J. L. (1997). Examination of age-related deficits on the Wisconsin Card Sorting Test. *Neuropsychology, 11*, 428–436.

Gadd, C., & Phipps, W. D. (2012). A preliminary standardisation of the Wisconsin Card Sorting Test for Setswana-speaking university students. *South African Journal of Psychology, 42*(3), 389–398.

Gamboz, N., Borella, E., & Brandimonte, M. A. (2009). The role of switching, inhibition and working memory in older adults' performance in the Wisconsin Card Sorting Test. *Aging, Neuropsychology, and Cognition, 16*(3), 260–284. http://doi.org/10.1080/13825580802573045

Garcia Espinosa, A., Andrade Machado, R., Borges González, S., García González, M. E., Pérez Montoto, A., & Toledo Sotomayor, G. (2010). Wisconsin Card Sorting Test performance and impulsivity in patients with temporal lobe epilepsy: Suicidal risk and suicide attempts. *Epilepsy & Behavior, 17*(1), 39–45. https://doi.org/10.1016/j.yebeh.2009.09.010

García-Molina, A., Tormos, J. M., Bernabeu, M., Junqué, C., & Roig-Rovira, T. (2012). Do traditional executive measures tell us anything about daily life functioning after traumatic brain injury in Spanish-speaking individuals? *Brain Injury, 26*(6), 864–874. http://doi.org/10.3109/02699052.2012.655362

Gasquoine, P., Croyle, K., Cavazosgonzalez, C., & Sandoval, O. (2007). Language of administration and neuropsychological test performance in neurologically intact Hispanic American bilingual adults. *Archives of Clinical Neuropsychology, 22*(8), 991–1001. http://doi.org/10.1016/j.acn.2007.08.003

Gibel, A., & Ritsner, M. S. (2008). Neurocognitive effects of ziprasidone and related factors in patients with chronic schizophrenia undergoing usual care: A 12-month, open-label, flexible-dose, naturalistic observational trial. *Clinical Neuropharmacology, 31*(4), 204–220. http://doi.org/10.1097/WNF.0b013e3181572781

Golden, C. J., Kushner, T., Lee, B., & McMorrow, M. A. (1997). Searching for the meaning of the Category Test and the Wisconsin Card Sort Test: A comparative. *International Journal of Neuroscience, 93*, 141–150.

Goldman, R. S., Axelrod, B. N., Heaton, R. K., Chelune, G. J., Curtiss, G., Kay, G. G., & Thompson, L. L. (1996). Latent structure of the WCST with the standardization samples. *Assessment, 3*, 73–78.

González-Ortega, I., de los Mozos, V., Echeburúa, E., Mezo, M., Besga, A., Ruiz de Azúa, S., . . . González-Pinto, A. (2013). Working memory as a predictor of negative symptoms and functional outcome in first episode psychosis. *Psychiatry Research, 206*(1), 8–16. http://doi.org/10.1016/j.psychres.2012.08.025

Grant, D. A., & Berg, E. A. (1948). A behavioral analysis of degree of impairment and ease of shifting to new responses in a Weigl-type card sorting problem. *Journal of Experimental Psychology, 39*, 404–411.

Grant, J. E., Odlaug, B. L., & Wozniak, J. R. (2007). Neuropsychological functioning in kleptomania. *Behaviour Research and Therapy, 45*(7), 1663–1670. https://doi.org/10.1016/j.brat.2006.08.013

Green, J., McDonald, W. M., Vitek, J. L., Evatt, M., Freeman, A., Haber, M., Bakay, R. A., Triche, S., Sirockman, B., & DeLong, M. R. (2002). Cognitive impairments in advanced PD without dementia. *Neurology, 59*, 1320–1324.

Greenwood, T. A., Light, G. A., Swerdlow, N. R., Radant, A. D., & Braff, D. L. (2012). Association analysis of 94 candidate genes and schizophrenia-related endophenotypes. *PloS One, 7*(1), e29630. http://doi.org/10.1371/journal.pone.0029630

Greve, K. W. (2001). The WCST-64: A standardized short-form of the Wisconsin Card Sorting Test. *The Clinical Neuropsychologist, 15*, 228–234.

Greve, K. W. (1993). Can perseverative responses on the Wisconsin Card Sorting Test be scored accurately? *Archives of Clinical Neuropsychology, 8*, 511–517.

Greve, K. W., Bianchini, K. J., Hartley, S. M., & Adams, D. (1999). The Wisconsin Card Sorting Test in stroke rehabilitation: Factor structure and relationship to outcome. *Archives of Clinical Neuropsychology, 14*, 497–509.

Greve, K. W., Bianchini, K. J., Mathias, C. W., Houston, R. J., & Crouch, J. A. (2002). Detecting malingered performance with the Wisconsin Card Sorting Test: A preliminary investigation in traumatic brain injury. *The Clinical Neuropsychologist, 16*(2), 179–191.

Greve, K. W., Brooks, J., Crouch, J., Rice, W. J., Cicerone, K., & Rowland, L. (1993). Factorial structure of the Wisconsin Card Sorting Test. *The Clinical Neuropsychologist, 7*, 350–351.

Greve, K. W., Heinly, M. T., Bianchini, K. J., & Love, J. M. (2009). Malingering detection with the Wisconsin Card Sorting Test in mild traumatic brain injury. *The Clinical Neuropsychologist, 23*(2), 343–362. http://doi.org/10.1080/13854040802054169

Greve, K. W., Ingram, F., & Bianchini, K. J. (1998). Latent structure of the Wisconsin Card Sorting Test in a clinical sample. *Archives of Clinical Neuropsychology, 13*, 597–609.

Greve, K. W., Love, J. M., Sherwin, E., Mathias, C. W., Houston, R. J., & Brennan, A. (2002). Temporal stability of the Wisconsin Card Sorting Test in a chronic traumatic brain injury sample. *Assessment, 9*, 271–277.

Greve, K. W., Love, J. M., Sherwin, E., Mathias, C. W., Ramzinski, P., & Levy, J. (2002). Wisconsin Card Sorting Test in chronic severe traumatic brain injury: Factor structure and performance subgroups. *Brain Injury, 16,* 29–40.

Greve, K. W., Stickle, T. R., Love, J. M., Bianchini, K. J., & Stanford, M. S. (2005). Latent structure of the Wisconsin Card Sorting Test: A confirmatory factor-analytic study. *Archives of Clinical Neuropsychology, 20,* 355–364.

Guo, W., Liu, F., Dai, Y., Jiang, M., Zhang, J., Yu, L., . . . Xiao, C. (2013). Decreased interhemispheric resting-state functional connectivity in first-episode, drug-naive major depressive disorder. *Progress in Neuro-Psychopharmacology and Biological Psychiatry, 41,* 24–29. http://doi.org/10.1016/j.pnpbp.2012.11.003

Hartman, M., Bolton, E., & Fehnel, S. E. (2001). Accounting for age differences on the Wisconsin Card Sorting Test: Decreased working memory, not inflexibility. *Psychology & Aging, 16,* 385–399.

Heaton, R. K. (1981). *Wisconsin Card Sorting Test manual.* Odessa, FL: Psychological Assessment Resources, Inc.

Heaton, R. K., Avitable, N., Grant, I., & Mathews, C. (1999). Further cross-validation of regression-based neuropsychological norms with an update for the Boston Naming Test. *Journal of Clinical and Experimental Neuropsychology, 21,* 572–582.

Heaton, R. K., Chelune, G. J., Talley, J. L., Kay, G. G., & Curtis, G. (1993). *Wisconsin Card Sorting Test (WCST) Manual, Revised and Expanded.* Odessa, FL: Psychological Assessment Resources.

Heinrichs, R. W. (1990). Variables associated with Wisconsin Card Sorting Test performance in neuropsychiatric patients referred for assessment. *Neuropsychiatry, Neuropsychology and Behavioral Neurology, 3,* 107–112.

Heinrichs, R. W., & Zakzanis, K. K. (1998). Neurocognitive deficit in schizophrenia: a quantitative review of the evidence. *Neuropsychology, 12,* 426–445.

Hellman, S. G., Green, M. F., Kern, R. S., & Christenson, C. D. (1992). Comparison of card and computer versions of the Wisconsin Card Sorting Test for psychotic patients. *International Journal of Methods in Psychiatric Research, 2,* 151–155.

Henry, J. D., & Crawford, J. R. (2004a). A meta-analytic review of verbal fluency performance following focal cortical lesions. *Neuropsychology, 18,* 284–295.

Henry, J. D., & Crawford, J. R. (2004b). A meta-analytic review of verbal fluency performance in patients with traumatic brain injury. *Neuropsychology, 18,* 621–628.

Henry, J. D., & Crawford, J. R. (2004c). Verbal fluency deficits in Parkinson's disease: A meta-analysis. *Journal of the International Neuropsychological Society, 10,* 608–622.

Henry, J. D., & Crawford, J. R. (2005). A meta-analytic review of verbal fluency deficits in schizophrenia relative to other neurocognitive deficits. *Cognitive Neuropsychiatry, 10,* 1–33.

Holmén, A., Juuhl-Langseth, M., Thormodsen, R., Sundet, K., Melle, I., & Rund, B. R. (2012). Executive function tests in early onset psychosis: which one to choose? Executive function tests in early onset psychosis. *Scandinavian Journal of Psychology, 53*(3), 200–205. http://doi.org/10.1111/j.1467-9450.2012.00940.x

Huang, S.-F., Liu, C.-K., Chang, C.-C., & Su, C.-Y. (2017). Sensitivity and specificity of executive function tests for Alzheimer's disease. *Applied Neuropsychology. Adult, 24*(6), 493–504. https://doi.org/10.1080/23279095.2016.1204301

Ingram, F., Greve, K. W., Fishel Ingram, P. T., & Soukup, V. M. (1999). Temporal stability of the Wisconsin Card Sorting Test in an untreated patient sample. *British Journal of Clinical Psychology, 38,* 209–211.

Iverson, G. L., Slick, D. J., & Franzen, M. D. (2000). Clinical normative data for the WCST-64 following uncomplicated mild head injury. *Applied Neuropsychology, 7,* 247–251.

Jodzio, K., & Biechowska, D. (2010). Wisconsin Card Sorting Test as a measure of executive function impairments in stroke patients. *Applied Neuropsychology, 17*(4), 267–277. http://doi.org/10.1080/09084282.2010.525104

Johnson-Selfridge, M., & Zalewski, C. (2001). Moderator variables of executive functioning in schizophrenia: Meta-analytic findings. *Schizophrenia Bulletin, 27,* 305–313.

Kantrowitz, J. T., Revheim, N., Pasternak, R., Silipo, G., & Javitt, D. C. (2009). It's all in the cards: Effect of stimulus manipulation on Wisconsin Card Sorting Test performance in schizophrenia. *Psychiatry Research, 168*(3), 198–204. http://doi.org/10.1016/j.psychres.2008.05.013

Kao, Y.-C., Liu, Y.-P., Lien, Y.-J., Lin, S.-J., Lu, C.-W., Wang, T.-S., & Loh, C.-H. (2013). The influence of sex on cognitive insight and neurocognitive functioning in schizophrenia. *Progress in Neuro-Psychopharmacology and Biological Psychiatry, 44,* 193–200. http://doi.org/10.1016/j.pnpbp.2013.02.006

Kim, S.-W., Shin, I.-S., Kim, J.-M., Lee, S.-H., Lee, Y.-H., Yang, S.-J., & Yoon, J.-S. (2009). Effects of switching to long-acting injectable risperidone from oral atypical antipsychotics on cognitive function in patients with schizophrenia. *Human Psychopharmacology: Clinical and Experimental, 24*(7), 565–573. http://doi.org/10.1002/hup.1057

King, J. H., Sweet, J. J., Sherer, M., Curtiss, G., & Vanderploeg, R. D. (2002). Validity indices within the Wisconsin Card Sorting Test: Application of new and previously researched multivariate procedures in multiple traumatic brain injury samples. *The Clinical Neuropsychologist, 16,* 506–523.

Klein, C., Foerster, F., & Hartnegg, K. (2007). Regression-based developmental models exemplified for Wisconsin Card Sorting Test parameters: Statistics and software for individual predictions. *Journal of Clinical and Experimental Neuropsychology, 29*(1), 25–35. http://doi.org/10.1080/13803390500276859

Kongs, S. K., Thompson, L. L., Iverson, G. L., & Heaton, R. K. (2000). *Wisconsin Card Sorting Test-64 Card Version.* Lutz, FL: Psychological Assessment Resources.

Koren, D., Seidman, L. J., Harrison, R. H., Lyons, M. J., Kremen, W. S., Caplan, B., Goldstein, J. M., Faraone, S. V., & Tsuang, M. T. (1998). Factor structure of the Wisconsin Card Sorting Test: Dimensions of deficit in schizophrenia. *Neuropsychology, 12,* 289–302.

Lacerda, A. L. T., Dalgalarrondo, P., Caetano, D., Haas, G. L., Camargo, E. E., Keshavan, M. S. (2003). Neuropsychological performance and regional cerebral blood flow in obsessive-compulsive disorder. *Progress in Neuro-Psychopharmacology & Biological Psychiatry, 27,* 657–665.

Laiacona, M., Inzaghi, M. G., De Tanti, A., & Capitani, E. (2000). Wisconsin Card Sorting Test: A new global score, with Italian norms and its relationship with the Weigl sorting test. *Neurological Science, 21,* 279–291.

Lange, F., Kröger, B., Steinke, A., Seer, C., Dengler, R., & Kopp, B. (2016). Decomposing card-sorting performance: Effects of working memory load and age-related changes. *Neuropsychology, 30*(5), 579–590. https://doi.org/10.1037/neu0000271

Larrabee, G. J. (2003). Detection of malingering using atypical performance patterns on standard neuropsychological tests. *The Clinical Neuropsychologist, 17,* 410–425.

Lee, S.-H., Kubicki, M., Asami, T., Seidman, L. J., Goldstein, J. M., Mesholam-Gately, R. I., . . . Shenton, M. E. (2013). Extensive white matter abnormalities in patients with first-episode schizophrenia: A diffusion tensor imaging (DTI) study. *Schizophrenia Research, 143*(2-3), 231–238. http://doi.org/10.1016/j.schres.2012.11.029

Lezak, M. D. (Ed.). (2012). *Neuropsychological assessment* (5th ed.). Oxford, New York: Oxford University Press.

Liebermann, D., Ploner, C. J., Kraft, A., Kopp, U. A., & Ostendorf, F. (2013). A dysexecutive syndrome of the medial thalamus. *Cortex, 49*(1), 40–49. http://doi.org/10.1016/j.cortex.2011.11.005

Lien, Y.-J., Liu, C.-M., Faraone, S. V., Tsuang, M. T., Hwu, H.-G., Hsiao, P.-C., & Chen, W. J. (2010). A genome-wide quantitative trait loci scan of neurocognitive performances in families with schizophrenia. *Genes, Brain and Behavior, 9*(7), 695–702. http://doi.org/10.1111/j.1601-183X.2010.00599.x

Lim, J., Oh, I. K., Han, C., Huh, Y. J., Jung, I.-K., Patkar, A. A., . . . Jang, B.-H. (2013). Sensitivity of cognitive tests in four cognitive domains in discriminating MDD patients from healthy controls: A meta-analysis. *International Psychogeriatrics, 25*(09), 1543–1557. http://doi.org/10.1017/S1041610213000689

Lin, S.-H., Liu, C.-M., Hwang, T.-J., Hsieh, M. H., Hsiao, P.-C., Faraone, S. V., . . . Chen, W. J. (2013). Performance on the Wisconsin Card Sorting Test in families of schizophrenia patients with different familial loadings. *Schizophrenia Bulletin, 39*(3), 537–546. http://doi.org/10.1093/schbul/sbs141

Liu, Y.-M., Tsai, S.-Y., Fleck, D. E., & Strakowski, S. M. (2011). Cross-cultural comparisons on Wisconsin Card Sorting Test performance in euthymic patients with bipolar disorder. *Psychiatry Research, 189*(3), 469–471. http://doi.org/10.1016/j.psychres.2011.05.038

Lombardi, W. J., Andreason, P. J., Sirocco, K. Y., Rio, D. E., Gross, R. E., Umhau, J. C., & Hommer, D. W. (1999). Wisconsin Card Sorting Test performance following head injury: Dorsolateral fronto-striatal circuit activity predicts perseveration. *Journal of Clinical and Experimental Neuropsychology, 21*, 2–16.

Lyvers, M., & Tobias-Webb, J. (2010). Effects of acute alcohol consumption on executive cognitive functioning in naturalistic settings. *Addictive Behaviors, 35*(11), 1021–1028. http://doi.org/10.1016/j.addbeh.2010.06.022

Marazziti, D., Catena Dell'Osso, M., Conversano, C., Consoli, G., Vivarelli, L., Mungai, F., . . . Golia, F. (2008). Executive function abnormalities in pathological gamblers. *Clinical Practice and Epidemiology in Mental Health, 4*(1), 7. https://doi.org/10.1186/1745-0179-4-7

Mathewson, K. J., Jetha, M. K., Goldberg, J. O., & Schmidt, L. A. (2012). Autonomic regulation predicts performance on Wisconsin Card Sorting Test (WCST) in adults with schizophrenia. *Biological Psychology, 91*(3), 389–399. http://doi.org/10.1016/j.biopsycho.2012.09.002

Matsui, H., Nishinaka, K., Oda, M., Niikawa, H., Komatsu, K., Kubori, T., & Udaka, F. (2007). Wisconsin Card Sorting Test in Parkinson's disease: Diffusion tensor imaging. *Acta Neurologica Scandinavica, 116*(2), 108–112. http://doi.org/10.1111/j.1600-0404. 2006.00795.x

Mattioli, F., Flavia, M., Stampatori, C., Zanotti, D., Parrinello, G., & Capra, R. (2010). Efficacy and specificity of intensive cognitive rehabilitation of attention and executive functions in multiple sclerosis. *Journal of the Neurological Sciences, 288*(1–2), 101–105. https://doi.org/10.1016/j.jns.2009.09.024

Mattioli, F., Stampatori, C., & Capra, R. (2011). The effect of natalizumab on cognitive function in patients with relapsing-remitting multiple sclerosis: Preliminary results of a 1-year follow-up study. *Neurological Sciences, 32*(1), 83–88. http://doi.org/10.1007/s10072-010-0412-4

McCormick, C. M., Lewis, E., Somley, B., & Kahan, T. A. (2007). Individual differences in cortisol levels and performance on a test of executive function in men and women. *Physiology & Behavior, 91*(1), 87–94. https://doi.org/10.1016/j.physbeh.2007.01.020

Merrick, E. E., Donders, J., & Wiersum, M. (2003). Validity of the WCST-64 after traumatic brain injury. *The Clinical Neuropsychologist, 17*, 153–158.

Meyer, S. E., Carlson, G. A., Wiggs, E. A., Martinez, P. E., Ronsaville, D. S., Kilmes-Dougan, B., . . . Radke-Yarrow, M. (2004). A prospective study of the association among impaired executive functioning, childhood attentional problems, and the development of bipolar disorder. *Development & Psychopathology, 16*, 461–476.

Milner, B. (1963). Effects of different brain lesions on card sorting. *Archives of Neurology, 9*, 90–100.

Minshew, N. J., Meyer, J., & Goldstein, G. (2002). Abstract reasoning in autism: A dissociation between concept formation and concept identification. *Neuropsychology, 16*, 327–334.

Miyake, A., Friedman, N. P., Emerson, M. J., Witzki, A. H., & Howerter, A. (2000). The unity and diversity of executive functions and their contributions to complex "frontal lobe" tasks: A latent variable analysis. *Cognitive Psychology, 41*, 49–109.

Monchi, O., Petrides, M., Doyon, J., Postuma, R. B., Worsley, K., & Dagher, A. (2004). Neural bases of set-shifting deficits in Parkinson's disease. *Journal of Neuroscience, 24*, 702–710.

Moritz, S., Birkner, C., Kloss, M., Jahn, H., Hand, I., Haasen, C., & Krausz, M. (2002). Executive functioning in obsessive-compulsive disorder, unipolar depression, and schizophrenia. *Archives of Clinical Neuropsychology, 17*, 477–483.

Nelson, H. E. (1976). A modified card sorting test sensitive to frontal lobe defects. *Cortex, 12*, 313–324.

Norman, M. A., Moore, D. J., Taylor, M., Franklin, D., Cysique, L., Ake, C., . . . the HNRC Group. (2011). Demographically corrected norms for African Americans and Caucasians on the Hopkins Verbal Learning Test–Revised, Brief Visuospatial Memory Test–Revised, Stroop Color and Word Test, and Wisconsin Card Sorting Test 64-Card Version. *Journal of Clinical and Experimental Neuropsychology, 33*(7), 793–804. http://doi.org/10.1080/13803395.2011.559157

Nowakowska, K., Jablkowska, K., & Borkowska, A. (2008). Cognitive dysfunctions in patients with alcohol dependence. *Archives of Psychiatry and Psychotherapy, 3*, 29–35.

Nybo, T., & Koskiniem, M. (1999). Cognitive indicators of vocational outcome after severe traumatic brain injury (TBI) in childhood. *Brain Injury, 13*, 759–766.

Nyhus, E., & Barceló, F. (2009). The Wisconsin Card Sorting Test and the cognitive assessment of prefrontal executive functions: A critical update. *Brain and Cognition, 71*(3), 437–451. https://doi.org/10.1016/j.bandc.2009.03.005

O'Donnell, J. P., MacGregor, L. A., Dabrowski, J. J., Oestreicher, J. M., & Romero, J. J. (1994). Construct validity of neuropsychological tests of conceptual and attentional abilities. *Journal of Clinical Psychology, 50*, 596–600.

O'Donnell, L. A., Deldin, P. J., Pester, B., McInnis, M. G., Langenecker, S. A., & Ryan, K. A. (2017). Cognitive flexibility: A trait of bipolar disorder that worsens with length of illness. *Journal of Clinical and Experimental Neuropsychology, 39*(10), 979–987. https://doi.org/10.1080/13803395.2017.1296935

Ord, J. S., Greve, K. W., Bianchini, K. J., & Aguerrevere, L. E. (2010). Executive dysfunction in traumatic brain injury: The effects of injury severity and effort on the Wisconsin Card Sorting Test. *Journal of Clinical and Experimental Neuropsychology, 32*(2), 132–140. http://doi.org/10.1080/13803390902858874

Osmon, D. C., & Suchy, Y. (1996). Fractionating frontal lobe functions: Factors of the Milwaukee Card Sorting Test. *Archives of Clinical Neuropsychology, 11*, 451–552.

Ozonoff, S. (1995). Reliability and validity of the Wisconsin Card Sorting Test in studies of autism. *Neuropsychology, 9*, 491–500.

Paolo, A. M., Axelrod, B. N., Ryan, J. J., & Goldman, R. S. (1994). Administration accuracy of the Wisconsin Card Sorting Test. *The Clinical Neuropsychologist, 8*, 112–116.

Paolo, A. M., Axelrod, B. N., & Troster, A. I. (1996a). Test-retest stability of the Wisconsin Card Sorting Test. *Assessment, 3*, 137–143.

Paolo, A. M., Axelrod, B. N., Troster, A. I., Blackwell, K. T., & Koller, W. C. (1996b). Utility of a Wisconsin Card Sorting Test short form in persons with Alzheimer's and Parkinson's disease. *Journal of Clinical and Experimental Neuropsychology, 18*, 892–897.

Paolo, A. M., Troster, A. I., Axelrod, B. N., & Koller, W. C. (1995). Construct validity of the WCST in normal elderly and persons with Parkinson's disease. *Archives of Clinical Neuropsychology, 10*, 463–473.

Parkin, A. J., Walter, B. M., & Hunkin, N. M. (1995). Relationships between normal aging, frontal lobe function, and memory for temporal and spatial information. *Neuropsychology, 9*, 304–312.

Peña, J., Ojeda, N., Segarra, R., Eguiluz, J. I., García, J., & Gutiérrez, M. (2011). Executive functioning correctly classified diagnoses in patients with first-episode psychosis: Evidence from a 2-year longitudinal study. *Schizophrenia Research, 126*(1-3), 77–80. http://doi.org/10.1016/j.schres.2010.09.019

Pendleton, M. G., & Heaton, R. K. (1982). A comparison of the Wisconsin Card Sorting Test and the Category Test. *Journal of Clinical Psychology, 38*, 392–396.

Perrine, K. (1993). Differential aspects of conceptual processing in the category test and Wisconsin Card Sorting Test. *Journal of Clinical and Experimental Neuropsychology, 15*, 461–473.

Pineda, D. A., & Merchan, V. (2003). Executive function in young Colombian adults. *International Journal of Neuroscience, 113*, 397–410.

Polgár, P., Réthelyi, J. M., Bálint, S., Komlósi, S., Czobor, P., & Bitter, I. (2010). Executive function in deficit schizophrenia: What do the dimensions of the Wisconsin Card Sorting Test tell us? *Schizophrenia Research, 122*(1-3), 85–93. http://doi.org/10.1016/j.schres.2010.06.007

Poreh, A., Pastel, D., Miller, A., & Levin, J. (2012). The Cleveland Sorting Test: A preliminary study of an alternate form of the Wisconsin Card-Sorting Test. *Applied Neuropsychology, 19*(2), 147–152. http://doi.org/10.1080/09084282.2011.643952

Pukrop, R., Matuschek, E., Ruhrmann, S., Brockhaus-Dumke, A., Tendolkar, I., Bertsch, A., & Klosterkotter, J. (2003). Dimensions of working memory dysfunction in schizophrenia. *Schizophrenia Research, 62*, 259–268.

Quan, M., Lee, S.-H., Kubicki, M., Kikinis, Z., Rathi, Y., Seidman, L. J., . . . Levitt, J. J. (2013). White matter tract abnormalities between rostral middle frontal gyrus, inferior frontal gyrus and striatum in first-episode schizophrenia. *Schizophrenia Research, 145*(1-3), 1–10. http://doi.org/10.1016/j.schres.2012.11.028

Rady, A., Elsheshai, A., el Wafa, H. A., & Elkholy, O. (2011). Wisconsin Card Sort Test (WCST) performance in schizophrenia and severe depression with psychotic features. *German Journal of Psychiatry, 14*(2).

Ragland, J. D., Yoon, J., Minzenberg, M. J., & Carter, C. S. (2007). Neuroimaging of cognitive disability in schizophrenia: Search for a pathophysiological mechanism. *International Review of Psychiatry, 19*(4), 417–427. http://doi.org/10.1080/09540260701486365

Rempfer, M., Hamera, E., Brown, C., & Bothwell, R. J. (2006). Learning proficiency on the Wisconsin Card Sorting Test in people with serious mental illness: What are the cognitive characteristics of good learners? *Schizophrenia Research, 87*(1-3), 316–322. http://doi.org/10.1016/j.schres.2006.05.012

Rey, G. J., Feldman, E., Rivas-Vazquez, R., Levin, B. E., & Benton, A. (1999). Neuropsychological test development and normative data on Hispanics. *Archives of Clinical Neuropsychology, 14*, 593–602.

Rhodes, M. G. (2004). Age-related differences in performance on the Wisconsin Card Sorting Test: A meta-analytic review. *Psychology and Aging, 19*, 482–494.

Robinson, A. L., Heaton, R. K., Lehman, R. A. W., & Stilson, D. W. (1980). The utility of the Wisconsin Card Sorting Test in detecting and localizing frontal lobe lesions. *Journal of Consulting and Clinical Psychology, 48*, 605–614.

Roca, M., Manes, F., Chade, A., Gleichgerrcht, E., Gershanik, O., Arévalo, G. G., . . . Duncan, J. (2012). The relationship between executive functions and fluid intelligence in Parkinson's disease. *Psychological Medicine, 42*(11), 2445–2452. http://doi.org/10.1017/S0033291712000451

Rocca, P., Montemagni, C., Castagna, F., Giugiario, M., Scalese, M., & Bogetto, F. (2009). Relative contribution of antipsychotics, negative symptoms and executive functions to social functioning in stable schizophrenia. *Progress in Neuro-Psychopharmacology and Biological Psychiatry, 33*(2), 373–379. http://doi.org/10.1016/j.pnpbp.2009.01.002

Salthouse, T. A., Atkinson, T. M., & Berish, D. E. (2003). Executive functioning as a potential mediator of age-related cognitive decline in normal adults. *Journal of Experimental Psychology: General, 132*, 566–594.

Salthouse, T. A., Fristoe, N., & Rhee, S. H. (1996). How localized are age-related effects on neuropsychological measures? *Neuropsychology, 10*, 272–285.

Sánchez, J. L., Martín, J., & López, C. (2017). Diagnostic utility of the shortened version of the Wisconsin Card Sorting Test in patients with sporadic late onset Alzheimer disease. *American Journal of Alzheimer's Disease and Other Dementias, 32*(8), 472–478. https://doi.org/10.1177/1533317517728334

Schretlen, D. J., Testa, S. M., & Pearlson, G. D. (2010). *Calibrated neuropsychological normative system.* Lutz, FL: PAR.

Sherer, M., Nick, T. G., Millis, S. R., & Novack, T. A. (2003). Use of the WCST and the WCST-64 in the assessment of traumatic brain injury. *Journal of Clinical and Experimental Neuropsychology, 25*, 512–520.

Sherman, E. M., Strauss, E., Spellacy, F., & Hunter, M. (1995). Construct validity of WAIS-R factors: Neuropsychological correlates in adults referred for possible head injury. *Psychological Assessment, 7*, 440–444.

Shim, J.-C., Jung, D.-U., Jung, S.-S., Seo, Y.-S., Cho, D.-M., Lee, J.-H., . . . others. (2012). Adjunctive varenicline treatment with antipsychotic medications for cognitive impairments in people with schizophrenia: A randomized double-blind placebo-controlled trial. *Neuropsychopharmacology, 37*(3), 660–668.

Stephan, R. A., Alhassoon, O. M., Allen, K. E., Wollman, S. C., Hall, M., Thomas, W. J., . . . Grant, I. (2017). Meta-analyses of clinical neuropsychological tests of executive dysfunction and impulsivity in alcohol use disorder. *American Journal of Drug and Alcohol Abuse, 43*(1), 24–43. https://doi.org/10.1080/00952990.2016.1206113

Su, C.-Y., Lin, Y.-H., Kwan, A.-L., & Guo, N.-W. (2008). Construct validity of the Wisconsin Card Sorting Test-64 in patients with stroke. *The Clinical Neuropsychologist, 22*(2), 273–287. http://doi.org/10.1080/13854040701220036

Somerville, J., Tremont, J., & Stern, R. A. (2000). The Boston Qualitative Scoring System as a measure of executive functioning in Rey-Osterrieth Complex Figure performance. *Journal of Clinical and Experimental Neuropsychology, 22*, 613–621.

Starchina, Y. A., Parfenov, V. A., Chazova, I. E., Sinitsyn, V. E., Pustovitova, T. S., Kolos, I. P., & Ustyuzhanin, D. V. (2007). Cognitive function and the emotional state of stroke patients on antihypertensive therapy. *Neuroscience and Behavioral Physiology, 37*(1), 13–17.

Steinmetz, J.-P., Brunner, M., Loarer, E., & Houssemand, C. (2010). Incomplete psychometric equivalence of scores obtained on the manual and the computer version of the Wisconsin Card Sorting Test? *Psychological Assessment, 22*(1), 199–202. http://doi.org/10.1037/a0017661

Steinmetz, J.-P., & Houssemand, C. (2011). What about inhibition in the Wisconsin Card Sorting Test? *The Clinical Neuropsychologist, 25*(4), 652–669. http://doi.org/10.1080/13854046.2011.568525

Suhr, J. A., & Boyer, D. (1999). Use of the Wisconsin Card Sorting Test in the detection of malingering in student simulator and patient sample. *Journal of Clinical and Experimental Neuropsychology, 21*, 701–708.

Sullivan, E. V., Mathalon, D. H., Zipursky, R. B., Kersteen-Tucker, Z., Knight, R. T., & Pfefferbaum, A. (1993). Factors of the Wisconsin Card Sorting Test as measures of frontal-lobe function in schizophrenia and in chronic alcoholism. *Psychiatry Research, 46*, 175–199.

Takeda, N., Terada, S., Sato, S., Honda, H., Yoshida, H., Kishimoto, Y., . . . Kuroda, S. (2010). Wisconsin Card Sorting Test and brain perfusion imaging in early dementia. *Dementia and Geriatric Cognitive Disorders, 29*(1), 21–27. http://doi.org/10.1159/000261645

Tate, R. L., Perdices, M., & Maggiotto, S. (1998). Stability of the Wisconsin Card Sorting Test and the determination of reliability of change in scores. *The Clinical Neuropsychologist, 12*, 348–357.

Tchanturia, K., Davies, H., Roberts, M., Harrison, A., Nakazato, M., Schmidt, U., . . . Morris, R. (2012). Poor cognitive flexibility in eating disorders: Examining the evidence using the Wisconsin Card Sorting Task. *PloS One, 7*(1), e28331. http://doi.org/10.1371/journal.pone.0028331

Terada, S., Sato, S., Honda, H., Kishimoto, Y., Takeda, N., Oshima, E., . . . Uchitomi, Y. (2011). Perseverative errors on the Wisconsin Card Sorting Test and brain perfusion imaging in mild Alzheimer's disease. *International Psychogeriatrics, 23*(10), 1552–1559. http://doi.org/10.1017/S1041610211001463

Teubner-Rhodes, S., Vaden, K. I., Dubno, J. R., & Eckert, M. A. (2017). Cognitive persistence: Development and validation of a novel measure from the Wisconsin Card Sorting Test. *Neuropsychologia, 102*, 95–108. https://doi.org/10.1016/j.neuropsychologia.2017.05.027

Tomida, K., Takahashi, N., Saito, S., Maeno, N., Iwamoto, K., Yoshida, K., . . . Ozaki, N. (2010). Relationship of psychopathological symptoms and cognitive function to subjective quality of life in patients with chronic schizophrenia. *Psychiatry and Clinical Neurosciences, 64*(1), 62–69. http://doi.org/10.1111/j.1440-1819.2009.02033.x

Turner, T. H., LaRowe, S., Horner, M. D., Herron, J., & Malcolm, R. (2009). Measures of cognitive functioning as predictors of treatment outcome for cocaine dependence. *Journal of Substance Abuse Treatment, 37*(4), 328–334. http://doi.org/10.1016/j.jsat.2009.03.009

Van Autreve, S., De Baene, W., Baeken, C., van Heeringen, C., & Vervaet, M. (2013). Do Restrictive and bingeing/purging subtypes of anorexia nervosa differ on central coherence and set shifting? Central coherence and set shifting in AN. *European Eating Disorders Review, 21*(4), 308–314. http://doi.org/10.1002/erv.2233

Van der Does, A. J. W., & Van den Bosch, R. J. (1992). What determines Wisconsin Card Sorting performance in schizophrenia? *Clinical Psychology Review, 12*, 567–583.

Van der Linden, D., Frese, M., & Meijman, T. F. (2003). Mental fatigue and the control of cognitive processes: Effects on perseveration and planning. *Acta Psychologia, 113*, 45–65.

Vanderploeg, R. D., Schinka, J. A., & Retzlaff, P. (1994). Relationships between measures of auditory verbal learning and executive functioning. *Journal of Clinical and Experimental Neuropsychology, 16*, 243–252.

Vasic, N., Walter, H., Höse, A., & Wolf, R. C. (2008). Gray matter reduction associated with psychopathology and cognitive dysfunction in unipolar depression: A voxel-based morphometry study. *Journal of Affective Disorders, 109*(1-2), 107–116. http://doi.org/10.1016/j.jad.2007.11.011

Vogel, S. J., Strauss, G. P., & Allen, D. N. (2013). Using negative feedback to guide behavior: Impairments on the first 4 cards of the Wisconsin Card Sorting Test predict negative symptoms of schizophrenia. *Schizophrenia Research, 151*(1-3), 97–101. http://doi.org/10.1016/j.schres.2013.07.052

Waford, R. N., & Lewine, R. (2010). Is perseveration uniquely characteristic of schizophrenia? *Schizophrenia Research, 118*(1-3), 128–133. http://doi.org/10.1016/j.schres.2010.01.031

Wagner, G. P., & Trentini, C. M. (2009). Assessing executive functions in older adults: A comparison between the manual and the computer-based versions of the Wisconsin Card Sorting Test. *Psychology & Neuroscience, 2*(2), 195–198. http://doi.org/10.3922/j.psns.2009.2.011

Withall, A., Harris, L. M., & Cumming, S. R. (2009). The relationship between cognitive function and clinical and functional outcomes in major depressive disorder. *Psychological Medicine, 39*(3), 393–402. https://doi.org/10.1017/S0033291708003620

Wiegner, S., & Donders, J. (1999). Performance on the Wisconsin Card Sorting Test after traumatic brain injury. *Assessment, 6*, 179–188.

Woicik, P. A., Urban, C., Alia-Klein, N., Henry, A., Maloney, T., Telang, F., . . . Goldstein, R. Z. (2011). A pattern of perseveration in cocaine addiction may reveal neurocognitive processes implicit in the Wisconsin Card Sorting Test. *Neuropsychologia, 49*(7), 1660–1669. http://doi.org/10.1016/j.neuropsychologia.2011.02.037

Woods, S. T., & Troster, A. I. (2003). Prodromal frontal/executive dysfunction predicts incident dementia in Parkinson's disease. *Journal of the International Neuropsychological Society, 9*, 17–24.

Xiang, Y.-T., Shum, D., Chiu, H. F., Tang, W.-K., & Ungvari, G. S. (2010). Association of demographic characteristics, symptomatology, retrospective and prospective memory, executive functioning and intelligence with social functioning in schizophrenia. *Australian and New Zealand Journal of Psychiatry, 44*(12), 1112–1117.

Yantz, C. J., & McCaffrey, R. J. (2007). Social facilitation effect of examiner attention or inattention to computer-administered neuropsychological tests: First sign that the examiner may affect results. *The Clinical Neuropsychologist, 21*(4), 663–671. http://doi.org/10.1080/13854040600788158

Yatham, L. N., Torres, I. J., Malhi, G. S., Frangou, S., Glahn, D. C., Bearden, C. E., . . . Chengappa, K. N. R. (2010). The International Society for Bipolar Disorders-Battery for Assessment of Neurocognition (ISBD-BANC): ISBD-BANC. *Bipolar Disorders, 12*(4), 351–363. http://doi.org/10.1111/j.1399-5618.2010.00830.x

Yuan, P., & Raz, N. (2014). Prefrontal cortex and executive functions in healthy adults: A meta-analysis of structural neuroimaging studies. *Neuroscience and Biobehavioral Reviews, 42*, 180–192. https://doi.org/10.1016/j.neubiorev.2014.02.005

Zimmermann, N., Cardoso, C. de O., Trentini, C. M., Grassi-Oliveira, R., & Fonseca, R. P. (2015). Brazilian preliminary norms and investigation of age and education effects on the Modified Wisconsin Card Sorting Test, Stroop Color and Word test and Digit Span test in adults. *Dementia & Neuropsychologia, 9*(2), 120–127. http://doi.org/10.1590/1980-57642015DN92000006

10 | MEMORY

BENTON VISUAL RETENTION TEST FIFTH EDITION (BVRT-5)

TEST NAME	**Benton Visual Retention Test Fifth Edition (BVRT-5)**
DOMAIN	Visual memory
AGE RANGE	In adults, to 80+ years
ADMINISTRATION TIME	5 to 10 minutes for each administration
SCORING FORMAT	Hand scored
REFERENCE	Sivan, A. B. (1992). *Benton Visual Retention Test* (5th ed.). San Antonio, TX: The Psychological Corporation. www.pearsonclinical.com

DESCRIPTION

The purpose of the Benton Visual Retention Test Fifth Edition (BVRT-5) is to assess visual memory, visual perception, and visual-constructive abilities. Other test names are the Visual Retention Test—Revised (VRT-5) and the Benton Test. There are two main administration modes for the BVRT requiring either drawing or multiple-choice responses from the examinee but the latter is only available in the German edition of the test (see Table 10–1). The drawing administrations of the BVRT have three alternate forms (C, D, and E) that are roughly of equivalent difficulty (see the section "Reliability" for details). Each form is composed of 10 designs: the first two designs in each form consist of one major geometric figure, and the other eight designs consist of two major figures and a smaller peripheral figure.

ADMINISTRATION

There are four main types of administration (see Table 10–1). Under Administration A, the standard (and most commonly used) procedure, each design is displayed for 10 seconds and then withdrawn. Immediately after this, the examinee is required to reproduce the design from memory at their own pace on a blank piece of paper. Administration B is similar to A except that each design is exposed for only five seconds. Administration C (copying) requires the examinee to copy each of the designs without removing the stimulus card from sight. In Administration D, each design is exposed for 10 seconds and the examinee must reproduce the design after a 15-second delay.

Two additional multiple-choice forms (F and G) are available only in the German edition of the test; they are used to measure the examinee's recognition, rather than reproduction ability (Administration M). Because of its minimal reliance on language, Administration M is also appropriate for non–English-speaking individuals. The multiple-choice administration can be used for people with or without motor handicaps to determine whether an individual's disability lies in the area of memory, perception, or drawing ability.

DRAWING ADMINISTRATIONS

See the manual. Drawings should be numbered in the right-hand corner by the examiner after completion to identify the spatial orientation of the drawing and the specific design that was drawn (Wellman, 1985).

MULTIPLE-CHOICE ADMINISTRATIONS

See manual (Sivan & Spreen, 1996). For Administration M, each of the 15 stimulus cards, consisting of one to three geometric figures, is exposed for 10 seconds. Immediately after each exposure, the stimulus card is withdrawn and the examinee is shown a multiple-choice card with four similar stimuli

TABLE 10–1 Administration Forms of the Benton Visual Retention Test Fifth Edition (BVRT-5)

MODE	ALTERNATE FORMS	ADMINISTRATION	EXPOSURE DURATION (S)	TASK	AGE RANGE (YEARS) FOR NORMS PROVIDED HERE	SIVAN (1992)
Drawing	C, D, E	A	10	After each exposure, examinee draws the design from memory	17–97	8–80+ years
Drawing	C, D, E	B	5	After each exposure, examinee draws the design from memory	—	16–60 years
Drawing	C, D, E	C	—	Examinee copies each design	—	Adults: ages not reported; Children: 5 years 6 months to 13 years
Drawing	C, D, E	D	10	Examinee reproduces design after 15-second delay	—	—
Multiple-Choice	F, G	M	10	Examinee chooses the design from a four-choice display	20–86	—

labeled A, B, C, and D; the examinee must choose (point to or name by letter) the one that is identical to the stimulus card.

There are also other administrations. In Administration O, the stimulus card is removed, and, after 15 seconds, the examinee is asked to make the choice. Administration P (form discrimination) is used primarily with children; the stimulus card is shown at the same time as the M-Choice card. In Administration PR, the examinee draws all 10 stimulus figures according to Administration C and then is shown the M-Choice cards and asked to indicate which of the figures the examinee has drawn.

Of note, some of the items on the multiple-choice version of the BVRT can be correctly completed without viewing the target stimuli, merely by solving the task as an oddity problem (Blanton & Gouvier, 1985). Therefore, the validity of the test may be compromised in examinees who respond strategically rather than by relying on visual memory. Franzen (1989) recommended that the examiner interview the examinee after the test to determine the type of strategy that was used.

SCORING

Scoring is accomplished according to explicit criteria that are detailed in the manual (Sivan, 1992; Sivan & Spreen, 1996). Briefly, two scoring systems (the number of correct reproductions and the error score) are available for the evaluation of an examinee's performance on the drawing forms (Administrations A through D).

The number correct score has a range of 0 to 10 because each of the 10 designs is scored on an all-or-none basis and given a credit of 1 or 0. Principles underlying the scoring of the designs, together with specific scoring samples illustrating correct and incorrect reproductions, are presented in the manual.

The scoring of errors allows for both quantitative and qualitative analysis of an examinee's performance. Six major types of errors are noted: (a) omissions (b) distortions (c) perseverations (d) rotations (e) misplacements, and (f) size. Each major category contains a variety of specific error subtypes. Provision is also made for noting right- and left-sided errors. Scoring is recorded and summarized on the record form. This form allows the examiner to indicate the correct designs and to summarize the types of errors made on each design.

For the multiple-choice administration, the number of correct choices (of a possible 15) is recorded.

DEMOGRAPHIC EFFECTS

ADMINISTRATION A

AGE

Age is the strongest predictor of performance on Administration A, accounting for 9–18% of the variance in test scores (Coman et al., 1999; Messinis et al., 2009; Youngjohn et al., 1993). Scores show a progressive rise from age 6 years (Rosselli et al., 2001) until a plateau is reached at the age of 14 or 15 years (Sivan, 1992). This plateau is maintained into the third decade of life, after which a progressive decline in performance occurs, beginning at age 40 to 50 years (Giambra et al., 1995; Resnick et al., 1995; Youngjohn et al., 1993; also see Coman et al., 2002, for a review). The threshold for marked decline in level of performance appears to be about age 75 years (Coman et al., 2002). Variability in BVRT performance increases with aging, although the increases are not significant (Coman et al., 2002).

GENDER

Most studies have found that gender has little effect on performance (Coman et al., 1999, 2002; Giambra et al.,

1995; Messinis et al., 2009; Resnick et al., 1995; Rosselli et al., 2001; Seo et al., 2007; Youngjohn et al., 1992). One study found that gender effects differed as a function of age and education. Poorly educated men obtained better scores than poorly educated women, and older men performed better than older women (Seo et al., 2007).

EDUCATION AND IQ

Performance on the BVRT shows a moderate to high correlation with intelligence (r = .30 to .70; Dougherty et al., 2003; Randall et al., 1988) and with education (Coman et al., 2002; Messinis et al., 2009; Youngjohn et al., 1993). The effects of education interact with those of age. For example, among older adults, the performance of highly educated individuals tends to decline less with age than that of examinees with limited education. One study suggested that education accounted for more variance than age on the BVRT (Seo et al., 2007). In older adults with moderate to severe cognitive deficits, however, the more generalized effects of neurological insult override any protective effect of education, so that BVRT performance is adversely affected regardless of age or educational level (Coman et al., 1999, 2002).

Occupational status is another important consideration. Dartigues et al. (1992) found that in 2,720 healthy community-dwelling older adults, BVRT results corresponded strongly with lifetime occupation regardless of education level; in particular, farmers, domestic service employees, and blue-collar workers showed poor memory two to three times more often than people with professional or managerial occupations.

ADMINISTRATION C

Findings are generally similar to Administration A. Gender differences depend on level of education, with men who have low education performing better than women with low education. Moreover, those with higher education perform the same with advancing age, but those with lower education perform worse with increasing age, particularly those with fewer than four years of education (Seo et al., 2007).

ADMINISTRATION M

AGE

Adult levels are obtained by about age 12 years (Sivan & Spreen, 1996). In general, adults tend to make two or fewer errors. Performance declines with advancing age (Miatton et al., 2004; Tuokko & Woodward, 1996).

GENDER

Gender effects tend to be minimal (Miatton et al., 2004; Tuokko & Woodward, 1996; Wagner, 1992).

EDUCATION AND IQ

Performance is affected by education (Le Carret et al., 2003; Miatton et al., 2004). Le Carret et al. (2003) suggested that the better performance of those with higher educational level is partly mediated by their ability to use a more strategic search of the targets in memory.

ETHNICITY, NATIONALITY, AND LINGUISTIC EFFECTS

Differences between older Caucasian and African-American adults (Manly et al., 1998) and between older Spanish-speaking and English-speaking adults (Jacobs et al., 1997) have been reported, with Caucasians and English speakers scoring higher even after education and various medical conditions are taken into account. However, if quality of education is taken into consideration, differences between Caucasians and African Americans are eliminated (Manly et al., 2002).

NORMATIVE DATA

ADMINISTRATION A

Data for adults (aged 15–69 years) are presented in the manual (Sivan, 1992). The norms are given by age and IQ level. Note that the data are based on the performance of 600 adults evaluated more than 50 years ago by Benton (1963), and no information is provided regarding their education, gender, or method of recruitment. The majority were inpatients and outpatients of hospitals in Iowa City, Iowa, with no evidence or history of psychosis, no evidence of cerebral injury or disease except for intellectual disability, and no serious physical depletion as a consequence of somatic disease. The manual includes additional normative information based on two studies (Arenberg, 1978; Benton et al., 1981) that extended the norms to old age. The Arenberg data are based solely on male adults, stratified by age group but not by education, and normative information is provided for mean number of errors only. The data from Benton et al. (1981) are presented in terms of means (M), standard deviations (SD), and range of scores for number of errors and number correct.

Coman et al. (1999) refined the norms collected by Benton in 1981 for the age range 55 to 97 years by providing adjustments for age and education (see Table 10–2). Note that the sample was largely female, and cell sizes were very small at the extremes of the age distributions (e.g., $N = 6$ for ages 55–64 years, N = 29 for ages 85+). The authors cautioned that the window of greatest accuracy encompasses ages 63 to 79 years and 11 to 17 years of education.

Similar results, shown in Table 10–3, were obtained in a study of 1,128 adults and older adults, aged 17 to 84 years, by Youngjohn et al. (1993).

The choice of which normative dataset to use for estimating the performance level of a given patient depends on

TABLE 10–2 Normative Expected Scores: Benton Visual Retention Test Fifth Edition (BVRT-5) Administration A, Number Correct (*N* = 156 Healthy Older Adults)

	YEARS OF EDUCATION (*SD* = 1.6 FOR EACH CELL)										
AGE (YEARS)	8	9	10	11	12	13	14	15	16	18	20
55	6.54	6.72	6.90	7.09	7.27	7.46	7.64	7.82	8.01	8.38	8.74
60	6.09	6.28	6.46	6.64	6.82	7.01	7.19	7.37	7.56	7.92	8.29
65	5.65	5.83	6.01	6.20	6.38	6.56	6.74	6.92	7.10	7.47	7.83
70	5.21	5.39	5.57	5.75	5.93	6.11	6.29	6.47	6.65	7.01	7.37
75	4.77	4.95	5.12	5.30	5.48	5.66	5.84	6.02	6.20	6.56	6.91
80	4.32	4.50	4.68	4.86	5.03	5.21	5.39	5.57	5.75	6.10	6.46
85	3.88	4.06	4.23	4.41	4.59	4.76	4.94	5.12	5.29	5.65	6.00
90	3.44	3.61	3.79	3.96	4.14	4.31	4.49	4.67	4.84	5.19	5.54
95	3.00	3.17	3.34	3.52	3.69	3.87	4.04	4.21	4.39	4.74	5.08

NOTE: *N* = 156; age *M* = 71 years, *SD* = 8.40; education *M* = 12.67, *SD* = 3.46, range = 4–20; 80% females; primarily Caucasian.

SOURCE: From Coman et al. (1999).

the patient's particular demographic characteristics. Where datasets overlap (ages 55–70 years), the set provided by Youngjohn et al. (1993) is preferred, given its larger sample size. In addition, their norms are preferred for relatively young, highly educated adults. The tables provided by Coman et al. (1999) may be more applicable to older adults with limited education. Of note, Coman et al. (1999) also provided expected scores for healthy older adults with memory concerns, as well as for a group with mixed neurological disorders.

Messinis et al. (2009) provide norms from a Greek sample Administration A, Form C. See Table 10–4.

ADMINISTRATION B

According to the manual (Sivan, 1992), the norms were generated from the performance of 103 medical patients with no evidence of neurological damage. The data probably date back to the 1960s. Based on these data, the manual suggests that one point should be subtracted from the expected number correct score for Administration A.

ADMINISTRATION C

Normative data, dating from the 1960s and derived from the performance of 200 medical patients with no history or evidence of cerebral disease, are provided in the manual (Sivan, 1992). For adults, only rounded error scores without *SDs* are provided. In general, adults of average intellectual ability are reported to make two or fewer errors on this form of the test. Robinson-Whelen (1992) reported means of 9.38 (number correct) and 0.65 (number of errors) for a group of 122 older adults with an average of 12.8 years of education (mean age, 72 years). This suggests that less than one error is made even in older adults.

TABLE 10–3 Mean Number of Correct Responses and Errors by Age and Education Level for Benton Visual Retention Test Fifth Edition (BVRT-5) Administration A

	EDUCATION 12–14 YEARS			EDUCATION 15–17 YEARS			EDUCATION 18+ YEARS		
AGE	*N*	*M*	*SD*	*N*	*M*	*SD*	*N*	*M*	*SD*
Number Correct									
18–39	29	7.59	1.52	27	8.04	1.19	18	8.11	1.28
40–49	18	7.11	1.53	23	7.78	1.54	19	7.42	1.22
50–59	130	6.66	1.47	146	7.08	1.70	133	7.55	1.53
60–69	129	6.18	1.67	159	6.70	1.47	134	6.80	1.55
70+	53	5.62	1.73	54	6.06	1.84	49	6.22	1.57
Number of Errors									
18–39	29	3.38	2.37	27	2.52	1.70	18	2.67	1.78
40–49	18	4.22	2.62	23	3.48	2.78	19	3.74	2.47
50–59	130	4.90	2.42	146	4.21	2.85	133	3.64	2.76
60–69	129	5.55	2.74	159	4.99	2.78	134	4.93	2.87
70+	53	7.28	3.55	54	7.74	4.34	49	6.33	3.63

NOTE: *N* = 1128; age range = 17–84 years; education M = 16.01 years, *SD* = 2.29, range = 12–25 years; 58.8% females. Screened for evidence or history of physical, psychiatric, or neurological conditions that would affect memory; average non-depressed range on self-report measure of mood.

SOURCE: Adapted from Youngjohn et al. (1993).

TABLE 10–4 Mean Number of Correct Responses and Errors as a Function of Age and Education for Administration A in a Greek Sample

	≤12 YEARS OF EDUCATION			13+ YEARS OF EDUCATION		
AGE (YEARS)	*N*	*M*	*SD*	*N*	*M*	*SD*
Number correct						
18–39	65	7.64	1.30	73	7.94	1.20
40–49	32	6.30	1.10	22	7.56	1.32
50–59	39	5.50	2.10	14	7.22	1.64
60–69	36	5.22	0.94	12	6.40	1.48
70–85	49	3.9	1.2	10	5.98	1.46
Number errors						
18–39	65	3.20	2.20	73	2.54	1.54
40–49	32	5.30	2.04	22	3.82	1.84
50–59	39	5.50	2.10	14	3.66	1.86
60–69	36	5.92	2.60	12	4.80	1.20
70–85	49	8.80	2.85	10	8.35	2.26

NOTE: *N* = 352 healthy adults age *M* = 37.9, *SD* = 17.72, range = 18–84; education *M* = 12.48, *SD* = 3.15, range = 6–21; 46.9% females; WASI *M* = 104.52, *SD* = 14.06, range = 78–132. Exclusion criteria include history of psychiatric, neurological, or cardiovascular disorders, substance abuse or dependence, and head injury or other medical condition.

SOURCE: Messinis et al. (2009).

ADMINISTRATION D

The manual (Sivan, 1992) indicates that healthy adults obtain number correct scores about 0.4 points less with Administration D (10-second exposure, 15-second delay) than with Administration A.

ADMINISTRATION M

Form G is easier than Form F, and the two forms are differentially affected by age and education (see "Evidence for Reliability"). On Form F, younger people and those with higher education perform better. Form G is affected only by age, with older adults performing worse (Lannoo & Vingerhoets, 1997; Miatton et al., 2004). Miatton et al. (2004) presented data for each form separately, using a sample of Flemish people (aged 20–86 years) who, based on a standardized interview, had no history of cardiovascular, neurological, or psychiatric disease and were taking no psychoactive medications. The data are shown in Tables 10–5 (Form F) and 10–6 (Form G).

EVIDENCE FOR RELIABILITY

EVIDENCE FOR INTERNAL RELIABILITY

Cronbach's alpha coefficients are adequate for Administration A (r = .76 to .79 for Form C, D, and E number correct; r = .71 to .82 for number of errors; Steck et al., 1990). Internal consistency rises to .91 when all 30 items (Form C + D + E) are administered. Steck (2005) developed two 20-item parallel forms (items taken from all three forms) that also show high reliability. Split-half reliability of the multiple-choice forms (Administration M) is adequate (r = .76; Sivan & Spreen, 1996).

EVIDENCE FOR TEST-RETEST RELIABILITY, MEASURING CHANGE, AND PRACTICE EFFECTS

Test-retest reliability for Administration A is reported to be high in adults (.85; Benton, 1974), although details regarding the sample and duration of retest interval are not provided. Three-week test-retest reliability of healthy volunteers aged 17 to 82 years appears low (r = .57 for number correct; r = .53 for number of errors; Youngjohn et al., 1992). In an acute stroke sample, four-week test-retest reliability was adequate (r = .78) for number correct but low for number errors (r = .59) (Messinis et al., 2009). Snow et al. (1988) also reported low one-year test-retest reliability coefficients in a sample of 100 older adults for both copy and multiple-choice versions (r = .52 and .53, respectively).

Practice effects after retesting are in dispute. Botwinick et al. (1986) found virtually no change in scores for 64- to 81-year-olds tested four times at 18-month intervals.

TABLE 10–5 Normative Data for Benton Visual Retention Test Fifth Edition (BVRT-5) Form F According to Age and Education in a Flemish Sample

	EDUCATION ≤ 12 YEARS			EDUCATION > 12 YEARS		
AGE	20 TO 30 (*N* = 22)	30 TO 50 (*N* = 21)	50+ (*N* = 22)	20 TO 30 (*N* = 42)	30 TO 50 (*N* = 30)	50+ (*N* = 14)
Mean (*SD*)	13.2 (1.3)	13.1 (1.5)	11.2 (2.3)	13.9 (1.2)	13.1 (1.3)	12.4 (2.1)
Percentile Rank						
10th	11.3	11	7	12.3	12	9
20th	12	12	9	13	12	11
30th	12	12	9.9	14	12	11
40th	13	12	11	14	13	12
50th	13.5	13	12	14	13	12.5
60th	14	14	12	14	13	13
70th	14	14	13	15	14	14
80th	14	15	13	15	14	15
90th	15	15	14	15	15	15

SOURCE: Adapted from Miatton et al. (2004).

TABLE 10-6 Normative Data for Benton Visual Retention Test Fifth Edition (BVRT-5) Form G According to Age in a Flemish Sample

	20 TO 30 (N = 35)	30 TO 50 (N = 38)	50+ (N = 60)
Mean (*SD*)	14.3 (0.7)	14.1 (0.9)	13.0 (1.9)
Percentile Rank			
10th	13	13	10
20th	14	13	11
30th	14	14	12
40th	14	14	13
50th	14	14	13
60th	14.6	15	14
70th	15	15	14
80th	15	15	15
90th	15	15	15

SOURCE: Adapted from Miatton et al. (2004).

Similarly, Lezak (cited in Lezak et al., 2004) gave three administrations to healthy controls six and 12 months apart and found no significant differences between either number correct or error score means. Coefficients of concordance between scores obtained for each administration were .74 for number correct and .77 for errors. By contrast, Larrabee et al. (1986) found an improvement of more than one point on retesting of 60- to 90-year-olds after 10 to 13 months. Similar findings were reported by Youngjohn et al. (1992) in their sample of adults (aged 17–82 years) retested after an interval of about three weeks. Messinis et al. (2009) reported minimal improvements in performance of healthy individuals from first ($M = 6.04$, $SD = 2.10$) to second administration ($M = 6.70$, $SD = 2.13$) retested over a four-week interval; however, no practice effect was noted for number of errors.

EVIDENCE FOR RELIABILITY OF ALTERNATE OR COMPUTER FORMS

Sivan (1992) reported correlation coefficients ranging from .79 to .84 among the three forms (C, D, and E) of the test. There is some evidence (Breidt, 1970) that Form D is slightly more difficult than Form C for the memory but not the copying task, with Form E occupying an intermediate position, although other studies found virtually no difference among these forms (Brown & Rice, 1967; Weiss, 1974). Updated data have not been reported.

For the multiple-choice administration (M), alternate-form reliability (Forms F and G) is reported to be good (.80, Sivan & Spreen, 1996). However, higher scores were reported for Form G in Flemish adults, and the two forms are differentially influenced by demographic factors (Lannoo & Vingerhoets, 1997; Miatton et al., 2004).

A computerized BVRT Administration A, in which the examinee draws the designs on a graphics tablet using a cordless pen, has been described (Thompson et al., 2007). Thompson et al. (2007) gave both the computerized and the traditional version of the BVRT Administration A to healthy adults and found that participants performed better (more correct responses and fewer errors) on the traditional version than the computerized version. Although participants found the computerized version more "fun," they preferred the traditional version because they found it more comfortable and easier to concentrate on. Attitude toward computers did not affect performance on the computerized version.

EVIDENCE FOR INTERRATER RELIABILITY

For the drawing administrations of the BVRT, interscorer agreement for number correct and the total error score is reportedly high ($r > .95$; Dougherty et al., 2003; Seo et al., 2007; Swan et al., 1990; Wahler, 1956), although interrater reliability for Administration C appears to be slightly lower ($r = .84$; Seo et al., 2007). Interrater agreement for some qualitative aspects of the scoring system is also good (omissions, $r = .96$; perseverations, $r = .88$; rotations, $r = .88$) but is less acceptable for scoring of misplacement and size errors (Swan et al., 1990). The introduction of augmented scoring rules and examples in the current edition of the manual may improve this situation. However, estimates based on the revised scoring guidelines are not yet available.

EVIDENCE FOR VALIDITY

RELATIONSHIPS AMONG FORMATS

As might be expected, number correct and error scores are highly correlated (Benton, 1974; Vakil et al., 1989). The various formats appear to be measuring similar, but not totally identical skills. There is a moderate relation ($r = .41$ to .52) between performance levels on the copying task (Administration C) and the memory task (Administration B; Benton, 1974). Positive correlations, ranging from .40 to .83, have also been reported between immediate reproduction (Administration A) and delayed reproduction (Administration D) versions (Benton, 1974). The correlation between the multiple-choice and reproduction forms is $r = .55$ (Sivan & Spreen, 1996).

FACTOR-ANALYTIC STUDIES

Moses (1986) showed that Administration A and the multiple-choice administration both loaded on a first factor representing primarily memory skills and on a second factor described as attention span and perceptual-analytic ability. The copying form (Form C) loaded primarily on the second factor. A replication study with 162 neuropsychiatric patients (Moses, 1989) confirmed that the BVRT copy and memory scores form separable factorial components. Executive control processes appear to play a role in BVRT performance. There is evidence that impulsivity (e.g., commission errors on continuous performance tasks) impairs performance on the BVRT (Administration A), at least in adolescents with disruptive behavior disorder (Dougherty et al., 2003).

Similarly, Lockwood et al. (2011) examined the factor structure of the BVRT in a sample of veterans with mixed neuropsychiatric diagnosis by submitting BVRT recall and multiple choice (BVRT-MC) to principal components analysis (PCA). The BVRT alone yielded two components, comprising items 5–10 for component 1 (hard items) and items 1–4 for component 2 (easy items), explaining 44% of the variance. Item difficulty analysis revealed that the first four items of the BVRT show high pass rates, whereas items 5–10 show lower pass rates. With BVRT-MC included in the PCA, BVRT-MC and BVRT items 1–4 loaded on the same component while BVRT items 3–10 loaded on the second component, suggesting that the BVRT-MC may be easy. Including Wechsler Adult Intelligence Scale—Revised (WAIS-R) components in the PCA yielded four components. Items in component 2 appear to be amenable to verbal mediation for recall, recognition, reproduction, and perception, while attention or executive functions affect the easy items in component 4, and the items with medium difficulty are affected by nonverbal reasoning. However, BVRT items 5–10 are not affected by intellectual or perceptual abilities and may be the most useful measure of complex immediate visual recall and reproduction (Lockwood et al., 2011).

RELATIONSHIPS WITH OTHER TESTS

Factor analyses have shown that the BVRT (Administration A) loads primarily on a visual-perceptual-motor factor and only secondarily on a memory-concentration-attention factor (Crook & Larrabee, 1988; Larrabee et al., 1985). A second factor-analytic study (Larrabee & Crook, 1989) found that the test loaded on two factors, "vigilance" and "psychomotor speed," when analyzed in the context of other memory tests and measures of everyday memory performance. Indeed, de Sousa et al. (2012) reported that Rey Auditory Verbal Learning Test (RAVLT) learning and delayed recall were moderately correlated with BVRT in healthy undergraduates ($r = .39$ for BVRT delayed and RAVLT delayed; $r = .44$ for BVRT immediate and RAVLT learning). However, in an Attention Deficit/Hyperactivity Disorder (ADHD) sample, when all tests were submitted to a PCA, three factors were obtained, with RAVLT total learning and delayed recall, and visual learning and delayed recall forming the learning and delayed recall factor, explaining 52% of the variance. BVRT number correct and errors formed its own factor named "visual short-term memory," explaining 17% of the variance. The third factor comprised of Digit Span explained 13% of the variance (Dige et al., 2008). These results suggest that the BVRT does not measure the same learning/memory processes as other list learning tasks. Among patients with schizophrenia or schizoaffective disorder, BVRT was moderately correlated with Wisconsin Card Sorting Test (WCST) Categories, Non-Perseverative Errors, Perseverative Errors, and Conceptual Level of Response ($r = .47$ to $.67$; Egan et al., 2011), suggesting an executive component to the BVRT.

CLINICAL STUDIES

Numerous studies have examined BVRT performance in various diagnostic groups (e.g., Bigras et al., 2013; Dige et al., 2008; Egan et al., 2011; Paweczyk et al., 2015; Raffaitin et al., 2011; Zonderman et al., 1995). Overall, these studies showed that the standard version of the test (Administration A) is sensitive to the presence of neurobehavioral disturbance, although its diagnostic ability is not high. For example, left and right temporal lobe epilepsy (TLE) patients are mildly impaired on the BVRT compared to published norms but no differences are seen between left and right TLE even though the right TLE patients show superior performance on Wechsler Memory Scale Third Edition (WMS-III) Word List delayed recall, indicating that the BVRT may not be useful as a measure for material-specific memory in presurgical TLE cases (Bigras et al., 2013). Steck et al. (1990) reported that a 30-item version did not show significant score or type-of-error differences among small groups of adults with depression, schizophrenia, alcoholism, or brain damage, although all groups showed error scores well above those of 145 healthy controls.

Impairment on the standard administration (Administration A) of the BVRT has been reported in adults with a variety of conditions thought to affect memory, including those with head injury (Levin et al., 1990), the relapsing-remitting form of multiple sclerosis (MS; Rugglieri et al., 2003), gene carriers of Huntington's disease (HD) not clinically diagnosed with the disorder (Witjes-Ane et al., 2003), postmenopausal women not treated with estrogen replacement therapy (Resnick et al., 1997), older men with both the apolipoprotein ε4 allele (APOE-ε4) and magnetic resonance imaging (MRI) signs of brain atrophy (Carmelli et al., 2000), and older adults with metabolic syndrome (Raffaitin et al., 2011). In particular, those with hypertension or diabetes have an increased risk of decline on the BVRT over four years, suggesting that the BVRT may be sensitive to vascular cognitive impairment (Raffaitin et al., 2011). In acute stroke samples, healthy adults outperform stroke patients on number correct but not errors, and stroke severity is associated with BVRT number correct but not errors (Messinis et al., 2009).

Patients with subcortical dementia (associated with Parkinson's disease [PD]) and cortical dementia (Alzheimer's disease [AD]) are impaired on the standard form (Administration A; Kuzis et al., 1999). However, there is only an isolated decline in WCST but no change in BVRT performance or other tests of executive function immediately following unilateral posteroventral stereotactic pallidotomy in patients with PD (Olzak et al., 2006). Of note, the test is sensitive to even mild forms of dementia. Robinson-Whelen (1992) reported significant differences between healthy controls and patients with very mild or moderate dementia for both Administration A and Administration C. Omission errors were significantly higher on both administrations in demented patients, although other error types also showed significant differences. Storandt et al. (1986) also reported that patients with mild AD showed significantly more errors on Administration C (M = 3.3, SD = 5.1) than did age-matched controls. Furthermore, 2½ years later, the error score had climbed rapidly (M = 13.5, SD = 11.7), whereas the scores of controls showed virtually no change.

There is evidence that performance on the BVRT (Administration A) can predict the development of AD more than a decade before diagnosis (Kawas et al., 2003; Zonderman et al., 1995). Kawas et al. (2003) reported that individuals who scored six or more errors on the BVRT had about twice the risk of developing AD than did those with zero to five errors, up to 15 years before the diagnosis of AD. No single error type was consistently associated with the risk of AD in the interval before diagnosis. However, others tasks (e.g., Letter Cancellation) appear to be better predictors of short-term (within two years) conversion to dementia (Amieva et al., 2004). Swan et al. (1996) found the BVRT to be a significant predictor of mortality in a follow-up study of older adults, in the context of a regression analysis including health factors such as cancer, cardiovascular disease, systolic blood pressure, and cholesterol level.

The BVRT has also been used to examine the protective effect of long-chain omega-3 fatty acids eicosapentaeoic acid (EPA) and docosahexaenoic acid (DHA) on cognitive functioning in APOE-ε4 allele carriers and those with depressive symptoms. Over seven years, baseline plasma EPA was related to slower BVRT decline in depressed individuals regardless of APOE-ε4 allele status. This relationship remained after excluding those who developed dementia at follow-up, suggesting that depression but not APOE-ε4 allele is related to baseline plasma EPA. Baseline plasma DHA was related to slower BVRT decline in APOE-ε4 allele carriers but not in noncarriers and the relationship disappeared in those who remained dementia-free at follow-up, suggesting that APOE-ε4 allele status but not depression is related to baseline plasma DHA (Samieri et al., 2011).

The BVRT is also sensitive to cognitive dysfunction in those with psychiatric conditions, including patients with posttraumatic stress disorder (PTSD; Emdad & Söndergaard, 2006a, 2006b), individuals who are considered ultra-high-risk for psychosis (Paweczyk et al., 2015), ADHD (Dige et al., 2008), opiate-dependent individuals (Pirastu et al., 2006), and polydrug abusers (Amir & Bahri, 1999). In fact, those with schizophrenia or schizoaffective disorder are impaired on the BVRT but not on the California Verbal Learning Test (CVLT-II) in one study (Egan et al., 2011).

Among those with ADHD, severe impairment on the BVRT has been reported in all three subtypes of ADHD (Predominantly Inattentive, Predominantly Hyperactive-Impulsive, and Combined subtypes), and the BVRT can differentiate among the three subtypes (Dige et al., 2008). Specifically, the Inattention subtype was the best in number of correct responses and errors of all three groups, followed by the Hyperactive-Impulsive subtype, and Combined subtype (Dige et al., 2008). Accordingly, this study suggests that the attentional demand of the BVRT may be low.

Baum et al. (1996) conducted a canonical analysis of a variety of measures of activities of daily living (ADLs) and a set of neuropsychological tests. The BVRT had a loading of .85 (memory) and .69 (copying) on the first canonical variate, indicating good ecological validity in this AD population. Poor performance on the BVRT may also signify problems in decision making (assessed via Bechara's Card Test) in patients with AD (Torralva et al., 2000), and the test is also related to problems in vocational outcome after severe traumatic brain injury (TBI) in childhood (Nybo & Koskiniem, 1999).

The test has also been used in case study designs to estimate the effect of memory training in patients with brain trauma (Kaschel, 1994) and in alcoholics (Unterholzner et al., 1992), and of cognitive/communicative training in people with schizophrenia (Roder et al., 1987). In a group design (N = 168), John et al. (1991) found that significant improvement compared with controls during an alcohol detoxification program occurred mainly during the first week, whereas subsequent weeks did not show further improvement. Interestingly, isometric exercise via handgrip following administration of the BVRT enhanced BVRT performance when tested two weeks later relative to those who did not undergo isometric exercise (Nielson et al., 2014).

By contrast, spaced retrieval training in those with mild and very mild AD shows improvement in retention span with training but no changes in BVRT performance following training (Lee et al., 2009). Adherence to the Mediterranean diet in French older adults over five years also did not alter performance on the BVRT despite slower overall cognitive decline (Feart et al., 2009). Similarly, the BVRT did not change despite six months of treatment in adults with vitamin B_{12} deficiency neurological syndrome, even though other tests such as the Mini-Mental State Examination (MMSE) and Trail Making Test (TMT) improved (Kalita et al., 2013).

Subjective memory complaint is associated with poorer BVRT delayed recall and TMT performance even after accounting for demographic background and depressive symptoms. However, social activity, education, or living alone does not modify the association (Genziani et al., 2013).

NEUROANATOMICAL CORRELATES AND IMAGING STUDIES

The clinical impression is that patients with right posterior lesions tend to be most impaired on the reproduction administrations of the BVRT, but the evidence is inconsistent (Sivan, 1992). For example, right and left TLE patients do not differ on the BVRT (Bigras et al., 2013). By contrast, in older adults with early or prodromal AD, BVRT copy is associated with regional cerebral glucose metabolism as measured by fluorodeoxyglucose positron emission tomography (FDG-PET) in bilateral posterior brain regions including parieto-temporo-occipital regions whereas recall is correlated with left parietal and temporo-occipital regions (Han et al., 2015).

In examining the hippocampus alone, Brickman et al. (2011) noted that different hippocampal region (i.e., entorhinal cortex and dentate gyrus) are associated with different memory tests in community-dwelling older adults. BVRT recognition was associated with the dentate gyrus specifically (Brickman et al., 2011).

PERFORMANCE VALIDITY

The test does not appear to have been well-validated as a performance validity test (PVT) as have other visual memory tests such as, notably, the WMS-IV, Continuous Visual Memory Test (CVMT), Rey-Osterrieth Complex Figure Test (RCFT), and BVMT-R. Of the few existing studies, results indicate that simulators and litigants suspected of malingering produce fewer correct responses and more errors than do brain-damaged patients, and more distortion errors than do brain-damaged patients, depressed patients, and patients with somatoform disorders (Benton & Spreen, 1961; Suhr et al., 1997).

COMMENT

This popular test has been in use since 1946 (Benton, 1946) and has stimulated numerous psychometric and clinical studies, although less so in recent years. The BVRT has a number of advantages (Wellman, 1985). These include short administration time, precise scoring criteria, excellent interrater reliability, acceptable internal reliability (at least for forms used with Administration A), and the availability of alternate forms. Furthermore, because of its multiple-choice, drawing from memory, and copying administrations, the examiner may be able to discriminate among perceptual, motor, and memory deficits. The test has been used not only with English-speaking populations but also in countries such as China, Egypt, Greece, India, and Venezuela. The reader is referred to Mitrushina et al. (2005) for normative reports for these and other countries.

Clinical studies have demonstrated the sensitivity of the BVRT (particularly Administration A) to age-related cognitive decline, dementia, head injury, and psychiatric conditions, although the test's sensitivity to right hemisphere lesions, such as in the case of material-specific memory in epilepsy, is less compelling. Examination of the pattern of errors may be useful in detecting neglect. Use of the BVRT to assess treatment effects may be effective in some conditions but insensitive in other conditions.

Users should be aware of the test's limitations. Availability of up-to-date norms appears to be the biggest shortcoming of the BVRT. Some of the normative data provided in the 1992 manual were compiled more than 50 years ago, and the most recent norms updates were collected more than 20 years ago. It is important to highlight that the breadth of normative data varies by administration type, and the most up-to-date and extensive norms are available only for Administration A. Adjustments for education have been proposed, but it is important to bear in mind that reliance on a simple measure of educational achievement such as highest grade attained does not capture the extent of discrepancies in educational experience between and within various ethnic groups. One way to avoid faulty interpretations may be to adjust for reading recognition (Manly et al., 2002).

Note that a ceiling effect appears evident on Administrations A and M in young and middle-aged adults of above-average education, and, therefore, results should be interpreted with caution in this group. Test-retest reliability information is conflicting. In addition, cultural effects have been examined systematically only for the multiple-choice format.

Finally, the specific construct measured by the BVRT remains to be determined. Although performance is intended to measure nonverbal memory, some of the geometric figures can be verbalized (Arenberg, 1978), and some items on the multiple-choice version can be solved strategically (Blanton & Gouvier, 1985). The BVRT has at most a 15-second delay interval for assessing memory recall. The lack of a longer delay may diminish its utility in milder cognitive disorders. Furthermore, the reproduction administrations may be more closely associated with visual-perceptual-motor ability than with visual memory. In fact, brain imaging studies show that BVRT performance seems to rely on greater left than right hemisphere involvement, particularly of the left parietal region, and may also involve the dentate gyrus in the hippocampus. Last, the BVRT-5 does not provide any validated embedded validity indicators to assess for invalid performance as do some other visual memory measures, notably the WMS-IV, CVMT, RCFT, and BVMT-R.

REFERENCES

Amieva, H., Letenneur, L., Dartigues, J. F., Rouch-Leroyer, I., Sourgen, C., D'Alchee-Biree, F., . . . Fabrigoule, C. (2004). Annual rate and predictors of conversion to dementia in subjects presenting Mild Cognitive Impairment criteria defined according to a population-based study. *Dementia and Geriatric Cognitive Disorders, 18,* 87–93.

Amir, T., & Bahri, T. (1999). Effect of polydrug abuse on sustained attention, visuographic function, and reaction time. *Social Behavior and Personality, 27,* 289–296.

Arenberg, D. (1978). Differences and changes with age in the Benton Visual Retention Test. *Journal of Gerontology, 33,* 534–540.

Baum, C., Edwards, D., Yonan, C., & Storandt, M. (1996). The relation of neuropsychological test performance to performance on functional tasks in dementia of the Alzheimer type. *Archives of Clinical Neuropsychology, 11,* 69–75.

Benton, A. L. (1946). *A visual retention test for clinical use.* New York: Psychological Corporation.

Benton, A. L. (1963). *Revised Visual Retention Test: Clinical and experimental applications* (3rd ed.). New York: Psychological Corporation.

Benton, A. L. (1974). *Revised Visual Retention Test* (4th ed.). New York: Psychological Corporation.

Benton, A. L., & Spreen, O. (1961). Visual Memory Test: The simulation of mental incompetence. *Archives of General Psychiatry, 4,* 79–83.

Benton, A. L., Eslinger, P. J., & Damasio, A. R. (1981). Normative observations on neuropsychological test performances in old age. *Journal of Clinical Psychology, 3,* 33–42.

Bigras, C., Shear, P. K., Vannest, J., Allendorfer, J. B., & Szaflarski, J. P. (2013). The effects of temporal lobe epilepsy on scene encoding. *Epilepsy & Behavior, 26*(1), 11–21.

Blanton, P. D., & Gouvier, W. D. (1985). A systematic solution to the Benton Visual Retention Test: A caveat to examiners. *International Journal of Clinical Neuropsychology, 7,* 95–96.

Botwinick, J., Storandt, M., & Berg, L. (1986). A longitudinal, behavioral study of senile dementia of the Alzheimer type. *Archives of Neurology, 43,* 1124–1127.

Breidt, R. (1970). Möglichkeiten des Benton-Tests in der Untersuchung psychoorganischer Störungen nach Hirnverletzungen. *Archiv für Psychologie, 122,* 314–326.

Brickman, A. M., Stern, Y., & Small, S. A. (2011). Hippocampal subregions differentially associate with standardized memory tests. *Hippocampus, 21*(9), 923–928.

Brown, L. F., & Rice, J. A. (1967). Form equivalence analysis of the Benton Visual Retention Test in children with low IQ. *Perceptual and Motor Skills, 24,* 737–738.

Carmelli, D., DeCarli, C., Swan, G. E. (2000). The joint effect of apolipoprotein E epsilon4 and MRI findings on lower-extremity function and decline in cognitive function. *Journals of Gerontology—Series A: Biological Sciences & Medical Sciences, 55A,* M103–M109.

Coman, E., Moses, J. A., & Kraemer, H. C. (1999). Geriatric performance on the Benton Test: Demographic and diagnostic considerations. *The Clinical Neuropsychologist, 13,* 66–77.

Coman, E., Moses, J. A., Kraemer, H. C., Friedman, L., Benton, A. L., & Yesavage, J. (2002). Interactive influences on BVRT performance level: Geriatric considerations. *Archives of Clinical Neuropsychology, 17,* 595–610.

Crook, T. H., & Larrabee, G. J. (1988). Interrelationship among everyday memory tests: Stability of factor structure with age. *Neuropsychology, 2,* 1–12.

Dartigues, J. F., Gagnon, M., Mazaux, J. M., & Barberger-Gateau, P. (1992). Occupation during life and memory performance in non-demented French elderly community residents. *Neurology, 42,* 1697–1701.

de Sousa Magalhães, S., Malloy-Diniz, L. F., & Hamdan, A. C. (2012). Validity convergent and reliability test-retest of the Rey Auditory Verbal Learning Test. *Clinical Neuropsychiatry, 9*(3), 129–137.

Dige, N., Maahr, E., & Backenroth-Ohsako, G. (2008). Memory tests in subgroups of adult attention deficit hyperactivity disorder reveals simultaneous capacity deficit. *International Journal of Neuroscience, 118*(4), 569–591.

Dougherty, D. M., Mathias, C. M., March, D. M., Greve, K. W., Bjork, J. M., & Moeller, F. G. (2003). Commission error rates on a continuous performance test are related to deficits measured by the Benton Visual Retention Test. *Assessment, 10,* 3–12.

Egan, G. J., Hasenkamp, W., Wilcox, L., Green, A., Hsu, N., Boshoven, W., . . . Duncan, E. (2011). Declarative memory and WCST-64 performance in subjects with schizophrenia and healthy controls. *Psychiatry Research 188*(2), 191–196.

Emdad, R., & Söndergaard, H. P. (2006a). General intelligence and short-term memory impairments in Post-Traumatic Stress Disorder patients. *Journal of Mental Health, 15*(2), 205–216.

Emdad, R., & Söndergaard, H. P. (2006b). Short communication: Visuoconstructional ability in PTSD patients compared to a control group with the same ethnic background. *Stress and Health, 22*(1), 35–43.

Féart, C., Samieri, C., Rondeau, V., Amieva, H., Portet, F., Dartigues, J., . . . Barberger-Gateau, P. (2009). Adherence to a Mediterranean diet, cognitive decline, and risk of dementia. *Journal of the American Medical Association, 302*(6), 638–648.

Franzen, M. D. (1989). *Reliability and validity in neuropsychological assessment.* New York: Plenum.

Genziani, M., Stewart, R., Béjot, Y., Amieva, H., Artero, S., & Ritchie, K. (2013). Subjective memory impairment, objective cognitive functioning and social activity in French older people: Findings from the three cities study. *Geriatrics & Gerontology International, 13*(1), 139–145.

Giambra, L. M., Arenberg, D., Zonerman, A. B., Kawas, C., & Costa, P. T. (1995). Adult life span changes in immediate visual memory and verbal intelligence. *Psychology and Aging, 10,* 123–139.

Han, J. Y., Byun, M. S., Seo, E. H., Yi, D., Choe, Y. M., Sohn, B. K., . . . Lee, D. Y. (2015). Functional neural correlates of figure copy and recall task performances in cognitively impaired individuals: An [1]8F-FDG-PET study. *NeuroReport, 26*(17), 1077–1082.

Jacobs, D. M., Sano, M., & Albert, S. (1997). Cross-cultural neuropsychological assessment: A comparison of randomly selected, demographically matched cohorts of English- and Spanish-speaking older adults. *Journal of Clinical and Experimental Neuropsychology, 19,* 331–339.

John, U., Veltrup, C., Schnofl, A., Wetterling, T., Kanitz, W. D., & Dilling, H. (1991). Gedächtnisdefizite Alkoholabhängiger in der ersten Woche der Abstinenz. *Zeitschrift für klinische Psychologie, Psychopathologie und Psychotherapie, 39,* 348–356.

Kalita, J., Agarwal, R., Chandra, S., & Misra, U. K. (2013). A study of neurobehavioral, clinical psychometric, and P3 changes in vitamin B12 deficiency neurological syndrome. *Nutritional Neuroscience, 16*(1), 39–46.

Kaschel, R. (1994). *Neuropsychologische rehabilitation von Gedächtnisleistungen.* Weinheim, Germany: Beltz Psychologie Verlags Union.

Kawas, C. H., Corrada, M. M., Brookmeyer, R., Morrison, A., Resnick, S. M., Zonderman, A. B., & Arenberg, D. (2003). Visual memory predicts Alzheimer's disease more than a decade before diagnosis. *Neurology, 60,* 1089–1093.

Kuzis, G., Sabem L., Tiberti, C., Merello, M., Leiguarda, R., & Stark-stein, S. E. (1999). Explicit and implicit learning in patients with Alzheimer's disease and Parkinson disease with dementia. *Neuropsychiatry, Neuropsychology, and Behavioral Neurology, 12,* 265–269.

Lannoo, E., & Vingerhoets, G. (1997). Flemish normative data on common neuropsychological tests: Influence of age, education, and gender. *Psychological Belgica, 37,* 141–155.

Larrabee, G. J., & Crook, T. H. (1989). Dimensions of everyday memory in age-associated memory impairment. *Psychological Assessment, 1,* 92–97.

Larrabee, G. J., Kane, R. L., Schuck, J. R., & Francis, D. J. (1985). Construct validity of various memory testing procedures. *Journal of Clinical and Experimental Neuropsychology, 7,* 239–250.

Larrabee, G. J., Levin, H. S., & High, W. M. (1986). Senescent forgetfulness: A quantitative study. *Developmental Neuropsychology, 2,* 373–385.

Le Carret, N., Rainville, C., Lechevaliier, N., Lafont, S., Letenneur, L., & Fabrigoule, C. (2003). Influence of education on the Benton Visual

Retention Test performance as mediated by a strategic search component. *Brain and Cognition, 53,* 408–411.

Lee, S. B., Park, C. S., Jeong, J. W., Choe, J. Y., Hwang, Y. J., Park, C., . . . Kim, K. W. (2009). Effects of spaced retrieval training (SRT) on cognitive function in Alzheimer's disease (AD) patients. *Archives of Gerontology and Geriatrics, 49*(2), 289–293.

Levin, H. S., Gary, H. E., & Eisenberg, H. M. (1990). Neurobehavioral outcome 1 year after severe head injury: Experience of the Traumatic Coma Data Bank. *Journal of Neurosurgery, 73,* 699–709.

Lezak, M. D., Howieson, D. B., & Loring, D. W. (2004). *Neuropsychological assessment* (4th ed.). New York: Oxford University Press.

Lockwood, C. A., Mansoor, Y., Homer-Smith, E., & Moses, J. A. J. (2011). Factor structure of the Benton Visual Retention Tests: Dimensionalization of the Benton Visual Retention Test, Benton Visual Retention Test-Multiple Choice, and the Visual Form Discrimination Test. *The Clinical Neuropsychologist, 25*(1), 90–107.

Manly, J. J., Jacobs, D. M., Sano, M., Bell, K., Merchant, C. A., Small, S., & Stern, Y. (1998). Cognitive test performance among nondemented elderly African Americans and Whites. *Neurology, 50,* 1238–1245.

Manly, J. J., Jacobs, D. M., Touradji, P., Small, S. A., & Stern, Y. (2002). Reading level attenuates differences in neuropsychological test performance between African American and White elders. *Journal of the International Neuropsychological Society, 8,* 341–348.

Messinis, L., Lyros, E., Georgiou, V., & Papathanasopoulos, P. (2009). Benton Visual Retention Test performance in normal adults and acute stroke patients: Demographic considerations, discriminant validity, and test–retest reliability. *The Clinical Neuropsychologist, 23*(6), 962–977.

Miatton, M., Wolters, M., Lannoo, E., & Vingerhoets, G. (2004). Updated and extended normative data of commonly used neuropsychological tests. *Psychologica Belgica, 44,* 189–216.

Mitrushina, M. M., Boone, K. B., Razani, J., & D'Elia, L. F. (2005). *Handbook of normative data for neuropsychological assessment* (2nd ed.). New York: Oxford University Press.

Moses, J. A. (1986). Factor structure of Benton's tests of visual retention, visual construction, and visual form discrimination. *Archives of Clinical Neuropsychology, 1,* 147–156.

Moses, J. A. (1989). Replicated factor structure of Benton's tests of visual retention, visual construction, and visual form discrimination. *International Journal of Clinical Neuropsychology, 11,* 30–37.

Nielson, K. A., Wulff, L. L., & Arentsen, T. J. (2014). Muscle tension induced after learning enhances long-term narrative and visual memory in healthy older adults. *Neurobiology of Learning and Memory, 109,* 144–150.

Nybo, T., & Koskiniem, M. (1999). Cognitive indicators of vocational outcome after severe traumatic brain injury (TBI) in childhood. *Brain Injury, 13,* 759–766.

Olzak, M., Laskowska, I., Jelonek, J., Michalak, M., Szolna, A., Gryz, J., . . . Gorzelanczyk, E. J. (2006). Psychomotor and executive functioning after unilateral posteroventral pallidotomy in patients with Parkinson's disease. *Journal of the Neurological Sciences, 248*(1-2), 97–103.

Pawelczyk, A., Kotlicka-Antczak, M., Rabe-Jablonska, J., Pawelczyk, T., Ruszpel, A., & Lojek, E. (2015). Figural fluency and immediate visual memory in patients with at-risk mental state for psychosis: Empirical study. *Early Intervention in Psychiatry, 9*(4), 324–330.

Pirastu, R., Fais, R., Messina, M., Bini, V., Spiga, S., Falconieri, D., & Diana, M. (2006). Impaired decision-making in opiate-dependent subjects: Effect of pharmacological therapies. *Drug and Alcohol Dependence, 83*(2), 163–168.

Raffaitin, C., Féart, C., Le Goff, M., Amieva, H., Helmer, C., Akbaraly, T. N., . . . Barberger-Gateau, P. (2011). Metabolic syndrome and cognitive decline in French elders: The three-city study. *Neurology, 76*(6), 518–525.

Randall, C. M., Dickson, A. L., & Plasay, M. T. (1988). The relationship between intellectual function and adult performance on the Benton Visual Retention Test. *Cortex, 24,* 277–289.

Resnick, S. M., Metterm J. E., & Zonderman, A. B. (1997). Estrogen replacement therapy and longitudinal decline in visual memory: A possible protective effect. *Neurology, 49*(6), 1491–1497.

Resnick, S. M., Trotman, K. M., Kawas, C., & Zonderman, A. B. (1995). Age-associated changes in specific errors on the Benton Visual Retention Test. *Journals of Gerontology: Psychological Sciences, 50B,* P171–P178.

Robinson-Whelen, S. (1992). Benton Visual Retention Test performance among normal and demented older adults. *Neuropsychology, 6,* 261–269.

Roder, V., Studer, K., & Brenner, H. (1987). Erfahrungen mit einem integrierten psychologischen therapieprogramm zum training kommunikativer und kognitiver fähigkeiten in der rehabilitation schwer chronisch schizophrener patienten. *Schweizer Archiv für Neurologie und Psychiatrie, 138,* 31–44.

Rosselli, M., Ardila, A., Bateman, J. R. (2001). Neuropsychological test scores, academic performance, and developmental disorders in Spanish-speaking children. *Developmental Neuropsychology, 20,* 355–373.

Rugglieri, R. M., Palermo, R., Vitello, G., Gennuso, M., Settipani, N., & Piccoli, F. (2003). Cognitive impairment in patients suffering from relapsing-remitting multiple sclerosis with EDSS <3.5. *Acta Neurological Scandinavica, 108,* 323–326.

Samieri, C., Féart, C., Proust-Lima, C., Peuchant, E., Dartigues, J., Amieva, H., & Barberger-Gateau, P. (2011). Omega-3 fatty acids and cognitive decline: Modulation by ApoEe4 allele and depression. *Neurobiology of Aging, 32*(12), e13–e22.

Seo, E. H., Lee, D. Y., Choo, I. H., Youn, J. C., Kim, K. W., Jhoo, J. H., . . . Woo, J. I. (2007). Performance on the Benton Visual Retention Test in an educationally diverse elderly population. *The Journals of Gerontology: Series B: Psychological Sciences and Social Sciences, 62*(3), P191–P193.

Sivan, A. B. (1992). *Benton Visual Retention Test* (5th ed.). San Antonio, TX: The Psychological Corporation.

Sivan, A. B., & Spreen, O. (1996). *Der Benton-Test* (7th ed.). Berne, Switzerland: Verlag Hans Huber.

Snow, J. (1998). Clinical use of the Benton Visual Retention Test for children and adolescents with learning disabilities. *Archives of Clinical Neuropsychology, 13,* 629–636.

Snow, W. G., Tierney, M. C., Zorzito, M. L., Fisher, R. H., & Reid, D. W. (1988). *One-year test-retest reliability of selected neuropsychological tests in older adults.* Paper presented to the International Neurological Society, New Orleans.

Steck, P., Beer, U., Frey, A., Frühschütz, H. G., & Körner, A. (1990). Testkritische Überprüfung einer 30-Item Version des Visual Retention Tests nach A. L. Benton. *Diagnostica, 36,* 38–49.

Steck, P. H. (2005). A revision of A. L. Benton's Visual Retention test (BVRT) in two parallel forms. *Archives of Clinical Neuropsychology, 20,* 409–416.

Storandt, M., Botwinick, J., & Danzinger, W. L. (1986). Longitudinal changes: Patients with mild SDAT and matched healthy controls. In L. W. Poon (Ed.), *Handbook for clinical memory assessment of older adults* (pp. 277–284). Washington, DC: American Psychological Association.

Suhr, J., Tranel, D., Wefel, J., & Barrash, J. (1997). Memory performance after head injury: Contributions of malingering, litigation status, psychological factors, and medication use. *Journal of Clinical and Experimental Neuropsychology, 19,* 500–514.

Swan, G. E., Carmelli, D., & Larue, A. (1996). *Psychomotor speed and visual memory as predictors of 7-year all-cause mortality in older adults.* Paper presented at the meeting of the International Neuropsychological Society, Chicago.

Swan, G. E., Morrison, E., & Eslinger, P. J. (1990). Interrater agreement on the Benton Visual Retention Test. *The Clinical Neuropsychologist, 4,* 37–44.

Thompson, S. B. N., Ennis, E., Coffin, T., & Farman, S. (2007). Design and evaluation of a computerised version of the Benton Visual Retention Test. *Computers in Human Behavior, 23*(5), 2383–2393.

Torralva, T., Dorrego, F., Sabe, L., Chemerinski, E., & Starkstein, S. E. (2000). Impairments of social cognition and decision making in Alzheimer disease. *International Psychogeriatrics, 12,* 359–368.

Tuokko, H., & Woodward, T. S. (1996). Development and validation of the demographic correction system for neuropsychological measures used in the Canadian Study of Health and Aging. *Journal of Clinical and Experimental Neuropsychology, 18,* 479–616.

Unterholzner, G., Sagstetter, E., & Bauer, M. G. (1992). Mehrstufiges Trainingsprogramm (MKT) zur verbesserung kognitiver funktionen bei chronischen alkoholikern. *Zeitschrift für klinische Psychologie, Psychopathologie und Psychotherapie, 40,* 378–395.

Vakil, E., Blachstein, H., Sheleff, P., & Grossman, S. (1989). BVRT-Scoring system and time delay in the differentiation of lateralized hemispheric damage. *International Journal of Clinical Neuropsychology, 11,* 125–128.

Wagner, H. (1992). The Benton test in school counselling diagnostics. *Acta Paedopsychiatrica, 55,* 179–181.

Wahler, H. J. (1956). A comparison of reproduction errors made by brain-damaged and control patients on a memory-for- designs test. *Journal of Abnormal and Social Psychology, 52,* 251–255.

Weiss, A. A. (1974). Equivalence of three alternate forms of Benton's Visual Retention Test. *Perceptual and Motor Skills, 38,* 623–635.

Wellman, M. M. (1985). Benton Revised Visual Retention Test. In D. J. Keyser & R. C. Sweetland (Eds.), *Test critiques* (pp. 58–67). Kansas City, MO: Test Corporation of America.

Witjes-Ane, M. N. W., Vegter-Vander Vlis, M., van Vugt, J. P. P., Lanser, J. B. K., Hermans, J., Zwinderman, A. H., . . . Roos, R. A. C. (2003). Cognitive and motor functioning in gene carriers for Huntington's disease: A baseline study. *Journal of Neuropsychiatry and Clinical Neuroscience, 15,* 7–16.

Youngjohn, J. R., Larrabee, G. J., & Crook, T. H. (1992). Test-retest reliability of computerized, everyday memory measures and traditional memory tests. *The Clinical Neuropsychologist, 6,* 276–286.

Youngjohn, J. R., Larrabee, G. J., & Crook, T. H. (1993). New adult-and education-correction norms for the Benton Visual Retention Test. *The Clinical Neuropsychologist, 7,* 155–160.

Zonderman, A. B., Giamba, L. M., Arenberg, D., Resnick, S. M., & Costa, P. T. (1995). Changes in immediate visual memory predict cognitive impairment. *Archives of Clinical Neuropsychology, 10,* 111–123.

BRIEF VISUOSPATIAL MEMORY TEST—REVISED (BVMT-R)

TEST NAME	**Brief Visuospatial Memory Test—Revised (BVMT-R)**
DOMAIN	Visual memory
AGE RANGE	18 to 79 years
ADMINISTRATION TIME	15 minutes plus 25-minute delay interval
SCORING FORMAT	Hand scored
REFERENCE	Benedict, R. H. B. (1997). *Brief Visuospatial Memory Test—Revised*. Odessa, FL: Psychological Assessment Resources. www.parinc.com

DESCRIPTION

The Brief Visuospatial Memory Test—Revised (BVMT-R) measures visual learning and memory using a multiple-trial list-learning paradigm devised by Benedict and colleagues (Benedict, 1997; Benedict & Groninger, 1995; Benedict et al., 1996) and modeled after the Visual Reproduction subtest of the WMS (Russell Revision), but with alternate forms. The test consists of six alternate forms that yield measures of immediate recall, rate of acquisition, delayed recall, and recognition. It is part of the Measurement and Treatment Research to Improve Cognition in Schizophrenia (MATRICS) Consensus Cognitive battery to assess cognitive functioning in schizophrenia, as well as the MS-Cog and Brief International Cognitive Assessment for Multiple Sclerosis (BICAMS) battery, both batteries to assess cognitive functioning in MS (see "Clinical Studies" for further discussion).

ADMINISTRATION

The instructions for administering the BVMT-R are provided in the manual. Briefly, the examiner presents the displays and reads the instructions. The examinee is briefly shown an 8 × 11-inch plate containing six simple geometric visual designs in a 2 × 3 matrix and asked to reproduce (on a blank sheet of paper) as many of the designs as possible in the same location as they appeared on the display. Two additional learning trials using the same plate are given, and the patient is encouraged to improve their performance. After 25 minutes of distracting tasks, the patient is asked to reproduce the designs again. This delayed recall trial is followed by a recognition trial in which the individual is shown 12 designs, one at a time. The patient is asked to respond "yes" only to those designs that were included in the original matrix. This yes/no delayed recognition task includes six targets and six nontargets. An optional copy trial can be given after the recognition trial. Recall performance is recorded on a scoring sheet for each of the immediate recall trials (Trials 1 to 3) and for the delayed recall and recognition trials. There is no time limit for recall.

SCORING

Each response is evaluated in terms of two dimensions: accuracy and location. Two points are awarded for each reproduction that is correct with regard to accuracy and location. One point is given if the reproduction is correct with regard to accuracy but incorrectly placed or is incorrect but recognizable as the target and correctly placed. If the drawing is incorrect (not present or present but not recognizable), 0 points are given. Scoring examples for each design are provided in the manual. The maximum total for each recall trial is 12.

As shown in Table 10–7, a number of different scores are derived. The recall scores are combined to form three additional measures of learning and memory. The total immediate recall score is the sum of Trials 1 to 3. The learning score is the best of Trials 2 and 3 minus the Trial 1 score. The percent retained after delay is calculated as Trial 4 recall divided by the best of Trials 2 and 3. Finally, measures of target discriminability and response bias are calculated from the total number of true- and false-positive responses obtained from the delayed recognition trial. Higher scores on the response bias measure reflect a liberal as opposed to a conservative response bias.

Raw scores on Trials 1 to 3, total recall, learning, and delayed recall are converted to T scores and percentile equivalents. Scores on percent retained, recognition hits, false alarms, discrimination index, and response bias all had highly skewed distributions in the normative sample, and only percentile rank ranges were calculated for these scores (e.g., 6th–10th percentile).

OTHER SCORING METHODS

Gaines et al. (2008) developed an alternative scoring method comprising qualitative error and recall consistency indices

TABLE 10-7 Overview of Brief Visuospatial Memory Test—Revised (BVMT-R) Scores

BVMT-R VARIABLE	DESCRIPTION
Trials 1 to 3	Raw scores range from 0 to 12 for each trial and reflect accuracy and correct placement
Total Learning	Sum of scores across the three trials
Learning	The best of Trial 2 or 3 minus the Trial 1 score
Delayed Recall	Raw scores range from 0 to 12 and reflect recall of designs after a 25-min delay
Percent Retained	Scores range from 1 to 100 and reflect the amount originally learned that was retained across the delay
Recognition Hits	Number of target figures correctly recognized; scores range from 0 to 6
Recognition False Alarms	Number of distractors incorrectly recognized as targets; scores range from 0 to 6
Recognition Discrimination Index	Recognition hits minus recognition false alarms; scores range from −6 to 6
Recognition Response Bias	Scores range from 0.00 to 1.00 and reflect the tendency to answer "yes" to a recognition item

for MS patients. In this scoring method, error types included configuration errors, location errors, rotation errors, perseverations, and intrusions. For the interested reader, please contact Dr. Benedict for specific scoring guidelines (personal communication, Dr. Ralph Benedict, October 28, 2016). The recall consistency index is as follows:

$$\text{Recall consistency} = \frac{\begin{array}{c}(\text{Trial 2 Consistency Points}) + \\ (\text{Trial 3 Consistency Points})\end{array}}{(\text{Standard Points Trials } 2+3)}$$

DEMOGRAPHIC EFFECTS

AGE

Small to moderate correlations with age are reported (Kane & Yochim, 2014; Kemmotsu et al., 2013; Miotto et al., 2012; Norman et al., 2011; Tam & Schmitter-Edgecombe, 2013). Benedict et al. (1996) reported that age was moderately correlated with single-trial recall scores (r = –.44 to –.50). Correlations between age and recognition performance are not significant. On average, age accounts for about 11% of the variance in BVMT-R scores (Benedict, 1997).

GENDER

Most studies report that gender does not influence most aspects of recall and recognition performance (Benedict, 1997; Kane et al., 2014; Kemmotsu et al., 2013; Miotto et al., 2012; Norman et al., 2011). Gale et al. (2007) noted that female older adults outperformed male older adults on learning and recall but not recognition trials. Specifically, gender differences were seen in healthy older adults but not mild cognitive impairment (MCI) or AD groups. Despite similar performance on Clinical Dementia Rating (CDR), MMSE, and Dementia Rating Scale (DRS), the degree of discrepancies in BVMT-R scores between females with MCI or AD and healthy females was remarkably larger than that of males (Gale et al., 2016).

EDUCATION AND IQ

Correlations with education are small to moderate (Benedict et al., 1996; Kane et al., 2014; Kemmotsu et al., 2013; Miotto et al., 2012; Norman et al., 2011). However, the proportion of variance in age-adjusted scores accounted for by years of education is only about 1% (Benedict, 1997). IQ shows a moderate relation with BVMT-R recall but not with recognition-discrimination measures (Diaz-Asper et al., 2004).

ETHNICITY, NATIONALITY, AND LINGUISTIC EFFECTS

Norman et al. (2011) reported that age and education but not gender were significant predictors of BVMT-R scores in Caucasians, whereas all three variables were predictive of BVMT-R scores in African Americans. Acculturation does not impact performance once demographic variables are controlled for (Kemmotsu et al., 2013). No differences in BVMT-R performance are found between Japanese Americans and non-Hispanic whites (Kemmotsu et al., 2013).

NORMATIVE DATA

STANDARDIZATION SAMPLE

Table 10–8 shows the characteristics of the standardization sample. Based on the significant relationships between age and BVMT-R scores and the insignificant relationships with other demographic variables (i.e., gender and years of education), normative values are provided in the manual subdivided according to age (Benedict, 1997). Normative tables were constructed using the method of overlapping-midpoint age cells. Separate normative data are also given for a subset of the normative sample (N = 377) selected to reflect the age distributions of the US population for the year 2000. Base-rate data are also provided that show the proportion of normal subjects and patients with neurological disorders who fall within the various score ranges.

To expand on the age range for the BVMT-R, additional norms have been reported in the literature. Gale et al. (2007) provide norms for older adults 60 to 89 years for both RAVLT and BVMT-R. Tables 10–9 and 10–10 present the normative data. Please see the RAVLT review elsewhere in this chapter for RAVLT norms in this volume. Kane et al. (2014) provide norms for older adults aged 80+ for 29 healthy individuals (Table 10–11).

TABLE 10-8 Characteristics of the Brief Visuospatial Memory Test—Revised (BVMT-R) Normative Sample

Sample size	588
Age (years)[a]	18 to 84 years (*M* = 38.6, *SD* = 18)
Sample Type	Two distinct samples: (a) 171 college students and (b) 417 community participants who responded to advertisements
Gender	64% Women 36% Men
Ethnicity	82% Caucasian 15% African American 4% Other
Education	*M* = 13.4, *SD* = 1.8
Screening	University students were not screened, but all were in acceptable academic standing; community participants were screened with structured interview, and those with neurological or psychiatric disorders or substance dependence were excluded; also, participants aged 60 years and older were required to score at least 25/30 on the MMSE

NOTE: Values are rounded.

[a]Age ranges: 18–22, 20–24, 22–26, 24–28, 26–30, 28–32, 30–34, 32–36, 34–38, 36–40, 38–42, 40–44, 42–46, 44–48, 46–50, 48–52, 50–54, 52–56, 54–58, 56–60, 58–62, 60–64, 62–66, 64–68, 66–70, 68–72, 70–74, and 72–79 years.

SOURCE: Adapted from Benedict (1997).

Schretlen, Testa, and Pearlson (2010) provide norms for 327 adults on the BVMT-R; these use the Calibrated Neuropsychological Normative System (CNNS) scoring to derive T scores and discrepancies based on a large sample of older adults from the northeastern United States. Characteristics of the normative sample are shown in Table

TABLE 10-9 Brief Visuospatial Memory Test—Revised (BVMT-R) Normative Data for 60- to 89-Year-Old Adults as a Function of Age and Gender

		MALE		FEMALE		TOTAL	
AGE	*SCORE*	*M*	*SD*	*M*	*SD*	*M*	*SD*
60–69		*N* = 20		*N* = 31		*N* = 51	
	Total Learning	16.5	4.2	18.7	6.5	18.2	5.8
	Delayed Recall	7.5	2.3	8.2	2.5	7.9	2.4
	Recognition	5.6	0.5	5.8	0.5	5.7	0.5
70–79		*N* = 20		*N* = 44		*N* = 64	
	Total Learning	15.3	5.2	16.8	6.0	16.4	5.8
	Delayed Recall	6.6	2.3	6.9	2.7	6.8	2.5
	Recognition	5.6	0.7	5.5	0.7	5.5	0.7
80–89		*N* = 19		*N* = 38		*N* = 57	
	Total Learning	13.5	5.1	15.0	6.1	14.6	5.8
	Delayed Recall	6.2	2.8	6.5	2.9	6.4	2.8
	Recognition	5.6	0.7	5.6	0.7	5.5	0.7

NOTE: Based on *N* = 172; mean age = 74.61, *SD* = 7.79; mean education = 15.48, *SD* = 3.02, range = 6–24; 65% females. The sample was determined to be healthy based on medical, neurologic, radiologic, and functional examinations. Total Learning = total score over Trials 1–3. Delayed Recall = score after the delay. Recognition = true positives on the recognition trial.

SOURCE: Adapted from Gale et al. (2007).

TABLE 10-10 Brief Visuospatial Memory Test—Revised (BVMT-R) Scores by Overlapping Age Groups

		BVMT-R TOTAL		DELAYED RECALL		RECOGNITION	
AGE	*N*	*M*	*SD*	*M*	*SD*	*M*	*SD*
60 to 64	37	20.1	5.4	8.9	2.0	5.6	0.5
62 to 66	14	18.4	5.4	8.6	2.3	5.9	0.5
64 to 68	21	17.0	4.6	7.7	2.1	5.8	0.5
66 to 70	17	17.1	4.9	7.5	2.2	5.8	0.6
68 to 72	23	16.0	6.0	6.8	2.4	5.6	0.7
70 to 74	31	16.7	6.2	6.8	2.5	5.5	0.8
72 to 76	40	17.3	5.9	7.1	2.5	5.6	0.6
74 to 78	39	16.5	5.8	6.9	2.5	5.5	0.7
76 to 80	33	14.8	6.3	6.4	2.7	5.5	0.7
78 to 82	36	14.3	6.4	6.3	3.1	5.6	0.6
80 to 84	41	14.8	6.0	6.5	2.8	5.5	0.7
82 to 86	29	14.6	6.0	6.3	2.7	5.3	0.8
84 to 88	16	13.1	5.0	5.4	2.7	5.7	0.5
86 to 89	19	14.2	5.2	6.3	2.7	5.8	0.4

NOTE: BVMT-R Total is the total score over Trials 1–3. Delayed Recall is the BVMT-R score after the delay. Recognition is the BVMT-R score (true positive) on the recognition trial.

Based on *N* = 172; mean age = 74.61, *SD* = 7.79; mean education = 15.48, *SD* = 3.02, range = 6–24; 65% females. The sample was determined to be healthy based on medical, neurologic, radiologic, and functional examinations.

SOURCE: From Gale et al. (2007).

TABLE 10-11 BVMT-R Norms for Older Adults Age 80+

	M	*SD*
Total Learning	15.52	5.40
Delayed Recall	6.41	2.01
Percent Retained	94.93	23.84
Discrimination Index	5.34	1.26

NOTE: *N* = 29; mean age = 83.2, *SD* = 2.3, range = 80–88; mean education = 14.4, *SD* = 2.6, range = 8–20; 51.7% females; all Caucasians. Screened for neurological disorder, and were independent in IADLS.

SOURCE: From Kane et al. (2014).

TABLE 10-12 Characteristics of the Brief Visuospatial Memory Test—Revised (BVMT-R) Normative Sample from the Calibrated Neuropsychological Normative System (CNNS)

Sample size	327
Age	18 to 92 years
Geographic location	Baltimore, MD, and Hartford, CT, USA
Sample type	Community sample
Education	14.2 (*SD* = 3.0), range 3 to 20 years
Gender	44% Men 56% Women
Ethnicity	80% Caucasian 18% African American 2% Hispanic, Asian, or Other
Screening	History of Alzheimer's disease, Parkinson's disease, stroke, brain injury, bipolar disorder, or substance abuse

SOURCE: Adapted from Schretlen et al. (2010).

10–12. The norms are available through Psychological Assessment Resources (PAR; www.parinc.com). A major advantage of these norms is the option to correct for demographic variables such as age, sex, education, and ethnicity. Several other commonly used neuropsychological tests are co-normed using this sample, which facilitates cross-test comparisons.

Brazilian norms are provided by Miotto et al. (2012) for both BVMT-R and Hopkins Verbal Learning Test-Revised (HVLT-R). Form 1 of both measures were administered. Table 10–13 presents the norms of ages 18 to 80+. Please refer to the HVLT-R review elsewhere in this chapter for HVLT-R norms. Note that some cell sizes are extremely small and should not be used.

Norman et al. (2011) present demographically corrected norms in a sample of 246 participants of which 103 were African Americans. In this sample, age and education but not gender were significant predictors of BVMT-R scores in Caucasians, whereas all three variables were predictive of BVMT-R scores in African Americans. Raw scores are converted to scaled scores using Table 10–14. T scores corrected for demographic variables are generated using the formula presented in Table 10–15. Application of the correction improved classification accuracy by half for African Americans, but no change in BVMT-R total recall was seen in Caucasians.

Goretti et al. (2014) provide Italian norms for the BVMT-R along with Symbol Digit Modalities Test (SDMT) and CVLT-II data in a cognitive test battery for MS (see other chapters for norms in this volume). The participants were drawn from the community in 10 representative Italian sites. Scaled scores are converted from raw scores using Table 10–16 and demographically corrected T scores are generated using the following formulae.

$$\text{BVMT-R T score} = \frac{\text{(actual scaled score converted using Table 10}-16) - \begin{pmatrix} 12.694 + \text{age}\,(-.039) + \text{age2}\,(-.001) \\ + \text{gender}\,(-.671) + \text{education}\,(.101) \end{pmatrix}}{3.133}$$

Note: 1 for male, 2 for female; age in years; education in years.

Vanotti et al. (2016) provide Spanish-Argentinian norms for the BVMT-R as part of the BICAMS comprising SDMT, Spanish CVLT, and BVMT-R Form 1 to assess cognitive function in MS patients (N = 100; mean age = 42.37, SD = 10.07; mean education = 14.94, SD = 2.49; 75% females). Demographically corrected z scores can be obtained using Table 10–17 and the following formula:

$$\text{BVMT-R SS}_{\text{predicted}} = 6.5162 + \text{age}\,(.1438) + \text{age}^2\,(-.0029) + \text{sex}\,(-.1892) + \text{education}\,(.2111)$$

where male = 1, female = 2.

$$\text{BVMT-R } z \text{ score} = (\text{SS}_{\text{actual}} - \text{SS}_{\text{predicted}})/2.8341$$

EVIDENCE FOR RELIABILITY

EVIDENCE FOR INTERNAL RELIABILITY

Not reported.

TABLE 10–13 Brazilian Brief Visuospatial Memory Test—Revised (BVMT-R) Means (Standard Deviations) as a Function of Age and Education

EDUCATION (YEARS)	SCORE	AGE (YEARS) 18–20	21–30	31–40	41–50	51–60	61–70	71–80	80+
0 to 4		N = 10	N = 55	N = 34	N = 50	N = 40	N = 80	N = 51	N = 15
	Total Learning	12.2 (8.27)	17.47 (10.21)	16.29 (8.35)	13.22 (7.90)	12.30 (7.75)	15.71 (9.61)	14.29 (7.79)	10.60 (6.91)
	Delayed Recall	5.1 (3.87)	7.33 (4.01)	7.00 (3.19)	5.36 (3.29)	5.08 (3.16)	6.13 (3.81)	6.00 (3.11)	4.56 (3.05)
	Recognition	4.8 (1.87)	5.31 (1.2)	5.50 (1.08)	5.16 (1.08)	4.95 (1.54)	4.89 (1.48)	5.08 (1.41)	5.17 (1.10)
5 to 8		N = 5	N = 53	N = 34	N = 29	N = 15	N = 70	N = 15	N = 4
	Total Learning	28.00 (10.98)	23.72 (7.22)	20.09 (8.71)	19.28 (9.29)	16.73 (7.46)	18.39 (8.23)	18.00 (7.92)	14.50 (4.73)
	Delayed Recall	10.20 (4.02)	9.51 (2.41)	7.62 (3.34)	8.00 (3.64)	7.60 (3.44)	7.30 (3.23)	8.47 (3.20)	5.00 (1.41)
	Recognition	5.80 (0.45)	5.64 (0.68)	5.74 (0.67)	5.21 (1.08)	4.87 (1.06)	5.36 (1.32)	6.13 (1.73)	5.15 (0.50)
9 to 11		N = 15	N = 31	N = 23	N = 36	N = 29	N = 29	N = 13	N = 7
	Total Learning	27.27 (5.90)	22.06 (8.85)	23.39 (6.46)	23.28 (8.77)	17.86 (8.85)	21.83 (7.52)	21.00 (7.63)	15.14 (4.91)
	Delayed Recall	10.87 (1.81)	10.23 (6.28)	9.00 (2.28)	9.14 (2.99)	7.62 (3.20)	8.07 (2.87)	7.92 (3.52)	5.57 (2.82)
	Recognition	5.80 (0.56)	5.52 (0.89)	5.52 (1.31)	5.86 (0.54)	5.41 (1.09)	5.86 (0.44)	5.38 (0.77)	5.43 (1.13)
12 to 17		N = 7	N = 74	N = 53	N = 52	N = 52	N = 91	N = 27	N = 9
	Total Learning	30.86 (3.02)	28.84 (5.58)	27.74 (6.28)	27.44 (6.56)	23.88 (7.16)	23.14 (6.72)	20.00 (8.70)	11.67 (2.35)
	Delayed Recall	12.00 (1.88)	11.03 (1.69)	11.00 (1.49)	10.48 (2.28)	9.52 (2.54)	9.29 (2.88)	7.26 (3.01)	2.67 (7.50)
	Recognition	5.86 (0.38)	5.85 (0.43)	6.00 (0.76)	5.83 (0.47)	5.65 (0.59)	5.81 (1.37)	5.33 (1.00)	5.56 (2.24)

NOTE: N = 1,108, age 18–85 years, education 0–17 years. Screened for neurologic and psychiatric disorder.

SOURCE: Adapted from Miotto et al. (2012).

TABLE 10–14 Raw Score to Scaled Score Conversion Based on Norman et al. (2011) Demographically Corrected Norms (BVMT-R)

SCALED SCORE	TOTAL RECALL RAW SCORE	DELAYED RECALL RAW SCORE
17	36	
16		
15	34–35	
14	33	12
13	32	
12	30–31	
11	28–29	11
10	26–27	
9	24–25	10
8	21–23	9
7	19–20	8
6	16–18	7
5	14–15	5–6
4	10–13	4
3	0–9	3
2		0–2
1		

SOURCE: Norman et al. (2011).

TABLE 10–16 Brief Visuospatial Memory Test—Revised (BVMT-R) Raw Score to Scaled Score Conversion

SCALED SCORE	BVMT-R RAW SCORE
18	36
17	
16	
15	35
14	34
13	33
12	32
11	30–31
10	28–29
9	25–27
8	23–24
7	20–22
6	17–19
5	14–16
4	12–13
3	11
<2	<11

NOTE: Based on N = 273, 66% females; mean age = 38.9, SD = 13; mean education = 14.9, SD =3.1. Screened for neurological and major psychiatric illness, history of LD, serious head trauma, alcohol or drug abuse and major medical illness.

SOURCE: Adapted from Goretti et al. (2014).

EVIDENCE FOR TEST-RETEST RELIABILITY, MEASURING CHANGE, AND PRACTICE EFFECTS

Test-retest reliability varies by measure and test form. One-year test-retest reliability of stable patients infected with human immunodeficiency virus (HIV-1) is low (r = .52 to .57; Woods et al., 2006). Combined across the six test forms, the manual reports that reliability coefficients for a retest interval of about 56 days are marginal to high, ranging from .60 for Trial 1 to .84 for Trial 3. The reliability coefficient for the total recall score is .80 (Benedict, 1997). Ceiling effects were found for the recognition task and for the percent retained score for both test sessions. Three-week test-retest reliability is adequate (r = .74; Goretti et al., 2014). Two-week test-retest reliability is high for the Spanish-Argentinian Brief International Cognitive Assessment for MS (BICAMS) version (r = .82; Vanotti et al., 2016), adequate for the Brazilian version (r = .77; Spedo et al., 2015), and marginal as reported in the Canadian BICAMS (r = .69; Walker et al., 2016). One-week test-retest reliability is adequate (r = .79; Duff, 2014).

Cysique et al. (2011) retested a sample of HIV-uninfected and neuromedically stable HIV-infected

TABLE 10–15 Formula to Generate Demographically Corrected T Scores for Caucasians and African Americans

T-SCORE FORMULAS	
Caucasian	
BVMT-R Total Recall	[(Total learning scaled score – (0.2589) × (edu – 14.11) + (–0.0515) × (age – 37.62) + 0.9276 × sex + 10.0712))/2.8912] × 10 + 50
BVMT-R Delayed Recall	[(Delayed recall scaled score – (0.2084 × (edu – 14.11) + (–0.0286) × (age – 37.62) + 10.3007))/ 2.6989] × 10 + 50
African American	
BVMT-R Total Recall	[Total learning scaled score – (0.2834 × (edu – 13.86) + (–0.1125) × (age – 40.63) + 1.0394 × sex + 8.0679))/2.570] × 10 + 50
BVMT-R Delayed Recall	[(Delayed recall scaled score – (0.2267 × (edu – 13.86) + (–0.12.62) × (age – 40.63) + 0.8593 × sex + 7.691))/2.5197] × 10 + 50

NOTE: Sex: male = 0, female = 1. Edu, education: years of education were determined using a previously defined and standardized procedure where education level ranges from 1–20 based on number of years of schooling completed (Heaton et al., 2004).

SOURCE: Adapted from Norman et al. (2011).

TABLE 10–17 Raw Score to Scaled Score (SS_{actual}) Conversion

SCALED SCORE	BVMT-R RAW SCORE
2	0–6
3	7–10
4	11
5	12
6	13–16
7	17–19
8	20–21
9	22
10	23–25
11	26
12	27–28
13	29
14	30–31
15	32
16	33
17	34–35
18	36

NOTE: Based on N = 100; mean age = 42.37, SD = 10.07; mean education = 14.94, SD = 2.49; 75% females.

SOURCE: Adapted from Vanotti et al. (2016).

individuals every 11 months for six cycles. Reliability coefficients using alternate forms remained generally stable in the marginal range for Total Learning (r = .63 to .67), and low for Delayed Recall (r = .48 to .55).

PRACTICE EFFECTS

Depending on the form, gains of two to four raw-score points are evident in total recall scores when healthy participants (age M = 43.5 years, SD = 9.6; education M = 13.6 years, SD = 1.7) are retested after an interval of about 56 days (SD = 10) (Benedict, 1997).

Duff et al. (2008) found that an amnestic MCI group improved 26% and 32% on the BVMT-R learning and delayed recall trials, respectively, when retested a week later, whereas a healthy group improved 30% and 13%, respectively. In a combined sample of community-dwelling older adults and those with amnestic MCI, a one-week retest period yielded an 8.2 (SD = 5.4) point improvement on the learning trial and a 2.3 (SD = 2.1) point improvement on the delayed recall trial. Benedict and Zgaljardic (1998) found that healthy older adults (aged 57–82 years, M = 63.3, SD = 6.8) who were administered the same form every two weeks improved significantly over four sessions, showing gains of about nine points in total recall.

There are also subtle practice effects with the use of alternate forms. Healthy college students, administered alternate forms at intervals of six weeks, improved their BVMT-R total recall scores from 28.9 (SD = 3.1) in session one to 30.8 (SD = 1.8) by session six, a difference of about five T scores (Benedict et al., 1996). Older adults improved their total recall from 18.8 (SD = 5.0) on session one to 22.1 (SD = 5.6) by session four (Benedict & Zgaljardic, 1998), a difference of about seven T scores.

Based on a sample of 167 community-dwelling older adults and those with amnestic MCI, Duff (2014) presents a variety of reliable change indices (RCIs) to evaluate cognitive change over a one-week interval (Table 10–18).

EVIDENCE FOR RELIABILITY OF ALTERNATE FORMS

Benedict et al. (1996) randomly assigned the six different test forms to a large sample of healthy individuals (N = 457) and a sample of 18 college students. Completed at weekly intervals, both between-groups and within-subjects analyses revealed equivalence of the alternate forms.

EVIDENCE FOR INTERRATER RELIABILITY

This is reported to be high (>.90; Benedict, 1997). Interrater reliability for the Gaines et al. (2008) qualitative error index ranges from adequate to excellent.

EVIDENCE FOR VALIDITY

RELATIONSHIPS WITH OTHER TESTS

In healthy older adults, moderate correlations with verbal memory (CVLT-II; r = .54 to .59) have been reported. Moderate to weak correlations with tests that measure other cognitive domains have also been reported, including with the Delis-Kaplan Executive Function System (D-KEFS) TMT switching condition (r = .57 to .63), DKEFS Category Fluency (r = .36 to .37), DKEFS Letter Fluency (r = .19 to .26), and Neuropsychological Assessment Battery (NAB) Naming (r = .38 to .40; Kane et al., 2014). Similar findings have been reported in patients with either nonlateralized cerebral pathology or psychiatric disease. Benedict et al. (1996) found that Total Learning and Delayed Recall correlated most strongly with other tests of explicit memory, such as the HVLT, WMS-R Visual Reproduction, and Rey Figure recall (r = .65 to .80); less strongly with a measure of visuospatial construction, the copy portion of the Rey figure (r = .65 to .66); and moderately with measures of expressive language, FAS word fluency, and the Boston Naming Test (BNT) (r = .24 to 54). Using hierarchical regression, SDMT-oral but not FAS was a unique predictor of BVMT-R learning and recall after controlling for age and visuocontructional ability (Tam & Schmitter-Edgecombe,

TABLE 10–18 Reliable Change Indices for One-Week Retest Interval in Older Adults

	SDI	RCI	RCI + PE	RCI + $PE_{IVERSON}$
Total Learning	$T_2 - T_1/7.0$	$T_2 - T_1/4.5$	$(T_2 - T_1) - 8.2/4.5$	$(T_2 - T_1) - 8.2/5.2$
Delayed Recall	$T_2 - T_1/3.4$	$T_2 - T_1/2.2$	$(T_2 - T_1) - 2.3/2.2$	$(T_2 - T_1) - 2.3/2.1$
	Simple standardized regression-based change scores			
	Predicted T_2			Reliable change score
Total Learning	$7.87 + (T_1 * 1.02)$			(Observed T_2 – Predicted T_2)/5.46
Delayed Recall	$3.71 + (T_1 * 0.72)$			(Observed T_2 – Predicted T_2)/1.95
	Complex standardized regression-based change scores			
	Predicted T_2			Reliable change score
Total Learning	$14.13 + (T_1 * 0.92) + (edu * 0.43) - (age * 0.14)$			(Observed T_2 – Predicted T_2)/5.29
Delayed Recall	$0.28 + (T_1 * 0.72) + (edu * 0.18) - (sex * 0.99)$			(Observed T_2 – Predicted T_2)/1.88

NOTE: SDI, standard deviation index; RCI, reliable change index; RCI+PE, reliable change index correcting for practice effects; RCI+$PE_{Iverson}$, reliable change index correcting for practice effects using Iverson (2001) modification; T_1, baseline score; T_2, one-week score. Based on N = 167; mean age = 78.6, SD = 7.8; mean education = 15.4, SD = 2.5; 81% females; and of average premorbid intellect.

SOURCE: Adapted from Duff (2014).

2013). The findings suggest that the BVMT-R, like other visual memory tests, involves both verbal and nonverbal processes. On the other hand, in a factor analysis that also included the TMT, COWAT, Visual-Motor Integration (VMI), and HVLT, the BVMT-R loaded on a separate factor, suggesting that it does measure visuospatial learning and memory in a mixed clinical sample with a reasonable degree of specificity (Benedict et al., 1996). However, support for this proposal is weakened because of the distortion introduced by the use of multiple scores from the same test (method variance problem; Larrabee, 2003).

Divergent validity of the Gaines et al. (2008) scoring method is demonstrated by the lack of correlation between the error scores and language (BNT), processing speed (SDMT), basic visuoperception (Judgment of Line Orientation [JLO]), verbal memory error measures (CVLT), and executive functions (D-KEFS Sorting), though some error scores are correlated with the Paced Auditory Serial Addition Test (PASAT). Recall consistency is moderately correlated with SDMT and BVMT-R learning and recall scores only (Gaines et al., 2008).

CLINICAL STUDIES

Impaired performance has been noted in a variety of conditions thought to affect memory, including HIV infection, MS, and various neurodegenerative disorders such as AD, dementia with Lewy bodies (DLB), and vascular dementia (VaD) (see later discussion; Benedict et al., 1996, 1999; Foster et al., 2010; McLaughlin et al., 2012; Okonkwo et al., 2014; Troyer et al., 2008). Those who are methamphetamine-dependent also perform significantly worse on the BVMT-R, likely due to deficient strategic encoding and retrieval related to dysfunction of frontostriatal circuit (Morgan et al., 2012). However, cognitive remediation interventions, such as those targeting self-initiation of semantic encoding strategies for improving episodic memory, do not improve BVMT-R performance, at least in those with schizophrenia (Guimond & Lepage, 2016). Abstinent smokers with schizophrenia perform worse on BVMT-R retention and show more recognition biases compared to those using nicotine patches or those who do not undergo smoking intervention (Ghiasi et al., 2013). Interestingly, exposure to stress during pregnancy also has long-term effects on visuospatial memory in adulthood. Li and colleagues (2015) studied the impact of exposure to the Tangshang earthquake, which impacted BVMT-R but not HVLT-R performance. Those exposed as infants obtained the worst scores, followed by the prenatal exposure group. In particular, exposure to the earthquake during the second and third trimesters yielded lower scores than exposure in the first trimester (Li et al., 2015). Subjective cognitive complaints in those with mild-to-moderate TBI tested six months post injury can be partially explained by performance on BVMT-R and CVLT-II over and above depression (Chamelian & Feinstein, 2006).

Neurodegenerative disorders. Among middle-aged adults at risk for AD over six years, baseline BVMT-R learning and delayed recall identifies decliners from those who remain stable (stables) even though no differences are seen on various brain imaging techniques including PET, functional MRI (fMRI), and FDG-PET. When contrasting imaging and cognitive measures, BVMT-R is better than all imaging measures in identifying decliners/stables (Okonkwo et al., 2014). Although the BVMT-R is sensitive to memory impairments seen in a variety of neurodegenerative disorders, none of the BVMT-R measures, however, discriminates between AD and VaD patients. AD and DLB groups obtain equally poor scores on the BVMT-R, suggesting that the visuospatial deficits in DLB extends into visuospatial memory to the magnitude of those with AD (McLaughlin et al., 2012). On the other hand, persons with amnestic MCI score worse than healthy controls on item recall and associative recall (more impaired than item recall) on a modified scoring procedure (Troyer et al., 2008).

Differences in memory performance have been found in PD patients with left hemibody onset of motor symptoms (LHO) and right hemibody onset of motor symptoms (RHO). While no LHO versus RHO group differences were seen in their immediate or delayed recall on HVLT-R and BVMT-R measures, the RHO group showed declines from HVLT-R immediate to delayed recall and improvements from BVMT-R immediate to delayed recall. In the RHO group, the Stroop task was positively correlated with HVLT-R change score and negatively correlated with BVMT-R change scores. The authors surmised that these findings may be related to the asymmetric distribution of dopaminergic and cholinergic systems in the cerebral hemispheres or the use of verbal encoding for visuospatial stimuli (Foster et al., 2010).

Epilepsy. Poor test performance has also been noted in patients with epilepsy (Barr et al., 2004). However, the test is not able to discriminate lateralized disturbances. That is, presurgical candidates with left or right temporal lobe seizures do not differ in their patterns of performance on the learning, delayed recall, or recognition trials (Barr et al., 2004).

MS. Poor test performance has also been noted in patients with MS (Benedict et al., 2001). Interestingly, aerobic capacity and muscular strength in MS are associated with SDMT performance but not CVLT-II or BVMT-R performance (Sandroff et al., 2015). Gromisch et al. (2016) reported that an abbreviated version of the BVMT-R may be useful to screen for visuospatial memory dysfunction in patients with MS. With −1.5 *SD* defined as impairment, administration of Trial 1 alone yielded a classification accuracy of 92%, a sensitivity of 85%, and a specificity of 85% at a cutoff of 3 or less correct for identifying visuospatial memory dysfunction on the full BVMT-R. Administration of both Trials 1 and 2 generated a classification accuracy of 98%, a sensitivity of 92%, and a specificity of 90% at a cutoff of 9. With −2.0 *SD* defined as impairment, administration of Trial 1 only yielded a classification accuracy of 90%, a sensitivity of 71%, and a specificity of 90% at a cutoff of 2. Administration of both Trials 1 and 2 generated a classification accuracy of 97%, a sensitivity of 94%, and a specificity of 89% at a cutoff of 8.5.

The Gaines et al. (2008) scoring method yielded intrusion errors in 80% of their MS sample, followed by rotation (73%), perseveration (18%), and location errors (14%). As expected in healthy adults, the recall consistency index was generally high. Location errors, rotations, intrusions, and total errors were negatively correlated with Total Learning and Delayed Recall. In terms of frequency of error type, 64% of healthy adults made at least one such error, followed by intrusions (55%). Other error types were infrequently made by healthy adults (3–8%). Using logistic regression, the new error types only modestly improved the classification accuracy of healthy adults versus MS patients.

The BVMT-R has been used in a number of batteries for assessing cognitive functioning in MS (Benedict et al., 2012; Dusankova et al., 2012; Goretti et al., 2014; Spedo et al., 2015; Vanotti et al., 2016; Walker et al., 2016) and to assess change in cognitive functioning for MS clinical trials (Erlanger et al., 2014). For example, the BVMT-R has been used in conjunction with the Buschke Selective Reminding Test, PASAT, and SDMT to form the MS-Cog as a sensitive and reliable test battery suitable as a cognitive endpoint in MS pharmaceutical trials (Erlanger et al., 2014).

In particular, the BICAMS, comprising the SDMT, CVLT-II, and BVMT-R, has been examined across multiple international samples with highly reliable and valid findings. Using the Canadian BICAMS data, Walker and colleagues (2016) found that an MS group performed worse than healthy controls on the BVMT-R and the SDMT, but no differences on the CVLT-II were found after accounting for depression and fatigue. More than half the patient group obtained at least one abnormal test result. Overall, MS patients were more likely to be impaired on the BVMT-R than on the other measures. The BVMT-R correctly classified 82% of participants as impaired, while the SDMT was the best, at 95% accuracy. The BVMT-R yielded an area under the curve (AUC) of .81 at a 23.5 cutoff score, with a sensitivity of 78%, and a specificity of 82% for identifying cognitive dysfunction. In fact, the BVMT-R predicted employment status over and above demographic variables and depression (Walker et al., 2016). On the Czech, Spanish-Argentinian, and Brazilian BICAMS, MS patients perform worse than healthy controls (Dusankova et al., 2012; Spedo et al., 2015; Vanotti et al., 2016). Based on a cutoff of impairment on one or more of the three tests, a sensitivity of 94% and a specificity of 86% on the Czech BICAMS were reported (Dusankova et al., 2012).

NEUROANATOMICAL CORRELATES AND IMAGING STUDIES

In PD patients, BVMT-R and CVLT-II delayed recall are correlated with left but not right hippocampal head and amygdala volume. In non-PD, the BVMT-R does not correlate with hippocampal or amygdala volume (Bouchard et al., 2008). The BVMT-R was found to be a better predictor of cognitive decline than brain imaging techniques (Okonkwo et al., 2014).

PERFORMANCE VALIDITY

A variety of BVMT-R indices have been used as embedded performance validity indicators, including Recognition Hits, Recognition Hits minus false positives, and Retention Percentage. Table 10–19 presents the cutoff score, sensitivity, specificity, positive predictive value (PPV), and negative predictive value (NPV) of the various indicators. It is of note that the values differ depending on the gold-standard measure used to determine performance validity and the population in question. BVMT-R Recognition appears to be one of the more sensitive scores compared to Finger Tapping, Wechsler Adult Intelligence Scale (WAIS-III) PSI, WAIS-III WMI, and CVLT Forced-Choice (CVLT-FC), at least when the MSVT is used to determine performance validity. Combining BVMT-R Recognition Hits with other embedded indices as continuous variables in a regression model improves the

TABLE 10–19 Sensitivity, Specificity, PPV, NPV, and LR of Various Brief Visuospatial Memory Test—Revised (BVMT-R) Embedded Measures of Performance Validity

	CUTOFF	SENSITIVITY (%)	SPECIFICITY (%)	PPV (%)	NPV (%)	LR
Recognition Hits (Denning et al., 2012)[a]	≤4	45	89	–	–	4.00
Recognition Hits (Shura et al., 2016)[b]	≤4	11	98	49	86	6.33
Recognition Hits minus false positives (Shura et al., 2016)	≤4	16	96	41	89	4.43
Retention Percentage (Sawyer et al., 2016)[c]	≤58	31	92	50	83	–

NOTE: PPV, positive predictive value; NPV, negative predictive value; LR, likelihood ratio.

[a]Failing MSVT constituted invalid performance in this sample of veterans with a variety of psychiatric diagnoses referred to an outpatient Veterans Affairs neuropsychology clinic from primary care clinics, psychiatry, neurology, and about 15% from compensation and pension disability evaluations mostly for TBI.

[b]Failing WMT constituted invalid performance in this sample of post-deployment veterans. Base rate of failure = 15%.

[c]Military veterans sample. Failing two or more of the following standalone/embedded PVTs constituted invalid performance: MSVT, WMT, TOMM, CVLT-II LD FCR < 15, WAIS-III RDS < 7, RCFT Effort Equation < 51, WMS-III LM Effort Equation ≤ 39.5, Rey-15 with Recognition < 20, Warrington Recognition Memory Test-Words < 43, RBANS Effort Scale < 120. Base rate of failure = 21%.

classification of passing or failing the MSVT, yielding a sensitivity of 58%, specificity of 94%, hit rate of 83%, and likelihood ratio of 9, suggesting that this indicator should be combined with other embedded measures (Denning, 2012). However, Recognition Hits performed worse than Recognition Hits minus false positives in another study, and both performed worse than CVLT-FC as embedded performance validity indicators (Shura et al., 2016).

COMMENT

This task has a number of advantages, including its brevity, the availability of six equivalent forms, and the inclusion of multitrial learning, delayed recall, and recognition components. Reliability is good, and the test has demonstrated validity in a number of clinical conditions, including neurodegenerative disorders, MS, schizophrenia, HIV, and drug dependency. In fact, in one study, the BVMT-R was found to be a better predictor of cognitive decline than brain imaging techniques (Okonkwo et al., 2014). Furthermore, normative data span the whole adult life span from 18 to 80+ years. The BVMT-R has also been combined with other measures to form batteries for assessing cognitive functioning in MS (MS-Cog, BICAMS) and schizophrenia (MATRICS); normative data for the BICAMS are available for international settings. Some components of the BVMT-R appear useful as embedded performance validity indicators; however, while specific, their sensitivities are variable and need replication in other studies. The BVMT-R indicators should be combined with other standalone and embedded indicators to improve identification of invalid performance.

Despite the advantages, a number of limitations bear mention. Motor (drawing) responses are required, limiting its use to those who do not have motor deficits. It may also be difficult to disentangle visual-constructional deficits from memory problems. An optional copy trial can be given after the recognition trial, but normative data are not provided. Furthermore, studies seem to suggest verbal and nonverbal components to the BVMT-R. Therefore, it has not been useful in predicting lateralized deficits in epilepsy surgical candidates, a situation that is not unique to the BVMT-R among visual memory tests.

Users should be aware of some limitations of the scoring system and normative data. First, responses are evaluated with regard to both accuracy and spatial location. These aspects are combined in the scoring (and in the normative data). Research is needed to determine whether separate consideration of these two dimensions would improve diagnostic accuracy. Second, the distribution of scores on some of the measures is skewed, rendering interpretation of some scores (e.g., the Recognition Discrimination Index) problematic. Third, the literature suggests that IQ is moderately related to most of the BVMT measures. Accordingly, poor performance must be interpreted with considerable caution in those with below-average IQ (Diaz-Asper et al., 2004).

The available evidence suggests that the BVMT-R is useful in detecting memory impairment in a variety of clinical groups. Qualitative scoring methods as outlined by Gaines et al. (2008) appears to hold promise in differentiating among various disorders. However, the ability of the test to characterize the unique learning and memory deficits associated with various disorders requires additional study.

REFERENCES

Barr, W., Morrison, C., Zaroff, C., & Devinsky, O. (2004). Use of the Brief Visuospatial Memory Test-Revised (BVMT-R) in neuropsychological evaluation of epilepsy surgery candidates. *Epilepsy and Behavior, 5,* 175–179.

Benedict, R. H. B. (1997). *Brief Visuospatial Memory Test—Revised.* Odessa, FL: Psychological Assessment Resources.

Benedict, R. H. B., Amato, M. P., Boringa, J., Brochet, B., Foley, F., Fredrikson, S., . . . Langdon, D. (2012). International Cognitive Assessment for MS (BICAMS): International standards for validation. *BMC Neurology, 12*(1), 55.

Benedict, R. H. B., Dobraski, M., & Goldstein, M. Z. (1999). A preliminary study of the association between changes in mood and cognition in a mixed geriatric psychiatry sample. *Journal of Gerontology: Psychological Sciences, 54B,* P94–P99.

Benedict, R. H. B., & Groninger, L. (1995). Preliminary standardization of a new visuospatial memory test with six alternate forms. *The Clinical Neuropsychologist, 9,* 11–16.

Benedict, R. H. B., Priore, R. L., Miller, C., Munschauer, F., & Jacobs, L. (2001). Personality disorder in multiple sclerosis correlates with cognitive impairment. *Journal of Neuropsychiatry and Clinical Neuroscience, 13,* 70–76.

Benedict, R. H. B., Schretlen, D., Groninger, L., Dobraski, M., & Shpritz, B. (1996). Revision of the Brief Visuospatial Memory Test: Studies of normal performance, reliability, and validity. *Psychological Assessment, 8,* 145–153.

Benedict, R. H. B., & Zgaljardic, D. J. (1998). Practice effects during repeated administrations of memory tests with and without alternate forms. *Journal of Clinical and Experimental Neuropsychology, 20,* 339–352.

Bouchard, T. P., Malykhin, N., Martin, W. R. W., Hanstock, C. C., Emery, D. J., Fisher, N. J., & Camicioli, R. M. (2008). Age and dementia-associated atrophy predominates in the hippocampal head and amygdala in Parkinson's disease. *Neurobiology of Aging, 29*(7), 1027–1039.

Chamelian, L., & Feinstein, A. (2006). The effect of major depression on subjective and objective cognitive deficits in mild to moderate traumatic brain injury. *The Journal of Neuropsychiatry and Clinical Neurosciences, 18*(1), 33–38.

Cysique, L. A., Franklin, D. J., Abramson, I., Ellis, R. J., Letendre, S., Collier, A., . . . Heaton, R. K. (2011). Normative data and validation of a regression based summary score for assessing meaningful neuropsychological change. *Journal of Clinical and Experimental Neuropsychology, 33*(5), 505–522.

Denning, J. H. (2012). The efficiency and accuracy of the Test of Memory Malingering Trial 1, errors on the first 10 items of the Test of Memory Malingering, and five embedded measures in predicting invalid test performance. *Archives of Clinical Neuropsychology, 27,* 417–432.

Diaz-Asper, C., Schretlen, D. J., & Pearlson, G. D. (2004). How well does IQ predict neuropsychological test performance in normal adults. *Journal of the International Neuropsychological Society, 10,* 82–90.

Duff, K. (2014). One-week practice effects in older adults: Tools for assessing cognitive change. *The Clinical Neuropsychologist, 28*(5), 714–725.

Duff, K., Beglinger, L. J., Van, D. H., Moser, D. J., Arndt, S., Schultz, S. K., & Paulsen, J. S. (2008). Short-term practice effects in amnestic mild cognitive impairment: Implications for diagnosis and treatment. *International Psychogeriatrics, 20*(5), 986–999.

Dusankova, J. B., Kalincik, T., Havrdova, E., & Benedict, R. H. B. (2012). Cross cultural validation of the Minimal Assessment of Cognitive Function in Multiple Sclerosis (MACFIMS) and the Brief International Cognitive Assessment for Multiple Sclerosis (BICAMS). *The Clinical Neuropsychologist, 26*(7), 1186–1200.

Erlanger, D. M., Kaushik, T., Caruso, L. S., Benedict, R. H. B., Foley, F. W., Wilken, J., . . . DeLuca, J. (2014). Reliability of a cognitive endpoint for use in a multiple sclerosis pharmaceutical trial. *Journal of the Neurological Sciences, 340*(1-2), 123–129.

Foster, P. S., Drago, V., Crucian, G. P., Skidmore, F., Rhodes, R. D., Shenal, B. V., . . . Heilman, K. M. (2010). Verbal and visuospatial memory in lateral onset Parkinson disease: Time is of the essence. *Cognitive and Behavioral Neurology, 23*(1), 19–25.

Gaines, J. J., Gavett, R. A., Lynch, J. J., Bakshi, R., & Benedict, R. H. B. (2008). New error type and recall consistency indices for the Brief Visuospatial Memory Test-Revised: Performance in healthy adults and multiple sclerosis patients. *The Clinical Neuropsychologist, 22*(5), 851–863.

Gale, S. D., Baxter, L., Connor, D. J., Herring, A., & Comer, J. (2007). Sex differences on the Rey Auditory Verbal Learning Test and the Brief Visuospatial Memory Test-Revised in the elderly: Normative data in 172 participants. *Journal of Clinical and Experimental Neuropsychology, 29*(5), 561–567.

Gale, S. D., Baxter, L., & Thompson, J. (2016). Greater memory impairment in dementing females than males relative to sex-matched healthy controls. *Journal of Clinical and Experimental Neuropsychology, 38*(5), 527–533.

Ghiasi, F., Farhang, S., Farnam, A., & Safikhanlou, S. (2013). The short term effect of nicotine abstinence on visuospatial working memory in smoking patients with schizophrenia. *Nordic Journal of Psychiatry, 67*(2), 104–108.

Goretti, B., Niccolai, C., Hakiki, B., Sturchio, A., Falautano, M., Minacapelli, E., . . . Amato, M. P. (2014). The Brief International Cognitive Assessment for Multiple Sclerosis (BICAMS): Normative values with gender, age and education corrections in the Italian population. *BMC Neurology, 14*(1), 171.

Gromisch, E. S., Zemon, V., Holtzer, R., Chiaravalloti, N. D., DeLuca, J., Beier, M., . . . Foley, F. W. (2016). Assessing the criterion validity of four highly abbreviated measures from the Minimal Assessment of Cognitive Function in Multiple Sclerosis (MACFIMS). *The Clinical Neuropsychologist, 30*(7), 1032–1049.

Guimond, S., & Lepage, M. (2016). Cognitive training of self-initiation of semantic encoding strategies in schizophrenia: A pilot study. *Neuropsychological Rehabilitation, 26*(3), 464–479.

Heaton, R. K., Miller, S. W., Taylor, M. J., & Grant, I. (2004). *Revised comprehensive norms for an Expanded Halstead-Reitan Battery: Demographically adjusted neuropsychological norms for African American and Caucasian adults.* Lutz, FL: PAR.

Kane, K. D., & Yochim, B. P. (2014). Construct validity and extended normative data for older adults for the Brief Visuospatial Memory Test, Revised. *American Journal of Alzheimer's Disease and Other Dementias, 29*(7), 601–606.

Kemmotsu, N., Enobi, Y., & Murphy, C. (2013). Performance if older Japanese American adults on selected cognitive instruments. *Journal of the International Neuropsychological Society, 19*(7), 773–781.

Larrabee, G. J. (2003). Lessons on measuring construct validity: A commentary on Delis, Jacobson, Bondi, Hamilton, and Salmon. *Journal of the International Neuropsychological Society, 9*, 947–954.

Li, N., Wang, Y., Zhao, X., Gao, Y., Song, M., Yu, L., . . . Wang, X. (2015). Long-term effect of early life stress from earthquake exposure on working memory in adulthood. *Neuropsychiatric Disease and Treatment, 11*, 2959.

McLaughlin, N. C. R., Chang, A. C., & Malloy, P. (2012). Verbal and nonverbal learning and recall in dementia with Lewy bodies and Alzheimer's disease. *Applied Neuropsychology: Adult, 19*(2), 86–89.

Miotto, E. C., Campanholo, K. R., Rodrigues, M. M., Serrao, V. T., de Lucia, Mara C. S., & Scaff, M. (2012). Hopkins Verbal Learning Test-Revised and Brief Visuospatial Memory Test-Revised: Preliminary normative data for the Brazilian population. *Arquivos De Neuro-Psiquiatria, 70*(12), 962–965.

Morgan, E. E., Woods, S. P., Poquette, A. J., Vigil, O., Heaton, R. K., & Grant, I. (2012). Visual memory in methamphetamine-dependent individuals: Deficient strategic control of encoding and retrieval. *Australian and New Zealand Journal of Psychiatry, 46*(2), 141–152.

Norman, M. A., Moore, D. J., Taylor, M., Franklin, D. J., Cysique, L., Ake, C., . . . Heaton, R. K. (2011). Demographically corrected norms for African Americans and Caucasians on the Hopkins Verbal Learning Test–Revised, Brief Visuospatial Memory Test–Revised, Stroop Color and Word Test, and Wisconsin Card Sorting Test 64-card version. *Journal of Clinical and Experimental Neuropsychology, 33*(7), 793–804.

Okonkwo, O. C., Oh, J. M., Koscik, R., Jonaitis, E., Cleary, C. A., Dowling, N. M., . . . Johnson, S. C. (2014). Amyloid burden, neuronal function, and cognitive decline in middle-aged adults at risk for Alzheimer's disease. *Journal of the International Neuropsychological Society, 20*(4), 422–433.

Sandroff, B. M., Pilutti, L. A., Benedict, R. H. B., & Motl, R. W. (2015). Association between physical fitness and cognitive function in multiple sclerosis: Does disability status matter? *Neurorehabilitation and Neural Repair, 29*(3), 214–223.

Sawyer, R. J., Testa, S. M., & Dux, M. (2016). Embedded performance validity tests within the Hopkins Verbal Learning Test–Revised and the Brief Visuospatial Memory Test–Revised. *The Clinical Neuropsychologist, 31*(1), 207–218.

Schretlen, D. J., Testa, S. M., & Pearlson, G. D. (2010). *Calibrated Neuropsychological Normative System*. Lutz, FL: PAR.

Shura, R. D., Miskey, H. M., Rowland, J. A., Yoash-Gantz, R. E., & Denning, J. H. (2016). Embedded performance validity measures with postdeployment veterans: Cross-validation and efficiency with multiple measures. *Applied Neuropsychology: Adult, 23*(2), 94–104.

Spedo, C. T., Frndak, S. E., Marques, V. D., Foss, M. P., Pereira, D. A., Carvalho, L. d. F., . . . Barreira, A. A. (2015). Cross-cultural adaptation, reliability, and validity of the BICAMS in Brazil. *The Clinical Neuropsychologist, 29*(6), 836–846.

Tam, J. W., & Schmitter-Edgecombe, M. (2013). The role of processing speed in the Brief Visuospatial Memory Test—Revised. *The Clinical Neuropsychologist, 27*(6), 962–972.

Troyer, A. K., Murphy, K. J., Anderson, N. D., Hayman-Abello, B. A., Craik, F. I., & Moscovitch, M. (2008). Item and associative memory in amnestic mild cognitive impairment: Performance on standardized memory tests. *Neuropsychology, 22*(1), 10.

Vanotti, S., Smerbeck, A., Benedict, R. H. B., & Caceres, F. (2016). A new assessment tool for patients with multiple sclerosis from Spanish-speaking countries: Validation of the Brief International Cognitive Assessment for MS (BICAMS) in Argentina. *The Clinical Neuropsychologist, 30*(7), 1023–1031.

Walker, L. A. S., Osman, L., Berard, J. A., Rees, L. M., Freedman, M. S., MacLean, H., & Cousineau, D. (2016). Brief International Cognitive Assessment for Multiple Sclerosis (BICAMS): Canadian contribution to the international validation project. *Journal of the Neurological Sciences, 362*, 147–152.

Woods, S. P., Childers, M., Ellis, R. J., Guaman, S., Grant, I., & Heaton, R. K. (2006). A battery approach for measuring neuropsychological change. *Archives of Clinical Neuropsychology, 21*(1), 83–89.

CALIFORNIA VERBAL LEARNING TEST—SECOND EDITION (CVLT-II)

TEST NAME	**California Verbal Learning Test—Second Edition (CVLT-II)**
DOMAIN	Verbal memory
AGE RANGE	16 to 89 years
ADMINISTRATION TIME	20 minutes plus 20-minute delay interval
SCORING FORMAT	Computerized
REFERENCE	Delis, D. C., Kramer, J. H., Kaplan, E., & Ober, B. A. (2000). *California Verbal Learning Test—Second Edition.* San Antonio, TX: The Psychological Corporation. www.pearsonclinical.com

DESCRIPTION

The California Verbal Learning Test—Second Edition (CVLT-II) measures verbal learning and memory using a multiple-trial word list-learning format. The original version (Delis et al., 1987) was developed using a process-oriented approach and proved very popular because of its ability to parse multiple components of learning and memory and to characterize distinct memory profiles associated with different disorders. The CVLT was revised to accommodate new developments in the field and address concerns raised about the first edition. The revised version includes new word lists that are easier to understand than those in the first edition, a larger normative database, new measures to analyze aspects of learning and memory (see also Stricker et al., 2002), an optional forced-choice recognition task, alternate and short forms, and updated scoring software.

The Standard Form of the CVLT-II assesses both recall and recognition of two word lists over immediate and delayed memory trials. In the first five learning trials, the examinee is asked to recall words from List A immediately after presentation of the list. List A is composed of 16 words, four from each of four semantic categories. Words from the same semantic category are never presented consecutively. A 16-word interference list (List B) is then presented for one trial, followed by Short-Delay Free Recall (SDFR) and Short-Delay Cued Recall (SDCR) trials of List A. A 20-minute delay occurs next, during which nonverbal testing takes place (see the sections "Administration" and "Comment" for further discussion). After the delay interval, Long-Delay Free Recall (LDFR), Long-Delay Cued Recall (LDCR), and Long-Delay Yes/No Recognition trials of List A are administered. Finally, an optional Long-Delay Forced-Choice Recognition (FC) trial is given about 10 minutes after the Long-Delay Yes/No Recognition trial. An Alternate Form is also available.

The CVLT-II Short Form (CVLT-II SF) is designed for examinees with severe cognitive dysfunction or as a screening instrument for memory impairment. Like the long form, it requires the person to learn and remember a list of words under various testing conditions, including free recall, cued recall, and recognition. It differs from the CVLT-II in several ways: a shorter list (nine words instead of 16), only one list of words instead of two, shorter delay intervals (10 and five minutes), and fewer recall trials (e.g., four instead of five learning trials).

ADMINISTRATION

See Source. The examiner reads the word list at a rate slightly slower than one second per word and records the examinee's oral responses verbatim in the order in which they are given. A prompt ("Anything else?") is to be given after every trial in which the examinee fails to recall all the words.

The manual states that nonverbal tasks should be administered during the delay interval. However, studies have found that administration of the WAIS-III Vocabulary or Peabody Picture Vocabulary Test (PPVT-IIIB) during the delay interval does not affect the recall scores in undergraduate volunteers (Williams & Donovick, 2008) or nondemented older adults (Williams et al., 2014). It is of note that if the CVLT-II is given before a verbal fluency task, examinees are likely to use the words from the CVLT-II, thereby resulting in higher scaled scores on category fluency tasks than if they were given the CVLT-II second to the verbal fluency tasks (Lloyd et al., 2012).

SCORING

Hand scoring of the CVLT-II is possible. However, the CVLT-II yields raw scores and standardized scores for more than 50 learning and memory variables. The depth of analysis provided by the software is superior and faster to that which can be computed practically by hand. The authors recommend that the test results be scored using the

CVLT-II scoring software. About 10 to 15 minutes is required to score the CVLT-II using the software.

The software can be used to score the Standard Form, the Alternate Form, and the Short Form. It computes all raw and standardized scores, corrected for the examinee's age and gender. The examiner can choose any combination of three different reports: the Core Report, the Expanded Report, or the Research Report. The Core Report provides raw and standardized scores for 27 of the most commonly used CVLT-II measures. The Expanded Report generates the same information, plus raw and standardized scores for 66 normed variables of the CVLT-II (51 for the Short Form), offering more in-depth analysis of an individual's verbal learning and memory performance. Finally, the Research Report provides raw scores for more than 260 non-normed variables that may be useful to researchers.

Primary measures include the following:

- List A Trials 1–5 Total Learning
- List B
- Short-Delay Free/Cued Recall (SDFR/SDCR)
- Long-Delay Free/Cued Recall (LDFR/LDCR)
- Yes/No Recognition Discriminability
- Forced-Choice Recognition (FC)

The test also provides a number of additional measures:

- Learning strategies (e.g., semantic clustering, serial clustering, subjective clustering)
- Primacy-recency effects in recall
- Rate of new learning per trial
- Consistency of item recall across trials
- Degree of vulnerability to proactive and retroactive interference
- Retention of information over short and longer delays
- Enhancement of recall performance by category cueing and recognition testing
- Breakdown of recognition performance (discriminability and response bias) derived from signal-detection theory
- Indices reflecting the relative integrity of encoding, storage, and retrieval processes
- Analysis of intrusion-error types in recall (e.g., semantically related, semantically unrelated, across-list intrusions)
- Repetition errors in recall
- Analysis of false-positive types in recognition testing
- Performance validity indices

In addition to the traditional computation of semantic clustering, a new list-based method was developed by Delis et al. (2010):

$$\text{Expected Semantic Clustering}_i = [(r - 1)(m - 1)]/(N_L - 1)]$$

where r = number of correct words on trial i, i = a given trial, m = number of members of each semantic category on the original list, N_L = total number of words on the original list.

Delis et al. (2010) examined the new equation in a sample of older adults with AD and healthy controls and found that healthy controls obtained higher semantic clustering scores than did the AD group using either traditional or new scoring methods. However, the new method accounted for more variance in predicting diagnostic group membership (84% vs. 76% overall percentage correct) and may be a better measure than the traditional semantic clustering method to assist in identifying AD.

DEMOGRAPHIC EFFECTS

AGE

Test scores are highly affected by age (r = –.51), with performance declining with advancing age (Delis et al., 2000; Fine et al., 2012). According to the test authors, age accounts for 26% of the variance, followed by gender (5%), and education (5%). The authors decided to correct for age and gender but not to stratify by education because doing so would have resulted in cell sizes as low as 10 cases per cell for some age groups.

GENDER

Gender affects most scores, with women tending to score an average of five words more than men across the five learning trials of List A (Delis et al., 2000; Lundervold et al., 2014; Vaskinn et al., 2011). Sunderaraman et al. (2013) noted that women score higher on Total Learning scores than men possibly because they are more likely to use semantic clustering. Similarly, Lundervold et al. (2014) stated that steeper age-related decline seen in males than females over time is possibly due to differences in learning strategies and accuracy. For some variables (e.g., FC Accuracy), gender differences are not significant (Delis et al., 2000).

EDUCATION AND IQ

Education also correlates with memory performance (r = .29 for the CVLT-II Total Learning; Delis et al., 2000; Fine et al., 2012). As might be expected, IQ shows a moderate relationship with CVLT-II performance (e.g., r = .40 between Full Scale IQ [FSIQ] and Total Learning; Delis et al., 2000).

ETHNICITY, NATIONALITY, AND LINGUISTIC EFFECTS

Ethnicity has a negligible impact, explaining 0.3% of the variance (Delis et al., 2000). However, age of language acquisition among immigrants predicts CVLT-II performance, particularly if the host language was acquired after age 16 (Poreh et al., 2015).

NORMATIVE DATA

STANDARDIZATION SAMPLE

The sample consisted of 1,087 healthy volunteers, ranging in age from 16 to 89 years and in education from less than nine to more than 16 years, matched to 1999 US Census data in terms of race/ethnicity, education, and region (see Table 10–20).

Norms were developed by converting raw scores on the List A Trials 1–5 Total Learning measure to age- and gender-corrected T scores, with a mean of 50 and a standard deviation of 10. Raw scores on the other CVLT-II measures varied in the extent to which they reflected normal distributions, so they were converted to age- and gender-corrected *z* scores, with a mean of 0 and a standard deviation of 1. The range of *z* scores is +5 to –5, reported in increments of 0.5.

For most of the CVLT-II *z* scores, higher values indicate better performance; however, there are exceptions, including the various error measures (i.e., repetitions, intrusions, and false positives) and the recency-recall index, for which higher *z* scores reflect greater deficits. For a few variables, higher positive *z* scores tend to reflect deficient performances but not always (e.g., serial clustering index).

The FC variable was designed to yield a high ceiling effect, precluding *z*-score transformation. For this reason, normative results are reported in frequency and cumulative frequency values by age only. In addition, three intrusion error types (non-category, across-list, and synonym/subordinate) were rare in the normative sample and therefore were also normed in terms of frequency and cumulative-frequency values by age only.

Raw scores on the Alternate Form were calibrated to the Standard Form using linear equating. The equating study was based on a sample of 288 nonclinical adults (106 men, 182 women) who were given both forms in a counterbalanced order. Raw scores on the Short Form were calibrated to raw scores on the Standard Form using equipercentile equating due to skewness of some variables on the Short Form. This equating study was based on a sample of 278 adults who were given both forms in a counterbalanced order.

Fine et al. (2012) provide CVLT-II Short Form normative data for older women aged 85 and older from the Study of Osteoporotic Fractures, an ongoing observational study of women aged 65 and older at baseline (Table 10–21). The sample was screened for 3MS of less than 88, Informant Questionnaire on Cognitive Decline in the Elderly (IQCODE) greater than 3.6, dementia, nursing home residence, late life depression (i.e., Geriatric Depression Scale [GDS] ≥6 or higher), and cognitive change over the 20-year period.

TABLE 10–20 Characteristics of the California Verbal Learning Test—Second Edition (CVLT-II) Standardization Sample

Sample size	1,087
Sample type	Based on 1999 US Census data
Age	16 to 89[a] years
Geographical location	65% California 30% Michigan 5% Eastern Seaboard
Education	34% 12 years 28% 13 to 15 years 20% >16 years 11% 9 to 11 years 7% <9 years
Gender	52% Women 48% Men
Ethnicity	75% Caucasian 11% African American 9% Hispanic 5% Other
Screening	Screened for self-reported neurologic, psychiatric, or debilitating medical disorder

NOTE: Values are rounded.

[a] Broken down into seven age groups: 16–19 (*n* = 150), 20–29 (*n* = 190), 30–44 (*n* = 200), 45–59 (*n* = 150), 60–69 (*n* = 145), 70–79 (*n* = 145), and 80–89 years (*n* = 107).

BASE RATES OF INDEX DISCREPANCIES

Donders (2006) examined the frequency of discrepancies in indices in the standardization sample. The following indices were examined: Proactive Interference Index (PI), Retroactive Interference Index (RI), First Rapid Forgetting Index (RF_1), Second Rapid Forgetting Index (RF_2), First Retrieval Problem Index (RP_1), and Second Retrieval Problem Index (RP_2). An unusually large discrepancy (i.e., occurring in less than 10% of the standardization sample) was defined as PI ≤ –1.5, RI ≤ –1, RF_1 ≤ –1, RF_2 ≤ –1, RP_1 ≥1.5, and RP_2 ≥1.5. Users may refer to Table 10–22 to determine the cumulative percentage of various discrepancy scores. In healthy people, at least one large discrepancy occurs in one in three persons and therefore should not be interpreted as pathological.

A sample comprised of consecutive referrals to a TBI rehabilitation facility was screened for complicated premorbid history, compensation-seeking status, and FC of at least 15/16. When the frequency of discrepancies on the CVLT-II indices was examined using the same definition as Donders (2006), 9% had PI ≤ –1.5, 12% had RI ≤ –1, 21% had RF_1 ≤ –1, 13% had RF_2 ≤ –1, 4% had RP_1 ≥1.5, and 3% had RP_2 ≥1.5 (Jacobs & Donders, 2008). In general, TBI patients showed a similar degree of performance discrepancies as the standardization sample. As such, the presence of

TABLE 10–21 California Verbal Learning Test—Second Edition (CVLT-II) Short Form Normative Data for Women Age 85 to 95 Stratified by Age and Education

		T1		T4		T1-4		SDFR		LDFR		REC-HITS		REC-FP		REC-DISC	
AGE	EDUCATION	M	*SD*	M	*SD*	M	*SD*	M	*SD*	M	*SD*	M	*SD*	M	*SD*	M	*SD*
85–86		4.8	1.2	7.7	1.2	26.3	3.9	7.1	1.4	6.5	1.7	8.4	1.0	1.0	1.0	2.9	.52
	≤12	4.8	1.2	7.6	1.3	26.0	4.2	6.9	1.4	6.4	1.8	8.5	.8	1.0	1.0	3.0	.48
	>12	4.9	1.1	7.7	1.1	26.7	3.7	7.2	1.3	6.6	1.7	8.2	1.2	.85	1.0	2.9	.55
87–89		4.6	1.4	7.5	1.2	25.5	4.3	7.1	1.5	6.4	1.8	8.4	.9	1.0	1.3	2.9	.50
	≤12	4.4	1.4	7.3	1.2	24.8	4.4	6.9	1.5	6.6	1.7	8.4	.8	1.0	1.1	2.9	.49
	>12	4.8	1.4	7.7	1.0	26.3	4.0	7.2	1.4	6.6	1.7	8.4	.9	1.1	1.4	2.9	.50
90–95		4.4	1.3	7.4	1.3	24.8	4.3	6.8	1.4	6.1	1.9	8.4	1.0	1.3	1.4	2.7	.58
	≤12	4.3	1.4	7.3	1.3	24.6	4.3	6.8	1.5	6.2	1.9	8.3	1.0	1.1	1.2	2.9	.53
	>12	4.5	1.3	7.4	1.3	25.0	4.3	6.7	1.4	5.9	2.0	8.4	1.3	1.5	1.6	2.8	.65

NOTE: *N* = 680, 98% non-Hispanic Caucasian. Sample comprised of 23% heart disease, 11% stroke, 13% diabetes, and 25% cancer. T1, Trial 1; T4, Trial 4; T1–4, sum of Trials 1–4; SDFR, Short-Delay Free Recall; LDFR, Long-Delay Free Recall; Rec-Hits, Recognition Hits; Rec-FP, Recognition False Positives; Rec-Disc, Recognition Discriminability.

SOURCE: Adapted from Fine et al. (2012).

one unusually large performance discrepancy should not be interpreted as pathological even in persons with TBI.

EVIDENCE FOR RELIABILITY

EVIDENCE FOR INTERNAL RELIABILITY

The authors note that tests of recall ability pose special difficulties for the estimation of internal consistency because of problems with item interdependence within and between trials. First, because of limitations in learning and memory capacity, recall of any one word on a trial decreases the likelihood that other items will be recalled on that same trial. Second, the process of recalling a word on one trial tends to increase the probability that the same word will be recalled on subsequent trials. Accordingly, the authors used three approaches to estimate the internal consistency for the CVLT-II (see manual).

TABLE 10–22 Cumulative Percentages of the California Verbal Learning Test—Second Edition (CVLT-II) Standardization Sample Obtaining Various Values of Specific Performance Discrepancies

Z	PI	RI	RF_1	RF_2	RP_1	RP_2
≤–3.0	1.01	0.28	0.29			0.09
–2.5	2.85	0.55	0.55		0.28	0.18
–2.0	5.70	1.93	1.38	0.18	0.83	0.83
–1.5	12.14	5.06	4.42	1.56	3.31	4.88
–1.0	24.10	12.97	13.43	9.84	11.41	17.11
–0.5	38.09	30.73	31.37	32.01	31.65	35.97
0.0	55.84	58.23	59.06	68.26	59.98	62.65
0.5	73.60	83.53	81.97	89.70	79.85	83.53
1.0	85.00	94.66	93.28	97.15	93.56	93.84
1.5	92.36	98.62	98.34	98.90	97.52	98.44
2.0	97.42	100.00	99.82	99.72	99.45	99.63
2.5	99.17		99.91	99.91	99.91	99.91
≥3.0	100.00		100.00	100.00	100.00	100.00

NOTE: PI, Proactive Interference Index; RI, Retroactive Interference Index; RF_1, First Rapid Forgetting Index; RF_2, Second Rapid Forgetting Index; RP_1, First Retrieval Problem Index; RP_2, Second Retrieval Problem Index. PI, List B vs. List A Trial 1; RI, SDFR vs. List A Trial 5; RF_1, LDRF vs. List A Trial 5; RF_2, LDFR vs. SDFR; RP_1, Recognition discriminability vs. LDFR; RP_2, Recognition discriminability vs. LDFR discriminability.

SOURCE: From Donders (2006).

The first approach analyzed total trial scores by splitting the immediate recall trials (Trials 1 + 3 versus Trials 2 + 4, and Trials 2 + 4 versus trials 3 + 5) and then applying the Spearman-Brown formula to the average of these correlations, with a lengthening factor of 2.5. Split-half reliability was very high for the total normative sample ($r = .94$), as well as for a mixed clinical sample ($r = .96$). The second method involved examination of performance in the four categories of words on List A across the five learning trials. Coefficient alphas calculated on word category scores across trials were high for the standardization sample and for the mixed clinical sample ($r = .82$ and .83, respectively). The third approach involved examining the number of times each of the 16 words on List A were recalled across the five learning trials. Reliability (split-half) was .79 for the standardization sample and .83 for the clinical sample. Similar values were obtained when coefficient alphas were computed. In short, these three approaches suggest that internal consistency is high for the five learning trials.

EVIDENCE FOR TEST-RETEST RELIABILITY, MEASURING CHANGE, AND PRACTICE EFFECTS

According to the test authors and shown in Table 10–23, three-week test-retest (range 9–49 days) reliability coefficients for some of the measures, in particular those measuring overall level of achievement (e.g., Total Learning, SDFR, LDFR, and Recognition Discrimination) are high; however, those measuring process/strategy aspects (e.g., Percent Recall, Total Learning Slope, Trial 1, Total Repetitions) are poor (Delis et al., 2000). This is based on a sample of 78 examinees (health status not reported), ranging in age from 16 to 88 years (mean = 46.9 years) given the Standard Form twice. On average, examinees recall about eight more words across the five learning trials on retesting. Whether these patterns apply equally for all age groups is not reported, nor are data reported for the Short Form.

Two-week test-retest reliability for a Spanish version of CVLT-II Total Learning is very high ($r = .87$)

TABLE 10–23 California Verbal Learning Test—Second Edition (CVLT-II) Test-Retest Correlations

MAGNITUDE OF COEFFICIENT	MEASURE
Very high (≥.90)	–
High (.80 to .89)	Trial 4 Correct Trials 1–5 Correct Short Delay Free Recall Long Delay Free Recall Recognition Discrimination
Adequate (.70 to .79)	Trial 5 Correct Semantic Clustering (Chance-Adjusted) Trials 1–5 Long-Delay Yes/No Recognition Hits Long-Delay Yes/No Recognition False Positives
Marginal (.60 to .69)	Trial 2 Correct Trial B Correct Total Intrusions (all recall trials, all types)
Low (≤.59)	Trial 1 Correct Trial 3 Correct Total Learning Slope, Trials 1–5 Percent Recall Primacy Region Percent Recall Middle Region Percent Recall Recency Region Total Repetitions (all recall trials) Total Response Bias

SOURCE: Adapted from Delis et al. (2000).

TABLE 10–24 California Verbal Learning Test—Second Edition (CVLT-II) Values for 68%, 90%, and 95% RCI Confidence Intervals when the Standard Form or Alternate Form is Given on Retest

	68% CI	90% CI	95% CI
Standard-Standard			
Total Trials 1–5	−.21 to 15.81	−5.38 to 20.98	−7.90 to 23.50
SDFR	−.89 to 3.61	−2.34 to 5.06	−3.05 to 5.77
SDCR	−.56 to 3.28	−1.80 to 4.52	−2.40 to 5.12
LDFR	−.54 to 3.42	−1.82 to 4.70	−2.44 to 5.32
LDCR	−.67 to 3.35	−1.97 to 4.65	−2.60 to 5.28
Recognition Discriminability	−.24 to .72	−.55 to 1.03	−.70 to 1.18
Standard-Alternate			
Total Trials 1–5	−7.38 to 10.04	−12.99 to 15.66	−15.74 to 18.40
SDFR	−2.19 to 3.53	−4.03 to 5.37	−4.97 to 6.28
SDCR	−2.05 to 3.03	−3.69 to 4.67	−4.49 to 5.47
LDFR	−2.24 to 3.18	−3.99 to 4.93	−4.84 to 5.78
LDCR	−2.23 to 3.01	−3.92 to 4.70	−4.75 to 5.53
Recognition Discriminability	−.70 to .68	−1.15 to 1.13	−1.36 to 1.34

NOTE: Based on N = 195 healthy adults screened for history of any condition that may adversely affect neurocognitive functions. Eighty of them received the same standard form on repeat assessment, whereas the rest of the 115 participants received the alternate form on retest. Values outside the ranges indicate significant reliable change. CI, confidence interval; SDFR, Short-Delay Free Recall; SDCR, Short-Delay Cued Recall; LDFR, Long-Delay Free Recall; LDCR, Long-Delay Cued Recall.

SOURCE: Adapted from Woods et al. (2006).

(Vanotti et al., 2016). One-month test-retest reliability of the Standard Form is high (ρ = .80 to .84) for the primary measures when the same form is given on retest, and marginal to adequate (ρ = .61 to .73) for the primary measures when the Alternate Form is given on retest (Woods et al., 2006). Significant practice effects are noted on 60% of the measures including primary indices when the same form is given on retest, whereas only 11% of the process measures show significant practice effects. Users may refer to Table 10–24 to determine reliable change when the Standard or Alternate Form is given on retest.

EVIDENCE FOR RELIABILITY OF ALTERNATE OR SHORT FORMS

Both the Standard Form and the Alternate Form were given to 288 nonclinical adults (106 men, 182 women; age M = 47.77, SD = 23.51; manual). The median interval between administrations was 21 days (range, 0–77 days). A total of 155 individuals received the Standard Form first, followed by the Alternate Form; the remainder were given the tests in the reverse order. Reliability coefficients were adequate for the primary measures (e.g., List A Trials 1–5 Total Learning, SDFR, LDFR, and Recognition Discriminability). Coefficients were low for variables that assess efficiency of learning characteristics and error types (see Table 10–25). The authors suggest that exposure to the first form may alert the examinee to other, potentially more efficient strategies at retest. Mean raw scores between the two forms were, however, quite similar, and there were no order effects, suggesting that performance changed in unsystematic ways across individuals. That is, some individuals may have discovered an optimal strategy, but others improved less or may even have deteriorated if a suboptimal strategy was attempted.

Reliability estimates for the Short Form are not reported.

EVIDENCE FOR INTERRATER RELIABILITY

Not reported, but the simplicity of administration and scoring should render interrater reliability high.

EVIDENCE FOR VALIDITY

FACTOR-ANALYTIC STUDIES

Factor analysis of the CVLT-II in the standardization sample and in a separate mixed clinical sample yields six and five factors, respectively (Delis et al., 2000), similar to what was found in the CVLT (Spreen & Strauss, 1998). The six factors are labeled general verbal learning (consisting of multiple measures of the level of immediate and delayed recall and recognition), response discrimination (consisting of Intrusion Errors and Recognition Response Bias), primacy-recency effects, organization strategies (consisting of Semantic and Serial Clustering), recall efficiency (consisting of Repetition Errors and Subjective Clustering), and acquisition rate (Total Learning Slope). Only acquisition rate is not obtained in the mixed clinical

TABLE 10–25 California Verbal Learning Test—Second Edition (CVLT-II) Alternate Form Reliability

MAGNITUDE OF COEFFICIENT	MEASURE
Very High (≥.90)	–
High (.80 to .89)	–
Adequate (.70 to .79)	Trial 3 Correct Trial 4 Correct Trial 5 Correct Trials 1–5 Correct Short-Delay Free Recall Long-Delay Free Recall
Marginal (.60 to .69)	Trial 2 Correct Semantic Clustering (Chance-Adjusted) Trials 1–5 Long-Delay Yes/No Recognition Hits Forced-Choice Recognition Percent Total Accuracy
Low (≤.59)	Trial 1 Correct Trial B Correct Serial Clustering Forward (Chance-Adjusted) Trials 1–5 Percent Recall Primacy Region Percent Recall Middle Region Percent Recall Recency Region Total Intrusions (all recall trials, all types) Total Repetitions (all recall trials) Long-Delay Yes/No Recognition Hits Total Response Bias

SOURCE: Adapted from Delis et al. (2000).

sample, although only 16, and not 19, scores were used in the factor analysis.

Donders (2008) conducted a confirmatory factor analysis (CFA) of the CVLT-II using 13 variables in the standardization sample. A four-factor solution best fits the data, representing attention span (List A Trial 1, List B, Middle Region Recall), learning efficiency (List A Trial 5, Semantic Clustering, Recall Consistency), delayed memory (SDFR, SDCR, LDFR, LDCR, Recognition Hits), and inaccurate memory (Total Intrusions, Recognition False Positives; Donders, 2008). Correlations between factors were generally moderate to high (r = –.39 to .85), with the lowest between inaccurate memory and other factors and the highest between learning efficiency and delayed memory. These solutions fit the age groups 16 to 30 and 31 to 60, but the structure was less robust for the adults older than 60. The four-factor solution was replicated in another study using a TBI sample screened for complicated premorbid or comorbid history and 12 variables from the CVLT-II (DeJong & Donders, 2009). Significant correlations were found between all factors and length of coma.

RELATIONSHIP TO THE CVLT

The CVLT-II correlates well with its predecessor. Correlation coefficients between variables of the CVLT and CVLT-II range from marginal (Free-Recall Intrusions) to high (Long-Delay Yes/No Recognition False Positives). Most of the coefficients are adequate to high (e.g., Total Learning, r = .76; Delis et al., 2000).

The CVLT normative data were known to be too stringent, probably because of the high education level of the sample. The CVLT-II normative sample is more representative of the educational level of the US population, resulting in less stringent norms and more accurate classification of an individual's performance (Delis et al., 2000). However, differences in the CVLT and CVLT-II raw scores are negligible; therefore, the authors suggest that the best method for comparing a person's relative performance on the two tasks is to examine changes in raw scores rather than in standardized scores.

CVLT-II SCORE INTERCORRELATIONS

Semantic Clustering and Total Learning are moderately correlated (r = .52) and explain 45% of variance in Total Learning (Sunderaraman et al., 2013).

RELATIONSHIPS WITH OTHER MEMORY TESTS

The CVLT-II Total Learning is not correlated with the WMS-IV Verbal Paired Associates (VPA I) whereas CVLT-II LDFR and VPA II are moderately correlated (r = .33) in university volunteers (Thiruselvam et al., 2015). Users may refer to the WMS-IV review elsewhere in this chapter for further discussion about the use of the CVLT-II as a substitute for the WMS-IV VPA (e.g., Miller et al., 2012a, 2012b).

Strong correlations are reported between the CVLT-II indices and Word Memory Test (WMT) memory subtests (r = .57 to .81), with the largest correlation seen between the CVLT-II Total Learning and the WMT Free Recall in outpatient referrals who passed the WMT validity indices (Davis & Wall, 2014). However, the WMT memory subtests appear more difficult as they yield more impaired scores (>1 *SD* below the mean) than the CVLT-II. See the WMT review for an in-depth discussion about the WMT memory subtests.

RELATIONSHIPS WITH OTHER NON-MEMORY TESTS

In a sample of older adults with MCI or probable mild dementia and nondemented older adults, the CVLT-II Total Learning and LDFR were positively correlated with TMT B (r = .34 and .23, respectively). In addition, CVLT-II SDFR, LDFR, Repetition, and Intrusion scores are positively correlated with the Controlled Oral Word Association Test (COWAT) (r = .24 to .29). WCST Perseverative Responses are not related to any memory scores (Brooks et al., 2006). These findings suggest that some executive functions may play a role in CVLT-II performance.

Executive functioning tests explain 24 to 31% of variance on recall trials and recognition discriminability in mixed neurologic samples. On the other hand, executive functions explain only 4 to 10% of variance on Total Learning, Semantic Clustering, Repetitions, Intrusions, and False Positives, suggesting that these scores are less likely affected by executive functioning problems but perhaps more so by attentional functions (Hill et al., 2012). In a sample of older adults with MCI or probable mild dementia and nondemented older adults, those with executive dysfunction (based on WCST-64, TMT-B, or COWAT) performed worse than those without executive dysfunction on the CVLT-II Total Learning and SDFR but not on other indices. Not unexpectedly, no differences were seen on immediate and delayed recall of WMS-R LM, a measure of memory minimally affected by executive dysfunction given the structured and meaningful nature of the stimuli (Brooks et al., 2006). In another study, executive measures (verbal fluency and Clock Drawing) predicted the CVLT-II Total Learning in PD but not in AD after controlling for DRS and WMS Logical Memory performance, suggesting that the contribution of executive dysfunction in memory impairment in AD is minimal, whereas executive dysfunction plays an important role in memory impairment in PD (O'Brien et al., 2009). Taken together, executive dysfunction should be considered when interpreting recall and discriminability scores.

Modest correlations between the CVLT-II Total Learning and the GDS and Geriatric Anxiety Scale-Affective are reported (r = –.24 and –.27, respectively), suggesting that the CVLT-II Total Learning scores may be somewhat related to mood disturbance in older adults (Yochim et al., 2013).

CLINICAL STUDIES

The CVLT-II provides multiple scores that are useful to differentiate among various memory processes and therefore has been used to measure memory in a number of conditions where memory may be affected, including MS (Stegen et al., 2010; Vanotti et al., 2016), chronic kidney disease (Thornton et al., 2007), breast cancer (Root et al., 2015), adult survivors of pediatric brain tumor (Jayakar et al., 2015), TBI (Donders & Nienhuis, 2007; Jacobs & Donders, 2007, 2008), and neurodegenerative disorders (Brooks et al., 2006; Fine et al., 2008; McLaughlin et al., 2014; O'Brien et al., 2009; Pike et al., 2013; Rabin et al., 2009). For example, adult survivors of pediatric brain tumor show lower Trial 1 and Trial 5 scores about 15 years post-diagnosis than typically developing adults, although the increase in number of words from Trial 1 to Trial 5 is similar in both groups (Jayakar et al., 2015). Breast cancer survivors show poor performance on attention only, and there is not a pattern of rapid forgetting over time, suggesting that attentional dysfunction and not a primary memory disorder is the reason for subjective memory complaint in this population (Root et al., 2015).

Neurodegenerative Disorders. The CVLT-II has been found to be sensitive to memory disturbance associated with MCI, AD, PD, and HD (Brooks et al., 2006; Fine et al., 2008; McLaughlin et al., 2014; O'Brien et al., 2009; Pike et al., 2013; Rabin et al., 2009). The CVLT-II consists of process measures that assess memory strategies and has been used to study the profile of memory strategy use in older adults with amnestic MCI, nonamnestic MCI, AD, and healthy controls (Delis et al., 2010; McLaughlin et al., 2014). Healthy controls show intact ability to utilize semantic clustering in their learning and recall of the word lists, somewhat similar to persons with nonamnestic MCI although to a lesser extent in the latter group. Not surprisingly, people with AD fail to utilize semantic clustering strategies and show greater recall impairment than persons with amnestic MCI. More importantly, those healthy adults who progress to amnestic MCI show lower baseline semantic clustering on the short delay than those who remain stable, suggesting that failure to implement memory strategies may be useful as an early marker of disease progression (McLaughlin et al., 2014).

Pike et al. (2013) compared the WMS-IV VPA with the CVLT-II in distinguishing amnestic MCI from healthy controls and found that the CVLT-II yielded higher classification accuracy rates than the VPA in general. Another study identified the CVLT-II Total Learning as better than Logical Memory in distinguishing MCI from normal aging, yielding a sensitivity of 90% and a specificity of 84% (Rabin et al., 2009). Combining CVLT-II LDFR and Logical Memory Recognition predicted progression from MCI to AD over four years, with an overall classification accuracy of 88% (Rabin et al., 2009).

Fine et al. (2008) reported that various recognition discriminability indices are able to distinguish between HD and AD even though the groups perform similarly on LDFR. These include (1) Total Recognition Discriminability (TRD), which is the ability to endorse all targets and reject all distractors; (2) Source Recognition Discriminability (SRD), which is the ability to endorse all List A targets and reject all List B targets; and (3) Novel Recognition Discriminability (NRD), which is the ability to endorse all List A targets and reject all distractors not on List B. They found that HD patients perform better than AD patients on NRD and TRD, but SRD does not differ between the patient groups. NRD appears to be the best recognition measure for differentiating between AD and HD (Fine et al., 2008).

Fazeli et al. (2014) reported that older adults who are dependent in instrumental ADLs (IADL) perform worse than those who are independent across all the CVLT-II primary measures, although this is dependent on age. CVLT-II indices predict IADL functions in older adults (>49 years) but not in younger adults (<50 years).

TBI. The pattern of performance on the CVLT-II may be useful in measuring different aspects of memory deficits in those with TBI. Patients with TBI generally make more intrusive errors and recall fewer words than healthy individuals (Donders & Nienhuis, 2007). Those with moderate to severe TBI perform worse than healthy controls on Total Recall Discriminability and Recognition Discriminability, while those with mild TBI perform worse on Recognition Discriminability only. The discriminability indices generally yield overall classification accuracies of 66 to 70%, with a sensitivity of 60 to 74%, specificity of 63 to 75%, and 49 to 53% false-positive rate. Total Recall Discriminability appears to have the best criterion validity for TBI severity but should not be used in isolation (Jacobs & Donders, 2007) because recall discriminability indices are not better than the traditional scores (e.g., SDFR, LDFR) in identifying the patient group (Donders & Nienhuis, 2007).

DeJong and Donders (2010) performed a cluster analysis using four CVLT-II factors in a TBI sample, yielding six clusters of varying performance patterns. Cluster 1 reflected performance above the mean; Cluster 2 reflected "slow to start"; Cluster 3 reflected below-mean performance on recall trials but at-mean performance for False Positives; Cluster 4 reflected below-mean performance on recall and false positive trials; Cluster 5 reflected above-mean List A Trial 1, below-mean List A Trial 5 and LDFR, and at-mean performance for False Positives; and Cluster 6 reflected performance below the mean. Those in Cluster 6 had the longest length of coma compared to the other clusters, although FSIQ mediated the effect of coma length on CVLT-II performance in this cluster. The authors noted that these clusters are similar to those found in the standardization sample but are simply lower in performance, not unexpected for a TBI sample.

Psychiatric Conditions. Self-reported depression and anxiety have an impact on CVLT-II scores (O'Jile et al., 2005). Among community-dwelling older adults, depression and anxiety predict poor CVLT-II Total Learning, partly due to reduced semantic clustering in those who are anxious but not depressed (Yochim et al., 2013). Similarly, depression as measured by the Personality Assessment Inventory (PAI) is associated with lower Trial 5, SDFR, SDCR, LDFR, LDCR, Recognition Discriminability, and Semantic Clustering scores on the CVLT-II but not on WMS-III VPA or LM after controlling for other motivation factors following TBI, suggesting that the CVLT-II is more demanding possibly due to the requirement to self-generate semantic organization and may be more sensitive to the effects of depression (Keiski et al., 2007).

Similarly, impairments on the CVLT-II have been reported in severe psychiatric illnesses. For example, individuals with schizophrenia or bipolar disorder generally perform worse than healthy controls (Vaskinn et al., 2011) and their biological siblings and parents (Stone et al., 2011). Specifically, patients with schizophrenia perform worse than healthy controls on Total Learning, SDFR and LDFR, and Recognition (d = .93, .84, and .40, respectively), and schizophrenia patients who smoke perform worse than those who do not (Stone et al., 2015). In fact, siblings and parents of schizophrenia probands have been found to perform worse than community comparisons on Recognition Discriminability (Stone et al., 2011). New-onset bipolar disorder with mania is associated with Total Learning, SDFR, and LDFR impairments (Chakrabarty et al., 2015). Negative symptoms in psychotic major depression predict CVLT-II Recognition but not Total Learning after controlling for depression (Che et al., 2012). Overall, studies suggest that the memory impairment in severe psychiatric illnesses may be due to learning inefficiency rather than an amnestic process.

When those with schizophrenia are divided into nonlearners, learners, and high achievers based on their Trial 1 and learning slope performance, high achievers utilize more semantic clustering than the other groups. Nonlearners show less consistency in recalling words over Trials 1 to 5 than the other groups (Vaskinn et al., 2008).

Impact of Cannabis Use. Cannabis use has been found to affect learning scores on the CVLT-II. As the amount of marijuana use increases, CVLT-II Trial 5, Total Learning, SDFR, and LDCR decrease (r = .22 to .25; Roebke et al., 2014). However, differences in scores are found in those who are early users (at or before age 16) and not late users (after age 16). Although no group effects on learning slope are found, early users obtain lower Total Learning scores than late users and nonusers, who do not differ in Total Learning scores. As a result of lower Total Learning scores, early users also have lower Delayed Recall scores compared to late users and nonusers, but the pattern is not suggestive of an amnestic process (Schuster et al., 2016).

Handedness. Mixed-handed undergraduate volunteers appear to perform better on the CVLT-II primary measures than those who are consistently right-handed (Chu et al., 2012).

NEUROANATOMICAL CORRELATES AND IMAGING STUDIES

Studies report that CVLT-II performance relates to brain regions important for verbal memory but also executive function. CVLT-II recall scores are associated with left hippocampal head volume (Bouchard et al., 2008; Chakrabarty et al., 2015; Jayakar et al., 2015), although other brain regions are also involved in CVLT-II performance. In adult survivors of pediatric brain tumors and in those who underwent radiation therapy, total hippocampal volume is moderately correlated with Trial 1 only (r = .43 and .50, respectively). Furthermore, in those who underwent radiation therapy, hippocampal volume is also moderately to highly correlated with Trial 5, LDFR, and Recognition (r = .46 to .62). In new-onset bipolar disorder with mania,

Trial 1 is correlated with left superior frontal gyrus volume. Total Learning and Recognition Discriminability are correlated with bilateral hippocampal volume, learning slope, and SDFR are correlated with left hippocampal volume, and LDFR is correlated with left hippocampal volume and right inferior frontal gyral volume. Number of intrusive errors is correlated with right rostral middle frontal gyrus volume. Retention scores are not correlated with any brain regions (Chakrabarty et al., 2015). In addition, recall scores are correlated with bilateral amygdala volume in PD without dementia (Bouchard et al., 2008).

Erickson et al. (2014) found that individuals with agenesis of the corpus callosum performed worse than healthy controls on the delayed memory factor identified by Donders (2008), including the primary recall measure, as well as Total Learning and Recognition Discriminability.

The impact of executive dysfunction on the CVLT-II is initially supported by a study that examined memory performance in patients with focal frontal lesions (Baldo et al., 2002). In comparison to age- and education-matched controls, patients showed poorer overall recall, an increased tendency to make intrusions, reduced Semantic Clustering, and impaired Yes/No Recognition but normal Forced-Choice Recognition. Further analysis of the error rates in the Yes/No Recognition task revealed that patients with focal frontal lesions were most likely to mistakenly endorse two types of distractors: semantically related words and words from the interference list. The findings were interpreted as being consistent with the role of the frontal lobes in the selection of relevant activations and the inhibition of irrelevant activations.

PERFORMANCE VALIDITY

A number of embedded performance validity indicators within the CVLT-II have been studied, including the CVLT-II Forced-Choice Recognition trial (FC), the Critical Item Analysis indices (CIA; manual), and the Wolfe et al. (2010) equation. By far, the FC is the most frequently used embedded PVT among CVLT-II indices and is therefore one of the more well-known of the embedded PVTs; many of the PVTs reviewed in this volume have used this measure in their validation studies.

There is evidence that those who are seeking financial compensation, litigating, or shown to be noncredible on PVTs perform worse on the CVLT-II than those with TBI or those with credible performance on PVTs (Moore & Donders, 2004; Sawyer et al., 2014; Wolfe et al., 2010). In fact, those with noncredible performance based on two or more failures on stand-alone or embedded PVTs obtain scores that are at least one to two standard deviations lower than credible groups, with effect sizes ranging from .63 (Recognition Discriminability) to 1.27 (LDFR; Sawyer et al., 2014).

FORCED-CHOICE RECOGNITION (FC)

The FC appears to show the most promise as an embedded performance validity indicator at a cutoff score of 14/16 or lower. Based on data presented in a systematic review of 37 studies with a large overall sample (N = 7,575; Schwartz et al., 2016), healthy individuals score at least 14/16 on FC. About 17% score 14 or less on FC, and 26% fail reference PVTs. Those without external incentives and those who pass reference PVTs generally perform well on the FC (4% and 6% FC failure rates, respectively). By contrast, those with external incentives and those who fail reference PVTs are more likely to also fail the FC (14% and 49%, respectively; Schwartz et al., 2016). Moore and Donders (2004) examined patients referred to a rehabilitation facility for TBI and found the FC and the Test of Memory Malingering (TOMM) to be equally sensitive to invalid test performance. Although the two instruments were strongly related, their agreement was not perfect.

There is evidence that a prior psychiatric history increases the risk of invalid test performance on the CVLT-II (Moore & Donders, 2004). Donders and Boonstra (2007) reported that in their sample comprised of consecutive referrals to a TBI rehabilitation facility, 24% obtained invalid performance based on either the CVLT-II FC or WMT. Prior psychiatric treatment, prior abuse, female gender, time post-injury, and lack of prolonged coma differentiated valid from invalid test performance. The authors concluded that individuals with long-standing emotional difficulties may engage in selective augmentation of cognitive and somatic symptoms, possibly as a result of a perception that dysfunction caused by physical trauma is more socially acceptable than that caused by emotional trauma (Moore & Donders, 2004).

Importantly, the CVLT-II FC appears insensitive to low intellectual functioning, a condition known to increase false positives on PVTs. Marshall and Happe (2007) reported that in their sample of 110 adults with FSIQ of less than 75 (mean = 63, range = 51–74) who were not seeking compensation or in litigation, more than 90% passed the CVLT-II FC. Those who failed the CVLT-II FC had poorer Spatial Span Forward and Logical Memory II performance than those who passed the task. As such, failure on the CVLT-II FC in those with intellectual disability appears rare.

CRITICAL ITEM ANALYSIS (CIA)

The CIA indices are (1) CIA-Recall, which is the recall of an item on any recall trial also recognized in the FC and (2) CIA-Recognition, which is the recognition of an item in Long-Delay Recognition also recognized in the FC.

Root et al. (2006) examined the utility of FC and CIA indices in differentiating among three groups: a clinically referred group, a forensically referred group not suspected of invalid performance, and a forensically referred group who failed standalone PVTs (TOMM or VIP). No one in

TABLE 10–26 California Verbal Learning Test—Second Edition (CVLT-II) Forced-Choice Recognition (FC) Classification Accuracy at Different Cutoffs for Forensic-Valid and Forensic-Invalid Performance

CUT SCORE	SENS (%)	SPEC (%)	PPV (%) 48/30/15	NPV (%) 48/30/15
9	4	100	100/100/100	53/71/86
10	8	100	100/100/100	54/72/86
11	12	100	100/100/100	54/73/87
12	20	96	83/68/47	57/74/87
13	36	96	90/79/61	62/78/89
14	44	93	85/73/53	64/79/90
15	60	81	75/58/36	69/83/92

NOTE: Invalid performance base rate = 48%, 30%, and 15%. SENS, sensitivity; SPEC, specificity; PPV, positive predictive value; NPV, negative predictive value.

SOURCE: From Root et al. (2006).

the clinical group obtained FC less than 15/16, including those who scored 1.5 *SD* or less below the mean on LDFR. About 90% of those forensic referrals with valid performance obtained more than 15/16 on FC, including those who scored 1.5 *SD* or less below the mean on LDFR, similar to the normative sample. In these groups, LDFR and FC were not correlated. As seen in Table 10–26, a FC cutoff of 14 or lower had at least 90% specificity, though sensitivity was lower, at 44%. A CIA-Recall and CIA-Recognition cutoff of one or more correctly identified 35% and 32% of persons with invalid performance, respectively. FC appears better than the CIA to measure invalid performance.

WOLFE ET AL. EQUATION

In one study (Wolfe et al., 2010), data from the CVLT-II (without FC) from litigating individuals for alleged TBI who met Slick et al. (1999) criteria for malingering and a TBI group with moderate to severe TBI were submitted to Bayesian model averaging. Total Recall Discriminability, d', and LDFR together distinguished between the TBI and litigating groups, with LDFR yielding the largest odds ratio (1.38). The litigating group performed worse than the TBI group in all recall and recognition measures, with d' disproportionately worse than recall measures.

Given these findings, Wolfe and colleagues (2010) provided an equation using these three variables to generate a probability of response bias (Wolfe et al., 2010). The Wolfe et al. (2010) equation is

$$\text{Probability of response bias} = \frac{e^{[-1.092+0.32(\text{LDFR raw score})-0.99(\text{d-prime raw score})-0.693(\text{Recall Discriminability standard score})]}}{1+e^{[-1.092+0.32(\text{LDFR raw score})-0.99(\text{d-prime raw score})-0.693(\text{Recall Discriminability standard score})]}}$$

The equation was cross-validated in an independent clinical sample of TBI patients from a general clinical practice by Donders and Strong (2011). Those who failed based on the original cutoff of .50 were three times more likely to fail the WMT than those who did not. The risk was higher when a cutoff of .62 was used. The sensitivity of this equation to identify invalid performance (against WMT) was in the 37 to 55% range, while specificity was in the 75 to 87% range. To achieve greater than 90% specificity, a cutoff of .67 is required, yielding 38% sensitivity and 78% classification accuracy. The CVLT-II composite scores vary with length of coma, whereas the CVLT-II FC does not (Donders & Strong, 2011). In light of the impact of injury severity on the equation as well as the high false-positive rate based on the original cutoff, the authors concluded that the Wolfe et al. (2010) equation must be used with caution in the clinical setting. As well, validation on a single PVT is not an optimal method, again supporting the value of the FC score above other CVLT-II embedded indices.

COMMENT

The CVLT-II is among the top memory assessment instruments used by neuropsychologists. The original version generated a wealth of research that has both theoretical and clinical relevance. Since its development, the CVLT-II has had a prominent role in neuropsychology and has proved valuable in characterizing the unique learning and memory profiles of various neurological and psychiatric disorders. One of its biggest strengths is the large variety of scores generated, which are useful to profile the varying memory deficits in different neurological and psychiatric conditions. It is also sensitive enough to identify more subtle memory impairments in neurological conditions such as MCI, and in fact predicts progression to AD over time.

In contrast to other verbal memory tests, the authors have thoroughly investigated the internal consistency of the CVLT-II and found it to be excellent. Test-retest and alternate form reliability estimates appear reasonable for the various measures tapping overall level of performance (e.g., Total Learning, SDFR, and LDFR). A large number of studies have also supported the use of the FC as an embedded performance validity indicator insensitive to low intellectual functioning and genuine memory impairments.

Unusually large performance discrepancies are not uncommon in the standardization sample or in TBI samples. As such, the presence of one unusually large discrepancy should not be taken as pathological. Users may wish to refer to Table 10–22 for the frequency of various discrepancy indices in the standardization sample when interpreting the performance discrepancy of their examinees.

Although the manual states that nonverbal tasks should be administered during the delay interval, studies have found that administration of verbal tasks during the delay interval does not affect the recall scores.

Users should be aware of the test's limitations. Reliability coefficients tend to be poor for some process-oriented variables, suggesting that users should be cautious in drawing inferences regarding certain strategic aspects of an individual's learning and memory abilities. Furthermore, given the lack of information regarding reliability or validity for the Short Form, this version should be regarded as experimental. Of note, interpretation of some of the test scores can be confusing. In most cases, a positive z score indicates intact performance; however, in other cases (e.g., error scores), higher z scores reflect greater deficits.

Users should bear in mind that executive functioning contributes a proportion of variance to CVLT-II performance. In addition to left hippocampal volume, this fits with neuroimaging research indicating that CVLT-II performance is related to other brain regions including the frontal lobes, thus providing further evidence of the contribution of executive functions to CVLT-II performance. Accordingly, an impaired CVLT-II may also in part reflect executive dysfunction rather than a primary memory disorder. Among process scores, the semantic clustering score may be of utility in profiling memory impairment. Last, more updated normative data would be of benefit; public-domain tests such as the RAVLT also appear equally effective at memory assessment..

REFERENCES

Baldo, J. V., Delis, D., Kramer, J., & Shimamura, A. P. (2002). Memory performance on the California Verbal Learning Test-II: Findings from patients with focal frontal lesions. *Journal of the International Neuropsychological Society, 8*, 539–546.

Bouchard, T. P., Malykhin, N., Martin, W. R. W., Hanstock, C. C., Emery, D. J., Fisher, N. J., & Camicioli, R. M. (2008). Age and dementia-associated atrophy predominates in the hippocampal head and amygdala in Parkinson's disease. *Neurobiology of Aging, 29*(7), 1027–1039.

Brooks, B. L., Weaver, L. E., & Scialfa, C. T. (2006). Does impaired executive functioning differentially impact verbal memory measures in older adults with suspected dementia? *The Clinical Neuropsychologist, 20*(2), 230–242.

Chakrabarty, T., Kozicky, J., Torres, I. J., Lam, R. W., & Yatham, L. N. (2015). Verbal memory impairment in new onset bipolar disorder: Relationship with frontal and medial temporal morphology. *The World Journal of Biological Psychiatry, 16*(4), 249–260.

Che, A. M., Gomez, R. G., Keller, J., Lembke, A., Tennakoon, L., Cohen, G. H., & Schatzberg, A. F. (2012). The relationships of positive and negative symptoms with neuropsychological functioning and their ability to predict verbal memory in psychotic major depression. *Psychiatry Research, 198*(1), 34–38.

Chu, O., Abeare, C. A., & Bondy, M. A. (2012). Inconsistent vs. consistent right-handers' performance on an episodic memory task: Evidence from the California Verbal Learning Test. *Laterality: Asymmetries of Body, Brain and Cognition, 17*(3), 306–317.

Davis, J. J., & Wall, J. R. (2014). Examining verbal memory on the Word Memory Test and California Verbal Learning Test–second edition. *Archives of Clinical Neuropsychology, 29*(8), 747–753.

DeJong, J., & Donders, J. (2009). A confirmatory factor analysis of the California Verbal Learning Test–second edition (CVLT-II) in a traumatic brain injury sample. *Assessment, 16*(4), 328–336.

DeJong, J., & Donders, J. (2010). Cluster subtypes on the California Verbal Learning Test–second edition (CVLT-II) in a traumatic brain injury sample. *Journal of Clinical and Experimental Neuropsychology, 32*(9), 953–960.

Delis, D. C., Fine, E. M., Stricker, J. L., Houston, W. S., Wetter, S. R., Cobell, K., . . . Bondi, M. W. (2010). Comparison of the traditional recall-based versus a new list-based method for computing semantic clustering on the California Verbal Learning Test: Evidence from Alzheimer's disease. *The Clinical Neuropsychologist, 24*(1), 70–79.

Delis, D. C., Kramer, J. H., Kaplan, E., & Ober, B. A. (1987). *California Verbal Learning Test.* San Antonio, TX: The Psychological Corporation.

Delis, D. C., Kramer, J. H., Kaplan, E., & Ober, B. A. (2000). *California Verbal Learning Test—Second Edition.* San Antonio, TX: The Psychological Corporation.

Donders, J. (2006). Performance discrepancies on the California Verbal Learning Test–second edition (CVLT-II) in the standardization sample. *Psychological Assessment, 18*(4), 458–463.

Donders, J. (2008). A confirmatory factor analysis of the California Verbal Learning Test–second edition (CVLT-II) in the standardization sample. *Assessment, 15*(2), 123–131.

Donders, J., & Boonstra, T. (2007). Correlates of invalid neuropsychological test performance after traumatic brain injury. *Brain Injury, 21*(3), 319–326.

Donders, J., & Nienhuis, J. B. (2007). Utility of California Verbal Learning Test–second edition, recall discriminability indices in the evaluation of traumatic brain injury. *Journal of the International Neuropsychological Society, 13*(2), 354–358.

Donders, J., & Strong, C. H. (2011). Embedded effort indicators on the California Verbal Learning Test–second edition (CVLT–II): An attempted cross-validation. *The Clinical Neuropsychologist, 25*(1), 173–184.

Erickson, R. L., Paul, L. K., & Brown, W. S. (2014). Verbal learning and memory in agenesis of the corpus callosum. *Neuropsychologia, 60*, 121–130.

Fazeli, P. L., Doyle, K. L., Scott, J. C., Iudicello, J. E., Casaletto, K. B., Weber, E., . . . Woods, S. P. (2014). Shallow encoding and forgetting are associated with dependence in instrumental activities of daily living among older adults living with HIV infection. *Archives of Clinical Neuropsychology, 29*(3), 278–288.

Fine, E. M., Delis, D. C., Wetter, S. R., Jacobson, M. W., Hamilton, J. M., Peavy, G., . . . Salmon, D. P. (2008). Identifying the 'source' of recognition memory deficits in patients with Huntington's disease or Alzheimer's disease: Evidence from the CVLT-II. *Journal of Clinical and Experimental Neuropsychology, 30*(4), 463–470.

Fine, E. M., Kramer, J. H., Lui, L., & Yaffe, K. (2012). Normative data in women aged 85 and older: Verbal fluency, digit span, and the CVLT-II short form. *The Clinical Neuropsychologist, 26*(1), 18–30.

Hill, B. D., Alosco, M., Bauer, L., & Tremont, G. (2012). The relation of executive functioning to CVLT-II learning, memory, and process indexes. *Applied Neuropsychology: Adult, 19*(3), 198–206.

Jacobs, M. L., & Donders, J. (2007). Criterion validity of the California Verbal Learning Test—second edition (CVLT-II) after traumatic brain injury. *Archives of Clinical Neuropsychology, 22*(2), 143–149.

Jacobs, M. L., & Donders, J. (2008). Performance discrepancies on the California Verbal Learning Test—second edition (CVLT-II) after traumatic brain injury. *Archives of Clinical Neuropsychology, 23*(1), 113–118.

Jayakar, R., King, T. Z., Morris, R., & Na, S. (2015). Hippocampal volume and auditory attention on a verbal memory task with adult survivors of pediatric brain tumor. *Neuropsychology, 29*(2), 303–319.

Keiski, M. A., Shore, D. L., & Hamilton, J. M. (2007). The role of depression in verbal memory following traumatic brain injury. *The Clinical Neuropsychologist, 21*(5), 744–761.

Lloyd, K. P., Higginson, C. I., Lating, J. M., & Coiro, M. J. (2012). Test-order effects: A measure of verbal memory influences performance on a measure of verbal fluency. *Applied Neuropsychology: Adult, 19*(4), 299–304. doi:10.1080/09084282.2012.670153

Lundervold, A. J., Wollschläger, D., & Wehling, E. (2014). Age and sex related changes in episodic memory function in middle aged and older adults. *Scandinavian Journal of Psychology, 55*(3), 225–232.

Marshall, P., & Happe, M. (2007). The performance of individuals with mental retardation on cognitive tests assessing effort and motivation. *The Clinical Neuropsychologist, 21*(5), 826–840.

McLaughlin, P. M., Wright, M. J., LaRocca, M., Nguyen, P. T., Teng, E., Apostolova, L. G., . . . Woo, E. (2014). The 'Alzheimer's type' profile of semantic clustering in amnestic mild cognitive impairment. *Journal of the International Neuropsychological Society, 20*(4), 402–412.

Miller, J. B., Axelrod, B. N., Rapport, L. J., Hanks, R. A., Bashem, J. R., & Schutte, C. (2012a). Substitution of California Verbal Learning Test—second edition for Verbal Paired Associates on the Wechsler Memory Scale, fourth edition. *The Clinical Neuropsychologist, 26*(4), 599–608.

Miller, J. B., Axelrod, B. N., Rapport, L. J., Millis, S. R., VanDyke, S., Schutte, C., & Hanks, R. A. (2012b). Parsimonious prediction of Memory Scale, fourth edition scores: Immediate and delayed memory indexes. *Journal of Clinical and Experimental Neuropsychology, 34*(5), 531–542.

Moore, B. A., & Donders, J. (2004). Predictors of invalid neuropsychological test performance after traumatic brain injury. *Brain Injury, 18*, 975–984.

O'Brien, T. J., Wadley, V., Nicholas, A. P., Stover, N. P., Watts, R., & Griffith, H. R. (2009). The contribution of executive control on verbal-learning impairment in patients with Parkinson's disease with dementia and Alzheimer's disease. *Archives of Clinical Neuropsychology, 24*(3), 237–244.

O'Jile, J. R., Schrimsher, G. W., & O'Bryant, S. E. (2005). The relation of self-report of mood and anxiety to CVLT-C, CVLT, and CVLT-2 in a psychiatric sample. *Archives of Clinical Neuropsychology, 20*, 547–553.

Pike, K. E., Kinsella, G. J., Ong, B., Mullaly, E., Rand, E., Storey, E., . . . Parsons, S. (2013). Is the WMS-IV Verbal Paired Associates as effective as other memory tasks in discriminating amnestic mild cognitive impairment from normal aging? *The Clinical Neuropsychologist, 27*(6), 908–923.

Poreh, A. M., Avital, R., Dines, P. L., & Levin, J. B. (2015). The effects of age of language acquisition on verbal memory tests in a sample of older adults immigrants. *Psychology & Neuroscience, 8*(1), 66–74.

Rabin, L. A., Barr, W. B., & Burton, L. A. (2005). Assessment practices of clinical neuropsychologists in the United States and Canada: A survey of INS, NAN, and APA Division 40 members. *Archives of Clinical Neuropsychology, 20*, 33–65.

Rabin, L. A., Paré, N., Saykin, A. J., Brown, M. J., Wishart, H. A., Flashman, L. A., & Santulli, R. B. (2009). Differential memory test sensitivity for diagnosing amnestic mild cognitive impairment and predicting conversion to Alzheimer's disease. *Aging, Neuropsychology, and Cognition, 16*(3), 357–376.

Roebke, P. V., Vadhan, N. P., Brooks, D. J., & Levin, F. R. (2014). Verbal learning in marijuana users seeking treatment: A comparison between depressed and non-depressed samples. *American Journal of Drug and Alcohol Abuse, 40*(4), 274–279. doi:10.3109/00952990.2013.875551

Root, J. C., Robbins, R. N., Chang, L., & Van Gorp, W. G. (2006). Detection of inadequate effort on the California Verbal Learning Test—Second Edition: Forced choice recognition and critical item analysis. *Journal of the International Neuropsychological Society, 12*(5), 688–696.

Root, J. C., Ryan, E., Barnett, G., Andreotti, C., Bolutayo, K., & Ahles, T. (2015). Learning and memory performance in a cohort of clinically referred breast cancer survivors: The role of attention versus forgetting in patient-reported memory complaints. *Psycho-Oncology, 24*(5), 548–555.

Sawyer, R. J., Young, J. C., Roper, B. L., & Rach, A. (2014). Are verbal intelligence subtests and reading measures immune to non-credible effort? *The Clinical Neuropsychologist, 28*(5), 756–770.

Schuster, R. M., Hoeppner, S. S., Evins, A. E., & Gilman, J. M. (2016). Early onset marijuana use is associated with learning inefficiencies. *Neuropsychology, 30*(4), 405–415.

Schwartz, E. S., Erdodi, L., Rodriguez, N., Ghosh, J. J., Curtain, J. R., Flashman, L. A., & Roth, R. M. (2016). CVLT-II forced choice recognition trial as an embedded validity indicator: A systematic review of the evidence. *Journal of the International Neuropsychological Society, 22*(8), 851–858.

Slick, D. J., Sherman, E. M., & Iverson, G. L. (1999). Diagnostic criteria for malingered neurocognitive dysfunction: Proposed standards for clinical practice and research. *The Clinical Neuropsychologist, 13*(4), 545–561.

Spreen, O., & Strauss, E. (1998). *A compendium of neuropsychological tests: Administration, norms and commentary.* New York: Oxford University Press.

Stegen, S., Stepanov, I., Cookfair, D., Schwartz, E., Hojnacki, D., Weinstock-Guttman, B., & Benedict, R. H. B. (2010). Validity of the California Verbal Learning Test–II in multiple sclerosis. *The Clinical Neuropsychologist, 24*(2), 189–202.

Stone, W. S., Giuliano, A. J., Tsuang, M. T., Braff, D. L., Cadenhead, K. S., Calkins, M. E., . . . Seidman, L. J. (2011). Group and site differences on the California Verbal Learning Test in persons with schizophrenia and their first-degree relatives: Findings from the consortium on the genetics of schizophrenia (COGS). *Schizophrenia Research, 128*(1-3), 102–110.

Stone, W. S., Mesholam-Gately, R., Braff, D. L., Calkins, M. E., Freedman, R., Green, M. F., . . . Seidman, L. J. (2015). California Verbal Learning Test–II performance in schizophrenia as a function of ascertainment strategy: Comparing the first and second phases of the consortium on the genetics of schizophrenia (COGS). *Schizophrenia Research, 163*(1-3), 32–37.

Stricker, J. L., Brown, G. G., Wixted, J., Baldo, J. V., & Delis, D. C. (2002). New semantic and serial clustering indices for the California Verbal Learning Test—second edition: Background, rationale, and formulae. *Journal of the International Neuropsychological Society, 8*, 425–435.

Sunderaraman, P., Blumen, H. M., DeMatteo, D., Apa, Z. L., & Cosentino, S. (2013). Task demand influences relationships among sex, cluster strategy, and recall: 16-word versus 9-word list learning tests. *Cognitive and Behavioral Neurology, 26*(2), 78–84.

Thiruselvam, I., Vogt, E. M., & Hoelzle, J. B. (2015). The interchangeability of CVLT-II and WMS-IV Verbal Paired Associates scores: A slightly different story. *Archives of Clinical Neuropsychology, 30*(3), 248–255.

Thornton, W. L., Shapiro, R. J., Deria, S., Gelb, S., & Hill, A. (2007). Differential impact of age on verbal memory and executive functioning in chronic kidney disease. *Journal of the International Neuropsychological Society, 13*(2), 344–353.

Vanotti, S., Smerbeck, A., Benedict, R. H. B., & Caceres, F. (2016). A new assessment tool for patients with multiple sclerosis from Spanish-speaking countries: Validation of the Brief International Cognitive Assessment for MS (BICAMS) in Argentina. *The Clinical Neuropsychologist, 30*(7), 1023–1031.

Vaskinn, A., Sundet, K., Friis, S., Ueland, T., Simonsen, C., Birkenaes, A. B., . . . Andreassen, O. A. (2008). Can learning potential in schizophrenia be assessed with the standard CVLT-II? An exploratory study. *Scandinavian Journal of Psychology, 49*(2), 179–186.

Vaskinn, A., Sundet, K., Simonsen, C., Hellvin, T., Melle, I., & Andreassen, O. A. (2011). Sex differences in neuropsychological performance and social functioning in schizophrenia and bipolar disorder. *Neuropsychology, 25*(4), 499–510.

Williams, B. R., & Donovick, P. J. (2008). Questioning the rule of thumb: Can verbal tasks be administered during the CVLT-II delay interval? *The Clinical Neuropsychologist, 22*(5), 807–812.

Williams, B. R., Sullivan, S. K., Morra, L. F., Williams, J. R., & Donovick, P. J. (2014). The similar effects of verbal and non-verbal intervening tasks on word recall in an elderly population. *The Clinical Neuropsychologist, 28*(3), 505–513.

Wolfe, P. L., Millis, S. R., Hanks, R., Fichtenberg, N., Larrabee, G. J., & Sweet, J. J. (2010). Effort indicators within the California Verbal Learning Test–II (CVLT-II). *The Clinical Neuropsychologist, 24*(1), 153–168.

Woods, S. P., Delis, D. C., Scott, J. C., Kramer, J. H., & Holdnack, J. A. (2006). The California Verbal Learning Test—second edition: Test-retest reliability, practice effects, and reliable change indices for the standard and alternate forms. *Archives of Clinical Neuropsychology, 21*(5), 413–420.

Yochim, B. P., Mueller, A. E., & Segal, D. L. (2013). Late life anxiety is associated with decreased memory and executive functioning in community dwelling older adults. *Journal of Anxiety Disorders, 27*(6), 567–575.

CONTINUOUS VISUAL MEMORY TEST (CVMT)

TEST NAME	**Continuous Visual Memory Test (CVMT)**
DOMAIN MEASURED	Visual memory
AGE RANGE	18 to 91 years
ADMINISTRATION TIME	15 minutes plus 30-minute delay interval
SCORING FORMAT	Hand scored
REFERENCE	Trahan, D. E., & Larrabee, G. J. (1988). *Continuous Visual Memory Test.* Lutz, FL: Psychological Assessment Resources. www.parinc.com

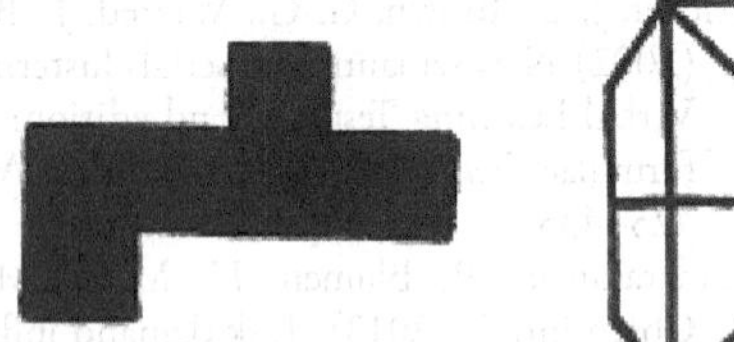
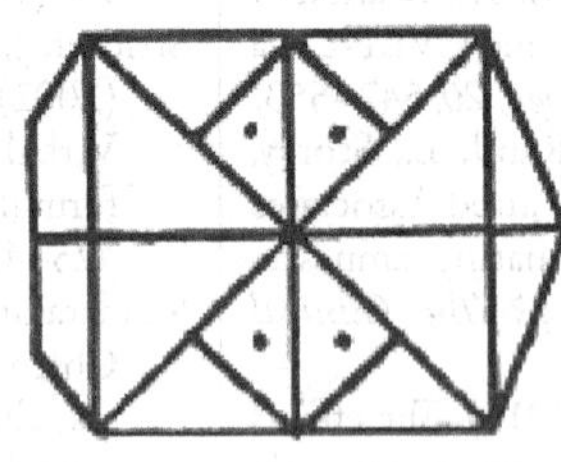
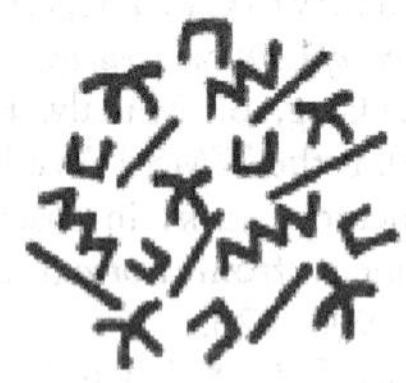

Example of items from the CVMT

Reproduced by special permission of the Publisher, Psychological Assessment Resources, Inc., 16204 North Florida Avenue, Lutz, Florida 33549, from the Continuous Visual Memory Test, by Donald E. Trahan, Ph.D. and Glenn J. Larrabee, Ph.D., Copyright 1983, 1988 by PAR, Inc. Further reproduction is prohibited without permission from PAR, Inc.

DESCRIPTION

The Continuous Visual Memory Test (CVMT) is a measure of visual learning and memory that was developed based on five principles: (1) recognition memory format (2) complex and ambiguous stimuli that minimized potential for verbal labeling (3) large number of stimuli across classes of perceptually similar stimuli (4) brief exposure time, and (5) inclusion of a delayed recognition trial. The authors posited that the use of a recognition format eliminates the limitations associated with motor and visuospatial deficits when examinees are required to draw the designs from memory. Moreover, unlike most other memory tests with long exposures, the brief exposure time and use of ambiguous line drawings reduces the potential for verbal encoding.

ADMINISTRATION

This test comprises three parts. In the acquisition task, a total of 112 complex ambiguous line-drawn designs are presented, one at a time, for a two-second exposure period. Following the presentation of each design, examinees indicate if the design was "new" or "old" based on whether or not they have seen the design in previous trials. In the series of designs, seven of the designs recur seven times. After a 30-minute delay, examinees are asked to identify previously viewed stimuli from a set of perceptually similar foils. In the final part, a visual discrimination task allows distinction between visual discrimination and visual memory problems.

SCORING

A total of six scores are calculated for the CVMT. From the acquisition trial, four scores are generated, three of which are based on signal detection theory (Hits, False Alarms, and d'). The Total score represents the total number of correct responses from items 17–112. The calculation of d' is based on several mathematical transformations and is interpreted as an overall measure of memory sensitivity in the acquisition phase. Both Total score and d' have shown similar effectiveness in differentiating between healthy samples from neurological samples, but in rare situations of extreme values, the Total score should be interpreted. Both the delayed recognition task and visual discrimination task generate a score each for the total number of correct responses. In general, Total, d', and Delayed scores are recommended for clinical interpretation by the authors. Interpretation of the visual discrimination task score is not described in the manual, although, given the simplicity of this task, healthy individuals are unlikely to obtain less than perfect scores. The manual presents cutoff scores for impaired performance stratified by age. In addition, a computer-assisted administration has also been developed (see later discussion).

DEMOGRAPHIC EFFECTS

The CVMT does not appear to be affected by education (Paolo et al., 1998a) or gender (Paolo et al., 1998a; Trahan & Quintana, 1990). This test appears most sensitive to age (Trahan et al., 1990). The manual cautions against interpreting the Delayed score in older adults (>60) because of considerable variability in test performance, with some healthy older adults performing at chance. This is supported by one study where a large percentage (63%) of healthy older adults aged 80 and older was misclassified as impaired on the Delayed score when the cutoff score in the manual was used (Hall et al., 1996). Within the age 60–69 and 70–79 groups, 21% and 25% of healthy individuals, respectively, were considered impaired on the Delayed score. These healthy individuals were misclassified despite their high education level and intact scores on the DRS (Mattis, 1988; range = 130–144). In a separate study, a significant number of healthy older adults screened for dementia and other neurological illnesses were considered impaired on the CVMT: one-third of the healthy adults aged 75 to 79 years were impaired on *d′* and Delayed scores, while 50% of those older than age 80 were impaired on the *d′* score (Paolo et al., 1998a).

NORMATIVE DATA

Since the publication of the test, the original normative data have been expanded to include older adults in a supplemental norms set. Characteristics of the original normative and supplemental samples are summarized in Table 10–27. The original normative sample comprises a small subset of older adults ($n = 88$). As such, the authors suggest that the supplemental normative data be used in place of the original norms for ages 50 and older. The authors caution against

TABLE 10–27 Characteristics of Standardization Samples for the Continuous Visual Memory Test (CVMT)

CHARACTERISTIC	ORIGINAL NORMATIVE SAMPLE	SUPPLEMENTAL OLDER ADULT SAMPLE
Reference	Trahan and Larrabee (1988)	Trahan and Larrabee (1997)
Sample size	310	165
Recruitment	US, unspecified	Combined data from studies of normal aging in Texas, Montana and Los Angeles
Age	18 to 91 years	50 to 80+ years
Education	13 to 15 years[a]	13 to 14 years[b]
Gender	55% Women 45% Men	73% Women 27% Men
Ethnicity	Not reported	Not reported
Socioeconomic status	Not reported	Not reported

[a] Education was reported according to age groups: age 18–29 = 13.24 years of education; age 30–49 = 14.11 years of education; age 50–69 = 13.60 years of education; age 70+ = 15.70 years of education.

[b] Education was reported according to age groups: age 50–64 = 13.34 years of education; age 65–79 = 14.92 years of education; age 80+ = 14.17 years of education.

SOURCE: Reproduced by special permission of the Publisher, Psychological Assessment Resources, Inc. (PAR), 16204 North Florida Avenue, Lutz, Florida 33549, from the Continuous Visual Memory Test, by Donald E. Trahan, Ph.D. and Glenn J. Larrabee, PhD, Copyright 1983, 1988 by PAR. Further reproduction is prohibited without permission from PAR.

TABLE 10–28 Continuous Visual Memory Test (CVMT) Demographic Background of Revised Normative Sample

AGE GROUP	*N*	M/F	AGE (*SD*)	EDUCATION (*SD*)	DRS TOTAL (*SD*)
60–64	25	8/17	62.32 (1.22)	14.64 (2.56)	138.60 (3.18)
65–69	48	19/29	67.40 (1.23)	14.90 (2.57)	138.63 (3.50)
70–74	58	28/30	72.10 (1.35)	14.60 (2.49)	138.17 (3.07)
75–79	30	15/15	76.53 (1.43)	14.73 (2.32)	136.70 (3.46)
80+	16	4/12	83.25 (3.87)	15.31 (2.57)	134.81 (2.81)

SOURCE: From Paolo et al. (1998).

the use of the CVMT with individuals aged 80 and older because of the poor performance of healthy older adults in this age group. Use of the CVMT in those with limited education (less than six years) should also be done with caution because data are lacking in this group.

Revised cutoff scores for older adults have been suggested since the initial publication of the test (Paolo et al., 1998a Trahan & Larrabee, 1997). The supplemental norms include revised cutoff scores for older adults (Trahan & Larrabee, 1997). Paolo, Tröster, and Ryan (1998a) also provide updated normative data based on an independent sample comprising community-dwelling volunteers recruited from community and retirement centers in the Midwestern United States. As seen in Table 10–28, their sample appears comparable in terms of age (range 60–94 years) and educational background (14–15 years) to Trahan and Larrabee's (1997) supplemental older adult sample. Means, *SD*s, and abnormal cutoff scores based on their sample are presented in Table 10–29. Delayed scores are not presented because there are no statistically significant differences among the age groups on this score in their sample. Information on how the revised cutoff scores in the supplemental and Paolo et al. study were derived is not reported. Studies also have not been done to validate these revised cutoff scores in clinical samples. Consequently, users may wish to refer to the supplemental normative data for norms and cutoffs.

Norms for the computer-administered version are not available. However, an equivalence study using healthy, undergraduate volunteers (Trahan et al., 1996) indicates adequate correlations between the traditional and computer-assisted formats for the Total score ($r = .70$) and False Alarms ($r = .79$). The correlations are very low for both Hits ($r = .25$) and Delayed ($r = .22$) scores as participants perform almost perfectly on these scores.

EVIDENCE FOR RELIABILITY

EVIDENCE FOR INTERNAL RELIABILITY

Evidence for internal reliability for the CVMT appears strong, but evidence for test-retest reliability is somewhat more limited. As reported in the manual, the Spearman-Brown split-half reliability coefficient (odd and even items) in a sample comprising 25 healthy individuals age- and gender-matched with the clinical sample is .80 for the

TABLE 10–29 Continuous Visual Memory Test (CVMT) Revised Normative Data and Cutoff Scores for Age 60 and Older

		CVMT SCORE							
		TOTAL SCORE				*D′*			
AGE GROUP	N	*M (SD)*	85%	90%	95%	*M (SD)*	85%	90%	95%
60–64	25	74.08 (5.70)	67	65	62	1.84 (0.54)	1.34	1.21	0.95
65–69	48	72.38 (7.66)	66	64	61	1.71 (0.50)	1.26	1.20	0.92
70–74	58	71.84 (7.08)	63	62	59	1.73 (0.47)	1.17	1.10	0.90
75–79	30	68.97 (5.97)	62	60	58	1.47 (0.41)	1.00	0.90	0.80
80+	16	65.44 (5.32)	58	56	53	1.24 (0.27)	0.86	0.74	0.70

NOTE: Scores below the cut-off values suggest possible impairment.

SOURCE: Paolo et al. (1998).

recurring items and .98 for the non-recurring items. In the clinical sample comprising 25 patients with severe traumatic head injuries, reliability coefficients are .98 and .90 for the recurring and non-recurring items, respectively (Trahan & Larrabee, 1988). Internal consistency coefficients of the computer-assisted version appear marginal to adequate ($r = .61$ to .70).

EVIDENCE FOR TEST-RETEST RELIABILITY, MEASURING CHANGE, AND PRACTICE EFFECTS

Test-retest reliability appears adequate to high (Total score, $r = .85$; d' score, $r = .80$; Delayed score, $r = .76$) based on the original sample of 12 healthy individuals over a seven-day retest interval reported in the manual (Trahan & Larrabee, 1988). Over a one-year retest interval, very low reliability coefficients (Total score, $r = .49$; d' score, $r = .44$; Delayed score, $r = .48$) have been reported in healthy older adults ($n = 92$; Paolo et al., 1998b). The authors recommend the use of Total, d', and Delayed scores for clinical interpretation; reliability data on some scores such as Hits, False Alarms, and Visual Discrimination have not been reported. No data are available on the test-retest reliability of the computer-administered version. No data are available on practice effects and measuring change.

EVIDENCE FOR RELIABILITY OF ALTERNATE FORM

An alternate form was developed by Trahan et al. (1996). In comparing the original and alternate forms (inter-test interval ranged from 1 to 10 days), variance estimates for the forms are close to zero. The generalizability coefficients range from .53 to .66 in a combined sample of healthy people and patients, and .45 to .72 in a patient group (neurologic/psychiatric patients aged 17–79 years). Similar to the original form, only age has major effects on the alternate form, but not gender or education. At present the alternate form is not available from a commercial source; however, PAR has authorized limited distribution of the alternate form for research purposes only, and interested researchers may contact the primary author directly for a copy of the alternate form (D. E. Trahan, personal communication, May 31, 2013).

EVIDENCE FOR VALIDITY

FACTOR-ANALYTIC STUDIES AND RELATIONSHIPS WITH OTHER TESTS

Larrabee, Trahan, and Curtiss (1992) examined the factor structure of the CVMT using d' and Delayed scores based on a sample of healthy adults. A three-factor solution was generated using the d' score. The d' score loaded on both the verbal (WAIS Information and Shipley Vocabulary) and visual/nonverbal (WAIS Block Design and Picture Completion, and WMS Visual Reproduction) intelligence factors, and it loaded minimally on the third factor representing verbal memory. Analysis using the Delayed score revealed a four-factor solution, with verbal and visual/nonverbal intelligence, and verbal memory factors as discussed earlier. The CVMT Delayed score and WMS Visual Reproduction loaded as a separate dimension of visual memory. These results suggest that d' is associated with verbal and nonverbal intellectual factors, whereas the Delayed score is a factorially pure measure of visual memory. Data on the Total score were not reported.

Overall, the relationship of the CVMT with other visual memory tests is not consistent, and it also appears to measure other domains such as general intellectual functioning and verbal memory. In a sample of patients with intractable TLE, moderately high correlations were reported between the Total score and the WAIS-R FSIQ, Verbal IQ (VIQ), Block Design, and Meier Visual Discrimination test, while the Delayed score also correlated with Performance IQ (PIQ); the CVMT did not show strong correlations with other visual memory tests such as WMS-R Visual Reproduction or RCFT in this sample. The CVLT did not provide additive information in a sample of patients with moderate-severe TBI once age, duration of coma, and PIQ are entered in the regression model to predict CVMT performance (Strong & Donders, 2008). However, relationships with other tests differed depending on the administration modality: on the traditional format, the Total score correlated significantly with CVLT-II Long-Delay

Free Recall and Recognition, but the computer-assisted administration format did not in a sample of healthy college-aged volunteers (Baños et al., 2001).

CLINICAL STUDIES

The CVMT demonstrates sensitivity to visual memory problems in patients with severe closed head injury, AD, and amnestic syndromes, according to data presented in the manual (Trahan & Larrabee, 1988). As a visual memory test, the CVMT appears to be sensitive to impairments associated with right cerebrovascular accidents (CVA). Patients with right CVA perform significantly worse than those with left CVA, and both groups perform worse than age-matched healthy controls on all scores (Trahan et al., 1990). In this study of patients with CVA, Total and *d'* scores were also correlated with WAIS-R Block Design. The Delayed score did not show significant correlation with Block Design, suggesting that the Delayed score may be a "pure" measure of visual memory, similar to results reported by Larrabee et al. (1992).

The CVMT differentiates between moderate-severe TBI and matched healthy controls (Strong & Donders, 2008). When tested within one-year post-injury, statistically significant differences on Total and Delayed scores have been reported. Hierarchical regression analysis revealed that older age and longer coma were associated with worse performance on the CVMT. The addition of PIQ into the model attenuated the relationship between Total score and coma, suggesting visuospatial skills as a mediating factor, though coma still predicted Delayed score. Total score correctly classified 76% of the TBI patients and controls (sensitivity 72%; specificity 81%). Interestingly, lower rates (classification 73%; sensitivity 66%; specificity 79%) were obtained when both Total and Delayed scores were entered into the logistic regression.

Patients with TLE who were medically intractable and being evaluated for surgical candidacy for resection of unilateral mesial temporal focus (hippocampal sclerosis) were given the CVMT to evaluate its utility to lateralize impairments. Results suggest that attentional, speed, and visuospatial processing factors may play a bigger role than memory (associated with mesial temporal structures) alone on CVMT performance, thus raising questions about its utility in this setting (Snitz et al., 1996).

NEUROANATOMICAL CORRELATES AND IMAGING STUDIES

Retzlaff and Morris (1996) conducted a study using event-related potentials to examine visual recognition processing. The old designs elicited higher P300 amplitude than new designs, and both types of designs elicited progressively greater electrocortical activity from occipital to frontal electrode sites. Greater amplitude increase in the frontal electrode site was also obtained when participants responded to old rather than new designs. Results suggest frontal involvement of recognition and decision-making processes of these ambiguous visual designs.

PERFORMANCE VALIDITY

A number of studies have developed embedded validity scales using the CVMT. Applying Slick et al. (1999) criteria for probable malingered neurocognitive dysfunction (MND), Henry and Enders (2007) developed cutoff scores on the CVMT based on logistic regression to identify malingerers using a known-group design. They retrospectively identified 27 malingerers out of 44 personal litigation cases and 10 disability claimants. The nonmalingering group had similar performance on all CVMT scores, whereas the probable malingering group obtained lower scores on Hits, Total, and Delayed scores and higher False Alarms compared to the nonmalingering group. Logistic regression revealed that all but Hits were significant predictors of group membership. Removing Hits from the predictor model, the following cutoff scores for each of the variables were obtained: False Alarm 21 or higher, Total score 72 or lower, and Delayed score less than 3. These cutoff scores correctly classified 70–74% of the sample, with specificity at 85–93%. Table 10–30 also presents the adjusted cutoff scores to obtain 100% positive predictive power. Given the findings from past studies, however, the authors cautioned against using the CVMT for assessing performance validity in older adults.

A CVMT symptom validity scale (CVMT SVT) has been derived by Larrabee (2009) based on a cross-validated known-group design using litigants meeting Slick et al. (1999) criteria for MND and contrasting with patients with moderate and severe TBI. The litigants performed significantly worse than chance on the Portland Digit Recognition Test. Items that showed significant differences between MND and TBI patients were identified using chi-square. The scale, which represents the number of correct responses over the 20 items, was cross-validated in a sample of neurologic and psychiatric patients. Table 10–31 presents data for the optimal cutoff score of less than 14 correct based on receiver operating characteristic (ROC) analysis. These results were comparable to that of stand-alone PVTs such as TOMM and WMT as reported by Greve and colleagues (2008). To obtain the CVMT Symptom Validity

TABLE 10–30 Optimal Cutoff Scores Based on Raw Scores to Identify Malingered Neurocognitive Dysfunction on the Continuous Visual Memory Test (CVMT)

	CUTOFF SCORE, 85–93% SPECIFICITY	CUTOFF SCORE, 100% SPECIFICITY
Total Score	≤72	<69
False Alarms	≥21	>22
Delayed Score	<3	<2

SOURCE: Henry and Enders (2007).

TABLE 10–31 Prediction of Malingered Neurocognitive Dysfunction in Two Clinical Samples for a Cutoff Score of <14 on the Continuous Visual Memory Test (CVMT) SVT

SAMPLE	AREA UNDER ROC CURVE	SENSITIVITY (%)	SPECIFICITY (%)	FALSE POSITIVE RATE (%)
Traumatic brain injury	.92	83	89	11
Neurologic/ psychiatric	.78	35	93	7

NOTE: ROC, Receiver Operating Characteristic.

SOURCE: Larrabee (2009).

Scale score, sum the number of correct responses for item numbers 19, 20, 23, 26, 30, 32, 37, 42, 50, 68, 75, 83, 88, 94, 97, 98, 107, 110, 111, and D7.

The CVMT SVT was also evaluated using a heterogeneous group of litigating TBI patients who failed or passed either TOMM or WMT (Krishnan & Donders, 2011). Invalid performance on the CVMT SVT was based on Larrabee's (2009) proposed cutoff score (<14 CVMT SVT correct responses). Lower CVMT SVT scores are associated with lower Total scores and Delayed scores, but the group differences between those who failed and passed the TOMM or WMT, although significant, were minimal. Those who failed the stand-alone PVTs were more likely to also fail the CVMT SVT using the proposed cutoff, although a number (5 out of 12) who failed the CVMT SVT did not fail either of the SVTs. As such, the authors suggested a lower cutoff score of less than 12, which yielded a better classification rate (Table 10–32). Only one potential false positive (i.e., failed CVMT SVT but passed both WMT/TOMM) was identified by this lower cutoff score. Given their findings, the authors caution against using CVMT SVT alone, but that its use along with stand-alone PVTs may improve diagnostic accuracy (Krishnan & Donders, 2011). However, it is noted that a criterion of single-PVT failure is not sufficient for validation of PVTs, and so the cutoffs provided by Henry and Enders (2007) and Larrabee (2009) may be preferred.

TABLE 10–32 Sensitivity and Specificity of Larrabee's (2009) Proposed Cutoff and Krishnan and Donders' (2011) Suggested Cutoff for the CVMT SVT

CVMT SVT CUTOFF	SENSITIVITY (%)	SPECIFICITY (%)	PPV (%)	NPV (%)	CLASSIFICATION RATE (%)
<14	42	93	42	94	88
<12	25	99	75	92	91

NOTE: Proposed cutoff <14 by Larrabee (2009); Suggested cutoff <12 by Krishnan and Donders (2011); PPV, positive predictive value; NPV, negative predictive value.

SOURCE: Krishnan and Donders (2011).

COMMENT

The CVMT offers a compelling way to assess visual memory in that it measures learning via the repetition of some items throughout the acquisition trial, unlike other visual memory tests with single-trial presentation of stimuli. It is also in a format that may be particularly useful for examinees who cannot draw or move objects because of physical limitations. The CVMT also appears useful as a measure of visual memory in specific adult patient populations such as TBI or CVA. In addition, unlike some other visual memory tests, it includes an embedded symptom validity scale that may help identify examinees who are not fully engaged in the task or attempting to exaggerate memory problems. Moreover, unlike many embedded PVTs and even fewer visual memory PVTs, it has been validated against multidimensional malingering criteria. Last, the computer version shows promise in enabling computer-based assessment of memory; further studies are needed to provide additional information about its psychometric properties and utility in clinical and older adult samples.

Users should be aware of the test's limitations. First, it is lengthy, and instructions may be too complicated for adults with significant impairments. Next, data on reliability appear limited. The test-retest reliability is based on a small sample, while the older adult data show poor reliability over long intervals.

The complex and ambiguous stimuli are purportedly difficult to encode verbally; however, research is conflicting in this regard. The CVMT appears to measure other cognitive aspects outside of visual memory, including attention and speed. Evidence that it taps hippocampal functions has not been established in TLE with unilateral mesial temporal sclerosis, while neuroimaging suggests a frontal component—although the latter is not unique among memory tests. The adequacy of the CVMT's recognition format in the assessment of memory disorders is brought into question as free recall procedures tend to be superior to recognition formats for detection of memory deficits. However, the test may be an adequate memory screen in populations where memory deficits are not a critical question.

The high rate of misclassification at older ages consistently reported in studies also raises concern about its use in older adults, and studies using the revised cutoff scores generated from the updated normative data have not been conducted. Finally, the CVMT would benefit from more independent validity studies in clinical samples, as well as studies examining practice effects, ways to measure change, and treatment sensitivity. Until such data are available, clinicians are advised to use the CVMT with caution in assessments where precise assessment of memory is necessary (e.g., dementia, TLE).

REFERENCES

Baños, H. J., Dickson, A. L., & Greer, T. (2001). A computer-assisted administration of the Continuous Visual Memory Test. *The Clinical Neuropsychologist, 15*(4), 551–555.

Greve, K. W., Ord, J., Curtis, K. L., Bianchini, K. J., & Brennan, A. (2008). Detecting malingering in traumatic brain injury and chronic pain: A comparison of three forced-choice symptom validity tests. *The Clinical Neuropsychologist, 22*(5), 896–918.

Hall, S., Pinkston, S. L., Szalda-Petree, A. C., & Coronis, A. R. (1996). The performance of healthy older adults on the Continuous Visual Memory Test and the Visual-Motor Integration Test: Preliminary findings. *Journal of Clinical Psychology, 52*(4), 449–454.

Henry, G. K., & Enders, C. (2007). Probable malingering and performance on the Continuous Visual Memory Test. *Applied Neuropsychology, 14*(4), 267–274.

Krishnan, M., & Donders, J. (2011). Embedded assessment of validity using the Continuous Visual Memory Test in patients with traumatic brain injury. *Archives of Clinical Neuropsychology, 26*(3), 176–183.

Larrabee, G. J. (2009). Malingering scales for the Continuous Recognition Memory Test and the Continuous Visual Memory Test. *The Clinical Neuropsychologist, 23*(1), 167–180.

Larrabee, G. J., Trahan, D. E., & Curtiss, G. (1992). Construct validity of the continuous visual memory test. *Archives of Clinical Neuropsychology, 7*(5), 395–405.

Mattis, S. (1988). *Dementia Rating Scale*. Odessa, FL: Psychological Assessment Resources.

Paolo, A. M., Tröster, A. I., & Ryan, J. J. (1998a). Continuous Visual Memory Test performance in healthy persons 60 to 94 years of age. *Archives of Clinical Neuropsychology, 13*(4), 333–337.

Paolo, A. M., Tröster, A. I., & Ryan, J. J. (1998b). Test-retest stability of the Continuous Visual Memory Test in elderly persons. *Archives of Clinical Neuropsychology, 13*(7), 617–621.

Retzlaff, P. D., & Morris, G. L. (1996). Event-related potentials during the Continuous Visual Memory Test. *Journal of Clinical Psychology, 52*(1), 43–47.

Slick, D. J., Sherman, E. M., & Iverson, G. L. (1999). Diagnostic criteria for malingered neurocognitive dysfunction: Proposed standards for clinical practice and research. *The Clinical Neuropsychologist, 13*(4), 545–561.

Snitz, B. E., Roman, D. D., & Beniak, T. E. (1996). Efficacy of the Continuous Visual Memory Test in lateralizing temporal lobe dysfunction in chronic complex-partial epilepsy. *Journal of Clinical and Experimental Neuropsychology, 18*(5), 747–754.

Strong, C. A. H., & Donders, J. (2008). Validity of the Continuous Visual Memory Test (CVMT) after traumatic brain injury. *Journal of Clinical and Experimental Neuropsychology, 30*(8), 885–891.

Trahan, D. E., & Larrabee, G. J. (1988). *Continuous Visual Memory Test.* Lutz, FL: Psychological Assessment Resources.

Trahan, D. E., Larrabee, G. J., Fritzsche, B., & Curtiss, G. (1996). Continuous Visual Memory Test: Alternate form and generalizability estimates. *The Clinical Neuropsychologist, 10*(1), 73–79.

Trahan, D. E., Larrabee, G. J., & Psychological Assessment Resources. (1997). *Continuous Visual Memory Test: Supplemental normative data for children and older adults.* Lutz, FL: Psychological Assessment Resources.

Trahan, D. E., Larrabee, G. J., & Quintana, J. W. (1990). Visual recognition memory in normal adults and patients with unilateral vascular lesions. *Journal of Clinical and Experimental Neuropsychology, 12*(6), 857–872.

Trahan, D. E., & Quintana, J. W. (1990). Analysis of gender effects upon verbal and visual memory performance in adults. *Archives of Clinical Neuropsychology, 5*(4), 325–334.

HOPKINS VERBAL LEARNING TEST—REVISED (HVLT-R)

TEST NAME	**Hopkins Verbal Learning Test—Revised (HVLT-R)**
DOMAIN	Verbal memory
AGE RANGE	In adults, to 92 years
ADMINISTRATION TIME	15 minutes plus 20- to 25-minute delay interval
SCORING FORMAT	Hand scored
REFERENCE	Brandt, J., & Benedict, R. H. B. (2001). *Hopkins Verbal Learning Test–Revised.* Odessa, FL: Psychological Assessment Resources. www.parinc.com

DESCRIPTION

The Hopkins Verbal Learning Test—Revised (HVLT-R) is used to provide a brief assessment of verbal learning and memory. The original version, the HVLT, was published by Brandt in 1991. It is identical to the HVLT-R, except that the original version had no Delayed Recall trial and the Recognition trial was given immediately after the three learning trials. The test was modeled after other word-list learning tasks (e.g., RAVLT, CVLT), but the list was shorter. When the Delayed Recall trial was introduced, the modified test was named the HVLT-R.

Devised by Brandt and Benedict (2001), the HVLT-R was designed to be methodologically similar to the BVMT-R (Benedict, 1997; see the review of the BVMT-R elsewhere in this chapter). Because it has few learning trials and a relatively short list of words, it was intended to be suitable for even moderately demented patients. It comprises six alternate forms, each consisting of a list of 12 nouns with four words drawn from each of three semantic categories (e.g., four-legged animals, precious stones, human dwellings). The semantic categories differ across the six forms. The HVLT-R includes three learning trials, a delayed recall trial (given without forewarning after a delay of 20–25 min), and a yes/no delayed recognition trial. This last trial consists of a randomized list of 12 target and 12 nontarget words, six of which are drawn from the same semantic categories as the targets. Because of the availability of six alternate forms, the HVLT-R is suitable for repeat testing.

ADMINISTRATION

See the manual. Briefly, the examiner reads the word list and asks the examinee to verbally repeat the list of words (immediately and after a 20- to 25-minute delay) in any order and to identify the words from a list that is presented orally. The interstimulus interval is 2 seconds. Recall performance is recorded verbatim on a scoring sheet for each of the immediate recall trials (Trials 1–3) and for the delayed recall and recognition trials. Examinees are not warned that delayed recall will be tested later. For selection of alternate forms when repeat testing is needed, see the section "Reliability."

A slightly modified administration, which allows derivation of cued-recall and learning scores, has also been used in older African Americans (Friedman et al., 2002; also see "Normative Data").

SCORING

Minor errors in pronunciation (e.g., "cimmonim" for "cinnamon") or pluralization (e.g., "rubies" for "ruby") are corrected and counted as correct. The maximum total for each recall trial (Learning Trials 1–3, Delayed Recall Trial 4) is 12. The recall scores are combined to form three additional measures of learning and memory. The Total Recall score is the sum of Learning Trials 1 to 3. The percentage retained after the delay (% Retention) is calculated as Trial 4 recall divided by the best of Trials 2 and 3 (×100). Finally, the Recognition Discrimination Index is the number of true positives minus the number of false positives on the Recognition Trial.

Raw scores for four HVLT-R measures (Total Recall, Delayed Recall, % Retention, and the Recognition Discrimination Index) are converted to T scores using age-based tables provided in the test manual. These four variables constitute the primary measures for the test. Four other scores are recorded on the score sheet: total number of true-positive hits, semantically related false-positive errors, semantically unrelated false-positive errors, and total number of false-positive errors.

A number of process scores have been reported in the literature. The traditional learning score is calculated by subtracting the Trial 1 score from the higher of Trial 2 or 3 and then age-corrected into a z score using norms provided by Benedict et al. (1998).

Cumulative Word Learning (CWL) is calculated by multiplying the traditional learning z score by the total number of words recalled across all learning trials. CWL may be more sensitive to mild memory changes than the traditional score (Foster et al., 2009).

The Semantic Clustering Ratio (SCR) is calculated by adding the number of times a correct word recalled is followed by another correct word from a similar category divided by the total number of correctly recalled words in the same trial (Gaines et al., 2006).

DEMOGRAPHIC EFFECTS

AGE

The test authors report that age has the largest effect on every variable, accounting for a high of 19% of the variance on Total Recall and a low of 3% on % Retention. Age effects were also reported in a large sample from Latin America (Arango-Lasprilla et al., 2015) as well as a sample of Spanish-speaking older adults from Spain (Gonzalez-Palau et al., 2013).

GENDER

No gender differences were found in an adolescent sample (Barr, 2003), in an Australian sample of older adults (Hester et al., 2004), in a Brazilian sample (Miotto et al., 2012), and in a large sample from 11 Latin-American countries except for a Guatemalan sample (Arango-Lasprilla et al., 2015). By contrast, in community-dwelling older African Americans (Friedman et al., 2002) and in Caucasians (Vanderploeg et al., 2000), gender was found to account for modest amounts of test score variance (<10%) in addition to other variables (age, education). According to Vanderploeg et al. (2000), women tended to outperform men by about three points on Total Recall. Brandt and Benedict (2001) report that, in adults, gender makes a statistically significant contribution to every variable. However, it accounts, at most, for only 2% of the remaining variance (on Total Recall).

EDUCATION AND IQ

According to the test authors, education (highest grade completed) accounts for an additional 5% of the remaining variance on Total Recall (beyond age) and less on the other variables. Others (Arango-Lasprilla et al., 2015; Friedman et al., 2002; Hester et al., 2004; Miotto et al., 2012) have also reported that education has a significant impact on test scores. However, Vanderploeg et al. (2000) found that educational attainment did not affect HVLT-R performance in a predominantly white, community-dwelling sample. IQ affected recall but not Recognition Discrimination scores (Diaz-Asper et al., 2004). Correlations between Total Recall and VIQ ($r = .52$) and PIQ ($r = .49$) are moderate in size.

ETHNICITY, NATIONALITY, AND LINGUISTIC EFFECTS

The normative sample was predominantly Caucasian (J. Brandt, personal communication, February 18, 2005), and the impact of ethnicity is not reported.

NORMATIVE DATA

STANDARDIZATION SAMPLE

The description of the standardization sample is provided in Table 10–33. The sample included 1,179 community-dwelling individuals who reported being free of neurological or psychiatric disorders. Their ages ranged from 16 to 92 years, with a mean age of 59 years (SD = 18.62). They had between two and 20 years of education, with a mean of 13.47 years (SD = 2.88). The majority (n = 798) were also given the MMSE, and their scores ranged from 22 to 30 (M = 28.31, SD = +1.65). Note that the inclusion of individuals with MMSE scores as low as 22 raises the concern that some cognitively compromised individuals may have been included in the normative base (G. Larrabee, personal communication, June 16, 2004). Race/ethnicity of participants was not reported.

As part of their participation in six different research protocols, healthy respondents were given one form of the HVLT-R. Normative data, subdivided according to age, are provided in the manual for use with any of the six forms. Normative tables were constructed using the method of overlapping-midpoint age cells. The authors note that, for most age groups, the distributions of the four primary scores (Total Recall, Delayed Recall, % Retention, and Recognition Discrimination Index) are restricted in range or significantly skewed or both. There are ceiling effects for some variables (e.g., Delayed Recall, Recognition), especially for the younger age groups. Accordingly, the authors recommend caution in assigning T scores in these cases. Rather, it may be more appropriate to report either T-score ranges (e.g., "T ≥70") or descriptive categories (e.g., "recognition discrimination was errorless") in these instances.

Means and SDs for a variety of other scores, including each of the three learning trials, total number of true-positive

TABLE 10–33 Characteristics of the Hopkins Verbal Learning Test—Revised (HVLT-R) Standardization Sample

Sample size	1,179
Age	16 to 92[a] years
Sample type	Standardization sample
Geographical location	Not reported
Education	2 to 20 years (M = 13.47, SD = 2.88)
Gender	75% Women 25% Men
Ethnicity	Not reported[b]
Screening	Self-reported as being free of neurological and psychiatric disorders

[a]Broken down into 13 age groups using the method of overlapping cells: (16–19, 20–29, 25–34, 30–39, 35–44, 45–54, 50–59, 55–64, 60–69, 65–74, 70–79, 75–84, and 80+ years).

[b]Predominantly Caucasian (J. Brandt, personal communication, February 18, 2005).

SOURCE: Adapted from Brandt and Benedict (2001). Reproduced by special permission of the Publisher, Psychological Assessment Resources, Inc. (PAR), 16204 North Florida Avenue, Lutz, Florida 33549, from the Hopkins Verbal Learning Test-Revised by Jason Brandt, PhD and Ralph H. B. Benedict, PhD, Copyright 1991, 1998, 2001 by PAR. Further reproduction is prohibited without permission from PAR.

TABLE 10–34 Characteristics of the Hopkins Verbal Learning Test—Revised (HVLT-R) Normative Sample from the Calibrated Neuropsychological Normative System (CNNS)

Sample size	327
Age	18 to 92 years
Geographic location	Baltimore, MD, and Hartford, CT
Sample type	Community sample
Education	14.2 (*SD* = 3.0), range 3 to 20 years
Gender	56% Women 44% Men
Ethnicity	80% Caucasian 18% African American 2% Hispanic, Asian, or Other
Screening	History of Alzheimer's disease, Parkinson's disease, stroke, brain injury, bipolar disorder, or substance abuse

SOURCE: Adapted from Schretlen et al. (2010). Reproduced by special permission of the Publisher, Psychological Assessment Resources, Inc. (PAR), 16204 North Florida Avenue, Lutz, Florida 33549, from the Calibrated Neuropsychological Normative System, by David J. Schretlen, PhD, ABPP, S Marc Testa, PhD and Godfrey D. Pearlson, MD, Copyright 2010 by PAR. Further reproduction is prohibited without permission from PAR.

hits, semantically related false-positive errors, and semantically unrelated false-positive errors, are provided in the test manual and are stratified by age group.

OTHER NORMATIVE DATA

Schretlen, Testa, and Pearlson (2010) provide norms for 327 adults on the HVLT-R; these use the CNNS scoring to derive T scores and discrepancies based on a large sample of older adults from the northeastern United States. Characteristics of the normative sample are shown in Table 10–34. The norms are available through PAR (www.parinc.com). A major advantage of these norms is the option to correct for demographic variables such as age, sex, education, and ethnicity. Several other commonly used neuropsychological tests are co-normed using this sample, which facilitates cross-test comparisons.

Vanderploeg et al. (2000) provided age- and gender-adjusted normative data based on a community-dwelling sample of 394 older adults (aged 60 to 84, mean education = 14.1 years) in Florida. Hester et al. (2004) provided age- and education-adjusted normative data for 203 older Australian adults (91 males, 112 females), aged 60 to 89 years. Comparison between the Florida and Australian samples indicates a generally comparable profile of performance, although scores were slightly lower than those reported by Brandt and Benedict (2001). The Australian sample had a lower level of education (M = 11.07 years, SD = 3.10), and therefore this study extends the clinical utility of the HVLT-R to those with lower levels of education. Participants with a history of psychiatric illness, neurological disorder, or drug abuse were excluded, as were those who were not fluent in English or who had an MMSE score of less than 25. The data for Form 1 are shown in Table 10–35. Note, however, that the cell sizes are quite small, particularly for the oldest age group (80–89 years).

For older African Americans, the data provided by Friedman et al. (2002) are preferred. These authors tested a population-based sample of 237 healthy African-American individuals (108 men, 129 women), living in Tampa, Florida, for Form 1 of the HVLT-R. Individuals who self-reported a history of neurological disorder were excluded from study. The data were stratified by age (60–71 years, n = 111; 72–80 years, n = 126), and score adjustments were given for education (<12 years, 12 years, >12 years) and gender. In addition to providing data on the standard indices, they also reported data for the Delayed Cued Recall and Learning measures. After Delayed Free Recall, examinees were given memory cues and asked, one subcategory at a time, to recall all words from the subcategories. The Learning measure is calculated as the higher of Trial 2 or Trial 3 recall, minus Trial 1 recall. The data are provided in Tables 10–36 (ages 60–71) and 10–37 (ages 72–84). Raw score adjustments (Table 10–38) are applied for the

TABLE 10–35 Normative Data for Hopkins Verbal Learning Test—Revised (HVLT-R) Performance of an Australian Sample, Subdivided by Education

	AGE 60 TO 69 YEARS						AGE 70 TO 79 YEARS						AGE 80 TO 89 YEARS					
	≤10			≥11			≤10			≥11			≤10			≥11		
MEASURE	*N*	*M*	*SD*	*N*	*M*	*SD*	*N*	*M*	*SD*	*N*	*M*	*SD*	*N*	*M*	*SD*	*N*	*M*	*SD*
Trial 1	29	5.2	1.5	35	6.4	1.7	63	4.7	1.9	45	5.3	1.5	15	4.2	1.5	16	5.1	1.3
Trial 2	29	6.7	2.2	35	8.5	2.0	63	6.8	2.0	45	6.7	1.9	15	6.1	1.8	16	7.4	1.6
Trial 3	29	8.1	2.3	35	9.8	1.6	63	7.8	2.5	45	8.2	2.0	15	7.1	2.5	16	8.6	2.1
Learning	29	2.9	1.8	35	3.5	1.5	63	3.2	1.8	45	3.1	1.8	15	3.2	1.6	16	3.8	1.3
Total	29	20.0	5.5	35	24.6	4.8	63	19.4	5.8	45	20.2	4.6	15	17.4	5.2	16	21.1	4.6
Delayed Recall	16	6.3	3.3	25	8.4	2.9	43	6.4	3.5	32	7.3	2.7	10	5.4	3.1	10	5.4	2.6
% Retention	16	73.7	34.8	25	82.9	23.3	43	80.4	36.3	32	83.6	23.9	10	78.3	48.8	10	57.9	23.6
Discrimination Index	16	8.4	2.3	25	9.9	1.8	43	8.9	2.2	32	9.4	2.0	10	9.0	2.3	10	8.6	3.1

SOURCE: Adapted from Hester et al. (2004).

TABLE 10–36 Normative Data for Hopkins Verbal Learning Test—Revised (HVLT-R) Performance for African-American Individuals 60–71 Years of Age

	CUMULATIVE PERCENTILE										
RAW SCORE	TRIAL 1	TRIAL 2	TRIAL 3	LEARNING	SUM (TRIALS 1–3)	DELAYED RECALL	CUED RECALL	TRUE POSITIVES	FALSE POSITIVES[a]	DISCRIMINATION	% RETENTION PERCENTILE
30					99						
29											
28											
27					97						
26					96						
25					96						
24					94						
23					90						
22					86						
21					79						
20					72						
19					61						
18					52						
17					38						
16					26						
15					16						
14					7						
13					5						
12					1		99			87	
11		99	98		<1	99	98			63	
10		98	95			96	95			47	
9		95	83			87	78			32	
8	97	88	64			72	59	44		16	
7	92	60	32			50	32	27		7	
6	84	29	9	99		29	14	15		2	
5	59	5	1	95		8	3	5		1	
4	23	<5	<1	74		2	1	1	95	<1	
3	5			38		<2	<1	<1	79		
2	<5			7					48		
1				2					15		
0				<2					<15		
% Retention											
140											99
117											96
114											95
113											93
111											91
100											53
89											51
88											45
86											30
83											21
82											20
80											16
78											14
71											9
67											5
63											3
50											<3
Mean	4.4	6.3	7.2	2.9	17.9	6.6	7.2	11.1	1.6	9.4	90.5
SD	1.3	1.3	1.4	1.1	3.5	1.6	1.6	1.3	1.1	1.9	15.0
Range	2–8	4–11	4–11	0–6	11–30	3–11	3–12	7–12	0–4	3–12	50–140

[a]Related false positives only. In this sample, there was only one unrelated false-positive response across groups. False positives are reversed scored; more false positives is an indication of poor performance.

SOURCE: From Friedman et al. (2002).

TABLE 10–37 Normative Data for Hopkins Verbal Learning Test—Revised (HVLT-R) Performance for African-American Individuals 72–84 Years of Age

	CUMULATIVE PERCENTILE										
RAW SCORE	TRIAL 1	TRIAL 2	TRIAL 3	LEARNING	SUM (TRIALS 1–3)	DELAYED RECALL	CUED RECALL	TRUE POSITIVES	FALSE POSITIVES[a]	DISCRIMINATION	% RETENTION PERCENTILE
28					99						
27											
26											
25					98						
24					96						
23					94						
22					90						
21					85						
20					81						
19					75						
18					70						
17					64						
16					57						
15					44						
14					29						
13					25						
12					21			55		89	
11			99		14		98	47		71	
10			96		8	98	96	38		60	
9		98	90		5	88	81	26		48	
8	98	91	78		2	79	69	13		37	
7	95	75	53		<2	65	52	5		25	
6	84	60	33			47	33	2	99	17	
5	75	29	15	97		27	18	1	98	10	
4	48	9	4	79		14	8	<1	90	5	
3	18	2	<4	39		6	2		71	2	
2	2	<2		17		1	<2		45	1	
1	2			3		<1			20	<1	
0	<2			2					<20		
−1				1							
−2				<1							
% Retention											
133											99
129											98
125											97
114											96
113											94
100											53
91											52
90											51
89											49
88											44
86											34
83											23
80											17
75											12
71											11
67											9
60											6
50											2
40											2
29											1
17											<1
Mean	3.8	5.4	6.3	1.2	15.5	5.8	6.4	10.1	1.8	8.4	88.8
SD	1.5	1.5	1.7	2.6	4.3	2	2	2.1	1.3	2.7	17.9
Range	0–8	2–9	3–11	−2–5	7–28	1–10	2–11	4–12	0–6	0–12	17–133

[a] Related false positives only. In this sample, there was only one unrelated false-positive response across groups. False Positives are reverse scored; more false positives is an indication of poor performance.

SOURCE: From Friedman et al. (2002).

TABLE 10–38 Education and Gender Adjustments to Hopkins Verbal Learning Test—Revised (HVLT-R) Raw Scores to Estimate Education and Gender-Based Level of Performance for Friedman et al. (2002) Norms

HVLT-R INDEX	EDUCATION (YEARS)	AGE 60 TO 71 YEARS MALE	AGE 60 TO 71 YEARS FEMALE	AGE 72 TO 84 YEARS MALE	AGE 72 TO 84 YEARS FEMALE
Trial 1	<12	0	0	1	0
	12	0	0	0	−1
	>12	−1	−1	−1	−1
Trial 2	<12	0	0	1	0
	12	0	−1	1	−1
	>12	0	−1	1	−1
Trial 3	<12	0	0	1	0
	12	0	−1	1	−2
	>12	0	−1	0	−1
Learning	<12	0	0	0	0
	12	0	0	1	0
	>12	1	0	2	0
Sum of Trials 1–3	<12	1	1	2	−1
	12	1	−2	1	−5
	>12	0	−4	0	−3
Delayed Recall	<12	0	0	1	0
	12	1	−1	1	−2
	>12	1	−1	3	0
Cued Recall	<12	0	0	1	0
	12	1	0	0	−2
	>12	0	−1	0	−1
% Retention	<12	−1	−2	0	−1
	12	5	−5	8	−8
	>12	10	6	39	17
True Positives	<12	0	0	0	0
	12	0	0	1	−2
	>12	0	0	−1	−1
False Positives[a]	<12	0	0	−1	0
	12	0	0	1	0
	>12	0	1	0	1
Discrimination Index	<12	1	0	1	0
	12	0	0	0	−3
	>12	0	−1	−1	−2

NOTE: The values in the table can be added to or subtracted from a raw score before looking up level of performance information in Tables 10–36 and 10–37. This would result in an education- and gender-adjusted score.

[a] Correction provided applies only to the Related False Positive score.

SOURCE: From Friedman et al. (2002).

effects of education and gender before the standardized performance associated with the score is obtained.

Users should bear in mind, however, that the number of participants with greater than 12 years of education was relatively small (n = 39), possibly affecting the reliability and generalizability of the normative values in this education group. Furthermore, only Form 1 was used, and the version differed from the standard protocol in that a cued-recall trial was included between the Delayed Free Recall and the Delayed Recognition trials. Therefore, recognition data with this version are not comparable to scores from the standard administration.

TABLE 10–39 Performance by 100 High School Athletes on the Hopkins Verbal Learning Test—Revised (HVLT-R)

VARIABLE	MEAN	SD
Total Recall (Trials 1–3)	25.8	4.8
Delayed Recall	9.4	1.9
Recognition Discrimination Index	11.7	0.7

NOTE: There were no gender differences.

SOURCE: Adapted from Barr (2003).

Barr (2003) tested a group of 100 high school athletes (60 males, 40 females; aged 13–17 years, M = 15.9, SD = .98). The ethnic composition of the sample was 88% Caucasian. All spoke English as their native language and were in good academic standing at their school. Three reported a history of ADHD, and three reported a history of dyslexia or learning disability. Means and *SDs* are shown in Table 10–39. Performance appeared comparable to that of adults.

Arango-Lasprilla et al. (2015) provide norms for 18- to 95-year-old, native Spanish-speaking adults from 11 Latin-American countries (Tables 10–40 to 10–50). Only Form 5 of the HVLT-R was administered. To be included in the normative sample, participants were native to the country where testing took place and had at least one year of formal education and the ability to read and write. All participants obtained MMSE scores of 23 or more, Patient Health Questionnaire (PHQ-9) scores of 4 or less, and 90 or more on the Barthel Index. Participants were excluded if they self-reported neurologic or psychiatric disorders. Note that the norms were generated using regression models that included age and education and/or gender. Given strong impact of age and education, users should use age- and education-adjusted norms for each country except on Delayed Recall for Bolivia (Table 10–41), where the impact of education was minimal.

Miotto et al. (2012) provide Brazilian co-normed data for Form 1 of the HVLT-R and BVMT-R for adults aged 18 to 85 years whose education spanned from 0 to 17 years. Table 10–51 presents the norms for ages 18 to 80+. Please refer to the BVMT-R review elsewhere in this chapter for BVMT-R norms. Users should be aware that some cell sizes are extremely small and should not be used for clinical decision making.

EVIDENCE FOR RELIABILITY

EVIDENCE FOR INTERNAL RELIABILITY

Not reported.

EVIDENCE FOR TEST-RETEST RELIABILITY, MEASURING CHANGE, AND PRACTICE EFFECTS

Benedict et al. (1998) reported that 40 older adults completed different forms of the test on two occasions, with a mean test-retest interval of six weeks. Reliability coefficients for the four primary HVLT-R variables were at least marginal for Total Recall and Delayed Recall and poor for %

TABLE 10–40 Norms for Hopkins Verbal Learning Test—Revised (HVLT-R) Total and Delayed Recall as a Function of Age and Education Levels for Argentina

EDUCATION (YEARS)	PERCENTILE	AGE (YEARS) 18–22		23–27		28–32		33–37		38–42		43–47	
>12		TR	DR	TR	DR	TR	DR	TR	DR	TR	DR	TR	DR
	95	34.6	–	34.3	–	33.9	–	33.6	–	33.2	–	32.9	12.0
	80	31.1	12.0	30.8	11.8	30.4	11.6	30.1	11.4	29.7	11.2	29.4	11.0
	50	27.5	10.4	27.1	10.1	26.8	9.9	26.4	9.7	26.1	9.5	25.7	9.3
	20	23.8	8.6	23.5	8.4	23.1	8.2	22.8	8.0	22.4	7.8	22.1	7.6
	10	21.9	7.8	21.6	7.5	21.2	7.3	20.9	7.1	20.5	6.9	20.2	6.7
	5	20.3	7.0	20.0	6.8	19.6	6.6	19.3	6.4	18.9	6.2	18.6	6.0
≤12		TR	DR	TR	DR	TR	DR	TR	DR	TR	DR	TR	DR
	95	31.9	12.0	31.5	12.0	31.2	11.7	30.8	11.5	30.5	11.3	30.1	11.1
	80	28.4	10.5	28.0	10.3	27.7	10.1	27.3	9.9	27.0	9.7	26.6	9.5
	50	24.7	8.8	24.4	8.6	24.0	8.4	23.7	8.2	23.3	8.0	23.0	7.8
	20	21.1	7.1	20.7	6.9	20.4	6.7	20.0	6.5	19.7	6.3	19.3	6.1
	10	19.1	6.2	18.8	6.0	18.4	5.8	18.1	5.6	17.8	5.4	17.4	5.2
	5	17.6	5.5	17.2	5.3	16.9	5.1	16.5	4.9	16.2	4.7	15.8	4.4

EDUCATION (YEARS)	PERCENTILE	AGE (YEARS) 48–52		53–57		58–62		63–67		68–72		73–77		>77	
>12		TR	DR	TR	DR	TR	DR	TR	DR	TR	DR	TR	DR	TR	DR
	95	32.5	12.0	32.2	12.0	31.8	12.0	31.5	11.8	31.1	11.6	30.8	11.3	30.4	11.1
	80	29.1	10.8	28.7	10.6	28.4	10.4	28.0	10.1	27.7	9.9	27.3	9.7	27.0	9.5
	50	25.4	9.1	25.0	8.9	24.7	8.7	24.3	8.4	24.0	8.2	23.7	8.0	23.3	7.8
	20	21.7	7.4	21.4	7.2	21.0	6.9	20.7	6.7	20.3	6.5	20.0	6.3	19.6	6.1
	10	19.8	6.5	19.5	6.3	19.1	6.1	18.8	5.8	18.4	5.6	18.1	5.4	17.7	5.2
	5	18.3	5.8	17.9	5.5	17.6	5.3	17.2	5.1	16.9	4.9	16.5	4.7	16.2	4.5
≤12		TR	DR	TR	DR	TR	DR	TR	DR	TR	DR	TR	DR	TR	DR
	95	29.8	10.9	29.4	10.7	29.1	10.5	28.7	10.3	28.4	10.0	28.0	9.8	27.7	9.6
	80	26.3	9.3	25.9	9.1	25.6	8.8	25.2	8.6	24.9	8.4	24.5	8.2	24.2	8.0
	50	22.6	7.6	22.3	7.4	21.9	7.1	21.6	6.9	21.2	6.7	20.9	6.5	20.5	6.3
	20	19.0	5.9	18.6	5.6	18.3	5.4	17.9	5.2	17.6	5.0	17.2	4.8	16.9	4.6
	10	17.1	5.0	16.7	4.8	16.4	4.5	16.0	4.3	15.7	4.1	15.3	3.9	15.0	3.7
	5	15.5	4.2	15.1	4.0	14.8	3.8	14.4	3.6	14.1	3.4	13.7	3.2	13.4	3.0

NOTE: TR, Total Recall; DR, Delayed Recall.

SOURCE: Adapted from Arango-Lasprilla et al. (2015).

TABLE 10–41 Norms for Hopkins Verbal Learning Test—Revised (HVLT-R) Total and Delayed Recall as a Function of Age and Education Levels for Bolivia

EDUCATION (YEARS)	PERCENTILE	AGE (YEARS) 18–22		23–27		28–32		33–37		38–42		43–47	
>12		TR	DR	TR	DR	TR	DR	TR	DR	TR	DR	TR	DR
	95	32.5	12.0	31.9	12.0	31.4	11.8	30.8	11.4	30.3	11.1	29.7	10.8
	80	29.1	10.5	28.6	10.1	28.0	9.8	27.4	9.5	26.9	9.2	26.3	8.8
	50	25.6	8.4	25.0	8.1	24.5	7.8	23.9	7.4	23.3	7.1	22.8	6.8
	20	22.0	6.4	21.5	6.0	20.9	5.7	20.4	5.4	19.8	5.1	19.2	4.8
	10	20.2	5.3	19.6	5.0	19.1	4.6	18.5	4.3	18.0	4.0	17.4	3.7
	5	18.7	4.4	18.1	4.1	17.6	3.8	17.0	3.4	16.4	3.1	15.9	2.8
≤12*		TR		TR		TR		TR		TR		TR	
	95	29.2		28.7		28.1		27.5		27.0		26.4	
	80	25.9		25.3		24.7		24.2		23.6		23.1	
	50	22.3		21.8		21.2		20.6		20.1		19.5	
	20	18.8		18.2		17.7		17.1		16.5		16.0	
	10	16.9		16.4		15.8		15.2		14.7		14.1	
	5	15.4		14.8		14.3		13.7		13.2		12.6	

TABLE 10–41 Continued

EDUCATION (YEARS)		AGE (YEARS)													
		48–52		53–57		58–62		63–67		68–72		73–77		>77	
>12	PERCENTILE	TR	DR	TR	DR	TR	DR	TR	DR	TR	DR	TR	DR	TR	DR
	95	29.1	10.5	28.6	10.2	28.0	9.8	27.5	9.5	26.9	9.2	26.3	8.9	25.8	8.5
	80	25.8	8.5	25.2	8.2	24.6	7.9	24.1	7.6	23.5	7.2	23.0	6.9	22.4	6.6
	50	22.2	6.5	21.7	6.2	21.1	5.8	20.5	5.5	20.0	5.2	19.4	4.9	18.9	4.5
	20	18.7	4.4	18.1	4.1	17.6	3.8	17.0	3.5	16.4	3.1	15.9	2.8	15.3	2.5
	10	16.8	3.4	16.3	3.0	15.7	2.7	15.2	2.4	14.6	2.1	14.0	1.7	13.5	1.4
	5	15.3	2.5	14.8	2.2	14.2	1.8	13.6	1.5	13.1	1.2	12.5	0.9	12.0	0.5
≤12		TR		TR		TR		TR		TR		TR		TR	
	95	25.9		25.3		24.8		24.2		23.6		23.1		22.5	
	80	22.5		21.9		21.4		20.8		20.3		19.7		19.1	
	50	19.0		18.4		17.8		17.3		16.7		16.2		15.6	
	20	15.4		14.9		14.3		13.7		13.2		12.6		12.1	
	10	13.6		13.0		12.4		11.9		11.3		10.8		10.0	
	5	12.1		11.5		10.9		10.4		9.8		9.3		8.7	

NOTE: TR, Total Recall; DR, Delayed Recall. *Use the >12 years education DR norms regardless of education.

SOURCE: Adapted from Arango-Lasprilla et al. (2015).

TABLE 10–42 Norms for Hopkins Verbal Learning Test—Revised (HVLT-R) Total and Delayed Recall as a Function of Age and Education Levels for Chile

EDUCATION (YEARS)		AGE (YEARS)											
		18–22		23–27		28–32		33–37		38–42		43–47	
>12	PERCENTILE	TR	DR	TR	DR	TR	DR	TR	DR	TR	DR	TR	DR
	95	35.9	–	35.2	–	34.5	–	33.9	–	33.2	–	32.5	12.0
	80	32.1	12.0	31.4	12.0	30.7	11.9	30.1	11.5	29.4	11.2	28.8	10.8
	50	28.1	10.6	27.4	10.3	26.8	9.9	26.1	9.6	25.4	9.2	24.8	8.9
	20	24.1	8.7	23.4	8.3	22.8	8.0	22.1	7.6	21.5	7.3	20.8	6.9
	10	22.0	7.6	21.4	7.3	20.7	6.9	20.0	6.6	19.4	6.3	18.7	5.9
	5	20.3	6.8	19.7	6.5	19.0	6.1	18.3	5.8	17.7	5.4	17.0	5.1
≤12		TR	DR	TR	DR	TR	DR	TR	DR	TR	DR	TR	DR
	95	31.7	–	31.1	12.0	30.4	12.0	29.7	12.0	29.1	11.7	28.4	11.4
	80	27.9	11.3	27.3	10.9	26.6	10.6	25.9	10.2	25.3	9.9	24.6	9.5
	50	23.9	9.3	23.3	9.0	22.6	8.6	22.0	8.3	21.3	7.9	20.6	7.6
	20	20.0	7.4	19.3	7.0	18.6	6.7	18.0	6.3	17.3	6.0	16.7	5.7
	10	17.9	6.4	17.2	6.0	16.6	5.7	15.9	5.3	15.2	5.0	14.6	4.6
	5	16.2	5.5	15.5	5.2	14.9	4.8	14.2	4.5	13.5	4.2	12.9	3.8

EDUCATION (YEARS)		AGE (YEARS)													
		48–52		53–57		58–62		63–67		68–72		73–77		>77	
>12	PERCENTILE	TR	DR	TR	DR	TR	DR	TR	DR	TR	DR	TR	DR	TR	DR
	95	31.9	12.0	31.2	12.0	30.6	11.6	29.9	11.3	29.2	10.9	28.6	10.6	27.9	10.3
	80	28.1	10.5	27.4	10.1	26.8	9.8	26.1	9.4	25.5	9.1	24.8	8.7	24.1	8.4
	50	24.1	8.5	23.5	8.2	22.8	7.8	22.1	7.5	21.5	7.1	20.8	6.8	20.1	6.5
	20	20.1	6.6	19.5	6.2	18.8	5.9	18.2	5.5	17.5	5.2	16.8	4.9	16.2	4.5
	10	18.1	5.6	17.4	5.2	16.7	4.9	16.1	4.5	15.4	4.2	14.7	3.8	14.1	3.5
	5	16.3	4.7	15.7	4.4	15.0	4.0	14.4	3.7	13.7	3.4	13.0	3.0	12.4	2.7
≤12		TR	DR	TR	DR	TR	DR	TR	DR	TR	DR	TR	DR	TR	DR
	95	27.7	11.1	27.1	10.7	26.4	10.4	25.8	10.0	25.1	9.7	24.4	9.3	23.8	9.0
	80	24.0	9.2	23.3	8.9	22.6	8.5	22.0	8.2	21.3	7.8	20.6	7.5	20.0	7.1
	50	20.0	7.3	19.3	6.9	18.7	6.6	18.0	6.2	17.3	5.9	16.7	5.5	16.0	5.2
	20	16.0	5.3	15.3	5.0	14.7	4.6	14.0	4.3	13.4	3.9	12.7	3.6	12.0	3.2
	10	13.9	4.3	13.3	4.0	12.6	3.6	11.9	3.3	11.3	2.9	10.6	2.6	9.9	2.2
	5	12.2	3.5	11.5	3.1	10.9	2.8	10.2	2.4	9.6	2.1	8.9	1.7	8.2	1.4

NOTE: TR, Total Recall; DR, Delayed Recall

SOURCE: Adapted from Arango-Lasprilla et al. (2015).

TABLE 10–43 Norms for Hopkins Verbal Learning Test—Revised (HVLT-R) Total and Delayed Recall as a Function of Age and Education Levels for Cuba

EDUCATION (YEARS)		AGE (YEARS)											
		18–22		23–27		28–32		33–37		38–42		43–47	
>12	PERCENTILE	TR	DR	TR	DR	TR	DR	TR	DR	TR	DR	TR	DR
	95	33.7	–	33.1	–	32.6	12.0	32.0	12.0	31.4	12.0	30.8	12.0
	80	30.3	11.4	29.7	11.1	29.2	10.9	28.6	10.7	28.0	10.5	27.4	10.3
	50	26.7	9.5	26.1	9.3	25.6	9.1	25.0	8.9	24.4	8.7	23.8	8.5
	20	23.1	7.7	22.6	7.5	22.0	7.3	21.4	7.1	20.8	6.9	20.3	6.6
	10	21.3	6.8	20.7	6.6	20.1	6.3	19.5	6.1	19.0	5.9	18.4	5.7
	5	19.7	6.0	19.2	5.8	18.6	5.6	18.0	5.3	17.4	5.1	16.8	4.9
≤12		TR	DR	TR	DR	TR	DR	TR	DR	TR	DR	TR	DR
	95	30.9	11.7	30.3	11.4	29.7	11.2	29.2	11.0	28.6	10.8	28.0	10.6
	80	27.5	9.9	26.9	9.7	26.3	9.5	25.8	9.3	25.2	9.1	24.6	8.8
	50	23.9	8.1	23.3	7.9	22.7	7.7	22.2	7.5	21.6	7.2	21.0	7.0
	20	20.3	6.3	19.7	6.1	19.2	5.9	18.6	5.6	18.0	5.4	17.4	5.2
	10	18.4	5.3	17.9	5.1	17.3	4.9	16.7	4.7	16.1	4.5	15.6	4.3
	5	16.9	4.6	16.3	4.4	15.7	4.1	15.2	3.9	14.6	3.7	14.0	3.5

EDUCATION (YEARS)		AGE (YEARS)													
		48–52		53–57		58–62		63–67		68–72		73–77		>77	
>12	PERCENTILE	TR	DR	TR	DR	TR	DR	TR	DR	TR	DR	TR	DR	TR	DR
	95	30.3	11.8	29.7	11.6	29.1	11.3	28.5	11.1	28.0	10.9	27.4	10.7	26.8	10.5
	80	26.9	10.1	26.3	9.8	25.7	9.6	25.1	9.4	24.6	9.2	24.0	9.0	23.4	8.7
	50	23.3	8.2	22.7	8.0	22.1	7.8	21.5	7.6	21.0	7.4	20.4	7.1	19.8	6.9
	20	19.7	6.4	19.1	6.2	18.5	6.0	18.0	5.8	17.4	5.5	16.8	5.3	16.2	5.1
	10	17.8	5.5	17.2	5.3	16.7	5.0	16.1	4.8	15.5	4.6	14.9	4.4	14.4	4.2
	5	16.3	4.7	15.7	4.5	15.1	4.3	14.5	4.0	14.0	3.8	13.4	3.6	12.8	3.4
≤12		TR	DR	TR	DR	TR	DR	TR	DR	TR	DR	TR	DR	TR	DR
	95	27.4	10.3	26.9	10.1	26.3	9.9	25.7	9.7	25.1	9.5	24.6	9.3	24.0	9.0
	80	24.0	8.6	23.4	8.4	22.9	8.2	22.3	8.0	21.7	7.7	21.1	7.5	20.6	7.3
	50	20.4	6.8	19.9	6.6	19.3	6.4	18.7	6.1	18.1	5.9	17.6	5.7	17.0	5.5
	20	16.9	5.0	16.3	4.8	15.7	4.6	15.1	4.3	14.6	4.1	14.0	3.9	13.4	3.7
	10	15.0	4.0	14.4	3.8	13.8	3.6	13.3	3.4	12.7	3.2	12.1	2.9	11.5	2.7
	5	13.4	3.3	12.9	3.0	12.3	2.8	11.7	2.6	11.1	2.4	10.6	2.2	10.0	1.9

NOTE: TR, Total Recall; DR, Delayed Recall.

SOURCE: Adapted from Arango-Lasprilla et al. (2015).

TABLE 10–44 Norms for Hopkins Verbal Learning Test—Revised (HVLT-R) Total and Delayed Recall as a Function of Age and Education Levels for El Salvador

EDUCATION (YEARS)		AGE (YEARS)											
		18–22		23–27		28–32		33–37		38–42		43–47	
>12	PERCENTILE	TR	DR	TR	DR	TR	DR	TR	DR	TR	DR	TR	DR
	95	33.6	–	33.1	12.0	32.5	12.0	32.0	12.0	31.4	11.8	30.8	11.5
	80	29.9	11.2	29.3	10.9	28.8	10.6	28.2	10.3	27.7	10.0	27.1	9.8
	50	26.0	9.3	25.4	9.0	24.9	8.8	24.3	8.5	23.8	8.2	23.2	7.9
	20	22.1	7.5	21.5	7.2	21.0	6.9	20.4	6.6	19.8	6.3	19.3	6.0
	10	20.0	6.5	19.5	6.2	18.9	5.9	18.4	5.6	17.8	5.3	17.2	5.0
	5	18.4	5.7	17.8	5.4	17.2	5.1	16.7	4.8	16.1	4.5	15.6	4.2
≤12		TR	DR	TR	DR	TR	DR	TR	DR	TR	DR	TR	DR
	95	28.3	11.0	27.8	10.7	27.2	10.4	26.7	10.1	26.1	9.8	25.6	9.5
	80	24.6	9.2	24.1	8.9	23.5	8.6	22.9	8.3	22.4	8.1	21.8	7.8
	50	20.7	7.3	20.1	7.1	19.6	6.8	19.0	6.5	18.5	6.2	17.9	5.9
	20	16.8	5.5	16.2	5.2	15.7	4.9	15.1	4.6	14.6	4.3	14.0	4.0
	10	14.7	4.5	14.2	4.2	13.6	3.9	13.1	3.6	12.5	3.3	11.9	3.0
	5	13.1	3.7	12.5	3.4	11.9	3.1	11.4	2.8	10.8	2.5	10.3	2.2

TABLE 10–44 Continued

EDUCATION (YEARS)		AGE (YEARS)													
		48–52		53–57		58–62		63–67		68–72		73–77		>77	
>12	PERCENTILE	TR	DR	TR	DR	TR	DR	TR	DR	TR	DR	TR	DR	TR	DR
	95	30.3	11.2	29.7	11.0	29.2	10.7	28.6	10.4	28.1	10.1	27.5	9.8	26.6	9.5
	80	26.6	9.5	26.0	9.2	25.4	8.9	24.9	8.6	24.3	8.3	23.8	8.0	23.2	7.7
	50	22.6	7.6	22.1	7.3	21.5	7.0	21.0	6.7	20.4	6.4	19.8	6.1	19.3	5.8
	20	18.7	5.7	18.2	5.4	17.6	5.1	17.1	4.8	16.5	4.5	15.9	4.2	15.4	3.9
	10	16.7	4.7	16.1	4.4	15.6	4.1	15.0	3.8	14.4	3.5	13.9	3.2	13.3	3.0
	5	15.0	3.9	14.4	3.6	13.9	3.3	13.3	3.0	12.8	2.7	12.2	2.4	11.6	2.2
≤12		TR	DR	TR	DR	TR	DR	TR	DR	TR	DR	TR	DR	TR	DR
	95	25.0	9.3	24.4	9.0	23.9	8.7	23.3	8.4	22.8	8.1	22.2	7.8	21.6	7.5
	80	21.3	7.5	20.7	7.2	20.2	6.9	19.6	6.6	19.0	6.3	18.5	6.0	17.9	5.7
	50	17.4	5.6	16.8	5.3	16.2	5.0	15.7	4.7	15.1	4.4	14.6	4.1	14.0	3.8
	20	13.4	3.7	12.9	3.4	12.3	3.1	11.8	2.8	11.2	2.5	10.6	2.2	10.1	1.9
	10	11.4	2.7	10.8	2.4	10.3	2.1	9.7	1.8	9.2	1.5	8.6	1.3	8.0	1.0
	5	9.7	1.9	9.2	1.6	8.6	1.3	8.0	1.0	7.5	0.7	6.9	0.4	6.4	0.2

NOTE: TR, Total Recall; DR, Delayed Recall.

SOURCE: Adapted from Arango-Lasprilla et al. (2015).

TABLE 10–45 Norms for Hopkins Verbal Learning Test—Revised (HVLT-R) Total and Delayed Recall as a Function of Age and Education Levels for Guatemala

EDUCATION (YEARS)		AGE (YEARS)											
		18–22		23–27		28–32		33–37		38–42		43–47	
>12	PERCENTILE	TR	DR	TR	DR	TR	DR	TR	DR	TR	DR	TR	DR
	95	33.7	–	33.2	–	32.8	–	32.3	–	31.8	–	31.4	12.0
	80	29.8	11.7	29.3	11.4	28.9	11.2	28.4	11.0	27.9	10.8	27.5	10.6
	50	25.7	9.4	25.2	9.2	24.8	9.0	24.3	8.7	23.9	8.5	23.4	8.3
	20	21.6	7.1	21.2	6.9	20.7	6.7	20.2	6.5	19.8	6.2	19.3	6.0
	10	19.5	5.9	19.0	5.7	18.6	5.5	18.1	5.3	17.6	5.0	17.2	4.8
	5	17.7	5.0	17.3	4.7	16.8	4.5	16.3	4.3	15.9	4.1	15.4	3.9
≤12		TR	DR	TR	DR	TR	DR	TR	DR	TR	DR	TR	DR
	95	30.7	12.0	30.2	12.0	29.7	12.0	29.3	11.8	28.8	11.6	28.4	11.4
	80	26.8	10.3	26.3	10.1	25.8	9.9	25.4	9.6	24.9	9.4	24.5	9.2
	50	22.7	8.0	22.2	7.8	21.8	7.6	21.3	7.4	20.8	7.1	20.4	6.9
	20	18.6	5.8	18.1	5.5	17.7	5.3	17.2	5.1	16.7	4.9	16.3	4.6
	10	16.4	4.6	16.0	4.3	15.5	4.1	15.1	3.9	14.6	3.7	14.1	3.5
	5	14.7	3.6	14.2	3.4	13.8	3.2	13.3	2.9	12.9	2.7	12.4	2.5

EDUCATION (YEARS)		AGE (YEARS)													
		48–52		53–57		58–62		63–67		68–72		73–77		>77	
>12	PERCENTILE	TR	DR	TR	DR	TR	DR	TR	DR	TR	DR	TR	DR	TR	DR
	95	30.9	12.0	30.5	12.0	30.0	12.0	29.5	11.8	29.1	11.6	28.6	11.4	28.2	11.2
	80	27.0	10.3	26.6	10.1	26.1	9.9	25.6	9.7	25.2	9.4	24.7	9.2	24.3	9.0
	50	22.9	8.1	22.5	7.8	22.0	7.6	21.6	7.4	21.1	7.2	20.6	7.0	20.2	6.7
	20	18.9	5.8	18.4	5.6	17.9	5.4	17.5	5.1	17.0	4.9	16.6	4.7	16.1	4.5
	10	16.7	4.6	16.3	4.4	15.8	4.2	15.3	3.9	14.9	3.7	14.4	3.5	13.9	3.3
	5	15.0	3.6	14.5	3.4	14.0	3.2	13.6	3.0	13.1	2.7	12.7	2.5	12.2	2.3
≤12		TR	DR	TR	DR	TR	DR	TR	DR	TR	DR	TR	DR	TR	DR
	95	27.9	11.1	27.4	10.9	27.0	10.7	26.5	10.5	26.1	10.2	25.6	10.0	25.1	9.8
	80	24.0	9.0	23.5	8.7	23.1	8.5	22.6	8.3	22.2	8.1	21.7	7.9	21.2	7.6
	50	19.9	6.7	19.5	6.5	19.0	6.3	18.5	6.0	18.1	5.8	17.6	5.6	17.2	5.4
	20	15.8	4.4	15.4	4.2	14.9	4.0	14.4	3.8	14.0	3.5	13.5	3.3	13.1	3.1
	10	13.7	3.2	13.2	3.0	12.8	2.8	12.3	2.6	11.8	2.4	11.4	2.1	10.9	1.9
	5	11.9	2.3	11.5	2.0	11.0	1.8	10.5	1.6	10.1	1.4	9.6	1.2	9.2	0.9

NOTE: TR, Total Recall; DR, Delayed Recall.

SOURCE: Adapted from Arango-Lasprilla et al. (2015).

TABLE 10–46 Norms for Hopkins Verbal Learning Test—Revised (HVLT-R) Total and Delayed Recall as a Function of Age and Education Levels for Honduras

EDUCATION (YEARS)		AGE (YEARS)											
		18–22		23–27		28–32		33–37		38–42		43–47	
>12	PERCENTILE	TR	DR	TR	DR	TR	DR	TR	DR	TR	DR	TR	DR
	95	29.7	12.0	29.2	12.0	28.7	11.9	28.2	11.6	27.7	11.4	27.2	11.1
	80	26.3	10.5	25.8	10.3	25.3	10.0	24.8	9.7	24.3	9.5	23.8	9.2
	50	22.8	8.5	22.3	8.3	21.8	8.0	21.3	7.8	20.8	7.5	20.3	7.3
	20	19.3	6.6	18.8	6.3	18.3	6.1	17.8	5.8	17.3	5.5	16.8	5.3
	10	17.5	5.5	17.0	5.3	16.5	5.0	16.0	4.8	15.5	4.5	15.0	4.3
	5	16.0	4.7	15.5	4.4	15.0	4.2	14.5	3.9	14.0	3.7	13.5	3.4
≤12		TR	DR	TR	DR	TR	DR	TR	DR	TR	DR	TR	DR
	95	25.9	10.5	25.4	10.3	24.9	10.0	24.4	9.8	23.9	9.5	23.4	9.3
	80	22.6	8.7	22.1	8.4	21.6	8.2	21.1	7.9	20.6	7.6	20.1	7.4
	50	19.1	6.7	18.6	6.4	18.1	6.2	17.6	5.9	17.1	5.7	16.6	5.4
	20	15.6	4.7	15.1	4.5	14.6	4.2	14.0	4.0	13.5	3.7	13.0	3.4
	10	13.7	3.7	13.2	3.4	12.7	3.2	12.2	2.9	11.7	2.7	11.2	2.4
	5	12.2	2.9	11.7	2.6	11.2	2.3	10.7	2.1	10.2	1.8	9.7	1.6

EDUCATION (YEARS)		AGE (YEARS)													
		48–52		53–57		58–62		63–67		68–72		73–77		>77	
>12	PERCENTILE	TR	DR	TR	DR	TR	DR	TR	DR	TR	DR	TR	DR	TR	DR
	95	26.7	10.8	26.2	10.6	25.7	10.3	25.2	10.1	24.7	9.8	24.2	9.6	23.7	9.3
	80	23.3	9.0	22.8	8.7	22.3	8.5	21.8	8.2	21.3	7.9	20.8	7.7	20.3	7.4
	50	19.8	7.0	19.3	6.7	18.8	6.5	18.3	6.2	17.8	6.0	17.3	5.7	16.8	5.5
	20	16.3	5.0	15.8	4.8	15.3	4.5	14.8	4.3	14.3	4.0	13.8	3.7	13.3	3.5
	10	14.5	4.0	14.0	3.7	13.5	3.5	13.0	3.2	12.5	3.0	12.0	2.7	11.4	2.5
	5	13.0	3.2	12.5	2.9	12.0	2.6	11.5	2.4	10.9	2.1	10.4	1.9	9.9	1.6
≤12		TR	DR	TR	DR	TR	DR	TR	DR	TR	DR	TR	DR	TR	DR
	95	22.9	9.0	22.4	8.7	21.9	8.5	21.4	8.2	20.9	8.0	20.4	7.7	19.9	7.5
	80	19.6	7.1	19.1	6.9	18.6	6.6	18.1	6.4	17.6	6.1	17.1	5.8	16.5	5.6
	50	16.1	5.2	15.5	4.9	15.0	4.6	14.5	4.4	14.0	4.1	13.5	3.9	13.0	3.6
	20	12.5	3.2	12.0	2.9	11.5	2.7	11.0	2.4	10.5	2.2	10.0	1.9	9.5	1.6
	10	10.7	2.2	10.2	1.9	9.7	1.6	9.2	1.4	8.7	1.1	8.2	0.9	7.7	0.6
	5	9.2	1.3	8.7	1.1	8.2	0.8	7.7	0.5	7.2	0.3	6.7	–	6.2	–

NOTE: TR, Total Recall; DR, Delayed Recall.

SOURCE: Adapted from Arango-Lasprilla et al. (2015).

TABLE 10–47 Norms for Hopkins Verbal Learning Test—Revised (HVLT-R) Total and Delayed Recall as a Function of Age and Education Levels for Mexico

EDUCATION (YEARS)		AGE (YEARS)											
		18–22		23–27		28–32		33–37		38–42		43–47	
>12	PERCENTILE	TR	DR	TR	DR	TR	DR	TR	DR	TR	DR	TR	DR
	95	33.1	–	32.5	–	32.0	12.0	31.4	12.0	30.8	12.0	30.3	11.7
	80	29.6	11.4	29.0	11.1	28.4	10.8	27.9	10.5	27.3	10.2	26.8	9.9
	50	25.8	9.5	25.3	9.2	24.7	8.9	24.2	8.7	23.6	8.4	23.0	8.1
	20	22.1	7.7	21.6	7.4	21.0	7.1	20.5	6.8	19.9	6.5	19.3	6.2
	10	20.2	6.7	19.6	6.4	19.1	6.1	18.5	5.8	17.9	5.6	17.4	5.3
	5	18.6	5.9	18.0	5.6	17.5	5.3	16.9	5.0	16.4	4.8	15.8	4.5
≤12		TR	DR	TR	DR	TR	DR	TR	DR	TR	DR	TR	DR
	95	30.9	12.0	30.4	12.0	29.8	11.7	29.3	11.4	28.7	11.1	28.1	10.8
	80	27.4	10.5	26.8	10.2	26.3	9.9	25.7	9.6	25.2	9.4	24.6	9.1
	50	23.7	8.7	23.1	8.4	22.6	8.1	22.0	7.8	21.4	7.5	20.9	7.2
	20	20.0	6.8	19.4	6.5	18.9	6.2	18.3	5.9	17.7	5.7	17.2	5.4
	10	18.0	5.8	17.5	5.5	16.9	5.3	16.3	5.0	15.8	4.7	15.2	4.4
	5	16.4	5.0	15.9	4.8	15.3	4.5	14.8	4.2	14.2	3.9	13.6	3.6

TABLE 10–47 Continued

EDUCATION (YEARS)		AGE (YEARS)													
		48–52		53–57		58–62		63–67		68–72		73–77		>77	
>12	PERCENTILE	TR	DR	TR	DR	TR	DR	TR	DR	TR	DR	TR	DR	TR	DR
	95	29.7	11.4	29.2	11.1	28.6	10.8	28.0	10.6	27.5	10.3	26.9	10.0	26.4	9.7
	80	26.2	9.7	25.6	9.4	25.1	9.1	24.5	8.8	24.0	8.5	23.4	8.2	22.8	7.9
	50	22.5	7.8	21.9	7.5	21.4	7.2	20.8	6.9	20.2	6.7	19.7	6.4	19.1	6.1
	20	18.8	5.9	18.2	5.7	17.7	5.4	17.1	5.1	16.5	4.8	16.0	4.5	15.4	4.2
	10	16.8	5.0	16.3	4.7	15.7	4.4	15.1	4.1	14.6	3.8	14.0	3.5	13.5	3.3
	5	15.2	4.2	14.7	3.9	14.1	3.6	13.6	3.3	13.0	3.0	12.4	2.8	11.9	2.5
≤12		TR	DR	TR	DR	TR	DR	TR	DR	TR	DR	TR	DR	TR	DR
	95	27.6	10.5	27.0	10.3	26.5	10.0	25.9	9.7	25.3	9.4	24.8	9.1	24.2	8.8
	80	24.0	8.8	23.5	8.5	22.9	8.2	22.4	7.9	21.8	7.6	21.2	7.4	20.7	7.1
	50	20.3	6.9	19.8	6.6	19.2	6.4	18.6	6.1	18.1	5.8	17.5	5.5	17.0	5.2
	20	16.6	5.1	16.1	4.8	15.5	4.5	14.9	4.2	14.4	3.9	13.8	3.6	13.3	3.4
	10	14.7	4.1	14.1	3.8	13.5	3.5	13.0	3.3	12.4	3.0	11.9	2.7	11.3	2.4
	5	13.1	3.3	12.5	3.0	12.0	2.7	11.4	2.5	10.8	2.2	10.3	1.9	9.7	1.6

NOTE: TR, Total Recall; DR, Delayed Recall.

SOURCE: Adapted from Arango-Lasprilla et al. (2015).

TABLE 10–48 Norms for Hopkins Verbal Learning Test—Revised (HVLT-R) Total and Delayed Recall as a Function of Age and Education Levels for Paraguay

EDUCATION (YEARS)		AGE (YEARS)											
		18–22		23–27		28–32		33–37		38–42		43–47	
>12	PERCENTILE	TR	DR	TR	DR	TR	DR	TR	DR	TR	DR	TR	DR
	95	30.6	11.6	30.0	11.3	29.5	11.1	28.9	10.8	28.4	10.5	27.8	10.2
	80	27.4	10.2	26.9	9.9	26.3	9.6	25.7	9.4	25.2	9.1	24.6	8.8
	50	24.1	8.7	23.5	8.4	23.0	8.1	22.4	7.9	21.8	7.6	21.3	7.3
	20	20.7	7.2	20.2	6.9	19.6	6.6	19.0	6.4	18.5	6.1	17.9	5.8
	10	19.0	6.4	18.4	6.1	17.9	5.9	17.3	5.6	16.7	5.3	16.2	5.0
	5	17.5	5.8	17.0	5.5	16.4	5.2	15.9	4.9	15.3	4.7	14.7	4.4
≤12		TR	DR	TR	DR	TR	DR	TR	DR	TR	DR	TR	DR
	95	24.9	8.7	24.4	8.5	23.8	8.2	23.2	7.9	22.7	7.6	22.1	7.4
	80	21.7	7.3	21.2	7.0	20.6	6.8	20.1	6.5	19.5	6.2	18.9	5.9
	50	18.4	5.8	17.8	5.5	17.3	5.3	16.7	5.0	16.2	4.7	15.6	4.4
	20	15.0	4.3	14.5	4.0	13.9	3.8	13.4	3.5	12.8	3.2	12.2	2.9
	10	13.3	3.5	12.7	3.3	12.2	3.0	11.6	2.7	11.1	2.4	10.5	2.2
	5	11.9	2.9	11.3	2.6	10.7	2.3	10.2	2.1	9.6	1.8	9.1	1.5

EDUCATION (YEARS)		AGE (YEARS)													
		48–52		53–57		58–62		63–67		68–72		73–77		>77	
>12	PERCENTILE	TR	DR	TR	DR	TR	DR	TR	DR	TR	DR	TR	DR	TR	DR
	95	27.3	10.0	26.7	9.7	26.1	9.4	25.6	9.1	25.0	8.9	24.5	8.6	23.9	8.3
	80	24.1	8.5	23.5	8.3	22.9	8.0	22.4	7.7	21.8	7.4	21.3	7.2	20.7	6.9
	50	20.7	7.0	20.2	6.8	19.6	6.5	19.0	6.2	18.5	6.0	17.9	5.7	17.4	5.4
	20	17.4	5.5	16.8	5.3	16.3	5.0	15.7	4.7	15.1	4.5	14.6	4.2	14.0	3.9
	10	15.6	4.8	15.1	4.5	14.5	4.2	13.9	3.9	13.4	3.7	12.8	3.4	12.3	3.1
	5	14.2	4.1	13.6	3.9	13.1	3.6	12.5	3.3	11.9	3.0	11.4	2.8	10.8	2.5
≤12		TR	DR	TR	DR	TR	DR	TR	DR	TR	DR	TR	DR	TR	DR
	95	21.6	7.1	21.0	6.8	20.5	6.5	19.9	6.3	19.3	6.0	18.8	5.7	18.2	5.5
	80	18.4	5.7	17.8	5.4	17.3	5.1	16.7	4.9	16.1	4.6	15.6	4.3	15.0	4.0
	50	15.0	4.2	14.5	3.9	13.9	3.6	13.4	3.4	12.8	3.1	12.2	2.8	11.7	2.5
	20	11.7	2.7	11.1	2.4	10.6	2.1	10.0	1.9	9.4	1.6	8.9	1.3	8.3	1.0
	10	9.9	1.9	9.4	1.6	8.8	1.3	8.3	1.1	7.7	0.8	7.1	0.5	6.6	0.3
	5	8.5	1.3	7.9	1.0	7.4	0.7	6.8	0.4	6.3	0.2	5.7	–	5.1	–

NOTE: TR, Total Recall; DR, Delayed Recall.

SOURCE: Adapted from Arango-Lasprilla et al. (2015).

TABLE 10-49 Norms for Hopkins Verbal Learning Test—Revised (HVLT-R) Total and Delayed Recall as a Function of Age and Education Levels for Peru

		AGE (YEARS)											
EDUCATION (YEARS)		18–22		23–27		28–32		33–37		38–42		43–47	
>12	PERCENTILE	TR	DR	TR	DR	TR	DR	TR	DR	TR	DR	TR	DR
	95	32.0	12.0	31.6	11.8	31.1	11.6	30.6	11.3	30.1	11.1	29.7	10.8
	80	28.5	10.5	28.1	10.2	27.6	10.0	27.1	9.7	26.6	9.5	26.1	9.3
	50	24.8	8.8	24.4	8.6	23.9	8.3	23.4	8.1	22.9	7.9	22.5	7.6
	20	21.2	7.2	20.7	6.9	20.2	6.7	19.7	6.4	19.2	6.2	18.8	6.0
	10	19.2	6.3	18.7	6.1	18.3	5.8	17.8	5.6	17.3	5.3	16.8	5.1
	5	17.6	5.6	17.2	5.4	16.7	5.1	16.2	4.9	15.7	4.6	15.3	4.4
≤12		TR	DR	TR	DR	TR	DR	TR	DR	TR	DR	TR	DR
	95	30.0	10.8	29.6	10.6	29.1	10.4	28.6	10.1	28.1	9.9	27.7	9.6
	80	26.5	9.3	26.1	9.0	25.6	8.8	25.1	8.6	24.6	8.3	24.1	8.1
	50	22.8	7.6	22.4	7.4	21.9	7.1	21.4	6.9	20.9	6.7	20.5	6.4
	20	19.2	6.0	18.7	5.7	18.2	5.5	17.7	5.3	17.2	5.0	16.8	4.8
	10	17.2	5.1	16.7	4.9	16.3	4.6	15.8	4.4	15.3	4.2	14.8	3.9
	5	15.6	4.4	15.2	4.2	14.7	3.9	14.2	3.7	13.7	3.4	13.3	3.2

		AGE (YEARS)													
EDUCATION (YEARS)		48–52		53–57		58–62		63–67		68–72		73–77		>77	
>12	PERCENTILE	TR	DR	TR	DR	TR	DR	TR	DR	TR	DR	TR	DR	TR	DR
	95	29.2	10.6	28.7	10.4	28.2	10.1	27.8	9.9	27.3	9.6	26.8	9.4	26.3	9.2
	80	25.7	9.0	25.2	8.8	24.7	8.5	24.2	8.3	23.8	8.1	23.3	7.8	22.8	7.6
	50	22.0	7.4	21.5	7.1	21.0	6.9	20.6	6.7	20.1	6.4	19.6	6.2	19.1	5.9
	20	18.3	5.7	17.8	5.5	17.3	5.3	16.9	5.0	16.4	4.8	15.9	4.5	15.4	4.3
	10	16.4	4.9	15.9	4.6	15.4	4.4	14.9	4.2	14.5	3.9	14.0	3.7	13.5	3.4
	5	14.8	4.2	14.3	3.9	13.8	3.7	13.4	3.4	12.9	3.2	12.4	3.0	11.9	2.7
≤12		TR	DR	TR	DR	TR	DR	TR	DR	TR	DR	TR	DR	TR	DR
	95	27.2	9.4	26.7	9.2	26.2	8.9	25.8	8.7	25.3	8.4	24.8	8.2	24.3	8.0
	80	23.7	7.8	23.2	7.6	22.7	7.4	22.2	7.1	21.8	6.9	21.3	6.6	20.8	6.4
	50	20.0	6.2	19.5	5.9	19.0	5.7	18.6	5.5	18.1	5.2	17.6	5.0	17.1	4.8
	20	16.3	4.5	15.8	4.3	15.3	4.1	14.9	3.8	14.4	3.6	13.9	3.3	13.4	3.1
	10	14.4	3.7	13.9	3.4	13.4	3.2	12.9	3.0	12.5	2.7	12.0	2.5	11.5	2.2
	5	12.8	3.0	12.3	2.7	11.8	2.5	11.4	2.3	10.9	2.0	10.4	1.8	9.9	1.5

NOTE: TR, Total Recall; DR, Delayed Recall.

SOURCE: Adapted from Arango-Lasprilla et al. (2015).

TABLE 10-50 Norms for Hopkins Verbal Learning Test—Revised (HVLT-R) Total and Delayed Recall as a Function of Age and Education Levels for Puerto Rico

		AGE (YEARS)											
EDUCATION (YEARS)		18–22		23–27		28–32		33–37		38–42		43–47	
>12	PERCENTILE	TR	DR	TR	DR	TR	DR	TR	DR	TR	DR	TR	DR
	95	34.1	–	33.3	–	32.5	–	31.8	–	31.0	12.0	30.2	12.0
	80	30.8	12.0	30.0	11.9	29.3	11.5	28.5	11.1	27.8	10.7	27.0	10.3
	50	27.4	10.4	26.6	10.0	25.9	9.6	25.1	9.2	24.4	8.8	23.6	8.4
	20	24.0	8.5	23.2	8.1	22.5	7.7	21.7	7.3	20.9	6.9	20.2	6.5
	10	22.2	7.5	21.4	7.1	20.7	6.7	19.9	6.3	19.2	5.9	18.4	5.5
	5	20.7	6.7	20.0	6.3	19.2	5.9	18.5	5.5	17.7	5.1	16.6	4.7
≤12		TR	DR	TR	DR	TR	DR	TR	DR	TR	DR	TR	DR
	95	32.8	–	32.0	–	31.3	12.0	30.5	12.0	29.7	11.7	29.0	11.3
	80	29.5	11.5	28.8	11.1	28.0	10.7	27.3	10.3	26.5	9.9	25.7	9.6
	50	26.1	9.7	25.4	9.3	24.6	8.9	23.9	8.5	23.1	8.1	22.3	7.7
	20	22.7	7.8	22.0	7.4	21.2	7.0	20.4	6.6	19.7	6.2	18.9	5.8
	10	20.9	6.8	20.2	6.4	19.4	6.0	18.7	5.6	17.9	5.2	17.1	4.8
	5	19.5	6.0	18.7	5.6	18.0	5.2	17.2	4.8	16.4	4.4	15.7	4.0

TABLE 10–50 Continued

EDUCATION (YEARS)		AGE (YEARS)													
		48–52		53–57		58–62		63–67		68–72		73–77		>77	
>12	PERCENTILE	TR	DR	TR	DR	TR	DR	TR	DR	TR	DR	TR	DR	TR	DR
	95	29.5	11.6	28.7	11.2	28.0	10.8	27.2	10.4	26.4	10.0	25.7	9.6	24.9	9.2
	80	26.2	9.9	25.5	9.5	24.7	9.1	24.0	8.7	23.2	8.3	22.4	7.9	21.7	7.5
	50	22.8	8.0	22.1	7.6	21.3	7.2	20.5	6.8	19.8	6.4	19.0	6.0	18.3	5.6
	20	19.4	6.1	18.7	5.7	17.9	5.3	17.1	4.9	16.4	4.5	15.6	4.1	14.8	3.7
	10	17.6	5.1	16.9	4.7	16.1	4.3	15.3	3.9	14.6	3.5	13.8	3.1	13.1	2.7
	5	16.2	4.3	15.4	3.9	14.6	3.5	13.9	3.1	13.1	2.7	12.4	2.3	11.6	1.9
≤12		TR	DR	TR	DR	TR	DR	TR	DR	TR	DR	TR	DR	TR	DR
	95	28.2	10.9	27.5	10.5	26.7	10.1	25.9	9.7	25.2	9.3	24.4	8.9	23.7	8.5
	80	25.0	9.2	24.2	8.8	23.5	8.4	22.7	8.0	21.9	7.6	21.2	7.2	20.4	6.8
	50	21.6	7.3	20.8	6.9	20.0	6.5	19.3	6.1	18.5	5.7	17.8	5.3	17.0	4.9
	20	18.2	5.4	17.4	5.0	16.6	4.6	15.9	4.2	15.1	3.8	14.3	3.4	13.6	3.0
	10	16.4	4.4	15.6	4.0	14.8	3.6	14.1	3.2	13.3	2.8	12.6	2.4	11.8	2.0
	5	14.9	3.6	14.1	3.2	13.4	2.8	12.6	2.4	11.9	2.0	11.1	1.6	10.3	1.2

NOTE: TR, Total Recall; DR, Delayed Recall.

SOURCE: Adapted from Arango-Lasprilla et al. (2015).

Retention and Recognition Discrimination Index (see Table 10–52). They noted that the restricted and nonnormal distribution of some of the test variables may have limited the range of possible reliability coefficients.

Others have reported noticeably lower reliability coefficients. In high-school athletes retested with an alternate form about 60 days after baseline testing, test-retest reliability coefficients were low (Barr, 2003; see Tables 10–52 and 10–53). Barr (2003) noted that variable motivation might play a role in the performance of the participants (e.g., some may not have taken the tests seriously).

In patients with TBI tested at least one-year post-injury, six- to eight-week test-retest reliability was generally high while test-retest coefficients for T scores were lower (O'Neil-Pirozzi et al., 2012; see Table 10–52).

Similarly, Woods et al. (2005) examined the reliability of standard as well as process measures of encoding (e.g., semantic and serial clustering), retrieval, and error rates in healthy young adults retested with an alternate form after an interval of about one year. Reliability coefficients were low for the various measures, with Total Recall showing the highest coefficient (r = .49). Woods et al. (2005) suggested that the low temporal stability of these measures (particularly component process variables) might relate in part to the low number of trials and list items on the HVLT. It should be noted, however, that the same pattern emerges when the 16-item version of the CVLT-II is used (see CVLT-II), so the low reliabilities are a function of these process scores, not of the number of items.

TABLE 10–51 Brazilian Norms for Hopkins Verbal Learning Test—Revised (HVLT-R) Form 1

EDUCATION (YEARS)	AGE (YEARS)							
	18–20	21–30	31–40	41–50	51–60	61–70	71–80	80+
0 to 4	N = 10	N = 55	N = 34	N = 50	N = 40	N = 80	N = 51	N = 15
Total Recall	17.6 (4.72)	18.56 (4.91)	19.82 (4.24)	17.76 (4.86)	18.83 (4.47)	19.00 (5.16)	18.96 (13.97)	18.53 (4.34)
Delayed Recall	6.3 (2.21)	6.51 (2.64)	6.91 (2.31)	5.84 (2.23)	5.90 (2.58)	6.28 (2.52)	6.25 (2.41)	6.13 (2.67)
Recognition	10.7 (2.67)	10.44 (2.11)	10.59 (1.48)	9.58 (2.47)	10.33 (1.91)	9.30 (2.42)	9.61 (2.43)	8.73 (3.10)
5 to 8	N = 5	N = 53	N = 34	N = 29	N = 15	N = 70	N = 15	N = 4
Total Recall	20.8 (2.59)	21.60 (4.52)	22.79 (4.37)	22.83 (5.61)	22.87 (5.76)	21.49 (4.52)	19.93 (4.95)	19.00 (5.80)
Delayed Recall	7.20 (4.44)	7.87 (1.74)	7.47 (2.14)	7.86 (3.06)	7.27 (3.10)	7.10 (2.15)	7.53 (1.68)	6.75 (3.30)
Recognition	10.40 (2.07)	10.55 (1.62)	10.91 (1.24)	9.79 (2.55)	10.27 (1.33)	9.81 (2.42)	9.53 (2.10)	8.50 (2.38)
9 to 11	N = 15	N = 31	N = 23	N = 36	N = 29	N = 29	N = 13	N = 7
Total Recall	26.80 (4.25)	23.90 (3.11)	22.00 (3.87)	23.64 (4.00)	23.17 (4.74)	24.97 (4.35)	22.62 (3.12)	19.20 (6.16)
Delayed Recall	9.87 (1.96)	8.10 (1.92)	7.70 (2.55)	8.83 (2.04)	8.59 (2.15)	8.72 (1.96)	8.77 (1.79)	6.86 (3.44)
Recognition	11.53 (0.74)	10.77 (1.31)	10.13 (1.98)	11.17 (1.28)	11.14 (1.09)	11.34 (1.14)	10.31 (1.75)	9.57 (1.62)
12 to 17	N = 7	N = 74	N = 53	N = 52	N = 52	N = 91	N = 27	N = 9
Total Recall	27.57 (4.08)	28.00 (3.58)	26.79 (3.88)	26.83 (5.66)	24.40 (4.58)	25.44 (5.42)	24.04 (4.42)	20.33 (0.83)
Delayed Recall	9.43 (1.62)	10.27 (1.75)	9.92 (1.77)	9.56 (1.87)	8.48 (2.60)	9.15 (2.62)	8.07 (2.25)	7.00 (4.64)
Recognition	11.57 (0.79)	11.38 (1.22)	11.70 (2.43)	11.38 (1.07)	10.68 (1.82)	10.64 (1.66)	10.30 (1.68)	10.00 (2.12)

NOTE: N = 1108. Screened for neurologic and psychiatric disorder.

SOURCE: Adapted from Miotto et al. (2012).

TABLE 10–52 Hopkins Verbal Learning Test—Revised (HVLT-R) Test-Retest Correlations

MAGNITUDE OF COEFFICIENT	MEASURE		
	ADULTS (BENEDICT ET AL., 1998)	ADOLESCENTS (BARR, 2003)	TBI (O'NEIL-PIROZZI ET AL., 2012)
Very high (≥.90)			
High (.80 to .89)			Total Recall Delayed Recall
Adequate (.70 to .79)	Total Recall		Total Recall T score Delayed Recall T score
Marginal (.60 to .69)	Delayed Recall		Recognition Discrimination Index % Retention % Retention T score
Low (≤.59)	% Retention Recognition Discrimination Index	Total Recall Delayed Recall Discrimination Index	Recognition Discrimination Index T score

PRACTICE EFFECTS AND MEASUREMENT OF CHANGE

Practice effects do emerge when healthy individuals are given the same form after a two-week interval (Benedict & Zgaljardic, 1998). Scores improve in the second test session (with gains of about three points in Total Recall), and less learning occurs in the subsequent two test sessions. However, when alternate forms are used, practice effects are minimal (less than one point in Total Recall on the second test session; Barr, 2003; Benedict & Zgaljardic, 1998), and the slopes of the learning curves appear similar (Benedict & Zgaljardic, 1998).

As noted previously, Barr (2003) retested high-school athletes with an alternate form after an interval of about 60 days. RCIs are shown in Table 10–54. Each RCI value is followed by the percentage of adolescents with change scores exceeding the lower limit. This value represents the level of raw score decline that is required to exceed what might be expected on the basis of normal error variance and the effects of practice. Upper limits are also listed to aid in interpretation of possible improvements. As an example of the use of this table, suppose an athlete obtains a baseline score of 27 on Total Recall. Repeat testing within 48 hours of a concussion reveals a score of 20. Table 10–54 shows that a drop of seven points exceeds the lower limit (−6) of the 90% confidence interval (CI), and so this would be considered true change.

Woods et al. (2005) retested healthy individuals after an interval of about one year. Form 1 was given at the first test session and Form 2 at the second. The *SD*s of the mean difference scores on Forms 1 and 2 and RCIs were derived for a number of HVLT-R variables (including process ones). These are shown in Table 10–55.

EVIDENCE FOR RELIABILITY OF ALTERNATE FORMS

The test manual (Brandt & Benedict, 2001) reports two studies of interform reliability. In the first (Benedict et al., 1998), 432 college students were given one form of the test selected at random. In the second study (Benedict et al., 1998), 18 students were administered a different form of the HVLT-R each week for six weeks. Results revealed that the six forms are equivalent for the recall trials. However, there were slight differences in the degree to which they elicited false-positive responses on the Delayed Recognition trial. More specifically, there were small but statistically significant differences among the six test forms on three of the HVLT-R variables: semantically related false-positive errors, semantically unrelated false-positive errors, and the Recognition Discrimination Index. Forms 1, 2, and 4 make a homogeneous subgroup, as do Forms 3, 5, and 6. Therefore, separate T-score conversion columns for the Recognition Discrimination Index for Forms 1, 2, and 4 and Forms 3, 5, and 6 are provided in each normative table in the test manual. The authors recommend that, when the HVLT-R is used in repeated examination, Forms 1, 2, and 4 be considered equivalent, and slightly more difficult on the Delayed Recognition trial than Forms 3, 5, and

TABLE 10–53 HVLT-R Test Scores (Mean and Standard Deviation [*SD*]) in 48 Adolescents at Baseline and at Retesting About 60 Days Later

	T1	T2	T2 − T1	*R*	*SEM*	^{S}DIFF
Total Recall (Trials 1–3)	27.0 (3.4)	27.3 (4.3)	0.27 (3.9)	.54	2.63	3.72
Delayed Recall	9.6 (1.8)	9.8 (2.1)	0.19 (1.9)	.56	1.21	1.71
Discrimination Index	11.6 (0.9)	11.7 (0.7)	−0.01 (0.9)	.39	0.73	1.03

NOTE: Based on 32 males, 16 females; aged 13–17 years, *M* = 15.96, *SD* = .94.

TABLE 10–54 HVLT-R Adjusted Reliable Change Indices (RCIs) calculated for 90%, 80%, and 70% Confidence Intervals (CI), Followed by the Percentage of the Sample of Adolescents with Scores Falling Below the Lower Limit

	90% CI	80% CI	70% CI
Total Recall (Trials 1–3)	−6, +6 (2.1)	−4, +5 (18.8)	−4, +4 (18.8)
Delayed Recall	−3, +3 (8.3)	−2, +2 (14.6)	−2, +2 (14.6)
Discrimination Index	−2, +2 (8.3)	−1, +1 (14.6)	−1, +1 (14.6)

SOURCE: Adapted from Barr (2003).

6, which are equivalent. However, it was reported in an AD and an amnestic MCI sample from Spain that Forms 1 and 4 were equivalent for Total Recall and Delayed Recall but not Recognition. More words were recognized in Form 4 than Form 1 (Gonzalez-Palau et al., 2013).

EVIDENCE FOR VALIDITY

FACTOR-ANALYTIC STUDIES

Gaines et al. (2006) conducted a factor analysis using the Semantic Clustering Ratio and all other recall trials. This yielded a two-factor solution with the Semantic Clustering Ratio loading on a factor separate from recall scores (Gaines et al., 2006).

RELATIONSHIPS WITH OTHER TESTS

The test has shown evidence of convergent validity with similar measures such as the CVLT. In a sample of patients with AD, Lacritz et al. (2001) found that Total Recall ($r = .36$), Delayed Recall ($r = .62$), intrusion errors ($r = .34$), and recognition hits ($r = .48$) were moderately related across tests. Learning curves and retention rates were quite similar, although patients recalled less information from the HVLT-R than from the CVLT on delayed recall. Both tasks were similarly related to severity of dementia ($r = .40$).

There also is evidence that the test correlates more strongly with verbal memory (e.g., WMS-R Logical Memory, $r = .65$ to .77) than with visual memory (WMS-R Visual Reproduction, $r = .54$ to .69; Shapiro et al., 1999).

In a sample of older adults referred to an outpatient memory disorder clinic, positive correlations with MMSE were seen for Total Recall, Delayed Recall, and Recognition Discriminability ($r = .43$ to .55). It is important to highlight that in this sample, patients who had an MMSE of greater than 25 obtained on average, HVLT-R scores in the mildly impaired range. More than half of those who obtained normal MMSE scores (>25) performed in the moderately impaired range on the HVLT-R, and a quarter scored in the severely impaired range. In fact, almost half of those who scored near perfect on the MMSE had moderately to severely impaired scores on the HVLT-R, suggesting that the HVLT-R may be more sensitive to dementia than the MMSE (Lacy et al., 2015). Hogervorst et al. (2002) also found that a combined memory score (sum of Total Recall and Discrimination Index) was more sensitive than the MMSE to the presence of dementia, whereas Gaines and colleagues (2006) reported that dementia status was best predicted by Delayed Recall scores over and above MMSE in a logistic regression using all recall and Semantic Clustering Ratio scores (Gaines et al., 2006).

Benedict et al. (1996) evaluated patients with either nonlateralized cerebral pathology or psychiatric disease and performed factor analysis on scores from the HVLT-R along with the TMT, COWA, VMI, and BVMT-R. The HVLT-R recall and recognition scores loaded on a separate factor, suggesting that, in a mixed clinical sample, the test

TABLE 10–55 Hopkins Verbal Learning Test—Revised (HVLT-R) Descriptive Statistics (Mean and Standard Deviation [*SD*]) Reliability Data, and Reliability[e] Change Indices (RCIs) in Healthy Adults Retested After About 12 Months

VARIABLE	TIME 1	TIME 2	*R*	M_{DIFF}	*SD*[a]	90% CI	95% CI
Total Recall	27.49 (4.12)	27.95 (4.05)	.49	.46	4.13	±6.77	±8.09
Delayed Recall	10.24 (1.20)	10.07 (1.81)	.36	.17	1.77	±2.90	±3.47
% Retention	95.24 (7.25)	91.46 (11.47)	0.14[d]	−3.78	12.49	±20.48	±24.48
Learning[c]	1.55 (.91)	1.46 (.88)	.15	−.09	1.16	±1.90	±2.27
Semantic Clustering	2.12 (1.72)	1.82 (1.64)	.31	−.30	1.98	±3.25	±3.88
Serial Clustering	.32 (.88)	1.63 (1.29)	−.25	1.31	1.74	±2.85	±3.41
Pair Frequency	4.68 (3.63)	4.39 (4.10)	.17	−.29	4.98	±8.17	±9.76
Intrusions	.46 (.89)	.66 (1.30)	.15[d]	.20	1.40	±2.30	±2.74
Repetitions	1.39 (1.52)	1.63 (2.20)	.14[d]	.24	2.67	±4.38	±5.23
Recognition Discriminability	11.15 (.73)	11.12 (1.10)	.27[d]	−.02	1.11	±1.82	±2.18
Recognition SFP[b]	.63 (.66)	.66 (1.01)	.35[d]	.02	1.01	±1.66	±1.98
Retrieval Index[e]	.90 (1.04)	1.05 (1.97)	.32[d]	.15	1.93	±3.17	±3.78

[a] The *SD* also serves as the 68% RCI confidence interval.
[b] Semantic false-positive errors.
[c] Average new correct words per trial.
[d] Spearman's rho.
[e] Delayed free recall vs. recognition discrimination.
SOURCE: From Woods et al. (2005).

does measure something distinct (Benedict et al., 1996). Similar findings were reported by Shapiro et al. (1999) in a heterogeneous group of older neuropsychiatric patients and healthy adults. However, support for this view is weakened because of the distortion introduced by using multiple scores from the same test (method variance problem; Larrabee, 2003).

Correlations between the Semantic Clustering Ratio and TMT-B, WAIS-R Digit Symbol, COWA, and Category Fluency range from .22 to .36, whereas correlations of these measures with Total Recall and Delayed Recall are higher (–.38 to .61; Malek-Ahmadi et al., 2011). Of note, Total Recall but not the learning measures (i.e., traditional and CWL; see "Scoring") is affected by language skills as measured by BNT and COWA in patients with mild AD (Foster et al., 2009).

CLINICAL STUDIES

AD and MCI. Impaired performance has been noted in patients with AD (Brandt & Benedict, 2001). In addition to producing few correct responses, AD patients, including those in the early stages of the disease, tend to make false-positive identifications on recognition testing, particularly of nontarget words that are semantically related to the targets. This is presumed to reflect the deterioration of semantic memory or impaired access to semantic representations, which was partially supported by the findings of Foster and colleagues (2013). They reported that when using COWA as measure of spreading activation, a negative correlation was found between average word frequency and HVLT-R performance in healthy older adults, suggesting that spreading activation helps with connections of concepts and therefore aids in free recall of verbal information (Foster et al., 2013).

There are suggestions that process scores may be more sensitive to mild memory problems than traditional scores such as Total Recall and Delayed Recall (Foster et al., 2009; Malek-Ahmadi et al., 2011). As CWL takes into account learning capacity as well as total recall and has a wider range, it is possibly less sensitive to floor and ceiling effects (Foster et al., 2009). For example, mild AD patients obtain average traditional learning z scores but notably different CWL scores compared to healthy controls, whereas moderate AD patients obtain poorer scores on both scores compared to healthy controls (Foster et al., 2009). Similarly, Malek-Ahmadi et al. (2011) found that Semantic Clustering Ratio for both Total Recall and Delayed Recall differed between healthy controls and amnestic MCI group. Semantic clustering was used by those with amnestic MCI but not to the same degree as cognitively healthy individuals (Malek-Ahmadi et al., 2011).

One study suggests that the HVLT-R appears superior to Logical Memory in identifying memory impairments in older adults. In comparing the impairment rates of classifying amnestic or amnestic-plus MCI using HVLT-R and WMS-III Logical Memory (LM I and LM II), Tremont and colleagues (2010) reported that HVLT-R Delayed Recall classified 80% in the MCI range whereas only 32% performed in the MCI range using LM II. About half of those intact on LM I were impaired on HVLT-R Total Recall; even greater proportion (78%) of those intact on LM II were impaired on HVLT-R Delayed Recall. Twice as many amnestic MCI were impaired on HVLT-R Delayed Recall as LM II. Comparable rates were obtained in the amnestic-plus MCI group. Patients with executive dysfunction performed worse on LM I and HVLT-R Total Recall than those without executive dysfunction; no differences were seen on delayed recall trials of both measures. In sum, the HVLT-R appears to be more demanding and more sensitive to early memory changes than Logical Memory; accordingly, patients are less likely to be classified as impaired on Logical Memory than on HVLT-R (Tremont et al., 2010).

The HVLT-R also appears useful to differentiate between AD, amnestic MCI (single and multiple domains), and healthy individuals (Gonzalez-Palau et al., 2013). In a Spanish sample, healthy controls outperformed AD and MCI groups on Total Recall, Delayed Recall, and Recognition. Table 10–56 shows the sensitivity and specificity of various HVLT-R trials in detecting the different groups. Recognition scores had lower sensitivity and specificity for identifying AD or amnestic MCI than Total Recall and Delayed Recall.

PD. Patients with PD with left or right hemibody motor-symptom onset were given the HVLT-R and BVMT-R to examine material-specific memory in this population (Foster et al., 2010). The authors found that those with right onset showed a drop in HVLT-R performance from the learning trials to Delayed Recall and improvement in BVMT-R from the learning trials to Delayed Recall, whereas no performance changes were seen in those with left onset (Foster et al., 2010). The presence of HVLT-R memory impairments in PD patients may be related to the presence of APOE-ε4 allele. Mata and colleagues (2014) found that among PD patients with and without dementia, the APOE-ε4 allele was associated with all indices on the HVLT-R. For every additional copy of the allele, a decrease of 1.55 words in Total Recall was found. Each allele had the same effect on the Total Recall score as 3.5 years less education or 6.0 years more in age. In those without dementia, the APOE-ε4 allele was associated with Total Recall scores only. Microtuble-associated protein tau (MAPT) and α-synuclein (SNCA) genes were not associated with performance on the HVLT-R (Mata et al., 2014).

HD. Individuals with HD show impaired Total Recall and Delayed Recall performance, like patients with AD (Brandt & Benedict, 2001). However, recognition performance is relatively impaired in AD but intact in HD. Among individuals with prodromal HD, a temporal gradient in the relationship between disease progression and

TABLE 10–56 Hopkins Verbal Learning Test—Revised (HVLT-R) Sensitivity and Specificity at Different Cutoffs for Different Samples

STUDY	SAMPLE	CUTOFF	AUC	SENSITIVITY (%)	SPECIFICITY (%)
Gonzalez-Palau et al. (2013)	AD, amnestic MCI, healthy controls from Spain	AD:			
		Total Recall <13	.95	96	85
		Delayed Recall <3	.95	89	81
		Amnestic MCI:			
		Total Recall <15	.84	84	65
		Delayed Recall <4	.84	88	70
Hogervorst et al. (2002)	AD	Total Recall 1 *SD* below norms	–	95	83
	Vascular dementia	Total Recall 1 *SD* below norms	–	85	76
Aretouli et al. (2010)	AD vs. HD	Total Recall <12.5	.77	97	52
		Delayed Recall <3.5	.91	83	83
		CWL <54	.67	43	90
	AD vs. PD	Total Recall <12.5	.64	72	52
		Delayed Recall <0.5	.79	89	62
		CWL <43.5	.64	44	86
	PD vs. HD	Total Recall <13.5	.66	87	44
		Delayed Recall <3.5	.70	60	83
		CWL <26.0	.54	73	50

NOTE: AD, Alzheimer's disease; amnestic MCI, amnestic mild cognitive impairment; AUC, area under the curve; HD, Huntington's disease; PD, Parkinson's disease; CWL, Cumulative Word Learning.

HVLT-R scores is found, with lower HVLT-R Total Recall, Delayed Recall, and Recognition Discriminability scores but not Retention scores associated with closer proximity to clinical diagnosis (Solomon et al., 2007). The presence of memory problems in prodromal HD may be related to a number of factors. Smith and colleagues (2012) reported that severity of depression is associated with HVLT-R Total Recall but not Delayed Recall performance. Those who endorsed minimal depressive symptoms on the BDI-II performed significantly better on HVLT-R Total Recall than those who endorsed moderate or severe depressive symptoms. However, whether one is positive for gene mutation contributed more to HVLT-R Total Recall and Delayed Recall performance than did depression status (Smith et al., 2012). Solomon and colleagues (2007) reported that those with cytosine-adenine-guanine (CAG) expansion (i.e., expansion of the DNA bases CAG in the gene coding for the Huntingtin protein) but minimal motor signs performed worse on the HVLT-R than a CAG-normative group; those with more motor signs performed worse on the HVLT-R than those with minimal motor signs.

In a Chinese sample, those with vascular cognitive impairment-no dementia performed better than those with amnestic MCI on HVLT-R Total Recall, Delayed Recall, Recognition, and Semantic Clustering Ratio, whereas, as expected, they performed worse on tests of executive functions (TMT-A, TMT-B, and WCST) and processing speed (PASAT, SDMT; Sun et al., 2016). However, Gaines et al. (2006) reported that healthy individuals obtained better recall and Semantic Clustering Ratio scores than patient groups (AD and VaD) and showed an improvement of Semantic Clustering Ratio over the trials, although, overall, VaD and AD patients did not differ on Semantic Clustering Ratio scores even though only the Semantic Clustering Ratio in the AD group showed a decline from learning to Delayed Recall. Shapiro et al. (1999) reported on the sensitivity/specificity of Total Recall in detecting AD and VaD (see Table 10–56). In a population with roughly equal numbers of AD patients and nondemented persons, the PPV of Total Recall was 84% (i.e., 84% of those who perform below the 1 *SD* criterion value have dementia), and the NPV was 94% (i.e., 94% of those who score at or above the criterion do not have dementia). In patients with VaD, a PPV of 76% and a NPV of 85% were obtained. The authors cautioned that the predictive power indices are highly dependent on estimated base rates. Therefore, in settings where the prevalence of dementia is low, a more stringent cutoff score of 2 or 3 *SDs* should be used to limit the number of false-positive results.

Aretouli and Brandt (2010) used the HVLT-R to distinguish between AD, PD, and HD. The HVLT-R CWL, Delayed Recall, and Discrimination Index were worse for AD than for the subcortical groups (HD and PD). AD performance was worse than PD on HVLT-R Total Recall, too. When HVLT-R and the Hopkins Board (HB), a measure of verbal and visuospatial learning and memory, were entered into a discriminant function after demographic variables and MMSE, HB Delayed Recall and HVLT-R Delayed Recall were the best predictors of cortical-subcortical group membership, although the addition of the memory measures contributed only about 5% of variance. Overall classification accuracy was about 91%. Similarly, for the prediction of disease-specific membership, HB Delayed Recall, HVLT-R Delayed Recall, and HVLT-R Total Recall added only 4% of classification accuracy over demographics and MMSE, giving rise to a classification accuracy of 78% (see Table 10–56). This suggests superior prediction of MMSE, demographics, and HVLT-R than use of the HVLT-R in isolation. In short, the HVLT-R appears to be a valid test for detecting memory impairment in various neurodegenerative disorders and may be useful in differentiating various dementias.

Left Versus Right-Sided Lesions. Lesion studies suggest greater impairment with left than right lesions. For example, older patients with left or right hemisphere stroke were compared to healthy controls on their performance on the HVLT-R, BNT, and letter-number sequencing about 84–89 months after stroke (Andrews et al., 2014). Those with left hemisphere stroke performed worse than those with right hemisphere stroke and healthy controls on the HVLT-R. No differences were seen in those with right hemisphere stroke and healthy controls. The left hemisphere stroke group did not improve from Trial 2 to Trial 3, unlike both the right hemisphere stroke and healthy control groups. Similarly, the former group performed worse than the right hemisphere stroke and healthy groups on Trials 2, 3, Delayed Recall, and Recognition. No differences were seen on the Retention score. Using BNT and letter-number sequencing as predictors of HVLT-R performance, BNT (13%) and letter-number sequencing (17%) were predictive of HVLT-R performance in the left hemisphere stroke group only. Only BNT was a predictor for the right hemisphere stroke group (56%) and healthy controls (9%; Andrews et al., 2014).

Noll et al. (2016) reported on HVLT-R performance of patients with left or right temporal lobe glioma. Greater memory impairment, including lower Semantic Clustering Ratio and Total Recall, was seen in the left temporal lobe glioma group compared to the right-sided group. Learning slope and CWL were similar for both groups (Foster et al., 2009). Large correlations were seen between semantic clusters and Total Recall and Delayed Recall, as well as Semantic Clustering Ratio and Total Recall and Delayed Recall. Moderate correlation was seen between CWL and Total Recall, Delayed Recall, and Recognition.

HIV. Carey et al. (2004) provided some support for use of the HVLT-R to detect neuropsychological impairment in persons with HIV infection, a disorder considered to produce a pattern of verbal learning and retrieval deficits consistent with prominent prefrontal-striatal pathophysiology. The HVLT-R Total Recall measure (especially in combination with the Grooved Pegboard Test nondominant hand or WAIS-III Digit Symbol score) demonstrated reasonably high degrees of diagnostic accuracy. Interestingly, individuals with subtype C HIV-positive status performed worse than HIV-negative individuals on HVLT-R Total Recall, but they were intact on Delayed Recall as well as on semantic clustering and serial clustering indices, contrary to the encoding and retrieval problems seen in subtype B HIV-positive individuals (Witten et al., 2015).

Psychiatric Conditions. The HVLT-R appears to be sensitive to verbal memory impairments in psychiatric disorders. Van Rheenen and Rossell (2014) found that the HVLT-R is sensitive to learning, recall, and recognition problems in those with bipolar disorder, although no differences were seen between bipolar disorder and healthy controls on process indices such as learning slope, retrieval, retention percentage, or Semantic Clustering Ratio. As such, the authors suggested that the HVLT-R may be used to assess treatment responsiveness in clinical trials for medications to improve verbal memory in bipolar disorder. Similarly, Czepielewski et al. (2015) reported that individuals with early stage bipolar disorder performed similarly to controls and better than those with late-stage bipolar disorder or schizophrenia (both recent onset or chronic) on the HVLT-R, whereas late-stage bipolar disorder and those with chronic schizophrenia performed worse than others on HVLT-R Retention. Among patients with first-episode schizophrenia, poor time-based prospective memory was associated with a longer period of untreated psychosis, lower HVLT-R scores, less categories completed on the WCST, and high scores on Color Trails 2. Worse performance on event-based prospective memory was associated with lower HVLT-R scores, higher WCST perseverative errors, and a longer period of untreated psychosis (Zhou et al., 2012).

Verbal memory impairments as measured by the HVLT-R are also seen in first-degree relatives of people with schizophrenia (Hou et al., 2016; Zhou et al., 2014). For example, in comparing HVLT-R performance, those with first-episode schizophrenia performed the worst, followed by ultra-high-risk first-degree relatives, followed by first-degree relatives without ultra-high-risk, and finally, by healthy controls (Hou et al., 2016). Poorer time-based prospective memory in first-degree relatives of people with schizophrenia was predicted by lower HVLT-R and Stroop Color-Word Interference scores, whereas poorer event-based prospective memory was predicted by lower education and better Color Trails 2 scores (Zhou et al., 2014).

Measuring Treatment Effects. Most research on the HVLT-R has evaluated its validity as a screening test for dementia. However, the HVLT-R has also been used to study the treatment effect of memory rehabilitation for older adults with memory/cognitive complaints (Craik et al., 2007), low-frequency repetitive transcranial magnetic stimulation for stroke patients (Carey et al., 2008), deep brain stimulation for PD patients (Mikos et al., 2010), and other drug treatments (Fan et al., 2009; Lawrence et al., 2016; Mahoney et al., 2014). In using the HVLT-R to assess the effect of memory rehabilitation on older adults with memory/cognitive complaints, Delayed Recall increased immediately after the training period and persisted even after six months, whereas Total Recall did not benefit from the training (Craik et al., 2007). By contrast, although benefits of low-frequency repetitive transcranial magnetic stimulation to the contralesional primary motor cortex of stroke patients were seen immediately after treatment, memory returned to baseline by the next day (Carey et al., 2008). The test is also sensitive to detection of memory deficits related to deep brain stimulation in PD (Mikos et al., 2010).

Among studies that examined the effect of drug treatment on cognitive functions, erythropoietin (a hormone that controls red blood cell production) did not appear to have a protective effect on the cognitive function of individuals with breast cancer undergoing chemotherapy. Decline in HVLT-R was seen regardless of treatment groups, though those who received epoetin-alfa, a drug used to stimulate the increase of red blood cell levels, reported better quality of life than those who received standard care (Fan et al., 2009). However, the HVLT-R, particularly Total Recall and Recognition Discriminability, was sensitive to the effect of treatment with acetylcholinesterase inhibitors among breast cancer survivors with cognitive complaints who received adjuvant chemotherapy, whereas other indicators such as objective measures of attention, language, visuomotor skills, processing speed, executive function, and motor dexterity as well as subjective reports of cognitive functions, fatigue, sleep, mood, and health-related quality of life were not improved by treatment (Lawrence et al., 2016). Interestingly, the cholinesterase inhibitor rivastigmine improved working memory but not HVLT-R performance of long-term cocaine users (Mahoney et al., 2014).

Englund et al. (2013) studied the effects of cannabidiol (CBD) and tetrahydrocannabinol (THC), both chemical compounds found in cannabis, on memory using the HVLT-R. Total and Delayed Recall were poorer after THC compared to baseline. However, pretreatment with CBD appeared to have a protective effect, although the effect was seen on Delayed Recall only.

With regard to benefits of exercise, HVLT-R performance is not affected by physical activity in sedentary older adults (Sink et al., 2015). Specifically, Sink et al. (2015) noted that at 24 months following a moderate-intensity physical activity program (walking, resistance training, and flexibility exercises) or a health education program (educational workshop and upper extremity stretching), no group differences were found on HVLT-R scores in their sample of community-dwelling sedentary older adults at risk for mobility disability. In fact, neither of the programs benefitted cognitive functions.

In treatment studies, the availability of multiple, equivalent test forms is a particular strength of the HVLT-R. For example, the test has proved useful in clinical studies requiring serial assessment, such as evaluations of the cognitive effects associated with head injury (Bruce & Echemendia, 2003), changes in mood (Benedict et al., 1999), nutritional deficits (Lambert et al., 2002), and drug treatments (Van Rheenen & Rossell, 2014; Womack & Heilman, 2003). The HVLT-R, along with Color Trails and Grooved Pegboard, is also useful for defining cognitive impairment in clinical trials of effectively treated HIV-infected adults (Arenas-Pinto et al., 2014).

Finally, the HVLT-R appears sensitive to exposure to traffic pollution. Wellenius et al. (2012) found that community-dwelling older adults who live a short distance to a major roadway, a marker of long-term exposure to traffic pollution, showed poor HVLT-R Total Recall and Delayed Recall scores even after adjusting for demographics, medical history, education, and socioeconomic status.

NEUROANATOMICAL CORRELATES AND IMAGING STUDIES

In a study examining venular density using 7T MRI and cognitive function using the HVLT-R in homozygous sickle cell anemia, patients were more likely than controls to have a low density of long venules and a high density of short venules (Novelli et al., 2015). HVLT-R Retention was negatively correlated with density of short venules and positively correlated with density of long venules. In those with prodromal HD, Total Recall and Recognition Discriminability are associated with smaller striatal volume on MRI (Solomon et al., 2007).

PERFORMANCE VALIDITY

Not reported.

COMMENT

This test is relatively brief for a list-learning test and appears well-tolerated and suitable for difficult-to-test or more severely impaired individuals. The availability of alternate forms facilitates serial or multiple testing such as to monitor treatment effects. Existing research suggests that Form 3 is less likely to produce false-positive recognition errors than Forms 1, 2, or 4. Although the degree of difference appears modest, the authors recommend that, when the HVLT-R is used in repeated examination, Forms 1, 2, and 4 or Forms 3, 5, and 6 be used together. Analyses of the recall trials indicate that all six forms are interchangeable (Benedict et al., 1998).

Numerous studies support the use of the HVLT-R to detect dementia, and it appears to be more sensitive than the MMSE or WMS Logical Memory in identifying dementia. Research has also supported its use to assess memory impairment in various conditions including psychiatric disorders and HIV, as well as to assess effects of drug treatment and rehabilitation programs. Co-normed with the BVMT-R, both the HVLT-R and BVMT-R can be used as measures of material-specific memory in left versus right temporal lobe lesions. The inclusion of learning, delayed recall, and recognition components allows characterization of the unique learning and memory deficits associated with various disorders and can also be used to differentiate among various degenerative disorders such as amnestic MCI, AD, PD, and HD with a relatively high degree of accuracy (e.g., Aretouli et al., 2010; Gonzalez-Palau et al., 2013). The addition of other tests, such as reading ability, may also improve discrimination of dementia subtypes (Kuslansky et al., 2004). Although a lengthier or more complex test, such as the CVLT-II, was suggested for the finer assessment of memory performance in patients with mild and/ or more complex disorders (Lacritz et al., 2001), studies indicate that process scores are sufficiently sensitive to milder memory impairment (e.g., Foster et al., 2009; Malek-Ahmadi et al., 2011).

In terms of limitations, it is important to note that young and middle-aged well-educated adults achieve ceiling scores on the test, and older well-educated adults approach ceiling by the last learning trial. Because of ceiling effects for Delayed Recall and Recognition Discriminability, the authors suggest the use of descriptives or T-score ranges. Users should note that women were overrepresented in the standardization sample, and the number of men in some of the cells was small (e.g., the 80+ age group included only 18 men). In addition, individuals with MMSE scores as low as 22 were included, raising concerns that some cognitively compromised individuals may have been included in the normative base. The availability of additional norms for older adults (e.g., Hester et al., 2004; Vanderploeg et al., 2000) is a positive feature.

It is also important to note that test-retest reliabilities for some of the variables (e.g., % Retention, Recognition Discrimination) are very low in adults, most likely as a reflection of their restricted range and non-normal distribution. Greater confidence can be had with the Total Recall score, although, even here, rather large gains or declines in performance may be needed before change can be reliably detected.

Kuslansky et al. (2004) reported that HVLT performance is compromised in persons with low reading ability, and clinicians needed to take reading performance into account when interpreting HVLT scores. This likely also holds for the HVLT-R.

There is some evidence that time of testing can affect performance in older adults. Older individuals evaluated at their nonpreferred time of day obtained slightly lower Total scores than when tested at their preferred time of day (Paradee et al., 2005). Furthermore, a subjective rating of sleep quality and efficiency was also negatively associated with Total Recall and Delayed Recall scores (Sun et al., 2016). Therefore, testing at the nonoptimal time may increase the relative difficulty of the task for older adults.

Finally, there is a lack of performance validity or malingering studies. Its use is not recommended in groups where malingering is expected to occur at high base rates (e.g., litigants, disability claimants, criminal defendants), and the addition of performance validity tests is recommended for all other examinees.

REFERENCES

Andrews, G., Halford, G. S., Shum, D. H. K., Maujean, A., Chappell, M., & Birney, D. P. (2014). Verbal learning and memory following stroke. *Brain Injury, 28*(4), 442–447.

Arango-Lasprilla, J., Rivera, D., Garza, M. T., Saracho, C. P., Rodríguez, W., Rodríguez-Agudelo, Y., . . . Perrin, P. B. (2015). Hopkins Verbal Learning Test-Revised: Normative data for the Latin American Spanish speaking adult population. *Neurorehabilitation, 37*(4), 699–718.

Arenas-Pinto, A., Winston, A., Stöhr, W., Day, J., Wiggins, R., Quah, S. P., . . . Paton, N. I. (2014). Neurocognitive function in HIV-infected patients: Comparison of two methods to define impairment. *Plos One, 9*(7), e103498.

Aretouli, E., & Brandt, J. (2010). Episodic memory in dementia: Characteristics of new learning that differentiate Alzheimer's, Huntington's, and Parkinson's diseases. *Archives of Clinical Neuropsychology, 25*(5), 396–409.

Barr, W. B. (2003). Neuropsychological testing of high school athletes: Preliminary norms and test-retest indices. *Archives of Clinical Neuropsychology, 18*, 91–101.

Benedict, R. H. B. (1997). *Brief Visuospatial Memory Test—Revised.* Odessa, FL: Psychological Assessment Resources.

Benedict, R. H. B., Dobraski, M., & Goldstein, M. Z. (1999). A preliminary study of the association between changes in mood and cognition in a mixed geriatric psychiatry sample. *Journal of Gerontology: Psychological Sciences, 54B*, P94–P99.

Benedict, R. H. B., Schretlen, D., Groninger, L., & Brandt, J. (1998). The Hopkins Verbal Learning Test-Revised: Normative data and analysis of interform and test-retest reliability. *The Clinical Neuropsychologist, 12*, 43–55.

Benedict, R. H. B., Schretlen, D., Groninger, L., Dobraski, M., & Shritz, B. (1996). Revision of the Brief Visuospatial Memory Test: Studies of normal performance, reliability, and validity. *Psychological Assessment, 8*, 145–153.

Benedict, R. H. B., & Zgaljardic, D. J. (1998). Practice effects during repeated administrations of memory tests with and without alternate forms. *Journal of Clinical and Experimental Neuropsychology, 20*, 339–352.

Brandt, J. (1991). The Hopkins Verbal Learning Test: Development of a new memory test with six equivalent forms. *The Clinical Neuropsychologist, 5*, 125–142.

Brandt, J., & Benedict, R. H. B. (2001). Hopkins Verbal Learning Test–Revised. Odessa, FL: PAR.

Bruce, J. M., & Echemendia, R. J. (2003). Delayed-onset deficits in verbal encoding strategies among patients with mild traumatic brain injury. *Neuropsychology, 17*, 622–629.

Carey, C. L., Woods, S. P., Rippeth, J. D., Gonzalez, R., Moore, D. J., Marcotte, T. D., . . . the HNRC Group. (2004). Initial validation of a screening battery for the detection of HIV-associated cognitive impairment. *Clinical Neuropsychologist, 18*, 234–248.

Carey, J. R., Evans, C. D., Anderson, D. C., Bhatt, E., Nagpal, A., Kimberley, T. J., & Pascual-Leone, A. (2008). Safety of 6-hz primed low-frequency rTMS in stroke. *Neurorehabilitation and Neural Repair, 22*(2), 185–192.

Craik, F. I. M., Winocur, G., Palmer, H., Binns, M. A., Edwards, M., Bridges, K., . . . Stuss, D. T. (2007). Cognitive rehabilitation in the elderly: Effects on memory. *Journal of the International Neuropsychological Society, 13*(1), 132–142.

Czepielewski, L. S., Massuda, R., Goi, P., Sulzbach-Vianna, M., Reckziegel, R., Costanzi, M., . . . Gama, C. S. (2015). Verbal episodic memory along the course of schizophrenia and bipolar disorder:

A new perspective. *European Neuropsychopharmacology, 25*(2), 169–175.

Diaz-Asper, C., Schretlen, D. J., & Pearlson, G. D. (2004). How well does IQ predict neuropsychological test performance in normal adults. *Journal of the International Neuropsychological Society, 10,* 82–90.

Englund, A., Morrison, P. D., Nottage, J., Hague, D., Kane, F., Bonaccorso, S., . . . Kapur, S. (2013). Cannabidiol inhibits THC-elicited paranoid symptoms and hippocampal-dependent memory impairment. *Journal of Psychopharmacology, 27*(1), 19–27.

Fan, H. G. M., Park, A., Xu, W., Yi, Q. –., Braganza, S., Chang, J., . . . Tannock, I. F. (2009). The influence of erythropoietin on cognitive function in women following chemotherapy for breast cancer. *Psycho-Oncology, 18*(2), 156–161.

Foster, P. S., Drago, V., Crucian, G. P., Rhodes, R. D., Shenal, B. V., & Heilman, K. M. (2009). Verbal learning in Alzheimer's disease: Cumulative word knowledge gains across learning trials. *Journal of the International Neuropsychological Society, 15*(5), 730–739.

Foster, P. S., Drago, V., Crucian, G. P., Skidmore, F., Rhodes, R. D., Shenal, B. V., . . . Heilman, K. M. (2010). Verbal and visuospatial memory in lateral onset Parkinson disease: Time is of the essence. *Cognitive and Behavioral Neurology, 23*(1), 19–25.

Foster, P. S., Roosa, K. M., Drago, V., Branch, K., Finney, G., & Heilman, K. M. (2013). Recall of word lists is enhanced with increased spreading activation. *Aging, Neuropsychology, and Cognition, 20*(5), 553–566.

Friedman, M. A., Schinka, J. A., Mortimer, J. A., & Graves, A. B. (2002). Hopkins Verbal Learning Test—Revised: Norms for elderly African Americans. *The Clinical Neuropsychologist, 16,* 356–373.

Gaines, J. J., Shapiro, A., Alt, M., & Benedict, R. H. B. (2006). Semantic clustering indexes for the Hopkins Verbal Learning Test-Revised: Initial exploration in elder control and dementia groups. *Applied Neuropsychology, 13*(4), 213–222.

González-Palau, F., Franco, M., Jiménez, F., Parra, E., Bernate, M., & Solis, A. (2013). Clinical utility of the Hopkins Verbal Learning Test-Revised for detecting Alzheimer's disease and mild cognitive impairment in Spanish population. *Archives of Clinical Neuropsychology, 28*(3), 245–253.

Hester, R. L., Kinsella, G. J., Ong, B., & Turner, M. (2004). Hopkins Verbal Learning Test: Normative data for older Australian adults. *Australian Psychologist, 39,* 251–255.

Hogervorst, E., Combrinck, M., Lapuerta, P., Rue, J., Swales, K., & Budge, M. (2002). The Hopkins Verbal Learning Test and screening for dementia. *Dementia and Geriatric Cognitive Disorders, 13,* 13–20.

Hou, C., Xiang, Y., Wang, Z., Everall, I., Tang, Y., Yang, C., . . . Jia, F. (2016). Cognitive functioning in individuals at ultra-high risk for psychosis, first-degree relatives of patients with psychosis and patients with first-episode schizophrenia. *Schizophrenia Research, 174*(1-3), 71–76.

Kuslansky, G., Katz, M., Verghese, J., Hall, C. B., Lapuerta, P., LaRuffa, G., & Lipton, R. B. (2004). Detecting dementia with the Hopkins Verbal Learning Test and the Mini-Mental State examination. *Archives of Clinical Neuropsychology, 19,* 89–104.

Lacritz, L. H., Cullum, M. C., & Weiner, M. F. (2001). Comparison of the Hopkins Verbal Learning Test-Revised to the California Verbal Learning Test in Alzheimer's disease. *Applied Neuropsychology, 8,* 180–184.

Lacy, M., Kaemmerer, T., & Czipri, S. (2015). Standardized Mini-Mental State Examination scores and verbal memory performance at a memory center: Implications for cognitive screening. *American Journal of Alzheimer's Disease and Other Dementias, 30*(2), 145–152.

Lambert, A., Knaggs, K., Scragg, R., Metcalf, P., & Schaaf, D. (2002). Effects of iron treatment on cognitive performance and working memory in non-anaemic, iron deficient girls. *New Zealand Journal of Psychology, 31,* 19–28.

Larrabee, G. J. (2003). Lessons on measuring construct validity: A commentary on Delis, Jacobson, Bondi, Hamilton, and Salmon. *Journal of the International Neuropsychological Society, 9,* 947–954.

Lawrence, J. A., Griffin, L., Balcueva, E. P., Groteluschen, D. L., Samuel, T. A., Lesser, G. J., . . . Rapp, S. R. (2016). A study of donepezil in female breast cancer survivors with self-reported cognitive dysfunction 1 to 5 years following adjuvant chemotherapy. *Journal of Cancer Survivorship, 10*(1), 176–184.

Mahoney, J. J. I., II, Kalechstein, A. D., Verrico, C. D., Arnoudse, N. M., Shapiro, B. A., & Garza, D. L. (2014). Preliminary findings of the effects of rivastigmine, an acetylcholinesterase inhibitor, on working memory in cocaine-dependent volunteers. *Progress in Neuro-Psychopharmacology & Biological Psychiatry, 50,* 137–142.

Malek-Ahmadi, M., Raj, A., & Small, B. J. (2011). Semantic clustering as a neuropsychological predictor for amnestic-MCI. *Aging, Neuropsychology, and Cognition, 18*(3), 280–292.

Mata, I. F., Leverenz, J. B., Weintraub, D., Trojanowski, J. Q., Hurtig, H. I., Van Deerlin, V. M., . . . Zabetian, C. P. (2014). ApoE, MAPT, and SNCA genes and cognitive performance in Parkinson disease. *JAMA Neurology, 71*(11), 1405–1412.

Mikos, A., Zahodne, L., Okun, M. S., Foote, K., & Bowers, D. (2010). Cognitive declines after unilateral deep brain stimulation surgery in Parkinson's disease: A controlled study using reliable change, part II. *The Clinical Neuropsychologist, 24*(2), 235–245.

Miotto, E. C., Campanholo, K. R., Rodrigues, M. M., Serrao, V. T., de Lucia, Mara C. S., & Scaff, M. (2012). Hopkins Verbal Learning Test-Revised and Brief Visuospatial Memory Test-Revised: Preliminary normative data for the Brazilian population. *Arquivos De Neuro-Psiquiatria, 70*(12), 962–965.

Noll, K. R., Weinberg, J. S., Ziu, M., & Wefel, J. S. (2016). Editor's choice: Verbal learning processes in patients with glioma of the left and right temporal lobes. *Archives of Clinical Neuropsychology, 31*(1), 37–46.

Novelli, E. M., Sarles, C. E., Aizenstein, H. J., Ibrahim, T. S., Butters, M. A., Ritter, A. C., . . . Rosano, C. (2015). Brain venular pattern by 7T MRI correlates with memory and haemoglobin in sickle cell anaemia. *Psychiatry Research: Neuroimaging, 233*(1), 18–22.

O'Neil-Pirozzi, T. M., Goldstein, R., Strangman, G. E., & Glenn, M. B. (2012). Test–re-test reliability of the Hopkins Verbal Learning Test-Revised in individuals with traumatic brain injury. *Brain Injury, 26*(12), 1425–1430.

Paradee, C. V., Rapport, L. J., Hanks, R. A., & Levy, J. A. (2005). Circadian preference and cognitive functioning among rehabilitation inpatients. *The Clinical Neuropsychologist, 19,* 55–72.

Schretlen, D. J., Testa, S. M., & Pearlson, G. D. (2010). Calibrated Neuropsychological Normative System. Lutz, FL: PAR.

Shapiro, A. M., Benedict, R. H. B., Schretlen, D., & Brandt, J. (1999). Construct and concurrent validity of the Hopkins Verbal Learning Test-Revised. *The Clinical Neuropsychologist, 13,* 348–358.

Sink, K. M., Espeland, M. A., Castro, C. M., Church, T., Cohen, R., Dodson, J. A., . . . Williamson, J. D. (2015). Effect of a 24-month physical activity intervention vs. health education on cognitive outcomes in sedentary older adults: The LIFE randomized trial. *JAMA: Journal of the American Medical Association, 314*(8), 781–790.

Smith, M. M., Mills, J. A., Epping, E. A., Westervelt, H. J., & Paulsen, J. S. (2012). Depressive symptom severity is related to poorer cognitive performance in prodromal Huntington disease. *Neuropsychology, 26*(5), 664–669.

Solomon, A. C., Stout, J. C., Johnson, S. A., Langbehn, D. R., Aylward, E. H., Brandt, J., . . . Paulsen, J. S. (2007). Verbal episodic memory declines prior to diagnosis in Huntington's disease. *Neuropsychologia, 45*(8), 1767–1776.

Sun, Q., Luo, L., Ren, H., Wei, C., Xing, M., Cheng, Y., & Zhang, N. (2016). Semantic clustering and sleep in patients with amnestic mild cognitive impairment or with vascular cognitive impairment-no dementia. *International Psychogeriatrics, 28*(9), 1493–1502.

Tremont, G., Miele, A., Smith, M. M., & Westervelt, H. J. (2010). Comparison of verbal memory impairment rates in mild cognitive impairment. *Journal of Clinical and Experimental Neuropsychology, 32*(6), 630–636.

Vanderploeg, R. D., Schinka, J. A., Jones, T., Small, B. J., Graves, A. B., & Mortimer, J. A. (2000). Elderly norms for the Hopkins Verbal Learning Test-Revised. *The Clinical Neuropsychologist, 14,* 318–334.

Van Rheenen, T. E., & Rossell, S. L. (2014). Investigation of the component processes involved in verbal declarative memory function in bipolar disorder: Utility of the Hopkins Verbal Learning Test-Revised. *Journal of the International Neuropsychological Society, 20*(7), 727–735.

Wellenius, G. A., Boyle, L. D., Coull, B. A., Milberg, W. P., Gryparis, A., Schwartz, J., . . . Lipsitz, L. A. (2012). Residential proximity to nearest major roadway and cognitive function in community-dwelling seniors: Results from the mobilize Boston study. *Journal of the American Geriatrics Society, 60*(11), 2075–2080.

Witten, J. A., Thomas, K. G. F., Westgarth-Taylor, J., & Joska, J. A. (2015). Executive dyscontrol of learning and memory: Findings from a clade C HIV-positive South African sample. *The Clinical Neuropsychologist, 29*(7), 956–984.

Womack, K. B., & Heilman, K. B. (2003). Tolterodine and memory: Dry but forgetful. *Archives of Neurology, 60,* 771–773.

Woods, S. P., Scott, J. C., Conover, E., Marcotte, T. D., Heaton, R. K., Grant, I., & HIV Neurobehavioral Research Center (HNRC) Group. (2005). Test-retest reliability of component process variables within the Hopkins Verbal Learning Test-Revised. *Assessment, 12,* 96–100.

Zhou, F., Hou, W., Wang, C., Ungvari, G. S., Chiu, H. F. K., Correll, C. U., . . . Xiang, Y. (2014). Prospective memory performance in non-psychotic first- degree relatives of patients with schizophrenia: A controlled study. *Plos One, 9*(11), e111562. doi:10.1371/journal.pone.0111562.

Zhou, F., Xiang, Y., Wang, C., Dickerson, F., Au, R. W. C., Zhou, J., . . . Ungvari, G. S. (2012). Characteristics and clinical correlates of prospective memory performance in first-episode schizophrenia. *Schizophrenia Research, 135*(1–3), 34–39.

REY AUDITORY VERBAL LEARNING TEST (RAVLT)

TEST NAME	**Rey Auditory Verbal Learning Test (RAVLT)**
DOMAIN	Verbal memory
AGE RANGE	Up to 89 years
ADMINISTRATION TIME	10 to 15 minutes plus 20-minute delay interval
SCORING FORMAT	Hand scored
REFERENCE	Rey, A. (1958). *L'examen clinique en psychologie*. Paris: Presse Universitaire de France.

DESCRIPTION

The Rey Auditory Verbal Learning Test (RAVLT) is a brief, easily administered, pencil-and-paper measure that assesses immediate memory span, new learning, susceptibility to interference, and recognition memory. Another name includes the Auditory Verbal Learning Test (AVLT). The original version, a one-trial word list memory test, was developed by the Swiss psychologist Édouard Claparède in the early 1900s, making it one of the oldest mental tests in continuous use, albeit in modified form (Boake, 2000). Another Swiss psychologist, André Rey, one of Claparède's doctoral students, modified the task by introducing five recall trials followed by a recognition trial in which the examinee was to identify the list words in a story that also contained an equal number of concrete nouns as distractors (Boake, 2000). Taylor (1959) and Lezak (1976, 1983) further altered the test and adapted it for use with English-speaking examinees.

There are many variants of the RAVLT (see Lezak et al., 2012; Mitrushina et al., 2005). The most commonly used version (see Figure 10–1) consists of 15 nouns (List A) that are read aloud for five consecutive trials, each trial followed by a free recall test. The order of presentation of words remains fixed across trials. Instructions are repeated before each trial to minimize forgetting. On completion of Trial 5, an interference list of 15 words (List B) is presented, followed by a free recall test of that list. Immediately after this, delayed recall of the first list is tested (Trial 6) without further presentation of those words. After a 20-minute delay period, the examinee is again required to recall words from List A (Trial 7). Finally, a story that uses all the words from List A is presented, either orally or in written form (depending on the examinee's reading ability), and the person must identify words recognized from List A. Alternatively, recognition can be tested with the use of a matrix array of words, in which the individual must identify List A words from a list of 50 words containing all items from Lists A and B and 20 words that are phonemically or semantically similar to those in Lists A and B. This is the more popular format.

Analysis of task performance yields considerable information, including acquisition, learning rate, susceptibility to proactive and retroactive interference, and retention/forgetting. Learning is operationalized by changes in the number of words recalled across the five trials. Acquisition is typically evaluated by summing the total number of words recalled across the first five recall trials, and learning rate is examined by comparing the number of words recalled on the first trial with the number of words recalled on the fifth recall trial. In this way, the examiner can determine whether repeated presentations of the word list contribute to gains in recall performance. Aspects of retention can be examined because the fifth trial is followed by the distractor list (List B), which in turn is followed by immediate (Trial 6) and delayed recall trials (Trial 7) of the primary list. Therefore, susceptibility to proactive interference (Trial 1 recall vs. List B recall) and retroactive interference (Trial 5 vs. Trial 6) can be assessed. Forgetting is typically assessed by comparing the number of words recalled on the fifth recall trial with the number of words recalled after the 20-minute delay (i.e., by calculating a "savings" score).

A more complete characterization of memory can be had by evaluating performance across various serial positions of the presentation items, including primacy (performance is collapsed across serial positions 1–3), middle (performance is collapsed across serial positions 5–11), and recency (performance is collapsed across serial positions 13–15). Finer-grained analysis of trial-by-trial performance can also be done by measuring the gains in access to items from one trial to the next ("gained access") and losses in access to items from one trial to the next ("lost access"); in this way deficits in

Name ____________________

Date ____________________

Examiner ____________________

(Note: Do not re-read List A for Recall Trial A6 or A7)										
List A	*A1*	*A2*	*A3*	*A4*	*A5*	*List B*	*B1*	*A6*	*A7*	
Drum						Desk				Drum
Curtain						Ranger				Curtain
Bell						Bird				Bell
Coffee						Shoe				Coffee
School						Stove				School
Parent						Mountain				Parent
Moon						Glasses				Moon
Garden						Towel				Garden
Hat						Cloud				Hat
Farmer						Boat				Farmer
Nose						Lamb				Nose
Turkey						Gun				Turkey
Color						Pencil				Color
House						Church				House
River						Fist				River
# Correct										

Total A1 to A5 ________

Trial A6 – A5 ________

Word List for Testing RAVLT Recognition

Bell (A)	Home (SA)	Towel (B)	Boat (B)	Glasses (B)
Window (SA)	Fish (B)	Curtain (A)	Hot (PA)	Stocking (SB)
Hat (A)	Moon (A)	Flower (SA)	Parent (A)	Shoe (B)
Barn (SA)	Tree (PA)	Color (A)	Water (SA)	Teacher (SA)
Ranger (B)	Balloon (PA)	Desk (B)	Farmer (A)	Stove (B)
Nose (A)	Bird (B)	Gun (B)	Rose (SPA)	Nest (SPB)
Weather (SB)	Mountain (B)	Crayon (SA)	Cloud (B)	Children (SA)
School (A)	Coffee (A)	Church (B)	House (A)	Drum (A)
Hand (PA)	Mouse (PA)	Turkey (A)	Stranger (PB)	Toffee (PA)
Pencil (B)	River (A)	Fountain (PB)	Garden (A)	Lamb (B)

Figure 10–1 *Rey Auditory Verbal Learning Test (RAVLT) sample scoring sheet. On the recognition list, A-words from list A; B-words from list B; S-words with a semantic association to a word on list A or B as indicated; P-words phonemically similar to a word on list A or B as indicated.*

SOURCE: From Lezak (1983).

intertrial acquisition and consolidation can be revealed (Woodard et al., 1999).

The addition of a recognition trial permits the identification of individuals with suspected retrieval problems who may score better on this trial than on free recall. In addition, comparison of recognition of the two lists permits the evaluation of words that have been studied five times (List A) versus words that were studied once only (List B), as well as source memory for which list contained the words (Schmidt, 1996).

OTHER FORMS

In addition to the standard form (Lists A and B), Lezak (1983) and Taylor (1959) provided an alternate list (List C) to be used as a substitute for either List A or List B. However, List C contains more low-frequency words and is more difficult than List A (Crawford et al., 1989; Ryan et al., 1986). Word frequencies also differ between Lists B and C, with List B containing more low-frequency words. The substitution of List C for B may lead to elevated interference trial scores and to superior recognition performance for List A relative to that expected when List B is used (Fuller et al., 1997). Several other investigators have provided alternate forms of the test (e.g., Crawford et al., 1989; Geffen et al., 1994; Lannoo & Vingerhoets, 1997; Majdan et al., 1996; Ryan et al., 1986; Shapiro & Harrison, 1990; Van den Burg & Kingma, 1999). The versions by Geffen et al. (1994) and Majdan et al. (1996) seem to produce comparable scores and are presented in Figures 10–2 and 10–3.

In order to reduce cultural bias, the World Health Organization/University of California Los Angeles (WHO/UCLA) version of the AVLT was developed (Maj et al., 1993; Ponton et al., 1996, 2000). The test is administered in the language of the examinee, and all test items were selected from five categories (body parts, animals, tools, household objects, and transportation vehicles) and presumably have universal familiarity. There are 15 items, including three examples from each category (see Figure 10–4). Note that this version differs from the standard one in that it does not consist of unrelated words.

The RAVLT has been adapted for use in a number of other languages including Arabic (Poreh et al., 2012), Chinese (Lee, 2003), Czech (Bezdicek et al., 2014), Dutch (Van den Burg & Kingma, 1999), Flemish (Lannoo & Vingerhoets, 1997), German (Helmstaedter & Durwen, 1990), Greek (Messinis et al., 2007), Hebrew (Vakil & Blachstein, 1994; Vakil et al., 1998), Portuguese (Fichman et al., 2010; Malloy-Diniz et al., 2007), and Spanish (Correia & Osorio, 2014; Miranda & Valencia, 1997). Please refer to Table 10-77 for more information about their normative data.

ADMINISTRATION

For specific instructions, see Figure 10–5. Administration of the WHO/UCLA form (Figure 10–4) is in the language of the examinee.

Some authors use a presentation rate of one word per second (e.g., Forrester & Geffen, 1991), whereas others (e.g., Van den Burg & Kingma, 1999) use a one-second interval between words. However, the various studies yield similar results, suggesting little effect in the range of rates considered here.

TIME OF ADMINISTRATION

Lehmann et al. (2013) reported that adults tested at their optimal time (synchrony effect) perform better than when they were tested at their nonoptimal time, more so for the younger adults than older adults on Total Learning and Delayed Recall. Younger adults perform better in the afternoon while older adults perform better in the morning. In fact, younger adults tested during their optimal time outperform older adults tested during their optimal time. However, no group differences are seen on Recognition and the Proactive Interference Index. These results suggest that the synchrony effect exists but it does not explain age-related differences.

SCORING

See sample scoring sheet for recording correct answers in Figure 10–1. Words that are repeated can be marked R; words that are repeated and self-corrected can be marked RC. If the examinee questions whether they have repeated a word but remains unsure, the word can be marked RQ. Words that are not on the list are errors and are marked E.

A number of different measures can be derived (see also Schmidt, 1996). Geffen et al. (1990) provided a list of scores of different aspects of memory function, only some of which are reported here. See Table 10–57 for a description of some of the scores.

Ivnik et al. (1992) also introduced a number of other measures to summarize the learning and retrieval processes, and these are shown in Table 10–58. In order to use the Mayo's Older Americans Normative Studies (MOANS) norms provided by Ivnik et al. (1992) for adults aged 55 to 97 years, the examiner must convert RAVLT scores to age-corrected and normalized MOANS Scaled Scores ($M = 10$, $SD = 3$). MOANS Scaled Scores are then grouped and summed within groups to allow derivation of three summary indices: the Mayo Auditory-Verbal Learning Efficiency Index (MAVLEI), the Mayo Auditory-Verbal Delayed Recall Index (MAVDRI), and the Mayo Auditory-Verbal Percent Retention Index (MAVPRI). These summary indices have means equal to 100 and *SD*s equal to 15. Note, however, that Ivnik

List A	Interference List B			
Pipe	Bench			
Wall	Officer			
Alarm	Cage			
Sugar	Sock			
Student	Fridge			
Mother	Cliff			
Star	Bottle			
Painting	Soap			
Bag	Sky			
Wheat	Ship			
Mouth	Goat			
Chicken	Bullet			
Sound	Paper			
Door	Chapel			
Stream	Crab			
Recognition List				
Alarm (A)	Eye (SA)	Soap (B)	Ship (B)	Bottle (B)
Aunt (SA)	Crab (B)	Wall (A)	Car (PA)	Seat (SB)
Bag (A)	Star (A)	Clock (SA)	Mother (A)	Sock (B)
Creek (SA)	Rag (PA)	Sound (A)	Duck (SA)	Tone (SA)
Officer (B)	Bun (PA)	Bench (B)	Wheat (A)	Fridge (B)
Mouth (A)	Cage (B)	Bullet (B)	Floor (SPA)	Rock (SPB)
Arrow (SB)	Cliff (B)	Night (SA)	Sky (B)	Bread (SA)
Student (A)	Sugar (A)	Chapel (B)	Door (A)	Pipe (A)
Hail (PA)	Cream (PA)	Chicken (A)	Bridge (PB)	Ball (PA)
Paper (B)	Stream (A)	Coat (PB)	Painting (A)	Goat (B)

Figure 10–2. *Alternate form of the Rey Auditory Verbal Learning Test (RAVLT) by Geffen et al. (1994). Abbreviations for the recognition list are the same as in Figure 10-1.*

SOURCE: Adapted from Geffen et al. (1994).

Form 1

LIST A	LIST B	RECOGNITION	BUFFERS:	BOTTLE	CALENDAR
Violin	Orange	**Scarf**	*Toad*	*Donkey*	Train
Tree	Table	Leaf	*Chin*	Pear	Uncle
Scarf	Toad	**Stairs**	**Ham**	**Cousin**	**Violin**
Ham	Corn	Frog	Piano	Grass	Stars
Suitcase	Bus	*Table*	**Field**	**Dog**	*Spider*
Cousin	Chin	**Banana**	*Soap*	Gloves	
Earth	Beach	Hospital	**Tree**	*Hotel*	
Stairs	Soap	**Suitcase**	City	**Bucket**	
Dog	Hotel	Peel	**Hunter**	Sofa	
Banana	Donkey	*Book*	*Orange*	**Town**	
Town	Spider	Blanket	*Money*	*Beach*	
Radio	Monkey	*Padlock*	Doctor	Cork	
Hunter	Book	**Earth**	*Soldier*	Corn	
Bucket	Soldier	Television	**Radio**	*Lunchbox*	
Field	Padlock	Rock	Chest	*Bus*	

Form 2

LIST A	LIST B	RECOGNITION	BUFFERS:	TELEPHONE	*ZOO*
Doll	Dish	**Nail**	*Hill*	*Foot*	*Fly*
Mirror	Jester	Stall	*Forest*	Bread	Dart
Nail	Hill	**Bed**	**Sailor**	**Desert**	**Doll**
Sailor	Coat	Engine	Pony	Street	Captain
Heart	Tool	*Jester*	**Road**	**Machine**	*Shield*
Desert	Forest	**Milk**	*Ladder*	Jail	
Face	Perfume	Soot	**Mirror**	*Girl*	
Letter	Ladder	Heart	Envelope	**Horse**	
Bed	Girl	Silk	**Music**	Joker	
Machine	Foot	*Insect*	*Dish*	**Letter**	
Milk	Shield	Screw	*Pie*	*Perfume*	
Helmet	Pie	*Car*	Song	Plate	
Music	Insect	**Face**	*Ball*	*Coat*	
Horse	Ball	Armour	**Helmet**	Sand	
Road	Car	Head	Pool	*Tool*	

Figure 10–3 *Two alternate forms of the Rey Auditory Verbal Learning Test (RAVLT) by Majdan et al. (1996). Words from principal list are in boldface; words from interference list are in italics.*

List A	*List B*	
Arm	Boot	
Cat	Monkey	
Axe	Bowl	
Bed	Cow	
Place	Finger	
Ear	Dress	
Dog	Spider	
Hammer	Cup	
Chair	Bee	
Car	Foot	
Eye	Hat	
Horse	Butterfly	
Knife	Kettle	
Clock	Mouse	
Bike	Hand	
Recognition Items		
Mirror	**Horse**	Truck
Hammer	Leg	**Eye**
Knife	**Dog**	Fish
Candle	Table	**Ear**
Motorcycle	**Cat**	**Bike**
Axe	Lips	Snake
Clock	Tree	Stool
Chair	**Arm**	Bus
Plane	Nose	**Bed**
Turtle	Sun	**Car**

Figure 10–4 *World Health Organization/University of California Los Angeles (WHO/UCLA) version of the Rey Auditory Verbal Learning Test (RAVLT). On the recognition list, boldface items are words from the principal list.*
SOURCE: Courtesy of P. Satz.

et al. (1992) used a 30-word list, as opposed to a 50-word list, for their recognition trial (see Figure 10–6). The Mayo's Older African American Normative Studies (MOAANS) uses the same procedure. Because the MOANS norms are more than 30 years old, they will not be presented here. Interested readers may refer to their article for the norms tables.

Ricci et al. (2012) developed a memory index to differentiate AD from behavioral variant-frontotemporal dementia:

RAVLT MEI = (Delayed Recall ÷ 15) ÷ (Trials 1–5 ÷ 75)
+ (Delayed Recognition Hits ÷ 15)
– (False Positives ÷ total number of distractors)

Please refer to the section "Clinical Studies" for more information about this memory index.

DEMOGRAPHIC EFFECTS

COMBINED EFFECTS OF DEMOGRAPHIC VARIABLES

Age affects performance on the RAVLT and has been reported to account for up to 10% of variance (Bezdicek et al., 2014); the influence of gender and intellectual/educational level is less consistent across studies and generally accounts for less variance than age (Bezdicek et al., 2014; Carstairs et al., 2012; Correia & Osorio, 2014; Fichman et al., 2010; Kurlyo et al., 2001; Magalhaes & Hamdan, 2010; Malloy-Diniz et al., 2007; Messinis et al., 2007, 2016; Poreh et al., 2012; Schoenberg et al., 2006;

TABLE 10–57 Description of Rey Auditory Verbal Learning Test (RAVLT) Scores

SCORE	DESCRIPTION
Trial 1	Number of List A words correctly recalled on the first trial
Trial 5	Number of List A words correctly recalled on the fifth trial
Total Learning (Trials 1 to 5)	Sum of List A Trials 1 to 5
List B (Interference trial)	Number of List B words recalled
Immediate Recall (Trial 6)	Number of List A words recalled immediately after List B
Delayed Recall (Trial 7)	Number of List A words recalled after a 20-minute delay
Repetitions	Sum of repeated words, Trials 1 to 5
Intrusions	Sum of non-List A words, Trials 1 to 5
Retroactive Interference	Percentage of words lost from Trial 5 to Trial 6
Proactive Interference	Interference from learning List A in the learning of List B
Recognition	Sum of recognition hits

For Trial 1, the examiner gives the following instructions: *I am going to read a list of words. Listen carefully, for when I stop you are to repeat back as many words as you can remember. It doesn't matter in what order you repeat them. Just try to remember as many as you can.*

The examiner reads the 15 words on List A, with a 1-s interval between words. Check off the words recalled, using numbers to keep track of the patient's order of word recall. No feedback should be given regarding the number of correct responses, repetitions, or errors.

After the patient indicates that they can recall no more words, the examiner rereads the list after giving a second set of instructions: *Now I am going to read the same words again, and once again when I stop I want you to tell me as many words as you can remember, including words you said the first time. It doesn't matter in what order you say them. Just say as many words as you can remember whether or not you said them before.*

The list is reread for Trials 3 through 5, using Trial 2 instructions each time. The examiner may praise the patient as they recall more words; the examiner may tell the patient the number of words already recalled, particularly if the patient is able to use the information for reassurance or as a challenge.

After Trial 5, the examiner reads List B with instructions to perform as on the first (A) list trial: *Now I'm going to read a second list of words. Listen carefully, for when I stop you are to repeat back as many words as you can remember. It doesn't matter in what order you repeat them. Just try to remember as many as you can.*

Immediately after the List B trial, the examiner asks the patient to recall as many words from the first list (List A) as they can (Trial 6) without further presentation of those words: *Now tell me all the words that you can remember from the first list.*

After a 20-min delay period filled with other activity, the subject is asked to recall the words from List A: *A while ago, I read a list of words to you several times, and you had to repeat back the words. Tell me the words from that list.*

On completion of the delay trial, the recognition test should be given. The recognition task requires the patient to identify as many of the list words as they can and, if possible, the specific list of origin. If the patient can read at least at grade 7 level, ask the patient to read the list and circle the correct words. If the patient has difficulty with reading, the examiner should read the list to the patient: *I will say some words that were on the word lists that I read to you, and some other words that were not on those lists. Tell me each time I say a word that was read to you. If you can remember that the word was from the word lists, tell me if the word was from the first or second list.*

Figure 10–5 *Administration instructions for the Rey Auditory Verbal Learning Test (RAVLT).*
SOURCE: Adapted from Geffen et al. (1990); Lezak (1976, 1983); Schmidt (1996); and Vakil and Blachstein (1994).

Teruya et al., 2009; Van der Elst et al., 2005; also see Mitrushina et al., 2005, for reviews).

TABLE 10–58 MOANS Summary Scores for the RAVLT

SCORE	DESCRIPTION	PROCEDURE
Learning Over Trials Score (LOT)	Sum of words learned across Trials 1–5, corrected for immediate word span	Total Learning over five trials − (5 × Trial 1 score)
Short-Term Percent Retention (STPR)	Trial 6 Recall expressed as a proportion of Trial 5 Recall	100 × (Trial 6 Recall ÷ Trial 5 Recall)
Long-Term Percent Retention (LTPR)	Delayed Recall score expressed a proportion of Trial 5 recall	100 × (Delayed Recall Score ÷ Trial 5 Recall)
Auditory Verbal Learning Efficiency Index (MAVLEI or LEI)	Sum of MOANS Scaled Score for Trial 1 and LOT scores; reflects learning process	Sum MOANS Trial 1 and LOT
Mayo Auditory-Verbal Delayed Recall Index (MAVDRI or DRI)	Sum of Trial 6 and 30-min Delayed Recall score; reflects absolute amount remembered	Sum MOANS Trial 6 and 30-min Delayed Recall
Mayo Auditory-Verbal Percent Retention Index (MAVPRI or PRI)	Sum of Trials A6 and A7 expressed as percent retention scores; reflects recall after a delay as a function of amount originally learned	Sum of STPR and LTPR

NOTE: STPR, Short-Term Percent Retention; LTPR, Long-Term Percent Retention.

AGE

The evidence indicates that certain RAVLT scores tend to decrease in adults with advancing age (Bennett et al., 2015). Two distinct segments can be distinguished as well: the age group 20 to 59 years is less distinguishable from itself than is the 60- to 90-year-old age range (Vakil & Blachstein, 1997). Rates of learning, proactive interference, and recognition show less change with age (Bennett et al., 2015), whereas the number of free-recall words on the learning and delay trials shows greater decline with advancing age (Bennett et al., 2015; Dunlosky & Salthouse, 1996; Mitrushina et al., 2005; Vakil & Blachstein, 1997). However, Uttl (2005) has argued that, when ceiling effects on preceding recall trials are minimized by administering only three learning trials, age-related declines on RAVLT Long Delay Recall and Recognition are comparable.

Most authors (Dunlosky & Salthouse, 1996; Vakil & Blachstein, 1997) have found that forgetting increases with advancing age. Some have observed an age-related decline in the primacy and middle portions, but not in the recency component of free recall (Graf & Uttl, 1995); others (Dunlosky & Salthouse, 1996) have reported a decline in the primacy component only. Graf and Uttl (1995) suggested that the age change in free recall reflects age changes in processing rate and capacity. Findings from studies by Salthouse et al. (1996) and Dunlosky and Salthouse (1996) indicate that speed of processing plays a central role in mediating age-related effects on free-recall

Teacher	Coffee
River	Road
Bridge	Hat
Farmer	Turkey
Pen	Minute
Forehead	Nose
Kerchief	School
House	Bell
Moon	Face
Color	Garden
Beat	Classroom
Curtain	Parent
Floor	Children
Soldier	Broomstick
Drum	Gun

Recognition instructions: "Sometimes people can remember more of the words if they see them. Read all these words, and circle the ones that you think were on that first list that I read . . . the list I read five times to you."

Recognition hits (REC) = ___
False-positive errors (ERR) = ___
RPC = [REC + (15 – ERR)] × 100 = ___

Figure 10–6 *Mayo's Older Americans Normative Studies (MOANS) 30-Word recognition list.*
SOURCE: Adapted from Ferman et al. (2005).

performance but that it is not the only factor contributing to those effects.

GENDER

Some authors have found that gender has no impact on test scores (e.g., Correia & Osorio, 2014; Fichman et al., 2010; Kurlyo et al., 2001; Magalhaes & Hamdan, 2010; Messinis et al., 2016; Mitrushina et al., 2005; Vogel et al., 2012). When gender differences do emerge, females outperform males on the recall trials by about one word per trial, but not on the recognition trials (Bezdicek et al., 2014; Carstairs et al., 2012; Gale et al., 2016; Malloy-Diniz et al., 2007; Messinis et al., 2007; Miatton et al., 2004; Miller et al., 2015; Poreh et al., 2012; Sunderman et al., 2016; Sziklas & Jones-Gotman, 2008; Teruya et al., 2009; but see Harris et al., 2002, and Van der Elst et al., 2005, who found that females outperformed males on recognition as well).

Gale et al. (2016) found that gender differences are seen in healthy older adults but not in those with MCI or AD. Moreover, despite similar performance on the CDR, MMSE, and DRS, the degree of discrepancies in RAVLT scores between females with MCI or AD and healthy females is remarkably larger than that of males. Sunderman et al. (2016) further reported that the gender differences on RAVLT are dependent on hippocampal volume/intracranial volume ratio. Women obtain higher RAVLT scores than men but only in those with moderate to large hippocampal volume/intracranial volume ratio, and particularly among those with amnestic MCI.

EDUCATION AND IQ

Most studies reported that performance is better at higher educational levels (Bezdicek et al., 2014; Correia & Osorio, 2014; Fichman et al., 2010; Kurlyo et al., 2001; Magalhaes & Hamdan, 2010; Malloy-Diniz et al., 2007; Messinis et al., 2007, 2016; Miatton et al., 2004; Poreh et al., 2012; Schoenberg et al., 2006; Van der Elst et al., 2005), and yet others note that education effects are seen in some indices but not others (Carstairs et al., 2012; Teruya et al., 2009; Vogel et al., 2012). Steinberg et al. (2005) argued that education does not account for RAVLT test score variance beyond that accounted for by IQ.

Recall tends to be better at higher IQ levels (Vakil et al., 1997; Vogel et al., 2012). It should be noted that relations with FSIQ are not uniform across scores within the test. For example, correlations between intelligence and RAVLT recognition tend to be about half as strong as those between intelligence and various indices of learning and recall (Schmidt, 1996; Steinberg et al., 2005). Furthermore, the strength of the RAVLT-FSIQ correlations appears greatest at moderate levels of intelligence (Steinberg et al., 2005).

ETHNICITY, NATIONALITY, AND LINGUISTIC EFFECTS

Among African Americans, lower levels of acculturation are linked to significantly poorer scores (Kennepohl et al., 2004). In comparing the French-Canadian version of the RAVLT to the English version, Sziklas and Jones-Gotman (2008) reported that francophones perform slightly worse than anglophones on the Immediate and Delayed Recall trials but not on Recognition, possibly due to the higher difficulty of the French-Canadian word list. Comparison among healthy individuals in Thailand, Zaire, Germany, and Italy suggests that the WHO/UCLA AVLT is freer of cultural influences than the traditional RAVLT (Maj et al., 1993).

NORMATIVE DATA

Mitrushina et al. (2005) compiled data from four to eight studies, comprising 453 to 1,910 participants aged 20 to 79 years for Trial 1, Trial 5, Recall after interference (Trial 6), Recognition, and Total Learning. The values match closely the metanorms provided by Schmidt (1996) for most variables (Trial 1, Trial 5, Trial 6) and are similar in the rate of age-related changes for most of the variables. Mean education levels were quite high (about 14 years), and the metanorms may overestimate expected scores for individuals with lower educational or intellectual levels. Therefore, the examiner can refer to specific reference studies recommended for various groups (see Mitrushina et al., 2005, and later discussion).

Given that IQ is more strongly related to performance than education, Steinberg et al. (2005) reanalyzed data from the MOANS project and provided age- (55+) and IQ-adjusted percentile equivalents of MOANS age-adjusted RAVLT scores. Readers should note that all FSIQs are age-adjusted scores, which are based on the WAIS-R, not the WAIS-III. Given the upward shift in scores (Flynn effect) with the passage of time, use of the WAIS-R FSIQ, rather than the WAIS-III, might result in a given RAVLT appearing less favorable. The interested reader is referred to their article for the relevant tables.

Ferman et al. (2005) provide age- and education-adjusted normative data based on 306 African-American community-dwelling participants from the MOAANS project in Jacksonville, Florida. Participants ranged in age from 56 to 94 years and varied in education from 0 to 20 years of formal education. They were screened to exclude those with active neurological, psychiatric, or other conditions that might affect cognition. The test administration procedure was identical to that used in the MOANS project (see Ivnik et al., 1992) and included the 30-item recognition task. Tables 10–59 through 10–65 convert RAVLT scores to age-corrected MOAANS Scaled Scores (M = 10, SD = 3) and summary Mayo Auditory-Verbal Indices (M = 100, SD = 15; Table 10–66). Note that the number of recognition hits (REC) and false positive errors (ERR) are also provided in Tables 10-59 through 10-65. As with the original MOANS project, the cells are based on the method of overlapping age intervals.

Age- and education-adjusted adult MOAANS scaled scores are obtained by applying the algorithms in Table 10–67 to each age-adjusted scaled score. Age- and education-corrected indices for learning (LEI), delayed recall (DRI), and percent retention (PRI) are computed in a two-step process. The MOAANS age- and education-adjusted scaled scores replace the MOAANS age-adjusted scaled scores. Once the appropriate sums are calculated, they can be transformed to their respective index scores by locating the values under the appropriate column in Table 10–68. The authors noted that one of the strengths

TABLE 10–59 MOAANS RAVLT Scaled Scores for Ages 56 to 62 Years (Midpoint Age = 61, Age Range for Norms = 56–66)

SCALED SCORE	TRIAL 1	LIST B	TRIAL 6	30-MIN DELAY	REC	ERR	RPC	LOT	STPR	LTPR	PERCENTILE RANGE
2	0	0	0–1	–	0–6	7+	–	<1	0–21	–	<1
3	1	–	–	–	7	–	<66	1	22–27	–	1
4	2	1	2	0	–	6	66–67	2	28–29	–	2
5	–	–	–	–	8	5	68–70	3–4	30–36	0	3–5
6	3	2	3	1	9	4	71–75	5–7	37–44	1–20	6–10
7	–	–	4	2–3	10	3	76–80	8–9	45–55	21–40	11–18
8	4	3	5	4	11–12	2	81–85	10	56–63	41–47	19–28
9	–	–	6	5	13	–	86–88	11–12	64–68	48–59	29–40
10	5	4	7	6–7	14	1	89–93	13–15	69–77	60–73	41–59
11	6	5	8	8	–	–	94–95	16–17	78–84	74–81	60–71
12	–	–	9	9	–	0	96–99	18–20	85–90	82–89	72–81
13	7	6	10–11	10	15	–	–	21–23	91–93	90–92	82–89
14	–	7	12	11	–	–	100	24–26	94+	93+	90–94
15	8	8	13	12	–	–	–	27–29	–	–	95–97
16	9	–	14	13	–	–	–	30–32	–	–	98
17	10+	9+	15	–	–	–	–	33+	–	–	99
18	–	–	–	14–15	–	–	–	–	–	–	>99

NOTE: ERR, false-positive errors; LOT, learning over trials; LTPR, long-term percent retention; REC, recognition hits; RPC, recognition percent correct; STPR, short-term percent retention. See Table 10–58 for definitions.

SOURCE: From Ferman et al. (2005).

TABLE 10–60 MOAANS RAVLT Scaled Scores for Age 63 to 65 Years (Midpoint Age = 64, Age Range for Norms = 59–69)

SCALED SCORE	TRIAL 1	LIST B	TRIAL 6	30-MIN DELAY	REC	ERR	RPC	LOT	STPR	LTPR	PERCENTILE RANGE
2	0	0	0–1	–	0–6	7+	–	<1	0–21	–	<1
3	1	–	–	–	7	–	<64	–	22–27	–	1
4	2	1	2	0	–	6	64–66	1	28–29	–	2
5	–	–	–	–	8	5	67–70	2–4	30–36	0	3–5
6	3	2	3	1	9	4	71–75	5–6	37–44	1–20	6–10
7	–	–	4	2–3	10–11	3	76–80	7–9	45–55	21–40	11–18
8	4	3	5	4	–	2	81–84	10	56–61	41–47	19–28
9	–	–	6	5	12	–	85–88	11–12	62–67	48–59	29–40
10	5	4	7	6–7	13–14	1	89–92	13–15	68–77	60–73	41–59
11	–	–	8	8	–	–	93–94	16–17	78–83	74–81	60–71
12	6	5	9	9	–	0	95–99	18–20	84–90	82–89	72–81
13	–	6	10	10	15	–	–	21–23	91–92	90–92	82–89
14	7	–	11	11	–	–	100	24–26	93+	93+	90–94
15	–	7–8	12	12	–	–	–	27–29	–	–	95–97
16	8	–	13	–	–	–	–	30–32	–	–	98
17	9	9+	14–15	13	–	–	–	33	–	–	99
18	10+	–	–	14–15	–	–	–	34+	–	–	>99

NOTE: ERR, false-positive errors; LOT, learning over trials; LTPR, long-term percent retention; REC, recognition hits; RPC, recognition percent correct; STPR, short-term percent retention. See Table 10–58 for definitions.

SOURCE: From Ferman et al. (2005).

of their normative sample is its inclusion of a wide range of educational levels; however, they cautioned that African Americans with qualitatively different educational backgrounds (e.g., those educated outside the segregated South) may perform differently. They also noted the presence of floor effects on the 30-minute Delayed Recall trial, raising concerns regarding the utility of this measure with regard to the information that it can provide about retention of information over time in this population. The RPC index appears to be more resistant to floor effects.

Carstairs et al. (2012) provide norms for 390 young adults aged 18–34 years from Sydney, Australia. A scoring program is provided for ease of scoring at https://www.mq.edu.au/__data/assets/excel_doc/0008/905282/RAVLT-1.xls. Tables 10–69 to 10–73 present the normative data.

TABLE 10–61 MOAANS RAVLT Scaled Scores for Age 66 to 68 Years (Midpoint Age = 67, Age Range for Norms = 62–72)

SCALED SCORE	TRIAL 1	LIST B	TRIAL 6	30-MIN DELAY	REC	ERR	RPC	LOT	STPR	LTPR	PERCENTILE RANGE
2	0	–	0	–	0–3	7+	–	<1	0–17	–	<1
3	1	0	1	–	4–6	–	<63	–	18–21	–	1
4	–	–	2	–	7	6	63–66	1	22–27	–	2
5	2	1	–	0	8	5	67–70	2–3	28–32	0	3–5
6	3	2	3	1	9	4	71–75	4–6	33–43	1–16	6–10
7	–	–	4	2–3	10	3	76–79	6–7	44–53	17–39	11–18
8	–	3	5	4	11	2	80–82	8–10	54–59	40–46	19–28
9	4	–	6	–	12	–	83–87	11–12	60–67	47–56	29–40
10	5	4	7	5–6	13	1	88–92	13–15	68–77	57–69	41–59
11	–	–	8	7–8	14	–	93–94	16–17	78–83	70–80	60–71
12	6	5	9	9	–	0	95–99	18–19	84–90	81–89	72–81
13	–	–	10	10	15	–	–	20–22	91–92	90–92	82–89
14	7	6	11	11	–	–	–	23–26	93+	93+	90–94
15	–	7	–	–	–	–	100	27–29	–	–	95–97
16	8	8	12	12	–	–	–	30–31	–	–	98
17	9	9+	13–14	13	–	–	–	32–33	–	–	99
18	10+	–	15	14–15	–	–	–	34+	–	–	>99

NOTE: ERR, false-positive errors; LOT, learning over trials; LTPR, long-term percent retention; REC, recognition hits; RPC, recognition percent correct; STPR, short-term percent retention. See Table 10–58 for definitions.

SOURCE: From Ferman et al. (2005).

TABLE 10-62 MOAANS RAVLT Scaled Scores for Age 69–71 Years (Midpoint Age = 70, Age Range for Norms = 65–75)

SCALED SCORE	TRIAL 1	LIST B	TRIAL 6	30-MIN DELAY	REC	ERR	RPC	LOT	STPR	LTPR	PERCENTILE RANGE
2	0	–	–	–	0–3	9+	–	<1	–	–	<1
3	1	0	0	–	4–6	7–8	<61	–	0–11	–	1
4	–	–	1	–	–	–	61–66	1	12–20	–	2
5	2	1	2	0	7	5–6	67–70	2	21–28	0	3–5
6	3	2	3	1	8–9	4	71–74	3–5	29–40	1–14	6–10
7	–	–	–	2–3	–	3	75–78	6–7	41–46	15–38	11–18
8	–	3	4	–	10–11	2	79–82	8–9	47–56	39–44	19–28
9	4	–	5	4	12	–	83–86	10–12	57–65	45–55	29–40
10	5	4	6–7	5–6	13	1	87–92	13–15	66–76	56–68	41–59
11	–	–	–	7	14	–	93–94	16–17	77–82	69–77	60–71
12	6	5	8	8	–	0	95	18–19	83–88	78–86	72–81
13	–	–	9	9–10	–	–	96–99	20–22	89–92	87–91	82–89
14	7	6	10	–	15	–	–	23	93+	92+	90–94
15	–	7	11	11	–	–	100	24–27	–	–	95–97
16	8	–	12	12	–	–	–	28–30	–	–	98
17	9	8	–	13	–	–	–	31–33	–	–	99
18	10+	9+	13+	14–15	–	–	–	34+	–	–	>99

NOTE: ERR, false-positive errors; LOT, learning over trials; LTPR, long-term percent retention; REC, recognition hits; RPC, recognition percent correct; STPR, short-term percent retention. See Table 10–58 for definitions.

SOURCE: From Ferman et al. (2005).

TABLE 10-63 MOAANS RAVLT Scaled Scores for Age 72 to 74 Years (Midpoint Age = 73, Age Range for Norms = 68–78)

SCALED SCORE	TRIAL 1	LIST B	TRIAL 6	30-MIN DELAY	REC	ERR	RPC	LOT	STPR	LTPR	PERCENTILE RANGE
2	0	–	–	–	0–2	9+	–	<1	–	–	<1
3	1	0	0	–	3–5	8	<61	–	0–5	–	1
4	–	–	–	–	6	7	61–66	1	6–11	–	2
5	2	1	1	0	7	5–6	67–70	2	12–28	0	3–5
6	–	2	2–3	1	8–9	4	71–74	3–5	29–40	1–14	6–10
7	3	–	–	2–3	10	3	75–78	6–7	41–46	15–38	11–18
8	–	3	4	–	11	2	79–82	8–9	47–56	39–44	19–28
9	4	–	5	4	12	–	83–86	10–12	57–65	45–55	29–40
10	5	4	6–7	5–6	13	1	87–92	13–15	66–74	56–68	41–59
11	–	–	–	7	14	–	93–94	16–17	75–81	69–77	60–71
12	–	5	8	8	–	0	95	18–19	82–88	78–86	72–81
13	6	–	9	9–10	–	–	96–99	20–22	89–92	87–91	82–89
14	7	6	10	–	15	–	–	23	93+	92+	90–94
15	–	7	11	11	–	–	100	24–26	–	–	95–97
16	8	–	12	12	–	–	–	27	–	–	98
17	9	8	–	13	–	–	–	28–30	–	–	99
18	10+	9+	13+	14–15	–	–	–	31+	–	–	>99

NOTE: ERR, false-positive errors; LOT, learning over trials; LTPR, long-term percent retention; REC, recognition hits; RPC, recognition percent correct; STPR, short-term percent retention. See Table 10–58 for definitions.

SOURCE: From Ferman et al. (2005).

TABLE 10-64 MOAANS RAVLT Scaled Scores for Age 75 to 77 Years (Midpoint Age = 76, Age Range for Norms = 71–81)

SCALED SCORE	TRIAL 1	LIST B	TRIAL 6	30-MIN DELAY	REC	ERR	RPC	LOT	STPR	LTPR	PERCENTILE RANGE
2	0	–	–	–	0–2	9+	–	<1	–	–	<1
3	1	0	0	–	3–5	8	<60	–	0–5	–	1
4	–	–	–	–	6	7	60–65	1	6–10	–	2
5	–	1	1	0	7	5–6	66–69	2	11–22	0	3–5
6	2	–	2	1	8	4	70–72	3–5	23–33	1–14	6–10
7	3	2	3	2	9	3	73–76	6–7	34–43	15–36	11–18
8	–	–	4	3	10–11	2	77–80	8	44–55	37–44	19–28
9	4	3	5	4	12	–	81–84	9–11	56–63	45–54	29–40
10	–	4	6	5	13	1	85–89	12–14	64–72	55–63	41–59
11	5	–	7	6	–	–	90–92	15–17	73–79	64–70	60–71
12	–	5	8	7–8	14	0	93–95	18–19	80–87	71–85	72–81
13	6	–	9	9	–	–	96–97	20–22	88–92	86–91	82–89
14	–	6	10	10	15	–	98–99	23	93+	92+	90–94
15	7	–	11	11	–	–	100	24–25	–	–	95–97
16	8	7	12	12	–	–	–	26	–	–	98
17	9	8	–	13	–	–	–	27–30	–	–	99
18	10+	9+	13+	14–15	–	–	–	31+	–	–	>99

NOTE: ERR, false-positive errors; LOT, learning over trials; LTPR, long-term percent retention; REC, recognition hits; RPC, recognition percent correct; STPR, short-term percent retention. See Table 10–58 for definitions.

SOURCE: From Ferman et al. (2005).

TABLE 10–65 MOAANS RAVLT Scaled Scores for Age 78+ Years (Midpoint Age = 79, Age Range for Norms = 74–94)

SCALED SCORE	TRIAL 1	LIST B	TRIAL 6	30-MIN DELAY	REC	ERR	RPC	LOT	STPR	LTPR	PERCENTILE RANGE
2	0	–	–	–	–	–	–	<1	–	–	<1
3	1	0	0	–	0–5	–	<60	–	0	–	1
4	–	–	–	–	6	9+	61–61	1	1–6	–	2
5	–	1	1	–	7	6–8	62–66	2	7–11	–	3–5
6	2	–	2	0	8	4–5	67–70	3–4	12–31	0–9	6–10
7	–	2	3	1	9	3	71–73	5–6	32–42	10–20	11–18
8	3	–	4	2–3	10	2	74–78	7–8	43–50	21–40	19–28
9	–	3	–	4	11	–	79–83	9–11	51–59	41–52	29–40
10	4	–	5–6	5	12–13	1	84–88	12–14	60–71	53–63	41–59
11	5	4	7	6	–	–	89–91	15–16	72–76	64–70	60–71
12	–	–	–	7	14	0	92–94	17–18	77–86	71–82	72–81
13	6	5	8–9	8–9	–	–	95	19–21	87–91	83–90	82–89
14	–	–	10	10	15	–	96–99	22–23	–	91+	90–94
15	–	6	11	–	–	–	100	24	92+	–	95–97
16	7	–	–	11	–	–	–	25	–	–	98
17	–	7+	12	12	–	–	–	26	–	–	99
18	8+	–	13+	13–15	–	–	–	27+	–	–	>99

NOTE: ERR, false-positive errors; LOT, learning over trials; LTPR, long-term percent retention; REC, recognition hits; RPC, recognition percent correct; STPR, short-term percent retention. See Table 10–58 for definitions.

SOURCE: From Ferman et al. (2005).

TABLE 10–66 MOAANS RAVLT Age-Adjusted Index Score Conversions

INDEX SCORE	MOAANS LEARNING EFFICIENCY INDEX (LEI)	MOAANS AUDITORY-VERBAL DELAYED RECALL INDEX (DRI)	MOAANS AUDITORY-VERBAL PERCENT RETENTION INDEX (PRI)	INDEX SCORE
≤65	<13	<9	<10	≤65
66		9		66
67			10	67
69	13	10		69
71			11	71
73	14	11	12	73
76	15		13	76
77		12		77
80		13		80
81			14	81
82	16			82
84		14		84
86		15	15	86
87	17			87
89		16	16	89
91	18			91
92		17	17	92
94		18	18	94
96	19			96
97		19	19	97
100	20	20	20	100
103		21	21	103
105	21	22		105
107			22	107
108		23		108
109	22		23	109
111		24		111
112			24	112
114	23	25		114
115			25	115
117		26		117
119	24	27	26	119
121		28		121
123			27	123
124	25			124
125		29		125
129	26	30		129
130			28	130
132		31		132
133	27			133
≥135	>27	>31	>28	≥135

SOURCE: From Ferman et al. (2005).

TABLE 10–67 RAVLT Computational Algorithm for Age- and Education-Corrected MOAANS Scores

RAVLT VARIABLE	K	W_1	W_2
Trial 1	1.06	1.11	0.17
List B	0.49	1.10	0.13
Trial 6	1.08	1.09	0.16
30-min delay	1.07	1.09	0.16
Recognition	0.40	1.10	0.11
False-positive errors	−1.43	1.30	0.09
Recognition percent correct (RPC)	0.77	1.10	0.15
Learning over trials (LOT)	−0.11	1.07	0.04
Short-term percent retention (STPR)	−0.10	1.13	0.09
Long-term percent retention (LTPR)	−0.08	1.17	0.12

NOTE: Age- and education-corrected MOAANS scaled scores ($MSS_{A\&E}$) are calculated using the age-corrected scaled score derived from Tables 10–59 through 10–65 (MSS_A) and the examinee's years of education using the formula:

$MSS_{A\&E} = K + (W_1 \times MSS_A) - (W_2 \times Educ)$

where K = a constant, W_1 = a regression-derived weight to be applied to MSS_A and W_2 = a regression-derived weight to be applied to education.

SOURCE: From Ferman et al. (2005).

Gale et al. (2007) provide updated norms for older adults aged 60–89 years for the RAVLT, co-normed with the BVMT-R (see Table 10–74; for BVMT-R norms, please refer to the BVMT-R review elsewhere in this chapter). The sample was determined to be healthy based on medical, neurologic, radiologic, and functional examinations.

Miller et al. (2015) provide norms for extended testing using the RAVLT to assess accelerated long-term forgetting (ALF). The Recognition trial was not administered but a telephone follow-up after seven days was arranged to assess longer term memory. ALF is defined as a normal 30-minute Delayed Recall score but impaired Percent Change score. ALF is seen more often in epilepsy patients than in healthy controls (47% vs. 17%), more so with the RAVLT than the Logical Memory or Aggies Figure Test. Table 10–75 presents the normative information for assessing ALF.

Vogel et al. (2012) provide RAVLT Danish norms using the Nielsen et al. (1989) version, co-normed with the RCFT. Table 10–76 presents the RAVLT norms. Please refer to the RCFT chapter in this volume for RCFT norms.

Many other normative studies based on large samples of healthy people are available. For the ease of clinicians, the references and relevant information are presented in Table 10–77. Users may refer to the table for the sample most appropriate for their evaluation purposes.

It is important to note that ceiling effects appear to be present on the later recall trials, with many young adults unable to demonstrate their true memory ability. Inferences made about the degree of memory deficits should take the raw scores into consideration.

EVIDENCE FOR RELIABILITY

EVIDENCE FOR INTERNAL RELIABILITY

Internal reliability (Cronbach's alpha) is adequate to very high, ranging from .78 to about .90 (Magalhaes et al., 2012; Van den Burg & Kingma, 1999).

EVIDENCE FOR TEST-RETEST RELIABILITY, MEASURING CHANGE, AND PRACTICE EFFECTS

Over a 35-day period, test-retest reliability ranges from low to adequate for the primary indices (r = .21 [Delayed Recall] to .76 [Total Learning]; Magalhaes et al., 2012). Over a one-year interval, the test has marginal/adequate test-retest reliability. Trial 5 and Delayed Recall trials are among the more reliable scores (r values about .60 to .70; Carstairs et al., 2012; Mitrushina & Satz, 1991b; Uchiyama et al., 1995).

Small, but significant improvements (on average one to two words per trial) can be expected on successive administrations of the same form of the RAVLT (Crawford et al., 1989; Uchiyama et al., 1995), although in older adults (aged 57–85 years) tested yearly for three years, the gains on Trials 5 and 7 tend to be negligible (Mitrushina & Satz, 1991a).

The literature suggests that practice effects are reduced when people are retested with a different RAVLT version (Crawford et al., 1989; Delaney et al., 1992; Geffen et al., 1994; Lemay et al., 2004; Moritz et al., 2003; Van den Burg & Kingma, 1999). For example, Lemay et al. (2004) evaluated middle-aged and older adults on three test occasions with intersession intervals of 14 days using the standard and two alternate forms. The Total Learning and Delayed Recall trials had acceptable reliability (r values >.70) whereas acquisition trials, recognition trials, and derived scores (except retrieval efficiency) showed unacceptably low reliabilities.

Moritz et al. (2003) tested 31 patients (20 males, 11 females) with schizophrenia (age M = 33.03 years, SD = 11.26; education M = 11.77 years, SD = 1.45) and 38 healthy controls (26 males, 12 females; age M = 32.45 years, SD = 9.98; education M = 11.47 years, SD = 1.48) on two occasions, spaced two weeks apart. The standard form was given at baseline and an alternate version (B) at retest. In both samples, reliability coefficients were generally higher for the Total Learning score (healthy examinees, r = .72; patients with schizophrenia, r = .69) than for the individual learning trials, and practice effects were absent. Reliable change estimates for the RAVLT Total Learning score were derived for each sample, and these are shown in Table 10–78. Therefore, when using alternate forms with patients with schizophrenia, clinicians can be 90% confident that a change of 16 or more points in the Total Learning score is not the result of measurement error

TABLE 10–68 MOAANS RAVLT Age- and Education-Adjusted Index Score Conversions

INDEX SCORE	MOAANS LEARNING EFFICIENCY INDEX (LEI)	MOAANS AUDITORY-VERBAL DELAYED RECALL INDEX (DRI)	MOAANS AUDITORY-VERBAL PERCENT RETENTION INDEX (PRI)	INDEX SCORE
≤65	<12	<9	<9	≤65
66	12		9	66
67		9		67
69	13			69
70			10	70
71		10		71
72	14			72
73			11	73
75		11		75
76			12	76
78	15	12		78
80			13	80
81	16	13		81
83			14	83
84		14		84
86	17		15	86
87		15		87
89			16	89
90	18	16		90
91			17	91
92		17		92
93		18		93
94			18	94
96	19	19	19	96
99		20	20	99
100	20			100
102		21	21	102
105	21	22	22	105
107			23	107
108	22	23		108
110		24	24	110
112	23	25	25	112
115	24	26	26	115
117		27		117
118			27	118
119		28		119
120	25			120
121		29		121
122			28	122
125		30	29	125
126	26			126
128		31		128
131	27	32	30	131
≥135	>27	>32	>30	≥135

SOURCE: From Ferman et al. (2005).

(for healthy participants, the corresponding value is nine points). The authors stressed that it is clearly possible for patients to experience real change even if their scores do not exceed the criterion. Clinicians simply should have less confidence in clinical inferences based on changes that fall within the probable range of measurement error, and they need to seek additional evidence to support or refute such an opinion.

However, there may be effects from proactive interference from repeating parallel forms over very short retest intervals. For example, Rahimi-Golkhandan et al. (2012) gave healthy adults parallel forms within minutes of each other and found a decrease of more than two words on Total Learning with each parallel form administered. Furthermore, rehearsal of the word list immediately after the examinee completed each recall trial has been found to improve performance by between 2.9 and 4.4 T-score points, respectively, suggesting that minor administration changes or use of strategy can affect performance on the RAVLT (Hessen, 2011).

Stålhammar et al. (2015) presented a case study of a 20-year-old top-ranking mnemonist who was not born

TABLE 10-69 Australian Rey Auditory Verbal Learning Test (RAVLT) Scaled Score Equivalents of Raw Scores for Total Sample

SCALED SCORE	TRIAL 1	TRIAL 2	TRIAL 3	TRIAL 4	TRIAL 5	LIST B	IR	DR	RM	TRIALS 1–5	SCALED SCORE
19	15					14+				75	19
18	14									74	18
17	13					13				*72–73*	17
16	12	15				11–*12*				70–71	16
15	11	14	15			10				69	15
14	10			15		9	15	15		66–68	14
13		13			15	8				64–65	13
12	9	12	14				14	14	15	62–63	12
11	8		13	14		7		13		59–61	11
10	7	11	12	13	14	6	13	12		56–58	10
9		10			13		*12*	11	14	53–55	9
8	6	9	11	12		5	11	10		50–52	8
7	5	8	10	11	12		9–10	9	13	47–49	7
6			9	10	11	4	8	8	12	44–46	6
5	4	7		9	10	3	7	7	11	41–43	5
4		6	8	*8*	9		6	*5–6*	10	39–40	4
3		5	7	7	*8*	2	5	4	9	36–38	3
2	3	4	6	6	*6–7*	1	4	3	*6–8*	30–35	2
1	*0–2*	*0–3*	*0–5*	*0–5*	*0–5*	0	*0–3*	*0–2*	*0–5*	0–29	1

NOTE: List B, recall for list B; IR, immediate recall for list A; DR, delayed recall for list A; RM, recognition memory list A. Interpolated or extrapolated values are presented in italics. Based on *N* = 390, age M = 25.6, *SD* = 5.0, range = 18–34; education M = 12.9, *SD* = 2.1; 52% female.

SOURCE: From Carstairs et al. (2012).

with superior memory but had been trained in memory techniques for about eight years prior to neuropsychological testing. He demonstrated ceiling effects on the first trial of the RAVLT and all subsequent learning and recall trials, but the ability was not transferred to other cognitive domains, including visual memory. Thus, memory training may be thought of as a type of practice effect; therefore, the authors suggested that the RAVLT may be susceptible to potential practice effects that are beyond two to three *SD*s, albeit these would be rare in clinical practice.

TABLE 10-70 RAVLT Scaled Score Equivalents of Raw Scores for Australian Males with 12 Years or Less of Education

SCALED SCORE	TRIAL 1	TRIAL 2	TRIAL 3	TRIAL 4	TRIAL 5	LIST B	IR	DR	RM	TRIALS 1–5	SCALED SCORE
19											19
18											18
17	13+					13+					17
16	11–12	14+	15			10–*12*				69+	16
15		13				9	15			66–68	15
14	10		14	15		8		15		64–65	14
13	9	12			15	7		14		61–63	13
12	8	11	13	14			14	13	15	59–60	12
11	7	10	12	13	14	6	13	12		55–58	11
10	6	9	11				12	11		52–54	10
9				12	13	5	11	10	14	49–51	9
8	5	8	10	11	12		10	9		46–48	8
7		7	9	10	11	4	9	8	13	43–45	7
6	4			9	10	3	8	7	11–*12*	41–42	6
5		6	8		9	2	7	6	10	39–40	5
4		5	7	8	*7–8*	1	5–6	5	*7–9*	36–38	4
3	3	4	6	*6–7*	6	0	4	*3–4*	6	27–35	3
2	*2*	*2–3*	*3–5*	*3–5*	*3–5*		*2–3*	2	*3–5*	*13–26*	2
1	*0–1*	*0–1*	*0–2*	*0–2*	*0–2*		*0–1*	*0–1*	*0–2*	*0–12*	1

NOTE: List B, recall for list B; IR, immediate recall for List A; DR, delayed recall for list A; RM, recognition memory list A. Interpolated or extrapolated values are presented in italics. Based on *N* = 87.

SOURCE: From Carstairs et al. (2012).

TABLE 10–71 Rey Auditory Verbal Learning Test (RAVLT) Scaled Score Equivalents of Raw Scores for Australian Females with 12 Years or Less of Education

SCALED SCORE	TRIAL 1	TRIAL 2	TRIAL 3	TRIAL 4	TRIAL 5	LIST B	IR	DR	RM	TRIALS 1–5	SCALED SCORE
19											19
18											18
17	12+					14+				72+	17
16						11–*13*				71	16
15	11	14+	15			10				67–70	15
14	10					9	15	15		65–66	14
13	9	13	14	15	15	8				63–64	13
12	8	12				7	14	14	15	61–62	12
11		11	13	14			13	13		59–60	11
10	7		12	13	14	6		12		55–58	10
9	6	10			13		12	11	14	54	9
8		9	11	12		5	11	10		51–53	8
7	5		10	11	12		9–*10*	9	13	48–50	7
6		8		10		4	8	8	12	47	6
5	4	6–7	9		11		6–7	7	11	44–46	5
4		5	*7–8*	9	10	3	5	4–6		39–43	4
3	3	4	6	8	8–9	*2*	4	*2–3*	10	30–38	3
2	*2*	*2–3*	*3–5*	*4–7*	*4–7*	*1*	*2–3*	*1*	*6–9*	*15–29*	2
1	*0–1*	*0–1*	*0–2*	*0–3*	*0–3*	*0*	*0–1*	*0*	*0–5*	*0–14*	1

NOTE: List B, recall for list B; IR, immediate recall for list A; DR, delayed recall for list A; RM, recognition memory list A. Interpolated or extrapolated values are presented in italics. Based on *N* = 91.

SOURCE: From Carstairs et al. (2012).

EVIDENCE FOR RELIABILITY OF ALTERNATE FORMS

Different studies yield a wide variety of reliability coefficients but generally fall above the marginal range (>.60; see the section "Practice Effects"). As noted earlier (see "Other Forms"), a number of authors have provided alternate forms of the test. The versions by Geffen et al. (1994; Figure 10–2) and Majdan et al. (1996; Figure 10–3) appear to produce comparable scores.

TABLE 10–72 Rey Auditory Verbal Learning Test (RAVLT) Scaled Score Equivalents of Raw Scores for Australian Males with More Than 12 Years of Education

SCALED SCORE	TRIAL 1	TRIAL 2	TRIAL 3	TRIA 4	TRIAL 5	LIST B	IR	DR	RM	TRIALS 1–5	SCALED SCORE
19											19
18	14+									74+	18
17	*12–13*									72–73	17
16	11	15				13+				71	16
15			15			11–*12*	15			70	15
14	10	14		15		10		15		65–69	14
13	9	13	14		15	9				63–64	13
12		12				8	14	14	15	61–62	12
11	8		13	14	14	7	13	13		58–60	11
10	7	11	12	13			12	12	14	55–57	10
9		10	11		13	6	11	11		53–54	9
8	6	9	10	12		5	10	10	13	50–52	8
7	5	8		11	11–12	4	9	9		47–49	7
6			9	10	10		8	*7–8*	11–12	43–46	6
5	4	7	8	9		3	7	6		40–42	5
4			*6–7*	7–8	8–9		6	5	9–10	37–39	4
3			*4–5*				*4–5*		*7–8*		3
2	3	6	*2–3*	6	7	2	3	4	6	36	2
1	*0–2*	*0–5*	*0–1*	*0–5*	*0–6*	*0–1*	*0–2*	*0–3*	*0–5*	*0–35*	1

NOTE: List B, recall for list B; IR, immediate recall for list A; DR, delayed recall for list A; RM, recognition memory list A. Interpolated or extrapolated values are presented in italics. Based on *N* = 101.

SOURCE: Carstairs et al. (2012).

TABLE 10–73 Rey Auditory Verbal Learning Test (RAVLT) Scaled Score Equivalents of Raw Scores for Australian Females with More Than 12 Years of Education

SCALED SCORE	TRIAL 1	TRIAL 2	TRIAL 3	TRIAL 4	TRIAL 5	LIST B	IR	DR	RM	TRIALS 1–5	SCALED SCORE
19											19
18	15									75	18
17	*13–14*					13+				72–74	17
16		15				12				71	16
15	12					11				70	15
14	11	14	15			10				68–69	14
13				15		9	15	15		66–67	13
12	10	13			15	8			15	65	12
11	9	12	14	14		7	14	14		62–64	11
10	8		13							61	10
9	7	11		13	14	6	13	13		57–60	9
8			12		13	5	12	12	14	55–56	8
7	6	10	11	12			11	11		53–54	7
6		9	10		12		10	10	13	51–52	6
5	5	8		11		4	9			48–50	5
4		7	9		11			9	12	47	4
3	4			10	10	3	8	8	11	43–46	3
2	*2–3*	6	8	9	9	*2*	*4–7*	*6–7*	10	*39–42*	2
1	*0–1*	*0–5*	*0–7*	*0–8*	*0–8*	*0–1*	*0–3*	*0–5*	*0–9*	*0–38*	1

NOTE: List B, recall for list B; IR, immediate recall for 1st A; DR, delayed recall for list A; RM, recognition memory list A. Interpolated or extrapolated values are presented in italics. Based on *N* = 111.

SOURCE: From Carstairs et al. (2012).

EVIDENCE FOR VALIDITY

FACTOR-ANALYTIC STUDIES

Factor-analytic studies indicate that the RAVLT loads primarily with other verbal memory tests, such as those found on the WMS (Anderson & Lajoie, 1996; Johnstone et al., 2000; Salthouse et al., 1996; Strauss et al., 1995). The RAVLT, however, may measure a construct that is not singularly verbal in nature. Some factor analyses of variable sets that include the RAVLT indicate that memory variables load together regardless of whether they are verbal or nonverbal measures, which tends to be the case for most memory tests (Malec et al., 1991; Smith et al., 1992). However, Johnstone et al. (2000) found that the RAVLT loaded with measures of verbal but not nonverbal memory.

With regard to the internal structure of the test, either one factor (Salthouse et al., 1996; Vakil & Blachstein, 1993), or two or three factors (Vakil & Blachstein, 1993) emerge in healthy adults, depending

TABLE 10–74 Rey Auditory Verbal Learning Test (RAVLT) Normative Data for 60- to 89-Year-Old Adults as a Function of Age and Gender

AGE	MALE M	MALE *SD*	FEMALE M	FEMALE *SD*	TOTAL M	TOTAL *SD*
60–69	*N* = 20		*N* = 31		*N* = 51	
Total Learning	42.3	8.6	49.5	9.6	46.8	9.8
Delayed Recall	7.8	2.8	10.8	2.6	9.5	3.3
Recognition	12.0	2.4	13.8	1.4	13.1	2.0
70–79	*N* = 20		*N* = 44		*N* = 64	
Total Learning	42.1	8.6	48.0	10.0	46.0	9.9
Delayed Recall	7.6	3.4	10.3	3.0	9.4	3.3
Recognition	13.3	1.3	13.7	2.0	13.5	1.9
80–89	*N* = 19		*N* = 38		*N* = 57	
Total Learning	37.6	7.6	44.7	7.8	42.4	8.4
Delayed Recall	7.4	2.4	9.5	2.7	8.8	2.8
Recognition	12.8	1.7	13.4	1.8	13.2	1.8

NOTE: Total Learning = total score over Trials 1-5. Delayed Recall = score after the delay. Recognition = true positives on the recognition trial.

Based on *N* = 172; mean age = 74.61, *SD* = 7.79; mean education = 15.48, *SD* = 3.02, range = 6–24; 65% females.

SOURCE: Adapted from Gale et al. (2007).

TABLE 10–75 Accelerated Long-Term Forgetting Norms for the Rey Auditory Verbal Learning Test (RAVLT)

	30-MIN DELAY (MAX = 15)		PERCENT CHANGE SCORE (MAX = 100)
Sex	Male	Female	Male + female
N	28	32	60
Mean score (SD)	10.5 (3.0)	12.3 (2.4)	36.3 (21.8)
Cutoff score (z = ± 1.64)	5.6	8.4	72.1
For ALF	Performs above this level		Shows greater change score

NOTE: Percent Change Score = [(30-min recall – 7-day recall)/30-min recall] × 100. Based on *N* = 60 healthy adults (convenience sample), aged 18–61, equal gender distribution screened for psychiatric or neurological history.

SOURCE: From Miller et al. (2015).

TABLE 10–76 Danish Norms for the Rey Auditory Verbal Learning Test (RAVLT)

EDUCATION	AGE		TRIAL 1–5	SHORT RECALL (A6)	LONG RECALL (A7)
8–11 years	60–70				
		N	18	18	18
		Mean	38.1	7.5	7.8
		SD	8.4	2.8	3.2
		Range	23–55	3–13	1–12
	71–87				
		N	30	30	30
		Mean	38.9	7.5	7.6
		SD	7.1	2.7	2.5
		Range	23–50	1–12	2–12
12–17 years	60–70				
		N	32	32	32
		Mean	45.3	8.7	8.8
		SD	8.8	3.0	3.0
		Range	31–65	3–15	2–15
	71–87				
		N	20	20	20
		Mean	42.8	7.8	7.6
		SD	9.4	3.3	3.5
		Range	21–51	1–13	1–14

NOTE: Based on *N* = 100; age mean = 70.9, *SD* = 6.4, range = 60–87; education mean = 11.9, *SD* = 2.6, range = 8–17; 56% female.

SOURCE: Adapted from Vogel et al. (2012).

on the particular combination of scores included in the analyses and the criteria used to determine the number of factors. Vakil and Blachstein (1993) identified two basic factors that they interpreted as reflecting acquisition (defined by variables such as Trial 1, List B trial, and Total Learning) and retention. The latter can be further subdivided into a storage component (defined primarily by recognition memory) and a retrieval component (defined by Trial 5, delayed-recall trials and temporal order). By contrast, Mueller et al. (1997) examined two heterogeneous clinical samples, one comprised mostly of people with AD or major depression and the other of patients with seizures, using a German version of the RAVLT. Structural equation modeling suggested that short-term memory and long-term latent memory variables provide a good explanation of the test in both clinical samples.

SCORE INTERCORRELATIONS

Total Learning scores show the highest correlations with all other trials (r = .52 to .88; Messinis et al., 2016; Van den Burg & Kingma, 1999). Delayed Recall is also highly correlated with Recognition (r = .61; Messinis et al., 2016). Other indices (e.g., percent recall from primacy, middle, and recency regions) also have significant correlations (r >.80) with the total number of words recalled and therefore are not pure measures of the qualitative traits that they purportedly assess (Schmidt, 1997). However, an index based on recency minus primacy (Gainotti & Marra, 1994) seems not to be substantially confounded with number of words recalled and therefore appears promising (Schmidt, 1997).

RELATIONSHIPS WITH OTHER TESTS

The RAVLT correlates moderately well with other measures of learning and memory such as the Wechsler Logical Memory subtest (Jafari et al., 2010; Johnstone et al., 2000) and the CVLT (Crossen & Wiens, 1994; Stallings et al., 1995). The RAVLT may be somewhat more difficult than the CVLT, requiring more effortful strategies for encoding and retrieval. The CVLT consists of words that can be categorized, with semantic clustering becoming the strategy of choice for healthy adults. The RAVLT words do not show a clear semantic relationship, and temporal tagging may become a more important strategy (Vakil & Blachstein, 1994; Vakil et al., 2004). When standard, as opposed to raw, scores are considered, CVLT scores are considerably lower than those of the RAVLT in head-injured patients (Stallings et al., 1995). The discrepancies may reflect differences in the composition of the standardization samples or the greater sensitivity of the CVLT to executive dysfunction (perhaps related to the requirement of semantic clustering), or both. Stallings et al. (1995) noted that use of the CVLT, as opposed to the RAVLT, results in a higher frequency of head-injury patients being classed as memory-impaired, and their memory impairments appear greater. If both tests are given within a few days of one another, there are no significant effects for order of presentation (Crossen & Wiens, 1994; Stallings et al., 1995). It will be important to compare the RAVLT with the CVLT-II in future studies.

On the other hand, RAVLT yields modest correlations with visual memory measures such as Wechsler Visual Reproduction, RCFT (r = .21 to .26), and BVRT (r = .37 to .44; Johnstone et al., 2000; Magalhaes et al., 2012; Vogel et al., 2012), suggesting that it measures overlapping but different aspects of memory. The correlation with TMT is not significant (Magalhaes et al., 2012), providing support for divergent validity.

CLINICAL STUDIES

The RAVLT is sensitive to neurological impairment and memory deficits in a variety of patient groups, including those with left TLE (see later discussion), ruptured aneurysm of the anterior communicating artery (Simard et al., 2003; Stefanova et al., 2002), unilateral middle cerebral artery (MCA) occlusion (Xie et al., 2011), specific language impairment (Records et al., 1995), MCI (see later discussion), AD (see later discussion), PD (Alegret et al., 2001), HD (Shimamura et al., 1987), Korsakoff's syndrome (Shimamura et al., 1987), amyotrophic lateral

TABLE 10–77 List of Rey Auditory Verbal Learning Test (RAVLT) Normative Studies from Various Countries and Languages

REFERENCE	LANGUAGE	COUNTRY/ REGION	POPULATION	*N*	AGE	EDUCATION	GENDER (% FEMALE)	NOTES
Ferman et al. (2005)	English	Jacksonville, Florida	Healthy African-American older adults	306	Range = 56–94	Range = 0–20	Not reported	Participants from the MOAANS project screened for active neurological, psychiatric, or other conditions that might affect cognition.
Gale et al. (2007)	English	Arizona, USA	Healthy older adults	172	*M* = 74.6, *SD* = 7.8, range = 60–89	*M* = 15.5, *SD* = 3.0, range = 6–24	65%	Health status determined using medical, neurological, radiologic, and functional examinations.
Carstairs et al. (2012)	English	Sydney, Australia	Healthy young adults	390	*M* = 25.6, *SD* = 5.0, range = 18–34	*M* = 12.9, *SD* = 2.1	52%	Scoring program available: http://www.psy.mq.edu.au/RAVLT
Miller et al. (2015)	English	Sydney, Australia	Healthy adults	60	Range = 18–61	Not reported	Equal distribution	Norms for Delayed Recall percent change at seven-day telephone follow-up.
Poreh et al. (2012)	Arabic	Oman	Healthy adults from university and surrounding community as well as inland small village	200	*M* = 25.46, *SD* = 6.2, range = 18–49	*M* = 10.48, *SD* = 21.29, range = 0–18	66%	Screened for history of psychiatric illness, head injury, and psychoactive drug use. Translated from French version of RAVLT.
Bezdicek et al. (2014)	Czech	Prague, Czech Republic	Healthy community-dwelling adults	306	*M* = 47.0, *SD* = 16.2, range = 20–85	*M* = 14.0, *SD* = 3.4, range = 8–26	60%	No recognition trial. Czech version wordlist provided.
Vogel et al. (2012)	Danish	Denmark	Healthy community-dwelling older adults	100	*M* = 70.9, *SD* = 6.4, range = 60–87	*M* = 11.9, *SD* = 2.6, range = 8–17	56%	Screened for history of neurological or psychiatric disease, alcohol consumption above recommended levels, and use of cognition-altering medication. Used the Nielsen et al. (1989) version.
Van der Elst et al. (2005)	Dutch	Maastricht, The Netherlands	Healthy adults	1780	*M* = 51.29, *SD* = 16.22, range = 24–81	Low, average, and high education corresponding to *M* = 8.60, 11.41, 15.25, *SD* = 1.95, 2.48, 3.31, respectively	50%	Screened for neurological conditions, intellectual disability, psychopathology, chronic psychotropic drug use, MMSE < 24, or hearing loss > 35dB.
Teruya et al. (2009)	Portuguese	Brazil	Healthy adults	130	*M* = 57.4, *SD* = 13.4, range = 34–85	*M* = 10.0, *SD* = 4.6, range = 4–25	75%	Screened for hearing impairment, neurological or psychiatric illnesses, chronic psychotropic drug use, TBI with LOC > 15, history of stroke or epilepsy.
Correia and Osorio (2014)	Spanish	Venezuela	Healthy adults	629	Range = 20–79	Range = 0–>16	52%	Screened for psychiatric, metabolic, immunologic, neurological illnesses, substance abuse, and psychotropic medication use history. Spanish version wordlist provided.

TABLE 10–78 Total Learning (Trials 1–5) in Healthy Adults and Individuals with Schizophrenia Retested with a Rey Auditory Verbal Learning Test (RAVLT) Alternate Form After 2 Weeks

MEASURE	T1 MEAN AND *SD*	T1 *SEM*	T2 MEAN AND *SD*	T2 *SEM*	*R*	S_{DIFF}	90% CI	80% CI
Healthy	59.2 (6.1)	3.22	57.8 (8.5)	4.50	.72	5.54	9.08	7.09
Patients	46.3	12.3	45.7	12.1	.69	9.58	15.70	12.26

NOTE: Mean age about 33 years. T1 = Baseline; T2 = Retest.

SOURCE: Adapted from Moritz et al. (2003).

sclerosis (ALS; Christidi et al., 2012), MS (Demers et al., 2011), TBI (see later discussion), AIDS (Messinis et al., 2007; Ryan et al., 1992), intellectual deficiency (Vakil et al., 1997), ADHD (Pollak et al., 2007), chronic fatigue syndrome (Crowe & Casey, 1999), idiopathic rapid eye movement sleep behavior disorder in older adults (Li et al., 2016), lead exposure (Stewart et al., 1999), and psychiatric disorders including depression and schizophrenia (Moritz et al., 2001; Seltzer et al., 1997; Torres et al., 2001; see later discussion). Schoenberg et al. (2006) compared the RAVLT Total Learning performance of numerous clinical groups and found that all patient groups performed below norms, not unexpectedly. Neurological groups performed worse than psychiatric group on all primary indices, whereas dementia groups performed worse than psychiatric and other neurological groups. Delayed Recall yields the best hit rate for AD (83%) among all neurological conditions relative to psychiatric groups using metanorms by Schmidt (1996).

Trial 1 may be considered an indication of immediate memory, with healthy young adults recalling seven words on average. Note, however, that it is not identical to Digit Span (Talley, 1986). In general, healthy people learn about five words from Trial 1 to Trial 5, and they recall one to two fewer words on the Recall Trial (Trial 6) than on Trial 5. There is little forgetting over a 30-minute delay. Forgetting does, however, occur after lengthier delay periods. Miller et al. (2015) noted that a decline of about 36% over seven days is normative, and decline greater than 72% may represent accelerated long-term forgetting, such as may be seen in TLE. Geffen et al. (1997) reported that adults lose about one word after a 24-hour delay, and over a period of seven days one additional word is forgotten. A proactive interference effect is observed for all adult groups; recall for the second word list is inferior to initial recall of the first word list. Finally, a high incidence of false positives on the recognition task is quite unusual in healthy adults.

Neurodegenerative Disorders. The RAVLT, particularly Total Learning and Delayed Recall, appears sensitive to AD and amnestic MCI (Balthazar et al., 2007; Consonni et al., 2017; Marchiani et al., 2008; Messinis et al., 2016; Meyer et al., 2016). However, Total Learning scores show a quadratic trend against global cognitive impairment as measured by the Cognitive Screening Test (CST), leveling off at a score of 29 or lower for 90% of amnestic MCI and 94% of AD patients. These results suggest that the RAVLT shows a floor effect and may not be suitable for monitoring disease progression once a diagnosis is established (Meyer et al., 2016). However, scores on the RAVLT also offer some predictive utility. AD patients who show a positive learning curve are more likely to benefit from rehabilitative group therapy than are patients who show little learning (Haddad & Nussbaum, 1989).

Evidence for the utility of the RAVLT to differentiate AD from behavioral variant frontotemporal dementia (bvFTD) appears conflicting. Flanagan et al. (2016) reported that the groups obtain similar scores on Delayed Recall and Recognition False Positives. By contrast, Ricci et al. (2012) found that Delayed Recall appears to best discriminate among AD, bvFTD, and healthy controls; AD patients obtain the lowest recognition scores of the groups (Consonni et al., 2017). Ricci and colleagues (2012) also developed a memory index using the RAVLT that appears to differentiate AD from bvFTD and healthy controls with a high degree of sensitivity and specificity. See "Scoring" for the equation. A cutoff score of 1.2 yielded a sensitivity and a specificity of 85% for distinguishing between AD and bvFTD. A cutoff score of 1.9 differentiated between bvFTD and healthy controls, yielding a sensitivity of 82% and a specificity of 73%.

Recall of the RAVLT word list is affected by the serial positioning of the words and executive dysfunction, and the pattern of memory recall may give clues to the etiology of the memory impairment (Consonni et al., 2017; Fernaeus et al., 2014). Using item response theory, Gavett and Horwitz (2012) found serial position effects on the RAVLT, with four of 15 items found to be misfits; removal of these items results in a better fit to the data. In particular, an inverse relationship between ability and probability of recall is found for items 14 and 15, such that 75% of individuals with severely poor memory (i.e., three *SD*s below the mean) will recall these last two items on the list.

In another study using patients with AD, VaD, MCI, and those with subjective cognitive impairments as well as healthy controls, serial position data (with the word list divided into five parts with three words in each part) and data from the five learning trials submitted to a factor analysis yield a three-factor solution representing Primacy, Recency, and Resistance to Interference factors (Fernaeus et al.,

2014). As expected, on the Primacy factor, healthy controls perform the best, followed by subjective cognitive impairment, MCI, and, finally, AD patients, who score lower than all other groups. On the Resistance to Interference factor, the opposite pattern was found, with AD, VaD, and MCI scoring worse than subjective cognitive impairment. On the Recency factor, AD and MCI score lower than subjective cognitive impairment, and no differences are seen between VaD and MCI.

Somewhat similar findings were reported in another study. AD patients showed impairment for words in the beginning and middle of the list (Primacy) during the learning trials and impairment across the list in the Delayed Recall and Recognition trials. ALS patients with executive dysfunction were impaired in recalling words in the middle of the list during the learning trials, and this score was highly correlated with phonemic fluency scores ($r = -.90$). Patients with bvFTD, on the other hand, were impaired in recalling words at the end of the list (Recency) during both learning and delayed recall trials. Based on the known pathology of these conditions, the authors surmised that the learning trials are impacted by frontal executive dysfunction, whereas Delayed Recall and Recognition trials are impacted by temporal lobe dysfunction.

PD patients do not show impairment across all RAVLT trials. PD patients also do not show change in RAVLT performance during their medication wearing-off period of motor fluctuations (Caillava-Santos et al., 2015).

The RAVLT is one of the most useful tests for predicting dementia. Of 12 neuropsychological tests, RAVLT Immediate Recall and WAIS-R Digit Symbol are the best tests for 10-year prediction of all-cause dementia in the Canadian Study of Health and Aging, yielding a sensitivity of 78%, specificity of 72%, and positive likelihood ratio of 2.81. Every additional word recalled on the RAVLT decreases the risk of developing dementia within 10 years by 18%, and every additional symbol copied on Digit Symbol decreases the risk by 5%. Within a five-year period, WMS Information, RAVLT Immediate Recall, animal fluency, and WAIS-R Digit Symbol are the best predictors of dementia, yielding a sensitivity of 75%, specificity of 74%, and positive likelihood ratio of 2.90. Every additional word recalled on the RAVLT decreases the risk of developing dementia within five years by 15% (Tierney et al., 2011). Even against cerebrospinal fluid (CSF) biomarkers and hippocampal volume, Eckerström et al. (2013) reported that RAVLT is the best predictor of conversion from MCI to dementia over two years.

APOE-ε4 status affects RAVLT performance. RAVLT scores are correlated with CSF markers (total tau, phosphor-tau, beta-amyloid) in ε4+ older adults, but not in those who are ε4−. Among the ε4+ older adults, those classified as having severely or moderately impaired RAVLT scores have lower beta-amyloid levels than all other groups. Those with severely impaired RAVLT scores who are ε4- show higher levels of total tau and phospho-tau compared to other groups. Those who have severely impaired RAVLT scores show cognitive decline on follow-up regardless of ε4 status (Andersson et al., 2007).

TBI. Patients with TBI show on average an improvement of 0.13 words annually on repeat testing of the RAVLT (Chu et al., 2007). Age at injury and posttraumatic amnesia (PTA) are negatively correlated with RAVLT performance at one year, with every one year in age associated with 0.29 fewer words recalled and every one day increment in PTA associated with 0.09 fewer words recalled. Interestingly, RAVLT performance at the acute stage is not predictive of performance at one-year post-injury, and none of the variables (age, education, gender, PTA length, or acute RAVLT scores) predicts trajectory of memory recovery after the first year (Chu et al., 2007). Even at 10 years post-TBI, RAVLT Total Learning remains impaired, with greater length of PTA associated with worse test scores (Draper & Ponsford, 2008).

In adult patients with TBI, performance on the RAVLT is predictive of psychosocial outcome (community integration) one year after injury (Millis et al., 1994). Changes in performance on the list-learning task from the acute inpatient rehabilitation time point to one-year follow-up predict functional status at two-year follow-up in those with moderate to severe TBI (Bercaw et al., 2011).

TLE. The RAVLT is a sensitive measure for the purpose of measuring material-specific memory in TLE presurgical evaluations. Numerous studies suggest that RAVLT Total Learning and Delayed Recall are sensitive to left-sided seizure focus (Boucher et al., 2015; Loring et al., 2008; Soble et al., 2016; Grammaldo et al., 2006, 2009; Passarelli et al., 2015). For example, using RAVLT Delayed Recall as a predictor for side of seizure focus yields 77% classification accuracy. A T-score cutoff of 36.5 provides the best balance between sensitivity and specificity while maintaining sensitivity above 80%. This cutoff yields a sensitivity of 81%, a specificity of 79%, and positive likelihood ratio of 3.85 for classifying left TLE. A T-score cutoff of 41.5 yields a sensitivity of 84%, specificity of 69%, and positive likelihood ratio of 2.69 for predicting right TLE (Soble et al., 2016). Accordingly, Soble et al. (2016) noted that scores falling between 36.5 and 41.5 may be less valuable for predicting seizure laterality. However, Grammaldo et al. (2006) found that the RAVLT is effective in lateralizing epileptogenesis in those with hippocampal sclerosis but not in those with tumors or other lesions relative to Story Recall, Digit Span, RCFT, and Corsi Blocks Sequence Learning Test. A RAVLT Delayed Recall cutoff score of 6.15 yields a sensitivity of 78%, specificity of 77%, PPV of 78%, NPV of 77%, and an overall classification rate of 78% for the identification of TLE due to hippocampal sclerosis.

The RAVLT outperforms other memory measures in predicting lateralized memory impairments or seizure focus (Loring et al., 2008; Soble et al., 2014, 2016). Soble and colleagues (2014) used hierarchical logistic regression to evaluate the predictive accuracy of WMS-IV against RAVLT in identifying lateralized memory impairments. The RAVLT appears to predict laterality with about 70% accuracy, but none of the WMS-IV subtests or verbal-visual memory difference scores added to the prediction model. The authors suggested that the insensitivity of the WMS-IV to seizure laterality may be due to the subtests containing verbal and visual components or because of the single-trial learning, which can be affected by poor attention or comprehension. Loring et al. (2008) reported that the magnitude of performance differences between left and right TLE patients is smaller on the CVLT compared to the RAVLT (Cohen's d = .30 and .47, respectively). Furthermore, once the RAVLT, CVLT, BNT, and MAE Visual Naming are entered into a logistic regression, the RAVLT and BNT both predict the side of seizure focus (Loring et al., 2008).

Passarelli et al. (2015) reported that medically refractory epilepsy patients with left mesial temporal sclerosis (MTS) and ictal electroencephalogram (EEG) abnormality involving the contralateral temporal region obtain lower RAVLT scores than controls and lower WMS-III Faces scores than those with ictal EEG involvement exclusively ipsilateral to the MTS. Those with contralateral ictal EEG involvement also show lower RAVLT seven-day performance than healthy controls. As such, the RAVLT appears sensitive not just to MTS but also to ictal EEG epileptiform activity.

Patients who have undergone left anterior temporal resection for TLE show decline on the RAVLT within the first year postsurgery compared to those patients who have had right-sided surgery (Boucher et al., 2015; Grammaldo et al., 2009; Sziklas & Jones-Gotman, 2008), although improvement in Delayed Recall by postsurgical year two has been reported (Grammaldo et al., 2009). The Total Learning decline is more prevalent after standard anterior temporal lobectomy than after selective amygdalohippocampectomy (Boucher et al., 2015). Interestingly, there is evidence that improvements in Trial 6 may be seen following right-sided surgery (Boucher et al., 2015; Grammaldo et al., 2009).

Psychiatric Conditions and Stress Effects. There are suggestions that the impact of psychiatric conditions such as depression, schizophrenia, and bipolar disorder on RAVLT performance is related to executive dysfunction seen in these conditions. Some studies suggest impairment in Total Learning only (Kulkarni et al., 2010; Mannie et al., 2009; Messinis et al., 2010; Miclutia & Popescu, 2008), whereas others suggest impairment in Delayed Recall (Gooren et al., 2013; Hurlemann et al., 2008; Paula et al., 2013; Yuan et al., 2008). Patients with schizophrenia who have better verbal memory on the RAVLT are more likely to perform better on tasks of independent living (e.g., shopping; Remfer et al., 2003).

In other studies, young women with a parent with depression but without a personal history of depression were impaired on RAVLT Total Learning, although memory was not related to allelic variation in the promotor region of the serotonin transporter gene, a genetic factor relevant to the development of depression (Mannie et al., 2009). Other studies do not find memory impairment in those with severe depression. For example, McClintock et al., 2010) reported that up to 71% of their patients with severe depression referred for electroconvulsive therapy (ECT) obtained normal scores on RAVLT Delayed Recall trials; the Hamilton Rating Scale for Depression did not predict RAVLT scores. However, in another study, severely depressed patients who underwent ECT showed decline in Immediate and Delayed Recall on the RAVLT after three ECT sessions but no changes were seen in 3MS or Digit Span (Porter et al., 2008).

Compared to patients with schizophrenia, those with depression recall 1.18 fewer words on Delayed Recall but no differences are seen in Total Learning or Immediate Recall (Trial 6), whereas the schizophrenia group obtains impaired scores across the RAVLT (Gooren et al., 2013; Hurlemann et al., 2008; Manglam & Das, 2013; Miclutia & Popescu, 2008), even after controlling for IQ, age, and gender (Badcock et al., 2011). Moreover, healthy siblings of probands with first-episode schizophrenia are impaired on RAVLT Total Learning, Proactive Interference, and Immediate Recall (Trial 6) but not Delayed Recall or Recognition (Miclutia & Popescu, 2008). Some improvements on the RAVLT with treatment (e.g., clozapine or ziprasidone, the latter yielding larger improvements; Harvey et al., 2008) may be seen in patients with schizophrenia in as little as six weeks of treatment (Manglam & Das, 2013).

Adults with ADHD do not show impairment on the RAVLT learning and recognition measures, but they are more prone to repetition and intrusive errors on recall trials. Repetition and intrusive errors are moderately correlated with TMT and Digit Span but not FSIQ, suggesting the influence of executive dysfunction on memory functioning rather than memory deficits per se (Pollak et al., 2007).

Personality factors also affect RAVLT performance, at least on Delayed Recall. For example, Allen et al. (2011) found that older adults with low scores on the NEO extraversion scale (i.e., reduced positive affect) obtain lower delayed scores than those with high extraversion scores (i.e., high positive affect), who obtain similar delayed scores as younger adults. No differences are seen in the Trial 1 scores of older adults regardless of extraversion scores.

Acute mental stress typical of everyday life appears to have little negative effect on test performance, but may in fact enhance memory in the short run (Hoffman & al'Absi, 2004; Nater et al., 2007). A number of studies have attempted to assess the impact of acute stress and corresponding cortisol levels on RAVLT performance by inducing stress (and consequently increasing cortisol level) prior to test administration (Espin et al., 2013; Hidalgo et al., 2014). Contrary to expectation, participants appear to benefit from pre-learning stress, as those who are in the stress induction condition obtain greater Immediate and Delayed Recall scores than those in the control condition (Espin et al., 2013). Notably, the effect is gender specific. Men exposed to pre-learning stress show better recall than men in the control condition, whereas no differences are seen among women regardless of exposure to pre-learning stress. Females in the control group outperformed males, but men's performance improved to the level of the women when they were exposed to stress prior to the learning trials. Only women in the luteal phase had negative correlations between peak cortisol level and all RAVLT trials, suggesting that sex hormones may modulate the relationship between cortisol and memory. Moreover, it has been reported that pre-learning stress affects only older adults but not young adults (Hidalgo et al., 2014).

Nater et al. (2007) noted that stress exposure itself does not affect memory performance on the RAVLT; however, high cortisol responders obtain better Total Learning after stress exposure but not on other trials. Similarly, Pulopulos et al. (2014) reported that hair cortisol level (reflecting long-term cortisol exposure) is associated with RAVLT scores, whereas diurnal salivary cortisol (measuring HPA-axis dysregulation) is not.

Substance Abuse. RAVLT performance is negatively impacted by drug use, including alcohol, cannabis, cocaine, heroin, and MDMA (Fox et al., 2009; Messinis et al., 2007, 2009; Parada et al., 2011; Quednow et al., 2006; Wagner et al., 2010). Adults who are long-term heavy cannabis users but who have been abstinent for at least 24 hours prior to testing perform worse than healthy controls on all trials except Trial B (Messinis et al., 2007). Age of first use, frequency, and duration of use interactions are predictive of test performance. Those with short duration of use obtain better scores than those with long duration of use on Trial 1 but show more word loss after the interference trial (Wagner et al., 2010). Undergraduate students who binge drink (defined as six or more alcoholic drinks on a single occasion one or more times a month, and three or more drinks per hour) obtain poorer List B scores and experience greater proactive interference than non-binge drinkers regardless of gender (Parada et al., 2011). Similarly, a dose-response relationship is seen between MDMA and memory performance ($r = -.56$ to $-.70$; Quednow et al., 2006).

Corticosteroids appear to affect RAVLT performance although the effects do not last. For example, healthy individuals given three days of 60 mg/day prednisone show decline in RAVLT Delayed Recall but not Immediate Recall (Trial 6) after the first prednisone exposure. Smaller declines than the first are observed after the second exposure, suggesting attenuation of memory response (Brown et al., 2006). Furthermore, patients given corticosteroid and adjunctive levetiracetam or lamotrigine show improvements in their RAVLT performance (Brown et al., 2007, 2008).

Health Factors. Reis et al. (2013) reported that cardiovascular metrics such as obesity, diet, smoking, physical activity, total cholesterol, blood pressure, and fasting glucose in young adulthood and middle age are associated with RAVLT scores 25 years later. Each ideal metric at baseline is associated with 0.12 more words recalled on the RAVLT in midlife. Those with five or more ideal metrics obtain better RAVLT performance than those with fewer than five. Smoking, blood pressure, and total cholesterol are particularly related to RAVLT performance. Similarly, poor health, history of stroke, alcohol consumption, low fruit and vegetable consumption, low multivitamin supplement consumption, and low level of physical activity are all related to worse RAVLT memory scores when reassessed 10 years later (Wu & Chiu, 2016). Furthermore, every minute of cardiorespiratory fitness at baseline in young adults is associated with 0.12 more words on Delayed Recall when tested 25 years later, and the relationship between baseline cardiorespiratory fitness and RAVLT performance remains even after adjusting for various lifestyle and health factors (Zhu et al., 2014). As such, effective management of these modifiable health factors has implications for memory functioning in the long term and demonstrate the utility of the RAVLT in tracking health at the population level over decades.

Of note, hearing impairment is associated with poor memory function, and in fact increases RAVLT age-related changes over time by 26% in older adults (Wu & Chiu, 2016).

NEUROANATOMICAL CORRELATES AND IMAGING STUDIES

Poor RAVLT performance has been associated with reduced hippocampal volume in amnestic MCI, AD, and schizophrenia (Balthazar et al., 2010; Hurlemann et al., 2008; Marchiani et al., 2008; Walhovd et al., 2009). The association of RAVLT and other brain regions is less consistent. One study reported that Total Learning, Delayed Recall, and Recognition are correlated with medial prefrontal cortex in amnestic MCI and AD; the relationship is strongest between Total Learning and medial prefrontal cortex and hippocampi structures than with other trials (Balthazar et al., 2010). Another study of amnestic MCI patients indicated that Delayed Recall is correlated with metabolism in bilateral posterior cingulate gyrus and left precuneus whereas Total Learning does not correlate with any brain areas (Brugnolo et al., 2014). A third study found that Delayed Recall was correlated with an amygdala functional connectivity network in the bilateral dorsolateral prefrontal cortex, dorsomedial and anterior prefrontal cortex, posterior cingulate cortex, middle occipital gyrus, right inferior parietal cortex, and left middle temporal gyrus (Xie et al., 2012). PD patients show decreased task-related deactivations in the default mode network on fMRI (Ibarretxe-Bilbao et al., 2011).

On the other hand, although patients with previous or current major depression show smaller bilateral hippocampal volume, this finding is associated with WCST perseverative errors and responses but not RAVLT (Frodl et al., 2006). Similarly, in patients with chronic severe TBI (average about four years post injury), the best predictors of RAVLT memory scores are the parietal-precuneus but not hippocampus volumes, suggesting that, in TBI patients, RAVLT memory deficits may be explained by aberration in cortico-subcortical connectivity instead of hippocampus atrophy (Palacios et al., 2013).

A number of white matter bundles have also been shown to be associated with RAVLT performance, including integrity of the fornix and uncinate fasciculus (Bennett et al., 2015; Christidi et al., 2014; Walhovd et al., 2009). In patients with ALS, Total Learning is moderately correlated with the left uncinate fasciculus, whereas Delayed Recall is correlated bilaterally (Christidi et al., 2014). In MCI patients, DTI fractional anisotropy of the retrosplenial white matter predicts Total Learning, accounting for 37% of the variance (Walhovd et al., 2009).

Finally, decreased qEEG activation in the left posterior temporoparietal region but not in the right is associated with decreased Total Learning (Foster et al., 2007).

PERFORMANCE VALIDITY

Individuals with noncredible memory problems often exhibit a pattern of excessive impairment on the RAVLT (Suhr, 2002; Sullivan et al., 2001). In particular, there is evidence that severe RAVLT recognition memory impairment (e.g., scores <7) most likely reflects exaggeration of deficits in patients with TBI (Binder et al., 2003; Chouinard & Rouleau, 1997; King et al., 1998; Meyers et al., 2001; Sherman et al., 2002). Recognition exhibits a high degree of specificity for noncredible performance, but only modest sensitivity (Whitney & Davis, 2015). For example, Binder et al. (2003) reported that 92% of patients with moderate to severe head injury obtain scores of more than five correct responses, whereas only 38% of patients failing the Portland Digit Recognition Test obtain such scores. Numerous indicators, including abnormal serial position effects (i.e., absence of primacy effects in recall), number of false positives on the Recognition trial, discrepancies in Recall-Recognition scores, and failure to recognize words recalled at least three times on the learning trials have been suggested, but subsequent studies have not supported their use for the purpose of identifying invalid performance (see Table 10–79; Bernard et al., 1993; Boone et al., 2005; Powell et al., 2004; Suhr & Gunstad, 2000; Sullivan et al., 2002).

For that reason, Boone et al. (2005) developed an Effort Equation which yields high sensitivity and specificity for identifying invalid performance (Table 10–79), as follows:

Effort Equation = True Recognition (Recognition – False Positives) + Primacy Recognition (number of words recognized from the first third of the test)

TABLE 10–79 Sensitivity, PPV, and NPV at Various Base Rates of Noncredible Performance for Rey Auditory Verbal Learning Test (RAVLT) Performance Validity Indices (≥90% Specificity)

		15% BASE RATE		30% BASE RATE		40% BASE RATE	
	SENSITIVITY (%)	PPV (%)	NPV (%)	PPV (%)	NPV %)	PPV (%)	NPV (%)
Effort Equation ≤ 12	74	55	95	75	89	83	83
True Recognition + Stem ≤ 2 + Temporal Order ≤ 22	76	65	96	83	90	82	90
Recognition ≤ 9	67	63	94	81	87	87	80
True Recognition ≤ 7	64	61	94	81	86	87	79
Recency Recognition ≤ 2	54						
Primacy Recall ≤ 10	54						
Index 1 ≥ 3	28						
Stem ≤ 4	26						
Index 2 ≥ 2	8						
Temporal Order ≤ 4	14						

NOTE: All presented cutoffs yielded ≥90% specificity. PPV, positive predictive value; NPV, negative predictive value.

Stem = number of RAVLT words produced on word stem. This implicit procedure was based on presentation of 12 three-letter word stems from an alternate list, and another 12 three-letter word stems from RAVLT List A.

Index 1 = failure to identify a word on the Recognition trial that had been recalled at least three times during learning trials (Suhr et al., 1997).

Index 2 = failure to identify a word on the Recognition trial that had been recalled during Trial 8 (Suhr et al., 1997).

Effort Equation = True Recognition (Recognition minus False Positives) + Primacy Recognition (number of words recognized from the first third of the test).

Data are based on 61 noncredible patients from medical centers or private practice who were in litigation or seeking compensation and showing noncredible performance on two or more stand-alone or embedded PVTs, 88 clinical patients with no motive to feign cognitive problems, and 25 healthy volunteers.

SOURCE: Adapted from Boone et al. (2005).

Boone et al. (2005) also developed implicit (i.e., "stem") and temporal order indices as add-ons to the RAVLT to measure performance validity. The implicit procedure was based on presentation of 12 three-letter word stems from an alternate list and another 12 three-letter word stems from RAVLT List A.

As can be seen in Table 10–79, the Boone et al. (2005) Effort Equation appears to yield the best sensitivity at 90% specificity and is modestly superior to the sensitivity obtained with the standard Recognition score. Addition of the implicit and temporal procedures also does not improve sensitivity to identifying noncredible performance and so does not justify the extra administration time.

The addition of a second Delayed Recall and Recognition trial after 60 minutes (referred to as the expanded AVLT or AVLTX) may also enhance diagnostic accuracy. Barrash et al. (2004) constructed an Exaggeration Index (EI) based on the notion that malingerers would have difficulty estimating their 30-minute performance and keeping track of the words that they reported and those that they feigned forgetting. The EI is a composite index reflecting the extent to which memory performance is characterized by inconsistencies that are atypical of brain-injured individuals. It comprises seven aspects of improbable performance: exceedingly poor learning, lack of primacy effect, worsening recall, worsening recognition, failure to recognize learned words, and exceedingly poor recognition (see Table 10–80). The total score for the EI is the sum of the scaled score for these seven inconsistencies.

The EI demonstrates good sensitivity, identifying two-thirds of the probable malingerers as such, and positive predictive accuracy was .84 with a base rate of malingering of 30%. In comparison to the EI, the Warrington Recognition Memory Test demonstrates a higher level of sensitivity but lower positive predictive accuracy (.67). Initial development of the EI-AVLTX was based on patient groups (brain-injured, psychiatric, probable malingerers) referred for neuropsychological assessment. Subsequent studies by these authors (Suhr et al., 2004), using a simulation paradigm, found the EI-AVLTX to be modestly sensitive and relatively specific to malingering, as well as robust to the effects of a warning about malingering detection. Scores of 2 are considered consistent with "probable malingering," and scores of 3 are "highly probable" of malingering (Barrash et al., 2004; Suhr et al., 2004).

Ashendorf and Sugarman (2016) developed a Forced-Choice trial to be administered 10 minutes after the administration of the 50-item yes/no Recognition trial to be used as an embedded performance validity indicator for the RAVLT. The Forced-Choice word list is presented in Table 10–81. In a sample of 122 veterans who underwent neuropsychological evaluation at a Veterans Affairs polytrauma clinic divided into valid and invalid groups based on failure on two or more independent embedded or stand-alone performance validity measures, a Forced-Choice cutoff of 13 or less yielded a sensitivity of 68% and a specificity of 93% for identifying invalid performance and was better than Recognition as a performance validity indicator. At the time of this writing, additional studies verifying the utility of the Forced-Choice trial in other clinical samples would be beneficial.

Smith et al. (2014) provide adjusted cutoff scores for using various RAVLT indices to identify invalid performance in those with low IQ based on archival data from an outpatient neuropsychology clinic and private forensic practice (Table 10–82). Differences in PVT performance are seen between credible and noncredible low-IQ groups on the RAVLT Effort Equation (Boone et al., 2005), which yields the highest sensitivity compared to primary RAVLT indices. The adjusted cutoff score for the Effort Equation

TABLE 10–80 Exaggeration Index for the Expanded Auditory Verbal Learning Test (EI-AVLTX)

INCONSISTENCY		SCALED SCORE 0	1	2	3
1. Exceedingly Poor Learning	Immediate Recall of 15-word list, summed across learning Trials 1–5	≥28	23–27	18–22	0–17
2. Lack of Primacy Effect	Immediate Recall of words 1–3, summed across learning Trials 1–5	≥4	1–3	0	—
3. Worsening Recall	Delayed Recall at 30-min minus Delayed Recall at 60 min	0–2	3	4	≥5
4. Worsening Recognition	Delayed Recognition at 30 min minus Delayed Recognition at 60 min	0–2	—	3	≥4
5. Learned Words Not Recognized (scored only if made ≥2 false positive responses)	Words recalled on ≥4 learning trials but not recognized at 30 min plus words recalled on ≥4 learning trials but not recognized at 60 min	0–2	3–4	5–8	≥9
6. Recalled Words Not Recognized	Words recalled at 30 min but not recognized at 60 min	0–4	5–6	7–8	≥9
7. Exceedingly Poor Recognition	Recognition of target words summed across 30- and 60-min delays	>20	14–19	11–13	0–10

NOTE: Total score for the index is calculated by summing the scaled scores for the seven inconsistencies. Based on administration of a second Delayed Recall and Recognition trial after 60 minutes.

SOURCE: From Suhr et al. (2004).

TABLE 10-81 Rey Auditory Verbal Learning Test (RAVLT) Forced-Choice Word List

NOSE	STADIUM
HAPPY	BELL
RIVER	TISSUE
SMART	PARENT
WHEEL	HAT
TURKEY	LEARN
CURTAIN	SLED
OBSERVE	FARMER
HOUSE	OSTRICH
SMALL	SCHOOL
GARLIC	COLOR
GARDEN	CLEAN
DRUM	DIRT
SWIM	MOON
COFFEE	CHISEL

SOURCE: From Ashendorf and Sugarman (2016).

increased the specificity from 65% (based on the original cutoff ≤12) to 90% in this low-IQ sample.

Sherman et al. (2002) reported yet another method to identify invalid performance using RAVLT Trial 1 and Recognition as well as RCFT delay scores, as follows:

Discriminant Function Equation
= .006 (RAVLT Trial 1) – .062 (RCFT Delayed Recall) + .354 (RAVLT Recognition) – 2.508

They conducted a discriminant analysis using three groups: a medical center or private practice sample with noncredible performance based on at least two failures on stand-alone or embedded performance validity indicators who were in litigation or seeking disability, neurological patients not in litigation/seeking disability, and healthy controls. The discriminant function analysis cutoff of –.40 or less yielded a sensitivity of 71% while maintaining the specificity above 90%. The cutoff may be adjusted further to maintain the specificity even higher than 90% for individuals with low intellectual functioning, though the sensitivity will be notably lower.

In terms of correlations with other PVTs, measures derived from the RAVLT (e.g., Recognition, Delayed Recall) show modest to moderate relations with other indices of motivational status (e.g., Warrington Recognition Memory Test, Rey Fifteen-Item; Nelson et al., 2003). The implication is that the RAVLT provides nonredundant information and can serve as a relatively independent source of information regarding the validity of neuropsychological test performance.

TABLE 10-82 Rey Auditory Verbal Learning Test (RAVLT) Adjusted Cutoff Scores, Sensitivity, and Specificity for Use with Low-IQ Samples (FSIQ ≤ 75)

	CUTOFF	SENSITIVITY (%)	SPECIFICITY (%)
Total Learning	≤25	46	92
Short Delay	≤3	42	90
Boone et al. (2005) Effort Equation	≤7	50	90
Recognition	≤7	48	90
Sherman et al. (2002) Equation	≤–0.21	53	92

NOTE: Only indices with sensitivity >40% are included.
SOURCE: Adapted from Smith et al. (2014).

COMMENT

The RAVLT has been an important test in the field of neuropsychology for many decades and is one of the first standard tests of multitrial list learning and memory to achieve widespread clinical use (Woodard et al., 1999). The test has been adapted and administered in multiple languages and cultures, and the convergence of findings contributes to the validity of the test. It provides a wealth of information to characterize memory functioning (e.g., learning rate, susceptibility to proactive and retroactive interference). Analysis of the indices provides information on the nature of memory dysfunction in various neurological and psychiatric conditions and may aid in differential diagnosis as well as rehabilitation planning. It appears particularly useful in epilepsy presurgical evaluations over and above other list-learning, story memory, and visual memory tasks in identifying seizure focus and predicting postsurgical memory outcome. It is also a strong predictor of impending dementia even when compared to other biomarkers. The RAVLT is also useful for tracking health at the population level over decades. Numerous embedded performance validity indicators, such as the Boone et al. (2005) and the Ashendorf and Sugarman (2016) Forced-Choice trial, have contributed even further to its clinical utility. Coupled with it being a well-researched public-domain test, it is no wonder the RAVLT is one of the more popular and impressive memory tests in clinical use.

In testing recognition, some authors use story formats and others use word list formats. The word list formats also differ from the story formats in terms of, for example, word list length, delay intervals, and whether an intervening delayed recall trial was administered. Based on his review of the available literature, Schmidt (1996) suggested that the recognition memory scores are quite robust with regard to these procedural permutations, with no systematic differences occurring for different recognition procedures.

Users should be aware of the test's limitations. The most reliable measures are the Total Learning score, the Delayed Recall score, and the Trial 5 score. Although other measures are interesting from a research perspective, their reliabilities tend to be low and caution is needed in interpreting other features (e.g., flatness of the learning curve, number of errors, number of repetitions), including those that rely on differences between scores.

Because of its popularity, most of the updated norms have been collected in international settings. The most comprehensive North-American norms from the

MOANS are decades old and updated norms are lacking. The availability of updated norms for the alternate forms is also unclear.

It is important to note that ceiling effects appear to be present on the later recall trials. Uttl (2005) noted that ceiling effects can negatively affect test reliability and validity because of attenuated variability in test scores. In addition, floor effects have been observed in those with more advanced AD. Once the diagnosis is established, the RAVLT is not useful to monitor disease progression; however, this is true of several similar list-learning paradigms.

REFERENCES

Alegret, M., Junque, C., Valleoriola, F., Vendrell, P., Pilleri, M., Rumia, J., & Tolosa, E. (2001). Effects of bilateral subthalamic stimulation on cognitive function in Parkinson disease. *Archives of Neurology, 58,* 1223–1227.

Allen, P. A., Kaut, K., Baena, E., Lien, M.-C., & Ruthruff, E. (2011). Individual differences in positive affect moderate age-related declines in episodic long-term memory. *Journal of Cognitive Psychology, 23*(6), 768–779.

Anderson, V. A., & Lajoie, G. (1996). Development of memory and learning skills in school-aged children: A neuropsychological perspective. *Applied Neuropsychology, 3/4,* 128–139.

Andersson, C., Blennow, K., Johansson, S.-E., Almkvist, O., Engfeldt, P., Lindau, M., & Eriksdotter-Jönhagen, M. (2007). Differential CSF biomarker levels in & ApoEε4-positive and -negative patients with memory impairment. *Dementia and Geriatric Cognitive Disorders, 23*(2), 87–95.

Ashendorf, L., & Sugarman, M. A. (2016). Evaluation of performance validity using a Rey Auditory Verbal Learning Test Forced-Choice trial. *The Clinical Neuropsychologist, 30*(4), 599–609.

Badcock, J. C., Dragovic, M., Dawson, L., & Jones, R. (2011). Normative data for Rey's Auditory Verbal Learning Test in individuals with schizophrenia. *Archives of Clinical Neuropsychology, 26*(3), 205–213.

Balthazar, M. L., Martinelli, J. E., Cendes, F., & Damasceno, B. P. (2007). Lexical semantic memory in amnestic mild cognitive impairment and mild Alzheimer's disease. *Arquivos de Neuro-Psiquiatria, 65*(3A), 619–622.

Balthazar, M. L. F., Yasuda, C. L., Cendes, F., & Damasceno, B. P. (2010). Learning, retrieval, and recognition are compromised in amnestic MCI and mild AD: Are distinct episodic memory processes mediated by the same anatomical structures? *Journal of the International Neuropsychological Society, 16*(01), 205.

Barrash, J., Suhr, J., & Manzel, K. (2004). Detecting poor effort and malingering with an expanded version of the Auditory Verbal Learning Test (AVLTX): Validation with clinical samples. *Journal of Clinical and Experimental Neuropsychology, 26,* 125–140.

Bennett, I. J., Huffman, D. J., & Stark, C. E. L. (2015). Limbic tract integrity contributes to pattern separation performance across the lifespan. *Cerebral Cortex, 25*(9), 2988–2999.

Bercaw, E. L., Hanks, R. A., Millis, S. R., & Gola, T. J. (2011). Changes in neuropsychological performance after traumatic brain injury from inpatient rehabilitation to 1-year follow-up in predicting 2-year functional outcomes. *The Clinical Neuropsychologist, 25*(1), 72–89.

Bernard, L. C., Houston, W., & Natoli, L. (1993). Malingering on neuropsychological memory tests: Potential objective indicators. *Journal of Clinical Psychology, 49,* 45–53.

Bezdicek, O., Stepankova, H., Moták, L., Axelrod, B. N., Woodard, J. L., Preiss, M., . . . Poreh, A. (2014). Czech version of Rey Auditory Verbal Learning test: Normative data. *Aging, Neuropsychology, and Cognition, 21*(6), 693–721.

Binder, L. M., Kelly, M. P., Villanueva, M. R., & Winslow, M. M. (2003). Motivation and neuropsychological test performance following mild head injury. *Journal of Clinical and Experimental Neuropsychology, 25,* 420–430.

Boake, C. (2000). Edouard Claparede and the Auditory Verbal Learning Test. *Journal of Clinical and Experimental Neuropsychology, 22,* 286–292.

Boone, K. B., Lu, P., & Wen, J. (2005). Comparison of various RAVLT scores in the detection of noncredible memory performance. *Archives of Clinical Neuropsychology, 20*(3), 301–319.

Boucher, O., Dagenais, E., Bouthillier, A., Nguyen, D. K., & Rouleau, I. (2015). Different effects of anterior temporal lobectomy and selective amygdalohippocampectomy on verbal memory performance of patients with epilepsy. *Epilepsy & Behavior, 52,* 230–235.

Brown, E. S., Beard, L., Frol, A. B., & Rush, A. J. (2006). Effect of two prednisone exposures on mood and declarative memory. *Neurobiology of Learning and Memory, 86*(1), 28–34.

Brown, E. S., Frol, A. B., Khan, D. A., Larkin, G. L., & Bret, M. E. (2007). Impact of levetiracetam on mood and cognition during prednisone therapy. *European Psychiatry, 22*(7), 448–452.

Brown, E. S., Wolfshohl, J., Shad, M. U., Vazquez, M., & Osuji, I. J. (2008). Attenuation of the effects of corticosteroids on declarative memory with lamotrigine. *Neuropsychopharmacology, 33*(10), 2376–2383.

Brugnolo, A., Morbelli, S., Arnaldi, D., De Carli, F., Accardo, J., Bossert, I., . . . others. (2014). Metabolic correlates of Rey Auditory Verbal Learning Test in elderly subjects with memory complaints. *Journal of Alzheimer's Disease, 39*(1), 103–113.

Caillava-Santos, F., Margis, R., & Rieder, C. (2015). Wearing-off in Parkinson's disease: Neuropsychological differences between on and off periods. *Neuropsychiatric Disease and Treatment,* 1175.

Carstairs, J. R., Shores, E. A., & Myors, B. (2012). Australian norms and retest data for the Rey Auditory and Verbal Learning Test: RAVLT Australian normative data. *Australian Psychologist, 47*(4), 191–197.

Chouinard, M. J., & Rouleau, I. (1997). The 48-Pictures Test: A two-alternative forced-choice recognition test for the detection of malingering. *Journal of the International Neuropsychological Society, 3,* 545–552.

Christidi, F., Zalonis, I., Kyriazi, S., Rentzos, M., Karavasilis, E., Wilde, E. A., & Evdokimidis, I. (2014). Uncinate fasciculus microstructure and verbal episodic memory in amyotrophic lateral sclerosis: A diffusion tensor imaging and neuropsychological study. *Brain Imaging and Behavior, 8*(4), 497–505.

Christidi, F., Zalonis, I., Smyrnis, N., & Evdokimidis, I. (2012). Selective attention and the three-process memory model for the interpretation of verbal free recall in amyotrophic lateral sclerosis. *Journal of the International Neuropsychological Society, 18*(05), 809–818.

Chu, B.-C., Millis, S., Arango-Lasprilla, J. C., Hanks, R., Novack, T., & Hart, T. (2007). Measuring recovery in new learning and memory following traumatic brain injury: A mixed-effects modeling approach. *Journal of Clinical and Experimental Neuropsychology, 29*(6), 617–625.

Consonni, M., Rossi, S., Cerami, C., Marcone, A., Iannaccone, S., Francesco Cappa, S., & Perani, D. (2017). Executive dysfunction affects word list recall performance: Evidence from amyotrophic lateral sclerosis and other neurodegenerative diseases. *Journal of Neuropsychology, 11*(1), 74–90.

Correia, A. F., & Osorio, I. C. (2014). The Rey Auditory Verbal Learning Test: Normative data developed for the Venezuelan population. *Archives of Clinical Neuropsychology, 29*(2), 206–215.

Crawford, J. R., Stewart, L. E., & Moore, J. W. (1989). Demonstration of savings on the AVLT and development of a parallel form. *Journal of Clinical and Experimental Neuropsychology, 11,* 975–981.

Crossen, J. R., & Wiens, A. N. (1994). Comparison of the Auditory-Verbal Learning Test (AVLT) and California Verbal Learning Test

(CVLT) in a sample of normal subjects. *Journal of Clinical and Experimental Neuropsychology, 16,* 190–194.

Crowe, S. F., & Casey, A. (1999). A neuropsychological study of the chronic fatigue syndrome: Support for a deficit in memory function independent of depression. *Australian Psychologist, 34,* 70–75.

Delaney, R. C., Prevey, M. L., Cramer, J., Mattson, R. H., & VA Epilepsy Cooperative Study 264 Research Group. (1992). Test-retest comparability and control subject data for the Rey-Auditory Verbal Learning Test and Rey-Osterrieth/Taylor Complex Figures. *Archives of Clinical Neuropsychology, 7,* 523–528.

Demers, M., Rouleau, I., Scherze, P., Ouellet, J., Jobin, C., & Duquette, P. (2011). Impact of the cognitive status on the memory complaints in MS patients. *Canadian Journal of Neurological Sciences, 38*(05), 728–733.

Draper, K., & Ponsford, J. (2008). Cognitive functioning ten years following traumatic brain injury and rehabilitation. *Neuropsychology, 22*(5), 618–625.

Dunlosky, J., & Salthouse, T. A. (1996). A decomposition of age-related differences in multitrial free recall. *Aging, Neuropsychology, and Cognition, 3,* 2–14.

Eckerström, C., Olsson, E., Bjerke, M., Malmgren, H., Edman, Å., Wallin, A., & Nordlund, A. (2013). A combination of neuropsychological, neuroimaging, and cerebrospinal fluid markers predicts conversion from mild cognitive impairment to dementia. *Journal of Alzheimer's Disease, 36*(3), 421–431.

Espin, L., Almela, M., Hidalgo, V., Villada, C., Salvador, A., & Gomez-Amor, J. (2013). Acute pre-learning stress and declarative memory: Impact of sex, cortisol response and menstrual cycle phase. *Hormones and Behavior, 63*(5), 759–765.

Ferman, T. J., Lucas, J. A., Ivnik, R. J., Smith, G. E., Willis, F. B., Petersen, R. C., & Graff-Radford, N. R. (2005). Mayo's Older African American Normative Studies: Auditory-Verbal Learning Test norms for African American elders. *The Clinical Neuropsychologist, 19,* 214–228.

Fernaeus, S.-E., Östberg, P., Wahlund, L.-O., & Hellström, Å. (2014). Memory factors in Rey AVLT: Implications for early staging of cognitive decline. *Scandinavian Journal of Psychology, 55*(6), 546–553.

Fichman, H. C., Teresa Dias, L. B., Fernandes, C. S., Lourenço, R., Caramelli, P., & Nitrini, R. (2010). Normative data and construct validity of the Rey Auditory Verbal Learning Test in a Brazilian elderly population. *Psychology & Neuroscience, 3*(1), 79–84.

Flanagan, E. C., Wong, S., Dutt, A., Tu, S., Bertoux, M., Irish, M., . . . Hornberger, M. (2016). False recognition in behavioral variant frontotemporal dementia and Alzheimer's Disease—Disinhibition or amnesia? *Frontiers in Aging Neuroscience, 8,* 177. doi:10.3389/fnagi.2016.00177.

Forrester, G., & Geffen, G. (1991). Performance measure of 7- to 15-year-old children on the Auditory Verbal Learning Test. *The Clinical Neuropsychologist, 5,* 345–359.

Foster, P. S., Harrison, D. W., Crucian, G. P., Drago, V., Rhodes, R. D., & Heilman, K. M. (2007). Reduced verbal learning associated with posterior temporal lobe slow wave activity. *Developmental Neuropsychology, 33*(1), 25–43.

Fox, H. C., Jackson, E. D., & Sinha, R. (2009). Elevated cortisol and learning and memory deficits in cocaine dependent individuals: Relationship to relapse outcomes. *Psychoneuroendocrinology, 34*(8), 1198–1207.

Frodl, T., Schaub, A., Banac, S., Charypar, M., & others. (2006). Reduced hippocampal volume correlates with executive dysfunctioning in major depression. *Journal of Psychiatry & Neuroscience: JPN, 31*(5), 316.

Fuller, K. H., Gouvier, W. D., & Savage, R. M. (1997). Comparison of List B and List C of the Rey Auditory Verbal Learning Test. *The Clinical Neuropsychologist, 11,* 201–204.

Gainotti, G., & Marra, C. (1994). Some aspects of memory disorders clearly distinguish dementia of the Alzheimer's type from depressive pseudodementia. *Journal of Clinical and Experimental Neuropsychology, 16,* 65–74.

Gale, S. D., Baxter, L., Connor, D. J., Herring, A., & Comer, J. (2007). Sex differences on the Rey Auditory Verbal Learning Test and the Brief Visuospatial Memory Test–Revised in the elderly: Normative data in 172 participants. *Journal of Clinical and Experimental Neuropsychology, 29*(5), 561–567.

Gale, S. D., Baxter, L., & Thompson, J. (2016). Greater memory impairment in dementing females than males relative to sex-matched healthy controls. *Journal of Clinical and Experimental Neuropsychology, 38*(5), 527–533.

Gavett, B. E., & Horwitz, J. E. (2012). Immediate list recall as a measure of short-term episodic memory: Insights from the serial position effect and item response theory. *Archives of Clinical Neuropsychology, 27*(2), 125–135.

Geffen, G. M., Butterworth, P., & Geffen, L. B. (1994). Test-retest reliability of a new form of the Auditory Verbal Learning Test (AVLT). *Archives of Clinical Neuropsychology, 9,* 303–316.

Geffen, G. M., Geffen, L., & Bishop, K. (1997). Extended delayed recall of AVLT word lists: Effects of age and sex on adult performance. *Australian Journal of Psychology, 49,* 78–84.

Geffen, G., Moar, K. J., O'Hanlon, A. P., Clark, C. R., & Geffen, L. B. (1990). Performance measures of 16- to 86-year-old males and females on the Auditory Verbal Learning Test. *The Clinical Neuropsychologist, 4,* 45–63.

Gooren, T., Schlattmann, P., & Neu, P. (2013). A comparison of cognitive functioning in acute schizophrenia and depression. *Acta Neuropsychiatrica, 25*(06), 334–341.

Graf, P., & Uttl, B. (1995). Component processes of memory: Changes across the adult lifespan. *Swiss Journal of Psychology, 54,* 113–130.

Grammaldo, L. G., Di Gennaro, G., Giampà, T., De Risi, M., Meldolesi, G. N., Mascia, A., . . . Picardi, A. (2009). Memory outcome 2 years after anterior temporal lobectomy in patients with drug-resistant epilepsy. *Seizure, 18*(2), 139–144.

Grammaldo, L. G., Giampa, T., Quarato, P. P., Picardi, A., Mascia, A., Sparano, A., . . . Di Gennaro, G. (2006). Lateralizing value of memory tests in drug-resistant temporal lobe epilepsy. *European Journal of Neurology, 13*(4), 371–376.

Haddad, L. B., & Nussbaum, P. (1989). Predictive utility of the Rey Auditory-Verbal Learning Test with Alzheimer's patients. *The Clinical Gerontologist, 9,* 53–59.

Harris, M. E., Ivnik, R. J., & Smith, G. E. (2002). Mayo's Older Americans Normative Studies: Expanded AVLT recognition trial norms for ages 57 to 98. *Journal of Clinical and Experimental Neuropsychology, 24,* 214–220.

Harvey, P. D., Sacchetti, E., Galluzzo, A., Romeo, F., Gorini, B., Bilder, R. M., & Loebel, A. D. (2008). A randomized double-blind comparison of ziprasidone vs. clozapine for cognition in patients with schizophrenia selected for resistance or intolerance to previous treatment. *Schizophrenia Research, 105*(1–3), 138–143.

Helmstaedter, C., & Durwen, H. F. (1990). VLMT: Verbaler Lern- und Merkfahigkeitstest (VLMT: Verbal Learning and Memory Test). *Schwietzer Archiv fur Nurologie und Psychiatrie, 141,* 21–30.

Hessen, E. (2011). Rehearsal significantly improves immediate and delayed recall on the Rey Auditory Verbal Learning Test. *Applied Neuropsychology, 18*(4), 263–268.

Hidalgo, V., Almela, M., Villada, C., & Salvador, A. (2014). Acute stress impairs recall after interference in older people, but not in young people. *Hormones and Behavior, 65*(3), 264–272.

Hoffman, R., & al'Absi, M. (2004). The effects of acute stress on subsequent neuropsychological test performance. *Archives of Clinical Neuropsychology, 19,* 497–506.

Hurlemann, R., Jessen, F., Wagner, M., Frommann, I., Ruhrmann, S., Brockhaus, A., . . . Maier, W. (2008). Interrelated neuropsychological and anatomical evidence of hippocampal pathology in the at-risk mental state. *Psychological Medicine, 38*(06).

Ibarretxe-Bilbao, N., Zarei, M., Junque, C., Marti, M. J., Segura, B., Vendrell, P., . . . Tolosa, E. (2011). Dysfunctions of cerebral networks precede recognition memory deficits in early Parkinson's disease. *NeuroImage, 57*(2), 589–597.

Ivnik, R. J., Malec, J. F., Tangalos, E. G., Petersen, R. C., Kokmen, E., & Kurland, L. T. (1992). Mayo's Older Americans Normative Studies: Updated AVLT norms for ages 56 to 97. *The Clinical Neuropsychologist, 6,* 83–104.

Jafari, Z., Steffen Moritz, P., Zandi, T., Aliakbari Kamrani, A., & Malyeri, S. (2010). Psychometric properties of Persian version of the Rey Auditory-Verbal Learning Test (RAVLT) among the elderly. *Iranian Journal of Psychiatry and Clinical Psychology, 16*(1), 56–64.

Johnstone, B., Vieth, A. Z., Johnson, J. C., & Shaw, J. A. (2000). Recall as a function of single versus multiple trials: Implications for rehabilitation. *Rehabiliation Psychology, 45,* 3–19.

Kennepohl, S., Shore, D., Nabors, N., & Hanks, R. (2004). African American acculturation and neuropsychological test performance following traumatic brain injury. *Journal of the International Neuropsychological Society, 10,* 566–577.

King, J. H., Gfeller, J. D., & Davis, H. P. (1998). Detecting simulated memory impairment with the Rey Auditory Verbal Learning Test: Implications of base rates and study generalizeability. *Journal of Clinical and Experimental Neuropsychology, 20,* 603–612.

Kulkarni, S., Jain, S., Janardhan Reddy, Y., Kumar, K. J., & Kandavel, T. (2010). Impairment of verbal learning and memory and executive function in unaffected siblings of probands with bipolar disorder: Cognitive endophenotypes in bipolar disorder. *Bipolar Disorders, 12*(6), 647–656.

Kurlyo, M., Temple, R. O., Elliott, T. R., & Crawford, D. (2001). Rey Auditory Verbal Learning Test (AVLT) performance in individuals with recent-onset spinal cord injury. *Rehabilitation Psychology, 46,* 247–261.

Lannoo, E., & Vingerhoets, G. (1997). Flemish normative data on common neuropsychological test: Influence of age, education, and gender. *Psychologica Belgica, 37,* 141–155.

Lee, T. M. C. (2003). *Normative data: Neuropsychological measures for Hong Kong Chinese.* Neuropsychology Laboratory, The University of Hong Kong, Hong Kong.

Lehmann, C. A., Marks, A. D. G., & Hanstock, T. L. (2013). Age and synchrony effects in performance on the Rey Auditory Verbal Learning Test. *International Psychogeriatrics, 25*(04), 657–665.

Lemay, S., Bedard, M. A., Rouleau, I., & Tremblay, P. L. G. (2004). Practice effect and test-retest reliability of attentional and executive tests in middle-aged to elderly subjects. *The Clinical Neuropsychologist, 18,* 284–302.

Lezak, M. D. (1976). *Neuropsychological assessment.* New York: Oxford University Press.

Lezak, M. D. (1983). *Neuropsychological assessment* (2nd ed.). New York: Oxford University Press.

Lezak, M., Howieson, D., & Loring, D. (2012). *Neuropsychological Assessment* (5th ed). New York: Oxford University Press.

Lezak, M. D., Howieson, D. B., Loring, D. W., Hannay, H. J., & Fischer, J. S. (2004). *Neuropsychological Assessment* (4th ed.). New York: Oxford University Press.

Li, X., Zhou, Z., Jia, S., Hou, C., Zheng, W., Rong, P., & Jiao, J. (2016). Cognitive study on Chinese patients with idiopathic REM sleep behavior disorder. *Journal of the Neurological Sciences, 366,* 82–86.

Loring, D. W., Strauss, E., Hermann, B. P., Barr, W. B., Perrine, K., Trenerry, M. R., . . . Bowden, S. C. (2008). Differential neuropsychological test sensitivity to left temporal lobe epilepsy. *Journal of the International Neuropsychological Society, 14*(03), 394–400.

Magalhães, S. S., & Hamdan, A. C. (2010). The Rey Auditory Verbal Learning Test: Normative data for the Brazilian population and analysis of the influence of demographic variables. *Psychology & Neuroscience, 3*(1), 85–91.

Magalhães, S., Fernandes Malloy-Diniz, L., & Cavalheiro Hamdan, A. (2012). Validity convergent and reliability test-retest of the Rey Auditory Verbal Learning Test. *Clinical Neuropsychiatry, 9*(3), 129–138.

Maj, M., D'Elia, L., Satz, P., Janssen, R., Zaudig, M., Uchiyama, C., Starace, F., Galderisi, S., & Chervinsky, A. (1993). Evaluation of two new neuropsychological tests designed to minimize cultural bias in the assessment of HIV-1 seropositive persons: A WHO study. *Archives of Clinical Neuropsychology, 8,* 123–135.

Majdan, A., Sziklas, V., & Jones-Gotman, M. (1996). Performance of healthy subjects and patients with resection from the anterior temporal lobe on matched tests of verbal and visuoperceptual learning. *Journal of Clinical and Experimental Neuropsychology, 18,* 416–430.

Malec, J. F., Ivnik, R. J., & Hinkeldey, N. S. (1991). Visual Spatial Learning Test. *Psychological Assessment, 3,* 82–88.

Malloy-Diniz, L. F., Lasmar, V. A. P., Gazinelli, L. de S. R., Fuentes, D., & Salgado, J. V. (2007). The Rey Auditory-Verbal Learning Test: Applicability for the Brazilian elderly population. *Revista Brasileira de Psiquiatria, 29*(4), 324–329.

Manglam, M. K., & Das, A. (2013). Verbal learning and memory and psychopathology in schizophrenia. *Asian Journal of Psychiatry, 6*(5), 417–420.

Mannie, Z. N., Barnes, J., Bristow, G. C., Harmer, C. J., & Cowen, P. J. (2009). Memory impairment in young women at increased risk of depression: Influence of cortisol and 5-HTT genotype. *Psychological Medicine, 39*(05), 757.

Marchiani, N. C. P., Balthazar, M. L. F., Cendes, F., & Damasceno, B. P. (2008). Hippocampal atrophy and verbal episodic memory performance in amnestic mild cognitive impairment and mild Alzheimer's disease: A preliminary study. *Dementia & Neuropsychologia, 2*(1), 37–41.

McClintock, S. M., Cullum, C. M., Husain, M. M., Rush, A. J., Knapp, R. G., Mueller, M., . . . Kellner, C. H. (2010). Evaluation of the effects of severe depression on global cognitive function and memory. *CNS Spectrums, 15*(05), 304–313.

Messinis, L., Lyros, E., Andrian, V., Katsakiori, P., Panagis, G., Georgiou, V., & Papathanasopoulos, P. (2009). Neuropsychological functioning in buprenorphine maintained patients versus abstinent heroin abusers on naltrexone hydrochloride therapy. *Human Psychopharmacology: Clinical and Experimental, 24*(7), 524–531.

Messinis, L., Nasios, G., Mougias, A., Politis, A., Zampakis, P., Tsiamaki, E., . . . Papathanasopoulos, P. (2016). Age and education adjusted normative data and discriminative validity for Rey's Auditory Verbal Learning Test in the elderly Greek population. *Journal of Clinical and Experimental Neuropsychology, 38*(1), 23–39.

Messinis, L., Tsakona, I., Malefaki, S., & Papathanasopoulos, P. (2007). Normative data and discriminant validity of Rey's Verbal Learning Test for the Greek adult population. *Archives of Clinical Neuropsychology, 22*(6), 739–752.

Messinis, L., Vlahou, C. H., Tsapanos, V., Tsapanos, A., Spilioti, D., & Papathanasopoulos, P. (2010). Neuropsychological functioning in postpartum depressed versus nondepressed females and nonpostpartum controls. *Journal of Clinical and Experimental Neuropsychology, 32*(6), 661–666.

Meyer, S. R. A., Spaan, P. E. J., Boelaarts, L., Ponds, R. W. H. M., Schmand, B., & de Jonghe, J. F. M. (2016). Visual associations cued recall a paradigm for measuring episodic memory decline in Alzheimer's disease. *Aging, Neuropsychology, and Cognition, 23*(5), 566–577.

Meyers, J. E., Morrison, A. L., & Miller, J. C. (2001). How low is too low, revisited: Sentence repetition and AVLT-recognition in the detection of malingering. *Applied Neuropsychology, 4,* 234–241.

Miatton, M., Wolters, M., Lannoo, E., & Vingerhoets, G. (2004). Updated and extended normative data of commonly used neuropsychological tests. *Psychologica Belgica, 44,* 189–216.

Miclutia, I., & Popescu, C. (2008). Working memory in first-episode schizophrenic patients and their healthy siblings. *Journal of Cognitive & Behavioral Psychotherapies, 8*(1).

Miller, L. A., Flanagan, E., Mothakunnel, A., Mohamed, A., & Thayer, Z. (2015). Old dogs with new tricks: Detecting accelerated long-term forgetting by extending traditional measures. *Epilepsy & Behavior, 45,* 205–211.

Millis, S. R., Rosenthal, M., & Lourie, I. F. (1994). Predicting community integration after traumatic brain injury with neuropsychological measures. *International Journal of Neuroscience, 79,* 165–167.

Miranda, J. P., & Valencia, R. R. (1997). English and Spanish versions of a memory test: Word-length effects versus spoken-duration effects. *Hispanic Journal of Behavioral Sciences, 19,* 171–181.

Mitrushina, M., & Satz, P. (1991a). Changes in cognitive functioning associated with normal aging. *Archives of Clinical Neuropsychology, 6,* 49–60.

Mitrushina, M., & Satz, P. (1991b). Effect of repeated administration of a neuropsychological battery in the elderly. *Journal of Clinical Psychology, 47,* 790–801.

Mitrushina, M. N., Boone, K. B., Razani, J., & D'Elia, L. F. (2005). *Handbook of normative data for neuropsychological assessment* (2nd ed.). New York: Oxford University Press.

Moritz, S., Heeren, D., Andresen, B., & Krausz, M. (2001). An analysis of the specificity and the syndromal correlates of verbal memory impairments in schizophrenia. *Psychiatry Research, 101,* 23–31.

Moritz, S., Iverson, G. L., & Woodward, T. S. (2003). Reliable change indexes for memory performance in schizophrenia as a means to determine drug-induced cognitive decline. *Applied Neuropsychology, 10,* 115–120.

Mueller, H., Hasse-Sander, R., Horn, C., Helmstaedter, C., & Elger, C. E. (1997). Rey-Auditory Verbal Learning Test: Structure of a modified German version. *Journal of Clinical Psychology, 53,* 663–671.

Nater, U. M., Moor, C., Okere, U., Stallkamp, R., Martin, M., Ehlert, U., & Kliegel, M. (2007). Performance on a declarative memory task is better in high than low cortisol responders to psychosocial stress. *Psychoneuroendocrinology, 32*(6), 758–763.

Nelson, N. W., Boone, K., Dueck, A., Wagener, L., Lu, P., & Grills, C. (2003). Relationships between eight measures of suspect effort. *The Clinical Neuropsychologist, 17,* 263–272.

Nielsen, H., Knudsen, L., & Daugbjerg, O. (1989). Normative data for eight neuropsychological tests based on a Danish sample. *Scandinavian Journal of Psychology, 30,* 37–45.

Palacios, E. M., Sala-Llonch, R., Junque, C., Fernandez-Espejo, D., Roig, T., Tormos, J. M., . . . Vendrell, P. (2013). Long-term declarative memory deficits in diffuse TBI: Correlations with cortical thickness, white matter integrity and hippocampal volume. *Cortex, 49*(3), 646–657.

Parada, M., Corral, M., Caamaño-Isorna, F., Mota, N., Crego, A., Holguín, S. R., & Cadaveira, F. (2011). Binge drinking and declarative memory in university students. *Alcoholism: Clinical and Experimental Research, 35*(8), 1475–1484.

Passarelli, V., Castro-Lima Filho, H., Adda, C. C., Preturlon-Santos, A. P., Valerio, R. M., Jorge, C. L., . . . Castro, L. H. (2015). Contralateral ictal electrographic involvement is associated with decreased memory performance in unilateral mesial temporal sclerosis. *Journal of the Neurological Sciences, 359*(1–2), 241–246.

Paula, J. J. de, Miranda, D. M., Nicolato, R., Moraes, E. N. de, Bicalho, M. A. C., & Malloy-Diniz, L. F. (2013). Verbal learning on depressive pseudodementia: Accentuate impairment of free recall, moderate on learning processes, and spared short-term and recognition memory. *Arquivos de Neuro-Psiquiatria, 71*(9A), 596–599.

Pollak, Y., Kahana-Vax, G., & Hoofien, D. (2007). Retrieval processes in adults with ADHD: A RAVLT Study. *Developmental Neuropsychology, 33*(1), 62–73.

Ponton, M. O., Gonzalez, J. J., Hernandez, I., Herrera, L., & Higareda, I. (2000). Factor analysis of the Neuropsychological Screening Battery for Hispanics (NeSBHIS). *Applied Neuropsychology, 7,* 32–39.

Ponton, M. O., Satz, P., Herrera, L., Ortiz, F., Urrutia, C. P., Young, R., . . . Namerow, N. (1996). Normative data stratified by age and education for the Neuropsychological Screening Battery for Hispanics (NeSBHIS): Initial report. *Journal of the International Neuropsychological Society, 2,* 96–104.

Poreh, A., Sultan, A., & Levin, J. (2012). The Rey Auditory Verbal Learning Test: Normative data for the Arabic-speaking population and analysis of the differential influence of demographic variables. *Psychology & Neuroscience, 5*(1), 57–61.

Porter, R., Heenan, H., & Reeves, J. (2008). Early effects of electroconvulsive therapy on cognitive function. *The Journal of ECT, 24*(1), 35–39.

Powell, M. R., Gfeller, J. D., Oliveri, M. V., Stanton, S., & Hendricks, B. (2004). The Rey AVLT serial position effect: A useful indicator of symptom exaggeration? *The Clinical Neuropsychologist, 18,* 465–476.

Pulopulos, M. M., Hidalgo, V., Almela, M., Puig-Perez, S., Villada, C., & Salvador, A. (2014). Hair cortisol and cognitive performance in healthy older people. *Psychoneuroendocrinology, 44,* 100–111.

Quednow, B. B., Jessen, F., Kühn, K.-U., Maier, W., Daum, I., & Wagner, M. (2006). Memory deficits in abstinent MDMA (ecstasy) users: Neuropsychological evidence of frontal dysfunction. *Journal of Psychopharmacology, 20*(3), 373–384.

Rahimi-Golkhandan, S., Maruff, P., Darby, D., & Wilson, P. (2012). Barriers to repeated assessment of verbal learning and memory: A comparison of International Shopping List Task and Rey Auditory Verbal Learning Test on build-up of proactive interference. *Archives of Clinical Neuropsychology, 27*(7), 790–795.

Records, N. L., Tomblin, J. B., & Buckwalter, P. R. (1995). Auditory verbal learning and memory in young adults with specific language impairment. *The Clinical Neuropsychologist, 9,* 187–193.

Reis, J. P., Loria, C. M., Launer, L. J., Sidney, S., Liu, K., Jacobs, D. R., . . . Yaffe, K. (2013). Cardiovascular health through young adulthood and cognitive functioning in midlife: Ideal Cardiovascular Health. *Annals of Neurology, 73*(2), 170–179.

Remfer, M. V., Hamera, E. K., Brown, C. E., Cromwell, R. L. (2003). The relations between cognition and the independent living skill of shopping in people with schizophrenia. *Psychiatry Research, 117,* 103–112.

Rey, A. (1958). *L'examen clinique en psychologie.* Paris: Presse Universitaire de France.

Ricci, M., Graef, S., Blundo, C., & Miller, L. A. (2012). Using the Rey Auditory Verbal Learning Test (RAVLT) to differentiate Alzheimer's dementia and behavioural variant fronto-temporal dementia. *The Clinical Neuropsychologist, 26*(6), 926–941.

Ryan, J. J., Geisser, M. E., Randall, D. M., & Georgemiller, R. J. (1986). Alternate form reliability and equivalency of the Rey Auditory Verbal Learning Test. *Journal of Clinical and Experimental Neuropsychology, 8,* 611–616.

Ryan, J. J., Paolo, A. M., & Skrade, M. (1992). Rey Auditory Verbal Learning Test performance of a federal corrections sample with acquired immunodeficiency syndrome. *International Journal of Neuroscience, 64,* 177–181.

Salthouse, T. A., Fristoe, N., & Rhee, S. H. (1996). How localized are age-related effects on neuropsychological measures? *Neuropsychology, 10,* 272–285.

Schmidt, M. (1996). *Rey Auditory-Verbal Learning Test.* Los Angeles: Western Psychological Services.

Schmidt, M. (1997). Some cautions on interpreting qualitative indices for word-list learning tests. *The Clinical Neuropsychologist, 11,* 81–86.

Schoenberg, M., Dawson, K., Duff, K., Patton, D., Scott, J., & Adams, R. (2006). Test performance and classification statistics for the Rey Auditory Verbal Learning Test in selected clinical samples. *Archives of Clinical Neuropsychology, 21*(7), 693–703.

Seltzer, J., Conrad, C., & Cassens, G. (1997). Neuropsychological profiles in schizophrenia: Paranoid versus undifferentiated distinctions. *Schizophrenia Research, 23,* 131–138.

Shapiro, D. M., & Harrison, D. (1990). Alternate forms of the AVLT: A procedure and test of form equivalency. *Archives of Clinical Neuropsychology, 5,* 405–410.

Sherman, D. S., Boone, K. B., Lu, P., & Razani, J. (2002). Reexamination of a Rey Auditory Verbal Learning Test/Rey Complex Figure discriminant function to detect suspect effort. *The Clinical Neuropsychologist, 16,* 242–250.

Shimamura, A. P., Salmon, D. P., Squire, L. R., & Butters, N. (1987). Memory dysfunction and word priming in dementia and amnesia. *Behavioral Neuroscience, 101,* 347–351.

Simard, S., Rouleauu, I., Brosseau, J., Laframboise, M., & Bojanowsky, M. (2003). Impact of executive dysfunctions on episodic memory abilities in patients with ruptured aneurysm of the anterior communicating artery. *Brain and Cognition, 53,* 354–358.

Smith, G. E., Malec, J. F., & Ivnik, R. J. (1992). Validity of the construct of nonverbal memory: A factor-analytic study in a normal elderly sample. *Journal of Clinical and Experimental Neuropsychology, 14,* 211–221.

Smith, K., Boone, K., Victor, T., Miora, D., Cottingham, M., Ziegler, E., . . . Wright, M. (2014). Comparison of credible patients of very low intelligence and non-credible patients on neurocognitive performance validity indicators. *The Clinical Neuropsychologist, 28*(6), 1048–1070.

Soble, J. R., Eichstaedt, K. E., Waseem, H., Mattingly, M. L., Benbadis, S. R., Bozorg, A. M., . . . Schoenberg, M. R. (2014). Clinical utility of the Wechsler Memory Scale—Fourth Edition (WMS-IV) in predicting laterality of temporal lobe epilepsy among surgical candidates. *Epilepsy & Behavior, 41,* 232–237.

Soble, J. R., Osborn, K. E., Mattingly, M. L., Vale, F. L., Benbadis, S. R., Rodgers-Neame, N. T., & Schoenberg, M. R. (2016). Utility of Green's Word Memory Test Free Recall subtest as a measure of verbal memory: Initial evidence from a temporal lobe epilepsy clinical sample. *Archives of Clinical Neuropsychology, 31*(1), 79–87.

Stålhammar, J., Nordlund, A., & Wallin, A. (2015). An example of exceptional practice effects in the verbal domain. *Neurocase, 21*(2), 162–168.

Stallings, G., Boake, C., & Sherer, M. (1995). Comparison of the California Verbal Learning Test and the Rey Auditory-Verbal Learning Test in head-injured patients. *Journal of Clinical and Experimental Neuropsychology, 17,* 706–712.

Stefanova, E. D., Kostic, V. S., Ziropadja, L., Markovic, M., & Ocic, G. (2002). Serial position learning effects in patients with aneurysms of the anterior communicating artery. *Journal of Clinical and Experimental Neuropsychology, 24,* 687–694.

Steinberg, B. A., Bieliauskas, L. A., Smith, G. E., Ivnik, R. J., & Malec, J. F. (2005). MAYO's Older Americans Normative Studies: Age- and IQ-adjusted norms for the Auditory Verbal Learning Test and Visual Spatial Learning Test. *The Clinical Neuropsychologist, 19,* 464–523.

Stewart, W. F., Schwartz, B. S., Simon, D., Bola, K. I., Todd, A. C., & Links, J. (1999). Neurobehavioral function and tibial and chelatable lead levels in 543 former organolead workers. *Neurology, 52,* 1610–1617.

Strauss, E., Hunter, M., & Wada, J. (1995). Risk factors for cognitive impairment in epilepsy. *Neuropsychology, 9,* 457–464.

Suhr, J. A. (2002). Malingering, coaching, and the serial position effect. *Archives of Clinical Neuropsychology, 17,* 69–78.

Suhr, J. A., & Gunstad, J. (2000). The effects of coaching on the sensitivity and specificity of malingering measures. *Archives of Clinical Neuropsychology, 15,* 415–424.

Suhr, J., Gunstad, J., Greub, B., & Barrash, J. (2004). Exaggeration Index for an expanded version of the Auditory Verbal Learning Test: Robustness to coaching. *Journal of Clinical and Experimental Neuropsychology, 26,* 416–427.

Sullivan, K., Deffenti, C., & Keane, B. (2002). Malingering on the RAVLT: Part II. Detection strategies. *Archives of Clinical Neuropsychology, 17*(3), 223–233.

Sullivan, K., Keane, B., & Deffenti, C. (2001). Malingering on the RAVLT: Part I. Deterrence strategies. *Archives of Clinical Neuropsychology, 16*(7), 627–641.

Sundermann, E. E., Biegon, A., Rubin, L. H., Lipton, R. B., Mowrey, W., Landau, S., . . . others. (2016). Better verbal memory in women than men in MCI despite similar levels of hippocampal atrophy. *Neurology, 86*(15), 1368–1376.

Sziklas, V., & Jones-Gotman, M. (2008). RAVLT and nonverbal analog: French forms and clinical findings. *The Canadian Journal of Neurological Sciences, 35*(03), 323–330.

Talley, J. L. (1986). Memory in learning disabled children: Digit span and the Rey Auditory Verbal Learning Test. *Archives of Clinical Neuropsychology, 1,* 315–322.

Taylor, E. M. (1959). *The appraisal of children with cerebral deficits.* Cambridge, MA: Harvard University Press.

Teruya, L. C., Ortiz, K. Z., & Minett, T. S. C. (2009). Performance of normal adults on Rey Auditory Learning Test: A pilot study. *Arquivos de Neuro-Psiquiatria, 67*(2A), 224–228.

Tierney, M. C., Moineddin, R., & McDowell, I. (2011). Prediction of all-cause dementia using neuropsychological tests within 10 and 5 years of diagnosis in a community-based sample. *Journal of Alzheimer's Disease, 22*(4), 1231–1240.

Torres, I. J., Flashman, L. A., O'Leary, D. S., & Andreasen, N. C. (2001). Effects of retroactive and proactive interference on word list recall in schizophrenia. *Journal of the International Neuropsychological Society, 7,* 481–490.

Uchiyama, C. L., D'Elia, L. F., Dellinger, A. M., Becker, J. T., Selnes, O. A., Wesch, J. E., . . . Miller, E. N. (1995). Alternate forms of the Auditory-Verbal Learning Test: Issues of test comparability, longitudinal reliability, and moderating demographic variables. *Archives of Clinical Neuropsychology, 10,* 133–146.

Uttl, B. (2005). Measurement of individual differences. *Psychologica Science, 16,* 460–467.

Vakil, E., & Blachstein, H. (1993). Rey Auditory Verbal Learning Test: Structure analysis. *Journal of Clinical Psychology, 49,* 883–890.

Vakil, E., & Blachstein, H. (1994). A supplementary measure in the Rey AVLT for assessing incidental learning of temporal order. *Journal of Clinical Psychology, 50,* 241–245.

Vakil, E., & Blachstein, H. (1997). Rey AVLT: Developmental norms for adults and the sensitivity of different memory measures to age. *The Clinical Neuropsychologist, 11,* 356–369.

Vakil, E., Blachstein, H., Rochberg, J., & Vardi, M. (2004). Characterization of memory impairment following closed-head injury in children using the Rey Auditory Verbal Learning Test. *Child Neuropsychology, 10,* 57–66.

Vakil, E., Blachstein, H., & Sheinman, M. (1998). Rey AVLT: Developmental norms for children and the sensitivity of different memory measures to age. *Child Neuropsychology, 4,* 161–177.

Vakil, E., Shelef-Reshef, E., & Levy-Shiff, R. (1997). Procedural and declarative memory processes: Individuals with and without mental retardation. *American Journal on Mental Retardation, 102,* 147–160.

Van den Burg, W., & Kingma, A. (1999). Performance of 225 Dutch school children on Rey's Auditory Verbal Learning Test: Parallel test-retest reliabilities with an interval of 3 months and normative data. *Archives of Clinical Neuropsychology, 14,* 545–559.

Van der Elst, W., van Boxtel, P. J., van Breukelen, J. P., & Jolles, J. (2005). Rey's Verbal Learning Test: Normative data for 1855 healthy participants aged 24–81 years and the influence of age, sex, education, and mode of presentation. *Journal of the International Neuropsychological Society, 11,* 290–302.

Vogel, A., Stokholm, J., & JøRgensen, K. (2012). Performances on Rey Auditory Verbal Learning Test and Rey Complex Figure Test in a healthy, elderly Danish sample—reference data and validity issues: Performances on RAVLT and RCFT. *Scandinavian Journal of Psychology, 53*(1), 26–31.

Wagner, D., Becker, B., Gouzoulis-Mayfrank, E., & Daumann, J. (2010). Interactions between specific parameters of cannabis use and verbal memory. *Progress in Neuro-Psychopharmacology and Biological Psychiatry, 34*(6), 871–876.

Walhovd, K. B., Fjell, A. M., Amlien, I., Grambaite, R., Stenset, V., Bjørnerud, A., . . . Due-Tønnessen, P. (2009). Multimodal imaging in mild cognitive impairment: Metabolism, morphometry and diffusion of the temporal–parietal memory network. *NeuroImage, 45*(1), 215–223.

Whitney, K. A., & Davis, J. J. (2015). The non-credible score of the Rey Auditory Verbal Learning Test: Is it better at predicting non-credible neuropsychological test performance than the RAVLT Recognition score? *Archives of Clinical Neuropsychology, 30*(2), 130–138.

Woodard, J. L., Dunlosky, J., & Salthouse, T. A. (1999). Task decomposition analysis of intertrial free recall performance on the Rey Auditory Verbal Learning Test in normal aging and Alzheimer's disease. *Journal of Clinical and Experimental Neuropsychology, 21,* 666–676.

Wu, S.-T., & Chiu, C.-J. (2016). Age-related trajectories of memory function in middle-aged and older adults with and without hearing impairment. *Neuroepidemiology, 46*(4), 282–289.

Xie, C., Goveas, J., Wu, Z., Li, W., Chen, G., Franczak, M., . . . Li, S.-J. (2012). Neural basis of the association between depressive symptoms and memory deficits in nondemented subjects: Resting-state fMRI study. *Human Brain Mapping, 33*(6), 1352–1363.

Xie, M., Yi, C., Luo, X., Xu, S., Yu, Z., Tang, Y., . . . Wang, W. (2011). Glial gap junctional communication involvement in hippocampal damage after middle cerebral artery occlusion. *Annals of Neurology, 70*(1), 121–132.

Yuan, Y., Zhang, Z., Bai, F., Yu, H., Shi, Y., Qian, Y., . . . Liu, Z. (2008). Abnormal neural activity in the patients with remitted geriatric depression: A resting-state functional magnetic resonance imaging study. *Journal of Affective Disorders, 111*(2–3), 145–152.

Zhu, N., Jacobs, D. R., Schreiner, P. J., Yaffe, K., Bryan, N., Launer, L. J., . . . Sternfel, B. (2014). Cardiorespiratory fitness and cognitive function in middle age The CARDIA Study. *Neurology, 82*(15), 1339–1346.

REY-OSTERRIETH COMPLEX FIGURE TEST (RCFT)

TEST NAME	**Rey-Osterrieth Complex Figure Test (RCFT)**
DOMAIN	Visuospatial ability and visual memory
AGE RANGE	In adults, to 89 years
ADMINISTRATION TIME	10 to 15 minutes, plus 3- to 45-minute delay interval depending on version
SCORING FORMAT	Hand scored
REFERENCE	Meyers, J., & Meyers, K. (1995b). *The Meyers Scoring System for the Rey Complex Figure and the Recognition Trial: Professional manual.* Odessa, FL: Psychological Assessment Resources. www.parinc.com

DESCRIPTION

The Rey-Osterrieth Complex Figure Test (RCFT) assesses visual-spatial constructional ability and visual memory. It was developed by Rey (1941) and elaborated by Osterrieth (1944). The two original key French papers have been translated into English by Corwin and Bylsma (1993). The RCFT is one of the most commonly used tests in the field (Camara et al., 2000), consistently ranking among the top 10 tests used by neuropsychologists (Rabin et al., 2005, 2016). Its popularity derives from the fact that it permits assessment of a variety of cognitive processes, including planning, organizational skills, and problem-solving strategies, as well as perceptual, motor, and episodic memory functions (Meyers & Meyers, 1995a, Waber & Holmes, 1985, 1986). Other names for the RCFT include the Rey Complex Figure Test, the Complex Figure Test (CFT), and the Rey Figure (RF).

The original test developed by Rey (1941) consisted of a copy trial followed by a recall trial three minutes later. Following the initial test development, a variety of administration procedures have been developed. Some procedures include both immediate and delayed recall trials whereas others measure only delayed recall. Please see Knight et al. (2003) or the third edition of the *Compendium* for descriptions of other procedures.

The amount of delay varies from three minutes (Bigler et al., 1989; Boone et al., 1993; Rey, 1941) to 45 minutes (Taylor, 1969, 1979). There is little difference in performance between Immediate and three-minute Delayed Recall scores (Meyers & Meyers, 1995a; Tremblay et al., 2015). The length of delay chosen (15, 30, 45, or 60 minutes) does not affect overall recall performance, provided the delay is no longer than one hour (Berry & Carpenter, 1992). Most forgetting tends to occur very quickly, within the first few minutes after copying (Berry & Carpenter, 1992; Chiulli et al., 1995; Delaney et al., 1992; Lezak et al., 2004). Because very little difference is observed in healthy individuals between Immediate and Delayed Recall trials (e.g., Chiulli et al., 1995, Loring et al., 1990; Mitrushina et al., 2005), a decline between the Immediate and Delayed Recall trials may be of clinical significance.

After the Delayed Recall trial, a Recognition subtest (Meyers & Lange, 1994; Meyers & Meyers, 1995a) can be given. The Recognition subtest was developed from elements of the Rey and Taylor figures. Twenty-four figures are randomly placed on four pages in two columns per page. The examinee is required to circle the 12 figures that were part of the original design drawn.

In a survey of members of the International Neuropsychology Society (INS) by Knight et al. (2003), the largest percentage of respondents (57%) reported typically administering a protocol that included a Copy trial, an Immediate Recall trial, and a Delayed Recall trial. The most frequently endorsed interval between the Copy and the Immediate Recall trial was 0 to 5 seconds. The average interval between the Immediate and Delayed Recall trials was 27 minutes (*SD* = 14 minutes), with the 16- to 30-minute range most frequently endorsed. The average interval between the Copy trial and the Delayed Recall trial was also 27 minutes (*SD* = 14 minutes), and 30 minutes was the most frequently reported delay interval.

OTHER VERSIONS AND VARIANTS

There are a number of alternate figures, such as the Taylor Figure (Taylor, 1969, 1979; Figure 10–7), the Modified Taylor Figure (Hubley & Tremblay, 2002; Figure 10–8), and the four Medical College of Georgia (MCG) complex figures (see Loring & Meador, 2003; Meador et al., 1991, 1993).

ADMINISTRATION

For instructions, see Meyers and Meyers (1995b). Alternatively, the examiner can use the instructions shown in Figure 10–9 or refer to Knight (2003) for a more extensive listing of administration procedures.

A couple of studies found no significant differences between dominant and non-dominant hand performance on the Copy portion of the task in an undergraduate volunteer sample and a sample of adults without neurological compromise (Budd et al., 2008; Bush & Martin, 2004). The implication is that use of the nondominant hand to complete the

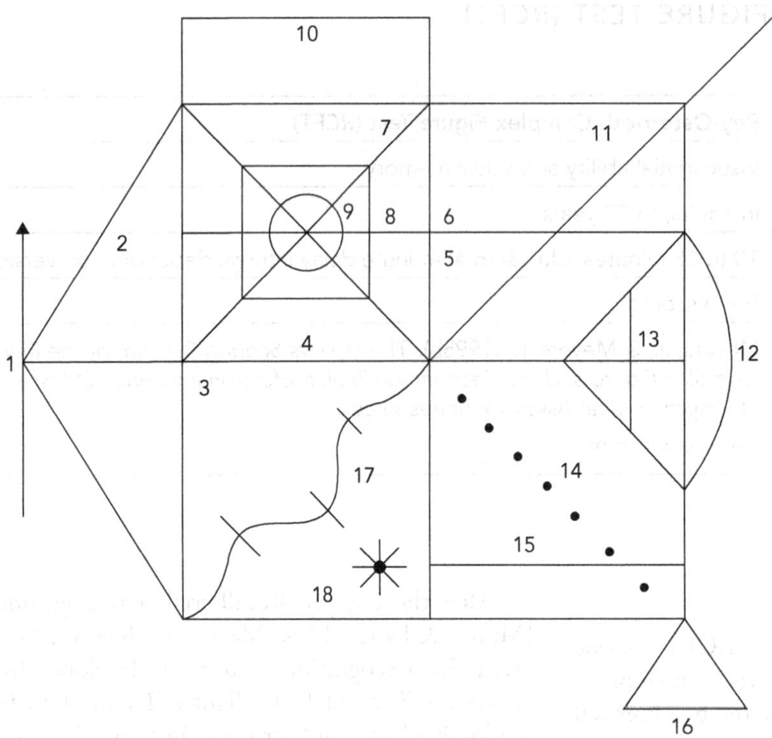

REY-OSTERRIETH COMPLEX FIGURE TEST
FORM B (Taylor Alternate Version)

Details:	COPY	DELAY
1. Arrow at left	____	____
2. Triangle at left	____	____
3. Square	____	____
4. Horizontal line	____	____
5. Vertical line	____	____
6. Horizontal in top half	____	____
7. Diagonals in top left quadrant	____	____
8. Square in top left quadrant	____	____
9. Circle	____	____
10. Rectangle	____	____
11. Arrow top right quadrant	____	____
12. Semicircle	____	____
13. Triangle line	____	____
14. Row of dots	____	____
15. Horizontal line between dots	____	____
16. Triangle at bottom of 3	____	____
17. Curves & cross bars	____	____
18. Star	____	____
TOTAL SCORE	____	

Scoring:
Consider each of the eighteen units separately. Appraise accuracy of each unit and relative position within the whole of the design.
For each unit count as follows:

Correct, placed properly	2 points
Correct, placed poorly	1 point
Distorted or incomplete but recognizable, placed properly	1 point
Distorted or incomplete but recognizable, placed poorly	½ point
Absent or not recognizable	0 points
Maximum	36 points

Figure 10–7 Rey-Osterrieth Complex Figure Test: Form B (Taylor Alternate Version) and legend.
SOURCE: Courtesy of L. Taylor.

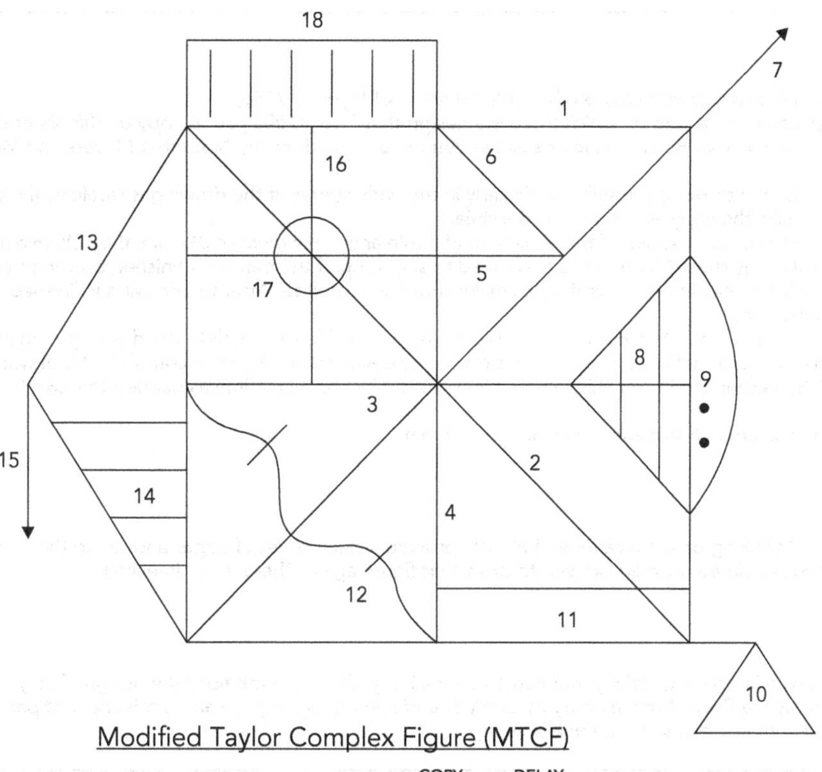

Component	COPY	DELAY
1. Large square	____	____
2. Crossed diagonal lines in 1	____	____
3. Horizontal midline of 1	____	____
4. Vertical midline of 1	____	____
5. Short horizontal line in upper right quadrant	____	____
6. Short diagonal line in upper right quadrant	____	____
7. Diagonal arrow attached to corner of 1	____	____
8. Triangle in 1 on right, two vertical lines included	____	____
9. Semicircle attached to right side of 1, two dots included	____	____
10. Triangle attached to 1 by horizontal line	____	____
11. Horizontal line in lower right quadrant	____	____
12. Wavy line, includes two short lines	____	____
13. Large triangle attached to left of 1	____	____
14. Four horizontal lines within 13	____	____
15. Arrow attached to apex of 13	____	____
16. Horizontal and vertical lines in upper left quadrant	____	____
17. Circle in upper left quadrant	____	____
18. Small rectangle above 1 on left, six lines included	____	____
TOTAL SCORE	____	____

Scoring:

Consider each of the eighteen units separately. Appraise accuracy of each unit and relative position within the whole of the design. For each unit count as follows:

Correct, placed properly	2 points
Correct, placed poorly	1 point
Distorted or incomplete but recognizable, placed properly	1 point
Distorted or incomplete but recognizable, placed poorly	½ point
Absent or not recognizable	0 points
Maximum	36 points

Figure 10–8 *Modified Taylor Complex Figure (MTCF) showing scoring components.*

SOURCE: © 1996, 1998: A. M. Hubley. Reproduced with kind permission from A. M. Hubley.

Copy portion may be an acceptable alternative if the dominant hand is nonfunctional. However, Yamashita (2010) reported that while hand use did not impact Copy scores, Recall scores were lower among those who copied the figure using their nondominant left hand than those using their dominant right hand. Hand use during the Recall trial itself had no effect on scores. The implication is that the use of the nondominant hand to complete the RCFT Copy trial may underestimate visual (recall) memory performance.

COPY

There are two methods for recording a patient's strategy: the colored pencil method and the flowchart method. One can use a system of colored pencils or pens to record the

Copy

Put a plain sheet of 8½ x 11-inch paper vertically on the table (Meyers & Meyers, 1995b).

Then say: *I am going to show you a card on which there is a design that I would like you to copy on this sheet of paper. Please copy the figure as carefully as you can.* Begin timing as soon as you expose the drawing. Note that Meyers and Meyers (1995b) allow erasing.

It is important to supervise the drawing carefully, particularly in the early stages. If the drawing is careless, the patient should be reminded that they are to make the copy as accurate as possible.

The card and the subject's copy are exposed for a maximum of 5 min and a minimum of 2½ min. If by 2½ min it is obvious that the patient is drawing too slowly, they should be told this and asked to speed up. If the patient is finished drawing before 2½ min, they should be told to check the drawing over carefully to make sure it is complete. After the drawing is finished, it is removed from sight along with the stimulus card.

Record the *total* time taken to complete the drawing. Subjects should be able to complete the drawing in no more than 5 min, unless they have considerable motor difficulty. It is more important, however, for a subject to complete the drawing as well as they can than it is to get it finished within 5 min. For this reason, allow the subject as much time as needed to make the best copy that they are capable of drawing.

Expose the card for a maximum of 5 min and a minimum of 2½ min.

3-Minute Recall

After a 3-min delay filled with talking or some other verbal task, provide a clean sheet of paper and say to the patient: *Remember a short time ago I had you copy a figure. I would like you to draw that figure again.* There is no time limit.

Delayed Recall

After a 30-min delay filled with interfering activity (not constructional), say: *Do you remember the design I had you copy a while ago? Now I would like you to draw the figure from memory as carefully and completely as you can on this sheet of paper. If you make a mistake, do not erase, just correct whatever you think is wrong.*

Figure 10–9 *Instructions for Administration of the Rey-Osterrieth Complex Figure Test (RCFT).*

SOURCE: Reproduced by special permission of the Publisher, Psychological Assessment Resources, Inc. (PAR), 16204 North Florida Avenue, Lutz, Florida 33549, from the Rey Complex Figure Test and Recognition Trial Professional Manual by John E. Meyers, PsyD and Kelly R. Meyers, Copyright 1995 by PAR. Further reproduction is prohibited without permission from PAR.

examinee's strategy while copying the figure. Each time the person completes a section of the drawing, the examiner hands the patient a different colored pencil and notes the order of the colors. The examiner uses three or four different colored pencils and switches pencils at approximately equal points in the construction of the figure. The examiner should not switch pencils while the patient is in the middle of drawing one of the standard 18 elements.

Alternatively, to use the flowchart method, the examiner can reproduce the examinee's drawing on a separate sheet, noting the order (by numbering) and directionality (by an arrow) of each line as it is drawn. The latter system is preferred by some authors (Meyers & Meyers, 1995b), including ourselves. When figures are scored using the traditional 36-point scoring system, the amount and quality (i.e., accuracy, placement) of information copied and recalled is not affected by the administration procedure (pencil-switching versus flowchart; Ruffolo et al., 2001). There is also no difference in administration time between the two procedures using the traditional 36-point system. However, when assessing *qualitative* aspects (see the section "Scoring"), there is evidence that pencil-switching results in better performance on qualitative scores, and the productions drawn with pencil-switching are also significantly faster to score (Ruffolo et al., 2001). Therefore, when scoring qualitative aspects, the pencil-switching method may be preferred.

THREE-MINUTE RECALL

There is no time limit on the three-minute recall task. As in the Copy trial, the order of approach may be recorded by using the system of colored pencils or by drawing along with the examinee on a separate sheet, noting the sequence and organization of the reproduction.

DELAYED RECALL

The examiner waits about 30 minutes after the first administration of the RCFT and then requests recall of the figure. The interposed tests should be quite different from the RCFT, to avoid interference. One should especially not give any tests of drawing (but see later discussion). There is no time limit, and the order of approach may be recorded by using the system of colored pencils or by drawing along on a separate sheet.

The nature of the task administered during the RCFT interval period can affect recall performance (Morra et al., 2013). In one study, an undergraduate volunteer group given the WAIS-III Vocabulary during the interval performed better on Delayed Recall than Immediate Recall while the groups given the Benton Facial Recognition Test or Taylor Figure performed better on Immediate Recall than Delayed Recall. Not unexpectedly, those given the Taylor Figure in the interval recalled less on delay than those given the Benton or Vocabulary, suggesting retroactive interference from a task of a very similar nature. In fact, only those given the Taylor figure in the interval obtained mildly impaired scores on Delayed Recall and Recognition. In sum, administration of a similar task during the interval negatively impacts later recall but there may be some flexibility in the types of intervening tasks.

RECOGNITION

After the 30-minute recall, the examinee is provided with stimulus sheets and is instructed to circle the figures that were part of the design that was copied and drawn.

SCORING

The measures of performance that are typically derived on the RCFT include a Copy score (which reflects the accuracy of the original copy and is a measure of visual-constructional ability), the time required to copy the figure, Immediate or three-minute and 30-minute Delayed Recall scores (which assess the amount of information retained over time), and the number of items correctly and incorrectly identified on the recognition task.

There are numerous scoring systems that provide various criteria for scoring the RCFT. Most of the systems provide criteria for assessing accuracy of copy and recall (i.e., quantity).

The most extensive quantitative scoring systems are the Meyers and Meyers (1995b) and the Extended Complex Figure Test (ECFT, Fastenau, 2002). Each of these scoring systems is available with a manual covering administration, scoring, and age-stratified norms for children and adults. Users may refer to the previous edition of this *Compendium* for details of other scoring systems.

Over time, the quantitative scoring systems have changed, mainly by elaboration of more specific scoring criteria for the original 18 elements developed by Osterrieth (Knight, 2003). Qualitative scoring systems have steadily evolved from single measures with a limited focus (e.g., segmentation/fragmentation, discontinuity/disjunction) to more comprehensive, multivariate measures of strategy and organization with established psychometric properties (Knight, 2003). The Boston Qualitative Scoring System (BQSS; Stern et al., 1999) and Developmental Scoring System for the Rey-Osterrieth Complex Figure (DSS-ROCF; Bernstein & Waber, 1996) are the most comprehensive qualitative scoring systems. The DSS-ROCF norms focus more on children, whereas the BQSS is normed for adults.

ACCURACY

Copy and Memory Trials. The figure is broken down into 18 scorable elements: between 0.5 and 2.0 points are awarded for each element, depending on the accuracy, distortion, and location of its reproduction. Two points are awarded if the unit is correct and is placed properly, 1 point if the unit is correct but placed poorly, 1 point if the unit is distorted but placed correctly, 0.5 points if the unit is distorted and placed poorly, and no points if the unit is absent or not recognizable. The highest possible score on each figure is 36.

It is important to be attentive to both the method of administration (e.g., whether an Immediate Recall trial is interposed between the Copy and 30-minute Delayed Recall trials) and the particular scoring criteria used to generate the norms. We generally use the normative data (ages 6–89 years) provided by Meyers and Meyers (1995b) for copy, three-minute recall, 30-minute recall, and recognition trials of the Rey Figure, and their explicit scoring guidelines are used for protocols within this age range.

Recognition. A correct response on the recognition subtest (Meyers & Meyers, 1995b) is credited if the patient correctly circles a figure as having been part of the RCFT; a correct response is also awarded if the figure was not part of the RCFT and was not circled. The maximum correct score is 24. False positives (if a figure that was not part of the RCFT was circled) and false negatives (if a figure that should have been circled was not) are also noted.

QUALITY

Interpretation of the RCFT should consider not only the actual score but also qualitative aspects of performance. For example, some examinees have difficulty with the organizational processes that are crucial for efficient encoding and retrieval of information, whereas others have trouble with the consolidation and storage of new memories. The RCFT is suited to address such distinctions. A number of qualitative scoring systems have been described, with the BQSS most commonly used by neuropsychologists.

BOSTON QUALITATIVE SCORING SYSTEM

The most comprehensive system, the BQSS, was developed by Stern et al. (1994, 1999). It was normed on 433 adults, aged 18 to 94 years. The BQSS divides the figure into three hierarchically arranged elements (i.e., Configurals, Clusters, and Details), each of which is scored according to its presence, accuracy (for Configurals and Clusters), and placement (for Clusters and Details). Scores range from 0 (poor) to 4 (good). In addition, several other scores based on the entire production (Fragmentation, Planning, Neatness, and Perseveration) and the Organization Summary Score (sum of Planning and Fragmentation) were developed to be sensitive to executive dysfunction. Scores for the Fragmentation, Planning, Neatness, and Perseveration variables range from 0 (poor) to 4 (good), whereas the Organization Summary Score ranges from 0 (poor) to 8 (good). Please refer to the manual for scoring criteria.

According to the authors, scoring takes five to 15 minutes for a single reproduction and decreases to about five minutes once the examiner is familiar with the method. However, others (Folbrecht et al., 1999; Hartman & Potter, 1998) have noted average scoring times of about 13 to 20 minutes per figure. Although scoring time decreased with experience, the scorers were never able to decrease scoring time to five minutes or less. One possibility might be to supplement more traditional scoring systems with the Organization Summary Score and/or the Planning score from the BQSS because these values can be calculated independently of the rest of the system and offer excellent reliability (Elderkin-Thompson et al., 2004a; Hartman & Potter, 1998).

SAVAGE SCORING SYSTEM

The system developed by Savage et al. (1999) evaluates five organizational units (the large rectangle, the diagonal cross, the vertical midline, the horizontal midline, and the vertex of the triangle on the right), each of which must be drawn as an unfragmented piece to receive credit for organization. Support for the validity of this system has been established in patients with obsessive-compulsive disorder and eating disorders (for review, see Deckersbach et al., 2000a; Lang et al., 2016; Sherman et al., 2006).

EXTENDED COMPLEX FIGURE TEST (ECFT)

Fastenau (1996) developed recognition and matching trials (the ECFT) to clarify contributions of perception and memory retrieval to defective memory recall performance. He has also provided norms for this extended version (Fastenau, 2002; Fastenau et al., 1999).

DEMOGRAPHIC EFFECTS

AGE

Age contributes to performance on the RCFT. Copy scores increase with age, with adult levels being reached at about age 17 years (Meyers & Meyers, 1996). Some suggest little decrement in Copy scores with advancing age (Hubley, 2010; Mitrushina et al., 1990). Others, however, have found that age influences Copy performance, particularly after age 50 years, although the changes are quite subtle (Casarotti et al., 2014; Dinn & Dinn, 2012; Gallagher & Burke, 2007; Kasai et al., 2006; Meyers & Meyers, 1995b; Miatton et al., 2004; Tremblay et al., 2015; Vogel et al., 2012). Mitrushina et al. (2005) in their meta-analysis, documented an age-related decline in Copy scores as well as an increase in variability with advancing age. Drawings are not less organized in older adults (aged 60+ years), although they are messier, reflecting minor inaccuracies in drawing (e.g., curved lines, rounded corners, gaps, overshoots) that are perhaps due to either mild visual-spatial deficiencies or motor problems (Hartman & Potter, 1998).

Scores on the Immediate and Delayed Recall trials also show a decline with advancing age (Anderson & Lajoie, 1996; Caffarra et al., 2002; Dinn & Dinn, 2012; Hartman & Potter, 1998; Kramer & Wells, 2004; Meyers & Meyers, 1995b, 1996; Miatton et al., 2004; Mitrushina et al., 1990, 2005; Ostrosky-Solis et al., 1998; Ponton et al., 1996). Advancing age is primarily associated with an increase in the number of omitted elements of the drawing, rather than distortion of the elements (Hartman & Potter, 1998; Mitrushina et al., 1990). Not only do mean scores decrease with aging, but also *SD*s increase with advancing age; that is, there is greater heterogeneity in the older age groups (Mitrushina et al., 2005; Ostrosky-Solis et al., 1998).

Rates of forgetting (Copy score minus Delay score) also show some relation with age (Ostrosky-Solis et al., 1998), suggesting that memory declines in older adults may be attributable, at least in part, to impaired storage. Young adults (aged 20–30 years) retain about 65% of the information they acquired on the Copy trial; individuals aged 70+ retain less than 40% of the information. Recognition performance shows a slight decline with advancing age (Meyers & Meyers, 1995b).

Recall of the figures is differentially influenced by demographic factors but age affects recall of both the Rey and Taylor figures.

GENDER

The importance of gender is controversial. Some have reported that males outperform females (Caffarra et al., 2002; Kramer & Wells, 2004; Sakamoto & Spiers, 2014), but the differences in performance have generally been small (about two points) or nonexistent (e.g., Casarotti et al., 2014; Demsky et al., 2000; Dinn & Dinn, 2012; Meyers & Meyers, 1995b, 1996). Some suggest that the ambiguous and contradictory data may reflect the fact that there is considerable variability within the sexes. They argue that, in addition to gender, handedness (Dinn & Dinn, 2012; Karapetsas & Vlachos, 1997), familial handedness (Weinstein et al., 1990), and academic concentration (e.g., mathematics/science or other; Vlachos et al., 2003; Weinstein et al., 1990) need to be taken into consideration.

Gender also contributes differently. Women perform better than men on the Taylor Figure Copy trial (Tremblay et al., 2015; Vingerhoets et al., 1998), whereas men outperform women on the Rey Delayed Recall trial (Vingerhoets et al., 1998). The Rey Immediate Recall is more impacted by the Copy score in men than in women, whereas the same is not found on the Taylor Figure (Tremblay et al., 2015).

EDUCATION AND IQ

The influence of education is less certain. A few authors (Caffarra et al., 2002; Casarotti et al., 2014; Dinn & Dinn, 2012; Kasai et al., 2006; Miatton et al., 2004; Tremblay et al., 2015; Vogel et al., 2012) have reported poorer scores in individuals with lower educational levels, with correlations in the moderate range ($r = .30$ to .46; Dinn & Dinn, 2012). Some, however, have found that RCFT measures are relatively unaffected by education (Ashton et al., 2005; Hubley, 2010; Meyers & Meyers, 1995b).

Scores on the RCFT show a modest correlation with measures of general intellectual ability (Diaz-Asper et al., 2004; Gallagher & Burke, 2007; Vogel et al., 2012), particularly with nonverbal reasoning ability. Ashton et al. (2005) reported that higher levels of WAIS-III perceptual organization skills were predictive of better performance on the Recall and Recognition trials. However, the modest correlations with IQ indicate that the RCFT provides a large amount of information not accounted for by IQ (Chervinsky et al., 1992).

ETHNICITY, NATIONALITY, AND LINGUISTIC EFFECTS

Cross-cultural differences have been reported (Rosselli & Ardila, 1991; Sakamoto & Spiers, 2014). For example, Native Japanese with Kanji education perform better than non–Japanese-speaking Japanese Americans and North Americans on RCFT Immediate and Delayed Recall, with the native Japanese using a more holistic copy strategy than other groups, suggesting that experience with pictorial written language may influence performance on the RCFT (Sakamoto & Spiers, 2014). However, Japanese undergraduate volunteers obtain scores comparable to North-American university volunteers (Hubley & Tremblay, 2002; Yamashita, 2006).

NORMATIVE DATA

With respect to norms for evaluating the accuracy of the figure, wide variability exists with regard to the type of administration. There is some evidence (Loring et al., 1990; Meyers & Meyers, 1995a) that inclusion of an Immediate Recall trial increases Delayed Recall performance by about 2 to 6 points in healthy young adults. Furthermore, diverse scoring systems complicate attempts to compile norms from different sources. Table 10–83 summarizes the most updated norms available for various RCFT versions. For norms of other scoring systems or delay intervals, please refer to the previous edition of the *Compendium*.

Mitrushina et al. (2005) compiled metanorms for adults aged 22 to 79 years, based on the standard 36-point scoring system on the Copy, Immediate Recall, and Delayed Recall conditions. Data for three-minute Delayed Recall was not examined. The Delayed Recall trial included studies varying in delay interval between 15 and 60 minutes and was preceded by an Immediate or a three-minute Delayed Recall trial but not both. Nine studies, comprising 1,340 participants, were analyzed for the Copy condition, and seven studies, based on a total of 1,056 participants, were analyzed for the Delayed Recall condition. Mitrushina et al. (2005) noted that the mean education of their sample was relatively high (about 14 years) and that their normative values may overestimate expected scores for individuals with lower educational levels. The values match closely the normative data provided in the manual by Meyers and Meyers (1995b). It should be noted that the educational achievement of the normative sample provided by Meyers and Meyers was similarly high.

MEYERS AND MEYERS (1995B) ADMINISTRATION

This administration comprises a Copy trial followed by three-minute and 30-minute Recall trials as well as a Recognition trial. Meyers and Meyers (1995b) provided

TABLE 10–83 Summary of Rey-Osterrieth Complex Figure Test (RCFT) Adult Norms Available for Various Versions

REFERENCE	VERSION	TRIALS	SAMPLE	AGE
Mitrushina et al. (2005)	Standard 36-point system	Copy Immediate Recall 15- to 60-minute Recall	Metanorms from nine studies for Copy trial, and seven studies for Delayed Recall trial	22–79
Meyers & Meyers (1995b)	Meyers & Meyers (1995b)	Copy 3-minute Recall 30-minute Recall Recognition	American adults	18–89
Kasai et al. (2006)	Meyers & Meyers (1995b)	Copy	Japanese older adults	65–91
Vogel et al. (2012)	Meyers & Meyers (1995b)	Copy 3-minute Recall	Danish older adults	60–87
Tremblay et al. (2015)[a]	Meyers & Meyers (1995b)	Copy Immediate or 3-minute Recall 20-minute Recall	French-Canadian older adults	50–91
	Taylor Figure	Copy 3-minute Recall 20-minute Recall		71–86
Casarotti et al. (2014)	Modified Taylor Complex Figure	Copy 15-minute Recall	Italian adults	19–98
Stern et al. (1999)	Boston Qualitative Scoring System (BQSS)	Copy Immediate Recall 20-minute Recall	American and Canadian adults	18–94
Fastenau et al. (1999)	Extended Complex Figure Test	Copy Immediate Recall Delayed Recall Recognition	American adults and older adults	30–85

[a] Demographically corrected equations.

TABLE 10–84 Characteristics of the Adult Normative Sample for Meyers and Meyers (1995b) Administration (Copy, 3-Minute Immediate Recall, Delayed Recall, and Recognition) for the Rey-Osterrieth Complex Figure Test (RCFT)

SAMPLE SIZE	601 ADULTS
Age	18 to 89[a] years
Geographic location	Majority of adults recruited from the north central and western areas of the United States; a subset of the adult normative sample n = (394) matched US Census data for age distribution for the year 2000
Sample type	University students, volunteers from suburban communities
Education	Approximately 14 years
Gender	Not reported
Ethnicity	Not reported
Screening	No history of neurological dysfunction, psychiatric disorder, learning disability, on alcohol or drug abuse or dependence

[a] Normative tables are grouped into a 2-year age span for 18- to 19-year-olds, 5-year spans for ages 20–79 years, and a 10-year span for ages 80–89 years.

SOURCE: Adapted from Meyers and Meyers (1995b).

normative data (see Table 10–84) based on a sample of 601 healthy adults, aged 18 to 89 years, and a sample of 505 normal children and adolescents, aged 6 to 17 years. Their explicit scoring guidelines must be used (see Source). Caution should be used when interpreting RCFT performance for older adults aged 80 to 89 years because of the small number of normative participants in this age range ($n = 15$). Age-corrected T scores and percentile equivalents are provided for three-minute (called "Immediate") Recall, Delayed Recall, and Recognition Total Correct. Normative data for Copy, Time to Copy, Recognition True and False Positives, and Recognition True and False Negatives are presented in five percentile ranges (e.g., >16th percentile, 16th to 11th percentile, etc). Note that this set of normative data is more than two decades old.

The frequency of occurrence of different scores for each scoring unit was examined in a heterogeneous sample of brain-injured patients ($n = 100$) and in a matched normative sample. This base rate information is provided in the test manual for the various drawing and recognition trials.

Schretlen, Testa, and Pearlson (2010) provide norms for 327 adults on the RCFT Copy (Meyers & Meyers, 1995b, administration); these use the CNNS scoring to derive T scores and discrepancies based on a large sample of older adults from the northeastern United States. Characteristics of the normative sample are shown in Table 10–85. The norms are available through PAR (www.parinc.com). A major advantage of these norms is the option to correct for demographic variables such as age, sex, education, and ethnicity. Several other commonly used neuropsychological tests are co-normed using this sample, which facilitates cross-test comparisons.

TABLE 10–85 Characteristics of the Rey-Osterrieth Complex Figure Test (RCFT) Normative Sample from the Calibrated Neuropsychological Normative System (CNNS)

Sample size	327
Age	18 to 92 years
Geographic location	Baltimore, MD, and Hartford, CT, USA
Sample type	Community sample
Education	14.2 (*SD* = 3.0), range 3–20 years
Gender	56% Women 44% Men
Ethnicity	80% Caucasian 18% African American 2% Hispanic, Asian, or Other
Screening	History of Alzheimer's disease, Parkinson's disease, stroke, brain injury, bipolar disorder, or substance abuse

SOURCE: Schretlen et al. (2010). Reproduced by special permission of the Publisher, Psychological Assessment Resources, Inc. (PAR), 16204 North Florida Avenue, Lutz, Florida 33549, from the Calibrated Neuropsychological Normative System, by David J. Schretlen, PhD, ABPP, S Marc Testa, PhD and Godfrey D. Pearlson, MD, Copyright 2010 by PAR. Further reproduction is prohibited without permission from PAR.

Vogel et al. (2012) provide RCFT (Meyers & Meyers, 1995b administration) norms for Danish older adults, aged 60 to 87. Only Copy and three-minute Immediate Recall trials were administered. Those who scored almost perfect on the Copy trial (score = 34–36) obtained much higher recall scores than those who scored poorly on the Copy trial. As such, the mean Recall scores for both groups are presented in Table 10–86 and may be used to

TABLE 10–86 Danish Norms for the RCFT [Meyers & Meyers (1995b) Administration]

EDUCATION	AGE		COPY	3-MINUTE RECALL	3-MINUTE RECALL (COPY SCORE 34–36)
8–11 years	60–70				
		N	18	17	13
		Mean	34.4	21.2	23.0
		SD	2.7	4.8	3.3
		Range	28–36	12–27	17–27
	71–87				
		N	30	30	18
		Mean	32.8	13.1	16.9
		SD	3.6	7.2	6.6
		Range	20.5–36	3.5–27	7–27
12–17 years	60–70				
		N	31	31	26
		Mean	35.1	21.1	22.0
		SD	1.37	5.4	4.8
		Range	31–36	8–32	10–32
	71–87				
		N	20	20	15
		Mean	34.3	17.6	20.4
		SD	2.6	7.5	6.4
		Range	26.5–36	6–31	6–31

NOTE: Based on *N* = 100; age mean = 70.9, *SD* = 6.4, range = 60–87; education mean = 11.9, *SD* = 2.6, range = 8–17; 56% females.

SOURCE: Adapted from Vogel et al. (2012).

evaluate the quality of the memory performance relative to visuoconstructional scores. The Danish sample obtained higher scores than the US standardization sample.

Kasai et al. (2006) provide RCFT (Meyers & Meyers, 1995b administration) Copy norms for healthy Japanese older adults from the Tajiri Project, a community-based study on stroke, dementia, and bed-confinement prevention (Table 10–87). All healthy participants were community-dwelling without any cognitive or physical problems (CDR 0).

Tremblay et al. (2015) provide demographically adjusted RCFT (Meyers & Meyers, 1995b administration) and Taylor Figure (Taylor, 1969) French-Canadian older adult norms. Their sample comprised community-dwelling, French-speaking older adults with MMSE or MoCA of greater than 26 and GDS of less than 11, screened for self-reported neurological or psychiatric illnesses. No time limit was set for the copy trial. As Copy Time and Accuracy also influenced Recall scores in addition to demographic background, these variables were included in the calculation of standard scores as seen in Table 10–88 for the RCFT and Table 10–89 for the Taylor Figure. The authors recommend using the expected score equations that include demographic and Copy scores to interpret memory performance on the RCFT. To apply demographic and Copy-score correction for the RCFT, calculate the expected score using the equations shown in Table 10–88, then apply the following z score equation. Use Table 10–89 to adjust for demographic and Copy scores for the Taylor figure and then apply the following z score equation.

$$\text{Z-score} = \frac{\text{raw score} - \text{expected score}}{\text{square root of the mean square residual}}$$

OTHER VERSIONS

Casarotti et al. (2014) provide norms for the Modified Taylor Complex Figure (MTCF) with 15-minute delay interval (see Figure 10–8 for scoring criteria) for healthy Italian adults, stratified by age and education. Raw scores are age- and education-adjusted using the correction grid showed in Table 10–90. An adjusted Copy score of 27.66 or less or a Recall score of 8.4 or less represents the bottom 5% of the normative sample and is considered abnormal. For example, an examinee age 25 with 12 years of education who obtained a raw score of 29 on MTCF Copy will have an adjusted score of 27 (i.e., 2 points taken off according to the correction grid), which is below the cutoff for abnormal scores. An examinee age 64 with 10 years of education who obtained the same raw score of 29 on the MTCF Copy will have an adjusted score of 29.30 (i.e., .30 points added

TABLE 10–87 RCFT Copy Trial Norms for Japanese Older Adults [Meyers & Meyers (1995b) Administration]

EDUCATION LEVEL	AGE (YEARS) 65–69 (N = 176)	70–74 (N = 74)	75–79 (N = 58)	80–91 (N = 73)
≤6 years (n = 42)	33.0 (n = 16)	34.0 (n = 10)	31.0 (n = 10)	33.1 (n = 6)
8 years (n = 256)	34.0 (n = 110)	33.0 (n = 47)	32.5 (n = 44)	32.3 (n = 55)
≥10 years (n = 83)	34.0 (n = 50)	34.0 (n = 17)	32.3 (n = 4)	34.0 (n = 12)

NOTE: Based on N = 381; age mean = 72.5 (age 65+); mean education = 8.4.

SOURCE: From Kasai et al. (2006).

TABLE 10–88 Demographically Corrected RCFT Expected Score Equation for Older Adults [Meyers & Meyers (1995b) Administration]

		SQUARE ROOT OF THE MEAN SQUARE RESIDUAL
Copy	$0.166E - 1.018S - 0.019A - 0.005CT + 31.673$	3.648
Immediate Recall	$0.243E + 0.966S - 0.095A - 0.021CT + 0.353(CS - 31.2955) + 0.941\ (S(CS - 31.2955)) + 23.147$	4.705
Delayed Recall	$0.010E - 0.280S - 0.030A + 0.006\ (CT - 238.1975) + 0.199CS + 0.868\ (IRS - 15.4114) + 0.001((IRS - 15.4114) \times (CT - 238.1975)) + 11.205$	2.289

NOTE: A, Age in years; E, Education in years; CT, Copy time in seconds; CS, Copy score (max = 36); IRS, Immediate Recall score (max = 36); S, Sex (1 = men, 0 = women).

Based on community-dwelling, French-speaking older adults from Quebec, Canada. N = 220; age mean = 67.56, SD = 7.51, range = 50–91; education mean = 14.43, SD = 3.69, range = 3–24; 70.9% females. MMSE or MoCA >26 and GDS <11, and screened for self-reported neurological or psychiatric illnesses.

SOURCE: Adapted from Tremblay et al. (2015).

TABLE 10–89 Demographically-Corrected Taylor Figure Score Equation for Older Adults (Taylor Figure Administration)

		SQUARE ROOT OF THE MEAN SQUARE RESIDUAL
Copy	$0.148E - 0.113A - 0.459S + 0.003\ (CT - 242.891475) + 36.624$	2.669
Immediate Recall	$-0.023E - 0.170A + 0.032S + 0.699CS + 0.002\ (CT - 242.891475) - 0.017\ ((CT - 242.891475)S) + 10.273$	4.627
Delayed Recall	$0.022E - 0.34A - 0.335S - 0.001CT + 0.074CS + 0.845IRS + 3.163$	1.988

NOTE: A, Age in years; E, Education in years; CT, Copy time in seconds; CS, Copy score (max = 36);
IRS, Immediate Recall score (max = 36); S, Sex (1 = men, 0 = women).

Based on community-dwelling, French-speaking older adults from Quebec, Canada. N = 432; age mean = 77.38, SD = 3.92, range = 71–86; education mean = 12.92, SD = 4.23, range = 3–23; 53.9% females. MMSE or MoCA >26 and GDS <11, and screened for self reported neurological or psychiatric illnesses.

SOURCE: Adapted from Tremblay et al. (2015).

TABLE 10–90 Correction Grid for the Modified Taylor Complex Figure (MTCF) Copy and 15-Minute Delayed Recall Trials

EDUCATION	AGE													
	19–25	26–30	31–35	36–40	41–45	46–50	51–55	56–60	61–65	66–70	71–75	76–80	81–85	86–98
COPY														
≤5	−.10	.30	.70	.90	1.20	1.50	1.80	2.00	2.30	2.60	2.90	3.20	3.40	4.60
6–8	−.80	−.40	0.00	.20	.40	.70	.90	1.30	1.60	1.80	2.20	2.40	2.60	2.90
9–13	−2.00	−1.70	−1.30	−1.00	−.80	−.60	−.30	0.00	.30	.60	.90	1.20	1.40	1.80
14–16	−2.70	−2.50	−2.10	−1.80	−1.60	−1.20	−1.00	−.70	−.50	0.00	.10	.50	.80	1.10
≥17	−2.80	−2.70	−2.40	−2.10	−1.80	−1.60	−1.20	−1.10	−.60	−.40	−.10	.20	.40	.70
RECALL														
≤5	0.00	.60	1.20	1.70	2.30	2.90	3.50	4.10	4.60	5.20	5.70	6.40	6.80	7.30
6–8	−1.80	−.90	−.30	.30	.70	1.30	1.80	2.60	3.30	3.70	4.30	4.80	5.50	5.90
9–13	−4.00	−3.40	−2.60	−2.10	−1.60	−1.20	−.60	.20	.70	1.30	1.80	2.50	3.00	3.70
14–16	−5.50	−5.00	−4.20	−3.60	−3.20	−2.40	−2.00	−1.40	−1.00	−.10	.30	.90	1.60	2.30
≥17	−5.70	−5.50	−4.80	−4.30	−3.70	−3.10	−2.40	−2.10	−1.20	−.80	−.10	.40	.90	1.30

NOTE: Based on N = 290 healthy Italians; 51% females; age mean = 54.10, SD = 19.2, range = 19–98; education mean = 12.26, SD = 4.26, range = 3–23. The sample was screened for self-reported history of neurological or psychiatric disease, substance abuse, potential organic causes for cognitive deficits, and significant sensory loss. Age- and education-adjusted value from the table are added or subtracted from raw scores. An adjusted Copy score of ≤27.66 or Recall score of ≤8.4 represents the bottom 5% of the normative sample and is considered abnormal.

SOURCE: Adapted from Casarotti et al. (2014).

according to the correction grid), which is above the cutoff for abnormal scores.

EVIDENCE FOR RELIABILITY

EVIDENCE FOR INTERNAL RELIABILITY

The internal consistency of the RCFT has been evaluated by treating each detail as an item and computing split-half and alpha coefficients (Berry et al., 1991; Fastenau et al., 1996). Both split-half and coefficient alpha reliabilities were greater than .60 for the Copy condition and greater than .80 for Recall conditions in adults, suggesting that all of the details tap into a common construct.

EVIDENCE FOR TEST-RETEST RELIABILITY, MEASURING CHANGE, AND PRACTICE EFFECTS

Some scores (e.g., Copy, Recognition) are restricted in range due to ceiling effects in healthy individuals, thereby artificially reducing the magnitude of the test-retest correlation coefficients (Meyers & Meyers, 1995b; see also Levine et al., 2004). Moreover, the incidental learning paradigm is contaminated when the examinee is retested after the original administration. Based on these considerations, Meyers and Meyers (1995b) evaluated test-retest reliability only for scores with sufficient range after a retest interval of about six months (Immediate Recall, $r = .76$; Delayed Recall, $r = .89$; Recognition Total Correct, $r = .87$). The percentage agreement in the clinical interpretation between the first and second testing sessions was high (92%) for these three measures. No significant differences for other RCFT variables (Copy, Time to Copy, Recognition True Positives, False Positives, True Negatives, False Negatives) across the retest interval were found (Meyers & Meyers, 1995b).

One-year test-retest reliability in older individuals has been reported as low for Copy ($r = .18$) and moderate for the Recall trials ($r = .47$ to .59; Berry et al., 1991). Others reported better reliabilities for adults assessed over three annual probes, ranging from .56 to .68 for Copy and .57 to .77 for three-minute Immediate Recall (Mitrushina & Satz, 1991; Levine et al., 2004).

Levine et al. (2004) reported gains for Immediate and Delayed Recall trials for 478 healthy men who were reassessed across a wide time interval of four to 24 months (M = 251 days, SD = 129). Table 10–91 shows change scores, SDs of the change scores, and test-retest reliability coefficients for use in RCI formulas. Table 10–92 shows the regression formulas that can be used to estimate Time 2 scores. The residual SDs for the regression formulas are also shown and can be used to establish the normal range for retest scores. For example, a 90% CI can be created around the scores by multiplying the residual SD by 1.645, which allows for 5% of people to fall outside of the upper and lower extremes. Individuals whose scores exceed the extremes are considered to have significant changes. Neither the length

TABLE 10–91 Change Scores, Standard Deviations (SDs), and Reliability Coefficients for the Rey-Osterrieth Complex Figure Test (RCFT)

MEASURE	TIME 1 (T1)		TIME 2 (T2)		T2 − T1		
	MEAN	SD	MEAN	SD	MEAN	SD	R
Copy	34.8	1.83	34.7	1.59	−0.03	1.76	.47
Immediate	22.8	6.25	25.3	6.0	2.48	4.51	.73
Delayed	22.5	6.2	24.8	6.01	2.30	4.32	.79

NOTE: Based on a sample of 478 well-educated (M = 16.4 years, SD = 2.3), mostly Caucasian men (age M = 42.2 years, SD = 8.6).

SOURCE: Adapted from Levine et al. (2004).

TABLE 10-92 Regression Equations for Estimating Retest Scores on the Rey-Osterrieth Complex Figure Test (RCFT)

MEASURE	REGRESSION EQUATION	RESIDUAL *SD*
Copy	20.57 + (.407 × Time 1 score)	1.41
Immediate	9.32 + (.701 × Time 1 score)	4.11
Delayed	8.27 + (.735 × Time 1 score)	3.99

NOTE: Based on a sample of 478 well-educated (*M* = 16.4 years, *SD* = 2.3), mostly Caucasian men (age *M* = 42.2 years, *SD* = 8.6).

SOURCE: Adapted from Levine et al. (2004).

of the retest interval nor educational level contributed significantly to prediction.

EVIDENCE FOR RELIABILITY OF ALTERNATE FORMS

Reliability coefficients are in the moderate range when the Rey and Taylor figures are evaluated (Berry et al., 1991; Delaney et al., 1992). In healthy young adults, the copy administrations of the various figures (Rey, Taylor, MCG) are of equivalent difficulty; however, recall of the Rey Figure is somewhat harder (about 2–4 points lower in healthy people) compared with the Taylor, MTCF, and MCG figures (Hubley, 2010; Miatton et al., 2004; Peirson & Jansen, 1997; Vingerhoets et al., 1998; Yamashita, 2006).

The MTCF appears to yield copy and memory scores that are comparable to those of the Rey Figure, with reliabilities reported in the moderate to very high range (r = .74 to .95) in mixed-age samples (Casarotti et al., 2014; Hubley & Jassal, 2006), though examinees took longer to copy the Rey figure when it was administered before the MTCF than when it was administered second (Hubley & Jassal, 2006). When both forms were given to the same individuals one week apart, alternate form reliability was adequate on all trials (>.65) except the copy trial (Hubley & Tremblay, 2002), suggesting that their use as matched forms to measure constructional ability requires some caution. There are no significant differences in test scores between the Taylor Figure and the four MCG figures (Meador et al., 1993).

In direct comparisons of the RCFT, Taylor Figure, and MTCF, Copy scores were equivalent for all three versions, but better recall of the Taylor Figure was found, whereas no differences were seen in recall of the Rey Figure and MTCF (Yamashita, 2006). The authors concluded that the MTCF is superior to the Taylor figure as a parallel version to the Rey Figure, at least in young adults. By contrast, Hubley (2010) reported that MTCF Copy scores were higher than RCFT Copy scores but no differences were seen on the Recall trials in older adults. Given these findings, Hubley (2010) stated that the RCFT and MTCF cannot be considered parallel forms for the purpose of measuring visuoconstructional ability in older adults, but they are interchangeable as recall measures.

TABLE 10-93 Sensitivity, Specificity, Positive Predictive Values (PPV), and Negative Predictive Values (NPV) for Invalid Rey-Osterrieth Complex Figure Test (RCFT) Scores at Base Rates of 15%, 30%, and 45% Invalid Performance

			15%		30%		45%	
SCORES	SENSITIVITY (%)	SPECIFICITY (%)	PPV (%)	NPV (%)	PPV (%)	NPV (%)	PPV (%)	NPV (%)
Copy								
≤27	50	91	53	92	70	81	83	69
≤25	45	96	64	91	81	80	90	68
Immediate Recall								
≤10	45	86	36	90	57	79	72	65
≤9	36	91	44	89	64	77	78	63
True-Positive Recognition								
≤5	52	93	56	92	77	82	86	70
≤4	38	96	58	90	78	78	88	65
≤3	24	99	71	88	90	75	93	61
False-Positive Errors								
>3	16	94	33	87	55	73	69	57
>4	7	100	100	86	100	72	100	57
Combination Score								
≤47	76	91	61	95	78	90	88	82
≤45	74	94	70	95	85	90	92	82
≤43	67	94	68	95	84	88	91	78
≤42	57	96	69	93	85	84	92	73

NOTE: The Recognition trial was given after the Immediate Recall trial. Combination score = Copy score + [(True-Positive Recognition - Atypical Recognition score) × 3]. Atypical Recognition Errors = sum of incorrect answer on items 1, 4, 6, 10, 11, 16, 18, and 21. The specificities presented in this table are based on a combined clinic patient group comprising those who are verbal memory impaired, visual memory impaired, or non–memory impaired. Values are rounded to the nearest percent.

SOURCE: Adapted from Lu et al. (2003).

EVIDENCE FOR INTERRATER RELIABILITY

Scoring according to the criteria of Osterrieth (1944) and E. M. Taylor (1959), or variants of these criteria, yield adequate to high interrater and intrarater reliability for total scores (>.80; Boone et al., 1993; Caffarra et al., 2002; Casarotti et al., 2014; Deckersbach et al., 2000a; Fastenau et al., 1996; Hubley, 2010; Tupler et al., 1995; Yamashita, 2006). Reliabilities for the 18 individual items, however, ranged from poor (.14) to excellent (.96), suggesting that the Osterrieth system would benefit from more detailed specification of quantitative decision rules (e.g., minimal angle size required for 1 point; Tupler et al., 1995). The strict scoring criteria described by others (Fastenau et al., 1996; Hubley & Tremblay, 2002; Meyers & Meyers, 1995a; Stern et al., 1994, 1999) also show high (>.90) interrater reliability for total scores.

Interrater reliability is high for most scores (>.80) for the BQSS but poor for others, such as asymmetry and confabulation (Folbrecht et al., 1999) or cluster placement and detail placement (Stern et al., 1999). Reliability coefficients are higher for two or more raters. Accordingly, it is recommended that more than one rater score the Rey Figure and that their average score be used for interpretation (Folbrecht et al., 1999). Internal consistency reliabilities are also high (>.70; Folbrecht et al., 1999).

EVIDENCE FOR VALIDITY

The precise cognitive operations required for adequate performance are thought to include visual perception, visual-spatial organization, motor functioning, and, on the recall condition, memory. Overall, the data from correlational and factor-analytic studies support the validity of the RCFT as a measure of visual-constructional ability (Copy) and memory (Recall and Recognition).

FACTOR-ANALYTIC STUDIES

Meyers and Meyers (1995b) conducted a principal components factor analysis of the data for healthy individuals. The analysis suggested a five-factor solution. The first factor was termed a Visuospatial Recall factor due to high loading from the three- and 30-minute Delay trials. Factor 2 reflected a Visuospatial Recognition factor. Factor 3, labeled a Response Bias factor, demonstrated a high loading of Recognition False Positives. Factor 4 was interpreted as a Processing Speed factor because of a high loading of Time to Copy. Finally, Factor 5 reflected Visuospatial Constructional Ability, with a high loading of the Copy score. Analysis of data from brain-injured patients (N = 100) revealed the same five factors, supporting the notion that the test measures different dimensions of cognition, not a unitary visual memory construct.

RELATIONSHIPS AMONG TEST MEASURES

Large correlations are found between Immediate (three-minute) Recall and Delayed Recall (r = .88 to .92; Dinn & Dinn, 2012; Meyers & Meyers, 1995b; Tremblay et al., 2015). Meyers and Meyers (1995b) reported that the Recall measures demonstrated lower but still significant correlations (r = .15) with Recognition Total Correct, suggesting that they are assessing different aspects of memory. Time to Copy had minimal relations to the accuracy of the Copy or the Recall (r = –.15; Tremblay et al., 2015). Moderate correlations are noted between Copy and Immediate (three-minute) Recall and Delayed Recall scores (r = .33 and .38, respectively), suggesting a relationship between the ability to copy the complex figure and the ability to later recall and draw the figure from memory (see also "Relationships Between Copy Strategy and Recall"). In fact, Copy time, Copy accuracy, and Immediate Recall are highly predictive of Delayed Recall (Tremblay et al., 2015).

RELATIONSHIPS BETWEEN COPY STRATEGY AND RECALL

Qualitative Copy scores tend to be correlated with both Copy and Recall accuracy scores. A strategy that involves clustering the elements into meaningful units is more effective than one that relies on the recall of isolated elements (e.g., Akshoomoff & Stiles, 1995; Anderson et al., 2001; Chiulli et al., 1995; Deckersbach et al., 2000a). Consequently, it is important to consider organizational strategy when assessing visual memory of the figure.

In this context, it is worth noting that perceptual bias (the tendency to allocate more attentional or perceptual resources to either the global or the local features of a stimulus) also affects performance. In healthy individuals, the tendency to view a stimulus from a global (as opposed to a local) vantage point is associated with better recall (Kramer & Wells, 2004). See "Clinical Studies" for further discussion.

According to Osterrieth (1944), 83% of adults adopt a conceptual or part-configurational approach, and only 15% use a piecemeal approach. Use of a configural approach shows little decline with advancing age (Chiulli et al., 1995). However, the role of organization differs between young and old adults. Hartman and Potter (1998) noted that, in comparison to younger adults (aged 18–32 years), older adults (aged 60–81 years) appear to rely more on the hierarchical structure of the figure to maintain accuracy of individual elements, with failures to organize resulting in reduced Copy scores. In contrast, younger adults are able to draw individual elements accurately even in the absence of a well-organized production. Therefore, the organizational abilities of older adults are not only well preserved but also appear important for maintaining a high level of performance. In the memory production, errors (typically in the form of omissions) are common in the Recall condition but rare in the Copy condition (Hartman & Potter, 1998; Mitrushina et al., 1990). In short, age-related differences in adults on the Copy condition are relatively minor. On the Recall trial, errors of omission are prominent with advancing age. Therefore, marked distortion or disorganization of the drawing elements in either the Copy or Recall condition may signify abnormality rather than normal aging (Hartman & Potter, 1998).

RELATIONSHIPS BETWEEN REY AND TAYLOR FIGURES

The Rey Figure takes more time to both copy and reproduce from memory than does the Taylor Figure (Peirson & Jansen, 1997; Tombaugh & Hubley, 1991). The Rey Figure appears to have a more complex organizational structure (Hamby et al., 1993), it contains a greater number and variety of lines (Hubley & Tremblay, 2002), and it does not lend itself readily to a verbal strategy (Casey et al., 1991). As a result, individuals with visual imagery problems cannot compensate by using a verbal strategy. With the Taylor Figure, in contrast, deficits in visual imagery may be circumvented and therefore obscured by the use of verbal strategies.

The greater recall difficulty of the Rey Figure suggests that this measure may be more sensitive than the alternate versions to the presence of memory deficits, particularly nonverbal ones (Strauss & Spreen, 1990; see also Hamby et al., 1993). Even though the Taylor Figure is easier to remember than the Rey Figure (Yamashita, 2006), parallel forgetting functions occur for both figures, indicating that both reflect comparable degrees of sensitivity when they are used to measure rates of forgetting (Tombaugh & Hubley, 1991).

RELATIONSHIPS WITH OTHER TESTS

Memory and visuomotor ability contribute to performance. In a heterogeneous sample of patients with neurological disorders, Meyers and Meyers (1995b) found that the Copy, three-minute Recall, 30-minute Recall, and Recognition Total Correct scores were significantly correlated with tasks requiring memory and constructional ability (BVRT Total Correct, RAVLT Trial 5, Benton Form Discrimination, Hooper, TMT-B, and the Token Test). Language measures (FAS, Sentence Repetition) had no significant relationships with any RCFT measures. Modest correlations were reported between RCFT Recall and the RAVLT (r = .36; Anderson & Lajoie, 1996).

Correlational analyses indicate that scores on the RCFT are moderately related to performance on visual-spatial subtests (Block Design and Object Assembly) of the Wechsler (e.g., Poulton & Moffitt, 1995; Tombaugh et al., 1992). Similarly, Sherman et al. (1995) found that scores on the RCFT (both Copy and 30-minute Delayed Recall) were moderately related to the Perceptual Organization factor of the WAIS-R. Scores on the RCFT were not related to the Verbal Comprehension and Freedom from Distractibility factors of the WAIS-R. Meyers and Meyers (1995b) also reported that, in a mixed sample of patients with neurological disorders, RCFT measures correlated more strongly with Performance subtests than with Verbal subtests. Recall of the RCFT shows a moderate relation to functional memory, assessed via the Rivermead Behavioural Memory Test (Ostrosky-Solis et al., 1998).

Factor-analytic studies of the RCFT and other neuropsychological tests suggest that RCFT scores load heavily on what appears to be a visual-spatial perceptual/memory factor, based on common loadings with the WMS Visual Reproduction (Berry et al., 1991; Ostrosky-Solis et al., 1998), Line Orientation (Berry et al., 1991), Hooper (Johnstone & Wilhelm, 1997), and Raven's Standard Progressive Matrices scores (Ponton et al., 2000).

Executive functions play a role, at least in the copying of the figure. In patients with AD, MCI, or dementia, cognitive flexibility and working memory (i.e., executive functions) but not inhibition mediate the relationship between planning and copying, suggesting some selectivity with respect to the types of executive functions underlying competent copying of the complex figure (Ávila et al., 2015; Freeman et al., 2000). In moderate to severe TBI patients, executive functions (FAS, TMT-B, and WCST) explain between 11% and 15% of the variance on the RCFT. Modest correlations are generally found between RCFT and executive tests (r = .12 to .35; Schwarz et al., 2009).

Organization scores on the RCFT appear to tap into different aspects of executive functioning compared to organization scores on other tests. Specifically, in one study utilizing undergraduate volunteers, CFA conducted on a variety of neuropsychological tests and their organization scores (i.e., CVLT-II cluster score, letter and category fluency cluster size and cluster ratio, RCFT organization, VPA pairs ratio, Ruff Figural Fluency cluster size and ratio) revealed modest to moderate correlations among the tests (r = .17 to .41). The one-factor model was nonsignificant, suggesting that the organization scores measured somewhat different aspects of organization. As such, the authors suggested that a variety of organizational processing strategies across different cognitive domains be included in test batteries (Banerjee & White, 2015).

Some support for the validity of the BQSS executive scores derives from studies of patient populations with known executive dysfunction (Schreiber et al., 1999; Somerville et al., 2000; Troyer & Wishart, 1997) and from the pattern of correlations with other executive and nonexecutive measures. For example, Sommerville et al. (2000) reported that the executive BQSS variables were more highly correlated with executive measures (r = .26; e.g., WCST perseverative responses, COWA) than with nonexecutive measures (r = .16; e.g., Digit Span, Logical Memory, and Visual Reproduction retention). In addition, the BQSS Organization Summary Score significantly differentiated patients with either no, mild, or severe executive dysfunction defined according to performance on other tests of executive function.

The advantage of the BQSS lies in its ability to characterize unique differences among patients that are not evident in the traditional 36-point scoring system. For example, the BQSS is more sensitive to aging effects than the traditional system is (Hartman & Potter, 1998), and it appears useful in determining whether poor organization could account for recall difficulties. Similarly, Elderkin-Thompson et al. (2004a, 2004b) found that the Planning score was particularly useful in understanding visual-spatial memory impairment in depressed elderly patients. These patients appear not to encode the figure in an organized manner, and this lack of structure seems to account for their poor memory.

CLINICAL STUDIES

The test is sensitive to central nervous system health problems known to affect memory and executive function, such as head injury (Berry et al., 1991; Poulton & Moffitt, 1995); medial temporal lobe damage (Kixmiller et al., 2000); seizure disorders (McConley et al., 2006; Poulton & Moffitt, 1995); MCI (Kasai et al., 2006); AD (Ardila et al., 2000; Freeman et al., 2000; Tei et al., 1997; Westervelt et al., 2016); PD (Freeman et al., 2000; Scarpina et al., 2016); ischemic VaD (Freeman et al., 2000); Korsakoff's disease (Kixmiller et al., 2000); systemic lupus erythematosus (Coín-Mejías et al., 2008); MDMA, cocaine, and polydrug abuse (Cuyàs et al., 2011; Rosselli & Ardila, 1996); and anterior communicating artery aneurysm (Diamond & DeLuca, 1996; Diamond et al., 1997; Kixmiller et al., 2000). In one study, patients with chronic renal failure who underwent peritoneal dialysis showed significantly higher recall performance than those who underwent hemodialysis (Kaya et al., 2013).

Dementia. The RCFT alone or in combination with other tests has utility in distinguishing between AD and DLB or PD. Westervelt et al. (2016) reported that using a RCFT Copy cutoff of less than 13 yielded 86% sensitivity and 45% specificity for identifying DLB from AD patients. If the Brief Smell Identification Test (cutoff of 6) was included, the specificity improved to 65% while sensitivity remained at 86%. Use of the HVLT (cutoff of 0) with RCFT Copy yielded a 70% sensitivity and an 85% specificity. A combination of all three tests yielded a sensitivity of 70% and a specificity of 91%.

PD patients score low on Planning, Neatness, Organization, and Rotation scores on the BQSS. A BQSS copy cutoff of 16 or lower yields a sensitivity of 70% and a specificity of 97% for identifying PD patients from healthy controls (Scarpina et al., 2016).

Lateralized Brain Dysfunction. Furthermore, information from the Copy portion of the test may be useful in differentiating different disorders. For example, a piecemeal approach to the copying of the RCFT is characteristic of patients with either left- or right-hemisphere lesions (Akshoomoff et al., 2002; Trojano et al., 2004). However, the drawings by patients with right-brain lesions tend to be less accurate (but see Rapport et al., 1995 and 1996, who found that this might apply only to patients who show neglect) and more distorted than those of their left-sided counterparts (Binder, 1982). Patients with left-hemisphere damage exhibited more difficulty copying right-sided local elements (Poreh & Shye, 1998).

The Copy task is also sensitive to hemispatial neglect. Patients with right CVAs who were identified as having neglect on a letter-cancellation task showed an increased incidence of omission of items on the left side of the figure, a rightward attentional bias (reflected in their starting point on the task), and a poorer accuracy of reproduction on the left side (Rapport et al., 1995, 1996). Furthermore, hemispatial deficits noted on the RCFT Copy trial are related to inpatient falls (Rapport et al., 1995). Interestingly, Global Processing Training (which trains global to local encoding) but not Rote Repetition Training (which does not provide encoding strategies) has been shown to improve RCFT Copy in patients with right-hemisphere stroke (Chen et al., 2012).

Differences between patients with parietal-occipital lesions and patients with frontal lobe lesions are also noted on the Copy trial. Patients with posterior lesions are more likely to have difficulty with the spatial organization of the figure. Patients with frontal lobe lesions are more likely to have difficulty planning their approach to the task. However, it is important to note that healthy individuals may exhibit a wide variety of approaches to copying the RCFT. For example, Wilson and Batchelor (2015) evaluated RCFT organization in a sample of healthy undergraduate volunteers and found a large variability in organization and global processing scores. Only half of this healthy sample started with the base rectangle first, and only 11–18% continued with drawing the diagonals or the bisectors using two consecutively drawn lines, respectively.

With regard to the memory trials, there is a tendency for adult patients with right-hemisphere lesions to perform more poorly than patients with left-hemisphere disturbances on the Recall trial (Loring et al., 1988). The test, however, is not a perfect predictor of side of lesion (Lee et al., 1989; Loring et al., 1988), and others have found the task to be insensitive to right-hemisphere lesions (Ashton et al., 2005; Barr et al., 1997; McConley et al., 2008). In one study, the task was not associated with seizure laterality or hippocampal pathology in patients with left or right TLE; the only association was between RCFT Delayed Recall and left hippocampal volume ($r = .20$; McConley et al., 2008).

Analysis of qualitative features (e.g., distortion of overall configuration, major mislocation, location of element) may be helpful in distinguishing laterality of dysfunction on Recall (Loring et al., 1988; Poreh & Shye, 1998). If the initial Copy is performed satisfactorily, misplacement and distortion on the Recall trial tend to be characteristic of patients with right-, as opposed to left-hemisphere dysfunction (Loring et al., 1988). Poreh and Shye (1998) found that patients with left-hemisphere damage randomly recalled the local elements of the right side of the figure, whereas the left side and middle (global) portions were copied and recalled as a separate class. Patients with right-hemisphere damage, on the other hand, showed no evidence of a tendency to exhibit either a left- or right-hemifield superiority.

TBI. The test's sensitivity to TBI has been questioned. Ashton et al. (2005) found that higher levels of (WAIS-III) perceptual organization skills and, to a lesser extent, the absence of a diffuse intracranial injury were predictive of better performance on the Recall and Recognition trials. Measures of injury severity proved unrelated to performance. Furthermore, a large proportion of the sample improved by at least one *SD* from Delayed Recall to Recognition, and this was mediated by perceptual organization skills but not by injury parameters. Given the limited sensitivity of the Recall and Recognition trials to injury severity, these authors concluded that performance on the RCFT after TBI was more affected by perceptual organization skills and that clinicians should supplement the RCFT with other measures of learning and memory.

Expectations regarding diagnosis (diagnosis threat) may negatively influence recall performance. Suhr and Gunstad (2005) reported that head-injured individuals exposed to diagnosis threat performed more poorly than matched controls on the recall portion, despite no differences in test validity (WMT), anxiety, or depression. The findings suggest that a person's knowledge and expectancies about neurological insult (e.g., head injury) and its cognitive consequences can affect performance, perhaps due to beliefs about distractibility and poor cognitive efficiency.

Alcohol Abuse. Chronic inpatients with alcohol dependence and detoxified alcoholics show impairments on RCFT Copy, Immediate and Delayed Recall, and Recognition, but performance is not associated with lifetime consumption of alcohol or other substance use or length of sobriety. The recall deficits are most likely because of inefficient learning (poor organizational and problem-solving skills) or retrieval problems as Copy strategy is correlated with Copy accuracy (rho = .30), which in turn affects Recall accuracy (Rosenbloom et al., 2009). Similarly, detoxified alcoholics also show impaired Recall and Recognition performance, most likely because of inefficient learning and retrieval strategies (Dawson & Grant, 2000; Paikkatt et al., 2014; Rosenbloom et al., 2009). This is supported by DTI studies, which find lower fractional anisotropy in the frontal forceps of alcoholics than controls, which may impact their planning ability (Rosenbloom et al., 2009).

Psychiatric Conditions. Extensive research has been conducted on the association between RCFT performance, particularly the copy approach using the Savage scoring system, and various psychiatric disorders, including eating disorders (Aloi et al., 2015; Heled et al., 2014; Lang et al., 2016; Lopez et al., 2008a, 2008b; Sherman et al., 2006; Zuchova et al., 2013), obsessive-compulsive disorder (OCD; Buhlmann et al., 2006; Hwang et al., 2007; Jang et al., 2010; Shin et al., 2010), schizophrenia (Kim et al., 2008; Seeck-Hirschner et al., 2010), depression (Behnken et al., 2010; Hinkelmann et al., 2012; Loo et al., 2007; Seeck-Hirschner et al., 2010), bipolar disorder (Seidman et al., 2003), body dysmorphic disorder (Deckersbach et al., 2000b), and borderline personality disorder (Harris et al., 2002). Most of these studies suggest that Copy organization plays a large role in later recall of the complex figure.

Symptoms of eating disorder are negatively correlated with the RCFT Copy and Recall (Aloi et al., 2015; Zuchova et al., 2013). In particular, people with eating disorders perform worse than healthy controls on BQSS Planning, Neatness, and Organization scores (Heled et al., 2014). Some studies find that those with anorexia bulimia (AN) and bulimia nervosa use different organizational strategies on the Copy trial compared to healthy controls, and their use of detail processing strategies rather than global processing on the Copy trial affects their performance on the Recall trial (Harrison et al., 2011; Lopez et al., 2008a; Sherman et al., 2006). Mothers of patients with AN also show lower levels of global processing strategies, suggesting a familial trait in cognitive processing style (Lang et al., 2016). In short, the RCFT may be useful to assess cognitive processing style in eating disorders, and the primary differences in RCFT memory performance may be due to cognitive processing style rather than memory dysfunction per se.

Similar to those with eating disorders, patients with OCD, whether medicated or not, also perform worse than healthy controls on BQSS organization scores and RCFT Recall accuracy (Deckersbach et al., 2000a; Jang et al., 2010; Mataix-Cols et al., 2003; Savage et al., 2000; Shin et al., 2004; Shin et al., 2010). One study found that the obsessions/checking dimension as measured by the Yale-Brown Obsessive-Compulsive Scale is related to organization scores (Jang et al., 2010). However, only those with late-onset OCD appear to have worse Recall scores than healthy controls (Hwang et al., 2007). Organizational strategy on RCFT Copy and, consequently, the recall of the figure may be improved by cognitive retraining. However, organization appears to improve on retest regardless of training, suggesting that those with OCD may have difficulty in utilizing strategies spontaneously but their ability to implement strategies when given a second trial is preserved (Buhlmann et al., 2006).

In schizophrenia, studies have suggested that initial organizational processing impairments are an important component of retention difficulties but do not fully account for recall difficulty. For example, Seidman et al. (2003) reported that patients with schizophrenia were impaired on Copy, Recall, and Recognition components and that Recall accuracy deficits remained significant after controlling for organizational approach on the copy portion. In another study, a piecemeal approach to copying the figure mediated Delayed Recall in schizophrenia (Kim et al., 2008).

Patients with remitted major depressive disorder perform worse than healthy controls on Recall accuracy, which also appears to be mediated by poor organization during the Copy trial even though the patients are not impaired on Copy accuracy (Behnken et al., 2010). In one study, following right unilateral ECT for depression, no changes in RCFT performance were seen six months later despite decreases in verbal list learning and letter fluency (Loo et al., 2007). Seeck-Hirschner et al. (2010) reported that patients with schizophrenia or depression who took a 40-minute daytime nap performed better on the RCFT Recall than those who did not nap, but the improvement was not observed in healthy controls. No differences as a result of napping were seen on the Copy trial. These studies suggest that poor RCFT recall performance in depression, schizophrenia, OCD, and eating disorders may be due to frontal systems dysfunction rather than to a primary memory disorder.

Other authors (Chiulli et al., 1995; Suhr & Gunstad, 2005; Vingerhoets et al., 1995) have noted that psychological distress (anxiety, depression) has no effect on recall of the RCFT. Acute mental stress, typical of everyday life, appears to have little impact on test performance (Hoffman & al'Absi, 2004).

In psychiatric patients, Recognition scores correlate with overall functional ability better than Recall scores do (Meyers & Lange, 1994). The higher the recognition trial score, the more independent functioning.

Other Conditions. Young adults who survive childhood brain tumor are poorer on BQSS planning and perseverative errors than healthy controls, and planning mediates community living skills as measured by the Scales of Independent Behavior-Revised (King et al., 2015). In criminal offenders, organizational quality is linked to self-reported impulsivity (Cornell et al., 1997). More impulsive individuals are less likely to follow a well-organized plan; however, self-reported impulsivity does not affect copy or recall accuracy.

NEUROANATOMICAL CORRELATES AND IMAGING STUDIES

Among alcoholics, DTI measurements of the occipital forceps and external capsule are significantly correlated with Copy accuracy (r = .29 and .36, respectively) while inferior cingulate fractional anisotropy is correlated with Recall accuracy (r = .32; Rosenbloom et al., 2009). In patients with subcortical VaD, the number of lenticulostriate artery branches as measured by 7T magnetic resonance angiography (MRA) is highly correlated with Delayed Recall scores (r = .77; Seo et al., 2012). Early changes in Recall and Recognition following aerobic exercise in older adults are moderately correlated with changes in $VO_{2\,VAT}$, hippocampal regional cerebral blood flow, hippocampal regional cerebral blood volume, and hippocampal head volume (Maass et al., 2015).

PERFORMANCE VALIDITY

The RCFT may also be useful in the detection of invalid performance. For example, Knight and Meyers (1995) found that individuals instructed to malinger could be distinguished from brain-injured individuals by a pattern of poorer level of accuracy, slower production speed, and poorer delayed and recognition memory (see also Meyers & Meyers, 1995b). Meyers and Volbrecht (1999) examined the concept of Memory Error Patterns in litigants, nonlitigants, suspected malingerers, and simulators. They reported that all of the malingerers and most (80%) of the simulators produced either a "storage" Memory Error Pattern (defined as a decline of more than 3 T scores from the three-minute Delayed Recall trial to the Recognition trial) or an "attention" Memory Error Pattern (achieved when three-minute Delayed Recall, 30-minute Delayed Recall, and Recognition scores all fell below a T score of 24).

Lu et al. (2003) examined litigating patients with suspect performance with various neurological and psychiatric disorders with or without memory impairment. They found that patients suspected of invalid performance displayed significantly lower Recognition scores than did patients with bona fide visual memory impairment. The presence of one or more Atypical Recognition Errors defined as incorrect answers on items 1, 4, 6, 10, 11, 16, 18, and 21, which are rarely answered incorrectly by healthy adults or brain-injured patients, was also more common among the patients with suspect performance. However, individual RCFT scores (Copy, Immediate Recall, True-Positive Recognition, False-Positive Errors) were not very sensitive in capturing noncredible performance, nor were particular configurations on the various test trials identified by Meyers and Volbrecht (1999) sensitive to noncredible performance.

Sensitivity, specificity, and positive and negative predictive values for various RCFT scores at differing base rate for the Lu et al. (2003) equation are shown in Table 10–93. To improve classification accuracy, the authors derived a combination score incorporating the Copy, True-Positive Recognition, and Atypical Recognition Errors scores. A cutoff score of 45 or less yielded a sensitivity of 74% while misclassifying only about 4% of patients with verbal memory impairment, 12% of those without visual memory impairment, and 3% of those with memory impairment, an acceptable level of false positives in most contexts. The equation for the combination score [also known as Lu et al. (2003) equation] is as follows:

TABLE 10–94 Cutoffs, Sensitivity, and Specificity of the Rey-Osterrieth Complex Figure Test (RCFT) Trials to Malingering in an Outpatient Neuropsychology Clinic Patient Sample

	CUTOFF	SENSITIVITY (%)	SPECIFICITY (%)
Copy	<26	47	92
3-minute Delay	<10	42	91
True-Positive Recognition	<7	61	93
Lu et al. (2003) Combination Score Equation	≤50	80	90

SOURCE: Adapted from Reedy et al. (2013).

$$\text{Combination score} = \text{Copy score} + [(\text{True-Positive Recognition} - \text{Atypical Recognition Errors}) \times 3]$$

Of note, even though individual RCFT test scores are not particularly sensitive to invalid performance, examination of individual scores may alert the clinician to the possibility of invalid performance (Lu et al., 2003). Therefore, when abnormal scores are obtained (e.g., True-Positive Recognition score ≤3, False-Positive Errors >4), they may be suggestive of invalid performance (see Table 10–93).

Indices derived from the RCFT show moderate correlations with other measures of invalid performance; however, none exceeds 50% shared score variance (Nelson et al., 2003). The RCFT thus contributes additional information that is helpful in evaluating performance validity and which is not redundant with other tests of performance validity.

Reedy et al. (2013) cross-validated the Lu et al. (2003) equation using outpatient neuropsychology clinic patients divided into credible and noncredible according to Slick et al. (1999) malingering criteria. As seen in Table 10–94, in this sample, a Copy score of less than 26 yielded a sensitivity of 47%, an Immediate Recall score of less than 10 yielded a sensitivity of 42%, and a True-Positive Recognition score of less than 7 yielded a sensitivity of 61% while maintaining specificity at a level of at least 90%. The Lu et al. (2003) formula appeared better than the other scores in identifying noncredible groups, yielding a sensitivity of 80% while maintaining specificity at 90% using a cutoff score of 50 or lower. Those in the credible group who obtained 50 or lower ($N = 12$) on the Lu et al. (2003) equation were identified to be older in age, lower in intellectual functioning, and to have a history of learning disability. Adjusting the cutoff to 49 or lower for those older than age 59 and 48 or lower for those of low-average intelligence (IQ = 80–89) yielded a specificity of 100%.

Blaskewitz et al. (2009) compared various indices of invalid performance including Atypical Recognition Errors, Recognition Failure Errors (defined as correctly recalling an item in the delayed recall trial but failing to recognize it in the recognition trial), and suspicious Memory Error Patterns (Meyers & Volbrecht, 1999) using a group of neurological patients with independently verified valid performance as well as a group of compensation-seeking forensic patients with independently verified invalid performance. The valid performance group was based on valid performance on the Medical Symptom Validity Test and Reliable Digit Span tested in the acute or subacute phase. The invalid performance group was defined by failure on the Computerized Assessment of Response Bias and WMT. Like Lu et al. (2003), Blaskewitz and colleagues (2009) found that Recall scores and Recognition Failure Errors were similar for both groups. However, the forensic group yielded lower Copy and Recognition scores and more Atypical Recognition Errors than the patients. The number of errors ranged from 0 to 2 in the patient group and 0 to 7 in the forensic group. Using the Atypical Recognition Errors, Recognition Failure Errors, or Memory Error Patterns, a specificity of 78% was obtained in the patient group and a sensitivity of 50% in the forensic group. Using the Lu et al. (2003) equation, a cutoff of 45 or lower yielded a sensitivity of 52% and a specificity of 95% for detecting noncredible performance.

Table 10–95 presents the PPV and NPV at various base rates. Meyers and Meyers criteria (based on a combination of two or more Atypical Recognition Errors or Recognition Failure Errors or Memory Error Patterns) showed very low PPV and acceptable NPV, while the Lu et al. (2003) equation yielded better classification rates. Use of two or more rare mistakes obtained low sensitivity (21%) and acceptable specificity (93%). Overall, the Lu et al. (2003) formula appeared more effective than the Meyers and Meyers criteria.

TABLE 10–95 Positive Predictive Values and Negative Predictive Values at Different Base Rates for Different Classification Systems for Detecting Noncredible Performance with the Rey-Osterrieth Complex Figure Test (RCFT)

	MEYERS AND MEYERS CRITERIA		LU ET AL. CRITERIA		MEMORY ERROR PATTERNS ONLY	
BASE RATE (%)	PPV (%)	NPV (%)	PPV (%)	NPV (%)	PPV (%)	NPV (%)
15	29	90	65	92	37	90
30	49	78	82	82	58	79
45	65	66	89	71	72	67

NOTE: PPV, positive predictive value; NPV, negative predictive value; Meyers and Meyers criteria = combination of two or more Atypical Recognition Errors or Recognition Failure Errors or Memory Error Patterns; Lu et al. criteria = Copy score + [(True-Positive Recognition – Atypical Recognition Errors) × 3]; Memory Error Patterns (Meyers & Volbrecht, 1999).

SOURCE: Blaskewitz et al. (2009).

COMMENT

The RCFT has a long history in neuropsychology. Over the years, a large body of research has supported its use as a measure of a variety of cognitive processes, including visual-spatial skills, visual-construction ability, visual memory, and executive function. The inclusion of the Recognition trial appears to be a useful addition to recall testing.

The test is useful for assessing a variety of neurological and psychiatric conditions. It is less useful for lateralizing impairments or predicting side of seizure focus, possibly due to the verbalizability of the items, a common shortcoming in many visual memory measures, and also because of the fact that visual memory is less clearly lateralized. Executive functioning components may also not permit easy lateralization based on test score patterns. Analysis of the profile or pattern of test scores on the various components (Copy, Recall, and Recognition trials) is recommended (e.g., Meyers & Meyers, 1995b) and may help to distinguish among disorders.

The RCFT affords the examinee multiple approaches and strategies. As Seidman et al. (2003) pointed out, there is no obvious beginning or end; there are many ways (more or less efficient) in which a person can arrive at an accurate rendition, and there are built-in visual components that lend themselves to being perceived as large-scale organization features or small details. These features allow measurement of strategic processes such as planning and monitoring because some approaches are more common and more efficient than others, thus providing sensitivity to unusual performance (Akshoomoff et al., 2002).

Numerous systems have been developed to assess accuracy and qualitative (e.g., planning, organizational) aspects. The most extensive quantitative and qualitative systems currently in use are those developed by Meyers and Meyers (1995b) and the BQSS by Stern and colleagues (1999). In general, the literature shows that qualitative Copy scores are correlated significantly with both Copy accuracy and Recall scores. Additionally, most of these qualitative Copy scores correlate moderately with measures of executive ability and appear to be useful in distinguishing patients from controls. Their advantage lies in their ability to characterize unique differences among examinees that are not evident when using the traditional 36-point scoring system.

A number of embedded indices have been developed to assist in identifying invalid performance, such as the use of Atypical Recognition Errors, suspicious Memory Error Patterns, and the Lu et al. (2003) combination score equation. The sensitivity and specificity data for these indices are encouraging in studies utilizing known-group designs and validated by established malingering criteria, with the Lu et al. (2003) cutoff appearing particularly useful for this purpose. However, users may have to make adjustments to the cutoff score of this equation for examinees who are older and of lower intellectual functioning (Reedy et al., 2013).

Users should be aware of the test's limitations. Multiple administration procedures with varying delay intervals as well as scoring systems have been developed over the years. Care must be taken to utilize the corresponding norms as the administration (or not) of the immediate recall trial affects later recall scores. It is noteworthy that the norms of several earlier administration procedures are a few decades old and have not been updated. We recommend using the Meyers and Meyers (1995b) administration and present some normative dataset that are more recent than the 1995 norms, which themselves could benefit from updating.

It should be noted that the distribution of scores for the Copy and Recognition conditions is not normal. The majority of healthy individuals are able to draw the figure without major distortions and obtain high scores on the Recognition trial. Therefore, a label of "superior" given to a high Copy or Recognition score is meaningless; on the other hand, low performance has clinical significance (see also Mitrushina et al., 2005). It has also been reported that a variety of copy strategies ranging from global to local processing may be seen even in healthy young adults (Wilson & Batchelor, 2015). As such, fragmentations in the copying of the figure do not necessarily imply constructional impairment, although qualitative scores may have implications for community living skills (King et al., 2015).

Furthermore, interpretation of the Recall scores (see also Meyers & Meyers, 1995b) must consider whether the initial copy is performed adequately. Organizational approach has been found to mediate recall of the figure (e.g., Kim et al., 2008). Familiarity with a pictorial writing system may also affect figure recall (Sakamoto & Spiers, 2014). Disrupted encoding due to visual-perceptual or organizational difficulties might be suggested if the initial copy is poor. Given the impact of the Copy trial on the interpretation of memory scores on the RCFT, Tremblay et al. (2015) developed equations taking demographic variables and Copy scores into consideration for French-Canadian older adults; use of these equations in other samples has not yet been verified.

A number of alternate figures have been developed; however, it is important to bear in mind that the Rey Figure is harder to recall than the alternate figures, and it may be more sensitive to the presence of visual memory deficits. Comparisons of the various alternate figures show that the MTCF is the most suitable as a parallel version, at least in young adults. In older adults, however, significant differences between the Rey Figure and MTCF copy trials have been found, indicating that the MTCF is not suitable as an alternate form for assessing visuoconstructional ability in this age group. Memory performance on the Taylor Figure should be evaluated against normative data that are specific to this figure and should never be compared against normative data for the Rey Figure.

REFERENCES

Akshoomoff, N. A., Feroleto, C. C., Doyle, R. E., & Stiles, J. (2002). The impact of early unilateral brain injury on perceptual organization and visual memory. *Neuropsychologia, 40,* 539–561.

Akshoomoff, N. A., & Stiles, J. (1995). Developmental trends in visuospatial analysis and planning: II. Memory for a complex figure. *Neuropsychology, 9,* 378–389.

Aloi, M., Rania, M., Caroleo, M., Bruni, A., Palmieri, A., Cauteruccio, M. A., . . . Segura-García, C. (2015). Decision making, central coherence and set-shifting: A comparison between binge eating disorder, anorexia nervosa and healthy controls. *BMC Psychiatry, 15*(1), 6.

Anderson, P., Anderson, V., & Garth, J. (2001). Assessment and development of organizational ability: The Rey Complex Figure Organizational Strategy Score (RCF-OSS). *The Clinical Neuropsychologist, 15,* 81–94.

Anderson, V. A., & Lajoie, G. (1996). Development of memory and learning skills in school-aged children: A neuropsychological perspective. *Applied Neuropsychology, 3/4,* 128–139.

Ardila, A., Lopera, F., Rosselli, M., Moreno, S., Madrigal, L., Arango-Lasprilla, J. C., . . . Ossa, J. (2000). Neuropsychological profile of a large kindred with familial Alzheimer's disease caused by the E280A single presenilin-1 mutation. *Archives of Clinical Neuropsychology, 15,* 515–528.

Ashton, V. L., Donders, J., & Hoffman, N. M. (2005). Rey Complex Figure test performance after traumatic brain injury. *Journal of Clinical and Experimental Neuropsychology, 27,* 55–64.

Ávila, R. T., de Paula, J. J., Bicalho, M. A., Moraes, E. N., Nicolato, R., Malloy-Diniz, L., & Diniz, B. S. (2015). Working memory and cognitive flexibility mediates visuoconstructional abilities in older adults with heterogeneous cognitive ability. *Journal of the International Neuropsychological Society, 21*(5), 392–398.

Banerjee, P., & White, D. A. (2015). Clinical assessment of organizational strategy: An examination of healthy adults. *Psychological Assessment, 27*(2), 726.

Barr, W. B., Chelune, G. J., Hermann, B. P., Loring, D., Perrine, K., Strauss, E., . . . Westerveld, M. (1997). The use of figural reproduction tests as measures of nonverbal memory in epilepsy surgery candidates. *Journal of the International Neuropsychological Society, 3,* 435–443.

Behnken, A., Schöning, S., Gerß, J., Konrad, C., de Jong-Meyer, R., Zwanzger, P., & Arolt, V. (2010). Persistent non-verbal memory impairment in remitted major depression—Caused by encoding deficits? *Journal of Affective Disorders, 122*(1-2), 144–148.

Bernstein, J. H., & Waber, D. P. (1996). *Developmental scoring system for the Rey-Osterrieth Complex Figure.* Odessa, FL: Psychological Assessment Resources.

Berry, D. T. R., Allen, R. S., & Schmitt, F. A. (1991). Rey-Osterrieth Figure: Psychometric characteristics in a geriatric sample. *The Clinical Neuropsychologist, 5,* 143–153.

Berry, D. T. R., & Carpenter, G. S. (1992). Effect of four different delay periods on recall of the Rey-Osterrieth Complex Figure by older persons. *The Clinical Neuropsychologist, 6,* 80–84.

Bigler, E. D., Rosa, L., Schultz, F., Hall, S., and Harris, J. (1989). Rey-Auditory Verbal Learning and Rey-Osterrieth Complex Figure Design test performance in Alzheimer's disease and closed head injury. *Journal of Clinical Psychology, 45,* 277–280.

Binder, L. M. (1982). Constructional strategies on complex figure drawing after unilateral brain damage. *Journal of Clinical Neuropsychology, 4,* 51–58.

Blaskewitz, N., Merten, T., & Brockhaus, R. (2009). Detection of suboptimal effort with the Rey Complex Figure Test and Recognition trial. *Applied Neuropsychology, 16*(1), 54–61.

Boone, K. B., Lesser, I. M., Hill-Gutierrez, E., Berman, N. G., & D'Elia, L. F. (1993). Rey-Osterrieth Complex Figure performance in healthy, older adults: Relationship to age, education, sex, and IQ. *The Clinical Neuropsychologist, 7,* 22–28.

Budd, M. A., Houtz, A., & Lambert, P. (2008). Comparison of nondominant- and dominant-hand performances on the copy portion of the Rey Complex Figure Test (RCFT). *Journal of Clinical and Experimental Neuropsychology, 30*(3), 380–386.

Buhlmann, U., Deckersbach, T., Engelhard, I., Cook, L. M., Rauch, S. L., Kathmann, N., . . . Savage, C. R. (2006). Cognitive retraining for organizational impairment in obsessive-compulsive disorder. *Psychiatry Research, 144*(2-3), 109–116.

Bush, S., & Martin, T. A. (2004). Intermanual differences on the Rey Complex Figure Test. *Rehabilitation Psychology, 49,* 76–78.

Caffarra, P., Vezzadini, G., Dieci, F., Zonato, F., & Venneri, A. (2002). Rey-Osterrieth Complex Figure: Normative values in an Italian population sample. *Neurological Science, 22,* 443–447.

Camara, W. J., Nathan, J. S., & Puente, A. E. (2000). Psychological test usage: Implications in professional psychology. *Professional Psychology: Research and Practice, 31,* 141–154.

Casarotti, A., Papagno, C., & Zarino, B. (2014). Modified Taylor Complex Figure: Normative data from 290 adults. *Journal of Neuropsychology, 8*(2), 186–198.

Casey, M. B., Winner, E., Hurwitz, I., & DaSilva, D. (1991). Does processing style affect recall of the Rey-Osterrieth or Taylor Complex Figures? *Journal of Clinical and Experimental Neuropsychology, 13,* 600–606.

Chen, P., Hartman, A. J., Galarza, C. P., & DeLuca, J. (2012). Global processing training to improve visuospatial memory deficits after right-brain stroke. *Archives of Clinical Neuropsychology, 27*(8), 891–905.

Chervinsky, A., Mitrushina, M., & Satz, P. (1992). Comparison of four methods of scoring the Rey-Osterrieth Complex Figure Drawing Test on four age groups of normal elderly. *Brain Dysfunction, 5,* 267–287.

Chiulli, S. J., Haaland, K. Y., LaRue, A., & Garry, P. J. (1995). Impact of age on drawing the Rey-Osterrieth figure. *The Clinical Neuropsychologist, 9,* 219–224.

Coín-Mejías, M. Á., Peralta-Ramírez, M. I., Santiago-Ramajo, S., Morente-Soto, G., Ortego-Centeno, N., Callejas Rubio, J., . . . Pérez-García, M. (2008). Alterations in episodic memory in patients with systemic lupus erythematosus. *Archives of Clinical Neuropsychology, 23*(2), 157–164.

Cornell, D. G., Roberts, M., & Oram, G. (1997). The Rey-Osterrieth Complex Figure Test as a neuropsychological measure in criminal offenders. *Archives of Clinical Neuropsychology, 12,* 47–56.

Corwin, J., & Bylsma, F. W. (1993). "Psychological Examination of Traumatic Encephalopathy" by A. Rey and "The Complex Figure Copy Test" by P. A. Osterrieth. *The Clinical Neuropsychologist, 7,* 3–21.

Cuyàs, E., Verdejo-García, A., Fagundo, A. B., Khymenets, O., Rodríguez, J., Cuenca, A., . . . de la Torre, R. (2011). The influence of genetic and environmental factors among MDMA users in cognitive performance. *Plos One, 6*(11), e27206. doi:10.1371/journal.pone.0027206.

Dawson, L. K., & Grant, I. (2000). Alcoholics' initial organizational and problem-solving skills predict learning and memory performance on the Rey-Osterrieth Complex Figure. *Journal of International Neuropsychological Society, 6,* 12–19.

Deckersbach, T., Savage, C. R., Henin, A., Mataix-Cols, D., Otto, M. W., Wilhelm, S., . . . Jenike, M. A. (2000a). Reliability and validity of a scoring system for measuring organizational approach in the Complex Figure Test. *Journal of Clinical and Experimental Neuropsychology, 22,* 640–648.

Deckersbach, T., Savage, C. R., Phillips, K. A., Wilhelm, S., Buhlmann, U., Rauch, S. L., . . . Jenike, M. A. (2000b). Characteristics of memory dysfunction in body dysmorphic disorder. *Journal of the International Neuropsychological Society, 6,* 673–681.

Delaney, R. C., Prevey, M. L., Cramer, J., Mattson, R. H., & VA Epilepsy Cooperative Study 264 Research Group. (1992). Test-retest comparability and control subject data for the Rey-Auditory Verbal Learning Test and Rey-Osterrieth/Taylor Complex Figures. *Archives of Clinical Neuropsychology, 7,* 523–528.

Demsky, Y., Carone, D. A., Burns, W. J., & Sellers, A. (2000). Assessment of visual-motor coordination in 6- to 11-yr-olds. *Perceptual and Motor Skills, 91,* 311–321.

Diamond, B. J., & DeLuca, J. (1996). Rey-Osterrieth Complex Figure Test performance following anterior communicating artery aneurysm. *Archives of Clinical Neuropsychology, 11,* 21–28.

Diamond, B. J., DeLuca, J., & Kelley, S. M. (1997). Memory and executive functions in amnesic and non-amnesic patients with aneurysms of the anterior communicating artery. *Brain, 120,* 1015–1025.

Diaz-Asper, C., Schretlen, D. J., & Pearlson, G. D. (2004). How well does IQ predict neuropsychological test performance in normal adults. *Journal of the International Neuropsychological Society, 10,* 82–90.

Dinn, A. A., & Dinn, W. M. (2012). Rey Complex Figure Test profile of Turkish adults. *Archives of Neuropsychiatry, 49*(2), 145–151.

Elderkin-Thompson, V., Boone, K. B., Kumar, A., & Minz, J. (2004a). Validity of the Boston Qualitative Scoring System for the Rey-Osterrieth Complex Figure among depressed elderly patients. *Journal of Clinical and Experimental Neuropsychology, 26,* 598–607.

Elderkin-Thompson, V., Kumar, A., Mintz, J., Boone, K., Bahng, E., & Lavretsky, H. (2004b). Executive dysfunction and visuospatial ability among depressed elders in a community setting. *Archives of Clinical Neuropsychology, 19,* 597–611.

Fastenau, P. S. (1996). Developmental and preliminary standardization of the Extended Complex Figure Test (ECFT). *Journal of Clinical and Experimental Neuropsychology, 18,* 63–76.

Fastenau, P. S. (2002). *The Extended Complex Figure Test (ECTF).* Los Angeles: Western Psychological Services.

Fastenau, P. S., Bennett, J. M., & Denburg, N. L. (1996). Application of psychometric standards to scoring system evaluation: Is "new" necessarily "improved"? *Journal of Clinical and Experimental Neuropsychology, 18,* 462–472.

Fastenau, P. S., Denburg, N. L., & Hufford, B. J. (1999). Adult norms for the Rey-Osterrieth Complex Figure Test and for supplemental recognition and matching trials from the Extended Complex Figure Test. *The Clinical Neuropsychologist, 13,* 30–47.

Folbrecht, J. R., Charter, R. A., Walden, D. K., & Dobbs, S. M. (1999). Psychometric properties of the Boston Qualitative Scoring System for the Rey-Osterrieth Complex Figure. *The Clinical Neuropsychologist, 13,* 442–449.

Freeman, R. Q., Giovannetti, T., Lamar, M., Cloud, B. S., Stern, R. A., Kaplan, E., & Libon, D. J. (2000). Visuoconstructional problems in dementia: Contribution of executive systems functions. *Neuropsychology, 14,* 415–426.

Gallagher, C., & Burke, T. (2007). Age, gender and IQ effects on the Rey–Osterrieth Complex Figure Test. *British Journal of Clinical Psychology, 46*(1), 35–45.

Hamby, S. L., Wilkins, J. W., & Barry, N. S. (1993). Organizational quality on the Rey-Osterrieth and Taylor Complex Figure tests: A new scoring system. *Psychological Assessment, 5,* 27–33.

Harris, C. L., Dinn, W. M., & Marcinkiewicz, J. A. (2002). Partial seizure-like symptoms in borderline personality disorder. *Epilepsy and Behavior, 3,* 433–438.

Harrison, A., Tchanturia, K., & Treasure, J. (2011). Measuring state trait properties of detail processing and global integration ability in eating disorders. *The World Journal of Biological Psychiatry, 12*(5-6), 462–472.

Hartman, M., & Potter, G. (1998). Sources of age differences on the Rey-Osterrieth Complex Figure Test. *The Clinical Neuropsychologist, 12,* 513–524.

Heled, E., Hoofien, D., Bachar, E., Cooper-Kazaz, R., Gur, E., & Ebstein, R. P. (2014). Employing executive functions of perceptual and memory abilities in underweight and weight-restored anorexia nervosa patients. *Eating and Weight Disorders, 19*(4), 479–487.

Hinkelmann, K., Moritz, S., Botzenhardt, J., Muhtz, C., Wiedemann, K., Kellner, M., & Otte, C. (2012). Changes in cortisol secretion during antidepressive treatment and cognitive improvement in patients with major depression: A longitudinal study. *Psychoneuroendocrinology, 37*(5), 685–692.

Hoffman, R., & al'Absi, M. (2004). The effects of acute stress on subsequent neuropsychological test performance. *Archives of Clinical Neuropsychology, 19,* 497–506.

Hubley, A. M. (2010). Using the Rey–Osterrieth and Modified Taylor complex figures with older adults: A preliminary examination of accuracy score comparability. *Archives of Clinical Neuropsychology, 25*(3), 197–203.

Hubley, A. M., & Jassal, S. (2006). Comparability of the Rey–Osterrieth and Modified Taylor Complex figures using total scores, completion times, and construct validation. *Journal of Clinical and Experimental Neuropsychology, 28*(8), 1482–1497.

Hubley, A. M., & Tremblay, D. (2002). Comparability of total score performance on the Rey-Osterrieth Complex Figure and a modified Taylor Complex Figure. *Journal of Clinical and Experimental Neuropsychology, 24,* 370–382.

Hwang, S. H., Kwon, J. S., Shin, Y., Lee, K. J., Kim, Y. Y., & Kim, M. (2007). Neuropsychological profiles of patients with obsessive-compulsive disorder: Early onset versus late onset. *Journal of the International Neuropsychological Society, 13*(1), 30–37.

Jang, J. H., Kim, H. S., Ha, T. H., Shin, N. Y., Kang, D., Choi, J., . . . Kwon, J. S. (2010). Nonverbal memory and organizational dysfunctions are related with distinct symptom dimensions in obsessive-compulsive disorder. *Psychiatry Research, 180*(2-3), 93–98.

Johnstone, B., & Wilhelm, K. L. (1997). The construct validity of the Hooper Visual Organization Test. *Assessment, 4,* 243–248.

Karapetsas, A. N., & Vlachos, F. M. (1997). Sex and handedness in development of visuomotor skills. *Perceptual and Motor Skills, 85,* 131–140.

Kasai, M., Meguro, K., Hashimoto, R., Ishizaki, J., Yamadori, A., & Mori, E. (2006). Non-verbal learning is impaired in very mild Alzheimer's disease (CDR 0.5): Normative data from the learning version of the Rey–Osterrieth Complex Figure Test. *Psychiatry and Clinical Neurosciences, 60*(2), 139–146.

Kaya, Y., Ozturkeri, O. A., Benli, U. S., & Colak, T. (2013). Evaluation of the cognitive functions in patients with chronic renal failure before and after renal transplantation. *Acta Neurologica Belgica, 113*(2), 147–155.

Kim, M., Namgoong, Y., & Youn, T. (2008). Effect of organizational strategy on visual memory in patients with schizophrenia. *Psychiatry and Clinical Neurosciences, 62*(4), 427–434.

King, T. Z., Smith, K. M., & Ivanisevic, M. (2015). The mediating role of visuospatial planning skills on adaptive function among young—Adult survivors of childhood brain tumor. *Archives of Clinical Neuropsychology, 30*(5), 394–403.

Kixmiller, J. S., Verfaellie, M., Mather, M. M., & Cermak, L. S. (2000). Role of perceptual and organizational factors in amnesics' recall of the Rey-Osterrieth Complex Figure: A comparison of three amnesic groups. *Journal of Clinical and Experimental Neuropsychology, 22,* 198–207.

Knight, J. A. (2003). ROCF administration procedures and scoring systems. In J. A. Knight (Ed.), *The handbook of Rey-Osterrieth Complex Figure Usage: Clinical and research application* (pp. 57–191). Lutz, FL: PAR.

Knight, J. A., Kaplan, E., & Ireland, L. D. (2003). Survey findings of Rey-Osterrieth Complex Figure usage. In J. A. Knight (Ed.), *The handbook of Rey-Osterrieth Complex Figure Usage: Clinical and research application* (pp. 45–56). Lutz, FL: PAR.

Knight, J. A., & Meyers, J. E. (1995). *Comparison of malingered and brain-injured productions on the Rey-Osterrieth Complex Figure Test.* Paper presented at the meeting of the International Neuropsychological Society, Seattle, Washington.

Kramer, J. H., & Wells, A. M. (2004). The role of perceptual bias in complex figure recall. *Journal of Clinical and Experimental Neuropsychology, 26,* 838–845.

Lang, K., Treasure, J., & Tchanturia, K. (2016). Is inefficient cognitive processing in anorexia nervosa a familial trait? A neuropsychological pilot study of mothers of offspring with a diagnosis of anorexia nervosa. *The World Journal of Biological Psychiatry, 17*(4), 258–265.

Lee, G. P., Loring, D. W., & Thompson, J. L. (1989). Construct validity of material-specific memory measures following unilateral temporal lobe ablations. *Psychological Assessment, 1,* 192–197.

Levine, A. J., Miller, E. N., Becker, J. T., Selnes, O. A., & Cohen, B. A. (2004). Normative data for determining significance of test-retest differences on eight common neuropsychological instruments. *The Clinical Neuropsychologist, 18,* 373–384.

Lezak, M. D., Howieson, D. B., & Loring, D. W. (2004). *Neuropsychological assessment* (4th ed.). New York: Oxford University Press.

Loo, C., Sheehan, P., Pigot, M., & Lyndon, W. (2007). A report on mood and cognitive outcomes with right unilateral ultra-brief pulse width (0.3 ms) ECT and retrospective comparison with standard pulse width right unilateral ECT. *Journal of Affective Disorders, 103*(1-3), 277–281.

Lopez, C., Tchanturia, K., Stahl, D., Booth, R., Holliday, J., & Treasure, J. (2008b). An examination of the concept of central coherence in women with anorexia nervosa. *International Journal of Eating Disorders, 41*(2), 143–152.

Lopez, C. A., Tchanturia, K., Stahl, D., & Treasure, J. (2008a). Central coherence in women with bulimia nervosa. *International Journal of Eating Disorders, 41*(4), 340–347.

Loring, D. W., Lee, G. P., & Meador, K. J. (1988). Revising the Rey-Osterrieth: Rating right hemisphere recall. *Archives of Clinical Neuropsychology, 3,* 239–247.

Loring, D. W., Martin, R. C., Meador, K. J., & Lee, G. P. (1990). Psychometric construction of the Rey-Osterrieth Complex Figure: Methodological considerations and interrater reliability. *Archives of Clinical Neuropsychology, 5,* 1–14.

Loring, D. W., & Meador, K. J. (2003). The Medical College of Georgia (MCG) complex Figures: Four forms for follow-up. In J. A. Knight (Ed.), *The handbook of Rey-Osterrieth Complex Figure Usage: Clinical and research application* (pp. 313–321). Lutz, FL: PAR.

Lu, P. H., Boone, K. B., Cozolino, L., & Mitchell, E. (2003). Effectiveness of the Rey-Osterrieth Complex Figure Test and the Meyers and Meyers Recognition Trial in the detection of suspect effort. *The Clinical Neuropsychologist, 17,* 426–440.

Maass, A., Düzel, S., Goerke, M., Becke, A., Sobieray, U., Neumann, K., . . . Düzel, E. (2015). Vascular hippocampal plasticity after aerobic exercise in older adults. *Molecular Psychiatry, 20*(5), 585–593.

Mataix-Cols, D., Alonso, P., Hernandez, R., Deckersbach, T., Savage, C. R., Menchon, J. M., & Vellejo, J. (2003). Relation of neurological soft signs to nonverbal memory performance in obsessive-compulsive disorder. *Journal of Clinical and Experimental Neuropsychology, 25,* 842–851.

McConley, R., Martin, R., Baños, J., Blanton, P., & Faught, E. (2006). Global/local scoring modifications for the Rey–Osterrieth Complex Figure: Relation to unilateral temporal lobe epilepsy patients. *Journal of the International Neuropsychological Society, 12*(3), 383–390.

McConley, R., Martin, R., Palmer, C. A., Kuzniecky, R., Knowlton, R., & Faught, E. (2008). Rey–Osterrieth Complex Figure Test spatial and figural scoring: Relations to seizure focus and hippocampal pathology in patients with temporal lobe epilepsy. *Epilepsy & Behavior, 13*(1), 174–177.

Meador, K. J., Loring, D. W., Allen, M. E., Zamrini, E. Y., Moore, E. E., Abney, O. L., & King, D. W. (1991). Comparative cognitive effects of carbamazepine and phenytoin in healthy adults. *Neurology, 41,* 1537–1540.

Meador, K. J., Moore, E. E., Nichols, M. E., Abney, O. L., Taylor, H. S., Zamrini, E. Y., & Loring, D. W. (1993). The role of cholinergic systems in visuospatial processing and memory. *Journal of Clinical and Experimental Neuropsychology, 15,* 832–842.

Meyers, J., & Meyers, K. (1995b). *The Meyers Scoring System for the Rey Complex Figure and the Recognition Trial: Professional manual.* Odessa, FL: Psychological Assessment Resources.

Meyers, J., & Meyers, K. (1996). *Rey Complex Figure and the Recognition Trial: Professional manual: Supplemental norms for children and adolescents.* Odessa, FL: Psychological Assessment Resources.

Meyers, J. E., & Lange, D. (1994). Recognition subtest for the Complex Figure. *The Clinical Neuropsychologist, 8,* 153–166.

Meyers, J. E., & Meyers, K. R. (1995a). Rey Complex Figure Test under four different administration procedures. *The Clinical Neuropsychologist, 9,* 63–67.

Meyers, J. E., & Volbrecht, M. (1999). Detection of malingerers using the Rey Complex Figure and Recognition Trial. *Applied Neuropsychology, 6,* 201–207.

Miatton, M., Wolters, M., Lannoo, E., & Vingerhoets, G. (2004). Updated and extended normative data of commonly used neuropsychological tests. *Psychologica Belgica, 44,* 189–216.

Mitrushina, M., & Satz, P. (1991). Effect of repeated administration of a neuropsychological battery in the elderly. *Journal of Clinical Psychology, 47,* 790–801.

Mitrushina, M., Satz, P., & Chervinsky, A. B. (1990). Efficiency of recall on the Rey-Osterrieth Complex Figure in normal aging. *Brain Dysfunction, 3,* 148–150.

Mitrushina, M. M., Boone, K. B., Razani, J., & D'Elia, L. F. (2005). *Handbook of normative data for neuropsychological assessment* (2nd ed.). New York: Oxford University Press.

Morra, L. F., Garcon, S. M., Lucas, M. E., & Donovick, P. J. (2013). Intervening tasks and visuospatial memory: The role of similarity in retroactive interference. *The Clinical Neuropsychologist, 27*(5), 818–826.

Nelson, N. W., Boone, K., Dueck, A., Wagener, L., Lu, P., & Grills, C. (2003). Relationships between eight measures of suspect effort. *The Clinical Neuropsychologist, 17,* 263–272.

Osterrieth, P. A. (1944). Le test de copie d'une figure complex: Contribution a l'étude de la perception et de la mémoire. *Archives de Psychologie, 30,* 286–356.

Ostrosky-Solis, F., & Jaine, R. M., & Ardila, A. (1998). Memory abilities during normal aging. *International Journal of Neuroscience, 93,* 151–162.

Paikkatt, B., Akhouri, S., Jahan, M., & Singh, A. R. (2014). Visuospatial constructional ability, visual memory and recognition ability among individuals with chronic alcohol dependence on the rey complex figure test (RCFT). *Acta Neuropsychologica, 12*(3), 319–328.

Peirson, A. R., & Jansen, P. (1997). Comparability of the Rey-Osterrieth and Taylor forms of the Complex Figure Test. *The Clinical Neuropsychologist, 11,* 244–248.

Ponton, M. O., Gonzalez, J. J., Hernandez, I., Herrera, L., & Higareda, I. (2000). Factor analysis of the Neuropsychological Screening Battery for Hispanics (NeSBHIS). *Applied Neuropsychology, 7,* 32–39.

Ponton, M. O., Satz, P., Herrera, L., Ortiz, F., Urrutia, C. P., Young, R., . . . Namerow, N. (1996). Normative data stratified by age and education for the Neuropsychological Screening Battery for Hispanics (NeSBHIS): Initial report. *Journal of the International Neuropsychological Society, 2,* 96–104.

Poreh, A., & Shye, S. (1998). Examination of the global and local features of the Rey Osterrieth Complex Figure using faceted smallest space analysis. *The Clinical Neuropsychologist, 12,* 453–467.

Poulton, R. G., & Moffitt, T. E. (1995). The Rey-Osterrieth Complex Figure Test: Norms for young adolescents and an examination of validity. *Archives of Clinical Neuropsychology, 10,* 47–56.

Rabin, L. A., Barr, W. B., & Burton, L. A. (2005). Assessment practices of clinical neuropsychologists in the United States and Canada: A survey of INS, NAN, and APA Division 40 members. *Archives of Clinical Neuropsychology, 20,* 33–65.

Rabin, L. A., Paolillo, E., & Barr, W. B. (2016). Stability in test-usage practices of clinical neuropsychologists in the united states and canada over a 10-year period: A follow-up survey of INS and NAN members. *Archives of Clinical Neuropsychology, 31*(3), 206–230. https://doi.org/10.1093/arclin/acw007

Rapport, L. J., Dutra, R. L., Webster, J. S., Charter, R., & Morrill, B. (1995). Hemispatial deficits on the Rey-Osterrieth Complex Figure drawing. *The Clinical Neuropsychologist, 9,* 169–179.

Rapport, L. J., Farchione, T. J., Dutra, R. L., Webster, J. S., & Charter, R. (1996). Measures of hemi-inattention on the Rey Figure copy by the Lezak-Osterrieth scoring method. *The Clinical Neuropsychologist, 10,* 450–454.

Reedy, S. D., Boone, K. B., Cottingham, M. E., Glaser, D. F., Lu, P. H., Victor, T. L., . . . Wright, M. J. (2013). Cross validation of the Lu and colleagues (2003) Rey–Osterrieth Complex Figure Test effort equation in a large known-group sample. *Archives of Clinical Neuropsychology, 28*(1), 30–37.

Rey, A. (1941). L'examen psychologique dans les cas d'encephalopathie traumatique. *Archives de Psychologie, 28,* 286–340.

Rosenbloom, M. J., Sassoon, S. A., Pfefferbaum, A., & Sullivan, E. V. (2009). Contribution of regional white matter integrity to visuospatial construction accuracy, organizational strategy, and memory for a complex figure in abstinent alcoholics. *Brain Imaging and Behavior, 3*(4), 379–390.

Rosselli, M., & Ardila, A. (1991). Effects of age, education, and gender on the Rey-Osterrieth Complex Figure. *The Clinical Neuropsychologist, 5,* 370–376.

Rosselli, M., & Ardila, A. (1996). Cognitive effects of cocaine and polydrug abuse. *Journal of Clinical and Experimental Neuropsychology, 18,* 122–135.

Ruffolo, J. S., Javorsky, D. J., Tremont, G., Westervelt, H. J., & Stern, R. A. (2001). A comparison of administration procedures for the Rey-Osterrieth Complex Figure: Flowcharts versus pen switching. *Psychological Assessment, 13,* 299–305.

Sakamoto, M., & Spiers, M. V. (2014). Sex and cultural differences in spatial performance between Japanese and North Americans. *Archives of Sexual Behavior, 43*(3), 483–491.

Savage, C. R., Baer, L., Keuthen, N. J., Brown, H. D., Rauch, S. L., & Jenike, M. A. (1999). Organizational strategies mediate nonverbal memory impairment in obsessive-compulsive disorder. *Biological Psychiatry, 45,* 905–916.

Savage, C. R., Deckersbach, T., Wilhelm, S., Rauch, S. L., Baer, L., Reid, T., & Jenicke, M. A. (2000). Strategic processing and episodic memory impairment in obsessive compulsive disorder. *Neuropsychology, 14,* 141–151.

Scarpina, F., Ambiel, E., Albani, G., Pradotto, L. G., & Mauro, A. (2016). Utility of Boston Qualitative Scoring System for Rey–Osterrieth Complex Figure: Evidence from a Parkinson's diseases sample. *Neurological Sciences, 37*(10), 1603–1611.

Schreiber, H. E., Javorsky, D. J., Robinson, J., & Stern, R. A. (1999). Rey-Osterrieth Complex Figure performance in adults with attention deficit hyperactivity disorder: A validation study of the Boston Qualitative Scoring System. *The Clinical Neuropsychologist, 13,* 509–520.

Schretlen, D. J., Testa, S. M., & Pearlson, G. D. (2010). *Calibrated Neuropsychological Normative System.* Lutz, FL: PAR.

Schwarz, L., Penna, S., & Novack, T. (2009). Factors contributing to performance on the Rey Complex Figure Test in individuals with traumatic brain injury. *The Clinical Neuropsychologist, 23*(2), 255–267.

Seeck-Hirschner, M., Baier, P. C., Sever, S., Buschbacher, A., Aldenhoff, J. B., & Göder, R. (2010). Effects of daytime naps on procedural and declarative memory in patients with schizophrenia. *Journal of Psychiatric Research, 44*(1), 42–47.

Seidman, L. J., Lanca, M., Kremen, W. S., Faraone, S. V., & Tsuang, M. T. (2003). Organizational and visual memory deficits in schizophrenia and bipolar psychoses using the Rey-Osterrieth Complex Figure: Effects of duration of illness. *Journal of Clinical and Experimental Neuropsychology, 25,* 949–964.

Seo, S. W., Kang, C., Kim, S. H., Yoon, D. S., Liao, W., Wörz, S., . . . Cho, Z. (2012). Measurements of lenticulostriate arteries using 7T MRI: New imaging markers for subcortical vascular dementia. *Journal of the Neurological Sciences, 322*(1-2), 200–205.

Sherman, B. J., Savage, C. R., Eddy, K. T., Blais, M. A., Deckersbach, T., Jackson, S. C., . . . Herzog, D. B. (2006). Strategic memory in adults with anorexia nervosa: Are there similarities to obsessive compulsive spectrum disorders? *International Journal of Eating Disorders, 39*(6), 468–476.

Sherman, E. M. S., Strauss, E., Spellacy, F., & Hunter, M. (1995). Construct validity of WAIS-R factors: Neuropsychological test correlates in adults referred for possible head injury. *Psychological Assessment, 7,* 440–444.

Shin, M. S., Park, S. J., Kim, M. S., Lee, Y. H., Ha, T. H., & Kwon, J. S. (2004). Deficits in organizational strategy and visual memory in obsessive-compulsive disorder. *Neuropsychology, 18,* 665–672.

Slick, D. J., Sherman, E. M., & Iverson, G. L. (1999). Diagnostic criteria for malingered neurocognitive dysfunction: Proposed standards for clinical practice and research. *The Clinical Neuropsychologist, 13*(4), 545–561.

Shin, N. Y., Kang, D., Choi, J., Jung, M. H., Jang, J. H., & Kwon, J. S. (2010). Do organizational strategies mediate nonverbal memory impairment in drug-naïve patients with obsessive-compulsive disorder? *Neuropsychology, 24*(4), 527–533.

Somerville, J., Tremont, J., & Stern, R. A. (2000). The Boston Qualitative Scoring System as a measure of executive functioning in Rey-Osterrieth Complex Figure performance. *Journal of Clinical and Experimental Neuropsychology, 22,* 613–621.

Stern, R. A., Javorsky, D. J., Singer, E. A., Singer Harris, N. G., Somerville, J. A., Duke, L. M., . . . Kaplan, E. (1999). *The Boston qualitative scoring system for the Rey-Osterrieth Complex Figure.* Odessa, FL: Psychological Assessment Resources.

Stern, R. A., Singer, E. A., Duke, L. M., Singer, N. G., Morey, C. E., Daughtrey, E. W., & Kaplan, E. (1994). The Boston qualitative scoring system for the Rey-Osterrieth Complex Figure: Description and interrater reliability. *The Clinical Neuropsychologist, 8,* 309–322.

Strauss, E., & Spreen, O. (1990). A comparison of the Rey and Taylor figures. *Archives of Clinical Neuropsychology, 5,* 417–420.

Suhr, J. A., & Gunstad, J. (2005). Further exploration of the effect of "diagnosis threat" on cognitive performance in individuals with mild head injury. *Journal of the International Neuropsychological Society, 11,* 23–29.

Taylor, E. M. (1959). *Psychological appraisal of children with cerebral defects.* Cambridge, MA: Harvard University Press.

Taylor, L. B. (1969). Localization of cerebral lesions by psychological testing. *Clinical Neurosurgery, 16,* 269–287.

Taylor, L. B. (1979). Psychological assessment of neurosurgical patients. In T. Rasmussen & R. Marino (Eds.), *Functional neurosurgery* (pp. 165–180). New York: Raven Press.

Tei, H., Miyazaki, A., Iwata, M., Osawa, M., Nagata, Y., & Maruyama, S. (1997). Early stage Alzheimer's disease and multiple subcortical infarction with mild cognitive impairment: Neuropsychological comparison using an easily applicable test battery. *Dementia & Geriatric Cognitive Disorders, 8,* 355–358.

Tombaugh, T. N., & Hubley, A. M. (1991). Four studies comparing the Rey-Osterrieth and Taylor complex figures. *Journal of Clinical and Experimental Neuropsychology, 13,* 587–599.

Tombaugh, T. N., Schmidt, J. P., & Faulkner, P. (1992). A new procedure for administering the Taylor Complex Figure: Normative data over a 60-year age span. *The Clinical Neuropsychologist, 6,* 63–79.

Tremblay, M., Potvin, O., Callahan, B. L., Belleville, S., Gagnon, J. F., Caza, N., . . . Macoir, J. (2015). Normative data for the Rey–Osterrieth and the Taylor Complex Figure tests in Quebec-French people. *Archives of Clinical Neuropsychology, 30*(1), 78–87.

Trojano, L., Fragassi, N. A., Chiacchio, L., Izzo, O., Izzo, G., Di Cesare, G., . . . Grossi, D. (2004). Relationships between constructional and visuospatial abilities in normal subjects and in focal brain-damaged patients. *Journal of Clinical and Experimental Neuropsychology, 26,* 1103–1112.

Troyer, A. K., & Wishart, H. (1997). A comparison of qualitative scoring systems for the Rey-Osterrieth Complex Figure test. *The Clinical Neuropsychologist, 11,* 381–390.

Tupler, L. A., Welsh, K. A., Asare-Aboagye, Y., & Dawson, D. V. (1995). Reliability of the Rey-Osterrieth Complex Figure in use with memory-impaired patients. *Journal of Clinical and Experimental Neuropsychology, 17,* 566–579.

Vingerhoets, G., De Soete, G., & Jannes, C. (1995). Relationship between emotional variables and cognitive test performance before and after open-heart surgery. *The Clinical Neuropsychologist, 9,* 198–202.

Vingerhoets, G., Lannoo, E., & Wolters, M. (1998). Comparing the Rey-Osterrieth and Taylor complex figures: Empirical data and meta-analysis. *Psychologica Belgica, 38-2,* 109–119.

Vlachos, F., Andeou, G., & Andreou, E. (2003). Biological and environmental influences in visuospatial abilities. *Learning and Individual Differences, 13,* 339–347.

Vogel, A., Stokholm, J., & Jørgensen, K. (2012). Performances on Rey Auditory Verbal Learning Test and Rey Complex Figure Test in a healthy, elderly Danish sample—reference data and validity issues. *Scandinavian Journal of Psychology, 53*(1), 26–31.

Waber, D. P., & Holmes, J. M. (1985). Assessing children's copy productions of the Rey-Osterrieth Complex Figure. *Journal of Clinical and Experimental Neuropsychology, 7,* 264–280.

Waber, D. P., & Holmes, J. M. (1986). Assessing children's memory productions of the Rey-Osterrieth Complex Figure. *Journal of Clinical and Experimental Neuropsychology, 8,* 565–580.

Weinstein, C. S., Kaplan, E., Casey, M. B., & Hurwitz, I. (1990). Delineation of female performance on the Rey-Osterrieth Complex Figure. *Neuropsychology, 4,* 117–127.

Westervelt, H. J., Bruce, J. M., & Faust, M. A. (2016). Distinguishing Alzheimer's disease and dementia with Lewy bodies using cognitive and olfactory measures. *Neuropsychology, 30*(3), 304–311.

Wilson, N., & Batchelor, J. (2015). Examining Rey Complex Figure Test organization in healthy adults. *Journal of Clinical and Experimental Neuropsychology, 37*(10), 1052–1061.

Yamashita, H. (2006). Comparability of the Rey–Osterrieth Complex Figure, the Taylor Complex Figure, and the Modified Taylor Complex Figure in a normal sample of Japanese speakers. *Psychological Reports, 99*(2), 531–534.

Yamashita, H. (2010). Right- and left-hand performance on the Rey–Osterrieth Complex Figure: A preliminary study in non-clinical sample of right handed people. *Archives of Clinical Neuropsychology, 25*(4), 314–317.

Zuchova, S., Kubena, A. A., Erler, T., & Papezova, H. (2013). Neuropsychological variables and clinical status in anorexia nervosa: Relationship between visuospatial memory and central coherence and eating disorder symptom severity. *Eating and Weight Disorders, 18*(4), 421–428.

RIVERMEAD BEHAVIOURAL MEMORY TEST—THIRD EDITION (RBMT-3)

TEST NAME	**Rivermead Behavioural Memory Test—Third Edition (RBMT-3)**
DOMAIN	Verbal and visual memory (including prospective memory)
AGE RANGE	16 to 89 years
ADMINISTRATION TIME	30 minutes including delay interval
SCORING FORMAT	Hand scored
REFERENCE	Wilson, B. A., Greenfield, E., Clare, L., Baddeley, A., Cockburn, J., Watson, P., . . . Nannery, R. (2008). *The Rivermead Behavioural Memory Test* (3rd ed.) (RBMT-3). London: Pearson Assessment. www.pearsonclinical.com

DESCRIPTION

The purpose of the Rivermead Behavioural Memory Test—Third Edition (RBMT-3) is to detect memory impairment and monitor change over time. The RBMT (Wilson et al., 1985) was originally designed to detect memory problems that might interfere with rehabilitation of adults with acquired neurological damage (Cockburn & Keene, 2001; Wilson et al., 1989b). The test does not adhere to any particular theoretical model of memory; instead, it attempts to mimic the demands made on memory by normal daily life (Aldrich & Wilson, 1991). It does this through the use of items that involve either remembering to carry out some everyday task or retaining the type of information needed for adequate everyday functioning. As the RBMT was designed as a screening test for memory impairment, it is not sufficiently sensitive to detect mild deficits. To enhance the test's sensitivity, Wilson and her colleagues devised a more sensitive measure by increasing the level of difficulty through doubling the amount of material to be remembered on some subtests and making modifications to reduce floor and ceiling effects. Versions A and B of the original test were combined to make Version 1 of the Rivermead Behavioural Memory Test-Extended Version (RBMT-E), and Versions C and D of the original test were combined to make Version 2 of the RBMT-E (Wilson et al., 1999). The second edition (RBMT-II; Wilson et al., 2003) involves only minor changes to the original: it includes an updated set of photographs that are more representative of the multiracial nature of society and a slight change in the scoring procedure for the Route task. The current third edition includes several changes to improve the clinical applicability and utility of the RBMT, including adjustment to the item difficulty and updates to the normative data (see Table 10–96 for specific changes). The manual provides intervention strategies using RBMT-3 test results to help plan rehabilitation. The original RBMT has been translated into 14 languages, including Dutch (Van Balen & Groot Zwaaftink, 1987), German (Markowitsch et al., 1993), Spanish (Perez & Godoy, 1998), Turkish (Küçükdeveci et al., 2008), Irish (Hynes & Shiel, 2014), and Chinese (Man & Li, 2001). To our knowledge, only a Dutch version is available for the RBMT-3.

STRUCTURE

The original RBMT consists of 11 subtests that were chosen based on a study of memory problems typically experienced by people with head injury (Sunderland et al., 1983). The original structure is retained on the RBMT-3. Four subtests (Story, Route, Messages, and the Novel Task) have an immediate and a delayed recall component.

Memory for common objects and for faces is assessed using a recognition paradigm in which subjects must identify the original items among distractors. Prospective memory is assessed by three tasks: (a) remembering at the end of the session to ask for a personal possession that was put away at the beginning of the session, (b) remembering when an alarm rings to ask a specific question that was assigned when the alarm was set 20 minutes earlier, and (c) remembering to take a message on a route around the room and deliver it at a specific point along the route. There are two parallel versions of the RBMT-3 (Version 1 and 2), so that some of the practice effects caused by repeated testing with the same test can be minimized.

ADMINISTRATION

See Source. Briefly, the examiner presents stimuli, asks questions, traces a route, and records responses.

The manual provides a modified procedure to administer the Route Recall task to immobile examinees. Specifically, a model route using toy houses, trees, a car, a small block, and a bridge may be given, where the car goes on a journey with the block on its roof. Other examples may include asking the examinee to move a small figure

TABLE 10–96 Rivermead Behavioural Memory Test—Third Edition (RBMT-3) Subtests and Changes Made

SUBTEST		DESCRIPTION	CHANGES IN RBMT-3
1	First and Second Names	Examinee is shown photographic portraits and asked to recall first and last names of people in the photographs after a delay	Materials were updated
2	Belongings	A possession of the examinee is borrowed and secreted; the examinee is requested to ask for the belonging at the end of the test session and remember where it is hidden	Unchanged
3	Appointments	An alarm is set, and the examinee is required to ask two specific questions when the alarm sounds	Examinee to ask two questions instead of one
4	Picture Recognition	Line drawings are shown, and the examinee must recognize them from distractors after a delay	Stimuli updated; number of items increased
5	Story (Immediate, Delay)	Examinee listens to a story and then recalls it immediately and after a delay	Difficulty, imageability, and number of concepts of stories were modified
6	Face Recognition	Examinee is shown a set of faces and must recognize them from distractors after a delay	Stimuli updated to expand the ethnic diversity; number of items increased
7	Route (Immediate, Delay)	Examinee must retrace a route shown by the examiner immediately and after a delay	Number of sections increased; removed option to retrace route on paper
8	Messages (Immediate, Delay)	Examinee must remember to retrieve a message left on the route	Unchanged
9	Orientation and Date	Examinee is asked a set of orientation questions to assess knowledge of time, place, and person	Unchanged
10	Novel Task (Immediate, Delay)	Examinee is shown a specific order to put together different colored puzzle pieces and then asked to recall it	New task

SOURCE: Adapted from Wilson et al. (2008).

around a line drawing of a room (Towle & Wilsher, 1989). Clare et al. (2000) suggested that the Route and Messages subtests could be replaced by other versions of the tasks (Model Route Immediate, Newspaper Immediate, Model Route Delayed, and Newspaper Delayed) in which small figures are moved around mockups of the tasks (examiners are referred to Clare et al., 2000, to set up their own display). Normative data have been provided for these tasks (see the section "Normative Data"). As with the standard version, the route is first demonstrated by the tester, and the examinee is then asked to demonstrate it both immediately and after a delay. However, whether the model route is equivalent to the real route in the RBMT-3 remains to be examined, but it is unlikely that these tasks tap similar aspects of topographical memory.

SCORING

See the manual for scoring guidelines. The sum of scaled scores is used to convert to the General Memory Index (GMI).

DEMOGRAPHIC EFFECTS

AGE

Information on age effects on the RBMT-3 is not reported. On the RBMT/RBMT-II, scores increase with age and reach adult levels at about age eight years. Some have reported that middle-aged adults show a decline in performance (Fraser et al., 1999; Martin et al., 2000), whereas others have reported that decline emerges only after age 70 years (see Source; Elfkides et al., 2002; Van Balen et al., 1996). On the RBMT-E, age affects performance on Story (delayed), Route (immediate and delayed), Messages (delayed), Appointments, and Belongings subtests, with younger adults performing better than older ones (Wilson et al., 1999).

GENDER

Information on gender effects on the RBMT-3 is not reported. On the RBMT/RBMT-II, gender has little influence on performance in adolescents or adults (Aldrich & Wilson, 1991; Man & Li, 2001; Wilson et al., 1990, 1991), although Elfkides et al. (2002) noted that men perform better than women on the Belongings and Immediate Route tasks. On the RBMT-E, gender affects scores on some subtests (Route delayed, Messages immediate and delayed, First Names, Appointments, and Belongings), with women performing better than men (Wilson et al., 1999).

EDUCATION AND IQ

Information on education/IQ effects the RBMT-3 is not available. Education appears to affect RBMT performance (Elfkides et al., 2002; Fennig et al., 2002). On the RBMT/RBMT-II, modest to moderate correlations with intelligence are reported ($r = .21$ to .58; Cockburn & Smith, 1989, 2003; Fennig et al., 2002; Wilson et al., 1990; Wilson et al., 2003). The influence of intelligence operates primarily through performance on the Orientation and Story recall components of the test (Wilson et al., 1989a). IQ affects scores on most RBMT-E subtests (Story, Picture Recognition, Route, Orientation, First and Second Names; Wilson et al., 1999).

ETHNICITY, NATIONALITY, AND LINGUISTIC EFFECTS

No information on ethnicity is available on the RBMT-3. On the RBMT-E, examinees of European, African-Caribbean, and Asian origin were evaluated, with no systematic differences reported (Wilson et al., 1999).

NORMATIVE DATA

Normative data for the RMBT-3 are available in the manual for ages 16 to 89 ($N = 333$, age mean = 44.3, $SD = 18.17$; Wilson et al., 2008). Characteristics of the standardization sample are presented in Table 10–97. Tables for raw score to scaled score conversion are provided in the manual according to the examinee's age band. In addition, a mixed clinical sample comprising 75 individuals [TBI ($N = 19$), stroke ($N = 24$), encephalitis ($N = 20$), and progressive conditions ($N = 12$)] is included.

MODIFIED PROCEDURE

The modified procedure for the Route and Newspaper tasks was given to 111 healthy adults (72 women, 39 men), ranging in age from 16 to 76 years ($M = 41.1$, $SD = 15.5$) with a mean NART score of 113 ($SD = 7.35$, range = 90–127; Clare et al., 2000). The participants were part of the standardization sample for the RBMT-E in Sydney and Cambridge, and the tasks were administered as part of the longer test session in which the full RBMT-E was given. The normative data are reported in Table 10–98.

TABLE 10–97 Characteristics of the Rivermead Behavioural Memory Test—Third Edition (RBMT-3) Standardization Sample

Sample size	333
Age[a]	16 to 89 years
Geographical region	Scotland, Northern Ireland, Wales, Northern England, Midlands and East Anglia, Southern England (including London)
Sample type	Based on 2001 Census data for England and Wales, and for Scotland
Education[b]	35% Level 0 16% Level 1 18% Level 2 9% Level 3 21% Level 4
Gender	52% Women 48% Men
Ethnicity	94% White 6% Non-white
Exclusion criteria	History of hospitalization or treatment for severe psychiatric disturbance, drug or alcohol abuse; inadequate spoken English; severe visual impairment; brain damage or loss of consciousness for ≥5 minutes

NOTE: Values are rounded. With the exception of characteristics that are relatively uniformly distributed, only the percentage of the majority is shown.

[a] Age bands: 16–24 years (N = 49), 25–34 years (N = 67), 35–44 years (N = 56), 45–54 years (N = 61), 55–64 years (N = 45), 65–75 years (N = 29), 75–89 years (N = 26).

[b] Education levels based on the following England/Wales and Scotland system or equivalent: Level 0 = no qualifications; Level 1 = ≥1 "O" level or CSE/GCSE passes for England/Wales, and O Grade, Standard Grade, Intermediate 1 & 2 for Scotland; Level 2 = ≥5 "O" level or CSE (grade 1) or GCSE (grade A to C) passes for England/Wales, and Higher Grade for Scotland; Level 3 = ≥2 "A" level, ≥4 "AS" level passes, Higher School Certification for England/Wales, and HND for Scotland; Level 4 = First Degree and above for England/Wales and Scotland.

SOURCE: Adapted from Wilson et al. (2008).

EVIDENCE FOR RELIABILITY

EVIDENCE FOR INTERNAL RELIABILITY

Alternate form reliability (see Table 10–99) was used as evidence of internal reliability for the RBMT-3 (Wilson et al., 2008). The authors note that the majority of the healthy population should obtain a maximum score because the RBMT-3 is designed for the impaired population and therefore the reliability coefficients are low. A much higher reliability estimate is obtained with a mixed sample comprising clinical and healthy individuals (Table 10–99; Wilson et al., 2008). A high value of Cronbach's alpha (.86) is demonstrated for the Chinese version of the RBMT (Man & Li, 2001). No information on other versions is available.

EVIDENCE FOR TEST-RETEST RELIABILITY, MEASURING CHANGE, AND PRACTICE EFFECTS

Man and Li (2001) administered the same form of the Chinese RBMT to stroke patients twice within a two-week period and reported high test-retest reliability ($r = .89$). No information is available for the RBMT-3 or other versions.

EVIDENCE FOR RELIABILITY OF ALTERNATE FORMS

Alternate form reliability of the RBMT-3 subtests ranges from low to adequate as presented in Table 10–99 (Wilson et al., 2008).

EVIDENCE FOR INTERRATER RELIABILITY

High interrater agreement ($r > .91$) is reported for all RBMT-3 subtests except Messages Delayed Recall ($r = .79$; Wilson et al., 2008). Man and Li (2001) also reported adequate to high interrater reliability (.74 to .95) when two raters evaluated stroke patients on the Chinese version of the RBMT.

EVIDENCE FOR VALIDITY

FACTOR-ANALYTIC STUDIES

Wilson and colleagues (2008) submitted the RBMT-3 subtests to principal components factor analysis using the core standardization sample. Version 1 yielded a general factor that accounted for 32% of the variance with moderate to high loadings on most subtests except Picture Recognition (Wilson et al., 2008). Version 2 yielded similar results with 31% of the variance accounted for by the general factor. Using a mixed sample, similar results but with higher percentage of variance accounted for (about 50%) were found for both versions (Wilson et al., 2008).

TABLE 10–98 Conversion of Raw Scores to Profile Scores for the Modified Administration of the Rivermead Behavioural Memory Test—Third Edition (RBMT-3) Model Route and Newspaper Tasks

		PROFILE SCORE				
TASK	SUBGROUPS (AGE IN YEARS)	0	1	2	3	4
Model Route Immediate	Version 1 (<30, 30–50)	0–10	11–13	14–17	18	19
	Version 1 (>50)	0–8	9–11	12–15	16–18	19
	Version 2 (all ages)	0–7	8–11	12–16	17–18	19
Model Route Delayed	Version1 (<30, 30–50)	0–8	9–12	13–16	17–18	19
	Version 1 (>50)	0–7	8–9	10–15	16–18	19
	Version 2 (all ages)	0–8	9–11	12–15	16–18	19
Newspaper Immediate	All	0–2	3	4	5	6
Newspaper Delayed	All	0–2	3	4	5	6

SOURCE: From Clare et al. (2000).

PRIOR VERSIONS

Wester and colleagues (2013a) gave both the RBMT and RBMT-3 to 25 individuals with alcohol-related memory impairment, including patients with Korsakoff's syndrome. They found that performance of patients and healthy controls differs on both RBMT versions but fewer ceiling effects were seen on the RBMT-3 (up to 32% of patients) than RBMT (up to 60% of patients) in all but Belongings and Messages subtests. Moreover, although floor effects are relatively rare for both versions, fewer floor effects were found on the RBMT-3 Names and Appointments subtests (20% and 24%, respectively) than on the RBMT (48% and 52%, respectively). Examining the frequency of impaired performance (<5th percentile) on both versions, 0 to 8% of healthy controls and 24 to 68% of patients obtained impaired scores on the RBMT-3. On the RBMT, between 4 and 20% of healthy controls and 40 to 84% of patients obtained impaired scores. Compared to the RBMT, fewer healthy controls are classified as impaired on the RBMT-3. The authors concluded that the RBMT-3 is an improvement over the previous version (Wester et al., 2013a).

RELATIONSHIPS WITH OTHER TESTS

No independent studies are available. The manual noted that, in a mixed clinical and healthy sample, the RBMT-3 GMI shows moderate correlation with the proxy rating of the Prospective and Retrospective Memory Questionnaire, a rating scale for everyday memory problems, whereas weak correlation is found with the self-rating (Wilson et al., 2008).

CLINICAL STUDIES

The RBMT-3 appears to be sensitive to memory impairments in individuals with alcohol-related disorders that affect memory, including chronic alcoholism and

TABLE 10–99 Alternate Form Reliabilities for the Rivermead Behavioural Memory Test—Third Edition (RBMT-3) Subtests

	HEALTHY SAMPLE	MIXED SAMPLE
High (.80 to .89)	GMI Version 1 GMI Version 2	Orientation and Date
Adequate (.70 to .79)	Story—Delayed Recall Orientation and Date	Novel Task—Immediate Recall Story—Delayed Recall Picture Recognition—Delayed Recognition
Marginal (.60 to .69)	Story—Immediate Recall Novel Task	Novel Task—Delayed Recall Messages—Delayed Recall Route—Delayed Recall Face Recognition—Delayed Recognition Story—Immediate Recall Belongings First and Second Names
Low (<.59)	Messages Route Picture Recognition—Delayed Recognition Belongings First and Second Names Appointments Face Recognition—Delayed Recognition	Appointments Route—Immediate Recall

SOURCE: Adapted from Wilson et al. (2008).

Korsakoff's syndrome (Altgassen et al., 2016; Rensen et al., 2015; Wester et al., 2013a; Wester et al., 2013b; Wester et al., 2013c), with individuals with chronic alcoholism performing better than those with Korsakoff's syndrome (Altgassen et al., 2016; Rensen et al., 2015). Interestingly, confabulation in Korsakoff's syndrome is associated with poorer RBMT-3 but not executive function scores (D-KEFS TMT and Tower, Stroop Color-Word, Wechsler Intelligence Scale for Children [WISC] Mazes; Rensen et al., 2015). Wester and colleagues reported that patients with Korsakoff's syndrome perform worse than healthy controls on all RBMT-3 subtests whereas those with chronic alcoholism perform worse than healthy controls on all but Picture Recognition, Story-Delayed Recall, Messages-Immediate Recall, and Orientation subtests (Wester et al., 2013b). In addition, patients with Korsakoff's syndrome perform worse than those with chronic alcoholism on all but Story-Immediate Recall subtests. The largest effect sizes are seen on delayed recall, orientation, and cued/uncued prospective memory tests in patients with Korsakoff's syndrome. Using ROC analysis, the RBMT-3 GMI yielded an AUC of .85, a sensitivity of 80%, and a specificity of 69% at a cutoff score of less than 67.5 for classifying Korsakoff's and chronic alcoholism patients. At a cutoff of less than 87.5, AUC was .83, sensitivity was 80%, and specificity was 62% to identify patients with chronic alcoholism from healthy controls. As such, the authors concluded that the RBMT-3 appears to be a valid measure for assessing those with alcohol-related disorders (Wester et al., 2013b).

The test battery has also been used to monitor memory functioning in intervention studies among patients with acquired brain injury (McDonald et al., 2011) and to assess memory functioning in MCA stroke patients who underwent decompressive craniectomy (McKenna et al., 2012). In the latter, a case series of five MCA stroke patients who had infarction in the left hemisphere performed at ceiling on the Picture Recognition subtest whereas those with right-hemisphere infarction committed low-average to borderline omission errors. By contrast, on the Story subtest, those with right-hemisphere infarction obtained better scores than those with left-hemisphere infarction. A majority of the patients obtained impaired scores on the Orientation subtest, but the impaired scores were not due to aphasia (McKenna et al., 2012). This case series suggested that the three RBMT-3 subtests have differential sensitivity to dysfunction in different brain regions. However, Mayer and colleagues (2012) reported in a single case study of a patient with cerebral autosomal dominant arteriopathy with subcortical infarcts and leukoencephalopathy (CADASIL) that the patient performed within normal limits on the RBMT-3 (Mayer et al., 2012).

NEUROANATOMICAL CORRELATES AND IMAGING STUDIES

None reported.

PERFORMANCE VALIDITY

None reported.

COMMENT

The RBMT-3 is designed as an ecologically valid memory measure, with test items designed to sample memory behaviors characteristic of everyday activities. The inclusion of prospective memory tasks (remembering to carry out actions) is unique among memory tests. One should bear in mind, however, that the interpretation of the Messages subtest as a measure of prospective memory is not universally accepted, and further empirical evidence of its use as a prospective memory measure would be useful. Modifications to the Route task are available for mobility-impaired individuals. However, a task based on remembering a route traced by a model figure will tap somewhat different aspects of memory than one that requires the individual to navigate around the room; in the latter case the person's own position is changing relative to the environment, whereas this does not occur in the model version (Clare et al., 2000).

Although it appears to be a complement to more traditional memory-assessment techniques, there is no empirical evidence to indicate that the RBMT-3 is actually better at tapping ecologically relevant aspects of memory than other tests. The current edition has undergone revisions to address issues related to ceiling and floor effects and to improve the ethnic diversity of the Faces subtest, but few studies have been conducted on the revised third edition. The ceiling effects, while improved over the original, remain very high. There is no research on demographic effects, including the impact of age, gender, education/IQ, and ethnicity. It is of note that the normative sample is from the UK only, almost completely Caucasian, and not well-described. Considerable additional research is also needed regarding the test's psychometric properties. The RBMT-3 demonstrates poor alternate form reliability for some subtests, and information regarding internal consistency and test-retest reliability is meager, particularly for a test aimed at tracking change. The lack of studies on the relationship with other neuropsychological tests, a critical aspect of validity, is also another major criticism of the RBMT-3. Scant research has been done to validate its use for diagnostic or tracking purposes. Future studies should aim to assess the performance of various clinical groups such as dementia, MCI, and TBI; provide further evidence of the utility of the RMBT-3 in rehabilitation or intervention; and develop embedded validity indicators. At this time, the limitations of the RMBT-3 restrict its clinical application.

REFERENCES

Aldrich, F. K., & Wilson, B. (1991). Rivermead Behavioural Memory Test for Children (RBMT-C): A preliminary evaluation. *British Journal of Clinical Psychology, 30,* 161–168.

Altgassen, M., Ariese, L., Wester, A. J., & Kessels, R. P. C. (2016). Salient cues improve prospective remembering in Korsakoff's syndrome. *British Journal of Clinical Psychology, 55*(2), 123–136.

Clare, L., Wilson, B. A., Emslie, H., Tate, R., & Watson, P. (2000). Adapting the Rivermead Behavioral Memory Test Extended Version (RBMT-E) for people with restricted mobility. *British Journal of Psychology, 39*, 363–369.

Cockburn, J., & Keene, J. (2001). Are changes in everyday memory over time in autopsy-confirmed Alzheimer's disease related to changes in reported behavior? *Neuropsychological Rehabilitation, 11*, 201–271.

Cockburn, J., & Smith, P. T. (1989, 2003). *The Rivermead Behavioural Memory Test. Supplement 3: Elderly people.* Bury St. Edmunds, UK: Thames Valley Test Company.

Elfkides, A., Yiultsi, E., Kangellidou, T., Kounti, F., Dina, F., & Tsolaki, M. (2002). Weschler Memory Scale, Rivermead Behavioral Memory Test, and Everyday Memory Questionnaire in healthy adults and Alzheimer's patients. *European Journal of Psychological Assessment, 18*, 63–77.

Fennig, S., Mottes, A., Ricter-Levin, G., Treves, I., & Levkovitz, Y. (2002). Everyday memory and laboratory memory tests: General function prediction in schizophrenia and remitted depression. *Journal of Nervous & Mental Disease, 190*, 677–682.

Fraser, S., Glass. J. N., & Leathem, J. M. (1999). Everyday memory in an elderly New Zealand population: Performance on the Rivermead Behavioral Memory Test. *New Zealand Journal of Psychology, 28*, 118–123.

Hynes, S., & Shiel, A. (2014). Validating an Irish-Language Version of the Rivermead Behavioural Memory Test—Second Edition. *The British Journal of Occupational Therapy, 77*(4), 198–204.

Küçükdeveci, A. A., Kutlay, Ş., Elhan, A. H., & Tennant, A. (2008). Construct validity and reliability of the Rivermead Behavioural Memory Test in the Turkish population. *Brain Injury, 22*(1), 75–82.

Man, D. W. K., & Li, R. (2001). Assessing Chinese adults' memory abilities: Validation of the Chinese version of the Rivermead Behavioral Memory Test. *The Clinical Gerontologist, 24*, 27–36.

Markowitsch, H. J., von Cramon, Y., & Schuri, U. (1993). Mnestic performance profile of a bilateral diencephalic infarct patient with preserved intelligence and severe amnestic disturbances. *Journal of Clinical and Experimental Neuropsychology, 15*, 627–652.

Martin, C., West, J., Cull, C., & Adams, M. (2000). A preliminary study investigating how people with mild intellectual disabilities perform on the Rivermead Behavioral Memory Test. *Journal of Applied Research in Intellectual Disabilities, 13*, 186–193.

Mayer, J. F., Bishop, L. A., & Murray, L. L. (2012). The feasibility of a structured cognitive training protocol to address progressive cognitive decline in individuals with vascular dementia. *American Journal of Speech-Language Pathology, 21*(2), 167–179.

McDonald, A., Haslam, C., Yates, P., Gurr, B., Leeder, G., & Sayers, A. (2011). Google calendar: A new memory aid to compensate for prospective memory deficits following acquired brain injury. *Neuropsychological Rehabilitation, 21*(6), 784–807.

McKenna, A., Wilson, F. C., Caldwell, S., Curran, D., Nagaria, J., & Convery, F. (2012). Long-term neuropsychological and psychosocial outcomes of decompressive hemicraniectomy following malignant middle cerebral artery infarctions. *Disability and Rehabilitation, 34*(17), 1444–1455.

Perez, M., & Godoy, J. (1998). Comparison between a "traditional" memory test and a "behavioral" memory battery in Spanish patients. *Journal of Clinical and Experimental Neuropsychology, 20*, 496–502.

Rensen, Y. C. M., Oosterman, J. M., van Damme, J. E., Griekspoor, S. I. A., Wester, A. J., Kopelman, M. D., & Kessels, R. P. C. (2015). Assessment of confabulation in patients with alcohol-related cognitive disorders: The Nijmegen–Venray confabulation list (NVCL-20). *The Clinical Neuropsychologist, 29*(6), 804–823.

Sunderland, A., Harris, B., & Baddeley, A. D. (1983). Do laboratory tests predict everyday behavior? A neuropsychological study. *Journal of Verbal Learning and Verbal Behavior, 22*, 341–357.

Towle, D., & Wilsher, C. R. (1989). The Rivermead Behavioural Memory Test: Remembering a short route. *British Journal of Clinical Psychology, 28*, 287–288.

Van Balen, H. G. G., & Groot Zwaftink, A. J. M. (1987). The Rivermead Behavioral Memory Test. Handleiding (The Rivermead Behavioral Memory Test Manual). Reading, UK: Thames Valley Test Company.

Van Balen, H. G. G., Westzaan, P. S. H., & Mulder, T. (1996). Stratified norms for the Rivermead Behavioral Memory Test. *Neuropsychological Rehabilitation, 6*, 203–217.

Wester, A. J., Leenders, P., Egger, J. I. M., & Kessels, R. P. C. (2013a). Ceiling and floor effects on the Rivermead Behavioural Memory Test in patients with alcohol-related memory disorders and healthy participants. *International Journal of Psychiatry in Clinical Practice, 17*(4), 286–291.

Wester, A. J., van Herten, J. C., Egger, J. I. M., & Kessels, R. P. C. (2013b). Applicability of the Rivermead Behavioural Memory Test—Third Edition (RBMT-3) in Korsakoff's syndrome and chronic alcoholics. *Neuropsychiatric Disease and Treatment, 9*, 875–881.

Wester, A. J., Westhoff, J., Kessels, R. P. C., & Egger, J. I. M. (2013c). The Montreal Cognitive Assessment (MoCA) as a measure of severity of amnesia in patients with alcohol-related cognitive impairments and Korsakoff syndrome. *Clinical Neuropsychiatry, 10*(3-4), 134–141.

Wilson, B. A., Baddeley, A., Cockburn, J., & Hiorns, R. (1989a, 1991). *Rivermead Behavioural Memory Test: Supplement Two.* Bury St. Edmunds, UK: Thames Valley Test Company.

Wilson, B. A., Baddeley, A., Cockburn, J., & Hiorns, R. (1989b). The development and validation of a test battery for detecting and monitoring everyday memory problems. *Journal of Clinical and Experimental Neuropsychology, 11*, 855–870.

Wilson, B. A., Clare, L., Cockburn, J. M., Baddeley, A. D., Tate, R., & Watson, P. (1999). *The Rivermead Behavioural Memory Test—Extended Version.* Bury St. Edmunds, UK: Thames Valley Test Company.

Wilson, B. A., Cockburn, J., & Baddeley, A. (1985). *The Rivermead Behavioural Memory Test.* Bury St. Edmunds, UK: Thames Valley Test Company.

Wilson, B. A., Cockburn, J., Baddeley, A., & Hiorns, R. (2003). The Rivermead Behavioral Memory Test-II Supplement Two. Bury St. Edmunds, UK: Thames Valley Test Company.

Wilson, B. A., Forester, S., Bryant, T., & Cockburn, J. (1990). Performance of 11–14 year olds on the Rivermead Behavioural Memory Test. *Clinical Psychology Forum, December, 30*, 8–10.

Wilson, B. A., Greenfield, E., Clare, L., Baddeley, A., Cockburn, J., Watson, P., Tate, R., Sopena, S., & Nannery, R. (2008). *The Rivermead Behavioural Memory Test* (3rd ed.) (RBMT-3). London: Pearson Assessment.

SELECTIVE REMINDING TEST (SRT)

TEST NAME	**Selective Reminding Test (SRT)**
DOMAIN	Verbal memory
AGE RANGE	18 to 91 years
ADMINISTRATION TIME	30 minutes plus 30-minute delay interval
SCORING FORMAT	Hand scored
REFERENCE	Buschke, H. (1973). Selective reminding for analysis of memory and learning. *Journal of Verbal Learning and Verbal Behavior, 12*, 543–550.

DESCRIPTION

The Selective Reminding Test (SRT; Buschke, 1973; Buschke & Fuld, 1974) measures verbal learning and memory using a multiple-trial list-learning paradigm. Other names for the test are the Buschke Selective Reminding Test (BSRT) and the Verbal Selective Reminding Test (VSRT). The test has interesting aspects because it purports to parcel verbal memory into distinct component processes. It involves reading to the examinee a list of words and then having the examinee recall as many of these words as possible. Each subsequent learning trial involves the selective presentation of only those items that were not recalled on the immediately preceding trial. The SRT distinguishes between short-term and long-term components of memory by measuring recall of items that were not presented on a given trial. The rate at which examinees learn can also be evaluated.

A number of different versions of the test exist. For adults, the version described here is the same as that developed by Hannay and Levin (1985; Hannay, 1986). Briefly, the test consists of a series of 12 unrelated words presented over 12 selective reminding (SR) trials, or until the examinee is able to recall the entire list on three consecutive trials. A cued-recall trial is presented after the 12th or last selective-reminding trial. The first two or three letters of each word are presented on an index card, and the examinee is asked to recall the corresponding list word. After the cued-recall trial, the examiner presents a multiple-choice recognition trial. Here, the examiner presents a series of 12 index cards, each consisting of a list word, a synonym, a homonym, and an unrelated distractor word. Finally, a delayed-recall trial is given without forewarning 30 minutes after the multiple-choice recognition trial. Therefore, several trials allow the examiner to identify the conditions that promote otherwise impaired memory (e.g., cueing, multiple-choice recognition) or forgetting (e.g., delayed recall; Hannay & Levin, 1985).

Four different forms of the test are available. Figure 10–10 provides the word lists and Figure 10–11 gives the multiple-choice and cued-recall items for the versions of the test used with adults. Other translated versions available includes Greek (Zalonis et al., 2009), Hebrew (Gigi et al., 1999), and Spanish (Campo & Morales, 2004; Campo et al., 2000, 2003; Morales et al., 2010).

ADMINISTRATION

There is no commercial source. Users may refer to this text to design their own materials. Figure 10–12 shows the specific instructions for administering the SRT. The materials include a list of words, index cards containing

Form 1	*Form 2*	*Form 3*	*Form 4*
Bowl	Shine	Throw	Egg
Passion	Disagree	Lily	Runway
Dawn	Fat	Film	Fort
Judgement	Wealthy	Discreet	Toothache
Grant	Drunk	Loft	Drown
Bee	Pin	Beef	Baby
Plane	Grass	Street	Lava
County	Moon	Helmet	Damp
Choice	Prepare	Snake	Pure
Seed	Prize	Dug	Vote
Wool	Duck	Pack	Strip
Meal	Leaf	Tin	Truth

Figure 10–10 *Word list for Forms 1 through 4 of the adult version of the Selective Reminding Test (SRT).*

SOURCE: From Hannay & Levin (1985). Reprinted with the kind permission of Psychology Press.

Form 1		Multiple-Choice Words	
1. bowl	dish	bell	view
2. love	poison	conform	passion
3. dawn	sunrise	bet	down
4. pasteboard	verdict	judgement	fudge
5. grand	grant	give	jazz
6. see	sting	fold	bee
7. pain	plane	pulled	jet
8. county	state	tasted	counter
9. voice	select	choice	cheese
10. flower	seed	herd	seek
11. date	sheep	wool	would
12. mill	queen	food	meal
Form 2			
1. shine	glow	chime	cast
2. dispute	disappear	contour	disagree
3. fat	oil	trail	fit
4. stopwatch	affluent	wealthy	worthy
5. trunk	drunk	stoned	blunt
6. fin	peg	wake	pin
7. glass	grass	plan	lawn
8. moon	beam	spark	noon
9. propose	ready	prepare	husband
10. award	prize	pot	size
11. bark	bird	duck	luck
12. leap	ranch	blade	leaf
Form 3			
1. throw	toss	through	plate
2. flower	lilt	intent	lily
3. film	movie	slave	kiln
4. waver	cautious	discreet	distinct
5. soft	loft	attic	tack
6. beet	meat	clue	beef
7. stream	street	speed	road
8. helmet	armor	bacon	velvet
9. smoke	serpent	snake	pool
10. hoed	dug	hay	dog
11. blank	bundle	pack	puck
12. ton	shirt	foil	tin
Form 4			
1. egg	shell	beg	source
2. airline	runner	darling	runway
3. fort	castle	sink	fork
4. boldness	dentist	toothache	headache
5. blown	drown	float	rib
6. body	infant	middle	baby
7. larva	lava	echo	rock
8. damp	moist	hook	stamp
9. purse	clean	pure	bare
10. ballot	vote	dish	note
11. chain	peal	strip	slip
12. trust	rise	fact	truth

Cued-Recall Words

Form 1	Form 2	Form 3	Form 4
BO	SH	TH	RU
PA	DI	LI	FO
DA	FA	FI	TO
JUD	WEA	DI	DR
GR	DR	LO	BA
PL	GR	BE	LA
COU	MO	ST	DA
CH	PRE	HE	PU
SE	PR	DU	VO
WO	DU	PA	ST
ME	LE	SN	TR
_	_	_	_

Figure 10–11 *Multiple-choice and cued-recall items for Forms 1 through 4 of the Selective Reminding Test (SRT).*

SOURCE: From Hannay (1986), and Hannay & Levin (1985).

"This test is to see how quickly you can learn a list of words. I am going to read you a list of words. I want you to listen carefully, because when I stop, I want you to tell me as many of the words as you can recall. The words do not have to be in any particular order. When you have given me all the words that you can recall, I will tell you the words that you didn't give me from the list; then I want you to give me the entire list all over again. We do this 12 times and each time I want you to try to give me all the words"

Read the list of words at a rate of one word every 2 s, and always present the words in order, beginning with the top of the list and working to the bottom. The presentation of words will, of course, skip over the words that were recalled correctly on the preceding trial. If the examinee is able to recall correctly all 12 words on three consecutive trials, discontinue, but score as if all trials had been given. If the examinee recalls words not on the list, inform the examinee, and note the extra words. The total number of words on the list is not disclosed.

For the cued-recall trial, the first two to three letters of each list word are presented on an index card and the examinee is asked to say the word from the list that would begin with the first two letters on the card. The cue cards are presented one at a time in the same order as the words on the list. There is no time limit, and the examinee is allowed to return to a previous card if they wish. Because one word on Form 1 (bee) can be clearly identified by the first two letters, it is omitted from cued recall, as are pin, tin, and egg on Forms 2, 3, and 4, respectively. Cues that fail initially to evoke the list word are presented a second time, after each cue has been given once. For the multiple-choice recognition trial, the examinee is shown each of the 12 index cards and is asked to identify the list word. Give the cued-recall and multiple-choice trials even if the examinee has recalled the entire list on the selective reminding trials. After a 30-min delay, ask the examinee to recall all 12 words. During the 30-min delay, the examinee should be given nonverbal tasks to perform.

Figure 10–12 *Instructions for administering the Selective Reminding Test (SRT).* Adapted from Hannay & Levin (1985), Clodfelter et al. (1987), and Morgan (1982).

the first two to three letters of each list word, and index cards containing the multiple-choice recognition items. Record by number the order of the examinee's recall on each trial. Intrusions of extra-list words are also recorded on each trial.

SCORING

See sample score sheet shown in Figure 10–13. A number of different scores are calculated (Buschke & Fuld, 1974; Hannay & Levin, 1985). These are shown in Figure 10–14. If a word is recalled on two consecutive trials, it is assumed to have entered long-term storage (LTS) on the first of these trials. Once a word enters LTS, it is considered to be in permanent storage, and it is scored as LTS on all following trials, regardless of the examinee's subsequent recall. When an examinee recalls a word that has entered LTS, it is scored as long-term retrieval (LTR). When an examinee begins to recall a word in LTS consistently on all subsequent trials, it is also scored as consistent long-term retrieval (CLTR) or list-learning, beginning on the first of the uninterrupted successful recall trials. Inconsistent LTR refers to recall of a word in LTS followed by subsequent failure to recall the word. It is scored as random long-term retrieval (RLTR) until it is recalled consistently. Short-term recall (STR) refers to recall of a word that has not entered LTS. The total recall (Sum Recall) on each trial is the sum of STR and LTR. The number of reminders given by the examiner before the next recall attempt is equal to 12 minus the Sum Recall of the previous trial.

The reader is directed to Levin et al. (1982, pp. 110–111) for two completely scored examples.

DEMOGRAPHIC EFFECTS

AGE

There is a decline on most SRT measures with advancing age (Campo & Morales, 2004; McGinnis, 2012; Morales et al., 2010; Sliwinski et al., 1997; Stricks et al., 1998; Wiederholt et al., 1993; Zalonis et al., 2009). Recognition scores tend to be less affected by aging, suggesting that this measure could be a potential marker of abnormality (Campo & Morales, 2004).

Various indices of acquisition (LTS, CLTR) decline with age, particularly after age 50 years. There are also age-related differences in rate of forgetting, but the effects tend to be quite modest and depend on the particular index used to measure what was stored in acquisition (Petersen et al., 1992; Trahan & Larrabee, 1993).

GENDER

Gender also affects scores, with females outperforming males (Bishop et al., 1990; Campo & Morales, 2004; Caselli et al., 2015; Morales et al., 2010; Trahan & Quintana, 1990; Wiederholt et al., 1993; Zalonis et al., 2009), although gender explains the least variance of all demographic variables (Zalonis et al., 2009). One study suggested that the performance of men declines more rapidly than that of women (Wiederholt et al., 1993). Another study of older adults did not find gender differences in the rate of memory decline (Caselli et al., 2015).

EDUCATION AND IQ

The influence of education is inconsistent, with some studies finding it to be relatively unimportant (Petersen et al., 1992; Trahan & Quintana, 1990), but with others (Campo & Morales, 2004; Morales et al., 2010; Scherl et al., 2004; Zalonis et al., 2009) noting significantly better performance for those with more education on all indices except the short-term memory index.

Intelligence is moderately related to SRT performance (Bishop et al., 1990; Sherman et al., 1995). Therefore, use of SRT normative data that do not consider intellectual level may put clinicians at risk of overestimating memory deficits in individuals with low-average IQs (Bishop et al., 1990).

Name____________ Date______________ Examiner_______________

	1	2	3	4	5	6	7	8	9	10	11	12	CR	MC	30 min
Bowl															
Passion															
Dawn															
Judgement															
Grant															
Bee															
Plane															
County															
Choice															
Seed															
Wool															
Meal															

Total Recall ____________________

LTR ____________________

STR ____________________

LTS ____________________

CLTR ____________________

RLTR ____________________

Reminders ____________________

Intrusions ____________________

Trial 1 _______

Total Recall _______ (Number recalled over 12 trials)

LTS _______ (Number recalled twice in a row, assumed to be in LTS from that point on. Mark with red underliner, counting blanks. Compute sum over the 12 trials.)

STR _______ (Words that are not underlined. Compute sum over the 12 trials.)

CLTR _______ (Words that are continuously recalled. Mark with highlighter. Compute sum across the 12 trials.)

RLTR _______ (Words that are underlined but NOT CLTR. Do not count blanks. Compute sum across 12 trials.)

Reminders _______ (Compute sum over 12 trials. Maximum = 144)

Intrusions _______ (Compute sum over 12 trials.)

Cued Recall _______ (Maximum = 11)

Mult. Choice _______ (Maximum = 12)

30-Min Recall _______ (Maximum = 12)

Figure 10–13 *Sample Selective Reminding Test (SRT) Score Sheet—Form 1.*

LTS	If a word is recalled on two consecutive trials, it is assumed to have entered long-term storage (LTS) on the first of these trials.
LTR	When an examinee recalls a word that has entered LTS, it is scored as long-term retrieval (LTR).
CLTR	When an examinee begins to recall a word in LTS consistently on all subsequent trials, it is also scored as consistent long-term retrieval (CLTR) or list-learning, beginning on the first of the uninterrupted successful recall trials.
RLTR	Inconsistent LTR refers to recall of a word in LTS followed by subsequent failure to recall the word. It is scored as random long-term retrieval (RLTR) until it is recalled consistently.
STR	Short-term recall refers to recall of a word that has not entered LTS.
Sum Recall	The total recall on each trial is the sum of STR and LTR.
Reminders	The number of reminders given by the examiner before the next recall attempt is equal to 12 minus the Sum Recall of the previous trial.

Figure 10–14 *Abbreviations and definitions of Selective Reminding Test scores.*

ETHNICITY, NATIONALITY, AND LINGUISTIC EFFECTS

Stricks et al. (1998) found that English speakers tended to score slightly higher than Spanish speakers, although any performance differences might have been related to translation issues or other factors (e.g., cultural differences, quality of education).

NORMATIVE DATA

Larrabee et al. (1988) provided norms for the adult version (Form 1) of the SRT, organized by age and gender, shown in Table 10–100. The reader should note that corrections need to be made for gender (see Note in Table 10–100). In addition, note that the mean values for LTR and STR do not sum to the exact value of the total correct score. The same is true for the relationship of the mean values for CLTR and RLTR to LTR. These small discrepancies appeared because different gender corrections were used for these respective scores. To measure forgetting, Trahan and Larrabee (1993) recommended use of the acquisition score (defined as the Trial 12 LTS) minus the Delayed Recall score.

Similar data have been reported for middle-aged adults by Ruff et al. (1989). Masur et al. (1989) also provided normative data for a large sample of older adults. Their sample, however, contained a large number of non-native English speakers. This may account for the fact that their scores were somewhat lower than those reported here.

SHORT FORM

Smith et al. (1995) pointed out that there is no theoretical rationale for choosing 12 as the requisite number of trials. They found that as few as six trials provided information highly consistent with that provided by 12 trials. The only score with consistently lower correlations with 12-trial scores was RLTR, a not surprising finding since it is a measure of random LTR and is not expected to be consistent across trials (see also Larrabee et al., 2000). Drane et al. (1998) also reported high ($r > .90$) correlations between six- and 12-trial LTS and CLTR in a sample of patients with TLE.

TABLE 10–100 Norms (Mean and *SD*) for the Buschke Verbal Selective Reminding Test (SRT)12-Trial Administration

	AGE RANGE						
VARIABLES	18–29	30–39	40–49	50–59	60–69	70–79	80–91
N	51	29	31	24	50	59	27
Age (years)	22.55 (3.30)	34.62 (2.69)	43.71 (2.91)	54.17 (2.74)	66.00 (2.47)	74.49 (2.92)	83.48 (3.10)
Education (years)	12.88 (1.73)	14.90 (2.47)	14.71 (2.72)	12.92 (1.98)	13.40 (3.57)	13.46 (3.78)	13.22 (3.76)
Female/Male	23/28	15/14	19/12	22/2	33/17	38/21	23/4
Total Recall	128.18 (9.16)	124.59 (13.40)	125.03 (12.00)	121.62 (10.46)	114.82 (15.77)	105.27 (16.67)	97.96 (17.49)
LTR	122.16 (13.12)	118.14 (20.64)	118.55 (17.96)	112.71 (16.10)	101.52 (24.68)	89.95 (29.23)	77.22 (26.26)
STR	6.14 (4.82)	6.72 (7.59)	6.48 (6.72)	8.96 (6.40)	13.52 (9.52)	17.47 (10.41)	20.74 (9.62)
LTS	124.00 (10.47)	121.62 (18.36)	122.45 (15.64)	116.67 (14.52)	107.00 (21.79)	95.54 (24.86)	87.48 (25.26)
CLTR	115.12 (19.67)	107.93 (27.62)	107.10 (26.62)	101.50 (22.39)	88.92 (35.85)	69.68 (35.96)	54.96 (29.04)
RLTR	8.12 (9.42)	10.12 (9.73)	11.19 (11.34)	10.79 (9.25)	14.66 (11.83)	20.71 (14.37)	22.19 (10.70)
Reminders	16.00 (8.42)	18.10 (13.12)	19.03 (11.26)	22.25 (10.06)	28.12 (15.16)	36.95 (15.17)	43.96 (15.77)
Intrusions	0.84 (.29)	0.97 (1.43)	1.81 (3.10)	1.17 (1.49)	3.90 (7.29)	4.22 (5.76)	3.30 (5.09)
Cued Recall	—	—	—	—	9.58[a] (1.93)	8.95[b] (2.12)	8.16[c] (2.22)
Multiple Choice	12.00 (0.00)	12.00 (0.00)	12.00 (0.00)	12.00 (0.00)	11.96 (0.20)	11.85 (0.58)	11.93 (0.27)
Delayed Recall	11.53 (0.83)	10.66 (1.97)	11.03 (1.43)	10.83 (1.40)	9.58 (2.46)	9.05 (2.62)	8.37 (2.45)

NOTE: Correction values for raw scores of males (calculate before entering normative tables): Total = +5; LTR = +9; STR = -4; LTS = +7; CLTR = +13; RLTR = -5; Reminders = -5; Intrusions = 0: Cued Recall = 0; Multiple Choice = 0; Delayed Recall = +1. Caution: Do not correct LTS or CLTR if raw score is 0. See text for definitions of Total, LTR, STR, LTS, CLTR, RLTR, Reminders, Intrusions, Cued Recall, Multiple Choice, and Delayed Recall.

[a] *n* = 31.

[b] *n* = 38.

[c] *n* = 19.

SOURCE: From Larrabee et al. (1988).

Moreover, the six- and 12-trial SRT administrations demonstrated comparable sensitivity and discrimination in patients with left versus right temporal lobe seizure focus, unless the six-trial score fell in the range between 1 and 2 *SDs* below the age-appropriate mean. A six- or eight-trial SRT would significantly reduce administration time and patient fatigue.

Larrabee et al. (2000) published normative data based on 267 neurologically healthy adults (172 females, 95 males; age range, 18–91 years) for a six-trial administration of Form 1 of the SRT. The data were constructed by rescoring SRT protocols of the healthy individuals upon whom the 12-trial normative data were based (Larrabee et al., 1988). All participants were interviewed before testing to exclude those with neurological or psychiatric disorders, a history of drug abuse, or evidence of intellectual disability based on educational and occupational attainment. Furthermore, participants aged 60 years and older had to achieve a passing score on a measure of temporal orientation. The data are shown in Table 10–101.

A regression-based procedure is also provided (Larrabee et al., 2000) so that existing delayed recall norms, based on a 12-trial administration, can be used after a six-trial administration. The regression equation for predicting 30-minute delayed recall by six-trial LTS is as follows:

$$\text{Estimated 30-minute delayed recall} = 0.124\,(\text{six-trial LTS}) + 4.676 \qquad SE_E = 1.595$$

Once the predicted score is obtained, a CI should be constructed around the predicted score, based on the SE_E, multiplied by the *z* scores for the desired CI (e.g., for a 90% CI, the range would be ±2.624). If the examinee's actual 30-minute delayed score falls within the CI, then the 30-minute delay norms presented by Larrabee et al. (1988) can be used. These norms require a gender correction.

If the examinee's 30-minute delayed recall score falls outside the CI, this suggests either (a) acceleration of forgetting if the score is below the CI cutoff or (b) motivational factors if the score is above the CI cutoff, in a pattern suggesting better memory than learning. In either case, the 30-minute delay norms cannot be used if performance falls outside the CI predicted on the basis of the six-trial LTS.

Six-trial SRT scores generally show comparable classification of healthy versus clinical group classification in most clinical settings, unless the six-trial score falls in the range of 1 to 2 *SDs* below the age-appropriate mean (Drane et al., 1998; Larrabee et al., 2000). Accordingly, Larrabee et al. (2000) cautioned that, for scores in this range in clinical settings, the clinician should consider a 12-trial SRT administration, particularly if the SRT is the only measure of verbal learning and memory. Alternatively, if other measures of verbal memory have also been administered, they can be used in conjunction with the six-trial SRT to more reliably assess the construct of verbal learning and memory.

The data provided by Larrabee et al. (2000) represent a fairly well-educated sample and are derived from the 12-trial version. Others have developed norms for the 12-word, six-trial version. For example, Scherl et al. (2004) recruited a random sample of community-dwelling participants in New York and reported slightly lower scores than those reported by Larrabee et al. (2000). However, their sample was small (*N* = 75) and was limited to those aged 30 to 59 years.

For individuals with more limited levels of education, the norms provided by Stricks et al. (1998) appear to be more appropriate. These authors used the six-trial SRT, with a 15-minute delayed recall trial followed by a multiple-choice recognition task. They provided norms based on a sample of 557 older, English-speaking adults living in the New York City area who were screened as nondemented by

TABLE 10–101 Norms (Mean and SD) for the Buschke Verbal Selective Reminding Test (SRT) 6-Trial Administration

	AGE RANGE						
	18–29	30–39	40–49	50–59	60–69	70–79	80–91
N	49	28	31	23	50	59	27
Age	22.53 (3.36)	34.54 (2.70)	43.71 (2.91)	54.00 (2.68)	66.00 (2.47)	74.49 (2.91)	83.48 (3.11)
Education	12.92 (1.75)	14.96 (2.49)	14.71 (2.72)	13.09 (1.83)	13.43 (3.54)	13.46 (3.78)	13.22 (3.76)
Female/Male	23/26	15/13	19/12	21/2	33/17	38/21	23/4
Total Recall	55.35 (5.01)	54.48 (8.58)	54.26 (7.90)	53.13 (5.99)	49.74 (8.11)	45.36 (8.62)	41.93 (7.71)
STR	7.29 (4.50)	6.18 (5.25)	7.16 (5.84)	8.26 (5.20)	10.96 (5.79)	13.07 (5.24)	14.70 (5.43)
LTR	49.12 (8.80)	49.18 (12.93)	47.84 (12.88)	44.96 (10.00)	39.44 (13.10)	33.02 (12.45)	27.48 (12.46)
LTS	50.86 (8.71)	51.46 (12.51)	50.48 (12.83)	47.35 (10.10)	41.54 (12.93)	35.02 (12.40)	30.67 (13.32)
CLTR	44.65 (9.85)	43.29 (15.20)	40.84 (14.65)	38.30 (11.18)	33.98 (14.01)	27.83 (12.94)	19.70 (10.84)
RLTR	4.43 (3.74)	5.89 (5.17)	7.00 (5.45)	6.57 (4.45)	5.44 (4.76)	5.32 (3.93)	7.74 (4.74)
Intrusions	0.65 (.99)	0.82 (1.25)	1.29 (2.18)	0.83 (1.03)	1.38 (2.81)	1.85 (2.41)	1.38 (1.81)
Delayed Recall[a]	11.53 (0.83)	10.66 (1.97)	10.03 (1.43)	10.83 (1.40)	9.58 (2.46)	9.05 (2.62)	8.37 (2.45)

NOTE: Correction values for raw scores of males (calculate before entering normative tables): LTR = +4; STR = −2; LTS = +4, CLTR = +4. Caution: do not correct LTS or CLTR if raw score is 0. See text for definition of Total Recall, STR, LTR, LTS, RLTR, CLTR, and Intrusions.

[a] Delayed recall data are based on a 12-trial administration from data reported by Larrabee et al. (1988). These norms should be used only after the regression procedure described in the norms section. The delayed recall correction for males is +1.

SOURCE: Larrabee et al. (2000).

TABLE 10–102 Normative Data (Mean and Standard Deviation [*SD*]) for English and Spanish Speakers on the Six-Trial Version of the Selective Reminding Test (SRT), Followed by a 15-Minute Delayed Recall Trial and a Recognition Trial, by Age and Education

		AGE 60–69		AGE 70–79		AGE 80+		GRAND MEAN
	EDUCATION	<9 YEARS	9+ YEARS	<9 YEARS	9+ YEARS	<9 YEARS	9+ YEARS	
English Speakers[a] *(n)*		*21*	*93*	*91*	*198*	*56*	*99*	*557*
	Total Recall	39.8 (10.3)	43.5 (9.3)	31.8 (9.5)	39.8 (9.8)	27.7 (10.7)	34.2 (11.9)	36.9 (11.3)
	LTR	26.6 (13.3)	31.7 (13.3)	18.6 (10.7)	25.9 (13.3)	14.1 (10.6)	20.2 (14.1)	23.5 (13.8)
	LTS	29.5 (14.2)	35.2 (13.6)	22.1 (11.9)	29.3 (14.0)	17.1 (11.5)	23.0 (14.7)	26.8 (14.5)
	CLTR	19.1 (12.1)	23.4 (12.8)	11.3 (9.7)	18.2 (12.5)	7.1 (8.0)	13.8 (12.5)	16.1 (12.7)
	Intrusions	1.6 (2.7)	0.9 (1.7)	1.3 (2.7)	0.6 (1.3)	1.3 (2.1)	1.1 (1.7)	1.0 (1.9)
	Delayed Recall	5.3 (2.8)	6.7 (2.8)	4.5 (2.6)	5.8 (2.7)	2.8 (2.5)	4.9 (2.9)	5.3 (2.9)
	Delayed Recognition	10.9 (1.9)	11.4 (1.2)	10.2 (2.0)	11.2 (1.4)	9.1 (2.3)	10.8 (2.1)	10.7 (1.8)
Spanish Speakers[b] *(n)*		*74*	*21*	*179*	*47*	*66*	*25*	*412*
	Total Recall	36.2 (7.7)	40.5 (7.7)	34.1 (8.3)	39.1 (9.8)	27.6 (7.4)	30.6 (9.2)	34.1 (9.0)
	LTR	22.8 (9.5)	27.2 (11.4)	21.3 (9.5)	26.0 (12.1)	14.8 (7.4)	16.1 (11.1)	21.0 (10.3)
	LTS	25.5 (10.6)	30.5 (12.0)	24.5 (10.2)	28.9 (12.6)	18.4 (8.6)	18.9 (11.7)	24.2 (11.0)
	CLTR	15.6 (8.9)	19.6 (11.8)	13.5 (8.9)	19.0 (11.0)	7.8 (8.6)	9.7 (9.5)	13.7 (9.9)
	Intrusions	1.2 (1.8)	0.7 (1.4)	1.3 (2.1)	1.3 (1.7)	1.8 (2.6)	0.9 (1.7)	1.3 (2.1)
	Delayed Recall	4.9 (2.1)	5.9 (2.3)	4.6 (1.9)	5.5 (2.5)	3.5 (2.1)	4.4 (2.2)	4.6 (2.2)
	Delayed Recognition	10.8 (1.7)	11.3 (1.1)	10.4 (1.8)	10.9 (1.8)	9.8 (2.6)	10.7 (1.7)	10.5 (1.9)

[a] <9 years of education: age, *M* = 77.5, *SD* = 6.8; education, *M* = 6.1, *SD* = 2.1; ethnicity = 76% Black, 4% Hispanic. 9+ years of education: age, *M* = 75.1, *SD* = 6.6; education, *M* = 12.7, *SD* = 2.6; ethnicity = 53% Black, 5% Hispanic.

[b] <9 years of education: age, *M* = 74.5, *SD* = 6.0; education, *M* = 4.5, *SD* = 2.7; ethnicity = 8% Black, 99% Hispanic. 9+ years of education: age, *M* = 75.4, *SD* = 7.0; education, *M* = 12.0, *SD* = 3.0; ethnicity = 6% Black, 96% Hispanic.

SOURCE: Adapted from Stricks et al. (1998).

a physician. Individuals with neurological conditions that might affect cognition were also excluded. Approximately 4% of the examinees were Hispanic, and 60% were African American. About 68% were female. The normative data are shown in Table 10–102. In addition, a group of 412 nondemented, disease-free Spanish speakers (largely of Caribbean origin) were tested in Spanish. These data are also provided in Table 10–102.

Zalonis et al. (2009) provide adult to older adult norms for the Greek version of the SRT. The word list is found in Table 10–103. Administration of this Greek version is based on the standard Buschke (1973) administration. Tables 10–104 to 10–106 present the normative data stratified by age and education (Age bands: 18–29 (*N* = 72), 30–39 (*N* = 75), 40–49 (*N* = 80), 50–59 (*N* = 79), 60–69 (*N* = 69), and 70–83 (*N* = 68). Education bands: 3–9 (*N* = 137), 10–12 (*N* = 145), 13–18 (*N* = 161)).

TABLE 10–103 Greek Selective Reminding Test (SRT) Word List

ENGLISH ORIGINAL LIST[a]	GREEK ADAPTED LIST[b]	GREEK WORD[b]
Bowl	Bowl	Koupa
Passion	Passion	Pathos
Dawn	Dawn	Anatoli
Judgement	Judgement	Krisi
Grant	Gift	Doro
Bee	Bee	Melissa
Plane	Boat	Varka
Country	Country	Chora
Choice	Choice	Eklogi
Seed	Seed	Sporos
Wool	Wool	Yfasma
Meal	Meal	Fagito

[a]Hannay and Levin (1985).

[b]Developed by Zalonis et al. (2007).

SOURCE: Zalonis et al. (2009).

Morales et al. (2010) provide adult to older adult norms for two Spanish six-trial SRT alternate versions as shown in Tables 10–107 to 10–118. The sample was drawn from two projects. A total of 884 individuals were included in this normative study: 451 from a previous normative study of the Spanish SRT, the others drawn from a longitudinal study of older adults. A total of 391 individuals completed Form 2 (203 from the previous normative study, the rest from the longitudinal study). Age groups included: 15–29, 30–39, 40–49, 50–59, 60–69, 70–79, and 80–95. Education groups were based on the International Standard Classification of Education (UNESCO, 1976): primary education (low; mean = 5.95 years, *SD* = 2.53), junior vocational training (average; mean = 10.85 years, *SD* = 1.05), and senior vocational or academic training (high; mean = 16.21 years, *SD* = 2.81). Inclusion criteria included no history of neuropathological conditions, no prior hospitalization due to psychopathology, no history of abnormal development, no substance abuse history, minimal psychotropic medication, Spanish as primary language, Spanish MMSE of greater than 24, and GDS of greater than 5. Correlations between this version and the 12-trial SRT are moderate to high ($r = .64$ to $.89$).

The six learning trials are administered based on the standard Buschke SRT instructions. The multiple-choice recognition trial (Table 10–108) is given immediately after the six learning trials. Four words (each row as shown

TABLE 10–104 Age and Education Stratified Normative Data for the Greek Version of the Selective Reminding Test (SRT) for Adults with 3 to 9 Years of Education

	18–29		30–39		40–49		50–59		60–69		70–83	
AGE	M	*SD*	M	*SD*	M	*SD*	M	*SD*	M	*SD*	M	*SD*
Trial 1 Recall	5.7	1.2	5.5	1.0	4.7	.9	4.1	1.1	3.7	0.9	3.7	0.9
Total Recall	117.0	9.2	109.4	11.0	108.1	13.8	100.7	14.3	82.4	17.0	78.7	14.5
LTR	106.7	12.7	97.0	16.4	90.6	25.2	84.1	19.3	60.4	22.9	52.9	23.7
STR	10.2	4.6	11.8	6.0	16.3	10.5	16.6	5.9	22.0	10.0	25.8	11.0
LTS	113.0	10.3	103.8	12.1	98.2	22.3	92.5	19.5	71.3	24.3	62.5	26.1
CLTR	89.3	20.8	72.5	28.7	73.3	29.6	61.9	21.7	36.4	21.1	31.5	22.4
RLTR	16.3	8.5	25.3	15.5	19.3	13.7	22.6	8.3	23.4	9.6	21.9	10.0
Intrusions	0.3	0.6	1.3	2.2	2.6	3.1	4.0	5.0	6.4	6.7	3.8	3.1
Cued Recall	11.6	0.7	10.8	1.6	10.4	1.5	10.6	1.6	9.4	1.8	9.4	1.5
Delayed Recall	10.1	0.8	9.8	1.6	9.1	1.9	9.1	1.9	7.0	2.5	6.7	1.5
N	22		18		25		27		21		24	

NOTE: Based on Greek sample recruited from a large metropolitan area in Greece. *N* = 443, 51% female, age mean = 49.2, *SD* = 16.9, range = 18–83, education mean = 11.8, *SD* = 3.5, range = 3–18. Screened for history of neurological or psychiatric illnesses, medical treatment that can cause cognitive impairment, substance abuse history, <2nd percentile on TMT, and MMSE <24.

SOURCE: Adapted from Zalonis et al. (2009).

TABLE 10–105 Age and Education Stratified Normative Data for the Greek Version of the Selective Reminding Test (SRT) for Adults with 10 to 12 Years of Education

	18–29		30–39		40–49		50–59		60–69		70–83	
AGE	M	*SD*	M	*SD*	M	*SD*	M	*SD*	M	*SD*	M	*SD*
Trial 1 Recall	6.3	1.0	5.3	1.0	5.6	1.0	5.2	0.9	4.6	0.9	4.3	0.9
Total Recall	122.0	10.5	113.7	12.5	111.0	8.4	108.5	12.4	103.9	11.7	90.9	12.2
LTR	112.4	17.0	104.9	15.5	97.4	14.4	91.3	23.3	87.3	18.9	66.6	19.1
STR	9.6	6.6	8.8	4.9	16.6	6.8	17.2	11.6	16.4	8.5	24.3	8.6
LTS	117.0	15.4	115.4	12.2	106.1	14.2	98.7	23.6	96.4	17.8	77.7	19.9
CLTR	97.2	25.3	85.2	28.2	71.3	25.4	67.6	27.2	65.4	22.6	38.0	16.4
RLTR	14.5	9.0	20.6	13.1	26.1	14.5	23.6	13.7	22.0	8.4	27.2	12.4
Intrusions	1.3	2.2	4.1	4.5	2.5	3.1	2.8	3.8	1.8	2.2	3.4	2.4
Cued Recall	11.7	0.7	11.9	0.3	11.2	1.1	10.6	1.5	11.0	1.3	9.9	1.1
Delayed Recall	11.1	0.8	10.6	1.3	10.0	1.6	9.9	1.3	9.4	1.5	6.6	1.7
N	23		25		27		23		25		22	

NOTE: Based on Greek sample recruited from a large metropolitan area in Greece. *N* = 443, 51% females, age mean = 49.2, *SD* = 16.9, range = 18–83, education mean = 11.8, *SD* = 3.5, range = 3–18. Screened for history of neurological or psychiatric illnesses, medical treatment that can cause cognitive impairment, substance abuse history, <2nd percentile on TMT, and MMSE <24.

SOURCE: Adapted from Zalonis et al. (2009).

TABLE 10–106 Age and Education Stratified Normative Data for the Greek Version of the Selective Reminding Test (SRT) for Adults with 13 to 18 Years of Education

	18–29		30–39		40–49		50–59		60–69		70–83	
AGE	M	*SD*	M	*SD*	M	*SD*	M	*SD*	M	*SD*	M	*SD*
Trial 1 Recall	6.4	0.9	6.8	1.3	6.3	1.2	5.6	1.1	5.6	1.3	4.5	0.9
Total Recall	126.6	7.0	124.4	10.9	119.9	11.6	108.9	16.3	112.3	13.2	101.8	11.2
LTR	121.4	10.5	116.3	17.8	110.9	18.2	92.8	25.5	98.4	20.7	86.5	15.9
STR	5.2	4.2	8.1	7.4	9.0	7.2	16.1	9.7	13.9	8.6	15.4	6.1
LTS	126.0	8.6	121.1	15.2	118.8	15.3	101.0	21.3	105.3	19.7	95.9	14.7
CLTR	107.8	21.7	100.6	29.4	87.1	28.7	66.8	39.6	78.8	26.5	56.1	17.7
RLTR	14.1	13.1	15.8	13.7	25.1	16.8	24.4	15.6	19.8	11.4	33.2	9.9
Intrusions	0.8	2.1	1.4	3.0	1.8	3.4	1.8	3.1	4.4	4.2	2.8	2.9
Cued Recall	11.8	0.5	11.7	1.0	11.7	0.5	11.4	1.0	11.4	0.8	10.7	1.2
Delayed Recall	11.8	0.5	11.1	1.0	11.0	1.2	10.0	1.5	9.6	1.7	8.5	1.5
N	27		32		28		29		23		22	

NOTE: Based on Greek sample recruited from a large metropolitan area in Greece. N = 443, 51% females, age mean = 49.2, *SD* = 16.9, range = 18–83, education mean = 11.8, *SD* = 3.5, range = 3–18. Screened for history of neurological or psychiatric illnesses, medical treatment that can cause cognitive impairment, substance abuse history, <2nd percentile on TMT, and MMSE <24.

SOURCE: Adapted from Zalonis et al. (2009).

TABLE 10–107 Words Comprising Forms 1 and 2 of the Spanish Six-Trial Selective Reminding Test (SRT)

FORM 1	FORM 2
Dado	Fácil
Cinta	Pipa
Norte	Bar
Jarro	Tiesto
Pollo	Duque
Frente	Costa
Llave	Sudor
Cruz	Perro
Fuego	Ley
Pena	Feliz
Modelo	Tía
Oído	Cierto

SOURCE: From Morales et al. (2010).

in Table 10–108) are shown to the examinee at once, and the examinee is to pick the target word out of the foils. Thirty minutes after the multiple-choice recognition trial, the delayed-recall trial is administered followed by the multiple-choice recognition trial again.

EVIDENCE FOR RELIABILITY

EVIDENCE FOR INTERNAL RELIABILITY

Information regarding internal reliability is not available.

TABLE 10–108 Words for the Recognition Trial of the Spanish Six-Trial Selective Reminding Test (SRT)

FORM 1			
Dado	Ficha	Lado	Moto
Reloj	Lazo	Pinta	Cinta
Norte	Cuadro	Oeste	Corte
Tinaja	Carro	Jarro	Lápiz
Espejo	Pollo	Bollo	Gallina
Fuente	Mapa	Cara	Frente
Cerradura	Título	Llave	Clave
Cruz	Luz	Puerta	Medalla
Incendio	Juego	Fuego	Flor
Vena	Pena	Niño	Llanto
Tigre	Patrón	Pomelo	Modelo
Caído	Oído	Olfato	Seta
FORM 2			
Fácil	Difícil	Cajón	Ágil
Revista	Pipa	Pita	Tabaco
Bar	Mar	Café	Pared
Jarrón	Puesto	Tiesto	Peine
Buque	Duque	Marqués	Cristal
Mosca	Playa	Betún	Costa
Sangre	Sudor	Prisa	Pudor
Perro	Santo	Cerro	Gato
Caja	Justicia	Ley	Rey
Licor	Perdiz	Alegría	Feliz
Día	Melón	Tía	Sobrino
Duda	Cactus	Puerto	Cierto

SOURCE: From Morales et al. (2010).

EVIDENCE FOR TEST-RETEST RELIABILITY, MEASURING CHANGE, AND PRACTICE EFFECTS

Information regarding test-retest reliability using the same form is not available.

One older study shows that there was no significant practice effect when patients with seizures underwent multiple administrations of alternate forms on four consecutive days (Westerveld et al., 1994). With healthy individuals, however, there appears to be a nonspecific practice effect with repeated administration of alternate forms based on old studies (Clodfelter et al., 1987; Hannay & Levin, 1985; Loring & Papanicolaou, 1987). There do not appear to be more recent studies on practice effects for the 12-trial version.

Practice effects are also noted when healthy individuals are given alternate forms of the six-trial SRT over a 12- to 16-week retest interval. Salinsky et al. (2001) tested a sample of 62 adults (age M = 34 years, range = 19–62; education M = 13.8 years, range 10–19) and reported Spearman correlations ranging from .55 (30-minute delayed recall) to .71 (CLTR). Practice effects were most pronounced for CLTR, Total Recall, and LTS but not on 30-minute delayed recall.

Dikmen et al. (1999) reported test-retest data for a 10-item, 10-trial version in a large group of neurologically healthy adults. Most were tested over an 11-month interval. Their findings were similar to those reported by Salinsky et al. (2001).

EVIDENCE FOR RELIABILITY OF ALTERNATE OR SHORT FORMS

Many of the existing studies on this question are quite dated. For example, in college students, Forms 2 to 4 are of equivalent difficulty, whereas Form 1 is about 10% harder than Forms 3, 4, and 5 (Hannay & Levin, 1985). However, the four forms appear to be of equivalent difficulty for older adults (Masur et al., 1989) and for patients with clinical memory disorders, at least for those with medically refractory epilepsy (Westerveld et al., 1994).

Other studies report that alternate form reliability coefficients tend to be variable (r = .48 to .85) in magnitude for both healthy and neurological samples (Clodfelter et al., 1987; Hannay & Levin, 1985; Westerveld et al., 1994), although values of .92 (for consistent retrieval) have been reported for patients with AD (Masur et al., 1989). Total Recall scores are the most stable, and STM scores are the least stable (Westerveld et al., 1994). Westerveld et al. (1994) suggested that use of the mean or the better of two baseline assessments minimizes error variance, thereby enhancing interpretation of change. Alternatively, given that Total Recall scores generally are less variable and that SRT scores appear to measure a single construct, examiners may choose to rely on Total Recall scores.

TABLE 10–109 Norms for Spanish Selective Reminding Test (SRT) Form 1 for TR and LTR Scores Stratified by Age and Education for Women

GROUP VARIABLES			TR							LTR						
			Z VALUES							Z VALUES						
AGE	EDUCATION	SEX	−1.64 (5%)	−1.28 (10%)	−0.84 (20%)	0 (50%)	0.84 (60%)	1.28 (90%)	1.64 (95%)	−1.64 (5%)	−1.28 (10%)	−0.84 (20%)	0 (50%)	0.84 (60%)	1.28 (90%)	1.64 (95%)
25	L	W	39.2	40.2	42.6	51.0	51.8	57.8	60.0	23.2	25.0	31.0	40.0	42.2	51.2	55.6
	A	W	43.3	44.0	47.2	53.0	54.6	59.8	62.7	24.3	26.2	34.0	46.0	48.0	56.2	60.4
	H	W	43.0	47.3	49.6	58.0	59.0	63.0	66.0	29.6	33.3	39.2	53.0	55.0	60.4	64.3
35	L	W	36.8	39.2	44.8	47.0	47.0	55.6	57.2	22.4	26.4	28.0	36.0	38.0	48.0	51.4
	A	W	43.0	43.0	43.4	51.0	52.0	54.9	57.7	25.9	29.7	36.2	43.0	45.2	48.9	53.0
	H	W	43.5	46.0	48.0	53.5	54.0	61.0	66.8	29.0	30.0	35.0	42.0	47.0	56.0	64.5
45	L	W	28.4	32.2	35.8	47.0	47.0	52.0	52.1	13.7	21.4	23.6	31.0	33.8	42.4	44.0
	A	W	38.8	41.2	43.2	45.5	47.8	55.6	57.8	18.8	21.4	25.8	32.0	33.2	51.4	53.3
	H	W	39.4	41.4	47.4	52.5	53.2	57.6	59.0	24.9	26.0	34.6	45.5	48.0	52.6	54.0
55	L	W	30.0	31.7	37.8	46.0	47.0	52.3	55.1	16.0	17.4	21.0	31.0	33.0	44.0	47.1
	A	W	31.8	35.8	39.4	48.0	49.0	59.0	60.6	18.2	19.8	26.6	38.0	39.4	54.6	58.2
	H	W	36.6	39.8	43.2	47.0	50.0	59.0	62.7	17.3	18.0	26.8	33.0	36.8	54.0	59.8
65	L	W	24.1	27.7	31.0	41.5	44.0	52.0	55.3	7.4	9.7	13.0	27.0	30.0	41.0	46.6
	A	W	32.0	35.0	38.0	42.5	45.0	52.5	58.2	10.5	13.5	21.0	28.5	32.0	47.5	51.8
	H	W	34.0	35.0	39.0	45.0	46.0	51.0	54.5	11.5	14.0	19.0	32.0	34.0	44.0	47.0
75	L	W	16.5	19.0	23.0	33.0	38.0	50.0	54.5	2.0	4.0	5.0	20.0	23.0	40.0	46.5
	A	W	27.6	29.0	29.4	34.0	35.0	44.2	48.1	6.2	8.2	10.0	12.5	18.8	27.8	34.7
	H	W	16.4	20.8	32.0	42.0	42.8	49.4	50.2	2.0	4.0	12.8	29.0	33.0	42.2	46.6
85	L	W	19.2	20.4	21.0	23.0	26.2	37.8	39.4	0.0	0.0	1.2	13.0	13.0	19.8	21.4
	A	W	34.0	34.0	34.0	34.0	34.0	34.0	34.0	8.0	8.0	8.0	8.0	8.0	8.0	8.0
	H	W	24.6	26.1	29.2	38.5	41.6	50.9	52.4	9.7	11.4	14.8	25.0	28.4	38.6	40.3

NOTE: The raw test score leading to a particular z value is given indicating the percentiles 5, 10, 20, 50, 60, 90, and 95. LTR, Long-Term Retrieval; TR, Total Recall; L, low; A, average; H, high; % = percentile

SOURCE: From Morales et al. (2010).

TABLE 10–110 Norms for Spanish Selective Reminding Test (SRT) Form 1 for LTS and STR Scores Stratified by Age and Education for Women

GROUP VARIABLES			LTS							STR						
			Z VALUES							*Z* VALUES						
AGE	EDUCATION	SEX	−1.64 (5%)	−1.28 (10%)	−0.84 (20%)	0 (50%)	0.84 (60%)	1.28 (90%)	1.64 (95%)	−1.64 (5%)	−1.28 (10%)	−0.84 (20%)	0 (50%)	0.84 (60%)	1.28 (90%)	1.64 (95%)
25	L	W	23.6	25.2	33.2	42.0	42.4	52.6	57.4	4.4	6.4	8.0	9.0	10.2	16.0	17.4
	A	W	26.2	29.6	35.0	49.0	50.6	59.8	62.7	2.3	3.0	4.0	8.0	10.0	17.4	18.0
	H	W	30.9	38.6	40.0	54.5	56.6	61.4	64.7	1.0	2.0	3.0	5.5	7.0	14.7	15.3
35	L	W	25.0	29.0	29.8	39.0	39.4	51.0	53.8	4.6	5.4	7.0	10.0	12.0	17.6	18.4
	A	W	28.0	32.7	39.8	47.0	48.2	57.6	59.3	3.0	3.3	6.2	7.5	8.0	13.5	17.1
	H	W	30.0	31.0	39.0	44.5	50.0	58.5	64.8	2.2	3.5	6.0	9.5	11.0	16.5	18.5
45	L	W	15.7	24.2	27.0	35.0	35.8	45.2	46.1	7.8	8.0	9.0	13.0	14.0	16.6	19.2
	A	W	19.8	22.4	27.2	34.0	36.8	55.8	56.5	4.5	5.1	7.2	15.0	16.6	20.0	20.4
	H	W	29.0	32.8	36.4	48.5	49.4	55.3	56.9	4.5	5.0	5.0	7.0	8.0	14.6	16.7
55	L	W	20.6	21.0	24.4	33.0	34.2	47.6	49.4	5.8	6.7	8.4	13.0	14.2	21.0	22.4
	A	W	16.8	22.4	29.8	41.0	43.8	56.6	58.6	3.2	4.4	6.0	10.0	12.0	17.0	21.0
	H	W	21.3	22.6	28.0	37.0	40.0	57.4	61.5	3.0	3.6	6.2	13.0	14.0	19.8	22.4
65	L	W	8.0	11.0	16.0	29.0	32.2	44.3	47.3	6.4	8.0	10.0	15.0	16.0	21.0	23.6
	A	W	14.2	19.0	22.0	32.0	36.0	52.5	56.8	4.0	6.0	8.0	15.0	17.0	23.5	24.5
	H	W	12.5	14.0	22.0	37.0	38.0	48.0	51.5	6.0	8.0	10.0	13.0	14.0	21.0	23.5
75	L	W	2.5	5.0	7.0	22.0	27.0	44.0	49.0	6.5	9.0	10.0	13.0	14.0	22.0	23.0
	A	W	7.3	10.1	11.4	15.5	19.6	33.7	39.4	9.0	9.4	13.0	18.0	19.6	24.8	25.0
	H	W	2.0	4.0	14.6	35.0	35.0	46.8	50.4	1.6	3.2	7.0	13.0	13.8	20.0	20.0
85	L	W	0.0	0.0	1.8	13.0	16.2	23.8	27.4	10.0	10.0	12.4	16.0	18.4	22.2	22.6
	A	W	11.0	11.0	11.0	11.0	11.0	11.0	11.0	26.0	26.0	26.0	26.0	26.0	26.0	26.0
	H	W	12.7	14.3	17.6	27.5	30.8	40.7	42.3	12.1	12.3	12.6	13.5	13.8	14.7	14.9

NOTE: The raw test score leading to a particular z value is given indicating the percentiles 5, 10, 20, 50, 60, 90, and 95. LTS, Long-Term Storage; STR, Short-Term Retrieval; L, low; A, average; H, high; % = percentile.

SOURCE: From Morales et al. (2010).

TABLE 10–111 Norms for Spanish Selective Reminding Test (SRT) Form 1 for CLTR and Delayed Recall Scores Stratified by Age and Education for Women

GROUP VARIABLES			CLTR							DELAYED RECALL						
			Z VALUES							*Z* VALUES						
AGE	EDUCATION	SEX	−1.64 (5%)	−1.28 (10%)	−0.84 (20%)	0 (50%)	0.84 (60%)	1.28 (90%)	1.64 (95%)	−1.64 (5%)	−1.28 (10%)	−0.84 (20%)	0 (50%)	0.84 (60%)	1.28 (90%)	1.64 (95%)
25	L	W	14.2	15.2	16.0	24.0	28.4	38.8	45.4	7.6	8.0	8.8	11	12.0	12.0	12.0
	A	W	8.0	12.2	17.2	32.0	37.2	51.4	57.8	7.0	8.6	10.0	11	11.0	12.0	12.0
	H	W	15.7	21.5	27.2	44.5	49.8	58.7	64.3	8.7	10.0	10.0	12	12.0	12.0	12.0
35	L	W	7.8	9.0	9.0	15.0	19.6	34.6	41.0	6.6	7.6	10.0	11	11.2	12.0	12.0
	A	W	17.6	19.3	22.0	28.0	31.4	35.9	45.9	6.7	8.1	9.0	11	11.0	12.0	12.0
	H	W	12.8	17.5	21.0	32.0	35.0	48.0	53.2	9.0	9.0	9.0	11	11.0	12.0	12.0
45	L	W	8.1	10.6	12.0	20.0	21.8	35.4	37.0	5.9	6.0	7.8	9	10.0	12.0	12.0
	A	W	8.6	9.4	14.2	20.0	23.6	39.9	43.2	6.0	6.1	7.0	11	11.0	11.0	11.4
	H	W	10.2	13.4	15.4	34.5	40.4	43.6	45.9	6.7	8.4	9.8	12	12.0	12.0	12.0
55	L	W	5.8	7.4	11.0	24.0	26.6	35.9	39.2	3.7	4.7	5.4	8	9.0	11.3	12.0
	A	W	3.0	5.8	12.8	26.0	28.8	48.4	51.6	4.4	6.0	6.0	9	10.0	11.6	12.0
	H	W	8.3	10.8	14.2	27.0	29.0	46.8	52.9	3.3	4.6	7.0	9	10.0	12.0	12.0
65	L	W	0.7	3.0	7.0	18.5	22.0	36.0	40.0	2.0	3.0	4.0	6	7.0	9.0	10.0
	A	W	1.5	7.5	11.0	21.5	23.0	36.0	38.8	2.0	3.0	5.0	6	8.0	10.5	11.0
	H	W	7.0	8.0	9.0	22.0	24.0	34.0	36.5	3.0	3.0	4.0	7	8.0	12.0	12.0
75	L	W	0.0	0.0	2.0	13.0	19.0	34.0	41.5	0.5	1.0	2.0	4	6.0	10.0	10.5
	A	W	1.1	2.2	4.0	10.5	11.6	21.9	28.7	1.1	2.1	3.0	4	4.6	6.0	6.9
	H	W	2.0	4.0	6.8	21.0	21.8	33.2	37.6	1.2	2.4	3.0	6	6.8	7.2	7.6
85	L	W	0.0	0.0	0.0	7.0	11.0	14.2	16.6	1.4	1.8	2.0	3	3.8	6.2	6.6
	A	W	2.0	2.0	2.0	2.0	2.0	2.0	2.0	0.0	0.0	0.0	0	0.0	0.0	0.0
	H	W	3.5	5.0	8.0	17.0	20.0	29.0	30.5	4.2	4.4	4.8	6	6.4	7.6	7.8

NOTE: The raw test score leading to a particular z value is given indicating the percentiles 5, 10, 20, 50, 60, 90, and 95. CLTR, Consistent Long-Term Retrieval; L, low; A, average; H, high; % = percentile.

SOURCE: From Morales et al. (2010).

TABLE 10–112 Norms for Spanish Selective Reminding Test (SRT) Form 1 for RLTR Score Stratified by Age and Education for Women and Men

GROUP VARIABLES		WOMEN							MEN						
		Z VALUES							*Z* VALUES						
AGE	EDUCATION	−1.64 (5%)	−1.28 (10%)	−0.84 (20%)	0 (50%)	0.84 (60%)	1.28 (90%)	1.64 (95%)	−1.64 (5%)	−1.28 (10%)	−0.84 (20%)	0 (50%)	0.84 (60%)	1.28 (90%)	1.64 (95%)
25	L	5.2	6.0	6.0	13.0	14.6	19.0	21.0	3.5	7.0	7.0	14.0	14.0	24.0	30.5
	A	0.0	0.0	5.0	9.0	11.2	23.4	27.7	2.0	2.4	4.8	11.0	14.4	18.0	20.2
	H	0.0	0.0	0.0	5.0	6.8	14.7	17.0	1.2	4.6	6.0	8.0	8.8	14.6	17.6
35	L	8.0	8.8	12.0	17.0	19.0	26.8	29.2	1.1	2.5	7.0	7.5	8.0	18.3	19.9
	A	1.7	3.4	7.4	12.0	13.6	16.9	18.8	6.7	7.4	8.8	16.0	16.4	22.6	29.9
	H	2.5	4.0	5.0	8.5	10.0	15.5	16.8	2.1	4.0	4.2	8.5	9.6	20.9	21.0
45	L	2.9	4.6	6.0	10.0	10.8	16.8	20.9	4.0	4.2	6.0	10.5	12.8	24.1	25.9
	A	3.6	5.1	6.4	9.5	10.6	17.7	21.6	1.5	3.0	3.0	6.0	9.0	16.0	21.0
	H	2.6	3.0	5.0	8.5	11.2	26.0	28.4	0.0	5.4	7.0	13.0	14.4	20.1	21.3
55	L	0.0	1.4	3.0	8.5	10.0	13.3	17.1	0.0	0.0	0.8	8.0	8.0	17.0	17.1
	A	0.0	0.8	4.0	9.0	9.4	18.6	22.2	0.0	0.0	2.0	7.0	8.0	17.0	17.0
	H	0.6	2.6	3.0	6.0	9.0	17.4	18.7	3.8	4.0	5.0	8.0	9.0	14.5	16.8
65	L	0.0	0.0	3.0	6.5	8.0	14.3	17.0	0.0	0.0	0.0	6.0	6.8	10.7	12.3
	A	1.5	3.5	4.0	8.0	9.0	15.5	17.2	1.8	2.0	3.6	8.0	8.0	14.0	14.5
	H	1.0	3.0	5.0	8.0	9.0	13.0	20.5	0.2	2.2	4.0	7.0	9.2	15.6	16.9
75	L	0.0	0.0	2.0	5.0	6.0	11.0	12.0	0.0	0.0	0.0	4.0	4.0	7.8	14.0
	A	0.0	0.0	0.6	6.5	7.0	9.9	10.9	4.3	4.7	5.4	10.0	11.2	14.0	14.0
	H	0.0	0.0	1.8	9.0	9.8	12.8	14.4	3.0	3.0	3.0	5.0	5.8	10.4	11.2
85	L	0.0	0.0	0.0	2.0	5.2	7.4	8.2	2.6	3.2	4.4	6.0	6.6	13.6	14.8
	A	5.0	5.0	5.0	5.0	5.0	5.0	5.0	0.4	0.8	1.6	4.0	4.8	7.2	7.6
	H	6.2	6.4	6.8	8.0	8.4	9.6	9.8	3.5	7.0	7.0	14.0	14.0	24.0	30.5

NOTE: The raw test score leading to a particular z value is given indicating the percentiles 5, 10, 20, 50, 60, 90, and 95. RLTR, Random Long-Term Retrieval; L, low; A, average; H, high; % = percentile.
SOURCE: From Morales et al. (2010).

TABLE 10–113 Norms for Spanish Selective Reminding Test (SRT) Form 1 for TR and LTR Scores Stratified by Age and Education for Men

GROUP VARIABLES			TR							LTR						
			Z VALUES							*Z* VALUES						
AGE	EDUCATION	SEX	−1.64 (5%)	−1.28 (10%)	−0.84 (20%)	0 (50%)	0.84 (60%)	1.28 (90%)	1.64 (95%)	−1.64 (5%)	−1.28 (10%)	−0.84 (20%)	0 (50%)	0.84 (60%)	1.28 (90%)	1.64 (95%)
25	L	M	38.0	39.0	46.0	51.0	54.0	60.0	65.0	20.0	23.0	37.0	43.0	45.0	58.0	63.5
	A	M	38.1	39.4	43.8	50.0	51.0	57.6	60.3	21.8	26.2	29.8	41.0	43.0	54.6	56.3
	H	M	44.8	46.8	49.0	53.0	55.0	62.4	64.0	29.8	31.8	37.0	47.0	49.6	59.0	59.6
35	L	M	35.9	39.2	41.2	44.0	44.0	57.8	60.4	19.8	22.1	23.0	31.5	32.6	48.9	53.6
	A	M	41.0	41.8	43.0	48.0	48.8	53.0	53.6	21.7	23.6	28.4	34.0	40.0	46.6	48.5
	H	M	33.3	39.7	49.2	56.0	57.6	60.9	61.0	10.7	25.5	31.8	49.0	51.2	56.0	56.0
45	L	M	29.5	30.1	31.8	40.5	41.6	50.0	51.3	12.7	14.0	15.4	24.5	29.2	41.2	43.8
	A	M	28.5	29.0	29.0	38.0	45.0	55.0	59.0	5.5	8.0	14.0	23.0	30.0	47.0	52.5
	H	M	37.0	37.9	43.8	48.5	50.0	57.1	58.3	11.9	21.0	28.8	35.5	41.8	51.2	53.4
55	L	M	30.0	33.6	37.6	43.0	44.0	47.0	47.4	2.0	14.6	18.0	26.0	29.2	37.0	37.4
	A	M	32.0	32.0	36.0	46.0	47.0	51.0	53.0	11.0	11.0	14.0	30.0	33.0	45.0	60.0
	H	M	34.0	36.0	39.0	41.0	42.0	50.5	52.2	13.8	14.0	15.0	24.0	32.0	46.0	48.8
65	L	M	26.0	27.0	31.6	37.5	40.0	46.0	50.5	4.3	6.6	9.6	19.0	20.8	30.0	39.0
	A	M	31.5	33.6	34.6	39.0	43.8	50.4	52.1	9.4	11.6	13.6	24.0	25.8	39.2	40.5
	H	M	32.4	36.2	38.0	43.0	44.0	49.0	50.8	10.0	10.4	16.8	24.0	25.6	40.8	42.8
75	L	M	12.6	15.2	25.4	32.0	35.2	45.8	46.4	0.0	1.2	6.4	14.0	16.4	30.4	31.0
	A	M	27.7	28.4	30.2	34.0	35.2	40.6	41.3	5.4	6.8	9.2	19.5	25.2	28.5	30.2
	H	M	21.0	23.0	25.8	31.0	31.8	40.8	48.4	6.4	6.8	7.0	11.0	11.0	25.8	37.4
85	L	M	16.6	17.2	19.4	27.0	28.2	35.4	35.7	4.6	5.2	6.0	9.0	12.6	18.8	20.9
	A	M	25.1	25.1	25.2	25.5	25.6	25.9	25.9	0.4	0.8	1.6	4.0	4.8	7.2	7.6

NOTE: The raw test score leading to a particular z value is given indicating the percentiles 5, 10, 20, 50, 60, 90, and 95. LTR, Long-Term Retrieval; TR, Total Recall; L, low; A, average; H, high; % = percentile.

SOURCE: From Morales et al. (2010).

TABLE 10–114 Norms for Spanish Selective Reminding Test (SRT) Form 1 for LTS and STR Scores Stratified by Age and Education for Men

GROUP VARIABLES			LTS							STR						
			Z VALUES							*Z* VALUES						
AGE	EDUCATION	SEX	−1.64 (5%)	−1.28 (10%)	−0.84 (20%)	0 (50%)	0.84 (60%)	1.28 (90%)	1.64 (95%)	−1.64 (5%)	−1.28 (10%)	−0.84 (20%)	0 (50%)	0.84 (60%)	1.28 (90%)	1.64 (95%)
25	L	M	27.0	31.0	39.0	49.0	50.0	63.0	66.0	1.5	2.0	8.0	9.0	9.0	16.0	18.0
	A	M	23.9	28.0	33.0	43.0	45.8	59.0	59.3	2.0	4.0	6.8	9.0	10.4	17.2	19.5
	H	M	31.4	32.8	40.2	51.0	51.8	60.0	61.2	3.0	3.0	4.0	8.0	9.8	14.6	17.0
35	L	M	21.6	22.4	26.6	32.0	33.2	48.8	53.6	6.8	9.0	9.2	12.5	13.6	19.8	20.9
	A	M	23.1	25.2	29.4	37.0	43.0	50.6	51.9	5.1	6.0	6.0	12.0	12.8	19.0	19.9
	H	M	13.7	27.4	33.0	52.5	54.6	57.9	58.0	4.0	5.0	5.0	6.0	8.2	18.6	19.0
45	L	M	15.2	17.1	19.2	26.5	30.0	42.4	46.6	5.7	7.3	10.2	14.5	15.0	19.0	19.9
	A	M	7.0	10.0	15.0	29.0	33.0	51.0	54.5	6.5	8.0	9.0	15.0	15.0	26.0	26.0
	H	M	11.9	24.6	31.6	38.5	46.4	55.3	58.2	3.0	4.8	5.8	9.0	14.8	17.8	25.2
55	L	M	3.0	14.7	18.8	30.0	31.2	40.3	43.0	8.8	10.8	11.8	16.5	17.0	26.2	28.0
	A	M	11.0	11.0	15.0	32.0	35.0	49.0	61.0	4.0	5.0	10.0	16.0	19.0	24.0	25.0
	H	M	16.8	18.0	19.0	26.5	36.0	50.0	50.8	5.8	6.5	9.0	16.5	17.0	22.5	23.8
65	L	M	8.0	9.3	13.2	21.0	24.6	34.0	42.3	9.6	12.0	14.0	17.0	18.8	24.0	27.3
	A	M	11.4	13.6	17.0	25.0	29.6	42.0	42.6	9.7	10.8	12.2	17.0	17.0	23.0	23.1
	H	M	10.2	12.4	17.6	27.0	29.2	45.8	48.7	6.2	8.4	11.4	18.0	20.2	24.0	25.8
75	L	M	0.0	1.2	8.4	17.0	21.0	31.6	35.0	9.2	11.0	14.0	17.0	18.0	23.8	25.8
	A	M	9.1	10.1	13.0	24.0	31.2	34.2	35.6	10.0	10.0	10.0	14.0	16.0	22.2	23.6
	H	M	7.8	8.6	9.6	14.0	14.8	26.8	38.4	7.8	8.6	13.2	16.0	16.8	24.4	25.2
85	L	M	6.3	6.6	8.0	17.0	17.0	24.0	25.5	12.0	12.0	12.0	13.0	16.0	19.8	20.4
	A	M	0.6	1.2	2.4	6.0	7.2	10.8	11.4	17.4	17.9	18.8	21.5	22.4	25.1	25.6

NOTE: The raw test score leading to a particular z value is given indicating the percentiles 5, 10, 20, 50, 60, 90, and 95. LTS, Long-Term Storage; STR, Short-Term Retrieval; L, low; A, average; H, high; % = percentile.

SOURCE: From Morales et al. (2010).

TABLE 10–115 Norms for Spanish Selective Reminding Test (SRT) Form 1 for CLTR and Delayed Recall Scores Stratified by Age and Education for Men

GROUP VARIABLES			CLTR Z VALUES							DELAYED RECALL Z VALUES						
AGE	EDUCATION	SEX	−1.64 (5%)	−1.28 (10%)	−0.84 (20%)	0 (50%)	0.84 (60%)	1.28 (90%)	1.64 (95%)	−1.64 (5%)	−1.28 (10%)	−0.84 (20%)	0 (50%)	0.84 (60%)	1.28 (90%)	1.64 (95%)
25	L	M	4.0	6.0	9.0	30.0	34.0	43.0	56.0	8.0	9.0	10.0	10.0	10.0	12.0	12.0
	A	M	11.4	14.6	22.6	27.0	29.0	40.6	49.0	7.4	8.4	9.0	11.0	11.0	12.0	12.0
	H	M	17.8	20.6	25.6	36.0	37.8	51.8	55.6	9.0	9.0	10.0	11.0	12.0	12.0	12.0
35	L	M	8.6	9.2	11.4	20.5	22.8	40.8	49.2	6.0	6.1	7.0	9.0	9.6	11.9	12.0
	A	M	5.6	8.8	11.6	17.0	20.8	35.2	38.7	8.0	8.0	8.0	10.0	10.0	10.6	11.3
	H	M	4.1	7.2	21.0	37.0	39.6	49.7	50.0	9.0	9.0	11.0	11.0	11.0	12.0	12.0
45	L	M	2.2	4.2	6.4	17.0	18.2	25.5	26.9	4.5	5.0	5.4	8.0	8.6	10.9	11.0
	A	M	3.0	6.0	8.0	12.0	20.0	27.0	42.5	6.0	6.0	7.0	9.0	9.0	11.0	11.5
	H	M	2.0	9.2	14.4	23.0	25.0	41.3	44.9	5.9	6.0	7.0	9.5	11.0	12.0	12.0
55	L	M	1.9	7.4	8.0	18.0	19.4	25.2	27.9	1.0	2.8	5.0	7.0	9.0	11.0	11.0
	A	M	7.0	8.0	11.0	16.0	19.0	37.0	58.0	3.0	4.0	5.0	7.0	8.0	10.0	10.0
	H	M	5.8	6.0	7.0	16.0	21.0	35.0	38.0	4.0	4.0	5.0	9.0	10.0	11.0	11.2
65	L	M	1.3	2.0	7.0	15.5	17.6	24.7	29.5	0.7	1.3	2.0	4.0	4.0	7.0	9.0
	A	M	0.0	1.6	7.0	16.0	20.8	31.4	33.0	3.8	4.0	4.0	5.0	5.0	8.4	10.0
	H	M	6.0	6.8	10.0	16.0	17.4	29.6	30.9	2.0	2.2	3.4	5.0	5.0	8.0	8.9
75	L	M	0.0	0.0	1.4	9.0	12.0	22.8	25.2	0.0	1.2	2.0	4.0	5.0	6.8	7.0
	A	M	0.7	1.4	2.0	10.0	11.2	17.2	18.6	1.4	1.7	2.4	4.0	5.0	7.3	7.6
	H	M	0.4	0.8	1.6	4.0	5.6	22.8	34.4	0.8	1.6	2.0	3.0	3.0	6.8	8.4
85	L	M	0.0	0.0	0.0	2.0	3.2	9.8	10.4	0.3	0.6	1.2	3.0	3.0	5.2	6.1
	A	M	0.0	0.0	0.0	0.0	0.0	0.0	0.0	1.0	1.0	1.0	1.0	1.0	1.0	1.0

NOTE: The raw test score leading to a particular z value is given indicating the percentiles 5, 10, 20, 50, 60, 90, and 95. CLTR, Consistent Long-Term Retrieval; L, low; A, average; H, high; % = percentile.

SOURCE: From Morales et al. (2010).

TABLE 10–116 Norms for Spanish Selective Reminding Test (SRT) Form 2 for TR and LTR Scores Stratified by Age and Education

GROUP VARIABLES		TR							LTR						
		Z VALUES							Z VALUES						
AGE	EDUCATION	−1.64 (5%)	−1.28 (10%)	−0.84 (20%)	0 (50%)	0.84 (60%)	1.28 (90%)	1.64 (95%)	−1.64 (5%)	−1.28 (10%)	−0.84 (20%)	0 (50%)	0.84 (60%)	1.28 (90%)	1.64 (95%)
25	L	41.7	42.4	43.4	44.0	44.4	51.4	54.2	23.8	25.5	27.8	31.0	32.0	41.4	47.7
	A	43.8	45.0	49.6	53.0	53.0	58.0	59.2	28.0	31.8	36.2	44.0	44.8	52.6	56.2
	H	46.0	48.0	50.0	56.0	58.0	64.0	65.0	31.0	35.0	38.0	47.0	51.0	60.0	62.0
35	L	33.0	35.0	39.0	50.0	53.0	55.5	55.8	15.0	19.0	27.0	42.0	44.0	50.0	50.5
	A	40.5	43.2	45.8	51.0	52.4	54.6	57.1	23.7	31.2	33.0	37.0	43.2	47.8	52.0
	H	43.5	44.0	48.0	54.0	55.0	59.0	59.5	25.0	28.0	33.0	46.0	48.0	56.0	57.0
45	L	33.4	37.4	39.0	44.0	46.2	53.2	55.2	11.8	16.2	22.6	28.0	28.8	42.8	47.2
	A	33.2	35.5	36.0	43.0	46.0	53.2	58.6	14.8	16.6	17.8	30.5	31.4	44.9	53.4
	H	40.1	41.0	44.2	49.5	51.6	58.4	59.0	14.4	23.2	29.0	38.0	38.0	53.7	54.9
55	L	33.0	34.8	36.4	42.0	43.6	49.2	51.0	18.6	19.6	20.0	28.0	29.8	37.2	39.0
	A	40.6	42.2	44.2	49.0	49.8	54.0	56.0	24.6	26.2	27.0	37.0	37.8	48.6	49.8
	H	34.1	37.0	44.0	47.0	47.8	58.2	61.4	10.7	15.6	22.8	35.0	39.2	54.8	58.4
65	L	26.0	29.9	30.8	40.0	42.4	49.1	52.2	7.9	12.5	14.8	26.5	29.8	39.0	41.3
	A	25.5	28.9	40.6	44.0	44.8	50.0	51.7	7.3	9.3	19.6	29.5	31.0	39.7	43.4
	H	34.0	36.0	40.4	47.0	49.0	57.0	59.6	16.2	18.2	21.6	34.0	39.0	52.6	55.2
75	L	19.9	25.5	28.4	35.5	37.0	45.0	45.1	5.7	7.0	11.0	20.5	23.2	34.3	35.0
	A	27.8	29.6	34.0	37.0	39.0	48.2	50.0	11.4	13.6	16.4	24.0	24.0	35 0	35.2
	H	25.0	25.6	32.0	46.0	46.0	55.8	57.8	4.8	7.2	16.4	32.0	33.4	49.0	52.6
85	L	16.8	18.5	24.0	32.0	33.2	36.8	38.9	4.8	6.5	10.8	19.0	20.2	25.1	27.5

NOTE: The raw test score leading to a particular z value is given indicating the percentiles 5, 10, 20, 50, 60, 90, and 95. TR, Total Recall; LTR, Long-Term Retrieval; L, low; A, average; H, high; % = percentile.

SOURCE: From Morales et al. (2010).

TABLE 10–117 Norms for Spanish Selective Reminding Test (SRT) Form 2 for LTS and STR Scores Stratified by Age and Education

		LTS							STR						
GROUP VARIABLES		*Z* VALUES							*Z* VALUES						
AGE	EDUCATION	−1.64 (5%)	−1.28 (10%)	−0.84 (20%)	0 (50%)	0.84 (60%)	1.28 (90%)	1.64 (95%)	−1.64 (5%)	−1.28 (10%)	−0.84 (20%)	0 (50%)	0.84 (60%)	1.28 (90%)	1.64 (95%)
25	L	24.4	26.9	29.8	33.0	34.6	46.2	51.1	5.5	7.9	10.4	13.0	15.4	18.5	20.2
	A	30.2	33.6	38.8	46.0	46.0	56.4	59.2	3.4	4.8	6.0	9.0	9.8	17.0	17.0
	H	36.0	39.0	40.0	51.0	55.0	62.0	63.0	1.0	3.0	3.0	7.0	9.0	13.0	14.0
35	L	16.2	20.5	29.0	44.5	47.0	51.5	51.8	5.2	5.5	6.0	8.0	9.0	16.0	18.0
	A	27.8	35.4	36.0	41.0	44.6	49.2	52.7	4.4	5.8	7.8	11.0	12.4	14.6	18.9
	H	26.5	30.0	35.0	49.0	51.0	57.0	60.0	2.0	2.0	5.0	9.0	10.0	18.0	18.5
45	L	14.6	19.8	24.6	30.0	30.6	44.0	48.0	8.0	12.2	13.0	14.0	15.2	20.6	21.4
	A	17.7	20.4	21.8	32.0	33.4	47.7	55.3	4.2	6.5	8.6	15.5	16.0	19.0	19.0
	H	16.1	28.0	32.2	40.5	41.8	56.4	57.8	4.2	5.0	8.6	12.5	13.8	18.4	25.8
55	L	22.8	23.0	23.0	30.0	31.0	39.4	40.4	11.6	12.0	12.0	14.0	15.2	18.8	20.0
	A	28.0	28.0	28.6	41.0	41.0	49.4	50.2	2.8	5.6	8.8	13.0	13.0	16.4	17.2
	H	13.4	17.8	25.4	38.0	42.8	58.0	60.1	3.0	3.4	4.0	11.0	13.8	21.6	24.1
65	L	9.9	14.6	17.0	29.5	32.0	39.3	43.3	8.0	10.8	11.0	14.5	16.0	23.0	23.0
	A	8.3	11.2	21.6	32.5	34.0	44.0	47.4	8.0	8.3	10.2	14.0	16.0	22.0	22.0
	H	18.2	19.0	24.8	38.0	42.6	56.0	61.8	3.6	5.0	6.4	11.0	13.2	18.8	19.8
75	L	6.0	8.7	12.4	21.0	25.2	36.0	37.1	7.8	8.7	10.4	15.0	16.2	22.3	24.4
	A	13.4	16.2	18.4	26.0	27.0	36.4	37.4	12.0	12.0	13.2	15.0	15.6	19.4	20.0
	H	5.6	7.4	17.4	35.0	38.2	51.0	53.6	4.6	5.2	7.2	14.0	14.2	21.8	22.0
85	L	5.8	8.6	13.4	23.0	23.6	27.8	29.9	8.1	9.1	10.4	11.5	12.4	17.6	18.3

NOTE: The raw test score leading to a particular *z* value is given indicating the percentiles 5, 10, 20, 50, 60, 90, and 95. LTS, Long-Term Storage; STR, Short-Term Retrieval; L, low; A, average; H, high; % = percentile.
SOURCE: From Morales et al. (2010).

TABLE 10–118 Norms for Spanish Selective Reminding Test (SRT) Form 2 for CLTR and Delayed Recall Scores Stratified by Age and Education

GROUP VARIABLES		CLTR Z VALUES							DELAYED RECALL Z VALUES						
AGE	EDUCATION	−1.64 (5%)	−1.28 (10%)	−0.84 (20%)	0 (50%)	0.84 (60%)	1.28 (90%)	1.64 (95%)	−1.64 (5%)	−1.28 (10%)	−0.84 (20%)	0 (50%)	0.84 (60%)	1.28 (90%)	1.64 (95%)
25	L	9.4	11.9	14.4	19.0	20.4	32.0	39.0	8.0	8.0	8.0	9.0	9.2	10.6	11.3
	A	8.6	19.4	21.6	30.0	31.8	44.2	50.4	7.4	8.0	10.0	11.0	11.0	12.0	12.0
	H	16.0	19.0	24.0	36.0	45.0	59.0	62.0	9.0	10.0	10.0	12.0	12.0	12.0	12.0
35	L	6.0	8.0	12.0	28.0	32.0	42.0	46.5	9.2	9.5	10.0	11.5	12.0	12.0	12.0
	A	4.8	8.4	12.8	27.0	28.8	40.8	49.9	5.1	6.8	8.0	11.0	11.4	12.0	12.0
	H	16.0	19.0	20.0	30.0	35.0	48.0	53.5	8.0	9.0	10.0	11.0	11.0	12.0	12.0
45	L	3.0	4.6	12.2	16.0	18.2	28.2	33.4	5.0	5.2	6.0	7.0	8.2	10.0	10.4
	A	5.9	6.8	7.8	14.0	16.0	31.0	44.5	3.9	4.8	5.8	8.5	9.4	12.0	12.0
	H	6.2	7.6	10.8	27.0	32.2	41.4	46.2	4.3	6.0	8.6	10.0	10.0	12.0	12.0
55	L	3.2	4.6	6.6	11.0	11.0	17.0	17.8	3.8	4.0	5.2	7.0	8.0	10.0	10.2
	A	9.4	13.8	16.6	25.0	29.8	46.2	48.6	6.4	6.8	7.0	9.0	9.0	12.0	12.0
	H	0.7	3.0	9.2	26.0	27.8	43.4	54.3	3.4	4.0	6.4	10.0	10.4	12.0	12.0
65	L	0.0	2.9	5.8	17.0	21.4	30.0	32.5	3.0	3.0	4.0	5.0	6.0	8.1	10.0
	A	2.0	2.9	8.4	20.5	22.8	30.7	35.2	2.2	3.3	4.0	6.0	6.8	10.1	11.0
	H	7.8	9.0	11.4	21.0	23.6	39.8	45.2	2.6	3.2	5.0	8.0	8.0	12.0	12.0
75	L	0.0	2.0	4.0	16.0	18.2	27.0	27.3	2.0	2.0	2.0	4.0	5.0	7.0	8.0
	A	1.6	2.6	11.4	17.0	18.6	27.6	30.6	2.8	3.0	3.0	5.0	6.6	8.4	9.4
	H	3.6	6.0	7.2	22.0	23.2	44.2	48.2	1.0	1.4	3.0	6.0	7.2	9.8	10.8
85	L	2.4	2.7	5.0	10.0	11.0	17.5	19.2	1.1	2.1	3.0	3.5	4.0	4.9	5.9

NOTE: The raw test score leading to a particular z value is given indicating the percentiles 5, 10, 20, 50, 60, 90, and 95. CLTR, Consistent Long-Term Retrieval; L, low; A, average; H, high; % = percentile.

SOURCE: From Morales et al. (2010).

EVIDENCE FOR VALIDITY

FACTOR-ANALYTIC STUDIES

Larrabee and Curtiss (1995) evaluated the factor structure of several tests of memory and information-processing ability in a mixed clinical group and found that the SRT loaded on a general verbal visual memory factor (along with the Expanded Paired Associates Test, Continuous Recognition Memory Test, and CVMT). By contrast, Allen and Ruff (1999) found that, in a healthy sample, the SRT loaded on a verbal memory factor along with WMS-R Logical Memory; visual memory tasks (RULIT, Rey Complex Figure) loaded on a separate factor. Davis et al. (2006) also found that the two-factor model (verbal and nonverbal memory) was a better fit than the one-factor model (general memory) in a CFA using WMS-R Logical Memory and Visual Reproduction as well as SRT and Nonverbal Selective Reminding Test (NVSRT) in a sample of patients with epilepsy.

WITHIN-TEST RELATIONSHIPS

The SRT purports to parcel verbal memory into distinct component processes (e.g., LTS, LTR, CLTR, STR). In support of this notion, Beatty et al. (1996a) reported that, in patients with MS and controls, the probability of recall or recognition varied in a consistent manner as a function of the status of the words (CLTR, RLTR, or STR) in the examinee's memory at the conclusion of training. For example, words that were being retrieved from CLTR at the end of acquisition were more likely to be recalled after a delay than were words that were not being consistently retrieved from LTS. Words that were being retrieved from STR were the least likely to be recalled after a delay. However, there is evidence that the numerous scores that can be derived from the test tend to be highly intercorrelated, suggesting that these measures are assessing similar constructs (Kenisten, cited in Kraemer et al., 1983; Larrabee et al., 1988; Loring & Papanicolaou, 1987; Smith et al., 1995; Westerveld et al., 1994). Furthermore, although the SR procedure offers information regarding short- and long-term memory, the operational distinction between LTS and LTR is problematic (Loring & Papanicolaou, 1987). According to Bushke's definition, a word has entered LTS if it has been successfully recalled on two successive trials. By definition, failure to recall is due to a retrieval difficulty. However, the item may have been stored in a weak or degraded form, after which, through the process of additional repetition by the examiner, the word is encoded more deeply and efficiently (Loring & Papanicolaou, 1987). Therefore, operationally defined retrieval may have little to do with retrieval itself (e.g., it may reflect storage functions).

A single index from among those obtained using standard scoring methods may adequately convey the SRT result, given the redundancy of the scores. The total number of words recalled on all trials throughout the test, a fairly reliable measure, is recommended by Westerveld et al. (1994) as a measure of learning. To measure forgetting, Trahan and Larrabee (1993) recommend computing a score based on the number of words in LTS on the final learning trial (Trial 12 LTS) minus the 30-minute delayed recall score.

RELATIONSHIPS WITH OTHER TESTS

Modest correlations have been demonstrated among the SRT and other tests of verbal learning and memory, such as the CVLT, RAVLT, and WMS (Shear & Craft, 1989). Larrabee and Curtiss (1995) reported that SRT CLTR was moderately correlated with Logical Memory and NVSRT CLTR ($r = .46$ to .51, and $r = .35$, respectively), and weakly to moderately correlated with Visual Reproduction ($r = .26$ to .38).

McGinnis (2012) reported that the six-trial SRT showed moderate correlations with MMSE, category fluency, and Stroop errors ($r = .59$, .53, and 38, respectively). The SRT was also correlated with WCST-Categories completed, WCST Perseverative Errors, COWAT, TMT-B, Figural Fluency unique designs, and WISC-III Mazes in a sample of patients with frontal lobe epilepsy and TLE ($r = .25$ to .41). In another study involving epilepsy, CLTR appeared most sensitive to frontal systems dysfunction and had the strongest correlations with executive measures (Johnson-Markve et al., 2011). These findings suggest a notable contribution of executive functions to SRT performance.

CLINICAL STUDIES

Neurodegenerative Disorders. The test is useful for distinguishing healthy adults from demented older individuals (Campo et al., 2003; Kuzis et al., 1999; Reitz et al., 2007, Sabe et al., 1995). For instance, patients with AD recall fewer words on Trial 1; they also recall fewer words overall and enter fewer items into long-term memory, and they are more likely to show inconsistent recall from long-term memory as well as increased forgetting rates (Campo et al., 2003).

Scores from the SRT may also be useful as preclinical indicators of the development of dementia. Masur et al. (1990), using a modified SRT procedure (six trials, delayed recall and recognition after a five-minute period of distraction), reported that the Total Recall and Delayed Recall scores obtained one to two years before diagnosis were the measures best able to predict dementia, with sensitivities of 47% and 44%, respectively, and predictive values of 37% and 40%, respectively. Over about 15 months, those with MCI who converted to AD recalled about 4.2 words less on SRT Delayed Recall at baseline than those who did not convert (Devanand et al., 2006). In fact, baseline SRT Total Recall was remarkably lower in MCI converters than nonconverters even as long as three years before conversion (Devanand et al., 2008).

Krinsky-McHale et al. (2002) noted that a modified version of the SRT is useful in detecting early dementia in adults with Down syndrome. However, the SRT is not as sensitive as the UPSIT in predicting cognitive decline in cognitively intact older adults (Devanand et al., 2015).

The addition of other tests appears to improve the prediction of MCI to AD conversion. Tabert et al. (2006) found that SRT Total Recall and WAIS-R Digit Symbol were the best predictors of time to conversion from MCI to AD, though SRT Delayed Recall and percent savings also differentiated those who converted from those who did not convert to AD. SRT Total Recall and Digit Symbol together yielded a sensitivity of 76%, specificity of 90%, PPV of 76%, and NPV of 90% for identifying conversion to AD in three years. Similarly, Devanand et al. (2008) found that SRT Total Recall along with age, MMSE, Functional Activities Questionnaire, and UPSIT yielded a sensitivity of 81% and specificity of greater than 90% for predicting conversion to AD.

Rate of decline on the SRT appears to be influenced by APOE ε4 status (Caselli et al., 2015) and estradiol level (Yaffe et al., 2007). APOE-ε4 carriers show a steeper age-related memory decline, with predicted annual change ranging from −0.72 in those aged 70 to +1.21 in those aged 50 on SRT Total Recall. Conversely, those who are APOE ε4-negative show predicted annual change ranging from 0.43 in those aged 70 to 1.08 in those aged 50 (Caselli et al., 2015). Older women with lower estradiol are more likely to show decline on the SRT over two years than those with higher estradiol; testosterone does not affect memory functioning in either gender (Yaffe et al., 2007). Interestingly, there is preliminary suggestion that men with MCI treated with estrogen for 12 weeks improve on SRT Total Recall immediately after treatment compared to baseline or placebo (Sherwin et al., 2011).

Doing crossword puzzles may delay memory decline as measured by the SRT (Pillai et al., 2011). Cognitively intact older adults who do crossword puzzles obtain higher SRT scores at baseline than those who do not do crossword puzzles. Among those who eventually develop dementia, those who do crossword puzzles show a delay in accelerated memory decline as measured by the SRT by 2.54 years compared to those who do not do crossword puzzles (Pillai et al., 2011).

TBI. The SRT has been used effectively to assess memory functioning after brain injury (e.g., McCauley et al., 2014; Paniak et al., 1989), with length of unconsciousness related to the level of memory performance. McCauley et al. (2014) reported that individuals with mild TBI (mTBI) tested within 96 hours of injury performed worse than those sustaining only orthopedic injury and healthy controls on the six-trial SRT CLTR and Delayed Recall. However, no impairments on the SRT are seen in adolescents with mTBI tested about three days post-injury (Wu et al., 2010) or in veterans who sustained blast-related TBI (Troyanskaya et al., 2015).

Levin et al. (1979) report that the degree of SRT long-term memory impairment one year after severe brain injury corresponds to the overall level of disability in survivors. Patients who attained good recovery (i.e., resumption of work and normal social functioning) consistently recall words without further reminding at a level comparable to that of healthy adults. In contrast, consistent recall is grossly impaired in patients who were moderately or severely disabled at the time of the study.

Epilepsy. Impairment has been noted in the context of left temporal lobe abnormality in patients with epilepsy (e.g., Bell et al., 2005; Breier et al., 1997; Drane et al., 1998; Dulay et al., 2009; Lencz et al., 1992; Loring et al., 1991). For example, Sass et al. (1990) showed that SRT scores correlated significantly with hippocampal pyramidal cell density obtained from pathologic analysis of excised tissue from the left but not the right hippocampus of left-speech dominant adults with epilepsy. Furthermore, left-speech dominant patients with severe hippocampal neuron loss experienced no significant decrement in SRT performance after total excision of the left hippocampus (Sass et al., 1994), whereas patients with mild or moderate neuron loss had significant decline. In another study, left-hemisphere language-dominant patients with epilepsy who underwent left anterior temporal lobectomy experienced a significant decline in SRT scores (63%) and also showed a reduced learning slope on verbal learning (Dulay et al., 2009). Notably, those with good seizure outcome maintained their verbal memory performance.

Johnson-Markve et al. (2011) found that patients with frontal lobe epilepsy (FLE) performed worse than those with TLE, and differences between the groups were greater for the SRT than for WMS-III Logical Memory. Surprisingly, those with right FLE performed worse than those with left TLE on SRT CLTR and Delayed Recall. In short, the SRT may be useful to differentiate FLE and TLE. The SRT should not be used by itself to predict left temporal lobe abnormality in epilepsy.

In the SRT, as in many other memory tests (e.g., RAVLT, CVLT-II), retention is typically evaluated after a 30-minute interval. The question arises as to whether impairment in consolidation over this relatively short delay is a good predictor of memory function after a longer delay period. Bell et al. (2005) examined patients with TLE with delays of 30 minutes and 24 hours. At the individual level, there was no difference in the percentage of patients versus controls who demonstrated isolated memory impairment after a 24-hour delay. That is, in the absence of overt seizure activity, accelerated forgetting over 24 hours appears to be uncommon in patients with TLE. Interestingly, sleep may have a role in the forgetting of patients with TLE. Deak et al. (2011) reported that patients with TLE recalled 3.1 fewer words on the SRT than healthy controls after 12 hours of daytime wakefulness; no differences in number of words recalled were found following 12 hours of sleep even though both groups showed similar sleep quality, sleep architecture, and total sleep time.

MS. Patients with relapsing-remitting MS and clinically isolated syndrome perform similarly on the SRT, but worse than healthy controls. Depression does not affect SRT performance in those with MS (Iaffaldano et al., 2014). MS patients who use cannabis and those who do not perform similarly on the SRT even though differences are found on other measures (PASAT, 10/36 Spatial Recall, and two-back tasks; Pavisian et al., 2014). In patients with MS, the SRT has served to emphasize the heterogeneity of the memory disturbances. Beatty et al. (1996b) found evidence of three distinct patterns of SRT performance in patients with MS: unimpaired, mildly impaired with mainly retrieval problems, and more severely impaired with encoding as well as retrieval difficulties. Patients with PD also have difficulty on the SRT (Kuzis et al., 1999), likely due to an impairment in retrieval (Faglioni et al., 2000; Stern et al., 1998).

Medical Conditions. The SRT is also sensitive to subtle memory deficits in medical conditions such as diabetes and chronic kidney disease (Luchsinger et al., 2015; Palta et al., 2014; Reitz et al., 2007; Yaffe et al., 2014). Older adults with diabetes mellitus show impaired SRT (Palta et al., 2014), and HbA1c, a marker of inflammation, is associated with poorer SRT performance even after demographic background and vascular risk factors are considered (Luchsinger et al., 2015). Similarly, higher levels of serum cystatin C in those with chronic kidney disease are associated with poorer SRT Delayed Recall scores even after adjusting for estimated glomerular filtration rate (Yaffe et al., 2014).

Medication Effects. Some medications have been found to affect SRT performance in older adults, perhaps due to their sedating effects (Pomara et al., 2006, 2008, 2010). In highly educated, cognitively intact older adults, administration of lorazepam results in better recall of pre-drug word lists (i.e., retrograde facilitation) than placebo. This phenomenon is dose-dependent, with those administered 1 mg lorazepam recalling more pre-drug words than those administered .5 mg lorazepam. Greater retrograde facilitation is associated with more sedation and greater anterograde amnesia as measured by the SRT (Pomara et al., 2006). Similar findings are seen with trihexyphenidyl, an antiparkinsonian agent of the antimuscarinic class (Pomara et al., 2010). Cognitively intact older adults who were APOE ε4 carriers reported more mental slowing after administration of trihexyphenidyl than those who were administered placebo; the increased rate of mental slowing was associated with poorer SRT performance (Pomara et al., 2008). However, APOE-ε4 does not influence the retrograde facilitation effect (Pomara et al., 2010).

Psychiatric Conditions and Substance Abuse. There is also evidence that individuals with mood or thought disorders (e.g., combat-related PTSD, schizophrenia, depression) perform poorly on the SRT (Bremner et al., 1993; Ruchinskas et al., 2000; Sabe et al., 1995; but see Gass, 1996). In fact, baseline depressive symptoms in older adults without dementia predict worse SRT scores at 18- to 24-month follow-up and greater memory decline over 12 years (Zahodne et al., 2014). However, various therapies appear to improve SRT scores in depressed individuals. For example, depressed adults who receive ECT exhibit worse SRT Delayed Recall immediately post-ECT compared to pre-ECT but improvements are seen six months post-ECT (Sackeim et al., 2007). Older depressed adults treated with sertraline improve on the SRT following a 12-week medication trial regardless of whether or not they respond to the medication, more so than those treated with nortriptyline (Culang-Reinlieb et al., 2012). As well, depressed older adults with cognitive impairment treated with escitalopram and memantine also show improved SRT Total Recall over a 48-week treatment period (Pelton et al., 2016). By contrast, those with late-life depression treated with citalopram perform worse on the SRT at the end of an eight-week, double-blind trial than those given placebo. Nonresponders score 3.64 points lower than placebo nonresponders at study endpoint (Culang et al., 2009). Greater impairments in SRT have also been found in depressed individuals who attempted suicide in the past compared to depressed nonattempters (Keilp et al., 2013, 2014b) regardless of depression severity (Keilp et al., 2014a). Alcoholics perform worse than healthy controls on the SRT (Schottenbauer et al., 2007).

NEUROANATOMICAL CORRELATES AND IMAGING STUDIES

SRT delayed recall but not total recall is associated with hippocampal volume (Bruno et al., 2015), specifically the entorhinal cortex (Brickman et al., 2011). Bruno et al. (2015) found that hippocampal volume was positively correlated with delayed recall of the first four words on the SRT; the correlation with the rest of the word list was significant but weaker. Delayed recall is also associated with fractional anisotropy of the left cingulum bundle in adolescents with mTBI tested three days post-injury (Wu et al., 2010).

In a study of blast-related TBI, SRT CLTR is positively correlated with fractional anisotropy of the left and right posterior internal capsule and left corticospinal tract, and negatively correlated with diffusion coefficients for the left and right uncinate fasiculi and left posterior internal capsule (Levin et al., 2010).

PERFORMANCE VALIDITY

No studies have been conducted to develop embedded performance validity indicators using the SRT, to our knowledge.

COMMENT

The SRT has been in use for many decades and has been used in a substantial number of research studies. These have shown its sensitivity to memory disturbance in a number of medical conditions, psychiatric conditions, and neurological disorders, and its treatment responsiveness. It also is sensitive to MCI and shows utility in predicting conversion to AD. Given its sensitivity to subtle memory deficits, it has been included in a cognitive test battery for MS (Rao et al., 1990). A number of translated versions (e.g., Greek, Hebrew, Spanish) are available with updated normative data.

The task allows the assessment of different aspects of memory (e.g., retrieval from short-term and long-term memory). It also distinguishes two qualitative aspects of retrieval from long-term memory, an inconsistent type (RLTR) and a consistent type (CLTR), a unique feature compared to other memory tests. However, some studies indicate that because these scores are all highly intercorrelated, they may not necessarily tap unique aspects of memory.

Although some literature suggests an absence of practice effects in patients with neurological disorders, there are practice effects in healthy individuals, and there is extreme variability in some scores in clinical groups, suggesting caution in interpreting retest data.

Despite its positive features, the norms are old and in need of updates. Users are cautioned that many versions with different numbers of words, learning trials, and administration procedures (i.e., with or without cued recall) are used in the literature. Care should be taken to select the appropriate norms for the version administered, in particular as to whether a cued recall trial was given, as this may affect subsequent delayed recall. Many studies use the six-trial version, which appears sufficient to measure memory deficits. There is also a major lack of cross-cultural studies compared to other memory tests, and it is a cumbersome process to correct for gender effects in scoring. Other major limitations include the lack of basic psychometric information on internal and test-retest reliability, and the lack of performance validity indices. Consequently, until these are remedied, other verbal memory tests are recommended in clinical settings for diagnostic decision making.

Although past studies suggest that the SRT is associated with left temporal abnormalities, there is evidence that the SRT is correlated with executive measures and may be sensitive to frontal lobe or right-hemisphere dysfunction. Accordingly, users should not assume that impairment on SRT indicates left temporal lobe dysfunction.

REFERENCES

Allen, C. C., & Ruff, R. M. (1999). Factorial validation of the Ruff-Light Trail Learning Test. *Assessment, 6,* 43–50.

Beatty, W. W., Krull, K. R., Wilbanks, S. L., Blanco, C. R., Hames, K. A., & Paul, R. H. (1996a). Further validation of constructs from the Selective Reminding Test. *Journal of Clinical and Experimental Neuropsychology, 18,* 52–55.

Beatty, W. W., Krull, K. R., Wilbanks, S. L., Blanco, C. R., Hames, K. A., Tivis, R., & Paul, R. H. (1996b). Memory disturbance in multiple sclerosis: Reconsideration of patterns of performance on the Selective Reminding Test. *Journal of Clinical and Experimental Neuropsychology, 18,* 56–62.

Bell, B. D., Fine, J., Dow, C., Seidenberg, M., & Hermann, B. P. (2005). Temporal lobe epilepsy and the Selective Reminding Test: The conventional 30-minute delay suffices. *Psychological Assessment, 17,* 103–109.

Bishop, E. G., Dickson, A. L., & Allen, M. T. (1990). Psychometric intelligence and performance on Selective Reminding. *The Clinical Neuropsychologist, 4,* 141–150.

Breier, J. I., Brookshire, B. L., Fletcher, J. M., Thomas, A. B., Plenger, P. M., Wheless, J. W., . . . Papanicolaou, A. (1997). Identification of side of seizure onset in temporal lobe epilepsy using memory tests in the context of reading deficits. *Journal of Clinical and Experimental Neuropsychology, 19,* 161–171.

Bremner, J. D., Scott, T. M., Delaney, R. C., Southwick, S. M., Mason, J. W., Johnson, D. R., . . . Charney, D. S. (1993). Deficits in short-term memory in posttraumatic stress disorder. *American Journal of Psychiatry, 150,* 1015–1019.

Brickman, A. M., Stern, Y., & Small, S. A. (2011). Hippocampal subregions differentially associate with standardized memory tests. *Hippocampus, 21*(9), 923–928.

Bruno, D., Grothe, M. J., Nierenberg, J., Zetterberg, H., Blennow, K., Teipel, S. J., & Pomara, N. (2015). A study on the specificity of the association between hippocampal volume and delayed primacy performance in cognitively intact elderly individuals. *Neuropsychologia, 69,* 1–8.

Buschke, H. (1973). Selective reminding for analysis of memory and learning. *Journal of Verbal Learning and Verbal Behavior, 12,* 543–550.

Buschke, H., & Fuld, P. A. (1974). Evaluating storage, retention, and retrieval in disordered memory and learning. *Neurology, 24,* 1019–1025.

Campo, P., & Morales, M. (2004). Normative data and reliability for a Spanish version of the verbal Selective Reminding Test. *Archives of Clinical Neuropsychology, 19,* 421–435.

Campo, P., Morales, M., & Juan-Malpartida, M. (2000). Development of two Spanish versions of the Verbal Selective Reminding Test. *Journal of Clinical and Experimental Neuropsychology, 22,* 279–285.

Campo, P., Morales, M., & Martinez-Castillo, E. (2003). Discrimination of normal from demented elderly on a Spanish version of the Verbal Selective Reminding Test. *Journal of Clinical and Experimental Neuropsychology, 25,* 991–999.

Caselli, R. J., Dueck, A. C., Locke, D. E. C., Baxter, L. C., Woodruff, B. K., & Geda, Y. E. (2015). Sex-based memory advantages and cognitive aging: A challenge to the cognitive reserve construct? *Journal of the International Neuropsychological Society, 21*(2), 95–104.

Clodfelter, C. J., Dickson, A. L., Newton Wilkes, C., & Johnson, R. B. (1987). Alternate forms of Selective Reminding for children. *The Clinical Neuropsychologist, 1,* 243–249.

Culang, M. E., Sneed, J. R., Keilp, J. G., Rutherford, B. R., Pelton, G. H., Devanand, D. P., & Roose, S. P. (2009). Change in cognitive functioning following acute antidepressant treatment in late-life depression. *The American Journal of Geriatric Psychiatry, 17*(10), 881–888.

Culang-Reinlieb, M. E., Sneed, J. R., Keilp, J. G., & Roose, S. P. (2012). Change in cognitive functioning in depressed older adults following treatment with sertraline or nortriptyline. *International Journal of Geriatric Psychiatry, 27*(8), 777–784.

Davis, R. N., Andresen, E. N., Witgert, M. E., & Breier, J. I. (2006). Is basic memory structure invariant across epilepsy patient subgroups? *Journal of Clinical and Experimental Neuropsychology, 28*(6), 987–997.

Deak, M. C., Stickgold, R., Pietras, A. C., Nelson, A. P., & Bubrick, E. J. (2011). The role of sleep in forgetting in temporal lobe epilepsy: A pilot study. *Epilepsy & Behavior, 21*(4), 462–466.

Devanand, D. P., Habeck, C. G., Tabert, M. H., Scarmeas, N., Pelton, G. H., Moeller, J. R., . . . Stern, Y. (2006). PET network abnormalities and cognitive decline in patients with mild cognitive impairment. *Neuropsychopharmacology, 31*(6), 1327–1334.

Devanand, D. P., Lee, S., Manly, J., Andrews, H., Schupf, N., Doty, R. L., . . . Mayeux, R. (2015). Olfactory deficits predict cognitive decline and Alzheimer dementia in an urban community. *Neurology, 84*(2), 182–189.

Devanand, D. P., Liu, X., Tabert, M. H., Pradhaban, G., Cuasay, K., Bell, K., . . . Pelton, G. H. (2008). Combining early markers strongly predicts conversion from mild cognitive impairment to Alzheimer's disease. *Biological Psychiatry, 64*(10), 871–879.

Dikmen, S. S., Heaton, R. K., Grant, I., & Temkin, N. R. (1999). Test-retest reliability and practice effects of expanded Halstead-Reitan neuropsychological test battery. *Journal of the International Neuropsychological Society, 5,* 346–356.

Drane, D. L., Loring, D. W., Lee, G. P., & Meador, K. J. (1998). Trial-length sensitivity of the Verbal Selective Reminding Test to lateralized temporal lobe impairment. *The Clinical Neuropsychologist, 12,* 68–73.

Dulay, M. F., Levin, H. S., York, M. K., Li, X., Mizrahi, E. M., Goldsmith, I., . . . Yoshor, D. (2009). Changes in individual and group spatial and verbal learning characteristics after anterior temporal lobectomy. *Epilepsia, 50*(6), 1385–1395.

Faglioni, P., Saetti, M. C., & Botti, C. (2000). Verbal learning strategies in Parkinson's disease. *Neuropsychology, 14,* 456–479.

Gass, C. S. (1996). MMPI-2 variables in attention and memory test performance. *Psychological Assessment, 8,* 135–138.

Gigi, A., Schnaider-Beeri, M., Davidson, M., & Prohovnik, I. (1999). Validation of a Hebrew Selective Reminding Test. *Israel Journal of Psychiatry and Related Sciences, 36,* 11–17.

Hannay, H. J. (1986). *Experimental techniques in human neuropsychology.* New York: Oxford University Press.

Hannay, H. J., & Levin, H. S. (1985). Selective Reminding Test: An examination of the equivalence of four forms. *Journal of Clinical and Experimental Neuropsychology, 7,* 251–263.

Iaffaldano, P., Viterbo, R. G., Goretti, B., Portaccio, E., Amato, M. P., & Trojano, M. (2014). Emotional and neutral verbal memory impairment in multiple sclerosis. *Journal of the Neurological Sciences, 341*(1-2), 28–31.

Johnson-Markve, B., Lee, G. P., Loring, D. W., & Viner, K. M. (2011). Usefulness of Verbal Selective Reminding in distinguishing frontal lobe memory disorders in epilepsy. *Epilepsy & Behavior, 22*(2), 313–317.

Keilp, J. G., Beers, S. R., Burke, A. K., Melhem, N. M., Oquendo, M. A., Brent, D. A., & Mann, J. J. (2014a). Neuropsychological deficits in past suicide attempters with varying levels of depression severity. *Psychological Medicine, 44*(14), 2965–2974.

Keilp, J. G., Gorlyn, M., Russell, M., Oquendo, M. A., Burke, A. K., Harkavy-Friedman, J., & Mann, J. J. (2013). Neuropsychological function and suicidal behavior: Attention control, memory and executive dysfunction in suicide attempt. *Psychological Medicine, 43*(3), 539–551.

Keilp, J. G., Wyatt, G., Gorlyn, M., Oquendo, M. A., Burke, A. K., & Mann, J. J. (2014b). Intact alternation performance in high lethality suicide attempters. *Psychiatry Research, 219*(1), 129–136.

Kraemer, H. C., Peabody, C. A., Tinklenberg, J. R., & Yesavage, J. A. (1983). Mathematical and empirical development of a test of memory for clinical and research use. *Psychological Bulletin, 94,* 367–380.

Krinsky-McHale, S. J., Devenny, D. A., & Silverman, W. P. (2002). Changes in explicit memory associated with early dementia in adults with Down's syndrome. *Journal of Intellectual Disability Research, 46,* 198–208.

Kuzis, G., Sabe, L., Tiberti, C., Merello, M., Leiguarda, R., & Starkstein, S. E. (1999). Explicit and implicit learning in patients with Alzheimer disease and Parkinson disease with dementia. *Neuropsychiatry, Neuropsychology, and Behavioral Neurology, 12,* 265–269.

Larrabee, G. J., & Curtiss, G. (1995). Construct validity of various verbal and visual memory tests. *Journal of Clinical and Experimental Neuropsychology, 17,* 536–547.

Larrabee, G. J., Trahan, D. E., Curtiss, G., & Levin, H. S. (1988). Normative data for the Verbal Selective Reminding Test. *Neuropsychology, 2,* 173–182.

Larrabee, G. J., Trahan, D. E., & Levin, H. S. (2000). Normative data for a six-trial administration of the Verbal Selective Reminding Test. *The Clinical Neuropsychologist, 14,* 110–118.

Lencz, T., McCarthy, G., Bronen, R. A., Scott, T. M., Insemi, J. A., Sass, K. J., . . . Spencer, D. D. (1992). Quantitative magnetic resonance imaging in temporal lobe epilepsy: Relationship to neuropathology and neuropsychological function. *Annals of Neurology, 31,* 629–637.

Levin, H. S., Benton, A. L., & Grossman, R. G. (1982). *Neurobehavioral consequences of closed head injury.* New York: Oxford University Press.

Levin, H. S., Grossman, R. G., Rose, J. E., & Teasdale, G. (1979). Long-term neuropsychological outcome of closed head injury. *Journal of Neurosurgery, 50,* 412–422.

Levin, H. S., Wilde, E., Troyanskaya, M., Petersen, N. J., Scheibel, R., Newsome, M., . . . Li, X. (2010). Diffusion tensor imaging of mild to moderate blast-related traumatic brain injury and its sequelae. *Journal of Neurotrauma, 27*(4), 683–694.

Loring, D. W., Lee, G. P., Meador, K. J., Smith, J. R., Martin, R. C., Ackell, A. B., & Flanigin, H. F. (1991). Hippocampal contribution to verbal recent memory following dominant-hemisphere temporal lobectomy. *Journal of Clinical and Experimental Neuropsychology, 13,* 575–586.

Loring, D. W., & Papanicolaou, A. C. (1987). Memory assessment in neuropsychology: Theoretical considerations and practical utility. *Journal of Clinical and Experimental Neuropsychology, 9,* 340–358.

Luchsinger, J. A., Cabral, R., Eimicke, J. P., Manly, J. J., & Teresi, J. (2015). Glycemia, diabetes status, and cognition in Hispanic adults aged 55–64 years. *Psychosomatic Medicine, 77*(6), 653–663.

Masur, D. M., Fuld, P. A., Blau, A. D., Crystal, H., & Aronson, M. K. (1990). Predicting development of dementia in the elderly with the Selective Reminding Test. *Journal of Clinical and Experimental Neuropsychology, 12,* 529–538.

Masur, D. M., Fuld, P. A., Blau, A. D., Thal, L. J., Levin, H. S., & Aronson, M. K. (1989). Distinguishing normal and demented elderly with the Selective Reminding Test. *Journal of Clinical and Experimental Neuropsychology, 11,* 615–630.

McCauley, S. R., Wilde, E. A., Barnes, A., Hanten, G., Hunter, J. V., Levin, H. S., & Smith, D. H. (2014). Patterns of early emotional and neuropsychological sequelae after mild traumatic brain injury. *Journal of Neurotrauma, 31*(10), 914–925.

McGinnis, D. (2012). Susceptibility to distraction during reading in young, young-old, and old-old adults. *Experimental Aging Research, 38*(4), 370–393.

Morales, M., Campo, P., Fernández, A., Moreno, D., Yáñez, J., & Sañudo, I. (2010). Normative data for a six-trial administration of a Spanish version of the verbal Selective Reminding Test. *Archives of Clinical Neuropsychology, 25*(8), 745–761.

Morgan, S. F. (1982). Measuring long-term memory, storage and retrieval in children. *Journal of Clinical Neuropsychology, 4,* 77–85.

Palta, P., Golden, S. H., Teresi, J., Palmas, W., Weinstock, R. S., Shea, S., . . . Luchsinger, J. A. (2014). Mild cognitive dysfunction does not affect diabetes mellitus control in minority elderly adults. *Journal of the American Geriatrics Society, 62*(12), 2363–2368.

Paniak, C. E., Shore, D. L., & Rourke, B. P. (1989). Recovery of memory after severe closed head injury: Dissociations in recovery of memory parameters and predictors of outcome. *Journal of Clinical and Experimental Neuropsychology, 11,* 631–644.

Pavisian, B., MacIntosh, B. J., Szilagyi, G., Staines, R. W., O'Connor, P., & Feinstein, A. (2014). Effects of cannabis on cognition in patients with MS: A psychometric and MRI study. *Neurology, 82*(21), 1879–1887.

Pelton, G. H., Harper, O. L., Roose, S. P., Marder, K., D'Antonio, K., & Devanand, D. P. (2016). Combined treatment with memantine/escitalopram for older depressed patients with cognitive impairment: A pilot study. *International Journal of Geriatric Psychiatry, 31*(6), 648–655.

Petersen, R. C., Smith, G., Kokmen, E., Ivnik, R. J., & Tangalos, E. G. (1992). Memory function in normal aging. *Neurology, 42,* 396–401.

Pillai, J. A., Hall, C. B., Dickson, D. W., Buschke, H., Lipton, R. B., & Verghese, J. (2011). Association of crossword puzzle participation with memory decline in persons who develop dementia. *Journal of the International Neuropsychological Society, 17*(6), 1006–1013.

Pomara, N., Belzer, K., Hernando, R., Pena, D. L., & Sidtis, J. J. (2008). Increased mental slowing associated with the ApoE ε4 allele after trihexyphenidyl oral anticholinergic challenge in healthy elderly. *The American Journal of Geriatric Psychiatry, 16*(2), 116–124.

Pomara, N., Facelle, T. M., Roth, A. E., Willoughby, L. M., Greenblatt, D. J., & Sidtis, J. J. (2006). Dose-dependent retrograde facilitation of verbal memory in healthy elderly after acute oral lorazepam administration. *Psychopharmacology, 185*(4), 487–494.

Pomara, N., Yi, L., Belzer, K., Facelle, T. M., Willoughby, L. M., & Sidtis, J. J. (2010). Retrograde facilitation of verbal memory by trihexyphenidyl in healthy elderly with and without the ApoE ε4 allele. *European Neuropsychopharmacology, 20*(7), 467–472.

Rao, S. M. (1990). *A manual for the brief repeatable battery of neuropsychological tests in multiple sclerosis.* Milwaukee, WI: Medical College of Wisconsin.

Reitz, C., Patel, B., Tang, M., Manly, J., Mayeux, R., & Luchsinger, J. A. (2007). Relation between vascular risk factors and neuropsychological test performance among elderly persons with Alzheimer's disease. *Journal of the Neurological Sciences, 257*(1-2), 194–201.

Ruchinskas, R. A., Brishek, D. K., Crews, W. D., Barth, J. T., Francis, J. P., & Robbins, M. K. (2000). A neuropsychological normative database for lung transplant candidates. *Journal of Clinical Psychology in Medical Settings, 7,* 107–112.

Ruff, R. M., Quayhagen, M., & Light, R. H. (1989). Selective reminding tests: A normative study of verbal learning in adults. *Journal of Clinical and Experimental Neuropsychology, 11,* 539–550.

Sabe, L., Jason, L., Juejati, M., Leiguarda, R., & Strakstein, S. E. (1995). Dissociation between declarative and procedural learning in dementia and depression. *Journal of Clinical and Experimental Neuropsychology, 17,* 841–848.

Sackeim, H. A., Prudic, J., Fuller, R., Keilp, J., Lavori, P. W., & Olfson, M. (2007). The cognitive effects of electroconvulsive therapy in community settings. *Neuropsychopharmacology, 32*(1), 244–254.

Salinsky, M. C., Storzbach, D., Dodrill, C. B., & Binder, L. M. (2001). Test-retest bias, reliability, and regression equations for neuropsychological measures repeated over a 12-16-week period. *Journal of the International Neuropsychological Society, 7,* 597–605.

Sass, K. J., Spencer, D. D., Kim, J. H., Westerveld, M., Novelly, R. A., & Lencz, T. (1990). Verbal memory impairment correlates with hippocampal pyramidal cell density. *Neurology, 40,* 1694–1697.

Sass, K. J., Westerveld, M., Buchanan, C. P., Spencer, S. S., Kim, J. H., & Spencer, D. D. (1994). Degree of hippocampal neuron loss determines verbal memory decline following left anteromedial temporal lobectomy. *Epilepsia, 35,* 1179–1186.

Scherl, W. F., Krupp, L. B., Christodoulou, C., Morgan, T. M., Hyman, L., Chandler, B., Coyle, P. K., MacAllister, W. S., & Lyme Study Group. (2004). Normative data for the Selective Reminding Test: A random digit dialing sample. *Psychological Reports, 95,* 593–603.

Schottenbauer, M. A., Hommer, D., & Weingartner, H. (2007). Memory deficits among alcoholics: Performance on a selective reminding task. *Aging, Neuropsychology, and Cognition, 14*(5), 505–516.

Shear, J. M., & Craft, R. B. (1989). Examination of the concurrent validity of the California Verbal Learning Test. *The Clinical Neuropsychologist, 3,* 162–168.

Sherman, E. M. S., Strauss, E., Spellacy, F., & Hunter, M. (1995). Construct validity of WAIS-R factors: Neuropsychological test correlates in adults referred for possible head injury. *Psychological Assessment, 7,* 440–444.

Sherwin, B. B., Chertkow, H., Schipper, H., & Nasreddine, Z. (2011). A randomized controlled trial of estrogen treatment in men with mild cognitive impairment. *Neurobiology of Aging, 32*(10), 1808–1817.

Sliwinski, M., Buschke, H., Stewart, W. F., Masur, D., & Lipton, R. B. (1997). The effect of dementia risk factors on comparative diagnostic Selective Reminding norms. *Journal of the International Neuropsychological Society, 3,* 317–326.

Smith, R. L., Goode, K. T., la Marche, J. A., & Boll, T. J. (1995). Selective Reminding Test Short Form administration: A comparison of two through twelve trials. *Psychological Assessment, 7,* 177–182.

Stern, Y., Tang, M. X., Jacobs, D. M., Sano, M., Marder, K., Bell, K., . . . Cote, L. (1998). Prospective comparative study of the evolution of probable Alzheimer's disease and Parkinson's disease dementia. *Journal of the International Neuropsychological Society, 4,* 279–284.

Stricks, L., Pittman, J., Jacobs, D. M., Sano, M., & Stern, Y. (1998). Normative data for a brief neuropsychological battery administered to English- and Spanish-speaking community-dwelling elders. *Journal of the International Neuropsychological Society, 4,* 311–318.

Tabert, M. H., Manly, J. J., Liu, X., Pelton, G. H., Rosenblum, S., Jacobs, M., . . . Devanand, D. P. (2006). Neuropsychological prediction of conversion to Alzheimer disease in patients with mild cognitive impairment. *Archives of General Psychiatry, 63*(8), 916–924.

Trahan, D. E., & Larrabee, G. J. (1993). Clinical and methodological issues in measuring rate of forgetting with the Verbal Selective Reminding Test. *Psychological Assessment, 5,* 67–71.

Trahan, D. E., & Quintana, J. W. (1990). Analysis of gender effects upon verbal and visual memory performance in adults. *Archives of Clinical Neuropsychology, 5,* 325–334.

Troyanskaya, M., Pastorek, N. J., Scheibel, R. S., Petersen, N. J., McCulloch, K., Wilde, E. A., . . . Levin, H. S. (2015). Combat exposure, PTSD symptoms, and cognition following blast-related traumatic brain injury in OEF/OIF/OND service members and veterans. *Military Medicine, 180*(3), 285–289.

Westerveld, M., Sass, K. J., Sass, A., & Henry, H. G. (1994). Assessment of verbal memory in temporal lobe epilepsy using the Selective Reminding Test: Equivalence and reliability of alternate forms. *Journal of Epilepsy, 7,* 57–63.

Wiederholt, W. C., Cahn, D., Butters, N. M., Salmon, D. P., Kritz-Silverstein, D., & Barrett-Connor, E. (1993). Effects of age, gender, and education on selected neuropsychological tests in an elderly community cohort. *Journal of the American Geriatrics Society, 41,* 639–647.

Wu, T. C., Wilde, E. A., Bigler, E. D., Yallampalli, R., McCauley, S. R., Troyanskaya, M., . . . Levin, H. S. (2010). Evaluating the relationship between memory functioning and cingulum bundles in acute mild traumatic brain injury using diffusion tensor imaging. *Journal of Neurotrauma, 27*(2), 303–307.

Yaffe, K., Barnes, D., Lindquist, K., Cauley, J., Simonsick, E. M., Penninx, B., . . . Cummings, S. R. (2007). Endogenous sex hormone levels and risk of cognitive decline in an older biracial cohort. *Neurobiology of Aging, 28*(2), 171–178.

Yaffe, K., Kurella-Tamura, M., Ackerson, L., Hoang, T. D., Anderson, A. H., Duckworth, M., . . . Townsend, R. R. (2014). Higher levels of cystatin C are associated with worse cognitive function in older adults with chronic kidney disease: The chronic renal insufficiency cohort cognitive study. *Journal of the American Geriatrics Society, 62*(9), 1623–1629.

Zahodne, L. B., Stern, Y., & Manly, J. J. (2014). Depressive symptoms precede memory decline, but not vice versa, in non-demented older adults. *Journal of the American Geriatrics Society, 62*(1), 130–134.

Zalonis, I., Kararizou, E., Christidi, F., Kapaki, E., Triantafyllou, N. I., Varsou, A., . . . Vassilopoulos, D. (2009). Selective Reminding Test: Demographic predictors of performance and normative data for the Greek population. *Psychological Reports, 104*(2), 593–607.

TACTUAL PERFORMANCE TEST (TPT)

TEST NAME	**Tactual Performance Test (TPT)**
DOMAIN	Tactile memory
AGE RANGE	In adults, to 85 years
ADMINISTRATION TIME	15 to 50 minutes
SCORING FORMAT	Hand scored
REFERENCES	Reitan, R. M., & Wolfson, D. (1985). *The Halstead-Reitan Neuropsychological Test Battery.* Tucson, AZ: Neuropsychology Press. Russell, E. W., & Starkey, R. I. (2001). *Halstead Russell Neuropsychological Evaluation System (HRNES) manual.* Los Angeles: Western Psychological Services. www.wpspublish.com

DESCRIPTION

The Tactual Performance Test (TPT) is a test of tactile memory. The examinee is blindfolded and presented with blocks of differing shapes and a matching formboard with holes and is instructed to insert the blocks into the board as quickly as possible, first with the preferred hand, then with the nonpreferred hand, and then using both hands together. After completion of these trials, the formboard is concealed, the blindfold is removed, and the examinee is asked to draw from memory, indicating both the shapes of the blocks and their placement relative to each other. TPT performance is reported in terms of either time to complete the task or minutes per block, for (a) the preferred hand (b) the nonpreferred hand (c) both hands, and (d) the total time for the three tactile trials; in addition (e) a memory score for the number of blocks correctly reproduced and (f) a location score for the number of blocks correctly located in the drawing are recorded.

A 10-hole formboard is used for examinees aged 15 years and older. In addition to the formboard material, a clean, comfortably fitting blindfold (eye mask or gauze pads) and a stopwatch are required. Scoring forms (see Figure 10–15) can be easily produced. The material is sturdy and rarely needs replacing.

The test is part of the Halstead-Reitan Neuropsychological Evaluation System, Revised (HRNES-R; Russell & Starkey, 2001) but can be purchased and administered on its own.

ADMINISTRATION

For patients 15 years and older, the 10-block board is mounted vertically in the stand with the cross in the upper right-hand corner.

The examinee is seated, near and squarely facing the table, asked to close their eyes, and a blindfold or eye mask is tied over the eyes. The examiner questions the examinee about their ability to see, especially downward. After the examiner is certain the examinee cannot see, the board is brought out. The blocks are placed on the table in random sequence between the board and the examinee. Blocks adjacent to each other on the board should not be placed next to each other on the table. For specific instructions, see Figure 10–16. Some examiners prefer to guide the examinee to each block presented in standardized order, whereas others allow the examinee to pick blocks in random order. Chavez et al. (1982) indicated that the two modes of presentation show no differences in results on the time trials of the test. However, a standardized

Trial	*Hand*	*Circle*	*Time*
1	Dominant	R L	________
2	Nondominant	R L	________
3	Both		________
Total time	________		
Memory	________		
Location	________		

Figure 10–15 *Tactual Performance Test (TPT) sample scoring sheet.*

Dominant Hand

Ask the subject to give you the preferred (dominant) hand. Take the subject's wrist and move the hand over the board and the pieces on the table while giving the following instructions: *In front of you on the table is a board. This is the size and shape of it.* (Move the subject's hand around the edge of the board). *On the face of the board are holes of various shapes and sizes* (move subject's hand around the face of the board), *and here in front of you are blocks of various shapes and sizes* (pass the subject's hand over the blocks, then place the subject's hand in their lap). *You are to fit the blocks into the spaces on the board. There is a place for each block and a block for each opening. Now I want you to do your best using only your right hand* (or left if that is the dominant hand). *You may begin whenever you are ready.*

Start the stopwatch when the subject first touches the board or blocks, and stop it when the last piece has been placed. Record the time for each hand in minutes and seconds. It is helpful to praise the subject for correctly placed blocks and to encourage the subject if they are not doing well. As the blocks in front of the subject are used up, push over the others to keep a supply ready at hand. When the subject has finished, ask them not to remove the blindfold and suggest that the subject relax for a minute or two.

Some patients spends a very long time trying to complete the tasks. The trial can continue up to 15 min and then be discontinued unless the patient is about to complete the task.

Nondominant Hand

After laying out the blocks in random order, say: *Now I want you to do the test again, and this time you are to use only your left hand* (or right hand, if that is the nondominant hand). *Begin whenever you are ready.* Record the time needed for this hand.

Both Hands

Lay out the blocks again and say: *This time you may use both hands for the test.* When the subject is finished, ask them to leave the blindfold on for a few minutes and put the board out of sight. Say: *Please remove the bindfold.*

Memory

Place a sheet of white paper and pencil in front of the subject and say: *On this sheet of paper I want you to draw an outline of the shape of the board. On your drawing, put in the shapes of the blocks in the same place as you remember them on the board. Note that there are three parts to your task: the shape of the board, the shape of the blocks, and their location on the board. Be sure to label the top of your drawing. There is no time limit on this.*

Figure 10–16 *Instructions for administering the Tactual Performance Test (TPT).*

block presentation was associated with higher memory scores, and a trend was noted for higher location scores. See the section "Comments" for a discussion of rules for discontinuation.

SCORING

There are a number of ways to score the test. It can be scored by calculating the total time for the three placement trials (Time right, left, and both hands), by counting the number of blocks correctly drawn (Memory), and by counting the number of blocks properly located in the drawings (Location). Differences between right- and left-hand performances can also be noted.

Some authors have adopted the use of a minutes-per-block score (i.e., number of minutes divided by number of blocks correctly placed) for each of the three timed trials and for the total time score (Heaton et al., 2004). In this way, the examiner has a rate score that can be interpreted regardless of the number of blocks correctly placed. For example, if an examinee places five blocks in five minutes, the rate is 5/5, or one block per minute.

In counting the blocks correctly reproduced, count only those that are fairly accurately drawn and indicate that the examinee had a true mental picture of the block. A star of four or five points is accepted as correct. The location score is obtained by counting the right place on the drawing in relation to the other blocks and the formboard.

Examinees who have difficulty reproducing a shape on the drawing part of the test are given credit if they can correctly name the shape. However, they should be urged to do their best at drawing the figures. If two figures on the drawing look very similar, the examiner should ask the examinee if they are the same figure. For example, the square and the rectangle are often drawn very much alike. If the examinee calls one a square and the other a rectangle (or a "long square"), the examinee is given credit for both. If two identical figures are drawn, the examiner should give credit to the one most correctly localized, even if it is not the most accurate drawing.

In scoring location, the relationship of the figure to the board as well as to the other shapes drawn should be considered. For example, if the triangle is drawn near the top of the board, and the cross and half-circle are placed on each side of it but another shape is drawn in above the triangle, then the triangle does not count as correctly localized. Reitan and Wolfson (1985) recommended dividing the page into nine segments for scoring. If the major portion of a block fits in its appropriate division, it is given credit for localization. No localization credit is given unless memory credit for the block has already been given. A scoring guide for TPT Location appears in the HRNES-R Manual (Russell & Starkey, 2001).

DEMOGRAPHIC EFFECTS

AGE

Age contributes significantly to performance, with scores improving in childhood and declining with advancing age (e.g., Heaton et al., 2004; Sweeney & Johnson, 2001). In adults aged 20 to 85 years, Heaton et al. (2004) reported that, in their Caucasian sample of adults, about 10% to 19% of the variance in scores on the TPT time trials was accounted for by age. In the African-American sample, the values were 18% to 25%. For the Memory and Location trials, age accounted for 21% and 26%, respectively, of the variance in test scores in the Caucasian sample, and 27% and 21%, respectively, in the African-American sample. The contribution of variables such as age is sufficiently large to invalidate the use of simple cutoff scores. Failure to take age into account results in an increased probability of misclassifying healthy older adults as impaired. For example, Heaton et al. (2004) noted that application of a single set of norms for the Location score results in correct classification of 65% of Caucasians younger than 40 years of age but only 11% of those older than 60 years of age.

GENDER

The effect of gender tends to be minimal, accounting for 1% or less of the variance in test scores (Heaton et al., 2004).

EDUCATION AND IQ

The influence of education is less than that of age. Some authors (e.g., Ernst, 1987; Yeudall et al., 1987) found no relationship between educational level and TPT scores, whereas others reported better TPT performance with increasing levels of education (e.g., Heaton et al., 2004; Russell & Starkey, 2001). Heaton et al. (2004) documented in their large sample of neurologically healthy individuals (N = 1,212) that, in Caucasians, only about 1% to 4% of the variance in Time scores was accounted for by education; for Memory and Location, the percentages were somewhat greater, 10% and 6%, respectively.

IQ shows a moderate relationship with TPT scores (Dodrill, 1997; Heilbronner et al., 1991), with PIQ showing more of a correlation than VIQ (Yeudall et al., 1987).

ETHNICITY, NATIONALITY, AND LINGUISTIC EFFECTS

A study comparing Anglo-American, Mexican-American, and Mexican adults (Arnold et al., 1994) revealed an acculturation effect (faster performance in Anglo Americans) only for Time scores (dominant, nondominant, total), but not for Location or Memory scores. Because the amount of variance accounted for by age, education, and gender may differ in Caucasians and African Americans, Heaton et al. (2004) developed separate demographic corrections for these two groups.

NORMATIVE DATA

A number of authors have published normative data for use with adults (e.g., Greer et al., 2010; Heaton et al., 2004; Russell & Starkey, 2001). Because of the effects of age, education, and ethnicity, we recommend the use of normative data provided by Heaton et al. (2004). As noted in Table 10–119, they provided norms separately for two ethnicity groups (Caucasians and African Americans) organized by age, gender, and education. The samples are large and cover a wide range in terms of age and education, and the exclusion criteria are specified. T scores lower than 40 are classed as impaired.

Greer et al. (2010) provide pooled norms by pooling normative data from 110 published studies on healthy controls (N = 8,131) including students, community volunteers, and medical patients. The data are stratified by age and education and are presented in Table 10–120. Note that the cell sizes for well-educated (>15 years), middle-aged adults are relatively small. When compared to a clinical sample, the authors note that the pooled norms yield fewer elevations and lower average T scores than the Heaton et al. (2004) norms but obtain more elevations and higher average T scores than the Russell and Starkey (2001) norms. The authors suggest the use of the pooled norms for most patient groups and the more stringent Russell norms for community-dwelling individuals.

TABLE 10–119 Characteristics of the Tactual Performance Test (TPT) Normative Sample Provided by Heaton et al. (2004)

Sample size	1,212
Age	20 to 85[a] years
Geographic location	Various states in the United States, and Manitoba, Canada
Sample type	Individuals recruited as part of multicenter studies
Education	0 to 20[b] years
Gender	57% Men 43% Women
Ethnicity	634 Caucasian 578 African American
Screening	No reported history of learning disability, neurological disorder, serious psychiatric disorder, or alcohol or drug abuse

[a] Age groups: 20–34, 35–39, 40–44, 45–49, 50–54, 55–59, 60–64, 65–69, 70–74, 75–79, and 80–89.

[b] Education groups: 7–8, 9–11, 12, 13–15, 16–17, and 18–20.

SOURCE: Adapted from Heaton et al. (2004).

TABLE 10–120 Pooled Norms for the Tactual Performance Test (TPT) Stratified by Age and Education

	EDUCATION (YEARS)											
	<12			12 TO 14			≥15			ALL		
AGE (YEARS)	N	M	*SD*	N	M	*SD*	N	M	*SD*	N	M	*SD*
<35 years												
TPT-Time	124	12.31	5.43	922	11.18	4.54	187	9.04	3.08	1233	10.97	4.45
TPT-Mem	159	7.31	1.65	1929	8.00	1.34	187	8.19	1.23	2275	7.97	1.36
TPT-Loc	159	4.64	2.33	1929	5.20	2.24	187	6.36	2.07	2275	5.26	2.24
35 to 64 years												
TPT-Time	211	18.57	9.51	1329	14.73	7.91	82	12.71	5.44	1622	15.13	8.03
TPT-Mem	186	6.49	1.92	1500	7.34	1.56	82	7.75	1.24	1768	7.27	1.59
TPT-Loc	186	2.78	2.24	1500	4.05	2.31	82	4.75	2.08	1768	3.95	2.29

NOTE: TPT-Time, Tactual Performance Test-Total Time; TPT-Mem, Tactual Performance Test-Memory; TPT-Loc, Tactual Performance Test-Location; M, Mean; *SD*, Standard Deviation.
SOURCE: Adapted from Greer et al. (2010).

DIFFERENCES BETWEEN HANDS

There is no difference in test scores between right- and left-handed adults (Thompson et al., 1987). However, it has been reported that, on average, healthy adults show about 30% improvement in performance across the first two trials of the TPT (Boll, 1981). A reversal of this pattern (second trial with the nondominant hand and third trial with both hands slower than the first trial) is found frequently, especially in healthy older adults, perhaps because of a reduced rate of learning (Thompson et al., 1987). Thomson and Heaton (1991) warned that such reversals should not be interpreted as evidence of acquired right-hemisphere lesions unless the differences are large and other evidence supports such an interpretation.

EVIDENCE FOR RELIABILITY

EVIDENCE FOR INTERNAL RELIABILITY

Internal reliability correlations, using either time in seconds to place each block or blocks-per-minute scores for the preferred hand, nonpreferred hand, both hands, and total time, have ranged from .61 to .90 in adults (Charter, 2000a; Charter et al., 1987, 2001). As shown in Table 10–121, the reliabilities of the preferred hand and memory are marginal, whereas the reliability coefficient for location is adequate (Charter et al., 2000). Reliabilities of difference scores (e.g., nonpreferred minus preferred) are low (<.65; Charter, 2001). Therefore, the examiner can have little confidence that an examinee's obtained difference score is close to their hypothetical true difference score.

TABLE 10–121 Tactual Performance Test (TPT) Internal Consistency

MAGNITUDE OF COEFFICIENT	MEASURE
Very High (≥.90)	Total Time
High (.80 to .89)	Nonpreferred Hand Both Hands
Adequate (.70 to .79)	Location
Marginal (.60 to .69)	Preferred Hand Memory
Low (≤ .59)	

EVIDENCE FOR TEST-RETEST RELIABILITY, MEASURING CHANGE, AND PRACTICE EFFECTS

In adults, reliability coefficients tend to be adequate for the Time scores but lower than desirable for the Memory and Location scores. For example, Schludermann and Schludermann (1983) reported retest coefficients of .76 for Time, .60 for Memory, and .55 for Location scores in a sample of 174 executives retested after two years, and coefficients of .91, .72, and .53, respectively, for 86 individuals in the same sample who were tested again after three years. Goldstein and Watson (1989) reported retest reliabilities after four to 469 weeks for 150 neuropsychiatric patients; these ranged from .66 to .74 for Time, from .46 to .72 for Memory, and from .32 to .69 for Location, with similar values for alcoholics, trauma patients, and patients with vascular disorders, and somewhat lower coefficients for those with schizophrenia. However, in healthy adults retested after an interval of three weeks, reliability coefficients are higher for Memory ($r = .80$) and Location ($r = .77$) than for Time ($r = .69$) scores (Bornstein et al., 1987).

Dikmen et al. (1999) reported improvement in scores in a sample of 384 healthy or neurologically stable individuals who were retested about nine months after initial testing. Table 10–122 provides information to determine whether there has been substantial change taking practice into account (but see Hinton-Bayre, 2000, and Maassen, 2004, who raised concerns about the RCI calculation procedure used by Dikmen et al. [1999] and suggested that the 90% prediction intervals should actually be smaller). One first subtracts the mean T2 - T1 change (column 3) from the difference between the two testings for the individual and then compares the resulting value with 1.64 times the

TABLE 10–122 Tactual Performance Test (TPT) Test-Retest Effects in 384 Healthy Individuals Assessed After Intervals of 2 to 16 Months

	TIME 1 (1)		TIME 2 (2)		T2–T1 (3)		T1, T2 (4)
MEASURE	MEAN	*SD*	MEAN	*SD*	MEAN	*SD*	*R*
Total [time per block (min)]	0.5	0.49	.43	0.33	−.09	.29	.83
Memory	7.71	1.59	7.97	1.56	.26	1.21	.71
Location	4.39	2.49	4.92	2.57	.53	2.27	.60

NOTE: Mean Age = 34.2, *SD* = 16.7, range = 15–83; Mean education = 12.1, *SD* = 2.6, range = 0–19; 66% male; retest interval mean = 9.1 months, *SD* = 3.0, range = 2.4–15.8. Hinton-Bayre (2000) has indicated that there is an error in these calculations. He notes that, using the Jacobson and Truax RCI formula, the 90% prediction interval (PI) for TPT total is ± 0.39.

SOURCE: Adapted from Dikmen et al. (1999).

standard deviation of the difference (column 4). The 1.64 comes from the normal distribution and is exceeded in the positive or negative direction only 10% of the time if indeed there is no real change in clinical condition.

EVIDENCE FOR INTERRATER RELIABILITY

Martin and Greene (1978; cited in Snow, 1987) reported that the percentage of agreement between judges on scoring of Memory ranged from 71% to 76%. Location was scored with 56–64% agreement. In some pairs of judges, the percentage of agreement in scoring Memory was as low as 36%; for Location, it was as low as 29%. However, another study comparing results from three scorers found excellent interscorer reliability coefficients for the Memory and Location scores (both .98; Charter et al., 1998).

EVIDENCE FOR VALIDITY

RELATIONS WITHIN TEST

In their review, Thompson and Parsons (1985) noted that the three different scores are related to one another. This is especially true for Memory and Location, with correlations ranging from .56 to .71. TPT Time and Memory correlations range from .32 to .72, and TPT Time and Location correlations range from .26 to .62. In general, those completing the timed tasks most rapidly are also those who most successfully recall the shapes and their locations (Dinkins & deFilippis, 1997). In short, increasing exposure during the problem-solving component of the task does not necessarily translate into better performance on the memory component.

RELATIONSHIPS WITH OTHER TESTS

Berger (1998) examined a heterogeneous clinical sample and reported moderate to high correlations (r = .48 to .63) between TPT Time, Memory, and Location scores and the Perceptual Organization factor of the WAIS-R, suggesting that nonverbal reasoning is important for task performance. Correlations with the Verbal Comprehension and Freedom from Distractibility factors were minimal (r < .30).

Factor-analytic findings point to considerable overlap in what the scores represent, although there is some individual contribution as well. For example, Bornstein (1990) found that all three TPT scores (Time, Memory, and Location) loaded on the same factor, with only minor loadings from a large number of other tests. However, Campbell et al. (1989) found that, in young adults, the Time scores loaded on a factor with other time-dependent scores (e.g., Picture Completion, Block Design); the Memory score loaded on an attention factor together with Digit Span, Digit Symbol, Seashore Rhythm, and Trails A; and the TPT Location score loaded on all three of the extracted factors. The authors concluded that the test is multifactorial in nature (see also Johnstone et al., 2000).

ITEM DIFFICULTY

Charter (2000b) reported that, on the time trials (preferred, nonpreferred, both hands), blocks at the top of the board are more difficult than blocks at the bottom of the board. They noted that examinee strategy may contribute to item difficulty. If examinees try to fill the spaces on the top first, these spaces may be difficult because there are more block shapes to discriminate. There does not appear to be an easily discernible pattern of item difficulty in relation to block placement on the TPT board for Memory or Location trials (Charter & Dutra, 2001).

CLINICAL STUDIES

Few contemporary studies have been reported in the literature. Chronic alcoholism and/or a history of TBI have been associated with poor TPT Time, Memory, and Location scores (Allen et al., 2009; Charter et al., 2001; Dikmen et al., 1995; Goldstein et al., 2010; Gurling et al., 1991; Ross et al., 2006). Older studies report that TPT Time has been found to be one of the best predictors of cognitive dysfunction in the Halstead-Reitan battery, though there are inconsistent findings on the sensitivity of the individual trials. Older studies also found that the TPT is sensitive to the effects of MS (Ivnik, 1978) and epilepsy (e.g., Dodrill, 1987) and is predictive of overall adjustment and independent living in a longitudinal investigation of high-school adolescents with epilepsy (Dodrill & Clemmons, 1984).

Impairment has also been reported in neuropsychiatric conditions, including schizophrenia (e.g., Goldstein et al., 1998) and depression (Harris et al., 1981), and is associated with poor driving performance (Rothke, 1989). Surprisingly, healthy volunteers with low trait anxiety perform poorly on the TPT (Horwitz et al., 2008). By contrast, in one study using an outpatient neuropsychology clinic sample referred for evaluation because of brain injury, TPT Memory and Location scores were not related to psychological disturbances as measured by the MMPI-2 (Ross et al., 2006).

Horwitz and colleagues (2008) reported that poor TPT Location was associated with the presence of a third-party observers in a study on the impact of third-party observer on neuropsychological test performance among undergraduate volunteers. The obtained scores were more than one standard deviation below published age- and education-adjusted norms (i.e., classified as mild to moderate impairment) in the observer group, whereas controls generally scored within one standard deviation of published norms (i.e., within normal limits).

NEUROANATOMICAL CORRELATES AND NEUROIMAGING STUDIES

Brescian et al. (2014) reported a case study of an 88-year-old man with agenesis of the corpus callosum and colpocephaly who generally performed in the normal range on an extensive neuropsychological test battery except for the TPT. He was notably impaired on the both-hands trial on the TPT, suggesting that interhemispheric transfer via the corpus callosum is needed to coordinate the action of both hands in completing the TPT. No studies have been done using contemporary neuroimaging techniques. Classical studies show that time using the right hand is slower for patients with left-hemisphere brain damage, and left-hand time is slower for those with right-hemisphere damage (Dodrill, 1978). Several studies have found that patients with right-hemisphere damage perform more slowly than do patients with left-hemisphere damage (Reitan, 1964), although Goldstein and Shelly (1972) reported that TPT Time did not differentiate these two groups. The Memory and Location scores do not appear to discriminate reliably between right- and left-hemisphere deficits (Heilbronner et al., 1991; Thompson & Parsons, 1985).

Early studies found that patients with frontal lesions perform poorly on some or all TPT measures (Halstead, 1947; Shure & Halstead, 1958), but subsequent studies found more impairment in patients with posterior damage (Chapman & Wolff, 1959; Reitan, 1964). Chapman and Wolff (1959) suggested that patients with frontal damage performed more poorly in the early studies because they had larger lesions than did the patients with nonfrontal damage.

PERFORMANCE VALIDITY

Silk-Eglit et al. (2013) reported that among those undergoing neuropsychological evaluation for medico-legal purposes, individuals who failed two or more stand-alone performance validity tests (based on standard cutoffs on the TOMM, WMT, Victoria Symptom Validity Test [VSVT], and the Rey-15) performed worse on the TPT Memory and TPT Location compared to those who showed valid performance. One older study (Goebel, 1983) found that individuals instructed to feign brain damage underestimate the difficulty of the task for brain-injured individuals and obtain scores more similar to those of healthy controls than to scores of actual brain-injured patients on all parts of the test.

COMMENT

Although the TPT has been in existence for decades, there have been limited studies done to address several criticisms. These include the lack of psychometric studies, lack of updated norms, and uncertainties about neuroanatomical correlates/meaning of test results. Both internal consistency and test-retest reliability are less than optimal in some studies, and more information on practice effects is needed.

Criticisms have also been raised regarding the lack of standardization of the procedure. Reitan (1979) suggested that termination is possible after 15 minutes if the examinee is "getting discouraged and is making very slow progress" (p. 36) but recommended allowing the examinee to continue if a correct performance appeared close. Others (e.g., Russell & Starkey, 1993) use a 10-minute cutoff. Snow (1987) noted that, by reducing the time the examinee spends on the test, one reduces the amount of exposure the examinee has to the blocks and their locations on the board. Differing amounts of exposure duration may affect Memory and Location scores (but see Dinkins & deFilippis, 1997, and the section "Relations Within Test"). Differences in block presentation (guided vs. unstructured; Chavez et al., 1982) and type of formboard (Kupke, 1983) also affect performance. Kupke (1983) found better total Time scores in undergraduates with the use of a portable TPT as opposed to the standard version. Kupke noted that the holes proved to be "looser" on the portable version that he constructed.

The scoring criteria for Memory and Location are also vague and may lead to differences in interpretations between examiners (but see Charter et al., 1998). In short, standardization of the administration and scoring procedures is needed (Snow, 1987; Mitrushina et al., 2005). By addressing these issues, it may be possible to obtain a clearer understanding of the utility of this task.

The precise meaning of the test scores is not certain as there is a lack of contemporary studies examining the relationship of the TPT with other tests as well as the performance of different patient groups. Nonverbal reasoning, attention, manual dexterity, and coordination appear to be important. TPT Time scores appear to be better indicators of brain dysfunction than Memory or Location scores, although Time, Memory, and Location scores do not reliably identify laterality or localization.

Users should also bear in mind that age, education, and ethnicity/cultural factors influence performance and that reference to appropriate normative data is critical. Although the availability of the large normative dataset for adults created by Heaton et al. (2004) is a strength, it should be noted that the data are old and they were collected over a lengthy

25-year period. Overall, the test has many limitations at present that limit its routine clinical usage.

REFERENCES

Allen, D. N., Goldstein, G., Caponigro, J. M., & Donohue, B. (2009). The effects of alcoholism comorbidity on neurocognitive function following traumatic brain injury. *Applied Neuropsychology, 16*(3), 186–192. https://doi.org/10.1080/09084280903098687

Arnold, B. R., Montgomery, G. T., Castaneda, I., & Longoria, R. (1994). Acculturation and performance of Hispanics on selected Halstead-Reitan neuropsychological tests. *Assessment, 1,* 239–248.

Berger, S. (1998). The WAIS-R factors: Usefulness and construct validity in neuropsychological assessments. *Applied Neuropsychol-ogy, 5,* 37–42.

Boll, T. J. (1981). The Halstead-Reitan Neuropsychology Battery. In S. B. Filskov & T. J. Boll (Eds.), *Handbook of clinical neuropsychology* (pp. 577–607). New York: Wiley.

Bornstein, R. A. (1990). Neuropsychological test batteries in neuropsychological assessment. In G. B. Baker & M. Hiscock (Eds.), *Neuromethods: Vol. 17. Neuropsychology* (pp. 281–310). Clifton, NJ: Humana.

Bornstein, R. A., Baker, G. B., & Douglas, A. B. (1987). Short-term retest reliability of the Halstead-Reitan Battery in a normal sample. *Journal of Nervous and Mental Disease, 175,* 229–232.

Brescian, N. E., Curiel, R. E., & Gass, C. S. (2014). Case study: A patient with agenesis of the corpus callosum with minimal associated neuropsychological impairment. *Neurocase, 20*(6), 606–614. https://doi.org/10.1080/13554794.2013.826690

Campbell, M. L., Drobes, D. J., & Horn, R. (1989). *Young adult norms, predictive validity, and relationship between Halstead-Reitan Tests and WAIS-R scores.* Paper presented at the 9th meeting of the National Academy of Neuropsychology, Washington, DC.

Chapman, L. F., & Wolff, H. G. (1959). The cerebral hemispheres and the highest integrative functions of man. *Archives of Neurology, 1,* 357–424.

Charter, R. A. (2000a). Internal consistency reliability of the Tactual Performance Test trials. *Perceptual & Motor Skills, 91,* 460–462.

Charter, R. A. (2000b). Item difficulty analysis of the Tactual Performance Test trials. *Perceptual and Motor Skills, 91,* 903–909.

Charter, R. A. (2001). Difference score reliability for Tactual Performance Test trials. *Perceptual and Motor Skills, 92,* 941–942.

Charter, R. A., Adkins, T. G., Alekoumbides, A., & Seacat, G. F. (1987). Reliability of the WAIS, WMS, and Reitan Battery: Raw scores and standardized scores corrected for age and education. *International Journal of Clinical Neuropsychology, 9,* 28–32.

Charter, R. A., & Dutra, R. L. (2001). Tactual Performance Test: Item analysis of the Memory and Location scores. *Perceptual and Motor Skills, 92,* 899–902.

Charter, R. A., Dutra, R. L., & Rapport, L. J. (2000). Tactual Performance Test: Internal consistency reliability of the memory and location scores. *Perceptual and Motor Skills, 91,* 143–146.

Charter, R. A., Lopez, M. N., Oh, S., & Lazar, M. D. (2001). Tactual Performance Test trials: Psychometric properties of the blocks-per-minute scores. *Perceptual and Motor Skills, 92,* 750–754.

Charter, R. A., Walden, D. K., & Hoffman, C. (1998). Interscorer reliabilities for Memory and Localization scores of the Tactual Performance Test. *The Clinical Neuropsychologist, 12,* 245–247.

Chavez, E. L., Schwartz, M. M., & Brandon, A. (1982). Effects of sex of subject and method of block presentation on the Tactual Performance Test. *Journal of Consulting and Clinical Psychology, 50,* 600–601.

Dikmen, S. S., Heaton, R. K., Grant, I., & Temkin, N. R. (1999). Test-retest reliability and practice effects of expanded Halstead-Reitan neuropsychological test battery. *Journal of the International Neuropsychological Society, 5,* 346–356.

Dikmen, S. S., Machamer, J. E., Winn, H. R., & Temkin, N. R. (1995). Neuropsychological outcome at 1-year post head injury. *Neuropsychology, 9,* 80–90.

Dinkins, H. E., & DeFilippis, N. A. (1997). The effects of time of exposure on Tactual Performance Test Memory and Location scores. *Applied Neuropsychology, 4,* 247–248.

Dodrill, C. B. (1978). The hand dynamometer as a neuropsychological measure. *Journal of Consulting and Clinical Psychology, 46,* 1432–1435.

Dodrill, C. B. (1987). *What's normal? Presidential Address.* Seattle: Pacific Northwest Neuropsychological Association.

Dodrill, C. B. (1997). Myths of neuropsychology. *The Clinical Neuropsychologist, 11,* 1–17.

Dodrill, C. B., & Clemmons, D. (1984). Use of neuropsychological tests to identify high school students with epilepsy who later demonstrate inadequate performances in life. *Journal of Consulting and Clinical Psychology, 52,* 520–527.

Ernst, J. (1987). Neuropsychological problem-solving skills in the elderly. *Psychology and Aging, 2,* 363–365.

Goebel, R. A. (1983). Detection of faking on the Halstead-Reitan neuropsychological test battery. *Journal of Clinical Psychology, 39,* 731–742.

Goldstein, G., Allen, D. N., & Caponigro, J. M. (2010). A retrospective study of heterogeneity in neurocognitive profiles associated with traumatic brain injury. *Brain Injury, 24*(4), 625–635. https://doi.org/10.3109/02699051003670882

Goldstein, G., Allen, D. N., & Seaton, B. E. (1998). A comparison of clustering solutions for cognitive heterogeneity in schizophrenia. *Journal of the International Neuropsychological Society, 4,* 353–362.

Goldstein, G., & Shelly, C. H. (1972). Statistical and normative studies of the Halstead Neuropsychological Test Battery relevant to a neuropsychiatric setting. *Perceptual and Motor Skills, 34,* 603–620.

Goldstein, G., & Watson, J. R. (1989). Test-retest reliability of the Halstead-Reitan battery and the WAIS in a neuropsychiatric population. *The Clinical Neuropsychologist, 3,* 265–273.

Greer, S. E., Brewer, K. K., Cannici, J. P., & Pennett, D. L. (2010). Level of performance accuracy for core Halstead-Reitan measures by pooling normal controls from published studies: Comparison with existing norms in a clinical sample. *Perceptual and Motor Skills, 111*(1), 3–18. https://doi.org/10.2466/03.22.27.PMS.111.4.3-18

Gurling, H. M. D., Curtis, D., & Murray, R. M. (1991). Psychological deficit from excessive alcohol consumption: Evidence from a co-twin control study. *British Journal of Addiction, 86,* 151–155.

Halstead, W. C. (1947). *Brain and intelligence; a quantitative study of the frontal lobes.* Chicago, IL: University of Chicago Press.

Harris, M., Cross, H. J., & Van Nieuwkerk, R. (1981). The effects of state depression and sex on the Finger Tapping and Tactual Performance tests. *Clinical Neuropsychology, 3,* 28–34.

Heaton, R. K., Miller, S. W., Taylor, M. J., & Grant, I. (2004). *Revised comprehensive norms for an Expanded Halstead-Reitan Battery: Demographically adjusted neuropsychological norms for African American and Caucasian adults.* Lutz, FL: PAR.

Heilbronner, R. L., Henry, G. K., Buck, P., Adams, R. L., & Fogle, T. (1991). Lateralized brain damage and performance on Trail Making A and B, Digit Span Forward and Backward, and TPT Memory and Location. *Archives of Clinical Neuropsychology, 6,* 252–258.

Hinton-Bayre, A. (2000). Reliable change formula query. *Journal of the International Neuropsychological Society, 6,* 362–363.

Horwitz, J. E., & McCaffrey, R. J. (2008). Effects of a third party observer and anxiety on tests of executive function. *Archives of Clinical Neuropsychology, 23*(4), 409–417.

Ivnik, R. J. (1978). Neuropsychological test performance as a function of the duration of MS-related symptomatology. *The Journal of Clinical Psychiatry, 39*(4), 304–312.

Johnstone, B., Vieth, A. Z., Johnson, J. C., & Shaw, J. A. (2000). Recall as a function of single versus multiple trials: Implications for rehabilitation. *Rehabilitation Psychology, 45,* 3–19.

Kupke, T. (1983). Effect of subject sex, examiner sex, and test apparatus on Halstead Category and Tactual Performance tests. *Journal of Consulting and Clinical Psychology, 51,* 624–626.

Maassen, G. H. (2004). The standard error in the Jacobson and Truax reliable change index: The classical approach to the assessment of reliable change. *Journal of the International Neuropsychological Society, 10,* 888–893.

Mitrushina, M. N., Boone, K. B., Razani, J., & D'Elia, L. F. (2005). *Handbook of normative data for neuropsychological assessment* (2nd ed.). New York: Oxford University Press.

Reitan, R. M. (1964). Psychological deficits resulting from cerebral lesions in man. In J. M. Warren & K. A. Akert (Eds.), *The frontal granular cortex and behavior* (pp. 295–312). New York: McGraw-Hill.

Reitan, R. M. (1979). *Manual for administration of neuropsychological test batteries for adults and children.* Tucson, AZ: Neuropsychology Laboratory.

Reitan, R. M., & Wolfson, D. (1985). *The Halstead-Reitan Neuropsychological Test Battery.* Tucson, AZ: Neuropsychology Press.

Rothke, S. (1989). The relationship between neuropsychological test scores and performance on a driving evaluation. *International Journal of Clinical Neuropsychology, 11,* 134–136.

Ross, S. R., Putnam, S. H., & Adams, K. M. (2006). Psychological disturbance, incomplete effort, and compensation-seeking status as predictors of neuropsychological test performance in head injury. *Journal of Clinical and Experimental Neuropsychology, 28*(1), 111–125.

Russell, E. W., & Starkey, R. I. (1993, 2001). *Halstead Russell Neuropsychological Evaluation System (HRNES) manual.* Los Angeles: Western Psychological Services.

Schludermann, E. H., & Schludermann, S. M. (1983). Halstead's studies in the neuropsychology of aging. *Archives of Gerontology and Geriatrics, 2,* 49–172.

Shure, G. H., & Halstead, W. C. (1958). Cerebral localization of intellectual processes. In N. L. Munn (Ed.), *Psychological Monographs General and Applied, 72*(12), No. 465.

Silk-Eglit, G. M., Stenclik, J. H., Miele, A. S., Lynch, J. K., & McCaffrey, R. J. (2013). The degree of conation on neuropsychological tests does not account for performance invalidity among litigants. *Archives of Clinical Neuropsychology, 28*(3), 213–221. https://doi.org/10.1093/arclin/act013

Snow, W. G. (1987). Standardization of test administration and scoring criteria: Some shortcomings of current practice with the Halstead-Reitan Battery. *The Clinical Neuropsychologist, 1,* 250–262.

Sweeney, J. E., & Johnson, A. M. (2001). Age and neuropsychological status following exposure to violent nonimpact acceleration forces in MVAs. *Journal of Forensic Neuropsychology, 2,* 31–40.

Thompson, L. L., & Heaton, R. K. (1991). Patterns of performance on the Tactual Performance Test. *The Clinical Neuropsychologist, 5,* 322–328.

Thompson, L. L., Heaton, R. K., Matthews, C. G., & Grant, I. (1987). Comparison of preferred and nonpreferred hand performance on four neuropsychological motor tasks. *The Clinical Neuropsychologist, 1,* 324–334.

Thompson, L. L., & Parsons, O. A. (1985). Contribution of the TPT to adult neuropsychological assessment. *Journal of Clinical and Experimental Neuropsychology, 7,* 430–444.

Yeudall, L. T., Reddon, J. R., Gill, D. M., & Stefanyk, W. O. (1987). Normative data for the Halstead-Reitan neuropsychological tests stratified by age and sex. *Journal of Clinical Psychology, 43,* 346–367.

WARRINGTON RECOGNITION MEMORY TEST (WRMT)

TEST NAME	**Warrington Recognition Memory Test (WRMT)**
DOMAIN	Verbal and visual memory
AGE RANGE	18 to 70 years for Words; 18 to 93 years for Faces
ADMINISTRATION TIME	15 minutes
SCORING FORMAT	Hand scored
REFERENCE	Warrington, E. K. (1984). *Recognition Memory Test manual.* Windsor, UK: NFER-Nelson.

DESCRIPTION

The original purpose of the Warrington Recognition Memory Test (WRMT) was to assess recognition memory for words and faces. It was developed to detect material-specific memory deficits across a wide age range. A recognition memory paradigm was chosen to provide comparable techniques for the assessment of verbal and nonverbal memory. Recognition memory tests have the advantage of being less vulnerable than recall tests to the effects of anxiety and depression. In addition, they lend themselves to the assessment of memory in patients with speech deficits. In recent years, it has also gained popularity as a measure of performance validity.

ADMINISTRATION

See manual. The examinee is told at the outset that this is a test of memory, is then presented with 50 stimulus pictures (words or unfamiliar male faces) at intervals of 3 seconds, and is required to respond "yes" or "no" to each item according to whether it is judged as pleasant or not pleasant. This ensures that the individual attends to each item. Following presentation of the 50 items, memory for words (or faces) is tested. For both words and faces, retention is tested by a two-choice recognition task, each of the stimuli being presented with one distractor item. The examinee is required to point to the stimulus item (or to read the item aloud, in the case of the word list). The examiner records recognition memory responses on the answer sheet.

SCORING

The raw score is the number of items correctly recognized on each task. Raw scores are converted to standard scores (M = 10, SD = 3) and percentiles. A Words/Faces Discrepancy score can also be calculated to provide an estimate of material-specific memory impairment.

DEMOGRAPHIC EFFECTS

AGE

Age is negatively correlated with performance (Bird et al., 2003; Harvey & Siegert, 1999; Warrington, 1984; but see Diesfeldt, 1990). The effect of age appears negligible up to the age of 40 years, at which point a decrement in scores emerges.

GENDER

Gender has no impact on test scores (Diesfeldt, 1990; Soukop et al., 1999).

EDUCATION AND IQ

Some relationships to education are expected. Among Dutch subjects, education did not affect performance (Diesfeldt, 1990; Diesfeldt & Vink, 1989). By contrast, Soukop et al. (1999) found a moderate relationship between Faces and education (r = .39). Harvey and Siegert (1999) reported a positive relation between years of education and scores on Words (r = .39); the correlation was not significant for Faces (r = .13).

Intelligence (e.g., NART, Raven's Progressive Matrices, Mill Hill Vocabulary Test) shows modest to moderate correlations with performance on both the Words and Faces subtests (r = .18 to .56; Diesfeldt, 1990; Diesfeldt & Vink, 1989; Harvey & Siegert, 1999; Warrington, 1984). Some authors, however, have found that the relation between the NART and Faces is not significant (Bird et al., 2003; Harvey & Siegert, 1999).

ETHNICITY, NATIONALITY, AND LINGUISTIC EFFECTS

Race of the examinee (Caucasian, African American) does not affect performance on the Faces subtest in American examinees, despite the fact that this subtest consists of white male faces only (O'Bryant et al., 2003). It is not known whether this also applies in other countries.

NORMATIVE DATA

STANDARDIZATION SAMPLE

To our knowledge, there exist no current normative datasets, with the most recent dataset from 1999 (see later discussion). According to Warrington (1984), the original data were collected from 310 inpatients with extracerebral disease, ranging in age from 18 to 70 years (see Table 10–123). The norms for each task are presented in the manual for three age groups: 18 to 39, 40 to 54, and 55 to 70 years. Users should note that test scores tend to be skewed toward the upper limits, particularly among young and middle-aged adults.

The frequency of occurrence of various Words/Faces discrepancies is also provided in the manual. A Words/Faces Discrepancy score is considered significant (i.e., a selective deficit) if it occurs in fewer than 5% of the standardization sample. For Words to be significantly greater than Faces, correct identification of 10 or more words than faces is required; for Faces to be significantly greater, 6 or more faces than words must be identified.

OTHER NORMATIVE REPORTS

Harvey and Siegert (1999) tested a sample of 139 older adults (94 women, 45 men) in New Zealand, aged 70 to 90 years (M = 77.24, SD = 4.8). Most were living independently, although some (14%) were receiving some community support (e.g., Meals on Wheels). The sample was of average to above-average intelligence (males, NART IQ = 110, SD = 11.2; females, NART IQ = 106.72, SD = 12.7). Table 10–124 presents the scores for three age groups (70–74, 75–79, and 80+ years) for the Words and Faces subtests as cumulative frequency tables. Because intellectual level affects performance, these authors also provided means (and SDs) for the WRMT tasks for the three age groups by NART score. However, some of the cell sizes are too small (e.g., n = 2) to be used for clinical purposes. They are provided here (see Table 10–125) to illustrate that there is a decline in performance with decreasing NART IQ score.

TABLE 10–123 Characteristics of the Warrington Recognition Memory Test (WRMT) Normative Sample

Sample size	310
Age[a]	18 to 70 years
Sample type	Mostly inpatients at three hospitals in England
Gender	57% Men 43% Women
Ethnicity	Not reported
Education	2 to 20 years (M = 13.47, SD = 2.88)
Socioeconomic status	Not reported
Screening	Any participant with a past history of cerebral disease was rejected, and only participant educated in the normal English system were included

[a] Based on three age groups: 18–39 (n = 98), 40–54 (n = 107), and 55–70 (n = 105) years.

SOURCE: Adapted from Warrington (1984).

Diesfeldt and Vink (1989) provided normative data for older adults aged 69 to 93 years for the Faces subtest. The data appear very similar to those provided by Harvey and Siegert (1999). Healthy older adults required about 4.3 minutes (SD = 1.3) to complete the word recognition task and about 5.4 minutes (SD = 1.7) for recognition of the faces (Diesfeldt, 1990).

Of note, O'Bryant et al. (2003) tested a sample of 60 undergraduates at a large southern American university on the Faces subtest and found that the mean score fell at about the 10th percentile according to norms provided in the test manual, despite average performance on other cognitive tasks. They urged re-examination of the norms for the Faces subtest.

EVIDENCE FOR RELIABILITY

EVIDENCE FOR INTERNAL RELIABILITY

The WRMT subtests were reported to have adequate internal consistency in a sample of 72 patients with TBI, with Cronbach's alpha of .86 for Words and .77 for Faces (Malina et al., 1998).

EVIDENCE FOR TEST-RETEST RELIABILITY, MEASURING CHANGE, AND PRACTICE EFFECTS

In young adults, two-week test-retest reliability tends to be marginal (r = .63 and .64 for Words and Faces, respectively; O'Bryant et al., 2003). In older adults and individuals with neurological disorders, coefficients are somewhat higher. Bird et al. (2003) reported one-month test-retest reliabilities of r = .69 for Words and .76 for Faces.

Practice effects (gains of about three to four raw score points) are present on retest in the Faces subtest in both young and older healthy adults (Bird et al., 2003; O'Bryant et al., 2003). On the Words task, gains of about one point have been noted (Bird et al., 2003; O'Bryant et al., 2003), although in young and middle-aged adults, practice effects may be masked by ceiling effects. IQ (as indexed by the NART) does not play a significant role in determining practice effects on this test (Bird et al., 2003).

Bird et al. (2003) calculated 90% RCIs corrected for practice for use when the WRMT is repeated (see Table 10–126). Overall, RCIs were larger for Faces than Words. In addition, RCIs were larger for older adults (55–70 years). Therefore, in this older group, large changes in raw test scores are needed to detect improvement on the Faces subtest, and relatively smaller changes in scores are needed to detect a decline in performance. To use Table 10–126, a raw score greater than the value with the minus sign is required for reliable decline, and a raw score greater than the value with the plus sign is required for reliable improvement.

TABLE 10–124 Cumulative Frequencies (%) for the Warrington Recognition Memory Test (WRMT) by Age (Years)

	WORDS			FACES		
AGE	70 TO 74 (*N* = 45)	75 TO 79 (*N* = 48)	80+ (*N* = 45)	70 TO 74 (*N* = 45)	75 TO 79 (*N* = 49)	80+ (*N* = 45)
Score						
22					2	
26		2				
29	2				4	
30	4					4
31					8	7
32			2			9
33					10	18
34	7	4	7	7	12	24
35			11			31
36		8	16		20	36
37	11			16		42
38		14	18	24	22	49
39			22	36	33	53
40	20		24	40	39	64
41	24	21	27	42	43	67
42		25	36	47	49	69
43	27	31	42	53	67	78
44	36	40	44	67	74	84
45	40	48	47	76	82	87
46	47	60	58	84	88	91
47	56	75	67	89	96	98
48	64	79	80	98	98	100
49	82	92	91	100	100	
50	100	100	100			

SOURCE: From Harvey and Seigert (1999).

EVIDENCE FOR VALIDITY

RELATIONSHIP BETWEEN WORDS AND FACES SUBTESTS

The Words subtest shows a moderate correlation with the Faces subtest ($r = .30$ to .57; Compton et al., 1992; Diesfeldt, 1990; Harvey & Siegert, 1999; Hunkin et al., 2000).

FACTOR-ANALYTIC STUDIES

Factor analysis of the WRMT along with the Doors and People Test (DPT) and the WMS-Revised (WMS-R) in a heterogeneous sample of neurologically-impaired patients suggests three factors: a general recall factor (with loadings from DPT People and Shapes as well as WMS-R verbal, visual, and delay indices) and separate visual recognition (DPT Doors, WRMT Faces) and verbal recognition (DPT Names, WRMT Words) factors (Hunkin et al., 2000).

RELATIONSHIPS WITH OTHER TESTS

Moderately strong correlations ($r = .42$ to .51) have been reported between the Faces subtest and other measures of visuospatial function (e.g., Block Design, Benton Face Recognition Test, RCFT; Soukop et al., 1999). The test

TABLE 10–125 Warrington Recognition Memory Test (WRMT) Means and Standard Deviations (*SDs*) for Each Age Group by National Adult Reading Test (NART) IQ Score

		NART IQ SCORE			
AGE GROUP (YEARS)	TEST	<100	100–110	111–120	>120
70 to 74 (*n*)		10	15	13	7
	Words	39.90 (5.8)	44.4 (5.0)	48.54 (2.5)	47.43 (3.1)
	Faces	40.5 (3.3)	43.27 (3.4)	41.39 (5.4)	43.14 (4.1)
75 to 79 (*n*)		12	9	19	9
	Words	41.46 (4.8)	43.89 (2.0)	44.79 (5.8)	47.78 (1.6)
	Faces	38.59 (5.2)	38.89 (5.9)	42.63 (5.7)	42.67 (2.7)
80+ (*n*)		9	17	17	2
	Words	39.56 (5.3)	43.47 (5.1)	46.24 (4.0)	47.50 (.7)
	Faces	37.78 (4.4)	39.65 (6.0)	38.41 (4.8)	41.50 (2.1)

SOURCE: Adapted from Harvey and Siegert (1999).

TABLE 10-126 90% Reliable Change Indices (RCIs) for the Warrington Recognition Memory Test (WRMT) Corrected for Practice Effects

	WORDS RCI	FACES RCI
Young group (40–54 years)	−4.4, +4.4	−1.5, +7.1
Old group (55–70 years)	−3.6, +5.4	−2.6, +7.2

SOURCE: From Bird et al. (2003).

does not appear to be significantly correlated with measures of verbal fluency, verbal reasoning (Similarities), or problem solving (WCST; Soukop et al., 1999).

CLINICAL STUDIES

Neurological Conditions. The WRMT has been used extensively in studies of amnesic syndromes (e.g., Aggleton & Shaw, 1996; Baddeley et al., 2001; Mullally et al., 2012; Reed & Squire, 1997). Baddeley et al. (2001) described a young adult patient, Jon, who developed memory impairment early in life as a result of damage to the hippocampal region. He scored at the 25th percentile for recognition of words and faces on the WRMT but below the 5th percentile on tests of recall. The relatively preserved recognition as opposed to recall performance of some amnesics (perhaps those, like Jon, with early-onset damage) on forced-choice tasks such as the WRMT may reflect the fact that such a procedure relies less on recollection and more on assessment of familiarity, a process that may be relatively preserved in patients whose brains have reorganized early in life. Similarly, Mullally et al. (2012) presented a case of a patient who showed dense amnesia and about 50% bilateral hippocampal volume loss. The patient performed in the above-average range for Words but was mildly impaired on Faces, suggesting that the recognition paradigm may not be sensitive enough to identify memory impairment. However, it has also been reported that some amnesics perform within normal limits on the WRMT but poorly on other recognition tasks (Reed & Squire, 1997). Accordingly, examiners should be cautious in assuming that WRMT scores in the normal range rule out memory deficit.

There is also evidence that substantial brain dysfunction is required to disrupt WRMT performance. For example, the WRMT's sensitivity to the effects of TBI is low (Millis, 2002). Millis and Dijkers (1993) reported that the sensitivity of the Words subtest to brain injury in a sample of patients with mild to severe traumatic brain injury was 63%. Valentine et al. (2006), on the other hand, reported that Faces was most sensitive to face recognition/learning deficits in individuals with acquired brain injury tested at least six months post injury. About 77% of the sample obtained two or more *SD*s below the healthy adult mean on Faces, contrasted with only about 20% who obtained two or more *SD*s below the healthy adult mean on the Learning New Faces Test and RBMT Faces subtest.

The WRMT does appear sensitive to the presence of brain impairment in older adults. Warrington (1984) reported that patients with mild brain atrophy showed impairment on the WRMT. The test is also sensitive to the memory impairment associated with MCI (Archer et al., 2006), AD, and DLB (Calderon et al., 2001), unmedicated PD (Monetta & Pell, 2007) but not medicated PD (Edelstyn et al., 2007), and the logopenic variant of primary progressive aphasia (PPA; Rohrer et al., 2013). Diesfeldt (1990) found that the test (especially the Faces subtest) is effective in identifying memory impairment in individuals with AD, particularly those younger than 80 years of age. At the 95% specificity level, the sensitivities of the Words and Faces subtests for the detection of memory impairment were 81% and 100%, respectively, for examinees younger than 80 years of age and less satisfactory, 59% and 76%, for those older than 80 years. Words/Faces Discrepancy scores did not differentiate between demented and nondemented adults. Fox et al. (1998) found that, in familial AD, verbal memory deficits on the WRMT precede by two to three years more widespread deterioration and predate by four to five years the fulfillment of criteria for probable AD. Furthermore, AD patients show decline in Faces scores over 24 months whereas other groups (those with subjective memory impairment, depressed, or healthy controls) remain stable; no decline or differences across groups are observed for Words (Chamberlain et al., 2011). Patients with the logopenic variant of PPA retested after about one year show impaired scores at retest despite normal scores at baseline (Rohrer et al., 2013).

Faces has been used as one of two recognition memory tests to define prosopagnosia (e.g., Grueter et al., 2007; Hills et al., 2015; Leib et al., 2012; Liu et al., 2015; Moroz et al., 2016; Pancaroglu et al., 2016; Rubino et al., 2016). However, whereas one study showed that Faces may be sensitive to face recognition issues in developmental prosopagnosia (Leib et al., 2012), another reported that individuals with hereditary prosopagnosia do not perform any differently than healthy controls (Grueter et al., 2007).

Perceptual abilities affect performance on the Faces subtest. Diesfeldt (1990) reported that performance on those items of Raven's Colored Progressive Matrices that require perceptual discrimination (more so than abstract reasoning) strongly predicted performance on the Faces subtest. It is worth noting in this context that the photographs in the WRMT include many noninternal facial features by which they can be recognized. The photographs consist of shots that display each model's hair, face, and approximately one-third of the upper body. The hair, clothing, head postures, and body positions vary greatly among the models. In addition, some photographs contain missing corners, low brightness levels, or developmental imperfections (Duchaine & Weidenfeld, 2003). In fact, examinees can score in the normal range without using internal facial features (e.g., eyes, nose, mouth regions). Therefore, normal scores on the

Faces subtest do not demonstrate normal unfamiliar face recognition abilities (Duchaine & Weidenfeld, 2003).

The WRMT is also sensitive to memory impairments in TLE (Hunkin et al., 2015; Muhlert et al., 2011). Muhlert et al. (2011) reported in their small samples that TLE patients performed worse than controls on both Faces and Words, but no differences were seen between those with idiopathic generalized epilepsy and healthy controls. Patients with mesial temporal lobe or diencephalic damage performed poorly on both the subtests, although left and right TLE patients performed differently on Faces (Kent et al., 2006; see later discussion about the WRMT's sensitivity to laterality of impairment). However, the WRMT was not sensitive to memory loss in transient epileptic amnesia, a syndrome that can be observed in those with TLE (Milton et al., 2010, 2012). This also raises questions about the test's sensitivity to some memory deficits.

Sensitivity to Laterality of Disturbance. Warrington (1984) suggested that the discrepancy between Words and Faces scores could be used to detect laterality of disturbance. She reported that patients with left-hemisphere damage performed significantly worse than patients with right-hemisphere damage on the Words task; conversely, patients with right-hemisphere lesions scored significantly worse than left-hemisphere groups on the Faces task.

Other studies have been less supportive of the test's sensitivity to lateralized impairment (Baxendale, 1997; Bigler et al., 1996; Cahn et al., 1998; Fargo et al., 2007; Hermann et al., 1995; Kneebone et al., 1997; Millis & Dijkers, 1993; Sweet et al., 2000). For example, in a sample of patients with epilepsy who received neuropsychological evaluation, Faces showed a PPV of 22% and an NPV of 63% for left TLE, PPV of 27% and NPV of 75% for right TLE, and PPV of 13% and NPV of 94% for bilateral TLE (Fargo et al., 2007). Hermann et al. (1995) found that only 15% of patients with left TLE and 10% of patients with right-sided disturbance were correctly classified based on the Words/Faces Discrepancy score. These rates improved to 42% and 31%, respectively, six to eight months after anterior temporal lobectomy. Specificity (true negatives) was high at about 90%. Similarly, Sweet et al. (2000) examined a large sample of neurological patients and found that the sensitivity of the Words/Faces Discrepancy score for right- and left-hemisphere damage (10% and 48%, respectively) was too low to use confidently in a clinical setting. They also found that the WRMT discrepancy score did not show the expected pattern of relationships with WMS-R subtests of similar material specificity.

There is some evidence that the diagnostic capabilities of the test improve when IQ is taken into account; ceiling effects are less likely to mask any relationships in those with low IQ. Testa et al. (2004) examined presurgical candidates for temporal lobe surgery and found a strong degree of diagnostic utility for the Faces task among patients with lower but not higher IQ levels. They found that a person in the average to high-average IQ range who scored at or below the 5th percentile on the Faces subtest was 3.3 times as likely to have a right-sided disturbance than a person who scored above this level on the task. The odds ratios among persons with borderline or low-average FSIQ indicated that a person who scored below the 5th percentile on the Faces task was 12.4 times more likely to have right-sided dysfunction than a person who scored above this level on the task.

Psychiatric Conditions. Whether psychological distress affects performance is uncertain. Contradictory findings have been reported (Kalska et al., 1999; Rund et al., 2006). No differences were seen between patients with major depression and controls on the Words and Faces subtest (Kalska et al., 1999). Impairments on the WRMT were also not seen in a nonpsychotic depression group (Rund et al., 2006). However, Rund et al. (2006) reported that individuals with schizophrenia performed worse than those with nonpsychotic depression and healthy controls on both Words and Faces. Similarly, schizophrenia or bipolar disorder probands performed worse than relatives of schizophrenia probands on Words but no differences were observed on Faces (Ivleva et al., 2012).

NEUROANATOMICAL CORRELATES AND IMAGING STUDIES

There are few studies on imaging correlates. Words appeared to be sensitive to focal lesions in the hippocampus based on MRI findings, whereas Faces was sensitive to broader mesial temporal lobe damage including perirhinal cortex and hippocampus in a sample of patients with focal temporal lobe lesions with mixed etiology (Taylor et al., 2007).

PERFORMANCE VALIDITY

Although not originally designed as a PVT, the WRMT appears to have considerable utility in the detection of exaggerated memory impairment. In fact, in a survey of 588 neuropsychologists in the United Kingdom, respondents indicated that the WRMT is used specifically as a PVT (McCarter et al., 2009). Modest to moderate correlations have been reported between the Words subtest and other PVTs (Nelson et al., 2003). In no case, however, did the amount of shared variance exceed 50%. The implication is that the WRMT offers nonredundant information regarding the validity of neuropsychological test results and supports the recommendation that examiners should use multiple nonredundant PVTs in forensic examinations (Nelson et al., 2003).

The test's forced two-choice procedure provides a known chance level of correct performance (i.e., 50%). Scores at or below chance (<19 correct on either task) suggest the possibility of invalid performance. However, use of this criterion may be too stringent and may result in a high false-negative rate. Indeed, studies suggest that examinees who are faking may obtain a wide range of scores, including scores that are above chance (Flowers et al., 2008).

As a result, cutoff values other than below chance have been proposed (for review, see Bianchini et al., 2001). Based on studies of patients with brain injuries, Millis (2002) suggested that a score of 32 correct or less on Words in patients with mild brain injury should raise the issue of noncredible performance. Iverson and Franzen (1998) suggested that a score lower than 38 on Words is questionable, less than 32 is suspicious, less than 28 is highly suspicious, and less than 20 is invalid. In the case of Faces, they proposed that a score of less than 30 is questionable, less than 28 is suspicious, less than 26 is highly suspicious, and less than 20 is invalid.

There is some evidence that the Words subtest is a better procedure than the Faces subtest for detecting exaggerated memory impairment (Cato et al., 2003; Millis, 1992). In fact, several studies have utilized the Words subtest (≤42, Kim et al., 2010, or <33, Iverson & Franzen 1994) to define noncredible performance in validation studies of other PVTs (e.g., Bell-Sprinkel et al., 2013; Nitch et al., 2006; Reedy et al., 2013). Whereas use of both tasks is recommended by Millis (1994), Kim et al. (2010) found high sensitivity using the Words total correct and response time to detect malingering defined by Slick et al. (1999) malingering criteria. A Words cutoff score of 42 or less yielded an impressive sensitivity of 92% and specificity of 89%. A Words time cutoff of 207 seconds or longer yielded a sensitivity of 66% and a specificity of 91%. When both number correct and time were used in combination, the sensitivity improved even further (Table 10–127).

Millis (2002) noted the possibility that other indices may also be useful. For example, based on his examination of patients with TBI of varying levels of severity, the longest run of incorrect responses was four on the Words subtest and five on the Faces subtest. With regard to infrequently missed items on Words, the following items on the answer sheet were passed by more than 90% of the TBI sample: items 2, 5, 6, 8, 14, 16, 19, 23, 26, and 29. Although cross-validation is needed, infrequently missed items may be a promising way to detect noncredible performance on the test.

With regard to comparison to similar PVT paradigms, Erdodi et al. (2014) used archival data of patients of mixed clinical conditions from a neurorehabilitation facility to compare the Words subtest of the WRMT and ACS Word Choice, a stand-alone PVT that employs a similar format. Words is a more difficult test than Word Choice, with patients generally obtaining three raw score points higher on Word Choice than on the WRMT. About 3% of the sample performed below chance on the WRMT. At a cutoff of 32 or less to define failure on the WRMT, there were 10 times more failures on the WRMT than on Word Choice. Conversely, perfect scores were 10 times more common on Word Choice. Nevertheless, using external PVTs as reference, both tests appeared to be comparable at identifying invalid performance. It appears that the WRMT may be more sensitive to cognitive impairment than Word Choice, but they may be equivalent as PVTs (see also the review of Word Choice, in Chapter 15 of this volume).

With regard to correlations with neuropsychological tests, Ross et al. (2006) defined failure on the WRMT as 32 or less on one subtest and less than 40 on the other subtest and found that WRMT failures accounted for only 2–13% of variance on test scores in the Halstead-Reitan Battery in a sample of individuals with brain injury.

Nevertheless, like all PVTs, performance on the test is affected by dementia. Using archival data from patients with dementia but without external incentive to feign cognitive problems, Dean et al. (2009) found that at a cutoff of less than 33, the specificity of Words was only 59%. When its specificity for invalid performance was evaluated based on MMSE score, a score of MMSE 15–20 was associated with a specificity of only 20%, and a score of MMSE of less than 15 with a specificity of only 0% (i.e., 100% false-positive rate). As such, the Words subtest should not be used as a PVT when dementia is suspected, including mild dementia. Similarly, an unusually high proportion of nonlitigating neurological patients have been reported to obtain scores of dubious validity, indicating problems using the test as a PVT in these groups (i.e., <38 and <30 on Words and Faces

TABLE 10–127 Words Classification Rates for Total Score, Time to Complete, and Combined Total and Time for Detection of Malingered Neurocognitive Dysfunction

				BASE RATE					
				15%		40%		50%	
WARRINGTON—WORDS	CUTOFF	SENSITIVITY (%)	SPECIFICITY (%)	PPP (%)	NPP (%)	PPP (%)	NPP (%)	PPP (%)	NPP (%)
Accuracy score	≤42	89	92	66	98	88	93	92	89
Time in seconds	≥207"	66	91	55	94	82	80	88	72
Combination of above		94	87	56	99	83	95	88	93

NOTES: BR = base rate, percentage of individuals in sample who were malingering; Sensitivity = percentage of malingering group falling below cutoff; Specificity = percentage of credible group falling above cutoff; PPP = Positive Predictive Power, percentage of those with positive test sign who were malingering; NPP = Negative Predictive Power, percentage of those with negative test sign who were not malingering. Values are rounded to nearest percent.

SOURCE: From Kim et al. (2010).

TABLE 10–128 Warrington Words Adjusted Cutoffs and Corresponding Specificities for Malingered Neurocognitive Dysfunction in Low-IQ Examinees

IQ BAND	<70	70–79	80–89
N	4	16	13
Cutoff	<32	<39	<40
Specificity (%)	100	94	92

SOURCE: Adapted from Dean et al. (2008).

subtests, respectively; Johnson & van den Brock, 2001; see also Barrash et al., 2004).

In contrast, there is evidence that the Words subtest may be suitable as a PVT in those with low IQ, even though, in general, low IQ raises the risk of false positives for most PVTs. Smith et al. (2014) classified credible and noncredible participants based on Slick et al. (1999) malingering criteria; a Words correct cutoff of 42 or less yielded a specificity of only 80%; specificity was lower, at 74%, for the time score. However, when the Words correct cutoff was adjusted to 38 or less, an acceptable sensitivity of 64% and specificity of 91% were achieved. Adjusting the time cutoff to 265 seconds or longer also improved prediction, with a sensitivity of 41% and an acceptable specificity of 90%. In another study that examined the relationship between IQ and nine PVTs in a non–compensation-seeking sample, all PVTs were correlated with FSIQ, although correlation between FSIQ and the WRMT was moderate (r = .31). The WRMT appeared to have the best specificity in low-IQ examinees, along with the Finger Tapping Test. Adjusted scores for those with FSIQ of less than 90 to maintain specificity over 90% were suggested by the authors (Table 10–128; Dean et al., 2008). Clinicians may use the data in Table 10–128 to adjust the cutoff score according to the IQ band of the examinee although it must be noted that the cell sizes are very small.

COMMENT

The WRMT has a number of positive characteristics. It measures a distinct aspect of memory function—namely recognition memory—that can be further fractionated into verbal and visual components. The test is useful for patients with motor problems. Furthermore, the recognition paradigm is less psychologically taxing to a patient than a free-recall procedure and therefore may be more resistant to psychiatric conditions such as depression (Bird et al., 2003; Rund et al., 2006; Warrington, 1984).

Its insensitivity to mild impairments as well as its two-choice recognition paradigm lends itself well to performance validity assessment. It has been extensively studied as a PVT, more so than many other memory tests, and studies focusing on its utility as a performance validity measure have been very promising. The face validity possessed by the WRMT as a challenging memory test lessens the transparency of its dual role and probably contributes to its sensitivity (Barrash et al., 2004). It is also a suitable PVT for those with low IQ, although the cutoff score needs to be adjusted for this population.

On the other hand, there are some significant weaknesses. Test-retest reliability coefficients are modest, and large changes in test scores are needed to detect a significant improvement or decline in performance. Therefore, the test may have limited use for monitoring change. Of note, because significant practice effects are seen in healthy adults, a lack of improvement on retest may signal neurological compromise.

The Words task has a relatively low ceiling, whereas the norms for the Faces task for young adults provided in the test manual may be too high (O'Bryant et al., 2003). It is possible that the cues offered by the faces stimuli (clothing, hair, posture) are more relevant to individuals in the United Kingdom than to those in the United States, making it an easier task for UK examinees. More importantly, norms were collected more than 30 years ago and the pictures from the Faces subtest are dated and have not been revised. Given the very outdated norms (e.g., inpatients from before 1984), it is not recommended for clinical assessment of memory disorders. As well, as a clinical tool, although the test may be useful for detecting dementia, it may be insufficient for measurement of mild memory deficits. In addition, the test's ability to classify individuals with regard to laterality of disturbance is poor, including identifying material-specific memory in presurgical evaluation for epilepsy surgery, although classification rates appear to improve substantially in those with lower levels of IQ where ceiling effects are less likely to be operating.

It is also important to bear in mind that a single administration of the WRMT may not always reveal impaired memory in a patient who is nevertheless amnesic on other tests, including on other recognition tests, but particularly on recall tests which are necessary to properly assess memory. Clinicians should also note that some studies indicate that normal scores on the Faces subtest do not imply intact face recognition abilities because noninternal feature information provided in the photographs is rich enough to support scores in the normal range (Duchaine & Weidenfeld, 2003). However, several other studies support the utility of the Faces subtest for assessment of prosopagnosia (Grueter et al., 2007; Hills et al., 2015; Leib et al., 2012; Liu et al., 2015; Moroz et al., 2016; Pancaroglu et al., 2016; Rubino et al., 2016).

Last, the test should not be used as a performance validity indicator in individuals suspected of dementia, and, like all PVTs, the WRMT should not be used on its own to infer invalid performance but should be used in conjunction with other sources of evidence including other PVTs and clinical information. Overall, given some of its weaknesses as a memory test, consideration should be given to shifting the WRMT's utility from memory test to PVT.

REFERENCES

Aggleton, J. P., & Shaw, C. (1996). Amnesia and recognition memory: A reanalysis of psychometric data. *Neuropsychologia, 34,* 51–62.

Archer, H. A., MacFarlane, F., Price, S., Moore, E. K., Pepple, T., Cutler, D., . . . Rossor, M. N. (2006). Do symptoms of memory impairment correspond to cognitive impairment: A cross sectional study of a clinical cohort. *International Journal of Geriatric Psychiatry, 21*(12), 1206–1212.

Baddeley, A., Vargha-Khadem, F., & Mishkin, M. (2001). Preserved recognition in a case of developmental amnesia: Implications for the acquisition of semantic memory? *Journal of Cognitive Neuroscience, 13,* 357–369.

Barrash, J., Suhr, J., & Manzel, K. (2004). Detecting poor effort and malingering with an expanded version of the Auditory Verbal Learning Test (AVLTX): Validation with clinical samples. *Journal of Clinical and Experimental Neuropsychology, 26,* 125–140.

Baxendale, S. A. (1997). The role of the hippocampus in recognition memory. *Neuropsychologia, 35,* 591–598.

Bell-Sprinkel, T., Boone, K. B., Miora, D., Cottingham, M., Victor, T., Ziegler, E., . . . Wright, M. (2013). Re-examination of the Rey Word Recognition Test. *The Clinical Neuropsychologist, 27*(3), 516–527.

Bianchini, K. J., Mathias, C. W., & Greve, K. W. (2001). Symptom validity testing: A critical review. *The Clinical Neuropsychologist, 15,* 19–45.

Bigler, E. D., Johnson, S. C., Anderson, C. V., Blatter, D. D., Gale, S. D., Russo, A. A., . . . Abildskov, T. J. (1996). Traumatic brain injury and memory: The role of hippocampal atrophy. *Neuropsychology, 10,* 333–342.

Bird, C. M., Papadopoulou, K., Ricciardelli, P., Rossor, M. N., & Cipolotti, L. (2003). Test-retest reliability, practice effects and reliable change indices for the recognition memory test. *British Journal of Clinical Psychology, 42,* 407–425.

Cahn, D. A., Sullivan, E. V., Shear, P. K., Marsh, L., Fama, R., Lim, K. O., . . . Pfefferbaum, A. (1998). Structural MRI correlates of recognition memory in Alzheimer's disease. *Journal of the International Neuropsychological Society, 4,* 106–114.

Calderon, J., Perry, R. J., Erzinclioglu, S. W., Berrios, G. E., Dening, T R., & Hodges, J. R. (2001). Perception, attention, and working memory are disproportionately impaired in dementia with Lewy bodies compared with Alzheimer's disease. *Journal of Neurology, Neurosurgery and Psychiatry, 70,* 157–164.

Cato, M. A., Brewster, J., Ryan, T., & Giuliano, A. J. (2003). Coaching and the ability to simulate mild traumatic brain injury symptoms. [Erratum.] *The Clinical Neuropsychologist, 17,* 285–286.

Chamberlain, S. R., Blackwell, A. D., Nathan, P. J., Hammond, G., Robbins, T. W., Hodges, J. R., . . . Sahakian, B. J. (2011). Differential cognitive deterioration in dementia: A two year longitudinal study. *Journal of Alzheimer's Disease, 24*(1), 125–136.

Compton, J. M., Sherer, M., & Adams, R. L. (1992). Factor analysis of the Wechsler Memory Scale and the Warrington Recognition Memory Test. *Archives of Clinical Neuropsychology, 7,* 165–173.

Dean, A. C., Victor, T. L., Boone, K. B., & Arnold, G. (2008). The relationship of IQ to effort test performance. *The Clinical Neuropsychologist, 22*(4), 705–722.

Dean, A. C., Victor, T. L., Boone, K. B., Philpott, L. M., & Hess, R. A. (2009). Dementia and effort test performance. *The Clinical Neuropsychologist, 23*(1), 133–152.

Diesfeldt, H., & Vink, M. (1989). Recognition memory for Words and Faces in the very old. *British Journal of Clinical Psychology, 28,* 247–253.

Diesfeldt, H. F. A. (1990). Recognition memory for Words and Faces in primary degenerative dementia of the Alzheimer type and normal old age. *Journal of Clinical and Experimental Neuropsychology, 12,* 931–945.

Duchaine, B. C., & Weidenfeld, A. (2003). An evaluation of two commonly used tests of unfamiliar face recognition. *Neuropsychologia, 41,* 713–720.

Edelstyn, N. M. J., Mayes, A. R., Condon, L., Tunnicliffe, M., & Ellis, S. J. (2007). Recognition, recollection, familiarity and executive function in medicated patients with moderate Parkinson's disease. *Journal of Neuropsychology, 1*(2), 131–147.

Erdodi, L. A., Kirsch, N. L., Lajiness-O'Neill, R., Vingilis, E., & Medoff, B. (2014). Comparing the Recognition Memory Test and the Word Choice Test in a mixed clinical sample: Are they equivalent? *Psychological Injury and Law, 7*(3), 255–263.

Fargo, J. D., Schefft, B. K., Kent, G. P., Szaflarski, J. P., Privitera, M. D., & Yeh, H. (2007). The prevalence of seizure types among individuals referred for phase I neuropsychological assessment: Demographic and neuropsychological characteristics. *The Clinical Neuropsychologist, 21*(3), 442–455.

Flowers, K. A., Bolton, C., & Brindle, N. (2008). Chance guessing in a forced-choice recognition task and the detection of malingering. *Neuropsychology, 22*(2), 273–277.

Fox, N. C., Warrington, E. K., Seiffer, A. L., Agnew, S. K., & Rossor, M. N. (1998). Presymptomatic cognitive deficits in individuals at risk of familial Alzheimer's disease: A longitudinal prospective study. *Brain, 121,* 1631–1639.

Grueter, M., Grueter, T., Bell, V., Horst, J., Laskowski, W., Sperling, K., . . . Kennerknecht, I. (2007). Hereditary prosopagnosia: The first case series. *Cortex: A Journal Devoted to the Study of the Nervous System and Behavior, 43*(6), 734–749.

Harvey, J. A., & Siegert, R. J. (1999). Normative data for New Zealand elders on the Controlled Oral Word Association Test, Graded Naming Test, and the Recognition Memory Test. *New Zealand Journal of Psychology, 28,* 124–132.

Hermann, B. P., Connell, B., Barr, W. B., & Wyler, A. R. (1995). The utility of the Warrington Recognition Memory Test for temporal lobe epilepsy: Pre- and postoperative results. *Journal of Epilepsy, 8,* 139–145.

Hills, C. S., Pancaroglu, R., Duchaine, B., & Barton, J. J. S. (2015). Word and text processing in acquired prosopagnosia. *Annals of Neurology, 78*(2), 258–271.

Hunkin, N. M., Awad, M., & Mayes, A. R. (2015). Memory for between-list and within-list information in amnesic patients with temporal lobe and diencephalic lesions. *Journal of Neuropsychology, 9*(1), 137–156.

Hunkin, N. M., Stone, J. V., Isaac, C. L., Holdstock, J. S., Butterfield, R., Wallis, L. I., & Mayes, A. R. (2000). Factor analysis of three standardized tests of memory in a clinical population. *British Journal of Psychology, 39,* 169–180.

Iverson, G. L., & Franzen, M. D. (1994). The Recognition Memory Test, Digit Span, and Knox Cube Test as markers of malingered memory impairment. *Assessment, 1,* 323–334.

Iverson, G. L., & Franzen, M. D. (1998). Detecting malingered memory deficits with the Recognition Remory Test. *Brain Injury, 12,* 275–282.

Ivleva, E. I., Shohamy, D., Mihalakos, P., Morris, D. W., Carmody, T., & Tamminga, C. A. (2012). Memory generalization is selectively altered in the psychosis dimension. *Schizophrenia Research, 138*(1), 74–80.

Johnson, Z., & van den Brock, M. D. (2001). Letter to the editor. *Brain Injury, 15,* 187–188.

Kalska, H., Punamaki, R. L., Makinen-Pelli, T., & Saarinen, M. (1999). Memory and metamemory functioning among depressed patients. *Applied Neuropsychology, 6,* 96–107.

Kent, G. P., Schefft, B. K., Howe, S. R., Szaflarski, J. P., Yeh, H., & Privitera, M. D. (2006). The effects of duration of intractable epilepsy on memory function. *Epilepsy & Behavior, 9*(3), 469–477.

Kim, M. S., Boone, K. B., Victor, T., Marion, S. D., Amano, S., Cottingham, M. E., . . . Zeller, M. A. (2010). The Warrington Recognition Memory

Test for words as a measure of response bias: Total score and response time cutoffs developed on 'real world' credible and noncredible subjects. *Archives of Clinical Neuropsychology, 25*(1), 60–70.

Kneebone, A. C., Chelune, G. J., & Lüders, H. O. (1997). Individual patient prediction of seizure lateralization in temporal lobe epilepsy: A comparison between neuropsychological memory measures and the intracarotid amobarbital procedure. *Journal of the International Neuropsychological Society, 3,* 159–168.

Leib, A. Y., Puri, A. M., Fischer, J., Bentin, S., Whitney, D., & Robertson, L. (2012). Crowd perception in prosopagnosia. *Neuropsychologia, 50*(7), 1698–1707.

Liu, R. R., Corrow, S. L., Pancaroglu, R., Duchaine, B., & Barton, J. J. S. (2015). The processing of voice identity in developmental prosopagnosia. *Cortex, 71,* 390–397.

Malina, A. C., Bowers, D. A., Millis, S. R., & Uekert, S. (1998). Internal consistency of the Warrington Recognition Memory Test. *Perceptual and Motor Skills, 86,* 1320–1322.

McCarter, R. J., Walton, N. H., Brooks, D. N., & Powell, G. E. (2009). Effort testing in contemporary UK neuropsychological practice. *The Clinical Neuropsychologist, 23*(6), 1050–1066.

Millis, S. R. (1992). The Recognition Memory Test in the detection of malingered and exaggerated memory deficits. *The Clinical Neuropsychologist, 6,* 404–414.

Millis, S. R. (1994). Assessment of motivation and memory with the Recognition Memory Test after financially compensable mild head injury. *Journal of Clinical Psychology, 50,* 601–605.

Millis, S. R. (2002). Warrington's Recognition Memory Test in the detection of response bias. *Journal of Forensic Neuropsychology, 2,* 147–166.

Millis, S. R., & Dijkers, M. (1993). Use of the Recognition Memory Test in traumatic brain injury. *Brain Injury, 7,* 53–58.

Milton, F., Butler, C. R., Benattayallah, A., & Zeman, A. Z. J. (2012). The neural basis of autobiographical memory deficits in transient epileptic amnesia. *Neuropsychologia, 50*(14), 3528–3541.

Milton, F., Muhlert, N., Pindus, D. M., Butler, C. R., Kapur, N., Graham, K. S., & Zeman, A. Z. J. (2010). Remote memory deficits in transient epileptic amnesia. *Brain, 133*(5), 1368–1379.

Monetta, L., & Pell, M. D. (2007). Effects of verbal working memory deficits on metaphor comprehension in patients with Parkinson's disease. *Brain and Language, 101*(1), 80–89.

Moroz, D., Corrow, S. L., Corrow, J. C., Barton, A. R. S., Duchaine, B., & Barton, J. J. S. (2016). Localization and patterns of cerebral dyschromatopsia: A study of subjects with prospagnosia. *Neuropsychologia, 89,* 153–160.

Muhlert, N., Grünewald, R. A., Hunkin, N. M., Reuber, M., Howell, S., Reynders, H., & Isaac, C. L. (2011). Accelerated long-term forgetting in temporal lobe but not idiopathic generalised epilepsy. *Neuropsychologia, 49*(9), 2417–2426.

Mullally, S. L., Hassabis, D., & Maguire, E. A. (2012). Scene construction in amnesia: An fMRI study. *The Journal of Neuroscience, 32*(16), 5646–5653.

Nelson, N. W., Boone, K., Dueck, A., Wagener, L., Lu, P., & Grills, C. (2003). Relationships between eight measures of suspect effort. *The Clinical Neuropsychologist, 17,* 263–272.

Nitch, S., Boone, K. B., Wen, J., Arnold, G., & Alfano, K. (2006). The utility of the Rey Word Recognition Test in the detection of suspect effort. *The Clinical Neuropsychologist, 20*(4), 873–887.

O'Bryant, S. E., Hilsabeck, R. C., McCaffrey, R. J., & Gouvrier, W. D. (2003). The Recognition Memory Test: Examination of ethnic differences and norm validity. *Archives of Clinical Neuropsychology, 18,* 135–143.

Pancaroglu, R., Hills, C. S., Sekunova, A., Viswanathan, J., Duchaine, B., & Barton, J. J. S. (2016). Seeing the eyes in acquired prosopagnosia. *Cortex, 81,* 251–265.

Reed, J. M., & Squire, L. R. (1997). Impaired recognition memory in patients with lesions restricted to the hippocampal formation. *Behavioral Neuroscience, 111,* 667–675.

Reedy, S. D., Boone, K. B., Cottingham, M. E., Glaser, D. F., Lu, P. H., Victor, T. L., . . . Wright, M. J. (2013). Cross validation of the Lu and colleagues (2003) Rey-Osterrieth Complex Figure Test effort equation in a large known-group sample. *Archives of Clinical Neuropsychology, 28*(1), 30–37.

Rohrer, J. D., Caso, F., Mahoney, C., Henry, M., Rosen, H. J., Rabinovici, G., . . . Gorno-Tempini, M. (2013). Patterns of longitudinal brain atrophy in the logopenic variant of primary progressive aphasia. *Brain and Language, 127*(2), 121–126.

Ross, S. R., Putnam, S. H., & Adams, K. M. (2006). Psychological disturbance, incomplete effort, and compensation-seeking status as predictors of neuropsychological test performance in head injury. *Journal of Clinical and Experimental Neuropsychology, 28*(1), 111–125.

Rubino, C., Corrow, S. L., Corrow, J. C., Duchaine, B., & Barton, J. J. S. (2016). Word and text processing in developmental prosopagnosia. *Cognitive Neuropsychology, 33*(5-6), 315–328.

Rund, B. R., Sundet, K., Asbjørnsen, A., Egeland, J., Landrø, N. I., Lund, A., . . . Hugdahl, K. (2006). Neuropsychological test profiles in schizophrenia and non-psychotic depression. *Acta Psychiatrica Scandinavica, 113*(4), 350–359.

Slick, D. J., Sherman, E. M., & Iverson, G. L. (1999). Diagnostic criteria for malingered neurocognitive dysfunction: Proposed standards for clinical practice and research. *The Clinical Neuropsychologist, 13*(4), 545–561.

Smith, K., Boone, K., Victor, T., Miora, D., Cottingham, M., Ziegler, E., . . . Wright, M. (2014). Comparison of credible patients of very low intelligence and non-credible patients on neurocognitive performance validity indicators. *The Clinical Neuropsychologist, 28*(6), 1048–1070.

Soukop, V. M., Bimbela, A., & Scheiss, M. C. (1999). Recognition memory for Faces: Reliability and validity of the Warrington Recognition Memory Test (RMT) in a neurological sample. *Journal of Clinical Psychology in Medical Settings, 6,* 287–293.

Sweet, J. J., Demakis, G. J., Ricker, J. H., & Millis, S. R. (2000). Diagnostic efficiency and material specificity of the Warrington Recognition Memory Test: A collaborative multisite investigation. *Archives of Clinical Neuropsychology, 15,* 301–309.

Taylor, K. J., Henson, R. N. A., & Graham, K. S. (2007). Recognition memory for faces and scenes in amnesia: Dissociable roles of medial temporal lobe structures. *Neuropsychologia, 45*(11), 2428–2438.

Testa, S. M., Schefft, B. K., Privatera, M. D., & Yeh, H. S. (2004). Warrington's Recognition Memory for faces: Interpretive strategy and diagnostic utility in temporal lobe epilepsy. *Epilepsy and Behavior, 5,* 236–243.

Valentine, T., Powell, J., Davidoff, J., Letson, S., & Greenwood, R. (2006). Prevalence and correlates of face recognition impairments after acquired brain injury. *Neuropsychological Rehabilitation, 16*(3), 272–297.

Warrington, E. K. (1984). *Recognition Memory Test manual.* Windsor, UK: NFER-Nelson.

WECHSLER MEMORY SCALE—FOURTH EDITION (WMS-IV)

TEST NAME	**Wechsler Memory Scale—Fourth Edition (WMS-IV)**
DOMAIN	Verbal and visual memory
AGE RANGE	16 to 90 years
ADMINISTRATION TIME	75 to 100 minutes, including 20- to 30-minute delay interval
SCORING FORMAT	Computerized or hand scored
REFERENCE	Wechsler D. (2009). *Wechsler Memory Scale—Fourth Edition*. San Antonio, TX: Psychological Corporation. www.pearsonclinical.com

DESCRIPTION

The Wechsler Memory Scale—Fourth Edition (WMS-IV) is designed to assess auditory and visual declarative memory and visual working memory abilities in adolescents, adults, and older adults. It is the latest version in the family of Wechsler Memory Scales. Like the third edition, it is co-normed with the WAIS-IV.

The original WMS (Wechsler, 1945) contained seven subtests and two forms, Form I (Wechsler, 1945) and Form II (Stone & Wechsler, 1946), although most of the published studies deal with Form I. The validity and psychometric properties of the WMS were extensively criticized (Butters et al., 1988; Erickson & Scott, 1977; Larrabee et al., 1985; Loring & Papanicolauo, 1987; Prigatano, 1977, 1978), prompting several variations (e.g., Milberg et al., 1986; Russell, 1975) and a revision. In 1987, the test was revised (WMS-R; Wechsler, 1987), broadening its coverage of nonverbal and visual memory and incorporating delayed recall procedures. The WMS-R was a significant improvement over its predecessor. However, it, too, had limitations (for review, see Lezak et al., 2004; Lichtenberger et al., 2002; Spreen & Strauss, 1998). Based on the published literature, solicited reviews of the WMS-R, and recommendations from an advisory panel, the Psychological Corporation developed the WMS-III (The Psychological Corporation, 1997, 2002). The test was also co-developed with the WAIS-III and WTAR, allowing for more precise and meaningful comparisons between memory and intellectual ability.

The WMS-III continued to face criticisms with regard to its factor structure, psychometric properties, and sensitivity of its subtests to clinical groups (for review, see Strauss et al., 2006). As such, the latest version attempted to address prior shortcomings identified through surveys of current WMS-III users and review of the research literature (Wechsler, 2009). As a result of these investigations, the index structure of WMS-IV was simplified. Following extensive pilot studies, the Faces and Family Pictures subtests were eliminated and replaced with the Designs subtest. Scoring for Visual Reproduction was simplified. The subtests comprising the Working Memory Index in the WMS-III were replaced by Spatial Addition and Symbol Span subtests and relabeled as the Visual Working Memory Index. A brief screen of general cognitive functioning, the Brief Cognitive Status Exam (BCSE), was also added as an optional subtest. Contrast scores at the subtest and index level were introduced (see the section "Scores"). A separate battery of tests was created for adults aged 65+. Descriptions of each subtest are presented in Table 10–129. Users may refer to the manual for a detailed description of the modifications from WMS-III to WMS-IV.

The WMS-IV also comes with a supplemental WMS-IV Flexible Approach kit (separate purchase) that contains alternate index and supplemental subtests. This battery provides shorter testing time and also allows the examiner to substitute alternate measures to assess memory not included in the core battery. Specifically, two new subtests were developed to assess auditory-visual association memory: Logos (LO) and Names (NA), which are also useful in combination as a screener for general memory. The Flexible Approach includes four short batteries that generate different index scores and can be used independently depending on the assessment needs (see the section "Scoring" and Table 10–131).

In addition to the core battery, additional index and process scores can be found in the Advanced Clinical Solutions (ACS) kit for WAIS-IV and WMS-IV (Pearson Assessment, 2009). An extensive review of the ACS is beyond the scope of this chapter. The interested reader may wish to refer to Holdnack et al. (2013) for an excellent guide to the ACS.

TABLE 10–129 Description and Age Range of Wechsler Memory Scale—Fourth Edition (WMS-IV) Subtests

SUBTEST	AGE RANGE	DESCRIPTION
Logical Memory I and II (LM I and II)	16–90	Examinee recalls two stories read aloud by the examiner, both immediately and after a delay; a yes/no recognition test follows the delay
Verbal Paired Associates I and II (VPA I and II)	16–90	Examiner presents a list of word pairs; then the examinee hears one word and must provide the word that went with it. There are four trials of the list. The pairs are also tested after a delay. A recognition trial is included; the examinee must identify the word pairs from a list of distractors. An optional word recall trial requires the examinee to recall as many of the word pairs as they can
Designs I and II (DE I and II)	16–69	Examiner briefly presents 4-8 designs on a grid; then the examinee picks the designs from a deck of cards and places them in the grid accordingly immediately and after a delay. A recognition trial is included; the examinee identifies the design in the correct location from a series of distractors
Visual Reproduction I and II (VR I and II)	16–90	The examinee reproduces figures both immediately after presentation and following a delay. Recognition and copying conditions are also provided
Spatial Addition (SA)	16–69	Examiner briefly presents two grids with red and blue circles sequentially; the examinee has to place circles on the grid immediately following presentation based on a set of rules
Symbol Span (SSP)	16–90	Examiner briefly presents a series of abstract symbols; the examinee picks out the same symbols from an array of distractors in the same order they were presented
Brief Cognitive Status Exam (BCSE; optional)	16–90	The examinee is asked to perform a variety of tasks including orientation, time estimate, naming (not scored), mental control, clock drawing, incidental recall of naming items, inhibition, and generative naming

SOURCE: Adapted from Wechlser (2009).

STRUCTURE

The WMS-IV contains six subtests and one optional subtest that assesses global cognitive functioning. The CVLT-II may be used as a substitute for VPA in the Auditory Memory Index. All memory subtests include a delayed recognition trial. Table 10–130 presents the composition of scores for each index. The BCSE is a separate optional subtest to screen for cognitive impairment. This subtest is weighted such that low scores are suggestive of processing difficulties. Table 10–131 presents the composition of scores for the WMS-IV Flexible Approach.

ADMINISTRATION

See the manual. Briefly, the examiner presents items to the examinee and records responses in an individual response booklet. Discontinuation and scoring rules as well as time limits are noted in the test manual and on the record form. Standardized order of subtest administration is recommended. The manual specifies that the Symbol Span subtest should not be administered during the delay interval of Visual Reproduction. Use of dominant or nondominant hand does not appear to impact Visual Reproduction copy and memory scores (Umfleet et al., 2013).

For examinees between ages 65 and 69, the examiner may choose between the Adult Battery or Older Adult Battery depending on the characteristics of the examinee. The manual suggests that the Adult Battery should be administered if the examinee is highly educated or if a comprehensive assessment is needed. The Older Adult battery is brief and has a lower floor, and it would be suitable for those with significant clinical diagnoses, suspected poor memory, or if fatigue is a concern.

The CVLT-II can be used as a substitute for the VPA to generate index scores. However, the substituted score may underestimate index scores (Miller et al., 2012a; Thiruselvam et al., 2015; see the "Evidence for Validity" section for further discussion). Users should note that if the WAIS-IV subtests are administered during the WMS-IV delay interval, interference effects have been reported (Ingram et al., 2016). Those who were administered WAIS-IV subtests during the WMS-IV delay interval performed worse than those who watched a documentary during the delay interval. As such, users may wish to administer the WAIS-IV before the WMS-IV.

SCORING

See the manual. The Adult Battery provides five index scores (each ranging from standard scores of 40 to 160) and three contrast scores (each ranging from scaled scores of 1 to 19) at the index level. The Older Adult Battery provides four index scores and two contrast scores at the index level. See Table 10–130 for the composition of the various scores. The WMS-IV also provides cumulative percentages for Recognition trials. Scoring for the Visual Reproduction subtest has been simplified with the goal to focus on memory rather than accuracy of the drawings. Demographically adjusted scores are found in the ACS and will not be described here.

To estimate premorbid memory functioning on the WMS-IV, please refer to Chapter 4 for a review of the ACS Test of Premorbid Functioning.

TABLE 10–130 Wechsler Memory Scale—Fourth Edition (WMS-IV) Index, Subtest, and Contrast Scores

INDEXES	SUBTESTS
Auditory Memory Index (AMI)	*Logical Memory I Scaled Score* *Logical Memory II Scaled Score* *(Logical Memory II Recognition Cumulative Percentage)* *Verbal Paired Associates I Scaled Score* *Verbal Paired Associates II Scaled Score* *(Verbal Paired Associates Recognition Cumulative Percentage)* *(Verbal Paired Associates II Word Recall Scaled Score)*
Visual Memory Index (VMI)	Designs I Scaled Score (Designs I Content Scaled Score) (Designs I Spatial Scaled Score) Designs II Scaled Score (Designs II Recognition Cumulative Percentage) (Designs II Content Scaled Score) (Designs II Spatial Scaled Score) *Visual Reproduction I Scaled Score* *Visual Reproduction II Scaled Score* *(Visual Reproduction II Recognition Cumulative Percentage)* *(Visual Reproduction II Copy Cumulative Percentage)*
Visual Working Memory Index (VWMI)	Spatial Addition Scaled Score *Symbol Span Scaled Score*
Immediate Memory Index (IMI)	*Logical Memory I Scaled Score* *Verbal Paired Associates I Scaled Score* Designs I Scaled Score *Visual Reproduction I Scaled Score*
Delayed Memory Index (DMI)	*Logical Memory II Scaled Score* *Verbal Paired Associates II Scaled Score* Designs II Scaled Score *Visual Reproduction II Scaled Score*
Contrast Scores	
Index Level	
Auditory Memory Index vs. Visual Memory Index	
Visual Working Memory Index vs. Visual Memory Index	
Immediate Memory Index vs. Delayed Memory Index	
Subtest Level	
Logical Memory II Recognition vs. Delayed Recall	
Logical Memory Immediate Recall vs. Delayed Recall	
Verbal Paired Associates II Recognition vs. Delayed Recall	
Verbal Paired Associates Immediate Recall vs. Delayed Recall	
Designs I Spatial vs. Content	
Designs II Spatial vs. Content	
Designs II Recognition vs. Delayed Recall	
Designs Immediate vs. Delayed Recall	
Visual Reproduction II Recognition vs. Delayed Recall	
Visual Reproduction Copy vs. Immediate Recall	
Visual Reproduction Immediate Recall vs. Delayed Recall	

NOTE: Italics represent scores in the Older Adult Battery. Scores in parentheses are not part of the primary scores used to derive the index scores.

SOURCE: Adapted from Wechsler (2009).

TABLE 10–131 Wechsler Memory Scale—Fourth Edition (WMS-IV) Flexible Approach Indexes and Subtest Composition

BATTERY	AGES	INDEXES	SUBTESTS
as with 10–130			
LMDE	16–69	Immediate Memory Index Delayed Memory Index	Logical Memory, Designs
		Auditory Memory Index	Logical Memory
		Visual Memory Index	Designs
OAA	16–69	Immediate Memory Index Delayed Memory Index	Logical Memory, Verbal Paired Associates, Visual Reproduction
		Auditory Memory Index	Logical Memory, Verbal Paired Associates
		Visual Memory Index	Visual Reproduction
LMVR	16–90	Immediate Memory Index Delayed Memory Index	Logical Memory, Visual Reproduction
		Auditory Memory Index	Logical Memory
		Visual Memory Index	Visual Reproduction
VRLO	16–90	Visual Memory Index Visual Immediate Memory Index Visual Delayed Memory Index	Visual Reproduction, Logos
LONA	16–90	Auditory-Visual Memory Index Auditory-Visual Immediate Memory Index Auditory-Visual Delayed Memory Index	Logos, Names

NOTE: Please refer to the manual for more details about the subtest composition.

SOURCE: Adapted from Wechsler (2009).

CONTRAST SCORES

Contrast scores were introduced in the WMS-IV as a method to adjust a subtest score based on the initial performance on another relevant subtest. The contrast score does not replace the age-adjusted score but adds to the interpretation of the primary scaled score. The first subtest represents the control measure for the adjusted score. The contrast scaled scores range from 1 to 19 and are interpreted in the same manner as the age-adjusted subtest scaled scores. Contrast scores between 8 and 12 indicate that the two scores do not differ.

WAIS-IV AND WMS-IV DISCREPANCY SCORES

One of the advantages of using the WMS-IV is its co-norming with the WAIS-IV. Direct comparisons may be made between intellectual and memory functioning to determine if memory functioning is at the expected level for intellectual ability. Three methods are described in the manual to assess the discrepancy between intellectual and memory functioning. The Simple-Difference method subtracts the WMS-IV index score from the WAIS-IV composite score to determine if the difference is statistically significant and how frequent the difference occurs in the standardization sample.

The Predicted-Difference method uses a regression equation that takes into account WAIS-IV scores to calculate the predicted score to determine the statistical significance and frequency of the difference between expected and actual scores in the standardization sample.

Finally, contrast scores provide adjusted scores for comparing WMS-IV and WAIS-IV performance. In this case, the WAIS-IV score acts as the control while the WMS-IV is the adjusted score. Contrast scores between 8 and 12 indicate that the two scores do not differ.

SHORT FORMS

The WMS-IV Flexible Approach provides four short batteries shown in Table 10–131. Each battery is called after the subtests that compose it (i.e., LMVR, OAA, etc). Recommendation for the administration order of the short batteries is found in the manual.

Short versions to estimate Immediate Memory Index (IMI) and Delayed Memory Index (DMI) comprising (1) Visual Reproduction and Logical Memory; (2) Visual Reproduction, Logical Memory, and VPA; or (3) Visual Reproduction, Logical Memory, and CVLT-II have also been reported by Miller et al. (2012b). The three-subtest version with VPA shows the best estimate of IMI and DMI. However, the authors noted that the two-subtest version may be sufficient to estimate IMI and DMI because the addition of CVLT-II does not increase accuracy by a significant degree. To predict IMI and DMI using these Short Forms, the data in Table 10–132 may be used (i.e., multiply age-adjusted scaled scores of each subtest by their respective *B*, sum the totals, and then add the constant). All correlations with the original IMI and DMI are high ($r > .92$).

If demographically-adjusted scores are desired, the following two- or three-subtest versions comprising (1) Visual Reproduction and Logical Memory; (2) Visual Reproduction and VPA; or (3) Visual Reproduction, Logical Memory, and VPA may be used (Miller et al., 2012c). The authors suggested using the Visual Reproduction and VPA regression-based model if only two subtests are used. To predict index scores, the data from Table 10–133 may be used (i.e., multiply demographically-adjusted T scores from the ACS by the respective *B*, sum the totals, and add the constant).

Similar to the Flexible Approach, Bouman et al. (2016c) developed the Dutch WMS-IV (WMS-IV-NL) Short Forms based on a three-subtest combination (Logical Memory, VPA, Visual Reproduction) only for ages 16–69 and labeled OAA, and two two-subtest combinations (Logical Memory and Visual Reproduction for ages 16–90 labeled LMVR, and Logical Memory and Designs for ages 16–69 labeled LMDE) using a mixed clinical sample. All Short Forms generated four index scores. Correlations between the short forms and original are high (greater than $r > .86$), with the highest seen in OAA index scores. The OAA yields predictive accuracy greater than 91% for all index scores except for the VMI, which is 73%. The two-subtest versions have accuracy in the 61–80% range, raising concern about their clinical utility. As such, users interested in using the Dutch Short Forms should use the OAA and are discouraged from using the two-subtest combinations because of their poor predictive utility.

DEMOGRAPHIC EFFECTS

AGE

Age effects are seen on the WMS-IV. Age shows weak correlations with Symbol Span, Visual Reproduction, and Designs ($r = -.24$, $-.13$, and $-.11$, respectively) and moderate correlations with Spatial Addition, VPA, and Logical Memory ($r = -.32$, $-.33$, and $.37$, respectively). Logical Memory shows a cubic age trend suggesting an initial dip followed by a rise and later decline (Salthouse, 2009). A modest correlation is seen between age and the Dutch BCSE ($r = -.22$; Bouman et al., 2015a).

TABLE 10–132 Wechsler Memory Scale—Fourth Edition (WMS-IV) Short Forms

	B		*B*
Immediate Memory Index-2 (IMI-2)		Delayed Memory Index-2 (DMI-2)	
Logical Memory I	2.78	Logical Memory II	2.76
Visual Reproduction I	2.61	Visual Reproduction II	2.55
Constant	43.76	Constant	46.55
Immediate Memory Index-3C (IMI-3C)		Delayed Memory Index-3C (DMI-3C)	
Logical Memory I	2.32	Logical Memory II	2.39
Visual Reproduction I	2.48	Visual Reproduction II	2.35
CVLT-II	1.13	CVLT-II	.85
Constant	39.48	Constant	44.43
Immediate Memory Index-3W (IMI-3W)		Delayed Memory Index-3W (DMI-3W)	
Logical Memory I	1.83	Logical Memory II	1.98
Visual Reproduction I	2.25	Visual Reproduction II	2.02
Verbal Paired Associates I	2.16	Verbal Paired Associates II	1.94
Constant	36.77	Constant	40.43

NOTE: CVLT-II, California Verbal Learning Test, 2nd Edition. To use the table, multiply age-adjusted scaled scores of each subtest by their respective *B*, sum the totals, and then add constant.

SOURCE: Adapted from Miller et al. (2012b).

TABLE 10–133 Demographically-Adjusted Wechsler Memory Scale—Fourth Edition (WMS-IV) Short Forms

	B		*B*
IMIt-2-LM		DMIt-2-LM	
Logical Memory I	.57	Logical Memory II	.58
Visual Reproduction I	.57	Visual Reproduction II	.51
Constant	−7.67	Constant	−3.80
IMIt-2-VPA		DMIt-2-VPA	
Verbal Paired Associates I	.59	Verbal Paired Associates II	.58
Visual Reproduction 1	.61	Visual Reproduction II	.51
Constant	−12.12	Constant	−6.06
IMIt-3		DMIt-3	
Logical Memory I	.38	Logical Memory II	.42
Visual Reproduction I	.49	Visual Reproduction II	.42
Verbal Paired Associates I	.44	Verbal Paired Associates II	.41
Constant	−16.14	Constant	−12.28

NOTE: IMIt, Demographically-adjusted Immediate Memory Index; DMIt, Demographically-adjusted Delayed Memory Index. To use the table, multiply demographically-adjusted T scores from the ACS by the respective *B*, sum the totals, and add the constant.

SOURCE: Adapted from Miller et al. (2012c).

GENDER

Females generally perform better than males on AMI, IMI, and DMI, while males perform better than females on VMI and Visual Working Memory Index (VWMI), though the differences are minimal (r = .00 to .12; Holdnack et al., 2013).

EDUCATION

Moderate correlations between education and VWMI and IMI are found but the correlations with AMI, VMI, and DMI are low (Holdnack et al., 2013). At the subtest level, education effects are generally low across all subtests (r < .28) except for Spatial Addition and Symbol Span, which are in the moderate range (r = .39 and .33, respectively; Holdnack et al., 2013). No correlation with education is found for the Dutch BCSE (Bouman et al., 2015a).

ETHNICITY, NATIONALITY, AND LINGUISTIC EFFECTS

Correlations between performance and ethnicity are similar for whites and African Americans (r = .11 to .26 and −.13 to −.24, respectively) and larger than for Hispanics and Asians (r = −.02 to −.12 and .02 to .11 respectively; Holdnack et al., 2013).

NORMATIVE DATA

The characteristics of the sample are shown in Table 10–134. The standardization group was based on a sample of 1,400 individuals aged 16–90 years, selected to match the 2005 US Census data on the basis of age, gender, race/ethnicity, education level, and geographic region. A total of 900 participants contributed to the normative data of the Adult Battery and 500 participants completed the Older Adult Battery. Given the overlap in the 65–69 age range for both batteries, two independent groups of participants in this age range completed each battery. Normative data from 14 age bands, each comprising 100 examinees, are provided. The WMS-IV is co-normed with the WAIS-IV but data collection for the WMS-IV continued after data collection for WAIS-IV stopped in order to achieve a normative sample with a General Ability Index score of 100 without weighting the sample. The ACS software provides demographically adjusted norms.

BASE RATES

Carrasco, Grups, Evans, Simco, and Mittenberg (2015) provide base rate data for discrepancies between WAIS-IV and WMS-IV scores in healthy populations. Please refer to the review of WAIS-IV in Chapter 5 of this volume for more information.

Base rates of WMS-IV low scores at various cutoff scores in 900 healthy adults aged 16–69 from the WAIS-IV/WMS-IV standardization sample are reported by Brooks et al. (2011). They found that almost half the sample have one or more index scores 1 *SD* below the mean. At this cutoff, 10–25% of the standardization sample have three to five low index scores, and 10% or less have six or more low index scores. Almost 88% of those with eight or fewer years of education, 82% of those with 9–11 years of education, 56% of those with high-school diploma, 45% of those with some college, and 20% of those with 16 or more years of education have at least one score below the 16th percentile, suggesting that low scores become more common with less education.

Notably, when stratified by intelligence, 45% of those with average intelligence obtain at least one score below the 16th percentile. Using the 5th percentile or lower as cutoff, 20% have one or more low index scores, although as the number of years of education increases, the chances of having one or more low index scores at this cutoff decrease (i.e., 61% of those with ≤8 years of education vs. about 5% of those with ≥16 years of education). In short, low scores are more common in those with fewer years of education or lower intelligence. Similar patterns are observed at the subtest level. Accordingly, multiple low scores in those with low education or low intelligence may not be uncommon; however, multiple low scores in those who are high functioning may be uncommon. Clinicians may wish to refer to Tables 10–135 and 10–136 for the base rates of low WAIS-IV/WMS-IV index and subtest scores.

EVIDENCE FOR RELIABILITY

EVIDENCE FOR INTERNAL RELIABILITY

As seen in Tables 10–137 and 10–138, all WMS-IV as well as Flexible Approach indices and primary subtests have high

TABLE 10–134 Characteristics of the Wechsler Memory Scale—Fourth Edition (WMS-IV) Standardization Sample

Sample size	1,400
Age	16 to 90[a] years
Sample type	Based on 2005 US Census
Geographic location	From geographic regions in proportions consistent with US Census data
Education	<8 to >16 years and consistent with US Census proportions; for examinees aged 16 to 19 years, parent education was used
Gender	An equal number of males and females in each age group from 16 to 64 years; the older age groups included more women than men, in proportions consistent with 2005 US Census data
Ethnicity	The proportions of whites, African Americans, Hispanics, and other racial/ethnic groups were based on the 2005 US Census data
Screening	Screened via self-report for primary language spoken, sensory, substance abuse, medical, psychiatric, or motor condition that could potentially affect performance, etc.[b]

[a] Broken down into 14 age groups: 16–17, 18–19, 20–24, 25–29, 30–34, 35–44, 45–54, 55–64, 65–69, 70–74, 75–79, 80–84, and 85–90 years; 100 individuals were included in each age group. Two groups of examinees ages 65–69 completed each of the Adult Battery and Older Adult Battery.

[b] See manual for detailed exclusion criteria.

SOURCE: Adapted from Wechsler (2009).

to very high internal consistency (Wechsler, 2009). In general, higher reliability coefficients are obtained with clinical groups. As seen in Table 10–137, subtests show a very high degree of decision consistency. Similar findings are seen for both the Adult Battery and Older Adult Battery. Internal consistency is high (r >.90) for all Dutch WMS-IV Short Forms (Bouman et al., 2016c).

STANDARD ERROR OF MEASUREMENT (SEM)

SEMs for each subtest average about .50 (Visual Reproduction II) to 1.17 (Logical Memory II, VPA II, Designs I, and Designs II) age-scaled score points. For the primary indices, *SEMs* across age groups range from 3.35 points (AMI) to 4.12 points (VWMI). For the Older Adult Battery, subtest *SEMs* range from .60 (Visual Reproduction II) to 1.53 (VPA II), and 2.77 (VMI) to 4.29 (DMI) for primary indices (Wechsler, 2009).

For the Flexible Approach, *SEMs* for the indices range from 2.60 for VMI (Visual Reproduction) to 5.48 for IMI (Logical Memory-Designs) across age groups; for the subtests, *SEMs* range from .81 for Names Proper Names to 1.17 for Logos II (Wechsler, 2009).

EVIDENCE FOR TEST-RETEST RELIABILITY, MEASURING CHANGE, AND PRACTICE EFFECTS

Test-retest reliability is based on a subset of participants from the standardization sample over a 14- to 84-day interval (M = 23 days). Primary subtests and indices had at least adequate stability except for Visual Reproduction as seen in Table 10–137 (Wechsler, 2009). Higher stability coefficients are seen in the Older Adult Battery (Wechsler, 2009). Several subtests have substantially skewed distribution and were reported as cumulative percentages; thus test-retest reliability is estimated based on decision-consistency, in which a 10% or less cutoff was used to create a classification for comparison across both measurement periods.

Bouman et al. (2015b) reported comparable test-retest reliabilities on the Dutch WMS-IV (WMS-IV-NL) compared to the US version over short (about 8.5 weeks) and long (about 18 months) retest intervals for 234 healthy individuals aged 16–90. All index scores improved on reevaluation except for the VWMI. Mean increases were 10 points for AMI, 9 points for VMI, 4 points for VWMI, 11 points for IMI, and 10 points for DMI for short intervals but no significant improvements were seen with long intervals. On the Older Adult battery, mean increases were 6 points for AMI, 9 points for VMI, 8 points for IMI, and 8 points for DMI after short intervals, and significant improvements were also not seen with long intervals. Base rates of change over short and long intervals are found in Table 10–139. Overall, these results suggest minimal practice effects on performance after 12 to 24 months.

The ACS software provides reliable change for the US version and will not be described here. To determine reliable change for the Dutch version, the interested user may use the regression equation in Table 10–140 to calculate predicted retest scores. Subsequently, the following equation may be used to determine the significance of the discrepancy:

$$\text{Z-score} = (Y_o - Y_p) / SE_{est}$$

where Y_o is the observed retest score and Y_p is the predicted retest score, and SE_{est} is the standard error of the estimate from the regression analysis.

Z scores greater than ±1.64 are significant at a 90% CI.
Z scores greater than ±1.96 are significant at a 95% CI.

EVIDENCE FOR INTERRATER RELIABILITY

Interrater reliability is generally high (r > .98) for most subtests with objective scoring criteria. Agreement for the more subjective Visual Reproduction is 97%, and agreement is 86% for Clock Drawing scoring on the BCSE.

EVIDENCE FOR VALIDITY

FACTOR-ANALYTIC STUDIES

As reported in the manual, CFA was conducted using WMS-IV delayed memory and visual working memory measures. Two models were tested and both were found to fit the data well. Hence, the three-factor model (auditory

TABLE 10–135 Prevalence of Low Wechsler Adult Intelligence Scale—Fourth Edition/Wechsler Memory Scale—Fourth Edition (WAIS-IV/WMS-IV) Index Scores

CUTOFF SCORES AND SAMPLES	*N*	% WITH 0 LOW SCORES	% WITH 1 OR MORE LOW SCORES	MEDIAN NUMBER OF LOW SCORES	BELOW EXPECTED NUMBER OF LOW SCORES (10% TO 25% OF SAMPLE)	WELL BELOW EXPECTED NUMBER OF LOW SCORES (<10% OF SAMPLE)
Cutoff: ≤25th percentile (Index ≤ 90)						
Total sample	900	38.7	61.3	1	5–8	9+
Education (years)						
8 or less	41	4.9	95.1	6	10	—
9–11	78	10.3	89.7	5	9	10
12	276	28.6	71.4	2	6–8	9+
13–15	266	39.1	60.9	1	3–7	8+
16+	239	64.9	35.1	0	2–4	5+
TOPF-Demographics Predicted WAIS-IV Full Scale IQ Score						
<80	22	0.0	100	10	10	—
80–89	95	8.4	91.6	5	9	10
90–109	478	37.0	63.0	1	5–6	7+
110–119	157	68.2	31.8	0	2	3+
120+	22	90.9	9.1	0	—	1+
Cutoff: ≤16th percentile (Index ≤85)						
Total Sample	900	52.8	47.2	0	3–5	6+
Education (years)						
8 or less	41	12.2	87.8	4	9–10	—
9–11	78	17.9	82.1	4	6–9	10
12	276	43.5	56.5	1	4–6	7+
13–15	266	54.9	45.1	0	3–4	5+
16+	239	79.5	20.5	0	1	2+
TOPF-Demographics Predicted WAIS-IV Full Scale IQ Score						
<80	22	0.0	100	8	10	—
80–89	95	15.8	84.2	3	6–9	10
90–109	478	54.8	45.2	0	3–4	5+
110–119	157	80.9	19.1	0	1	2+
120+	22	90.9	9.1	0	—	1+
Cutoff: ≤9th percentile (Index ≤80)						
Total sample	900	70.1	29.1	0	2–3	4+
Education (years)						
8 or less	41	26.8	73.2	3	6–8	9+
9–11	78	38.5	61.5	1	5–6	7+
12	276	61.2	38.8	0	2–3	4+
13–15	266	74.8	25.2	0	1–2	3+
16+	239	92.9	7.1	0	—	1+
TOPF-Demographics Predicted WAIS-IV Full Scale IQ Score						
<80	22	0.0	100	6	8–9	10
80–89	95	36.8	63.2	1	4–7	8+
90–109	478	73.8	26.2	0	1	2+
110–119	157	93.6	6.4	0	—	1+
120+	22	95.5	4.5	0	—	1+
Cutoff: ≤5th percentile (Index ≤76)						
Total sample	900	79.2	20.8	0	1–2	3+
Education (years)						
8 or less	41	39.0	61.0	1	5–6	7+
9–11	78	47.4	52.6	1	3–5	6+
12	276	74.3	25.7	0	1–2	3+
13–15	266	85.3	14.7	0	1	2+
16+	239	95.4	4.6	0	—	1+
TOPF-Demographics Predicted WAIS-IV Full Scale IQ Score						
<80	22	4.5	95.5	3.5	6–8	9+
80–89	95	53.7	46.3	0	2–5	6+
90–109	478	85.1	14.9	0	1	2+
110–119	157	94.9	5.1	0	—	1+
120+	22	95.5	4.5	0	—	1+
Cutoff: ≤2nd percentile (Index ≤70)						
Total sample	900	89.3	10.7	0	—	1+
Education (years)						
8 or less	41	56.1	43.9	0	3–4	5+
9–11	78	67.9	22.1	0	1–2	3+

TABLE 10–135 Continued

CUTOFF SCORES AND SAMPLES	N	% WITH 0 LOW SCORES	% WITH 1 OR MORE LOW SCORES	MEDIAN NUMBER OF LOW SCORES	BELOW EXPECTED NUMBER OF LOW SCORES (10% TO 25% OF SAMPLE)	WELL BELOW EXPECTED NUMBER OF LOW SCORES (<10% OF SAMPLE)
12	276	89.5	10.5	0	—	1+
13–15	266	92.9	7.1	0	—	1+
16+	239	97.9	2.1	0	—	1+
TOPF-Demographics Predicted WAIS-IV Full Scale IQ Score						
<80	22	31.8	68.2	1	4	5+
80–89	95	72.6	27.4	0	2–3	4+
90–109	478	93.9	6.1	0	—	1+
110–119	157	97.5	2.5	0	—	1+
120+	22	100	0.0	0	—	1+

NOTE: WAIS-IV, Wechsler Adult Intelligence Scale—Fourth Edition; WMS-IV, Wechsler Memory Scale—Fourth Edition; TOPF, Test of Premorbid Functioning; FSIQ, Full Scale IQ. There are 10 Index scores from the WAIS-IV and WMS-IV that were considered simultaneously for these analyses (Full Scale IQ, Verbal Comprehension, Perceptual Reasoning, Working Memory, and Processing Speed from the WAIS-IV, and Visual Working Memory Auditory Memory, Visual Memory, Immediate Memory, and Delayed Memory from the WMS-IV). "Below expected" is defined as the bottom 25% of the sample, based on frequency distributions. "Well below expected" is defined as the bottom 10% of the sample, based on frequency distributions. Standardization data from the WAIS-IV copyright © 2008 NCS Pearson, Inc. and standardization data for the WMS-IV copyright © 2009 NCS Pearson, Inc. Used with permission. All rights reserved

SOURCE: From Brooks et al. (2011).

TABLE 10–136 Prevalence of Low Wechsler Adult Intelligence Scale—Fourth Edition/Wechsler Memory Scale—Fourth Edition (WAIS-IV/WMS-IV) Subtest Scores

CUTOFF SCORES AND SAMPLES	N	% WITH 0 LOW SCORES	% WITH 1 OR MORE LOW SCORES	MEDIAN NUMBER OF LOW SCORES	BELOW EXPECTED NUMBER OF LOW SCORES (~10% TO 25% OF SAMPLE)	WELL BELOW EXPECTED NUMBER OF LOW SCORES (<10% OF SAMPLE)
Cutoff: ≤25th percentile (scaled score ≤8)						
Total sample	900	10.9	89.1	5	10–14	15+
Education (years)						
8 or less	41	0.0	100	12	18–19	20
9–11	78	2.6	97.4	11	15–18	19+
12	276	5.1	94.9	6	11–14	15+
13–15	266	10.5	89.5	5	9–12	13+
16+	239	22.6	77.4	2	5–8	9+
TOPF-Demographics Predicted WAIS-IV Full Scale IQ Score						
<80	22	0.0	100	17	19	20
80–89	95	1.1	98.9	11	15–17	18+
90–109	478	7.1	92.9	5	10–12	13+
110–119	157	27.4	72.6	1	5–6	7+
120+	22	50.0	50.0	0.5	3	4+
Cutoff: ≤16th percentile (scaled score ≤7)						
Total sample	900	23.0	77.0	3	7–11	12+
Education (years)						
8 or less	41	0.0	100	10	16–17	18+
9–11	78	6.4	93.6	7.5	12–15	16+
12	276	13.4	86.6	4	8–11	12+
13–15	266	22.6	77.4	2	6–9	10+
16+	239	43.9	56.1	1	3–5	6+
TOPF-Demographics Predicted WAIS-IV Full Scale IQ Score						
<80	22	0.0	100	14.5	17–18	19+
80–89	95	1.1	98.9	7	12–16	17+
90–109	478	17.8	81.2	3	6–8	9+
110–119	157	49.7	50.3	1	3	4+
120+	22	68.2	31.8	0	2	3+
Cutoff: ≤9th percentile (scaled score ≤6)						
Total sample	900	39.8	60.2	1	4–7	8+
Education (years)						
8 or less	41	7.3	92.7	7	12–14	15+
9–11	78	10.3	89.7	4.5	8–11	12+
12	276	29.7	70.3	2	5–7	8+
13–15	266	42.1	58.9	1	4–6	7+
16+	239	64.0	36.0	0	2–3	3+

(continued)

TABLE 10–136 Continued

CUTOFF SCORES AND SAMPLES	N	% WITH 0 LOW SCORES	% WITH 1 OR MORE LOW SCORES	MEDIAN NUMBER OF LOW SCORES	BELOW EXPECTED NUMBER OF LOW SCORES (~10% TO 25% OF SAMPLE)	WELL BELOW EXPECTED NUMBER OF LOW SCORES (<10% OF SAMPLE)
TOPF-Demographics Predicted WAIS-IV Full Scale IQ Score						
<80	22	0.0	100	11	13–14	15+
80–89	95	10.5	89.5	4	8–13	14+
90–109	478	38.1	61.9	1	3–5	6+
110–119	157	66.2	33.8	0	2	3+
120+	22	77.3	22.7	0	1	2+
Cutoff: ≤5th percentile (scaled score ≤5)						
Total sample	900	56.6	44.4	0	3–4	5+
Education (years)						
8 or less	41	19.5	80.5	3	8–9	10+
9–11	78	20.5	79.5	3	5–8	9+
12	276	46.7	53.3	1	3–4	5+
13–15	266	63.9	36.2	0	2–3	4+
16+	239	77.8	22.2	0	1	2+
TOPF-Demographics Predicted WAIS-IV Full Scale IQ Score						
<80	22	0.0	100	6	10–11	12+
80–89	95	28.4	71.6	2	5–8	9+
90–109	478	57.9	42.1	0	2–3	4+
110–119	157	79.6	20.4	0	1	2+
120+	22	86.4	13.6	0	1	2+
Cutoff: ≤2nd percentile (scaled score ≤4)						
Total sample	900	73.7	26.3	0	2	3+
Education (years)						
8 or less	41	34.1	65.9	1	5–6	7+
9–11	78	47.4	52.6	1	3–4	5+
12	276	67.4	32.6	0	2	3+
13–15	266	78.9	21.1	0	1	2+
16+	239	90.4	9.6	0	—	1+
TOPF-Demographics Predicted WAIS-IV Full Scale IQ Score						
<80	22	9.1	90.9	3	6–7	8+
80–89	95	48.4	51.6	1	2–4	5+
90–109	478	77.0	23.0	0	1	2+
110–119	157	91.1	8.9	0	—	1+
120+	22	90.9	9.1	0	—	1+

NOTE: WAIS-IV, Wechsler Adult Intelligence Scale—Fourth Edition; WMS-IV = Wechsler Memory Scale—Fourth Edition; TOPF = Test of Premorbid Functioning; FSIQ = Full Scale IQ. There are slight variations due to rounding. There are 20 primary subtests from the WAIS-IV and WMS-IV that were simultaneously considered for these analyses (Vocabulary, Information, Similarities, Digit Span, Arithmetic, Block Design. Matrix Reasoning, Visual Puzzles, Coding, and Symbol Search from the WAIS-IV, and Logical Memory I and II, Verbal Paired Associates I and II, Designs I and II, Visual Reproduction I and II, Spatial Addition, and Symbol Span from the WMS-IV). "Below expected" is defined as the bottom 25% of the sample, based on frequency distributions, "Well below expected" is defined as the bottom 10% of the sample, based on frequency distributions. Standardization data from the WAIS-IV copyright © 2008 NCS Pearson. Inc. and standardization data for the WMS-IV copyright © 2009 NCS Pearson. Inc. Used with permission. All rights reserved.
SOURCE: From Brooks et al. (2011).

memory, visual memory, and visual working memory) was chosen to represent the WMS-IV. Subsequent CFAs using an independent healthy adult sample and clinical depression sample supported the original three-factor model, although factor loadings for the Symbol Span subtest were lower in the clinical than control sample (Pauls et al., 2013). Furthermore, when both WMS-III and WMS-IV were tested using the same samples, the WMS-IV yielded two components, representing auditory learning/memory and visual attention/memory. WMS-III, however, yielded a single component, confirming that WMS-IV may be more reflective of the underlying memory structures than the WMS-III (Hoelzle et al., 2011).

Holdnack et al. (2011) conducted CFAs to test 13 models for the WAIS-IV and WMS-IV using the standardization sample and found two models that appear to fit the data. One model was a seven-factor solution comprising Verbal Comprehension, Perceptual Reasoning, Processing Speed, Auditory Working Memory, Visual Working Memory, Auditory Memory, and Visual Memory, with a first-order General Ability factor. Model 2 was a five-factor model comprising Verbal Comprehension, Perceptual Reasoning, Processing Speed, Working Memory, and Memory. Miller et al. (2013) replicated the study in an independent sample of older adults and concluded that the WAIS-IV and WMS-IV factor structure

TABLE 10–137 Magnitude of Reliability Coefficients of Wechsler Memory Scale—Fourth Edition (WMS-IV) Subtests and Indices

	INTERNAL RELIABILITY	TEST-RETEST RELIABILITY	PERCENTAGE DECISION CONSISTENCY
Very High (.90+)	Auditory Memory Index Visual Memory Index Visual Working Memory Index (except ages 16–17) Immediate Memory Index Delayed Memory Index Verbal Paired Associates I Visual Reproduction Spatial Addition		Logical Memory II Recognition Verbal Paired Associates II Recognition Designs II Recognition Visual Reproduction II Recognition Visual Reproduction II Copy
High (.80 to .89)	Logical Memory Verbal Paired Associates II (ages 16–69) Designs Symbol Span	Auditory Memory Index Visual Memory Index Visual Working Memory Index Immediate Memory Index Delayed Memory Index	
Adequate (.70 to .79)	Verbal Paired Associates II Word Recall Designs Content Designs Spatial Dutch Brief Cognitive Status Exam	Logical Memory Verbal Paired Associates Designs Spatial Addition Symbol Span	
Marginal (.60 to .69)		Visual Reproduction Designs Content Designs II Spatial	
Low (≤.59)		Designs I Spatial	

TABLE 10–138 Magnitude of Reliability Coefficients of Wechsler Memory Scale—Fourth Edition (WMS-IV) Flexible Approach Subtests and Indices

	INTERNAL RELIABILITY
Very High (.90+)	Immediate Memory Index (OAA) Delayed Memory Index (OAA) Visual Memory Index (Visual Reproduction) Immediate Memory Index (LMVR) Delayed Memory Index (LMVR) Auditory Memory Index (Logical Memory) Visual Memory Index (Designs) Visual Memory Index (VRLO) Visual Immediate Memory Index (VRLO) VDMI (VRLO) Auditory Immediate Memory Index (LONA) Auditory-Visual Immediate Memory Index (LONA) Auditory-Visual Delayed Memory Index (LONA) Logos I Names I Names Proper Names Names Activity
High (.80–.89)	Immediate Memory Index (LMDE) Delayed Memory Index (LMDE) Logos II Names II
Adequate (.70–.79)	
Marginal (.60–.69)	
Low (≤.59)	

appears stable in aging despite the expected cognitive decline with age.

PRIOR VERSIONS

According to the manual, the composition of the VMI and VWMI has been dramatically changed in the WMS-IV compared to WMS-III, whereas the AMI is only slightly modified. Within this context, correlations between WMS-IV AMI and WMS-III Auditory Immediate Index and Auditory Delayed Index are strong, whereas the correlations between WMS-IV VMI and the WMS-III visual indices are moderate. Correlations between the Immediate Memory Index and Delayed Memory Index of both versions are strong. Given the different composition of the WMS-IV VWMI and WMS-III WMI, their correlation is surprisingly high (r = .67). At the subtest level, both versions of Logical Memory and VPA yield high correlations (r = .75 to .76 and .69 to .74, respectively). WMS-IV Designs shows moderate correlations with WMS-III visual subtests (r = .35 to .43). WMS-III Spatial Span is also moderately correlated to WMS-IV visual working memory subtests (r = .52 to .55; manual). With changes to the scoring criteria, WMS-IV Visual Reproduction is now moderately correlated with its prior version. In sum, despite the major changes to the WMS-IV, it appears to measure similar constructs to the WMS-III.

INDEX/SUBTEST INTERCORRELATIONS

Similar to the WMS-III, strong correlations are generally observed between immediate and delayed

TABLE 10–139 Base Rates of Change (Time 2—Time 1) for the Dutch Wechsler Memory Scale—Fourth Edition (WMS-IV) After Short and Long Intervals

	SHORT RETEST INTERVAL						LONG RETEST INTERVAL					
	≥5	≥10	≥15	≥20	≥25	≥30	≥5	≥10	≥15	≥20	≥25	≥30
Adult Battery			(*n* = 66)						(*n* = 52)			
AMI (%)	70.8	50.8	33.8	13.8	7.7	1.5	27.5	23.5	21.6	11.8	2.0	0
VMI (%)	62.5	46.9	31.36	14.1	3.1	3.1	43.1	23.5	7.8	0	0	0
VWMI (%)	46.2	32.3	16.9	10.8	4.6	3.1	42.3	17.3	9.6	7.7	3.8	1.9
IMI (%)	76.6	60.9	3.4	12.5	7.8	3.1	35.3	23.5	5.9	2.0	0	0
DMI (%)	72.3	40.0	27.7	18.5	10.8	4.6	33.3	25.5	19.6	2.0	0	0
Older Adult Battery			(*n* = 68)						(*n* = 48)			
AMI (%)	57.4	32.4	13.2	5.9	1.5	1.5	22.7	15.9	4.5	4.5	2.3	2.3
VMI (%)	73.5	50.0	22.1	7.4	4.4	1.5	37.5	29.2	22.9	12.5	8.3	4.2
IMI (%)	61.8	41.2	25.0	13.2	5.9	1.5	27.3	11.4	2.3	2.3	0	0
DMI (%)	64.7	42.6	25.0	14.7	2.9	1.5	31.8	20.5	13.6	4.5	2.3	2.3

NOTE: AMI, Auditory Memory Index; VMI, Visual Memory Index; VWMI, Visual Working Memory Index; IMI, Immediate Memory Index; DMI, Delayed Memory Index.
SOURCE: From Bouman et al. (2015b).

conditions for the subtests and index scores, except for Visual Reproduction, which has moderate correlations (Wechsler, 2009). Strong correlations are also seen between subtests and the index scores to which they contribute. As expected, the correlations between visual subtests and visual working memory subtests are moderate and generally higher for immediate than for delayed conditions. Moderate correlations are also observed between AMI and both the VMI and VWMI, suggesting that these latter indices may be verbally mediated. The relationship appears to be driven by Visual Reproduction because, at the subtest level, Visual Reproduction appears to correlate moderately with Designs as well as all auditory and visual working memory subtests, whereas correlations between Designs and auditory memory subtests are generally low. Similar findings are reported for the Older Adult Battery. The findings are similar in clinical groups, though the correlations are generally higher than in the standardization sample (manual).

TABLE 10–140 Equations to Generate Predicted Scores for the Dutch Wechsler Memory Scale—Fourth Edition (WMS-IV)

SHORT INTERVAL	EQUATION FOR PREDICTED SCORE
Adult Battery	
AMI	33.138 + (baseline AMI x .774)
VMI	36.284 + (baseline VMI x .731)
VWMI	47.982 + (baseline VWMI x .575)
IMI	37.172 + (baseline IMI x .745)
DMI	41.684 + (baseline DMI x .769) + (age x −.177)
Older Adult Battery	
AMI	46.042 + (baseline AMI x .863) + (age x −.345)
VMI	36.482 + (baseline VMI x .720)
IMI	25.652 + (baseline IMI x .816)
DMI	23.751 + (baseline DMI x .844)
LONG INTERVAL	
Adult Battery	
AMI	40.493 + (baseline AMI x .625)
VMI	21.201 + (baseline VMI x .781)
VWMI	31.065 + (baseline VWMI x .588) + (gender x 6.12)
IMI	26.989 + (baseline IMI x .734)
DMI	32.171 + (baseline DMI x .696)
Older Adult Battery	
AMI	26.354 + (baseline AMI x .725)
VMI	45.435 + (baseline VMI x .571)
IMI	33.984 + (baseline IMI x .661)
DMI	25.901 + (baseline DMI x .745)

NOTE: Age in years; gender: 1 = male, 2 = female. Age-adjusted standard scores used in all equations. AMI, Auditory Memory Index; VMI, Visual Memory Index; VWMI, Visual Working Memory Index; IMI, Immediate Memory Index; DMI, Delayed Memory Index.
SOURCE: Adapted from Bouman et al. (2015b).

In one study using university volunteers, Thiruselvam and colleagues (2015) reported that the VPA I is not correlated with CVLT-II Trials 1–5 Total whereas VPA II and CVLT-II Long Delay Free Recall are moderately correlated (r = .33). The substitute VPA scores are lower than the actual VPA scores for both CVLT-II conditions, resulting in lower AMI scores than when the VPA is used. Miller and colleagues (2012a) also found that using the CVLT-II to substitute for VPA results in lower AMI but not IMI or DMI scores. These findings suggest that the CVLT-II and VPA may not be equivalent and raise doubts on the use of the CVLT-II as a substitute for VPA on the WMS-IV.

RELATIONSHIPS WITH OTHER MEMORY TESTS

The manual indicates that WMS-IV subtests and index scores are moderately correlated with the CVLT-II, although visual subtests and index scores generally show weaker relationship with the CVLT-II than auditory subtests and index scores (r = .39 for Designs to .65 for the IMI). In short, WMS-IV auditory subtests appear to measure similar constructs as other verbal memory tests, but Designs and Visual Reproduction subtests overlap with verbal memory measures to some degree, raising doubt about their divergent validity.

RELATIONSHIPS WITH WECHSLER INTELLIGENCE SCALES

The manual reports that IQ is moderately related to memory scores (r = .54 to .71 between FSIQ/General Ability Index and WMS-IV index scores), supporting the association between intelligence and memory and the potential utility of discrepancy analyses for determining weaknesses in memory relative to general intellectual ability. The highest correlation is seen between VWMI and FSIQ (r = .71). The relationship between auditory memory measures and WAIS-IV Verbal Comprehension Index and Perceptual Reasoning Index appears equivalent (r = .38 to .47 and r = .32 to .40, respectively). On the other hand, visual memory measures show higher correlations to the WAIS-IV Perceptual Reasoning Index than to the Verbal Comprehension Index (r = .40 to .60 and r = .27 to .46, respectively). As expected, moderate correlations are observed between visual working memory measures and the WAIS-IV Working Memory Index (r = .52 and .54), suggesting that they measure a similar construct.

The relationship between WMS-IV and WISC-IV was examined in a sample of youth aged 16 who were administered both the test batteries. WISC-IV IQ was moderately correlated to memory scores though the relationship was small (r = .44 to .68 between FSIQ/General Ability Index and WMS-IV index scores). The highest correlation was seen between WMS-IV IMI and FSIQ (r = .68). Unlike the WAIS-IV, WMS-IV subtests show the expected relationship with corresponding WISC-IV index scores. Specifically, auditory memory measures show higher correlations with the WISC-IV Verbal Comprehension Index than Perceptual Reasoning Index (r = .32 to .54 vs. r = .32 to .49) whereas visual memory measures show higher correlations with the WISC-IV Perceptual Reasoning Index than the Verbal Comprehension Index (r = .47 to .53 vs. r = .18 to .42). Similar to the WAIS-IV, moderate relationships are seen between visual working memory measures and the Working Memory Index (r = .50 and .59; manual). In short, intelligence appear to have a moderate relationship with memory as measured by the WMS-IV across the life span.

RELATIONSHIPS WITH OTHER NEUROPSYCHOLOGICAL TESTS

The BCSE is highly correlated with the MMSE (r = .79; manual). WMS-IV subtests show moderate to high relationships with the RBANS Total Scale (r = .37 to .65). In particular, Visual Reproduction and Symbol Span appear to have the highest correlations with RBANS Total (r > .60), although it is of note that both subtests show moderate relationships across all RBANS domains. In fact, the VMI is moderately correlated with all memory, non-memory, and verbal, as well as nonverbal domains, suggesting that visual memory subtests on the WMS-IV may be tapping broad neuropsychological functions. On the other hand, AMI appears to strictly measure memory as correlations with non-memory domains are all low (r < .30). The highest correlation is observed between RBANS Delayed Memory and WMS-IV DMI (r = .71), followed by RBANS Immediate Memory and WMS-IV IMI (r = .64; manual). To summarize, AMI appears to assess only memory functions whereas VMI may be measuring broad cognitive functions. IMI and DMI appear to measure what they purport to measure.

Not surprisingly, the WMS-IV contains some frontal executive components as reported in the manual. For example, all index scores are moderately correlated with the D-KEFS TMT Switching condition. In fact, VWMI is moderately correlated with D-KEFS TMT, as well as Category Fluency and Category Switching. IMI and DMI are also moderately correlated with all the D-KEFS subtests sampled. At the subtest level, VPA I shows minimal correlation with the D-KEFS whereas Designs shows the highest correlation with the D-KEFS TMT. The relationship between the WMS-IV and the D-KEFS was stronger in a sample of individuals with TBI given the impairments in memory and executive functions often seen in this population (see manual).

The manual notes that the WMS-IV is moderately to strongly correlated with tests of academic achievement such as the Wechsler Individual Achievement Test (WIAT-II). VWMI shows the strongest relationship to WIAT-II Total Composite, followed by the AMI (r = .75 and .70, respectively). The VWMI also shows the strongest relationship to Mathematics while both the IMI and the DMI are strongly correlated to Oral Language. At the subtest level, the AMI and the VWMI are moderately correlated with all WIAT-II subtests, whereas correlations between the VMI and Word Reading, Pseudoword Decoding, Spelling, and Written Expression are weak. Overall, memory as measured by the WMS-IV appears important for academic skills.

RELATIONSHIPS WITH RATING SCALES

Low to high negative correlations have been reported in the manual between WMS-IV and the Brown ADD Scales in a sample of adults with ADHD (r = –.22 to –.54). Correlations with the BDI-II and BDI-II Fast Screen are low in a sample of older adults with MCI or AD (see manual).

In the standardization sample, WMS-IV Older Adult Battery index scores are moderated related to Independent Living Scales except for the Social Adjustment subscale, which had low to negligible correlations across all WMS-IV subtests and index scores. The ABAS-II, a measure of adaptive functioning, also has low to negligible relationships to the WMS-IV Older Adult Battery performance in healthy older adults as well as those with MCI. However, the WMS-IV and ABAS-II are moderately correlated in TBI, mild intellectual disability, and moderate intellectual disability groups, indicating that the WMS-IV may be useful for treatment planning in these samples.

The ecological validity of the WMS-IV was examined using the Texas Functional Living Scale (TFLS) in healthy individuals aged 16–90 years as well as in a sample of clinical patients with diagnoses including AD, mild intellectual disability, moderate intellectual disability, major depressive disorder (MDD), and autism (manual). Correlations were small to moderate in the range of .20 (Designs II) to .40 (VWMI) in the healthy sample while correlations were higher in the clinical sample (range = .52 to .80), particularly in the AD and TBI samples (manual). There were small correlations between TFLS and BCSE (r = .21; manual). The results were consistent with the fact that, with declining memory, functional capacity appears to decline (Drozdick & Cullum, 2011).

CLINICAL STUDIES

The manual reports that the WMS-IV is sensitive to a variety of conditions, including AD, MCI (except Designs II), TBI, schizophrenia, mild and moderate intellectual disability, and autism (but not Asperger's disorder). The WMS-IV also appears to be sensitive to the treatment effect of olanzapine on cognitive functions in patients with first-episode schizophrenia (Wang et al., 2013). However, only Visual Reproduction I and Spatial Addition are affected by MDD in adults, while Visual Reproduction I and Symbol Span are affected by anxiety in adults, suggesting that visual memory and visual working memory are particularly sensitive to mood and anxiety disorders. Those with mathematics disorder also perform worse than matched controls on visual memory and visual working memory subtests, while individuals with ADHD perform worse than matched controls on VPA and Designs II (Wechsler, 2009). By contrast, the WMS-IV does not appear to be affected by MDD in older adults or those with reading disorder (Wechsler, 2009). Laboratory-induced pain also does not affect Symbol Span, Spatial Addition, Logical Memory I, or VPA I performance in nonclinical volunteers (Etherton & Tapscott, 2015).

Among patients who have undergone temporal lobectomy for epilepsy, those with right temporal lobectomy perform worse than matched controls on visual memory and visual working memory subtests, but their performance on verbal memory measures do not differ from matched controls. On the other hand, verbal memory subtests do not yield the expected results among patients who have undergone left temporal lobectomy, though the sample (N = 8) is likely too small to detect an effect (Wechsler, 2009). Bouman et al. (2016a) reported that the index scores and subtest scores of the WMS-IV Dutch version (WMS-IV-NL) are lower in those with TLE compared to healthy controls, but not on VWMI, Logical Memory I, VPA I, and Designs II. In addition, Logical Memory I, Designs II, and all indices except AMI and VWMI are lower in TLE patients with mesiotemporal abnormalities (MTS) compared to those with lateral temporal abnormalities. However, there are no difference in side of seizure focus on all indices and subtests as well as on Auditory-Visual (AV) discrepancy scores. Overall, there was a poor classification rate for identifying left versus right TLE using the WMS-IV (AUC < .56 for all). Similar to the lobectomy patients, the study by Bouman et al. (2016a) suggests that the WMS-IV is sensitive to memory impairments in TLE but does not show material-specific memory impairment for the purposes of presurgical evaluation.

The insensitivity of the WMS-IV to material-specific memory in epilepsy was further demonstrated by Soble and colleagues (2014), who used hierarchical logistic regression to evaluate the predictive accuracy of WMS-IV against RAVLT in identifying lateralized memory impairments. The RAVLT appears to predict laterality with about 70% accuracy but none of the WMS-IV subtests or Auditory-Visual discrepancy scores adds to the prediction model. The authors suggested that the insensitivity of the WMS-IV to seizure laterality may be due to the subtests containing both verbal and visual components or because of the use of single-trial learning, which can be affected by poor attention or comprehension in those with TLE.

Several other independent studies also raise concern about the sensitivity of various WMS-IV scores to memory impairment in clinical samples. For example, one independent study compared VPA to CVLT-II, Logical Memory, and RCFT. While the VPA yielded similar classification accuracy in identifying amnestic MCI from healthy controls as the Logical Memory and RCFT, the CVLT-II yielded higher classification rates. Notably, the VPA II exhibited a smaller effect size than the CVLT-II delayed recall and failed to classify 70% of amnestic MCI as impaired (Pike et al., 2013). Other studies reported that although patients with TBI, TLE, or right MCA stroke perform worse than healthy controls on the WMS-IV subtests, index scores are in the average range for complicated mild/moderate TBI, average to low average for TLE, and low average for severe TBI and stroke (Bouman et al., 2016a; Carlozzi et al., 2013; Spedo et al., 2013).

With regard to the BCSE, the manual reports a sensitivity of 77%, specificity of 98%, PPV of 97%, and NPV of 81% for identifying AD. Using the Dutch version of the BCSE, Bouman et al. (2015a) reported that a dementia group performed worse than MCI and healthy groups while the MCI group performed worse than healthy controls. At a cutoff score of 42 or less, the BCSE yielded a sensitivity of 96%, specificity of 92%, PPV of 86%, and NPV of 97% to identify dementia. A BCSE cutoff score of 46 or less yielded a sensitivity of 81%, specificity of 80%, PPV of 61%, and NPV of 92%. These results are comparable to the MMSE. Table 10–141 shows the sensitivity and specificity of different BCSE cutoffs for identifying MCI and dementia.

Some data presented in the manual support the validity of the short forms. As reported in the manual, LMVR as well as LONA are sensitive to AD and TBI but not to left or right temporal lobectomy. Patients with moderate to severe TBI perform worse than healthy matched controls

TABLE 10–141 Brief Cognitive Status Exam (BCSE) Sensitivity, Specificity, and Predictive Values at Different Cutoff Scores to Identify Mild Cognitive Impairment (MCI) and Dementia

CUTOFF SCORE	MCI				DEMENTIA			
	SENSITIVITY (%)	SPECIFICITY (%)	PPV (%)	NPV (%)	SENSITIVITY (%)	SPECIFICITY (%)	PPV (%)	NPV (%)
36					78	96	91	89
37					82	95	89	91
38					84	95	90	92
39					92	93	87	96
40					92	92	86	96
41					94	92	86	97
42	70	92	77	88	96	92	86	98
43	73	91	76	89	96	91	85	97
44	73	88	70	88	96	88	80	98
45	73	82	62	88	96	82	74	98
46	81	80	61	92	96	80	72	98
47	86	75	58	92	96	75	67	97
48	86	67	51	91	96	67	61	97
49	89	64	49	92	98	64	56	98
50	92	59	47	93				

NOTE: BCSE, Brief Cognitive Status Exam; PPV, positive predictive value; NPV, negative predictive value.
SOURCE: Bouman et al. (2015a).

on OAA, VMI (Visual Reproduction), AMI (Logical Memory), LMDE, and VMI (Designs). Among those with right temporal lobectomy, performance on most of the batteries was significantly lower than in healthy matched controls except for the AMI (Logical Memory). The opposite was true among those who had left temporal lobectomy, suggesting utility of some of the short forms in assessing material-specific memory (Wechsler, 2009).

The Designs subtest may be susceptible to chance performance. Using a random number generator, Martin and Schroeder (2014) simulated random placement of cards on the Designs subtest for 100 "patients." Based on the simulation, scaled scores of 1 to 2 across all ages on Designs I were obtained; however, low average to average scaled scores in the older age groups (aged 45+) were obtained on Designs II. In particular, random selection of cards in the 65- to 69-year age group resulted in scaled scores of 7 or more greater than 50% of the time. Based on chance alone, those who are older than 65 years would obtain a low average or average score. The authors also noted that the probability of chance performance increases as the examinee's raw score approaches 36 (Martin & Schroeder, 2014).

NEUROANATOMICAL CORRELATES AND IMAGING STUDIES

The only study to our knowledge that examined the neuroanatomical correlates of the WMS-IV reported that Logical Memory is correlated with hippocampal head and dentate gyrus volume while Designs is correlated with dentate gyrus, and hippocampal body and tail volumes. Visual working memory measures (i.e., Spatial Addition and Symbol Span) are not associated with MRI hippocampal volume (Travis et al., 2014). Interestingly, Logical Memory is correlated with left hippocampal volumes while Designs is correlated bilaterally (Travis et al., 2014).

PERFORMANCE VALIDITY

The ACS is a complement to the WMS-IV that provides a number of embedded WMS-IV and WAIS-IV indices for identifying noncredible performance, including Visual Reproduction Recognition, Logical Memory Recognition, VPA Recognition, WAIS-IV Reliable Digit Span, and a new external measure, Word Choice. Readers may wish to refer to the review of Word Choice in Chapter 15 of this volume and in the excellent book by Holdnack and colleagues (2013) for guidelines on the use of the ACS performance validity indices.

Miller and colleagues (2011) examined the utility of the ACS indices in identifying TBI and healthy volunteers simulating impairments in an analog study. Logistic regression using all indices was "outstanding" for classifying simulators except for the Logical Memory Recognition (see the ACS Word Choice review for more information). Overall, use of the ACS in assessing performance validity is supported, although more research is needed.

Other studies have examined the utility of specific subtests. For example, Logical Memory and Designs are sensitive to noncredible performance among veterans attending a VA Medical Center (Sawyer et al., 2014). On Logical Memory, the noncredible group performs significantly lower than the credible group, with effect sizes ranging from .80 (Logical Memory I) to .94 (Logical Memory II). A similar pattern is seen on the Designs subtest, with

TABLE 10–142 Sensitivity and Specificity of Wechsler Adult Intelligence Scale—Fourth Edition (WAIS-IV) Spatial Addition in Identifying Noncredible Performance at Different Cutoff Scores

CUTOFF VALUE	SENSITIVITY (%)	SPECIFICITY (%)
<2	10	100
<3	30	96
<4	52	93
<5	62	89
<6	74	80
<7	80	70
<8	94	50
<9	96	43
<10	98	26
<11	100	17

NOTE: Extreme values for the curve were omitted.

SOURCE: From Bouman et al. (2016b).

effect sizes ranging from .84 (Designs II) to .90 (Designs Recognition).

Bouman et al. (2016b) examined performance validity using experimental malingerers and a sample of patients with mixed etiology using the Dutch WMS-IV in an analog study. Experimental malingerers were asked to simulate cognitive impairment due to TBI while healthy controls were asked to perform validly. Patients performed worse than controls on all subtests except the Visual Reproduction Copy. Experimental malingerers performed worse than healthy controls on all subtests and worse than patients on Logical Memory, Visual Reproduction I, Spatial Addition, Symbol Span, BCSE, Logical Memory Recognition, VPA Recognition, and Visual Reproduction Recognition. Submitting Spatial Addition, Symbol Span, Logical Memory Recognition, VPA Recognition, Designs Recognition, and Visual Reproduction Recognition into a logistic regression distinguished patients from experimental malingerers with 78% accuracy. Spatial Addition explained the greatest variance, with an odds ratio of 0.60. Using Spatial Addition alone, 77% classification accuracy was obtained. For every one scaled-score point increase on the Spatial Addition, the examinees were 0.58 times less likely to malinger. Spatial Addition may thus be useful to identify invalid performance. As such, sensitivity and specificity at various Spatial Addition cutoff scores are presented in Table 10–142. Note that simulation paradigms will tend to inflate sensitivity, and validation is required in verified malingerers.

COMMENT

The WMS-IV is a sophisticated battery for the assessment of memory functioning. It has undergone extensive revision in an attempt to address shortcomings of prior versions following surveys of users and the research literature. The test administration time has been shortened, the scoring is simplified, and the stimuli booklets are updated. The battery contains a variety of primary and process scores that are helpful to address various clinical questions, and the scores are easily generated by the accompanying scoring software. In addition to the core battery, which includes an Older Adult Battery that allows the assessment of low-functioning older adults, a number of supplemental materials including the ACS (Holdnack et al., 2013; Pearson Assessment, 2009) are available to maximize the flexibility of the WMS-IV for use in various settings. For instance, when there are time constraints, users may utilize one of the many short batteries to good effect (e.g., the Dutch OAA or the two- or three-subtest short forms by Miller et al., 2012). One of the main advantages of the WMS-IV is the large normative dataset, which is co-normed with the WAIS-IV, allowing direct comparison of intellectual ability and memory functioning. The structure of this revision appears to be an improvement over the WMS-III, with the indexes reflecting what they purport to measure. Internal consistencies of the indexes and subtests are high, and test-retest correlations are adequate to high for the verbal subtests. In addition, when used with information provided in the ACS, the WMS-IV appears to be an effective PVT, although more independent studies are needed on the WMS-IV embedded validity indexes in different populations.

The WMS-IV continues to face a number of criticisms. Loring and Bauer (2010) commented that the manual did not provide justification for changes, such as the change from two learning trials for one of the stories in WMS-III to single presentation for both stories in WMS-IV. The elimination of the Faces subtest from WMS-III due to its susceptibility to guessing also removed one important aspect of visual memory rarely examined in other memory tests. Although the Designs subtest replaced Faces in the WMS-IV, it, too, appears susceptible to chance performance (Martin & Schroeder, 2014).

As of this writing, much of the existing research on the WMS-IV utilizes the standardization sample. Few independent studies have been completed to examine its psychometric properties in other normative samples. Thus, despite the WMS-IV's popularity in clinical settings, limited independent studies have been conducted using clinical samples to examine its sensitivity to various neurological or psychiatric conditions.

The Flexible Approach is valuable for shortening testing time; however, very few independent studies have been completed to evaluate its predictive validity. In fact, one study that utilized the Dutch WMS-IV found that only the OAA short battery had adequate predictive validity in clinical samples (Bouman et al., 2016c).

Furthermore, the visual memory and visual working memory subtests and indices correlate with both verbal and visual tests, suggesting that these subtests continue to be verbally mediated like their predecessors. In fact, the Visual Reproduction subtest seems to be most problematic, possibly due to its simplified scoring procedure. Not only does it demonstrate low test-retest reliability, it is highly correlated with auditory tests and with the RBANS, a general neuropsychological screening battery, suggesting that Visual Reproduction may measure broad cognitive functioning. Finally, in our experience, the Spatial Addition subtest is challenging to administer because the instructions are confusing for patients.

The WMS-IV is also not useful as a battery to assess material-specific memory to predict side of seizure focus or risk of postsurgical memory deficit among those undergoing epilepsy presurgical evaluation, possibly because the index scores combine immediate and delayed conditions into one score or because visual subtests are verbally mediated. Although the Flexible Battery provides index scores that separate auditory immediate, auditory delayed, visual immediate, and visual delayed, no independent information is available about its utility for the purposes of epilepsy presurgical investigation. Compared to other memory tests, independent research is also very scant on important conditions associated with memory impairment, including dementia, MCI, and TBI. Users may prefer other tests when assessing these conditions, particularly dementia.

It is important to note that the WMS-IV is sensitive to demographic effects. Users should be aware that multiple low scores are common, especially among those with low education or low intellectual functioning (Brooks et al., 2011). When interpreting test performance, users should take the prevalence of low scores into consideration.

Finally, there are problems with the CVLT-II substitution yielding underestimation of index scores. Users should also note that if the WAIS-IV subtests are administered during the WMS-IV delay interval, interference effects are possible (Ingram et al., 2016). As such, users may wish to administer the WAIS-IV before the WMS-IV.

REFERENCES

Bouman, Z., Elhorst, D., Hendriks, M. P. H., Kessels, R. P. C., & Aldenkamp, A. P. (2016a). Clinical utility of the Wechsler Memory Scale—Fourth Edition (WMS-IV) in patients with intractable temporal lobe epilepsy. *Epilepsy & Behavior, 55*, 178–182.

Bouman, Z., Hendriks, M. P. H., Aldenkamp, A. P., & Kessels, R. P. C. (2015a). Clinical validation of the WMS-IV-NL brief cognitive status exam (BCSE) in older adults with MCI or dementia. *International Psychogeriatrics, 27*(2), 221–229.

Bouman, Z., Hendriks, M. P. H., Aldenkamp, A. P., & Kessels, R. P. C. (2015b). Temporal stability of the Dutch version of the Wechsler Memory Scale—Fourth Edition (WMS-IV-NL). *The Clinical Neuropsychologist, 29*, S30–S46.

Bouman, Z., Hendriks, M. P. H., Schmand, B. A., Kessels, R. P. C., & Aldenkamp, A. P. (2016b). Indicators of suboptimal performance embedded in the Wechsler Memory Scale—Fourth Edition (WMS–IV). *Journal of Clinical and Experimental Neuropsychology, 38*(4), 455–466.

Bouman, Z., Hendriks, M. P. H., Van, D. V., Aldenkamp, A. P., & Kessels, R. P. C. (2016c). Clinical validation of three short forms of the Dutch Wechsler Memory Scale—Fourth Edition (WMS-IV-NL) in a mixed clinical sample. *Assessment, 23*(3), 386–394.

Brooks, B. L., Holdnack, J. A., & Iverson, G. L. (2011). Advanced clinical interpretation of the WAIS-IV and WMS-IV: Prevalence of low scores varies by level of intelligence and years of education. *Assessment, 18*(2), 156–167.

Butters, N., Salmon, D. P., Cullum, C. M., Cairns, P., Tröster, A. I., Jacobs, D., et al. (1988). Differentiation of amnestic and demented patients with the Wechsler Memory Scale-revised. *The Clinical Neuropsychologist, 2*, 133–148.

Carlozzi, N. E., Grech, J., & Tulsky, D. S. (2013). Memory functioning in individuals with traumatic brain injury: An examination of the Wechsler Memory Scale—Fourth Edition (WMS–IV). *Journal of Clinical and Experimental Neuropsychology, 35*(9), 906–914.

Carrasco, R. M., Grups, J., Evans, B., Simco, E., & Mittenberg, W. (2015). Apparently abnormal Wechsler Memory Scale Index score patterns in the normal population. *Applied Neuropsychology: Adult, 22*(1), 1–6.

Drozdick, L. W., & Cullum, C. M. (2011). Expanding the ecological validity of WAIS-IV and WMS-IV with the texas functional living scale. *Assessment, 18*(2), 141–155.

Erickson, R. A., & Scott, M. L. (1977). Clinical memory testing: A review. *Psychological Bulletin, 84*, 1130–1149.

Etherton, J. L., & Tapscott, B. E. (2015). Performance on selected visual and auditory subtests of the Wechsler Memory Scale—Fourth Edition during laboratory-induced pain. *Journal of Clinical and Experimental Neuropsychology, 37*(3), 243–252.

Hoelzle, J. B., Nelson, N. W., & Smith, C. A. (2011). Comparison of Wechsler Memory Scale—Fourth Edition (WMS–IV) and Third edition (WMS–III) dimensional structures: Improved ability to evaluate auditory and visual constructs. *Journal of Clinical and Experimental Neuropsychology, 33*(3), 283–291.

Holdnack, J. A., Whipple Drozdick, L., Weiss, L. G., & Iverson, G. (Eds.). (2013). *WAIS-IV, WMS-IV, and ACS: Advanced clinical interpretation*. Waltham, MA: Academic.

Holdnack, J. A., Zhou, X., Larrabee, G. J., Millis, S. R., & Salthouse, T. A. (2011). Confirmatory factor analysis of the WAIS-IV/WMS-IV. *Assessment, 18*(2), 178–191.

Ingram, N. S., Diakoumakos, J. V., Sinclair, E. R., & Crowe, S. F. (2016). Material-specific retroactive interference effects of the Wechsler Adult Intelligence Scale–Fourth edition on Wechsler Memory Scale—Fourth Edition in a nonclinical sample. *Journal of Clinical and Experimental Neuropsychology, 38*(4), 371–380.

Larrabee, G. J., Kane, R. L., Schuck, J. R., & Francis, D. J. (1985). Construct validity of various memory test procedures. *Journal of Clinical and Experimental Neuropsychology, 7*, 497–504.

Lezak, M. D., Howieson, D. B., & Loring, D. W. (2004). *Neuropsychological assessment* (4th ed.). New York: Oxford University Press.

Lichtenberger, E. O., Kaufman, A. S., & Lai, Z. C. (2002). *Essentials of WMS-III assessment*. New York: Wiley.

Loring, D. W., & Bauer, R. M. (2010). Testing the limits: Cautions and concerns regarding the new Wechsler IQ and memory scales. *Neurology, 74*(8), 685–690.

Loring, D. W., & Papanicolauo, A. C. (1987). Memory assessment in neuropsychology: Theoretical considerations and practical utility. *Journal of Clinical and Experimental Neuropsychology, 9*, 340–358.

Martin, P. K., & Schroeder, R. W. (2014). Chance performance and floor effects: Threats to the validity of the Wechsler Memory Scale—Fourth Edition Designs subtest. *Archives of Clinical Neuropsychology, 29*(4), 385–390.

Milberg, W. P., Hebben, N., & Kaplan, E. (1986). The Boston process approach to neuropsychological assessment. In I. Grant & K. M. Adams (Eds.), *Neuropsychiatric disorders* (pp. 42–65). New York: Oxford University Press.

Miller, D. I., Davidson, P. S. R., Schindler, D., & Messier, C. (2013). Confirmatory factor analysis of the WAIS-IV and WMS-IV in older adults. *Journal of Psychoeducational Assessment, 31*(4), 375–390.

Miller, J. B., Axelrod, B. N., Rapport, L. J., Hanks, R. A., Bashem, J. R., & Schutte, C. (2012a). Substitution of California Verbal Learning Test, for Paired Associates on the Wechsler Memory Scale. *The Clinical Neuropsychologist, 26*(4), 599–608.

Miller, J. B., Axelrod, B. N., Rapport, L. J., Millis, S. R., VanDyke, S., Schutte, C., & Hanks, R. A. (2012b). Parsimonious prediction of Wechsler Memory Scale—Fourth Edition scores: Immediate and delayed memory indexes. *Journal of Clinical and Experimental Neuropsychology, 34*(5), 531–542.

Miller, J. B., Axelrod, B. N., & Schutte, C. (2012c). Parsimonious estimation of the Wechsler Memory Scale—Fourth Edition demographically adjusted index scores: Immediate and delayed memory. *The Clinical Neuropsychologist, 26*(3), 490–500.

Miller, J. B., Millis, S. R., Rapport, L. J., Bashem, J. R., Hanks, R. A., & Axelrod, B. N. (2011). Detection of insufficient effort using the advanced clinical solutions for the Wechsler Memory Scale—Fourth Edition. *The Clinical Neuropsychologist, 25*(1), 160–172.

Pauls, F., Petermann, F., & Lepach, A. C. (2013). Memory assessment and depression: Testing for factor structure and measurement invariance of the Wechsler Memory Scale—Fourth Edition across a clinical and matched control sample. *Journal of Clinical and Experimental Neuropsychology, 35*(7), 702–717.

Pearson Assessment. (2009). *Advanced Clinical Solutions for the WAIS-IV/WMS-IV*. San Antonio, TX: Author.

Pike, K. E., Kinsella, G. J., Ong, B., Mullaly, E., Rand, E., Storey, E., . . . Parsons, S. (2013). Is the WMS-IV Verbal Paired Associates as effective as other memory tasks in discriminating amnestic mild cognitive impairment from normal aging? *The Clinical Neuropsychologist, 27*(6), 908–923.

Prigatano, G. P. (1977). Wechsler Memory Scale is a poor screening test for brain dysfunction. *Journal of Clinical Psychology, 33,* 772–777.

Prigatano, G. P. (1978). Wechsler Memory Scale: A selective review of the literature. *Journal of Clinical Psychology, 34,* 816–832.

The Psychological Corporation. (1997, 2002). *WAIS-III/WMS-III Technical Manual.* San Antonio, TX: Author.

Russell, E. W. (1975). A multiple scoring method for the assessment of complex memory functions. *Journal of Consulting and Clinical Psychology, 43,* 800–809.

Salthouse, T. A. (2009). Decomposing age correlations on neuropsychological and cognitive variables. *Journal of the International Neuropsychological Society, 15*(5), 650–661.

Sawyer, R. J., Young, J. C., Roper, B. L., & Rach, A. (2014). Are verbal intelligence subtests and reading measures immune to non-credible effort? *The Clinical Neuropsychologist, 28*(5), 756–770.

Soble, J. R., Eichstaedt, K. E., Waseem, H., Mattingly, M. L., Benbadis, S. R., Bozorg, A. M., . . . Schoenberg, M. R. (2014). Clinical utility of the Wechsler Memory Scale—Fourth Edition (WMS-IV) in predicting laterality of temporal lobe epilepsy among surgical candidates. *Epilepsy & Behavior, 41,* 232–237.

Spedo, C. T., Foss, M. P., Elias, A. H. N., Pereira, D. A., Santos, P. L. d., de, A. R., . . . Barreira, A. A. (2013). Cross-cultural adaptation of visual reproduction subtest of Wechsler Memory Scale—Fourth Edition (WMS-IV) to a Brazilian context. *Clinical Neuropsychiatry, 10*(2), 111–119.

Spreen, O., & Strauss, E. (1998). *A compendium of neuropsychological tests: Administration, norms and commentary.* New York: Oxford University Press.

Stone, C., & Wechsler, D. (1946). *Wechsler Memory Scale form II.* San Antonio, TX: The Psychological Corporation.

Strauss, E., Sherman, E. M., & Spreen, O. (2006). *A compendium of neuropsychological tests: Administration, norms, and commentary.* New York: Oxford University Press.

Thiruselvam, I., Vogt, E. M., & Hoelzle, J. B. (2015). The interchangeability of CVLT-II and WMS-IV Verbal Paired Associates scores: A slightly different story. *Archives of Clinical Neuropsychology, 30*(3), 248–255.

Travis, S. G., Huang, Y., Fujiwara, E., Radomski, A., Olsen, F., Carter, R., . . . Malykhin, N. V. (2014). High field structural MRI reveals specific episodic memory correlates in the subfields of the hippocampus. *Neuropsychologia, 53,* 233–245.

Umfleet, L. G., Ryan, J. J., Morris, J., & Pliskin, N. (2013). Comparison of nondominant and dominant hand performances on the Wechsler Memory Scale–Fourth Edition Visual Reproduction subtest copy and memory components. *Journal of Clinical and Experimental Neuropsychology, 35*(5), 480–488.

Wang, C., Li, Y., Yang, J., Su, L., Geng, Y., Li, H., . . . Mu, J. (2013). A randomized controlled trial of olanzapine improving memory deficits in Han Chinese patients with first-episode schizophrenia. *Schizophrenia Research, 144*(1-3), 129–135.

Wechsler, D. (1945). A standardized memory scale for clinical use. *Journal of Psychology, 19,* 87–95.

Wechsler, D. (1987). *Wechsler Memory Scale-Revised.* San Antonio, TX: The Psychological Corporation.

Wechsler D. (2009). *Wechsler Memory Scale–Fourth Edition.* San Antonio, TX: Psychological Corporation.

11 | LANGUAGE

BOSTON DIAGNOSTIC APHASIA EXAMINATION THIRD EDITION (BDAE-3)

TEST NAME	**Boston Diagnostic Aphasia Examination Third Edition (BDAE-3)**
DOMAIN	Language
AGE RANGE	18 to 79 years
ADMINISTRATION TIME	90 minutes
SCORING FORMAT	Hand scored
REFERENCE	Goodglass, H., Kaplan, E., & Barresi, B. (2001b). *Boston Diagnostic Aphasia Examination* (3rd ed.). Philadelphia: Lippincott Williams & Wilkins.

DESCRIPTION

The Boston Diagnostic Aphasia Examination (BDAE) is a battery of tests designed to meet three goals: to enable diagnosis of aphasia syndromes, to measure the breadth and severity of aphasic disturbance, and to provide a comprehensive assessment of language to guide therapy (Goodglass et al., 2001a). The BDAE was initially published by Goodglass and Kaplan in 1972; it was revised in 1983 (Goodglass & Kaplan, 1983b) and again in 2001 (third edition, BDAE-3; Goodglass et al., 2001a, 2001b).

The third edition was substantially revised. Changes from the previous edition include the addition of abbreviated and expanded testing formats, the incorporation of the Boston Naming Test (BNT; Kaplan et al., 1983) as a subtest, the addition of a Language Competence Index, and clarification of scoring procedures and definitions. The revision was also designed to integrate neurolinguistics research, including methods to assess narrative and discourse complexity, category-specific dissociations in lexical production/comprehension, syntax comprehension, and analysis of grapheme-phoneme conversion during reading. However, the ultimate goal of the authors in developing the test was clinical utility (Goodglass et al., 2001a). The authors note that, like all methods for evaluating aphasia, the test has limitations. For instance, the score profile does not automatically produce a diagnosis, nor does it indicate the most suitable therapy. Examiners should use the test as a framework for sampling language performance and should feel free to build on this framework to further explore the examinee's abilities (Goodglass et al., 2001a).

The BDAE-3 includes more than 50 subtests and can be administered in three different formats: Standard, Short, and Extended. The Standard format is most closely related to earlier versions of the BDAE. The Short Form of the test provides "a brief, no-frills assessment," whereas the Extended version offers a fuller neurolinguistic assessment that includes evaluation of free narrative, processing of word categories, syntax comprehension, and reading/writing (Goodglass et al., 2001a). The BDAE-3 allows both a quantitative and a qualitative evaluation of language. For example, although several scores are based on pass/fail criteria, rating scales allow a qualitative evaluation of language aspects such as speech melody, fluency, anomia, syntactic organization, and paraphasia types.

Like earlier versions, the standard BDAE-3 is divided into five language-related sections and an additional section on praxis. The five language domains include conversational and expository speech, auditory comprehension, oral expression, reading, and writing. These are assessed by a number of different subtests, which are shown in Table 11–1, along with the specific subtests from the Standard and Extended Battery. In addition to individual subtest scores, the test also provides three main scoring methods (see the section "Scoring"): the Severity Rating Scale (a rating of the severity of observed language/speech disturbance), the Rating Scale Profile of Speech

TABLE 11–1 Boston Diagnostic Aphasia Exam Third Edition (BDAE-3) Domains and Subtests for the Standard and Extended Battery

DOMAIN	STANDARD BATTERY	EXTENDED BATTERY
Conversational and Expository Speech	Simple Social Responses[a] Free Conversation[a] Picture Description (Cookie Theft)[a]	Aesop's Fables[a]
Auditory Comprehension	Basic Word Discrimination Commands Complex Ideational Material	Word Comprehension by Categories—Tools/Implements Word Comprehension by Categories—Foods Word Comprehension by Categories—Animals Word Comprehension by Categories—Body Parts Word Comprehension by Categories—Comprehension Word Comprehension by Categories—Map Locations Semantic Probe Syntactic Processing—Touch A with B Reversible Possessives Embedded Sentences
Oral Expression	Nonverbal Agility Verbal Agility Automatized Sequences Recitation Melody Rhythm Single Word Repetition Repetition of Sentences Responsive Naming Boston Naming Test Screening for Naming of Special Categories (Letters, Numbers, Colors)	Repetition of Nonsense Words Naming in Categories—Colors Naming in Categories—Actions Naming in Categories—Animals Naming in Categories—Tools/Implements
Reading	Matching Across Cases and Scripts[b] Number Matching (three subtasks) Picture-Word Match Lexical Decision[b] Homophone Matching[b] Free Grammatical Morphemes[b] Basic Oral Word Reading Oral Reading of Sentences with Comprehension Reading Comprehension—Sentences and Paragraphs	Advanced Phonic Analysis—Pseudohomophone Matching Bound Grammatical Morphemes Derivational Morphemes Oral Reading of Special Word Lists—Mixed Morphological Types Oral Reading of Special Word Lists—Semantic Paralexia Prone Words
Writing	Mechanics of Writing Primer Word Vocabulary Regular Phonics Common Irregular Forms Written Picture Naming (Objects, Actions, Animals) Narrative Writing (Cookie Theft)[b]	Uncommon Irregularities Oral Spelling Nonsense Words Cognitive/Grammatical Influences—Part of Speech (Functors, Derivational Affixes, Verb Forms) Loaded Sentences
Praxis	—	Natural Gestures Conventional Gestures Use of Pretended Objects Bucco-Facial Respiratory Movements

NOTE: Extended subtests are administered in addition to Standard subtests.

[a] Provide basis for the Severity Rating and the Profile of Speech Characteristics.

[b] Includes an extended testing option.

SOURCE: Adapted from Goodglass et al. (2001a).

Characteristics (a rating of observed speech characteristics and of scores in two main language domains), and the Language Competency Index (a composite score of language performance on BDAE-3 subtests).

The extended version of the BDAE-3 includes a sixth section, "Praxis," which examines natural and conventional gestures, use of pretended objects, and buccofacial and respiratory movements (Table 11–1).

Supplementary nonlanguage tests (previously called the *Boston Parietal Lobe Battery* but now referred to as the *Spatial-Quantitative Battery*) were included as a separate adjunct in earlier versions of the BDAE and remain an option for the BDAE-3 (Table 11–2).

The BDAE-3 has also been adapted into other languages including Greek (Tsapkini et al., 2009) and Spanish (Pineda et al., 2000).

TABLE 11–2 The Spatial-Quantitative Battery

Constructional Deficits	Drawing To Command Stick Construction Memory Three-Dimensional Blocks
Finger Agnosia	Verbal: Comprehension Visual: Finger Naming Verbal-Visual: Paired-Finger Identification Visual-Visual: Matching Two Finger Positions Tactile-Visual
Acalculia	Arithmetic Clock Setting
Right-Left Orientation	Double-Other Person Double-Own Body Single-Other Person Single-Self

SOURCE: Adapted from Goodglass et al. (2001a).

ADMINISTRATION

See the manual. The 44-page test booklet serves as the guide for administration. Subtests appear in the same order in the booklet and in the stimulus card book. Short Form items are presented in bold typeface, and Extended Form items appear in italics. The abbreviated administration can also be given using a separate Short Form test booklet. For the Standard administration, all the Short Form items in boldface are administered, in addition to items in regular typeface.

SCORING

See the manual. Scoring instructions are provided in the manual and answer booklet. The profile summary automatically translates raw scores into percentile ranks. The Score Summary Sheet provides a visual profile of performance across all the BDAE-3 subtests grouped by domain.

The Severity Rating Scale (p. 9 of the test booklet) is designed to provide an estimate of the severity of impairment; this need not be specific to aphasia but can also include other speech disorders, such as dysarthria. The rating ranges from 0 (neither useful comprehension nor speech output is possible) to 5 (normal comprehension and speech output).

The Rating Scale Profile of Speech Characteristics is a profile form that includes aspects of speech that are not easily objectively quantified: articulatory agility, phrase length, grammatical facility, melodic line (prosody), and extent of word-finding difficulties. Each dimension is rated on a seven-point scale by the examiner. In addition, the profile includes mean percentile scores from two objective domains considered crucial to diagnostic differentiation (Sentence Repetition and Auditory Comprehension). At the bottom of the profile, the examiner may also provide ratings for rate, volume, and voice quality.

The Language Competency Index provides a percentile-based global measure of aphasia severity based on a combination of fluency, auditory comprehension, and naming subtest scores (according to the authors, reading and writing performance are not included because they can be disproportionally affected compared with spoken language). The formula for calculating this index is presented on the last page of the test booklet and is computed as shown in Figure 11–1.

Language Competence Index: (*Expression Component* + *Auditory Comprehension Component*)/2

Expression Component **= mean of percentiles for two expression subtests (Boston Naming Test and Grammatical Form rating from the Severity Rating)**

Auditory Comprehension Component **= mean of the percentiles for three auditory comprehension subtests (Word Discrimination, Commands, and Complex Ideational Material)**

Figure 11–1 Computation of language competency index for the Boston Diagnostic Aphasia Exam (BDAE-3).

DEMOGRAPHIC EFFECTS

AGE

The influence of age is controversial. Some authors (Heaton et al., 2004) have found little impact of age on performance, whereas others have reported that age affects performance on at least some of the BDAE and Parietal Lobe Battery tasks (Farver & Farver, 1982; Pineda et al., 2000; Radanovic & Mansur, 2002; Rosselli et al., 1990; Tsapkini et al., 2009). The younger the participants, the better the performance.

GENDER

The influence of gender appears to be small (Pineda et al., 2000; Rosselli et al., 1990) or nonexistent on the BDAE (Heaton et al., 2004; Radamovic & Mansur, 2002; Tsapkini et al., 2009) and on the Parietal Lobe Battery (Farver & Farver, 1982). For example, gender explained 0% unique variance on all subtests except the writing subtest (2%) in Tsapkini et al.'s (2009) healthy Greek sample.

EDUCATION

Education has a stronger effect on test scores, with lower academic achievement associated with lower scores, but the effect varies across subtests and studies (Jacobs et al., 1997; Pineda et al., 2000; Radanovic & Mansur, 2002; Rosselli et al., 1990; Tsapkini et al., 2009). For example, Heaton et al. (2004) examined the Complex Ideational subtest in 326 healthy individuals and found that only 7% of the variance in test scores was accounted for by education. Pineda et al. (2000) examined 156 individuals, aged 19 to 60 years in Colombia and noted that education was a low (<15%) to modest (>17%) predictor of variance in BDAE scores. Tsapkini et al. (2009) gave the Greek adaptation of the BDAE Short Form to 129 community-dwelling adults aged

18 to 81 years and reported that education has the most effect across all subtests and accounted for a minimum of 8% (auditory comprehension subtest) to 50% (writing subtest) of unique variance.

ETHNICITY, NATIONALITY, AND LINGUISTIC EFFECTS

Pineda et al. (2000) found that occupational status and socioeconomic status were low but significant predictors of performance on some subtests (Comprehension of Commands, Body-Part Naming).

For most expressive subtests of the BDAE, there are no significant differences in scores obtained by upper- and middle-status African-American and Caucasian adults (Molrine & Pierce, 2002). Ethnicity, however, can affect performance. Jacobs et al. (1997) compared the performance of English- and Spanish-speaking older adults (matched for age and education) on two of the tasks of the BDAE (repetition of high frequency phrases and an abbreviated version of the Complex Ideational Material subtest). Spanish speakers obtained lower scores on the auditory comprehension task. Level of acculturation was an important determinant of test performance because examinees tested in Spanish who reported that they could speak English well did not differ from participants tested in English.

NORMATIVE DATA

STANDARDIZATION SAMPLE

Unlike norms for previous test versions, which originated from inpatient data accumulated over time at the Boston Veterans Administration Medical Center, the patients with aphasia for the BDAE-3 were referred concurrently by field examiners at different testing sites; they also represented a wider range of severity because they came from inpatient, outpatient, and private practice sources. The normative data are therefore less skewed toward severely impaired patients compared with previous editions of the test; specifically, they are evenly distributed across severity ratings on the Aphasia Severity Rating Scale. As a result, a given BDAE-3 score corresponds to a lower percentile than it would have in previous editions. Tables to convert 1983 edition scores to 1999 scores are provided in the manual.

The test manual provides means and standard deviations (*SD*) for the BDAE-3 subtests for patients with aphasia. The number of patients varies from a maximum of 85 to a low of 31, depending on the subtest. Means are also provided for 15 healthy adults. In most cases, healthy adults, on average, failed less than one item per subtest. One exception was the "Touch A with B" subtest, on which one healthy individual failed more than half of the items.

Normative data for the Spatial-Quantitative Battery are provided in the manual based on data collected by Borod et al. (1980) on 147 neurologically healthy men (aged 25 to 85 years, education ranging from <8 years to college-level). These are provided because ceiling scores are not necessarily obtained for healthy individuals on these subtests, as is the case for the language subtests of the BDAE-3.

OTHER NORMATIVE DATA

Norms for the Complex Ideational Material subtest are provided by Heaton et al. (2004) for individuals aged 20 to 85 years. They are based on a sample of 326 Caucasian individuals with a mean (*M*) age of 52.0 years (*SD* = 18.6). Pineda et al. (2000) provide normative data, broken down by age (19–35 and 36–50 years) and education (1–9, 10–15, and >16 years) on the Spanish version of the BDAE (Goodglass & Kaplan, 1986), based on a sample of 156 healthy participants living in Medellin, Colombia. These are reproduced in Table 11–3. Norms for Spanish-speaking individuals are also provide by Rosselli et al. (1990). Tsapkini et al. (2009) provide normative data on the Greek adaptation of the BDAE Short Form based on 129 community-dwelling healthy adults aged 18 to 81 years from a large metropolitan area in Northern Greece, broken down by age and education, but note small *Ns* (Tables 11–4 and 11–5).

Norms (means but no *SDs*) for the Parietal Lobe Battery in older adults (aged 40 to 89 years) are presented by Farver and Farver (1982).

EVIDENCE FOR RELIABILITY

EVIDENCE FOR INTERNAL RELIABILITY

Although reliability coefficients are for the most part acceptable to high, there is variability across subtests (Goodglass et al., 2001a). For example, alpha coefficients presented in the manual range from very high for Sentence Repetition and the Boston Naming Test (>.95) to low for Auditory Comprehension—Foods—Extended and Reading—Picture-Word Match (<.65). No information is provided on the internal consistency of the rating scores, language competency index, praxis assessment, or Spatial-Quantitative Battery.

EVIDENCE FOR TEST-RETEST RELIABILITY, MEASURING CHANGE, AND PRACTICE EFFECTS

Stability coefficients are not presented in the manual. The authors state that repeatability varies among aphasics to a greater degree than among other populations, but that once recovery has stabilized, retest performance should fairly closely approximate baseline performance. No data are provided to support these claims. No stability information is provided for the ratings, language competency index, praxis assessment, or Spatial-Quantitative Battery.

TABLE 11–3 Age- and Education-Corrected Normative Data (Mean and *SD*) for the Boston Diagnostic Aphasia Exam (BDAE)—Spanish Version

	AGE 19–35 YEARS			AGE 36–50 YEARS		
	EDUCATION			EDUCATION		
	1–9	10–15	>16	1–9	10–15	>16
Word Discrimination	70.1 (2.0)	70.7 (2.5)	71.1 (1.9)	68.9 (3.8)	71.1 (1.3)	71.4 (1.3)
Body-Part Identification	18.1 (1.5)	18.6 (1.5)	19.3 (1.2)	18.4 (1.3)	19.0 (0.9)	19.3 (1.7)
Commands	14.0 (1.1)	14.5 (1.0)	14.3 (1.0)	14.0 (1.4)	14.6 (1.0)	14.6 (0.7)
Complex Ideational Material	8.3 (2.3)	8.9 (1.4)	9.2 (1.5)	7.9 (2.0)	9.4 (1.4)	9.5 (1.7)
Automatic Speech						
Automated Sentences	13.8 (0.7)	13.8 (0.4)	13.8 (0.4)	13.0 (1.5)	13.8 (0.6)	13.8 (0.8)
Singing and Rhyming	1.8 (0.7)	1.9 (0.3)	1.9 (0.4)	1.8 (0.6)	1.9 (0.5)	1.8 (0.6)
Repetition						
Words	10.0 (0)	9.9 (0.2)	10.0 (0)	10.0 (0)	10.0 (0)	30.0 (0)
High Probability	7.6 (0.7)	7.9 (0.4)	8.0 (0)	7.5 (0.9)	7.9 (0.3)	7.9 (0.3)
Low Probability	7.7 (0.7)	9.9 (0.3)	8.0 (0)	7.6 (0.5)	7.9 (0.4)	7.9 (0.4)
Oral Reading						
Words	28.2 (5.0)	30.0 (0)	30.0 (0)	29.9 (0.4)	30.0 (0)	30.0 (0)
Oral Sentences	8.8 (3.0)	10.0 (0)	9.9 (0.2)	10.0 (0)	10.0 (0)	9.9 (0.2)
Naming						
Responsive Naming	27.8 (6.0)	29.9 (0.4)	29.1 (4.2)	30.0 (0)	29.2 (3.8)	29.9 (0.6)
Confrontation Naming	93.8 (3.2)	95.7 (0.9)	95.8 (0.7)	91.1 (5.5)	94.7 (3.0)	95.5 (2.3)
Body-Part Naming	26.6 (2.4)	27.1 (2.5)	28.1 (1.9)	26.4 (2.7)	28.0 (2.2)	28.5 (2.2)
Animal Naming	21.3 (6.0)	26.4 (5.8)	29.6 (4.8)	21.0 (4.2)	24.0 (6.9)	28.5 (2.2)
Reading Comprehension						
Symbol Discrimination	8.8 (2.9)	9.9 (0.2)	10.0 (0)	9.4 (1.1)	9.7 (1.0)	9.9 (0.4)
Word Recognition	7.9 (0.3)	7.8 (1.2)	7.9 (0.3)	8.0 (0)	8.0 (0)	7.9 (0.2)
Oral Spelling	5.6 (2.1)	6.6 (1.6)	7.3 (1.1)	5.3 (2.1)	6.5 (1.5)	7.2 (1.0)
Word-Picture Matching	9.9 (0.3)	10.0 (0)	10.0 (0)	10.0 (0)	10.0 (0)	10.0 (0)
Sentences—Paragraphs	8.3 (1.3)	9.4 (0.9)	9.7 (0.5)	9.1 (1.3)	9.6 (0.8)	9.6 (0.5)
Writing						
Mechanics	5.0 (0)	5.0 (0)	4.9 (0.3)	5.0 (0)	4.9 (0.2)	4.9 (0.2)
Serial Writing	44.7 (7.2)	47.2 (1.5)	47.6 (0.9)	42.3 (6.8)	47.8 (1.5)	47.4 (1.2)
Primer-Level Dictation	13.3 (1.1)	13.7 (1.7)	14.0 (0)	13.5 (0.9)	13.9 (0.3)	13.6 (1.9)
Written Confrontation Naming	8.9 (2.6)	9.9 (0.2)	10.0 (0)	9.8 (0.5)	9.9 (0.2)	9.9 (0.4)
Spelling to Dictation	9.2 (2.3)	9.9 (0.2)	9.9 (0.2)	9.4 (1.0)	9.9 (0.3)	9.9 (0.2)
Sentences to Dictation	10.7 (3.6)	12.0 (0)	12.0 (0)	12.0 (0)	12.0 (0)	11.8 (0.7)
Narrative Writing	4.8 (0.7)	4.9 (0.3)	4.9 (0.3)	5.0 (0)	5.0 (0)	4.8 (0.7)

SOURCE: From Pineda et al. (2000).

EVIDENCE FOR RELIABILITY OF SHORT FORMS

For most subtests, correlations between the Short and Standard Forms are very high ($r > .90$; Goodglass et al., 2001a). Two exceptions are the Word Discrimination and Matching Numbers subtests, which have slightly lower correlations between Standard and Short Forms ($r = .77$ and .76, respectively). No information is provided for the ratings, language competency index, praxis assessment, or Spatial-Quantitative Battery.

EVIDENCE FOR INTERRATER RELIABILITY

The reliability of the Speech Characteristics Profile (melodic line, phrase length, articulatory agility, grammatical form, paraphasias, word finding, auditory comprehension) was first examined for the original BDAE, employing three judges who rated the tape-recorded speech samples of 99 patients. The lowest interjudge correlations were .78 and .79 for word-finding difficulties and paraphasias, respectively; the other dimensions had coefficients of at least .85. Other interrater agreement studies have also shown satisfactory results (Davis, 1993; Molrine & Pierce, 2002). In contrast, Gordon (1998) investigated fluency-nonfluency judgments of 24 experienced speech therapists listening to spontaneous speech and sentence repetition of 10 aphasic patients. She found only two-thirds agreement among raters for half of the patients even though the therapists reported that they used such ratings all the time. High variability was also found for individual adults, especially on articulation and paraphasia ratings.

EVIDENCE FOR VALIDITY

RELATIONSHIPS WITH OTHER TESTS

With regard to relations with other measures, Love and Oster (2002) supported the validity of syntactic auditory

TABLE 11–4 Normative Data for Auditory Comprehension (AC) and Oral Expression (OE) Subtests on the Greek Boston Diagnostic Aphasia Exam (BDAE) Short Form Stratified by Age and Education

	AGE 18 TO 39 YEARS EDUCATION (YEARS)						AGE 40 TO 59 YEARS EDUCATION (YEARS)						AGE 60 TO 81 YEARS EDUCATION (YEARS)					
	1 TO 9 (*N* = 0)		10 TO 12 (*N* = 17)		13 TO 21 (*N* = 20)		1 TO 9 (*N* = 8)		10 TO 12 (*N* = 18)		13 TO 21 (*N* = 17)		1 TO 9 (*N* = 17)		10 TO 12 (*N* = 17)		13 TO 21 (*N* = 15)	
%ILE	AC	OE	AC	OE	AC	OE	AC	OE	AC	OE	AC	OE	AC	OE	AC	OE	AC	OE
100			32.0	48.0	32.0	48.0	32.0	48.0	32.0	48.0	32.0	48.0	32.0	46.0	32.0	47.0	32.0	48.0
90	–	–	32.0	48.0	32.0	48.0	32.0	48.0	32.0	48.0	32.0	48.0	32.0	45.0	32.0	47.0	32.0	48.0
80	–	–	32.0	48.0	32.0	48.0	32.0	46.4	32.0	47.2	32.0	47.4	32.0	45.0	32.0	46.4	32.0	47.0
70	–	–	32.0	47.0	32.0	48.0	32.0	46.0	32.0	47.0	32.0	47.0	32.0	44.0	32.0	46.0	32.0	47.0
60	–	–	32.0	47.0	32.0	48.0	32.0	45.4	32.0	46.4	32.0	47.0	31.4	44.0	32.0	46.0	32.0	47.0
50	–	–	32.0	47.0	32.0	48.0	31.8	45.0	32.0	46.0	32.0	46.0	31.0	44.0	32.0	46.0	32.0	47.0
40	–	–	32.0	46.0	32.0	47.0	31.1	45.0	32.0	46.0	32.0	46.0	30.6	44.0	32.0	45.3	32.0	46.0
30	–	–	32.0	46.0	32.0	47.0	30.4	44.7	32.0	46.0	31.5	46.0	30.2	43.0	32.0	45.0	32.0	46.0
20	–	–	30.5	44.6	32.0	47.0	29.8	44.0	31.4	45.0	30.6	44.6	29.0	43.0	32.0	45.0	32.0	46.0
10	–	–	28.4	45.6	31.0	47.0	29.0	44.0	30.5	44.0	29.9	42.8	28.5	42.0	31.5	45.0	32.0	45.0
M	–	–	31.2	46.3	31.9	47.5	31.1	45.4	31.7	46.2	31.5	46.1	30.1	43.9	31.1	45.8	32.0	46.5
SD	–	–	2.0	1.2	0.3	0.76	1.6	1.3	0.6	1.2	0.85	1.7	1.3	1.1	0.2	0.75	0.0	0.9

SOURCE: From Tsapkini et al. (2009).

comprehension by examining correlations with a specific test assessing syntactic complexity (subject-relative, object-relative, active, and passive [SOAP]). However, a relationship between syntax comprehension and working memory/executive functioning has also been suggested (Giovannetti et al., 2008). Specifically, moderate correlations are reported between the Syntax subtest and Wechsler Memory Scale (WMS) Mental Control and FAS whereas low correlation is found with the Philadelphia (Repeatable) Verbal Learning Test (PrVLT; r = .39, .44, and –.27, respectively). When all neuropsychological measures (Mini-Mental State Examination [MMSE], WMS Mental Control, FAS, BNT, Animal naming, PrVLT) are included in a regression equation to predict Syntax Comprehension performance, only FAS is a significant predictor (Giovannetti et al., 2008).

The BDAE oral apraxia task specifically was related to other articulation tasks in one study (Sussman et al., 1986). Divenyi and Robinson (1989) reported correlations of r = .86 and .93 for the auditory comprehension measure in the BDAE with the Token Test and with the respective part of the Porch Index of Communicative Ability (PICA; Porch, 1971). However, the BDAE auditory comprehension subtest was not an adequate predictor of auditory paragraph comprehension when independent standardized material was used (Brookshire & Nicholas, 1984). With regard to the reading test items, Nicholas et al. (1986) showed that both aphasic and healthy individuals were able

TABLE 11–5 Normative Data for Reading (R) and Writing (WR) Subtests on the Greek Boston Diagnostic Aphasia Exam (BDAE) Short Form Stratified by Age and Education

	AGE 18 TO 39 YEARS EDUCATION (YEARS)						AGE 40 TO 59 YEARS EDUCATION (YEARS)						AGE 60 TO 81 EDUCATION (YEARS)					
	1 TO 9 (*N* = 0)		10 TO 12 (*N* = 17)		13 TO 21 (*N* = 20)		1 TO 9 (*N* = 8)		10 TO 12 (*N* = 18)		13 TO 21 (*N* = 17)		1 TO 9 (*N* = 17)		10 TO 12 (*N* = 17)		13 TO 21 (*N* = 15)	
%ILE	R	WR	R	WR	R	WR	R	WR	R	WR	R	WR	R	WR	R	WR	R	WR
100	–	–	39.0	84.0	39.0	84.0	39.0	84.0	39.0	84.0	39.0	84.0	39.0	83.0	39.0	84.0	39.0	84.0
90	–	–	39.0	84.0	39.0	84.0	39.0	84.0	39.0	84.0	39.0	84.0	39.0	81.4	39.0	84.0	39.0	84.0
80	–	–	39.0	84.0	39.0	84.0	39.0	83.2	39.0	84.0	39.0	84.0	39.0	80.4	39.0	84.0	39.0	84.0
70	–	–	39.0	84.0	39.0	84.0	39.0	82.3	39.0	84.0	39.0	84.0	39.0	79.6	39.0	84.0	39.0	84.0
60	–	–	39.0	84.0	39.0	84.0	38.4	80.2	39.0	84.0	39.0	84.0	39.0	79.0	39.0	84.0	39.0	84.0
50	–	–	39.0	84.0	39.0	84.0	38.0	78.5	39.0	84.0	39.0	84.0	39.0	78.0	39.0	84.0	39.0	84.0
40	–	–	39.0	84.0	39.0	84.0	38.0	77.6	39.0	84.0	39.0	83.2	38.2	75.4	39.0	84.0	39.0	84.0
30	–	–	39.0	83.4	39.0	84.0	37.7	76.7	39.0	84.0	39.0	83.0	38.0	74.4	39.0	83.4	39.0	84.0
20	–	–	39.0	83.0	39.0	84.0	36.8	75.8	39.0	83.0	38.0	83.0	38.0	71.4	39.0	83.0	39.0	84.0
10	–	–	39.0	82.2	39.0	84.0	36.0	75.0	39.0	81.8	38.0	81.0	36.6	68.6	37.8	82.0	39.0	84.0
M	–	–	39.0	83.5	39.0	83.9	38.0	79.3	39.0	83.5	38.8	83.4	38.4	76.4	38.8	83.6	39.0	84.0
SD	–	–	0.0	1.2	0.2	0.5	1.1	3.4	0.0	1.0	0.44	1.0	1.1	4.7	0.5	0.7	0.0	0.0

SOURCE: From Tsapkini et al. (2009).

to answer a similar number of questions about the items without having actually read the passage, suggesting a high passage dependency of this test. This dependency applied not only to the BDAE but also to similar tasks in aphasia batteries such as the Western Aphasia Battery (WAB).

CLINICAL STUDIES

Aphasia. According to Goodglass and Kaplan (1983a), discriminant validity between cases of Broca's, Wernicke's, conduction, and anomic aphasia is optimal if the following tests are entered into the equation: Body-Part Identification, Repetition of High-Probability Sentences, Paraphasia Rating, Word-Finding Rating, Phrase-Length Rating, and Verbal Paraphasias. Li and Williams (1990) showed that, in the Repeating Phrases and Sentences subtest, conduction aphasics showed a greater number of phonemic attempts, word revisions, and word and phrase repetitions; Broca's aphasics showed more phonemic errors and omissions; and Wernicke's aphasics produced more unrelated words and jargon.

It is important to note that decision rules for the "diagnosis" of the individual subtypes are not always clearly defined, although Reinvang and Graves (1975) attempted such clarification. Crary et al. (1992) tried to isolate subtypes of aphasia empirically by means of a Q-type factor analysis for the BDAE and the closely related Western Aphasia Battery (WAB). The resulting seven patient clusters (labeled Broca, anomic, global, Wernicke, conduction, and two unclassified clusters) agreed only poorly (in 38% of 47 patients) using the classification rules of the test itself; the results were even worse for the WAB. The study, although based on a limited number of participants and the use of a somewhat dated cluster-analysis technique, suggested that BDAE classification rules are based on clinical rather than construct validity. Similarly, Naeser and Hayward (1978) and Reinvang (1985) pointed out that scale profiles can aid in the classification but do not firmly classify patients into subtypes of aphasia. The test authors acknowledge that 30–80% of aphasic patients are not classifiable; this is also consistent with the clinical experience that a majority of aphasic patients show mixed rather than pure symptomatology.

Dementia. The sensitivity of earlier versions of the test has been explored in dementia patients. In persons with Alzheimer's disease (AD), Kirshner (1982) found language to be fluent, with normal prosody, syntax, and phrase length; few paraphasias were found, but word-finding problems and poor repetition of low-probability phrases were present. Sentence comprehension, but not letter or word reading, were found to be related to severity of AD (Cummings et al., 1986). Whitworth and Larson (1989) compared 25 AD patients, 25 patients with other dementias, and 58 age-matched controls. They found significant differences compared with controls on all but 4 of 38 BDAE scores (the exceptions were paraphasias, articulation, primer dictation, and word reading). Discriminant function analysis produced correct classification for 95% of the three patient groups. Nineteen test scores contributed to the discrimination of four levels ("stages") of severity of dementia, resulting in correct classification of 100% of 22 patients with dementia. Gorelick et al. (1993) found also that scores on the BDAE Commands and Responsive Naming subtests were lower in 66 patients with multi-infarct dementia, compared with a group of 86 patients who had infarcts without dementia. In a comparison of patients with multi-infarct dementia, AD patients, and healthy controls, Mendez and Ashla-Mendez (1991) found that the unstructured Cookie Theft card description discriminated better between groups than structured tests. In this study, the multi-infarct group produced fewer words per minute and fewer constructional assemblages. In a Greek sample of amnestic mild cognitive impairment (MCI) and mild AD patients, Tsantali et al. (2013) found that verbal fluency, auditory comprehension, reading comprehension, and narrative ability as measured by the Greek adaptation of the BDAE-2 were less affected in amnestic MCI than in mild AD, yielding a classification accuracy of 85%. Patients with AD also performed better than those with vascular dementia (VaD) on the Syntax subtest while no differences were seen in Complex Ideation Material (Giovannetti et al., 2008). Patients with Huntington's disease performed worse than healthy controls on the Comprehension Component, Expression Component, and Language Competency Index; no differences were found on the BNT (Azambuja et al., 2012).

Stroke. The BDAE can also be used to predict burden of stroke in the long run. For example, Doyle et al. (2006) found that BDAE Severity Scale (BDAE SS) obtained at three-months post-stroke was moderately correlated with the Burden of Stroke Scale (BSS) at 12-month post-stroke ($r = -.495$ for Communication Difficulty, $r = .518$ for Communication Distress) among stroke patients with aphasia of mild to moderate severity. In fact, BDAE SS predicted BSS scores over and above depression and social support. By contrast, the Token Test and the PICA (Porch, 1971) were not significant predictors of BSS.

Brain Injury. Using an earlier version of the test, 218 patients with closed head injury showed significantly poorer word fluency skills than healthy individuals. Although their strategies were similar to those used by the healthy examinees, some qualitative differences in semantic associations were found that were related to severity of cognitive disruption (Gruen et al., 1990).

Treatment Studies. Predictive validity has also been examined with earlier BDAE versions. The BDAE appears to predict progress in speech therapy (Helm-Estabrooks et al., 1989). Additionally, Marshall and Neuberger (1994) found that measured pretreatment effort in self-correction (but not success of self-correction) and good auditory comprehension were related to improvement during treatment as measured by the BDAE.

Some authors have examined the utility of the BDAE-3 in assessing language disturbances over telerehabilitation. In comparing face-to-face administration and telerehabilitation administration, Theodoros et al. (2008) did not find any differences in the scores obtained via both modalities. Interrater reliability remained high (r = .89) with telerehabilitation administration. In-depth examination of the subtests administered over telerehabilation compared to face-to-face administration in a sample of individuals with aphasia due to CVA or TBI revealed exact agreement ranging from 30% to 90% and greater than 90% clinical agreement except for melodic line in the mild aphasia group, which was still in the high 80%. There were no differences in scores between the two modalities except on the Naming and Paraphasia clusters as a function of aphasia severity; however, there were good agreements within each aphasia severity levels, suggesting that aphasia severity may affect assessment in these two clusters but that the challenge of telerehabilitation does not impact the accuracy of the assessment (Hill et al., 2009).

NEUROANATOMICAL CORRELATES AND IMAGING STUDIES

Goodglass and Kaplan (1972) based the design of their instrument on the observation that various components of language function may be selectively damaged by central nervous system (CNS) lesions. This selectivity is an indication of the neuroanatomical organization of language, the localization of the lesion causing the observed deficit, and the functional interactions of various parts of the language system. A number of studies have validated this stated purpose (e.g., Naeser & Hayward, 1978; Naeser et al., 1981, 1987).

In explorations of the role of subcortical structures in cognition, greater aphasia severity among chronic stroke patients was associated with fractional anisotropy abnormalities in the posterior arm of the internal capsule, posterior portion of the external capsule, and white matter underlying supramarginal cortex and temporoparietal junction (Rosso et al., 2015). Naming and auditory comprehension were specifically impaired in patients with thalamic lesions, whereas motor-articulatory problems predominated in patients with basal ganglia lesions (Radanovic & Scaff, 2003). Among those with VaD or AD, moderate to severe white matter alteration was associated with lower Syntax scores whereas no differences in Complex Ideation Material scores were found regardless of white matter alteration burden (Giovannetti et al., 2008).

On the Parietal Lobe Battery, impairment is strongest in patients with lesions in both left parietal and frontal areas (Borod et al., 1984). The Spatial-Quantitative tests (formerly called the Parietal Lobe Battery), together with the Wechsler Adult Intelligence Scale (WAIS), were applied to right- and left-handed patients with aphasia: left-handed aphasic patients performed significantly more poorly on both, especially on tasks involving visual-spatial construction, suggesting that, in left-handers, the left hemisphere is typically dominant for tasks usually considered as right-hemisphere specific (Borod et al., 1985).

PERFORMANCE VALIDITY

Use of BDAE Complex Ideational Material as a performance validity indicator was examined by Erdodi et al. (2016) using a sample with neurological (epilepsy) or other conditions (postconcussive disorder, psychiatric, psychogenic nonepileptic seizures) without reported or observed aphasia. All individuals passed the Test of Memory Malingering (TOMM) and a language-based embedded performance validity index (EI-5; interested readers can refer to the Erdodi et al., 2016, article for details about this language-based embedded performance validity index). In this sample, the mean raw score was 10.2 (SD = 1.8, range = 3–12) in which about 8% scored less than a raw score of 8 and 4% scored less than raw score of 7. Psychiatric history contributed to a higher rate of failure on Complex Ideational Material; however, performance on Complex Ideational Material did not differentiate between psychogenic non-epileptic seizures and epilepsy groups. Table 11–6 shows the classification accuracy of Complex Ideational Material as a performance validity test (PVT) against various performance validity indicators based on different cutoff scores. Although sensitivity was low to moderate (ranging from 17% to 40%), specificity was generally greater than 82%. The authors stated that individuals with epilepsy may be at risk of being falsely classified as invalid performers and as such, conservative cutoffs should be applied to these individuals. Poor performance (i.e., raw score ≤9 or ≤8; T score ≤29 or ≤23) on Complex Ideational Material without bona fide aphasia appears useful in identifying invalid performance.

COMMENT

The BDAE is one of the most popular batteries for use in aphasia settings. Studies have also suggested the BDAE's potential for assessing language disturbances via telerehabilitation. However, the test is lengthy (90 minutes), and it is probably more useful for assessments in the context of detailed studies of aphasia and aphasia rehabilitation than as a routine language test. Administration time may be reduced with the use of the BDAE-3 Short Form. The Extended format, in turn, provides an even more extensive examination than the Standard administration. In addition, the BDAE has always included useful directions for observing and recording many specific types of errors (e.g., paraphasias) found in individuals with aphasia, reflecting the Boston Process Approach. This applies to both the Speech Characteristics Profile and the Aphasia Severity Rating Scale, which are central to diagnostic decision making with the BDAE—especially its fluency-nonfluency

TABLE 11-6 Classification Accuracy of Boston Diagnostic Aphasia Exam (BDAE) Complex Ideational Material Raw and T-Score Cutoffs Against Reference Performance Validity Tests

		EI-5				HYPOTHETICAL BASE RATES (%)					
CIM	AUC (95% CI)	SENS (%)	SPEC (%)	+LR	–LR		10	20	30	40	50
Raw score ≤ 9	.72 (.60 to .83)	39	85	2.6	.72	PPP (%)	22	39	52	63	72
						NPP (%)	93	85	76	67	58
Raw score ≤ 8		18	92	2.4	.88	PPP (%)	20	36	49	60	69
						NPP (%)	91	82	72	63	53
T score ≤ 29	.66 (.54 to .78)	37	85	2.4	.75	PPP (%)	22	38	51	62	71
						NPP (%)	92	84	76	67	57
T score ≤ 23		18	90	1.8	.91	PPP (%)	17	31	44	55	64
						NPP (%)	91	81	72	62	52
		TOMM									
Raw score ≤ 9	66 (.53 to .76)	40	82	2.2	.74	PPP (%)	20	36	49	60	69
						NPP (%)	93	85	76	67	58
Raw score ≤ 8		17	95	3.2	.88	PPP (%)	27	46	59	69	77
						NPP (%)	91	82	73	63	53
T score ≤ 29	.62 (.60 to .82)	37	82	2.0	.78	PPP (%)	19	34	47	58	67
						NPP (%)	92	84	75	66	57
T score ≤ 23		20	92	2.5	.87	PPP (%)	22	39	52	63	71
						NPP (%)	91	82	73	63	54

NOTE: CIM, Complex Ideational Material; SENS, sensitivity; SPEC, Specificity; NPP, negative predictive power; PPP, positive predictive power. Classification accuracy against the Suhr & Boyer (1999) equation and King et al. (2002) equation is available in Erdodi et al. (2016).

SOURCE: From Erodi et al. (2016).

dimension. More detailed diagnoses may incorporate corroborative information from the profile sheet delineating subtest performances. The test manual provides profiles for classic and rarer aphasic subtypes. Note, however, that despite the term "diagnostic" in the title of the test, the classification of aphasia subtypes has so far shown only limited success, mostly because aphasic disorders are typically of a mixed rather than a pure type.

The detailed examination of conversational and expository speech has always been an important and relatively unique aspect of the BDAE; the BDAE-3 offers an even more extensive procedure for this assessment than earlier versions of the test. With its wealth of subtests, the BDAE-3 allows examiners to assess a wide variety of types of language disorders, including very specific deficits, with a great deal of flexibility. The use of short subtests comprised of few items makes it ideal for assessing deficits in the acute phase such as after cerebrovascular accident or acute brain injury and in low-functioning patients such as those with dementia, particularly when the Short Form is used. In addition, low scores on the Complex Ideation Material subtest are exceedingly rare and may be useful as an embedded performance validity indicator when assessing those without reported or observed aphasia, although more research is needed to validate proposed cutoffs.

Nevertheless, the test suffers from a number of significant limitations. The aphasic sample on which percentiles are based is not well described, particularly with regard to basic demographic information such as age, gender, and education. The same can be said for the very small healthy sample ($N = 15$). This is a major limitation, given that educational and ethnicity/acculturation effects were reported for previous editions, with a risk of overdiagnosis of impairment in individuals with low education. Users who assess Spanish-speaking or Greek-speaking individuals may want to employ other versions such as the BDAE-Spanish Version (Goodglass & Kaplan, 1986) or the Greek adaptation BDAE Short Form, with the age- and education-corrected norms shown in Tables 11–3 to 11–5.

Although this revision has been published for more than a decade, to our knowledge, no reliability information is available for the Praxis or Spatial-Quantitative subtests or for the Language Competency Index. Furthermore, the manual does not include any information on test-retest reliabilities of any of its scores, despite the test's obvious potential in tracking language disorders over time. Additionally, some studies have documented limited interrater reliability. Finally, much of the existing research on the BDAE is based on previous editions of the tests. Studies evaluating the validity and clinical utility of this version are needed.

REFERENCES

Azambuja, M. J., Radanovic, M., Haddad, M. S., Adda, C. C., Barbosa, E. R., & Mansur, L. L. (2012). Language impairment in Huntington's disease. *Arquivos de Neuro-Psiquiatria, 70*(6), 410–415.

Borod, J. C., Carper, M., Goodglass, H., & Naeser, M. (1984). Aphasic performance on a battery of constructional, visuo-spatial, and qualitative tasks: Factorial structure and CT scan localization. *Journal of Clinical Neuropsychology, 6*, 189–204.

Borod, J. C., Carper, M., & Naeser, M. (1985). Left-handed and right-handed aphasics with left hemisphere lesions compared on non-verbal performance measures. *Cortex, 21*, 81–90.

Borod, J. C., Goodglass, H., & Kaplan, E. (1980). Normative data on the Boston Diagnostic Aphasia Examination, Parietal Lobe Battery, and the Boston Naming Test. *Journal of Clinical Neuropsychology, 2*, 209–215.

Brookshire, R. H., & Nicholas, L. E. (1984). Comprehension of directly and indirectly stated main ideas and details in discourse by brain-damaged and non-brain-damaged listeners. *Brain and Language, 21*, 21–36.

Crary, M. A., Wertz, R. T., & Deal, J. L. (1992). Classifying aphasias: Cluster analysis of Western Aphasia Battery and Boston Diagnostic Aphasia Examination. *Aphasiology, 6*, 29–36.

Cummings, J. L., Houlihan, J. P., & Hill, M. A. (1986). The pattern of reading deterioration in dementia of the Alzheimer type: Observations and implications. *Brain and Language, 29*, 315–323.

Davis, A. G. (1993). *A Survey of Adult Aphasia* (2nd ed.). Englewood Cliffs, NJ: Prentice-Hall.

Divenyl, P. L., & Robinson, A. J. (1989). Nonlinguistic auditory capabilities in aphasia. *Brain and Language, 37*, 290–326.

Doyle, P. J., Matthews, C., Mikolic, J. M., Hula, W., & McNeil, M. R. (2006). Do measures of language impairment predict patient-reported communication difficulty and distress as measured by the burden of stroke scale (BOSS)? *Aphasiology, 20*(2-4), 349–361.

Erdodi, L. A., Tyson, B. T., Abeare, C. A., Lichtenstein, J. D., Pelletier, C. L., Rai, J. K., & Roth, R. M. (2016). The BDAE Complex Ideational Material—A measure of receptive language or performance validity? *Psychological Injury and Law, 9*(2), 112–120.

Farver, P. F., & Farver, T. B. (1982). Performance of normal older adults on tests designed to measure parietal lobe function (constructional apraxia, Gerstmann syndrome, visuospatial organization). *American Journal of Occupational Therapy, 36*, 444–449.

Giovannetti, T., Hopkins, M. W., Crawford, J., Bettcher, B. M., Schmidt, K. S., & Libon, D. J. (2008). Syntactic comprehension deficits are associated with MRI white matter alterations in dementia. *Journal of the International Neuropsychological Society, 14*(4), 542–551.

Goodglass, H., & Kaplan, E. (1972). *Boston Diagnostic Aphasia Examination (BDAE)*. Philadelphia: Lea & Febiger.

Goodglass, H., & Kaplan, E. (1983a). *The assessment of aphasia and related disorders* (2nd ed.). Philadelphia: Lea & Febiger.

Goodglass, H., & Kaplan, E. (1983b). *Boston Diagnostic Aphasia Examination (BDAE)*. Philadelphia: Lea & Febiger.

Goodglass, H., & Kaplan, E. (1986). *La Evaluacion de la Afasia y de Transfornos Relacionados* (2nd ed.). Madrid: Editorial Medica Panamericana.

Goodglass, H., Kaplan, E., & Barresi, B. (2001a). *The assessment of aphasia and related disorders* (3rd ed.). Philadelphia: Lippincott Williams & Wilkins.

Goodglass, H., Kaplan, E., & Barresi, B. (2001b). *Boston Diagnostic Aphasia Examination* (3rd ed.). Philadelphia: Lippincott Williams & Wilkins.

Gordon, J. K. (1998). The fluency dimension in aphasia. *Aphasiology, 12*, 673–688.

Gorelick, P. B., Brody, J., Cohen, D., & Freels, S. (1993). Risk factors for dementia associated with multiple cerebral infarcts: A case-control analysis in predominantly African American hospital-based patients. *Archives of Neurology, 50*, 714–720.

Gruen, A. K., Frankle, B. C., & Schwartz, R. (1990). Word fluency generation skills of head-injured patients in an acute trauma center. *Journal of Communication Disorders, 23*, 163–170.

Heaton, R. K., Miller, S. W., Taylor, M. J., & Grant, I. (2004). *Revised comprehensive norms for an expanded Halstead-Reitan Battery: Demographically adjusted neuropsychological norms for African American and Caucasian adults.* Lutz, FL: PAR.

Helm-Estabrooks, N., Ramsberger, G., Morgan, A. R., & Nicholas, M. (1989). *BASA: Boston Assessment of Severe Aphasia.* Chicago: Riverside Publishing Company.

Hill, A. J., Theodoros, D. G., Russell, T. G., Ward, E. C., & Wootton, R. (2009). The effects of aphasia severity on the ability to assess language disorders via telerehabilitation. *Aphasiology, 23*(5), 627–642.

Jacobs, D. M., Sano, M., Albert, S., & Schofield, P. (1997). Cross-cultural neuropsychological assessment: A comparison of randomly selected demographically matched cohorts of English- and Spanish-speaking older adults. *Journal of Clinical and Experimental Neuropsychology, 19*, 331–339.

Kaplan, E., Goodglass, H., & Weintraub, S. (1983). *The Boston Naming Test.* Philadelphia: Lea & Febiger.

Kirshner, H. S. (1982). Language disorders in dementia. In F. Freeman & H. S. Kirshner (Eds.), *Neurolinguistics: Vol. 12. Neurology of Aphasia* (pp. 187–196). Amsterdam: Swets & Zeitlinger.

Li, E. C., & Williams, S. E. (1990). Repetition deficits in three aphasic syndromes. *Journal of Communication Disorders, 23*, 77–88.

Love, T., & Oster, E. (2002). On the categorization of aphasic typologies: The SOAP (a test of syntactic complexity). *Journal of Psycholinguistic Research, 31*, 503–529.

Marshall, R. C., & Neuburger, S. I. (1994). Verbal self-correction and improvement in treated aphasia clients. *Aphasiology, 8*, 535–547.

Mendez, M. F., & Ashla-Mendez, M. (1991). Differences between multi-infarct dementia and Alzheimer's disease on unstructured neuropsychological tasks. *Journal of Clinical and Experimental Neuropsychology, 13*, 923–932.

Molrine, C. J., & Pierce, R. S. (2002). Black and White adults' expressive language in three tests of aphasia. *Journal of Speech-Language Pathology, 11*, 139–150.

Naeser, M. A., & Hayward, R. W. (1978). Lesion localization in aphasia with cranial computed tomography and the Boston Diagnostic Aphasia Exam. *Neurology, 28*, 545–551.

Naeser, M. A., Hayward, R. W., Laughlin, S. A., & Zatz, L. M. (1981). Quantitative CT scan studies in aphasia 1: Infarct size and CT numbers. *Brain and Language, 12*, 140–164.

Naeser, M. A., Mazurski, P., Goodglass, H., & Peraino, M. (1987). Auditory syntactic comprehension in nine aphasia groups (with CT scans) and children: Differences in degree but not order of difficulty observed. *Cortex, 23*, 359–380.

Nicholas, L. E., MacLennan, D. L., & Brookshire, R. H. (1986). Validity of multiple-sentence reading comprehension tests for aphasic adults. *Journal of Speech and Hearing Disorders, 51*, 83–87.

Pineda, D. A., Rosselli, M., Ardila, A., Mejia, S. E., Romero, M. G., & Perez, C. (2000). The Boston Diagnostic Aphasia Examination-Spanish version: The influence of demographic variables. *Journal of the International Neuropsychological Society, 6*, 802–814.

Porch, B. (1971). *The Porch index of communicative ability. Vol. 2: Administration and scoring.* Palo Alto, CA: Consulting Psychologists Press.

Radanovic, M., & Mansur, L. L. (2002). Performance of a Brazilian population sample on the Boston Diagnostic Aphasia Examination: A pilot study. *Brazilian Journal of Medical and Biological Research, 35*, 305–317.

Radanovic, M., & Scaff, M. (2003). Speech and language disturbances due to subcortical lesions. *Brain and Language, 84*, 337–352.

Reinvang, I. (1985). *Aphasia and brain organization.* New York: Plenum Press.

Reinvang, I., & Graves, R. (1975). A basic aphasia examination: Description with discussion of first results. *Scandinavian Journal of Rehabilitation Medicine, 7*, 129–135.

Rosselli, M., Ardila, A., Florez, A., & Castro, C. (1990). Normative data on the Boston Diagnostic Aphasia Evaluation in a Spanish-speaking population. *Journal of Clinical and Experimental Neuropsychology, 12*, 313–322.

Rosso, C., Vargas, P., Valabregue, R., Arbizu, C., Henry-Amar, F., Leger, A., . . . Samson, Y. (2015). Aphasia severity in chronic stroke patients: A combined disconnection in the dorsal and ventral language pathways. *Neurorehabilitation and Neural Repair, 29*(3), 287–295.

Suhr, J. A., & Boyer, D. (1999). Use of the Wisconsin card sorting test in the detection of malingering in student simulator and patient samples. *Journal of Clinical and Experimental Psychology, 21*(5), 701–708.

Sussman, H., Marquardt, T., Hutchinson, J., & MacNeilage, P. (1986). Compensatory articulation in Broca's aphasia. *Brain and Language, 27*, 56–74.

Theodoros, D., Hill, A., Russell, T., Ward, E., & Wootton, R. (2008). Assessing acquired language disorders in adults via the internet. *Telemedicine and e-Health, 14*(6), 552–559.

Tsantali, E., Economidis, D., & Tsolaki, M. (2013). Could language deficits really differentiate mild cognitive impairment (MCI) from mild Alzheimer's disease? *Archives of Gerontology and Geriatrics, 57*(3), 263–270.

Tsapkini, K., Vlahou, C. H., & Potagas, C. (2009). Adaptation and validation of standardized aphasia tests in different languages: Lessons from the Boston Diagnostic Aphasia Examination—Short form in Greek. *Behavioural Neurology, 22*(3-4), 111–119.

Whitworth, R. H., & Larson, C. M. (1989). Differential diagnosis and staging of Alzheimer's disease with an aphasia battery. *Neuropsychiatry, Neuropsychology, and Behavioral Neurology, 1*, 255–265.

BOSTON NAMING TEST, SECOND EDITION (BNT-2)

TEST NAME	**Boston Naming Test, Second Edition (BNT-2)**
DOMAIN	Language
AGE RANGE	In adults, to 95 years
ADMINISTRATION TIME	10 to 20 minutes
SCORING FORMAT	Hand scored
REFERENCE	Kaplan, E. F., Goodglass, H., & Weintraub, S. (2001). *The Boston Naming Test, Second Edition*. Philadelphia: Lippincott Williams & Wilkins.

DESCRIPTION

The purpose of the Boston Naming Test, Second Edition (BNT-2) is to assess visual naming using line drawings of common objects. This popular test, originally published by Kaplan et al. (1978) as an experimental version with 85 items, was revised to a 60-item test (Kaplan et al., 1983). The current version (BNT-2) retains the same 60 items and includes a short 15-item version as well as a multiple-choice version (see later discussion).

The stimuli for the BNT-2 are line drawings of objects with increasing difficulty, ranging from simple, high-frequency vocabulary words (e.g., *comb*) to more difficult words (see Figure 11–2).The BNT-2 and its short forms have been used with various populations and languages including Chinese (Cheung & Chan, 2004; Tsang & Lee, 2003), Italian (Riva et al., 2000), Jamaican (Unverzagt et al., 1999), Dutch (Marien et al., 1998; Storms et al., 2004), Greek (Patricacou et al., 2007), Korean (Kim & Na, 1999), Brazilian Portuguese (Miotto et al., 2010), Spanish (Casals-Coll et al., 2014; Olabarrieta-Landa et al., 2015; Pena-Casanova et al., 2009; Silvestre et al., 2017), and French Canadian (Morrison et al., 1996; Roberts et al., 2002). A 30-item adaptation is available for Spanish-speaking people in the United States (Ponton et al., 1996). See the section "Administration" for specific short-form items.

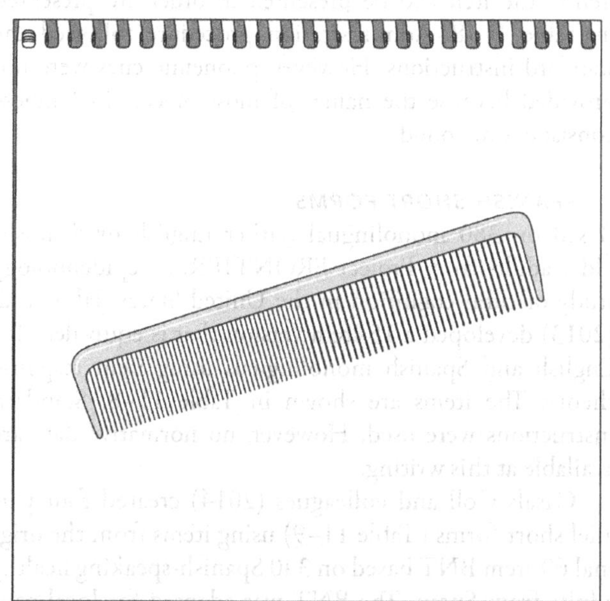

Figure 11–2 *Example of Boston Naming Test (BNT-2) item.* Boston Diagnostic Aphasia Examination–Third Edition (BDAE-3) Naming Test by Harold Goodglass with the collaboration of Edith Kaplan and Barbara Barresi, 2001, Austin: PRO-ED. Reproduced with permission.

ADMINISTRATION

STANDARD FORM (BNT-2)

For aphasic patients, begin with item 1 and discontinue after eight successive failures (in previous versions of this test, the discontinuation rule was six consecutive errors). For all other adults, begin with item 30 (*harmonica*). If any of the next eight items are failed, proceed backward from item 29 until eight consecutive preceding items are passed without assistance (i.e., without provision of a stimulus or phonemic cue); then resume in a forward direction and discontinue the test when the examinee makes eight consecutive errors.

Credit is given if the item is correctly named within 20 seconds. If (and only if) the examinee clearly misperceived the picture, the examinee is told that the picture represents something else and is supplied with the bracketed stimulus cues on the record form. A phonemic cue is given after every failure to respond correctly, whether spontaneously or after a stimulus cue. For example, if the response given for *mushroom* is "umbrella," the examinee is given the stimulus cue ("something to eat") and is given an additional 20 seconds to name the picture. If the examinee then correctly names the item within 20 seconds, a check is entered in the stimulus cue correct column. If the examinee is unable to name the picture correctly within 20 seconds after the stimulus cue is given, a second (phonemic) cue is offered (i.e., the underlined initial phoneme of the name of the item, "m").

The rules for discontinuation and for entry into the test at an advanced level save considerable time for examinees without obvious impairment. However, the rules for discontinuation are not clearly stated in the test manual. Correct responses provided after a phonemic cue are not included in the total score. The test manual is not clear as to whether such responses should be used to determine test discontinuation. S. Weintraub (personal communication, April 9, 2003) uses a rigorous interpretation that includes correct responses to phonemic cues in the count of errors (see "Comments" section for further discussion on this issue).

MULTIPLE-CHOICE FORM

After the test is completed, the examiner returns to each item not correctly named after a phonemic cue and presents the card with that item and four printed choices. The examiner reads each word and asks the examinee to indicate the correct choice.

BRAZILIAN PORTUGUESE FORM

Miotto et al. (2010) adapted the BNT for Portuguese-speaking Brazilians. Items were translated and back-translated. Twenty words that were less frequently used in Brazil were identified and replaced with words that were similar in terms of semantics and complexity (see Table 11–7). Normative data for both the original BNT and adapted BNT are out of a total of 60 (Table 11–21). Note that all original and new items were given, with the new items presented immediately after the original items.

TABLE 11–7 Items Replaced on the Brazilian-Portuguese Boston Naming Test (BNT)

ORIGINAL ITEM	BRAZILIAN-PORTUGUESE REPLACEMENT
19	Bolo (Cake)
28	Buquê (Bouquet)
29	Tamanduá (Tamandua)
31	Elefante (Elephant)
32	Cajú (Cashew)
38	Violino (Violin)
40	Cuco (Cuckoo)
41	Peru (Turkey)
42	Termômetro (Thermometer)
43	Cristo Redentor (Christ the Redeemer)
45	Saci-Pererê (Character from Brazilian folklore)
49	Beterraba (Beetroot)
50	Grampeador (Stapler)
52	Trena (Measuring tape)
53	Lupa (Magnifying glass)
55	Pão de Açúcar (Sugarloaf)
56	Estribo (Stirrup)
58	Estojo/Caixa de Lapis (Pencil box)
59	Furadeira (Drill)
60	Ampulheta (Hourglass)

NOTE: Numbers refer to the item numbers in the 60-item BNT.
SOURCE: From Miotto et al. (2010).

SHORT FORMS

Several short forms have been developed (e.g., Fastenau et al., 1998; Graves et al., 2004; Jahn et al., 2013; Lansing et al., 1999; Mack et al., 1992; Saxton et al., 2000) to reduce test time for examinees. One 15-item version, developed by Mack et al. (1992), known as Short Form 4 (Mack SF4), was adopted by the authors of the BNT-2. This short form precedes the standard 60 items in both the stimulus booklet and the answer sheet. The BNT-2 also includes a multiple-choice version to better assess the integrity of the lexicon. Following the standard presentation, the examiner returns to those items initially failed. The examinee then chooses one of four choices read aloud by the examiner. Short forms using alternate items have also been used (see "Normative Data").

Graves et al. (2004) used item response theory to develop two 15- and 30-item short forms that have high internal reliability, high correlations with the long form, and high classification agreement with the full BNT for Alzheimer's disease (AD) and vascular dementia (VaD) patient classification. The authors also developed an adaptive form in which the examiner first gives the 15-item version. If the score is 12 or greater, the examinee is given credit for 13 additional items; if the score is 3 or less, the examiner stops and uses the score obtained. Otherwise, the examiner administers the remaining items to complete the 30-item test. The various items in these short forms are shown in Table 11–8.

CHINESE SHORT FORM

Cheung et al. (2004) developed a Chinese short version suitable for individuals from Hong Kong. They selected the culturally relevant items from the original 60 English items. The items to be presented in order are presented in Table 11–8. Administration procedure followed the standard instructions. However, phonemic cues were not provided because the names of most objects in Chinese consist of one sound.

SPANISH SHORT FORMS

Based on 380 monolingual (either English or Spanish) older adults from Project FRONTIER, an epidemiology study of rural cognition in the United States, Jahn et al. (2013) developed a 15-item version that is equivalent for English and Spanish monolinguals using item response theory. The items are shown in Table 11–8. Standard instructions were used. However, no normative data are available at this writing.

Casals-Coll and colleagues (2014) created four parallel short forms (Table 11–9) using items from the original 60-item BNT based on 340 Spanish-speaking healthy adults from Spain. The BNT was adapted for local context, with "magdalena" added as an alternative to "pretzel." Standard instructions were used. Norms are presented in Tables 11–43 to 11–50.

TABLE 11-8 Boston Naming Test (BNT) Short-Form Items in the Graves et al. (2004), Jahn et al. (2013), and Cheung et al. (2004) Versions

GRAVES ET AL. BNT 30	GRAVES ET AL. BNT 15	JAHN ET AL. BNT 15[a]	CHEUNG ET AL. BNT 30 (CHINESE)
13	19	5	2
17	24	11	3
19	31	13	6
21	32	14	8
22	35	16	9
23	41	18	15
24	42	19	17
25	44	31	46
28	45	36	60
29	48	46	21
31	53	52	37
32	54	53	12
33	55	55	16
34	57	57	24
35	58	58	50
36			22
38			36
41			42
42			25
43			30
44			43
45			31
48			54
53			47
54			14
55			52
57			38
58			57
59			59
60			33

NOTE: Numbers refer to the item numbers in the published 60-item BNT.

[a] Based on N = 253 normal cognition, N = 81 MCI, N = 35 cognitive dysfunction without dementia, N = 8 AD, and N = 3 other dementia. Mean age = 64.12, SD = 13.01, range = 40–96; females = 70%; mean education = 11.49 years, SD = 3.96. Note that the Jahn et al. version can be administered in English or Spanish.

SCORING

Scores include the number of spontaneously produced correct responses, the number of cues given, the number of correct responses given after semantic cueing, and the number given after phonemic cueing. The total correct is the sum of the number of spontaneously given correct responses and the number of correct responses given after a stimulus cue. However, some norms were collected using different scoring procedures, which should be adhered to when interpreting scores.

Certain responses scored as incorrect on the BNT-2 are in fact commonly used synonyms in certain geographical regions. Patients with AD also use more synonyms. Adjustment of scores for these variants lead to minimal changes which, according to the authors, are "unlikely to change quantitative interpretations"; however, they warn that clinicians should be careful to avoid labeling such synonyms as paraphasias. Tombaugh and Hubley (1997) also noted that "mouth organ" and other incorrect responses ("lock" or "bolt" for *latch*, "dice" for *dominoes*, "toadstool" for *mushroom*) often occur in Canada and suggested that, in these and similar cases, a follow-up question should be asked: "What is another name for this?"

Heaton et al. (1999) provided a method to convert the original 85-item BNT to the BNT 60, and vice versa. Raw scores are first converted to scaled scores ($M = 10$, $SD = 3$). A prediction equation is then used to convert the scaled scores into demographically (age, education, and gender) corrected T scores.

DEMOGRAPHIC EFFECTS

AGE

Cross-sectional studies suggest that age affects performance. Correlations between the BNT and age are generally in the

TABLE 11-9 BNT Casals-Coll et al. Spanish Parallel Short Forms

A	B	C	D
Cama (bed)	Árbol (tree)	Casa (house)	Tijeras (scissors)
Escoba (broom)	Flor (flower)	Cepillo de dientes (toothbrush)	Peine (comb)
Banco (bench)	Silbato (whistle)	Caracol (snail)	Sierra (saw)
Pulpo (octopus)	Escalera mecánica (escalator)	Silla de ruedas (wheelchair)	Camello (camel)
Seta (mushroom)	Percha (hanger)	Lápiz (pencil)	Embudo (funnel)
Helicóptero (helicopter)	Bozal (muzzle)	Máscara (mask)	Raqueta (racquet)
Corona de flores (wreath)	Volcán (volcano)	Acordeón (accordion)	Espárragos (asparagus)
Pinzas (tongs)	Bellota (acorn)	Pirámide (pyramid)	Dominó (dominoes)
Compás (compass)	Cactus (cactus)	Harmónica (harmonica)	Rinoceronte (rhinoceros)
Magdalena (muffin)	Arpa (harp)	Globo terráqueo (globe)	Caballito de mar (seahorse)
Aldaba (knocker)	Dardo (dart)	Trípode (tripod)	Hamaca (hammock)
Canoa (canoe)	Soga (noose)	Pergamino (scroll)	Paleta (palette)
Pelícano (pelican)	Zancos (stilts)	Yugo (yoke)	Pestillo (latch)
Unicornio (unicorn)	Esfinge (sphinx)	Estetoscopio (stethoscope)	Iglú (igloo)
Transportador (protractor)	Pérgola (trellis)	Ábaco (abacus)	Castor (beaver)

NOTE: Based on N = 340 healthy adults from Spain with mean age = 65 years, SD = 9.3, range = 50–85; females = 59%; mean education = 10.5 years, SD = 5.5. 20% have <6 years of education, 44% have 6–12 years of education, the rest have >12 years. Clinical sample comprised of N = 172 older adults with amnestic MCI or AD.

SOURCE: Adapted from Casals-Coll et al. (2014).

moderate range (Pena-Casanova et al., 2009; Zec et al., 2007a). According to Heaton et al. (2004), in adults ranging in age from 20 to 85 years, age accounts for 9% of the variance in test scores in Caucasians (3% in African Americans). Scores increase in childhood, improve up to about the fourth decade of life, and subsequently decline, particularly after about 70 years of age (MacKay et al., 2005; Marien et al., 1998; Mitrushina et al., 2005; Randolph et al., 1999; Riva et al., 2000; Saxton et al., 2000; Storms et al., 2004; Tombaugh & Hubley, 1997; Tsang & Lee, 2003; Zec et al., 2007a). Compared to 50- to 59-year-olds, the 80–89 age group scores 4.43 fewer words, and significant declines are seen starting at age 70–79 (Zec et al., 2007a). Low scores (<45) are more frequent with increasing age and decreasing education (Zec et al., 2007a). There is also an increase in the *SDs* for older groups, suggesting that some people maintain high BNT performance with advancing age while others decline (Mitrushina & Satz, 1995; Mitrushina et al., 2005; Zec et al., 2007a).

Longitudinal analyses produce lesser estimates of age-related change than cross-sectional analyses do (Connor et al., 2004). A longitudinal study revealed no age-related change in healthy older adults (aged 59–96 years) over a four-year period (Cruice et al., 2000), although with longer intervals such as seven years (Au et al., 1995) or 20 years (Connor et al., 2004), subtle decline has been reported (about 2% per decade between ages 30 and 94), accelerating with advancing age (Connor et al., 2004). Individuals who have high levels of performance show less decline over time (Connor et al., 2004), consistent with the cognitive reserve hypothesis (Satz, 1993) that some combination of high level of intelligence, education, and a cognitively active lifestyle offers a neuroprotective effect.

Naming ability declines with increasing age on short forms as well (Casals-Coll et al., 2014; Fastenau et al., 1998; Graves et al., 2004; Kent & Luszcz, 2002). Longitudinal analyses suggest that the decline is greatest for individuals aged 80 years and older (Kent & Luszcz, 2002).

GENDER

Some authors have reported that gender is unrelated to BNT performance (e.g., Henderson et al., 1998; Lucas et al., 2005; Pena-Casanova et al., 2009; Riva et al., 2000; Silvestre et al., 2018; Zec et al., 2007a). Others, however, have found that men outperform women in older samples (Connor et al., 2004; Hall et al., 2012; Heaton et al., 1999; Marien et al., 1998; Randolph et al., 1999; Ripich et al., 1995; Ross & Lichtenberg, 1998; Welch et al., 1996), even after controlling for IQ, age, education, and the presence of hyperlipidemia and hypertension (Hall et al., 2012), perhaps because of a preponderance of male-biased items (e.g., compass, tripod, yoke; Randolph et al., 1999). Heaton et al. (2004) noted that about 1% of the variance in test scores of African Americans was accounted for by gender; in Caucasians, the amount was nil.

The effect of gender is inconsequential on short versions (Casals-Coll et al., 2014; Jefferson et al., 2007; Kent & Luszcz, 2002). For example, although the 30-item abbreviated BNT is impacted by ethnicity (white > African American), education (college+ > high school), and gender (male > female), the gender differences disappeared once education was accounted for (Jefferson et al., 2007). Casals-Coll et al. (2014) also reported that no effect of gender was found in their Spanish 15-item short form.

EDUCATION AND IQ

Verbal intelligence affects BNT scores (Killgore & Adams, 1999; Steinberg et al., 2005; Tombaugh & Hubley, 1997) as does Full Scale IQ (FSIQ; Diaz-Asper et al., 2004). Educational achievement also affects scores (Heaton et al., 1999; Jefferson et al., 2007; Lucas et al., 2005; Pena-Casanova et al., 2009; Randolph et al., 1999; Saxton et al., 2000; Tombaugh & Hubley, 1997), although less so than does IQ (Steinberg et al., 2005). Whereas IQ accounts for about 37% of the variance in test scores (Steinberg et al., 2005), education accounts for about 10–11% of the variance in test scores in Caucasians (13% in African Americans; Heaton et al., 2004; Steinberg et al., 2005). Steinberg et al. (2005) have reported that education was wholly redundant with the larger contributions of intelligence to test scores. Individuals with higher IQ (more years of education) are likely to have had exposure to a wider vocabulary, resulting in higher test scores. There is also an interaction of age and education, such that there is less of an age effect in more highly educated individuals (Connor et al., 2004; Neils et al., 1995; Welch et al., 1996).

Education also affects naming ability on the short forms, with higher education associated with better naming ability (Casals-Coll et al., 2014; Fastenau et al., 1998; Kent & Luszcz, 2002).

ETHNICITY, NATIONALITY, AND LINGUISTIC EFFECTS

Geographic region, ethnicity, and level of acculturation can affect performance (Azrin et al., 1996; Fillenbaum et al., 1997; Heaton et al., 2004; Lucas et al., 2005; Manly et al., 1998; Roberts et al., 2002; Ross & Lichtenberg, 1998; Welsh et al., 1995; but see Henderson et al., 1998; Manly et al., 2002). Even within a particular ethnic group, those who are more familiar with the dominant American culture score higher than those who are less acculturated (Manly et al., 1998; Touradji et al., 2001). Using differential item functioning, Pedraza et al. (2009) identified 12 items that differentiated between Caucasian and African-American older adults, including *rhinoceros, muzzle, unicorn, noose, latch, tripod, scroll, tongs, palette,* and *protractor*.

Not all minority groups perform poorly on the BNT. Native Americans reportedly perform as well as non-Native American older adults (Ferraro et al., 2002). There is also no difference in BNT scores of Caucasian Americans and second- or third-generation Japanese Americans (Kemmotsu et al., 2013). With regard to other populations, Canadians (Tombaugh & Hubley, 1997) score slightly higher than Americans (e.g., Ivnik et al., 1996; Mitrushina & Satz, 1995), and both tend to score higher than Australians (Cruice et al., 2000; Worrall et al., 1995), New Zealanders (Barker-Collo, 2002), and Dutch-speaking Belgians (Storms et al., 2004; also see Marien et al., 1998, who showed that the percentages correct per item differed in Dutch-speaking and Australian English-speaking populations), suggesting that norms for the BNT may differ considerably according to populations, languages, and cultural relevance.

Linguistic background also affects test scores. Roberts et al. (2002) compared 42 monolingual English individuals, 32 Spanish-English bilinguals, and 49 French-English bilinguals and found that BNT scores were similar for both sets of bilingual participants; however, both groups scored far lower than the English monolinguals. They concluded that English language norms cannot be used for bilingual speakers, even proficient ones. In Canada, monolingual English speakers perform better than French-English bilinguals, who perform better than monolingual French-speaking individuals. Bilinguals scored lower on the French administration (Sheppard et al., 2016). The authors also found that the French version is not equivalent to the English version, especially on *cactus, seahorse, knocker, tongs, mask, hammock, escalator, mushroom, snail, camel,* and *harmonica*. Accordingly, caution is needed when testing French-English bilinguals using the French version. Similarly, Gollan and colleagues (2012) indicated that the BNT is a poor tool for assessing naming in English-Spanish bilinguals as it tends to underestimate ability in Spanish and should not be used to assess bilinguals (Gollan et al., 2012). This is especially critical for balanced bilinguals, who obtain fewer items correct in their dominant language than unbalanced bilinguals (Gollan et al., 2007). Instead, the Multilingual Naming Test (MINT) appears to be a better test for assessing naming abilities in English-Spanish bilinguals (Gollan et al., 2012).

Findings on the advantage of allowing responses from either language when testing bilinguals are inconsistent. Sheppard and colleagues (2016) administered the BNT to French-English bilinguals from Canada. The majority of French-English bilingual Canadians benefitted from either-language scoring. A small subset of bilinguals performed worse with this scoring but this finding was not due to balance of bilingualism; rather it was due to overall naming abilities. By contrast, Gollan et al. (2007) administered the BNT to older adults who were balanced and unbalanced Spanish-English bilinguals. They found that those who were balanced bilinguals obtained higher scores when correct responses in either language were accepted whereas unbalanced bilinguals did not benefit from this scoring procedure. The either-language advantage may depend on language, acculturation, or object familiarity.

Misdraji-Hammond et al. (2015) investigated whether acculturation and object familiarity explains the bilingual disadvantage on the BNT using a sample of well-acculturated Spanish-English bilinguals and English monolinguals. Although the groups were comparable in their ratings of BNT object familiarity, bilinguals performed lower than monolinguals, even for those who were born and raised in the United States and obtained mainly English instructions in school. The authors concluded that the BNT may not be suitable for testing bilinguals (Misdraji-Hammond et al., 2015).

Reading vocabulary (from the Spot-the-Word, Gates-MacGinitie Reading Tests, Wechsler Abbreviated Scale of Intelligence [WASI] Vocabulary, and Peabody Picture Vocabulary Test [PPVT-R]) is strongly correlated (r = .61 to .81) with BNT performance (Graves & Carswell, 2003; Hawkins et al., 1993; Senior et al., 2001; Simos et al., 2011). Similarly, those with high-average Wide Range Achievement Test (WRAT-3) reading scores obtain higher BNT scores than those with average scores (Jefferson et al., 2007). Therefore, limited vocabulary may represent a substantial risk for misdiagnosis of anomia (see later discussion).

NORMATIVE DATA

STANDARD FORM (BNT OR BNT-2)

The BNT and BNT-2 contain the same items and so norms are interchangeable. Note that no normative data are available for the Multiple-Choice Form. Table 11–10 provides a list of BNT normative studies in various countries and languages.

Standardization Sample. The norms accompanying the BNT-2 60-item test (see Table 11–11) are based on small groups of adults (cell sizes of 11 to 56 individuals, depending on the age group), aged 18 to 79 years (N = 178), who were of above-average education (M = about 14 years). No information is provided regarding geographical region or ethnicity of the sample or in what year these data were collected. This is important given the general rise in ability over time (e.g., Flynn effect) and because norms may change over time as some objects represented come into disuse or change in form (Storms et al., 2004). Consequently, other normative datasets are preferred.

Other Normative Data. A variety of normative reports have appeared in the literature for English speakers (Boone et al., 1995; Heaton et al., 2004; Ivnik et al., 1996; Mitrushina & Satz, 1995; Neils et al., 1995; Ross et al., 1995, Ross & Lichetenberg, 1998; Saxton et al., 2000; Tombaugh & Hubley, 1997). Given the importance of age, geographical region, ethnicity, and education, several larger scale normative sets are discussed here (see Source for use with other language communities).

United States. Heaton et al. (2004) compiled data from multicenter studies conducted over a period of about

TABLE 11–10 List of Boston Naming Test (BNT) Normative Studies from Various Countries/Regions and Languages

REFERENCE	LANGUAGE	COUNTRY/ REGION	N	AGE	EDUCATION	GENDER (% FEMALE)	VERSION	NOTES
Kaplan et al. (2001)	English	Not reported	178	18–79	M = 14	Not reported	Standard	Original BNT-2
Heaton et al. (2004)	English	USA	1000	20–85	0–20	48	Standard	Caucasians and African Americans
Mitrushina et al. (2005)	English	–	1684	25–84	M = 13.79, *SD* = 1.5	Not reported	Standard	Compilation of data from 14 studies
Lucas et al. (2005)	English	Jacksonville, Florida	304	56–94	M = 12.2, *SD* = 3.48	75	Standard	African Americans
Zec et al. (2007b)	English	USA	1019	50–92	Not reported	Not reported	Standard	
Martielli et al. (2016)	English	St. Louis, Missouri	200	15–18	Parental education M = 15.8	50	Standard	
O'Bryant et al. (2018)	Spanish or English	Texas	797	>40	M = 9.9, *SD* = 4.6	73	Standard	Texas-based Mexican Americans
Tombaugh & Hubley (1997)	English	Ottawa, Canada	219	25–88	M = 12.9 (range = 9–21)	Not reported	Standard	
Miotto et al. (2010)	Portuguese	Brazil	739	6–77	0–17	Not reported	Adapted and Standard	Standard administration procedure not used
Pena-Casanova et al. (2009)	Spanish	Spain	340	50+	Not reported	59	Standard	All items administered
Aranciva et al. (2012)	Spanish	Spain	179	18–49	8–20	64	Standard	
Olabarrieta-Landa et al. (2015)	Spanish	10 Latin American countries	3779	18–95	1–12+	67	Standard	Rigorous administration
Silvestre et al. (2018)	Spanish	Dominican Republic	239	16–80	1–13+	51	Standard	All items of the Kaplan et al. (2005) version were administered
Patricacou et al. (2007)	Greek	Greece	100	20 to 71+	0 to 13+	Not reported	Adapted 60-item	Four items were replaced
Elkadi et al. (2006)	English	Australia	250	56–67	45% with >12 years	100	30-item even number Short Form	
Graves et al. (2004)	English	Canada	62	38–83	Not reported	Not reported	30-item and 15-item Short Forms	
Jefferson et al. (2007)	English	USA	219	55+	M = 16.4, *SD* = 2.7	66	30-item even number Short Form	
Casals-Coll et al. (2014)	Spanish	Spain	340	50+	M = 10.5, *SD* = 5.5	59	15-item Short Forms	Four parallel short forms are available
Cheung et al. (2004)	Chinese	Hong Kong	77	23–79	M = 9.73, *SD* = 4.35	53	30-item Short Form	

25 years and presented norms separately for two ethnicity groups (Caucasians, African Americans) organized by age, gender, and education. The samples were large and covered a wide range in terms of age and education; exclusion criteria were specified (see Table 11–12). T scores lower than 40 were classed as impaired. Note that regionally correct answers, such as "tom walkers" for *stilts,* were not given credit in the norms.

Mitrushina et al. (2005) compiled data for the 60-item version from 14 studies, comprising a total of 1,684

TABLE 11–11 Characteristics of the Boston Naming Test (BNT-2) Normative Sample Provided by Kaplan et al. (2001)

Sample size	178
Age	18 to 79[a] years
Sample type	Standardization
Geographical region	Not specified
Stratification	None
Education	Mean of about 14 years
Gender	Not specified
Ethnicity	Not specified
Screening	Not reported

[a]18–39 *N* = 21; 40–49 *N* = 11; 50–59 *N* = 49; 60–69 *N* = 56; 70–79 *N* = 41.

participants. The data are presented in five-year increments, from ages 25 to 84 years. Note that their sample was highly educated (*M* = 13.79 years, *SD* = 1.5) and of above-average IQ (*M* = 116.1, *SD* = 2.6). The data are very similar to those provided by Kaplan et al. (2001); the educational achievement of their sample was also above average. Given the influence of education and IQ on test scores, the values provided by both Mitrushina et al. (2005) and Kaplan et al. (2001) are likely to overestimate expected performance for individuals with lower educational/intellectual levels.

Lucas et al. (2005) provide age- and education-adjusted normative data based on 304 African-American, community-dwelling participants from the Mayo's Older African American Normative Studies (MOAANS) project in Jacksonville, Florida. Participants were predominantly female (75%), ranged in age from 56 to 94 years (*M* = 69.6, *SD* = 6.87), and varied in education from 0 to 20 years of formal education (*M* = 12.2, *SD* = 3.48). Examinees were screened to exclude those with active neurological, psychiatric, or other conditions that might affect cognition. These authors administered the BNT using the lenient interpretation of the discontinuation rule (i.e., items correctly named after presentation of phonemic cues were not counted as failures), making it possible to score and derive normative data for both the rigorous administration (counting items named correctly with a phonemic cue as errors) and the lenient administration. They accepted "Tom Walkers" or "Tommy Walkers" as correct for *stilts* and "mouth harp" as a correct response for *harmonica*. Mispronunciations of words (e.g., "stedascope" for *stethoscope*, "spinx" for *sphinx*, "tressle" for *trellis*) were considered incorrect. Age-corrected MOAANS scaled scores and percentile ranks for BNT data scored using both the lenient and the rigorous interpretation are presented in Table 11–13. Age- and education-corrected MOAANS scaled scores can also be computed using the formula provided in Table 11–14.

TABLE 11–12 Characteristics of the Boston Naming Test (BNT) Normative Sample Provided by Heaton et al. (2004)

Sample size	1,000
Age	20 to 85[a] years
Geographical region	Various states in the United States, and Manitoba, Canada
Sample type	Standardization
Stratification	None
Education	7 to 20[b] years
Gender	52% Men 48% Women
Ethnicity	65% African American 35% Caucasian
Screening	No reported history of learning disability, neurological disorder, serious psychiatric disorder, or alcohol or drug abuse

[a] Age groups: 20–34, 35–39, 40–44, 45–49, 50–54, 55–59, 60–64, 65–69, 70–74, 75–79, and 80–89 years.

[b] Education groups: 7–8, 9–11, 12, 13–15, 16–17, and 18–20.

Lucas et al. (2005) also provide cumulative frequency data for the number of correct responses to phonemic cues administered under each discontinuation rule. They reported that it was fairly common for African-American older adults to get eight additional BNT items correct with phonemic cueing under both rigorous (frequency = 28%) and lenient (frequency = 32%) administrations. They also noted that, depending on which discontinuation rule was used, 20–28% of the sample were administered 20 or more phonemic cues, indicating incorrect spontaneous responses to items and failure of stimulus cues (when given) to facilitate naming on at least one-third of the test items. These findings raise concerns regarding the equivalence of BNT item familiarity across ethnic groups and geographic regions and suggest caution in the interpretation of BNT performance in African Americans (see also the section "Demographic Effects").

Zec et al. (2007b) provide norms for English-speaking Caucasians based on 1,019 adults aged 50 to 92 (Tables 11–15 to 11–17). Their rigorous screening excluded those with neurological/psychiatric conditions that are high risk for cognitive impairment, including dementia, amnestic MCI, non-AD dementia, Pick's disease, multiple sclerosis (MS), Parkinson's disease (PD), chronic alcoholism, brain surgery, bipolar disorder, depression, brain injuries, and strokes. All 60 items were given to the participants *without cueing* and the total number of spontaneous correct responses were summed. The authors did not strictly adhere to the 20-second time limit for responding. Regional substitutes for harmonica ("French harp") and mask ("false face") were accepted as correct.

Martielli and Blackburn (2016) provide adolescent norms based on 200 Caucasian adolescents aged 15 to 18 from St. Louis, Missouri. Half the sample was female. Of the 18-year-olds, 42% of males and 80% of females were university students. Parental education of the sample was 15.8 years. The sample were of average estimated intelligence (Wechsler Test of Adult Reading [WTAR] estimated IQ mean = 102.52, *SD* = 8.23). The sample was screened for history of neurological disease, motor disorder, head injury with loss of consciousness, learning disability, Attention-Deficit/Hyperactivity Disorder (ADHD),

TABLE 11–13 MOAANS Age-Based Boston Naming Test (BNT) Norms in African-American Adults Using Rigorous (R) and Lenient (L) Administration Rules

SCALED SCORE	AGE RANGE 56 TO 62 R	L	63 TO 65 R	L	66 TO 68 R	L	69 TO 71 R	L	72 TO 74 R	L	75 TO 77 R	L	78+ R	L	PERCENTILE RANGES
N	108	105	130	127	165	162	180	177	156	154	119	117	78	76	
2	0–16	0–17	0–16	0–14	0–15	0–14	0–15	0–14	0–14	0–14	0–14	0–14	0–14	0–14	<1
3	17–18	18–21	17	15–17	16	15–17	16	15–17	15–16	15–17	15–16	15–17	15–16	15–17	1
4	19–21	22	18–19	18–19	17–19	18	17–18	18	17–18	18	17–18	18	17–18	18	2
5	22–23	23–27	20–21	20–23	20–21	19–23	19–20	19–23	19–20	19–23	19–20	19–23	19–20	19–23	3–5
6	24–30	28–34	22–24	24–28	22–24	24–28	21–24	24–27	21–24	24–27	21–24	24–27	21–22	—	6–10
7	31–37	35–38	25–33	29–35	25–32	29–34	25–32	28–33	25–32	28–32	25–32	28–32	23–29	24–30	11–18
8	38–40	39–41	34–39	36–40	33–37	35–38	33–36	34–36	33–36	33–36	33–36	33–36	30–32	31–33	19–28
9	41–44	42–45	40–43	41–43	38–42	39–43	37–41	37–41	37–41	37–40	37–41	37–40	33–37	34–38	29–40
10	45–50	46–50	44–48	44–49	43–47	44–47	42–47	42–47	42–47	41–44	42–47	41–47	38–44	39–45	41–59
11	51–52	51–52	49–51	50–51	48–50	48–50	48–50	48–50	48–50	48–50	48–50	48–50	45–49	46–50	60–71
12	53–54	53–54	52–53	52–54	51–52	51–52	51–52	51–52	51–52	51–52	51–52	51–52	50–52	51–52	72–81
13	55	55	54–55	55	53–54	53–54	53–54	53–54	53–54	53–54	53–54	53–54	53–54	53–54	82–89
14	56–57	56–57	56–57	56–57	55–56	55–56	55–56	55–56	55–56	55	55–56	55	55	55	90–94
15	58	58	58	58	57	57	57	57	57	56–57	57	56–57	56	56	95–97
16	—	—	—	—	58	58	58	58	—	—	—	—	—	—	98
17	59	59	59	—	59	—	59	—	58	58	58	58	57–58	57	99
18	60	60	60	59–60	60	59–60	60	59–60	59–60	59–60	59–60	59–60	59–60	58–60	>99

NOTE: R, rigorous administration; L, lenient administration.

SOURCE: Adapted from Lucas et al. (2005). Reprinted with the permission of the Mayo Foundation for Medical Education and Research.

developmental disability, psychiatric illness, or current medications with possible motor or cognitive side effects. Standard instructions were used: all participants started at item 30 to establish an eight-consecutive-correct basal level, and the test was discontinued after eight consecutive errors. The total score was based on the sum of correct spontaneous responses and correct responses after the provision of stimulus cues. Because of a non-normal distribution of scores, the authors recommend reporting whether the score is within normal limits using cumulative percentage instead of standard score or percentile (see Table 11–18).

O'Bryant et al. (2018) provide normative data from the Texas Mexican American Adult Normative Study, which combined the data from multiple Texas-based research studies, including Project FRONTIER, Texas Alzheimer's Research and Care Consortium, and the Health and Aging Brain Among Latino Elders study (Table 11–19). The norms are based on $N = 797$, mean age of 60.4 ($SD = 8.6$), mean education of 9.9 ($SD = 4.6$), and 73% females. A total of 412 participants opted to test in Spanish. All 60 items were administered starting from item 1.

Canada. Tombaugh and Hubley (1997) present age- and education-stratified norms based on a sample of 219 healthy, relatively well-educated (M = 12.9 years) volunteers residing in Ottawa, Canada. None of the individuals had less than nine years of education. The data are shown in Table 11–20.

Brazil. Miotto et al. (2010) adapted the BNT for Portuguese-speaking Brazilians ($N = 739$, age range 6 to 77, education range = 0 to 17 years). Normative data for both the original BNT and adapted BNT are provided in Table 11–21 and are out of a total of 60. As the standard administration procedure was not used, the data from Table 11–21 should be used with caution for clinical decision making.

Spain. Pena-Casanova et al. (2009) provide Spanish norms from the NEURONORMA project ($N = 340$, 59% female, age 50+ from various regions in Spain). Standard instructions were used and *magdalena* was added as alternative to *pretzel* for the Spanish population. The total score was calculated based on correct spontaneous response and correct response after stimulus cue. Norms are presented in Tables 11–22 and 11–23. All items were administered. As with the standard procedure, a stimulus cue was provided if the examinee did not give a response within 20 seconds, if the examinee stated that they did not know the name, or if the item was misperceived. The examinee was given another

TABLE 11–14 Computational Formula for Age- and Education-Corrected MOAANS Boston Naming Test (BNT) Scaled Scores

	K	W_1	W_2
BNT "Rigorous" Administration	3.53	1.20	0.44
BNT "Lenient" Administration	3.49	1.21	0.46

NOTE: Age- and education-corrected MOAANS Scaled Scores ($MSS_{A\&E}$) can be calculated for BNT scores by using age-corrected MOAANS Scaled Scores (MSS_A) and education (years completed) in the following formula: $MSS_{A\&E} = K + (W_1 * MSS_A) - (W_2 * EDUC)$.

Rigorous administration = counting items named correctly with a phonemic cue as errors.

Lenient administration = items correctly named after presentation of phonemic cues were not counted as failures.

SOURCE: Adapted from Lucas et al. (2005). Reprinted with the permission of the Mayo Foundation for Medical Education and Research.

TABLE 11–15 Boston Naming Test (BNT) Scaled Scores for Ages 50 to 92 Years and 12 Years or Less of Education

AGE RANGE	50 TO 56	53 TO 59	56 TO 62	59 TO 65	62 TO 68	65 TO 71	68 TO 74	71 TO 77	74 TO 80	77 TO 83	80 TO 86	83 TO 89	86 TO 92
Age mid–point	53	56	59	62	65	68	71	74	77	80	83	86	89
Scaled score	Raw score												
2	–	–	–	–	41	42–44	–	28–33	–	–	–	–	–
3	–	–	44	41	42	45	39	34	28	37	–	–	–
4	–	45	45–46	42–43	43–44	–	40–45	35–39	29–34	38	37	–	–
5	45–49	46–49	47–49	44–46	45–47	46–47	46	40–46	35–39	39	38	43–44	–
6	50–52	50–52	50–52	47–48	48	48	47–48	47–48	40–46	40–44	39–42	45–46	43–49
7	53	–	53	49–52	49–51	49–51	49–50	49	47	45–46	43–45	47–49	–
8	54	53	54	53	52–53	52	51–52	50–51	48–49	47	46–47	50	50–51
9	55	54	–	54	54	53–54	53	52	50–52	48–49	48–50	51	–
10	56	55–56	55–56	55–56	55–56	55	54–55	53–54	53–54	50–52	51–52	52	–
11	57	57	57	57	57	56–57	56	55	55	53–54	53	–	52–54
12	–	–	58	58	58	58	57	56–57	56–57	55–56	54–57	53–54	–
13	58	58	–	–	–	59	58	58	58	57–58	58	–	55
14	59–60	59	59	59	59	–	59	59	–	–	–	55	56–59
15	–	60	60	–	–	60	60	–	59	–	59	56–59	–
16	–	–	–	60	60	–	–	–	–	–	–	–	–
17	–	–	–	–	–	–	–	60	60	59	–	–	–
18	–	–	–	–	–	–	–	–	–	–	–	–	–

SOURCE: Adapted from Zec et al. (2007b).

20 seconds to respond; if a wrong answer was given, the phonemic cue was given. Multiple-choice items were given for all wrong responses after the test was completed. The total score is the sum of the number of correct spontaneous responses and after stimulus cueing. To use this set of norms, first look up the age-adjusted scaled score (NSS_A) using Table 11–22 and then apply the education adjustment to the age-adjusted scaled score (NSS_A) using Table 11–23.

Aranciva et al. (2012) provide Spanish norms from the young adult expansion of the NEURONORMA project (N = 179, age range = 18 to 49, education range 8 to 20, 64% female, 46% bilingual). Item 19 (*pretzel*) was replaced with *magdalena*. Standard instructions were used. The examinee was allowed 20 seconds to give a spontaneous answer. A semantic cue was given if an erroneous response was due to perceptual error. Incorrect spontaneous response or following semantic cueing was followed by phonemic cueing. The multiple-choice trial was administered if the examinee still did not get the right answer. Only correct responses given either spontaneously or after semantic cueing were summed to obtain the total score. Table 11–24 presents the normative data. To use this set of norms, first look up the scaled score (NSS) using Table 11–24 and then apply the education adjustment to the scaled score (NSS) using Table 11–25.

Latin America. Olabarrieta-Landa et al. (2015) provide norms for 18- to 95-year-old native Spanish-speaking

TABLE 11–16 Boston Naming Test (BNT) Scaled Scores for Ages 50 to 92 Years and 12 Years of Education

AGE RANGE	50 TO 56	53 TO 59	56 TO 62	59 TO 65	62 TO 68	65 TO 71	68 TO 74	71 TO 77	74 TO 80	77 TO 83	80 TO 86	83 TO 89	86 TO 92
Age mid–point	53	56	59	62	65	68	71	74	77	80	83	86	89
Scaled score	Raw score												
2	–	–	–	–	42–43	–	–	–	–	–	–	–	–
3	–	–	44	42	44	42	–	28	28	–	–	–	–
4	–	46	45–46	43–44	45	43–45	39	29–39	29–39	39	–	–	–
5	49–52	47–50	47–52	45–47	46–48	46–49	40–45	40–46	40–46	40–43	39–42	–	–
6	53	51–52	–	48–49	49	50	46–50	47–48	47	44–46	43–44	43–44	–
7	–	–	53	50–52	50–52	51–52	51	49–50	48–49	47	45–47	45–46	43–49
8	54	53–54	54	53	53–54	53–54	52	51–52	50–52	48–50	48–49	47–50	–
9	55	–	55	54–55	–	–	53–54	53	–	51	50–51	–	50–51
10	56	55–56	56	56	55–56	55–56	55	54–55	53–55	52–54	52	51	–
11	57	57	57	57	57	57	56	56	56	55–56	53	–	–
12	–	58	58	58	58	58	57	57	57	57–58	54–58	52	–
13	58	59	59	59	–	59	58	58	58	–	–	–	–
14	59–60	–	–	–	59	60	59	59	–	–	–	53	–
15	–	60	60	60	–	–	60	–	59	–	59	–	–
16	–	–	–	–	60	–	–	60	–	59	–	–	–
17	–	–	–	–	–	–	–	–	60	–	–	–	–
18	–	–	–	–	–	–	–	–	–	–	–	–	–

SOURCE: Adapted from Zec et al. (2007b).

TABLE 11–17 Boston Naming Test (BNT) Scaled Scores for Ages 50 to 92 Years and Greater Than 12 Years of Education

AGE RANGE	50 TO 56	53 TO 59	56 TO 62	59 TO 65	62 TO 68	65 TO 71	68 TO 74	71 TO 77	74 TO 80	77 TO 83	80 TO 86	83 TO 89	86 TO 92
Age mid–point	53	56	59	62	65	68	71	74	77	80	83	86	89
Scaled score	Raw score												
2	–	–	40	40–41	40–41	42–43	44	37–41	37	–	–	–	–
3	45	45	41–48	42	42	44	45	42	38	34	34	–	–
4	46	46–48	49–50	43–48	43–48	45–48	46–48	–	39–42	35–38	35–37	–	–
5	47–50	49–51	51–25	49–51	49–50	49	49	43–48	43–44	39–43	38–43	27–34	27
6	51–53	52–53	53	52	51–52	50–51	50–52	49–50	45–48	44–46	44–45	35–42	28–50
7	54–55	54	54	53–54	53–54	52–53	53	51–53	49–50	47–48	46–47	43–47	51
8	56	55–56	55–56	55	55	54–55	54	54	51–53	49–51	48–50	48–51	52
9	57	57	57	56	56	56	55–56	55	54	52–53	51–52	52	53–54
10	58	58	58	57–58	57–58	57	57	56–57	55–56	54–55	53–55	53–55	55–57
11	–	–	–	–	–	58	58	58	57	56	–	56–57	58–59
12	59	59	59	59	59	59	59	–	58	57	56–57	58–59	–
13	60	60	60	–	60	–	–	59	59	58	58	–	60
14	–	–	–	60	–	60	60	60	60	59	–	60	–
15	–	–	–	–	–	–	–	–	–	60	59–60	–	–
16	–	–	–	–	–	–	–	–	–	–	–	–	–
17	–	–	–	–	–	–	–	–	–	–	–	–	–
18	–	–	–	–	–	–	–	–	–	–	–	–	–

SOURCE: Adapted from Zec et al. (2007b).

adults from 10 Latin-American countries (Tables 11–26 to 11–35). The standard BNT procedure was used with rigorous administration; synonyms were not accepted as correct responses. To be included in the normative sample, participants were native to the country where testing took place and had at least one year of formal education and the ability to read and write. All participants obtained MMSE scores of 23 or more, Patient Health Questionnaire (PHQ-9) scores of 4 or less, and 90 or more on the Barthel Index. Participants were excluded if they self-reported neurologic or psychiatric disorders. Note that the norms were generated using regression models that included age, education, and/or gender.

Dominican Republic. Silvestre, Iglesias, and Silvestre (2018) provide norms for native Spanish-speaking Dominicans (N = 239; mean age = 47.87, SD = 18.86, range 16 to 80; mean education = 10.37, SD = 5.10; 51% female). To be included in the normative sample, participants were born and raised in the Dominican Republic, literate, obtained an MMSE of greater than 21, and self-reported no history of neurological or psychological problems or alcohol or substance abuse. The Kaplan et al. (2005) version of the BNT was used. All 60 items were administered using standard instructions. Acceptable alternative answers are presented in Table 11–36. In addition, regionalism and typical idiosyncrasies were also accepted if they could be found in the Dominican Spanish dictionary. Although they suggested an item administration order based on item difficulty, these norms were collected based on standard item order. Norms stratified by education are presented in Table 11–37.

TABLE 11–18 Cumulative Percentages for Boston Naming Test (BNT) Scores for Adolescents Aged 15 to 18

SCORE	CUMULATIVE PERCENT
38	0.5
39	1.0
40	3.0
41	3.5
42	4.0
43	5.0
44	6.0
45	10.5
46	14.0
47	19.0
48	22.5
49	31.5
50	37.5
51	46.0
52	55.5
53	63.5
54	74.5
55	84.5
56	92.5
57	96.5
58	98.5
59	100

NOTE: Standard instructions were used. The total score was based on the sum of correct spontaneous responses and correct responses after the provision of stimulus cues.

SOURCE: Martielli et al. (2016).

SHORT FORM NORMATIVE DATA

Elkadi et al. (2006) provide norms for Australian-born women enrolled in the Melbourne Women's Midlife Health Project (N = 250, mean age = 60, range = 56 to 67 years) on a BNT Short Form that uses 30 even-numbered items from the original 60-item BNT. This version used standard instructions, except that administration started at item 1 (Table 11–38).

Graves et al. (2004) recommend a cutoff of less than 25 on their own 30-item version and of less than 11 on their 15-item form. These cutoff points represent values set at the

TABLE 11–19 Boston Naming Test (BNT) Norms for Texas-Based Mexican Americans Age >40

AGE (YEARS)	40 TO 60				61+			
EDUCATION (YEARS) SCALED SCORE	0 TO 6 (*N* = 120)	3 TO 9 (*N* = 171)	6 TO 12 (*N* = 211)	12+ (*N* = 108)	0 TO 6 (*N* = 91)	3 TO 9 (*N* = 98)	6 TO 12 (*N* =113)	12+ (*N* = 73)
19	–	–	–	–	–	–	–	–
18	58–60	58–60	59–60	60	54–60	55–60	58–60	–
17	55–57	55–56	56–58	59	52–53	52–54	56–57	60
16	–	–	55	–	51	–	55	58–59
15	52–54	52–54	54	57–58	48–50	51	53–54	57
14	49–51	50–51	52–53	55–56	47	48–50	51–52	55–56
13	46–48	48–49	50–51	54	45–46	46–47	50	54
12	43–45	45–47	48–49	52–53	40–44	42–45	46–49	52–53
11	40–42	43–44	45–47	50–51	37–39	39–41	43–45	49–51
10	38–39	40–42	43–44	49	34–36	36–38	41–42	47–48
9	36–37	37–39	40–42	47–48	29–33	33–35	37–40	43–46
8	34–35	35–36	39	44–46	27–28	27–32	34–36	41–42
7	32–33	33–34	36–38	43	22–26	23–26	30–33	35–40
6	26–31	29–32	33–35	40–42	20–21	21–22	27–29	30–34
5	20–25	23–28	31–32	39	19	19–20	22–26	29
4	19	20–22	29–30	37–38	16–18	16–18	20–21	–
3	17–18	17–19	20–28	32–36	15	15	0–19	20–28
2	0–16	0–16	0–19	0–31	0–14	0–14	–	0–19
1	–				–	–	–	–

SOURCE: Adapted from O'Bryant et al. (2017).

20th percentile for 62 healthy adults, aged 38 to 83 years ($M = 59.2$, $SD = 10.5$) attending a memory disorders clinic who were found to have no significant medical or neurological complications. Using a value set at the 10th percentile, the cutoff points would be less than 22 on their 30-item form and less than 10 on their 15-item forms (Table 11–39).

Jefferson et al. (2007) provide norms (Tables 11–40 and 11–41) for an abbreviated BNT made up of 30 even items from the original BNT based on 219 cognitively healthy older adults age 55+ from the Boston University Alzheimer's Disease Core Center registry (mean age = 71.9, $SD = 8.4$, 55+ years; mean education = 16.4, $SD = 2.7$; 66% females). Total score was based on correct spontaneous responses and correct responses after stimulus cues. Cutoff scores reflect −1.5 *SD* or −2.0 *SD* below the mean.

Schretlen, Testa, and Pearlson (2010) provide norms for 325 adults on the BNT-30 Short Form; these use the Calibrated Neuropsychological Normative System (CNNS) scoring to derive T scores and discrepancies based on a large sample of older adults from the northeastern United States. Characteristics of the normative sample are shown in Table 11–42. The norms are available through Psychological Assessment Resources (PAR; www.parinc.com). A major advantage of these norms is the option to correct for demographic variables such as age, sex, education, and ethnicity. Several other commonly used neuropsychological tests are co-normed using this sample, which facilitates cross-test comparisons.

CHINESE SHORT FORM

Cheung et al. (2004) provide Chinese norms from 77 healthy adults aged 23 to 79 (mean age = 50.43, $SD = 11.59$; mean education = 9.73, $SD = 4.35$; 53% female). Participants were spouses or family members of

TABLE 11–20 Boston Naming Test (BNT) Normative Data Expressed as Percentiles for Age and Education Based on a Canadian Sample

	AGE 25 TO 69		AGE 70 TO 88		TOTAL
EDUCATION (YEARS)	9 TO 12 (*N* = 78)	13 TO 21 (*N* = 70)	9 TO 12 (*N* = 45)	13 TO 21 (*N* = 26)	(*N* = 219)
Percentile					
90	59	60	59	59	60
75	58	60	58	58	58
50	56	58	55	56	57
25	54	56	52	53	54
10	51	53	47	49	51
Mean education (years)	11.3	15.1	11.2	14.9	12.9

SOURCE: Adapted from Tombaugh and Hubley (1997).

TABLE 11–21 Portuguese-Brazilian Normative Data for the Original Boston Naming Test (BNT) and Adapted BNT as a Function of Age and Education

	ORIGINAL BNT																	
	EDUCATION (YEARS)																	
AGE GROUP	NONE			1 TO 6			7 TO 9			10 TO 12			13+			ALL		
(YEARS)	MEAN	*SD*	*N*	MEAN	*SD*	*N*	MEAN	*SD*	*N*	MEAN	*SD*	*N*	MEAN	*SD*	*N*	MEAN	*SD*	*N*
15–19	–	–	–	39.9	9.6	24	38.1	10.6	25	48.1	3.9	16	–	–	–	41.5	9.9	65
20–24	–	–	–	24.5	15.7	13	32.9	14.3	9	46.3	10.0	8	48.1	10.4	20	38.9	16.0	50
25–34	–	–	–	23.4	16.1	39	44.2	7.0	12	47.3	8.0	16	51.2	8.5	33	39.0	17.2	100
35–44	–	–	–	33.0	10.8	25	41.3	8.3	21	51.5	7.3	13	54.9	4.5	30	45.0	12.0	89
45–54	–	–	–	19.2	18.4	50	43.0	9.3	20	51.6	6.6	10	52.6	4.6	18	35.5	20.5	98
55–64	31.0	–	1	37.6	12.1	55	48.9	3.4	16	51.8	2.9	9	50.9	5.3	22	43.4	11.3	102
65–74	34.0	9.9	2	34.0	8.6	41	39.3	5.1	16	49.2	5.2	6	53.4	4.5	24	41.2	10.8	95
75+	30.0	–	1	28.4	11.2	10	37.0	6.9	3	47.0	1.4	2	–	–	–	32.4	11.2	11
All	29.6	6.2	9	32.0	14.1	370	40.3	10.4	133	49.2	6.6	80	52.0	6.9	147	39.3	14.3	739
	ADAPTED BNT																	
	EDUCATION (YEARS)																	
AGE GROUP	NONE			1 TO 6			7 TO 9			10 TO 12			13+			ALL		
(YEARS)	MEAN	*SD*	*N*	MEAN	*SD*	*N*	MEAN	*SD*	*N*	*MEAN*	*SD*	*N*	MEAN	*SD*	*N*	MEAN	*SD*	*N*
15–19	–	–	–	46.9	9.2	24	43.2	15.5	25	55.8	2.5	16	–	–	–	47.8	12.1	65
20–24	–	–	–	29.5	21.2	13	28.8	22.7	9	50.8	14.5	8	53.1	12.9	20	42.2	20.6	50
25–34	–	–	–	28.2	19.9	39	52.3	5.0	12	51.4	12.3	16	56.0	8.1	33	44.2	19.0	100
35–44	–	–	–	32.5	17.9	25	49.5	11.8	21	56.6	4.1	13	57.6	2.5	30	48.5	15.3	89
45–54	–	–	–	35.0	19.9	50	50.3	13.8	20	57.1	2.6	10	56.9	3.2	18	44.4	18.4	98
55–64	29.0	–	1	47.9	9.7	55	57.3	2.3	16	57.2	1.5	9	55.9	4.1	22	51.7	8.9	102
65–74	40.5	14.8	2	42.5	10.4	41	49.0	4.6	16	54.8	3.1	6	57.7	2.3	24	48.6	10.0	95
75+	42.0	–	1	37.7	12.8	10	40.7	9.3	3	55.5	0.7	2	–	–	–	40.8	12.1	11
All	31.1	9.6	9	39.5	16.1	370	46.3	15.6	133	54.8	7.7	80	56.3	6.6	147	45.6	15.6	739

Note that all original and new items were given, with the new items presented immediately after the original items. The adapted version uses alternate items as shown in Table 11–7.

SOURCE: Miotto et al. (2010).

TABLE 11–22 Age-Adjusted NEURONORMA Scores (NSS_A) for the Spanish Boston Naming Test (BNT)

SCALED SCORE	PERCENTILE RANGE	AGE RANGE (YEARS)									
		50 TO 56	57 TO 59	60 TO 62	63 TO 65	66 TO 68	69 TO 71	72 TO 74	75 TO 77	78 TO80	81+
2	<1	≤34	≤31	≤31	≤30	≤30	≤30	≤30	≤29	≤29	≤29
3	1	–	–	–	31	–	31	–	30	30	–
4	2	35–37	32–33	32–33	–	31	32	–	–	–	30
5	3–5	38	34–36	34–36	32–35	32–36	33–36	31–35	31–32	31	–
6	6–10	39–41	37–39	37–38	36–38	37–38	37–39	36–37	34–35	32–35	31–32
7	11–18	42–44	40–42	39–42	39–42	39–41	40–42	38–40	36–40	36	33–34
8	19–28	45	43–45	43–44	43–44	42–44	43	41–43	41–42	37–41	35–37
9	29–40	46–49	46–48	45–47	45–46	45–46	44–46	44–45	43–44	42–43	38–43
10	41–59	50–52	49–51	48–51	47–51	47–51	47–49	46–48	45–48	44–46	44–45
11	60–71	53–54	52–53	52–53	52	52–53	50–52	49–50	49–50	47–48	46–47
12	72–81	55	54–55	54	53–54	54	53–54	51–52	51–52	49–51	48–51
13	82–89	56	56	55	55	55	55	53–54	53–54	52	52
14	90–94	57	–	56	56	56	56	55–56	55–56	53	53
15	95–97	–	57	57	57	57–58	57–58	57	57	54	54–55
16	98	58–59	58	58	58–59	–	–	58	–	55	56
17	99		59	59	–	59	59	59	58	56	–
18	>99	60	60	60	60	60	60	60	59–60	57–60	57–60
Age range		50–60	53–63	56–66	59–69	62–72	65–75	68–78	71–81	74–84	77+ (77–90)
Sample size		136	132	123	105	118	124	123	97	62	38

NOTE: All items were administered. The total score is the sum of the number of correct spontaneous responses and after stimulus cues. *N* = 340, 59% female, age 50+ from various regions in Spain.

SOURCE: Pena-Casanova et al. (2009).

TABLE 11–23 Education Adjustment from Age-Adjusted Scaled Score for the Spanish Boston Naming Test (BNT)

	EDUCATION (YEARS)																				
SSS_A	0	1	2	3	4	5	6	7	8	9	10	11	12	13	14	15	16	17	18	19	20
2	5	5	4	4	4	3	3	3	3	2	2	2	2	1	1	1	0	0	0	0	−1
3	6	6	5	5	5	4	4	4	4	3	3	3	3	2	2	2	1	1	1	1	0
4	7	7	6	6	6	5	5	5	5	4	4	4	4	3	3	3	2	2	2	2	1
5	8	8	7	7	7	6	6	6	6	5	5	5	5	4	4	4	3	3	3	3	2
6	9	9	8	8	8	7	7	7	7	6	6	6	6	5	5	5	4	4	4	4	3
7	10	10	9	9	9	8	8	8	8	7	7	7	7	6	6	6	5	5	5	5	4
8	11	11	10	10	10	9	9	9	9	8	8	8	8	7	7	7	6	6	6	6	5
9	12	12	11	11	11	10	10	10	10	9	9	9	9	8	8	8	7	7	7	7	6
10	13	13	12	12	12	11	11	11	11	10	10	10	10	9	9	9	8	8	8	8	7
11	14	14	13	13	13	12	12	12	12	11	11	11	11	10	10	10	9	9	9	9	8
12	15	15	14	14	14	13	13	13	13	12	12	12	12	11	11	11	10	10	10	10	9
13	16	16	15	15	15	14	14	14	14	13	13	13	13	12	12	12	11	11	11	11	10
14	17	17	16	16	16	15	15	15	15	14	14	14	14	13	13	13	12	12	12	12	11
15	18	18	17	17	17	16	16	16	16	15	15	15	15	14	14	14	13	13	13	13	12
16	19	19	18	18	18	17	17	17	17	16	16	16	16	15	15	15	14	14	14	14	13
17	20	20	19	19	19	18	18	18	18	17	17	17	17	16	16	16	15	15	15	15	14
18	21	21	20	20	20	19	19	19	19	18	18	18	18	17	17	17	16	16	16	16	15

SOURCE: From Pena-Casanova et al. (2009).

brain-injured patients participating in the same research study. All examinees reported no history of head injury, alcohol abuse, or neurological or psychiatric conditions. In this sample, the healthy individuals obtained a mean score of 24.92 (SD = 3.04) for spontaneous naming. Total score after semantic cueing was M = 26.65 (SD = 2.75).

SPANISH SHORT FORM

Casals-Coll et al. (2014) provide normative data for four parallel Spanish Short Form from the NEURONORMA project (N = 340; mean age = 65, SD = 9.3; 59% female; mean education = 10.5, SD = 5.5). The BNT was adapted for local context, with *magdalena* added as an alternative to *pretzel*. The four parallel forms are presented in Table 11–9. Standard instructions were used. The data are presented in Tables 11–43 to 11–50. To use this set of norms, first look up the age-adjusted scaled score (NSS_A) using Tables 11–43 to 11–46 and then apply the education adjustment to the age-adjusted scaled score (NSS_A) using Tables 11–47 to 11–50.

TABLE 11–24 Spanish Boston Naming Test (BNT) Scaled Scores for Young Adults from Spain

NSS	RAW SCORE
2	≤38
3	39
4	40–42
5	43–44
6	45–46
7	47–49
8	50
9	51–52
10	53–54
11	55
12	56
13	–
14	57
15	58
16	–
17	–
18	59–60

NOTE: N = 179.

SOURCE: Adapted from Aranciva et al. (2012).

BNT SCORES IN PREMORBID ESTIMATION

The distribution of BNT scores for healthy people deviates from the normal bell curve in that BNT scores are skewed toward the high end of the range, and most scores cluster very closely around this ceiling (Hawkins & Bender, 2002). These properties of negative skew (asymmetry) and extreme kurtosis (peakedness) mean that the test does not discriminate well at the average and higher levels. Furthermore, healthy individuals with limited vocabularies score substantially below the mean. Because small SDs are associated with extreme kurtosis, even a small deviation will suggest pathology if corrections for vocabulary and education are inadequate (Hawkins & Bender, 2002).

TABLE 11–25 Education Adjustment Table for the Aranciva et al. (2012) Spanish Boston Naming Test (BNT)

EDUCATION	ADJUSTMENT
8	+1
9	+1
10	0
11	0
12	0
13	0
14	0
15	0
16	0
17	−1
18	−1
19	−1
20	−1

NOTE: The point corresponding to the examinee's education in years is added to or subtracted from the NSS obtained from Table 11-18.

SOURCE: Adapted from Aranciva et al. (2012).

TABLE 11–26 Spanish Boston Naming Test (BNT) Norms Stratified by Education Levels for Argentina

PERCENTILE	1 TO 12 YEARS OF EDUCATION	>12 YEARS OF EDUCATION
95	57.6	–
90	55.8	60.0
85	54.5	59.3
80	53.5	58.3
70	51.8	56.6
60	50.4	55.2
50	49.1	53.9
40	47.8	52.6
30	46.4	51.2
20	44.8	49.5
15	43.7	48.5
10	42.5	47.3
5	40.6	45.4

SOURCE: From Olabarrieta-Landa et al. (2015). Reprinted from *NeuroRehabilitation, 37*, Olabarrieta-Landa, L., Rivera, D., Morlett-Paredes, A., Jaimes-Bautista, A., Garza, M. T., Galarza-del-Angel, J., ... Arango-Lasprilla, J. C, Standard form of the Boston Naming Test: Normative data for the Latin American Spanish speaking adult population, 501–513, Copyright 2015, with permission from IOS Press. The publication is available at IOS Press through http://dx.doi.org/10.3233/NRE-151278

In fact, studies generating BNT norms have generally not been adequately representative of the population, with most featuring a disproportionate representation of highly educated individuals. Hawkins and Bender (2002) recommend that BNT norms should be finely stratified by education (the norms presented by Heaton et al. [2004] are an important contribution) and that, whenever possible, the clinical interpretation of BNT scores should be further moderated by estimations of premorbid verbal ability that are fairly resistant to cerebral damage. Table 11–51 gives some performance expectations based on Gates-MacGinitie reading level (Hawkins et al., 1993).

Graves and Carswell (2003) used a sample of 98 healthy older Canadians (age $M = 71.9$ years) to develop a regression equation to predict BNT scores from the Spot-the-Word Test of the Speed and Capacity of Language Processing Test (SCOLP). The predicted premorbid BNT score is determined as follows ($r = .61$, $SEE = 2.72$ items):

$$\text{Predicted BNT} = 33.668 + 0.423(\text{STW Raw Score})$$

Table 11–52 shows the discrepancy score distributions. Discrepancies below a chosen cutoff point (which establishes the specificity for healthy individuals) can be considered abnormal (e.g., below the 5th percentile). Senior et al. (2001) also developed a regression equation to predict BNT scores using the Spot-the-Word Test in a healthy sample of individuals living in Australia. The equation is similar to the one provided by Graves and Carswell (2003).

TABLE 11–27 Spanish Boston Naming Test (BNT) Norms Stratified by Education Levels for Bolivia

PERCENTILE	1 TO 12 YEARS OF EDUCATION	>12 YEARS OF EDUCATION
95	59.4	–
90	56.3	60.0
85	54.2	57.9
80	52.4	56.2
70	49.6	53.4
60	47.3	51.0
50	45.1	48.8
40	42.9	46.7
30	40.6	44.3
20	37.8	41.5
15	36.0	39.8
10	33.9	37.7
5	30.8	34.5

SOURCE: From Olabarrieta-Landa et al. (2015). Reprinted from *NeuroRehabilitation, 37*, Olabarrieta-Landa, L., Rivera, D., Morlett-Paredes, A., Jaimes-Bautista, A., Garza, M. T., Galarza-del-Angel, J., ... Arango-Lasprilla, J. C, Standard form of the Boston Naming Test: Normative data for the Latin American Spanish speaking adult population, 501–513, Copyright 2015, with permission from IOS Press. The publication is available at IOS Press through http://dx.doi.org/10.3233/NRE-151278

EVIDENCE FOR RELIABILITY

EVIDENCE FOR INTERNAL RELIABILITY

Internal consistency (coefficient alpha) for the 60-item form is generally high, ranging between .78 and .96 (Graves et al., 2004; Fastenau et al., 1998; Franzen et al., 1995; Saxton et al., 2000; Tombaugh & Hubley, 1997; Silvestre et al., 2018; Storms et al., 2004).

EVIDENCE FOR TEST-RETEST RELIABILITY, MEASURING CHANGE, AND PRACTICE EFFECTS

Over short intervals, reliability is high. For example, Flanagan and Jackson (1997) reported that the test exhibits acceptable score stability in older, healthy, right-handed adults (aged 50–76 years) when administered with an interval of approximately one to two weeks ($r = .91$; standard error of measurement [*SEM*] = 1.02). A gain of about one point is noted on the second test session. The *SEM* of 1.02 indicates that the chances are 95 in 100 that a non–brain-injured older adult would score, on the second administration, within ± 2.04 points of the first score.

Over longer intervals, findings are mixed. Mitrushina and Satz (1995) tested 122 healthy, older Caucasian adults between the ages of 57 and 85 years on three occasions, each spaced about one year apart. Test-retest reliability coefficients were marginal to high (.62 to .89), depending on the interval, with good consistency in mean scores over the three test intervals. Lower correlations ($r = .59$) were reported by Kent and Luszcz (2002) in a community sample of older adults ($N = 326$) in Australia tested over eight years, but these are still impressive considering the time interval.

Stability has also been investigated in patients with epilepsy. A test-retest reliability of .94 was found by Sawrie et al. (1996) after eight months in 51 adults with intractable epilepsy (age $M = 31.53$, $SD = 8.09$; FSIQ $M = 90.9$, $SD = 11.25$). To detect meaningful change after epilepsy surgery, Sawrie et al. (1996) provided 90% confidence intervals (CI; ± 5 points), adjusted for expected practice effects. This interval represents a statistically derived cutoff value within which 90% of the BNT change scores theoretically reside.

TABLE 11–28 Spanish Boston Naming Test (BNT) Norms Stratified by Age and Education Levels for Chile

		AGE (YEARS)												
	PERCENTILE	18–22	23–27	28–32	33–37	38–42	43–47	48–52	53–57	58–62	63–67	68–72	73–77	>77
> 12 years of education	95	–	–	–	–	–	–	–	–	–	–	–	60.0	60.0
	90	–	–	–	–	–	–	–	60.0	60.0	60.0	60.0	59.9	59.5
	85	–	–	–	–	60.0	60.0	60.0	59.9	59.5	59.1	58.7	58.3	57.9
	80	60.0	60.0	60.0	60.0	59.8	59.4	59.0	58.6	58.2	57.8	57.4	57.0	56.6
	70	59.3	58.9	58.5	58.1	57.7	57.3	56.9	56.5	56.1	55.7	55.3	54.9	54.4
	60	57.5	57.1	56.7	56.3	55.9	55.5	55.1	54.7	54.3	53.9	53.5	53.1	52.6
	50	55.9	55.5	55.1	54.7	54.2	53.8	53.4	53.0	52.6	52.2	51.8	51.4	51.0
	40	54.2	53.8	53.4	53.0	52.6	52.2	51.8	51.4	50.9	50.5	50.1	49.7	49.3
	30	52.4	52.0	51.6	51.2	50.8	50.4	50.0	49.6	49.1	48.7	48.3	47.9	47.5
	20	50.3	49.9	49.5	49.1	48.6	48.2	47.8	47.4	47.0	46.6	46.2	45.8	45.4
	15	48.9	48.5	48.1	47.7	47.3	46.9	46.5	46.1	45.7	45.3	44.9	44.5	44.0
	10	47.3	46.9	46.5	46.1	45.7	45.3	44.9	44.5	44.1	43.7	43.3	42.9	42.5
	5	44.9	44.5	44.1	43.7	43.3	42.9	42.5	42.1	41.7	41.3	40.9	40.5	40.1
1 to 12 years of education	95	60.0	60.0	60.0	59.7	59.3	58.9	58.5	58.1	57.7	57.3	56.9	56.5	56.1
	90	58.6	58.2	57.7	57.3	56.9	56.5	56.1	55.7	55.3	54.9	54.5	54.1	53.7
	85	57.0	56.6	56.2	55.7	55.3	54.9	54.5	54.1	53.7	53.3	52.9	52.5	52.1
	80	55.6	55.2	54.8	54.4	54.0	53.6	53.2	52.8	52.4	52.0	51.6	51.1	50.7
	70	53.5	53.1	52.7	52.3	51.9	51.5	51.1	50.6	50.2	49.8	49.4	49.0	48.6
	60	51.7	51.3	50.9	50.5	50.1	49.7	49.3	48.8	48.4	48.0	47.6	47.2	46.8
	50	50.0	49.6	49.2	48.8	48.4	48.0	47.6	47.2	46.8	46.4	46.0	45.5	45.1
	40	48.4	48.0	47.6	47.1	46.7	46.3	45.9	45.5	45.1	44.7	44.3	43.9	43.5
	30	46.6	46.2	45.8	45.3	44.9	44.5	44.1	43.7	43.3	42.9	42.5	42.1	41.7
	20	44.4	44.0	43.6	43.2	42.8	42.4	42.0	41.6	41.2	40.8	40.4	40.0	39.5
	15	43.1	42.7	42.3	41.9	41.5	41.1	40.7	40.3	39.8	39.4	39.0	38.6	38.2
	10	41.5	41.1	40.7	40.3	39.9	39.5	39.1	38.7	38.2	37.8	37.4	37.0	36.6
	5	39.1	38.7	38.3	37.9	37.5	37.1	36.7	36.3	35.8	35.4	35.0	34.6	34.2

SOURCE: From Olabarrieta-Landa et al. (2015). Reprinted from *NeuroRehabilitation, 37*, Olabarrieta-Landa, L., Rivera, D., Morlett-Paredes, A., Jaimes-Bautista, A., Garza, M. T., Galarza-del-Angel, J., ... Arango-Lasprilla, J. C, Standard form of the Boston Naming Test: Normative data for the Latin American Spanish speaking adult population, 501–513, Copyright 2015, with permission from IOS Press. The publication is available at IOS Press through http://dx.doi.org/10.3233/NRE-151278

TABLE 11–29 Spanish Boston Naming Test (BNT) Norms Stratified by Age and Education Levels for Cuba

		AGE (YEARS)												
	PERCENTILE	18–22	23–27	28–32	33–37	38–42	43–47	48–52	53–57	58–62	63–67	68–72	73–77	>77
> 12 years of education	95	–	–	–	–	–	–	–	60.0	60.0	60.0	60.0	60.0	59.5
	90	–	–	–	–	60.0	60.0	60.0	59.9	59.2	58.6	58.0	57.4	56.8
	85	–	–	60.0	60.0	59.9	59.2	58.6	58.0	57.4	56.8	56.2	55.6	54.9
	80	60.0	60.0	59.6	59.0	58.3	57.7	57.1	56.5	55.9	55.3	54.6	54.0	53.4
	70	58.4	57.7	57.1	56.5	55.9	55.3	54.7	54.0	53.4	52.8	52.2	51.6	51.0
	60	56.3	55.7	55.1	54.4	53.8	53.2	52.6	52.0	51.4	50.8	50.1	49.5	48.9
	50	54.4	53.8	53.2	52.5	51.9	51.3	50.7	50.1	49.5	48.8	48.2	47.6	47.0
	40	52.5	51.9	51.2	50.6	50.0	49.4	48.8	48.2	47.6	46.9	46.3	45.7	45.1
	30	50.4	49.8	49.2	48.6	48.0	47.3	46.7	46.1	45.5	44.9	44.3	43.6	43.0
	20	48.0	47.4	46.7	46.1	45.5	44.9	44.3	43.7	43.0	42.4	41.8	41.2	40.6
	15	46.4	45.8	45.2	44.6	44.0	43.4	42.7	42.1	41.5	40.9	40.3	39.7	39.1
	10	44.6	44.0	43.4	42.8	42.1	41.5	40.9	40.3	39.7	39.1	38.5	37.8	37.2
	5	41.9	41.2	40.6	40.0	39.4	38.8	38.2	37.6	36.9	36.3	35.7	35.1	34.5
1 to 12 years of education	95	–	–	–	–	60.0	60.0	60.0	60.0	59.7	59.0	58.4	57.8	57.2
	90	–	60.0	60.0	60.0	59.4	58.8	58.1	57.5	56.9	56.3	55.7	55.1	54.4
	85	60.0	59.4	58.8	58.2	57.5	56.9	56.3	55.7	55.1	54.5	53.8	53.2	52.6
	80	58.5	57.9	57.2	56.6	56.0	55.4	54.8	54.2	53.5	52.9	52.3	51.7	51.1
	70	56.0	55.4	54.8	54.2	53.6	52.9	52.3	51.7	51.1	50.5	49.9	49.3	48.6
	60	54.0	53.3	52.7	52.1	51.5	50.9	50.3	49.7	49.0	48.4	47.8	47.2	46.6
	50	52.1	51.4	50.8	50.2	49.6	49.0	48.4	47.7	47.1	46.5	45.9	45.3	44.7
	40	50.1	49.5	48.9	48.3	47.7	47.1	46.5	45.8	45.2	44.6	44.0	43.4	42.8
	30	48.1	47.5	46.9	46.2	45.6	45.0	44.4	43.8	43.2	42.5	41.9	41.3	40.7
	20	45.6	45.0	44.4	43.8	43.2	42.6	41.9	41.3	40.7	40.1	39.5	38.9	38.3
	15	44.1	43.5	42.9	42.3	41.7	41.0	40.4	39.8	39.2	38.6	38.0	37.3	36.7
	10	42.3	41.7	41.0	40.4	39.8	39.2	38.6	38.0	37.4	36.7	36.1	35.5	34.9
	5	39.5	38.9	38.3	37.7	37.1	36.5	35.8	35.2	34.6	34.0	33.4	32.8	32.1

SOURCE: Olabarrieta-Landa et al. (2015). Reprinted from *NeuroRehabilitation, 37*, Olabarrieta-Landa, L., Rivera, D., Morlett-Paredes, A., Jaimes-Bautista, A., Garza, M. T., Galarza-del-Angel, J., ... Arango-Lasprilla, J. C, Standard form of the Boston Naming Test: Normative data for the Latin American Spanish speaking adult population, 501–513, Copyright 2015, with permission from IOS Press. The publication is available at IOS Press through http://dx.doi.org/10.3233/NRE-151278

TABLE 11–30 Spanish Boston Naming Test (BNT) Norms Stratified by Age and Education Levels for El Salvador

		AGE (YEARS)												
	PERCENTILE	18–22	23–27	28–32	33–37	38–42	43–47	48–52	53–57	58–62	63–67	68–72	73–77	>77
> 12 years of education	95	–	–	–	–	–	–	–	–	–	–	–	–	–
	90	–	–	–	–	–	–	–	–	–	–	–	60.0	60.0
	85	–	–	–	–	–	–	–	60.0	60.0	60.0	60.0	59.7	59.3
	80	–	60.0	60.0	60.0	60.0	60.0	60.0	59.8	59.4	58.9	58.5	58.1	57.7
	70	60.0	59.8	59.3	58.9	58.5	58.1	57.6	57.2	56.8	56.3	55.9	55.5	55.1
	60	58.0	57.6	57.1	56.7	56.3	55.9	55.4	55.0	54.6	54.2	53.7	53.3	52.9
	50	56.0	55.5	55.1	54.7	54.3	53.8	53.4	53.0	52.6	52.1	51.7	51.3	50.8
	40	53.9	53.5	53.1	52.7	52.2	51.8	51.4	51.0	50.5	50.1	49.7	49.2	48.8
	30	51.8	51.3	50.9	50.5	50.0	49.6	49.2	48.8	48.3	47.9	47.5	47.1	46.6
	20	49.2	48.7	48.3	47.9	47.5	47.0	46.6	46.2	45.7	45.3	44.9	44.5	44.0
	15	47.5	47.1	46.7	46.3	45.8	45.4	45.0	44.5	44.1	43.7	43.3	42.8	42.4
	10	45.6	45.2	44.7	44.3	43.9	43.5	43.0	42.6	42.2	41.7	41.3	40.9	40.5
	5	42.7	42.3	41.8	41.4	41.0	40.5	40.1	39.7	39.3	38.8	38.4	38.0	37.5
1 to 12 years of education	95	59.3	58.8	58.4	58.0	57.5	57.1	56.7	56.3	55.8	55.4	55.0	54.6	54.1
	90	56.3	55.9	55.5	55.1	54.6	54.2	53.8	53.3	52.9	52.5	52.1	51.6	51.2
	85	54.4	54.0	53.5	53.1	52.7	52.3	51.8	51.4	51.0	50.5	50.1	49.7	49.3
	80	52.8	52.3	51.9	51.5	51.1	50.6	50.2	49.8	49.4	48.9	48.5	48.1	47.6
	70	50.2	49.8	49.3	48.9	48.5	48.0	47.6	47.2	46.8	46.3	45.9	45.5	45.0
	60	48.0	47.6	47.1	46.7	46.3	45.9	45.4	45.0	44.6	44.1	43.7	43.3	42.9
	50	46.0	45.5	45.1	44.7	44.3	43.8	43.4	43.0	42.5	42.1	41.7	41.3	40.8
	40	43.9	43.5	43.1	42.7	42.2	41.8	41.4	40.9	40.5	40.1	39.7	39.2	38.8
	30	41.7	41.3	40.9	40.5	40.0	39.6	39.2	38.8	38.3	37.9	37.5	37.0	36.6
	20	39.2	38.7	38.3	37.9	37.4	37.0	36.6	36.2	35.7	35.3	34.9	34.4	34.0
	15	37.5	37.1	36.7	36.2	35.8	35.4	35.0	34.5	34.1	33.7	33.3	32.8	32.4
	10	35.6	35.2	34.7	34.3	33.9	33.4	33.0	32.6	32.2	31.7	31.3	30.9	30.4
	5	32.7	32.2	31.8	31.4	31.0	30.5	30.1	29.7	29.2	28.8	28.4	28.0	27.5

SOURCE: From Olabarrieta-Landa et al. (2015). Reprinted from *NeuroRehabilitation*, 37, Olabarrieta-Landa, L., Rivera, D., Morlett-Paredes, A., Jaimes-Bautista, A., Garza, M. T., Galarza-del-Angel, J., … Arango-Lasprilla, J. C, Standard form of the Boston Naming Test: Normative data for the Latin American Spanish speaking adult population, 501–513, Copyright 2015, with permission from IOS Press. The publication is available at IOS Press through http://dx.doi.org/10.3233/NRE-151278

Therefore, any change score equaling or exceeding this cutoff value at either end of the distribution would constitute significant change. They also derived a regression equation to predict a patient's retest score ($SEE = 2.63$):

$$Y_{predicted} = 7.61 + 0.87\ (\text{Baseline Score})$$

TABLE 11–31 Spanish Boston Naming Test (BNT) Norms Stratified by Education Levels for Guatemala

PERCENTILE	1 TO 12 YEARS OF EDUCATION	>12 YEARS OF EDUCATION
95	52.1	60.0
90	49.2	58.6
85	47.3	56.6
80	45.7	55.0
70	43.1	52.5
60	40.9	50.3
50	38.9	48.3
40	36.9	46.3
30	34.8	44.1
20	32.2	41.6
15	30.6	40.0
10	28.7	38.0
5	25.8	35.1

SOURCE: From Olabarrieta-Landa et al. (2015). Reprinted from *NeuroRehabilitation*, 37, Olabarrieta-Landa, L., Rivera, D., Morlett-Paredes, A., Jaimes-Bautista, A., Garza, M. T., Galarza-del-Angel, J., … Arango-Lasprilla, J. C, Standard form of the Boston Naming Test: Normative data for the Latin American Spanish speaking adult population, 501–513, Copyright 2015, with permission from IOS Press. The publication is available at IOS Press through http://dx.doi.org/10.3233/NRE-151278

The predicted value can be compared to the patient's observed score to quantify the magnitude and direction of change. The difference between the predicted score and the observed retest score is transformed into a standardized *z* score using the following equation:

$$z\ \text{score} = (Y_{observed} - Y_{predicted})/SEE$$

Statistically meaningful and significant change ($p < .05$) can be identified when the standardized change score exceeds ± 1.64 *SDs*.

A reliable change index (RCI) for the BNT based on healthy adults older than age 56 years tested between nine to 24 months after baseline was provided by Sachs et al. (2012) as seen in Table 11–53. Family history of dementia did not change the RCI. At the respective cutoff RCI score, 6% of the healthy sample declined four or more points over nine to 15 months and 7% improved at least by five points. Over 16–24 months, 7% declined at least six points and 5% improved by at least seven points. These data also show that practice effects are negligible.

EVIDENCE FOR RELIABILITY OF ALTERNATE AND SHORT FORMS

Reliability is high for the versions developed by Graves et al. (2004), with alphas of .84 for the 15-item form and .90 for the 30-item form (Graves et al., 2004; Tombaugh & Hubley, 1997). Cronbach's alphas of the Chinese Short

TABLE 11–32 Spanish Boston Naming Test (BNT) Norms Stratified by Age and Education Levels for Mexico

		AGE (YEARS)												
	PERCENTILE	18–22	23–27	28–32	33–37	38–42	43–47	48–52	53–57	58–62	63–67	68–72	73–77	>77
> 12 years of education	95	–	–	–	–	–	–	–	60.0	60.0	60.0	60.0	60.0	60.0
	90	–	–	–	60.0	60.0	60.0	60.0	59.9	59.5	59.1	58.7	58.3	57.9
	85	60.0	60.0	60.0	59.9	59.5	59.1	58.7	58.3	57.9	57.5	57.1	56.7	56.3
	80	59.8	59.4	59.0	58.5	58.1	57.7	57.3	56.9	56.5	56.1	55.7	55.3	54.9
	70	57.6	57.2	56.8	56.4	56.0	55.6	55.2	54.8	54.3	53.9	53.5	53.1	52.7
	60	55.7	55.3	54.9	54.5	54.1	53.7	53.3	52.9	52.5	52.1	51.7	51.3	50.9
	50	54.0	53.6	53.2	52.8	52.4	52.0	51.6	51.2	50.8	50.4	50.0	49.6	49.2
	40	52.3	51.9	51.5	51.1	50.7	50.3	49.9	49.5	49.1	48.7	48.3	47.9	47.5
	30	50.5	50.1	49.7	49.3	48.9	48.5	48.1	47.7	47.3	46.9	46.4	46.0	45.6
	20	48.3	47.9	47.5	47.1	46.7	46.3	45.9	45.5	45.1	44.7	44.3	43.9	43.5
	15	46.9	46.5	46.1	45.7	45.3	44.9	44.5	44.1	43.7	43.3	42.9	42.5	42.1
	10	45.3	44.9	44.5	44.1	43.7	43.3	42.9	42.5	42.1	41.7	41.3	40.9	40.5
	5	42.8	42.4	42.0	41.6	41.2	40.8	40.4	40.0	39.6	39.2	38.8	38.4	38.0
1 to 12 years of education	95	60.0	60.0	59.8	59.4	59.0	58.6	58.2	57.8	57.4	57.0	56.6	56.2	55.8
	90	58.2	57.8	57.4	57.0	56.6	56.2	55.7	55.3	54.9	54.5	54.1	53.7	53.3
	85	56.5	56.1	55.7	55.3	54.9	54.5	54.1	53.7	53.3	52.9	52.5	52.1	51.7
	80	55.2	54.8	54.4	54.0	53.6	53.1	52.7	52.3	51.9	51.5	51.1	50.7	50.3
	70	53.0	52.6	52.2	51.8	51.4	51.0	50.6	50.2	49.8	49.4	48.9	48.5	48.1
	60	51.1	50.7	50.3	49.9	49.5	49.1	48.7	48.3	47.9	47.5	47.1	46.7	46.3
	50	49.4	49.0	48.6	48.2	47.8	47.4	47.0	46.6	46.2	45.8	45.4	45.0	44.6
	40	47.7	47.3	46.9	46.5	46.1	45.7	45.3	44.9	44.5	44.1	43.7	43.3	42.9
	30	45.9	45.5	45.1	44.7	44.3	43.9	43.5	43.1	42.7	42.3	41.9	41.5	41.0
	20	43.7	43.3	42.9	42.5	42.1	41.7	41.3	40.9	40.5	40.1	39.7	39.3	38.9
	15	42.3	41.9	41.5	41.1	40.7	40.3	39.9	39.5	39.1	38.7	38.3	37.9	37.5
	10	40.7	40.3	39.9	39.5	39.1	38.7	38.3	37.9	37.5	37.1	36.7	36.3	35.9
	5	38.3	37.9	37.4	37.0	36.6	36.2	35.8	35.4	35.0	34.6	34.2	33.8	33.4

SOURCE: From Olabarrieta-Landa et al. (2015). Reprinted from *NeuroRehabilitation, 37*, Olabarrieta-Landa, L., Rivera, D., Morlett-Paredes, A., Jaimes-Bautista, A., Garza, M. T., Galarza-del-Angel, J., ... Arango-Lasprilla, J. C, Standard form of the Boston Naming Test: Normative data for the Latin American Spanish speaking adult population, 501–513, Copyright 2015, with permission from IOS Press. The publication is available at IOS Press through http://dx.doi.org/10.3233/NRE-151278

Form (Cheung et al., 2004) are adequate to high, ranging from .70 in healthy individuals to .83 in brain-injured patients. Cronbach's alphas of all four Casals-Coll et al. (2014) Spanish Short Forms are satisfactory (.74 to .78).

EVIDENCE FOR INTERRATER RELIABILITY

Inconsistency in administration and scoring is a major criticism of the BNT. See the "Comments" section for further discussion.

TABLE 11–33 Spanish Boston Naming Test (BNT) Norms Stratified by Education Levels for Paraguay

PERCENTILE	1 TO 12 YEARS OF EDUCATION	>12 YEARS OF EDUCATION
95	60.0	–
90	59.7	–
85	58.9	–
80	58.2	60.0
70	57.1	59.3
60	56.1	58.3
50	55.2	57.4
40	54.3	56.6
30	53.4	55.6
20	52.3	54.5
15	51.6	53.8
10	50.7	52.9
5	49.4	51.7

SOURCE: Olabarrieta-Landa et al. (2015). Reprinted from *NeuroRehabilitation, 37*, Olabarrieta-Landa, L., Rivera, D., Morlett-Paredes, A., Jaimes-Bautista, A., Garza, M. T., Galarza-del-Angel, J., ... Arango-Lasprilla, J. C, Standard form of the Boston Naming Test: Normative data for the Latin American Spanish speaking adult population, 501–513, Copyright 2015, with permission from IOS Press. The publication is available at IOS Press through http://dx.doi.org/10.3233/NRE-151278

EVIDENCE FOR VALIDITY

RELATIONSHIPS BETWEEN THE STANDARD FORM AND SHORT FORMS

Correlations among the various short forms tend to be moderate to high (e.g., $r = .42$ to .62 for the 15-item Mack SF4 [Mack et al., 1992]) when the various short forms are given in counterbalanced order (rather than extrapolating data

TABLE 11–34 Spanish Boston Naming Test (BNT) Norms Stratified by Education Levels for Peru

PERCENTILE	1 TO 12 YEARS OF EDUCATION	>12 YEARS OF EDUCATION
95	54.2	–
90	52.1	60.0
85	50.8	59.0
80	49.6	57.8
70	47.8	56.0
60	46.3	54.5
50	44.8	53.1
40	43.4	51.6
30	41.9	50.1
20	40.0	48.3
15	38.9	47.1
10	37.5	45.8
5	35.5	43.7

SOURCE: From Olabarrieta-Landa et al. (2015). Reprinted from *NeuroRehabilitation, 37*, Olabarrieta-Landa, L., Rivera, D., Morlett-Paredes, A., Jaimes-Bautista, A., Garza, M. T., Galarza-del-Angel, J., ... Arango-Lasprilla, J. C, Standard form of the Boston Naming Test: Normative data for the Latin American Spanish speaking adult population, 501–513, Copyright 2015, with permission from IOS Press. The publication is available at IOS Press through http://dx.doi.org/10.3233/NRE-151278

TABLE 11–35 Spanish Boston Naming Test (BNT) Norms Stratified by Age and Education Levels for Puerto Rico

		AGE (YEARS)												
	PERCENTILE	18–22	23–27	28–32	33–37	38–42	43–47	48–52	53–57	58–62	63–67	68–72	73–77	>77
> 12 years of education	95	–	–	–	–	–	–	60.0	60.0	60.0	60.0	60.0	59.5	58.9
	90	–	–	–	60.0	60.0	60.0	59.5	58.9	58.3	57.8	57.2	56.6	56.0
	85	60.0	60.0	60.0	59.4	58.8	58.2	57.6	57.0	56.4	55.8	55.2	54.6	54.0
	80	59.6	59.0	58.4	57.8	57.2	56.6	56.0	55.4	54.8	54.2	53.2	53.0	52.4
	70	57.0	56.4	55.8	55.2	54.6	54.0	53.4	52.8	52.2	51.6	51.0	50.4	49.8
	60	54.8	54.2	53.6	53.0	52.4	51.8	51.2	50.6	50.0	49.4	48.8	48.2	47.6
	50	52.8	52.2	51.6	51.0	50.4	49.8	49.2	48.6	48.0	47.4	46.8	46.2	45.6
	40	50.7	50.1	49.5	48.9	48.3	47.7	47.1	46.5	45.9	45.4	44.8	44.2	43.6
	30	48.5	47.9	47.3	46.7	46.2	45.6	45.0	44.4	43.8	43.2	42.6	42.0	41.4
	20	45.9	45.4	44.8	44.2	43.6	43.0	42.4	41.8	41.2	40.6	40.0	39.4	38.8
	15	44.3	43.7	43.1	42.5	41.9	41.3	40.7	40.1	39.5	38.9	38.3	37.8	37.2
	10	42.4	41.8	41.2	40.6	40.0	39.4	38.8	38.2	37.6	37.0	36.4	35.8	35.2
	5	39.5	38.9	38.3	37.7	37.1	36.5	35.9	35.3	34.7	34.1	33.5	32.9	32.3
1 to 12 years of education	95	–	–	60.0	60.0	60.0	60.0	60.0	59.4	58.8	58.2	57.6	57.0	56.4
	90	60.0	60.0	59.4	58.8	58.2	57.6	57.0	56.4	55.8	55.2	54.6	54.0	53.5
	85	58.7	58.1	57.5	56.9	56.3	55.7	55.1	54.5	53.9	53.3	52.7	52.1	51.5
	80	57.1	56.5	55.9	55.3	54.7	54.1	53.5	52.9	52.3	51.7	51.1	50.5	49.9
	70	54.5	53.9	53.3	52.7	52.1	51.5	50.9	50.3	49.7	49.1	48.5	47.9	47.3
	60	52.3	51.7	51.1	50.5	49.9	49.3	48.7	48.1	47.5	46.9	46.3	45.7	45.1
	50	50.3	49.7	49.1	48.5	47.9	47.3	46.7	46.1	45.5	44.9	44.3	43.7	43.1
	40	48.2	47.6	47.0	46.4	45.8	45.2	44.6	44.0	43.4	42.8	42.2	41.6	41.1
	30	46.0	45.4	44.8	44.2	43.6	43.0	42.4	41.9	41.3	40.7	40.1	39.5	38.9
	20	43.4	42.8	42.2	41.6	41.1	40.5	39.9	39.3	38.7	38.1	37.5	36.9	36.3
	15	41.8	41.2	40.6	40.0	39.4	38.8	38.2	37.6	37.0	36.4	35.8	35.2	34.6
	10	39.9	39.3	38.7	38.1	37.5	36.9	36.3	35.7	35.1	34.5	33.9	33.3	32.7
	5	37.0	36.4	35.8	35.2	34.6	34.0	33.4	32.8	32.2	31.6	31.0	30.4	29.8

SOURCE: Olabarrieta-Landa et al. (2015). Reprinted from *NeuroRehabilitation, 37*, Olabarrieta-Landa, L., Rivera, D., Morlett-Paredes, A., Jaimes-Bautista, A., Garza, M. T., Galarza-del-Angel, J., … Arango-Lasprilla, J. C, Standard form of the Boston Naming Test: Normative data for the Latin American Spanish speaking adult population, 501–513, Copyright 2015, with permission from IOS Press. The publication is available at IOS Press through http://dx.doi.org/10.3233/NRE-151278

for shortened versions after the entire 60-item test is given; Fastenau et al., 1998; Kent & Luszcz, 2002). Correlations between the Mack SF4 and the full BNT 60 tend to be high (r = .62 to .98; Mack et al., 1992; Graves et al., 2004; Fastenau et al., 1998; Franzen et al., 1995), although agreement between the tests regarding abnormality is not guaranteed (Franzen et al., 1995; Graves et al., 2004). Better agreement with the full BNT is obtained with the 30-item version developed by Graves et al. (2004). The Graves et al. (2004) 15-item short form also agrees well with the classifications made by the full BNT (e.g., kappa > .80). Moderate to high correlations are reported among the four Casals-Coll et al. (2014) short forms (r = .78 to .81) and correlations with the full version are very high (r = .92 to .93; Casals-Coll et al., 2014).

Hobson et al. (2011) examined the ability of short forms (30-item, even and odd forms) to estimate full BNT score using a clinical database of patients with AD (N = 120) and healthy controls (N = 29). The 30-item form was multiplied by two to obtain a BNT estimate. Both 30-item forms were highly correlated with the original for the total sample (r = .98) and subgroups (r > .92). The diagnostic utility based on the receiver operating curve (ROC) yielded comparable results to the original

TABLE 11–36 Alternative BNT Spanish Responses Accepted in Silvestre et al. (2018)

ORIGINAL	SPANISH COMMON NAME	ALTERNATIVE NAME
Tree	Árbol	Mata
Whistle	Silbato	Pito
Saw	Serrucho	Sierra
Toothbrush	Cepillo de dientes	Cepillo dental
Hanger	Percha	Gancho
Camel	Camello	Dromedario
Mask	Máscara	Careta
Cupcake	Bizcocho	Bizcochito, Helado
Seahorse	Caballito de mar	Caballo de mar
Canoe	Canoa	Bote
Globe	Globo	Globo terraqueo, Mapamundi
Harmonica	Armónica	Acordeón de boca
Igloo	Iglú	Horno
Domino	Dominó	Dominós
Cactus	Cactus	Cayuco, Tuna, Alquitira
Escalator	Escalera mecánica	Escalera eléctrica
Lock	Cerradura	Llavín
Pacifier	Chupete	Bobo
Tongs	Pinzas	Tenaza
Yoke	Yugo	Yunta
Watering can	Regadera	Regador
Abacus	Ábaco	Contador

SOURCE: Adapted from Silvestre et al. (2018).

TABLE 11–37 Dominican Spanish Boston Naming Test (BNT) Norms Stratified by Education Level

EDUCATION (YEARS)	*N*	MEAN	*SD*
0 to 6	77	34.78	6.76
7 to 12	80	39.09	7.45
13+	82	46.71	6.82

SOURCE: Silvestre et al. (2018).

TABLE 11–38 Boston Naming Test (BNT) 30-Item Short Form Norms for Australian-Born Women

	EDUCATION						
	<12 YEARS			≥ 12 YEARS			
	56–59 (*N* = 76)	60–67 (*N* = 53)	OVERALL (*N* = 129)	56–59 (*N* = 70)	60–67 (*N* = 51)	OVERALL (*N* = 121)	OVERALL (*N* = 250)
M	26.63	26.70	26.67	27.68	27.80	27.73	27.18
SD	0.28	0.28	0.20	0.23	0.29	0.12	0.14

NOTE: This version used standard instructions except that items were administered starting at item 1.

SOURCE: From Elkadi et al. (2006).

BNT in this sample, with an area under the curve (AUC) of .93 for the 30-item (even) and an AUC of .95 for the 30-item (odd). For the 30-item (odd), a cutoff of 51/52 yielded a sensitivity of 89% and a specificity of 84%. For the 30-item (even), a cutoff of 49/50 yielded a sensitivity and a specificity of 83%. For the 15-item, cutoffs of 49/50/51/52 all yielded a sensitivity of 86% and a specificity of 84% for the identification of AD. Given the comparable findings between the 30-item and original version, norms for the original version can be used in clinical settings to interpret estimated scores from the 30-item forms (Hobson et al., 2011).

RELATIONSHIPS WITH OTHER TESTS

Several studies have related scores on the BNT with those on other language-related measures. For example, the BNT correlates highly ($r = .76$ to .86) with the Visual Naming Test of the Multilingual Aphasia Examination (Axelrod et al., 1994; Schefft et al., 2003), and moderately with the Pyramids and Palm Trees test ($r = .60$; Rami et al., 2008). The Spanish BNT is moderately correlated with animal fluency ($r = .50$) in healthy older adults age 60+ (Rami et al., 2008).

The BNT is also related to measures of intelligence. In the Mayo's Older American Normative Studies (MOANS) sample of older adults, the BNT loaded onto a Verbal Comprehension factor in a five-factor model along with WAIS-III Vocabulary, Information, and Similarities, as well as WRAT-3 Reading and the Controlled Oral Word Association Test [COWAT] (Greenaway et al., 2009). Axelrod et al. (1994) reported that, in their mixed clinical sample, the BNT was highly dependent on verbal intellectual ability (Verbal Comprehension Factor of the WAIS-R) and negligibly influenced by perceptual organization skills and distractibility. Schefft et al. (2003) reported that, in patients with seizures, the BNT showed stronger relations with Verbal IQ (VIQ; $r = .61$) than with Performance IQ (PIQ; $r = .43$). However, in healthy, older adults, BNT scores show moderate relations (.41) with both verbal (VIQ) and nonverbal (PIQ) ability (Mitrushina & Satz, 1995), though a more recent study reported that the relationship between PRI and BNT performance was fully mediated by verbal comprehension (Soble et al., 2016).

TABLE 11–39 Recommended Cutoff Scores for Boston Naming Test (BNT) Short Forms by Graves et al. (2004)

	20TH PERCENTILE	10TH PERCENTILE
Graves et al. BNT 30	<25	<22
Graves et al. BNT 15	<11	<10

SOURCE: Adapted from Graves et al. (2004).

There is some suggestion that the strategies older individuals use to retrieve names may change with time, with predominantly verbal processing on the first occasion shifting to predominantly visual-spatial processing later on (Mitrushina & Satz, 1995). Visual acuity has been shown to be negatively correlated with BNT performance (Worrall et al., 1995), but only to a small extent (Kent & Luszcz, 2002).

The interchangeability of the BNT, Neuropsychological Assessment Battery (NAB) Naming, Repeatable Battery for the Assessment of Neuropsychological Status (RBANS) Naming subtest, and Auditory Naming Test (Hamberger & Seidel, 2003; Brandt et al., 2010) for assessing word-finding difficulty appears to be affected by the frequency of everyday use of the words in each test. Yochim et al. (2013) compared these naming measures using results from the Elexicon Project, a study that assembled a corpus of words extracted from films and television in order to examine how well these naming tests tap into everyday language and, consequently, how sensitive they are to word-finding problems in everyday spoken language. From highest to lowest mean spoken-word frequency, the Brandt et al. (2010) Auditory Naming Test was found to contain words with the highest spoken-word frequency, followed by the Hamberger and Seidel (2003) Auditory Naming Test, RBANS Naming Form B, BNT items 1-60, RBANS Form A, NAB Form 2, NAB Form 1, and finally, BNT items 30–60. Not surprisingly, they found that the word order of BNT items 1–60 was negatively correlated with frequency of spoken word usage, and items 30–60 were the most difficult. These results indicated high variability in word frequency among these various naming tests, suggesting differential sensitivity to word-finding difficulty. As such, different diagnostic impressions may be elicited depending on the naming test used and whether it taps auditory or visual naming.

CLINICAL STUDIES

Poor performance on the BNT can occur in a variety of clinical conditions, including left-hemisphere cerebrovascular

TABLE 11-40 Boston Naming Test (BNT 30) Norms as a Function of Age and Education Using the Jefferson et al. (2007) Short Form

AGE AND EDUCATION	N	MIN	MAX	M (SD)	CUTOFF (-1.5 SD)	CUTOFF (-2.0 SD)
55 to 64 years old						
High school or less	3	26	28	27.3 (1.2)	26	25
Some college	7	28	30	29.3 (0.8)	28	28
College graduate	10	28	30	29.6 (0.7)	29	28
Less than graduate degree	16	24	30	28.8 (1.6)	26	26
Graduate degree	11	26	30	28.9 (1.4)	27	26
65 to 74 years old						
High school or less	10	22	30	27.1 (3.1)	22	21
Some college	13	24	30	28.3 (1.7)	26	25
College graduate	14	25	30	28.5 (1.8)	26	25
Less than graduate degree	24	26	30	29.5 (0.9)	28	28
Graduate degree	22	25	30	29.3 (1.2)	28	27
75 to 84 years old						
High school or less	12	22	29	27.0 (1.9)	24	23
Some college	17	22	30	27.9 (2.2)	25	24
College graduate	13	25	30	28.6 (1.6)	26	25
Less than graduate degree	22	23	30	28.6 (2.1)	25	24
Graduate degree	9	28	30	29.0 (0.9)	28	27
85+ years old						
High school or less	4	27	30	28.5 (1.7)	26	25
Some college	3	26	30	28.0 (2.0)	25	24
College graduate	3	29	30	29.7 (0.6)	29	29
Less than graduate degree	1	30	30	30.0 (0.0)	–	–
Graduate degree	5	27	30	29.0 (1.2)	27	27

NOTE: Cutoff scores are intended to reflect values where at least mild (–1.5 *SD*) or moderate (–2.0 *SD*) impairment is present in reference to the normative sample.

NOTE: The Jefferson et al. Short Form is made up of 30 even items from the original BNT. Total score was based on correct spontaneous responses and correct responses after stimulus cues.

SOURCE: From Jefferson et al. (2007).

accidents (CVAs; e.g., Kohn & Goodglass, 1985), anoxia (Tweedy & Schulman, 1982), subcortical disease (MS and PD; Henry & Crawford, 2004; Lezak et al., 1990; Locascio et al., 2003), small white matter infarcts in the brainstem (van Zandvoort et al., 2003), and prenatal exposure (Debes et al., 2016). The BNT is also sensitive as a tool to the effects of six weeks of treatment using epidural cortical stimulation plus language treatment or language treatment alone in stroke survivors with nonfluent aphasia (Cherney et al., 2012). By contrast, patients with Huntington's disease do not show BNT impairments even though they differ from healthy controls on other language tasks (e.g., BDAE subtests; Azambuja et al., 2012).

AD. The presence of anomia in AD is well documented. Patients with AD tend to show impairment on the BNT (Henry et al., 2004; Lansing et al., 1999; Mack et al., 1992; Testa et al., 2004), more so than patients with VaD (Barr et al., 1992; Lukatela et al., 1998). BNT impairment occurs regardless of disease severity in AD; however, it is ubiquitous only in moderate to severe dementia (Testa et al.,

TABLE 11-41 Boston Naming Test (BNT 30) Short Form Norms as a Function of Reading Level (WRAT-3 Reading)

AGE RANGE	N	MIN	MAX	M (SD)	CUTOFF (-1.5 SD)	CUTOFF (-2.0 SD)
Average reading level						
55 to 64 years old	21	26	30	28.8 (1.3)	27	26
65 to 74 years old	15	23	30	27.4 (2.1)	24	23
75 to 84 years old	11	22	29	26.7 (2.1)	26	25
85+ years old	–	–	–	–	–	–
High-average or better reading level						
55 to 64 years old	25	26	30	29.3 (0.9)	28	28
65 to 74 years old	67	22	30	29.1 (1.6)	27	26
75 to 84 years old	61	22	30	28.5 (1.8)	26	25
85+ years old	15	26	30	29.0 (1.4)	27	26

NOTE: **n* = 215; 4 participants did not complete the WRAT-3; cutoff scores are intended to reflect values where at least mild (–1.5 *SD*) or moderate (–1.5 *SD*) or severe (–2.0 *SD*) impairment is present in reference to the normative sample.

NOTE: The Jefferson et al. Short Form is made up of 30 even-items from the original BNT. Total score was based on correct spontaneous responses and correct responses after stimulus cues. WRAT, Wide Range Achievement Test.

SOURCE: From Jefferson et al. (2007).

TABLE 11–42 Characteristics of the Boston Naming Test (BNT 30) Short Form Normative Sample from the Calibrated Neuropsychological Normative System (CNNS)

Sample size	325
Age	18 to 92 years
Geographic location	Baltimore, MD, and Hartford, CT
Sample type	Community sample
Education	14.2 (*SD* = 3.0), range 3 to 20 years
Gender	56% Women 44% Men
Race/Ethnicity	80% Caucasian 18% African American 2% Hispanic, Asian, or Other
Screening	History of Alzheimer's disease, Parkinson's disease, stroke, brain injury, bipolar disorder, or substance abuse

SOURCE: Adapted from Schretlen, Testa, and Pearlson (2010).

2004). Therefore, impairment does not appear to be necessary for a diagnosis of AD. Furthermore, BNT impairment is not particularly useful in discriminating individuals at baseline who are subsequently diagnosed with AD, and measures of delayed recall (e.g., percent retention on the Rey Auditory Verbal Learning Test [RAVLT]) prove more useful in predicting conversion to AD (Testa et al., 2004). Finally, BNT scores are not especially useful in predicting rates of cognitive deterioration in AD. Beatty et al. (2002) found that poor performance on the BNT and young age identified AD patients at greater risk for cognitive decline (as measured with the Dementia Rating Scale one year later), although this accounted for only 6% of the variance.

The mechanism underlying naming deficits in AD is controversial. Most investigations rule out disruption in the perceptual stage as a primary cause of this breakdown; however, the relative contributions of disturbance in lexical retrieval and content and organization of the semantic system are issues of debate (Mitrushina et al., 2005). Similar controversy surrounds the nature of the age-related decline in BNT performance (Mitrushina et al., 2005). One study may provide some insight into this. Balthazar and colleagues (2008) reported that a mild AD group obtained impaired scores while an amnestic MCI group obtained normal scores and were helped by semantic cues. The mild AD group on the other hand did not benefit from semantic cues to the same degree as amnestic MCI and healthy groups. However, with phonemic cues, all three groups performed similarly.

Interestingly, Karrasch and colleagues (2010) developed a novel approach using the Finnish BNT (memo-BNT) to assess incidental memory. They administered the Finnish BNT with only the last 31 items given. Correct answers were given if the examinee failed to name the item despite phonemic cueing. Whereas no difference in memo-BNT scores were found between the healthy young (mean age 21.7) and healthy old (mean age 70.6), memo-BNT scores differentiated among mild AD and healthy groups. Incidental free recall was best at discriminating the AD and healthy old controls, and it was also better than naming itself. Incidental memory after administration of

TABLE 11–43 Age-Adjusted Scaled Scores (NSS_A) for the BNT A Short Form

SCALED SCORE	PERCENTILE RANGE	AGE RANGE 50–56	57–59	60–62	63–65	66–68	69–71	72–74	75–77	78–80	81+
2	<1	≤7	≤6	≤6	≤6	≤6	≤6	≤5	≤4	≤4	≤4
3	1		7	7					5	5	
4	2						7	6			5
5	3–5	8	8	8	7–8	7–8	8	7	6		
6	6–10	9					9	8	7	6	6
7	11–18	10	9	9	9	9–10	10	9	8–9	7	7
8	19–28		10	10	10			10		8–9	8–9
9	29–40	11	11	11	11	11	11		10	10	10
10	41–59	12	12	12	12	12	12	11–12	11	11	11
11	60–71	13	13	13	13	13	13		12		
12	72–81							13	13	12	12
13	82–89	14									13
14	90–94		14	14	14					13	
15	95–97					14	14	14			
16	98								14		14
17	99									14	
18	>99	15	15	15	15	15	15	15	15	15	15
Age range[a]		50–60	53–63	56–66	59–69	62–72	65–75	68–78	71–81	74–84	77–90
Sample size		134	132	123	105	118	124	125	100	67	42

NOTE: Based on *N* = 340 healthy adults from Spain with mean age = 65 years, *SD* = 9.3, range = 50–85; females = 59%; mean education = 10.5 years, *SD* = 5.5; 20% had <6 years of education, 44% had 6–12 years of education, and the rest had >12 years of education. The items can be found in Table 11-9.

[a] This is the range of ages contributing to each normative subsample.

SOURCE: From Casals-Coll et al. (2014).

TABLE 11-44 Age-Adjusted Scaled Scores (NSS$_A$) for the BNT B Short Form

SCALED SCORE	PERCENTILE RANGE	AGE RANGE									
		50–56	57–59	60–62	63–65	66–68	69–71	72–74	75–77	78–80	81+
2	<1	≤7	≤7	≤7	≤6	≤6	≤6	≤5	≤5	≤5	≤5
3	1	8			7	7		6			
4	2										
5	3–5	9	8	8			7	7	6	6	6
6	6–10	10	9	9	8	8	8	8	7	7	
7	11–18		10	10	9	9	9	9	8	8	7
8	19–28	11	11	11	10	10	10		9	9	8
9	29–40				11	11		10	10	10	9–10
10	41–59	12	12	12	12	12	11	11	11	11	11
11	60–71						12	12	12		
12	72–81	13	13	13	13	13	13			12	12
13	82–89							13	13		
14	90–94									13	13
15	95–97	14	14	14			14				
16	98				14	14		14	14		14
17	99									14	
18	>99	15	15	15	15	15	15	15	15	15	15
Age range[a]		50–60	53–63	56–66	59–69	62–72	65–75	68–78	71–81	74–84	77–90
Sample size		134	132	123	105	118	124	125	100	67	42

NOTE: Based on N = 340 healthy adults from Spain with mean age = 65 years, SD = 9.3, range = 50–85; females = 59%; mean education = 10.5 years, SD = 5.5; 20% had <6 years of education, 44% had 6–12 years of education, and the rest had >12 years of education. The items can be found in Table 11-9.

[a] This is the range of ages contributing to each normative subsample.

SOURCE: From Casals-Coll et al. (2014).

BNT naming may have clinical utility in identifying AD, though this is a preliminary finding because of the small sample size.

BNT scores given in both dominant and nondominant languages to bilinguals are predictive of age of diagnosis of AD, not self-reported degree of bilingualism, and the benefits of bilingualism in delaying AD onset are only seen in those with low education (Gollan et al., 2011). Spanish-English bilinguals with AD perform worse than matched bilingual controls on the BNT using their dominant language, whereas better BNT performance is obtained using their nondominant language. It may be that the

TABLE 11-45 Age-Adjusted Scaled Scores (NSS$_A$) for the BNT C Short Form

SCALED SCORE	PERCENTILE RANGE	AGE RANGE									
		50–56	57–59	60–62	63–65	66–68	69–71	72–74	75–77	78–80	81+
2	<1	≤9	≤6	≤6	≤6	≤6	≤6	≤5	≤5	≤5	≤5
3	1							6	6	6	
4	2		7				7				6
5	3–5		8–9	7	7	7	8	7	7		
6	6–10			8–9	8	8	9	8		7	7
7	11–18	10	10		9	9–10		9	8–9		
8	19–28			10	10		10	10	10	8–9	8
9	29–40	11	11	11	11	11				10	9–10
10	41–59	12	12	12	12		11	11	11	11	11
11	60–71	13				12	12	12	12		
12	72–81		13	13	13		13			12	12
13	82–89	14	14	14		13–14	14	13	13	13	
14	90–94				14			14	14		13
15	95–97									14	
16	98										14
17	99										
18	>99	15	15	15	15	15	15	15	15	15	15
Age range[a]		50–60	53–63	56–66	59–69	62–72	65–75	68–78	71–81	74–84	77–90
Sample size		134	132	123	105	118	124	125	100	67	42

NOTE: Based on N = 340 healthy adults from Spain with mean age = 65 years, SD = 9.3, range = 50–85; females = 59%; mean education = 10.5 years, SD = 5.5; 20% had <6 years of education, 44% had 6–12 years of education, and the rest had >12 years of education. The items can be found in Table 11-9.

[a] This is the range of ages contributing to each normative subsample.

SOURCE: Casals-Coll et al. (2014).

TABLE 11-46 Age-Adjusted Scaled Scores (NSS_A) for the BNT D Short Form

SCALED SCORE	PERCENTILE RANGE	AGE RANGE									
		50–56	57–59	60–62	63–65	66–68	69–71	72–74	75–77	78–80	81+
2	<1	≤7	≤6	≤7	≤6	≤6	≤5	≤5	≤4	≤4	≤4
3	1		7				6		5	5	
4	2				7	7					5
5	3–5	8					7	6–7	6–7		
6	6–10	9	8	8	8	8	8	8	8	6–7	6–7
7	11–18	10	9	9	9	9	9	9		8	8
8	19–28	11	10	10	10	10	10		9	9	
9	29–40	12	11	11	11	11	11	10–11	10		9
10	41–59		12	12	12	12	12	12	11	10–11	10–11
11	60–71	13	13	13	13	13			12	12	12
12	72–81	14					13	13			
13	82–89		14	14	14	14			13		13
14	90–94						14			13	
15	95–97							14	14		
16	98										
17	99										
18	>99	15	15	15	15	15	15	15	15	14	14
Age range[a]		50–60	53–63	56–66	59–69	62–72	65–75	68–78	71–81	74–84	77–90
Sample size		134	132	123	105	118	124	125	100	67	42

NOTE: Based on N = 340 healthy adults from Spain with mean age = 65 years, SD = 9.3, range = 50–85; females = 59%; mean education = 10.5 years, SD = 5.5; 20% had <6 years of education, 44% had 6–12 years of education, and the rest had >12 years of education. The items can be found in Table 11–9.

[a] This is the range of ages contributing to each normative subsample.

SOURCE: From Casals-Coll et al. (2014).

nondominant language is less vulnerable than the dominant language to dementia (Gollan et al., 2010).

Finally, improvement in BNT scores of about 1.6 points among older adults with probable AD after memantine treatment has been reported (Weiner et al., 2011).

Error Types. Verbal semantic paraphasias and "don't know" responses are the most common types of errors in adults (Marien et al., 1998; Tombaugh & Hubley, 1997). Neologisms, delayed responses, empty words, and phonemic paraphasias are rare in healthy individuals. Among patients with amnestic MCI and mild AD, coordinate errors (incorrect responses in the same category as correct answer) are the most frequent, followed by superordinate errors (responses belonging to a broader category than the correct answer) and circumlocutory errors (describing responses or function of item; Balthazar et al., 2008). Patients with AD are more likely to make associative and semantic errors whereas patients with dementia with Lewy bodies (DLB)

TABLE 11-47 Education Adjustment for the BNT A Short Form

NSS_A	EDUCATION (YEARS) 0	1	2	3	4	5	6	7	8	9	10	11	12	13	14	15	16	17	18	19	20
2	5	4	4	4	4	3	3	3	3	2	2	2	2	1	1	1	0	0	0	0	–1
3	6	5	5	5	5	4	4	4	4	3	3	3	3	2	2	2	1	1	1	1	0
4	7	6	6	6	6	5	5	5	5	4	4	4	4	3	3	3	2	2	2	2	1
5	8	7	7	7	7	6	6	6	6	5	5	5	5	4	4	4	3	3	3	3	2
6	9	8	8	8	8	7	7	7	7	6	6	6	6	5	5	5	4	4	4	4	3
7	10	9	9	9	9	8	8	8	8	7	7	7	7	6	6	6	5	5	5	5	4
8	11	10	10	10	10	9	9	9	9	8	8	8	8	7	7	7	6	6	6	6	5
9	12	11	11	11	11	10	10	10	10	9	9	9	9	8	8	8	7	7	7	7	6
10	13	12	12	12	12	11	11	11	11	10	10	10	10	9	9	9	8	8	8	8	7
11	14	13	13	13	13	12	12	12	12	11	11	11	11	10	10	10	9	9	9	9	8
12	15	14	14	14	14	13	13	13	13	12	12	12	12	11	11	11	10	10	10	10	9
13	16	15	15	15	15	14	14	14	14	13	13	13	13	12	12	12	11	11	11	11	10
14	17	16	16	16	16	15	15	15	15	14	14	14	14	13	13	13	12	12	12	12	11
15	18	17	17	17	17	16	16	16	16	15	15	15	15	14	14	14	13	13	13	13	12
16	19	18	18	18	18	17	17	17	17	16	16	16	16	15	15	15	14	14	14	14	13
17	20	19	19	19	19	18	18	18	18	17	17	17	17	16	16	16	15	15	15	15	14
18	21	20	20	20	20	19	19	19	19	18	18	18	18	17	17	17	16	16	16	16	15

NOTE: Education adjustment by applying the following formula: $NSS_{A\&E} = NSS_A - (\beta \times [\text{education (years)} - 12])$, where $\beta = 0.25243$.

SOURCE: From Casals-Coll et al. (2014).

TABLE 11-48 Education Adjustment for the BNT B Short Form

	EDUCATION (YEARS)																				
NSS_A	0	1	2	3	4	5	6	7	8	9	10	11	12	13	14	15	16	17	18	19	20
2	2	5	4	4	4	4	3	3	3	3	2	2	2	2	1	1	1	0	0	0	0
3	3	6	5	5	5	5	4	4	4	4	3	3	3	3	2	2	2	1	1	1	1
4	4	7	6	6	6	6	5	5	5	5	4	4	4	4	3	3	3	2	2	2	2
5	5	8	7	7	7	7	6	6	6	6	5	5	5	5	4	4	4	3	3	3	3
6	6	9	8	8	8	8	7	7	7	7	6	6	6	6	5	5	5	4	4	4	4
7	7	10	9	9	9	9	8	8	8	8	7	7	7	7	6	6	6	5	5	5	5
8	8	11	10	10	10	10	9	9	9	9	8	8	8	8	7	7	7	6	6	6	6
9	9	12	11	11	11	11	10	10	10	10	9	9	9	9	8	8	8	7	7	7	7
10	10	13	12	12	12	12	11	11	11	11	10	10	10	10	9	9	9	8	8	8	8
11	11	14	13	13	13	13	12	12	12	12	11	11	11	11	10	10	10	9	9	9	9
12	12	15	14	14	14	14	13	13	13	13	12	12	12	12	11	11	11	10	10	10	10
13	13	16	15	15	15	15	14	14	14	14	13	13	13	13	12	12	12	11	11	11	11
14	14	17	16	16	16	16	15	15	15	15	14	14	14	14	13	13	13	12	12	12	12
15	15	18	17	17	17	17	16	16	16	16	15	15	15	15	14	14	14	13	13	13	13
16	16	19	18	18	18	18	17	17	17	17	16	16	16	16	15	15	15	14	14	14	14
17	17	20	19	19	19	19	18	18	18	18	17	17	17	17	16	16	16	15	15	15	15
18	18	21	20	20	20	20	19	19	19	19	18	18	18	18	17	17	17	16	16	16	16

NOTE: Education adjustment by applying the following formula: $NSS_{A\&E} = NSS_A - (\beta \times [\text{education (years)} - 12])$, where $\beta = 0.26599$.

SOURCE: Casals-Coll et al. (2014).

are more likely to make visuoperceptual errors (Olszewski et al., 2011; Williams et al., 2007).

Differentiating Among Neurodegenerative Disorders. The BNT may have some utility in differentiating among various neurodegenerative disorders (Amici et al., 2007; Heyanka et al., 2010; Olszewski et al., 2011; Williams et al., 2007). Those with semantic dementia perform lower on the BNT compared to primary progressive aphasia, primary nonfluent aphasia, and logopenic progressive aphasia (Amici et al., 2007). BNT scores are lower for AD than for DLB, but DLB patients make more visuoperceptual errors while AD patients make more semantic errors. Phonemic errors do not differentiate between the two groups. These errors result in a classification accuracy of 86%, and an increase of one perceptual error increases DLB diagnosis likelihood by 30% (Williams et al., 2007). On the other hand, although frontotemporal dementia (FTD) and AD patients perform similarly on the BNT, FTD patients benefit from phonemic cueing but not AD patients, whose errors are primarily perceptual and associative (Olszewski et al., 2011). These qualitative differences likely reflect the semantic network breakdown and visual agnosia in AD and frontal-executive retrieval deficits in FTD. However, it is important to note that BNT performance is not different between

TABLE 11-49 Education Adjustment for the BNT C Short Form

	EDUCATION (YEARS)																				
NSS_A	0	1	2	3	4	5	6	7	8	9	10	11	12	13	14	15	16	17	18	19	20
2	6	5	5	5	4	4	4	3	3	3	2	2	2	1	1	0	0	0	−1	−1	−1
3	7	6	6	6	5	5	5	4	4	4	3	3	3	2	2	1	1	1	0	0	0
4	8	7	7	7	6	6	6	5	5	5	4	4	4	3	3	2	2	2	1	1	1
5	9	8	8	8	7	7	7	6	6	6	5	5	5	4	4	3	3	3	2	2	2
6	10	9	9	9	8	8	8	7	7	7	6	6	6	5	5	4	4	4	3	3	3
7	11	10	10	10	9	9	9	8	8	8	7	7	7	6	6	5	5	5	4	4	4
8	12	11	11	11	10	10	10	9	9	9	8	8	8	7	7	6	6	6	5	5	5
9	13	12	12	12	11	11	11	10	10	10	9	9	9	8	8	7	7	7	6	6	6
10	14	13	13	13	12	12	12	11	11	11	10	10	10	9	9	8	8	8	7	7	7
11	15	14	14	14	13	13	13	12	12	12	11	11	11	10	10	9	9	9	8	8	8
12	16	15	15	15	14	14	14	13	13	13	12	12	12	11	11	10	10	10	9	9	9
13	17	16	16	16	15	15	15	14	14	14	13	13	13	12	12	11	11	11	10	10	10
14	18	17	17	17	16	16	16	15	15	15	14	14	14	13	13	12	12	12	11	11	11
15	19	18	18	18	17	17	17	16	16	16	15	15	15	14	14	13	13	13	12	12	12
16	20	19	19	19	18	18	18	17	17	17	16	16	16	15	15	14	14	14	13	13	13
17	21	20	20	20	19	19	19	18	18	18	17	17	17	16	16	15	15	15	14	14	14
18	22	21	21	21	20	20	20	19	19	19	18	18	18	17	17	16	16	16	15	15	15

NOTE: Education adjustment applying the following formula: $NSS_{A\&E} = NSS_A - (\beta \times [\text{education (years)} - 12])$, where $\beta = 0.34083$.

SOURCE: From Casals-Coll et al. (2014).

TABLE 11-50 Education Adjustment for the BNT D Short Form

	EDUCATION (YEARS)																				
NSS_A	0	1	2	3	4	5	6	7	8	9	10	11	12	13	14	15	16	17	18	19	20
2	4	4	4	4	3	3	3	3	2	2	2	2	2	1	1	1	1	0	0	0	0
3	5	5	5	5	4	4	4	4	3	3	3	3	3	2	2	2	2	1	1	1	1
4	6	6	6	6	5	5	5	5	4	4	4	4	4	3	3	3	3	2	2	2	2
5	7	7	7	7	6	6	6	6	5	5	5	5	5	4	4	4	4	3	3	3	3
6	8	8	8	8	7	7	7	7	6	6	6	6	6	5	5	5	5	4	4	4	4
7	9	9	9	9	8	8	8	8	7	7	7	7	7	6	6	6	6	5	5	5	5
8	10	10	10	10	9	9	9	9	8	8	8	8	8	7	7	7	7	6	6	6	6
9	11	11	11	11	10	10	10	10	9	9	9	9	9	8	8	8	8	7	7	7	7
10	12	12	12	12	11	11	11	11	10	10	10	10	10	9	9	9	9	8	8	8	8
11	13	13	13	13	12	12	12	12	11	11	11	11	11	10	10	10	10	9	9	9	9
12	14	14	14	14	13	13	13	13	12	12	12	12	12	11	11	11	11	10	10	10	10
13	15	15	15	15	14	14	14	14	13	13	13	13	13	12	12	12	12	11	11	11	11
14	16	16	16	16	15	15	15	15	14	14	14	14	14	13	13	13	13	12	12	12	12
15	17	17	17	17	16	16	16	16	15	15	15	15	15	14	14	14	14	13	13	13	13
16	18	18	18	18	17	17	17	17	16	16	16	16	16	15	15	15	15	14	14	14	14
17	19	19	19	19	18	18	18	18	17	17	17	17	17	16	16	16	16	15	15	15	15
18	20	20	20	20	19	19	19	19	18	18	18	18	18	17	17	17	17	16	16	16	16

NOTE: Education adjustment applying the following formula: $NSS_{A\&E} = NSS_A - (\beta \times [\text{education (years)} - 12])$, where $\beta = 0.24325$.

SOURCE: From Casals-Coll et al. (2014).

healthy illiterate older adults and literate patients with mild AD (Youn et al., 2011). Moreover, although the BNT is sensitive to progression to AD in all groups over and above other tests (e.g., Wisconsin Card Sorting Test [WCST], phonemic fluency, visual memory), Hispanics (many bilinguals) score lower than non-Hispanics (mostly monolingual English-speaking) on the BNT despite matching on age, gender, and education (Weissberger et al., 2013).

Epilepsy. Scores tends to be reduced in patients with temporal lobe epilepsy (TLE) but are better than for patients with AD (Randolph et al., 1999). The BNT is more sensitive than the Visual Naming subtest of the Multilingual Aphasia Examination (MAE) in identifying left temporal lobe dysfunction (78% vs. 18%), particularly in those with FSIQs of 90 or higher (Scheffl et al., 2003). Within this FSIQ group, a person scoring at or below the 5th percentile on the BNT was four times as likely to have left TLE than someone who scored above the 5th percentile. The presence of phonemic paraphasias (which tend to be elicited by the BNT but not the MAE) is also useful in lateralizing the side of seizure origin. The differential patterns of classification rates in lateralizing side of dysfunction probably reflect the more demanding nature of the BNT, compared with the Visual Naming subtest of the MAE (Scheffl et al., 2003).

TABLE 11-51 Adult Norms Corrected for Reading Vocabulary Level

READING LEVEL[a]	PERCENTILE RANK[b]	ESTIMATED BNT TOTAL
4.1	01	34.4
5.0	03	37.2
6.1	05	39.9
7.0	08	42.0
8.0	13	44.7
9.2	21	47.5
10.1	29	49.6
11.1	40	51.6
12.2	45	52.3
Post high school	58	53.7
	66	54.3
	82	55.7
	90	56.4

NOTE: Based on a mixed psychiatric and healthy sample (N = 88).

[a] Estimated on the basis of Gates-MacGinitie Reading Vocabulary.

[b] Based on Gates-MacGinitie Reading Vocabulary, Level 7–9, Form K.

SOURCE: Adapted from Hawkins et al. (1993), with permission of the authors and Elsevier Science Ltd.

Ramirez et al. (2008) reported that interictal phonemic paraphasias on the BNT may be used to identify the laterality of seizure onset. At 53% base rate of dominant TLE, presence of interictal phonemic paraphasias on the BNT yielded a sensitivity of 97%, specificity of 86%, positive predictive value (PPV) of 89%, and negative predictive value (NPV) of 96% for identifying dominant TLE (Ramirez et al., 2008). When entered into a stepwise regression to predict seizure laterality along with verbal comprehension, visual matching, and Grooved Pegboard, only the BNT was a significant predictor (Lancman et al., 2012). In another study, RAVLT and BNT together predicted seizure laterality in a logistic regression analysis. Using BNT alone, the model yielded a sensitivity of 58% and a specificity of 70% (Loring et al., 2008).

The BNT has historically been used in TLE to assess naming decline after anterior temporal lobectomy (Janecek et al., 2013; Kovac et al., 2010). Declines after left anterior temporal lobectomy were more common than after right temporal lobectomy (Bell et al., 2000; Hermann et al., 1999). For example, in a series of Wada-determined bilateral language TLE surgical patients who

TABLE 11–52 Actual Minus Predicted Boston Naming Test (BNT) Discrepancy Based on the SCOLP Spot-the-Word Test

DISCREPANCY	PERCENTILE	DISCREPANCY	PERCENTILE
−10.71	1	.219	49.0
−7.94	2	.334	50.0
−6.67	3.1	.373	54.1
−5.24	4.1	.642	56.1
−4.51	5.1	.796	60.2
−4.36	6.1	.911	62.2
−4.13	7.1	.950	63.3
−3.94	8.2	1.03	65.3
−3.24	9.2	1.07	66.3
−3.20	10.2	1.22	68.4
−2.59	11.2	1.30	69.4
−2.51	13.3	1.33	70.4
−2.36	16.3	1.37	73.5
−2.21	18.4	1.49	74.5
−2.13	19.4	1.60	75.5
−2.09	21.4	1.80	76.5
−2.01	22.4	1.91	77.6
−1.67	23.5	2.07	80.6
−1.63	24.5	2.22	83.7
−1.51	25.5	2.33	84.7
−1.40	26.5	2.60	85.7
−1.36	30.6	2.64	88.8
−1.01	31.6	2.76	89.8
−.78	32.7	2.91	91.8
−.71	33.7	2.99	92.9
−.67	34.7	3.30	93.9
−.55	35.7	3.49	94.9
−.20	38.8	3.76	95.9
−.09	41.8	4.18	96.9
−.05	42.9	4.26	98.0
.065	43.9	6.03	100.0

SOURCE: Graves and Carswell (personal communication, R. Graves, January 2003).

were tested presurgically and six-months post-surgery, greater risk for decline in naming as measured by the BNT was seen among those who underwent left versus right anterior temporal lobectomy (Janecek et al., 2013), but more so among those with atypical language representation than those who were left-language dominant (Kovac et al., 2010). Although no differences in BNT scores were seen at baseline, the group that underwent nondominant temporal lobectomy improved by 2.03 points at six-month post-surgery whereas the dominant group declined by 6.72 points. Greater BNT declines were seen in those with late-onset seizures compared to those with early-onset seizures (Ruff et al., 2007). However, Drane and colleagues (2008) noted that the BNT may not be as sensitive to language deficits compared to category-specific naming and recognition tasks (famous faces, man-made objects, and living things). In their sample of TLE patients who underwent temporal lobectomy, almost 70% showed at least mild deficits on category-specific naming tasks but only 31% showed at least mild impairment on the BNT (Drane et al., 2008).

Among those TLE patients who demonstrate statistically meaningful decline, age at acquisition of a word is a significant predictor of performance; that is, words acquired early in childhood are less affected than words acquired late (Bell et al., 2000). The pattern differs as a function of side of TLE surgery. In the nondominant group, improvements in BNT occur for words acquired later in life, whereas the BNT declines after dominant anterior temporal lobectomy for words acquired later in life (Ruff et al., 2007).

TABLE 11–53 Boston Naming Test (BNT) Raw Score Points Required for Statistically Significant Change Based on Reliable Change Index in Healthy Older Adults

	N	R_{XY}	SE_{DIFF}	90% PI	PRACTICE EFFECT	RCI CUTOFF
All participants (9–24 months)	844	.86	2.94	±4.82	.56	−4 ≥ RC ≥ +5
Time interval (9–15 months)						
All participants	632	.84	2.66	±4.36	.61	−4 ≥ RC ≥ +5
Age at baseline						
<75	316	.78	2.32	±3.80	.72	−4 ≥ RC ≥ +5
≥75	316	.86	2.95	±4.84	.49	−5 ≥ RC ≥ +6
Family history of dementia						
Yes	409	.83	2.57	±4.22	.59	−4 ≥ RC ≥ +5
No	199	.86	2.78	±4.56	.59	−4 ≥ RC ≥ +6
Time interval (16–24 months)						
All participants	212	.86	3.64	±5.97	.43	−6 ≥ RC ≥ +7
Age at baseline						
<81	106	.84	3.14	±5.14	.77	−5 ≥ RC ≥ +6
≥81	106	.84	4.06	±6.66	.08	−7 ≥ RC ≥ +7
Family history of dementia						
Yes	95	.87	3.49	±5.72	.53	−6 ≥ RC ≥ +7
No	115	.87	3.48	±5.70	.16	−6 ≥ RC ≥ +6

NOTE: r_{xy}=test-retest reliability; SE_{diff} = standard error of the difference; Practice effect = (BNT time 2 mean score - BNT time 1 mean score); PI = 90% prediction interval; RCI = reliable change index adjusted for practice effect. Age at baseline based on median split.

SOURCE: From Sachs et al. (2012).

Decline in BNT scores is also associated with postsurgical seizure control. Poor postsurgical seizure control is more common in atypical language dominance than in left-language dominant patients. Anterior displacement of language may explain the BNT decline in atypical language patients while altered connectivity may explain the poor postsurgical seizure control in these patients (Kovac et al., 2010).

The BNT has also been used to measure the naming outcome of gamma knife radiosurgery for mesial TLE (Quigg et al., 2011). In the study, all but one patient ($N = 30$) were seizure-free post-surgery. Those who underwent high-dose radiosurgery in the dominant temporal lobe experienced mild decreases in BNT scores (average of three raw-score points after 12 and 24 months) and verbal memory (as measured by California Verbal Learning Test [CVLT]. Those who underwent low-dose dominant temporal lobe radiosurgery or nondominant temporal lobe radiosurgery experienced no declines in BNT scores.

The BNT and RAVLT have also been used to monitor the cognitive effects of long-term responsive neurostimulation over two years. BNT improvements are noted for those with neocortical seizure onset but not for those with mesial temporal lobe seizure onset. The reverse is seen for RAVLT performance (Loring et al., 2015).

Psychiatric Disorders. Impairment has also been reported in patients with psychiatric conditions, including schizophrenia (Landre et al., 1992) and depression (Hill et al., 1992; Ferraro et al., 1997; but see Boone et al., 1995).

NEUROANATOMICAL CORRELATES AND IMAGING STUDIES

BNT performance appears to correlate with left temporal gray matter volume more so than right (Alessio et al., 2006; Amici et al., 20007; Apostolova et al., 2008; Arlt et al., 2013; Balthazar et al., 2010). Circumlocutory and coordinate errors are weakly correlated with left more than right anterior and lateral temporal lobe atrophy (Balthazar et al., 2010), and the strongest rate of change in the left hippocampus is correlated with rate of decline in BNT performance among those with mild AD/MCI (Arlt et al., 2013). BNT performance is correlated with medial temporal atrophy but not white matter hyperintensities in AD as measured by MRI (Shim et al., 2011).

In patients with progressive language impairment including primary progressive aphasia, primary nonfluent aphasia, semantic dementia, and logopenic progressive aphasia, BNT impairment is correlated with inferior temporal gyri, fusiform gyri, temporal poles, and hippocampi and left parahippocampal gyrus and middle temporal gyrus volume as measured using voxel-based morphometry (Amici et al., 2007). Using voxel-based lesion mapping in patients with single-left hemisphere stroke, BNT performance was associated with perisylvian cortex volume, including left anterior to posterior middle temporal gyrus, superior temporal gyrus, and underlying white matter, extending into left inferior parietal cortex (Baldo et al., 2013). In one study on chronic mesial TLE, degree of left hippocampal atrophy (HA) and asymmetry of perirhinal cortex volume were correlated with BNT scores, verbal fluency, and general memory. The left HA group performed significantly worse than the right HA group on these neuropsychological measures (Alessio et al., 2006).

Involvement of other brain regions has also been reported. Using surface-based computational anatomy techniques to evaluate brain magnetic resonance imaging (MRI) in probable AD and multidomain amnestic MCI patients, BNT performance was strongly correlated with gray matter atrophy in the posterior middle and inferior temporal gyri, temporo-occipital and parieto-occipital association cortices, and posterior middle and superior frontal gyri bilaterally, as well as left inferior sensorimotor strips, left fusiform gyrus, right temporal pole, bilateral entorhinal, anterior cingulate, and mesial orbitofrontal cortex (Apostolova et al., 2008).

PERFORMANCE VALIDITY

The BNT may have some promise as a performance validity estimate, at least in the one study that examined this question. Whiteside et al. (2015) compared the performance of a compensation-seeking mild TBI group and a non-compensation-seeking moderate to severe TBI group on embedded performance validity indicators. No one in either group obtained T scores of less than 18 on the BNT based on standardized T scores (Heaton et al., 2004 norms), indicating minimal chance of false positives in a non-neurological population using this cutoff. The authors calculated a language performance validity indicator formula using standardized T scores from Heaton et al. (2004) norms that combine the test with other language measures:

$$\text{BNT} \times 0.05 - \text{FAS} \times 0.06 + \text{Animal Fluency} \times 0.06 - 2.11$$

Table 11–54 presents sensitivity/specificity data for this language performance validity indicator, which yielded acceptable classification accuracy for the combined scores. Note that the BNT, FAS, and Animal Fluency alone did not yield acceptable classification accuracy. Low sensitivity with adequate specificity was seen in this embedded performance validity indicator.

COMMENT

The BNT is a very well-known, popular test of visual confrontation naming. With the exception perhaps of word fluency, there is no test of verbal function that has received as much use in neuropsychology as the BNT. It is sensitive for identifying naming changes in a variety of

TABLE 11–54 Area Under Curve (AUC), Sensitivity, and Specificity for the Boston Naming Test (BNT), FAS, Animal Fluency, and Regression-Based Combined Language Performance Validity Indicator in Traumatic Brain Injury

VARIABLE	AUC	CUTOFF[a]	SENSITIVITY (%)	SPECIFICITY (%)
LANGPVT	.72*	−1.05	14	100
		−0.93	26	90
		−0.63	32	89
		−0.53	35	88
BNT	.65	18	2	100
		30	14	92
		31	18	90
		32	21	89
FAS	.53	17	2	100
		23	5	92
		24	5	90
		25	9	87
Animal Fluency	.65	13	5	100
		23	19	94
		24	23	91
		25	25	89

NOTE: AUC = area under the curve; LANGPVT = regression-derived language performance validity tests; BNT = Boston Naming; Test.

[a] T scores for Boston Naming Test, FAS, and Animal Fluency.

$*p < .01$.

SOURCE: Whiteside et al. (2015).

neurodegenerative and neurological disorders with language disturbances. A large body of research has also provided evidence for its use in epilepsy.

Despite its popularity, several criticisms were highlighted in Harry and Crowe's (2014) review of the literature on the BNT. First, the BNT shows notable ceiling effects and is not normally distributed. Most healthy adults obtain high scores on the BNT. The test is, therefore, most valuable in identifying low performers.

Interpretation must be moderated by estimation of premorbid ability, a variable that appears to be more important than age in evaluating BNT performance. Hawkins and Bender (2002) recommend that premorbid vocabulary or verbal IQ provides the best basis for BNT performance expectations. In the absence of such data, reading vocabulary tests (e.g., Gates-MacGinitie, Spot-the-Word) may provide guidance for BNT expectations. The alternative measure, years of education completed, bears a lesser relationship to BNT performance but should also be considered.

Next, differences in administration and scoring pose a critical problem when interpreting BNT scores (Harry & Crowe, 2014). The Bortnik et al. (2013) survey revealed that only about half of the respondents followed published discontinuation rules and there was inconsistency in operational definitions of failure: about half consider the item failed if the examinee is unable to name spontaneously or after a stimulus cue, whereas the other half consider the item failed only if the response remains incorrect after phonemic cues. Moreover, a majority of respondents do not wait for 20 seconds to elapse before providing feedback, and most give credit if the patient self-corrected without a phonemic cue (Bortnik et al., 2013).

Differences in administration may also affect scores. For example, automatically crediting 29 points based on standard administration procedure inflates the score by as much as 3.4 points in those with mild dementia, even though both full (starting at item 1) and standard administrations are effective in distinguishing among cognitive impairment groups (Stålhammar et al., 2016). Use of a "lenient" discontinuation method (excluding phonemically correct responses in the count of errors for the "six consecutive failures" tally) leads to score changes in 31% of AD patients. Among healthy examinees, discrepant scores are most often found in persons aged 80 years and older, and scores differ by up to 16 points. Because different interpretations of the discontinuation rule may alter test scores, it is important that users employ the same administration procedures as were used in the norms they are using.

Finally, there is a restricted range in the demographic background of norms despite sensitivity to these factors (Harry & Crowe, 2014). Bortnik and colleagues (2013) reported that almost half of the respondents in their survey do not consider linguistic and ethnic background when interpreting BNT scores, and a quarter do not consider educational level. Given the significant impact of individual difference variables (e.g., ethnicity, level of acculturation, regional differences, linguistic background) on BNT performance, clinicians should use language- and culture-specific normative data such as the ones presented in this review. However, caution should be used when a translated version of the test is employed in non-English-speaking populations because item difficulty may vary in different languages.

The issue of bilingualism bears discussion. Research conducted thus far indicates that age of second-language acquisition, frequency of use of language, balance between the two languages, proficiency in the nondominant language, context of each language use (formal vs. informal settings), cultural factors, and degree of immersion in both language environments may explain differences more so than bilingualism alone.

The "aging" of the norms should also be considered, given the general rise in ability (Flynn effect) and the possibility that some of the items represented in the tasks may have fallen into disuse (Storms et al., 2004). As with other tests relying on pictorial material (e.g., PPVT-4), visual-perceptual integrity should be checked if errors occur.

A number of short forms have been developed, but some of the norms are outdated and not included in this review. Although they tend to provide relatively homogeneous tests of naming ability, the forms are not interchangeable. In addition, differences in classification arise between short (particularly 15-item) and long forms of the test. The BNT 15 and BNT 30 forms developed by Graves et al. (2004) appear very promising with regard to reliability and classification agreement accuracy with the full BNT. The Spanish short forms show promise, although additional psychometric data are needed.

REFERENCES

Alessio, A., Bonilha, L., Rorden, C., Kobayashi, E., Min, L. L., Damasceno, B. P., & Cendes, F. (2006). Memory and language impairments and their relationships to hippocampal and perirhinal cortex damage in patients with medial temporal lobe epilepsy. *Epilepsy & Behavior, 8*(3), 593–600.

Amici, S., Ogar, J., Brambati, S. M., Miller, B. L., Neuhaus, J., Dronkers, N. L., & Gorno-Tempini, M. L. (2007). Performance in specific language tasks correlates with regional volume changes in progressive aphasia. *Cognitive and Behavioral Neurology, 20*(4), 203–211.

Apostolova, L. G., Lu, P., Rogers, S., Dutton, R. A., Hayashi, K. M., Toga, A. W., . . . Thompson, P. M. (2008). 3D mapping of language networks in clinical and pre-clinical Alzheimer's disease. *Brain and Language, 104*(1), 33–41.

Aranciva F., Casals-Coll, M., Sanchez-Benavides, G., Quintana, M., Manero, R. M., Rognoni, T., Calvo, L., . . . Pena-Casanova, J. (2012). Estudios normativos españoles en población adulta joven (Proyecto NEURO-NORMA jóvenes): Normas para el Boston Naming Test y el Token Test. *Neurología, 27,* 394–400.

Arlt, S., Buchert, R., Spies, L., Eichenlaub, M., Lehmbeck, J. T., & Jahn, H. (2013). Association between fully automated MRI-based volumetry of different brain regions and neuropsychological test performance in patients with amnestic mild cognitive impairment and Alzheimer's disease. *European Archives of Psychiatry and Clinical Neuroscience, 263*(4), 335–344.

Au, R., Joung, P. C., Nicholas, M., Obler, L. K., Kass, R., & Albert, M. L. (1995). Naming ability across the adult life span. *Aging and Cognition, 2,* 300–311.

Axelrod, B. N., Ricker, J. H., & Cherry, S. A. (1994). Concurrent validity of the MAE Visual Naming Test. *Archives of Clinical Neuropsychology, 9,* 317–321.

Azambuja, M. J., Radanovic, M., Haddad, M. S., Adda, C. C., Barbosa, E. R., & Mansur, L. L. (2012). Language impairment in Huntington's disease. *Arquivos de Neuro-psiquiatria, 70*(6), 410–415.

Azrin, R. L., Mercury, M. G., Millsaps, C., Goldstein, D., Trejo, T., & Pliskin, N. H. (1996). Cautionary note on the Boston Naming Test: Cultural considerations [Abstract]. *Archives of Clinical Neuropsychology, 11,* 365–366.

Baldo, J. V., Arévalo, A., Patterson, J. P., & Dronkers, N. F. (2013). Grey and white matter correlates of picture naming: Evidence from a voxel-based lesion analysis of the Boston Naming Test. *Cortex, 49*(3), 658–667.

Balthazar, M. L. F., Cendes, F., & Damasceno, B. P. (2008). Semantic error patterns on the Boston Naming Test in normal aging, amnestic mild cognitive impairment, and mild Alzheimer's disease: Is there semantic disruption? *Neuropsychology, 22*(6), 703.

Balthazar, M. L. F., Yasuda, C. L., Pereira, F. R. S., Bergo, F. P. G., Cendes, F., & Damasceno, B. P. (2010). Coordinated and circumlocutory semantic naming errors are related to anterolateral temporal lobes in mild AD, amnestic mild cognitive impairment, and normal aging. *Journal of the International Neuropsychological Society, 16*(6), 1099–1107.

Barker-Collo, S. L. (2002). The 60-item Boston Naming Test: Cultural bias and possible adaptations for New Zealand. *Aphasiology, 15,* 85–92.

Barr, A., Benedict, R., Tune, L., & Brandt, J. (1992). Neuropsychological differentiation of Alzheimer's disease from vascular dementia. *International Journal of Geriatric Psychiatry, 7,* 621–627.

Beatty, W. W., Salmon, D. P., Troester, A. I., & Tivis, R. D. (2002). Do primary and supplementary measures of semantic memory predict cognitive decline by patients with Alzheimer's disease? *Aging, Neuropsychology, and Cognition, 9,* 1–10.

Bell, B. D., Davies, K. G., Hermann, B. P., & Walters, G. (2000). Confrontation naming after anterior temporal lobectomy is related to age of acquisition of the object names. *Neuropsychologia, 38,* 83–92.

Boone, K. B., Lesser, I. M., Miller, B. L., Wohl, M., Berman, N., Lee, A., Palmer, B., & Back, C. (1995). Cognitive functioning in older depressed outpatients: Relationship of presence and severity of depression to neuropsychological test scores. *Neuropsychology, 9,* 390–398.

Bortnik, K. E., Boone, K. B., Wen, J., Lu, P., Mitrushina, M., Razani, J., & Maury, T. (2013). Survey results regarding use of the Boston Naming Test: Houston, we have a problem. *Journal of Clinical and Experimental Neuropsychology, 35*(8), 857–866.

Brandt, J., Bakker, A., & Maroof, D. A. (2010). Auditory confrontation naming in Alzheimer's disease. *The Clinical Neuropsychologist, 24*(8), 1326–1338.

Casals-Coll, M., Sánchez-Benavides, G., Meza-Cavazos, S., Manero, R. M., Aguilar, M., Badenes, D., . . . Pena-Casanova, J. (2014). Spanish multicenter normative studies (NEURONORMA project): Normative data and equivalence of four BNT short-form versions. *Archives of Clinical Neuropsychology, 29*(1), 60–74.

Cherney, L. R., Harvey, R. L., Babbitt, E. M., Hurwitz, R., Kaye, R. C., Lee, J. B., & Small, S. L. (2012). Epidural cortical stimulation and aphasia therapy. *Aphasiology, 26*(9), 1192–1217.

Cheung, M. C., & Chan, A. S. (2004). Confrontation naming in Chinese patients with left, right, or bilateral brain damage. *Journal of the International Neuropsychological Society, 10,* 46–53.

Connor, L. T., Spiro III, A., Oblerm L. K., & Albert, M. L. (2004). Change in object naming ability during adulthood. *Journal of Gerontology: Psychological Sciences, 59B,* P203–P209.

Cruice, M. N., Worrall, L. E., & Hickson, L. M. H. (2000). Boston Naming Test results for healthy older Australians: A longitudinal and cross-sectional study. *Aphasiology, 14,* 143–155.

Debes, F., Weihe, P., & Grandjean, P. (2016). Cognitive deficits at age 22 years associated with prenatal exposure to methylmercury. *Cortex, 74,* 358–369.

Diaz-Asper, C., Schretlen, D. J., & Pearlson, G. D. (2004). How well does IQ predict neuropsychological test performance in normal adults. *Journal of the International Neuropsychological Society, 10,* 82–90.

Drane, D. L., Ojemann, G. A., Aylward, E., Ojemann, J. G., Johnson, L. C., Silbergeld, D. L., . . . Tranel, D. (2008). Category-specific naming and recognition deficits in temporal lobe epilepsy surgical patients. *Neuropsychologia, 46*(5), 1242–1255.

Elkadi, S., Clark, M. S., Dennerstein, L., Guthrie, J. R., Bowden, S. C., & Henderson, V. W. (2006). Normative data for Australian midlife women on category fluency and a short form of the Boston Naming Test. *Australian Psychologist, 41*(1), 37–42.

Fastenau, P. S., Denburg, N. L., & Mauer, B. A. (1998). Parallel short forms for the Boston Naming Test: Psychometric properties and norms for older adults. *Journal of Clinical and Experimental Neuropsychology, 20,* 828–834.

Ferraro, F. R., Bercier, B., & Chelminski, I. (1997). Geriatric Depression Scale—Short Form in Native American elderly adults. *Clinical Gerontologist, 17,* 58–60.

Ferraro, F. R., Bercier, B. J., Holm, J., & McDonald, J. D. (2002). Preliminary normative data from a brief neuropsychological test battery in a sample of Native American elderly. In F. R. Ferraro (Ed.), *Minority and cross-cultural aspects of neuropsychological assessment: Studies on neuropsychology, development, and cognition* (pp. 227–240). Bristol, PA: Swets & Zeitlinger.

Fillenbaum, G. G., Huber, M., & Taussig, I. M. (1997). Performance of elderly white and African American community residents on the abbreviated CERAD Boston Naming Test. *Journal of Clinical and Experimental Neuropsychology, 19,* 204–210.

Flanagan, J. L., & Jackson, S. T. (1997). Test-retest reliability of three aphasia tests: Performance of non-brain-damaged older adults. *Journal of Communication Disorders, 30,* 33–43.

Franzen, M. D., Haut, M. W., Rankin, E., & Keefover, R. (1995). Empirical comparison of alternate forms of the Boston Naming Test. *The Clinical Neuropsychologist, 9,* 225–229.

Gollan, T. H., Fennema-Notestine, C., Montoya, R. I., & Jernigan, T. L. (2007). The bilingual effect on Boston Naming Test performance. *Journal of the International Neuropsychological Society, 13*(02), 197–208.

Gollan, T. H., Salmon, D. P., Montoya, R. I., & da Pena, E. (2010). Accessibility of the nondominant language in picture naming: A counterintuitive effect of dementia on bilingual language production. *Neuropsychologia, 48*(5), 1356–1366.

Gollan, T. H., Salmon, D. P., Montoya, R. I., & Galasko, D. R. (2011). Degree of bilingualism predicts age of diagnosis of Alzheimer's disease in low-education but not in highly educated Hispanics. *Neuropsychologia, 49*(14), 3826–3830.

Gollan, T. H., Weissberger, G. H., Runnqvist, E., Montoya, R. I., & Cera, C. M. (2012). Self-ratings of spoken language dominance: A multi-lingual naming test (MINT) and preliminary norms for young and aging Spanish-English bilinguals. *Bilingualism (Cambridge, England), 15*(3), 594.

Graves, R. E., Bezeau, S. C., Fogarty, J., & Blair, R. (2004). Boston Naming Test Short Forms: A comparison of previous forms with new item response theory based forms. *Journal of Clinical and Experimental Neuropsychology, 26,* 891–902.

Graves, R. E., & Carswell, L. (2003). *Prediction of Premorbid Boston Naming and California Verbal Learning Test scores.* Paper presented to the International Neuropsychological Society, Honolulu, Hawaii.

Greenaway, M. C., Smith, G. E., Tangalos, E. G., Geda, Y. E., & Ivnik, R. J. (2009). Mayo older Americans normative studies: Factor analysis of an expanded neuropsychological battery. *The Clinical Neuropsychologist, 23*(1), 7–20.

Hall, J. R., Vo, H. T., Johnson, L. A., Wiechmann, A., & O'Bryant, S. E. (2012). Boston Naming Test: Gender differences in older adults with and without Alzheimer's dementia. *Psychology, 3*(6), 485.

Hamburger, M. J., & Seidel, W. T. (2003). Auditory and visual naming tests: Normative and patient data for accuracy, response time, and tip-of-the-tongue. *Journal of the International Neuropsychological Society, 9*(03), 479–489.

Harry, A., & Crowe, S. F. (2014). Is the Boston Naming Test still fit for purpose? *The Clinical Neuropsychologist, 28*(3), 486–504.

Hawkins, K. A., & Bender, S. (2002). Norms and the relationship of Boston Naming Test performance to vocabulary and education: A review. *Aphasiology, 16,* 1143–1153.

Hawkins, K. A., Sledge, W. H., Orleans, J. F., Quinland, D. M., Rakfeldt, J., & Hoffman, R. E. (1993). Normative implications of the relationship between reading vocabulary and Boston Naming Test performance. *Archives of Clinical Neuropsychology, 8,* 525–537.

Heaton, R. K., Avitable, N., Grant, I., & Mathews, C. G. (1999). Further crossvalidation of regression-based neuropsychological norms with an update for the Boston Naming Test. *Journal of Clinical and Experimental Neuropsychology, 21,* 572–582.

Heaton, R. K., Miller, S. W., Taylor, M. J., & Grant, I. (1991, 1992, 2004). Revised comprehensive norms for an expanded Halstead-Reitan Battery: Demographically adjusted neuropsychological norms for African American and Caucasian adults. Lutz, FL: PAR.

Henderson, L. W., Frank, E. W., Pigatt, T., Abramson, R. K., & Houston, M. (1998). Race, gender and educational level effects on Boston Naming Test scores. *Aphasiology, 12,* 901–911.

Henry, J. D., & Crawford, J. R. (2004). Verbal fluency deficits in Parkinson's disease: A meta-analysis. *Journal of the International Neuropsychological Society, 10,* 608–622.

Henry, J. D., Crawford, J. R., & Phillips, L. H. (2004). Verbal fluency performance in dementia of the Alzheimer's type: A meta-analysis. *Neuropsychologia, 42,* 1212–1224.

Hermann, B. P., Perrine, K., Chelune, G. J., Barr, W., Loring, D. W., Strauss, E., . . . Westerveld, M. (1999). Visual confrontation naming following left anterior temporal lobectomy: A comparison of surgical approaches. *Neuropsychology, 13,* 3–9.

Heyanka, D. J., Mackelprang, J. L., Golden, C. J., & Marke, C. D. (2010). Distinguishing Alzheimer's disease from vascular dementia: An exploration of five cognitive domains. *International Journal of Neuroscience, 120*(6), 409–414.

Hill, C. D., Stoudemire, A., Morris, R., Martino-Saltzman, D., Mark-Walter, H. R., & Lewison, B. J. (1992). Dysnomia in the differential diagnosis of major depression, depression-related cognitive dysfunction, and dementia. *Journal of Neuropsychiatry and Clinical Neuroscience, 4,* 64–69.

Hobson, V. L., Hall, J. R., Harvey, M., Cullum, C. M., Lacritz, L., Massman, P. J., . . . O'Bryant, S. E. (2011). An examination of the Boston Naming Test: Calculation of 'estimated' 60-item score from 30- and 15-item scores in a cognitively impaired population. *International Journal of Geriatric Psychiatry, 26*(4), 351–355.

Ivnik, R. J., Malec, J. F., Smith, G. E., Tangalos, E. G., & Peterson, R. C. (1996). Neuropsychological test norms above age 55: COWAT, BNT, MAE Token, WRAT-R Reading, AMNART, Stroop, TMT, and JLO. *The Clinical Neuropsychologist, 10,* 262–278.

Jahn, D. R., Mauer, C. B., Menon, C. V., Edwards, M. L., Dressel, J. A., & O'Bryant, S. E. (2013). A brief Spanish–English equivalent version of the Boston Naming Test: A project FRONTIER study. *Journal of Clinical and Experimental Neuropsychology, 35*(8), 835–845.

Janecek, J. K., Swanson, S. J., Sabsevitz, D. S., Hammeke, T. A., Raghavan, M., Mueller, W., & Binder, J. R. (2013). Naming outcome prediction in patients with discordant Wada and fMRI language lateralization. *Epilepsy & Behavior, 27*(2), 399–403.

Jefferson, A. L., Wong, S., Gracer, T. S., Ozonoff, A., Green, R. C., & Stern, R. A. (2007). Geriatric performance on an abbreviated version of the Boston Naming Test. *Applied Neuropsychology, 14*(3), 215–223.

Kaplan, E., Goodglass, H., & Weintraub, B. (2005). Test de Vocabulario de Boston (2a ed.) [*Boston Naming Test* (2nd Ed.)]. Madrid: Editorial Médica Panamericana.

Kaplan, E. F., Goodglass, H., & Weintraub, S. (1978, 1983). *The Boston Naming Test: Experimental Edition (1978).* Boston: Kaplan & Goodglass. Philadelphia: Lea & Febiger.

Kaplan, E. F., Goodglass, H., & Weintraub, S. (2001). *The Boston Naming Test* (2nd Ed.). Philadelphia: Lippincott Williams & Wilkins.

Karrasch, M., Myllyniemi, A., Latvasalo, L., Söderholm, C., Ellfolk, U., & Laine, M. (2010). The diagnostic accuracy of an incidental memory modification of the Boston Naming Test (memo-BNT) in differentiating between normal aging and mild Alzheimer's disease. *The Clinical Neuropsychologist, 24*(8), 1355–1364.

Kemmotsu, N., Enobi, Y., & Murphy, C. (2013). Performance of older Japanese American adults on selected cognitive instruments. *Journal of the International Neuropsychological Society, 19*(07), 773–781.

Kent, P. S., & Luszcz, M. A. (2002). Review of the Boston Naming Test and multiple-occasion normative data for older adults on 15-item versions. *The Clinical Neuropsychologist, 16,* 555–574.

Killgore, W. D. S., & Adams, R. L. (1999). Prediction of Boston Naming Test performance from vocabulary scores: Preliminary guidelines for interpretation. *Perceptual and Motor Skills, 89,* 327–337.

Kim, H. L., & Na, D. L. (1999). Normative data on the Korean version of the Boston Naming Test. *Journal of Clinical and Experimental Neuropsychology, 21,* 127–133.

Kohn, S. E., & Goodglass, H. (1985). Picture-naming in aphasia. *Brain and Language, 24,* 266–283.

Kovac, S., Möddel, G., Reinholz, J., Alexopoulos, A. V., Syed, T., Koubeissi, M. Z., . . . Loddenkemper, T. (2010). Visual naming performance after ATL resection: impact of atypical language dominance. *Neuropsychologia, 48*(7), 2221–2225.

Lancman, G., Vazquez-Casals, G. A., Perrine, K., Feoli, E., & Myers, L. (2012). Predictive value of Spanish neuropsychological testing for laterality in patients with epilepsy. *Epilepsy & Behavior, 23*(2), 142–145.

Landre, N. A., Taylor, M. A., & Kearns, K. P. (1992). Language functioning in schizophrenic and aphasic patients. *Neuropsychiatry, Neuropsychology, and Behavioral Neurology, 5,* 7–14.

Lansing, A. E., Ivnik, R. J., Cullum, C. M., & Randolph, C. (1999). An empirically derived short form of the Boston Naming Test. *Archives of Clinical Neuropsychology, 14,* 481–487.

Lezak, M. D., Whitham, R., & Bourdette, D. (1990). Emotional impact of cognitive insufficiencies in multiple sclerosis (MS) [Abstract]. *Journal of Clinical and Experimental Neuropsychology, 12,* 50.

Locascio, J. J., Corkin, S., & Growde, J. H. (2003). Relation between clinical characteristics of Parkinson's disease and cognitive decline. *Journal of Clinical and Experimental Neuropsychology, 25,* 94–109.

Loring, D. W., Kapur, R., Meador, K. J., & Morrell, M. J. (2015). Differential neuropsychological outcomes following targeted responsive neurostimulation for partial-onset epilepsy. *Epilepsia, 56*(11), 1836–1844.

Loring, D. W., Strauss, E., Hermann, B. P., Barr, W. B., Perrine, K., Trenerry, M. R., . . . Bowden, S. C. (2008). Differential neuropsychological test sensitivity to left temporal lobe epilepsy. *Journal of the International Neuropsychological Society, 14*(3), 394–400.

Lucas, J. A., Ivnik, R. J., Smith, G. E., Ferman, T. J., Willis, F. B., Petersen, R. C., & Graff-Radford, N. R. (2005). Mayo's older African Americans normative studies: Norms for Boston Naming Test, controlled oral word association, category fluency, animal naming, Token Test, WRAT-3 Reading, Trail Making Test, Stroop Test, and Judgment of Line Orientation. *The Clinical Neuropsychologist, 19,* 243–269.

Lukatela, K., Malloy, P., Jenkins, M., & Cohen, R. (1998). The naming deficit in early Alzheimer's and vascular dementia. *Neuropsychology, 12,* 565–572.

Mack, W. J., Freed, D. M., Williams, B. W., & Henderson, V. W. (1992). Boston Naming Test: Shortened version for use in Alzheimer's disease. *Journal of Gerontology, 47,* 164–168.

MacKay, A., Connor, L. T., & Storandt, M. (2005). Dementia does not explain correlation between age and scores on Boston Naming Test. *Archives of Clinical Neuropsychology, 20,* 129–133.

Manly, J. J., Jacobs, D. M., Touradji, P., Small, S. A., & Stern, Y. (2002). Reading level attenuates differences in neuropsychological test performance between African American and White elders. *Journal of the International Neuropsychological Society, 8,* 314–348.

Manly, J. J., Miller, S. W., Heaton, R. K., Byrd, D., Reilly, J., Velasquez, R. J., . . . the HIV Neurobehavioral Research Center (HNRC) group. (1998). The effect of African American acculturation on neuropsychological test performance in normal and HIV-positive individuals. *Journal of the International Neuropsychological Society, 4,* 291–302.

Marien, P., Mampaey, E., Vervaet, A., Saerens, J., & De Deyn, P. P. (1998). Normative data for the Boston Naming Test in native Dutch-speaking Belgian elderly. *Brain and Language, 65,* 447–467.

Martielli, T. M., & Blackburn, L. B. (2016). When a funnel becomes a martini glass: Adolescent performance on the Boston Naming Test. *Child Neuropsychology, 22*(4), 381–393.

Miotto, E. C., Sato, J., Lucia, M. C. S., Camargo, C. H. P., & Scaff, M. (2010). Development of an adapted version of the Boston Naming Test for Portuguese speakers. *Revista Brasileira De Psiquiatria, 32*(3), 279–282.

Misdraji-Hammond, E., Lim, N. K., Fernandez, M., & Burke, M. E. (2015). Object familiarity and acculturation do not explain performance difference between Spanish–English bilinguals and English monolinguals on the Boston Naming Test. *Archives of Clinical Neuropsychology, 30*(1), 59–67.

Mitrushina, M., & Satz, P. (1995). Repeated testing of normal elderly with the Boston Naming Test. *Aging Clinical and Experimental Research, 7,* 123–127.

Mitrushina, M. M., Boone, K. B., Razani, J., & D'Elia, L. F. (2005). *Handbook of normative data for neuropsychological assessment* (2nd ed.) New York: Oxford University Press.

Morrison, L. E., Smith, L. A., & Sarazin, F. F. A. (1996). Boston Naming Test: A French-Canadian normative study (preliminary analyses) [Abstract]. *Journal of the International Neuropsychological Society, 2,* 4.

Neils, J., Baris, J. M., Carter, C., Dell'aira, A. L., Nordloh, S. J., Weiler, E., & Weisiger, B. (1995). Effects of age, education, and living environment on BNT performance. *Journal of Speech and Hearing Research, 38,* 1143–1149.

O'Bryant, S. E., Edwards, M., Johnson, L., Hall, J., Gamboa, A., & O'jile, J. (2018). Texas Mexican American adult normative studies: Normative data for commonly used clinical neuropsychological measures for English- and Spanish-speakers. *Developmental Neuropsychology, 43*(1), 1–26. https://doi.org/10.1080/87565641.2017.1401628

Olabarrieta-Landa, L., Rivera, D., Morlett-Paredes, A., Jaimes-Bautista, A., Garza, M. T., Galarza-del-Angel, J., . . . Arango-Lasprilla, J. C. (2015). Standard form of the Boston Naming Test: Normative data for the Latin American Spanish speaking adult population. *NeuroRehabilitation, 37*(4), 501–513. https://doi.org/10.3233/NRE-151278

Olszewski, H., Lukaszewska, B., & Tlokinski, W. (2011). The effects of phonemic cueing on confrontation naming in frontotemporal dementia and Alzheimer's disease: Evidence from the Polish version of the Boston Naming Test. *Acta Neuropsychologica, 9*(2), 155–165.

Patricacou, A., Psallida, E., Pring, T., & Dipper, L. (2007). The Boston Naming Test in Greek: Normative data and the effects of age and education on naming. *Aphasiology, 21*(12), 1157–1170. https://doi.org/10.1080/02687030600670643

Pedraza, O., Graff-Radford, N., Smith, G. E., Ivnik, R. J., Willis, F. B., Petersen, R. C., & Lucas, J. A. (2009). Differential item functioning of the Boston Naming Test in cognitively normal African American and Caucasian older adults. *Journal of the International Neuropsychological Society, 15*(5), 758–768.

Peña-Casanova, J., Quiñones-Úbeda, S., Gramunt-Fombuena, N., Aguilar, M., Casas, L., Molinuevo, J. L., . . . Martínez-Parra, C. (2009). Spanish multicenter normative studies (NEURONORMA Project): Norms for Boston Naming Test and Token Test. *Archives of Clinical Neuropsychology, 24*(4), 343–354.

Ponton, M. O., Satz, P., Herrera Ortiz, F., Urrutia, C. P., Young, R., D'Elia, L. F., . . . Namerow, N. (1996). Normative data stratified by age and education for the Neuropsychological Screening Battery for Hispanics (NESBHIS): Initial report. *Journal of the International Neuropsychological Society, 2,* 96–104.

Quigg, M., Broshek, D. K., Barbaro, N. M., Ward, M. M., Laxer, K. D., Yan, G., & Lamborn, K. (2011). Neuropsychological outcomes after Gamma Knife radiosurgery for mesial temporal lobe epilepsy: A prospective multicenter study. *Epilepsia, 52*(5), 909–916.

Rami, L., Serradell, M., Bosch, B., Caprile, C., Sekler, A., Villar, A., . . . Molinuevo, J. L. (2008). Normative data for the Boston Naming Test and the Pyramids and Palm Trees Test in the elderly Spanish population. *Journal of Clinical and Experimental Neuropsychology, 30*(1), 1–6.

Ramirez, M. J., Schefft, B. K., Howe, S. R., Hwa-Shain, Y., & Privitera, M. D. (2008). Interictal and postictal language testing accurately lateralizes language dominant temporal lobe complex partial seizures. *Epilepsia, 49*(1), 22–32.

Randolph, C., Lansing, A., Ivnick, R. J., Cullum, C. M., & Hermann, B. P. (1999). Determinants of confrontation naming performance. *Archives of Clinical Neuropsychology, 14,* 489–496.

Ripich, D. N., Petrill, S. A., Whitehouse, P. J., & Ziol, E. W. (1995). Gender differences in language of AD patients: A longitudinal study. *Neurology, 45,* 299–302.

Riva, D., Nichelli, F., & Devoti, M. (2000). Developmental aspects of verbal fluency and confrontation naming in children. *Brain and Language, 71,* 267–284.

Roberts, P. M., Garcia, L. J., Desrochers, A., & Hernandez, D. (2002) English performance of proficient bilingual adults on the Boston Naming Test. *Aphasiology, 16,* 635–645.

Ross, T. P., & Lichtenberg, P. A. (1998). Expanded normative data for the Boston Naming Test with urban, elderly medical patients. *The Clinical Neuropsychologist, 12,* 475–481.

Ross, T. P., Lichtenberg, P. A., & Christensen, K. (1995). Normative data on the Boston Naming Test for elderly adults in a demographically diverse medical sample. *The Clinical Neuropsychologist, 9,* 321–325.

Ruff, I. M., Swanson, S. J., Hammeke, T. A., Sabsevitz, D., Mueller, W. M., & Morris, G. L. (2007). Predictors of naming decline after dominant temporal lobectomy: Age at onset of epilepsy and age of word acquisition. *Epilepsy & Behavior, 10*(2), 272–277.

Sachs, B. C., Lucas, J. A., Smith, G. E., Ivnik, R. J., Petersen, R. C., Graff-Radford, N. R., & Pedraza, O. (2012). Reliable change on the Boston Naming Test. *Journal of the International Neuropsychological Society, 18*(02), 375–378.

Satz, P. (1993). Brain reserve capacity on symptom onset after brain injury: A formulation and review of evidence for threshold theory. *Neuropsychology, 7,* 273–295.

Sawrie, S. M., Chelune, G. J., Naugle, R. I., & Luders, H. O. (1996). Empirical methods for assessing meaningful change following epilepsy surgery. *Journal of the International Neuropsychological Association, 2,* 556–564.

Saxton, J., Ratcliff, G., Munro, C. A., Coffey, C. E., Becker, J. E., Fried, L., & Kuller, L. (2000). Normative data on the Boston Naming Test and two equivalent 30-item short-forms. *The Clinical Neuropsychologist, 14,* 526–534.

Schefft, B. K., Testa, S. M., Dulay, M. F., Privitera, M. D., & Yeh, H. S. (2003). Preoperative assessment of confrontation naming ability and interictal paraphasia production in unilateral temporal lobe epilepsy. *Epilepsy and Behavior, 4,* 161–168.

Schretlen, D. J., Testa, M., & Pearlson, G. D. (2010). *Calibrated neuropsychological normative system: Professional manual.* Lutz, FL: Psychological Assessment Resources.

Senior, G., Douglas, L., & Dawes, S. (2001). *Discrepancy analysis: A new/old approach to psychological test data interpretation.* Presentation at the 21st annual conference of the National Academy of Neuropsychology, San Francisco, California.

Sheppard, C., Kousaie, S., Monetta, L., & Taler, V. (2016). Performance on the Boston Naming Test in bilinguals. *Journal of the International Neuropsychological Society, 22*(3), 350–363.

Shim, Y. S., Youn, Y. C., Na, D. L., Kim, S. Y., Cheong, H. K., Moon, S. Y., . . . Kang, H. (2011). Effects of medial temporal atrophy and white matter hyperintensities on the cognitive functions in patients with Alzheimer's disease. *European Neurology, 66*(2), 75–82.

Silvestre, G., Iglesias, R. M., & Silvestre, E. (2018). Boston Naming Test norms for the Dominican population. *Aphasiology, 32*(3), 340–365. https://doi.org/10.1080/02687038.2017.1338662

Simos, P. G., Kasselimis, D., & Mouzaki, A. (2011). Effects of demographic variables and health status on brief vocabulary measures in Greek. *Aphasiology, 25*(4), 492–504.

Soble, J. R., Marceaux, J. C., Galindo, J., Sordahl, J. A., Highsmith, J. M., O'Rourke, J. J., . . . McCoy, K. J. (2016). The effect of perceptual reasoning abilities on confrontation naming performance: An examination of three naming tests. *Journal of Clinical and Experimental Neuropsychology, 38*(3), 284–292.

Stålhammar, J., Rydén, I., Nordlund, A., & Wallin, A. (2016). Boston Naming Test automatic credits inflate scores of nonaphasic mild dementia patients. *Journal of Clinical and Experimental Neuropsychology, 38*(4), 381–392.

Steinberg, B. A., Bieliauskas, L. A., Smith, G. E., Langellotti, C., & Ivnik, R. J. (2005). MAYO's older Americans normative studies: Age- and IQ-adjusted norms for the Boston Naming Test, the MAE Token Test, and the Judgement of Line Orientation Test. *The Clinical Neuropsychologist, 19,* 280–328.

Storms, G., Saerens, J., & De Deyn, P. P. (2004). Normative data for the Boston Naming Test in native Dutch-speaking Belgian children and the relation with intelligence. *Brain and Language, 91,* 274–281.

Testa, J. A., Ivnik, R. J., Boeve, B., Pedersen, R. C., Pankratz, V. S., Knopman, D., . . . Smith, G. E. (2004). Confrontation naming does not add incremental diagnostic utility in MCI and Alzheimer's disease. *Journal of the International Neuropsychological Society, 10,* 504–512.

Tombaugh, T. N., & Hubley, A. (1997). The 60-item Boston Naming Test: Norms for cognitively intact adults aged 25 to 88 years. *Journal of Clinical and Experimental Neuropsychology, 19,* 922–932.

Touradji, P., Manly, J. J., Jacobs, D. M., & Stern, Y. (2001). Neuropsychological test performance: A study of non-Hispanic white elderly. *Journal of Clinical and Experimental Neuropsychology, 23,* 643–649.

Tsang, H. L., & Lee, T. M. C. (2003). The effect of aging on confrontational naming ability. *Archives of Clinical Neuropsychology, 18,* 81–89.

Tweedy, J. R., & Schulman, P. D. (1982). Toward a functional classification of naming impairment. *Brain and Language, 15,* 193–206.

Unverzagt, F. W., Morgan, O. S., & Thesiger, C. H. (1999). Clinical utility of CERAD neuropsychological battery in elderly Jamaicans. *Journal of International Neuropsychological Society, 5,* 255–259.

Van Zandvoort, M., de Haan, E., van Gijn, J., & Kappelle, L. J. (2003). Cognitive functioning in patients with a small infarct in the brainstem. *Journal of the International Neuropsychological Society, 9,* 490–494.

Weiner, M. W., Sadowsky, C., Saxton, J., Hofbauer, R. K., Graham, S. M., Yu, S. Y., . . . Perhach, J. L. (2011). Magnetic resonance imaging and neuropsychological results from a trial of memantine in Alzheimer's disease. *Alzheimer's & Dementia, 7*(4), 425–435.

Weissberger, G. H., Salmon, D. P., Bondi, M. W., & Gollan, T. H. (2013). Which neuropsychological tests predict progression to Alzheimer's disease in Hispanics? *Neuropsychology, 27*(3), 343.

Welsh, K. A., Fillenbaum, G., Wilkinson, W., Heyman, A., Mohs, R. C., Stern, Y., Harrell, L., Edland, S. D., & Beekly, D. (1995). Neuropsychological test performance in African American and white patients with Alzheimer's disease. *Neurology, 45,* 2207–2211.

Welch, L. W., Doineau, D., Johnson, S., & King, D. (1996). Education and gender normative data for the Boston Naming Test in a group of older adults. *Brain and Language, 53,* 260–266.

Whiteside, D. M., Kogan, J., Wardin, L., Phillips, D., Franzwa, M. G., Rice, L., . . . Roper, B. (2015). Language-based embedded performance validity measures in traumatic brain injury. *Journal of Clinical and Experimental Neuropsychology, 37*(2), 220–227.

Williams, V. G., Bruce, J. M., Westervelt, H. J., Davis, J. D., Grace, J., Malloy, P. F., & Tremont, G. (2007). Boston Naming performance distinguishes between Lewy body and Alzheimer's dementias. *Archives of Clinical Neuropsychology, 22*(8), 925–931.

Worrall, L. E., Yiu, E. M. L., Hickson, L. M. H., & Barnett, H. M. (1995). Normative data for the Boston Naming Test for Australian elderly. *Aphasiology, 9,* 541–551.

Yochim, B. P., Rashid, K., Raymond, N. C., & Beaudreau, S. A. (2013). How frequently are words used on naming tests used in spoken conversation? *The Clinical Neuropsychologist, 27*(6), 973–987.

Youn, J. H., Siksou, M., Mackin, R. S., Choi, J. S., Chey, J., & Lee, J. Y. (2011). Differentiating illiteracy from Alzheimer's disease by using neuropsychological assessments. *International Psychogeriatrics, 23*(10), 1560–1568.

Zec, R. F., Burkett, N. R., Markwell, S. J., & Larsen, D. L. (2007a). A cross-sectional study of the effects of age, education, and gender on the Boston Naming Test. *The Clinical Neuropsychologist, 21*(4), 587–616.

Zec, R. F., Burkett, N. R., Markwell, S. J., & Larsen, D. L. (2007b). Normative data stratified for age, education, and gender on the Boston Naming Test. *The Clinical Neuropsychologist, 21*(4), 617–637.

MULTILINGUAL APHASIA EXAMINATION THIRD EDITION (MAE)

TEST NAME	**Multilingual Aphasia Examination Third Edition (MAE)**
DOMAIN	Language
AGE RANGE	In adults, to 69 years
ADMINISTRATION TIME	40 minutes
SCORING FORMAT	Hand scored
REFERENCE	Benton, A. L., Hamsher, K. de S., Rey, G. J., & Sivan, A. B. (1994). *Multilingual Aphasia Examination* (3rd Ed.). Iowa City, IA: AJA Associates. www.parinc.com

DESCRIPTION

The Multilingual Aphasia Examination Third Edition (MAE) provides a relatively brief examination of the presence, severity, and qualitative aspects of aphasic language disorders. It does not claim to follow a specific model of language function, although it covers the most common aspects of language function affected in aphasia. It includes nine subtests and two rating scales (see Table 11–55). An alternate version of Sentence Repetition, COWA, and the Token Test is available for repeat assessment. As its name implies, the MAE was conceived as a test battery consisting of functionally equivalent forms in different languages. The Spanish version (Rey & Benton, 1991; Rey et al., 1999) contains the same subtests, but items and wordings are rephrased appropriately for individuals of Cuban, Mexican, and Puerto Rican origin. For example, COWA uses the letters P, T, and M, reflecting similar levels of difficulty in Spanish. Hence, performance of the task in each language is functionally equivalent; that is, the different language versions of the MAE are functionally equivalent in content rather than being simple translations.

Two MAE subtests (COWA and the Token Test) have generated considerable literature in their own right and have also been incorporated into other cognitive batteries (e.g., Mayo norms; Ivnik et al., 1996). The reader is referred to descriptions of the COWA and Token Test elsewhere in this volume (see the sections "Verbal Fluency" and "Token Test").

ADMINISTRATION

See the manual.

SCORING

Scoring is fully described in the source and is relatively simple and straightforward. Of the nine tests, two (Sentence Repetition, COWA) require corrections for age and educational level and six require correction for education only. The MAE Token Test does not require corrections, according to the authors. The test comes with scoring sheets for each subtest and a summary sheet that provides space for percentiles compared to healthy controls and to patients with aphasia.

DEMOGRAPHIC EFFECTS

AGE

Borderline adult performance is reached at about age 12 years 3 months, although values for the Token Test and COWA approach plateau values starting at age 10 years (Schum et al., 1989). The manual discusses studies of norms for older adults and concludes that no noteworthy decline in performance has been found up to age 79 years, but that subnormal performance, especially on the Sentence Repetition and the Token Test, is "not rare" for individuals 80 to 89 years of age, perhaps because of the demands of these tests on memory (see also Schum & Sivan, 1997). In older adults, correlations with age tend to be small (< .30) for both COWA and the Token Test (Ivnik et al., 1996; Lucas et al., 2005).

GENDER

Schum and Sivan (1997) found no gender differences among older adults on the MAE. Similarly, Ivnik et al. (1996) and Lucas et al. (2005) reported little effect of gender on COWA and Token Test scores. Elias et al. (1997) found that gender accounted for only 1% of the variance for COWA in a sample of 1,893 community residents. In this sample, the oldest participants with the fewest years of education had the lowest performance on COWA, with lower levels for men than for women.

EDUCATION AND IQ

Education has a stronger effect than age on COWA scores (r = .38 to .42) and Token Test scores (r = .24 to .32; Elias

TABLE 11–55 Description of Multilingual Aphasia Examination Third Edition (MAE) Subtests and Rating Scales

AREA	SUBTEST/SCALE	DESCRIPTION
Oral Expression	Visual Naming	Requires naming of line drawings or parts thereof (e.g., telephone, telephone dial); 30 items, each scored as 0, 1, or 2 points
	Sentence Repetition	Requires the repetition of 14 sentences of increasing length up to 22 syllables; vocabulary and syntax are deliberately simple, but interrogative, negative, and other forms are included
	Controlled Oral Word Association	Word generation to three letters (CFL, PRW, see "Verbal Fluency" for a detailed discussion of this subtest)
Spelling	Oral Spelling	The word is presented, then presented again in a sentence, and the examinee must spell it orally (11 words)
	Written Spelling (to dictation)	The word is presented, then presented again in a sentence, and the examinee must write it (11 words)
	Block Letter Spelling	Plastic letters are spread in front of the examinee, who then must use these letters to spell the word (11 words)
Verbal Comprehension of Commands	Token Test	Consists of 22 commands at two levels of complexity (e.g., "Point to a large yellow square"), each scored as 0, 1, or 2 points
Comprehension	Aural Comprehension of Words and Phrases	The examinee must point to one of four choices of line drawings on six plates corresponding to the word or phrase (e.g., "dog under the table"); 18 items
	Reading Comprehension of Words and Phrases	Reading Comprehension is also administered in a multiple-choice format: a set of words and phrases is presented in written form (capital block letters), the examinee must point to the appropriate choice on the same six plates used in the previous test
Rating of Articulation and Writing Praxis	Rating of Articulation	Articulation is rated immediately on completion of the other tests on a 9-point scale, ranging from 0 ("speechless or usually unintelligible speech") to 8 ("normal speech")
	Rating of Praxis Features of Writing	Praxis features of writing are rated after completion of the written spelling test for imprecision, distortion, and legibility on a 9-point scale; scores range from 0 ("illegible scrawl") to 8 ("good penmanship")

SOURCE: Benton et al. (1994). Reproduced by special permission of the Publisher, Psychological Assessment Resources, Inc. (PAR), 16204 North Florida Avenue, Lutz, Florida 33549, from the Multilingual Aphasia Examination by Arthur L. Benton, PhD, Kerry deS. Hamsher, PhD, and Abigail Sivan, PhD. Copyright 1978, 2001 by PAR. Further reproduction is prohibited without permission from PAR.

et al., 1997; Ivnik et al., 1996; Lucas et al., 2005; Steinberg et al., 2005), with performance improving at higher educational levels. For the Token Test, education becomes redundant when IQ is taken into account (Steinberg et al., 2005). IQ and test scores are less strongly associated at the higher ends of the IQ continuum (Steinberg et al., 2005).

ETHNICITY, NATIONALITY, AND LINGUISTIC EFFECTS

Ethnicity affects test scores. Roberts and Hamsher (1984) found lower norm values for Visual Naming in an urban inner-city African-American population. They argued that Visual Naming may be especially sensitive to cultural experience and that separate normative data should be obtained for this population. Kennepohl et al. (2004) found that lower levels of acculturation were linked to lower scores on the Token Test among African Americans who had sustained a traumatic brain injury.

There do not appear to be nationality effects (i.e., Puerto Rican vs. Mexican) on the Spanish version of the test (MAE-S; Rey et al., 1999).

NORMATIVE DATA

STANDARDIZATION SAMPLE

The MAE manual provides normative data in the form of percentiles based on a sample of 360 healthy Iowa adults whose native language was English (see Table 11–56). Data from a sample of patients with aphasia are presented in the manual for various subtests to be used in cases where precise estimate of performance level is required among those with very low scores.

The MAE-S Manual includes normative information from a sample of 234 healthy Spanish-speaking adults from Texas and Puerto Rico (aged 18 to 70 years) without history or evidence of neurological or psychiatric disability. Cutoff values based on this normative group are

TABLE 11–56 Characteristics of the Multilingual Aphasia Examination Third Edition (MAE) Standardization Sample

Sample size	360
Age	16 to 69 years
Sample type	Standardization sample
Gender	Not reported
Ethnicity	Not reported
Education	Not reported
Socioeconomic status	Not reported
Screening	No evidence of history of neurological disease, intellectual disability, or hospitalization for psychiatric disorder

SOURCE: Benton et al. (1994). Reproduced by special permission of the Publisher, Psychological Assessment Resources, Inc. (PAR), 16204 North Florida Avenue, Lutz, Florida 33549, from the Multilingual Aphasia Examination by Arthur L. Benton, PhD, Kerry deS. Hamsher, PhD, and Abigail Sivan, PhD. Copyright 1978, 2001 by PAR. Further reproduction is prohibited without permission from PAR.

reported to be quite comparable to those of the English version (Rey et al., 1999).

OTHER NORMATIVE DATA

Schum and Sivan (1997) examined 54 older adult volunteers, residing in a college community in Iowa, who had above-average education (about 15 years) and self-ratings of good or very good health. Individual MAE subtest scores were adjusted for education levels when necessary, in accordance with specifications in the MAE manual (Benton et al., 1994). For Sentence Repetition and COWA, adjustments were made using the highest available age category (60–69 years) and educational level. Only Sentence Repetition showed a significant decline across the four age groups. There was also a slight, but not statistically significant, decline in performance on the Token Test. Note, however, that the cell sizes were very small and the participants reflected a highly selected group of older adults.

More extensive normative data are available for the COWA and the Token Test. The reader is referred to the section "Verbal Fluency" with regard to the COWA. Ivnik et al. (1996) provided age- and education-corrected scores for the Token Test for use with older adults aged 56 to 95+ years. Note that these norms were derived from a large sample (399) of Caucasian individuals living in an economically advantaged region of the United States. Their data are shown in Table 11–57, along with an equation to adjust scores for education level. Midpoint intervals were used to maximize the available information. The MOANS norms have a mean of 10 and an *SD* of 3. The authors cautioned that the validity of these norms for persons of other ethnic/cultural or socioeconomic backgrounds is questionable.

Steinberg et al. (2005) have expanded the utility of the MOANS project by providing age- and IQ-adjusted percentile equivalents of MOANS age-adjusted Token Test scores, for use with individuals aged 55+. Users should note that all FSIQs are MOANS age-adjusted scores, which are based on the WAIS-R, not the WAIS-IV, making these of limited utility.

Lucas et al. (2005) provide age- and education-adjusted normative data based on 289 African-American, community-dwelling participants from the MOAANS project in Jacksonville, Florida. Participants were predominantly female (74%), ranged in age from 56 to 94 years (M = 69.6, SD = 6.87) and varied in education from 0 to 20 years of formal education (M = 12.2, SD = 3.48). They were screened to exclude those with active neurological, psychiatric, or other conditions that might affect cognition. Table 11–58 presents their data, and Table 11–59 provides the computational formula used to calculate age- and education-adjusted MOAANS scaled scores. The authors urged that their data be used with caution because the number of very old adults is somewhat small and they used a sample of convenience that may not represent the full range of cultural and educational experiences of the African-American community.

EVIDENCE FOR RELIABILITY

EVIDENCE FOR INTERNAL RELIABILITY

This is not reported.

TABLE 11–57 Token Test MOANS Norms for Persons (Predominantly Caucasian) Aged 56 to 97 Years

PERCENTILE RANGES	56–62	63–65	66–68	69–71	72–74	75–77	78–80	81–83	84–86	87–89	90–97	SCALED SCORE
n	94	94	94	94	130	178	227	230	204	140	88	
<1	<29	<29	<29	<29	<29	<29	<24	<19	<18	<18	<17	2
1	29–30	29–30	29–30	29–30	29–30	29–30	24–28	19–23	18–22	18–20	17	3
2	31–32	31–32	31–32	31–32	31	31	29	24–28	23–27	21–27	18–19	4
3–5	33–35	33–35	33–35	33–35	32–35	32–34	30–33	29–31	28–30	28–29	20–25	5
6–10	36	36	36	36	36	35	34	32–33	31–33	30–32	26–32	6
11–18	37–38	37–38	37–38	37–38	37	36–37	35–36	34–35	34–35	33–34	33–34	7
19–28	39	39	39	39	38–39	38	37	36–37	36	35–36	35–36	8
29–40	40–41	40–41	40–41	40–41	40	39–40	38	38	37	37	37	9
41–59	42	42	42	42	41–42	41–42	39–41	39–41	38–41	38–40	38–40	10
60–71	43	43	43	43	43		42	42	42	41–42	41	11
72–81	44	44	44	44	44	43–44	43	43	43	—	42	12
82–89							44	44	44	43	43	13
90–94										44	44	14
95–97												15
98												16
99												17
>99												18

NOTE: Based on Mayo's Older Americans Normative Studies (MOANS). Age- and education-corrected MOANS Scaled Score ($MSS_{A\&E}$) is calculated from a person's age-corrected MOANS Scaled Score (MSS_A) and that person's education expressed in years of formal schooling completed as follows: $MSS_{A\&E} = 0.47 + (1.33 \times MSS_A) - (0.31 \times \text{Education})$. Mean FSIQ about 106, range: 76–138.

SOURCE: Adapted from Ivnik et al. (1996).

TABLE 11–58 Token Test MOAANS Age-Based Norms for African-American Adults

SCALED SCORE	56–62	63–65	66–68	69–71	72–74	75–77	78+	PERCENTILE RANGES
2	0–19	0–19	0–19	0–19	0–19	0–19	0–19	<1
3	20–26	20–25	20–25	20–25	20–25	20–25	20–25	1
4	27–29	26–27	26–27	26–27	26–27	26–27	26–27	2
5	30–32	28–30	28–30	28–30	28–30	28–30	28–30	3–5
6	33–36	31–35	31–35	31–34	31–34	31–34	31–34	6–10
7	37–38	36–38	36–37	35–37	35–37	35–37	35–37	11–18
8	39–40	39–40	38–39	38–39	38	38	38	19–28
9	41	41	40–41	40	39–40	39–40	39	29–40
10	42–43	42	42	41–42	41–42	41	40	41–59
11	–	43	43	43	43	42	41–42	60–71
12	–	–	–	–	–	43	43	72–81
13	44	44	44	44	44	–	–	82–89
14	–	–	–	–	–	44	44	90–94
15	–	–	–	–	–	–	–	95–97
16	–	–	–	–	–	–	–	98
17	–	–	–	–	–	–	–	99
18	–	–	–	–	–	–	–	>99
n	101	121	157	172	147	113	76	

SOURCE: Adapted from Lucas et al. (2005).

EVIDENCE FOR TEST-RETEST RELIABILITY, MEASURING CHANGE, AND PRACTICE EFFECTS

Test-retest reliability data were not reported in the manual. Test-retest reliability in cardiac patients who underwent cardiac procedures are adequate over three weeks (r = .80) and low over four months and one year (r = .59 and .59, respectively) for MAE Visual Naming (Sweet et al., 2008).

EVIDENCE FOR RELIABILITY OF ALTERNATE FORMS

There are no differences between Forms A and B for Sentence Repetition, COWA, or the Token Test (Schum & Sivan, 1997). There are also no differences for the three alternate spelling lists for the Oral, Written, and Block Spelling tests (Benton & Hamsher, 1989; Schum et al., 1989; Schum & Sivan, 1997).

EVIDENCE FOR VALIDITY

FACTOR-ANALYTIC STUDIES

A factor analysis of 16 aphasia battery subtests (including subtests of the MAE, Neurosensory Center Comprehensive Examination for Aphasia [NCCEA], and the WAB), given to healthy Taiwanese volunteers (Hua et al., 1997), suggested a major factor of verbal comprehension (including Token Test, Sentence Repetition, Digit Repetition, Visual Naming, Reading, and Aural Comprehension). A second factor was labeled "effortful writing." A third factor involved mainly verbal expression and word production.

TABLE 11–59 Computational Formula for Age- and Education-Corrected MOAANS Scaled Scores

	K	W_1	W_2
Token Test	0.67	1.23	0.23

NOTE: Age- and education-corrected MOAANS Scaled Scores ($MSS_{A\&E}$) can be calculated for Token Test scores by using age-corrected MOAANS Scaled Scores (MSS_A) and education (expressed in years completed) in the following formula: $MSS_{A\&E} = K + (W_1 \times MSS_A) - (W_2 \times EDUC)$.

SOURCE: From Lucas et al. (2005).

RELATIONSHIPS WITH OTHER TESTS

The Visual Naming subtest correlates highly with the 60-item Boston Naming Test (BNT; r = .76 to .86; Axelrod et al., 1994; Schefft et al., 2003). Axelrod et al. (1994) reported that Visual Naming showed strong relations to the WAIS-R verbal-comprehension factor but only minimal relations to the perceptual-organization and distractibility factors. Lincoln et al. (1994) used test performances on the MAE to better understand performance on the WAIS-R in a sample of patients with closed-head injury. WAIS-R Verbal subtests were correlated most strongly with MAE Visual Naming, with the exception of Digit Span and Arithmetic, which were correlated more closely with performance on MAE Sentence Repetition. As might be anticipated, WAIS-R Performance subtests showed lesser degrees of correlation with the MAE, but they showed modest correlations with the MAE Token Test and COWA.

CLINICAL STUDIES

Aphasia. The MAE (particularly the Token Test) is sensitive to language disorders. Jones and Benton (1995) evaluated the sensitivity of the MAE in aphasics with focal left hemisphere lesions and healthy controls. The aphasic group performed poorly on all subtests of the MAE relative to the controls. Using the suggested cutoffs, between 3% and 7%

of healthy controls and between 14% and 65% of aphasics were misclassified by individual subtests. All aphasics and 15% of controls performed poorly on at least one MAE subtest. Using a cutoff of two defective performances, 96% of aphasics but only 3% of controls performed poorly. The implication is that diagnosis should not be based on individual subtests.

Dementia. MAE subtests are sensitive to aphasia in various dementing disorders with language disturbances as their primary symptoms and may be useful to distinguish among various subgroups. In one study, patients with logopenic variant of primary progressive aphasia performed significantly lower than matched controls on MAE Sentence Repetition. However, the differences were due to a subgroup of patients with logopenic variant primary progressive aphasia who exhibited impaired single-word repetition and cortical thinning of the left superior temporal gyrus. MAE Sentence Repetition performance of this subgroup was remarkably worse than the other subgroups (i.e., a group with pure anomia and left-sided atrophy in the posterior inferior parietal lobe and lateral temporal cortex, and a second group with mild single-word comprehension deficits and bilateral thinning of the fusiform gyrus), suggesting that Sentence Repetition deficits are not uniform across all patients with logopenic variant primary progressive aphasia (Leyton et al., 2015). By contrast, patients with aphasia and AD pathology, aphasia and FTD pathology, and typical AD clinical features and AD pathology were equally impaired on the MAE Token Test (Josephs et al., 2008). The MAE Token Test may therefore not be useful in distinguishing among different dementias presenting with language disturbances. Similarly, whether low verbal fluency forecasts a diagnosis of probable AD is uncertain (Elias et al., 2000). Measures of retention of information (e.g., Logical Memory) and abstract reasoning (WAIS Similarities) are more powerful predictors (Elias et al., 2000).

TLE. As might be expected, patients with left TLE show significant impairment on the MAE (and on tests of verbal learning) compared with those with right TLE (Hermann & Wyler, 1988; Hermann et al., 1992). However, the BNT is diagnostically more superior to the Visual Naming subtest of the MAE in identifying left TLE (Schefft et al., 2003; Loring et al., 2008) perhaps because the latter is considerably easier and shorter than the BNT and also tends not to elicit paraphasias. For example, comparing the utility of BNT and MAE Visual Naming to predict side of seizure onset in TLE patients who subsequently underwent anterior temporal lobectomy, Loring and colleagues (2008) reported a sensitivity of 58%, specificity of 70%, positive likelihood ratio (LR+) of 1.91, and negative likelihood ratio (LR−) of .60 using the BNT, and a sensitivity of 75%, specificity of 39%, LR+ of 1.23, and LR− of .65 using MAE Visual Naming. O'Shea et al. (1996) found that self-report of memory problems in patients with TLE was related only to COWA, not to other MAE subtests.

Traumatic Brain Injury. Patients who have sustained head injuries also show language difficulties on the MAE. Levin et al. (1976, 1981) examined the linguistic performance of patients with closed head injuries, reporting a high frequency of naming errors, defective associative word finding, and impaired comprehension on the Token Test; these findings were correlated with severity of head injury. Millis et al. (2001) described similar findings in a longitudinal study of persons with TBI who received inpatient rehabilitation, and Rey et al. (2001) reported similar findings in Hispanics after TBI using the Spanish version of the MAE. Articulatory difficulties were also noted after TBI (Levin et al., 1981; Rey et al., 2001).

Language-related difficulties evident on the MAE may affect memory performance. Crosson et al. (1993) reported that, in patients who sustained head injury, visual object naming (Visual Naming) and auditory comprehension (Token Test) were predictive of total number of words recalled (but not percent retained) on the California Verbal Learning Test. The implication is that examiners should explore language deficits as a cause of performance deficits on verbal memory tasks.

Other Findings. The MAE Token Test has also been shown to be a sensitive indicator of acute confusional states (delirium) in nonaphasic medical patients (Lee & Hamsher, 1988). There is some preliminary evidence that the MAE Token Test administered via telemedicine to assess language deficits in mild AD is comparable to in-person assessment and that telemedicine was generally acceptable to participants (Vestal et al., 2006).

NEUROANATOMICAL CORRELATES AND IMAGING STUDIES

Not reported.

PERFORMANCE VALIDITY

Not reported.

COMMENT

The MAE is a relatively short aphasia battery, and each subtest may be used independently. In fact, most studies have utilized individual subtests (e.g., COWA, Visual Naming, Sentence Repetition, Token Test) rather than the MAE in its entirety. One strength of the MAE is the availability of a carefully constructed Spanish version.

Few recent studies have utilized the MAE and perhaps for good reasons. The limited reliability information presents a serious obstacle for use of the MAE in clinical diagnosis. In addition, there are ceiling effects for most of the tasks, and misclassifications regarding the presence or absence of language disturbance do occur when using individual subtests. Greater confidence is justified when the tests are used in combination or along with clinical features of aphasic speech (e.g., paraphasias).

More importantly for everyday clinical purposes, the original normative group is poorly described, and the information is more than two decades old (but see "Verbal Fluency" for additional COWA normative data). For most of the tasks, the normative sample was small, very well educated, and from the midwestern United States. Lack of updated norms from a diverse sample undermines the utility of clinical data obtained using the MAE. Caution is advised in applying these norms, particularly to individuals whose characteristics differ.

There are some preliminary data suggesting equivalence of MAE Token Test administered via telemedicine and in-person. Although these data address an important question about the contemporary use of the MAE, other relevant questions such as its correlates to brain imaging studies and availability of embedded performance validity indicators remain unanswered.

REFERENCES

Axelrod, B. N., Ricker, J. H., & Cherry, S. A. (1994). Concurrent validity of the MAE Visual Naming Test. *Archives of Clinical Neuropsychology, 9,* 317–321.

Benton, A. L., & Hamsher, K. (1989). *Multilingual Aphasia Examination—Second Edition.* Iowa City, IA: AJA Associates.

Benton, A. L., Hamsher, K. de S., Rey, G. J., & Sivan, A. B. (1994). *Multilingual Aphasia Examination* (3rd Ed.). Iowa City, IA: AJA Associates.

Crosson, B., Cooper, P. V., Lincoln, R. K., & Bauer, R. M. (1993). Relationship between verbal memory and language performance after blunt head injury. *The Clinical Neuropsychologist, 7,* 250–267.

Elias, M. F., Beiser, A., Wolf, P. A., Au, R., White, R. F., & D'Agostino, R. B. (2000). The preclinical phase of Alzheimer disease: A 22-year prospective study of the Framingham cohort. *Archives of Neurology, 57,* 808–813.

Elias, M. F., Elias, P. K., D'Agostino, R. B., Silbershatz, H., & Wolf, P. A. (1997). Role of age, education, and gender on cognitive performance in the Framingham Heart Study: Community-based norms. *Experimental Aging Research, 23,* 201–235.

Hermann, B. P., Seidenberg, M., Haltiner, A., & Wyler, A. R. (1992). Adequacy of language function and verbal memory performance in unilateral temporal lobe epilepsy. *Cortex, 28,* 423–433.

Hermann, B. P., & Wyler, A. R. (1988). Effects of anterior temporal lobectomy on language function. *Annals of Neurology, 23,* 585–588.

Hua, M. S., Chang, S. H., & Chen, S. T. (1997). Factor structure and age effects with an aphasia test battery in normal Taiwanese adults. *Neuropsychology, 11,* 156–162.

Ivnik, R. J., Malec, J. F., & Smith, G. E. (1996). Neuropsychological tests' norms above age 55: COWAT, BNT, MAE, WRAT-R Reading, AMNART, STROOP, TMT and JLO. *The Clinical Neuropsychologist, 10,* 262–278.

Jones, R. D., & Benton, A. L. (1995). Use of the Multilingual Aphasia Examination in the detection of language disorders [Abstract]. *Journal of the International Neuropsychological Society, 1,* 364.

Josephs, K. A., Whitwell, J. L., Duffy, J. R., Vanvoorst, W. A., Strand, E. A., Hu, W. T., ... Dickson, D. W. (2008). Progressive aphasia secondary to Alzheimer disease vs FTLD pathology. *Neurology, 70*(1), 25–34.

Kennepohl, S., Shore, D., Nobors, N., & Hanks, R. (2004). African American acculturation and neuropsychological test performance following traumatic brain injury. *Journal of the International Neuropsychological Society, 10,* 566–577.

Lee, G. P., & Hamsher, K. (1988). Neuropsychological findings in toxicometabolic confusional states. *Journal of Clinical and Experimental Neuropsychology, 10,* 769–778.

Levin, H., Grossman, R. G., & Kelly, P. J. (1976). Aphasic disorders in patients with closed-head injury. *Journal of Neurology, Neurosurgery, and Psychiatry, 39,* 1062–1070.

Levin, H., Grossman, R. G., Sarwar, M., & Meyers, C. A. (1981). Linguistic recovery after closed head injury. *Brain and Language, 12,* 360–374.

Leyton, C. E., Hodges, J. R., McLean, C. A., Kril, J. J., Piguet, O., & Ballard, K. J. (2015). Is the logopenic-variant of primary progressive aphasia a unitary disorder? *Cortex, 67,* 122–133.

Lincoln, R. K., Crosson, B., Bauer, R. M., Cooper, P. V., & Velozo, C. A. (1994). Relationship between WAIS-R subtests and language measures after blunt head injury. *The Clinical Neuropsychologist, 8,* 140–152.

Loring, D. W., Strauss, E., Hermann, B. P., Barr, W. B., Perrine, K., Trenerry, M. R., ... Bowden, S. C. (2008). Differential neuropsychological test sensitivity to left temporal lobe epilepsy. *Journal of the International Neuropsychological Society, 14*(3), 394–400.

Lucas, J. A., Ivnik, R. J., Smith, G. E., Ferman, T. J., Willis, F. B., Petersen, R. C., & Graff-Radford, N. R. (2005). Mayo's older African Americans normative studies: Norms for Boston Naming Test, controlled oral word association, category fluency, animal naming, Token Test, WRAT-3 Reading, Trail Making Test, Stroop Test, and judgment of line orientation. *The Clinical Neuropsychologist, 19,* 243–269.

Millis, S. R., Rosenthal, M., Novack, T. A., Sherer, M., Nick, T. G., Kreutzer, J. S., ... Ricker, J. H. (2001). Long-term neuropsychological outcome after traumatic brain injury. *Journal of Head Trauma Rehabilitation, 16,* 343–355.

O'Shea, M. F., Saling, M. M., Bladin, P. F., & Berkovic, S. F. (1996). Does naming contribute to memory self-report in temporal lobe epilepsy? *Journal of Clinical and Experimental Neuropsychology, 18,* 98–109.

Rey, G. J., & Benton, A. L. (1991). *Examen de Afasia Multilingue.* Iowa City, IA: AJA Associates.

Rey, G. J., Feldman, E., Hernandez, D., Levin, B. E., Rivas-Vasques, R., Nedd, K. J., & Benton, A. L. (2001). Application of the Multilingual Aphasia Examination—Spanish in the evaluation of Hispanic patients post closed-head trauma. *The Clinical Neuropsychologist, 15,* 13–18.

Rey, G. J., Feldman, E., Rivas-Vasques, R., Levin, B. E., & Benton, A. (1999). Neuropsychological test development and normative data on Hispanics. *Archives of Clinical Neuropsychology, 14,* 593–601.

Roberts, R. J., & Hamsher, K. (1984). Effects of minority status on facial recognition and naming performance. *Journal of Clinical Psychology, 40,* 539–545.

Schefft, B. K., Testa, S. M., Dulay, M. F., Privitera, M. D., & Yeh, H. S. (2003). Preoperative assessment of confrontation naming ability and interictal paraphasia in unilateral temporal lobe epilepsy. *Epilepsy and Behavior, 4,* 161–168.

Schum, R. L., & Sivan, A. B. (1997). Verbal abilities in healthy elderly adults. *Applied Neuropsychology, 4,* 130–134.

Schum, R. L., Sivan, A. B., & Benton, A. L. (1989). Multilingual Aphasia Examination: Norms for children. *The Clinical Neuropsychologist, 3,* 375–383.

Steinberg, B. A., Bieliauskas, L. A., Smith, G. E., Langellotti, C., & Ivnik, R. J. (2005). MAYO's older Americans normative studies: Age- and IQ-adjusted norms for the Boston Naming Test, the MAE Token Test, and the Judgement of Line Orientation Test. *The Clinical Neuropsychologist, 19,* 280–328.

Sweet, J. J., Finnin, E., Wolfe, P. L., Beaumont, J. L., Hahn, E., Marymont, J., ... Rosengart, T. K. (2008). Absence of cognitive decline one year after coronary bypass surgery: comparison to nonsurgical and healthy controls. *The Annals of thoracic surgery, 85*(5), 1571–1578.

Vestal, L., Smith-Olinde, L., Hicks, G., Hutton, T., & Hart, J. (2006). Efficacy of language assessment in Alzheimer's disease: Comparing in-person examination and telemedicine. *Clinical interventions in aging, 1*(4), 467.

TOKEN TEST

TEST NAME	**Token Test**
DOMAIN	Language
AGE RANGE	In adults, to 75 years
ADMINISTRATION TIME	10 minutes
SCORING FORMAT	Hand scored
REFERENCE	Spreen, O., & Benton, A. L. (1969, 1977). *The Neurosensory Center Comprehensive Examination for Aphasia.* Neuropsychology Laboratory, University of Victoria, Victoria, B.C., Canada. See text for other versions.

DESCRIPTION

The Token Test (TT) assesses comprehension of verbal commands of increasing complexity. The test was originally developed by De Renzi and Vignolo (1962) and by Boller and Vignolo (1966) and included 62 commands. A number of different versions have appeared, including short forms (De Renzi & Faglioni, 1978; Spellacy & Spreen, 1969; Van Harskamp & Van Dongen, 1977) and the Revised Token Test (RTT; McNeil & Prescott, 1978). Some versions are part of a larger test battery, such as the Indiana University Token Test (IUTT; Unverzagt et al., 1999), which is part of the Consortium to Establish a Registry for Alzheimer's Disease (CERAD), and a 22-item version, which is part of the MAE (Benton et al., 1989; Benton et al., 1994; see the section "Multilingual Aphasia Examination"). This latter version has become a part of test batteries designed for purposes other than traditional aphasia assessment. For example, it is part of the Traumatic Brain Injury Model Systems neuropsychology battery (Millis et al., 2001), and it was one of the tests used to create the extended neuropsychological normative dataset for older individuals used in the MOANS project (Ivnik et al., 1996).

The version presented here is part of the NCCEA (Test 11; Spreen & Benton, 1969, 1977). It can be used with children as well as adults, but only information on adults is presented here. It has also been included as part of the Meyers Short Battery (MSB; Volbrecht et al., 2000).

Computer-generated versions of the TT have been created (e.g., D'Arcy & Connolly, 1999; D'Arcy et al., 2000; Odell et al., 1996). Translated versions of the TT are available in several languages, including German (Orgass, 1976), Polish (Kosciesca, 1995), and Brazilian (de Araújo Carvalho et al., 2009). The German Aachen Aphasia Test (AAT) includes a version of the TT.

ADMINISTRATION

The NCCEA version of the TT uses 20 plastic tokens in five colors (red, white, yellow, blue, and green), two sizes (small, approximately 2 cm in diameter; large, approximately 3 cm in diameter), and two shapes (circles and squares—squares replacing the rectangles in the original De Renzi and Vignolo version), arranged in a fixed order in front of the examinee (Figure 11–3). The test involves 39 commands of increasing length and complexity (Figure 11–4). The Spellacy and Spreen (1969) short form uses the following 16 items from Figure 11–4: items 6, 10, 12, 16, 17, 19, 20, 21, 22, 23, 24, 26, 27, 29, 33, and 35.

Present tokens in the order shown in Figure 11–3, and ask the first question: "Show me a circle." Say the questions clearly and slowly, but take care not to deliberately stretch speech during the presentation of the test, because this may lead to improvement of test performance in aphasics (Poeck & Pietron, 1981). Instructions for parts A and B may be repeated once. No other instructions may be repeated. If the examinee makes no response, the examinee should be encouraged to give at least a partial response. For

Examiner

Row 1: Large circles in order: red, blue, yellow, white, green

Row 2: Large squares in order: blue, red, white, green, yellow

Row 3: Small circles in order: white, blue, yellow, red, green

Row 4: Small squares in order: yellow, green, red, blue, white

Examinee

Figure 11–3 *Token arrangement in front of examinee.*

Name ____________________ Date____________ Age ______ Examiner__________________

Score Sheet

IDENTIFICATION BY SENTENCE (TOKEN TEST)

A. Present tokens as in Figure 11–3. Instructions may be repeated once	
1. Show me a circle	
2. Show me a square	
3. Show me a yellow one	
4. Show me a red one	
5. Show me a blue one	
6. Show me a green one	
7. Show me a white one	
TOTAL A(7)	

B. Present only large tokens. Instructions may be repeated once	
8. Show me the **yellow** **square**	
9. Show me the **blue** **circle**	
10. Show me the **green** **circle**	
11. Show me the **white** **square**	
TOTAL B(8)	

C. Present all tokens as in Figure 11–3. Do not repeat instructions	
12. Show me the **small** **white** **circle**	
13. Show me the **large** **yellow** **square**	
14. Show me the **large** **green** **square**	
15. Show me the **small** **blue** **square**	
TOTAL C(12)	

D. Present large tokens only. Do not repeat instructions	
16. Take the **red** **circle** and the **green** **square**	
17. Take the **yellow** **square** and the **blue** **square**	
18. Take the **white** **square** and the **green** **circle**	
19. Take the **white** **circle** and the **red** **circle**	
TOTAL D(16)	

Figure 11–4 Neurosensory Center Comprehensive Examination for Aphasia (NCCEA) Subtest 11 (Token Test) sample scoring sheet. The initial order of token presentation is shown in Figure 11–3.

E. Present all tokens as in Figure 11–3. Do not repeat instructions	
20. Take the **large white circle** and the **small green square**	
21. Take the **small blue circle** and the **large yellow square**	
22. Take the **large green square** and the **large red square**	
23. Take the **large white square** and the **small green circle**	
TOTAL E(24)	

F. Present large tokens only. Do not repeat instructions	
24. Put the **red circle on** the **green square**	
25. Put the **white square behind** the **yellow circle**	
26. Touch the **blue circle with** the **red square**	
27. Touch the **blue circle and** the **red square**	
28. Pick up the **blue circle OR** the **red square**	
29. Move the **green square away from** the **yellow square**	
30. Put the **white circle in front of** the **blue square**	
31. If there is a **black circle, pick up** the **red square**	
32. Pick up all squares except the **yellow one**	
33. Put the **green square beside** the **red circle**	
34. Touch the **squares slowly and** the **circles quickly**	
35. Put the **red circle between** the **yellow square** and the **green square**	
36. Touch all circles, except the **green one**	
37. Pick up the **red circle – no** – the **white square**	
38. Instead of the **white square, pick up** the **yellow circle**	
39. Together with the **yellow circle, pick up** the **blue circle**	
TOTAL F(96)	

TOTAL A-F(163)

Figure 11–4 Continued

example, if the examinee says that they do not remember or asks for repetition of instructions, say: "Do it as I said. Do as much as you remember." Discontinue after three consecutive failures (i.e., on sections A, B, and C, if no part of the question received credit; on section D, if only one part received credit; and on sections E and F if only two parts received credit).

The first section (questions 1 through 7) also provides a gross check on color blindness, which could affect performance on this test. If difficulties in color recognition are noticed, further examination with the Ishihara plates or a similar test of color blindness is necessary. If gross color blindness is established both on this test and by a color-vision test, the test should be discontinued.

SCORING

The questions are listed on the score sheet (Figure 11–4). The TT uses a scoring system that credits almost *every word* of each item, rather than assigning a score of one point for the *entire item*. Give one-point credit for each part of a question correctly performed. For example, the correct performance of questions 1 through 7 receives one credit each, and the correct performance of questions 12 through 15 ("*small, white circle*") receives three credits each. For questions 24 to 39, the verb and the preposition as well as the correct token receive credit (e.g., "*Put* the *red circle on* the *green square*" = six credits). Occasionally a preposition may be interpreted in several ways, such as item 25, "*Put* the *white square behind* the *yellow circle*" (i.e., "behind" may be viewed as away from the examinee or as to the right of the yellow circle). In these instances, any reasonable interpretation of the preposition is accepted and scored as correct. Similarly, if the examinee puts the green circle behind the red square, the examinee receives five points, because the performance shows that five parts of the command (i.e., put, red, green, circle, and square) were comprehended, but the relationship ("on") was not. If the test is discontinued, prorate the remaining items of that section on the basis of the person's performance on the administered items. For example, if the test is discontinued after item 26 (third item of part F), and items 24 through 26 received two points each, the remaining 13 items would also receive two points each, for a total of 32 points for part F. If all or most of the items of sections B, C, D, E, and/or F were not given because of earlier failures, add a score of three points for part B, five points for Part C, six points for Part D, nine points for Part E, and 18 points for part F. No correction for age or educational level is necessary (but see later discussion of age effects). The maximum score is 163.

DEMOGRAPHIC EFFECTS

AGE

Performance improves in childhood, reaching adult levels by about age 11 years, and shows little decline with advancing age (Rich, 1993) until about age 30, when age-related decline has been reported (Emery, 1986). The IUTT version shows an age association among adults older than age 65; that is, greater age is associated with lower IUTT score and being older than 80 is associated with a 50% higher probability of a low or medium score than a high score (Snitz et al., 2009). Others have reported few age-related effects on other versions of the TT (De Renzi & Faglioni, 1978; Ivnik et al., 1996; Swisher & Sarno, 1969).

GENDER

No information on gender effects is available for the NCCEA version. No effect of gender is seen on the Brazilian short version (de Araújo Carvalho et al., 2009). Older women tend to obtain higher scores on the IUTT than older men (Snitz et al., 2009).

EDUCATION AND IQ

General conceptual ability plays a role. There is a high correlation between the TT and the MMSE ($r = .74$; Swihart et al., 1989), though the correlation between the MMSE and the Brazilian short version is moderate ($r = .40$; Paula et al., 2012). Higher education is associated with higher scores on the IUTT (Snitz et al., 2009). De Renzi and Faglioni (1978) recommended a correction for education, +2.36 – (.30 × Years of schooling), for an item-by-item scoring, but such a correction is not needed for the NCCEA version with individuals who have a grade eight education or higher. In those who have less than eight years of education, there is a four-point difference in performance compared to those with higher education (nine or more years of education) on the MAE version (Brewster et al., 2014). Specifically, TT performance corresponds more to verbal ability in the low education group than in the higher education group, suggesting that greater verbal demands may be required in those with less education (Brewster et al., 2014). Correlation between education and the Brazilian short version is at least moderate ($r = .53$; de Araújo Carvalho et al., 2009; Paula et al., 2012).

ETHNICITY, NATIONALITY, AND LINGUISTIC EFFECTS

Ethnicity does not appear to affect performance. Ripich et al. (1997) used the NCCEA short form (Spellacy & Spreen, 1969) to compare 11 African Americans and 32 white patients with early or mid-stage AD; they found no differences based on ethnicity. However, performance differences were related to acculturation on the MAE Token Test and IUTT among African Americans (Kennepohl et al., 2004; Snitz et al., 2009).

NORMATIVE DATA

Table 11–60 provides NCCEA TT normative data for 82 adult volunteers residing in Victoria, British Columbia, Canada, aged 25 to 75 years. The mean score for adults is 161. Scores lower than 157 are virtually absent in a healthy adult population. Tuokko and Woodward (1996) reported that this cutoff value also holds for older adults between 60 and 85 years of age. Normative data for older adults on the IUTT can be found in Snitz et al. (2009).

TABLE 11–60 Percentile Ranks for the Token Test for Healthy Adults (N = 82)

SCORE	PERCENTILE RANK
162	70
161	50
158	30
157	18
156	14
154	10
153	6
151	–

SOURCE: Spreen and Benton (1969, 1977).

EVIDENCE FOR RELIABILITY

EVIDENCE FOR INTERNAL RELIABILITY

The Kuder-Richardson internal reliability coefficient for the NCCEA 39-item version is very high (r = .92; Spellacy & Spreen, 1969). Van Harskamp and Van Dongen (1977) reported an internal reliability of .90 for Part E scored on a pass-fail basis.

EVIDENCE FOR TEST-RETEST RELIABILITY, MEASURING CHANGE, AND PRACTICE EFFECTS

For adults with average intelligence, ceiling scores can be expected. For this reason, one-year test-retest reliability in healthy older adults has been reported as only .50 (Snow et al., 1988). In a general clinical sample of patients screened for invalid performance, test-retest reliability was marginal (r = .68) after a retest interval of six months (Meyers & Rohling, 2004). Gains of about 2.75 points (SD = 11.29, SEM = 1.42) are noted on retest.

EVIDENCE FOR SHORT FORM RELIABILITY

Internal consistency of the Brazilian short version is adequate to high (healthy older adults: alpha = .75; AD patients: alpha = .81; Paula et al., 2012). In 41 patients with dementia who were reassessed with the NCCEA version of the TT short form after a 10-month interval, test-retest reliability was high (r = .85; Taylor, 1998).

EVIDENCE FOR INTERRATER RELIABILITY

None reported.

EVIDENCE FOR VALIDITY

WITHIN-TEST RELATIONSHIPS

There is evidence that the various parts of the NCCEA TT do not measure the same general language factor. Solving the first four parts requires a single uniform mode of processing; the last part is different because it incorporates items of greater syntactic/semantic variability (Orgass, 1976; Willmes, 1981). A two-factor solution was found in the Brazilian short version based on a sample of healthy older adults and AD patients, with one reflecting verbal comprehension and the other related to attention (Paula et al., 2012).

RELATIONSHIPS WITH OTHER TESTS

The test correlates highly with other measures of receptive ability, such as the Peabody Picture Vocabulary Test (r = .71; Lass & Golden, 1975). General cognitive ability appears to be important in task performance (McNeil, 1983; Riedel & Studdert-Kennedy, 1985). As might be expected, there is a high correlation between the TT and the MMSE (r = .74; Swihart et al., 1989), except for the Brazilian short version (Paula et al., 2012). Coupar (1976) reported a moderate correlation between the NCCEA version of the TT and the Raven's Progressive Matrices for brain-damaged patients (r = .35).

The TT embodies a variety of cognitive processes in addition to auditory comprehension, including analysis of the whole into a series of elements, the ability to generate a visual image of the verbal information, short-term memory (Lesser, 1976), and the ability to effectively ignore the automatically evoked, distracting stimulus (Winer et al., 2004). Working memory capacity has also been found to affect TT performance. In one study that examined the impact of working memory on TT performance in persons with aphasia, those with low working memory performed worse on TT than those with high working memory, particularly on the items with syntactically more complex structures (Sung et al., 2009). Therefore, performance on the TT can be affected by difficulties other than "pure" deficits in auditory comprehension.

The test correlates with the WAB aphasia quotient (r = .55), but appears unrelated to other aphasia tests such as the Functional Assessment of Communication Skills (ASHA; r = .14). Performance is inversely correlated to discourse quantity (r = –.30) and positively correlated with discourse quality (r = .46; Ulatowska et al., 2003). In short, performance on the TT appears to be only a modest predictor of some but not all aspects of functional language competence.

CLINICAL STUDIES

Dementia. Deficits on TT can be seen in those with MCI, in addition to memory deficits (Ribeiro et al., 2006). Rich (1993) reported severe impairment in AD patients compared with healthy older adults. For this patient group, the TT measures not only auditory comprehension but also severity of cognitive impairment (Swihart et al., 1989). In cases of dementia, TT performance may predict changes in dementia status as measured by the CDR (Ganguli et al.,

2010). In fact, the NCCEA 16-item short form proved to be one of the best indicators of overall level of cognitive functioning and was very sensitive to cognitive decline over a 10-month period in probable AD and multi-infarct dementia (Taylor, 1998). The Brazilian short version also yielded a decent balance of sensitivity (73%) and specificity (64%) for identifying AD at a raw score cutoff of 28 or lower (Paula et al., 2012).

Aphasia. The TT, in its original version by De Renzi and Vignolo (1962), as well as in various modifications, has proved useful for discriminating between aphasic and nonaphasic brain-injured patients (Boller & Dennis, 1979; Gallaher, 1979; Orgass, 1976; Ulatowska et al., 2001). Ulatowska et al. (2001) examined 30 African-American aphasics with left-hemisphere stroke (mean age = 51 years) and 30 matched healthy African Americans and found a highly significant difference (M = 106.8 and 152.3, respectively). However, when the TT was used to predict communication difficulty, Doyle et al. (2006) reported that performance on the RTT at three months post-stroke did not predict self-reported communication difficulty at 12 months among community-dwelling stroke patients with mild to moderate aphasia.

Brain Injury. As noted earlier, the NCCEA version of the TT is included as part of the MSB (Volbrecht et al., 2000). Meyers and Rohling (2004) reported that the battery distinguishes patients with mild TBI from healthy controls, chronic pain patients, and depressed patients, with a 96% correct classification rate. Other versions of the TT also appear to be sensitive to brain injury. For example, in a five-year follow-up of 90 patients with TBI who received inpatient rehabilitation, the MAE version of the TT found impairment in 22% of cases with no significant improvement over time (Millis et al., 2001). The Spanish MAE version is also sensitive to language difficulties occurring after brain injury. Furthermore, scores decline with increasing severity of injury as determined by the Glasgow Coma Scale (GCS) score (Rey et al., 2001).

NEUROANATOMICAL CORRELATES AND IMAGING STUDIES

A variety of imaging techniques have been used to study the neuroanatomical correlates of the TT, including structural MRI, DTI, functional MRI (fMRI), and fluorodeoxyglucose positron emission tomography (FDG-PET). In general, TT performance has been associated with frontal, temporal, and parietal regions. The studies also suggest bihemispheric involvement in TT performance (Frings et al., 2013; van Oers et al., 2010; Whitwell et al., 2013). In a sample of patients with AD, MCI, behavioral variant FTD (bvFTD), and primary progressive aphasia (PPA), baseline TT performance was associated with increased DTI mean diffusivity in the left inferior frontal gyrus, left middle frontal gyrus, bilateral superior frontal gyrus, left posterior parietal, and right postcentral/supramarginal gyrus. Over 14 months, declines in performance were linked to mean diffusivity increases in bilateral fronto-polar superior frontal gyrus, left caudate, and bilateral supplementary motor area and superior frontal gyrus, as well as to gray matter volume decline in left and right posterior parietal cortex (Frings et al., 2013). Among right-handed, left middle cerebral artery (MCA) stroke patients who underwent fMRI to examine the relative contribution of dominant and nondominant language networks to recovery from aphasia, recovery of TT scores over 10 months was positively correlated with activation in both left and right inferior frontal gyrus during semantic decision and verb generation tasks, but lesion volume was not associated with change on the TT (van Oers et al., 2013). Among patients with progressive apraxia of speech and agrammatic aphasia, performance was correlated with FDG-PET hypometabolism in the inferior orbitalis, inferior triangularis, inferior opercularis, middle frontal gyrus, and inferior parietal lobe, greater in the left than right hemisphere; 3T MRI findings showed correlations with the left inferior orbitalis and left superior temporal lobe values (Whitwell et al., 2013). Taken together, imaging studies suggest a verbal and nonverbal component to TT performance.

The TT has also been used for extraoperative language mapping in patients who are undergoing epilepsy surgery. Comparing six different tasks (counting, sentence reading, repetition of orally presented sentences, visual confrontation naming, body command, and TT), the authors concluded that visual confrontation naming of everyday items was the most sensitive task for language testing in the frontal and temporoparietal region, followed by the TT (Wellmer et al., 2009). However, the test is not useful in differentiating between left and right mesial TLE and frontal lobe epilepsy (Ramirez et al., 2010).

PERFORMANCE VALIDITY

There are few studies on the use of the test to detect invalid performance. Meyers et al. (1999) suggested that standard neuropsychological measures such as the TT can do double duty, not only as clinically useful neuropsychological tests but also to detect feigned deficits. They compared the NCCEA TT in 27 patients with moderate to severe brain injury, 35 nonlitigating patients with mild brain injury, 49 litigating patients with mild brain injury, 20 malingering "actors," and 30 healthy controls, all with a mean age of approximately 30 years. They found that the lowest TT score in the severe brain injury group was 151. Using a cutoff of 150 (one less than the lowest expected score), no one in the nonlitigating mild brain injury or healthy groups obtained scores below this cutoff, yielding 100% sensitivity and specificity. On the other hand, 8% of litigating mild brain injury patients and 45% of malingering "actors" fell below this cutoff. Accordingly, they recommended a cutoff score of 150, with scores at that level or lower raising the index of suspicion.

COMMENT

The TT and its variants have a long history in neuropsychology. The advantages of the TT lie in sound discriminative validity, reasonable reliability, and portability. It is also cost-effective in terms of material, time, and expertise required in administration and scoring. In addition, it is sensitive to all forms of aphasia, but especially to receptive aphasia. The latter parts of the test (parts E and F) have been shown to differ from the first four parts because they require complex auditory/cognitive processing as well as short-term memory and working memory, making the test useful in a variety of other conditions (e.g., dementia, brain injury) as well.

On the other hand, there are a number of limitations. First, the normative samples are poorly described, and the NCCEA data were collected more than 40 years ago, with very few updates reported in the past decade. Therefore, caution is advised in relying on the norms provided here. The clinician/researcher might consider other measures with stronger psychometric properties. Second, there are different versions of the TT, and this can be confusing. However, it should be remembered that all are adaptations of the original test items and wordings by De Renzi and Vignolo (1962) and that only the number of items and the scoring differ; hence, validity studies with different versions tend to support the validity of others. In fact, even short versions tend to show discriminant validity similar to that of the long version.

Imaging studies suggest bihemispheric involvement in TT performance. As such, the TT cannot be assumed to map only to the dominant hemisphere. It has not been helpful to differentiate between left and right TLE within the context of outpatient neuropsychological evaluation (Ramirez et al., 2010); however, the TT is useful for extraoperative language mapping, second only to visual confrontation naming (Wellmer et al., 2009).

Brookshire's (1973) early advice remains valid: the clinician should keep in mind that, although it is a sensitive indicator of comprehension deficits, the TT relies on a limited stimulus array. Other tests of auditory comprehension should be used to supplement the TT. Note that there are many reasons for poor performance other than simple comprehension per se, such as poor working memory (Sung et al., 2009).

REFERENCES

Benton, A. L., Hamsher, K. D., & Sivan, A. (1989). *Multilingual Aphasia Examination*. Iowa City, IA: AJA Associates.

Benton, A. L., Hamsher, K. de S., & Sivan, A. B. (1994). *Multilingual Aphasia Examination* (3rd Ed.). Iowa City, IA: AJA Associates.

Boller, F., & Dennis, M. (1979). *Auditory comprehension: Clinical and experimental studies with the Token Test.* New York: Academic.

Boller, F., & Vignolo, L. (1966). Latent sensory aphasia in hemisphere-damaged patients: An experimental study with the Token-Test. *Brain, 89,* 815–831.

Brewster, P. W., Tuokko, H., & MacDonald, S. W. (2014). Measurement equivalence of neuropsychological tests across education levels in older adults. *Journal of Clinical and Experimental Neuropsychology, 36*(10), 1042–1054.

Brookshire, R. H. (1973). The use of consequences in speech pathology: Incentive and feedback functions. *Journal of Communication Disorders, 6,* 88–92.

Coupar, M. (1976). Detection of mild aphasia: A study using the Token Test. *British Journal of Medical Psychology, 49,* 141–144.

D'Arcy, R. C. N., & Connolly, J. F. (1999). An event-related brain potential study of receptive speech comprehension using a modified Token Test. *Neuropsychologia, 37,* 1477–1489.

D'Arcy, R. C. N., Connolly, J. F., & Crocker, S. F. (2000). Latency shifts in the N2b component track phonological deviations in spoken words. *Clinical Neurophysiology, 111,* 40–44.

de Araújo Carvalho, S., Barreto, S. M., Guerra, H. L., & Gama, A. C. C. (2009). Oral language comprehension assessment among elderly: a population based study in Brazil. *Preventive Medicine, 49*(6), 541–545.

De Renzi, E., & Faglioni, P. (1978). Development of a shortened version of the Token Test. *Cortex, 14,* 41–49.

De Renzi, E., & Vignolo, L. (1962). The Token Test: A sensitive test to detect receptive disturbances in aphasics. *Brain, 85,* 665–678.

Doyle, P. J., Matthews, C., Mikolic, J. M., Hula, W., & McNeil, M. R. (2006). Do measures of language impairment predict patient-reported communication difficulty and distress as measured by the Burden of Stroke Scale (BOSS)? *Aphasiology, 20*(02–04), 349–361.

Emery, O. B. (1986). Linguistic decrement in normal aging. *Language and Communication, 6,* 47–64.

Frings, L., Dressel, K., Abel, S., Mader, I., Glauche, V., Weiller, C., & Hüll, M. (2013). Longitudinal cerebral diffusion changes reflect progressive decline of language and cognition. *Psychiatry Research: Neuroimaging, 214*(3), 395–401.

Gallaher, A. J. (1979). Temporal reliability of aphasic performance on the Token Test. *Brain and Language, 7,* 34–41.

Ganguli, M., Vander Bilt, J., Lee, C. W., Snitz, B. E., Chang, C. C. H., Loewenstein, D. A., & Saxton, J. A. (2010). Cognitive test performance predicts change in functional status at the population level: The MYHAT Project. *Journal of the International Neuropsychological Society, 16*(05), 761–770.

Ivnik, R. J., Malec, J. F., & Smith, G. E. (1996). Neuropsychological tests norms above age 55: COWAT, MAE Token, WRAT-R Reading, AMNART, Stroop, TMT and JLO. *The Clinical Neuropsychologist, 10,* 262–278.

Kennepohl, S., Shore, D., Nobors, N., & Hanks, R. (2004). African American acculturation and neuropsychological test performance following traumatic brain injury. *Journal of the International Neuropsychological Society, 10,* 566–577.

Kosciesza, M. (1995). Polish adaptation of the "Token Test" for children and its practical application. *Psychologia Wychowawcza, 38,* 350–358.

Lass, N. J., & Golden, S. S. (1975). A comparative study of children's performance on three tests for receptive language abilities. *Journal of Auditory Research, 15,* 177–182.

Lesser, R. (1976). Verbal and non-verbal memory components in the Token Test. *Neuropsychologia, 14,* 79–85.

McNeil, M. R. (1983). Aphasia: Neurological considerations. *Topics in Language Disorders, 3,* 1–19.

McNeil, M. R., & Prescott, T. E. (1978). *Revised Token Test.* Austin, TX: Pro-ed.

Meyers, J. E., Galinsky, A. M., & Volbrecht, M. (1999). Malingering and mild brain injury: How low is too low? *Applied Neuropsychology, 6,* 208–216.

Meyers, J. E., & Rohling, M. L. (2004). Validation of the Meyers Short Battery on mild TBI patients. *Archives of Clinical Neuropsychology, 19,* 637–651.

Millis, S. R., Rosenthal, M., Novack, T. A., Sherer, M., Nick, T. G., Kreutzer, J. S., . . . M., & Ricker, J. H. (2001). Long-term neuropsychological outcome after traumatic brain injury. *Journal of Head Trauma Rehabilitation, 16,* 343–355.

Odell, K. H., Miller, S. B., & Lee, C. (1996). A Comparison of aphasic performance on the standard and an experimental computerized version of the revised Token Test. *Clinical Aphasiology, 24,* 145–158.

Orgass, B. (1976). Eine revision des Token Tests II: Validitaetsnachweis, normierung und standardisierung. *Diagnostica, 22,* 141–156.

Paula, J. J. D., Bertola, L., Nicolato, R., Moraes, E. N. D., & Malloy-Diniz, L. F. (2012). Evaluating language comprehension in Alzheimer's disease: The use of the Token Test. *Arquivos de Neuro-psiquiatria, 70*(6), 435–440.

Poeck, K., & Pietron, H. P. (1981). The influence of stretched speech presentation on Token Test performance in aphasic and right brain damaged patients. *Neuropsychologia, 19,* 133–136.

Ramirez, M. J., Schefft, B. K., Howe, S. R., Hovanitz, C., Yeh, H. S., & Privitera, M. D. (2010). The effects of perceived emotional distress on language performance in intractable epilepsy. *Epilepsy & Behavior, 18*(1), 64–73.

Rao, P. (1990). Functional communication assessment of the elderly. In E. Cherov (Ed.), *Proceedings of the research symposium on communication sciences and disorders and aging* (pp. 28–34). Rockville, MD: American Speech and Hearing Association.

Rey, G. J., Feldman, E., Hernandez, D., Levin, B. E., Rivas-Vazquez, R., Nedd, K. J., & Benton, A. L. (2001). Application of the Multilingual Aphasia Examination–Spanish in the evaluation of Hispanic patients post closed-head trauma. *The Clinical Neuropsychologist, 15,* 13–18.

Ribeiro, F., De Mendonça, A., & Guerreiro, M. (2006). Mild cognitive impairment: deficits in cognitive domains other than memory. *Dementia and Geriatric Cognitive Disorders, 21*(5-6), 284–290.

Rich, J. B. (1993). *Pictorial and verbal implicit and recognition memory in aging and Alzheimer's disease: A transfer-appropriate processing account.* PhD. dissertation, University of Victoria, Victoria, BC, Canada.

Riedel, K., & Studdert-Kennedy, M. (1985). Extending formant transitions may not improve aphasic's perception of stop consonant place of articulation. *Brain and Language, 24,* 223–232.

Ripich, D. N., Carpenter, B., & Ziol, E. (1997). Comparison of African American and white persons with Alzheimer's disease on language measures. *Neurology, 48,* 781–783.

Semel, E., Wiig, E. H., & Secord, W. A. (2003). *CELF-4.* San Antonio, TX: The Psychological Corporation.

Snitz, B. E., Unverzagt, F. W., Chang, C. C. H., Vander Bilt, J., Gao, S., Saxton, J., . . . Ganguli, M. (2009). Effects of age, gender, education and race on two tests of language ability in community-based older adults. *International Psychogeriatrics, 21*(06), 1051–1062.

Snow, W. G., Tierney, M. C., Zorzitto, M. L., Fisher, R. H., & Reid, D. W. (1988). One-year test-retest reliability of selected neuropsychological tests in older adults. Paper presented at the International Neuropsychological Society Meeting, New Orleans [Abstract]. *Journal of Clinical and Experimental Neuropsychology, 10,* 60.

Spellacy, F., & Spreen, O. (1969). A short form of the Token Test. *Cortex, 5,* 390–397.

Spreen, O., & Benton, A. L. (1969, 1977), *The Neurosensory Center Comprehensive Examination for Aphasia.* Neuropsychology Laboratory, University of Victoria, Victoria, BC, Canada.

Sung, J. E., McNeil, M. R., Pratt, S. R., Dickey, M. W., Hula, W. D., Szuminsky, N. J., & Doyle, P. J. (2009). Verbal working memory and its relationship to sentence-level reading and listening comprehension in persons with aphasia. *Aphasiology, 23*(7-8), 1040–1052.

Swihart, A. A., Panisset, M., Becker, J. T., Beyer, J. T., Beyer, J. R., & Boller, F. (1989). The Token Test: Validity and diagnostic power in Alzheimer's disease. *Developmental Neuropsychology, 5,* 71–80.

Swisher, L. P., & Sarno, M. T. (1969). Token Test scores of three matched patient groups: Left brain-damaged with aphasia; right brain-damaged without aphasia; non brain-damaged. *Cortex, 5,* 264–273.

Taylor, R. (1998). Indices of neuropsychological functioning and decline over time in dementia. *Archives of Gerontology and Geriatrics, 27,* 165–170.

Tuokko, H., & Woodward, T. S. (1996). Development and validation of a demographic system for neuropsychological measures used in the Canadian Study of Health and Aging. *Journal of Clinical and Experimental Neuropsychology, 18,* 479–616.

Ulatowska, H. K., Olness, G. S., Wertz, R. T., Samson, A. G., Keebler, M. W., & Goins, K. E. (2003). Relationship between discourse and Western Aphasia Battery performance in African Americans with aphasia. *Aphasiology, 17,* 511–521.

Ulatowska, H. K., Olness, G. S., Wertz, R. T., Thompson, J., Keebler, M. W., Hill, C. L., & Auther, L. L. (2001). Comparison of language impairment, functional communication, and discourse measures in African American aphasic and normal adults. *Aphasiology, 15,* 2007–2016.

Unverzagt, F. W., Morgan, O. S., Thesiger, C. H., Eldemire, D. A., Luseko, J., Pokuri, S., . . . Hendrie, H. C. (1999). Clinical utility of CERAD neuropsychological battery in elderly Jamaicans. *Journal of the International Neuropsychological Society, 5*(03), 255–259.

Van Harskamp, F., & Van Dongen, H. R. (1977). Construction and validation of different short forms of the Token Test. *Neuropsychologia, 15,* 467–470.

van Oers, C. A., Vink, M., van Zandvoort, M. J., van der Worp, H. B., de Haan, E. H., Kappelle, L. J., . . . Dijkhuizen, R. M. (2010). Contribution of the left and right inferior frontal gyrus in recovery from aphasia. A functional MRI study in stroke patients with preserved hemodynamic responsiveness. *Neuroimage, 49*(1), 885–893.

Volbrecht, M., Meyers, J. E., & Kaster-Bundgaard, J. (2000). Neuropsychological outcome of head injury using a short battery. *Archives of Clinical Neuropsychology, 15,* 251–265.

Wellmer, J., Weber, C., Mende, M., Von Der Groeben, F., Urbach, H., Clusmann, H., . . . Helmstaedter, C. (2009). Multitask electrical stimulation for cortical language mapping: hints for necessity and economic mode of application. *Epilepsia, 50*(10), 2267–2275.

Whitwell, J. L., Duffy, J. R., Strand, E. A., Xia, R., Mandrekar, J., Machulda, M. M., . . . Josephs, K. A. (2013). Distinct regional anatomic and functional correlates of neurodegenerative apraxia of speech and aphasia: An MRI and FDG-PET study. *Brain and Language, 125*(3), 245–252.

Willmes, K. (1981). A new look at the Token Test using probabilistic test models. *Neuropsychologia, 19,* 631–645.

Winer, D. A., Connor, L. T., & Obler, L. K. (2004). Inhibition and auditory comprehension in Wernicke's aphasia. *Aphasiology, 18,* 599–609.

12 | VISUAL-SPATIAL SKILLS

BENTON FACIAL RECOGNITION TEST (FRT)

TEST NAME	**Benton Facial Recognition Test (FRT)**
DOMAIN	Visual perception
AGE RANGE	16 to 90 years
ADMINISTRATION TIME	10 minutes
SCORING FORMAT	Hand scored
REFERENCE	Benton, A. L., Sivan, A. B., Hamsher, K. de S., Varney, N. R., & Spreen, O. (1994). *Contributions to neuropsychological assessment: A clinical manual* (2nd ed.). New York: Oxford University Press.

DESCRIPTION

The Benton Facial Recognition Test (FRT) was developed by Benton and Van Allen (1968) to assess the ability to discriminate photographs of unfamiliar human faces. In the FRT, clothing and hair are shaded out so that only facial features can be seen. The full test (Long Form) consists of 54 items, whereas the Short Form (Levin et al., 1975) is an abbreviated version consisting of the first 27 items from the Long Form. A different short form was also created by Christensen et al. (2002).

The FRT consists of three parts:

1. Matching of identical front-view photographs (see Figure 12–1). The examinee is presented with a single front-view photograph of a single face (male or female) and is instructed to identify it in a display of six front-view photographs (the target and five distractors) that appears below the single photograph. There are six target faces, calling for a total of six responses.
2. Matching of front-view with three-quarter-view photographs (see Figure 12–2). The examinee is presented with a single front-view photograph of a face and is instructed to locate it three times in a display of six three-quarter views, three of which are views of the presented face and three views of other faces. There are eight target faces, calling for a total of 24 responses.

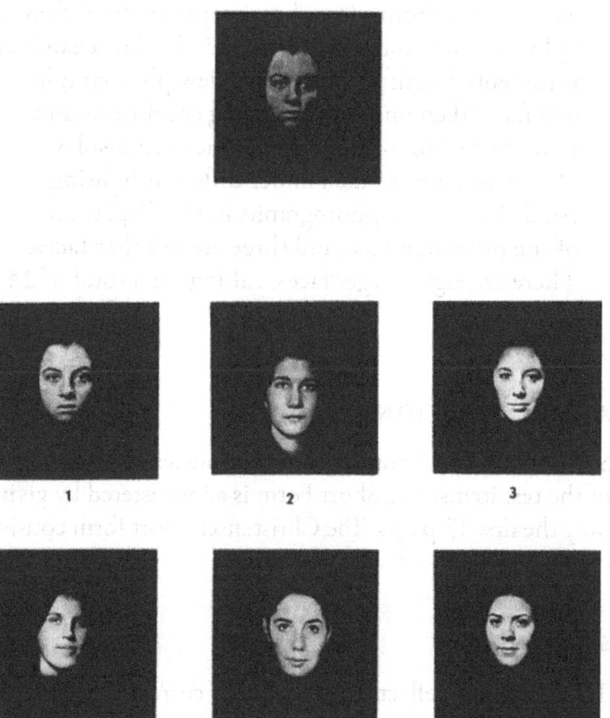

Figure 12–1 *Sample item from the Facial Recognition Test—identical front view.*
SOURCE: Reproduced by special permission of the Publisher, Psychological Assessment Resources, Inc. (PAR), 16204 North Florida Avenue, Lutz, Florida 33549, from the Benton Facial Recognition by Arthur L. Benton, PhD and Colleagues. Copyright 1978, 1983 by PAR. Further reproduction is prohibited without permission of PAR.

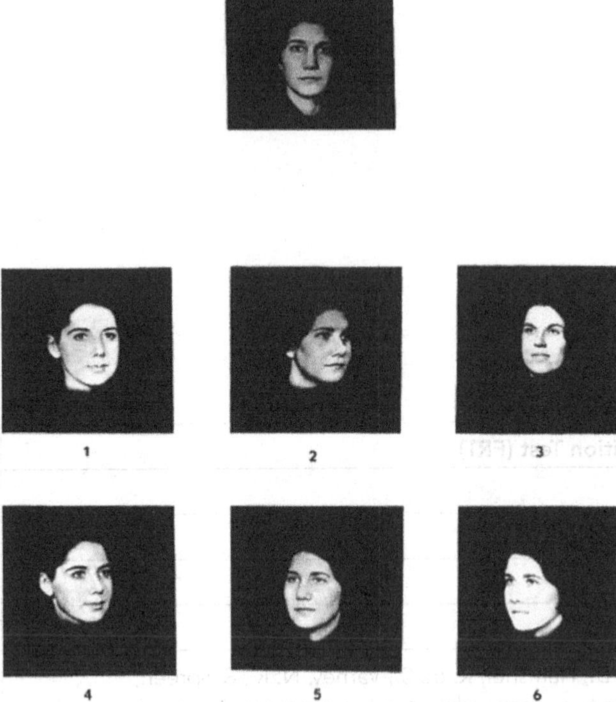

Figure 12–2 Sample item from the Facial Recognition Test—three-quarter view.

SOURCE: Reproduced by special permission of the Publisher, Psychological Assessment Resources, Inc. (PAR), 16204 North Florida Avenue, Lutz, Florida 33549, from the Benton Facial Recognition by Arthur L. Benton, PhD and Colleagues. Copyright 1978, 1983 by PAR. Further reproduction is prohibited without permission of PAR.

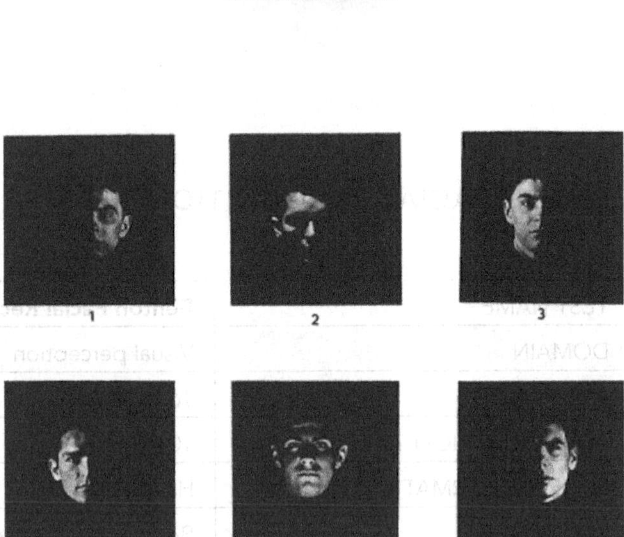

Figure 12–3 Sample item from the Facial Recognition Test—different lighting conditions.

SOURCE: Reproduced by special permission of the Publisher, Psychological Assessment Resources, Inc. (PAR), 16204 North Florida Avenue, Lutz, Florida 33549, from the Benton Facial Recognition by Arthur L. Benton, PhD and Colleagues. Copyright 1978, 1983 by PAR. Further reproduction is prohibited without permission of PAR.

3. Matching of front-view photographs under different lighting conditions (see Figure 12–3). The examinee is presented with a single front-view photograph of a face taken under full lighting conditions and is instructed to locate it three times in a display of six front views taken under different lighting conditions; three photographs in the display are of the presented face, and three are of other faces. There are eight target faces, calling for a total of 24 responses.

ADMINISTRATION

See Source. The Long Form is administered by giving all of the test items. The Short Form is administered by giving only the first 13 pages. The Christensen short form consists of pages 7, 8, 10–12, 14–19, and 22.

SCORING

The total score reflects the number of correct responses for the three different item types. For the Long Form, the maximum score is 54. For the Short Form, the maximum score is 27. The maximum score for the Christensen short form is 36. On the Long Form, a minimum score of 25 may be expected on the basis of chance alone. Hence, the effective range of Long Form scores may be considered to be 25 to 54 points. For the Short Form, the effective range may be considered to be 11 to 27 points.

According to the test manual, if the Short Form is used, the number of correct responses needs to be converted to Long Form scores following a conversion table in the manual. The test manual also provides age and education corrections for the Long Form and the converted Short Form scores (see the section "Standardization Sample"; Benton et al., 1994).

DEMOGRAPHIC EFFECTS

AGE

Age affects performance (Benton et al., 1994; Christensen et al., 2002; Schretlen et al., 2001). According to Benton et al. (1994), scores improve in childhood, with adult levels reached by about age 14 years. Test scores show some decline in old age.

EDUCATION AND IQ

Education also affects performance (Benton et al., 1994; Christensen et al., 2002; but see Schretlen et al., 2001, who found no significant effect for education). Scores increase with increasing FSIQ (Diaz-Asper et al., 2004).

GENDER

No gender-related differences have been reported (Benton et al., 1994; Christensen, 2002; Schretlen et al., 2001).

ETHNICITY, NATIONALITY, AND LINGUISTIC EFFECTS

Results for Hispanics appear to be equivalent to those obtained with primarily English-speaking individuals (Rey et al., 1999). Similar test scores have also been obtained in Italian adults (Ferracuti & Ferracuti, 1992) and in inner-city African Americans (Roberts & Hamsher, 1984), suggesting that the test is relatively independent of ethnic/cultural factors.

NORMATIVE DATA

STANDARDIZATION SAMPLE

Benton et al. (1994) provide score distributions for a standardization sample of 286 adults (age range, 16–74 years). The characteristics of the sample are shown in Table 12–1. The standardization sample consisted of two groups. One group comprised 196 patients without evidence of neurological or psychiatric disease or evidence of intellectual disability. The other group consisted of 90 volunteers in a study of aging. Age and education corrections are provided for participants older than 54 years of age and are based on a division between participants with less than a twelfth-grade education and those with an education of grade 12 or higher. Corrected scores of 40 or lower on the Long Form (20 or lower on the Short Form) raise the concern of abnormality. Note that the data were collected more than 40 years ago from a restricted region of the United States, with ethnicity not reported.

TABLE 12–1 Characteristics of the Adult Standardization Sample for the Facial Recognition Test (FRT)

Sample size	286
Age	16 to 74 years (mean age not reported)
Sample type	One sample (N = 196) consisted of patients from the neurological, neurosurgical, and medical services of the University of Iowa Hospital; a second sample consisted of 90 volunteers in a study of aging, aged 60 to 74 years
Education	6 to 12+ years
Gender	175 Women 111 Men
Ethnicity	Not reported
Socioeconomic status	Not reported
Screening	No evidence or history of neurological disease, intellectual disability, or hospitalization for psychiatric disorder

OTHER NORMATIVE DATA

Long Form. Christensen et al. (2002) provide more extensive normative data on the Long Form based on a sample of 346 healthy older adults aged between 60 and more than 90 years (M = 74.8, SD = 8.9; education M = 11.6, SD = 2.6). Participants were recruited from Minneapolis and St. Paul, Minnesota, based on age, gender, and education according to 1990 US Census characteristics for that geographical area. Participants were screened to exclude conditions that might affect cognition. The majority of the participants were Caucasian.

Application of Benton et al.'s (1994) age and education corrections to participants in the Christensen study who were aged 60 to 69 years yield mean scores and variability consistent with those of the Benton sample. However, scores for older participants are considerably lower than those suggested by Benton et al. (1994). The data of Christensen et al. (2002) are shown in Table 12–2 and are preferred for evaluation of older adults. The authors also found that other demographic data (highest education of daughter) and oral reading performance (Wide Range Achievement Test—Revised [WRAT-R] Reading) improved prediction of an individual's score based on age alone. They provided a prediction equation to aid interpretation (see Table 12–2). Comparison of obtained versus predicted FRT scores may be useful in determining whether there has been significant decline.

TABLE 12–2 Benton Facial Recognition Test (FRT) Normative Estimates for Facial Recognition Long Form

AGE (YEARS)	60–69	70–79	80–89	90+	ALL
N	101	99	96	50	346
Mean (SD)	42.8 (4)	40.6 (4)	38.3 (4.3)	36.4 (4.5)	40 (4.7)
Cut scores derived from age-based means					
95% probability defective	30.7	28.5	25.6	23.3	
95% probability nondefective	38.9	36.7	33.8	31.5	

NOTE: Regression equation for estimated long form score = (-22) Age + (.12) Reading + (.12) Daughter's education + 48.31 (R = .60; SE = 3.78), where Age is in years, Reading is the Wide Range Achievement Test (WRAT-R) Reading Level 2 Performance, and Daughter's education is in years, not including vocational school (e.g., 8th grade = 8, bachelor's degree = 16, master's degree = 18, doctorate = 20 (maximum level)).

SOURCE: Adapted from Christensen et al. (2002).

TABLE 12–3 Characteristics of the Facial Recognition Test (FRT) Normative Sample from the Calibrated Neuropsychological Normative System (CNNS)

Sample size	326
Age	18 to 92 years
Geographic location	Baltimore, MD, and Hartford, CT
Sample type	Community sample
Education	14.2 (*SD* = 3.0), range 3–20 years
Gender	56% Women 44% Men
Ethnicity	80% Caucasian 18% African American 2% Hispanic, Asian, or Other
Screening	History of Alzheimer's disease, Parkinson's disease, stroke, brain injury, bipolar disorder, or substance abuse

SOURCE: Adapted from Schretlen et al. (2010). Reproduced by special permission of the Publisher, Psychological Assessment Resources, Inc. (PAR), 16204 North Florida Avenue, Lutz, Florida 33549, from the Calibrated Neuropsychological Normative System, by David J. Schretlen, PhD, ABPP, S Marc Testa, PhD and Godfrey D. Pearlson, MD. Copyright 2010 by PAR. Further reproduction is prohibited without permission from PAR.

Schretlen, Testa, and Pearlson (2010) provide norms for 326 adults on the FRT; these use the Calibrated Neuropsychological Normative System (CNNS) scoring to derive T scores and discrepancies based on a large sample of older adults from the northeastern United States. Characteristics of the normative sample are shown in Table 12–3. The norms are available through Psychological Assessment Resources (PAR; www.parinc.com). A major advantage of these norms is the option to correct for demographic variables such as age, sex, education, and ethnicity. Several other commonly used neuropsychological tests are co-normed using this sample, which facilitates cross-test comparisons.

Short Forms. Dixon (personal communication, March 18, 2005) gave the Benton short form to a typically aging sample of 457 older, community-dwelling adults participating in the Victoria Longitudinal Study. Exclusion criteria included Mini-Mental State Examination (MMSE) scores of 24 or lower, moderate or very serious visual or auditory impairment even with corrective aids, history of major neurological disease (e.g., stroke, Parkinson's disease [PD], meningitis), history of severe depression, insulin-controlled diabetes, history of moderate or serious head injury, and diagnosed substance abuse within the past five years. The data are presented in Table 12–4. In order to maximize the amount of information available, overlapping-midpoint age ranges were used.

Christensen et al. (2002) provide normative data by age group for their short form, and these are shown in Table 12–5. The data are derived from the sample described earlier (see "Long Form").

EVIDENCE FOR RELIABILITY

EVIDENCE FOR INTERNAL RELIABILITY

Coefficient alpha for the Long Form in 206 undergraduates is only .57 (Hoptman & Davidson, 1993); however, internal reliability is higher when the first six items of the test (identity matches) are omitted (r = .66). In 346 healthy older adults, Christensen et al. (2002) found an internal consistency of .72 for the Long Form and .53 for the Short Form. In response to the poor internal consistency of the Short Form, Christensen et al. (2002) developed a new short form that yielded a coefficient alpha of .69 (item numbers 7, 8, 10–12, 14–19, and 22). The standard error of measurement was 2.0. The norms of the Christensen et al. (2002) short form are presented in Table 12–5.

EVIDENCE FOR TEST-RETEST RELIABILITY, MEASURING CHANGE, AND PRACTICE EFFECTS

Test-retest reliability after one year in older adults has been reported to be between .60 (Short Form) and .71 (Long Form; Christensen et al., 2002; Levin et al., 1991), with no significant change in mean scores. Scores on the modified short form by Christensen et al. (2002) have a stability coefficient of .71 over a one-year interval with no practice effect (N = 100).

EVIDENCE FOR INTERRATER RELIABILITY

Not reported.

EVIDENCE FOR VALIDITY

RELATIONSHIP BETWEEN LONG AND SHORT FORMS

Correlations between the Long and Short forms range from .88 in healthy adults to .92 in brain-injured examinees (Benton et al., 1994). Christensen and colleagues' (2002)

TABLE 12–4 Benton Facial Recognition Short Form Normative Data

AGE RANGE (MIDPOINT)	53 TO 60 (57)	55 TO 65 (60)	60 TO 70 (65)	65 TO 75 (70)	70 TO 80 (75)	75 TO 85 (80)	80 TO 90 (85)
N	92	180	172	145	135	112	58
Gender (F/M)	71/21	138/42	121/51	93/52	88/47	74/38	39/19
Mean education (*SD*)	15.72 (2.72)	15.68 (2.77)	15.50 (2.96)	15.13 (2.84)	14.95 (2.85)	14.66 (2.91)	14.34 (2.85)
Mean Benton score (*SD*)	22.90 (2.18)	22.87 (2.12)	22.65 (2.07)	22.20 (2.15)	21.84 (2.30)	21.40 (2.32)	20.57 (2.47)

SOURCE: R. Dixon, personal communication, March 18, 2005.

TABLE 12–5 Mean Scores for Christensen et al. (2002) Benton Facial Recognition Test (FRT) Short Form

AGE (YEARS)	60 TO 69	70 TO 79	80 TO 84	85 TO 89	90+
Mean	28.8	27.3	26.0	25.7	24.4
SD	3.1	3.2	3.7	3.3	3.50

NOTE: Item numbers for this short form: 7, 8, 10, 11, 12, 14, 15, 16, 17, 18, 19, 22.
SOURCE: Adapted from Christensen et al. (2002).

modified short form correlates highly with the Long Form ($r > .90$) in healthy older adults (Christensen et al., 2002).

RELATIONSHIPS WITH OTHER TESTS

Correlations between FRT scores and VIQ are not significant in patients with cerebrovascular accidents (CVAs) (Trahan, 1997). However, Performance IQ (PIQ) and FRT are highly correlated in patients with right CVAs with neglect and in those without neglect ($r = .60$ and .62, respectively; Trahan, 1997), suggesting a significant visual-perceptual component. Similarly, Larrabee (2000) found that the FRT loaded on a visual-perceptual reasoning factor defined by tests such as WAIS Picture Completion, Picture Arrangement, Block Design, Object Assembly, and Digit Symbol, as well as Wisconsin Card Sorting Test (WCST) perseverative errors and Trails B. By contrast, Hermann et al. (1993) reported that the FRT loaded with the Hooper Visual Organization Test but not with WAIS-R subtests or the Judgment of Line Orientation Test (JLO), which loaded together, suggesting that the FRT is more sensitive to object recognition than to spatial localization abilities.

CLINICAL STUDIES

The test is most sensitive to right posterior damage (e.g., Mulder et al., 1995; Trahan, 1997), though impairment has also been reported in left-sided lesions (Mattson et al., 2000; Trahan, 1997). Declines in FRT have also been reported following right or left anterior temporal lobectomy despite normal performance on the JLO, the Hooper, or the WAIS-R Performance subtests (Hermann et al., 1993), and the declines are not related to memory functioning (Botez-Marquand & Botez, 1992). With advancing age, normal age-related decrements in processing speed as well as atrophic brain changes may be associated with decline in face processing (Schretlen et al., 2001).

Migraineurs show a deficit in facial recognition compared to healthy controls even during the interictal period, but the deficit is not related to duration or frequency of attacks or lateralization of headaches (Yetkin-Ozden et al., 2015). In Williams syndrome, the trajectory of development appears to be atypical (delayed; Karmiloff-Smith et al., 2004; see "Neuroanatomical Correlates and Imaging Studies"). Deficits in face recognition have also been reported in patients with PD (Beatty et al., 1989; Levin et al., 1991), multiple sclerosis (MS; Beatty et al., 1989), alcoholism (Schwartz et al., 2002), AD (Andrikopoulos, 1997), moderate to severe closed head injury (Peck et al., 1992; Risser & Andrikopoulos, 1997), and in amateur soccer players (Matser et al., 1999). The findings in psychiatric patients are mixed, with some reporting normal face recognition scores in psychiatric patients (Risser & Andrikopulos, 1997), but others reporting more defective scores in patients with schizophrenia (e.g., Borod et al., 1993; Kucharska-Pietura et al., 2005). Hence, impaired performance on this test should not be interpreted, in and of itself, as evidence of focal neurological disturbance.

Intact vision is important for this test. Kempen et al. (1994) reported significantly poorer scores on this test with patients whose Jaeger near-vision was J5 (equivalent to 20/50) or worse due to refractory error, compared with examinees with normal vision. For this reason, a standard vision test should be administered before an interpretation of the results is attempted in patients with suspected visual disturbance. Interestingly, those who have been treated for congenital bilateral cataracts remain impaired in their facial recognition in the orientation and lighting conditions compared to sighted controls. This impairment is not related to duration of early visual deprivation or reduced visual acuity (Putzar et al., 2009).

Examinees commonly rely on feature-matching strategies using the hairline and eyebrows rather than recognizing the facial configuration. In fact, just the presence of the eyebrows and hairline is sufficient to support normal performance (Duchaine & Weidenfeld, 2003). Therefore, a normal score on the FRT does not demonstrate normal unfamiliar face recognition abilities.

NEUROANATOMICAL CORRELATES AND IMAGING STUDIES

As stated earlier, most studies suggest right-hemisphere correlation with the FRT. In a study using a lesion-deficit analysis method along with MRI, neurological patients with focal brain injury were retrospectively studied. Overall, the lowest FRT score was obtained by the bilateral group, and the left hemisphere group performed best. Among the impaired groups, the subgroup scores were not different from each other. Failure on the FRT was associated with MRI findings of right inferior posterior parietal and right inferior occiptotemporal lesions, specifically the angular gyrus with extension into adjacent lateral superior occipital cortices, as well as the fusiform gyrus. Some correlates were also seen in the right superior temporal gyrus and right inferior precentral gyrus (motor face area). There were no significant findings in the left hemisphere (Tranel et al., 2009).

Patients without dementia and MRI abnormality who demonstrate vertebrobasilar insufficiency as measured by

Doppler sonography obtain lower FRT scores than those with normal flow volume (Koçer et al., 2013).

Among people with Williams syndrome, the average right fusiform face area is twice as large as in typically developing individuals, though on the FRT there are no group differences. In people with Williams syndrome, there is a positive correlation between the right fusiform face area size and FRT performance. This correlation is independent of IQ (Golarai et al., 2010).

PERFORMANCE VALIDITY

Whiteside and colleagues (2011) reviewed the FRT performance of patients from a clinical practice and university training clinic referred by physicians, attorneys, and university disability offices. The most common diagnosis was mild TBI, and other diagnoses included seizure disorders, sleep apnea, fibromyalgia, mild dementia, diabetes, MCI, PD, and anoxia as well as psychological diagnosis. Participants were divided into biased responding and unbiased responding groups based on the Test of Memory Malingering (TOMM) and California Verbal Learning Test—Second Edition, Forced-Choice Recognition [CVLT-II FC]. The authors reported that a raw score of 39 achieved the best specificity for identifying noncredible performance with acceptable sensitivity (AUC = .75, 90% and 40%, respectively; Whiteside et al., 2011).

COMMENT

The FRT has a number of positive features. First, it is relatively brief and portable and can be administered at the bedside. Furthermore, it lends itself for use with a wide variety of patients because it is untimed and requires little motor involvement, although adequate vision is important. Moreover, unlike tests such as the Warrington Recognition Memory for Faces, target faces and test items are presented simultaneously, so that patients are not required to rely on a memory trace.

The FRT appears to tap object recognition more so than spatial localization abilities. However, normal scores on this test may not reflect intact face recognition processes because examinees may be able to score in the normal range without recognizing the facial configuration. That is, they may rely on feature-based procedures such as matching the eyebrows or hairlines, as opposed to configural processing (Duchaine & Weidenfeld, 2003). Therefore, impaired performance does indicate impaired face recognition and is informative, but examiners cannot rely on normal FRT performance to reflect intact face recognition processes. In a similar vein, models of face processing that are supported by dissociations involving normal performance on this task (i.e., normal unfamiliar face recognition and impaired familiar face recognition) must be questioned (Duchaine & Weidenfeld, 2003). Duchaine and Weidenfeld (2003) noted that reliance on a feature-based strategy requires more time. They suggested that it may be possible to test configural processing with the FRT by adding time norms or by limiting the amount of time allowed for each item, although research is needed to verify this method.

Users should bear in mind, however, that the stimuli are very dated, and much of the normative data stem from studies conducted by Benton and his colleagues more than 40 years ago. More current norms are preferred, although it should be noted that these are beginning to be dated, cover a limited age range from restricted geographical regions, and are not derived from national, randomly stratified samples. Overall, the test is in need of restandardization. Findings on the test's ability to identify noncredible performance are preliminary and require validation.

The Long Form has shown adequate internal consistency in some studies (i.e., Christensen et al., 2002) but not in others (Hoptman & Davidson, 1993). Accordingly, use of the *SEM* for computation of confidence intervals is important (Christensen et al., 2002). The internal consistency of the Short Form is poor, and the form should not be used clinically. The Christensen modified short form has slightly better psychometric properties. Accordingly, diagnostic decisions using the FRT should be limited unless supported by other measures with stronger psychometric properties.

REFERENCES

Andrikopoulos, J. (1997). Qualitative facial recognition test performance in Alzheimer's disease [Abstract]. *Archives of Clinical Neuropsychology, 12,* 282.

Beatty, W. W., Goodkin, D. E., & Weir, W. S. (1989). Affective judgements by patients with Parkinson's disease or chronic progressive multiple sclerosis. *Bulletin of the Psychonomic Society, 27,* 361–364.

Benton, A. L., Sivan, A. B., Hamsher, K. de S., Varney, N. R., & Spreen, O. (1994). *Contributions to neuropsychological assessment: A clinical manual* (2nd ed.). New York: Oxford University Press.

Benton, A. L., & Van Allen, M. W. (1968). Impairment in facial recognition in patients with cerebral disease. *Cortex, 4,* 344–358.

Borod, J. C., Martin, C. C., Alpert, M., & Brozgold, A. (1993). Perception of facial emotion in schizophrenic and right brain-damaged patients. *Journal of Nervous and Mental Disease, 181,* 494–502.

Botez-Marquand, T., & Botez, M. I. (1992). Visual memory deficits after damage to the anterior commissure and right fornix. *Archives of Neurology, 49,* 321–324.

Christensen, K. J., Riley, B. E., Hefferman, K. A., Love, S. B., & McLaughlin, M. E. (2002). Facial recognition test in the elderly: Norms, reliability and premorbid estimation. *The Clinical Neuropsychologist, 16,* 51–56.

Diaz-Asper, C., Schretlen, D. J., & Pearlson, G. D. (2004). How well does IQ predict neuropsychological test performance in normal adults. *Journal of the International Neuropsychological Society, 10,* 82–90.

Duchaine, B. C., & Weidenfeld, A. (2003). An evaluation of two commonly used tests of unfamiliar face recognition. *Neuropsychologia, 41,* 713–720.

Ferracuti, F., & Ferracuti, S. (1992). Taratura del campione Italiano. In *Test de Riconoscento di Volti Ignoti* (pp. 26–29). Florence: Organizzazione Speciali.

Golarai, G., Hong, S., Haas, B. W., Galaburda, A. M., Mills, D. L., Bellugi, U., ., &... Reiss, A. L. (2010). The fusiform face area is enlarged in Williams syndrome. *The Journal of Neuroscience, 30*(19), 6700–6712.

Hermann, B. P., Seidenberg, M., Wyler, A., & Haltiner, A. (1993). Dissociation of object recognition and spatial localization abilities following temporal lobe lesions in humans. *Neuropsychology, 7,* 343–350.

Hoptman, M. J., & Davidson, R. J. (1993). *Benton's Facial Recognition Task: A psychometric evaluation.* Paper presented at the meeting of the International Neuropsychological Society, Galveston, TX.

Karmiloff-Smith, A., Thomas, M., Annaz, D., Humphreys, K., Ewing, S., Brace, N., ... Campbell, R. (2004). Exploring the Williams syndrome face-processing debate: The importance of building developmental trajectories. *Journal of Child Psychology and Psychiatry, 45,* 1258–1274.

Kempen, J. H., Kritchevsky, M., & Feldman, S. T. (1994). Effect of visual impairment on neuropsychological test performance. *Journal of Clinical and Experimental Neuropsychology, 16,* 223–231.

Koçer, A., Koçer, E., Beşir, H., Dikici, S., Domaç, F., & Ercan, N. (2013). Low scores on the Benton Facial Recognition Test associated with vertebrobasilar insufficiency. *Medical Hypotheses, 80*(5), 527–529.

Kucharska-Pietura, K., David, A. S., Masiak, M., & Phillips, M. L. (2005). Perception of facial and vocal affect by people with schizophrenia in early and late stages of illness. *The British Journal of Psychiatry, 187*(6), 523–528.

Larrabee, G. J. (2000). Association between IQ and neuropsychological test performance: Commentary on Tremont, Hoffman, Scott, and Adams (1998). *The Clinical Neuropsychologist, 14,* 139–145.

Levin, B. E., Llabre, M. M., & Reisman, S. (1991). Visuospatial impairment in Parkinson's disease. *Neurology, 41,* 365–369.

Levin, H. S., Hamsher, K. de S., & Benton, A. L. (1975). A short form of the test of facial recognition for clinical use. *Journal of Psychology, 91,* 223–228.

Matser, E. J. T., Kessels, A. G., Lezak, M. D., Jordan, B. D., & Troost, J. (1999). Neuropsychological impairment in amateur soccer players. *Journal of the American Medical Association, 282,* 971–973.

Mattson, A. J., Levin, H. S., & Grafman, J. (2000). A case of prosopagnosia following moderate closed head injury with left hemisphere focal lesion. *Cortex, 36,* 125–137.

Mulder, J. L., Bouma, A., & Ansink, J. J. (1995). The role of visual discrimination disorders and neglect in perceptual categorization deficits in right and left hemisphere damaged patients. *Cortex, 31,* 487–501.

Peck, E. A., Mitchell, S. A., Burke, E. A., & Schwartz, S. M. (1992). *Post head injury normative data for selected Benton Neuropsychological Tests.* Paper presented at the meeting of the American Psychological Association, Washington, DC.

Putzar, L., Hötting, K., & Röder, B. (2009). Early visual deprivation affects the development of face recognition and of audio-visual speech perception. *Restorative Neurology and Neuroscience, 28*(2), 251–257.

Rey, G. J., Feldman, E., Rivas-Vazquez, R., Levin, B. E., & Benton, A. (1999). Neuropsychological test development and normative data on Hispanics. *Archives of Clinical Neuropsychology, 14,* 593–601.

Risser, A. H., & Andrikopoulos, J. (1997). *Facial recognition test performance in traumatic brain injury.* Paper presented at the meeting of the International Neuropsychological Society, Orlando, FL.

Roberts, R. J., & Hamsher, K. (1984). Effects of minority status on facial recognition and naming performance. *Journal of Clinical Psychology, 40,* 539–545.

Schretlen, D. J., Pearlson, G. D., Anthony, J. C., & Yates, K. O. (2001). Determinants of Benton Facial Recognition Test performance in normal adults. *Neuropsychology, 15,* 405–410.

Schretlen, D. J., Testa, S. M., & Pearlson, G. D. (2010). *Calibrated neuropsychological normative system.* Lutz, FL: PAR.

Schwartz, B. L., Parker, E. S., Deutsch, S. I., Rosse, R. B., Kaushik, M., & Isaac, A. (2002). Source monitoring in alcoholism. *Journal of Clinical and Experimental Neuropsychology, 24,* 806–817.

Trahan, D. E. (1997). Relationship between facial discrimination and visual neglect in patients with unilateral vascular lesions. *Archives of Clinical Neuropsychology, 12,* 57–62.

Tranel, D., Vianna, E., Manzel, K., Damasio, H., & Grabowski, T. (2009). Neuroanatomical correlates of the Benton Facial Recognition Test and Judgment of Line Orientation Test. *Journal of Clinical and Experimental Neuropsychology, 31*(2), 219–233.

Whiteside, D., Wald, D., & Busse, M. (2011). Classification accuracy of multiple visual spatial measures in the detection of suspect effort. *The Clinical Neuropsychologist, 25*(2), 287–301.

Yetkin-Ozden, S., Ekizoglu, E., & Baykan, B. (2015). Face recognition in patients with migraine. *Pain Practice, 15*(4), 319–322.

HOOPER VISUAL ORGANIZATION TEST (HVOT)

TEST NAME	**Hooper Visual Organization Test (HVOT)**
DOMAIN	Visuospatial skills
AGE RANGE	In adults, to 91 years
ADMINISTRATION TIME	15 minutes
SCORING FORMAT	Hand scored
REFERENCE	Hooper, H. E. (1958). *The Hooper Visual Organization Test: Manual.* Beverly Hills, CA: Western Psychological Services. www.wpspublish.com

DESCRIPTION

The Hooper Visual Organization Test (HVOT) was originally designed to differentiate adults with and without brain damage (Hooper, 1958). It consists of 30 drawings of common objects on 4 × 4-inch cards in a ring binder (test booklet). Each object is cut into two or more parts and illogically arranged in the drawing (see Figure 12–4). The task is to name the object, either orally or in writing. The 1983 edition, developed by the staff of Western Psychological Services (no author credited), is based on Hooper's original studies but adds references to other studies, age- and education-corrected raw score tables, and a T-score conversion table.

The task can be time-consuming for some patients. Accordingly, Merten (2002, 2004a) presented a shortened 15-item version based on an empirical and rational item analysis (Merten & Beal, 1999). Items with insufficient discriminant power, inappropriate cultural dependence, or questionable scoring rules and those otherwise maladaptive were eliminated. The short form was developed on a sample of 320 unselected neurological patients and a cross-validation sample of another 320 neurological patients. A practice item (horse) was also added to assist understanding of the task demands.

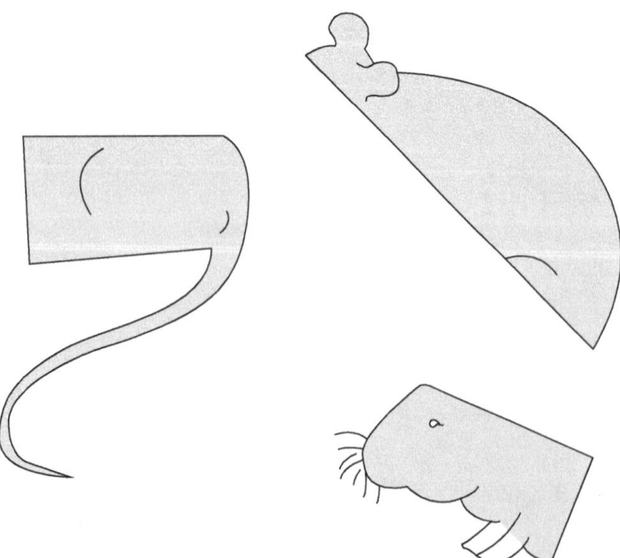

Figure 12–4 This Hooper Visual Organization Test (HVOT) figure, properly integrated, depicts a "mouse" or "guinea pig."

SOURCE: Hooper (1958). Sample item from the Hooper Visual Organization Test copyright © 1957, renewed 1985 by H. Elston Hooper. Reprinted by permission of Western Psychological Services (rights@wpspublish.com). Not to be reprinted in whole or in part for any additional purpose without the expressed, written permission of the publisher. All rights reserved.

ADMINISTRATION

See Source. With individual administration, the correct naming of each object is required. Group administration relies on written responses.

Merten (2002) formulated clearer administration rules. He recommended that the examiner do the following:

1. Ask for specification if a category answer is given (e.g., if the examinee says "fruit" for number 3, say: "What fruit do you mean?"). Guessing is encouraged.
2. If necessary, remind the examinee of the task to be fulfilled.
3. If different answers are proposed, assist the examinee to make a decision (e.g., if the examinee states, "This might be a rabbit or a horse," say: "Which one of the two do you think it is?").
4. Assist persons with anomic symptoms to name objects or animals if they seem to have recognized them.

Wetzel and Murphy (1991) found that discontinuing the test after five consecutive failures did not significantly change the scoring of this test. However, Merten and Beal (1999) cautioned against such a procedure because item ranking in the current form does not adequately reflect the order of item difficulty.

SCORING

STANDARD VERSION

The score is simply the total number of correct responses, although half-credit is given for some of the items for partially correct responses (e.g., "tower" or "castle" instead of lighthouse). At the examiner's discretion, other answers may be given full credit, but only if they are actual synonyms or closely resemble the correct answers.

Raw scores can be adjusted for age and education, and raw or corrected scores can be transformed to a T score by means of tables provided in the test manual. Higher T scores imply lower raw scores. Qualitative scoring includes the distinction between isolate, perseverative, bizarre, and neologistic responses.

15-ITEM SHORT FORM

Scoring rules for the short form are shown in Table 12–6 (Merten, 2002). Merten (2002) proposed additional scoring rules for both the long and short forms. He recommended that the examiner do the following:

1. Allow subspecification (e.g., "Cheshire cat" for cat).
2. Allow colloquial, regional, or infantile expressions.
3. Not penalize answers such as "an apple, cut into slices."

DEMOGRAPHIC EFFECTS

AGE

Performance follows a U-shaped function, with scores improving during childhood and declining with advancing age (e.g., Source; Giannakou & Kosmidis, 2006; Kirk, 1992; Libon et al., 1994; Mason & Ganzler, 1964; Merten, 2002; Nabors et al., 1997; Seidel, 1994; Walsh et al., 1997).

TABLE 12–6 Modified Scoring Rules for the Hooper Short Form Items

NO.	CONTENT	ORIGINAL ITEM NO.	MODIFIED OR SPECIFIED SCORING RULES
1	Table/bench	3	
2	Teakettle	16	Teapot, coffeepot, and so on are given full credit
3	Apple	11	No other fruits allowed; no half-credits
4	Airplane	4	
5	Scissors	13	
6	Chair/sofa	17	Sofa, settee, couch, and so on are given full credit
7	Book	23	
8	Cat	20	No half-credits
9	Sailboat	15	Boat, ship, vessel, and so on are given full credit
10	Mouse/rat	22	Full credit is given for naming other rodents, such as rat or guinea pig; no half-credits
11	Cane/walking stick	14	Hockey stick is not accepted as correct
12	Rabbit/hare	24	No half-credits
13	Block	25	
14	Key	28	
15	Ring	29	

SOURCE: Adapted from Merten (2002).

For example, Merten (2002) reported a correlation of −.50 in examinees ranging in age from 15 to 87 years who were seen for neuropsychological examination.

GENDER

There is no systematic relationship to gender (see Source; Giannakou & Kosmidis, 2006; Merten & Beal, 1999; Nabors et al., 1997; Seidel, 1994).

EDUCATION AND IQ

Examinees with more formal education obtain higher raw scores (see Source; Giannakou & Kosmidis, 2006; Merten & Beal, 1999; Merten, 2002; Nabors et al., 1997; Richardson & Marottoli, 1996; Walsh et al., 1997). However, correlations with age tend to be larger than those for education (e.g., $r = .21$, Merten & Beal, 1999), and most of the shared variance with education is attributable to general intelligence (Mason & Ganzler, 1964; also see Source). The test manual recommends that the task not be used with individuals with IQs lower than about 75.

ETHNICITY, NATIONALITY, AND LINGUISTIC EFFECTS

There is little evidence of ethnic bias in US samples (see Source; Lewis et al., 1997; Nabors et al., 1997), although the test manual does suggest that the examiner should be sensitive to cultural and regional variations in language. Kosmidis and colleagues (2010) reported that healthy Greek community-living adults (aged 16–74) performed significantly lower than their American counterparts (mean score of 18.3 vs. 26.2, respectively). When some modifications to the acceptable responses (see Table 12–7) were made, the mean score of healthy Greeks was 21.3 points (Giannakou & Kosmidis, 2006).

NORMATIVE DATA

STANDARDIZATION SAMPLE

The norms published with the test manual rely on data collected several decades ago by Mason and Ganzler (1964)

TABLE 12–7 Modified Scoring Rules for the Greek Version of the HVOT

ITEM	ADDITIONAL ACCEPTABLE ANSWERS
8. truck	semi-truck (νταλίκα, φορτηγό με καρότσα)
15. sailboat	ship (πλοίο), boat with sails (βάρκα με πανιά), vessel with sails (σκαφος με πανιά)
16. teapot	coffeepot (καφετιέρα)
17. chair	armchair (πολυθρόνα)
18. candle	candlestick (κηροπήγιο)
22. mouse	rat (αρουραίος), guinea pig (ινδικό χοιρίδιο)
24. rabbit	hare (λαγὸς), bunny (κουνέλι)

SOURCE: Giannakou and Kosmidis (2006). Reprinted with the kind permission of Taylor & Francis Ltd. www.tandfonline.com

TABLE 12-8 Characteristics of the HVOT Standardization Sample

Sample size	231
Age	<30 = 22 30 to 39 = 59 40 to 49 = 59 50 to 59 = 38 60 to 69 = 40 70 to 75 = 13
Geographical location	Long Beach, California
Sample type	Largely patients at a Veterans Administration hospital with pulmonary disease or requiring surgery for disorders such as fracture, infection, or hernia; also, a few (<15) nonprofessional hospital personnel and volunteer hospital workers were tested
Education	Not reported
Gender	100% Men 0% Women
Ethnicity	Exclusively or predominantly Caucasian
Socioeconomic status	Not reported
Screening	Screened to exclude those with history of psychiatric or neurological disorder or alcoholism

SOURCE: Mason and Ganzler (1964).

(see Table 12–8). Most of the testing was completed in small groups, but some was done individually, sometimes without supervision and all examinees were male (see Mason & Ganzler, 1964; also see Source). There was no time limit. Note that the normative scores tend to be quite skewed, meaning that the HVOT is not very sensitive to impairment at the upper score range.

OTHER NORMATIVE DATA

In addition to using the T-score table, a number of different cutoff points have been proposed for the long form (see Source). Based on the high correlation (r = .95) between short and long forms in a large sample of neurological patients (N = 640), Merten (2002) used linear regression analysis to develop cutoffs for the short form. The cutoff values for the long and short forms are shown in Table 12–9.

TABLE 12-9 Selected Cutoff Values for the Long and Short Forms of the HVOT

SOURCE	DESCRIPTION	LONG FORM	SHORT FORM
Test manual (1983), Merten (2002)	Suggestion of further assessment	<24	<13
Test manual (1983), Merten (2002)	Probable visual-spatial deficits, minimizing false positives	<21	<11
Merten (2002)	Probable visual-spatial deficits in geriatric patients		<8

TABLE 12-10 Means and Standard Deviations (*SDs*) for the Hooper Visual Organization Test (HVOT) in Older Adults, by Education

AGE 76 TO 80 YEARS		AGE 81 TO 91 YEARS	
<12 YEARS (*N* = 26)	≥12 YEARS (*N* = 24)	<12 YEARS (*N* = 18)	≥12 YEARS (*N* = 33)
17.90 (4.01)	21.69 (4.09)	17.62 (6.17)	19.71 (2.97)

NOTE: Community-dwelling older adults *N* = 101; 48% males; predominantly Caucasian; age range = 76–91; education range = 4–16 years.
SOURCE: Adapted from Richardson and Marattoli (1996).

Users should bear in mind, however, that no single cutoff point is appropriate for all individuals in all settings. For example, Nabors et al. (1997) reported that a lower cutoff value (15) may be needed with older, urban, medical populations to avoid false-positive results. Similarly, Richardson and Marattoli (1996) evaluated older individuals and noted that the ability to adjust for education is particularly important when testing older adults. Failure to do so will result in false-positive findings, particularly for examinees who are poorly educated. Data are presented in Table 12–10 for two age groups (76–80 and 81–91 years), each of which is broken down into two education groups (<12 years and ≥12 years of formal education). Data were excluded for participants who reported a history of neurological disease or excessive use of alcohol or scored below education-adjusted cutoffs for dementia on the MMSE. The older, more educated participants appeared to perform more poorly than the younger, similarly educated individuals. No obvious age effect was observed between the two less educated groups.

Giannakou and Kosmidis (2006) reported Greek normative data based on healthy individuals from the community. The data, stratified by age and education levels, are presented in Table 12–11.

EVIDENCE FOR RELIABILITY

EVIDENCE FOR INTERNAL RELIABILITY

Internal reliability is reported to be high ($r \geq .80$; see Source; Lopez et al., 2003; Merten & Beal, 1999). Estimates of internal consistency for the Merten 15-item short form yield coefficients of .84 (Cronbach's alpha) and .85 (split-half; Merten, 2004a) in neurological patients. The Greek version yields a similar Cronbach's alpha (.85; Giannakou & Kosmidis, 2006).

The item order of the standard form appears to have been established a priori, without empirical testing. Several authors have found the item ranking to deviate from the order of difficulty (e.g., Kirk, 1992; Merten & Beal, 1999). In addition, some items do not possess sufficient discriminatory power. For example, Lopez et al. (2003) reported that items 1, 2, 15, and 27 provided poor

TABLE 12–11 Greek Normative Data Stratified by Age and Education

	AGE (YEARS)								
	18 TO 39			40 TO 59			60+		
	EDUCATION (YEARS)			EDUCATION (YEARS)			EDUCATION (YEARS)		
PERCENTILE	1–9	10–12	13+	1–9	10–12	13+	1–9	10–12	13+
90	26.1	28.5	28.1	23.9	26.3	27.0	23.0	24.6	25.4
80	24.9	27.5	27.5	22.5	25.5	26.4	18.5	22.5	23.3
70	23.8	25.5	27.2	22.0	24.3	25.4	16.5	21.5	22.5
60	23.4	25.0	26.5	20.3	23.5	25.0	16.0	19.9	22.1
50	21.0	23.3	25.5	20.0	22.8	24.5	15.0	19.0	21.0
40	20.5	22.7	25.0	19.2	22.0	23.4	13.9	16.9	20.4
30	20.0	22.0	24.0	18.0	21.3	22.2	12.5	16.5	19.2
20	19.0	21.2	22.9	17.1	19.0	20.8	12.0	14.5	14.8
10	14.4	20.0	22.0	14.6	15.0	20.5	7.9	13.0	13.2
M	21.26	23.97	25.43	19.5	22.10	23.88	15.06	18.81	20.19
SD	4.14	3.09	2.17	3.56	3.76	2.60	4.46	4.40	4.10

NOTE: Greek sample N =206, 47% male; mean age = 47.78, SD = 18.30, range 18–79 years; mean education = 11.4, SD = 3.94, range = 2–21 years.
SOURCE: Giannakou and Kosmidis (2006). Reprinted with the kind permission of Taylor & Francis Ltd. www.tandfonline.com

discrimination between cognitively intact and cognitively impaired individuals.

EVIDENCE FOR TEST-RETEST RELIABILITY, MEASURING CHANGE, AND PRACTICE EFFECTS

Lezak (1982; Lezak et al., 2004, 2012) reported a coefficient of concordance of .86, indicating good test-retest reliability after six months and again after 12 months (sample composition not reported). Similarly, reliability at eight months in 51 adults with intractable epilepsy was .75 (Sawrie et al., 1996).

In an AD sample with mean MMSE of 22.27 (SD = 2.92) at baseline and 21.23 (SD = 4.10) at one-year follow-up, mean HVOT change was less than one point. Healthy older adults also showed minimal change over one year (Paxton et al., 2007).

EVIDENCE FOR RELIABILITY OF ALTERNATE OR SHORT FORMS

With the 15-item short form, test-retest reliability in a sample of neurological patients with an interval of 203 days is very high (r = .93) and with a mean increase of 0.6 points (Merten, 2004a). Seven-day retest reliability for a subgroup of 36 patients is reported as high (r = .93), with a mean increase of 1.1 points (Merten, 2004b). However, one-year retest reliability in healthy older adults is lower using a shortened 10-item version (r = .68; Levin et al., 1991).

EVIDENCE FOR INTERRATER RELIABILITY

The scoring instructions allow the examiner to give credit (1 or 1½ points) for answers that are synonyms or closely resemble the correct answers. Nonetheless, interrater reliabilities are high (>.95) for three and two raters (Lopez et al., 2003).

EVIDENCE FOR VALIDITY

RELATIONSHIPS WITH OTHER TESTS

Successful performance appears to depend primarily on visual-spatial abilities of the sort measured by the Wechsler IQ tests and less so on the capacity to label objects. For example, a study by Paolo et al. (1996) found that Wechsler performance subtests accounted for 44% of the variance, whereas the Boston Naming Test (BNT) accounted for only 5% of HVOT variance. Similarly, Ricker and Axelrod (1995) reported that object naming accounted for 11% of the variance in HVOT performance, whereas WAIS-R perceptual organization accounted for 48%. Johnstone and Wilhelm (1997) conducted a principal components factor analysis of the HVOT, WAIS-R, and other tasks (e.g., Rey-Osterrieth, BNT, Controlled Oral Word Association Test [COWA], Wechsler Memory Scale—Revised [WMS-R] Visual Reproduction) in a heterogeneous sample of patients (15 to 69 years old) who were referred for neuropsychological evaluation. They found that the HVOT loaded primarily on a global visual-spatial intelligence factor and had its highest correlates with PIQ subtests.

Hermann et al. (1993) gave the HVOT along with a battery of other tests to patients with temporal lobe epilepsy preoperatively. The HVOT loaded equally on two visual factors, one defined by the WAIS-R Performance subtests and the other by the Facial Recognition Test. Merten (2005) conducted a principal axis factor analysis of the HVOT with 20 other tests based on 200 neurological patients in Berlin; he found that the HVOT loaded primarily on a global nonverbal performance factor, together with the WAIS Block Design, TMT, Raven's Progressive Matrices, the Line Orientation Test, and Visual Object and Space Perception Battery (VOSP) Silhouettes, among others. Similarly, Paul et al. (2001) reported that in patients with vascular dementia, more than 60% of the variance in

HVOT performance was accounted for by WAIS-R Block Design; performance on the BNT did not make a significant contribution. In a PD sample, there were moderate correlations with Block Design ($r = .43$), and Trail Making Test (TMT) Part B minus Part A ($r = -.53$), while correlation with BNT was weaker ($r = .27$). When regressed with demographic variables, TMT Part B minus Part A was the only significant predictor of HVOT performance in this PD sample (Higginson et al., 2011).

Although perceptual organization skill is critical for success, object naming does play a role. Ricker and Axelrod (1995) gave the HVOT along with a naming test consisting of the HVOT figures to a group of 50 patients seen for neuropsychological evaluation. The ability to name the stimuli was unrelated to the ability to synthesize the fragmented parts. However, the extent of any language disorder in these patients was not described. To further explore the relationship between naming ability and HVOT performance, Schultheis et al. (2000) examined 14 stroke or TBI patients (mean age = 35 years) with anomia, defined as scoring in the lower 10% of norms for the BNT. The standard HVOT and a multiple-choice version of the HVOT that required the examinee to choose one of four words printed below each picture were administered. The patients obtained a significantly greater number of correct responses for the multiple-choice version compared with the standard HVOT. This improvement applied equally to those with right- and left-hemisphere lesions, although the former group had a greater error score overall. The authors concluded that naming ability does play a role in HVOT performance. Similarly, in a sample of probable AD patients, the HVOT loaded most heavily on a language factor and had strong secondary loading on a visuospatial processing factor (Paxton et al., 2007). In MCI, moderate to high correlations ($r = .34$ to $.69$) were seen with TMT-B, COWA, and BNT, with the BNT accounting for 43% of the variance on the HVOT (Jefferson et al., 2006).

CLINICAL STUDIES

Impairment has been reported in a number of conditions, including autism (Jolliffe & Baron-Cohen, 2001), dementia (Nabors et al., 1997; Paul et al., 2001; Walsh et al., 1997; Zec et al., 1992), AD (Paxton et al., 2007), PD (Gollaher, 1996; Higginson et al., 2011; Levin et al., 1991; Relja & Klepac, 2006), and MS (Giannakou & Kosmidis, 2006). For example, the HVOT provided moderate discrimination between probable AD and healthy controls, yielding a sensitivity of 81% and a specificity of 80% at an optimal cutoff score of 21.5 (Paxton et al., 2007). The higher the DRS score, the better the HVOT score.

The validity of this test for "general screening for brain damage" has been hotly debated in the past (Boyd, 1982a, 1982b; Rathbun & Smith, 1982; Woodward, 1982). For example, correct classification rates of 74% between unselected brain-damaged patients and healthy controls with a cutoff score of 25 have been reported (Boyd, 1981). However, Wetzel and Murphy (1991) found that many brain-injured persons perform well on the HVOT, raising the concern of a high rate of false-negative results. Such a screening function has become increasingly obsolete with the advent of other neuroimaging and neuropsychological tools. In a study of 305 neurological patients, Merten and Beal (1999) found that, although the concordance between the HVOT, the MMSE, and another German screening test was significant (contingency coefficient C = .40, Kendall's tau = .39, $p < .001$), discrepancies on the level of individual classification were considerable.

Psychiatric Conditions. Gerson (1974) concluded that the test is "not sensitive to . . . thought disorders" (p. 98) and that neologisms and bizarre responses did not occur in this population at all. However, others have reported that scores are lower in psychiatric inpatients (e.g., Tamkin & Jacobsen, 1984) and patients with schizophrenia (Giannakou & Kosmidis, 2006). Lee and Cheung (2005) reported poor performance on the HVOT in patients with schizophrenia, perhaps reflecting difficulties with attention. Zakzanis et al. (2001) noted that the HVOT contributed significantly to the differentiation between patients with late-onset schizophrenia and those with frontotemporal dementia. Performance was more impaired in those with schizophrenia.

Daily Living Skills. Whether the HVOT predicts functional ability is uncertain. Richardson et al. (1995) found that it was the best of five neuropsychological tests in the prediction of performance-based ratings of activities of daily living in a geriatric population. In contrast, Greve et al. (2000) found that, in patients with cardiovascular accidents, the relationship between HVOT scores and functional independence measures was not significant. Performance on the HVOT appears somewhat related to driving performance in older adults; however, other tasks (e.g., reaction time, useful field of view) are stronger predictors (Myers et al., 2000).

SHORT FORM

Merten (2002) reported that the short form correlates highly with WAIS Block Design ($r = .71$), as does the long form ($r = .75$). Correlations with other screening instruments (e.g., MMSE, Raven's) were similar and high for both forms. Patients with lateralized right-hemisphere damage scored significantly lower on this version than did those with left-hemisphere damage (Merten, 2004b).

NEUROANATOMICAL CORRELATES AND IMAGING STUDIES

Given the high visual-spatial demands of the task, one might expect right posterior involvement. Although some authors (Boyd, 1981; Schultheis et al., 2000; Wang, 1977; Wetzel & Murphy, 1991; York & Cermak, 1995) have been unable to demonstrate performance differences between patients with left- or right-hemisphere damage, trends have often been evident (Fitz et al., 1992; Schultheis et al., 2000; York & Cermak, 1995) and suggest impairment in the context of right-hemisphere disturbance.

One study (Moritz et al., 2004) adapted the task to functional MRI (fMRI) analysis and suggested an extensive bilateral response across all brain lobes, predominantly in the posterior brain, in regions of superior parietal lobules, ventral temporooccipital cortex, posterior visual association areas, and, to a lesser extent, the frontal eye fields bilaterally and left dorsolateral prefrontal cortex. Presumably these clusters reflect brain regions subserving visual-spatial processes, object identification, and covert naming.

PERFORMANCE VALIDITY

Whiteside and colleagues (2011) reviewed the HVOT performance of patients from a clinical practice and university training clinic referred by physicians, attorneys, and university disability offices. The most common diagnosis was mild TBI, with other diagnoses including seizure disorders, sleep apnea, fibromyalgia, mild dementia, diabetes, MCI, PD, and anoxia as well as psychological diagnosis. Participants were divided into biased responding and unbiased responding groups based on TOMM and CVLT-II Forced-Choice Recognition. The HVOT yielded an AUC of .71 for identifying biased responding, which indicates that the HVOT yields poor classification accuracy for identifying biased responding. Table 12–12 presents the classification accuracy data as a function of cutoff score of the HVOT. The authors reported that a raw score of 21.5 achieved the best balance of sensitivity and specificity for identifying noncredible performance (Whiteside et al., 2011). However, it is only moderately sensitive and should therefore be supplemented by other tests (Whiteside et al., 2011).

COMMENT

This test is brief and easy to administer. It can be given individually or in a group setting. In addition, it can be used with a variety of populations, and it may be particularly useful in those compromised by limited motor ability other than speech.

TABLE 12–12 Sensitivity and Specificity of the Hooper Visual Organization Test (HVOT) at Various Cutoff Scores

RAW SCORE	SENSITIVITY (%)	SPECIFICITY (%)
18	18	97
19	18	95
19.5	21	95
20	27	92
20.5	27	92
21	45	88
21.5	46	88
22	52	83
22.5	52	82
23	52	77

SOURCE: Adapted from Whiteside et al. (2011).

Although reliability appears satisfactory, other psychometric properties are not. Users should note that normative information for adults is dated, deriving from a sample of individuals, most with medical disorders, by poorly standardized procedures. The task requires clearer administration rules to advise the examiner how to assist people with anomic disorders, when and how to demand response specification, how to treat multiple responses, and so on (Merten, 2002). Scoring rules also appear to be arbitrary and need to be revised (Merten, 2002; Seidel, 1994). Contemporary normative data, stratified by age and IQ, also need to be provided.

Merten (2002) developed a short version and clarified instructions and scoring in an attempt to improve the internal consistency of the test. His 15-item version shows validity and reliability similar to the full-length version in neurological patients and may be a suitable substitute for the full HVOT.

The HVOT is not an adequate screening device of cognitive deficit because of its high rate of false-negative classifications. Although it may serve as a screen for visual-perceptual dysfunction, its ability to contribute additional information to the diagnostic process beyond that provided by other visual-spatial tasks (e.g., Wechsler performance subtests) is uncertain. In fact, Johnstone and Wilhelm (1997) considered the HVOT to be another measure of visual-spatial intelligence, not distinct from abilities tapped by Wechsler performance subtests. Furthermore, the HVOT lacks the capacity to provide differential diagnosis with respect to the location of functional deficits.

Users should also note that, although the test mainly measures visual-spatial/perceptual ability, the task does require naming. Accordingly, results in even mildly aphasic patients may be questionable. Merten (Merten, 2002; Merten & Beal, 1999) recommended that anomic patients should be assisted to maximize their HVOT scores as an adequate measure of their visual-perceptual abilities.

The validity of the test requires additional study. Whether the task predicts functional outcome above and beyond that provided by other standard tests (e.g., Wechsler performance subtests) also remains to be determined. Although some limited data are available to assess performance validity on the HVOT, it should not be used independently as an indicator of performance validity (Whiteside et al., 2011).

REFERENCES

Boyd, J. L. (1981). A validity study of the Hooper Visual Organization Test. *Journal of Consulting and Clinical Psychology, 49,* 15–19.

Boyd, J. L. (1982a). Reply to Rathbun and Smith: Who made the Hooper blooper? *Journal of Consulting and Clinical Psychology, 50,* 284–285.

Boyd, J. L. (1982b). Reply to Woodward. *Journal of Consulting and Clinical Psychology, 50,* 289–290.

Farver, P. F., & Farver, T. B. (1982). Performance of normal older adults on tests designed to measure parietal lobe functions. *American Journal of Occupational Therapy, 36,* 444–449.

Fitz, A. G., Conrad, P. M., Hom, D. L., & Sarff, P. L. (1992). Hooper Visual Organization Test performance in lateralized brain injury. *Archives of Clinical Neuropsychology, 7,* 243–250.

Gerson, A. (1974). Validity and reliability of the Hooper Visual Organization Test. *Perceptual and Motor Skills, 39,* 95–100.

Giannakou, M., & Kosmidis, M. H. (2006). Cultural appropriateness of the Hooper Visual Organization Test? Greek normative data. *Journal of Clinical and Experimental Neuropsychology, 28*(6), 1023–1029.

Gollaher, K. K. (1996). Visuospatial and visuo-constructional functioning in Parkinson's disease. *Dissertation Abstracts International, 56*(11-B), 6427.

Greve, K. W., Lindberg, R. F., Bianchini, K. J., & Adams, D. (2000). Construct validity and predictive value of the Hooper Visual Organization Test in stroke rehabilitation. *Applied Neuropsychology, 7,* 515–522.

Hermann, B. P., Seidenberg, M., Wyler, A., & Haltiner, A. (1993). Dissociation of object recognition and spatial localization abilities following temporal lobe lesions in humans. *Neuropsychology, 7,* 343–350.

Higginson, C. I., Wheelock, V. L., Levine, D., Pappas, C. T., & Sigvardt, K. A. (2011). Predictors of HVOT performance in Parkinson's disease. *Applied neuropsychology, 18*(3), 210–215.

Hooper, H. E. (1958). *The Hooper Visual Organization Test: Manual.* Beverly Hills, CA: Western Psychological Services.

Jefferson, A. L., Wong, S., Bolen, E., Ozonoff, A., Green, R. C., & Stern, R. A. (2006). Cognitive correlates of HVOT performance differ between individuals with mild cognitive impairment and normal controls. *Archives of Clinical Neuropsychology, 21*(5), 405–412.

Johnstone, B., & Wilhelm, K. L. (1997). The construct validity of the Hooper Visual Organization Test. *Assessment, 4,* 243–248.

Jolliffe, T., & Baron-Cohen, R. (2001). A test of central coherence theory: Can adults with high-functioning autism or Asperger syndrome integrate fragments of an object? *Cognitive Neuropsychiatry, 6,* 193–216.

Kirk, U. (1992). Evidence for early acquisition of visual organization ability: A developmental study. *The Clinical Neuropsychologist, 6,* 171–177.

Kosmidis, M. H., Tsotsi, S., Karambela, O., Takou, E., & Vlahou, C. H. (2010). Cultural factors influencing performance on visuoperceptual neuropsychological tasks. *Behavioural Neurology, 23*(4), 245–247.

Lee, T. M. C., & Cheung, P. P. Y. (2005). The relationship between visual-perception and attention in Chinese with schizophrenia. *Schizophrenia Research, 72,* 185–193.

Levin, B. E., Llabre, M. M., & Reisman, S. (1991). Visuospatial impairment in Parkinson's disease. *Neurology, 41,* 365–369.

Lewis, S., Campbell, A., & Takushi-Chinen, R., Brown, A., Dennis, G., Wood, D., & Weir, R. (1997). Visual Organization Test performance in an African American population with acute unilateral cerebral lesions. *International Journal of Neuroscience, 91,* 295–302.

Lezak, M. D. (1982). *The test-retest stability and reliability of some tests commonly used in neuropsychological assessment.* Paper presented at the meeting of the International Neuropsychological Society, Deauville, France.

Lezak, M. D., Howieson, D. B., Bigler, E. D., & Tranel, D. (2012). *Neuropsychological assessment* (5th ed.). New York: Oxford University Press.

Lezak, M. D., Howieson, D. B., & Loring, D. W. (2004). *Neuropsychological assessment* (4th ed.). New York: Oxford University Press.

Libon, D. J., Glosser, G., Malamut, B. L., Kaplan, E., Goldberg, E., Swenson, R., & Sands, L. P. (1994). Age, executive functions, and visuospatial functioning in healthy older adults. *Neuropsychology, 8,* 38–43.

Lopez, M. N., Lazar, M. D., & Oh, S. (2003). Psychometric properties of the Hooper Visual Organization Test. *Assessment, 10,* 66–70.

Mason, C. F., & Ganzler, H. (1964). Adult norms for the Shipley Institute of Living Scale and Hooper Visual Organization test based on age and education. *Journal of Gerontology, 19,* 419–424.

Merten, T. (2002). A short version of the Hooper Visual Organization Test: Development and validation. *The Clinical Neuropsychologist, 16,* 136–144.

Merten, T. (2004a). A short version of the Hooper Visual Organization Test: Reliability and validity. *Applied Neuropsychology, 11,* 99–102.

Merten, T. (2004b). Eine kurzform des Hooper Visual Organization Test. *Zeitschrift fur Neuropsychologie, 15,* 303–311.

Merten, T. (2005). Factor structure of the Hooper Visual Organization Test: A cross-cultural replication and extension. *Archives of Clinical Neuropsychology, 20,* 123–128.

Merten, T., & Beal, C. (1999). An analysis of the Hooper Visual Organization Test with neurological patients. *The Clinical Neuropsychologist, 13,* 521–529.

Moritz, C. H., Johnson, S. C., McMillan, K. M., Haughton, V. M., & Meyerand, M. E. (2004). Functional MRI neuroanatomic correlates of the Hooper Visual Organization Test. *Journal of the International Neuropsychological Society, 10,* 939–947.

Myers, R. S., Ball, K. K., Kalina, T. D., Roth, D. L., & Goode, K. T. (2000). Relation of useful field of view and other screening tests to on-road driving performance. *Perceptual and Motor Skills, 91,* 279–290.

Nabors, N. A., Vangel, S. J., Lichtenberg, P. A., & Walsh, P. (1997). Normative and clinical utility of the Hooper Visual Organization Test with geriatric medical inpatients. *Journal of Clinical Geropsychology, 3,* 191–198.

Nadler, J. D., Grace, J., White, D. A., Butters, M. A., & Malloy, P. F. (1996). Laterality differences in quantitative and qualitative Hooper performance. *Archives of Clinical Neuropsychology, 11,* 223–229.

Paolo, A. M., Cluff, R. B., & Ryan, J. J. (1996). Influence of perceptual organization and naming abilities on the Hooper Visual Organization Test. *Neuropsychiatry, Neuropsychology, and Behavioral Neurology, 9,* 254–257.

Paul, R., Cohen, R., Moser, D., Ott, B., Zawacki, T., & Gordon, N. (2001). Performance on the Hooper Visual Organization Test in patients diagnosed with subcortical vascular dementia: Relation to naming performance. *Neuropsychiatry, Neuropsychology and Behavioral Neurology, 14,* 93–97.

Paxton, J. L., Peavy, G. M., Jenkins, C., Rice, V. A., Heindel, W. C., & Salmon, D. P. (2007). Deterioration of visual-perceptual organization ability in Alzheimer's disease. *Cortex, 43*(7), 967–975.

Rathbun, J., & Smith, A. (1982). Comment on the validity of Boyd's validation study of the Hooper Visual Organization Test. *Journal of Consulting and Clinical Psychology, 50,* 281–283.

Relja, M., & Klepac, N. (2006). A dopamine agonist, pramipexole, and cognitive functions in Parkinson's disease. *Journal of the Neurological Sciences, 248*(1), 251–254.

Richardson, E. D., & Marottoli, R. A. (1996). Education-specific normative data on common neuropsychological indices for individuals older than 75 years. *The Clinical Neuropsychologist, 10,* 375–381.

Richardson, E. D., Nadler, J. D., & Malloy, P. F. (1995). Neuropsychologic prediction of performance measures of daily living skills in geriatric patients. *Neuropsychology, 9,* 565–572.

Ricker, J. H., & Axelrod, B. N. (1995). Hooper Visual Organization Test: Effects of object naming ability. *The Clinical Neuropsychologist, 9,* 57–62.

Sawrie, S. M., Chelune, G. J., Naugle, R. I., & Luders, H. O. (1996). Empirical methods for assessing meaningful neuropsychological changes following epilepsy surgery. *Journal of the International Neuropsychological Society, 2,* 556–564.

Schultheis, M. T., Caplan, B., Ricker, J. H., & Woessner, R. (2000). Fractioning the Hooper: A multiple-choice response format. *The Clinical Neuropsychologist, 14,* 196–201.

Seidel, W. T. (1994). Applicability of the Hooper Visual Organization Test to pediatric populations: Preliminary findings. *The Clinical Neuropsychologist, 8,* 59–68.

Tamkin, A. S., & Hyer, L. A. (1984). Testing for cognitive dysfunction in the aging population. *Military Medicine, 149,* 397–399.

Tamkin, A. S., & Jacobsen, R. (1984). Age-related norms for the Hooper Visual Organization Test. *Journal of Clinical Psychology, 40,* 1459–1463.

Walsh, P. F., Lichtenberg, P. A., & Rowe, R. J. (1997). Hooper Visual Organization Test performance in geriatric rehabilitation patients. *Clinical Gerontologist, 17,* 3–11.

Wang, P. L. (1977). Visual organization ability in brain-damaged adults. *Perceptual and Motor Skills, 45,* 723–728.

Wetzel, L., & Murphy, S. G. (1991). Validity of the use of a discontinuation rule and evaluation of discriminability of the Hooper Visual Organization Test. *Neuropsychology, 5,* 119–122.

Whiteside, D., Wald, D., & Busse, M. (2011). Classification accuracy of multiple visual spatial measures in the detection of suspect effort. *The Clinical Neuropsychologist, 25*(2), 287–301.

Woodward, C. A. (1982). The Hooper Visual Organization Test: A case against its use in neuropsychological assessment. *Journal of Consulting and Clinical Psychology, 50,* 286–288.

York, C. D., & Cermak, S. A. (1995). Visual perception and praxis in adults after stroke. *American Journal of Occupational Therapy, 49,* 543–550.

Zakzanis, K. K., Kielar, A., Young, D., & Boulos, M. (2001). Neuropsychological differentiation of late onset schizophrenia and frontotemporal dementia. *Cognitive Neuropsychiatry, 6,* 63–77.

Zec, R. F., Vicari, S., Kocis, M., & Reynolds, T. (1992). Sensitivity of different neuropsychological tests to very mild DAT [Abstract]. *The Clinical Neuropsychologist, 6,* 327.

JUDGMENT OF LINE ORIENTATION (JLO)

TEST NAME	**Judgment of Line Orientation (JLO)**
DOMAIN	Visual perception
AGE RANGE	In adults, to 90 years
ADMINISTRATION TIME	15 minutes
SCORING FORMAT	Hand scored
REFERENCE	Benton, A. L., Sivan, A. B., Hamsher, K. de S., Varney, N. R., & Spreen, O. (1994). *Contributions to neuropsychological assessment* (2nd ed.). Orlando, FL: Psychological Assessment Resources.

DESCRIPTION

A large number of tests have been devised to assess various aspects of spatial ability. The impetus for the development of the Judgment of Line Orientation (JLO) task as a clinical instrument came in part from findings of a left visual field/right-hemisphere superiority among right-handed university students in identifying the direction of lines presented tachistoscopically to the left and right visual fields (see Benton et al., 1994, for a history of the task). In addition, patients with right-hemisphere pathology performed defectively on such tasks (Benton et al., 1994).

There are two forms of the task, Form H and Form V, each consisting of the same 30 items, presented in a somewhat different order. In each form, items are presented in a generally ascending order of difficulty (but see Qualls et al., 2000). The test materials for each form are spiral-bound in a single booklet and consist of 35 stimuli appearing in the upper part of the booklet and a multiple-choice card (the same for all stimuli) appearing in the lower part (see Figure 12–5). The first five items are practice items. The multiple-choice response card consists of an array of lines, labeled "1" through "11" and drawn at 18-degree intervals from the point of origin. The respondent is required to identify which two lines, from the multiple-choice array, match the directions of the lines on the stimulus card. The lines on the stimulus card are shorter than the ones on the response card.

SHORT FORMS

A number of short forms have been presented: Odd (Form O) and Even (E) 15-item short forms (Vanderploeg et al., 1997; Woodard et al., 1996, 1998) have been proposed for Form V. Another pair of 15-item, internally consistent short forms (Forms Q and S) was developed by Qualls et al. (2000); they used item analysis to ensure equivalence of the two forms. Winegarden et al. (1998) described a 20-item short form consisting of items 11 through 30 from Form V. In a more recent revision, a short form based on item response theory (IRT), with number of items administered according to basal and ceiling rules, has also been described (see Table 12–13; Calamia et al., 2011).

ADMINISTRATION

See manual. Briefly, the test booklet and the multiple-choice card are placed flat on the table in front of the

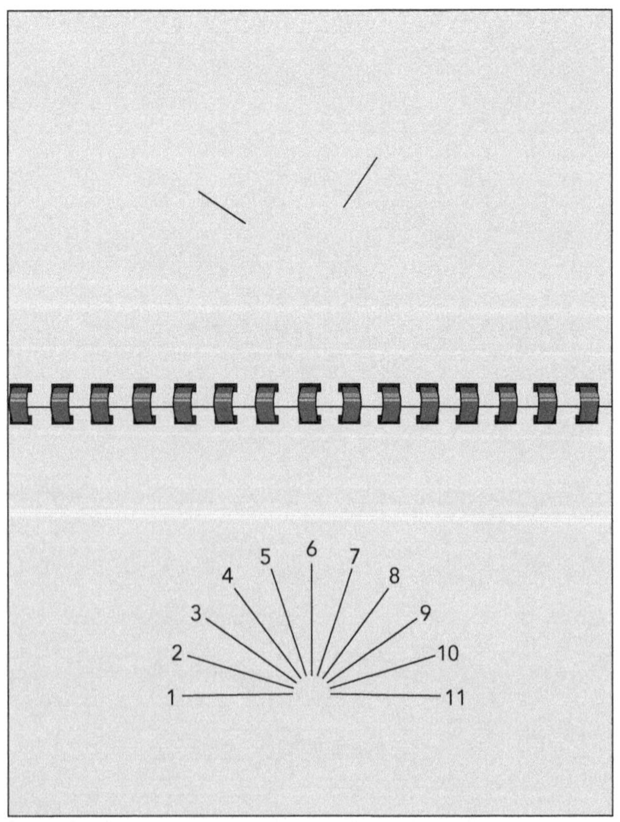

Figure 12–5 *Example of Judgment of Line Orientation (JLO) item.*

SOURCE: Reproduced by special permission of the Publisher, Psychological Assessment Resources, Inc. (PAR), 16204 North Florida Avenue, Lutz, Florida 33549, from the Judgment of Line Orientation by Arthur L. Benton, PhD. Copyright 1983 by PAR. Further reproduction is prohibited without permission of PAR.

TABLE 12–13 Items on the Judgment of Line Orientation (JLO) Short Form Based on Item Response Theory (IRT) Using Form V

NEW ITEM NUMBER	ORIGINAL FORM V ITEM NUMBER
1	4
2	11
3	3
4	6
5	5
6	16
7	9
8	2
9	12
10	17
11	10
12	13
13	7
14	30
15	8
16	19
17	20
18	14
19	15
20	1
21	21
22	22
23	18
24	23
25	26
26	28
27	25
28	29
29	27
30	24

SOURCE: From Calamia et al. (2011). Reprinted with the kind permission of Taylor & Francis Ltd. www.tandfonline.com

examinee and at a 45-degree angle to the multiple-choice array, in such a way that both are in an area of preserved vision. The examinee is instructed to look at the two lines of the stimulus card and to find "which of the lines below are in exactly the same position and point in the same direction," and "Tell me the number of the lines." If the examinee has difficulty comprehending the instructions, the examiner may proceed by asking the examinee to show the corresponding direction for just one line. Instructions and practice items may be repeated until the examinee gives two correct responses for the practice items. If this criterion is not met, the test is discontinued. There is no time limit for responding.

The 15-item short form developed by Qualls et al. (2000; Form Q) is comprised of Form V items 16, 9, 6, 2, 12, 30, 7, 17, 19, 28, 20, 21, 26, 24, and 22 administered in that order.

The Calamia et al. IRT form (Calamia et al., 2011) is administered starting from item 16 of the new item number (Table 12–13). If a basal of six consecutive correct responses is not established, the test is administered in reverse order until the basal rule is achieved. The test is discontinued once a ceiling of six consecutive incorrect responses is established.

SCORING

For the standard 30-item form and Calamia et al. (2011) short form, the score is the total number of correct responses. If the norms in the manual are used, corrections for age and gender consist of adding one point to the obtained scores of individuals in the 50- to 64-year-old age bracket, three points to the obtained scores of individuals in the 65-to 74-year-old age bracket, and an additional two points to the obtained scores of women in all age brackets.

For the 15-item O and E short forms, the score is the total number correct. One point should be added to scores of females before the score is looked up in the table for the short form (Woodard et al., 1998). Simple doubling of the score, so as to use standard long-form normative data, is not advised because such a practice can produce erroneous results (Woodard et al., 1996); rather, appropriate normative data should be used (Woodard et al., 1998).

Ska et al. (1990) introduced a qualitative scoring system that distinguishes four main error types: (a) misplacement of lines within the same quadrant (e.g., line confused with another from the same quadrant), (b) misperception of vertical and/or horizontal lines (e.g., incorrect identification of lines 1, 11, and 6), (c) displacement of a line from one quadrant to the other, and (d) displacement of a line to the opposite quadrant in combination with vertical or horizontal errors.

DEMOGRAPHIC EFFECTS

AGE

Age shows a curvilinear relationship with test scores (Benton et al., 1994). Scores increase during childhood, reaching adult levels by about age 13 years in both girls and boys. In adults, beginning at about 50 years of age, scores decline slightly with advancing age on the long form (Benton et al., 1994; Ivnik et al., 1996; Montse et al., 2001) and on the 15-item short form (Woodard et al., 1996).

GENDER

Males tend to score about two points higher than females on the long form (Basso & Lowery, 2004; Basso et al., 2000; Benton et al., 1994; Ferracuti & Ferracuti, 1992; Glamser & Turner, 1995; Riva & Benton, 1993; Spencer et al., 2013) and on the 15-item short form (Vanderploeg et al., 1997; Woodard et al., 1996). Sexual orientation has a strong effect on performance (Rahman & Wilson, 2003; Rahman et al., 2004). Although men perform better overall, there are large, significant differences between heterosexual and homosexual men in favor of the heterosexual group; the scores of heterosexual and homosexual women do not differ (Rahman & Wilson, 2003).

EDUCATION AND IQ

Benton et al. (1994) noted a trend for less well-educated individuals to score lower than the better-educated on the long form. Others (Ivnik et al., 1996; Lucas et al., 2005) have also observed a modest impact of education on test scores in older adults (r = .21 to .33). Higher scores are also associated with increasing levels of education on the 15-item short form (Woodard et al., 1996).

IQ has a moderate to large effect on performance (Rahman et al., 2004; Steinberg et al., 2005; Trahan, 1998; Woodard et al., 1996). In fact, education becomes redundant when IQ is taken into account (Steinberg et al., 2005). IQ and JLO test scores are less strongly associated at the higher ends of the IQ continuum (Steinberg et al., 2005).

ETHNICITY, NATIONALITY, AND LINGUISTIC EFFECTS

Trahan (1998) observed no score differences between Caucasian and African-American stroke patients, although the sample was very small. Similarly, there was no difference between Greek and US/UK samples (Kosmidis et al., 2010). Lucas et al. (2005), however, noted relatively poor performance in older African Americans. Rey et al. (1999) reported median scores and cutoff points for defective performance between Hispanic and English-speaking samples in the United States. The distribution for Hispanic participants (median JLO score = 24, cutoff = 17) was comparable to that reported by Benton et al. (1983) for English-speaking individuals (median JLO score = 25, cutoff = 15).

NORMATIVE DATA

STANDARDIZATION SAMPLE

The characteristics of the adult sample are shown in Table 12–14. Benton et al. (1994) noted that the test has a relatively low ceiling. In their sample of 137 "normal subjects or control patients," scores (corrected for age and gender) of 21 or higher were made by 93% of the sample. Accordingly, the authors recommended a cutoff of 19 to 20 points (after correction) as borderline.

TABLE 12–14 Judgment of Line Orientation (JLO): Characteristics of the Adult Normative Sample

Sample size	137
Age (years)	16 to 74
Geographic location	Iowa (USA)
Sample type	Healthy individuals or control patients
Education	Not reported
Gender	72 Women 65 Men
Ethnicity	Not reported
Screening	Patients with neurological disease excluded

SOURCE: Adapted from Benton et al. (1994).

OTHER NORMATIVE DATA

Glamser and Turner (1995) evaluated a sample of 167 college students (109 women, 58 men), ranging in age from 18 to 30 years, using a group-administered version of the JLO (via an overhead projector) with no time pressure. Approximately 23% of the sample were African Americans. The scores were very similar to those reported by Benton et al. (1994) for adults aged 16 to 49 years (men, M = 26.6; women, M = 23.3). However, readers are discouraged from using this set of norms because the JLO was administered in a group setting and not in the standard manner.

Ivnik et al. (1996) provide normative information for use with persons aged 55 to 97 years (see Table 12–15). Midpoint age intervals were used to maximize the information available at each age. Note that Mayo's Older Americans Normative Studies (MOANS) aged-corrected scaled scores have a mean of 10 and a standard deviation of 3. A computational formula is also provided in Table 12–15 to derive age- and education-corrected MOANS scaled scores. Although the sample size was relatively large (N = 216), it consisted almost exclusively of Caucasian older adults living in an economically stable region of the United States. Accordingly, Ivnik et al. (1996) urged caution in the use of these norms for persons of other ethnic, cultural, or socioeconomic backgrounds. Of note, scores for individuals aged 65 to 74 years appeared to be consistent with those reported by Benton et al. (1994).

Steinberg et al. (2005) expanded the utility of the MOANS project by providing age- and IQ-adjusted percentile equivalents of MOANS age-adjusted JLO scores for use with individuals aged 55+. Users should note that all FSIQs are Mayo age-adjusted scores that are based on the WAIS-R, not the WAIS-IV.

Lucas et al. (2005) provide normative data derived from African-American community-dwelling participants from the Mayo's Older African American Normative Studies (MOAANS) project in Jacksonville, Florida. Participants were predominantly female (75%), ranged in age from 56 to 94 years (mean age = 69.6, SD = 6.87), and varied in education from 0 to 20 years of formal education (mean education = 12.2, SD = 3.48). They were screened to exclude those with active neurological, psychiatric, or other conditions that might affect cognition. The authors note that more than 10% of the normative group failed the sample items, which would result in discontinuation of the test and interpretation of severe visual impairment (Benton et al., 1994). To improve the clinical utility of the JLO, they provide separate MOAANS norms for the subsample of individuals who passed the sample items and were administered the 30 test items. These data are provided in addition to norms for the entire sample (i.e., including those who received scores of zero due to failure of sample test items). Table 12–16a presents

TABLE 12–15 Judgment of Line Orientation (JLO) MOANS Norms for Persons Aged 56 to 97 Years

PERCENTILE RANGES	56–62	63–65	66–68	69–71	72–74	75–77	78–80	81–83	84–86	87–89	90–97	SCALED SCORE
N	119	119	119	119	119	119	119	127	113	82	82	
<1	–	–	–	–	–	–	–	–	–	–	–	2
1	–	–	–	–	–	–	–	–	–	–	–	3
2	0–7	0–7	0–7	0–7	0–7	0–7	–	–	–	–	–	4
3–5	8–11	8–11	8–11	8–11	8–11	8–11	0–10	0–10	0–8	–	–	5
6–10	12–14	12–14	12–14	12–14	12–14	12–14	11–13	11–13	9–12	0–9	0–9	6
11–18	15–17	15–17	15–17	15–17	15–17	15–17	14–16	14–16	13–15	10–14	10–14	7
19–28	18–19	18–19	18–19	18–19	18–19	18–19	17–18	17–18	16–17	15–16	15–16	8
29–40	20	20	20	20	20	20	19–20	19	18	17–18	17–18	9
41–59	21–22	21–22	21–22	21–22	21–22	21–22	21–22	20–21	19–21	19–21	19–21	10
60–71	23	23	23	23	23	23	–	22	22	22	22	11
72–81	24	24	24	24	24	24	23–24	23–24	23–24	23	23	12
82–89	25–26	25–26	25–26	25–26	25–26	25–26	25	–	–	24	24	13
90–94	27–28	27–28	27–28	27–28	27–28	27–28	26	25–26	25	25	25	14
95–97	29	29	29	29	29	29	27–28	27–28	26–28	26–27	26–27	15
98	30	30	30	30	30	30	29	29	29	28–29	28–29	16
99	–	–	–	–	–	–	30	30	30	30	30	17
>99	–	–	–	–	–	–	–	–	–	–	–	18

NOTE: Based on Mayo's Older Americans Normative Studies (MOANS). Age- and education-corrected MOANS Scaled Score ($MSS_{A\&E}$) is calculated from a person's age-corrected MOANS Scaled Score (MSS_A) and that person's education expressed in years of formal schooling completed, as follows: $MSS_{A\&E} = 1.54 + (1.10 \times MSS_A) - (0.23 \times \text{Education})$.

SOURCE: Adapted from Ivnik et al. (1996).

the age-scaled scores and Table 12–16b provides the computational formula used to calculate age- and education-adjusted MOAANS scaled scores. The authors urge that their data should be used with caution since the number of very old adults is relatively small, and they used a sample of convenience which may not represent the full range of cultural and educational experiences of the African-American community.

Tables 12–17 and 12–18 present normative data collected from a sample of midlife women in Australia enrolled in the Melbourne Women's Midlife Health Project, a prospective population-based longitudinal study of Australian-born women designed to assess health and lifestyle factors relative to menopausal transition and postmenopausal years (Elkadi et al., 2006). Eligibility criteria included having menstruated within the prior three months, having a uterus and at least one ovary, and not taking menopausal hormone therapy or hormonal contraceptive medication. This sample is highly educated, with 45% having more than 12 years of education, 3% having 12 years of education, and

TABLE 12–16A MOAANS Judgment of Line Orientation (JLO) Scaled Scores in African Americans: Sample Failures Included and Sample Failures Excluded, by Age

SCALED	56–62		63–65		66–68		69–71		72–74		75–77		78+		PERCENTILE
SCORES	INCL	EXCL	INCL	EXCL	INCL	EXCL	INCL	EXCL	INCL	EXCL	INCL	EXCL	INCL	EXCL	RANGES
N	108	98	130	114	166	144	181	158	157	139	119	105	79	71	
2	–	0–5	–	0–5	–	0–5	–	0–5	–	0–5	–	0–5	–	0–5	<1
3	–	–	–	–	–	–	–	–	–	–	–	–	–	–	1
4	–	6	–	6	–	6	–	6	–	6	–	6	–	6	2
5	0	7–8	–	7–8	–	7–8	–	7–8	–	7–8	–	7–8	–	–	3–5
6	1–5	9–10	0–5	9–10	0–5	9–10	0–5	9–10	0–5	9–10	0–5	9	0–1	7–9	6–10
7	6–10	11–12	6–9	11–12	6–9	11–12	6–9	11–12	6–9	11–12	6–9	10–12	2–8	10–12	11–18
8	11–13	13–14	10–12	13–14	10–12	13–14	10–12	13–14	10–12	13–14	10–12	13–14	9–11	13	19–28
9	14–15	15–16	13–15	15–16	13–15	15–16	13–15	15–16	13–15	15–16	13–14	15	12–13	14–15	29–40
10	16–18	17–18	16–18	17–18	16–18	17–18	16–17	17–18	16–17	17–18	15–17	16–17	14–16	16–17	41–59
11	19–20	19–20	19–20	19–20	19	19–20	18–19	19	18	19	18	18	17	18	60–71
12	21	21–22	21	21–22	20–21	21	20	20–21	19–20	20	19	19–20	18–19	19	72–81
13	22–24	23–24	22–23	23–24	22–23	22–23	21–22	22	21	21–22	20	21	20	20	82–89
14	25	25	24–25	25	24	24	23	23	22–23	23	21	22	21	21	90–94
15	26	26–27	–	26	25	25	24–25	24–25	24–25	24	22–23	23	22	22	95–97
16	27	28	26	27	26	26	26	26	26	25–26	24–26	24–26	23	23	98
17	28+	29	27–28	28	27–28	27–28	27–28	27–28	27–28	27	27	27	24	24–25	99
18	–	30	29+	29+	29+	29+	29+	29+	29+	28+	28+	28+	25+	26+	>99

SOURCE: Adapted from Lucas et al. (2005). Reprinted with the kind permission of Taylor & Francis Ltd. www.tandfonline.com

TABLE 12–16B Computational Formula for Age- and Education-Corrected Judgment of Line Orientation (JLO) MOAANS Scaled Scores

	K	W_1	W_2
JLO (excl. failures)	2.11	1.14	0.28
JLO (incl. failures)	1.45	1.20	0.29

NOTE: Age- and education-corrected MOAANS Scaled Scores ($MSS_{A\&E}$) can be calculated for JLO scores by using age-corrected MOAANS Scaled Scores (MSS_A) and education (expressed in years completed) in the following formula: $MSS_{A\&E} = K + (W_1 \times MSS_A) - (W_2 \times EDUC)$.

SOURCE: From Lucas et al. (2005). Reprinted with the kind permission of Taylor & Francis Ltd. www.tandfonline.com

TABLE 12–17 JLO Norms for Australian Midlife Women

	EDUCATION		
AGE	<12 YEARS	12+ YEARS	TOTAL
55 to 59 years			
M	53.35	55.54	54.49
SD	4.57	3.33	4.19
60 to 67 years			
M	52.55	54.27	53.31
SD	3.98	4.07	4.13
Total			
M	52.98	55.01	53.96
SD	4.32	3.74	4.19

NOTE: 0 point is allocated if the participant failed to get any line correct; one point for correct match of one line; and two points for correct match of two lines. Based on Australian women, N = 256; age M = 60 years, range 56–67; education not reported; estimated IQ based on NART = 116 (SD = 6.6).

SOURCE: Adapted from Elkadi et al. (2006).

TABLE 12–18 Judgment of Line Orientation (JLO) Raw Score to Scaled Score Conversion for Australian Midlife Women

	EDUCATION				
	<12 YEARS		12+ YEARS		
SCALED SCORES	55–59	60–65	55–59	60–65	SCALED SCORES
1	–	–	–	–	1
2	–	–	–	–	2
3	–	–	–	–	3
4	–	–	–	–	4
5	40–45	44–46	47–49	44–47	5
6	46–49	47–48	50–52	48–51	6
7	50–51	49	53	–	7
8	52	–	54	52	8
9	53	51	55	53–54	9
10	54	52	56–57	55	10
11	55	53–54	–	56	11
12	56	55	58	57–58	12
13	57–58	56	–	–	13
14	59	57–58	59–60	59–60	14
15	60	59	–	–	15

NOTE: Based on combination of percentile and z-score data as described by Clark et al. (2004).

SOURCE: Elkadi et al. (2006).

52% having less than 12 years of education. It is important to note that the scoring of the JLO is slightly different for this sample: 0 point is allocated if the participant failed to get any line correct, one point for correct match of one line, and two points for correct match of two lines.

Peña-Casanova et al. (2009) present normative data for a large sample of Spanish-speaking adults from nine different Spanish regions recruited as part of the NEURONORMA project (see Table 12–19). Of note, participants need not be completely medically healthy to participate in the NEURONORMA project as long as their active, chronic medical, psychiatric, neurological conditions, or physical disabilities were deemed correctly controlled or resolved and did not cause cognitive impairment. A total of 341 individuals were included in the JLO norms, with 41% males and about half with less than 10 years of education. Education-adjusted scores from age-adjusted scaled scores are presented in Tables 12–20 and 12–21, stratified by gender.

SHORT FORM NORMATIVE DATA

Woodard et al. (1998) presented norms for the two short forms (O and E) based on a sample of 131 healthy, community-living older individuals between 55 and 84 years of age (M = 65.8, SD = 6.7). The mean educational level was 14 years (SD = 2.3, range = 9–20), and the mean MMSE score was 27.5 (SD = 2.0, range = 21–30). The sample was predominantly female (87%), Caucasian (98%), and right-handed (94%). They also included a cross-validation sample of 49 similar participants between 55 and 79 years of age, predominantly Caucasian (98%), but more balanced with respect to gender (53% females). Scores lower than eight were quite rare in either sample and for either form. Based on findings from both samples, they recommended that short form scores of 10 be considered as borderline, and those of eight and nine as indicating mild deficit; for females, one point should be added to the score. The interpretation of scores for JLO short forms O and E, the frequency of individuals obtaining each score in the derivation sample, and the percentile ranges encompassed by each score are shown in Table 12–22.

EVIDENCE FOR RELIABILITY

EVIDENCE FOR INTERNAL RELIABILITY

As seen in Table 12–23, split-half reliability for the standard 30-item version is high (Benton et al., 1994; Qualls et al., 2000; Vanderploeg et al., 1997; Winegarden et al., 1998; Woodard et al., 1996).

EVIDENCE FOR TEST-RETEST RELIABILITY, MEASURING CHANGE, AND PRACTICE EFFECTS

Woodard et al. (1996) argued that Forms V and H are not really alternate forms because they use the same stimuli

TABLE 12–19 Judgment of Line Orientation (JLO) Age-Adjusted NEURONORMA Scores (NSS_A)

AGE		50 TO 56	57 TO 59	60 TO 62	63 TO 65	66 TO 68	69 TO 71	72 TO 74	75 TO 77	78 TO 80	>80
AGE RANGE FOR NORMS		50 TO 60	53 TO 63	56 TO 66	59 TO 69	62 TO 72	65 TO 75	68 TO 78	78 TO 81	74 TO 84	77 TO 90
SCALED SCORE	PERCENTILE RANGE										
2	<1	12	8	8	8	8	12	12	–	–	–
3	1	14	–	–	–	–	–	–	–	12	–
4	2	15	10	10	10	10	–	–	12	–	12
5	3–5	–	12–14	12–15	12–15	12–13	13–14	13–14	–	–	13
6	6–10	16–17	15–16	16–17	16–17	15–16	15–16	15–16	13–14	13	15
7	11–18	18–19	17–18	18	18	17–18	17–18	17	15–16	15–16	16
8	19–28	20	19	19–20	19–20	19–20	19–20	18–19	17–18	17	17
9	29–40	21–22	20–21	21	21	21	21–22	20	19–20	18–19	18–19
10	41–59	23–24	22–23	22–23	22–23	22–24	23–24	21–23	21–22	20–21	20
11	60–71	25–26	24–25	24–25	24–25	25	25	24–25	23–24	22–23	21–22
12	72–81	27	26	26–27	26–27	26–27	26	26	25–26	24	23–24
13	82–89	28	27	28	28	28	27–28	27	27	25	25
14	90–94	–	28	–	–	29	29	28–29	28	27	27
15	95–97	29	29	29	29	–	–	–	29	28	28
16	98	–	–	–	–	–	–	–	–	–	–
17	99	–	–	–	–	–	–	–	–	–	–
18	>99	30	30	30	30	30	30	30	30	30	30
Sample Size		135	131	119	103	119	125	125	100	131	40

SOURCE: Adapted from Peña-Casanova et al. (2009).

with only a subtle difference in the order of presentation. Benton et al. (1994) reported that a sample of 37 patients was given both forms of the test, with the test-retest interval ranging from six hours to 21 days. The reliability coefficient was .90 (*SEM* = 1.8 points) and there was no evidence of a systematic practice effect. Montse et al. (2001) gave Form H twice, with a 20-minute test-retest interval, to a sample of patients with PD and to controls. There were no effects of practice. Levin et al. (1991) retested healthy older adults with a 15-item version (form not specified) after a one-year interval and reported a correlation coefficient of only .59.

EVIDENCE FOR RELIABILITY OF ALTERNATE OR SHORT FORMS

Table 12–23 shows that the reliability coefficients for the short forms are lower than the full versions (Vanderploeg

TABLE 12–20 Judgment of Line Orientation (JLO) NEURONORMA Age-Adjusted Scaled Scores to Education-Adjusted Scaled Scores for Males

	EDUCATION YEARS																				
NSS_A	0	1	2	3	4	5	6	7	8	9	10	11	12	13	14	15	16	17	18	19	20
2	4	4	3	3	3	3	3	2	2	2	2	2	2	1	1	1	1	1	0	0	0
3	5	5	4	4	4	4	4	3	3	3	3	3	3	2	2	2	2	2	1	1	1
4	6	6	5	5	5	5	5	4	4	4	4	4	4	3	3	3	3	3	2	2	2
5	7	7	6	6	6	6	6	5	5	5	5	5	5	4	4	4	4	4	3	3	3
6	8	8	7	7	7	7	7	6	6	6	6	6	6	5	5	5	5	5	4	4	4
7	9	9	8	8	8	8	8	7	7	7	7	7	7	6	6	6	6	6	5	5	5
8	10	10	9	9	9	9	9	8	8	8	8	8	8	7	7	7	7	7	6	6	6
9	11	11	10	10	10	10	10	9	9	9	9	9	9	8	8	8	8	8	7	7	7
10	12	12	11	11	11	11	11	10	10	10	10	10	10	9	9	9	9	9	8	8	8
11	13	13	12	12	12	12	12	11	11	11	11	11	11	10	10	10	10	10	9	9	9
12	14	14	13	13	13	13	13	12	12	12	12	12	12	11	11	11	11	11	10	10	10
13	15	15	14	14	14	14	14	13	13	13	13	13	13	12	12	12	12	12	11	11	11
14	16	16	15	15	15	15	15	14	14	14	14	14	14	13	13	13	13	13	12	12	12
15	17	17	16	16	16	16	16	15	15	15	15	15	15	14	14	14	14	14	13	13	13
16	18	18	17	17	17	17	17	16	16	16	16	16	16	15	15	15	15	15	14	14	14
17	19	19	18	18	18	18	18	17	17	17	17	17	17	16	16	16	16	16	15	15	15
18	20	20	19	19	19	19	19	18	18	18	18	18	18	17	17	17	17	17	16	16	16

NOTES: Education adjustment applying the following formula: $NSS_{A\&E} = NSS_A - (\beta * [Education_{(years)} - 12])$, where $\beta = 0.19405$.

SOURCE: From Peña-Casanova et al. (2009).

TABLE 12–21 Judgment of Line Orientation (JLO) NEURONORMA Age-Adjusted Scaled Scores to Education-Adjusted Scaled Scores for Females

	EDUCATION YEARS																				
NSS_A	0	1	2	3	4	5	6	7	8	9	10	11	12	13	14	15	16	17	18	19	20
2	5	5	5	5	4	4	4	4	4	3	3	3	3	3	2	2	2	2	2	2	1
3	6	6	6	6	5	5	5	5	5	4	4	4	4	4	3	3	3	3	3	3	2
4	7	7	7	7	6	6	6	6	6	5	5	5	5	5	4	4	4	4	4	4	3
5	8	8	8	8	7	7	7	7	7	6	6	6	6	6	5	5	5	5	5	5	4
6	9	9	9	9	8	8	8	8	8	7	7	7	7	7	6	6	6	6	6	6	5
7	10	10	10	10	9	9	9	9	9	8	8	8	8	8	7	7	7	7	7	7	6
8	11	11	11	11	10	10	10	10	10	9	9	9	9	9	8	8	8	8	8	8	7
9	12	12	12	12	11	11	11	11	11	10	10	10	10	10	9	9	9	9	9	9	8
10	13	13	13	13	12	12	12	12	12	11	11	11	11	11	10	10	10	10	10	10	9
11	14	14	14	14	13	13	13	13	13	12	12	12	12	12	11	11	11	11	11	11	10
12	15	15	15	15	14	14	14	14	14	13	13	13	13	13	12	12	12	12	12	12	11
13	16	16	16	16	15	15	15	15	15	14	14	14	14	14	13	13	13	13	13	13	12
14	17	17	17	17	16	16	16	16	16	15	15	15	15	15	14	14	14	14	14	14	13
15	18	18	18	18	17	17	17	17	17	16	16	16	16	16	15	15	15	15	15	15	14
16	19	19	19	19	18	18	18	18	18	17	17	17	17	17	16	16	16	16	16	16	15
17	20	20	20	20	19	19	19	19	19	18	18	18	18	18	17	17	17	17	17	17	16
18	21	21	21	21	20	20	20	20	20	19	19	19	19	19	18	18	18	18	18	18	17

NOTES: Education adjustment applying the following formula: $NSS_{A\&E} = NSS_A - (\beta * [Education_{(years)} - 12])$, where $\beta = 0.19405$.

SOURCE: From Peña-Casanova et al. (2009).

et al., 1997; Winegarden et al., 1998; Woodard et al., 1996), an expected effect given the decrease in the number of items (Woodard et al., 1996). Nevertheless, most of the short forms show at least adequate reliabilities.

The correlation between the IRT short form and the full form is high (r = .96; Calamia et al., 2011). Classification differences occur in 2–3% of neurological and older adult samples when short versus long forms are contrasted using a cutoff of 21 for impairment (Calamia et al., 2011; Spencer et al., 2013). Based on a study that compared available short forms to the full JLO among young adults, older adults, and chronic kidney disease patients, the IRT form appears superior (Spencer et al., 2013; see Table 12–24).

TABLE 12–22 Judgment of Line Orientation (JLO) Normative Table for Short Forms O and E Derived from Form V

SCORE	FREQUENCY	CUMULATIVE %	INTERPRETATION
0–5	0	0	Severe deficit
6	1	1	Moderate deficit
7	2	2	Moderate deficit
8	7	8	Mild deficit
9	6	12	Mild deficit
10	9	19	Borderline
11	20	34	Normal
12	19	49	Normal
13	25	68	Normal
14	16	80	Normal
15+	26	100	Normal

NOTE: Based on Total N = 131, overall Mean = 12.3, SD = 2.3, range 6–16. One point should be added to scores of females before looking up the score on this table, producing a maximum possible score of 16.

SOURCE: From Woodard et al. (1998). Reprinted with the kind permission of Taylor & Francis Ltd. www.tandfonline.com

EVIDENCE FOR VALIDITY

RELATIONSHIPS WITH OTHER TESTS

Correlations tend to be higher with Wechsler visual-spatial subtests (Block Design r = .68; Object Assembly r = .69) compared to verbal ones (Information r = .45; Vocabulary r = .28; Trahan, 1998). Factor-analytic findings in patients with temporal lobe epilepsy (Hermann et al., 1993) and outpatient neuropsychiatric patients (Larrabee, 2000) suggest that the test loads with the Wechsler performance subtests and taps abilities somewhat separate from that of facial recognition. Global-local perceptual biases are associated with perception of visual-spatial orientation. Basso and Lowery (2004) found that scores on JLO increased with an increasing global (configural vs. local/detail) perceptual bias. In PD patients, JLO was not correlated with a Global Deterioration Scale, functional ability, or disease severity (Sabbagh et al., 2007).

The 15-item short forms (O and E) have been shown to correlate highly with one another (r = .71 to .81), producing similar mean scores and distributions (Vanderploeg et al., 1997; Woodard et al., 1996, 1998). There appears to be no effect of administration order, suggesting that these forms are useful for serial examinations. The forms also were shown to be equivalent to the full 30-item version in heterogeneous samples of patients with psychiatric or neurological disease (Vanderploeg et al., 1997; Woodard et al., 1996), geriatric populations (Woodard et al., 1998), and patients with TBI (Mount et al., 2002). That is, the short forms correlated highly (r = .90 to .95) with the long form (Mount et al., 2002; Vanderploeg et al., 1997; Winegarden et al., 1998; Woodard et al., 1996). The 15-item short form developed by Qualls et al. (2000; Form Q) correlates highly with the full test (r = .94) and agrees relatively well with the long

TABLE 12–23 Judgment of Line Orientation (JLO) Internal Consistency of Various Full Versions and Short Forms

JLO VERSION	SOURCE	SAMPLE	RELIABILITY
Form H Full	Benton et al. (1978)	General medical and neurologic patients	.84[a]
Form V Full	Benton et al. (1978)	General medical and neurologic patients	.84[a]
	Qualls et al. (2000)	Mixed neurologic patients	.90
	Vanderploeg et al. (1997)	Neurologic and psychiatric patients	.87
	Winegarden et al. (1998)	Neurologic and psychiatric patients	.84
	Woodard et al. (1996)	Neurologic and psychiatric patients	.85
	Spencer et al. (2013)	Young adults	.84
		Older adults	.81
		CKD patients	.81
Form V Odd	Mount et al. (2002)	TBI patients	.71[a]
	Vanderploeg et al. (1997)	Neurologic and psychiatric patients	.76
	Woodard et al. (1996)	Neurologic and psychiatric patients	.72
	Woodard et al. (1998)	Healthy older adults	.55[a]
	Spencer et al. (2013)	Young adults	.76
		Older adults	.68
		CKD patients	.69
Form V Even	Vanderploeg et al. (1997)	Neurologic and psychiatric patients	.77
	Woodard et al. (1996)	Neurologic and psychiatric patients	.75
	Spencer et al. (2013)	Young adults	.65
		Older adults	.65
		CKD patients	.65
Form V items 11–30	Winegarden et al. (1998)	Neurologic and psychiatric patients	.80
	Spencer et al. (2013)	Young adults	.75
		Older adults	.77
		CKD patients	.76
Form V items 1–20	Winegarden et al. (1998)	Neurologic and psychiatric patients	.75
	Spencer et al. (2013)	Young adults	.77
		Older adults	.70
		CKD patients	.75
Form V items 1–10	Winegarden et al. (1998)	Neurologic and psychiatric patients	.61
	Spencer et al. (2013)	Young adults	.74
		Older adults	.60
		CKD patients	.64
Form Q	Qualls et al. (2000)	Mixed neurologic patients	.82
	Spencer et al. (2013)	Young adults	.67
		Older adults	.65
		CKD patients	.66
Form S	Qualls et al. (2000)	Mixed neurologic patients	.81
	Spencer et al. (2013)	Young adults	.74
		Older adults	.69
		CKD patients	.72

[a] Split-half correlation; all others Cronbach's alpha. CKD, chronic kidney disease.

Form Q comprises Form V items 2, 6, 7, 9, 12, 16, 17, 19, 20, 21, 22, 24, 26, 28, 30.

Form S comprises Form V items 1, 3, 4, 5, 8, 10, 11, 13, 14, 15, 18, 23, 25, 27, 29.

form in detecting the presence of impairment (kappa = .85). However, agreement is not sufficiently high in classifying patients as normal, mild, moderate, or severely impaired. Winegarden et al. (1998) reported a correlation of $r = .97$ between the full-length JLO and a 20-item short form. Short-form scores have been equated with long-form scores (Winegarden et al., 1998), although normative data remain to be provided.

CLINICAL STUDIES

Impairment on the JLO task has been reported in a variety of conditions known to affect visual-spatial ability, including left visual neglect (Trahan, 1998), AD (Ska et al., 1990; but see Finton et al., 1998), Turner syndrome (Kesler et al., 2004), and PD (e.g., Finton et al., 1998; Levin et al., 1991; Montse et al., 2001; Sabbagh et al., 2007). Neither Form Q nor the long form discriminated between left-hemisphere and right-hemisphere stroke patients (Qualls et al., 2000). The ability of the O and E short forms to distinguish individuals with focal right-hemisphere and left-hemisphere damage remains to be evaluated.

Of note, most studies have examined the number correct. A few studies have evaluated error types. Whether patients with AD make specific types of errors is uncertain.

TABLE 12–24 Correlations Between Judgment of Line Orientation (JLO) Short and Full Forms and Misclassification Rates

	YOUNG ADULTS		OLDER ADULTS		CKD PATIENTS		TOTAL SAMPLE	
SHORT FORM	CORRELATION	MISCLASSIFICATION RATE (%)	CORRELATION	MISCLASSIFICATION RATE (%)	CORRELATION	MISCLASSIFICATION RATE (%)	CORRELATION	MISCLASSIFICATION RATE (%)
1–10	.85	*n/a*	.71	*n/a*	.79	*n/a*	.81	*n/a*
1–20	.94	*n/a*	.89	*n/a*	.94	*n/a*	.93	*n/a*
11–30[a]	.97	7.8	.97	6.4	.95	5.5	.97	6.7
Form Q	.93	9.4	.92	9.9	.91	16.4	.93	10.6
Form S	.94	8.6	.93	10.8	.92	10.9	.94	10.1
Odd[b]	.95	11.7	.93	10.3	.94	7.3	.94	10.4
Even[b]	.93	6.3	.92	7.4	.93	12.7	.936	7.8
IRT form	.98	3.1	.98	2.5	.98	3.8	.982	2.8

NOTE: CKD = chronic kidney disease; IRT = item response theory; *n/a* = not applicable.

[a] Cutoff of ≥13 as unimpaired (Winegarden et al., 1998).

[b] Score doubled before applying cutoff of ≥21 as unimpaired.

SOURCE: Spencer et al. (2013). Reprinted with the kind permission of Taylor & Francis Ltd. www.tandfonline.com

Ska et al. (1990) found that several error types (e.g., judging a line to be in one quadrant when it was in the other) tended to occur in patients with AD but not in healthy controls. By contrast, Finton et al. (1998) found no specific error that characterized patients with AD. Differences in severity of the disorder may explain these conflicting results. There is evidence that patients with PD tend to make a greater proportion of complex intraquadrant errors and horizontal line errors but fewer simple intraquadrant errors than controls, suggesting a visual-spatial deficit (Finton et al., 1998; Montse et al., 2001).

Depression can affect test scores (Kronfol et al., 1978; Culang et al., 2009), as do bipolar disorder, cognitive endophenotypes for bipolar disorder, and psychotic disorder (e.g., schizophrenia; Frantom et al., 2008; Hardoy et al., 2004; Lee & Cheung, 2005; Silver & Goodman, 2008). Older adults with late-life depression who respond to citalopram show improvements in JLO performance over nonresponders, although not significantly better than responders on placebo (Culang et al., 2009). A follow-up study of 39 patients with schizophrenia in a nonacute period found significant normalization of JLO scores, in line with scores presented in normative samples (Sweeney et al., 1991).

The JLO appears to be one of the best predictors of neurofibromatosis in adults along with the VMI and Peabody Picture Vocabulary Test—Revised (PPVT-R) in a battery of neuropsychological tests (Pavol et al., 2006). These predictors together correctly classified 75% of adults with neurofibromatosis and 84% of healthy controls.

Impact of Vision. Decreased visual acuity does not significantly affect performance (Kempen et al., 1994). The stimuli have a high degree of contrast without fine details. Blurring and loss of contrast sensitivity are expected to have little impact because information about global configuration is still available. Other types of visual disorders (e.g., macular degeneration) may well affect test performance.

Time of Day. Time of testing may affect performance in older adults. Older individuals obtain slightly lower scores when tested at their nonpreferred, rather than their preferred time of day (Paradee et al., 2005).

NEUROANATOMICAL CORRELATES AND IMAGING STUDIES

Benton's classic studies (Benton et al., 1978, 1994; Hamsher et al., 1992) demonstrated that patients with right posterior damage perform worse than those with left-hemisphere damage. Follow-up work (Trahan, 1998) has shown that patients with right-hemisphere lesions, particularly those with visual neglect, have a much higher incidence of defective performance relative to their left-sided counterparts (Trahan, 1998; but see Qualls et al., 2000). Furthermore, although impairment can occur in patients with left parietal dysfunction, right parietal damage is associated with the more severe deficit (Ng et al., 2000). These findings are corroborated by fMRI studies, which suggest a more dominant role of the right posterior hemisphere in this task (Gur et al., 2000; Ng et al., 2000, 2001), possibly leading the way and "kick-starting" the spatial processing. This may involve initial perception of lower spatial contrast frequencies, supporting global (gestalt, configural) features of the complex stimulus array before more local, detailed analysis by left-hemisphere regions (Ng et al., 2000).

Additional hypotheses regarding the specialized contributions of each hemisphere to line orientation were provided by Mehta and Newcombe (1996). The authors concluded based on their small experimental study that both the right hemisphere and the left hemisphere contribute to JLO performance, speculating that the left hemisphere contributes by "keeping track of decisions and updating decisions in more complex aspects" (p. 338). That is, in the standard JLO, it is necessary to keep simultaneous account of decisions and update decisions arising from at least three comparisons: a comparison between the target angle and its matched counterpart in the array and two further comparisons between the target angle and the two nearest alternative responses on either side of the correct angle in the array.

In another study (Tranel et al., 2009), JLO performance was most associated with right posterior parietal lesions using lesion-deficit mapping in a sample of 181 patients. According to the authors, they found evidence of the sensitivity of the JLO to right-hemisphere lesions and the importance of the right posterior structures in visuospatial processing. However, Treccani and Cubelli (2011) argued that the left-right structural asymmetry of the stimuli affects performance of patients with brain lesions. They tested patients with left-hemisphere or right-hemisphere lesions on both the original items and their mirror-reversed versions. Both groups of patients performed similarly once performance on both versions was considered, whereas differences emerged only when the versions were considered separately. These authors indicated that the standard scoring method may be impacted by attentional biases (Treccani & Cubelli, 2011).

PERFORMANCE VALIDITY

Whiteside and colleagues (2011) reviewed the JLO performance of patients from a clinical practice and university training clinic referred by physicians, attorneys, and university disability offices. The most common diagnosis was mild TBI, and other diagnoses included seizure disorders, sleep apnea, fibromyalgia, mild dementia, diabetes, MCI, PD, and anoxia as well as psychological diagnoses. Participants were divided into biased responding and unbiased responding groups based on TOMM and CVLT-II Forced Choice. The JLO had an AUC = .73 for biased responding. Table 12–25 provides the sensitivity/specificity data for various cutoff scores reflecting biased

TABLE 12–25 Classification Accuracy of the Judgment of Line Orientation (JLO)

RAW SCORE	SENSITIVITY (%)	SPECIFICITY (%)	PPP (%)	NPP (%)
11	11	98	38	91
12	11	97	29	91
13	14	97	34	91
14	20	95	31	91
15	23	95	34	92
16	23	94	30	92
17	28	92	28	92
18	31	90	26	92
19	31	87	21	92
20	40	85	23	93
21	51	81	23	94
22	60	76	22	94

NOTE: PPP, positive predictive power; NPP, negative predictive power. Base rate = 10%.
SOURCE: Whiteside et al. (2011). Reprinted with the kind permission of Taylor & Francis Ltd. www.tandfonline.com

responding (Whiteside et al., 2011). Note that the sensitivity rates are low to moderate despite high specificity.

Meyers et al. (1999) suggested that a score of 12 or less on the standard JLO is sufficiently rare in patients with moderate to severe TBI to raise the concern of noncredible performance. Iverson (2001) evaluated the utility of this cutoff in a large sample of individuals involved in head injury litigation. Patients identified as biased in their responses on two other tests (Word Memory Test [WMT], CARB) also showed poor performance on the JLO. However, the cutoff on the JLO was not sufficiently sensitive to detect exaggeration in most cases. In this sample, 88% of those who obtained suspicious scores on either the CARB or the WMT scored higher than the cutoff for suspicion on the JLO. Iverson (2001) concluded that the JLO should not be used to assess exaggeration of deficits; rather, it should be simply interpreted with caution if a patient's score falls in a range that does not make neuropsychological sense. Taken together, these studies indicate that the JLO as an embedded performance validity indicator shows modest-to-low sensitivity at appropriate specificity cutoffs of 90% or higher.

COMMENT

The JLO test has a number of advantages. It requires minimal motor skills, demands little or no verbal mediation, and appears to tap a relatively low-level skill (Collaer & Nelson, 2002). In addition, the test produces similar normative standards in North America and Europe, supporting its use in Western countries. Reliability generally appears high, and the test appears to be free of practice effects.

Note, too, that the test has a low ceiling in the healthy population, with many individuals earning perfect or near-perfect scores, thus restricting the range of performance. Therefore, a "normal" score may not reflect intact visual-spatial ability. By the same token, very low scores among older African Americans may not reflect cognitive dysfunction but rather culturally related factors such as test relevance, task familiarity, motivation/level of comfort in the test situation, and quality of educational experience (Lucas et al., 2005; Manly, 2005). The JLO also yields high specificity as an embedded performance validity indicator but users should note that the sensitivity is relatively low, suggesting that the JLO should be used as one of many indicators of performance invalidity.

It is notable that the original norms are really old and poorly described and probably should be avoided. Moreover, despite its demonstrated validity and reliability, the test can be frustrating for the older adult or severely impaired patient, who often take a considerable amount of time to make decisions about the slope of line angles. Short forms correlate highly with the long forms. However, the short forms do not categorize severity of impairment in the same way as the standard JLO (Qualls et al., 2000). In addition, information on test-retest reliability of short forms is limited, and further research is needed to determine their efficacy in detecting lateralized disturbance as well as perceptual impairments (defined by independent criteria; Qualls et al., 2000; Spencer et al., 2013). Therefore, the short forms are probably most useful for screening purposes when patient fatigue is a concern; if severity of impairment is an issue, the full form should be given. Alternatively, the Calamia et al. (2011) IRT form appears promising as a standalone measure, although interpretation guidelines are lacking (Spencer et al., 2013). Finally, users should not simply double the score and apply standard JLO normative data.

REFERENCES

Basso, M. R., Harrington, K., Matson, M., Lowery, N. (2000). Sex differences on the WMS-III: Findings concerning verbal paired associates and faces. *The Clinical Neuropsychologist, 14,* 231–245.

Basso, M. R., & Lowery, N. (2004). Global-local visual biases correspond with visual-spatial orientation. *Journal of Clinical and Experimental Neuropsychology, 26,* 24–30.

Benton, A. L., Sivan, A. B., Hamsher, K. de S., Varney, N. R., & Spreen, O. (1983). *Contributions to neuropsychological assessment.* Orlando, FL: Psychological Assessment Resources.

Benton, A. L., Sivan, A. B., Hamsher, K. de S., Varney, N. R., & Spreen, O. (1994). *Contributions to neuropsychological assessment* (2nd ed.). Orlando, FL: Psychological Assessment Resources.

Benton, A. L., Varney, N. R., & Hamsher, K. (1978). Visuospatial judgment: A clinical test. *Archives of Neurology, 35,* 364–367.

Calamia, M., Markon, K., Denburg, N. L., & Tranel, D. (2011). Developing a short form of Benton's Judgment of Line Orientation Test: An item response theory approach. *The Clinical Neuropsychologist, 25*(4), 670–684. doi:10.1080/13854046.2011.564209

Clark, M. S., Dennerstein, L., Elkadi, S., Guthrie, J. R. Bowden, S. C., & Henderson, V. W. (2004). Normative verbal and non-verbal memory test scores for Australian women aged 56–67. *Australian and New Zealand Journal of Psychiatry, 38,* 532–540.

Collaer, M. L., & Nelson, J. D. (2002). Large visuospatial sex difference in line judgment: Possible role of attentional factors. *Brain and Cognition, 49,* 1–12.

Culang, M. E., Sneed, J. R., Keilp, J. G., Rutherford, B. R., Pelton, G. H., Devanand, D. P., & Roose, S. P. (2009). Change in cognitive functioning following acute antidepressant treatment in late-life depression. *The American Journal of Geriatric Psychiatry, 17*(10), 881–888.

Elkadi, S., Clark, M. S., Dennerstein, L., Guthrie, J. R., Bowden, S. C., & Henderson, V. W. (2006). Normative visuospatial performance in Australian midlife women. *Australian Psychologist, 41*(1), 43–47.

Ferracuti, F., & Ferracuti, S. (1992). Taratura del compione italiano. In A. L. Benton, N. R. Varney, & K. Hamsher (Eds.), *Test di Guidatione di Orientamenta de Linee* (pp. 23–26). Firenze: Organizzioni Speciali.

Finton, M. J., Lucas, J. A., Graff-Radford, N. R., & Uitti, R. J. (1998). Analysis of visuospatial errors in patients with Alzheimer's disease or Parkinson's disease. *Journal of Clinical and Experimental Neuropsychology, 20,* 138–193.

Frantom, L. V., Allen, D. N., & Cross, C. L. (2008). Neurocognitive endophenotypes for bipolar disorder. *Bipolar Disorders, 10*(3), 387–399.

Glamser, F. D., & Turner, R. W. (1995). Youth sport participation and associated sex differences on a measure of spatial ability. *Perceptual and Motor Skills, 81,* 1099–1105.

Gur, R. C., Aslop, D., Glahn, D., Petty, R., Swanson, C. L., Maldjian, J. A., . . . Gur, R. E. (2000). An fMRI study of sex differences in regional activation to a verbal and a spatial task. *Brain and Language, 74,* 157–170.

Hamsher, K., Capruso, D. X., & Benton, A. L. (1992). Visual spatial judgment and right hemisphere disease. *Cortex, 23,* 493–496.

Hardoy, M. C., Carta, M. G., Catena, M., Hardoy, M. J., Cadeddu, M., Dell'Osso, L., . . . Carpiniello, B. (2004). Impairment in visual and spatial perception in schizophrenia and delusional disorders. *Psychiatry Research, 127,* 163–166.

Hermann, B. P., Seidenberg, M., Wyler, A., & Haltiner, A. (1993). Dissociation of object recognition and spatial localization abilities following temporal lobe lesions in humans. *Neuropsychology, 7,* 343–350.

Iverson, G. L. (2001). Can malingering be identified with the Judgment of Line Orientation Test? *Applied Neuropsychology, 8,* 167–173.

Ivnik, R. J., Malec, J. F., Smith, G. E., Tangalos, E. G., & Petersen, R. C. (1996). Neuropsychological tests' norms above age 55: COWAT, BNT, MAE Token, WRAT-R Reading, AMNART, Stoop, TMT, and JLO. *The Clinical Neuropsychologist, 10,* 262–278.

Kempen, J. H., Kritchevsky, M., & Feldman, S. T. (1994). Effect of visual impairment on neuropsychological test performance. *Journal of Clinical and Experimental Neuropsychology, 16,* 223–231.

Kesler, S. R., Haberecht, M. F., Menon, V., Warsofsky, I. S., Dyer-Friedman, J., Neely, E. K., & Reiss, A. L. (2004). Functional neuroanatomy of spatial orientation processing in Turner syndrome. *Cerebral Cortex, 14,* 174–180.

Kosmidis, M. H., Tsotsi, S., Karambela, O., Takou, E., & Vlahou, C. H. (2010). Cultural factors influencing performance on visuoperceptual neuropsychological tasks. *Behavioural Neurology, 23*(4), 245–247.

Kronfol, Z., Hamsher, K., Digre, K., & Waziri, R. (1978). Depression and hemispheric functions. *British Journal of Psychiatry, 132,* 560–567.

Larrabee, G. J. (2000). Association between IQ and neuropsychological test performance: Commentary on Tremont, Hoffman, Scott, and Adams (1998). *The Clinical Neuropsychologist, 14,* 139–145.

Lee, T. M. C., & Cheung, P. P. Y. (2005). The relationship between visual-perception and attention in Chinese with schizophrenia. *Schizophrenia Research, 72,* 185–193.

Levin, B. E., Llabre, M. M., Weiner, W. J., Sanchez-Ramos, J., Singer, C., & Brown, M. C. (1991). Visuospatial impairment in Parkinson's disease. *Neurology, 41,* 365–369.

Lucas, J. A., Ivnik, R. J., Smith, G. E., Ferman, T. J., Willis, F. B., Petersen, R. C., & Graff-Radford, N. R. (2005). Mayo's Older African Americans Normative Studies: Norms for Boston Naming Test, Controlled Oral Word Association, Category Fluency, Animal Naming, Token Test, WRAT-3 Reading, Trail Making Test, Stroop Test, and Judgement of Line Orientation. *The Clinical Neuropsychologist, 19,* 243–269.

Manly, J. J. (2005). Advantages and disadvantages of separate norms for African Americans. *The Clinical Neuropsychologist, 19,* 270–275.

Mehta, Z., & Newcombe, F. (1996). Dissociable contributions of the two hemispheres to judgments of line orientation. *Journal of the International Neuropsychological Society, 2,* 335–339.

Meyers, J. E., Galinsky, A. M., & Volbrecht, M. (1999). Malingering and mild brain injury: How low is low? *Applied Neuropsychology, 6,* 208–216.

Montse, A., Pere, V., Carme, J., Francesc, V., & Eduardo, T. (2001). Visuospatial deficits in Parkinson's disease assessed by Judgment of Line Orientation Test: Error analysis and practice effects. *Journal of Clinical and Experimental Neuropsychology, 23,* 592–598.

Mount, D. L., Hogg, J., & Johnstone, B. (2002). Applicability of the 15-item versions of the Judgment of Line Orientation Test for individuals with traumatic brain injury. *Brain Injury, 16,* 1051–1055.

Ng, V. W. K., Bullmore, E. T., de Zubicaray, G. I., Cooper, A., Suckling, J., & Williams, S. C. R. (2001). Identifying rate-limiting nodes in large-scale cortical networks for visuospatial processing: An illustration using fMRI. *Journal of Cognitive Neuroscience, 13,* 537–545.

Ng, V. W. K., Eslinger, P. J., Williams, S. C. R., Brammer, M. J., Bullmore, E. T., Andrew, C. M., . . . Benton, A. L. (2000). Hemispheric preference in visuospatial processing: A complementary approach with fMRI and lesion studies. *Human Brain Mapping, 10,* 80–86.

Paradee, C. V., Rapport, L. J., Hanks, R. A., & Levy, J. A. (2005). Circadian preference and cognitive functioning among rehabilitation inpatients. *The Clinical Neuropsychologist, 19,* 55–72.

Pavol, M., Hiscock, M., Massman, P., Moore, B. I., II, Foorman, B., & Meyers, C. (2006). Neuropsychological function in adults with von Recklinghausen's neurofibromatosis. *Developmental Neuropsychology, 29*(3), 509–526.

Peña-Casanova, J., Quintana-Aparicio, M., Quiñones-Úbeda, S., Aguilar, M., Molinuevo, J. L., Serradell, M., . . . Blesa, R. (2009). Spanish multicenter normative studies (NEURONORMA project): Norms for the Visual Object and Space Perception battery-abbreviated, and Judgment of Line Orientation. *Archives of Clinical Neuropsychology, 24*(4), 355–370.

Qualls, C. E., Bliwise, N. G., & Stringer, A. Y. (2000). Short forms of the Benton Judgment of Line Orientation Test: Development and psychometric properties. *Archives of Clinical Neuropsychology, 15,* 159–163.

Rahman, Q., & Wilson, G. D. (2003). Large sexual-orientation-related differences in performance on mental rotation and judgment of line orientation tasks. *Neuropsychology, 17,* 25–31.

Rahman, Q., Wilson, G. D., & Abrahams, S. (2004). Biosocial factors, sexual orientation and neurocognitive functioning. *Psychoneuroendocrinology, 29,* 867–881.

Rey, G. J., Feldman, E., Rivas-Vazquez, R., Levin, B. E., & Bentin, A. (1999). Neuropsychological test development and normative data on Hispanics. *Archives of Clinical Neuropsychology, 14,* 593–601.

Riva, D., & Benton, A. L. (1993). Visuospatial judgment: A crossnational comparison. *Cortex, 29,* 141–143.

Sabbagh, M. N., Lahti, T., Connor, D. J., Caviness, J. N., Shill, H., Vedders, L., . . . Adler, C. H. (2007). Functional ability correlates with cognitive impairment in Parkinson's disease and Alzheimer's disease. *Dementia and Geriatric Cognitive Disorders, 24*(5), 327–334.

Silver, H., & Goodman, C. (2008). Verbal as well as spatial working memory predicts visuospatial processing in male schizophrenia patients. *Schizophrenia Research, 101*(1-3), 210–217.

Ska, B., Poissant, A., & Joanette, Y. (1990). Line orientation judgment in normal elderly and subjects with dementia of the Alzheimer's type. *Journal of Clinical and Experimental Neuropsychology, 12,* 695–702.

Spencer, R. J., Wendell, C. R., Giggey, P. P., Seliger, S. L., Katzel, L. I., & Waldstein, S. R. (2013). Judgment of Line Orientation: An examination of eight short forms. *Journal of Clinical and Experimental Neuropsychology, 35*(2), 160–166.

Steinberg, B. A., Bieliauskas, L. A., Smith, G. E., Langellotti, C., & Ivnik, R. J. (2005). MAYO's Older Americans Normative Studies: Age- and IQ-adjusted norms for the Boston Naming Test, the MAE Token Test, and the Judgement of Line Orientation Test. *The Clinical Neuropsychologist, 19,* 280–328.

Sweeney, J. A., Haas, G. L., Keilp, J. G., & Long, M. (1991). Evaluation of the stability of neuropsychological functioning after acute episodes of schizophrenia: One-year followup study. *Psychiatry Research, 38,* 63–76.

Trahan, D. E. (1998). Judgment of Line Orientation in patients with unilateral cerebrovascular lesions. *Assessment, 5,* 227–235.

Tranel, D., Vianna, E., Manzel, K., Damasio, H., & Grabowski, T. (2009). Neuroanatomical correlates of the Benton Facial Recognition Test and Judgment of Line Orientation Test. *Journal of Clinical and Experimental Neuropsychology, 31*(2), 219–233.

Treccani, B., & Cubelli, R. (2011). The need for a revised version of the Benton Judgment of Line Orientation test. *Journal of Clinical and Experimental Neuropsychology, 33*(2), 249–256.

Vanderploeg, R. D., LaLone, L. V., Greblo, P., & Schinka, J. A. (1997). Odd-even short forms of the Judgment of Line Orientation Test. *Applied Neuropsychology, 4,* 244–246.

Whiteside, D., Wald, D., & Busse, M. (2011). Classification accuracy of multiple visual spatial measures in the detection of suspect effort. *The Clinical Neuropsychologist, 25*(2), 287–301.

Winegarden, B. J., Yates, B. L., Moses, J. A., Benton, A. L., & Faustman, W. O. (1998). Development of an optimally reliable short form for Judgment of Line Orientation. *The Clinical Neuropsychologist, 12,* 311–314.

Woodard, J. L., Benedict, R. H. B., Roberts, V. J., Goldstein, F. C., Kinner, K. M., Capruso, D. X., & Clark, A. N. (1996). Short-form alternatives to the Judgment of Line Orientation test. *Journal of Clinical and Experimental Neuropsychology, 18,* 898–904.

Woodard, J. L., Benedict, R. H. B., Salthouse, T. A., Toth, J. P., Zgaljardic, D. J., & Hancock, H. E. (1998). Normative data for equivalent, parallel forms of the Judgment of Line Orientation Test. *Journal of Clinical and Experimental Neuropsychology, 20,* 457–462.

13 | SENSORY FUNCTION

BELLS CANCELLATION TEST

TEST NAME	**Bells Cancellation Test**
DOMAIN	Neglect
AGE RANGE	18+ years
ADMINISTRATION TIME	5 minutes
SCORING FORMAT	Hand scored
REFERENCE	Gauthier, L., DeHaut, F., & Joanette, Y. (1989). The Bells Test: A quantitative and qualitative test for visual neglect. *International Journal of Clinical Neuropsychology, 11*, 49–54.

DESCRIPTION

The purpose of the Bells Test (Gauthier et al., 1989) is to detect visual inattention/neglect. It consists of a 21.5 × 28 cm sheet of paper on which seven lines of 35 distractor figures (e.g., bird, key, apple, mushroom, car) and five target figures (bells) are presented (see Figures 13–1 through 13–3). The target figures are arranged so that five each appear in seven equal columns on the page. The number of distractor figures in each column also remains constant.

ADMINISTRATION

The examinee is seated at a table across from the examiner with both forearms placed comfortably on the table. They are presented with a demonstration sheet that includes the target figure at the center and all distractors (see Figure 13–1). The examinee is asked to name the items as the examiner points to them. If unable to name the items because of language problems, they are asked to place cards representing each object on top of the object to ensure proper object recognition. The examiner then presents the test copy (see Figure 13–2) and provides the following instructions: "Your task consists of circling with the pencil all the bells that you can find on this sheet. Start when I say 'GO' and stop when you have circled all the bells" (adapted from Gauthier et al., 1989, pp. 49–50). There is no time limit.

If the examinee stops before all bells are circled, the examiner gives the following reminder only once: "Are you sure that all bells are now circled? Please check again." The examiner continues to check bells circled after this admonition but marks them by underlining or circling the numbers for later identification.

Care should be taken that the sheet is placed in the center of the patient's view and that they do not lean to the right or left of the sheet.

SCORING

The examiner keeps the score sheet (Figure 13–3) away from the view of the examinee and records the results by successively numbering the circling of bells by the examinee as well as the circling of other elements in the approximate location. This allows analysis of the scanning pattern of the examinee after the test is completed. The score consists of the number of bells correctly circled.

Gauthier et al. (1989) recommended scoring only the errors in the right and left sides of the visual field and scoring omissions in the center separately. For this type of scoring, the test sheet is divided lengthwise into seven sectors (three left, three right, and one center; see Figure 13–3). The total correct is 30 (omitting the center).

The Gauthier (1989) scoring system provides a binary outcome. It does not provide an index of neglect severity.

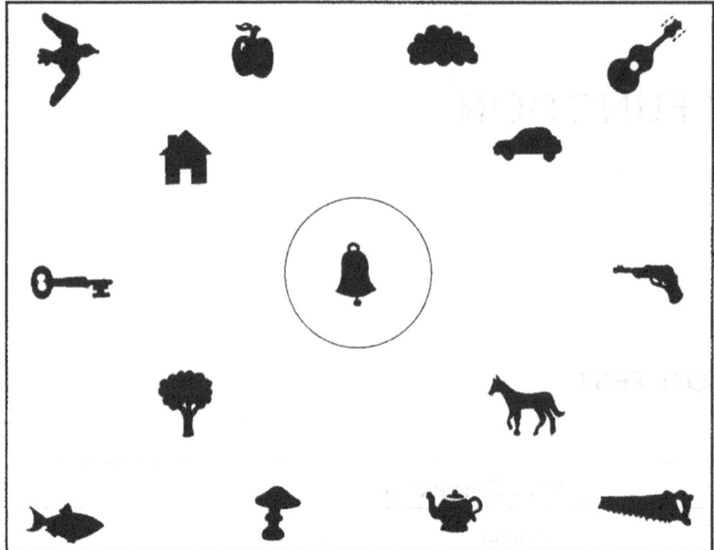

Figure 13–1 Demonstration sheet for the Bells Test, used to familiarize the examinee with the bell figure and distractor figures.
SOURCE: Gauthier et al. (1989).

Another scoring system, Center of Cancellation (CoC), has been developed by Rorden and Karnath (2010) to measure the severity of neglect by measuring the mean horizontal location of the cancelled stimuli. Free software is available for scoring ease (https://github.com/neurolabusc/Cancel). In this scoring system, a score of zero reflects unbiased spatial distribution. Scores approaching positive or negative 1 indicate left- or right-sided neglect, respectively (see the section "Clinical Studies" for details). In the original studies, high classification rate for neglect was seen with

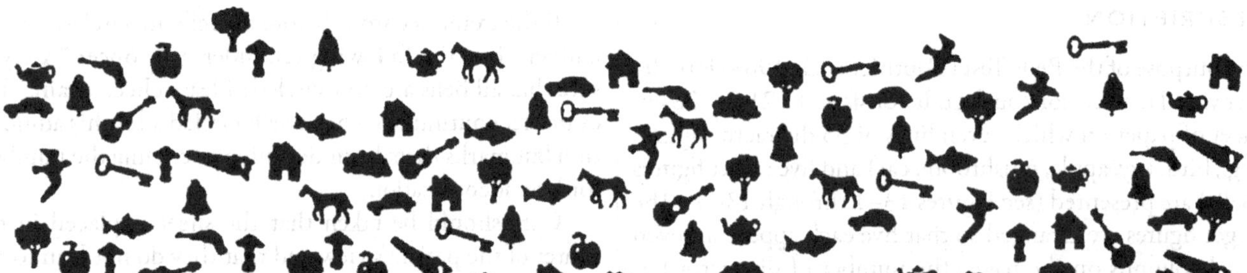

Figure 13–2 Bells Test for visual neglect.
SOURCE: Gauthier et al. (1989).

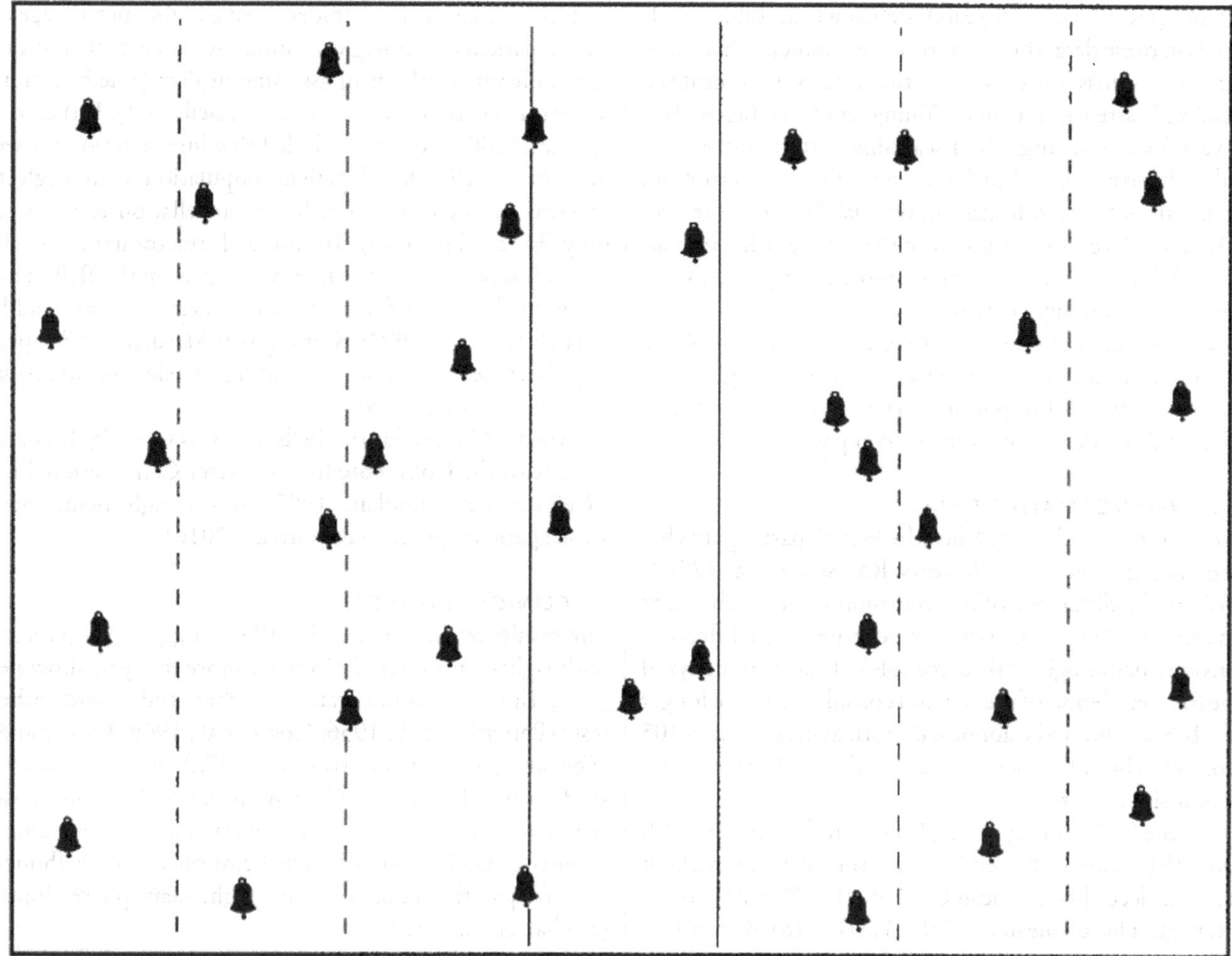

Figure 13–3 Scoring sheet for the Bells Test, indicating bells in central location and in three left and three right sectors of the visual field.
SOURCE: From Gauthier et al. (1989).

scores greater than .08 for right-hemisphere stroke and –.09 for left-hemisphere stroke (Rorden & Karnath, 2010; Suchan et al., 2012).

DEMOGRAPHIC EFFECTS

AGE

Gauthier et al. (1989) and de Oliveira et al. (2012) reported no effects of age. Rousseaux et al. (2001) noted only small increases in the incidence of omissions with advancing age.

GENDER

Gauthier et al. (1989) and Rousseaux et al. (2002) reported no significant effects of gender in adults.

EDUCATION

Education has only a small impact on scores, with increasing education linked to better performance (Rousseaux et al., 2002).

ETHNICITY, NATIONALITY, AND LINGUISTIC EFFECTS

Dawson (1997) noted that fewer adult Chinese examinees started their search with the left-top or left-middle orientation than was reported by Gauthier et al. (1989), and fewer used a systematic search pattern. The search approach may be influenced by the examinee's writing system (right-to-left) and should not be taken as pathological.

NORMATIVE DATA

STANDARDIZATION DATA

The number of errors in the three left and the three right segments of the Bells Test for older hospitalized controls (mean age = 71 years) without neurological deficit and for older right- and left-cerebrovascular accident (CVA)

TABLE 13–1 Distribution of Participants According to the Number of Omitted Bells in Each Half of Visual Space

		CVA PATIENTS	
	CONTROLS (*N* = 20)	RIGHT (*N* = 19)	LEFT (*N* = 20)
Left Omissions			
0	11	1	10
1–3	9	8	8
4–35	0	10	2
Right Omissions			
0	11	5	10
1–3	9	13	7
4–35	0	1	3

SOURCE: From Gauthier et al. (1989).

patients (mean age = 68 years) are shown in Table 13–1. Based on these data, the test authors recommend that more than three omissions on one or the other side indicates a lateralized attention deficit. Young controls (aged 18–28 years) show an organized scanning pattern, either vertical or horizontal, and make no more than two errors on either half of the test; healthy individuals between the ages of 50 and 81 years omit no more than three bells; in contrast, CVA patients tend to show a more disorganized scanning pattern and higher error scores.

The authors consider total time for completion of the test to be irrelevant to the measurement of neglect, although it may be of importance when test performance at different times during recovery are compared.

OTHER NORMATIVE DATA

Based on their study of 576 healthy French participants between the ages of 20 and 80 years, Rousseaux et al. (2002) considered a difference of one omission between the right and the left side as normal (95th percentile) and a difference of five as pathologic (5th percentile). They also analyzed time for completion of the test and considered a time longer than 183 seconds to be abnormal (normal mean time = 105 seconds). The difference between right- and left-handers was not significant.

For the CoC scoring system, Rorden and Karnath (2010) report that acute right-hemisphere stroke patients without spatial neglect obtain a mean CoC of .01 (*SD* = .03). Those with neglect have a mean CoC of .63 (*SD* = .28). By contrast, left-hemisphere stroke patients without spatial neglect obtain a mean CoC of –.003 (*SD* = 0.36). Those showing neglect have a mean CoC of –.36 (*SD* = .30; Suchan et al., 2012).

EVIDENCE FOR RELIABILITY

EVIDENCE FOR INTERNAL RELIABILITY

Not reported.

EVIDENCE FOR TEST-RETEST RELIABILITY, MEASURING CHANGE, AND PRACTICE EFFECTS

Two-week test-retest reliability is marginal (*r* = .69; Gauthier et al., 1989). However, Vanier et al. (1990) emphasize that hemineglect is a fluctuating deficit; therefore, a perfect correspondence of results between two performances on the test should not be expected.

EVIDENCE FOR INTERRATER RELIABILITY

Not reported.

EVIDENCE FOR VALIDITY

RELATIONSHIPS WITH OTHER TESTS

To establish concurrent validity, Vanier et al. (1990) compared the Bells Test with Albert's (1973) line-crossing task and found that the former identified a higher percentage of stroke patients with neglect. Similarly, in an evaluation of four different methods of assessing neglect (line bisection, letter cancellation, star cancellation, Bells Test), Ferber and Karnath (2001, 2002) concluded that line bisection missed 40% of a well-defined patient population with neglect, whereas the Bells Test and letter cancellation test missed only 6% (2/35 patients). The use of distractor items ("background noise") instead of line crossing, as in the Bells Test, tends to detect mild and moderate neglect more readily (Marsh & Kersel, 1993; Weintraub & Mesulam, 1985) perhaps because it is more demanding of selective attention (Ferber & Karnath, 2002).

The CoC score for the Bells Test was very highly correlated with the CoC score for the Letter Cancellation Task (Weintraub & Mesulam, 1985) in 110 right-hemisphere stroke patients (Rorden & Karnath, 2010).

CLINICAL STUDIES

The results by Gauthier et al. (1985) suggest that patients with right-hemisphere lesions are more likely to show neglect. This was demonstrated in other studies with other tests (Battersby et al., 1956; Costa et al., 1969; Friedland & Weinstein, 1977; Gainotti et al., 1972). A more updated study using the new CoC score, purportedly more sensitive than traditional binary classifiers, showed that similar severity of neglect occurs in left-hemisphere stroke, though less frequently, compared to right-hemisphere injury (Suchan et al., 2012).

In a study of the acute post-stroke period (both left and right ischemic and primary intracerebral hemorrhage), most patients did not miss any stimuli on the Bells Test. At a cutoff score of 3 or more bells, a quarter showed left visual inattention while 14% showed right visual inattention. Only 2% showed both left and right inattention. Bells Test score was correlated with functional independence (Barthel Index) and Mini-Mental State Examination (MMSE) scores. Better Bells Test scores are also associated with better Medical Short Form-36 Physical Component scores (Barker-Collo et al., 2010).

Azouvi et al. (2002) examined 206 consecutive patients with a right-hemisphere stroke with the Bells Test. They found an average of 8.4 omissions, with an average of 3.1 more omissions on the left compared with the right side; moreover, the starting point of the search tended to be in the fourth vector (from left to right). These three variables correlated significantly with omissions during the reading of 12 lines, writing (expanded left margin), omissions in the detection of overlapping figures, the tendency to omit figures on the left side, and, to a lesser extent, line bisection, figure copying, and clock drawing. The Bells Test variables loaded on a separate factor together with figure copying, reading, and writing. Behavioral neglect was assessed by 10 observations on grooming, dressing, eating, mouth cleaning, gaze orientation, and other activities in the Catherine Bergego scale (Bergego et al., 1995); this scale correlated with the total number of omissions ($r = .77$), with right minus left omissions ($r = .62$), and with the starting point ($r = .57$). The authors concluded that the Bells Test and the reading test were the most sensitive tests to detect neglect. They suggested a cutoff point of six omissions, two more omissions on the left side than the right side, and a starting point more to the left than sector five. Sensitivity increased up to 85% when several measures of neglect were used. Hence, normal performance on a single measure does not rule out spatial neglect in a given patient. Personal and extrapersonal neglect were found to be significantly more severe in patients with lesions located posterior to the Rolandic sulcus. However, the authors also found a small number of patients with lesions in the prefrontal region.

The CoC score yields a very good area under the curve (AUC) compared against traditional scoring methods. Classification accuracy is 98% for scores greater than .08 for neglect in right-hemisphere stroke. For left-hemisphere stroke, there is 96% classification accuracy for neglect at scores greater than -.09 (Rorden & Karnath, 2010; Suchan et al., 2012).

Tant et al. (2002) recommended the Bells Test as a screening task for measuring driving behavior in patients with hemianopia.

NEUROANATOMICAL CORRELATES AND IMAGING STUDIES

None reported.

PERFORMANCE VALIDITY

None reported.

COMMENT

The Bells Test has established itself as a sensitive measure of visual neglect, especially with the CoC score of neglect severity. It is easy to administer and is well tolerated by examinees. Because targets are embedded within numerous distractors (increasing the demands on visual selective attention), the task appears to be more useful for the detection of neglect than are line-crossing tasks. In line-crossing tasks, all given stimuli serve as targets, and the examinees do not have to segregate distractors from target stimuli (Ferber & Karnath, 2002). As a consequence, the Bells Test is more likely than simple cancellation tasks to reflect examinees' visual exploratory deficits (Ferber & Karnath, 2002). Yet it should not be used as a single method to measure visual neglect; other tests, especially behavioral inattention measures, should be used to confirm the results. It is of note that many of the studies on the Bells Test were conducted many years ago. Moreover, the CoC has not been independently validated.

REFERENCES

Albert, M. C. (1973). A simple test of visual neglect. *Neurology, 23,* 558–664.

Azouvi, P., Samuel, C., Louis-Dreyfus, A., Bernati, T., Bartolomeo, P., Beis, J. M., . . . French Collaborative Study Group on Assessment of Unilateral Neglect (GEREN/GRECO). (2002). Sensitivity of clinical and behavioral tests of spatial neglect after right hemisphere stroke. *Journal of Neurology, Neurosurgery and Psychiatry, 73,* 160–166.

Barker-Collo, S. L., Feigin, V. L., Lawes, C. M., Parag, V., & Senior, H. (2010). Attention deficits after incident stroke in the acute period: Frequency across types of attention and relationships to patient characteristics and functional outcomes. *Topics in Stroke Rehabilitation, 17*(6), 463–476.

Battersby, W. S., Bender, M. B., & Pollack, M. (1956). Unilateral spatial agnosia (inattention) in patients with cerebral lesions. *Brain, 79,* 68–93.

Bergego, C., Azouvi, P., Samuel, C., Marchal, F., Louis-Dreyfus, A., Jokic, C., et al. (1995). Validation d'une echelle d'evaluation functionelle de hemineglience dans la vie quotidienne: l'echelle CB. *Annales de Readaptation et de Medicine Physique, 38,* 183–189.

Costa, L. D., Vaughan, H. G., Horwitz, M., & Ritter, W. (1969). Patterns of behavior deficit associated with visual spatial neglect. *Cortex, 5,* 242–263.

Dawson, D. R. (1997). Visual scanning patterns in an adult Chinese population: Preliminary normative data. *Occupational Therapy Journal of Research, 17,* 264–279.

de Oliveira, C. R., Pedron, A. C., Gurgel, L. G., & Reppold, C. T. (2012). Executive functions and sustained attention: Comparison between age groups of 19–39 and 40–59 years old. *Dementia & Neuropsychologia, 6*(1).

Ferber, S., & Karnath. H. O. (2001). How to assess spatial neglect: Line bisection or cancellation tasks? *Journal of Clinical and Experimental Neuropsychology, 23,* 599–607.

Ferber, S., & Karnath, H. O. (2002). Neglect-tests im Vergleich: Welche sind geeignet? *Zeitschrift fuer Neuropsychologie, 13,* 39–44.

Friedland, R. P., & Weinstein, E. A. (1977). Hemi-inattention and hemisphere specialization: Introduction and historical review. In E. A. Weinstein & R. P. Friedland (Eds.), *Advances in neurology: Vol. 18. Hemi-inattention and hemisphere specialization* (pp. 1–31). New York: Raven Press.

Gainotti, G., Messerli, P., & Tissot, R. (1972). Qualitative analysis of unilateral spatial neglect in relation to laterality of cerebral lesions. *Journal of Neurology, Neurosurgery, and Psychiatry, 35,* 545–550.

Gauthier, L., DeHaut, F., & Joanette, Y. (1989). The Bells Test: A quantitative and qualitative test for visual neglect. *International Journal of Clinical Neuropsychology, 11,* 49–54.

Gauthier, L., Gauthier, F., & Joanette, Y. (1985). Visual neglect in left, right and bilateral Parkinsonism [Abstract]. *Journal of Clinical and Experimental Neuropsychology, 7,* 145.

Marsh, N. V., & Kersel, D. A. (1993). Screening tests for visual neglect following stroke. *Neuropsychological Rehabilitation, 3,* 245–257.

Rorden, C., & Karnath, H. O. (2010). A simple measure of neglect severity. *Neuropsychologia, 48*(9), 2758–2763.

Rousseaux, M., Beis, J. M., Pradat-Diehl, P., Martin, Y., Bartolomeo, P., Bernati, T., et al. (2001). Presentation d'une batterie de depistage de la negligence spatiale: Normes et effets de l'age, du niveau d'education, du sexe, de la main et de la lateralité. *Revue Neurologique, 157,* 1385–1400.

Suchan, J., Rorden, C., & Karnath, H. O. (2012). Neglect severity after left and right brain damage. *Neuropsychologia, 50*(6), 1136–1141.

Tant, M. L. M., Brouwer, M. L. M., Cornelissen, F. W., & Koojman, A. C. (2002). Driving and visuospatial performance in people with hemianopia. *Neuropsychological Rehabilitation, 12,* 419–437.

Vanier, M., Gauthier, L., Lambert, J., Pepin, E. P., Robillard, A., Dubouloz, C. J., et al. (1990). Evaluation of left visuospatial neglect: Norms and discrimination power of two tests. *Neuropsychology, 4,* 87–96.

Weintraub, S., & Mesulam, M. M. (1985). Mental state assessment of young and elderly adults in behavioral neurology. In M. M. Mesulam (Ed.), *Contemporary neurology series: Vol. 26. Principles of behavioral neurology* (pp. 71–123). Philadelphia: F. A. Davis.

FINGER LOCALIZATION

TEST NAME	**Finger Localization**
DOMAIN	Sensory function
AGE RANGE	16 to 65 years
ADMINISTRATION TIME	10 minutes
SCORING FORMAT	Hand scored
REFERENCE	Benton, A. L., Sivan, A. B., Hamsher, K. de S., Varney, N. R., & Spreen, O. (1994). *Contributions to neuropsychological assessment: A clinical manual* (2nd ed.). Orlando, FL: Psychological Assessment Resources.

DESCRIPTION

The Finger Localization test assesses the identification, naming, and localization of fingers. Attention to finger recognition and its pathological counterpart, finger agnosia, gained prominence after Gerstmann's (1924) and Head's (1920) descriptions. The finger agnosia described by Gerstmann involved a bilateral impairment in recognition that extended to the fingers of the examiner as well those of the examinee's hands. He interpreted the performance failure as an expression of a limited disorder of body schema. He coined the term "finger agnosia" and ascribed its occurrence to focal disease in the territory of the left angular gyrus. However, Head (1920) described unilateral impairment as a form of sensory defect resulting from parietal lobe disease (Benton et al., 1994). This form of defective finger recognition is quite different in nature from the bilateral disturbances in naming and identifying by name to which Gerstmann referred (Benton et al., 1994). Therefore, multiple tasks are required to probe for the presence of all the disabilities that have been designated by the term "finger agnosia."

Benton's 60-item test (Benton et al., 1994) consists of three parts (see Figure 13–4): Part A requires examinees to identify their fingers when touched by the examiner, B requires examinees to identify their fingers with the hand hidden from view, and C requires examinees to identify pairs of their fingers touched simultaneously with their hands hidden from view.

The mode of response is left up to the examinee. The examinee may name the fingers, point to them on an outline (see Figure 13–5), or call out their numbers.

OTHER VERSIONS

Another version of finger gnosis is included as part of the Parietal Lobe Battery (see the review of the Boston Diagnostic Aphasia Examination in Chapter 11). A shorter examination is offered by Reitan and Wolfson (1985) and Russell and Starkey (1993).

ADMINISTRATION

In all parts of the test, the examinee's hand rests on the table, palms up, fingers extended and slightly separated. In examinees with spastic hemiplegia who cannot assume this positioning, assessment of finger recognition is restricted to the unaffected hand. Instructions are provided in Figure 13–6.

SCORING

Correct responses are checked, and incorrect responses should be recorded by number. Responses on Part C are counted as correct only if both fingers are accurately identified. A total score for the whole test (maximum = 60) and separate scores for the right and left hands (30 for each) are computed.

DEMOGRAPHIC EFFECTS

AGE

Finger localization develops steadily and rapidly with age before age six and continues to develop up to age 12 years, when adult levels are reached (Benton et al., 1994; De Agostini & Dellatolas, 2001). Benton et al. (1994) found no effect of age in hospitalized individuals without evidence of brain or psychiatric disorder, aged 16 to 65 years.

GENDER

No relationship with gender has been reported (Benton et al., 1994; De Agostini & Dellatolas, 2001). However, gender effects (favoring females) and gender-by-age effects were found on a modified version (Yeudall et al., 1987).

Name ______________________ No. ______________________ Date ______________________

Age __________ Sex __________ Education __________ Handedness __________ Examiner __________

Finger Localization (Form B)*

A. Identification of Single Fingers—Hand Visible

Tips of fingers are touched in the following order (1 = thumb; 5 = little finger):

Score											
R_____	Right Hand	2____	5____	3____	1____	4____	3____	5____	2____	4____	1____
L_____	Left Hand	1____	4____	2____	5____	3____	4____	1____	3____	5____	2____

B. Identification of Single Fingers—Hand Hidden

Tips of fingers are touched in the following order:

Score											
R_____	Right Hand	5____	1____	3____	2____	4____	3____	5____	1____	4____	2____
L_____	Left Hand	2____	4____	1____	5____	3____	4____	2____	3____	1____	5____

C. Identification of Two Simultaneously Touched Fingers—Hand Hidden

Score											
R_____	Right Hand	1-4____	2-3____	2-4____	3-5____	3-4____	2-3____	2-5____	1-2____	3-4____	1-3____
L_____	Left Hand	1-3____	3-4____	1-2____	2-5____	2-3____	3-4____	3-5____	2-4____	2-3____	1-4____

Total Score_____ R Score_____ L Score_____

*Form A consists of the identical sequences of trials with the difference that the right-hand sequences are presented to the left hand and vice versa.

Figure 13–4 Finger Localization: Record form.

SOURCE: Benton et al. (1994).

EDUCATION AND IQ

Benton et al. (1994) reported that education did not influence performance.

HANDEDNESS

De Agostini and Dellatolas (2001) noted that increasing dextrality was associated with slightly higher scores on an abbreviated version of the task.

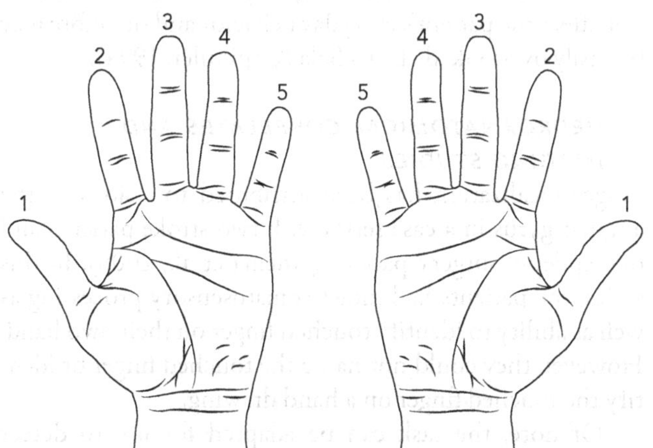

Figure 13–5 Outline drawings of the right and left hands on which the examinee identifies stimulated fingers by pointing to them or calling their number.

SOURCE: Benton et al. (1994).

Part A

Say: I am going to touch different fingers on your hand; you tell me which finger I touch. You can name the fingers, if you wish, or you can point on this card.

The fingertip should be touched firmly with the pointed end of a pencil for about 2 s. There should be no question that the patient feels the stimulation. In patients with sensory defect or disturbed attention, the stimulation may be prolonged to 3–4 s to ensure adequate reception of the stimulus. Some patients with severe sensory defect cannot be tested on the affected hand.

Part B

Say: Now put your (right, left) hand under this curtain. You won't see me touching your finger but you will feel it.

Guide the patient's hand, palm up, into the box; have patient extend and slightly separate the fingers. *Say: Tell me which finger I touch. You can name the finger or point to it on this card or call the number of the card.*

Part C

Say: Now I am going to touch two of your fingers at the same time. Tell me which fingers I touch. Again, either name the fingers or point to them on the card or call their numbers on the card.

Figure 13–6 Instructions for Finger Localization.

SOURCE: Adapted from Benton et al. (1994).

TABLE 13–2 Characteristics of the Finger Localization Standardization Sample

Sample size	104
Age	16 to 65 years
Geographic location	United States
Sample type	Hospital patients
Education	5 to 16+ years
Gender	64 Men 40 Women
Ethnicity	Not reported
Screening	No history or evidence of brain disease or psychiatric illness

NORMATIVE DATA

STANDARDIZATION SAMPLE

The standardization sample consists of 104 medical patients who had no evidence of brain disease or psychiatric illness (see Table 13–2). Errors were few, with 60% of the sample making two or fewer errors (Benton et al., 1994; see Table 13–3). When errors did occur, they tended to be made on Part C of the test (localization of simultaneously touched fingers out of view).

The distributions of scores for the right and left hands are very similar (M = 28.65 and 28.84, respectively). Differences between hands usually did not exceed one or two points; in fact, a difference score of two points or less is shown by 94% of patients (Benton et al., 1994).

EVIDENCE FOR RELIABILITY

EVIDENCE FOR INTERNAL RELIABILITY

This is not reported.

TABLE 13–3 Finger Localization: Distribution of Scores in Right and Left Hands

	RIGHT HAND		LEFT HAND		
SCORE	*N*	PERCENTILE	*N*	PERCENTILE	CLASSIFICATION
30	38	82+	45	78+	Normal
29	28	63	29	57	Normal
28	18	37	16	29	Normal
27	12	19	7	13	Normal
26	4	8	3	7	Borderline
25	2	4	2	4	Moderately defective
24	—	—	—	—	Moderately defective
23	2	2	—	—	Moderately defective
22	—	—	2	2	Moderately defective
<22	—	—	—	—	

SOURCE: From Benton et al. (1994).

EVIDENCE FOR TEST-RETEST RELIABILITY, MEASURING CHANGE, AND PRACTICE EFFECTS

This is not reported.

EVIDENCE FOR RELIABILITY OF ALTERNATE FORMS

This is not reported.

EVIDENCE FOR INTERRATER RELIABILITY

This is not reported.

EVIDENCE FOR VALIDITY

RELATIONSHIPS WITH OTHER TESTS

This is not reported.

CLINICAL STUDIES

Benton et al. (1994) noted that it is important to distinguish between bilateral and unilateral defects in finger localization. Gerstmann's bilateral "finger agnosia" and Head's unilateral impairment are different conditions, each with their own correlates and diagnostic implications. Although bilateral impairment is generally associated with both aphasic disorders and general mental impairment, the deficit may also be shown by patients who are neither aphasic nor demented (Della Sala & Spinnler, 1994; Gainotti et al., 1972; see Benton et al., 1994, for review). Relatively small lesions in the left posterior perisylvian region have been identified as the pathological basis for the deficit (Benton et al., 1994).

Gainotti and Tiacci (1973) investigated unilateral impairment and reported that contralateral impairment was more frequent in those with right- as opposed to left-hemisphere lesions. However, Benton et al. (1994) did not find this difference in their small series.

In instances of isolated finger agnosia, the deficit does not affect the patient's everyday behavior and therefore may be easily overlooked (Della Sala & Spinnler, 1994).

NEUROANATOMICAL CORRELATES AND IMAGING STUDIES

Finger localization has been attributed to lesions in the angular gyrus in a case series with two stroke patients and one epilepsy surgery patient (Anema et al., 2008). In this series, the patients had intact somatosensory processing as well as ability to identify touched finger on their own hand. However, they could not name the touched finger or identify the touched finger on a hand drawing.

Of note, the task can be adapted for use to detect callosal dysfunction, as in multiple sclerosis (Brown, 2003). Performance on finger localization tasks have also been correlated with corpus callosum volume deficits in recent-onset psychosis (Chaim et al., 2010) and schizophrenia (Rushe et al., 2007), as well as in young adults with moderate in-utero alcohol exposure, especially in the isthmus and splenium of the corpus callosum (Dodge et al., 2009). The examiner may stimulate the finger on one hand and ask the examinee to indicate the corresponding finger on the other hand. Interhemispheric transfer is implicated in crossed but not uncrossed localization because tactile information from the stimulated hand must be transferred across the corpus callosum in order for the other hand to respond.

PERFORMANCE VALIDITY

Simulators (nurses) performed well below brain-injured patients (Hayward et al., 1987). In addition, their performances included bizarre errors that were not made by patients.

COMMENT

Finger gnosis is an important aspect of various neurological disorders. It can occur as an isolated phenomenon and has also been described as one of the core features of Gerstmann's syndrome, along with right-left disorientation, dysgraphia, and dyscalculia. Benton's task recognizes that there may be different causes of finger recognition deficits. The availability of different response formats makes it unlikely that performance will be affected by even mild forms of aphasia. However, normative studies are dated and derived from samples of medical patients. Limited psychometric studies have been reported to date, especially regarding the various aspects of reliability, clinical validity, and performance validity. Regardless, this task may be useful as a bedside tool for finger agnosia.

REFERENCES

Anema, H. A., Kessels, R. P. C., de Haan, Edward H. F., Kappelle, L. J., Leijten, F. S., . . . Dijkerman, H. C. (2008). Differences in finger localisation performance of patients with finger agnosia. *NeuroReport: For Rapid Communication of Neuroscience Research, 19*(14), 1429–1433.

Benton, A. L., Sivan, A. B., Hamsher, K. de S., Varney, N. R., & Spreen, O. (1994). *Contributions to neuropsychological assessment: A clinical manual.* New York: Oxford University Press.

Brown, W. S. (2003). Clinical neuropsychological assessment of callosal dysfunction: Multiple sclerosis and dyslexia. In E. Zaidel & M. Iacoboni (Eds.), *The parallel brain: The cognitive neuroscience of the corpus callosum.* Cambridge, MA: MIT Press.

Chaim, T. M., Schaufelberger, M. S., Ferreira, L. K., Duran, F. L. S., Ayres, A. M., Scazufca, M., . . . Busatto, G. F. (2010). Volume reduction of the corpus callosum and its relationship with deficits in interhemispheric transfer of information in recent-onset psychosis. *Psychiatry Research: Neuroimaging, 184*(1), 1–9.

De Agostini, M., & Dellatoals, G. (2001). *Developmental Neuropsychology, 20,* 429–444.

Della Sala, S., & Spinnler, H. (1994). Finger agnosia: Fiction or reality. *Archives of Neurology, 51,* 448–449.

Dodge, N. C., Jacobson, J. L., Molteno, C. D., Meintjes, E. M., Bangalore, S., Diwadkar, V., . . . Jacobson, S. W. (2009). Prenatal alcohol exposure and interhemispheric transfer of tactile information: Detroit and Cape Town findings. *Alcoholism: Clinical and Experimental Research, 33*(9), 1628–1637.

Gainotti, G., Cianchetti, C., & Tiacci, C. (1972). The influence of hemispheric side of lesions on non-verbal tasks of finger localization. *Cortex, 8,* 364–381.

Gainotti, G., & Tiacci, C. (1973). The unilateral forms of finger agnosia. *Confinia Neurologica, 35,* 271–284.

Gerstmann, J. (1924). Fingeragnosie: eine umschriebene Storung der Orientierung am eigener Korper. *Wiener klinische Wochenschrift, 37,* 1010–1012.

Hayward, L., Hall, W., Hunt, M., & Zubrick, S. R. (1987). Can localized brain impairment be simulated on neuropsychological test profiles? *Australian and New Zealand Journal of Psychiatry, 21,* 87–93.

Head, H. (1920). *Studies in neurology.* London: Oxford University.

Reitan, R. M., & Wolfson, D. (1985). *The Halstead-Reitan Neuropsychological Test Battery: Theory and clinical interpretation.* Tucson, AZ: Neuropsychology Press.

Rushe, T. M., O'Neill, F. A., & Mulholland, C. (2007). Language and crossed finger localization in patients with schizophrenia. *Journal of the International Neuropsychological Society, 13*(5), 893–897.

Russell, E. W., & Starkey, R. I. (1993). *Halstead Russell Neuropsychological Evaluation System (HRNES-R).* Los Angeles: Western Psychological Services.

Yeudall, L. T., Reddon, J. R., Gill, D. M., & Stefanyk, W. O. (1987). Normative data for the Halstead-Reitan neuropsychological tests stratified by age and sex. *Journal of Clinical Psychology, 43,* 346–367.

UNIVERSITY OF PENNSYLVANIA SMELL IDENTIFICATION TEST (UPSIT)

TEST NAME	**University of Pennsylvania Smell Identification Test (UPSIT)**
DOMAIN	Olfaction
AGE RANGE	In adults, to 99 years
ADMINISTRATION TIME	Standard version: 10 to 15 minutes Brief versions: <5 minutes
SCORING FORMAT	Hand scored
REFERENCE	Doty, R. L. (1995). *The Smell Identification Test administration manual* (3rd ed.). Haddon Heights, NJ: Sensonics.

DESCRIPTION

The University of Pennsylvania Smell Identification Test (UPSIT) is the most widely used tool for measuring olfactory dysfunction. The 40-item standard version of the test (Doty, 1995) consists of a set of four envelope-sized booklets, each containing 10 "scratch and sniff" above-threshold odorants embedded on brown strips. The stimuli are released by scratching the strips with a pencil tip. Above each odorant is a multiple-choice array with four alternative responses. For example, one of the items reads: "This odor smells most like: (a) chocolate; (b) banana; (c) onion; or (d) fruit punch." The respondent marks one of the four alternatives, even if no smell sensation is perceived. The score is the number of items correctly answered. Translations are available in Arabic, Chinese, Dutch, French, German, Italian, Japanese, Portuguese, and Spanish.

According to Doty (1995), the standard version allows for detection of more extreme as well as subtle impairments. The briefer 12-item Brief Smell Identification Test (B-SIT) is useful for screening smell impairments in less than five minutes. The B-SIT was designed to include odors that are easily recognized by persons from a variety of cultures. Accordingly, it is also the version more appropriate for use outside North America. Alternatively, a Brazilian version (UPSIT-Br2; Silveira-Moriyama et al., 2010), where items unfamiliar to Brazilians are replaced, is also available. A three-item Pocket Smell Test (PST) provides for a very gross screen. Doty (1995) recommends that, if an examinee fails one or more of the three PST items, the standard UPSIT should be given to more accurately quantify the degree of loss.

ADMINISTRATION

The test was designed to be self-administered. Instructions are printed on the face page of the first of four booklets and should be read by or to the examinee before beginning the test. In order to release stimuli, it is important to emphasize to the examinee that the strip should be marked with a few strong strokes of the pencil tip across the strip's entire width (e.g., wide letter "z") and that the label should be sniffed immediately after it has been scratched to ensure that the odor has not significantly dissipated. Individuals are allowed unlimited time to respond. The test booklets should be given in chronological order. Although the test is typically administered to both nostrils, unilateral olfactory testing may be of value, such as in the detection of some types of tumors or in temporal lobe epilepsy (TLE). Normative data for such an administration are available (see the section "Normative Data"). For unirhinal UPSIT administration, one nostril is occluded using a suitably sized piece of tape (3M Company) across that nostril. Two books (20 items) are presented to each nostril, leading to two scores, each out of a possible 20.

SCORING

See the Manual. The maximum possible score is 40 on the standard UPSIT. Test scores are converted to percentiles. General interpretation of UPSIT raw scores according to the manual is shown on Table 13–4.

TABLE 13–4 Classification of University of Pennsylvania Smell Identification Test (UPSIT) Raw Scores for Age 15 Years and Older

UPSIT SCORE	CLASSIFICATION
>34 (men) >35 (women)	Normal
30–33 (men) 31–34 (women)	Mild microsmia
26–29 (men) 26–30 (women)	Moderate microsmia
19–25	Severe microsmia
≤5	Concern of malingering

DEMOGRAPHIC EFFECTS

AGE

Performance improves during childhood, with adult levels appearing at about age 15 years. Performance is generally stable through middle adulthood, with scores declining after about age 60 years on both the standard (Doty, 1995; Doty et al., 1984a, 1984b; Frank et al., 2003; Minor et al., 2004; Ship & Weiffenbach, 1993) and the B-SIT (Doty, 2001) versions. Over a three-year period, scores begin to worsen significantly by age 55 (particularly in men), reaching an estimated decrease of one UPSIT point per year in both men and women in their 80s (Ship et al., 1996). The age-related declines occur even in the absence of overt medical conditions. The age-related decline is more marked among males (Doty et al., 1984b).

TABLE 13–5 Characteristics of the 40-Item University of Pennsylvania Smell Identification Test (UPSIT) Normative Sample

Sample size	3,928
Age	5 to 85+[a] years
Geographic location	USA; region not reported
Sample type	Not reported
Education	Not reported
Gender	1,819 Men 2,109 Women
Ethnicity	Not reported
Screening	Not reported

[a] Grouped by gender and age; there are 17 five-year age bands, with 60 to 232 individuals per age band.

SOURCE: Adapted from Doty (1995).

GENDER

Females perform better than males on both the standard and brief versions (Doty, 1995, 2001; Doty et al., 1984a, 1985; Good et al., 2007; Ship & Weiffenbach, 1993; Ship et al., 1996; but see Frank et al., 2003) by as much as about two points in one study (Devanand et al., 2010). The gender effect transcends cultural differences. Gender effects have not been detected on unirhinal performance (Good et al., 2003).

EDUCATION

Education shows a small correlation with UPSIT scores ($r = .18$, Devanand et al., 2010; Good et al., 2003). Those with no secondary education identify about one odor less per nostril.

ETHNICITY, NATIONALITY, AND LINGUISTIC EFFECTS

Korean Americans outperform African and Caucasian Americans who, in turn, outperform Native Japanese on the UPSIT (Doty et al., 1985). However, once education and age are accounted for, the ethnic differences disappear (Devanand et al., 2010).

NORMATIVE DATA

STANDARD VERSION: STANDARDIZATION SAMPLE

Percentile norms are based on the administration of the UPSIT to 1,819 males and 2,109 females ranging in age from five to 85+. The description of the normative sample is sparse (see Table 13–5).

OTHER NORMATIVE DATA

Lower scores emerge when the test is given unirhinally. Good et al. (2003) provides unirhinal norms, as shown in Table 13–6. Because of the effects of education and smoking on performance (see "Clinical Studies"), Good et al. (2003) recommended adding one point to raw scores for each nostril for nonsmokers with no postsecondary education and two points for smokers with no postsecondary education before classifying performance according to these norms.

Table 13–7 presents data summarizing the distribution of internostril discrepancies (left minus right) within each age group. No correction is necessary in employing these norms. A laterality quotient was also computed to examine nostril asymmetry in order to correct for baseline effects (Left UPSIT − Right UPSIT)/(Left UPSIT + Right UPSIT). Despite a right-nostril/right-hemisphere advantage for olfactory discrimination (Good et al., 2002; Zatorre & Jones-Gotman, 1991), no lateral asymmetry was observed in unirhinal UPSIT scores.

B-SIT: STANDARDIZATION SAMPLE

The standardization sample for the B-SIT includes 198 healthy adults (83 men, mean age about 41 years; 115 women, mean age about 44 years). Mean responses on the 12 B-SIT items were compared with the mean of the 12 analogous UPSIT items. Because the means and distributions of test scores were comparable, Doty (2001) employed the UPSIT database to establish B-SIT norms. Percentile ranks are provided for males and females for each five-year age category ranging from age five to more than 84 years. In general, scores lower than 9 suggest abnormality for individuals 10 years and older.

EVIDENCE FOR RELIABILITY

EVIDENCE FOR INTERNAL RELIABILITY

According to the test author (Doty, 1995, 2001; Doty et al., 1989), split-half reliability coefficients are high for the standard version (about $r = .93$) and acceptable for the B-SIT ($r = .71$). The four booklets of the UPSIT correlate highly with one another (median $r = .92$) and with the overall UPSIT score (median $r = .85$), suggesting that they can be used, in appropriate instances, independently (Doty et al., 1989).

Using item response theory, Minor et al. (2004) found that the items of the UPSIT measured a single construct

TABLE 13–6 Descriptive Statistics for Unirhinal Performance on the University of Pennsylvania Smell Identification Test (UPSIT) by Age

	15–24		25–34		35–44		45–54		55–64		ALL EXAMINEES	
	RIGHT	LEFT	RIGHT	LEFT	RIGHT	LEFT	RIGHT	LEFT	RIGHT	LEFT	RIGHT	LEFT
Mean[a]	16.9	17.0	17.5	17.7	16.8	17.4	16.9	16.9	16.0	16.4	16.9	17.2
SEM	0.21	0.29	0.22	0.20	0.30	0.33	0.26	0.26	0.45	0.35	0.13	0.13
Median	17	18	18	18	17	18	17	17	16	17	17	18
SD	1.62	2.26	1.91	1.68	2.07	2.32	1.81	1.80	2.83	2.19	2.06	2.06
Percentiles												
5	14	13	13	15	13	12	13	14	10	12	13	13
10	15	14	15	16	13	13	15	14	11	12	14	14
25	16	16	17	17	15	16	16	16	14	16	16	16
50	17	18	18	18	17	18	17	17	16	17	17	18
75	18	19	19	19	18	19	18	18	18	18	18	19
90	19	19	19	20	19	20	19	19	19	19	19	19
95	19	19	20	20	20	20	19	20	20	19	20	20

NOTE: *N* = 270 healthy individuals, aged 15 to 64. Approximately 60% were male, 90% were right-handed, and 17% were current smokers. The mean education level was 15 years.
Adjustment formula for raw scores:

Education	Smoker	Nonsmoker
≤12 years	+2	+1
≥13 years	0	0

[a] Mean score out of a possible 20.

SOURCE: Good et al. (2003).

of olfactory ability in healthy controls and in chronically medicated outpatients with schizophrenia. Examination of item difficulty, however, revealed that the test did not incorporate enough difficult items to obtain accurate measurement in the upper range of olfactory identification. On the other hand, healthy controls showed a highly skewed distribution, supporting the test's utility in detecting odor-identification deficits in otherwise healthy populations.

EVIDENCE FOR TEST-RETEST RELIABILITY, MEASURING CHANGE, AND PRACTICE EFFECTS

For the standard version, this is reported to be high, both over short intervals of two weeks or less (r = .91 to .95; Doty, 1995; Frank et al., 2003) and for tests administered six or more months apart (r = .92; Doty, 1995). UPSIT scores are reported to decrease by 3.2 points every 10 years in older adults based on general linear modeling (McKinnon et al., 2010).

TABLE 13–7 Distribution of Internostril Discrepancy Scores with Recommended Cutoffs for the University of Pennsylvania Smell Identification Test (UPSIT) by Age

	15–24	25–34	35–44	45–54	55–64	ALL EXAMINEES
Mean (L-R)	0.03	0.23	0.63	0	0.44	0.25
SE of mean	0.30	0.23	0.32	0.30	0.39	0.13
SD	2.32	2.00	2.27	2.12	2.49	2.22
LQ[a]	−0.019	0.007	0.017	0.0001	0.0168	0.0073
L > R, 5%[b]	4	3	5	4	4	4
L > R, 10%[b]	4	3	4	3	3	3
R > L, 5%[b]	4	3	3	3	3	3
R > L, 10%[b]	3	2	2	3	3	2

[a] LQ (Laterality Quotient) = [Left UPSIT – Right UPSIT]/[Left UPSIT + Right UPSIT].

[b] Percentiles denoting impaired (5%) or borderline (10%) performance.

SOURCE: Good et al. (2003).

EVIDENCE FOR RELIABILITY OF ALTERNATE OR SHORT FORMS

For the B-SIT, test-retest reliability is adequate (r = .71) when the test is given on two test occasions separated by at least one week (Doty, 2001).

EVIDENCE FOR VALIDITY

RELATIONSHIPS BETWEEN THE UPSIT AND SHORT FORMS

The short form (B-SIT) correlates highly with the long form in patients with schizophrenia (r = .85) and in controls (r = .83; Goudsmit et al., 2004).

RELATIONSHIPS WITH OTHER TESTS

Correlations between scores on the UPSIT and detection threshold tests are in the order of .80 and higher (Doty, 1995; Doty et al., 1984b). The UPSIT also shows moderate to large correlation with other olfactory detection measures (Fortin et al., 2010; Frank et al., 2003). However, the UPSIT identified more individuals with impaired olfaction in a sample of traumatic brain injury (TBI) patients of varying severity than the Alberta Smell Test (Fortin et al., 2010). It should also be noted that UPSIT impairment (i.e., identification deficits) can occur in the context of normal detection ability (e.g., Jones-Gotman & Zatorre, 1988).

Odor identification deficits may not only indicate olfactory dysfunction but may also signify general cognitive disturbance. For example, Schmitt and colleagues (2010) reported moderate correlation between UPSIT performance and Repeatable Battery for the Assessment of Neuropsychological Status (RBANS) total scores in a healthy aging center sample of mild to moderate cognitively impaired older adults referred by physicians because of concerns about dementia. UPSIT scores were also moderately correlated with all RBANS index scores as well as with subtest scores except Digit Span (range $r = .36$ to $.64$).

Specifically, odor identification deficits appear to signify memory deficits (e.g., Devanand et al., 2010; Good et al., 2002; Gray et al., 2001; Royall et al., 2002; Stedman & Clair, 1998). Past studies found an association between UPSIT and memory test scores (e.g., Rey Auditory Verbal Learning Test [RAVLT], Benton Visual Retention Test [BVRT]) in patients with schizophrenia (Good et al., 2002) and their relatives (Compton et al., 2006). In older retirees, verbal memory impairment is associated with anosmia as defined by the UPSIT, consistent with a mesiotemporal disorder (Royall et al., 2002). Weak correlations with other temporal lobe functions such as category fluency and 15-item BNT have also been reported in older adults without dementia (Devanand et al., 2010).

A relationship between executive function and odor identification has been observed less consistently. Brewer et al. (1996) noted a relationship between UPSIT ability and performance on the modified Wisconsin Card Sorting Test (WCST) in patients with schizophrenia and controls. Others, however, have failed to find a relationship between olfactory deficits and executive dysfunction (verbal and design fluency; e.g., Good et al., 2002). Thus, odor identification may relate to certain executive processes and not others.

Given the association between olfaction and cognitive functions, Dulay and colleagues (2008) conducted a structural equation modeling analysis using a sample of older adults living in retirement communities. They found that verbal retrieval, working memory, and cognitive speed directly affected performance on the UPSIT. As such, the authors raised concerns that nonolfactory factors may inflate olfactory losses (Dulay et al., 2008).

The UPSIT relies on lexical functioning because the person must recognize and select the name of the previously smelled odor from a list—a task that requires semantic categorization (Nagy & Loveland, 2001). However, odor identification deficits do not appear to be entirely due to cognitive problems (Doty et al., 1984b; Frank et al., 2003; Kamath et al., 2013). For example, Morgan et al. (1995) investigated the impact of lexical functioning on odor identification in patients with probable AD. They showed that patients obtained poorer scores on the UPSIT than on the Picture Identification Test, a task identical to the UPSIT except that the examinee is required to match a picture instead of an odor to one of four verbal descriptors. Furthermore, the odor identification deficit in patients was evident when a picture-based odor identification task was used; that is, odor identification continued to be poor even when lexical demands were eliminated. Similarly, impairment in olfactory functioning in schizophrenia does not appear to be due to semantic processing deficits (Kamath et al., 2013).

CLINICAL STUDIES

Olfactory deficits, as measured by the UPSIT, have been found in a number of disorders. Deficits have been reported in schizophrenia (e.g., Doop et al., 2006; Good et al., 2002, 2010; Goudsmit et al., 2004; Ishizuka et al., 2010; Kohler et al., 2001; Malaspina & Coleman, 2003; Minor et al., 2004; Moberg et al., 1997; Stedman & Clair, 1998), multiple sclerosis (MS; Doty et al., 1984b, 1999), Kallman's syndrome (Doty et al., 1984b; Koenigkam-Santos et al., 2011), Parkinson's disease (PD; e.g., Bohnen et al., 2007; Doty et al., 1988, 1991, 1995; Goldstein et al., 2008; Hawkes et al., 1997; Shah et al., 2009; Silveira-Moriyama et al., 2009a, 2009b; Wenning et al., 1995), cerebellar hereditary ataxia (Fernandez-Ruiz et al., 2004), essential tremor (Louis et al., 2002; but see Busenbark et al., 1992; McKinnon et al., 2010; Quagliato et al., 2009; Shah et al., 2008), Huntington's disease (HD; Bylsma et al., 1997), Korsakoff's syndrome (Doty et al., 1984b), chronic alcohol use (Ditraglia et al., 1991), vascular dementia (Gray et al., 2001), Down's syndrome (Hemdal et al., 1993), Attention-Deficit/Hyperactivity Disorder (ADHD)-inattentive type (Gansler et al., 1998), and in individuals testing positive for human immunodeficiency virus (HIV; Brody et al., 1991; Westervelt et al., 1997).

According to the UPSIT manual, scores can separate individuals into five levels: normosmia, mild microsmia, moderate microsmia, severe microsmia, and total anosmia (see "Scoring"). However, Minor et al. (2004) evaluated healthy individuals and patients with schizophrenia using Rasch analysis and found support for only three ability levels, roughly corresponding to Doty's normosmia (normal olfactory ability), microsmia (decreased olfactory ability), and anosmia (complete inability to perceive qualitative odors).

AD/Mild Cognitive Impairment (MCI). Olfactory impairments are prominent in patients with AD (e.g., Doty et al., 1987, 1988; Gray et al., 2001; Moberg et al., 1997; Morgan et al., 1995), as might be expected given the temporal-limbic involvement in this condition. The ability to identify odors is affected early in AD, whereas the ability to detect odors is affected later (Serby et al., 1991). AD patients who have lower UPSIT scores are more likely to be rapid cognitive decliners (defined as ≥2 MMSE-point decline over the previous six months) than those who are non-rapid cognitive decliners. Lower MMSE, as well as more functional deficits and noncognitive symptoms are also observed in those who are classified as rapid olfactory progressers (UPSIT ≤15) compared to the slow olfactory progressers (UPSIT

>15). However, baseline UPSIT score does not predict progression of AD over shorter periods such as three months (Velayudhan et al., 2013).

Olfactory identification deficits are also evident in MCI. Specifically, those with amnestic MCI perform worse on the UPSIT than those with non-amnestic MCI, who in turn perform worse than those with no MCI (Devanand et al., 2010). MCI with olfactory deficits is predictive of the development of AD over a two-year interval (Devanand et al., 2000; see also Royall et al., 2002). In such individuals, olfactory loss accompanied by lack of awareness of olfactory identification deficits predicts AD independent of measures of attention, memory, and general cognitive status (e.g., modified MMSE; Devanand et al., 2000).

Impairment on the short form (B-SIT) has also been demonstrated in MCI, particularly in MCI patients with the APOE ε4 allele (Wang et al., 2002). The implication is that the decreased olfactory functioning in MCI may be a marker for the early diagnosis of AD, and the APOE genotype may be part of the basis of olfactory identification decline. In line with this proposal (and consistent with the literature for the UPSIT), there is evidence that olfactory impairment assessed on the B-SIT increases the risk of future cognitive decline in healthy older adults. B-SIT scores predict decline in verbal memory in nondemented older adults two to 4.5 years after initial testing (Graves et al., 1999; Swan & Carmelli, 2002). Those with a combination of being anosmic at testing and carrying the APOE ε4 allele appear to be at particularly high risk of cognitive decline. Healthy older adults who are anosmic at baseline and carry at least one ε4 allele have been shown to have almost five times greater risk of developing cognitive decline over two years compared with controls without these risk factors (Graves et al., 1999). The B-SIT classified people with cognitive decline better than did a global cognitive test (Graves et al., 1999).

The UPSIT has also been used as an olfactory stress test, where a nostril is tested with the first 20 items prior to intranasal administration of the anticholinergic drug atropine and the last 20 items given after the atropine administration. This is based on the idea that atropine concentrated at the olfactory bulb will exaggerate reduction in olfactory performance via compromised cholinergic pathways in incipient AD. Change in the scores has been found to correlate significantly with episodic memory and left hippocampal volume in a mixed sample of AD, Cognitive Impairment-No Dementia (CIND), and cognitively intact older adults. The atropine effect explained more variance in memory than did left hippocampal volume, suggesting that the UPSIT may be more sensitive to underlying AD pathology than structural brain imaging (Schofield et al., 2012).

PD, Parkinson-Plus Syndromes, and Essential Tremor. PD patients show severe impairment on the UPSIT and B-SIT (Bohnen et al., 2007; Double et al., 2003; Goldstein et al., 2008; Shah et al., 2009; Silveira-Moriyama et al., 2009a, 2009b). Impaired olfactory functions appear to be associated with impaired verbal and nonverbal memory but not attention/executive functions, visuoconstruction, and MMSE in PD (Postuma & Gagnon, 2010). Olfactory deficits progress with PD progression, correlating moderately with disease duration ($r = -.33$) and disease severity (UPDRS motor score; $r = -.34$; Berendse et al., 2011). With treatment, however, smell identification appears to improve along with motor symptoms. Alvarez and Grogan (2012) reported that the use of rasagiline as an adjunctive therapy for PD resulted in improved median UPSIT scores and motor symptoms at three-month follow-up in 82% of the patients (Alvarez & Grogan, 2012).

A number of studies have examined olfactory identification in Parkinson-plus syndromes with the goal of using olfactory deficits to aid in differential diagnosis. For example, multisystem atrophy (MSA) does not present with UPSIT impairments (Garland et al., 2011; Goldstein et al., 2008; Goldstein & Sewell, 2009). In one study comparing frontal-variant frontotemporal dementia (FTD) and corticobasal syndrome (CBS), almost all patients with frontal-variant FTD showed impairment on the UPSIT whereas about 70% of those with CBS showed UPSIT impairment (Pardini et al., 2009). The UPSIT performance of those with pure autonomic failures (PAF) are less consistent, with some suggesting similar performance to those with MSA (Silveira-Moriyama et al., 2009a) while others suggest impaired UPSIT scores in PAF at a level similar to PD (Garland et al., 2011; Goldstein & Sewell, 2009).

The UPSIT appears useful as a tool for differentiating essential tremor from PD. Unlike PD, essential tremor is not associated with olfactory identification deficits (McKinnon et al., 2010; Quagliato et al., 2009; Shah et al., 2008). For example, in the Sun Health Research Institute Brain and Body Donation Program, only those with clinically probable PD had olfactory deficits but not essential tremor, restless leg syndrome, or MCI (McKinnon et al., 2010).

Olfactory identification deficits have been reported in PD due to certain mutations, including leucine-rich repeat kinase G2019S (LRRK2) mutation (Saunders-Pullman et al., 2011; Silvera-Moriyama et al., 2008) and Parkin heterozygous mutation (Alcalay et al., 2011), although findings are inconsistent with regard to the severity of the smell deficits compared to idiopathic PD. One study indicated that the olfactory identification deficits in PD-manifesting LRRK2 G2019S mutation carriers appear less severe than in idiopathic PD (Saunders-Pullman et al., 2011), while another reported that LRRK2 G2019S mutation carriers who showed parkinsonism performed similarly on the UPSIT to patients with idiopathic PD (Silvera-Moriyama et al., 2008). On the other hand, early-onset PD patients who are glucocerebrosidase (GBA) mutation carriers and those who are noncarriers do not differ on their UPSIT scores even though the former have lower MMSE, verbal memory, and visuospatial skills (Alcalay et al., 2012). When LRRK2 G2019S mutation-related PD, PD without mutation, non-PD-manifesting carrier family members, and healthy controls were compared, deficits in olfactory identification in those with PD regardless of mutation status as well as in a subgroup of non–PD-manifesting mutation carriers have been reported. Interestingly, noncarriers with PD obtained worse scores than the PD-manifesting carriers. Given these findings, the subgroup of non–PD-manifesting carriers with olfactory deficits may need to be followed-up longitudinally to see if they are more likely to develop PD than those without olfaction deficits (Saunders-Pullman et al., 2011).

Bohnen and colleagues (2007) reported a diagnostic accuracy of greater than 75% for PD in each of the items banana, licorice, and dill pickle. Combining these items for a PD-specific score (UPSIT-PD3) yielded a sensitivity of 70% and a specificity of 96% for PD using a cutoff of one point or less (Bohnen et al., 2007). Tabert and colleagues (2005) reported that any incorrect response on 10 items making up the UPSIT-AD10, including menthol, clove, leather, strawberry, lilac, pineapple, smoke, soap, natural gas, and lemon identified patients with AD as well as predicted conversion from MCI to AD at two-year follow-up. However, different odorants have been identified in other studies involving PD or AD (e.g., Hawkes & Shephard, 1993), highlighting the need for further independent replication. Moreover, when both UPSIT-PD3 and UPSIT-AD10 were administered to PD patients, the tests were significantly correlated, and scores on both tests were lower for the patients than controls. These results suggest that the UPSIT-AD10 is not specific to AD (Chou & Bohnen, 2009).

Idiopathic REM Sleep Behavior Disorder. In one study, among those with idiopathic REM sleep behavior disorder (IRBD), baseline UPSIT scores were lower than in healthy controls (Iranzo et al., 2013). UPSIT scores were generally lower in patient than controls across three measurement periods (1.5, three, and four years), although the rate of change of UPSIT scores over four years did not differ between the patient and control groups (Iranzo et al., 2013). Of the patient group, three developed PD and one developed MSA but none had significant declines from baseline UPSIT at year 4. The authors indicated that the UPSIT is not useful as an outcome measure in IRBD (Iranzo et al., 2013). In another study, however, 86% of patients with IRBD who had normal olfactory functions at baseline remained disease-free (parkinsonism and/or dementia) over five years, compared to 35% with olfactory deficits at baseline (Postuma et al., 2011).

Temporal/Frontal Lobectomy. Olfactory impairment is evident in patients who have undergone unilateral temporal or frontal lobectomy, but not after a frontal lobe excision sparing the orbital cortex nor after left parietal or central area lesions (Jones-Gotman & Zatorre, 1988). The impairment is greater after frontal versus temporal lobectomy, emphasizing the importance of the orbitofrontal cortex to complex olfactory processing (Jones-Gotman & Zatorre, 1988). In nonoperated cases, patients with right-sided (but not left-sided) TLE exhibit significant impairment on the UPSIT, consistent with the notion of greater reliance of olfactory processing on right-hemisphere structures (Kohler et al., 2001).

TBI. A number of authors have reported an increased incidence of anosmia after head trauma (Callahan & Hinkebein, 2002), while others have not found a relationship between injury severity and UPSIT performance possibly because of the higher proportion of mild TBI in some samples (Fortin et al., 2010). For example, Callahan and Hinkebein (2002) gave the UPSIT to 122 adults diagnosed with TBI (49% severe, 16% moderate, 35% mild) and found that 56% exhibited impairment on the UPSIT. In addition, the risk of postinjury anosmia increased with injury severity: the more severe the injury, the more severe the olfactory deficit. Furthermore, about 40% of patients were unaware of their deficit.

In another study with 49 TBI patients of varying severity (29% severe; 18% moderate; 53% mild), 69% exhibited impaired olfaction. In this study, injury severity did not determine performance on the UPSIT once age was accounted for (Fortin et al., 2010). However, those with frontal lesions obtained worse scores on both tests than those with other lesions after controlling for age effects. Similar to the prior study, about 40–44% of participants showing impaired olfaction were unaware of their deficits.

Although some (Martzke et al., 1991; Varney, 1988) have asserted that anosmia (tested coarsely) after TBI is predictive of vocational dysfunction, Correia et al. (2001) failed to confirm the claim. Only 7% of their sample of patients with mild to moderate TBI and UPSIT scores indicative of anosmia (and nonmalingering) were vocationally dysfunctional.

On the three-item screening measure, missing even one item was associated with a 2:1 likelihood of being anosmic in a sample of individuals with TBI (Callahan & Hinkbein, 2002). However, Callahan and Hinkebein advised caution in the use of this screening measure because almost 20% of patients performing perfectly on the three-item screen scored in the anosmic range on the full UPSIT.

Psychosis and Schizophrenia. A number of studies have reported UPSIT deficits in schizophrenia (e.g., Doop et al., 2006; Good et al., 2002, 2010; Goudsmit et al., 2004; Ishizuka et al., 2010; Kohler et al., 2001; Kopala et al., 1994; Malaspina & Coleman, 2003; Minor et al., 2004; Moberg et al., 1997; Stedman & Clair, 1998), which appear to improve after three weeks of treatment with adjunctive intranasal oxytocin (Lee et al., 2013), but which are not associated with schizotypy in first-degree relatives (Compton

& Chien, 2008). Although patients with schizophrenia and bipolar disorder obtain lower scores than healthy controls, patients with schizophrenia show more deficits than those with bipolar disorder (Cumming et al., 2011).

However, not all symptoms of schizophrenia are correlated with UPSIT performance. For example, Ishizuka and colleagues (2010) found that negative symptoms, especially blunted affect, apathy, and anhedonia in schizophrenia, are associated with impaired olfactory functioning but not positive symptoms. Interestingly, patients with schizophrenia are more likely to rate the odorant as more pleasant than healthy controls, though they are more likely to show a restricted range of pleasantness ratings than healthy controls, who span the entire five-point range. Pleasantness ratings are related to affective flattening, in that those who display flat affect are more likely to rate odorants as pleasant (Doop et al., 2006).

UPSIT performance has also been used to predict treatment and functional outcome. In one study, patients with schizophrenia were assessed one year after treatment. Baseline UPSIT was similar between the remitters and nonremitters on the Positive and Negative Syndrome Scale (PANSS) positive and anxiety/depressive factor. However, baseline UPSIT was higher in those who showed remission of PANSS negative symptoms and cognitive/disorganized symptoms than in nonremitters (Good et al., 2006). About 80% who did not have olfactory deficits at baseline showed remission on PANSS negative symptoms one year post-treatment and 68% showed remission on PANSS cognitive/disorganized symptoms as compared to 56% and 33%, respectively, of those with impaired UPSIT at baseline (Good et al., 2006). Similarly, patients with first-episode psychosis who had impaired UPSIT at baseline were more likely to have worse functional outcome (as assessed by the Social and Occupational Functioning Assessment Scale and Levels of Functioning Scale) six months post-treatment than those who were normosmic at baseline in spite of similar premorbid adjustment (Good et al., 2010). These latter findings suggest that more intensive intervention may be required for those who are tested as microsmic at first diagnosis.

Olfactory deficits on the UPSIT (as well as the B-SIT) are linked to social dysfunction in schizophrenia, suggesting that they may share a common pathophysiology (Goudsmit et al., 2004). There is also evidence that deficits in grooming and hygiene (including poor body odor) observed in patients experiencing a first episode of schizophrenia are associated with an impairment in left-nostril (possibly left-hemisphere) olfactory processing (Szezko et al., 2004).

Depression. Whether olfactory performance is affected by depression is uncertain. Some find no deficits in those diagnosed with depression (e.g., Fortin et al., 2010; Kopala et al., 1994; Postolache et al., 1999). However, a negative relationship has also been reported between severity of depression and right nostril olfactory performance (Postolache et al., 1999). UPSIT scores were also weakly to moderately correlated with Beck Depression Inventory (BDI) and Beck Anxiety Inventory (BAI) scores in a sample of patients with PD (Berendse et al., 2011).

Smoking. Some studies report that smoking impairs performance (Doty et al., 1984b; Good et al., 2003; McLean et al., 2004; Minor et al., 2004), although it may have a "normalizing" effect in some patients with psychosis (McLean et al., 2004). In an epidemiologic study of older adults without dementia, UPSIT scores were not associated with history of smoking or current smoking (Devanand et al., 2010). Smoking interacts with educational status. Among individuals with no secondary education, smokers on average identify one odor less per nostril (Good et al., 2003).

Pregnancy. The effect of pregnancy on UPSIT performance appears small and inconsistent. UPSIT scores were similar among women who were pregnant, postpartum, or who had never been pregnant. Interestingly, ratings of odor pleasantness were reported as more intense and less pleasant in the first trimester than during the remainder of the pregnancy (Cameron, 2007).

NEUROANATOMICAL CORRELATES AND IMAGING STUDIES

The olfactory system is unique in that primary afferents from the olfactory bulb synapse directly on cortical processing areas within the pyriform and entorhinal cortices (Fulbright et al., 1998). The vast majority of the projections remain ipsilateral (Cinelli & Kauer, 1992; Doty & Snow, 1987). Secondary projections reach orbital frontal regions either directly or indirectly through the mediodorsal nucleus of the thalamus (Qureshy et al., 2000). Other brain regions associated with olfactory processing include the anterior cingulate (Qureshy et al., 2000), the insula (Delmaire et al., 2013; Zatorre et al., 1992), the amygdala (Segura et al., 2013; Zald & Pardo, 1997), the cuneus (Royet et al., 1999), and possibly the cerebellum (Dade et al., 1998; Yousem et al., 1997). It should be noted that olfactory projections are not completely unilateral: smell information arriving at one hemisphere crosses to the other via the anterior commissure, the corpus callosum, and possibly the hippocampal commissure (Postolache et al., 1999).

Studies using diffusion tensor magnetic resonance imaging (MRI) and functional MRI (fMRI) have demonstrated the relationship between UPSIT performance and specific areas in various conditions. For example, in nondemented older volunteers, associations with fractional anisotropy and mean diffusivity in the splenium of the corpus callosum and superior longitudinal fasciculi have been reported (Segura et al., 2013). In patients with HD, significant correlations are reported between UPSIT scores and diffusion tensor MRI mean diffusivity in the parietal, medial temporal lobes, cingulum, insula, anterior putamen, and caudate nucleus, as well as fractional anisotropy in the insula and external capsule (Delmaire et al., 2013). In PD, UPSIT scores are correlated to striatal dopamine transporter single-proton emission computed tomography (DAT-SPECT) binding (Berendse et al., 2011) but not to cerebral DAT binding (Chou et al., 2009). Given the identification component of the UPSIT, fMRI studies also show that blood oxygen level-dependent (BOLD) signals in the hippocampus are moderately correlated with UPSIT scores (Wang et al., 2010) and are generally weaker in AD than in healthy controls (Wang et al., 2010). A weak correlation with hippocampal volume has also been reported for older adults without dementia (Devanand et al., 2010).

Finally, UPSIT scores are highly correlated with MRI-identified presence of bulb aplasia in Kallman's syndrome, an idiopathic hypogonadotropic hypogonadism combined with complete or incomplete olfaction disturbance (Koenigkam-Santos et al., 2011), as well as right olfactory bulb volume in chronic schizophrenia (Nguyen et al., 2011).

PERFORMANCE VALIDITY

Doty et al. (1984b) asked 158 healthy individuals to feign total anosmia on the UPSIT. The modal number correct was zero. Because one fourth of the items should be correctly identified on the basis of chance alone, an anosmic should score on average 10/40 on the test. Therefore, based on simple probability, the chance of an anosmic obtaining a score of 5 or less is .05. Based on the interpretation suggested in the manual (see Table 13–4), those who successfully malingered correctly identified between six and 18 odors (anosmic range). Individuals who identified more than 18 odors were likely unsuccessful in their malingering attempt to feign deficits; those who obtained less than six odors correct were thus probable malingerers (Doty, 1995). Doty et al. (1998) suggested that the density of marking of the sandpaper may also prove useful in detecting malingerers. This proposal remains to be evaluated.

Coaching affects an individual's ability to feign deficits on the UPSIT. Bailie and colleagues (Bailie et al., 2008) provided undergraduates with varying degrees of coaching (Naïve, Informed, Coached) to feign olfactory deficits on the UPSIT and Smell Magnitude Test (SMT), a measure of sniff suppression to odor. They found that the coached group was more successful than the naïve group in feigning deficits on the UPSIT, but not on the SMT. The majority (55%) of the participants were not successful at feigning on the SMT because they performed in the normal range, while 23% were identified as probable feigners on the SMT (i.e., ratios >1.26). On the other hand, 62% of the participants successfully feigned on the UPSIT, but a slightly higher proportion (37%) than on the SMT was identified as probable feigners based on published criteria (i.e., score of less than six correct). As such, the authors suggested that a combination of UPSIT and SMT may be helpful to detect attempts to fake olfactory deficits.

COMMENT

The UPSIT is a widely used tool for the assessment of olfactory function. It is portable, rapid, and easy to administer and to score, and it can be used with a wide spectrum of patients. The reagents are relatively stable, and, as a result, the test booklets have a reasonably long shelf-life. Doty (1995) recommended that test booklets more than two years old not be used in order to ensure that test validity is maintained. An additional feature of the UPSIT is that it provides a gross index of suspect performance. Furthermore, the normative sample is large, although the description of the sample is sparse. Unirhinal normative data also exist (e.g., Good et al., 2003), allowing assessment of lateralized dysfunction.

Reliability is high for the standard version and adequate for the B-SIT. The UPSIT correlates well with other measures of olfactory function and appears to be useful in identifying impairments in a variety of populations, including schizophrenia. In neurodegenerative disorders such as PD and AD, research suggests early and significant olfactory dysfunction. It has utility as a tool to aid in the differential diagnosis of PD, MSA, and essential tremor (McKinnon et al., 2010; Quagliato et al., 2009; Shah et al., 2008) and as a marker of disease progression (Berendse et al., 2011). Importantly, disturbance is not strongly related to education and is not observed consistently in patients with depression. However, ceiling effects are present, limiting the capacity of the UPSIT to distinguish average from superior olfactory ability. In addition, the test may only be able to separate individuals into three ability levels (normal, decreased, complete inability to identify smells), rather than the five suggested by Doty (1995).

The test also has predictive validity, at least in older adults. Low scores may herald cognitive decline in otherwise healthy individuals, and those with MCI and olfactory deficits are at a higher risk of developing AD than MCI without olfactory deficits. Furthermore, the test may be more useful than measures of global cognition to predict impending cognitive decline (e.g., Graves et al., 1999). However, anosmia in association with head injury does not appear to be a bleak prognostic indicator for vocational adjustment (Correia et al., 2001).

It should be noted that disturbances can occur as a result of numerous causes, including upper respiratory tract infections, degenerative disorders, and neuropathological processes. Therefore, its utility in distinguishing among conditions is somewhat limited. In combination with other tests (e.g., APOE genotyping, neuropsychological assessment), however, specificity may be enhanced.

Clinicians are also advised to consider the possible contribution of peripheral olfactory functioning when olfactory deficits emerge.

The sensitivity and reliability of the 12-item B-SIT are lower than those of the standard UPSIT. In addition, missing data on the B-SIT have more of an impact than on the UPSIT because of the UPSIT's greater range of possible scores (Graves et al., 1999). The three-item screen provides a gross indication of olfactory ability; missing even one item on this test is suggestive of abnormality. However, caution is advised because many patients perform normally on the screen yet poorly on the complete test. Accordingly, the full or B-SIT version is recommended.

The task does make cognitive and linguistic demands. Similarly, cognitive dysfunction in patient populations can affect UPSIT performance. Cultural factors also play a role due to the lack of familiarity with some of items. The UPSIT has been translated into several languages, and it and the B-SIT appear very promising in this context.

REFERENCES

Alcalay, R. N., Caccappolo, E., Mejia-Santana, H., Tang, M. -, Rosado, L., Reilly, M. O., . . . Marder, K. (2012). Cognitive performance of GBA mutation carriers with early onset PD: The CORE-PD study. *Neurology, 78*(18), 1434–1440.

Alcalay, R. N., Siderowf, A., Ottman, R., Caccappolo, E., Mejia-Santana, H., Tang, M. -, . . . Marder, K. (2011). Olfaction in parkin heterozygotes and compound heterozygotes: The CORE-PD study. *Neurology, 76*(4), 319–326.

Alvarez, M. V., & Grogan, P. M. (2012). Hyposmia in Parkinson's disease. *Psychiatry and Clinical Neurosciences, 66*(4), 370–370.

Bailie, J. M., Rybalsky, K. A., Griffith, N. M., Horning, S. M., Gesteland, R. C., & Frank, R. A. (2008). The susceptibility of olfactory measures to malingering. *Chemosensory Perception, 1*(3), 168–173.

Berendse, H. W., Roos, D. S., Raijmakers, P., & Doty, R. L. (2011). Motor and non-motor correlates of olfactory dysfunction in Parkinson's disease. *Journal of the Neurological Sciences, 310*(1-2), 21–24.

Bohnen, N. I., Gedela, S., Kuwabara, H., Constantine, G. M., Mathis, C. A., Studenski, S. A., & Moore, R. Y. (2007). Selective hyposmia and nigrostriatal dopaminergic denervation in Parkinson's disease. *Journal of Neurology, 254*(1), 84–90.

Brewer, W. J., Edwards, J., Anderson, V., Robinson, T., & Pantelis, C. (1996). Neuropsychological, olfactory, and hygiene deficits in men with negative symptom schizophrenia. *Biological Psychiatry, 40,* 1021–1031.

Brody, D., Serby, M., Etienne, N., & Kalkstein, D. (1991). Olfactory identification deficits in HIV infection. *American Journal of Psychiatry, 148,* 248–250.

Busenbark, K. L., Huber, S. J., Greer, G., Pahwa, R., & Koller, W. C. (1992). Olfactory function in essential tremor. *Neurology, 42,* 1631–1632.

Bylsma, F. W., Moberg, P. J., Doty, R. L., & Brandt, J. (1997). Odor identification in Huntington's disease patients and asymptomatic gene carriers. *Journal of Neuropsychiatry and Clinical Neurosciences, 9,* 598–600.

Callahan, C. D., & Hinkebein, J. H. (2002). Assessment of anosmia after traumatic brain injury: Performance characteristics of the University of Pennsylvania Smell Identification Test. *Journal of Head Trauma Rehabilitation, 17,* 251–256.

Cameron, E. L. (2007). Measures of human olfactory perception during pregnancy. *Chemical Senses, 32*(8), 775–782.

Chou, K. L., & Bohnen, N. I. (2009). Performance on an Alzheimer-selective odor identification test in patients with Parkinson's disease and its relationship with cerebral dopamine transporter activity. *Parkinsonism & Related Disorders, 15*(9), 640–643.

Cinelli, A. R., & Kauer, J. S. (1992). Voltage-sensitive dyes and functional activity in the olfactory pathway. *Annual Review of Neuroscience, 15,* 321–351.

Compton, M. T., & Chien, V. H. (2008). No association between psychometrically determined schizotypy and olfactory identification ability in first-degree relatives of patients with schizophrenia and non-psychiatric controls. *Schizophrenia Research, 100*(1-3), 216–223.

Compton, M. T., Mack, L. M., Esterberg, M. L., Bercu, Z., Kryda, A. D., Quintero, L., . . . Walker, E. F. (2006). Associations between olfactory identification and verbal memory in patients with schizophrenia, first-degree relatives, and non-psychiatric controls. *Schizophrenia Research, 86*(1-3), 154–166.

Correia, S., Faust, D., & Doty, R. L. (2001). A re-examination of the rate of vocational dysfunction among patients with anosmia and mild to moderate closed head injury. *Archives of Clinical Neuropsychology, 16,* 477–488.

Cumming, A. G., Matthews, N. L., & Park, S. (2011). Olfactory identification and preference in bipolar disorder and schizophrenia. *European Archives of Psychiatry and Clinical Neuroscience, 261*(4), 251–259.

Dade, L., Jones-Gotman, M., Zatorre, R., & Evans, A. (1998). Human brain function during odor encoding and recognition. *Annals of the New York Academy of Sciences, 855,* 572–574.

Delmaire, C., Dumas, E. M., Sharman, M. A., den Bogaard, Simon J. A., Valabregue, R., Jauffret, C., . . . Lehéricy, S. (2013). The structural correlates of functional deficits in early Huntington's disease. *Human Brain Mapping, 34*(9), 2141–2153.

Devanand, D. P., Michaels-Marsten, K. S., Liu, X., Pelton, G. H., Padilla, M., Marder, K., . . . Brook, J. S. (2000). Olfactory deficits in patients with mild cognitive impairment predict Alzheimer's disease at follow-up. *American Journal of Psychiatry, 157,* 1399–1405.

Devanand, D. P., Tabert, M. H., Cuasay, K., Manly, J. J., Schupf, N., Brickman, A. M., . . . Mayeux, R. (2010). Olfactory identification deficits and MCI in a multi-ethnic elderly community sample. *Neurobiology of Aging, 31*(9), 1593–1600.

Ditraglia, G. M., Press, D. S., Butters, N., Jernigan, T. L., et al. (1991). Assessment of olfactory deficits in detoxified alcoholics. *Alcohol, 8,* 109–115.

Doop, M. L., & Park, S. (2006). On knowing and judging smells: Identification and hedonic judgment of odors in schizophrenia. *Schizophrenia Research, 81*(2-3), 317–319.

Doty, R. L. (1995). *The Smell Identification Test Administration Manual* (3rd ed.). Haddon Heights, NJ: Sensonics.

Doty, R. L. (2001). *The Brief Smell Identification Test Administration Manual.* Haddon Heights, NJ: Sensonics.

Doty, R. L., Applebaum, S., Zusho, H., & Settle, G. (1985). Sex differences in odor identification ability: A cross-cultural analysis. *Neuropsychologia, 23,* 667–672.

Doty, R. L., Bromley, S. M., & Stern, M. B. (1995). Olfactory testing as an aid in the diagnosis of Parkinson's disease: Development of optimal discrimination criteria. *Neurodegeneration, 4,* 93–97.

Doty, R. L., Deems, D. A., & Stellar, S. (1988). Olfactory dysfunction in parkinsonism: A general deficit unrelated to neurologic signs, disease state, or disease duration. *Neurology, 38,* 1237–1244.

Doty, R. L., Frye, R. E., & Agrawal, U. (1989). Internal consistency reliability of the fractionated and whole University of Pennsylvania Smell Identification Test. *Perception and Psychophysics, 45,* 381–384.

Doty, R. L., Genow, A., & Hummel, T. (1998). Scratch density differentiates microsmic from normosmic and anosmic subjects on the University of Pennsylvania Smell Identification Test. *Perceptual and Motor Skills, 86,* 211–216.

Doty, R. L., Li, C., Mannon, L. J., & Yousem, D. M. (1999). Olfactory dysfunction in multiple sclerosis: Relation to longitudinal changes in plaque numbers in central olfactory structures. *Neurology, 53,* 880–882.

Doty, R. L., Perl, D. P., Steele, J. C., Chen, K. M., Pierce, J. D., Reyes, P., & Kurland, L. T. (1991). Odor identification deficit of the parkinsonism-dementia complex of Guam: Equivalence to that of Alzheimer's and idiopathic Parkinson's disease. *Neurology, 41*(Suppl. 2), 77–80.

Doty, R. L., Reyes, P. F., & Gregor, T. P. (1987). Presence of both odor identification and detection deficits in Alzheimer's disease. *Brain Research Bulletin, 18,* 597–600.

Doty, R. L., Shaman, P., Applebaum, S. L., Giberson, R., Siksorski, L., & Rosenberg, L. (1984a). Smell identification ability: Changes with age. *Science, 226,* 1441–1443.

Doty, R. L., Shaman, P., & Dann, M. (1984b). Development of the University of Pennsylvania Smell Identification Test: A standardized microencapsulated test of olfactory function. *Physiology and Behavior, 32,* 489–502.

Doty, R. L., & Snow, J. B. (1987). Olfaction. In J. Goldman, *The principles and practice of rhinology* (pp. 761–785). New York: Wiley.

Double, K. L., Rowe, D. B., Hayes, M., Chan, D. K., Blackie, J., Corbett, A., . . . Halliday, G. M. (2003). Identifying the pattern of olfactory deficits in Parkinson disease using the Brief Smell Identification Test. *Archives of Neurology, 60,* 545–549.

Dulay, M. F., Gesteland, R. C., Shear, P. K., Ritchey, P. N., & Frank, R. A. (2008). Assessment of the influence of cognition and cognitive processing speed on three tests of olfaction. *Journal of Clinical and Experimental Neuropsychology, 30*(3), 327–337. doi:10.1080/13803390701415892

Fernandez-Ruiz, J., Diaz, R., Hall-Haro, C., Vergara, P., Fiorentini, A., Nunnez, L., . . . Alonso, M. E. (2004). Olfactory dysfunction in hereditary ataxia and basal ganglia disorders. *Neuroreport: For Rapid Communication of Neuroscience Research, 14,* 1339–1341.

Fortin, A., Lefebvre, M. B., & Ptito, M. (2010). Traumatic brain injury and olfactory deficits: The tale of two smell tests! *Brain Injury, 24*(1), 27–33.

Frank, R. A., Dulay, M. F., & Gesteland, R. C. (2003). Assessment of the Sniff Magnitude Test as a clinical test of olfactory function. *Physiology and Behavior, 78,* 195–204.

Fulbright, R., Skudlarski, P., Lacadie, C., Warrenbeurg, S., Bowers, A., Gore, J., & Wexler, B. (1998). Functional MR imaging of regional brain responses to pleasant and unpleasant odors. *American Journal of Neuroradiology, 19,* 1721–1726.

Gansler, D. A., Fucetola, R., Krengel, M., Stetson, S., Zimering, R., & Makary, C. (1998). Are there cognitive subtypes in adult attention deficit/hyperactivity disorder? *The Journal of Nervous and Mental Disease, 186,* 776–781.

Garland, E. M., Raj, S. R., Peltier, A. C., Robertson, D., & Biaggioni, I. (2011). A cross-sectional study contrasting olfactory function in autonomic disorders. *Neurology, 76*(5), 456–460.

Goldstein, D. S., Holmes, C., Bentho, O., Sato, T., Moak, J., Sharabi, Y., . . . Eldadah, B. A. (2008). Biomarkers to detect central dopamine deficiency and distinguish Parkinson disease from multiple system atrophy. *Parkinsonism & Related Disorders, 14*(8), 600–607.

Goldstein, D. S., & Sewell, L. (2009). Olfactory dysfunction in pure autonomic failure: Implications for the pathogenesis of Lewy body diseases. *Parkinsonism & Related Disorders, 15*(7), 516–520.

Good, K. P., Leslie, R. A., McGlone, J., Milliken, H. I., & Kopala, L. C. (2007). Sex differences in olfactory function in young patients with psychotic disorders. *Schizophrenia Research, 97*(1-3), 97–102.

Good, K. P., Martzke, J. S., Daoud, M. A., & Kopala, L. C. (2003). Unirhinal norms for the University of Pennsylvania Smell Identification Test. *The Clinical Neuropsychologist, 17,* 226–234.

Good, K. P., Martzke, J. S., Milliken, H. J., Honer, W. G., & Kopala, L. C. (2002). Unirhinal olfactory identification deficits in young male patients with schizophrenia and related disorders: Association with impaired memory function. *Schizophrenia Research, 56,* 211–223.

Good, K. P., Tibbo, P., Milliken, H., Whitehorn, D., Alexiadis, M., Robertson, N., & Kopala, L. C. (2010). An investigation of a possible relationship between olfactory identification deficits at first episode and four-year outcomes in patients with psychosis. *Schizophrenia Research, 124*(1-3), 60–65.

Good, K. P., Whitehorn, D., Rui, Q., Milliken, H., & Kopala, L. C. (2006). Olfactory identification deficits in first-episode psychosis may predict patients at risk for persistent negative and disorganized or cognitive symptoms. *The American Journal of Psychiatry, 163*(5), 932–933.

Goudsmit, N., Coleman, E., Seckinger, R. A., Wolitzky, R., Stanford, A. D., Corcoran, C., . . . Malaspina, D. (2004). A brief smell identification test discriminates between deficit and non-deficit schizophrenia. *Psychiatry Research, 120,* 155–164.

Graves, A. B., Bowen, J. D., Rajaram, L., McCormick, W. C., McCurry, S. M., Schellenberg, G. D., & Larson, E. B. (1999). Impaired olfaction as a marker for cognitive decline. *Neurology, 53,* 1480–1487.

Gray, A. J., Staples, V., Murren, K., Dhariwal, A., & Bentham, P. (2001). Olfactory identification is impaired in clinic-based patients with vascular dementia and senile dementia of Alzheimer type. *International Journal of Geriatric Psychiatry, 16,* 513–517.

Hawkes, C. H., & Shephard, B. C. (1993). Selective anosmia in Parkinson's disease? *The Lancet, 341*(8842), 435–436.

Hawkes, C. H., Shepard, B. C., & Daniel, S. E. (1997). Olfactory dysfunction in Parkinson's disease. *Journal of Neurology, Neurosurgery and Psychiatry, 62,* 436–446.

Hemdal, P., Corwin, J., & Oster, H. (1993). Olfactory identification deficits in Down's syndrome and idiopathic mental retardation. *Neuropsychologia, 31,* 977–984.

Iranzo, A., Serradell, M., Vilaseca, I., Valldeoriola, F., Salamero, M., Molina, C., . . . Tolosa, E. (2013). Longitudinal assessment of olfactory function in idiopathic REM sleep behavior disorder. *Parkinsonism & Related Disorders, 19*(6), 600–604.

Ishizuka, K., Tajinda, K., Colantuoni, C., Morita, M., Winicki, J., Le, C., . . . Cascella, N. G. (2010). Negative symptoms of schizophrenia correlate with impairment on the University Of Pennsylvania Smell Identification Test. *Neuroscience Research, 66*(1), 106–110.

Jones-Gotman, M., & Zatorre, R. J. (1988). Olfactory identification deficits in patients with focal cerebral excision. *Neuropscyhologia, 26,* 387–400.

Kamath, V., Turetsky, B. I., Seligman, S. C., Marchetto, D. M., Walker, J. B., & Moberg, P. J. (2013). The influence of semantic processing on odor identification ability in schizophrenia. *Archives of Clinical Neuropsychology, 28*(3), 254–261.

Koenigkam-Santos, M., Santos, A. C., Versiani, B. R., Diniz, P. R. B., Junior, J. E., & de Castro, M. (2011). Quantitative magnetic resonance imaging evaluation of the olfactory system in Kallmann syndrome: Correlation with a clinical smell test. *Neuroendocrinology, 94*(3), 209–217.

Kohler, C. G., Moberg, P. J., Gur, R. E., O'Connor, M. J., Sperling, M. R., & Doty, R. L. (2001). Olfactory dysfunction in schizophrenia and temporal lobe epilepsy. *Neuropsychiatry, Neuropsychology, and Behavioral Neurology, 14,* 83–88.

Kopala, L. C., Good, K. P., & Honer, W. G. (1994). Olfactory hallucinations and olfactory identification ability in patients with schizophrenia and other psychiatric disorders. *Schizophrenia Research, 12,* 205–211.

Lee, M. R., Wehring, H. J., McMahon, R. P., Linthicum, J., Cascella, N., Liu, F., . . . Kelly, D. L. (2013). Effects of adjunctive intranasal oxytocin on olfactory identification and clinical symptoms in schizophrenia: Results from a randomized double blind placebo controlled pilot study. *Schizophrenia Research, 145*(1-3), 110–115.

Louis, E. D., Bromley, S. M., Jurewicz, E. C., & Watner, D. (2002). Olfactory dysfunction in essential tremor: A deficit unrelated to disease duration or severity. *Neurology, 59,* 1631–1633.

Malaspina, D., & Coleman, E. (2003). Olfaction and social drive in schizophrenia. *Archives of General Psychiatry, 60,* 578–584.

Martzke, J. S., Swan, C. S., & Varney, N. R. (1991). Posttraumatic anosmia and orbital frontal damage: Neuropsychological and neuropsychiatric correlates. *Neuropsychology, 5,* 213–225.

McKinnon, J., Evidente, V., Driver-Dunckley, E., Premkumar, A., Hentz, J., Shill, H., . . . Adler, C. (2010). Olfaction in the elderly: A cross-sectional analysis comparing Parkinson's disease with controls and other disorders. *International Journal of Neuroscience, 120*(1), 36–39.

McLean, D., Feron, F., MacKay-Sim, A., McCurdy, R., Chant, D., & McGrath, J. (2004). Paradoxical association between smoking and olfactory identification in psychosis versus controls. *Australian and New Zealand Journal of Psychiatry, 38,* 81–83.

Minor, K. L., Wright, B. D., & Park, S. (2004). The Smell Identification Test as a measure of olfactory identification ability in schizophrenia and healthy populations: A Rasch psychometric study. *Journal of Abnormal Psychology, 113,* 207–216.

Moberg, P. J., Doty, R. L., Mahr, R. N., Mesholam, R. I., Arnold, S. E., Turetsky, B. I., & Gur, R. E. (1997). Olfactory identification in elderly schizophrenia and Alzheimer's disease. *Neurobiology of Aging, 18,* 163–167.

Morgan, C. D., Nordin, S., & Murphy, C. (1995). Olfactory identification as an early marker for Alzheimer's disease: Impact of lexical functioning and detection sensitivity. *Journal of Clinical and Experimental Neuropsychology, 17,* 793–803.

Nagy, E., & Loveland, K. A. (2001). Olfactory deficit in Alzheimer's disease? *American Journal of Psychiatry, 158,* 1533.

Nguyen, A. D., Pelavin, P. E., Shenton, M. E., Chilakamarri, P., McCarley, R. W., Nestor, P. G., & Levitt, J. J. (2011). Olfactory sulcal depth and olfactory bulb volume in patients with schizophrenia: An MRI study. *Brain Imaging and Behavior, 5*(4), 252–261.

Pardini, M., Huey, E. D., Cavanagh, A. L., & Grafman, J. (2009). Olfactory function in corticobasal syndrome and frontotemporal dementia. *Archives of Neurology, 66*(1), 92–96.

Postolache, T. T., Doty, R. L., Wehr, T. A., et al. (1999). Monorhinal odor identification and depression scores in patients with seasonal affective disorder. *Journal of Affective Disorders, 56,* 27–35.

Postuma, R., & Gagnon, J. (2010). Cognition and olfaction in Parkinson's disease. *Brain: A Journal of Neurology, 133*(12), 1–2.

Postuma, R. B., Gagnon, J., Vendette, M., Desjardins, C., & Montplaisir, J. Y. (2011). Olfaction and color vision identify impending neurodegeneration in rapid eye movement sleep behavior disorder. *Annals of Neurology, 69*(5), 811–818.

Quagliato, L. B., Viana, M. A., Quagliato, E. M. A. B., & Simis, S. (2009). Olfaction and essential tremor. *Arquivos De Neuro-Psiquiatria, 67*(1), 21–24.

Qureshy, A., Kawashima, R., Imran, M., et al. (2000). Functional mapping of human brain in olfactory processing: A PET study. *Journal of Neurophysiology, 84,* 1656–1666.

Royall, D. R., Chiodo, L. K., Polk, M. J., & Jaramillo, C. J. (2002). Severe dysosmia is specifically associated with Alzheimer-like memory deficits in nondemented elderly retirees. *Neuroepidemiology, 21,* 68–73.

Royet, J. P., Koenig, O., Gregoire, M. C., Cinotti, L., Lavenne, F., Bars, D. L., . . . Holley, A. (1999). Functional anatomy of perceptual and semantic processing for odours. *Journal of Cognitive Neuroscience, 11,* 94–109.

Saunders-Pullman, R., Stanley, K., Wang, C., Luciano, M. S., Shanker, V., Hunt, A., . . . Bressman, S. B. (2011). Olfactory dysfunction in LRRK2 G2019S mutation carriers. *Neurology, 77*(4), 319–324.

Schmitt, A. L., Livingston, R. B., Reese, E. M., & Davis, K. M. (2010). The relationship between the repeatable battery for the assessment of neuropsychological status (RBANS) and olfaction in patients referred for a dementia evaluation. *Applied Neuropsychology, 17*(3), 163–171.

Schofield, P. W., Ebrahimi, H., Jones, A. L., Bateman, G. A., & Murray, S. R. (2012). An olfactory 'stress test' may detect preclinical Alzheimer's disease. *BMC Neurology, 12.* doi:10.1186/1471-2377-12-24

Segura, B., Baggio, H. C., Solana, E., Palacios, E. M., Vendrell, P., Bargalló, N., & Junqué, C. (2013). Neuroanatomical correlates of olfactory loss in normal aged subjects. *Behavioural Brain Research, 246,* 148–153.

Serby, M., Larson, P., & Kalkstein, D. (1991). The nature and course of olfactory deficits in Alzheimer's disease. *American Journal of Psychiatry, 148,* 357–360.

Shah, M., Deeb, J., Fernando, M., Noyce, A., Visentin, E., Findley, L. J., & Hawkes, C. H. (2009). Abnormality of taste and smell in Parkinson's disease. *Parkinsonism & Related Disorders, 15*(3), 232–237.

Shah, M., Muhammed, N., Findley, L. J., & Hawkes, C. H. (2008). Olfactory tests in the diagnosis of essential tremor. *Parkinsonism & Related Disorders, 14*(7), 563–568.

Ship, J. A., Pearson, J. D., Cruise, L. J., Brant, L. J., & Metter, E. J. (1996). Longitudinal changes in smell identification. *Journal of Gerontology, 51A,* M86–M91.

Ship, J. A., & Weiffenbach, J. M. (1993). Age, gender, medical treatment, and medication effects on smell identification. *Journals of Gerontology, 48,* M26–M32.

Silveira-Moriyama, L., Azevedo, A. M. S., Ranvaud, R., Barbosa, E. R., Doty, R. L., & Lees, A. J. (2010). Applying a new version of the Brazilian-Portuguese UPSIT smell test in Brazil. *Arquivos De Neuro-Psiquiatria, 68*(5), 700–705.

Silveira-Moriyama, L., Guedes, L. C., Kingsbury, A., Ayling, H., Shaw, K., Barbosa, E. R., . . . Lees, A. J. (2008). Hyposmia in G2019S LRRK2-related parkinsonism: Clinical and pathologic data. *Neurology, 71*(13), 1021–1026.

Silveira-Moriyama, L., Mathias, C., Mason, L., Best, C., Quinn, N. P., & Lees, A. J. (2009a). Hyposmia in pure autonomic failure. *Neurology, 72*(19), 1677–1681.

Silveira-Moriyama, L., Schwingenschuh, P., O'Donnell, A., Schneider, S. A., Mir, P., Carrillo, F., . . . Lees, A. J. (2009b). Olfaction in patients with suspected parkinsonism and scans without evidence of dopaminergic deficit (SWEDDs). *Journal of Neurology, Neurosurgery & Psychiatry, 80*(7), 744–748.

Stedman, T. J., & Clair, A. L. (1998). Neuropsychological, neurological and symptom correlates of impaired olfactory identification in schizophrenia. *Schizophrenia Research, 32,* 23–30.

Swan, G. E., & Carmelli, D. (2002). Impaired olfaction predicts cognitive decline in nondemented older adults. *Neuroepidemiology, 21,* 58–67.

Szeszko, P. R., Bates, J., Robinson, D., et al. (2004). Investigation of unirhinal olfactory identification in antipsychotic-free patients experiencing a first-episode schizophrenia. *Schizophrenia Research, 67,* 219–225.

Tabert, M. H., Liu, X., Doty, R. L., Serby, M., Zamora, D., Pelton, G. H., . . . Devanand, D. P. (2005). A 10-item smell identification scale related to risk for Alzheimer's disease. *Annals of Neurology, 58*(1), 155–160.

Varney, N. (1988). Prognostic significance of anosmia in patients with closed-head trauma. *Journal of Clinical and Experimental Neuropsychology, 10,* 250–254.

Velayudhan, L., Pritchard, M., Powell, J. F., Proitsi, P., & Lovestone, S. (2013). Smell identification function as a severity and progression marker in Alzheimer's disease. *International Psychogeriatrics, 25*(7), 1157–1166.

Wang, J., Eslinger, P. J., Doty, R. L., Zimmerman, E. K., Grunfeld, R., Sun, X., . . . Yang, Q. X. (2010). Olfactory deficit detected by fMRI in early Alzheimer's disease. *Brain Research, 1357,* 184–194.

Wang, Q-S., Tian, L., Huang, Y-L., Qin, S., He, L-Q., & Zhou, J-N. (2002). Olfactory identification and apoliprotein E ε4 allele in mild cognitive impairment. *Brain Research, 951,* 77–81.

Wenning, G. K., Shephard, B., Hawkes, C., Petuckevitch, A., et al. (1995). Olfactory function in atypical parkinsonian syndromes. *Acata Neurologica Scandinavica, 91,* 247–250.

Westervelt, H. J., McCaffrey, R. J., Cousings, J. P., Wagle, W. A., & Haase, R. F. (1997). Longitudinal analysis of olfactory deficits in HIV infection. *Archives of Clinical Neuropsychology, 12,* 557–565.

Yousem, D. M., Williams, S. C., Howard, R. O., Andrew, C., Simmons, A., Allin, M., . . . Doty, R. L. (1997). Functional MR imaging during odor stimulation: Preliminary data. *Radiology, 204,* 833–838.

Zald, D., & Pardo, J. (1997). Emotion, olfaction, and the human amygdala: Amygdala activation during aversive olfactory stimulation. *Proceedings from the National Academy of Sciences, 94,* 4119–4124.

Zatorre, R., Jones-Gotman, M., Evans, A., & Myer, E. (1992). Functional localization and lateralization of human olfactory cortex. *Nature, 360,* 339–340.

Zatorre, R. J., & Jones-Gotman, M. (1991). Human olfactory discrimination after unilateral frontal or temporal lobectomy. *Brain, 114,* 71–84.

14 | MOTOR FUNCTION

FINGER TAPPING TEST (FTT)

TEST NAME	**Finger Tapping Test (FTT)**
DOMAIN	Fine motor speed
AGE RANGE	Up to 85 years
ADMINISTRATION TIME	15 minutes
SCORING FORMAT	Hand scored
REFERENCE	Reitan, R. M., & Wolfson, D. (1985). *The Halstead-Reitan Neuropsychological Test Battery: Theory and interpretation.* Tucson, AZ: Neuropsychology Press.

DESCRIPTION

The Finger Tapping Test (FTT) measures self-directed manual motor speed. The FTT (Reitan, 1969) was originally called the Finger Oscillation Test (FOT) and was part of Halstead's (1947) test battery. Professional surveys have indicated that the test is commonly used by neuropsychologists.

Using a specially adapted tapper and counter, the examinee is instructed to tap as rapidly as possible using the index finger of the preferred hand. A comparable set of measurements is then obtained with the nonpreferred hand. The procedure calls for five consecutive trials within a five-point range with each hand (Reitan & Wolfson, 1985). This procedure is used to avoid undue influence of single deviant scores on total performance. There are other variants of the procedure. For example, Russell and Starkey (1993) ask the examinee to perform six trials with each hand, in sets of three, alternating hands between sets. Ashendorf et al. (2015) also provide information on an abbreviated version (see the section "Evidence for Reliability of Alternate, Short, or Computer Forms"). Computer variants have also been developed (see Hubel et al., 2013a, 2013b), and the FTT is part of the CNS Vital Signs computerized test battery (see review elsewhere in this volume). However, the most commonly used method is the one described by Reitan and Wolfson (1985).

ADMINISTRATION

The instructions derive from Reitan and Wolfson (1985). The examinee places the preferred hand palm down, with fingers extended and the index finger placed on the key. The individual is asked to tap as quickly as possible, moving only the index finger, not the whole hand or arm. A practice trial is given before the test begins to enable the examinee to become familiar with the apparatus. Begin timing when you hear the first "click" of the counter. In addition, listen for extra taps after you ask the examinee to stop. Record the number on the counter when the examiner says stop, rather than when the examinee stops.

The examinee is given five consecutive 10-second trials with the preferred hand. The procedure is then repeated with the nonpreferred hand. Five 10-second trials are given for each hand except when the results are too variable from one trial to another. Specifically, the test procedure requires that the five consecutive trials for each hand be within a five-point range from fastest to slowest. If one or more of the trials exceed this range, additional trials are given and the scores of the deviant trials are discarded. A maximum of ten trials with each hand is allowed. Do *not* alternate hand trials. Do not allow the examinee to move the whole hand from the wrist. With adults who struggle with coordination, this requirement can be unrealistic and may be relaxed. However, the score obtained should reflect index finger oscillation and not movement of the whole hand.

Fatigue may affect performance, particularly with the nondominant hand (Hubel et al., 2013a), and a brief rest period should be given after each trial. Even if no sign of fatigue is apparent, a rest period of 1–2 minutes is required after the third trial. Third-party observation was not noted to significantly affect performance in a group of people with traumatic brain injury (TBI; Lynch, 2005).

SCORING

The finger tapping score is computed for each hand separately and is the mean of five consecutive 10-second trials within a range of five taps. A maximum of 10 trials with each hand is allowed, and, if this criterion is not met, the score is the mean of the total number of trials. The performance between the preferred and nonpreferred hand is also frequently compared (see "Hand Preference and Intermanual Differences" and "Clinical Studies").

DEMOGRAPHIC EFFECTS

AGE

In adults, performance declines with advancing age (Ashendorf et al., 2009; Bornstein, 1985; Goldstein & Braun, 1974; Heaton et al., 1991; Hubel et al., 2013a; Leckliter & Matarazzo, 1989; McCurry et al., 2001; Mitrushina et al., 2005; Ott et al., 1995; Shimoyama et al., 1990; Trahan et al., 1987; Ylikoski et al., 1998). Variability also increases with older age (Hubel et al., 2013a; Mitrushina et al., 2005). Heaton et al. (2004) reported that in their large normative sample (aged 20–85 years), about 12–18% of the variance in finger tapping scores was accounted for by age.

GENDER

Most studies suggest that men tend to outperform women (Ashendorf et al., 2009; Bornstein, 1985; Carlier et al., 1993; Fromm-Auch & Yeudall, 1983; Harris et al., 1981; Heaton et al., 1991; Leckliter & Matarazzo, 1989; Mitrushina et al., 2005; Nagasaki et al., 1988; Ruff & Parker, 1993; Shimoyama et al., 1990; Trahan et al., 1987; Yamashita, 2014; Ylikoski et al., 1998). Heaton et al. (2004) reported that, in adults, about 16–20% of the variance in test scores was accounted for by gender. Ashendorf et al. (2009) reported that in their older adult sample, the difference in favor of men was large according to Cohen's conventions (d = 1.01, .93).

Dodrill (1979) suggested that the observed gender difference for finger tapping may be attributed to sexual dimorphism in body and hand size rather than a neuropsychological mechanism. However, Schmidt et al. (2000) noted that controlling for finger and hand size did not eliminate the main effect of gender on finger tapping. Similarly, Hubel et al. (2013a) found that men tapped faster than women on a computerized variant of finger tapping, which was not accounted for by age, fatigue, or kinetics of movement. However, a review by Roivainen (2011) suggests that there is a female advantage in processing speed that involves digits, alphabets, and rapid naming, with a male advantage on reaction time and finger tapping.

EDUCATION AND IQ

Ashendorf et al. (2009) reported that, in their older adult sample, individuals with an education level that exceeded high school performed better than adults with fewer years of education. However, age and gender have stronger effects than education on performance in adults (Bornstein, 1985). According to Heaton et al. (2004), education accounts for only about 2–4% of the variance in tapping scores.

Performance tends to be better with increasing IQ (Leckliter & Matarazzo, 1989; but see Horton, 1999) and with more years of education (Bornstein, 1985; Heaton et al., 1991; but see McCurry et al., 2001; Ruff & Parker, 1993; Ylikoski et al., 1998).

ETHNICITY, NATIONALITY, AND LINGUISTIC EFFECTS

Performance tends to be somewhat better in Caucasians than in African Americans (Heaton et al., 2004). No differences have been reported between Mexican-American, Anglo-American, and Mexican individuals (Arnold et al., 1994).

HAND PREFERENCE AND INTERMANUAL DIFFERENCES

Age and years of education do not have a strong relationship with measures of intermanual differences in adults (Bornstein, 1986b; Heaton et al., 1991; Ruff & Parker, 1993; Thompson et al., 1987). The findings regarding gender differences in intermanual difference scores are inconsistent; some studies report greater differences between hands for males than for females (Bornstein, 1986b; Fromm-Auch & Yeudall, 1983), and others do not (Ruff & Parker, 1993; Thompson et al., 1987). There is evidence that right-handers show larger intermanual differences than left-handers (Thompson et al., 1987).

Typically, the performances of the preferred and nonpreferred hands are compared on motor tasks to determine whether there is consistent evidence of poor performance with one hand relative to the other. In general, finger tapping performance with the preferred hand is superior to that with the nonpreferred hand (Bornstein, 1985, 1986a; Corey et al., 2001; Finlayson & Reitan, 1976; Heaton et al., 2004; Peters, 1990; Shimoyama et al., 1990; Thompson, et al., 1987; Triggs et al., 2000; but see Ruff & Parker, 1993). The most frequently reported guideline is that the preferred hand should perform about 10% better than the nonpreferred hand (Reitan & Wolfson, 1985). On a computerized variant, Hubel et al. (2013a) reported that the nondominant hand was relatively poorer than the dominant hand on a number of variables, including median tapping rate, tap kinetics (relative time button is closed), and variability of rate of tapping.

However, there is considerable variability in the healthy population, and the preferred hand is not necessarily the faster one, especially when left-handed people are considered (Bornstein, 1986a; Corey et al., 2001; Thompson et al., 1987). Patterns of performance indicating equal or better performance with the nonpreferred hand occur with considerable regularity in the healthy population (about 30%), and neurological involvement should not be inferred from an isolated lack of concordance. Fairly large discrepancies between the hands on the FTT alone also cannot be used to suggest unilateral impairment (Bornstein, 1986a; Thompson et al., 1987). Greater confidence in the clinical judgment of impaired motor function with one or the other hand can be gained from consideration of the consistency of intermanual discrepancies across several motor tasks because truly consistent, deviant performances are quite rare in the healthy population (Bornstein, 1986a, 1986b; Thompson et al., 1987).

It is also important to note that there could be reasons other than a lateralized motor defect for an individual with a neurologic condition to perform poorly with the nonpreferred hand on skilled motor tasks. For example, if cognitive efficiency is reduced, perhaps as a result of cortical and/or subcortical involvement in both hemispheres, then performance with the nonpreferred (less practiced) hand may be affected on tasks that require adaptation and skilled movement, such as finger tapping (Lewis & Kupke, 1992).

TABLE 14–1 Characteristics of the Finger Tapping Normative Sample Provided by Heaton et al. (2004)

Number	1,212
Age (years)	20 to 85[a]
Geographic location	Various states in the United States, and Manitoba, Canada
Sample type	Individuals recruited as part of multicenter studies
Education (years)	0 to 20[b]
Gender (%)	
Male	56.8
Female	43.2
Race/Ethnicity	
Caucasian	634
African American	578
Screening	No reported history of learning disability, neurological disorder, serious psychiatric disorder, or alcohol or drug abuse

[a]Age groups: 20 to 34, 35 to 39, 40 to 44, 45 to 49, 50 to 54, 55 to 59, 60 to 64, 65 to 69, 70 to 74, 75 to 79, and 80 to 89 years.

[b]Education groups: 7 to 8, 9 to 11, 12, 13 to 15, 16 to 17, and 18 to 20 years.

SOURCE: Reproduced by special permission of the Publisher, Psychological Assessment Resources, Inc. (PAR), 16204 North Florida Avenue, Lutz, FL 33549, from *Revised Comprehensive Norms for an Expanded Halstead-Reitan Battery Professional Manual*, Copyright 1991, 1992, 2004 by Psychological Assessment Resources, Inc. All rights reserved.

NORMATIVE DATA

Normative data, rather than conventional cutoff scores (Reitan & Wolfson, 1985), should be used because high false-positive rates are likely to occur with use of cutoff scores (Bernard, 1989; Bornstein, 1986c). Cutoffs were based on the performance of individuals who were largely middle-aged and above average intellectually. For example, among Bornstein's sample of 365 healthy volunteers with a mean age of 43 years, use of conventional cutoff scores resulted in 80% of subjects being misclassified as impaired on preferred hand finger tapping scores.

A number of normative datasets are available. Heaton et al. (2004) offers a large normative database spanning a broad age and education range, and stratified by relevant demographic variables. Greer et al. (2010) offer normative data for a large sample, but many of the studies included did not report important demographic characteristics. Additionally, these data are adjusted for age and education, not gender. Ashendorf et al. (2009) provide a dataset for older adults that may be useful when working with this population.

Heaton et al. (2004; Table 14–1) provide norms separately for two ethnic groups (Caucasians and African Americans), organized by age, gender, and education. The sample is large and covers a wide range in terms of age (20 to 85 years) and education (0 to 20 years), and the exclusion criteria are specified. T scores lower than 40 are classified as impaired. According to Heaton et al. (2004), the procedure used was the one specified by Reitan and Wolfson (1985).

A number of other investigators have provided norms for specific groups, including Bornstein (1985, for 20–69 years), Fromm-Auch and Yeudall (1983, for 15–64 years), Goldstein and Braun (1974, for 20–79 years), Ruff and Parker (1993, for 16–70 years), and Trahan et al. (1987, for 18–91 years). Mitrushina et al. (2005) compiled data from eight studies for men and four for women, comprising 530 to 963 participants (depending on hand preference and gender), aged 20 to 74 years. They noted that the integrity of their meta-analysis was undermined by the lack of consistency in reporting data regarding handedness. Their data appear fairly similar to those reported by Heaton et al. (2004).

Ruff and Parker (1993) provided cross-sectional normative data for 358 adult volunteers, aged 16 to 70 years. Their education level ranged from 7 to 22 years, and they resided in California (65%), Michigan (30%), and the US Eastern seaboard (5%). All participants were screened to exclude those with a positive history of psychiatric hospitalization, chronic polydrug abuse, or neurological disorders. Hand preference was determined by both questionnaire

TABLE 14–2 Mean Performance of Adults for Finger Tapping

AGE GROUP	DOMINANT			NONDOMINANT	
	N	*M*	*SD*	*M*	*SD*
Women					
16–24	45	49.5	5.1	45.6	5.1
25–39	45	49.0	4.1	44.6	4.6
40–54	44	47.0	5.6	43.5	5.2
55–70	45	45.7	5.5	40.4	5.2
Men					
16–24	45	52.9	5.1	48.2	4.4
25–39	44	52.7	6.8	48.7	5.7
40–54	45	54.3	5.7	48.9	5.8
55–70	45	53.5	6.4	48.3	5.0

SOURCE: From Ruff and Parker (1993). © Perceptual and Motor Skills 1993. Reprinted with permission.

and performance on a series of tasks. Note that the method of administration differed somewhat from that of Reitan and Wolfson (1985). That is, participants were given a brief opportunity to practice with either hand, after which five 10-second trials were alternatively administered to the dominant and then the nondominant hand. If there was a spread of more than five taps between any two trials of one hand, then two additional trials were required for that hand. If seven trials were necessary, both the highest and lowest scores were eliminated, and the mean was calculated using the remaining five scores. Despite the differences, their data agree fairly well with those of Heaton et al. (2004) and Mitrushina et al. (2005). Table 14–2 provides their data (means and standard deviations) for both dominant and nondominant hands, stratified by age and gender.

McCurry et al. (2001) presented data based on a sample of Japanese Americans, aged 70 years and older, who were enrolled in a prospective study of aging and dementia in King County, Washington. None of the participants was classified as presenting with dementia based on clinical and screening neuropsychological examinations. The data are provided in Table 14–3 and represent an important source of information for this understudied segment of the US population.

Greer et al. (2010) provide pooled normative data amalgamated across 96 studies for 153 samples (n = 9,489) for the FTT. Data for other Halstead-Reitan tests were also included. Of note, the studies were published from 1950 to 2003. Studies varied in data reported, with few reporting occupation. Ethnicity was reported in 30 studies, with an overall proportion of Caucasian participants (85%), with a male majority (58%). Normative data by education and age grouping are provided in Table 14–4.

Ashendorf, Vanderslice-Barr, and McCaffrey (2009) present normative data for the FTT and the Grooved Pegboard for more than 300 older (55 to 74 years old) community-dwelling individuals (Table 14–5). Participants were a mean age of 63.9 years (standard deviation [*SD*] = 6.0), 51% female, with an average education level of 13.8 (*SD* = 2.6 years). North American Adult Reading Test (NAART) mean score was 107.3 (*SD* = 8.9). All participants were Caucasian and lived in New York. Exclusion criteria were current treatment for depression, current excessive alcohol or drug use, neurodegenerative or neurological condition, human immunodeficiency virus (HIV) infection, AIDS, or severe arthritis prohibiting completion of motor tests. The FTT was administered according to the Reitan and Wolfson approach.

EVIDENCE FOR RELIABILITY

EVIDENCE FOR TEST-RETEST RELIABILITY, MEASURING CHANGE, AND PRACTICE EFFECTS

Reliability coefficients range from .58 to .93 in healthy and clinical samples (Bornstein et al., 1987; Dikmen et al., 1999; Dodrill & Troupin, 1975; Gill et al., 1986; Goldstein & Watson, 1989; Morrison et al., 1979; Provins & Cunliffe, 1972; Ruff & Parker, 1993; Sjogren et al., 2000; but see

TABLE 14–3 Finger Tapping Means, Standard Deviations (*SD*s), and Quartiles by Age for Japanese Americans

AGE AND GENDER	*N*	MEAN	*SD*	25TH PERCENTILE	MEDIAN	75TH PERCENTILE
Men 70–79 years						
Dominant	58	42.96	8.3	35	45	49
Nondominant	57	39.63	4.67	35	40	42
Women 70–79 years						
Dominant	44	42.77	7.88	40	42	47
Nondominant	43	39.27	7.01	36	40	42
Men 80–89 years						
Dominant	18	35.81	9.27	31	33	45
Nondominant	18	35.09	8.05	29	36	42
Women 80–89 years						
Dominant	37	36.62	9.28	30	36	44
Nondominant	35	33.78	7.63	28	37	41

NOTE: The sample consisted of 160 adults. Mean education about 11.0 (*SD* = 3.0); 72.9% born in the United States (94.9% in the age group 70 to 79; 35.7% in the age group 80+), 94% right-handed. Age but not gender, education, or language spoken significantly affected test scores.

SOURCE: S. McCurry, personal communication with previous authors, May 17, 2004.

TABLE 14–4 Normative Data Adjusted for Age and Education for the Finger Tapping Test

	<12 YEARS EDUCATION		12 TO 14 YEARS EDUCATION		≥15 YEARS EDUCATION	
	<35	35 TO 64	<35	35 TO 64	<35	35 TO 64
Dominant hand	49.05 (6.57)	40.73 (8.00)	51.15 (6.60)	48.44 (7.44)	51.15 (6.22)	47.99 (6.98)
Nondominant hand	43.85 (5.43)	37.31 (6.72)	45.06 (6.37)	45.47 (7.37)	45.00 (5.39)	41.43 (6.24)

SOURCE: Adapted from Greer et al. (2010).

Matarazzo et al., 1974, for values < .50). A computerized variant of finger tapping suggested high test-retest reliability (i.e., .81 to .82 for dominant and nondominant index; Hubel et al., 2013b). Some investigators have reported that the differences between hands are reliable ($r > .70$; Massman & Doody, 1996; Provins & Cunliffe, 1972), whereas others have reported low reliability ($r = .50$; Morrison et al., 1979).

Practice effects tend to be minimal in both healthy (e.g., Bornstein et al., 1987; Salinsky et al., 2001) and clinical populations (e.g., Dodrill & Troupin, 1975). Haaland et al. (1994) noted a slight improvement, two taps per 10 seconds for healthy people and those with mild TBI who were tested at one month and again at one year post-injury. The similar, though subtle, improvement in finger tapping should alert clinicians to overinterpreting tapping improvement as evidence of recovery.

Dikmen et al. (1999) reported slight improvement in scores in a sample of 384 healthy or neurologically stable individuals (aged 15–83 years, $M = 34.2$, $SD = 16.7$) who were retested about nine months after initial testing. Table 14–6 provides information to determine whether there has been significant change taking practice into account. One first subtracts the mean T2 – T1 change (column 3) from the difference between the two testing sessions for the individual and then compares the resulting value with 1.64 times the *SD* of the difference (column 4). The 1.64 comes from the healthy distribution and is exceeded in the positive or negative direction only 10% of the time if indeed there is no real change. Dikmen et al. (1999) also noted that those with better initial scores have bigger improvements in test scores. Factors such as the length of retest interval, age, and education of the individual had little effect on change.

EVIDENCE FOR RELIABILITY OF ALTERNATE, SHORT, OR COMPUTER FORMS

Ashendorf, Horwitz, and Gavett (2015) evaluated abbreviated procedures (12 permutations of consecutive three-, four-, and five-trial combinations from among the first five trials of the FTT, involving average and maximum performance, resulting in 12 permutations) of the FTT in a sample of 71 people (predominantly male, mean age approximately 37 years, mean education approximately 13 years; 82% white) who presented to Veterans' Affairs hospital for neuropsychological assessment, typically related to TBI (79% of sample). Seventeen percent of the sample scored below cutoffs on the Test of Memory Malingering (TOMM). The authors noted a shortened version that involved the mean score of trials three to five accounted for the largest amount of variance in total tests scores, with the lowest error among versions examined. This version had strong reliability (intraclass correlation [*ICC*] = .90), even more so than the full version (*ICC* = .66), with sensitivity values exceeding 91%. The authors reported that when Trials three to five differ by 15 taps or more, administration of the conventional FTT would be required.

EVIDENCE FOR INTERRATER RELIABILITY

Information regarding interrater reliability is not available.

TABLE 14–5 Normative Data Adjusted by Age, Gender, and Education for Older Adults

		MEN				WOMEN			
		EDUC. ≤ 12 YEARS		EDUC. > 12 YEARS		EDUC. ≤ 12 YEARS		EDUC. > 12 YEARS	
		AGE 55–64 N = 35	AGE 65–74 N = 34	AGE 55–64 N = 55	AGE 65–74 N = 25	AGE 55–64 N = 42	AGE 65–74 N = 23	AGE 55–64 N = 51	AGE 65–74 N = 39
Dom	*M*	46.3	44.7	47.9	45.6	37.7	36.8	42.5	39.0
	SD	5.5	8.4	6.8	5.7	6.6	7.0	5.3	8.0
NDom	*M*	42.3	41.2	43.7	43.2	36.7	34.3	39.9	36.9
	SD	5.5	6.3	5.1	6.3	5.3	5.6	4.5	6.2
Ratio	*M*	1.11	1.08	1.10	1.07	1.03	1.08	1.07	1.06
	SD	0.15	0.13	0.12	0.13	0.14	0.13	0.12	0.18

NOTE: Educ. = education; Dom = dominant hand; NDom = nondominant hand; Ratio = dominant ÷ nondominant hand performance; *M* = mean, *SD* = standard deviation.

SOURCE: Ashendorf et al. (2009).

TABLE 14–6 Finger Tapping Test-Retest Effects in 384 Healthy or Neurologically Stable Individuals Assessed After Intervals of About 2–16 Months

	TIME 1		TIME 2		T2 - T1		T1, T2
MEASURE	(1) *M*	*SD*	(2) *M*	*SD*	(3) *M*	(4) *SD*	*R*
Dominant	50.88	6.59	51.36	6.46	.48	4.39	.77
Nondominant	47.02	6.39	47.87	6.47	.85	4.31	.78

NOTE: Mean Age = 34.2, *SD* = 16, 7, range = 15 to 83; Mean education = 12.1, *SD* = 2.6, range = 0 to19; 66% male; retest interval mean = 9.1 months, *SD* = 3.0, range = 2.4 to 15.8.

SOURCE: Adapted from Dikmen et al. (1999).

EVIDENCE FOR VALIDITY

FACTOR-ANALYTIC STUDIES AND RELATIONSHIPS WITH OTHER TESTS

Finger tapping dominant and nondominant hand performance are highly related (.70; Ashendorf et al., 2009). Austin et al. (2011) described that a novel method of measuring motor speed (keystroke intervals of a participant's routine computer use at home) correlated with the FTT at .70 (dominant) and .77 (nondominant hand), providing support for ecological validity of the test.

Factor-analytic findings suggest that finger tapping and pegboard dexterity measure independent dimensions of manual proficiency (Fleishman & Hempel, 1954; Stanford & Barratt, 1996). Ashendorf et al. (2009) reported generally nonsignificant correlations between the FTT and the Grooved Pegboard Test (GPT). Yamashita (2014) reported a small but significant correlation with GPT and their variant of the FTT (.19). Duffield et al. (2013), however, reported moderate correlations between FTT and GPT in typically-developing adults (.42) and those with autism spectrum disorder (ASD; .49).

However, when between-hand asymmetry is considered, finger tapping correlates highly (.78) in healthy adults with the Purdue Pegboard, a task that requires independent, precise finger movement. This suggests that both tasks depend at least in part on a common neural substrate; namely, asymmetry in the corticospinal system (Triggs et al., 2000). The correlation, however, is lower between finger tapping and Grip Strength asymmetry (.41). Notably, Grip Strength does not require independent or precise control of the fingers (Triggs et al., 2000). Similar size correlations have been reported in other studies (e.g., *rs* = .40 to .56; Duffield et al., 2014; Yamashita, 2014).

The test shows relationships with handedness. A variant of the FTT correlates significantly with a questionnaire of hand preference (Edinburgh Handedness Inventory; Spearman rank correlation = .43; Yamashita, 2014).

In one study, the Wechsler Adult Intelligence Scale (WAIS-III) Full Scale IQ (FSIQ) and the FTT correlated mildly in a mixed clinical sample of neuropsychology outpatients (r = .21; Dean et al., 2008). Both the dominant and nondominant FTT are correlated significantly with Block Design (*rs* = .20, .16) and WMS Visual Reproduction (*rs* = .17 to .20; Ashendorf et al., 2009), although correlations are small. It shows only a small correlation (r = .25) with the Processing Speed Index of the WAIS-III, suggesting that the FTT involves only minimal amounts of the type of central resources required in more complex measures of speeded perceptual processing (Kennedy et al., 2003).

Minimal to negligible relationships have been reported between the FTT and attention/executive functioning (e.g., Digit Span, Trail Making Test [TMT-B], Wisconsin Card Sorting Test [WCST]; Ashendorf et al., 2009, Sánchez-Cubillo et al., 2009) and memory tests (Ashendorf et al., 2009).

CLINICAL STUDIES

There is evidence that tapping speed is sensitive to a wide variety of conditions, including chronic alcoholism (Leckliter & Matarazzo, 1989), Korsakoff's syndrome (Welch et al., 1997), chronic pain (Sjogren et al., 2000), the mild stages of degenerative dementias (Muller et al., 1991; Ott et al., 1995; see also Massman & Doody, 1996; Wefel et al., 1999), and sleep apnea–hypopnea syndrome (Neu et al., 2011). The FTT is sensitive to multiple sclerosis (MS; Chipchase et al., 2003) and correlates with disability and T2 lesion load (Bergendal et al., 2013). The FTT has been used as an outcome measure in many clinical groups, including studies of the effect of sertraline on depression in Alzheimer's disease (AD; Munro et al., 2012) and studies of hormone replacement for individuals with posttraumatic hypopituitarism after TBI (High et al., 2010). Modafinil in cancer patients is associated with improved FTT performance (Lundorff et al., 2009). In addition to direct motoric effects, the speed, coordination, and pacing requirements of Finger Tapping can be affected by varying levels of alertness, impaired ability to focus and maintain attention, problems with generating responses, or generalized slowing of responses.

Motor Conditions. The test can distinguish patients with motor dysfunctions of cerebellar, basal ganglia, and cerebral origin from healthy controls (Shimoyama et al., 1990). However, tapping frequency cannot distinguish between clinical groups (Shimoyama et al., 1990). Other measures (e.g., intertap variability, time in flexion and extension in the tap cycle, time-sequential histograms of tapping intervals) may be able to differentiate between groups and identify motor impairments that are not apparent in tapping rate (Roy et al., 1992; Shimoyama et al., 1990).

Variants of the FTT have been used to study movement in PD (e.g., Ariaset al., 2012; Chen et al., 2012; Khan et al., 2014; Yokoe et al., 2009) and orthostatic hypotension in PD (Hohler et al., 2012).

TBI. The FTT is sensitive to TBI (Dikmen et al., 1995; Haaland et al., 1994; Prigatano & Borano, 2003). It is worth noting that although most investigators evaluate speed of finger tapping, qualitative features of the task may also have diagnostic value. For example, Prigatano and Borgaro (2003) reported that abnormal finger tapping patterns (e.g., failure to inhibit movement of fingers other than the index finger) are more common in individuals with TBI than healthy controls and that the frequency of abnormal finger movements may relate to the severity of the injury.

Psychiatric Conditions. FTT performance improves after quetiapine in schizophrenia (Kivircik Akdede et al., 2005). Variants of the FTT have been used to study procedural learning in schizophrenia (Da Silva et al., 2012).

Lim et al. (2013) reported in a meta-analysis of patients with major depressive disorder that the FTT failed to differentiate people with major depressive disorder from controls. In bipolar disorder, lithium negatively impacted FTT speed in euthymic patients, and levels of thyroid stimulating hormone correlated with performance in medication-free patients (Atagun et al., 2013).

Daily Function. The FTT has a number of correlates with daily function. Performance on the FTT is related to rehabilitation outcome after stroke (Prigatano & Wong, 1997) and also to employment status after various brain disorders (Dikmen & Morgan, 1980; Heaton et al., 1978), with faster tapping related to better outcome. Performance on the test is moderately predictive of daily living skills in geriatric patients (Searight et al., 1989) and in patients with TBI (Prigatano et al., 1990).

NEUROANATOMICAL CORRELATES, LESION STUDIES, AND IMAGING STUDIES

The FTT is sensitive to the presence and laterality of brain lesions (e.g., Barnes & Lucas, 1974; Bigler & Tucker, 1981; Dodrill, 1978; Dufouil et al., 2003; Finlayson & Reitan, 1980; Haaland & Delaney, 1981; Hom & Reitan, 1982, 1990; Reitan & Wolfson, 1994, 1996; Ylikoski et al., 1998). Given the crossed nature of the motor system, performance tends to be worse in the hand contralateral to the lesion.

In a functional magnetic resonance imaging (fMRI) study with the right hand (Johnson & Prigatano, 2000), activations in regions of the contralateral and ipsilateral primary motor cortex, left lateral premotor cortex, left dorsolateral prefrontal cortex, and ipsilateral cerebellum were noted in healthy individuals' performance on the FTT. Prigatano, Johnson, and Gale (2004) reported that fMRI showed greater bilateral frontal activation in healthy controls compared to patients with TBI, with activation differences especially in the supplementary motor cortex. The FTT is negatively related to motor cortex volume (Duffield et al., 2014). Tobe et al. (2010) reported that reduced bilateral cerebellar volume (particularly in crus I and lobules VI, VIIB, and VIIIA) was related to performance on a variant of FTT in people with Tourette syndrome (Tobe et al., 2010). Therefore, although motor regions are implicated, disturbances in a variety of brain regions and circuits may be associated with slow finger tapping.

Central dopamine plays a role in motor activity. Consistent with this notion, there is a relationship between performance and striatal D_2 receptor density (Yang et al., 2003, 2004), suggesting that the FTT may be sensitive to monitoring various diseases (e.g., those affecting extrapyramidal systems) and medication effects across a variety of conditions. Furthermore, the sensitivity of the task to aging may be explained in part by a decline in dopamine D_2 density.

PERFORMANCE VALIDITY

The FTT has been used in a number of studies evaluating performance validity, in a number of groups. The Arnold index is typically used (see later discussion), and, typically, malingerers are found to perform worse than controls (e.g., Hubel et al., 2013b on a computerized variant; although see Greiffenstein et al., 1996; Trueblood & Schmidt, 1993). Greiffenstein and Baker (2008) reported that nearly 38% of individuals with disability claims related to mild TBI and posttraumatic stress disorder (PTSD) were found to have FTT scores associated with a high likelihood of noncredibility.

Larrabee (2003) found that a raw score of less than 63 on combined (right plus left) finger tapping correctly identified 10/25 (40%) of individuals meeting criteria for definite malingered neurocognitive dysfunction and 29/31 (94%) of individuals with moderate/severe TBI. This cutoff, however, appears to require adjustment for gender.

Arnold et al. (2005) evaluated FTT performance in seven groups: noncredible patients and credible patients with head injury, dementia, intellectual disability, psychosis, or depression, and healthy older adults. Dominant-hand scores proved to be more sensitive to noncredible performance than other scores such as nondominant hand, sum of both hands, or difference between hands. With specificity set at an optimal level of 90% to minimize false positives, sensitivity estimates were moderate, similar to most performance validity tests (PVTs): a dominant-hand cutoff score of 35 for men yielded 50% sensitivity, and a cutoff of 28 for women yielded 61% sensitivity.

However, specificity values for cutoffs varied considerably across the comparison groups, indicating that the cutoff should be selected based on gender and claimed diagnosis. Positive and negative predictive power for the

TABLE 14–7 Positive Predictive Values (PPV) and Negative Predictive Values (NPV) for Dominant-Hand Finger Tapping for Different Base Rates

CUTOFF VALUE	15% BASE RATE		30% BASE RATE		50% BASE RATE	
	PPV (%)	NPV (%)	PPV (%)	NPV (%)	PPV (%)	NPV (%)
WOMEN						
15	75	87	86	74	91	55
28	63	93	80	85	87	70
32	48	94	68	87	83	73
35	39	94	60	87	78	85
38	28	94	48	86	69	73
MEN						
21	80	88	89	74	93	55
33	53	90	76	79	87	62
35	50	91	68	80	84	64
38	45	91	67	82	83	65
40	35	92	58	82	77	67

SOURCE: Arnold et al. (2005). Reprinted with the kind permission of Psychology Press.

dominant-hand scores with the highest sensitivity/specificity rates at varying base rates of suspect performance are shown in Table 14–7. With a base rate of 30% noncredible subjects, a dominant-hand cutoff of 28 or lower for women resulted in a positive predictive value (PPV) of 80% with a negative predictive value (NPV) of 85%. Using the same base rate of 30% for men, a cutoff score of 35 or lower resulted in a PPV of 68% and an NPV of 80%. These data suggest that the FTT may be a more effective measure of performance validity in women than in men.

Greiffenstein et al. (1996) reported that compensation-seeking patients with postconcussion syndrome demonstrated a nonphysiologic profile (Grip Strength < FTT < Grooved Pegboard). However, Rapport et al. (1998) observed that the presence of nonphysiologic configurations showed poor predictive accuracy among simulators and controls.

Axelrod, Meyers, and Davis (2014) assessed three scoring systems to detect invalid performance on FTT: the raw score for the dominant hand (Arnold et al., 2005), the raw scores combined for both hands (Larrabee, 2003), and the estimated finger tapping difference score (Meyers & Volbrecht, 2003). The sample comprised clinical Veterans' Affairs and compensation-seeking patients, typically with TBI. Credible performance was defined as passing scores on other PVTs, and noncredible performance was defined as failing two or more other PVTs. The Fail group had fewer taps in the dominant hand and a lower combined score. Each method yielded moderate sensitivity rates for the Fail group (24 to 55%) and high specificity rates for the Pass group (88 to 94%). The authors then identified optimal cutoffs in their samples to achieve a 90% specificity rate to minimize false positives. These cutoffs included a dominant hand score of less than 37 for Veterans' Affairs patients and less than 32 for compensation-seeking patients, and a combined score of less than 69 and less than 65.

In dementia, the test yields a high number of false positives, a problem not unique to the FTT. For example, Dean, Victor, Boone, Philpott, and Hess (2009) evaluated dementia patients on 18 embedded performance validity indices, including the FTT. For cutoffs of men at 35 and lower and women at 28 and lower, the authors reported 69% specificity, which although indicating an unacceptable number of false positives, was one of the highest among embedded indices. False positives increased as Mini-Mental State Examination (MMSE) scores decreased and were best in frontotemporal and Alzheimer's dementias and poorest in vascular dementia. It is important to note that the subsamples were small and groups were heterogeneous in terms of age, education, and MMSE score. An adjusted cutoff score attaining an acceptable false-positive rate with 90% specificity was less than 21 taps.

The FTT has been examined in low-IQ samples, with promising results. Dean, Victor, Boone, and Arnold (2008) examined a number of validity indicators in their mixed clinical sample of nonlitigating neuropsychology clinic outpatients, noting high rates of failure in those with the lowest IQs on a number of validity indicators. Among indicators examined, the FTT using the Arnold et al. (2005) indicator (men ≤35, women ≤28) was among the most accurate indicators in the low-IQ subsamples, with a specificity of 83% in people with IQs ranging from 70 to 79. To maintain a 90% specificity, cutoffs of lower than 29 were suggested in low-IQ groups, with a cutoff of less than 34 in people with IQ scores in the range of 80 to 89. Smith et al. (2014) examined tests and scores that differentiated credible from noncredible patients with FSIQs 75 or lower, as well as a noncredible sample unselected for IQ. Credible women had faster tapping speed than noncredible women, but differences were not found between males of each group. Scores of less than 24 (dominant) and less than 20 (nondominant) in the noncredible group were associated with sensitivity scores of 37% and 31%, respectively, at a specificity of 90%.

The FTT has also been used to evaluate performance validity in psychiatric populations, with better utility in movement disorders than schizophrenia. Criswell, Sterling, Swisher, Evanoff, and Racette (2010) reported that a six-trial variant of the FTT was particularly effective in detection of psychogenic movement disorders; the FTT ratio had nearly 80% sensitivity and 89% specificity. Whearty, Allen, Lee, and Strauss (2015) reported nearly 36% of schizophrenia patients failing the FTT effort index by Arnold et al. (2005; average dominant hand score across trials; cutoffs for men ≤35, women ≤28). Furthermore, a high proportion (35%) of patients with IQs in the 70 to 79 range had scores below cutoff, suggesting caution in interpreting this index in this group.

COMMENT

The FTT measures motor speed of the preferred and nonpreferred hands. Although several variants exist, the most commonly used method is that described by Reitan and Wolfson (1985). Computer variants also have promise for use clinically in measuring a broader range of variables.

Perhaps unsurprisingly, the performance of the preferred hand is typically better than that of the nonpreferred hand; however, a high rate of variability exists in the population, and thus superior performance of the nonpreferred hand should not necessarily be interpreted as indicative of neurological impairment. The FTT correlates moderately with Grip Strength and relatively little with Grooved Pegboard, suggesting relative independence of the motor functions measured by FTT and pegboard tasks. This may reflect the notion that FTT is a relatively pure measure of motor speed, whereas pegboard tasks likely involve a number of other cognitive processes. In support of this concept, the FTT shows relatively small relationships with other cognitive measures and is related modestly to moderately with fluid intelligence and minimally with attention, executive tasks, and memory tasks.

Neuroanatomically, the test is associated with frontal activation, and there is also evidence that a larger circuit of primarily motor and learning areas (e.g., cerebellum) are also activated. The test has been used in a variety of clinical groups and appears to have maximal utility in motor conditions, although it also correlates with daily functional outcomes and can be useful in this regard.

Demographic effects influence performance, especially age and gender. Education appears relatively less influential. Although data are limited, ethnicity affected performance in one large-scale normative study (Heaton et al., 2004). Test-retest reliability is quite variable, ranging from marginal to very high. Practice effects tend to be small. Ashendorf et al. (2015) have introduced an abbreviated form that appears to be quite promising.

Heaton et al. (2004) offer a large normative database spanning a broad age and education range and stratified by relevant demographic variables. Greer et al. (2010) offer normative data for a large sample, but many of the studies included did not report important demographic characteristics. Additionally, these data are adjusted for age and education, not gender. Ashendorf et al. (2009) provide a dataset for older adults that may be useful when working with this population.

The test has been used rather extensively in research on performance validity. Like many embedded indicators, the FTT overall has medium sensitivity; note, however, that detection accuracy is variable depending on base rate of impairment and context of assessment (e.g., litigating vs. clinical), diagnosis, IQ, and gender and also shows interactions among these variables in research. The appropriate cutoff score may thus vary depending on the specific clinical population. Overall, like all PVTs, the FTT is most useful in combination with other PVTs, with caveats regarding its use in dementia and certain psychiatric disorders.

REFERENCES

Arias, P., Robles-García, V., Espinosa, N., Corral, Y., & Cudeiro, J. (2012). Validity of the Finger Tapping Test in Parkinson's disease, elderly and young healthy subjects: Is there a role for central fatigue? *Clinical Neurophysiology, 123*(10), 2034–2041. http://doi.org/10.1016/j.clinph.2012.04.001

Arnold, B. R., Montgomery, G. T., Castaneda, I., & Longoria, R. (1994). Acculturation and performance of Hispanics on selected Halstead-Reitan neuropsychological tests. *Assessment, 1,* 239–248.

Arnold, G., Boone, K. B., Lu, P., Dean, A., Wen, J., Nitch, S., & McPherson, S. (2005). Sensitivity and specificity of Finger Tapping Test scores for the detection of suspect effort. *The Clinical Neuropsychologist, 19,* 105–120.

Ashendorf, L., Horwitz, J. E., & Gavett, B. E. (2015). Abbreviating the Finger Tapping Test. *Archives of Clinical Neuropsychology, 30*(2), 99–104. http://doi.org/10.1093/arclin/acu091

Ashendorf, L., Vanderslice-Barr, J. L., & McCaffrey, R. J. (2009). Motor tests and cognition in healthy older adults. *Applied Neuropsychology, 16*(3), 171–176. http://doi.org/10.1080/09084280903098562

Atagun, M., Balaban, O., Lordoglu, D., & Evren, E. (2013). Lithium and Valproate may effect motor and sensory speed in patients with bipolar disorder. *Bulletin of Clinical Psychopharmacology,* 1. http://doi.org/10.5455/bcp.20130304010158

Austin, D., Jimison, H., Hayes, T., Mattek, N., Kaye, J., & Pavel, M. (2011). Measuring motor speed through typing: a surrogate for the Finger Tapping Test. *Behavior Research Methods, 43*(4), 903–909. http://doi.org/10.3758/s13428-011-0100-1

Axelrod, B. N., Meyers, J. E., & Davis, J. J. (2014). Finger Tapping Test performance as a measure of performance validity. *The Clinical Neuropsychologist, 28*(5), 876–888. http://doi.org/10.1080/13854046.2014.907583

Barnes, G. W., & Lucas, G. J. (1974). Cerebral dysfunction vs. psychogenesis in Halstead-Reitan tests. *The Journal of Nervous and Mental Disease, 158,* 50–60.

Bergendal, G., Martola, J., Stawiarz, L., Kristoffersen-Wiberg, M., Fredrikson, S., & Almkvist, O. (2013). Callosal atrophy in multiple sclerosis is related to cognitive speed. *Acta Neurologica Scandinavica, 127*(4), 281–289. http://doi.org/10.1111/ane.12006

Bernard, L. C. (1989). Halstead-Reitan neuropsychological test performance of Black, Hispanic, and White young adult males from poor academic backgrounds. *Archives of Clinical Neuropsychology, 4,* 267–274.

Bigler, E. D., & Tucker, D. M. (1981). Comparison of Verbal IQ, Tactual Performance, Seashore Rhythm and Finger Oscillation tests in the blind and brain damaged. *Journal of Clinical Psychology, 37,* 849–851.

Bornstein, R. A. (1985). Normative data on selected neuropsychological measures from a nonclinical sample. *Journal of Clinical Psychology, 41,* 651–659.

Bornstein, R. A. (1986a). Normative data on intermanual differences on three tests of motor performance. *Journal of Clinical and Experimental Neuropsychology, 8,* 12–20.

Bornstein, R. A. (1986b). Consistency of intermanual discrepancies in normal and unilateral brain lesion patients. *Journal of Consulting and Clinical Psychology, 54,* 719–723.

Bornstein, R. A. (1986c). Classification rates obtained with "standard" cut-off scores on selected neuropsychological measures. *Journal of Clinical and Experimental Neuropsychology, 8,* 413–420.

Bornstein, R. A., Baker, G. B., & Douglas, A. B. (1987). Short-term retest reliability of the Halstead-Reitan Battery in a normal sample. *Journal of Nervous and Mental Disease, 175,* 229–232.

Camara, W. J., Nathan, J. S., & Puente, A. E. (2000). Psychological test usage: Implications in professional psychology. *Professional Psychology: Research and Practice, 31,* 141–154.

Carlier, M., Dumont, A. M., Beau, J., & Michel, F. (1993). Hand performance of French children on a Finger Tapping Test in relation to handedness, sex and age. *Perceptual and Motor Skills, 76,* 931–940.

Chen, C., Cowles, V. E., Sweeney, M., Stolyarov, I. D., & Illarioshkin, S. N. (2012). Pharmacokinetics and pharmacodynamics of gastroretentive delivery of levodopa/carbidopa in patients with Parkinson disease: *Clinical Neuropharmacology, 35*(2), 67–72. http://doi.org/10.1097/WNF.0b013e31824523de

Chipchase, S. Y., Lincoln, N. B., & Radford, K. A. (2003). Measuring fatigue in people with multiple sclerosis. *Disability and Rehabilitation: An International Multidisciplinary Journal, 25,* 778–784.

Corey, D. M., Hurley, M. M., & Foundas, A. L. (2001). Right and left handedness defined. *Neuropsychiatry, Neuropsychology, and Behavioral Neurology, 14,* 144–152.

Criswell, S., Sterling, C., Swisher, L., Evanoff, B., & Racette, B. A. (2010). Sensitivity and specificity of the Finger Tapping task for the detection of psychogenic movement disorders. *Parkinsonism & Related Disorders, 16*(3), 197–201. http://doi.org/10.1016/j.parkreldis.2009.11.007

Da Silva, F. N., Irani, F., Richard, J., Brensinger, C. M., Bilker, W. B., Gur, R. E., & Gur, R. C. (2012). More than just tapping: Index finger-tapping measures procedural learning in schizophrenia. *Schizophrenia Research, 137*(1-3), 234–240. http://doi.org/10.1016/j.schres.2012.01.018

Dean, A. C., Victor, T. L., Boone, K. B., & Arnold, G. (2008). The Relationship of IQ to effort test performance. *The Clinical Neuropsychologist, 22*(4), 705–722. http://doi.org/10.1080/13854040701440493

Dean, A. C., Victor, T. L., Boone, K. B., Philpott, L. M., & Hess, R. A. (2009). Dementia and effort test performance. *The Clinical Neuropsychologist, 23*(1), 133–152. http://doi.org/10.1080/13854040701819050

Dikmen, S. S., Machamer, J. E., Winn, H. R., & Temkin, N. R. (1995). Neuropsychological outcome at 1-year post head injury. *Neuropsychology, 9,* 80–90.

Dikmen, S., & Morgan, S. F. (1980). Neuropsychological factors related to employability and occupational status in person with epilepsy. *Journal of Nervous and Mental Disease, 168,* 236–240.

Dikmen, S. S., Heaton, R. K., Grant, I., & Temkin, N. R. (1999). Test-retest reliability and practice effects of the expanded Halstead-Reitan neuropsychological test battery. *Journal of the International Neuropsychological Society, 5,* 346–356.

Dodrill, C. B. (1978). A neuropsychological battery for epilepsy. *Epilepsia, 19,* 611–623.

Dodrill, C. B. (1979). Sex differences on the Halstead-Reitan Neuropsychological Battery and on other neuropsychological measures. *Journal of Clinical Psychology, 35,* 236–241.

Dodrill, C. B., & Troupin, A. S. (1975). Effects of repeated administrations of a comprehensive neuropsychological battery among chronic epileptics. *Journal of Nervous and Mental Disease, 161,* 185–190.

Duffield, T. C., Trontel, H. G., Bigler, E. D., Froehlich, A., Prigge, M. B., Travers, B., . . . Lainhart, J. (2013). Neuropsychological investigation of motor impairments in autism. *Journal of Clinical and Experimental Neuropsychology, 35*(8), 867–881. http://doi.org/10.1080/13803395.2013.827156

Dufouil, C., Alperovitch, A., & Tzourio, C. (2003). Influence of education on the relationship between white matter lesions and cognition. *Neurology, 60,* 831–836.

Finlayson, M. A., & Reitan, R. M. (1976). Handedness in relation to measures of motor and tactile-perceptual function in normal children. *Perceptual and Motor Skills, 43,* 475–481.

Finlayson, M. A. J., & Reitan, R. M. (1980). Effect of lateralized lesions on ipsilateral and contralateral motor functioning. *Journal of Clinical Neuropsychology, 2,* 237–243.

Fleishman, E. A., & Hempel, W. E. (1954). A factor analysis of dexterity tests. *Personnel Psychology, 7,* 15–32.

Fromm-Auch, D., & Yeudall, L. T. (1983). Normative data for the Halstead-Reitan neuropsychological tests. *Journal of Clinical Neuropsychology, 5,* 221–238.

Gill, D. M., Reddon, J. R., Stefanyk, W. O., & Hans, H. S. (1986). Finger Tapping: Effects of trials and sessions. *Perceptual and Motor Skills, 62,* 674–678.

Goldstein, S. G., & Braun, L. S. (1974). Reversal of expected transfer as a function of increased age. *Perceptual and Motor Skills, 38,* 1139–1145.

Goldstein, G., & Watson, J. R. (1989). Test-retest reliability of the Halstead-Reitan battery and the WAIS in a neuropsychiatric population. *The Clinical Neuropsychologist, 3,* 265–273.

Greer, S. E., Brewer, K. K., Cannici, J. P., & Pennett, D. L. (2010). Level of performance accuracy for core Halstead-Reitan measures by pooling normal controls from published studies: Comparison with existing norms in a clinical sample. *Perceptual and Motor Skills, 111*(1), 3–18. http://doi.org/10.2466/03.22.27.PMS.111.4.3-18

Greiffenstein, M. F., & Baker, W. J. (2008). Validity testing in dually diagnosed post-traumatic stress disorder and mild closed head injury. *The Clinical Neuropsychologist, 22*(3), 565–582. http://doi.org/10.1080/13854040701377810

Greiffenstein, M. F., Baker, W. J., & Gola, T. (1996). Motor dysfunction profiles in traumatic brain injury and postconcussion syndrome. *Journal of the International Neuropsychological Society, 2,* 477–485.

Haaland, K. Y., & Delaney, H. D. (1981). Motor deficits after left or right hemisphere damage due to stroke or tumor. *Neuropsychologia, 19,* 17–27.

Haaland, K. Y., Temkin, N., Randahl, G., & Dikmen, S. (1994). Recovery of simple motor skills after head injury. *Journal of Clinical and Experimental Neuropsychology, 16,* 448–456.

Halstead, W. C. (1947). *Brain and Intelligence.* Chicago: University of Chicago Press.

Harris, M., Cross, H., Van Nieuwkerk, R. (1981). The effects of state depression, induced depression and sex on the Finger Tapping and Tactual Performance tests. *Clinical Neuropsychology, 3,* 28–34.

Heaton, R. K., Chelune, G. J., & Lehman, R. A. W. (1978). Using neuropsychological and personality tests to assess the likelihood of patients employment. *Journal of Nervous and Mental Disease, 166,* 408–516.

Heaton, R. K., Grant, I., & Mathews, C. G. (1991). *Comprehensive Norms for an Expanded Halstead-Reitan Battery.* Odessa, Fla.: Psychological Assessment Resources.

Heaton, R. K., Miller, S. W., Taylor, M. J., & Grant, I. (2004). *Revised comprehensive norms for an expanded Halstead-Reitan Battery: Demographically adjusted neuropsychological norms for African American and Caucasian adults.* Lutz, FL: PAR.

Heaton, R. K., Smith, H. H., Lehman, R. A., & Vogt, A. T. (1978). Prospects for faking believable deficits on neuropsychological testing. *Journal of Consulting and Clinical Psychology, 46,* 892–900.

High Jr, W. M., Briones-Galang, M., Clark, J. A., Gilkison, C., Mossberg, K. A., Zgaljardic, D. J., . . . Urban, R. J. (2010). Effect of growth hormone replacement therapy on cognition after traumatic brain injury. *Journal of Neurotrauma, 27*(9), 1565–1575.

Hohler, A. D., Zuzuárregui, J. R. P., Katz, D. I., DePiero, T. J., Hehl, C. L., Leonard, A., . . . Saint-Hilaire, M. (2012). Differences in motor and cognitive function in patients with Parkinson's disease with and without orthostatic hypotension. *International Journal of Neuroscience, 122*(5), 233–236.

Hom, J., & Reitan, R. M. (1982). Effect of lateralized cerebral damage upon contralateral and ipsilateral sensorimotor performances. *Journal of Clinical Neuropsychology, 4,* 249–268.

Hom, J., & Reitan, R. M. (1990). Generalized cognitive function after stroke. *Journal of Clinical and Experimental Neuropsychology, 12,* 644–655.

Horton, A. M. (1999). Above-average intelligence and neuropsychological test score performance. *International Journal of Neuroscience, 99,* 221–231.

Hubel, K. A., Reed, B., Yund, E. W., Herron, T. J., & Woods, D. L. (2013a). Computerized measures of Finger Tapping: Effects of hand dominance, age, and sex. *Perceptual and Motor Skills, 116*(3), 929–952. http://doi.org/10.2466/25.29.PMS.116.3.929-952

Hubel, K. A., Yund, E. W., Herron, T. J., & Woods, D. L. (2013b). Computerized measures of Finger Tapping: Reliability, malingering and traumatic brain injury. *Journal of Clinical and Experimental Neuropsychology, 35*(7), 745–758. http://doi.org/10.1080/13803395.2013.824070

Johnson, S. C., & Prigatano, G. P. (2000). Functional MR imaging during finger tapping. *BNI Quarterly, 16,* 155–158.

Kennedy, J. E., Clement, P. F., & Curtiss, G. (2003). WAIS-III Processing Speed Index scores after TBI: The influence of working memory, psychomotor speed and perceptual processing. *The Clinical Neuropsychologist, 17,* 303–307.

Khan, T., Nyholm, D., Westin, J., & Dougherty, M. (2014). A computer vision framework for finger-tapping evaluation in Parkinson's disease. *Artificial Intelligence in Medicine, 60*(1), 27–40. http://doi.org/10.1016/j.artmed.2013.11.004

Kivircik Akdede, B. B., Alptekin, K., Kitiş, A., Arkar, H., & Akvardar, Y. (2005). Effects of quetiapine on cognitive functions in schizophrenia. *Progress in Neuro-Psychopharmacology and Biological Psychiatry, 29*(2), 233–238. http://doi.org/10.1016/j.pnpbp.2004.11.005

Larrabee, G. J. (2003). Detection of malingering using atypical performance patterns on standard neuropsychological tests. *The Clinical Neuropsychologist, 17,* 410–425.

Leckliter, I. N., & Matarzazzo, J. D. (1989). The influence of age, education, IQ, gender, and alcohol abuse on Halstead-Reitan neuropsychological test battery performance. *Journal of Clinical Psychology, 45,* 484–512.

Lewis, R., & Kupke, T. (1992). Intermanual differences on skilled and unskilled motor tasks in nonlateralized brain dysfunction. *The Clinical Neuropsychologist, 6,* 374–382.

Lim, J., Oh, I. K., Han, C., Huh, Y. J., Jung, I.-K., Patkar, A. A., . . . Jang, B.-H. (2013). Sensitivity of cognitive tests in four cognitive domains in discriminating MDD patients from healthy controls: A meta-analysis. *International Psychogeriatrics, 25*(09), 1543–1557. http://doi.org/10.1017/S1041610213000689

Lundorff, L., Jonsson, B., & Sjogren, P. (2009). Modafinil for attentional and psychomotor dysfunction in advanced cancer: A double-blind, randomised, cross-over trial. *Palliative Medicine, 23*(8), 731–738. http://doi.org/10.1177/0269216309106872

Lynch, J. K. (2005). Effect of a third party observer on neuropsychological test performance following closed head injury. *Journal of Forensic Neuropsychology, 4*(2), 17–25. http://doi.org/10.1300/J151v04n02_02

Massman, P. J., & Doody, R. S. (1996). Hemispheric asymmetry in Alzheimer's disease is apparent in motor functioning. *Journal of Clinical and Experimental Neuropsychology, 18,* 110–121.

Matarazzo, J. D., Wiens, A. N., Matarazzo, R. G., & Goldstein, S. G. (1974). Psychometric and clinical test-retest reliability of the Halstead Impairment Index in a sample of healthy, young, normal men. *Journal of Nervous and Mental Disease, 158,* 37–49.

McCurry, S. M., Gibbons, L. E., Uomoto, J. M., Thompson, M. L., Graves, A. B., Edland, S. D., Bowne, J., McCormick, W. C., & Larson, E. B. (2001). Neuropsychological test performance in a cognitively intact sample of older Japanese American adults. *Archives of Clinical Neuropsychology, 16,* 447–459.

Meyers, J. E., & Volbrecht, M. E. (2003). A validation of multiple malingering detection methods in a large clinical sample. *Archives of Clinical Neuropsychology, 18*(3), 261–276.

Mitrushina, M. M., Boone, K. B., Razani, J., & D'Elia, L. F. (2005). *Handbook of normative data for neuropsychological assessment* (2nd Ed.) New York: Oxford University Press.

Morrison, M. W., Gregory, R. J., & Paul, J. J. (1979). Reliability of the Finger Tapping Test and a note on sex differences. *Perceptual and Motor Skills, 48,* 139–142.

Muller, G., Weisbrod, S., & Klingberg, F. (1991). Finger tapping frequency and accuracy are decreased in early stage primary degenerative dementia. *Dementia, 2,* 169–172.

Munro, C. A., Longmire, C. F., Drye, L. T., Martin, B. K., Frangakis, C. E., Meinert, C. L., . . . Schneider, L. S. (2012). Cognitive outcomes after sertaline treatment in patients with depression of Alzheimer disease. *The American Journal of Geriatric Psychiatry, 20*(12), 1036–1044.

Nagasaki, H., Itoh, H., Maruyama, H., & Hashizume, K. (1988). Characteristic difficulty in rhythmic movement with aging and its relation to Parkinson's disease. *Experimental Aging Research, 14,* 171–176.

Neu, D., Kajosch, H., Peigneux, P., Verbanck, P., Linkowski, P., & Le Bon, O. (2011). Cognitive impairment in fatigue and sleepiness associated conditions. *Psychiatry Research, 189*(1), 128–134. http://doi.org/10.1016/j.psychres.2010.12.005

Ott, B. R., Ellias, S. A., & Lannon, M. C. (1995). Quantitative assessment of movement in Alzheimer's disease. *Journal of Geriatric Psychiatry and Neurology, 8,* 71–75.

Peters, M. (1990). Subclassification of non-pathological left-handers poses problems for theories of handedness. *Neuropsychologia, 28,* 279–289.

Prigatano, G. P., Altman, I. M., & O'Brien, K. P. (1990). Behavioral limitations that traumatic brain-injured patients tend to underestimate. *The Clinical Neuropsychologist, 4,* 163–176.

Prigatano, G. P., & Borgano, S. R. (2003). Qualitative features of finger movement during the Halstead Finger Oscillation Test following traumatic brain injury. *Journal of the International Neuropsychological Society, 9,* 128–133.

Prigatano, G. P., Johnson, S. C., & Gale, S. D. (2004). Neuroimaging correlates of the Halstead Finger Tapping Test several years post-traumatic brain injury. *Brain Injury, 18*(7), 661–669. http://doi.org/10.1080/02699050310001646170

Prigatano, G., & Wong, J. L. (1997). Speed of finger tapping and goal attainment after unilateral cerebral vascular accident. *Archives of Physical Medicine and Rehabilitation, 78,* 847–852.

Provins, K. A., & Cunliffe, P. (1972). The reliability of some motor performance tests of handedness. *Neuropsychologia, 10,* 199–206.

Rabin, L. A., Barr, W. B., & Burton, L. A. (2005). Assessment practices of clinical neuropsychologists in the United States and Canada: A survey of INS, NAN, and APA Division 40 members. *Archives of Clinical Neuropsychology, 20,* 33–65.

Rapport, L. J., Farchione, T. J., Coleman, R. D., & Axelrod, B. N. (1998). Effects of coaching on malingered motor function profiles. *Journal of Clinical and Experimental Neuropsychology, 20,* 89–97.

Reitan, R. M. (1969). *Manual for administration of neuropsychological test batteries for adults and children.* Indianapolis, Ind.

Reitan, R. M., & Wolfson, D. (1985). *The Halstead-Reitan Neuropsychological Test Battery: Theory and interpretation.* Tucson, AZ: Neuropsychology Press.

Reitan, R. M., & Wolfson, D. (1994). Dissociation of motor impairment and higher-level brain deficits in strokes and cerebral neoplasms. *The Clinical Neuropsychologist, 8,* 193–208.

Reitan, R. M., & Wolfson, D. (1996). Relationships between specific and general tests of cerebral functioning. *The Clinical Neuropsychologist, 10,* 37–42.

Roivainen, E. (2011). Gender differences in processing speed: A review of recent research. *Learning and Individual Differences, 21*(2), 145–149. http://doi.org/10.1016/j.lindif.2010.11.021

Roy, E. A., Clark, P., Aigbogun, S., & Quare-Storer, P. A. (1992). Ipsilesional disruptions to reciprocal finger tapping. *Archives of Clinical Neuropsychology, 7,* 213–219.

Ruff, R. M., & Parker, S. B. (1993). Gender- and age-specific changes in motor speed and eye-hand coordination in adults: Normative values for the Finger Tapping and Grooved Pegboard tests. *Perceptual and Motor Skills, 76,* 1219–1230.

Russell, E. W., & Starkey, R. (1993). *Halstead-Russell Neuropsychological Evaluation System—Revised (HRNES-R).* Los Angeles: Western Psychological Services.

Salinsky, M. C., Storzbach, D., Dodrill, C. B., & Binder, L. M. (2001). Test-retest bias, reliability, and regression equations for neuropsychological measures repeated over a 12–16-week period. *Journal of the International Neuropsychological Society, 7,* 597–605.

Sánchez-Cubillo, I., Periáñez, J. A., Adrover-Roig, D., Rodríguez-Sánchez, J. M., Ríos-Lago, M., Tirapu, J., & Barceló, F. (2009). Construct validity of the Trail Making Test: Role of task-switching, working memory, inhibition/interference control, and visuomotor abilities. *Journal of the International Neuropsychological Society, 15*(03), 438. http://doi.org/10.1017/S1355617709090626

Searight, H. R., Dunn, E. J., Grisso, T., Margolis, R. B., et al. (1989). The relation of the Halstead-Reitan neuropsychological battery to ratings of everyday functioning in a geriatric sample. *Neuropsychology, 3,* 135–145.

Schmidt, S. L., Oliveira, R. M., Krahe, T. E., & Filgueiras, C. C. (2000). The effect of hand preference and gender on finger tapping performance asymmetry by the use of an infra-red light measurement device. *Neuropsychologia, 38,* 529–534.

Shimoyama, I., Ninchoji, T., & Uemura, K. (1990). The Finger Tapping Test: A quantitative analysis. *Archives of Neurology, 47,* 681–684.

Sjogren, P., Thomsen, A., & Olsen, A. K. (2000). Impaired neuropsychological performance in chronic non-malignant pain patients receiving long-term oral opioid therapy. *Journal of Pain and Symptom Management, 19,* 100–108.

Smith, K., Boone, K., Victor, T., Miora, D., Cottingham, M., Ziegler, E., . . . Wright, M. (2014). Comparison of credible patients of very low intelligence and noncredible patients on neurocognitive performance validity indicators. *The Clinical Neuropsychologist, 28*(6), 1048–1070. http://doi.org/10.1080/13854046.2014.931465

Stanford, M. S., & Barratt, E. S. (1996). Verbal skills, finger tapping, and cognitive tempo define a second-order factor of temporal information processing. *Brain and Cognition, 31,* 35–45.

Thompson, L. L., Heaton, R. K., Mathews, C. G., & Grant, I. (1987). Comparison of preferred and nonpreferred hand performance on four neuropsychological motor tasks. *The Clinical Neuropsychologist, 1,* 324–334.

Tobe, R. H., Bansal, R., Xu, D., Hao, X., Liu, J., Sanchez, J., & Peterson, B. S. (2010). Cerebellar morphology in Tourette syndrome and obsessive-compulsive disorder. *Annals of Neurology, 67*(4), 479–487. http://doi.org/10.1002/ana.21918

Trahan, D. E., Patterson, J., Quintana, J., & Biron, R. (1987). *The Finger Tapping Test: A re-examination of traditional hypotheses regarding normal adult performance.* Paper presented at the International Neuropsychological Society, Washington, D.C.

Triggs, W. J., Calvanio, R., Levine, M., Heaton, R. K., & Heilman, K. M. (2000). Predicting hand preference with performance on motor tasks. *Cortex, 36,* 679–689.

Trueblood, W., & Schmidt, M. (1993). Malingering and other validity considerations in the neuropsychological evaluation of mild head injury. *Journal of Clinical and Experimental Neuropsychology, 15,* 578–590.

Wefel, J. S., Hoyt, B. D., & Massman, P. J. (1999). Neuropsychological functioning in depressed versus nondepressed participants with Alzheimer's disease. *The Clinical Neuropsychologist, 13,* 249–257.

Welch, L. W., Cunningham, A. T., Eckardt, M. J., & Martin, P. R. (1997). Fine motor speed deficits in alcoholic Korsakoff 's syndrome. *Alcoholism: Clinical and Experimental Research, 21,* 134–139.

Whearty, K. M., Allen, D. N., Lee, B. G., & Strauss, G. P. (2015). The evaluation of insufficient cognitive effort in schizophrenia in light of low IQ scores. *Journal of Psychiatric Research, 68,* 397–404. http://doi.org/10.1016/j.jpsychires.2015.04.018

Yamashita, H. (2014). Intermanual differences on neuropsychological motor tasks in a Japanese university student sample: Neuropsychological motor tasks: Intermanual difference. *Japanese Psychological Research, 56*(2), 103–113. http://doi.org/10.1111/jpr.12039

Yang, Y. K., Chiu, N. T., Chen, C. C., Chen, M., Yeh, T. L., & Lee, I. H. (2003). Correlation between fine motor activity and striatal dopamine D_2 receptor density in patients with schizophrenia and healthy controls. *Psychiatry Research: Neuroimaging, 123,* 191–197.

Yang, Y. K., Yeh, T. L., Chiu, N. T., Lee, I. H., Chen, P. S., Lee, L.-C., & Jeffries, K. J. (2004). Association between cognitive performance and striatal dopamine binding is higher in timing and motor tasks in patients with schizophrenia. *Psychiatry Research: Neuroimaging, 131*(3), 209–216. http://doi.org/10.1016/j.pscychresns.2003.07.002

Ylikoski, R., Ylikoski, A., Erkinjuntti, T., Sulkava, R., Keskivaara, P., Raininko, R., & Tilvis, R. (1998). Differences in neuropsychological functioning associated with age, education, neurological status, and magnetic resonance imaging findings in neurologically healthy elderly individuals. *Applied Neuropsychology, 5,* 1–4.

Yokoe, M., Okuno, R., Hamasaki, T., Kurachi, Y., Akazawa, K., & Sakoda, S. (2009). Opening velocity, a novel parameter, for finger tapping test in patients with Parkinson's disease. *Parkinsonism & Related Disorders, 15*(6), 440–444. http://doi.org/10.1016/j.parkreldis.2008.11.003

GRIP STRENGTH

TEST NAME	**Grip Strength**
DOMAIN	Fine motor strength
AGE RANGE	Up to 85 years
ADMINISTRATION TIME	5 minutes
SCORING FORMAT	Hand scored
REFERENCE	Reitan, R. M., & Wolfson, D. (1985). *The Halstead-Reitan Neuropsychological Test Battery: Theory and interpretation*. Tucson, AZ: Neuropsychology Press.

DESCRIPTION

The purpose of Grip Strength is to measure the strength of voluntary grip movements of each hand, which serves as an index of the integrity of motor function (Reitan & Davison, 1974; Reitan & Wolfson, 1985). The test requires the examinee to hold the upper part of the dynamometer in the palm of their hand and squeeze the stirrup with the fingers as hard as they possibly can (Smedley version). According to Reitan and Wolfson (1985), two measurements within 5 kilograms of each other are recorded for each hand. The mean is calculated for each hand separately.

ADMINISTRATION

The procedure proposed by Reitan and Wolfson (1985), shown in Figure 14–1, is typically used, which involves a Smedley (spring) dynamometer. A Jamar dynamometer, which is a hydraulic hand dynamometer, has also been used, typically in the occupational and ergonomic literature (see the section "Normative Data"). Influences on performance have been reported in the literature. As might be expected, pain is associated with decreased strength (Pienimaeki et al., 2002). Some research has reported that fatigue associated with cognitive effort does not affect Grip Strength (Paul et al., 1998); however, others have reported negative impacts of fatigue on performance in older adults following multiple measurements (Abizanda et al., 2012). Wu, Wu, Liang, Wu, and Huang (2009) reported that palm length was related to Grip Strength, and others have reported relationships between physical parameters (e.g., body mass index) and performance (see discussion by Ekşioğlu, 2016; Werle et al., 2009). Occupation may also be influential, with manual workers exhibiting better Grip Strength in some studies (see Anakwe et al., 2007; Ekşioğlu, 2016; Werle et al., 2009). Observation by a third party was associated with a facilitation effect on Grip Strength, in the range of a small to medium effect size (Lynch, 2005). Finally, Shapiro, Crews, Harrison, and Everhart (1996) reported that ambient sensory conditions (e.g., bright light, noise) exert a minimal effect on Grip Strength.

> Ask the examinee to stand, if able. The length of the dynamometer stirrup should be adjusted to the size of the subject's hand (see Instrument Manual). Demonstrate the use of the instrument to the subject. Indicate that the lower pointer will register the grip, so that the subject does not have to continue gripping while the scale is read. Then place the dynamometer in the subject's preferred hand (palm down) and instruct the subject to hold their arm down at the side and away from the body. The subject is then told to squeeze the dynamometer as hard as possible, taking as much time as needed to squeeze to the maximum. Allow two recorded trials with each hand, preferred and nonpreferred alternately, with pauses between each trial to avoid excessive fatigue. If either an increase or a decrease of more than 5 kg occurs on the second trial for either hand, wait a few moments and provide a third trial.

Figure 14–1 *Instructions for grip strength.*

DEMOGRAPHIC EFFECTS

AGE

Grip Strength declines with advancing age in adults (e.g., Bornstein, 1985; Christensen et al., 2001, 2004; Ernst, 1988; Ekşioğlu, 2016; Heaton et al., 2004; MacDonald et al., 2004; Mitrushina et al., 2005), and approximately 5–7% of the variance in tests scores is accounted for by age (Heaton et al., 2004).

Individuals with weaker Grip Strength tend to score lower on cognitive tests (e.g., slowed reaction times; Anstey et al., 2005). Changes in Grip Strength over a three- to four-year period also correlate moderately with changes in cognitive functioning (e.g., information processing speed and memory); that is, they tend to move together longitudinally to some extent (Christensen et al., 2001, 2004). A longitudinal relationship has also been reported between Grip Strength and spatial ability and verbal reasoning in older adults, in addition to memory

(Sternäng et al., 2016). The decline may be due to common factors (e.g., vascular disease, decreased metabolic rate, programmed cell death, age-related myelin degeneration, dopaminergic depletion) that, along with specific processes, underlie age-related deterioration in cognitive and noncognitive processes (Christensen et al., 2001, 2004; Sternäng et al., 2016). Of note, poor performance is predictive of cognitive decline in older adults over a 12-year period (MacDonald et al., 2004). Poor performance also predicts mortality, even after controlling for health and demographic factors (e.g., Anstey et al., 2001; see also Cooper, Kuh, & Hardy, 2010).

GENDER

Men tend to obtain better scores than women (e.g., Bornstein, 1985; Christensen et al., 2001, 2004; Deary et al., 2011; Ernst, 1988; Ekşioğlu, 2016; Heaton et al., 2004; Mitrushina et al., 2005; Wang, 2010). In fact, gender accounts for 55 to 60% of the variance in scores (Heaton et al., 2004).

EDUCATION AND IQ

Although some have reported a positive relationship between Grip Strength and education (Bornstein, 1985), others have reported minimal education effects (Christensen et al., 2004; Heaton et al., 2004; Mitrushina et al., 2005).

ETHNICITY, NATIONALITY, AND LINGUISTIC EFFECTS

African-American women have been found to have better Grip Strength than their Caucasian peers (Rantanen et al., 1998). Northern continental European countries reportedly have higher Grip Strength than other European countries, even when other variables (e.g., age, gender, height, weight, education, health, socioeconomic status) are controlled (Andersen-Ranberg et al., 2009).

HANDEDNESS AND INTERMANUAL DIFFERENCES

Age and education do not affect the magnitude of intermanual differences (Bornstein, 1986a; Ernst, 1988). The findings regarding gender differences in intermanual difference scores are inconsistent; some studies find gender-related differences (i.e., greater between-hand differences for males than for females; Bornstein, 1986a), and others do not (Ernst, 1988; Fromm-Auch & Yeudall, 1983; Mitrushina et al., 2005; Thompson et al., 1987).

Performance tends to be better with the preferred than with the nonpreferred hand (e.g., Bornstein, 1985; Heaton et al., 2004), with estimates suggesting an approximate 10% difference in favor of the preferred hand (Bornstein, 1985, 1986a; Mitrushina et al., 2005; Triggs et al., 2000). However, there is considerable variability in the general population, and the preferred hand is not necessarily the stronger one, especially when left-handed people are considered (Bohannon, 2003; Koffler & Zehler, 1985).

Equal or better performance with the nonpreferred hand occurs with considerable regularity in the healthy population, and neurological involvement should not be inferred from an isolated lack of concordance. Even fairly large discrepancies between the hands on Grip Strength alone cannot be used to suggest unilateral impairment (Bornstein, 1986a; Koffler & Zehler, 1985; Thompson et al., 1987). Large discrepancies (i.e., more than 1 *SD* from the mean) occur in approximately 25% of the general population. Thus, the consistency of intermanual discrepancies across several motor tasks should be considered prior to determining the presence of unilateral motor impairment (Bornstein, 1986b; Thompson et al., 1987). Consistent deviant performances are infrequent in the healthy population and therefore, in the absence of musculoskeletal injury, may indicate lateralized brain dysfunction (Bornstein, 1986b; Thompson et al., 1987).

NORMATIVE DATA

Because of demographic influences on performance, the normative data provided by Heaton et al. (2004; see Table 14–8) have considerable utility. Regression-based norms are provided separately for two ethnic groups (Caucasians and African Americans) and are organized by age, gender, and education. The samples are large and cover a wide range in terms of age (20 to 85 years) and education (0 to

TABLE 14–8 Characteristics of the Heaton et al. (2004) Grip Strength Normative Sample

Number	1,482
Age (years)	20 to 85[a]
Geographic location	Various states in the United States, and Manitoba, Canada
Sample type	Individuals recruited as part of multicenter studies
Education (years)	0 to 20[b]
Gender (%)	
Male	60
Female	40
Race/Ethnicity (%)	
Caucasian	56
African American	44
Screening	No reported history of learning disability, neurological disorder, serious psychiatric disorder, or substance abuse.

[a]Age groups: 20 to 34, 35 to 39, 40 to 44, 45 to 49, 50 to 54, 55 to 59, 60 to 64, 65 to 69, 70 to 74, 75 to 79, and 80 to 89.

[b]Education groups: 7 to 8, 9 to 11, 12, 13 to 15, 16 to 17, and 18 to 20.

SOURCE: Adapted from Heaton et al. (2004). Reproduced by special permission of the Publisher, Psychological Assessment Resources, Inc. (PAR), 16204 North Florida Avenue, Lutz, FL 33549, from *Revised Comprehensive Norms for an Expanded Halstead-Reitan Battery Professional Manual*, Copyright 1991, 1992, 2004 by Psychological Assessment Resources, Inc. All rights reserved.

TABLE 14–9 Performance of Adults for Grip Strength (Kilograms), by Education, Age, and Gender

	<GRADE 12			≥GRADE 12		
AGE GROUP (YEARS)	*N*	*M*	*SD*	*N*	*M*	*SD*
Males, Preferred hand						
20–39	21	50.8	11.5	86	49.9	8.4
40–59	13	39.8	6.0	17	48.2	7.3
60–69	16	38.7	5.9	22	44.5	5.6
Males, Nonpreferred hand						
20–39	21	47.7	11.7	86	46.4	7.6
40–59	13	38.2	6.5	17	46.4	9.1
60–69	16	37.2	5.4	22	39.3	5.5
Females, Preferred hand						
20–39	13	32.7	8.7	50	31.0	5.4
40–59	22	27.7	5.9	43	29.8	5.8
60–69	22	25.6	5.3	34	25.0	4.9
Females, Nonpreferred hand						
20–39	13	31.2	8.0	50	28.7	5.0
40–59	22	24.9	6.7	43	26.9	5.4
60–69	22	24.0	6.0	34	22.8	4.8

SOURCE: From Bornstein (1985).

20 years); exclusion criteria are specified. T scores lower than 40 are classified as impaired. According to Heaton et al. (2004), the procedure used was as specified by Reitan and Wolfson (1985). It is unclear how hand preference was determined, and the data were collected over a lengthy period (25 years).

Mitrushina et al. (2005) also provide data for a large sample, compiled from five to nine studies, including 407 to 713 men and women (25 to 69 years). They noted that the integrity of their metanorms was undermined by the lack of consistency in reporting hand preference.

Table 14–9 shows norms (Bornstein, 1985) for adults 20 to 69 years of age. These are based on a sample of 365 individuals from the general population living in a large western Canadian city. They appear to be fairly similar to those provided by Heaton et al. (2004) and Mitrushina et al. (2005). The preferred hand was determined to be the hand used for signing the consent form. Unfortunately, some cell sizes were quite small (e.g., $n = 13$). Although the health status and exclusion criteria were not reported, other reports (e.g., Bornstein, 1986b) with the same sample indicated that individuals with a history of neurological or psychiatric illness were excluded from the study.

For adults aged 53–90 years, Dixon (personal communication with previous authors, April 5, 2005) provides normative data derived from a large sample of 457 typically aging, older, community-dwelling adults who participated in the Victoria Longitudinal Study (VLS), in Victoria, Canada. The sample was well-educated ($M = 15.23$ years, $SD = 2.86$), predominantly female (70%), Caucasian (98%), and considered English their primary language (90%). Individuals with MMSE scores of 24 or less, moderate/severe visual or auditory impairment even with corrective aids, or a history of significant neurological or psychiatric disorders were excluded. Hand preference was self-reported, and the test was administered with the participant standing and alternating hands. The values shown in Table 14–10 reflect the average of two trials.

Of note, a Jamar dynamometer, rather than a Smedley dynamometer, has also been used. Turkish normative data are provided for 211 (39% female) persons ages 18 to 69 years (Ekşioğlu, 2016). Values for dominant and nondominant hands were 455.2 ± 73.6 and 441.5 ± 72.6 for males and 258 ± 46.1 and 246.2 ± 49.1 for females (see Table 14–11). A sample from Scotland using the Jamar dynamometer is also provided for 250 individuals (31% female) from various occupations (Anakwe et al., 2007). The mean age of men in the study was 44.3 (range 18 to 83) years and the mean age of women was 41.6 (range 18 to 78) years. Males had a dominant hand performance mean of 48.6 ($SD = 10.96$) and nondominant mean of 44.8 ($SD = 9.81$), whereas females had a dominant hand performance mean of 28.5 ($SD = 4.6$) and nondominant mean of 26.6 ($SD = 4.9$). Normative data are also available for 1,023 Swiss participants (50% female, aged 18 to 96 years), as listed in Table 14–12 (Werle et al., 2009).

TABLE 14–10 Grip Strength (Mean and Standard Deviation [*SD*]) by Age Range (Midpoint) and Gender

	53–60 (57)	55–65 (60)	60–75 (65)	65–75 (70)	70–80 (75)	75–85 (80)	80–90 (85)
N	92	180	172	145	135	112	58
F/M	71/21	138/42	121/51	93/52	88/47	74/38	39/19
Males							
Dominant hand	44.79 (8.79)	44.15 (7.93)	42.71 (6.58)	41.79 (6.35)	39.07 (6.27)	36.27 (5.08)	34.82 (4.36)
Nondominant hand	43.26 (7.19)	42.58 (7.00)	40.72 (7.32)	39.66 (6.82)	37.06 (6.40)	33.43 (4.79)	31.81 (4.57)
Discrepancy	5.08 (4.14)	4.46 (3.19)	4.16 (3.24)	3.66 (3.17)	3.31 (2.48)	3.70 (2.76)	3.90 (2.60)
Females							
Dominant hand	27.08 (5.20)	27.10 (5.02)	26.73 (4.63)	25.31 (5.26)	23.19(5.61)	21.17 (4.30)	20.30 (3.76)
Nondominant hand	25.86 (5.43)	25.34 (5.40)	24.29 (4.87)	22.94 (4.88)	21.38 (5.39)	19.84 (4.34)	19.22 (3.36)
Discrepancy	2.22 (1.62)	2.74 (1.84)	3.16 (2.28)	3.03 (2.49)	2.65 (1.85)	2.31 (1.50)	2.20 (1.54)

NOTE: Dominance self-reported; participant standing, alternating hands, average of two trials with Smedley dynamometer.

SOURCE: R. Dixon, personal communication with previous authors, April 5, 2005.

TABLE 14–11 Grip Strength (Percentiles and Standard Deviation [*SD*]) by Age Group, Gender, and Occupation (Jamar Dynamometer)

	MALE (*N* = 128)								FEMALE (*N* = 83)							
	DOMINANT				NONDOMINANT				DOMINANT				NONDOMINANT			
	Percentile				Percentile				Percentile				Percentile			
Age-group (yrs)	5	50	95	sd	5	50	95	sd	5	50	95	sd	5	50	95	sd
18–29	333.5	463.0	591.5	78.5	326.7	451.3	575.8	75.5	185.4	253.1	320.8	41.2	162.8	242.3	321.8	48.1
30–39	357.1	467.9	577.8	66.7	350.2	447.3	544.5	58.9	228.6	299.2	369.8	43.2	216.8	287.4	358.1	43.2
40–49	364.9	453.2	542.0	54.0	348.3	453.2	558.2	63.8	229.6	284.5	339.4	33.4	204.0	268.8	333.5	39.2
50–59	349.2	431.6	514.0	50.0	301.2	398.3	495.4	58.9	216.8	249.2	281.5	19.6	185.4	235.4	285.5	30.4
(NME only) 60–69	306.1	364.9	422.8	35.3	279.6	360.0	440.5	49.1	138.3	195.2	252.1	34.3	153.0	185.4	217.8	19.6
Overall (18–69)	**334.5**	**455.2**	**575.8**	**73.6**	**321.8**	**441.5**	**561.1**	**72.6**	**182.5**	**258.0**	**333.5**	**46.1**	**165.8**	**246.2**	**326.7**	**49.1**
ME* (25–58)	386.5	477.7	569.7	55.9	372.0	464.0	556.0	55.9	–	–	–	–	–	–	–	–
NME (18–69)																
ns-NME (18–69)	325.0	444.4	563.8	72.6	282.7	419.9	557.0	83.4	190.6	264.9	339.1	45.1	178.2	254.1	329.9	46.1
s-NME (18–27)	324.7	461.1	596.4	82.4	319.6	450.3	581.0	79.5	173.3	249.2	325.0	46.1	146.3	233.5	320.6	53.0

NOTE: *ME: Manual employees, NME: Non-manual employees, ns-NME: non-student NME, s-NME: student NME.

SOURCE: Ekşioğlu (2016).

TABLE 14–12 Grip Strength by Age Group and Gender (Jamar Dynamometer)

	MEN (*N* = 496)							WOMEN (*N* = 482)						
AGE	*N*	HAND	MEAN	*SD*	SEM	MIN	MAX	*N*	HAND	MEAN	*SD*	SEM	MIN	MAX
18–19	33	D	51.2	6.6 (12.9)	1.15	33.7	64.0	31	D	32.0	4.8 (15.1)	0.87	22.7	42.7
		ND	48.3	7.7 (15.8)	1.33	28.7	63.3		ND	30.7	4.1 (13.3)	0.73	24.0	38.0
20–24	29	D	53.9	8.7 (16.2)	1.62	40.7	79.0	31	D	33.4	5.4 (16.2)	0.97	23.7	42.3
		ND	51.2	8.5 (16.6)	1.58	34.3	72.7		ND	31.5	4.8 (15.3)	0.87	19.0	38.3
25–29	30	D	53.0	7.5 (14.1)	1.36	40.7	74.3	30	D	34.3	5.7 (16.5)	1.04	22.0	45.0
		ND	50.4	7.5 (14.9)	1.37	40.0	73.3		ND	33.6	6.1 (18.1)	1.1	23.3	45.7
30–34	28	D	55.0	7.1 (12.9)	1.33	42.0	68.0	30	D	33.8	5.9 (17.3)	1.07	20.3	45.7
		ND	52.5	7.3 (13.9)	1.38	40.0	68.3		ND	32.6	4.6 (14.2)	0.85	22.3	40.0
35–39	41	D	55.9	7.9 (14.1)	1.23	36.0	73.0	42	D	35.8	6.7 (18.7)	1.02	18.7	50.0
		ND	53.6	8.7 (16.2)	1.36	37.3	73.3		ND	34.6	5.9 (17.0)	0.91	18.7	50.0
40–44	37	D	54.2	8.1 (15.0)	1.33	40.0	78.0	39	D	34.0	6.0 (16.7)	0.96	24.3	51.3
		ND	53.4	8.5 (15.9)	1.39	36.7	83.7		ND	34.7	5.3 (15.4)	0.85	25.3	45.7
45–49	31	D	51.8	8.3 (16.0)	1.49	30.7	64.0	40	D	34.1	5.3 (15.5)	0.83	24.3	47.7
		ND	60.0	7.2 (14.5)	1.3	32.3	62.7		ND	33.7	4.6 (13.7)	0.86	24.0	47.3
50–54	40	D	50.8	9.1 (17.8)	1.43	26.3	73.3	34	D	33.7	4.5 (13.2)	0.77	24.0	42.0
		ND	59.2	8.9 (18.0)	1.4	28.3	72.3		ND	33.7	4.6 (13.7)	0.79	22.7	42.7
55–59	30	D	53.6	8.6 (16.1)	1.58	35.7	72.0	28	D	31.9	4.9 (15.3)	0.92	25.3	48.0
		ND	51.1	8.0 (15.6)	1.45	37.7	69.0		ND	31.5	5.9 (18.6)	1.11	25.0	55.3
60–64	33	D	47.9	6.4 (13.3)	1.11	33.7	62.7	30	D	28.7	5.5 (19.1)	1.0	13.3	37.0
		ND	47.6	6.5 (13.7)	1.14	30.7	58.7		ND	28.3	5.3 (18.7)	0.96	15.3	35.3
65–69	46	D	43.0	6.8 (15.8)	1.0	25.3	57.0	34	D	29.5	3.6 (12.2)	0.62	23.3	36.7
		ND	42.3	6.4 (15.2)	0.95	24.0	54.0		ND	27.8	4.5 (16.1)	0.77	20.0	36.7
70–74	33	D	41.7	8.9 (21.3)	1.54	22.7	61.0	27	D	26.4	6.8 (25.6)	1.3	10.3	40.7
		ND	40.8	8.6 (21.2)	1.5	21.3	61.3		ND	26.0	5.5 (21.1)	1.06	14.3	38.0
75–79	28	D	36.8	9.7 (26.5)	1.84	19.3	52.7	26	D	25.0	4.5 (17.9)	0.88	16.7	34.7
		ND	30.7	8.9 (24.2)	1.67	19.3	52.7		ND	23.7	4.8 (20.1)	0.93	14.3	30.7
80–84	29	D	30.7	9.1 (29.5)	1.68	12.3	54.0	32	D	19.2	5.2 (27.3)	0.93	9.3	30.3
		ND	29.4	8.7 (29.6)	1.62	11.3	47.0		ND	19.7	5.1 (25.7)	0.9	9.7	29.0
>85	28	D	22.4	6.2 (27.6)	1.17	11.3	36.3	28	D	16.9	4.8 (28.1)	0.9	9.3	27.0
		ND	23.2	5.9 (25.3)	1.11	9.7	34.3		ND	16.7	4.9 (29.4)	0.93	7.7	25.7

NOTE: D, dominant hand; ND, nondominant hand.

SOURCE: Werle et al. (2009).

EVIDENCE FOR RELIABILITY

EVIDENCE FOR INTERNAL RELIABILITY

Christensen et al. (2001) reported that Cronbach's alpha was high ($r = .82$) in 838 older adults tested over four trials for each hand.

EVIDENCE FOR TEST-RETEST RELIABILITY, MEASURING CHANGE, AND PRACTICE EFFECTS

Performance of each hand is fairly reliable over test sessions, even with lengthy intervals between retest sessions (e.g., 30 months). Reliability coefficients range from .52 to .96, with most greater than .70 in both healthy individuals and those with neurologic conditions (Anstey et al., 1997; Dikmen et al., 1999; Dodrill & Troupin, 1975; Reddon et al., 1985; Thomas & Hageman, 2002; though see Burton et al., 2002).

Within a session, Grip Strength may deteriorate after an extended number of trials when brief (e.g., 15–30 seconds) intertrial intervals are used (Montazer & Thomas, 1992; Reddon et al., 1985). Performance drops significantly after two trials, with Grip Strength decreasing to about 80% with 10 trials and to about 40% in 100 trials (Montazer & Thomas, 1992). However, with longer intertrial intervals (e.g., 120 seconds), performance improves across trials (at least over a series of four trials), with the greatest increase evident after the first trial (Dunwoody et al., 1996).

In healthy young adults, performance improves to a minor extent with repeated practice over short intervals (Bornstein et al., 1987; Reddon et al., 1985). Dikmen et al. (1999) reported slight declines in scores in a sample of 384 healthy or neurologically stable individuals (aged 15–83 years, $M = 34.2$, $SD = 16.7$) retested after a nine-month interval. Table 14–13 provides information to determine whether there has been significant change, taking practice into account. One first subtracts the mean T2–T1 change (column 3) from the difference between the two testing sessions for the individual and then compares the result with 1.64 times the *SD* of the difference (column 4). The 1.64 is derived from the healthy distribution and is exceeded in the positive or negative direction only 10% of the time if indeed there is no real change in clinical condition.

EVIDENCE FOR VALIDITY

FACTOR-ANALYTIC STUDIES AND RELATIONSHIPS WITH OTHER TESTS

Factor analysis of a variety of motor and sensory tasks in older, community-dwelling adults revealed a three-factor solution (MacDonald et al., 2004). Grip Strength loaded on a sensorimotor factor, along with measures of close and distance vision, hearing in the speech frequency range, and peak expiratory flow. Grip and knee extension strength were demonstrated to reflect a common factor and are thought to be a valid indicator of limb muscle strength in older adults (Bohannon, 2012). Grip Strength relates to reasoning according to a longitudinal study, although these were not found to be casually related (Deary et al., 2011). Grip Strength was moderately related to performance in a number of cognitive domains, including working memory, semantic and episodic memory, processing, and motor speed, with relationships intensifying prior to death (Praetorius Björk et al., 2016). Also see the section "Age" for relationships between this test and variables related to health and biological aging.

CLINICAL STUDIES

TBI. Haaland, Temkin, Randahl, and Dikmen (1994) found that Grip Strength was sensitive to recovery in the first year after TBI. Healthy individuals showed no change, whereas patients with TBI improved from the one-month to the one-year evaluation. Burton et al. (2002) compared individuals with TBI and healthy controls, noting no differences between groups. However, the right-hand performance of patients with TBI was more variable, suggesting that measures taken at a single time point may not provide an accurate reflection of a patient's functioning.

Mood Disorders. Lower Grip Strength is related to depression and anxiety (Lever-van Milligen et al., 2017; van Milligen et al., 2012), and lower scores predicted persistence of anxiety and depressive symptoms in one study (van Milligen et al., 2012). Greater asymmetry between hands has also been linked to depressive and anxiety symptoms (Yu et al., 2017). Specific personality characteristics are related to Grip Strength in older adults, specifically lower Grip Strength associated with higher neuroticism and

TABLE 14–13 Grip Strength Test-Retest Effects in 384 Healthy or Neurologically Stable Individuals Assessed After a Nine-Month Mean Interval

	TIME 1		TIME 2		T2 - T1		T1, T2
MEASURE	(1) *M*	*SD*	(2) *M*	*SD*	(3) *M*	(4) *SD*	*R*
Dominant	43.34	13.33	42.41	13.44	–.93	6.09	.90
Nondominant	40.60	12.89	39.65	13.19	–.96	5.67	.91

NOTE: Interval range 2 to 16 months, *SD* = 3.0.

SOURCE: Adapted from Dikmen et al. (1999).

lower levels of openness, extraversion, agreeableness, and conscientiousness (Mueller et al., 2016).

Other Populations. Reduced Grip Strength has also been reported in a variety of other conditions, including mild cognitive impairment (Fujiwara et al., 2013), AD (Fujisawa et al., 2017), autism (Hardan et al., 2003), MS (Paul et al., 1998), chemical exposure (Ames et al., 2018; Dick et al., 2002), nonepileptic seizures (Sackellares & Sackellares, 2001), outcome post-stroke (Di Cesare et al., 2016), following rehabilitation post-stroke (Rice et al., 2016), and after unilateral posterior ventral pallidotomy in the treatment of Parkinson's disease (PD; Cahn et al., 1998). A variant of the dynamometer was used in a mixed sample of homecare patients, and a high level of weakness was noted (e.g., nearly 71% bilaterally; Bohannon, 2010). After controlling for multiple demographic and health factors, Grip Strength was independently associated with dementia in a Korean sample (Shin et al., 2012), with every 8-kilogram decrease associated with an increased risk of dementia (odds ratio 1.59).

Functional Activities. Grip Strength is related to everyday functioning. Impaired Grip Strength in older adults is related to reduced levels of daily function (e.g., Femia et al., 2001; Judge et al., 1996) and, in conjunction with other measures, is a predictor of fall risk in older adults (Bauermeister et al., 2017), especially in those with cognitive impairment (Welmer et al., 2017). The test is predictive of functional decline over a three-year period (Ishizaki et al., 2000). Grip Strength demonstrated small associations with progression to disability in older adults in a systematic review (den Ouden et al., 2011). As noted earlier, poor performance is also predictive of cognitive decline (MacDonald et al., 2004) and mortality (Anstey et al., 2001) in older adults. As part of the African American Health Project, Miller et al. (2010) reported that decreases in Grip Strength were more likely in men with cardiovascular disease, limited activities of daily living (ADLs), lower body functional limitations, high blood pressure, and high body mass.

A variant of Grip Strength was one of the predictors of driving cessation in older adults, along with age and residency type (e.g., living in care vs. at home; Carr et al., 2006). Grip Strength is one of the measures used to index frailty in older adults (Chen et al., 2016; Heuberger, 2011; Woo et al., 2012). The hand dynamometer was identified as a suitable measure for evaluating physical fitness in older adults with intellectual disabilities (Hilgenkamp et al., 2010).

In stroke patients, Grip Strength can be used as a gross index of recovery of arm function and has some prognostic value. Sunderland, Tinson, Bradley, and Langton-Hewer (1989) noted that the absence of measureable Grip Strength one month after stroke indicated that there would be poor outcome with regard to motor function. If there was detectable grip at one month, then there would likely be at least a rudimentary level of function five months later. A variant of Grip Strength, along with other variables, was one of the best predictors of functional outcome and ADLs six months post-stroke (Woldag et al., 2006).

NEUROANATOMICAL CORRELATES, LESION STUDIES, AND IMAGING STUDIES

The midbody corpus callosal area was associated with Grip Strength via MRI in older adults, consistent with relations between this region and motor cortex (Anstey et al., 2007). Grip Strength is useful in differentiating individuals with neurologic conditions and healthy controls and in detecting the laterality of brain lesions (Bornstein, 1986b; Dodrill, 1978; Hom & Reitan, 1982; Lewis & Kupke, 1990). As expected, right-hemisphere lesions tend to depress performance on the left hand, and left-hemisphere lesions tend to lower performance on the right hand. Dodrill (1978) reported that the dynamometer correctly identified the side of brain lesions with higher accuracy than either the Finger Tapping Test or the Tactual Performance Test, which may be due to its simplicity and low demands on skill and adaptation (Haaland et al., 1994; Lewis & Kupke, 1990). Reduced Grip Strength was related to reduced thalamic and caudate volume in older adults with human immunodeficiency virus (HIV) infection (Kallianpur et al., 2016). Grip Strength was related to gamma-aminobutyric acid (GABA) decrease in patients with MS (Cawley et al., 2015).

PERFORMANCE VALIDITY

A number of investigators (e.g., Greiffenstein et al., 1996; Heaton et al., 1978; Rapport, Farchione, Coleman, & Axelrod, 1998) have reported that Grip Strength may be useful as an index of performance validity; however, the data at present are mixed.

For example, Greiffenstein et al. (1996) observed that compensation-seeking patients with postconcussion syndrome demonstrated a nonphysiological profile (Grip Strength < Finger Tapping < Grooved Pegboard Test) compared with a group of patients with TBI whose performance followed a gradient of increasing impairment corresponding to the complexity of these tasks. However, Rapport et al. (1998) found that the presence of nonphysiological configurations showed poor predictive accuracy among simulators and controls. The authors also found that a significant proportion of healthy individuals show poorer performance on Grip Strength compared with fine motor tasks and cautioned that the motor dysfunction profile does not appear to be a reliable or valid decision-making tool that can be used independently in performance validity assessment. Note that Davis, Wall, Ramos, Whitney, and Barisa (2010) reported that variables measured by force curve analysis via a digital variant of the dynamometer (average to peak ratio) discriminated between controls and simulators; no differences in performance were found on the Smedley dynamometer. This may suggest some promise for variables

TABLE 14–14 Sensitivity and Specificity of Grip Strength Estimates in Detection of Credible and Noncredible Performance

AUTHOR	CV CUTOFF VALUE	SENSITIVITY	PERCENT OF MISCLASSIFIED SUBMAXIMAL EFFORTS	SPECIFICITY	PERCENT OF MISCLASSIFIED MAXIMAL EFFORTS
Dvir, 1990	95% Level of Confidence	.44	66%	NS	NC
Hamilton-Farifax, 1995	15%	.39	61%	.92	8%
	7.5%	.78	22%	.19	81%
Mitterhauser, 1997	15%	.74	26%	.98	2%
Robinson, 1993	15%	.31	69%	NS	NC
	11%	.45	55%	NS	NC
Shechtman, 2001	15%	.55	45%	.94	6%
	11%	.69	31%	.82	18%

Abbreviation: Not specified in article; NC = Not calculated.

SOURCE: Shechtman et al. (2006).

measured via digital variants of Grip Strength in performance validity assessment.

The coefficient of variation (CV) is one metric that has been used to evaluate performance validity using Grip Strength. The CV reflects variability and is computed by dividing the standard deviation (*SD*) of three or more consecutive trials by the mean and multiplying by 100 [CV = (*SD*/Mean) × 100]. The CV is expressed as a percentage, with greater CV reflecting larger variability. In their meta-analysis, Shechtman, Anton, Kanasky, and Robinson (2006) reported variable but overall poor sensitivity (31–78%) and specificity (19–98%) for the CV in the detection of noncredible performance, with misclassifications ranging from 2% to 81%. See Table 14–14 for estimates by study. Test-retest reliability of the CV was also very poor (.02 to .25). Given these findings, the CV for Grip Strength is not recommended as a measure of performance validity.

COMMENT

Reitan and Wolfson's (1985) procedure is commonly used, although other variants exist. There are a number of influences on performance that are relevant for clinical settings: pain can decrease performance, as can fatigue, particularly in older adults across multiple measurements. Performance can decrease across many trials, especially with brief intertrial intervals, and a rest time of one minute between trials is recommended. Although the preferred hand is typically stronger than the nonpreferred hand, the opposite pattern is not uncommon in healthy populations. Additionally, the difference score has been associated with weak reliability in some research. Therefore, an isolated finding of a pattern of superior nonpreferred hand performance should not be interpreted as reflecting neurologic impairment.

Grip Strength correlates with many physical parameters and general health variables and is related to age. Gender appears highly influential, with men performing better than women. Education effects appear to be relatively small. There appear to be differences regionally and ethnically. The normative data provided by Heaton et al. (2004) are large and adjusted for important demographic variables. The data provided by Dixon et al. also have many strengths and utility for older adults. There are also normative data available for the Jamar version of the instrument.

In terms of reliability, internal reliability is high. Test-retest reliability is variable, but adequate overall. There are relatively small practice effects. Clinically, the test has been used in a fairly heterogeneous group of clinical populations and has shown utility in lateralization and lesion studies. Grip Strength is related to a wide range of functional outcomes, which may reflect the test's association with general health and biological aging variables, as discussed in "Demographic Effects." Performance validity research is mixed, and the coefficient of variation, derived as a possible performance validity estimate, is not recommended for use.

REFERENCES

Abizanda, P., Navarro, J. L., García-Tomás, M. I., López-Jiménez, E., Martínez-Sánchez, E., & Paterna, G. (2012). Validity and usefulness of hand-held dynamometry for measuring muscle strength in community-dwelling older persons. *Archives of Gerontology and Geriatrics*, *54*(1), 21–27. http://doi.org/10.1016/j.archger.2011.02.006

Ames, J., Warner, M., Brambilla, P., Mocarelli, P., Satariano, W. A., & Eskenazi, B. (2018). Neurocognitive and physical functioning in the Seveso Women's Health Study. *Environmental Research*, *162*, 55–62. https://doi.org/10.1016/j.envres.2017.12.005

Anakwe, R. E., Huntley, J. S., & McEachan, J. E. (2007). Grip strength and forearm circumference in a healthy population. *The Journal of Hand Surgery, European Volume*, *32*(2), 203–209. https://doi.org/10.1016/J.JHSB.2006.11.003

Andersen-Ranberg, K., Petersen, I., Frederiksen, H., Mackenbach, J. P., & Christensen, K. (2009). Cross-national differences in grip strength among 50+ year-old Europeans: results from the SHARE study. *European Journal of Ageing*, *6*(3), 227–236.

Anstey, K. J., Luszcz, M. A., Giles, L. C., & Andrews, G. R. (2001). Demographic, health, cognitive, and sensory variables as predictors of mortality in very old adults. *Psychology and Aging*, *16*(1), 3.

Anstey, K. J., Dear, K., Christensen, H., & Jorn, A. F. (2005). Biomarkers, health, lifestyle, and demographic variables as correlates of reaction time performance in early, middle, and late adulthood. *The Quarterly Journal of Experimental Psychology, 58A,* 5–21.

Anstey, K. J., Mack, H. A., Christensen, H., Li, S.-C., Reglade-Meslin, C., Maller, J., . . . Sachdev, P. (2007). Corpus callosum size, reaction time speed and variability in mild cognitive disorders and in a normative sample. *Neuropsychologia, 45*(8), 1911–1920. http://doi.org/10.1016/j.neuropsychologia.2006.11.020

Anstey, K. J., Smith, G. A., & Lord, S. (1997). Test-retest reliability of a battery of sensory, motor and physiological measures of aging. *Perceptual and Motor Skills, 84,* 831–834.

Bauermeister, S., Sutton, G., Mon-Williams, M., Wilkie, R., Graveson, J., Cracknell, A., . . . Bunce, D. (2017). Intraindividual variability and falls in older adults. *Neuropsychology, 31*(1), 20.

Bohannon, R. W. (2003). Grip strength: A summary of studies comparing dominant and nondominant limb measurements. *Perceptual and Motor Skills, 96,* 728–730.

Bohannon, R. W. (2010). Grip strength impairments among older adults receiving physical therapy in a home-care setting. *Perceptual and Motor Skills, 111*(3), 761–764. http://doi.org/10.2466/03.10.15.PMS.111.6.761-764

Bohannon, R. W. (2012). Are hand-grip and knee extension strength reflective of a common construct?. *Perceptual and Motor Skills, 114*(2), 514–518. http://doi.org/10.2466/03.26.PMS.114.2.514-518

Bornstein, R. A. (1985). Normative data on selected neuropsychological measures from a nonclinical sample. *Journal of Clinical Psychology, 41,* 651–659.

Bornstein, R. A. (1986a). Normative data on intermanual differences on three tests of motor performance. *Journal of Clinical and Experimental Neuropsychology, 8,* 12–20.

Bornstein, R. A. (1986b). Consistency of intermanual discrepancies in normal and unilateral brain lesion patients. *Journal of Consulting and Clinical Psychology, 54,* 719–723.

Bornstein, R. A., Baker, G. B., & Douglas, A. B. (1987). Short-term retest reliability of the Halstead-Reitan Battery in a normal sample. *Journal of Nervous and Mental Disease, 175,* 229–232.

Burton, C. L., Hultsch, D. F., Strauss, E., & Hunter, M. A. (2002). Intraindividual variability in physical and emotional functioning: Comparison of adults with traumatic brain injuries and healthy adults. *The Clinical Neuropsychologist, 16,* 264–279.

Cahn, D. A., Sullivan, E. V., Shear, P. K., Heit, G., Lim, K. O., Marsh, L., Lane, B., Wasserstein, P., & Silverberg, G. D. (1998). Neuropsychological motor functioning after unilateral anatomically guided posterior ventral pallidotomy: Preoperative performance and three-month follow-up. *Neuropsychiatry, Neuropsychology, & Behavioral Neurology, 11,* 136–145.

Carr, D. B., Flood, K. L., Steger-May, K., Schechtman, K. B., & Binder, E. F. (2006). Characteristics of frail older adult drivers. *Journal of the American Geriatrics Society, 54*(7), 1125–1129. http://doi.org/10.1111/j.1532-5415.2006.00790.x

Cawley, N., Solanky, B. S., Muhlert, N., Tur, C., Edden, R. A. E., Wheeler-Kingshott, C. A. M., . . . Ciccarelli, O. (2015). Reduced gamma-aminobutyric acid concentration is associated with physical disability in progressive multiple sclerosis. *Brain, 138*(9), 2584–2595. https://doi.org/10.1093/brain/awv209

Chen, S., Honda, T., Narazaki, K., Chen, T., Nofuji, Y., & Kumagai, S. (2016). Global cognitive performance and frailty in non-demented community-dwelling older adults: Findings from the Sasaguri Genkimon Study: Global cognitive performance and frailty. *Geriatrics & Gerontology International, 16*(6), 729–736. https://doi.org/10.1111/ggi.12546

Christensen, H., Mackinnon, A. J., Korten, A., & Jorm, A. F. (2001). The "Common Cause Hypothesis" of cognitive aging: Evidence for not only a common factor but also specific associations of age with vision and grip strength in a cross-sectional analysis. *Psychology and Aging, 16,* 588–599.

Christensen, H., Mackinnon, A. J. Jorm, A. F., Korten, A., Jacomb, P., Hofer, S. M., & Henderson, S. (2004). The Canberra Longitudinal Study: Design, aims, methodology, outcomes and recent empirical investigations. *Aging, Neuropsychology and Cognition, 11,* 169–195.

Cooper, R., Kuh, D., & Hardy, R. (2010). Objectively measured physical capability levels and mortality: systematic review and meta-analysis. *BMJ, 341,* c4467.

Davis, J. J., Wall, J. R., Ramos, C. K., Whitney, K. A., & Barisa, M. T. (2010). Using grip strength force curves to detect simulation: A preliminary investigation. *Archives of Clinical Neuropsychology, 25*(3), 204–211. http://doi.org/10.1093/arclin/acq002

Deary, I. J., Johnson, W., Gow, A. J., Pattie, A., Brett, C. E., Bates, T. C., & Starr, J. M. (2011). Losing one's grip: A bivariate growth curve model of grip strength and nonverbal reasoning from age 79 to 87 years in the lothian birth cohort 1921. *The Journals of Gerontology Series B: Psychological Sciences and Social Sciences, 66B* (6), 699–707. http://doi.org/10.1093/geronb/gbr059

den Ouden, M. E. M., Schuurmans, M. J., Arts, I. E. M. A., & van der Schouw, Y. T. (2011). Physical performance characteristics related to disability in older persons: A systematic review. *Maturitas, 69*(3), 208–219. http://doi.org/10.1016/j.maturitas.2011.04.008

Di Cesare, F., Mancuso, J., Silver, B., & Loudon, P. T. (2016). Assessment of Cognitive and Neurologic Recovery in Ischemic Stroke Drug Trials: Results from a Randomized, Double-blind, Placebo-controlled Study. *Innovations in Clinical Neuroscience, 13*(9–10), 32.

Dick, F., Semple, S., Osborne, A., Soutar, A., Seaton, A., Cherrie, J. W., Walker, L. G., & Haites, N. (2002). Organic solvent exposure, genes, and risk of neuropsychological impairment. *QJM: Monthly Journal of the Association of Physicians, 95,* 379–387.

Dikmen, S. S., Heaton, R. K., Grant, I., & Temkin, N. R. (1999). Test-retest reliability and practice effects of expanded Halstead-Reitan neuropsychological test battery. *Journal of the International Neuropsychological Society, 5,* 346–356.

Dodrill, C. B. (1978). The hand dynamometer as a neuropsychological measure. *Journal of Consulting and Clinical Psychology, 46,* 1432–1435.

Dodrill, C. B., & Troupin, A. S. (1975). Effects of repeated administrations of a comprehensive neuropsychological battery among chronic epileptics. *Journal of Nervous and Mental Disease, 161,* 185–190.

Dunwoody, L., Tittmar, H. G., & McClean, W. S. (1996). Grip strength and intertrial rest. *Perceptual & Motor Skills, 83,* 275–278.

Dvir, Z. (1999). Coefficient of variation in maximal and feigned static and dynamic grip efforts. *American Journal of Physical Medicine & Rehabilitation, 78*(3), 216–221.

Ernst, J. (1988). Language, grip strength, sensory-perceptual, and receptive skills in a normal elderly sample. *The Clinical Neuropsychologist, 2,* 30–40.

Ekşioğlu, M. (2016). Normative static grip strength of population of Turkey, effects of various factors and a comparison with international norms. *Applied Ergonomics, 52,* 8–17. https://doi.org/10.1016/j.apergo.2015.06.023

Fairfax, A. H., Balnave, R., & Adams, R. D. (1995). Variability of grip strength during isometric contraction. *Ergonomics, 38*(9), 1819–1830.

Femia, E. E., Zarit, S. H., & Johansson, B. (2001). The disablement process in very late life. *Journal of Gerontology Series B: Psychological Sciences and Social Sciences, 56,* P12–P23.

Fromm-Auch, D., & Yeudall, L. T. (1983). Normative data for the Halstead-Reitan Neuropsychological Tests. *Journal of Clinical Neuropsychology, 5,* 221–238.

Fujisawa, C., Umegaki, H., Okamoto, K., Nakashima, H., Kuzuya, M., Toba, K., & Sakurai, T. (2017). Physical function differences between the stages from normal cognition to moderate Alzheimer disease. *Journal of the American Medical Directors Association, 18*(4), 368–e9.

Fujiwara, Y., Suzuki, H., Kawai, H., Hirano, H., Yoshida, H., Kojima, M., . . . Obuchi, S. (2013). Physical and sociopsychological characteristics of older community residents with mild cognitive impairment as assessed by the Japanese version of the Montreal Cognitive

Assessment. *Journal of Geriatric Psychiatry and Neurology, 26*(4), 209–220. https://doi.org/10.1177/0891988713497096

Greiffenstein, M. F., Baker, W. J., & Gola, T. (1996). Motor dysfunction profiles in traumatic brain injury and postconcussion syndrome. *Journal of the International Neuropsychological Society, 2,* 477–485.

Haaland, K. Y., Temkin, N., Randahl, G., & Dikmen, S. (1994). Recovery of simple motor skills after head injury. *Journal of Clinical and Experimental Neuropsychology, 16,* 448–456.

Hardan, A. Y., Kilpatrick, M., Keshavan, M. S., & Minshew, N. J. (2003). Motor performance and anatomic Magnetic Resonance Imaging (MRI) of the basal ganglia in autism. *Journal of Child Neurology, 18,* 317–324.

Heaton, R. K., Miller, S. W., Taylor, M. J., & Grant, I. (2004). *Revised comprehensive norms for an expanded Halstead-Reitan Battery: Demographically adjusted neuropsychological norms for African American and Caucasian adults.* Lutz, FL: PAR.

Heaton, R. K., Smith, H. H., Lehman, R. A., & Vogt, A. T. (1978). Prospects for faking believable deficits on neuropsychological testing. *Journal of Consulting and Clinical Psychology, 46,* 892–900.

Heuberger, R. A. (2011). The Frailty Syndrome: A comprehensive review. *Journal of Nutrition in Gerontology and Geriatrics, 30*(4), 315–368. http://doi.org/10.1080/21551197.2011.623931

Hilgenkamp, T. I. M., van Wijck, R., & Evenhuis, H. M. (2010). Physical fitness in older people with ID—Concept and measuring instruments: A review. *Research in Developmental Disabilities, 31*(5), 1027–1038. http://doi.org/10.1016/j.ridd.2010.04.012

Hom, J., & Reitan, R. M. (1982). Effect of lateralized cerebral damage upon contralateral and ipsilateral sensorimotor performances. *Journal of Clinical Neuropsychology, 4,* 249–268.

Ishizaki, T., Watanabe, S., Suzuki, T., Shibata, H., & Haga, H. (2000). Predictors of functional decline among nondisabled older Japanese living in a community during a 3-year follow-up. *Journal of the American Geriatrics Society, 48,* 1424–1429.

Judge, J. O., Schechtman, K., & Cress, E. (1996). The relationship between physical performance measures and independence in instrumental activities of daily living. *Journal of the American Geriatrics Society, 44,* 1332–1341.

Kallianpur, K. J., Sakoda, M., Gangcuangco, L. M. A., Ndhlovu, L. C., Umaki, T., Chow, D., . . . Shikuma, C. M. (2016). Frailty characteristics in chronic HIV patients are markers of white matter atrophy independently of age and depressive symptoms: A pilot study. *Open Medicine Journal, 3,* 138–152. https://doi.org/10.2174/1874220301603010138

Koffler, S. P., & Zehler, D. (1985). Normative data for the hand dynamometer. *Perceptual and Motor Skills, 61,* 589–590.

Lever-van Milligen, B. A., Lamers, F., Smit, J. H., & Penninx, B. W. J. H. (2017). Six-year trajectory of objective physical function in persons with depressive and anxiety disorders. *Depression and Anxiety, 34*(2), 188–197. https://doi.org/10.1002/da.22557

Lewis, R., & Kupke, T. (1990). Intermanual differences on skilled and unskilled motor tasks in nonlateralized brain dysfunction. *The Clinical Neuropsychologist, 6,* 374–382.

Lynch, J. K. (2005). Effect of a Third Party Observer on Neuropsychological Test Performance Following Closed Head Injury. *Journal of Forensic Neuropsychology, 4*(2), 17–25. http://doi.org/10.1300/J151v04n02_02

MacDonald, S. W. S., Dixon, R. A., Cohen, A-L., & Hazlitt, J. E. (2004). Biological age and 12-year cognitive change in older adults: Findings from the Victoria Longitudinal Study. *Gerontology, 50,* 64–81.

Miller, D. K., Malmstrom, T. K., Miller, J. P., Andresen, E. M., Schootman, M., & Wolinsky, F. D. (2010). Predictors of Change in Grip Strength Over 3 Years in the African American Health Project. *Journal of Aging and Health, 22*(2), 183–196. http://doi.org/10.1177/0898264309355816

Mitrushina, M. N., Boone, K. B., Razani, J., *&* d'Elia, L. F. (2005). *Handbook of Normative data for neuropsychological assessment* (2nd Ed.) New York: Oxford University Press.

Montazer, M. A., & Thomas, J. G. (1992). Grip strength as a function of 200 repetitive trials. *Perceptual and Motor Skills, 75,* 1320–1322.

Mueller, S., Wagner, J., Drewelies, J., Duezel, S., Eibich, P., Specht, J., . . . Gerstorf, D. (2016). Personality development in old age relates to physical health and cognitive performance: Evidence from the Berlin Aging Study II. *Journal of Research in Personality, 65,* 94–108. https://doi.org/10.1016/j.jrp.2016.08.007

Paul, R. H., Beatty, W. W., Schneider, R., Blanco, C. R., & Hames, K. A. (1998). Cognitive and physical fatigue in multiple sclerosis: Relations between self-report and objective performance. *Applied Neuropsychology, 5,* 143–148.

Pienimaeki, T., Tarvainen, T., Siira, P., Malmivaara, A., & Vanharanta, H. (2002). Associations between pain, grip strength, and manual tests in the treatment evaluation of chronic tennis elbow. *Clinical Journal of Pain, 18,* 164–170.

Praetorius Björk, M., Johansson, B., & Hassing, L. B. (2016). I forgot when I lost my grip—strong associations between cognition and grip strength in level of performance and change across time in relation to impending death. *Neurobiology of Aging, 38,* 68–72. https://doi.org/10.1016/j.neurobiolaging.2015.11.010

Rantanen, T., Guralnik, J. M., Leveille, S., Izmirlian, G., Simonsick, E., Ling, S., & Fried, L. P. (1998). Racial differences in muscle strength in disabled older women. *Journal of Gerontology: Series A: Biological Sciences and Medical Sciences, 53A,* B355–B361.

Rapport, L. J., Farchione, T. J., Coleman, R. D., & Axelrod, B. N. (1998). Effects of coaching on malingered motor function profiles. *Journal of Clinical and Experimental Neuropsychology, 20,* 89–97.

Reddon, J. R., Stefanyk, W. O., Gill, D. M., & Renney, C. (1985). Hand dynamometer: Effects of trials and sessions. *Perceptual and Motor Skills, 61,* 1195–1198.

Reitan, R. M., & Davison, L. A. (1974). *Clinical Neuropsychology: Current Status and Applications.* Washington, DC: V. H. Winston.

Reitan, R. M., & Wolfson, D. (1985). *The Halstead-Reitan Neuropsychological Test Battery: Theory and interpretation.* Tucson, AZ: Neuropsychology Press.

Rice, D., Janzen, S., McIntyre, A., Vermeer, J., Britt, E., & Teasell, R. (2016). Comprehensive outpatient rehabilitation program: hospital-based stroke outpatient rehabilitation. *Journal of Stroke and Cerebrovascular Diseases, 25*(5), 1158–1164. https://doi.org/10.1016/j.jstrokecerebrovasdis.2016.02.007

Robinson, M. E., Geisser, M. E., Hanson, C. S., & O'Connor, P. D. (1993). Detecting submaximal efforts in grip strength testing with the coefficient of variation. *Journal of Occupational Rehabilitation, 3*(1), 45–50.

Sackellares, D. K., & Sackellares, J. C. (2001). Impaired motor function in patients with psychogenic pseudoseizures. *Epilepsia, 42,* 1600–1606.

Shapiro, D. M., Crews, W. D., Harrison, D. W., & Everhart, D. E. (1996). Age differences in hemispheric activation to sensory condition. *International Journal of Neuroscience, 87,* 249–256.

Shechtman, O. (2001). The coefficient of variation as a measure of sincerity of effort of grip strength, Part II: sensitivity and specificity. *Journal of Hand Therapy, 14*(3), 188–194.

Shechtman, O., Anton, S. D., Kanasky Jr, W. F., & Robinson, M. E. (2006). The use of the coefficient of variation in detecting sincerity of effort: a meta-analysis. *Work, 26*(4), 335–341.

Shin, H.-Y., Kim, S.-W., Kim, J.-M., Shin, I.-S., & Yoon, J.-S. (2012). Association of grip strength with dementia in a Korean older population: Grip strength and dementia. *International Journal of Geriatric Psychiatry, 27*(5), 500–505. http://doi.org/10.1002/gps.2742

Sternäng, O., Reynolds, C. A., Finkel, D., Ernsth-Bravell, M., Pedersen, N. L., & Dahl Aslan, A. K. (2016). Grip Strength and Cognitive Abilities: Associations in Old Age. *The Journals of Gerontology Series B: Psychological Sciences and Social Sciences, 71*(5), 841–848. https://doi.org/10.1093/geronb/gbv017

Sunderland, A., Tinson, D., Bradley, L., & Langton-Hewer, R. (1989). Arm function after stroke. An evaluation of grip strength as a measure of recovery and a prognostic indicator. *Journal of Neurology, Neurosurgery, and Psychiatry, 52,* 1267–1272.

Thomas, V. S., & Hageman, P. A. (2002). A preliminary study on the reliability of physical performance measures in older day-care center clients with dementia. *International Psychogeriatrics, 14,* 17–23.

Thompson, L. L., Heaton, R. K., Mathews, C. G., & Grant, I. (1987). Comparison of preferred and nonpreferred hand performance on four neuropsychological motor tasks. *The Clinical Neuropsychologist, 1,* 324–334.

Triggs, W. J., Calvanio, R., Levine, M., Heaton, R. K., & Heilman, K. M. (2000). Predicting hand preference with performance on motor tasks. *Cortex, 36,* 679–689.

van Milligen, B. A., Vogelzangs, N., Smit, J. H., & Penninx, B. W. J. H. (2012). Physical function as predictor for the persistence of depressive and anxiety disorders. *Journal of Affective Disorders, 136*(3), 828–832. http://doi.org/10.1016/j.jad.2011.09.030

Wang, C. Y. (2010). Hand dominance and grip strength of older Asian adults. *Perceptual and Motor Skills, 110*(3), 897–900.

Welmer, A.-K., Rizzuto, D., Laukka, E. J., Johnell, K., & Fratiglioni, L. (2017). Cognitive and physical function in relation to the risk of injurious falls in older adults: A population-based study. *The Journals of Gerontology. Series A, Biological Sciences and Medical Sciences, 72*(5), 669–675. https://doi.org/10.1093/gerona/glw141

Werle, S., Goldhahn, J., Drerup, S., Simmen, B. R., Sprott, H., & Herren, D. B. (2009). Age-and gender-specific normative data of grip and pinch strength in a healthy adult Swiss population. *Journal of Hand Surgery (European Volume), 34*(1), 76–84.

Woldag, H., Gerhold, L. L., de Groot, M., Wohlfart, K., Wagner, A., & Hummelsheim, H. (2006). Early prediction of functional outcome after stroke. *Brain Injury, 20*(10), 1047–1052. http://doi.org/10.1080/02699050600915422

Woo, J., Leung, J., & Morley, J. E. (2012). Comparison of frailty indicators based on clinical phenotype and the multiple deficit approach in predicting mortality and physical limitation. *Journal of the American Geriatrics Society, 60*(8), 1478–1486. http://doi.org/10.1111/j.1532-5415.2012.04074.x

Wu, S.-W., Wu, S.-F., Liang, H.-W., Wu, Z.-T., & Huang, S. (2009). Measuring factors affecting grip strength in a Taiwan Chinese population and a comparison with consolidated norms. *Applied Ergonomics, 40*(4), 811–815. https://doi.org/10.1016/j.apergo.2008.08.006

Yu, J., Rawtaer, I., Mahendran, R., Kua, E.-H., & Feng, L. (2017). Degree, but not direction of grip strength asymmetries, is related to depression and anxiety in an elderly population. *Laterality: Asymmetries of Body, Brain and Cognition, 22*(3), 268–278. https://doi.org/10.1080/1357650X.2016.1184677

GROOVED PEGBOARD TEST

TEST NAME	**Grooved Pegboard Test**
DOMAIN	Fine motor dexterity
AGE RANGE	In adults, to 85 years
ADMINISTRATION TIME	5 minutes
SCORING FORMAT	Hand scored
REFERENCE	Matthews, C. G., & Klove, K. (1964). *Instruction manual for the Adult Neuropsychology Test Battery.* Madison: University of Wisconsin Medical School.

DESCRIPTION

The Grooved Pegboard Test (GPT; Matthews & Klove, 1964) measures eye-hand coordination and motor speed. The GPT consists of a metal board with a matrix of 25 holes with randomly positioned slots (see Figure 14–2). Pegs have a ridge along one side and must be rotated to match the hole before they can be inserted. The examinee's task is to insert metal pegs as quickly as possible into the slots in sequence, first with the dominant hand and then with the nondominant hand. The examinee continues until all pegs have been placed. The score is the time in seconds required to complete the array with each hand.

The test is also part of the Halstead-Russell Neuropsychological Evaluation System (HRNES; Russell & Starkey, 1993). The score is computed for each hand separately, as is the time required to place the pegs. Some researchers also record the number of pegs not placed and the number of pegs dropped. Although some research suggests that dropping errors are rarely seen in neurologically healthy individuals (Heaton et al., 2004), in Ashendorf, Vanderslice-Barr, and McCaffrey's (2009) sample of older individuals, 59% of examinees dropped at least one peg with either hand, and almost 16% dropped at least one peg with each hand (see the section "Normative Data").

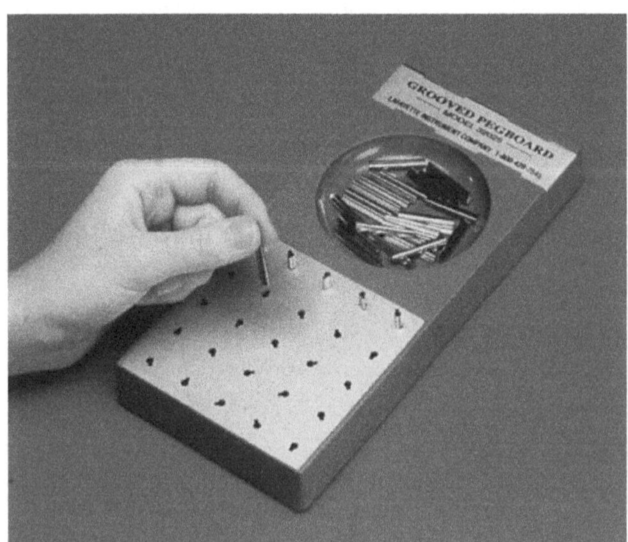

Figure 14–2 Grooved Pegboard Test (GPT).

The standard version of the GPT involves speeded placement of the pegs (Place task). Bryden, Roy, Rohr, and Eglio (2007) created a novel variant (Remove task), which involves removing pegs under timed conditions. Remove versions of the task are completed considerably faster than Place versions of the task.

ADMINISTRATION

The instructions are provided in the manual. Briefly, the apparatus is placed with the peg tray oriented above the pegboard. The examinee is instructed to insert the pegs, matching the groove of the peg with the groove of the hole, filling the rows in a given direction as quickly as possible, without skipping any slots. Using the right hand, the examinee is asked to work from left to right and, with the left hand, in the opposite direction. The dominant hand is tested first. The examinee is instructed that only one peg should be picked up at a time and that only one hand is to be used. If a peg is dropped, the examiner does not retrieve it; rather, one of the pegs correctly placed (usually, the first or second peg) is taken out and used again.

The examiner demonstrates one row before the examinee begins. A practice trial is not given, and a trial may discontinue after five minutes. In the HRNES version (Russell & Starkey, 1993), the examinee continues until all pegs have been placed or until a time limit of three minutes has been reached. In both versions, the examiner begins timing after cueing the examinee to begin. Directionality of peg placement for the left-hand condition (right to left vs. left to right) did not affect performance (Fouty et al., 2015). Of note, third-party observation has not been noted to affect test scores on this task (Lynch, 2005), nor has rapport (Barnett et al., 2017). However, poor performance can relate to non-neurologic factors, such as deficits in tactile acuity (Tremblay et al., 2002). See also "Clinical Studies."

DEMOGRAPHIC EFFECTS

AGE

Performance declines with advancing age (e.g., Ashendorf et al., 2009; Bornstein, 1985; Mitrushina et al., 2005; Ruff & Parker, 1993). In their study of older adults, Ashendorf et al. (2009) noted that the younger group in their sample (55- to 64-year-olds) performed better than the older group. According to Heaton et al. (2004), about 30 to 34% of the variance in test scores is accounted for by age.

GENDER

Some have found significant gender differences in performance, with women outperforming men (Ashendorf et al., 2009; Bornstein, 1985; Bryden & Roy, 2005; Fouty et al., 2015; Ruff & Parker, 1993), perhaps reflecting differences in finger size (Peters et al., 1990). However, others have noted that gender has little effect on performance (Ayesa-Arriola et al., 2016; Mitrushina et al., 2005), accounting for less than 1% of the variance in test scores (Heaton et al., 2004).

EDUCATION AND IQ

Some have reported that individuals with more years of education perform faster (Ruff & Parker, 1993). However, others report that education has minimal effect (Ashendorf et al., 2009; Bornstein, 1985; Mitrushina et al., 2005), accounting for about 3 to 6% of the variance in test scores (Heaton et al., 2004).

ETHNICITY, NATIONALITY, AND LINGUISTIC EFFECTS

The impact of ethnicity and other sociodemographic variables has not been reported.

HAND PREFERENCE AND INTERMANUAL DIFFERENCES

Age, education, and hand preference are not related to intermanual differences scores (Bornstein, 1986c; Ruff & Parker, 1993; Thompson et al., 1987); however, intermanual differences may be larger for women than men (Thompson et al., 1987; but see Bornstein, 1986c). Handedness does not affect test scores (Ruff & Parker, 1993).

Typically, performance of the preferred and nonpreferred hands is compared on motor tasks to determine whether there is consistent evidence of poor performance with one hand relative to the other. Performance is typically faster with the dominant/preferred hand (Bryden & Roy, 2005; Bryden et al., 2007; Heaton et al., 2004), with estimates of nearly a four-second difference in right-handed participants for right versus left hand performance (Bryden et al., 2007) or as much as seven seconds in other studies (Bryden & Roy, 2005). Others have reported that performance with the preferred hand is superior (by about 10%) compared to that of the nonpreferred hand (Mitrushina et al., 2005; Thompson et al., 1987).

However, like other motor tests reviewed in this volume, there is considerable variability in the healthy population, and the preferred hand is not necessarily the faster one (Bornstein, 1986c; Corey et al., 2001), especially when left-handed people are considered (Corey et al., 2001; Thompson et al., 1987). Equal or better performance with the nonpreferred hand occurs in a quarter of the healthy population, and neurological involvement should not be inferred from an isolated lack of concordance. Furthermore, discrepancies of a large magnitude on the test are not uncommon (about 20%) in the healthy population (Bornstein, 1986b; Thompson et al., 1987). In addition, intermanual discrepancies are imperfect predictors of the side of lesion (Bornstein, 1986a). Thus, the consistency of intermanual discrepancies across several motor tasks should be considered prior to determining the presence of unilateral motor impairment (Bornstein, 1986b; Thompson et al., 1987).

NORMATIVE DATA

The use of simple cutoff scores is not recommended because reliance on simple cutoff scores yields a high rate of misclassification (Bornstein, 1986b). Normative data provided by Trites (1977) are available in the manual; however, the sample is not well-described, and the data are not stratified by gender. Heaton et al. (2004) provide normative data based on a large sample of Caucasians and African Americans (see Table 14–15). They provide norms separately for these two ethnicity groups, organized by age, gender, and education. The dataset covers a wide range in terms of age (20 to 85 years) and education (0 to 20 years), and exclusion criteria are specified. T scores lower than 40 are classed as impaired. According to Heaton et al. (2004), the procedure used was the one specified by the Lafayette Instrument Company. The method for determining hand preference was not described.

Hamby, Bardy, and Wilkins (1997) examined performance in individuals with HIV and reported that the GPT may not be well-suited for identifying subtle deficits or making fine discriminations because of ceiling effects. The restriction in range complicates conversions between one score to the other (e.g., to z scores and percentiles) and can decrease accuracy in determining level of performance. For example, a dominant hand GPT score of 74.1 seconds yields a z score of −.5 (using the Hamby mean and *SD*). If the data were normally distributed, this would convert to a percentile score of 31% (average range). However, the actual percentile for that score, according to the sample distribution, is 13% (below average). Therefore, an examinee's performance may be determined to be within healthy limits when it actually indicates some degree of impairment. As a result, Hamby et al. (1997) recommend that norms for the test include true percentiles, not merely the mean and *SD*.

TABLE 14–15 Characteristics of the Heaton et al. (2004) Grooved Pegboard Normative Sample

Number	1,482
Age (years)	20 to 85[a]
Geographic location	Various states in the United States, and Manitoba, Canada
Sample type	Individuals recruited as part of multicenter studies
Education (years)	0 to 20[b]
Gender (%)	
Male	60
Female	40
Ethnicity (%)	
Caucasian	56
African American	44
Screening	No reported history of learning disability, neurological disorder, serious psychiatric disorder, or substance abuse.

[a]Age groups: 20 to 34, 35 to 39, 40 to 44, 45 to 49, 50 to 54, 55 to 59, 60 to 64, 65 to 69, 70 to 74, 75 to 79, and 80 to 89 years.

[b]Education groups: 7 to 8, 9 to 11, 12, 13 to 15, 16 to 17, and 18 to 20 years.

SOURCE: Adapted from Heaton et al. (2004). Reproduced by special permission of the Publisher, Psychological Assessment Resources, Inc. (PAR), 16204 North Florida Avenue, Lutz, FL 33549, from *Revised comprehensive norms for an expanded Halstead-Reitan Battery professional manual*, Copyright 1991, 1992, 2004 by Psychological Assessment Resources, Inc. All rights reserved.

Mitrushina et al. (2005) provide metanorms based on six studies and representing 2,382 participants, 20–64 years of age. They note that the integrity of the results is undermined by the lack of consistency in the method of reporting hand preference. Table 14–16 provides data (Ruff & Parker, 1993) based on a sample of 357 individuals 16 to 70 years of age, with education levels ranging from 7 to 22 years. Participants were screened to exclude those with a history of psychiatric hospitalization, chronic polysubstance abuse, or neurological disorders. Hand preference was evaluated using a lateral dominance examination. The data are relatively consistent with those provided by Mitrushina et al. (2005).

TABLE 14–16 Mean Performance of Adults for the Grooved Pegboard Test (GPT), by Education, Age, and Gender

AGE GROUP (YEARS)	≤GRADE 12 *N*	*M*	*SD*	>GRADE 12 *N*	*M*	*SD*
Females, Preferred hand						
16–39	30	62.8	8.9	60	57.8	6.2
40–54	14	63.1	4.4	30	63.3	7.4
55–70	15	78.6	11.7	29	75.3	11.3
Females, Nonpreferred hand						
16–39	29	66.8	10.7	60	65.2	10.3
40–54	14	69.6	6.5	30	70.8	8.9
55–70	13	84.3	15.3	29	82.0	12.5
Males, Preferred hand						
16–39	29	67.8	9.2	60	64.7	10.9
40–54	15	71.9	15.1	30	70.4	10.9
55–70	15	83.7	10.2	30	74.1	13.0
Males, Nonpreferred hand						
16–39	29	74.5	10.9	59	67.8	10.8
40–54	15	79.1	14.9	30	73.7	9.9
55–70	15	91.0	12.7	28	83.5	13.4

NOTE: Based on a sample of 357 healthy participants.

SOURCE: From Ruff and Parker (1993).

TABLE 14–17A Mean Performance of Adults by Age and Gender

		MEN AGE 55–64 N = 79	MEN AGE 65–74 N = 65	WOMEN AGE 55–64 N = 78	WOMEN AGE 65–74 N = 71
Dom	*M*	78.0	90.0	74.7	83.9
	SD	14.5	19.5	11.4	18.1
NDom	*M*	83.5	98.8	80.9	89.2
	SD	17.8	21.4	15.0	18.2
Ratio	*M*	0.95	0.92	0.94	0.95
	SD	0.14	0.15	0.12	0.13

NOTE: Ratio = dominant ÷ nondominant hand performance; *M* = mean, *SD* = standard deviation.

SOURCE: Ashendorf et al. (2009).

Ashendorf et al. (2009) present normative data for the GPT and the Finger Tapping Test for more than 300 older (55- to 74-year-old) community-dwelling adults. Participants were a mean age of 63.9 years (*SD* = 6.0), 51% female, with an average education level of 13.8 (*SD* = 2.6 years). The North American Adult Reading Test (NAART) mean score was 107.3 (*SD* = 8.9). All participants were Caucasian and lived in New York. Exclusion criteria were: current treatment for depression, current alcohol or substance abuse, neurodegenerative or neurological condition, HIV or AIDS, or severe arthritis prohibiting completion of motor tests. Table 14–17a presents age- and gender-adjusted data, and the cumulative percentage for the number of pegs dropped is shown in Table 14–17b.

Bryden and Roy (2005) provided normative data for two GPT versions: Place, the conventional task involving speeded placement of pegs, and Remove, the novel task involving speeded removal of pegs. Participants included more than 150 (71% female) undergraduate students ranging in age from 18 to 24 years. Approximately 11% of the sample was left-handed, with more male left-handers than female left-handers (17% vs. 9%). Normative data are provided in Table 14–18.

Last, Schretlen, Testa, and Pearlson (2010) provide norms for 297 adults as part of the Calibrated

TABLE 14–17B Cumulative Percentage of Pegs Dropped

# DROPS	DOMINANT HAND (%)	NONDOMINANT HAND (%)
0	100.0	100.0
1	38.6	34.5
2	15.0	6.8
3	3.8	3.1
4+	<1.0	<1.0

NOTE: Cumulative percentages represent the percent of individuals who dropped the given number of pegs or more (e.g., 15% dropped at least two pegs with their dominant hand).

SOURCE: Ashendorf et al. (2009).

TABLE 14–18 Mean Performance on the GPT Place and Remove Task by Gender

		PLACE TASK		REMOVE TASK		LATERALITY QUOTIENT	
	WHQ	PREFERRED HAND	NONPREFERRED HAND	PREFERRED HAND	NONPREFERRED HAND	PLACE TASK	REMOVE TASK
Left-handers							
Male	1.76 (0.67)	55.2 (4.7)	64.1 (6.7)	17.2 (1.5)	17.8 (2.1)	1.5 (3.4)	7.4 (4.8)
Female	1.45 (0.69)	50.9 (3.3)	55.1 (5.2)	17.8 (3.2)	16.9 (2.6)	–2.2 (6.8)	3.8 (6.2)
Total	1.59 (0.68)	52.9 (4.5)	59.3 (7.4)	17.6 (2.5)	17.4 (2.4)	–0.5 (5.6)	5.5 (5.6)
Right-handers							
Male	3.31 (0.48)	56.7 (6.7)	65.5 (10.1)	16.7 (1.9)	18.4 (2.5)	4.8 (5.3)	6.9 (5.6)
Female	3.38 (0.48)	50.3 (4.1)	58.3 (5.9)	15.9 (1.8)	16.9 (1.9)	3.6 (5.3)	7.4 (4.6)
Total	3.36 (0.48)	52.2 (5.7)	60.5 (8.0)	16.0 (1.7)	17.4 (2.2)	3.9 (5.3)	7.3 (4.9)
Total	3.16 (0.76)	52.3 (5.6)	60.4 (7.9)	16.2 (1.9)	17.4 (2.2)	3.4 (5.5)	7.1 (5.0)

NOTE: WHQ, Waterloo Handedness Questionnaire.

SOURCE: Bryden and Roy (2005).

Neuropsychological Normative System (CNNS) available through Psychological Assessment Resources (PAR; www.parinc.com). These provide T scores and discrepancies based on a large sample of older adults from the northeastern United States. A major advantage of these norms is the option to correct for demographic variables such as age, sex, education, and ethnicity. Several other commonly used neuropsychological tests are co-normed using this sample, which facilitates cross-test comparisons.

EVIDENCE FOR RELIABILITY

EVIDENCE FOR TEST-RETEST RELIABILITY, MEASURING CHANGE, AND PRACTICE EFFECTS

With retest intervals of 4 to 24 months, reliability coefficients range from marginal to high (.67 to .86) in healthy individuals (Dikmen et al., 1999; Levine et al., 2004; Ruff & Parker, 1993). Test-retest reliability for the GPT ranged from $r = .69$ to .83 in a sample of people with intellectual disabilities (Carmeli et al., 2008).

When repeated trials are administered within a session, performance improves particularly after the first trial (Schmidt et al., 2000). With two or more administrations at different time points over weeks and months, performance steadily improves (McCaffrey et al., 1993; but see Bornstein et al., 1987). When examinees are retested after intervals ranging from 2 to 24 months, practice effects are evident (Dikmen et al., 1999; Levine et al., 2004; Ruff & Parker, 1993).

Dikmen et al. (1999) examined a sample of 121 healthy adults (age $M = 43.6$, $SD = 19.6$; education $M = 12.0$, $SD = 3.3$) after retest intervals of about 2 to 16 months ($M = 5.4$, $SD = 2.5$). Table 14–19 provides information to assess change, taking practice effects into account (reliable change indices [RCI-PE]). Using values in Table 14–19, one first subtracts the mean T2–T1 change (column 3) from the difference between the two testing sessions for the individual and then compares the result with 1.64 times the standard deviation of the difference (column 4). The 1.64 is derived from the healthy distribution and is exceeded in the positive or negative direction only 10% of the time if there is no actual change in clinical condition.

Drawing from a database of 605 well-educated men (education $M = 16.4$, $SD = 2.3$), mostly Caucasian (age $M = 39.5$, $SD = 8.7$), Levine and colleagues (2004) used both RCI-PE and simple linear regression approaches to derive estimates of change. The retest interval ranged from 4 to 24 months ($M = 218$ days, $SD = 95$). The length of retest interval did not contribute significantly to the regression equation. Table 14–20 shows the means, *SD*s of the change scores, and test-retest correlations for use in RCI equations. Table 14–21 shows the regression formulas used to estimate scores at the second time point. The residual *SD*s for the regression formulas are also shown and can be used to establish the healthy range for retest scores.

TABLE 14–19 Grooved Pegboard Test (GPT) Test-Retest Effects in 121 Healthy Individuals

	TIME 1		TIME 2		T2–T1		T1, T2
MEASURE	(1) *M*	*SD*	(2) *M*	*SD*	(3) *M*	(4) *SD*	*R*
Dominant	69.66	19.27	68.68	21.04	–.98	10.03	.86
Nondominant	75.80	21.56	73.70	19.69	–2.09	11.11	.86

NOTE: Based on a sample of 121 healthy individuals (mean age = 43.6, SD = 19.6; mean education = 12.0, SD = 3.3) after retest intervals of about 2–16 months (mean = 5.4, SD = 2.5). One first subtracts the mean T2-T1 change (column 3) from the difference between the two testing points for the individual and then compares it to 1.64 times the standard deviation of the difference (column 4). The 1.64 is from the healthy distribution and is exceeded in the positive or negative direction only 10% of the time if indeed there is no real change in clinical condition.

SOURCE: Adapted from Dikmen et al. (1999).

TABLE 14–20 Grooved Pegboard Test (GPT) Test-Retest Effects in 605 Healthy Men

	TIME 1		TIME 2		T2–T1		T1, T2
MEASURE	(1) *M*	*SD*	(2) *M*	*SD*	(3) *M*	(4) *SD*	*R*
Dominant	64.2	8.94	61.7	8.16	−2.50	7.01	.67
Nondominant	69.1	10.39	66.5	9.55	−2.61	7.37	.73

NOTE: Based on a sample of 605 healthy males, mostly Caucasian (mean age = 39.5, *SD* = 8.5; mean education = 16.4, *SD* = 2.3) after retest intervals of about 2 to 24 months (mean = 218 days, *SD* = 95).

SOURCE: Adapted from Levine et al. (2004).

For example, a 90% confidence interval (CI) can be created around the scores by multiplying the residual *SD* by 1.645, which allows for 5% of people to fall outside of both the upper and lower extremes. Individuals whose scores exceed the extremes are considered to have significant changes. Of note, Levine et al. (2007) evaluated the generalizability of data based on a healthy sample in detecting change among persons with HIV; the reader is referred to their paper for additional details.

EVIDENCE FOR VALIDITY

FACTOR-ANALYTIC STUDIES AND RELATIONSHIPS WITH OTHER TESTS

Dominant hand performance shows a moderate relationship with tapping speed (−.35; Schear & Sato, 1989). Examination of relationships between fine motor tests in healthy individuals suggests that Finger Tapping and pegboard tasks are more closely related to one another than to Grip Strength (Corey et al., 2001). For example, Finger Tapping and Grip Strength were correlated with the GPT in healthy controls (*rs* = .42, .35) and people with ASD (*rs* = .49, .28; Duffield et al., 2013). In addition to requiring motor execution, the GPT also requires adequate vision. Schear and Sato (1989) found a moderately strong correlation ($r = -.62$) between near visual acuity and time to complete the GPT (dominant hand).

Moderate associations overall (range of absolute value *rs* = .24 to .60) have been reported with measures of attention and executive function (Ashendorf et al., 2009; Schear & Sato, 1989; Strenge et al., 2002), speed (Ashendorf et al., 2009; Schear & Sato, 1989), and nonverbal reasoning, as measured by tasks with a motor component (Ashendorf et al., 2009; Haaland & Delaney, 1981; Schear & Sato, 1989). A factor analysis involving GPT, Symbol Digit Modalities Test (SDMT), Coding, and Category Fluency yielded two factors, with GPT, SDMT, and Coding loading on one factor (thought to reflect a motor component) and Category Fluency and Coding on another (Kochunov et al., 2010). Grip Strength predicted Montreal Cognitive Assessment scores in PD (Bezdicek et al., 2014). Memory shows relatively small relationships with GPT performance (*rs* = Logical Memory −.14 to −.20; Visual Reproduction −.28 to −.33).

TABLE 14–21 Regression Equations for Estimating Retest Scores

MEASURE	REGRESSION EQUATION	REGRESSION *SD*
Dominant	22.57 + (.609 × Time 1 score)	6.08
Nondominant	20.15 + (.671 × Time 1 score)	6.53

NOTE: Based on a sample of 605 healthy males, mostly Caucasian (mean age = 39.5, *SD* = 8.5; mean education = 16.4, *SD* = 2.3) after retest intervals of about 2 to 24 months (mean = 218 days, *SD* = 95).

SOURCE: Adapted from Levine et al. (2004).

CLINICAL STUDIES

GPT performance is reduced in a number of conditions, including stroke (Dacosta-Aguayo et al., 2014; Haaland & Delaney, 1981), tumor (Haaland & Delaney, 1981), multiple sclerosis (Almuklass et al., 2017), ASD (Duffield et al., 2013; Hardan et al., 2003), bipolar disorder (Wilder-Willis et al., 2001), first-episode psychosis (Ayesa-Arriola et al., 2016), end-stage heart disease (Putzke et al., 2000), spinocerebellar ataxia (Rentiya et al., 2017), toxic exposure (Bleecker et al., 1997; Grashow et al., 2013; Mathiesen et al., 1999), very low birthweight (Husby et al., 2013), and chronic low back pain (Weiner et al., 2006). People with greater waist circumference perform more poorly on the GPT, particularly with the dominant hand (Waldstein & Katzel, 2006), as do those with hypertension, particularly when inadequately managed (Waldstein et al., 2005). Antiepileptic medication (carbamazepine, phenytoin) also impairs performance (Meador et al., 1991).

The GPT has been used in PD research (Bohnen et al., 2008), including evaluation of various treatments, such as levodopa (L-DOPA; Kwak et al., 2013), deep brain stimulation (Heo et al., 2008), and vibration therapy (King et al., 2009). The Place procedure of the GPT (conventional task) was found to show moderate to large correlations between upper limb control, rigidity, and bradykinesia in PD, with weaker associations for the Remove variant of the task (Sage et al., 2012). The GPT shows moderate to large correlations with other measures of motor function in PD, especially in early stages of the disease (Sage et al., 2012).

The GPT does not significantly differ between older individuals who sustained a TBI compared to those who did not (Ashman et al., 2008). The GPT has been found to be one of the tests that best differentiated a mixed neurologic population from medical controls (Cohen's $d = 1.08$;

Larrabee et al., 2008). Persons who sustained a moderate to severe TBI and carried the APOE-Ɛ4 allele performed worse on the GPT and other cognitive measures compared to persons who sustained a severe TBI without the APOE-Ɛ4 allele (Ariza et al., 2006).

The GPT is sensitive to HIV (Behrman-Lay et al., 2016; Carey et al., 2004; Hestad et al., 1993; Kamminga et al., 2017) and is part of the HIV-associated neurocognitive disorder (HAND) screening protocol (see Antinori et al., 2007), with strong diagnostic accuracy reported (de Almeida et al., 2017). Carey et al. (2004) identified nondominant GPT scores in combination with the Hooper Visual Learning Test as particularly effective in detecting neuropsychological impairment in persons with HIV, with 78% sensitivity, 85% specificity, and an odds ratio of nearly 21. The GPT was related to cytokines concentration level in persons with HIV (Cohen et al., 2011; Nolting et al., 2012). The GPT has been identified as a potentially useful assessment tool in HIV populations internationally where limited resources may exist (Holguin et al., 2011; Parsons et al., 2007). In those with HIV, poor performance may represent an early sign of a dementing process: defective performance on the GPT was linked with an increased risk of developing dementia over a 30-month follow-up period (Stern et al., 2001).

The test is also a sensitive, but not totally accurate, indicator of lateralized disturbance (Bornstein, 1986a; Haaland & Delaney, 1981). Left cerebral lesions tend to attenuate the relatively more typical pattern of manual asymmetry; right lesions move the discrepancies in the opposite direction. However, ipsilateral impairment is also seen—perhaps a reflection of the significant sequencing, visuospatial, and monitoring requirements of the tasks (Haaland & Delaney, 1981). Lewis and Kupke (1992) also suggested that difficulty adapting to the novelty of the task, especially with the nonpreferred hand, may affect performance.

The GPT correlates with some aspects of daily function, particularly driving. The GPT was a significant predictor of safety errors in older drivers (Dawson et al., 2010). For example, an increase of approximately three years in age, a decrease of five points on Block Design, and an increase of seven seconds on the GPT jointly predicted an increase of one driving error. The GPT was identified as a significant predictor (along with simple reaction time and the Trail Making Test, Part A) of on-road driving performance in patients with TBI or stroke (Aslaksen et al., 2013). The GPT was an individual predictor of driving cessation in older adults (Emerson et al., 2012).

NEUROANATOMICAL CORRELATES AND IMAGING STUDIES

Although limited data exist, neuroimaging studies suggest that not only frontal activation, but also a range of white matter tracts are involved in performance. Amplitude of low frequency blood oxygen-level dependent (BOLD) signal fluctuations in the premotor cortex predicts PD patients' performance on the GPT (Kwak et al., 2012). Patients with first-episode psychosis and GPT impairment show reduced fractional anisotropy in the forceps minor, inferior frontooccipital fasciculus, anterior thalamic radiation, and corticospinal and corticopontine tracts (Pérez-Iglesias et al., 2010). Projection tracts are also related to GPT performance in patients with stroke, such as the left superior corona radiata and left anterior thalamic radiation, as well as the right inferior longitudinal fasciculus and right posterior corona radiata, depending on subgroup (Dacosta-Aguayo et al., 2014). In one study, predictors of GPT performance included age, systolic blood pressure, striatal gray matter volume, and striatal glutamate in a model that accounted for approximately 45% of the variance (Zahr et al., 2013). GPT performance is correlated with gray matter density in patients with spinocerebellar ataxia type 6, particularly in medial superior hemispheric regions (Rentiya et al., 2017).

PERFORMANCE VALIDITY

Individuals simulating TBI tend to suppress their performance on the GPT (Johnson & Lesniak-Karpiak, 1997; Rapport et al., 1998; but see Wong et al., 1998). Greiffenstein, Baker, and Gola (1996) examined the average performance of the dominant and nondominant hands on tests of motor functioning and reported that compensation-seeking patients with postconcussion syndrome demonstrated a nonphysiologic profile on Grip Strength, Finger Tapping, and the GPT (Grip Strength < Finger Tapping < GPT). However, Rapport et al. (1998) found that nonphysiologic configurations showed poor predictive accuracy for feigning among simulators.

An analysis of studies that have used the GPT in the assessment of performance validity suggested that the dominant hand of the GPT is associated with effect sizes ranging from medium to large in differentiating between credible and noncredible groups, with most studies reporting greater within-group variability in the noncredible group (Erdődi et al., 2017). Based on their mixed clinical sample of 190 patients referred for neuropsychological assessment, Erdődi et al. (2017) identified optimal cutoff scores for maximizing differentiation of credible and noncredible performers using failure on other PVTs as the reference standard. As depicted in Table 14–22, sensitivity estimates were comparatively smaller than specificity estimates, with positive and negative predictive power strongest overall at a hypothetical base rate of 20% or more. They also reported that failure on the dominant hand cutoff was associated with higher self-reported anxiety and depressive symptoms, with associations with the Personality Assessment Inventory (e.g.,

TABLE 14–22 Optimal Cutoff Scores for Differentiating Between Credible and Noncredible Performance on the Grooved Pegboard Test (GPT)

HAND	CUTOFF	SENS	SPEC[a]	PREDICTIVE POWER	HYPOTHETICAL BASE RATE OF INVALID PERFORMANCE 10%	20%	30%	40%	50%
DOM	≤29	.42	.87	Pos	.26	.45	.58	.68	.76
				Neg	.93	.86	.78	.69	.60
Non-DOM	≤29	.45	.88	Pos	.29	.48	.62	.71	.78
				Neg	.94	.86	.79	.71	.62
COMB	≤31	.42	.89	Pos	.30	.49	.62	.72	.79
				Neg	.93	.86	.78	.70	.61

NOTE: Sens = sensitivity; Spec = specificity; DOM = dominant hand (demographically adjusted *T* score); Non-DOM = nondominant hand (demographically adjusted *T* score); COMB = combined (with *Pass* defined as a score below cutoff on either or neither hand and *Fail* defined as a score below cutoff on both hands; demographically adjusted *T* scores); Pos = positive; Neg = negative.

[a]Ipsative analyses revealed that these cutoffs were associated with perfect specificity. Therefore, positive predictive power is estimated to be 1.00 across all hypothetical base rates on invalid performance.

SOURCE: Erdődi et al. (2017).

scales related to somatic complaints, borderline personality, antisocial, and substance use dimensions).

COMMENT

The GPT requires manual precision, eye-hand coordination, and motor speed. Age appears to be the most influential demographic variable, with mixed findings with respect to gender and education. Limited findings regarding ethnicity are available. Although the preferred hand is typically stronger than the nonpreferred hand, the opposite pattern is not uncommon in healthy populations. Therefore, an isolated finding of better performance with the nonpreferred hand should not be interpreted as reflective of neurologic impairment.

Normative data provided by Heaton et al. (2004) offer several strengths, including a large sample size spanning many ages and adjustment for relevant demographic variables. The normative data provided by Ashendorf et al. (2009) for older adults also has strengths, including normative data for the number of pegs dropped.

Test-retest reliability is marginal to high. There are practice effects, even after test-retest intervals that exceed a year. Reliable change calculations are available to assess the significance of change. GPT performance is moderately associated with a number of tests, especially those with a speeded component, including tapping, attention and executive function, processing speed, and visual reasoning, and less so with memory. The test has been used in a number of clinical populations, and impairment has been associated with both neurologic and nonneurologic conditions, demonstrating that impairment on this task is not specific to neurological involvement but other factors must also be considered (e.g., medication use, anxiety, visual and tactile abilities). The GPT has shown particular utility in research on PD, HIV, and driving safety. More information is needed with respect to neural correlates, although available research suggests involvement of a number of areas beyond frontal cortex. Information on the test for assessment of performance validity is promising.

REFERENCES

Almuklass, A. M., Feeney, D. F., Mani, D., Hamilton, L. D., & Enoka, R. M. (2017). Peg-manipulation capabilities during a test of manual dexterity differ for persons with multiple sclerosis and healthy individuals. *Experimental Brain Research*, *235*(11), 3487–3493. https://doi.org/10.1007/s00221-017-5075-4

Antinori, A., Arendt, G., Becker, J. T., Brew, B. J., Byrd, D. A., Cherner, M., . . . Wojna, V. E. (2007). Updated research nosology for HIV-associated neurocognitive disorders. *Neurology*, *69*(18), 1789–1799. https://doi.org/10.1212/01.WNL.0000287431.88658.8b

Ariza, M., Pueyo, R., Matarín, M. d. M., Junqué, C., Mataró, M., Clemente, I., . . . Sahuquillo, J. (2006). Influence of APOE polymorphism on cognitive and behavioural outcome in moderate and severe traumatic brain injury. *Journal of Neurology, Neurosurgery & Psychiatry*, *77*(10), 1191–1193. https://doi.org/10.1136/jnnp.2005.085167

Ashendorf, L., Vanderslice-Barr, J. L., & McCaffrey, R. J. (2009). Motor tests and cognition in healthy older adults. *Applied Neuropsychology*, *16*(3), 171–176. http://doi.org/10.1080/09084280903098562

Ashman, T. A., Cantor, J. B., Gordon, W. A., Sacks, A., Spielman, L., Egan, M., & Hibbard, M. R. (2008). A comparison of cognitive functioning in older adults with and without traumatic brain injury. *The Journal of Head Trauma Rehabilitation*, *23*(3), 139–148.

Aslaksen, P. M., Ørbo, M., Elvestad, R., Schäfer, C., & Anke, A. (2013). Prediction of on-road driving ability after traumatic brain injury and stroke. *European Journal of Neurology*, *20*(9), 1227–1233. http://doi.org/10.1111/ene.12172

Ayesa-Arriola, R., Rodríguez-Sánchez, J. M., Suero, E. S., Reeves, L. E., Tabarés-Seisdedos, R., & Crespo-Facorro, B. (2016). Diagnosis and neurocognitive profiles in first-episode non-affective psychosis patients. *European Archives of Psychiatry and Clinical Neuroscience*, *266*(7), 619–628. https://doi.org/10.1007/s00406-015-0667-0

Barnett, M. D., Parsons, T. D., Reynolds, B. L., & Bedford, L. A. (2017). Impact of rapport on neuropsychological test performance. *Applied Neuropsychology: Adult*, 1–8. https://doi.org/10.1080/23279095.2017.1293671

Behrman-Lay, A. M., Paul, R. H., Heaps-Woodruff, J., Baker, L. M., Usher, C., & Ances, B. M. (2016). Human immunodeficiency virus has similar effects on brain volumetrics and cognition in males and females. *Journal of NeuroVirology*, *22*(1), 93–103. https://doi.org/10.1007/s13365-015-0373-8

Bezdicek, O., Nikolai, T., Hoskovcová, M., Štochl, J., Brožová, H., Dušek, P., . . . Růžička, E. (2014). Grooved pegboard predicates more of cognitive than motor involvement in Parkinson's disease. *Assessment, 21*(6), 723–730.

Bleecker, M. L., Lindgren, K. N., & Ford, D. P. (1997). Differential contribution of current and cumulative indices of lead dose to neuropsychological performance by age. *Neurology, 48,* 639–645.

Bohnen, N. I., Studenski, S. A., Constantine, G. M., & Moore, R. Y. (2008). Diagnostic performance of clinical motor and non-motor tests of Parkinson disease: A matched case-control study: Diagnosis of Parkinson disease based on motor and non-motor symptoms. *European Journal of Neurology, 15*(7), 685–691. http://doi.org/10.1111/j.1468-1331.2008.02148.x

Bornstein, R. A. (1985). Normative data on selected neuropsychological measures from a nonclinical sample. *Journal of Clinical Psychology, 41,* 651–658.

Bornstein, R. A. (1986a). Classification rates obtained with "standard" cut-off scores on selected neuropsychological measures. *Journal of Clinical and Experimental Neuropsychology, 8,* 413–420.

Bornstein, R. A. (1986b). Normative data on intermanual differences on three tests of motor performance. *Journal of Clinical and Experimental Neuropsychology, 8,* 12–20.

Bornstein, R. A., Baker, G. B., & Douglas, A. B. (1987). Short-term test-retest reliability of the Halstead-Reitan Battery in a normal sample. *The Journal of Nervous and Mental Disease, 175,* 229–232.

Bryden, P. J., & Roy, E. A. (2005). A new method of administering the Grooved Pegboard Test: Performance as a function of handedness and sex. *Brain and Cognition, 58*(3), 258–268. http://doi.org/10.1016/j.bandc.2004.12.004

Bryden, P. J., Roy, E. A., Rohr, L. E., & Egilo, S. (2007). Task demands affect manual asymmetries in pegboard performance. *Laterality: Asymmetries of Body, Brain and Cognition, 12*(4), 364–377. http://doi.org/10.1080/13576500701356244

Carey, C. L., Woods, S. P., Rippeth, J. D., Gonzalez, R., Moore, D. J., Marcotte, T. D., . . . the HNRC Group. (2004). Initial validation of a screening battery for the detection of HIV-associated cognitive impairment. *The Clinical Neuropsychologist, 18,* 234–248.

Carmeli, E., Bar-Yossef, T., Ariav, C., Levy, R., & Liebermann, D. G. (2008). Perceptual-motor coordination in persons with mild intellectual disability. *Disability and Rehabilitation, 30*(5), 323–329. http://doi.org/10.1080/09638280701265398

Cohen, R. A., de la Monte, S., Gongvatana, A., Ombao, H., Gonzalez, B., Devlin, K. N., . . . Tashima, K. T. (2011). Plasma cytokine concentrations associated with HIV/hepatitis C coinfection are related to attention, executive and psychomotor functioning. *Journal of Neuroimmunology, 233*(1-2), 204–210. http://doi.org/10.1016/j.jneuroim.2010.11.006

Corey, D. M., Hurley, M. M., & Foundas, A. L. (2001). Right and left handedness defined. *Neuropsychiatry, Neuropsychology, and Behavioral Neurology, 14,* 144–152.

Dacosta-Aguayo, R., Graña, M., Fernández-Andújar, M., López-Cancio, E., Cáceres, C., Bargalló, N., . . . Mataró, M. (2014). Structural integrity of the contralesional hemisphere predicts cognitive impairment in ischemic stroke at three months. *PLoS ONE, 9*(1), e86119. https://doi.org/10.1371/journal.pone.0086119

Dawson, J. D., Uc, E. Y., Anderson, S. W., Johnson, A. M., & Rizzo, M. (2010). Neuropsychological predictors of driving errors in older adults. *Journal of the American Geriatrics Society, 58*(6), 1090–1096. http://doi.org/10.1111/j.1532-5415.2010.02872.x

de Almeida, M., Kamat, R., Cherner, M., Umlauf, A., Ribeiro, C. E., de Pereira, A. P., . . . Ellis, R. J. (2017). Improving detection of HIV-associated cognitive impairment: Comparison of the International HIV Dementia Scale and a brief screening battery. *JAIDS Journal of Acquired Immune Deficiency Syndromes, 74*(3), 332–338.

Dikmen, S. S., Heaton, R. K., Grant, I., & Temkin, N. R. (1999). Test-retest reliability and practice effects of expanded Halstead-Reitan neuropsychological test battery. *Journal of the International Neuropsychological Society, 5,* 346–356.

Duffield, T. C., Trontel, H. G., Bigler, E. D., Froehlich, A., Prigge, M. B., Travers, B., . . . Lainhart, J. (2013). Neuropsychological investigation of motor impairments in autism. *Journal of Clinical and Experimental Neuropsychology, 35*(8), 867–881. http://doi.org/10.1080/13803395.2013.827156

Emerson, J. L., Johnson, A. M., Dawson, J. D., Uc, E. Y., Anderson, S. W., & Rizzo, M. (2012). Predictors of driving outcomes in advancing age. *Psychology and Aging, 27*(3), 550–559. https://doi.org/10.1037/a0026359

Erdődi, L. A., Seke, K. R., Shahein, A., Tyson, B. T., Sagar, S., & Roth, R. M. (2017). Low scores on the Grooved Pegboard Test are associated with invalid responding and psychiatric symptoms. *Psychology & Neuroscience, 10*(3), 325–344. https://doi.org/10.1037/pne0000103

Fouty, H. E., McWaters, A. R., Sanchez, H. C., Mills, R. A., Brandon, B. M., & Weitzner, D. S. (2015). Effect of left-hand peg placement direction on the Grooved Pegboard Test. *Applied Neuropsychology: Adult, 22*(5), 332–334. https://doi.org/10.1080/23279095.2014.930039

Grashow, R., Spiro, A., Taylor, K. M., Newton, K., Shrairman, R., Landau, A., . . . Weisskopf, M. (2013). Cumulative lead exposure in community-dwelling adults and fine motor function: Comparing standard and novel tasks in the VA Normative Aging Study. *NeuroToxicology, 35,* 154–161. https://doi.org/10.1016/j.neuro.2013.01.005

Greiffenstein, M. F., Baker, W. J., & Gola, T. (1996). Motor dysfunction profiles in traumatic brain injury and postconcussion syndrome. *Journal of the International Neuropsychological Society, 2,* 477–485.

Haaland, K. Y., & Delaney, H. D. (1981). Motor deficits after left or right hemisphere damage due to stroke or tumor. *Neuropsychologia, 19,* 17–27.

Hamby, S. L., Bardi, C. A., & Wilkins, J. W. (1997). Neuropsychological assessment of relatively intact individuals: Psychometric lessons from an HIV+ sample. *Archives of Clinical Neuropsychology, 12,* 545–556.

Hardan, A. Y., Kilpatrick, M., Keshavan, M. S., & Minshew, N. J. (2003). Motor performance and anatomic magnetic resonance imaging (MRI) of the basal ganglia in autism. *Journal of Child Neurology, 18,* 317–324.

Heaton, R. K., Miller, S. W., Taylor, M. J., & Grant, I. (2004). *Revised comprehensive norms for an expanded Halstead-Reitan Battery: Demographically adjusted neuropsychological norms for African American and Caucasian adults.* Lutz, FL: PAR.

Heo, J.-H., Lee, K.-M., Paek, S. H., Kim, M.-J., Lee, J.-Y., Kim, J.-Y., . . . Jeon, B. S. (2008). The effects of bilateral Subthalamic Nucleus Deep Brain Stimulation (STN DBS) on cognition in Parkinson disease. *Journal of the Neurological Sciences, 273*(1-2), 19–24. http://doi.org/10.1016/j.jns.2008.06.010

Hestad, K., McArthur, J. H., Dal Pan, G. J., Selnes, O. A., et al. (1993). Regional brain atrophy in HIV-1 infection: Association with specific neuropsychological test performance. *Acta Neurological Scandinavica, 88,* 112–118.

Holguin, A., Banda, M., Willen, E. J., Malama, C., Chiyenu, K. O., Mudenda, V. C., & Wood, C. (2011). HIV-1 effects on neuropsychological performance in a resource-limited country, Zambia. *AIDS and Behavior, 15*(8), 1895–1901. http://doi.org/10.1007/s10461-011-9988-9

Husby, I. M., Skranes, J., Olsen, A., Brubakk, A.-M., & Evensen, K. A. I. (2013). Motor skills at 23 years of age in young adults born preterm with very low birth weight. *Early Human Development, 89*(9), 747–754. http://doi.org/10.1016/j.earlhumdev.2013.05.009

Johnson, J. L., & Lesniak-Karpiak, K. (1997). The effect of warning on malingering on memory and motor tasks in college samples. *Archives of Clinical Neuropsychology, 12,* 231–238.

Kamminga, J., Lal, L., Wright, E. J., Bloch, M., Brew, B. J., & Cysique, L. A. (2017). Monitoring HIV-associated neurocognitive disorder using screenings: a critical review including guidelines for clinical and research use. *Current HIV/AIDS Reports, 14*(3), 83–92.

King, L. K., Almeida, Q. J., & Ahonen, H. (2009). Short-term effects of vibration therapy on motor impairments in Parkinson's disease. *NeuroRehabilitation, 25*(4), 297–306.

Kochunov, P., Coyle, T., Lancaster, J., Robin, D. A., Hardies, J., Kochunov, V., . . . Fox, P. T. (2010). Processing speed is correlated with cerebral health markers in the frontal lobes as quantified by neuroimaging. *NeuroImage, 49*(2), 1190–1199. http://doi.org/10.1016/j.neuroimage.2009.09.052

Kwak, Y., Bohnen, N. I., Müller, M. L. T. M., Dayalu, P., Burke, D. T., & Seidler, R. D. (2013). Task-dependent interactions between dopamine D2 receptor polymorphisms and L-DOPA in patients with Parkinson's disease. *Behavioural Brain Research, 245,* 128–136. http://doi.org/10.1016/j.bbr.2013.02.016

Kwak, Y., Peltier, S. J., Bohnen, N. I., Müller, M. L. T. M., Dayalu, P., & Seidler, R. D. (2012). L-DOPA changes spontaneous low-frequency BOLD signal oscillations in Parkinson's disease: a resting state fMRI study. *Frontiers in Systems Neuroscience, 6.* http://doi.org/10.3389/fnsys.2012.00052

Larrabee, G. J., Millis, S. R., & Meyers, J. E. (2008). Sensitivity to brain dysfunction of the Halstead-Reitan vs an ability-focused neuropsychological battery. *The Clinical Neuropsychologist, 22*(5), 813–825. http://doi.org/10.1080/13854040701625846

Levine, A. J., Hinkin, C. H., Miller, E. N., Becker, J. T., Selnes, O. A., & Cohen, B. A. (2007). The generalizability of neurocognitive test/retest data derived from a nonclinical sample for detecting change among two HIV+ cohorts. *Journal of Clinical and Experimental Neuropsychology, 29*(6), 669–678. http://doi.org/10.1080/13803390600920471

Levine, A. J., Miller, E. N., Becker, J. T., Selnes, O. A., & Cohen, B. A. (2004). Normative data for determining significance of test-retest differences on eight common neuropsychological instruments. *The Clinical Neuropsychologist, 18,* 373–384.

Lewis, R., & Kupke, T. (1992). Intermanual differences on skilled and unskilled motor tasks in nonlateralized brain dysfunction. *The Clinical Neuropsychologist, 6,* 374–382.

Lynch, J. K. (2005). Effect of a third party observer on neuropsychological test performance following closed head injury. *Journal of Forensic Neuropsychology, 4*(2), 17–25. http://doi.org/10.1300/J151v04n02_02

Mathiesen, T., Ellingsen, D. G., & Kjuus, H. (1999). Neuropsychological effects associated with exposure to mercury vapor among former chloralkali workers. *Scandinavian Journal of Work, Environment and Health, 25,* 342–250.

Matthews, C. G., & Klove, K. (1964). *Instruction manual for the Adult Neuropsychology Test Battery.* Madison: University of Wisconsin Medical School.

McCaffrey, R. J., Ortega, A., & Haase, R. F. (1993). Effects of repeated neuropsychological assessments. *Archives of Clinical Neuropsychology, 8,* 519–524.

Meador, K. J., Loring, D. W., Allen, M. E., Zamini, E. Y., et al. (1991). Comparative cognitive effects of carbamazepine and phenytoin in healthy adults. *Neurology, 41,* 1537–1540.

Mitrushina, M. N., Boone, K. B., Razani, J., & d'Elia, L. F. (2005). *Handbook of normative data for neuropsychological assessment* (2nd ed.). New York: Oxford University Press.

Nolting, T., Lindecke, A., Hartung, H.-P., Koutsilieri, E., Maschke, M., . . . Arendt, G. (2012). Cytokine levels in CSF and neuropsychological performance in HIV patients. *Journal of NeuroVirology, 18*(3), 157–161. http://doi.org/10.1007/s13365-012-0091-4

Parsons, T. D., Rogers, S., Hall, C., & Robertson, K. (2007). Motor based assessment of neurocognitive functioning in resource-limited international settings. *Journal of Clinical and Experimental Neuropsychology, 29*(1), 59–66. http://doi.org/10.1080/13803390500488538

Pérez-Iglesias, R., Tordesillas-Gutiérrez, D., McGuire, P. K., Barker, G. J., Roiz-Santiañez, R., Mata, I., . . . others. (2010). White matter integrity and cognitive impairment in first-episode psychosis. *American Journal of Psychiatry, 167*(4), 451–458.

Peters, M., Servos, P., & Day, R. (1990). Marked sex difference between right-handers and left-handers disappear when finger size is used as a covariate. *Journal of Applied Psychology, 75,* 87–90.

Putzke, J. D., Williams, M. A., Daniel, F. J., Foley, B. A., Kirklin, J. K., & Boll, T. J. (2000). Neuropsychological functioning among heart transplant candidates: A case control study. *Journal of Clinical and Experimental Neuropsychology, 22,* 95–103.

Rapport, L. J., Farchione, T. J., Coleman, R. D., & Axelrod, B. N. (1998). Effects of coaching on malingered motor function profiles. *Journal of Clinical and Experimental Neuropsychology, 20,* 89–97.

Rentiya, Z., Khan, N.-S., Ergun, E., Ying, S. H., & Desmond, J. E. (2017). Distinct cerebellar regions related to motor and cognitive performance in SCA6 patients. *Neuropsychologia, 107,* 25–30. https://doi.org/10.1016/j.neuropsychologia.2017.10.036

Ruff, R. M., & Parker, S. B. (1993). Gender- and age-specific changes in motor speed and eye hand coordination in adults: Normative values for the Finger Tapping and Grooved Pegboard tests. *Perceptual and Motor Skills, 76,* 1219–1230.

Russell, E. W., & Starkey, R. I. (1993). *Halstead Russell Neuropsychological Evaluation System (HRNES).* Los Angeles: Western Psychological Services.

Sage, M. D., Bryden, P. J., Roy, E. A., & Almeida, Q. J. (2012). The relationship between the grooved pegboard test and clinical motor symptom evaluation across the spectrum of Parkinson's disease severity. *Journal of Parkinson's Disease, 2*(3), 207–213. https://doi.org/10.3233/JPD-2012-012093

Schear, J. M., & Sato, S. D. (1989). Effects of visual acuity and visual motor speed and dexterity on cognitive test performance. *Archives of Clinical Neuropsychology 4,* 25–32.

Schmidt, S. L., Oliveira, R. M., Rocha, F. R., & Abreu-Villaca, Y. (2000). Influences of handedness and gender on the Grooved Pegboard Test. *Brain and Cognition, 44,* 445–454.

Schretlen, D. J., Testa, S. M., & Pearlson, G. D. (2010). *Calibrated neuropsychological normative system.* Lutz, FL: PAR.

Stern, Y., McDermott, M. P., Albert, S., Palumbo, D., Selnes, O. A., McArthur, J., . . . Dana Consortium on the Therapy of HIV-Dementia and Related Cognitive Disorders. (2001). Factors associated with incident human immunodeficiency virus-dementia. *Archives of Neurology, 58,* 473–479.

Strenge, H., Niedenberger, U., & Seelhorst, U. (2002). Correlation between tests of attention and performance on Grooved and Purdue Pegboards in normal subjects. *Perceptual and Motor Skills, 95,* 507–514.

Thompson, L. L., Heaton, K. R., Matthews, C. G., & Grant, I. (1987). Comparison of preferred and nonpreferred hand performance on four neuropsychological motor tasks. *The Clinical Neuropsychologist, 1,* 324–334.

Tremblay, F., Wong, K., Sanderson, R., & Cote, L. (2002). Tactile spatial acuity in elderly persons: Assessment with grating domes and relationship with manual dexterity. *Somatosensory and Motor Research, 20,* 127–132.

Trites, R. (1977). *Neuropsychological test manual.* Ottawa, Ontario, Canada: Royal Ottawa Hospital (available from Lafayette Instrument Company).

Waldstein, S. R., Brown, J. R., Maier, K. J., & Katzel, L. I. (2005). Diagnosis of hypertension and high blood pressure levels negatively affect cognitive function in older adults. *Annals of Behavioral Medicine, 29*(3), 174–180.

Waldstein, S. R., & Katzel, L. I. (2006). Interactive relations of central versus total obesity and blood pressure to cognitive function. *International Journal of Obesity, 30*(1), 201–207.

Weiner, D. K., Rudy, T. E., Morrow, L., Slaboda, J., & Lieber, S. (2006). The relationship between pain, neuropsychological performance, and physical function in community-dwelling older adults with chronic low back pain. *Pain Medicine, 7*(1), 60–70.

Wilder-Willis, K. E., Sax, K., Rosenberg, H. L., Fleck, D. E., Shear, P. K., & Strakowski, S. M. (2001). Persistent attentional dysfunction in remitted bipolar disorder. *Bipolar Disorders, 3,* 58–62.

Wong, J. L., Lerrner-Poppen, L., & Durham, J. (1998). Does warning reduce obvious malingering on memory and motor tasks in college samples? *International Journal of Rehabilitation and Health, 4,* 153–165.

Zahr, N. M., Mayer, D., Rohlfing, T., Chanraud, S., Gu, M., Sullivan, E. V., & Pfefferbaum, A. (2013). In vivo glutamate measured with magnetic resonance spectroscopy: Behavioral correlates in aging. *Neurobiology of Aging, 34*(4), 1265–1276. http://doi.org/10.1016/j.neurobiolaging.2012.09.014

PURDUE PEGBOARD TEST

TEST NAME	**Purdue Pegboard Test**
DOMAIN	Fine motor dexterity
AGE RANGE	In adults, to 89 years
ADMINISTRATION TIME	5 to 10 minutes
SCORING FORMAT	Hand scored
REFERENCE	Tiffin, J. (1968). *Purdue Pegboard: Examiner manual.* Chicago: Science Research Associates.

DESCRIPTION

The purpose of the Purdue Pegboard Test is to measure unimanual and bimanual finger and hand dexterity. The Purdue Pegboard was developed in the 1940s as a test of fine motor dexterity for use in personnel selection (Tiffin, 1968; Tiffin & Asher, 1948) and has also been used historically in neuropsychological assessment to assist in localizing cerebral lesions (Reddon et al., 1988).

ADMINISTRATION

The instructions are described in the manual. The board consists of two parallel columns of 25 holes each (see Figure 14–3). Pegs (also called pins) are located at the extreme right- and left-hand cups at the top of the board. Collars and washers occupy the two middle cups. In the first three subtests, the examinee places as many pins as possible in the holes, first with the preferred hand, then with the nonpreferred hand, and finally with both hands, within a 30-second interval. When using only the right hand, the examinee inserts as many pins as possible in the holes, starting at the top right. When using only the left hand, the examinee starts at the top left. Both hands then are used together to fill both columns top to bottom. In the fourth subtest, the examinee uses both hands alternately to construct "assemblies," which consist of a pin, a washer, a collar, and another washer. The examinee must complete as many assemblies as possible within one minute. Demonstration and practice are provided before each subtest. Each task may be repeated three times. The right-hand test is administered three times before proceeding to the left-hand test, and so on, throughout the series of tests.

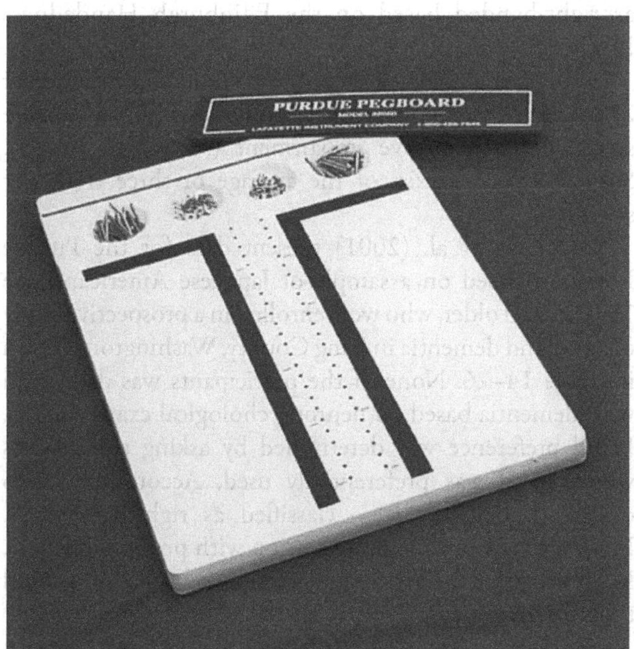

Figure 14–3 Purdue Pegboard.

SCORING

Scores are derived for each part of the test. The scores for the pin placement subtests consist of the number of pins inserted in the time period for each hand. The score for the bimanual condition consists of the total number of pairs of pins inserted. The assembly score reflects the number of parts assembled.

DEMOGRAPHIC EFFECTS

AGE

Performance declines with advancing age (Agnew et al., 1988; DesRosiers et al., 1995; McCurry et al., 2001; Wittich & Nadon, 2017).

GENDER

Females tend to perform better than males (e.g., Agnew et al., 1988; DesRosiers et al., 1995; Nilsson et al., 2005; Peters, 1990; Soer et al., 2006; Yeudall et al., 1986). Gender differences in fine motor dexterity may be confounded by differences in finger size (Peters et al., 1990).

EDUCATION AND IQ

Education appears unrelated to performance (McCurry et al., 2001; Yeudall et al., 1986). In a sample of people with Tourette's syndrome, the Kaufman Brief Intelligence Test was moderately correlated with performance (r = .38 to .42; Bloch et al., 2006).

ETHNICITY, NATIONALITY, AND LINGUISTIC EFFECTS

Primary language spoken (English, Japanese) among older Japanese adults did not affect scores (McCurry et al., 2001). Margolis et al. (2006) reported that socioeconomic status was related to dominant hand performance in their study of adults with Tourette's syndrome.

HANDEDNESS

In general, performance is better with the preferred hand than with the nonpreferred hand (e.g., DesRosiers et al., 1995; Judge & Stirling, 2003; Margolis et al., 2006; Noguchi et al., 2006; Triggs et al., 2000). Left-handers may perform better on the assembly component (Judge & Stirling, 2003). The unimanual condition is faster than the bimanual condition (Margolis et al., 2006).

NORMATIVE DATA

Table 14–23 provides normative data for adults stratified on the basis of age (15 to 40 years) and gender (Yeudall et al., 1986). Exclusion criteria included evidence from the interview of medicolegal involvement, prenatal or birth complications, psychiatric disorders, or substance abuse. Hand preference was determined by the hand the participants used to write with. Administration was one trial per subtest.

TABLE 14–23 Mean Performance of Young Adults for the Purdue Pegboard (One Trial per Subtest)

	AGE GROUPS				
	15–20	21–25	26–30	31–40	15–40
Females					
N	30	36	16	16	98
Preferred hand	16.69	16.64	17.25	15.94	16.64
SD	2.16	2.31	1.38	1.61	2.10
Nonpreferred hand	16.10	15.89	16.13	15.63	15.95
SD	1.57	1.79	1.50	1.89	1.68
Both hands	13.76	13.75	13.31	13.13	13.58
SD	1.41	1.54	1.45	1.31	1.45
Assemblies	41.83	42.47	40.44	41.44	41.77
SD	5.08	5.43	5.90	5.75	5.42
Males					
N	32	37	32	26	127
Preferred hand	15.56	15.44	16.22	15.35	15.65
SD	1.52	1.71	1.81	1.72	1.71
Nonpreferred hand	15.09	15.08	15.41	15.12	15.17
SD	1.42	1.98	2.08	1.77	1.82
Both hands	12.59	12.97	12.94	12.42	12.75
SD	1.56	1.18	1.29	1.65	1.42
Assemblies	40.25	38.89	39.13	37.50	39.01
SD	4.64	6.60	3.58	3.64	4.92

NOTE: Data were compiled from 225 healthy adults, largely right-handed (88%), with above-average IQ, residing in a large city in Western Canada.

SOURCE: Adapted from Yeudall et al. (1986).

TABLE 14–24 Performance on the Purdue Pegboard in Older Adults, by Age and Gender (One Trial)

	MALES		FEMALES	
	MEAN	*SD*	MEAN	*SD*
60–69 years				
Right	12.7	1.5	14.3	1.3
Left	12.7	1.5	13.7	1.3
Both	10.2	1.3	10.9	1.5
Assembly	27.6	5.1	30.6	5.3
70–79 years				
Right	11.2	1.9	12.7	1.8
Left	10.7	2.1	11.8	1.8
Both	8.2	2.0	9.7	1.7
Assembly	23.1	5.5	25.0	5.8
80+ years				
Right	10.1	2.0	11.5	1.8
Left	9.8	1.7	10.7	2.1
Both	7.4	1.6	8.3	1.9
Assembly	18.5	5.2	21.8	5.5

NOTE: Each age group contained 60 males and 60 females.

SOURCE: Adapted from DesRosiers et al. (1995).

Table 14–24 shows normative data (DesRosiers et al., 1995) based on a random sample of 360 older adults, stratified by age and gender, drawn from the electoral pool of a city in Quebec, Canada. All participants were 60 to 89 years of age and independent in ADLs; all could see sufficiently well and had no impairment affecting upper limb functioning. Most (92%) were classed as right-handed based on the Edinburgh Handedness Inventory.

Agnew et al. (1988) provide data based on a sample of 212 healthy, well-educated 40- to 85-year-olds who were screened for cognitive impairment (see Table 14–25). Subtest scores consist of the average of three trials per subtest.

McCurry et al. (2001) present data for the Purdue Pegboard based on a sample of Japanese Americans, age 70 years and older, who were enrolled in a prospective study of aging and dementia in King County, Washington, as seen in Table 14–26. None of the participants was diagnosed with dementia based on neuropsychological examinations. Hand preference was determined by asking participants which hand was preferentially used. Accordingly, 94% of the participants were classified as right-handed (S. McCurry, personal communication with previous authors, May 11, 2004). Participants completed two 30-second trials for each hand.

Normative data are available for 134 patients with low vision, typically related to macular degeneration

TABLE 14–25 Mean Performance of Adults for the Purdue Pegboard (Three Trials per Subtest)

	AGE GROUPS				
	40–49	50–59	60–69	70–79	80–89
Males					
N	19	20	24	17	11
Preferred hand	14.6	14.4	13.6	13.0	10.8
SD	2.08	2.15	1.74	1.90	1.33
Nonpreferred hand	14.4	13.9	13.1	12.4	10.6
SD	2.35	2.19	1.56	1.48	1.84
Both hands	12.2	11.9	10.9	10.4	8.5
SD	2.43	2.22	1.46	1.27	1.21
Purdue Assembly	34.9	33.8	28.0	27.5	21.5
SD	7.66	9.66	5.06	5.06	4.81
Pref. minus nonpref.	0.16	0.23	0.44	0.59	0.18
SD	1.19	1.21	1.86	0.93	1.46
Females					
N	21	27	29	31	13
Preferred hand	15.9	15.0	14.6	13.8	12.9
SD	1.45	1.56	2.03	1.27	1.80
Nonpreferred hand	15.2	14.4	13.9	12.9	11.3
SD	1.48	1.69	1.78	1.52	2.05
Both hands	13.1	12.1	11.6	10.5	9.2
SD	1.56	1.30	1.87	1.19	1.92
Purdue Assembly	39.8	34.6	31.7	29.1	21.9
SD	4.54	8.21	6.83	4.85	4.54
Pref. minus nonpref.	0.73	0.63	0.71	0.94	1.56
SD	1.05	1.31	1.23	1.39	1.24

SOURCE: Agnew et al. (1988).

or glaucoma, recruited from a rehabilitation center in Canada as presented in Table 14–27 (Wittich & Nadon, 2017). Participants were eligible for inclusion if they were at least 60 years old and had a measurable level of vision; age ranged from 60 to 97 years (M = 82.6 years, SD = 9.0 years). The sample was predominantly female (72%) and right-handed (90%). Visual acuity of the eye with the highest acuity ranged from 20/30 to 20/604.

EVIDENCE FOR RELIABILITY

EVIDENCE FOR TEST-RETEST RELIABILITY, MEASURING CHANGE, AND PRACTICE EFFECTS

The number of trials per subtest affects reliability, with multiple trials related to higher reliability coefficients. For one-trial administrations over intervals of one to two weeks, variable correlation coefficients have been reported (*rs* = .37 to .82; Buddenberg & Davis, 2000; DesRosiers et al., 1995; Reddon et al., 1988; Tiffin, 1968). Reliability values are high for the dominant and nondominant hand in adults tested twice within a 10-day interval (intraclass correlation coefficients [ICCs] = .72 to .76; Soer et al., 2006). Compared to single-trial administrations, three-trial administrations yield higher reliabilities after retest intervals of one week (r = .81 to .89; Buddenberg & Davis, 2000) and six months (r = .76; Doyen & Carlier, 2002).

Comparisons of administrations across five trials yield reliabilities ranging from ICCs of .69 to .71 for the dominant hand and ICCs ranging from .44 to .67 for the nondominant hand (Noguchi et al., 2006). ICCs of the Purdue Pegboard are slightly lower than other motor tests used in the evaluation of a hand function protocol (ICCs = .80 to .82), with recommendations that more than one trial be administered in order to increase reliability (Hollak et al., 2014).

The bimanual score is associated with an ICC of .66 in patients with schizophrenia (Sota & Heinrichs, 2004). After cold exposure, reliabilities range from *rs* = .49 to .84 (ICCs .65 to .89) for the dominant hand and *rs* = .49 to .62 (ICCs .63 to .76) bimanually (Muller et al., 2011).

It is important to note that right-left difference scores or ratios tend to be associated with low reliability estimates (r = .22 to .61, Reddon et al., 1988; Sappington, 1980). Reddon et al. (1998) noted that when right-handed adults

TABLE 14–26 Purdue Pegboard Means, Standard Deviations (*SDs*), and Quartiles by Age and Gender for Japanese Americans (Two Trials per Subtest)

	MEAN	*SD*	25TH PERCENTILE	MEDIAN	75TH PERCENTILE
Males 70–79 years					
Dominant hand (*n* = 52)	12.96	2.30	11	13	14.5
Nondominant hand (*n* = 52)	11.85	2.08	10	11.5	14.0
Females 70–79 years					
Dominant (*n* = 39)	14.17	1.55	13	13.5	15
Nondominant hand (*n* = 38)	13.31	2.14	12	13	14
Males 80–89 years					
Dominant hand (*n* = 17)	11.41	1.79	11	12	12.5
Nondominant hand (*n* = 17)	11.47	2.52	9.5	12.5	13.5
Females 80–89 years					
Dominant (*n* = 26)	13.08	2.34	11.5	12.5	14.5
Nondominant hand (*n* = 25)	11.28	1.49	11.0	11.5	12.5

NOTE: Age and gender, but not education or language spoken, significantly affected test scores.
SOURCE: From McCurry et al., personal communication with previous authors (May 10, 2004).

TABLE 14–27 Purdue Pegboard Means and Standard Deviations by Age and Gender for Older Adults with Low Vision

GENDER	AGE	N	HAND	MEAN	SD
Women	60–69	9	D	9.63	2.70
			ND	8.85	2.58
			Both	7.50	2.36
	70–79	18	D	8.66	2.35
			ND	7.47	2.29
			Both	5.72	2.05
	80–89	43	D	7.33	2.74
			ND	6.95	2.47
			Both	4.95	2.16
	90–100	21	D	6.06	2.49
			ND	5.33	2.49
			Both	3.77	2.22
Men	60–69	7	D	7.10	2.17
			ND	7.67	2.13
			Both	5.21	2.21
	70–69	5	D	9.80	1.92
			ND	9.13	2.36
			Both	7.50	2.24
	80–89	16	D	6.67	2.64
			ND	5.85	2.71
			Both	4.24	2.25
	90–100	10	D	6.10	1.98
			ND	5.47	2.02
			Both	4.15	1.70

NOTE: D = dominant; ND = nondominant; SD = standard deviation.

SOURCE: Wittich and Nadon (2017).

were tested weekly over five occasions, the right-hand score was greater than the left-hand score 50% (men) to 63% (women) of the time, with a wide range observed. Because between-hand changes in performance occur commonly in healthy adults, caution should be exercised in interpreting any changes in between-hand asymmetry as clinically significant.

There are practice effects, with scores improving on subsequent trials (DesRosiers et al., 1995; Feinstein et al., 1994; Reddon et al., 1988; Soer et al., 2006). In a small sample of young men who completed the test five times, the first trial had lower means than the subsequent fourth and fifth trials, and with the dominant hand the first trial was lower than the fifth trial. Unsurprisingly, trials were correlated with one another, with correlations among trials for dominant and nondominant hands averaging $r = .41$ (Noguchi et al., 2006). Feinstein et al. (1994) examined the effects of practice in healthy volunteers tested at two- to four-week intervals over eight test sessions. Performance improved with time, and a practice effect was discernible at the eighth session. Age also appears to interact with practice, with younger examinees showing a more pronounced improvement.

EVIDENCE FOR INTERRATER RELIABILITY

Intrarater reliability was scored by a blinded assessor on a small number of cases two weeks apart and yielded excellent ICCs of 1.0 (Bitter et al., 2011).

EVIDENCE FOR VALIDITY

FACTOR-ANALYTIC STUDIES AND RELATIONSHIPS WITH OTHER TESTS

The test loads on a finger dexterity factor, with the assembly condition also loading on a manual dexterity factor (Fleishman & Ellison, 1962; Fleishman & Hempel, 1954), as well as on an attention factor (Strenge et al., 2002). Pegboard dexterity and Finger Tapping measure independent dimensions of manual proficiency (Fleishman & Hempel, 1954; Stanford & Barratt, 1996). However, when between-hand asymmetry is considered, Purdue Pegboard placement correlates highly in healthy adults with Finger Tapping ($r = .78$; Triggs et al., 2000). Laterality indices derived from the Purdue Pegboard also correlate moderately well ($r = .52$ to .68) with those from other manual dexterity tasks (e.g., Doyen & Carlier, 2002).

Correlations between hand preference and relative manual proficiency on the Purdue Pegboard are high ($r = .70$; Triggs et al., 2000). However, left-handers have a smaller mean between-hand discrepancy score in Purdue Pegboard performance (Judge & Stirling, 2003; Verdino & Dingman, 1998) and greater variance in performance than right-handed individuals (Verdino & Dingman, 1998). Left-handers, however, perform more proficiently than right-handers on the assembly component, a task that requires timely coordination of both hands, which may be due to more proficient use of the nonpreferred hand overall in left-handed people (Judge & Stirling, 2003). The test correlates moderately with measures of executive function in older adults, with planning (Stockings of Cambridge) significantly predicting performance in both younger and older adults (Corti et al., 2017).

CLINICAL STUDIES

The Purdue Pegboard has been included in batteries in several studies, including the Cardiovascular Determinants of Dementia (CASCADE) study (Nilsson et al., 2005) and the European First Episode Schizophrenia Trial (EUFEST; Wobrock et al., 2013). Impairment has been noted in a variety of conditions, including progressive supranuclear palsy (Zakzanis et al., 1998), Huntington's disease (Brown et al., 1993), cerebellar disease (Brown et al., 1993), and schizophrenia (Flyckt et al., 1999; Molina et al., 2016; Roy et al., 2003). Improvement on the Purdue Pegboard has been reported in patients with stroke who completed modified constraint-induced movement therapy (Kim et al., 2008). The Purdue Pegboard is associated with vocational outcome in TBI (Asikainen et al., 1999; Nybo & Koskiniem, 1999).

Lesion Studies. The peg placement portion of the Purdue Pegboard may provide information of lateralizing significance (Costa et al., 1983; Vaughan & Costa, 1962). Right-hemisphere lesions tend to impair left-hand scores, whereas left-hemisphere lesions may result in a right-sided decrement.

PD. The Purdue Pegboard has shown promise as one means to detect PD. Postuma, Lang, Gagnon, Pelletier, and Montplaisir (2012) identified patients with idiopathic rapid-eye movement (REM) sleep behavior disorder, which is associated with an elevated risk of Parkinsonism. The test detected PD with 71% sensitivity and 82% specificity three years prior to diagnosis. The test was reported to be the most useful measure among motor tests examined in differentiating patients with PD from controls, with a sensitivity of 68% and a specificity of 82% (Růžička et al., 2016).

The test has been used to study outcomes of treatment in patients with PD, including after repetitive transcranial magnetic stimulation (Rothkegel et al., 2008), pallidotomy (Uitti et al., 1997), and motor training with visual cuing (Mak & Hallett, 2013). Performance improves in patients with PD after levodopa administration (Fregni et al., 2006). Performance is related to speech impairment in PD (Rusz et al., 2017).

Tourette's Syndrome and Tic Disorders. People with Tourette's syndrome show lower performance than controls on the test (Margolis et al., 2006). In addition to group differences between people with tic disorders and healthy controls (O'Connor et al., 2008), the Purdue Pegboard shows evidence of predictive validity in this group. Poor performance on the Purdue Pegboard (dominant hand) during childhood predicted adulthood tic severity at nearly eight-year follow-up; along with Beery Visual Motor Integration (VMI) performance, Purdue Pegboard performance in childhood was also found to be a significant predictor of adult psychosocial function (Bloch et al., 2006). Improvements in performance were found subsequent to cognitive-behavioral treatment (O'Connor et al., 2008).

Psychiatric Conditions. Sasayama et al. (2012) reported that people with bipolar disorder obtain lower scores than people with depression and healthy controls. Furthermore, the dosage of lithium and chlorpromazine was negatively correlated with aspects of performance. Poor performance on the Purdue Pegboard along with Block Design in childhood relates to obsessive-compulsive disorder symptom persistence at nearly eight-year follow-up (Bloch et al., 2011).

Fine motor dexterity is important for nearly all tasks of daily living. In schizophrenia, the Purdue Pegboard was one variable that significantly predicted quality of life at three-year follow-up (Sota & Heinrichs, 2004) and performance has been associated with better social functioning in this population (Lehoux et al., 2003).

Other Studies. There are influences on performance. Berger, Krul, and Daanen (2009) reported that wearing gloves decreased performance on the Purdue Pegboard by approximately 9%. Bitter, Hillier, and Civetta (2011) reported that training in sensory awareness (e.g., spatial relations between digits, sense of motion, ease of motion) in healthy adults improves performance. Visual acuity is moderately related to performance (Wittich & Nadon, 2017). Sleep deprivation may also affect performance (Bougard et al., 2016).

NEUROANATOMICAL CORRELATES AND IMAGING STUDIES

Schmidt et al. (1993) reported that healthy individuals who showed MRI white matter hyperintensities obtained lower scores on the assembly condition than did other subjects. White matter alterations as measured via mean diffusivity indices in diffusion tensor imaging in projection tracts including the posterior thalamic radiation are related to poorer performance on the Purdue Pegboard as well as on a number of attention tasks in older adults (Cremers et al., 2016). Lower scores on the test were associated with cerebral microbleeds (Akoudad et al., 2016).

PERFORMANCE VALIDITY

No information is available.

COMMENT

The Purdue Pegboard measures unimanual and bimanual finger and hand dexterity. It was originally devised for vocational selection purposes and subsequently used in neuropsychology for localization and lateralization. Of the motor tasks reviewed in this volume, this task is the most complex, incorporating not only peg placement but also the construction of "assemblies." The test shows moderate to large correlations overall with other tasks of fine motor speed, yet factor-analytic studies suggest that the Purdue Pegboard also measures skills beyond finger dexterity.

Demographic effects exist; age is related to performance, and women are generally found to perform better than men. There is some evidence this is related to finger size. Education appears to not be highly influential. There is limited information on the effects of ethnicity and other sociodemographic variables. The preferred hand tends to perform faster than the nonpreferred hand, although this is not a consistent finding and discrepancies between hands do not appear to be reliably interpretable. There are a number of normative studies available, especially for older adults, all of which adjust for age and gender. Of note, a number of these are quite dated, and each uses somewhat different numbers of trials.

Test-retest reliability is variable (poor to high), although reliability coefficients tend to improve after multiple (i.e., three-trial) administrations, suggesting multiple trials may be desirable in clinical practice to bolster the psychometric integrity of the task. Practice effects are found on this test over multiple trials. Interrater reliability is excellent. Clinically, the test has been used in a number of groups, showing particular utility in motor conditions such as PD and Tourette's syndrome and to predict functional correlates in daily life. Limited information is available on neuroanatomical correlates and performance validity, unlike other motor dexterity and speed tasks reviewed in this volume (e.g., Finger Tapping, Grooved Pegboard Test).

REFERENCES

Agnew, J., Bolla-Wilson, K., Kawas, C. H., & Bleeker, M. L. (1988). Purdue Pegboard age and sex norms for people 40 years old and older. *Developmental Neuropsychology, 4,* 29–35.

Akoudad, S., Wolters, F. J., Viswanathan, A., de Bruijn, R. F., van der Lugt, A., Hofman, A., . . . Vernooij, M. W. (2016). Association of cerebral microbleeds with cognitive decline and dementia. *JAMA Neurology, 73*(8), 934. https://doi.org/10.1001/jamaneurol.2016.1017

Asikainen, L., Nybo, T., Mueller, K., Sarna, S., & Kaste, M. (1999). Speed performance and long-term functional and vocational outcome in a group of young patients with moderate or severe traumatic brain injury. *European Journal of Neurology, 6,* 179–185.

Berger, M. A. M., Krul, A. J., & Daanen, H. A. M. (2009). Task specificity of finger dexterity tests. *Applied Ergonomics, 40*(1), 145–147. http://doi.org/10.1016/j.apergo.2008.01.014

Bitter, F., Hillier, S., & Civetta, L. (2011). Change in dexterity with sensory awareness training: A randomised controlled trial. *Perceptual and Motor Skills, 112*(3), 783–798. http://doi.org/10.2466/15.22.PMS.112.3.783-798

Bloch, M. H., Sukhodolsky, D. G., Dombrowski, P. A., Panza, K. E., Craiglow, B. G., Landeros-Weisenberger, A., . . . Schultz, R. T. (2011). Poor fine-motor and visuospatial skills predict persistence of pediatric-onset obsessive-compulsive disorder into adulthood: Poor fine-motor skills and persistence of pediatric-onset OCD. *Journal of Child Psychology and Psychiatry, 52*(9), 974–983. http://doi.org/10.1111/j.1469-7610.2010.02366.x

Bloch, M. H., Sukhodolsky, D. G., Leckman, J. F., & Schultz, R. T. (2006). Fine-motor skill deficits in childhood predict adulthood tic severity and global psychosocial functioning in Tourette's syndrome. *Journal of Child Psychology and Psychiatry, 47*(6), 551–559. http://doi.org/10.1111/j.1469-7610.2005.01561.x

Bougard, C., Moussay, S., Espié, S., & Davenne, D. (2016). The effects of sleep deprivation and time of day on cognitive performance. *Biological Rhythm Research, 47*(3), 401–415. https://doi.org/10.1080/09291016.2015.1129696

Brown, R. G., Jahanshahai, M., & Marsden, D. C. (1993). The execution of bimanual movements in patients with Parkinson's, Huntington's, and cerebellar disease. *Journal of Neurology, Neurosurgery and Psychiatry, 56,* 295–297.

Buddenberg, L. A., & Davis, C. (2000). Test-retest reliability of the Purdue Pegboard Test. *American Journal of Occupational Therapy, 54,* 555–558.

Corti, E. J., Johnson, A. R., Riddle, H., Gasson, N., Kane, R., & Loftus, A. M. (2017). The relationship between executive function and fine motor control in young and older adults. *Human Movement Science, 51,* 41–50. https://doi.org/10.1016/j.humov.2016.11.001

Costa, L. D., Scarola, L. M., & Rapin, I. (1983). Purdue Pegboard scores for normal grammar school children. *Perceptual and Motor Skills, 18,* 748.

Cremers, L. G. M., de Groot, M., Hofman, A., Krestin, G. P., van der Lugt, A., Niessen, W. J., . . . Ikram, M. A. (2016). Altered tract-specific white matter microstructure is related to poorer cognitive performance: The Rotterdam Study. *Neurobiology of Aging, 39,* 108–117. https://doi.org/10.1016/j.neurobiolaging.2015.11.021

DesRosiers, J., Hebert, R., Bravo, G., & Dutil, E. (1995). The Purdue Pegboard Test: Normative data for people aged 60 and over. *Disability and Rehabilitation, 17,* 217–224.

Doyen, A-L., & Carlier, M. (2002). Measuring handedness: A validation study of Bishop's Reaching Card Test. *Laterality, 7,* 115–130.

Feinstein, A., Brown, R., & Ron, M. (1994). Effects of practice of serial tests of attention in healthy subjects. *Journal of Clinical and Experimental Neuropsychology, 16,* 436–447.

Fleishman, E. A., & Ellison, G. D. (1962). A factor analysis of fine manipulative tests. *Journal of Applied Psychology, 46,* 96–105.

Fleishman, E. A., & Hempel, W. E., Jr. (1954). A factor analysis of dexterity tests. *Personnel Psychology, 7,* 15–32.

Flyckt, L., Sydow, O., Bjerkenstedt, L., Edman, G., Rydin, E., & Wiesel, F-A. (1999). Neurological signs and psychomotor performance in patients with schizophrenia, their relatives and healthy controls. *Psychiatry Research, 86,* 113–129.

Fregni, F., Boggio, P. S., Bermpohl, F., Maia, F., Rigonatti, S. P., Barbosa, E. R., & Pascual-Leone, A. (2006). Immediate placebo effect in Parkinson's disease – is the subjective relief accompanied by objective improvement? *European Neurology, 56*(4), 222–229. http://doi.org/10.1159/000096490

Hollak, N., Soer, R., van der Woude, L. H., & Reneman, M. F. (2014). Towards a comprehensive functional capacity evaluation for hand function. *Applied Ergonomics, 45*(3), 686–692. http://doi.org/10.1016/j.apergo.2013.09.006

Judge, J., & Stirling, J. (2003). Fine motor skill performance in left-and right-handers: Evidence of an advantage for left-handers. *Laterality, 8,* 297–306.

Kim, D. G., Cho, Y. W., Hong, J. H., Song, J. C., Chung, H., Bai, D., . . . Jang, S. H. (2008). Effect of constraint-induced movement therapy with modified opposition restriction orthosis in chronic hemiparetic patients with stroke. *NeuroRehabilitation, 23*(3), 239–244.

Lehoux, C., Everett, J., Laplante, L., Emond, C., Trepanier, J., Brassard, A., . . . Roy, M.A. (2003). Fine motor dexterity is correlated to social functioning in schizophrenia. *Schizophrenia Research, 62,* 269–273.

Mak, M., & Hallett, M. (2013). Effect of cued training on motor evoked potential and cortical silent period in people with Parkinson's disease. *Clinical Neurophysiology, 124*(3), 545–550. http://doi.org/10.1016/j.clinph.2012.08.017

Margolis, A., Donkervoort, M., Kinsbourne, M., & Peterson, B. S. (2006). Interhemispheric connectivity and executive functioning in adults with Tourette syndrome. *Neuropsychology, 20*(1), 66–76. http://doi.org/10.1037/0894-4105.20.1.66

McCurry, S. M., Gibbons, L. E., Uomoto, J. M., Thompson, M. L., Graves, A. B., Edland, S. D., . . . Larson, E. B. (2001). Neuropsychological test performance in a cognitively intact sample of older Japanese American adults. *Archives of Clinical Neuropsychology, 16,* 447–459.

Molina, J. L., González Alemán, G., Florenzano, N., Padilla, E., Calvó, M., Guerrero, G., . . . de Erausquin, G. A. (2016). Prediction of neurocognitive deficits by parkinsonian motor impairment in schizophrenia: A study in neuroleptic-naïve subjects, unaffected first-degree relatives and healthy controls from an indigenous population. *Schizophrenia Bulletin, 42*(6), 1486–1495. https://doi.org/10.1093/schbul/sbw023

Muller, M. D., Ryan, E. J., Kim, C.-H., Muller, S. M., & Glickman, E. L. (2011). Test–retest reliability of Purdue Pegboard performance in thermoneutral and cold ambient conditions. *Ergonomics, 54*(11), 1081–1087. http://doi.org/10.1080/00140139.2011.620178

Nilsson, L.-G., Söderlund, H., Berger, K., Breteler, M., de Ridder, M., Dufouil, C., . . . Launer, L. J. (2005). Cognitive Test Battery of Cascade: Tasks and data. *Aging, Neuropsychology, and Cognition, 12*(1), 32–56. http://doi.org/10.1080/13825580590925099

Noguchi, T., Demura, S., Nagasawa, Y., & Uchiyama, M. (2006). An examination of practice and laterality effects on the Purdue Pegboard and Moving Beans with Tweezers. *Perceptual and Motor Skills, 102*(1), 265–274.

Nybo, T., & Koskiniem, M. (1999). Cognitive indicators of vocational outcome after severe traumatic brain injury (TBI) in childhood. *Brain Injury, 13,* 759–766.

O'Connor, K. P., Lavoie, M. E., Stip, E., Borgeat, F., & Laverdure, A. (2008). Cognitive-behaviour therapy and skilled motor performance in adults with chronic tic disorder. *Neuropsychological Rehabilitation, 18*(1), 45–64. http://doi.org/10.1080/09602010701390835

Peters, M. (1990). Subclassification of non-pathological left-handers poses problems for theories of handedness. *Neuropsychologia, 28,* 279–289.

Peters, M., Servos, P., & Day, R. (1990). Marked sex differences on a fine motor skill task disappear when finger size is used as a covariate. *Journal of Applied Psychology, 75,* 87–90.

Postuma, R. B., Lang, A. E., Gagnon, J. F., Pelletier, A., & Montplaisir, J. Y. (2012). How does parkinsonism start? Prodromal parkinsonism motor changes in idiopathic REM sleep behaviour disorder. *Brain, 135*(6), 1860–1870. http://doi.org/10.1093/brain/aws093

Reddon, J. R., Gill, D. M., Gauk, S. E., & Maerz, M. D. (1988). Purdue Pegboard: Test-retest estimates. *Perceptual and Motor Skills, 66,* 503–506.

Rothkegel, H., Sommer, M., Rammsayer, T., Trenkwalder, C., & Paulus, W. (2008). Training effects outweigh effects of single-session conventional rTMS and Theta Burst Stimulation in PD patients. *Neurorehabilitation and Neural Repair, 23*(4), 373–381. http://doi.org/10.1177/1545968308322842

Roy, M-A., Lehoux, C., Emond, C., Laplante, L., Bouchard, R. H., Everett, J., . . . Maziade, M. (2003). A pilot neuropsychological study of Kraepelinian and non-Kraepelinian schizophrenia. *Schizophrenia Research, 62,* 155–163.

Rusz, J., Tykalová, T., Krupička, R., Zárubová, K., Novotný, M., Jech, R., . . . Růžička, E. (2017). Comparative analysis of speech impairment and upper limb motor dysfunction in Parkinson's disease. *Journal of Neural Transmission, 124*(4), 463–470. https://doi.org/10.1007/s00702-016-1662-y

Růžička, E., Krupička, R., Zárubová, K., Rusz, J., Jech, R., & Szabó, Z. (2016). Tests of manual dexterity and speed in Parkinson's disease: Not all measure the same. *Parkinsonism & Related Disorders, 28,* 118–123. https://doi.org/10.1016/j.parkreldis.2016.05.009

Sappington, T. J. (1980). Measures of lateral dominance: Interrelationships and temporal stability. *Perceptual and Motor Skills, 50,* 783–790.

Sasayama, D., Hori, H., Teraishi, T., Hattori, K., Ota, M., Matsuo, J., . . . Kunugi, H. (2012). More severe impairment of manual dexterity in bipolar disorder compared to unipolar major depression. *Journal of Affective Disorders, 136*(3), 1047–1052. http://doi.org/10.1016/j.jad.2011.11.031

Schmidt, R., Fazekas, F., Offenbacher, H., Dusek, T., Zac, E., Reinhart, B., . . . Lechner, H. (1993). Neuropsychologic correlations of MRI white matter hyperintensities: A study of 150 normal volunteers. *Neurology, 43,* 2490–2492.

Soer, R., Gerrits, E. H. J., & Reneman, M. F. (2006). Test-retest reliability of a WRULD functional capacity evaluation in healthy adults. *Work, 26*(3), 273–280.

Sota, T. L., & Heinrichs, R. W. (2004). Demographic, clinical, and neurocognitive predictors of quality of life in schizophrenia patients receiving conventional neuroleptics. *Comprehensive Psychiatry, 45*(5), 415–421. http://doi.org/10.1016/j.comppsych.2004.06.010

Strenge, H., Niederberger, U., & Seelhorst, U. (2002). Correlation between tests of attention and performance on Grooved and Purdue Pegboards in normal subjects. *Perceptual and Motor Skills, 95,* 507–514.

Tiffin, J. (1968). *Purdue Pegboard: Examiner manual.* Chicago: Science Research Associates.

Tiffin, J., & Asher, E. J. (1948). The Purdue Pegboard: Norms and studies of reliability and validity. *Journal of Applied Psychology, 32,* 234–247.

Triggs, W. J., Calvanio, R., Levine, M., Heaton, R. K., & Heilman, K. M. (2000). Predicting hand preference with performance on motor tasks. *Cortex, 36,* 679–689.

Uitti, R. J., Wharen, R. E., Turk, M. F., Lucas, J. A., Finton, M. J., Graff-Radford, N. R., . . . Atkinson, E. J. (1997). Unilateral pallidotomy for Parkinson's disease: Comparison of outcome in younger versus elderly patients. *Neurology, 49,* 1072–1077.

Vaughan, H. G., & Costa, L. D. (1962). Performance of patients with lateralized cerebral lesions: II. Sensory and motor tests. *Journal of Nervous and Mental Disease, 134,* 237–243.

Verdino, M., & Dingman, S. (1998). Two measures of laterality in handedness: The Edinburgh Handedness Inventory and the Purdue Pegboard test of manual dexterity. *Perceptual and Motor Skills, 86,* 476–478.

Wittich, W., & Nadon, C. (2017). The Purdue Pegboard test: Normative data for older adults with low vision. *Disability and Rehabilitation: Assistive Technology, 12*(3), 272–279. https://doi.org/10.3109/17483107.2015.1129459

Wobrock, T., Falkai, P., Schneider-Axmann, T., Hasan, A., Galderisi, S., Davidson, M., . . . Fleischhacker, W. W. (2013). Comorbid substance abuse in first-episode schizophrenia: Effects on cognition and psychopathology in the EUFEST study. *Schizophrenia Research, 147*(1), 132–139. http://doi.org/10.1016/j.schres.2013.03.001

Yeudall, L. T., Fromm, D., Reddon, J. R., & Stefanyk, W. O. (1986). Normative data stratified by age and sex for 12 neuropsychological tests. *Journal of Clinical Psychology, 42,* 918–946.

Zakzanis, K. K., Leach, L., & Freedman, M. (1998). Structural and functional meta-analytic evidence for fronto-subcortical system deficit in progressive supranuclear palsy. *Brain and Cognition, 38,* 283–296.

15 | PERFORMANCE VALIDITY

b TEST

TEST NAME	**b Test**
DOMAIN	Performance validity
AGE RANGE	17+ years
ADMINISTRATION TIME	15 minutes
SCORING FORMAT	Hand scored
REFERENCE	Boone, K., Lu, P., & Herzberg, D. S. (2002). *The b Test*. Los Angeles: Western Psychological Services. www.wpspublish.com

DESCRIPTION

The b Test (Boone et al., 2000, 2002) is a letter-recognition task that is designed to detect suspect test-taking via assessment of an overlearned skill that is fairly resistant to acquired brain injury. Because individuals who feign or exaggerate cognitive deficits may not be aware of this relative preservation, they may be flagged by the test. Anecdotally, Boone assessed several malingerers who stated that they had become dyslexic (i.e., seeing letters upside down and backward) after an equivocal head injury, a complaint not reported in most head-injured patients. This experience led to the development of this measure.

ADMINISTRATION

Details on administration, items, and format are not provided to preserve test security. Please see test manual for details. The authors caution that the test should not be given to those who have significant visual or motor impairments, moderate to severe dementia, acute psychosis, or substance intoxication.

SCORING

See the manual. The error and time scores are used to compute the E-score, which is the primary score required for interpretation. In the equation used to calculate the E-score, commission errors are given added weight to reflect their importance as signs of suspect performance. The examinee's performance can be evaluated against that of honest respondents and respondents whose performance is known to be suspect.

Although the E-score is the primary score used to interpret performance, clinicians can also examine the component scores (commission errors, "d" commission errors, omission errors, total time) to evaluate whether an examinee chose inaccurate or slowed responding as the method of symptom fabrication. Appendix B in the test manual provides sensitivity and specificity values for b Test component scores. See the sections "Normative Data" and "Clinical Studies" for additional information.

DEMOGRAPHIC EFFECTS

AGE

Boone et al. (2002) reported that age does not affect test scores.

GENDER

Gender has no effect on E-scores (Boone et al., 2002).

EDUCATION

Education does affect E-scores, although the amount of variance accounted for by education is reported to be very small

(R^2 = .03; Boone et al., 2002). However, low to moderate correlations between the b Test and education were found in a sample of male US monolingual Spanish speakers from Los Angeles or Mexico with less than seven years of education (r = –.25 to –.40); higher E-scores were found in those with less than seven years of education (Robles et al., 2015).

ETHNICITY, NATIONALITY, AND LINGUISTICS EFFECTS

Spanish examinees appear to perform similarly to their North-American counterparts on the b Test (Vilar-Lopez et al., 2007; 2008). Data from low-education, low-acculturation US Spanish-speaking examinees shows that most cutoffs correspond generally well with the recommended cutoffs for the test, but some scores require higher cutoffs to avoid false positives (Robles et al., 2015; see also "Normative Data").

NORMATIVE DATA

Performance is evaluated relative to an invalid performance group and a valid performance group that corresponds most closely to the complaint of the examinee. As shown in Table 15–1, 161 individuals were included in the valid performance group. None was involved in litigation or seeking disability benefits. The invalid performance group consisted of 91 individuals, 88 of whom were in personal injury litigation or seeking disability benefits associated with alleged medical or psychiatric disorders (37% head injury; 27% stress/chronic pain). One was diagnosed with a factitious disorder, and two were inmates in a county jail seeking to obtain more lenient sentences.

Data on a number of honest-responder groups are provided in the test manual, including a non-neurological group and patients with a variety of neurological and psychiatric conditions (depression, schizophrenia, head injury, stroke, learning disability; Table 15–1). The examiner selects a group whose clinical status best matches the presenting complaint of the examinee. The test authors indicate that the combined comparison group should be used only if the examinee's presenting complaint does not match well with any of the specific comparison groups.

A table is provided (table 5 in the test manual) that presents recommended cutoffs and the associated values for four indices of classification accuracy: sensitivity, specificity, positive predictive values (PPV), and negative predictive values (NPV). PPV and NPV are calculated using three hypothetical base rates: 15%, 30%, and 45%. If the E-score is less than the specified cutoff, the examinee's performance is considered to fall within the range of valid performance. The recommended cutoffs were chosen to minimize false positives while maintaining adequate sensitivity for invalid performance. Appendix A in the test manual includes tables showing other cutoff scores with associated values of sensitivity, specificity, PPV, and NPV. These tables allow the examiner to opt for different cutoff scores in order to maximize sensitivity or specificity in various situations. As the cutoff score is raised, specificity and PPV increase, and sensitivity and NPV decrease. This occurs because a higher cutoff reduces the likelihood of false-positive errors but reduces the detection of individuals with invalid performance.

Boone et al. (2002) found that only 3% of the invalid performance participants produced E-scores of 50 or less, whereas 32% of all the valid performance participants produced such scores. Accordingly, based on their analysis of invalid and valid performance groups, they suggested that an E-score of 50 or less is very likely to represent credible performance. Only 7% of the valid performance participants produced E-scores of 160 or greater. By contrast, 58% of the invalid performance individuals produced such scores. Accordingly, E-scores of 160 or greater are typically associated with invalid performance. The test authors found that "d" commission errors are highly suggestive of invalid performance. Only 3% of the honest responders committed three or more such errors.

TABLE 15–1 b test Honest Responder Comparison Groups

HONEST RESPONDER GROUPS	DESCRIPTION	N (GENDER)	MEAN AGE IN YEARS (RANGE)	MEAN EDUCATION IN YEARS (RANGE)
Nonclinical	No psychiatric disorder, substance abuse, or neurological disorders	26 (8 M, 18 F)	73.1 (52–84)	14.5 (10–21)
Depression	Met DSM-III-R criteria for Major Depression	38 (18 M, 20 F)	60.9 (51–81)	14.3 (10–21)
Schizophrenia	Met DSM-III-R criteria for Schizophrenia	28 (18 M, 10 F)	35.3 (22–56)	13.1 (6–21)
Head Injury	Head trauma with brain lesion documented with CT or MRI	20 (14 M, 6F)	34.6 (18–56)	12.9 (10–17)
Stroke	CVA with brain lesion documented with CT or MRI	18 (10 M, 8 F)	63.2 (35–81)	15.9 (12–22)
Learning Disability	LD documented by cognitive testing; receiving special services	31 (14 M, 17 F)	31.0 (19–72)	15.6 (13–18)
Combined Group	All of above	161 (82 M, 79 F)	49.8 (18–84)	14.4 (6–22)

NOTE: CT, computed tomography; CVA, cerebrovascular accident, LD, learning disability; MRI, magnetic resonance imaging.
SOURCE: Adapted from Boone et al. (2002).

TABLE 15–2 b Test Scores for a Mixed Neuropsychological Sample

	CREDIBLE (*N* = 103)		NONCREDIBLE (*N* = 212)	
	MEAN (SD)	RANGE	MEAN (SD)	RANGE
Age	40.79 (13.07)		44.19 (11.19)	
Education	13.47 (2.56)		12.96 (2.78)	
E-score	66.67 (153.56)	23 to 1,588	343.44 (677.34)	26 to 5,360
Total Time (seconds)	492.78 (156.27)	287 to 1,237	749.39 (804.10)	272 to10,760
Omissions	13.04 (12.63)	0 to 73	47.66 (77.92)	0 to 944
Commissions	1.96 (15.17)	0 to 154	17.72 (44.86)	0 to 371
"d" Commission Errors	.09 (.32)	0 to 2	7.94 (22.64)	0 to 157

SOURCE: Adapted from Roberson et al. (2013).

There is evidence that other cutoffs may maximize sensitivity and specificity for identifying malingering. Roberson et al. (2013) cross-validated the b Test in a heterogeneous neuropsychology clinic sample. The sample was divided into credible and noncredible groups based on Slick et al. (1999) malingering criteria. The groups differed on all individual scores. The recommended E-score cutoff yielded a sensitivity of 41% and a specificity of 99% in this sample but lowering the E-score cutoff to 82 or higher maintained the specificity above 90% while improving sensitivity to 68%, suggesting utility of a lower E-score to capture more malingerers. Means (*M*) and standard deviations (*SDs*) are shown in Table 15–2 for information purposes.

Robles et al. (2015) provide US data from a sample of healthy male monolingual Spanish speakers from Los Angeles and Mexico with low education (age mean = 28.23, *SD* = 8.74, range = 18–49; education mean = 6.66, *SD* = 2.54, range = 0–10). Most had low levels of acculturation to the US. Adjusted cutoff scores recommended for monolingual Spanish-speakers with low education are presented in Table 15–3. Note that these cutoffs have not been tested in clinical patients and examinees who meet Slick et al. (1999) criteria for malingering, but they indicate that higher cutoffs are needed in groups with differing cultural, linguistic, and educational backgrounds for some scores. Notably, the b Test Total Time score cutoff was similar to that recommended in the manual, appearing relatively robust to cultural, language, and educational factors (Robles et al., 2015).

TABLE 15–3 Individual b Test Cutoff Scores Associated with ≥90% Specificity in Monolingual US Spanish Speakers

	EDUCATION	
	0–6 YEARS	7–10 YEARS
E-score	≥204 (92%)	≥142 (90%)
Total time (seconds)	≥588 (92%)	≥542 (90%)
Omissions	≥100 (92%)	≥63 (90%)
Commissions	≥7 (92%)	≥4 (93%)
"d" Commission Errors	≥3 (92%)	≥3 (93%)

NOTE: Values in parentheses represent specificity.
SOURCE: Adapted from Robles et al. (2015).

EVIDENCE FOR RELIABILITY

Boone et al. (2002) did not provide data on reliability, arguing that credibility of responding is not a stable trait or skill; rather "it is a capacity that responds to the external contingencies of the assessment setting. When the test-taking situation itself introduces a variable effect on the construct being measured, traditional reliability statistics have little meaning" (p. 23). They argued that the best evidence for the reliability of a PVT is that the test can discriminate among groups whose performance validity has been established by other means and that it can do so consistently across groups representing different problems and clinical states. Our view on test-retest reliability is that it is important to know that persons with legitimate injuries reliably produce valid scores on PVTs (see "Comments").

EVIDENCE FOR INTERNAL RELIABILITY

Not reported.

EVIDENCE FOR TEST-RETEST RELIABILITY, MEASURING CHANGE, AND PRACTICE EFFECTS

Not reported.

EVIDENCE FOR VALIDITY

CORRELATIONS WITH AND COMPARISONS TO OTHER PVTS

The test shows modest to moderate correlations with other PVTs (e.g., Dot Counting $r = .60$, Rey Fifteen-Item $r = -.42$, Warrington Recognition Memory Test [WRMT] $r = -.18$; Nelson et al., 2003). Reliable Digit Span (RDS) and b Test E-score were moderately correlated ($r = -.34$) in a sample referred for ADHD assessment (Marshall et al., 2010). The elapsed time variables from the Dot Counting and b Test were highly correlated, sharing about 42% of the variance. This finding suggests that these two scores may provide some, but not total, overlapping information regarding validity of performance.

In comparison with other stand-alone performance validity measures (i.e., Victoria Symptom Validity Test

TABLE 15–4 Sensitivity and Specificity of the b Test Compared to Other Performance Validity Tests (PVTs) in a Spanish Sample

REFERENCE	PVT	SENSITIVITY (%)		SPECIFICITY (%)	
Vilar-Lopez et al. (2007)		PCS-Litigation		Analog Malingerers	PCS-No Litigation
	N	14		35	12
	b Test E-score	33		80	92
	VSVT Total	50		97	100
	TOMM Trial 2	41		86	100
Vilar-Lopez et al. (2008)		Malingering based on Slick Criteria[a]	Analog Malingerers	Non–Compensation Seeking	Compensation-Seeking but Not Malingering
	N	10	54	30	14
	b Test E-score	100	78	90	81
	VSVT Difficult items	63	83	95	100
	VSVT Total	38	36	100	100
	Rey Fifteen-Item	56	11	85	82

NOTE: PCS-No Litigation, postconcussive syndrome not in litigation; PCS-Litigation, postconcussive syndrome in litigation. All examinees from Spain.

[a]Based on Slick et al. (1999) malingering criteria.

SOURCE: Adapted from Vilar-Lopez et al. (2007, 2008).

[VSVT] and Rey Fifteen-Item) in Spanish speakers with mild brain injury or postconcussive syndrome (PCS), Vilar-Lopez et al. (2008) found that the b Test E-score yielded the largest effect size for differentiating between non–compensation-seeking and compensation-seeking groups (whether suspected or not of malingering). The VSVT was, on the other hand, best for differentiating between non–compensation-seeking and invalid performance groups. As can be seen in Table 15–4, the Rey Fifteen-Item was the least sensitive of the three PVTs in detecting noncredible performance in this sample. However, the b Test appeared to perform less well in detecting noncredible performance in a Spanish population with PCS and in analog malingerers when compared against the VSVT and Test of Memory Malingering (TOMM; Vilar-Lopez et al., 2007). Group differences were seen in VSVT Total Correct, TOMM Trial 2, and b Test E-score, with the analog malingerer group performing the worst while no group differences were observed in the PCS groups regardless of litigation status (Table 15–4).

CLINICAL STUDIES

In support of the validity of the task, Boone et al. (2002) found that it was able to discriminate an invalid performance group of personal-injury claimants from seven honest responder groups (see Table 15–1). In order to be included in the invalid performance group, examinees had to show noncredible performance on two other tasks and behavioral features consistent with invalid performance (e.g., implausible self-reported symptoms). None of the individuals in the honest responder groups was involved in litigation or seeking compensation. The invalid performance group made more errors and took significantly longer to complete the task than did the honest responders. Data from this study were used to calculate sensitivity, specificity, PPV, and NPV over a range of possible cutoff scores (see "Scoring"). The primary criterion for selecting the cutoff score was to obtain a specificity of at least 85%. The recommended cutoff scores yielded sensitivities of about 70% for all comparison groups except schizophrenia and stroke, for which sensitivity was lower, at 56%.

Boone et al. (2002) reported that the b Test performed best when used with a head-injury comparison group. The recommended cutoff score of 90 had a sensitivity of 77% and a specificity of 90% in detecting invalid performance. PPVs were 58% with a base rate of invalid performance of 15%, 77% with a base rate of 30%, and 86% with a base rate of 45%. Therefore, the use of the b Test appears limited when the base rate of invalid performance is about 30% or less because the likelihood of a false-positive error is high (more than two of 10 claimants would be incorrectly labeled as noncredible responders). This problem is, of course, not specific to the b Test but would be expected in the case of most PVTs and SVTs.

As already noted, cutoffs may be adjusted to maximize sensitivity while retaining acceptable specificity (i.e., false-positive rate). Roberson et al. (2013) cross-validated the b Test in a heterogeneous neuropsychology clinic sample. The sample was divided into malingering and nonmalingering groups based on Slick et al. (1999) criteria (Table 15–5). The recommended E-score cutoff yielded a sensitivity of 41% and a specificity of 99% in this sample. However, lowering the E-score cutoff to 82 or higher maintained the specificity above 90% while the sensitivity improved to 68%.

Other individual scores are presented in Table 15–5 along with their sensitivity and specificity data. As can be seen, the E-score appears to be more sensitive than all other scores when specificity is held at an optimal level of .90 or higher. It is of note that failures were common in those with somatoform disorders.

Vilar-Lopez et al. (2008) also provide data on sensitivity and specificity to detecting malingering based on Slick et al.

TABLE 15–5 b Test Classification Accuracy of Cutoffs for Prediction of Malingered Neurocognitive Dysfunction (MND) in a Mixed Neuropsychology Sample

	SENSITIVITY (%)				SPECIFICITY (%)	
	TOTAL (*N* = 211)	MILD TRAUMATIC BRAIN INJURY (*N* = 71)	DEPRESSION (*N* = 21)	PSYCHOSIS (*N* = 21)	CREDIBLE (*N* = 102)	SOMATOFORM (*N* = 15)
E-score ≥82	68	58	76	67	90	53
Time ≥682 seconds	36	24	48	43	90	67
Omissions ≥32	45	44	19	43	90	93
Commissions ≥3	48	40	57	52	92	53
"d" Commission Errors ≥1	48	38	62	67	92	73

SOURCE: Adapted from Roberson et al. (2013).

(1999) malingering criteria, indicating good classification accuracy statistics compared to PVTs such as the VSVT and Rey Fifteen-Item test in Spanish examinees (Table 15–4). Smith et al. (2014) also provide data on detection of Slick et al. (1999) malingering criteria using the b Test (see "Low IQ," in this review).

Stroke. With regard to stroke, recommended cutoffs had to be set substantially higher than the other groups to avoid false positives, suggesting that the cognitive impairments associated with stroke may affect test performance independent of credibility of responding. The test authors recommend that scores be interpreted cautiously when assessing such patients.

Dementia. Dean et al. (2009) examined the utility of various performance validity indicators in a sample of nonlitigating patients with dementia of mixed etiology (Table 15–6). At a cutoff of 160 or higher, the b Test yielded a specificity of 47%, comparable to other stand-alone PVTs such as TOMM Trial 2 (45%) and Dot Counting (50%), but worse than RDS (70%). As the severity of dementia increased, the specificity of the b Test to noncredible performance decreased (Table 15–6). Again, this problem is not specific to the b Test; failures on stand-alone and embedded PVTs are common in those with moderate to severe dementia (Dean et al., 2009).

Low IQ. Smith et al. (2014) provide adjusted cutoff scores calibrated for the detection of malingering based on Slick et al. criteria in low-IQ examinees (Full Scale IQ [FSIQ] <75) that minimize false positives by maintaining a specificity of 90% or higher. As can be seen from Table 15–7, sensitivity varied across scores; omissions appeared promising with good sensitivity, but other scores exhibited limited sensitivity to malingering (i.e., E-score, Commissions). As expected, higher cutoffs are needed in low-IQ examinees to prevent false-positive identification of noncredible performance.

Psychiatric Conditions. The b Test appears to be less useful in patients with schizophrenia than in other clinical groups. The recommended cutoffs had to be set substantially higher than the other groups to avoid false positives, suggesting that cognitive impairment associated with schizophrenia may affect test performance independent of credibility of responding. The test authors recommend that the test findings be interpreted cautiously when assessing such patients.

ADHD. The b Test may have some utility in identifying feigning of ADHD (Jasinski et al., 2011; Marshall et al., 2010). Using archival data from patients referred for ADHD assessment in a university neuropsychology practice, the b Test showed a sensitivity of 47% and at least 90% specificity in differentiating among those with and without ADHD and suspect or credible performance on cognitive tests (Marshall et al., 2010). Detection using the b Test was somewhat comparable to that of the TOMM (Jasinski et al., 2011) and Dot Counting Test (DCT), but not as good as that of the Word Memory Test (WMT;

TABLE 15–6 Specificity of the b Test in Dementia According to Mini-Mental State Examination (MMSE) Scores

SAMPLE	SPECIFICITY (%)
Total sample	47
MMSE <15 (*N* = 2)	0
MMSE 15–20 (*N* = 8)	38
MMSE 21–30 (*N* = 10)	50

SOURCE: Adapted from Dean et al. (2009).

TABLE 15–7 b Test Classification Accuracy for Cutoffs with Acceptable Specificities (≥90%) for Prediction of Malingered Neurocognitive Dysfunction (MND) in Examinees with Low Intelligence (FSIQ ≤ 75)

	CUTOFF	SENSITIVITY (%)	SPECIFICITY (%)
E-score	≥409	28	90
Omissions	≥46	43	90
Commissions	≥33	25	90
"d" Commission errors	≥3	35	92

NOTE: Malingering group: age mean = 35.60 (*SD* = 13.13), *N* = 55; education mean = 11.78 (*SD* = 2.20), *N* = 54; gender = 60% female, *N* = 55; Wechsler Adult Intelligence Scale (WAIS-III) FSIQ mean = 69.20 (*SD* = 5.45), *N* = 55

Nonmalingering group: age mean = 41.93 (*SD* = 10.03), *N* = 74; education mean = 11.08 (*SD* = 2.12), *N* = 74; gender = 42% female, *N* = 74; WAIS-III FSIQ mean = 63.05 (*SD* = 7.16), *N* = 74

SOURCE: Adapted from Smith et al. (2014).

TABLE 15–8 b Test Sensitivity, Specificity, PPV, and NPV for Identifying Noncredible Performance in the Assessment of ADHD

				15% BASE RATE		30% BASE RATE	
	CUTOFF	SENSITIVITY (%)	SPECIFICITY (%)	PPV (%)	NPV (%)	PPV (%)	NPV (%)
E-score	≥70	47	93	56	91	75	80
E-score	≥90	36	96	61	90	79	78
E-score	≥120	22	97	61	88	76	74
Commissions	≥2	34	90	39	89	61	76
Commissions	≥5	17	97	55	87	74	73
Omissions	≥25	24	92	35	87	56	74
Omissions	≥30	17	94	35	87	57	73
Total Time	≥550	34	93	46	89	68	77
Total Time	≥600	22	97	57	88	76	74
"d" Commission Errors	≥2	33	90	38	88	59	76

NOTE: PPV, positive predictive value; NPV, negative predictive value.

SOURCE: Adapted from Marshall et al. (2010).

Marshall et al., 2010). Clinicians may use the information found in Table 15–8 to adjust the cutoff scores for their setting.

By contrast, Jasinski et al. (2011), in their simulation study, found that those with ADHD who were instructed to feign their symptoms performed similarly on the b Test as those with ADHD instructed to try their best. A group without ADHD instructed to feign performed the worst on all the PVTs administered. Although more research in clinical patients is needed, while the b Test may have some utility in detecting noncredible performance in ADHD, use of the b Test alone may not be sufficient in ADHD assessments.

Learning Disorders. The test can distinguish individuals with invalid performance from those with bona fide learning disabilities (Boone et al., 2002). Note that, in this case, the learning-disabled individuals comprised a highly educated group of university students (mean education, 13–18 years). Whether the task will prove equally effective with a more diverse group of learning-disabled individuals remains to be determined.

A case study of a litigating woman who sustained minor head trauma and developed delayed onset of language and speech problems suggests utility of the b Test in detecting feigned language disturbance. She performed in the normal range on several cognitive domains except language and processing speed tasks, and she obtained valid performance on almost all PVTs except for language-based tasks such as the b Test (Cottingham et al., 2010).

NEUROANATOMICAL CORRELATES AND IMAGING STUDIES

Not available.

COMMENT

Because malingerers may be selective as to which impairments they choose to feign (e.g., memory, mental speed, reading), it is important to have tools such as the b Test that capture differing approaches to deficit exaggeration, including feigning of dyslexia. In this way, the b Test is quite unique. Other strengths of the test include the availability of different honest-responder reference groups and the provision of sensitivity, specificity, and predictive accuracy scores corresponding to different base rates of invalid performance in various groups, as well as classification accuracy data in brain injury, low intelligence, dementia, and ADHD. The test's cutoffs have also been validated against Slick et al. (1999) malingering criteria in at least three studies, including one in Spanish examinees and another in low-IQ examinees. The test has been studied in diverse groups including a sample from Spain and Spanish-speaking groups in the United States with low education and acculturation.

In the few studies comparing it against other PVTs, the test performs generally well against established stand-alone PVTs such as the TOMM and VSVT. Data provided by the test authors suggest that the b Test is a useful addition to complement other measures of performance validity. The task is moderately but not highly correlated with other PVTs, suggesting that it provides relatively independent information. Additional studies are needed to confirm these findings.

Boone et al. (2002) do not provide information on reliability, arguing that PVTs are state measures, reflecting behavioral responses to environmental contingencies. Nevertheless, evidence for score stability in healthy controls is important, as is knowing that persons with legitimate injuries reliably produce valid scores.

The b Test is based on the notion that certain skills are highly resistant to the effects of brain injury and neurological diseases. Although the test authors present data showing that the task is minimally affected by the presence of neurological, psychiatric, or learning disabilities, users should note that cognitive impairments can affect test performance such as in the case of schizophrenia, stroke, and dementia. This is unsurprising and the case for most PVTs. At present, the instrument should be used with caution in people with lower educational achievement, particularly in those with less than seven years of education (Robles et al., 2015).

The b Test appears to be particularly effective in the assessment of brain injury and ADHD. Clinicians should note, however, that its utility appears most evident in settings where the base rate of invalid performance exceeds 30%; that is, practices that specialize primarily in medical-legal evaluations. In clinical settings with base rates of 30% and lower, the risk of false positives may be unacceptably high. This is also the case for many PVTs, which is mitigated to some extent by administering multiple PVTs. Evidence for the use of the b Test in criminal, military, and chronic pain samples is scant as of this writing, and more data on somatoform disorders would be of benefit. Finally, users should bear in mind that determination of malingering should not be based solely on the results of any single test, but rather must rely on a comprehensive assessment in which the clinician evaluates multiple aspects of the patient's performance, history, and behavior.

REFERENCES

Boone, K., Lu, P., & Herzberg, D. S. (2002). *The b Test.* Los Angeles: Western Psychological Services.

Boone, K. B., Lu, P., Sherman, D., Palmer, B., Back, C., Warner-Chacon, K., & Berman, N. G. (2000). Validation of a new technique to detect malingering of cognitive symptoms: The b Test. *Archives of Clinical Neuropsychology, 15,* 227–241.

Cottingham, M. E., & Boone, K. B. (2010). Noncredible language deficits following mild traumatic brain injury. *The Clinical Neuropsychologist, 24*(6), 1006–1025.

Dean, A. C., Victor, T. L., Boone, K. B., Philpott, L. M., & Hess, R. A. (2009). Dementia and effort test performance. *The Clinical Neuropsychologist, 23*(1), 133–152.

Jasinski, L. J., Harp, J. P., Berry, D. T. R., Shandera-Ochsner, A., Mason, L. H., & Ranseen, J. D. (2011). Using symptom validity tests to detect malingered ADHD in college students. *The Clinical Neuropsychologist, 25*(8), 1415–1428.

Marshall, P., Schroeder, R., O'Brien, J., Fischer, R., Ries, A., Blesi, B., & Barker, J. (2010). Effectiveness of symptom validity measures in identifying cognitive and behavioral symptom exaggeration in adult Attention Deficit Hyperactivity Disorder. *The Clinical Neuropsychologist, 24*(7), 1204–1237.

Nelson, N. W., Boone, K., Dueck, A., Wagener, L., Lu, P., & Grills, C. (2003). Relationships between eight measures of suspect effort. *The Clinical Neuropsychologist, 17,* 263–272.

Roberson, C. J., Boone, K. B., Goldberg, H., Miora, D., Cottingham, M., Victor, T., . . . Wright, M. (2013). Cross validation of the b test in a large known groups sample. *The Clinical Neuropsychologist, 27*(3), 495–508.

Robles, L., López, E., Salazar, X., Boone, K. B., & Glaser, D. F. (2015). Specificity data for the b Test, Dot Counting Test, Rey-15 Item plus recognition, and Rey Word Recognition Test in monolingual Spanish-speakers. *Journal of Clinical and Experimental Neuropsychology, 37*(6), 614–621.

Slick, D. J., Sherman, E. M. S., & Iverson, G. L. (1999). Diagnostic criteria for malingered neurocognitive dysfunction: Proposed standards for clinical practice and research. *The Clinical Neuropsychologist, 13,* 545–561.

Smith, K., Boone, K., Victor, T., Miora, D., Cottingham, M., Ziegler, E., . . . Wright, M. (2014). Comparison of credible patients of very low intelligence and noncredible patients on neurocognitive performance validity indicators. *The Clinical Neuropsychologist, 28*(6), 1048–1070.

Vilar-López, R., Gómez-Río, M., Caracuel-Romero, A., Llamas-Elvira, J., & Pérez-García, M. (2008). Use of specific malingering measures in a Spanish sample. *Journal of Clinical and Experimental Neuropsychology, 30*(6), 710–722.

Vilar-López, R., Santiago-Ramajo, S., Gómez-Río, M., Verdejo-García, A., Llamas, J. M., & Pérez-García, M. (2007). Detection of malingering in a Spanish population using three specific malingering tests. *Archives of Clinical Neuropsychology, 22*(3), 379–388.

DOT COUNTING TEST (DCT)

TEST NAME	**Dot Counting Test (DCT)**
DOMAIN	Performance validity
AGE RANGE	17+ years
ADMINISTRATION TIME	10 minutes
SCORING FORMAT	Hand scored
REFERENCE	Boone, K., Lu, P., & Herzberg, D. S. (2002a). *The Dot Counting Test.* Los Angeles: Western Psychological Services. www.wpspublish.com

DESCRIPTION

The Dot Counting Test (DCT) is a measure of performance validity. Unlike most PVTs that use a forced-choice memory paradigm, the DCT taps attention and speed of processing (Boone, 2013). The DCT was originally developed as two separate tasks by Andre Rey (1941; described in Frederick, 2002) and adapted by Lezak (1983; Lezak et al., 2004, 2012) to detect invalid performance; the tasks are used in tandem. Details on administration, items, and format are not provided to preserve test security; please see original source for details. Performance can be evaluated in terms of the difference between the time required to perform each task, with deviations from expectation raising the index of suspicion for invalid performance.

The version offered by Boone et al. (2002a) is similar to the original, but the cards are enlarged to facilitate ease of handling. Furthermore, both accuracy (errors) and speed (counting time) are considered in the Effort Index score (E-score), which is the primary measure on this version of the DCT.

ADMINISTRATION

See manual.

SCORING

Scoring of the original DCT involves recording the response time for each item. Some clinicians also record errors.

For the Boone et al. (2002a) version, both time and errors are recorded for each card, and these are used to compute the E-score. The E-score consists of the sum of the total number of counting errors, the mean ungrouped time (first set of cards), and the mean grouped time (second set of cards).

A table is provided (table 5 in the test manual) that presents recommended cutoffs and the associated values for four indexes of classification accuracy: sensitivity, specificity, PPV, and NPV. PPV and NPV are calculated using three hypothetical base rates: 15% (general clinical assessment setting), 30% (practices in which a mixture of clinical and medical-legal referrals is seen), and 45% (practices that specialize in medical-legal evaluations). If the E-score is less than the specified cutoff, the examinee's performance is considered to be valid. The recommended cutoff points were chosen to minimize false positives while maintaining adequate sensitivity for noncredible performance. Appendix A in the test manual includes tables showing other cutoff scores with associated values of sensitivity, specificity, PPV, and NPV. These tables allow the examiner to opt for different cutoff scores in order to maximize sensitivity or specificity in various situations. As the cutoff score is raised, specificity and PPV increase, and sensitivity and NPV decrease. This occurs because a higher cutoff reduces the likelihood of false-positive errors.

DEMOGRAPHIC EFFECTS

AGE

Age is related to performance (Arnett & Franzen, 1997; Back et al., 1996); however, the impact appears to be minimal. Boone et al. (2002a) reported that correlations with age are less than .20.

GENDER

Gender has no effect on E-scores (Boone et al., 2002a; Weiss & Rosenfeld, 2010).

EDUCATION AND IQ

Education does affect E-scores, although the amount of variance accounted for by education is reported to be small ($R^2 = .04$; Boone et al., 2002a; Weiss & Rosenfeld, 2010). Among those with low education (≤10 years), the impact of education is minimal (Robles et al., 2015). Moderate to high correlations with estimated FSIQ have been reported ($r = -.59$; Green et al., 2012).

ETHNICITY, NATIONALITY, AND LINGUISTIC EFFECTS

Findings on the impact of ethnicity are inconsistent but suggest caution in some groups. Vilar-Lopez et al. (2008) found that the DCT yielded an unacceptably high rate of misclassification of individuals with genuine impairment in a sample from Spain. Similarly, individuals from rural India obtain unexpectedly high DCT E-scores despite clinician ratings of credible symptom reporting (Weiss & Rosenfeld, 2010), as do honestly-responding African immigrants (Weiss & Rosenfeld, 2016). By contrast, Robles et al. (2015) reported that the measure appears robust to cultural/language factors in monolingual Spanish-speakers from Los Angeles and Mexico with low acculturation to the United States.

NORMATIVE DATA

ORIGINAL VERSION

Lezak et al. (2004, 2012) provide percentile norms for the time (in seconds) to count ungrouped and grouped dots on each card. The data appear quite dated because they are based on work published more than 70 years ago (Rey, 1941). Others have described different cutoffs. For example, Paul et al. (1992) recommended the following cutoff points: (a) longer than 130 seconds total time on grouped dots, (b) longer than 180 seconds total time for ungrouped dots, (c) less than three correct responses on grouped-dot cards, (d) less than one correct response on ungrouped-dot cards, and (e) more than four trend reversals (instances in which the respondent fails to show the expected pattern of requiring more time to count larger arrays of dots). However, the sensitivity of these cutoffs is poor (Boone et al., 2002a; Rose et al., 1998).

BOONE ET AL. (2002A) VERSION

In the Boone et al. version, the examinee's performance can be evaluated against that of honest respondents and respondents whose performance credibility is known to be suspect based on other cognitive and behavioral criteria. A number of honest-responder groups are provided in the manual, including a non-neurological group and patients with a variety of neurological and psychiatric conditions (depression, schizophrenia, head injury, stroke, learning disability, mild dementia). A total of 228 individuals were included (see Table 15–9). None was involved in litigation or seeking disability payments.

The noncredible performance group consisted of 99 individuals, 85 of whom were in personal injury litigation or seeking disability benefits associated with alleged medical or psychiatric disorders. All were suspected of noncredible performance based on other behavioral and cognitive criteria. Data from this study were used to calculate sensitivity, specificity, PPV, and NPV over a range of possible cutoff scores (see the section "Scoring"). The primary criterion for selecting the cutoff score was a specificity of at least 90% (achieved for all but the stroke group). The recommended cutoff scores achieved a PPV of at least 80% (except for stroke cases), using a base rate assumption of 30% for noncredible performance.

The examiner selects an honest-responder group whose clinical status best matches the presenting complaint of the examinee. The authors indicate that the combined honest-responder comparison should be used only if the examinee's presenting complaint does not match well with any of the specific honest-responder comparison groups.

Boone et al. (2002a) found that only 4% of all the noncredible performance participants produced E-scores of 9 or less, whereas 51% of all the honest responders produced such scores. Accordingly, based on their analysis of noncredible performance and honest-responder groups, they suggested that an E-score of 9 or less is very likely to represent credible performance. Fewer than 10% of the honest responders produced E-scores of 22 or greater, but 55% of individuals with noncredible

TABLE 15–9 Honest-Respondent Comparison Groups for the Dot Counting Test (DCT)

HONEST RESPONDER GROUP	DESCRIPTION	*N* (GENDER)	MEAN AGE IN YEARS (RANGE)	MEAN EDUCATION IN YEARS (RANGE)
Nonclinical	No psychiatric disorder, substance abuse, or neurological disorder; age > 45	51 (16 M, 35 F)	65.3 (46–80)	15.3 (12–20)
Depression	Met DSM-III-R criteria for Major Depression; age > 45	64 (30 M, 34 F)	59.8 (50–85)	15.1 (11–20)
Schizophrenia	Met DSM-III-R criteria for schizophrenia	28 (18 M, 10 F)	35.3 (22–56)	13.1 (6–21)
Head injury	Head trauma with brain lesion documented with CT or MRI	20 (14 M, 6 F)	34.6 (18–56)	12.9 (10–17)
Stroke	CVA with brain lesion documented with CT or MRI	18 (10 M, 8 F)	61.2 (35–81)	15.9 (12–22)
Learning disability	LD documented by cognitive testing; receiving special services	31 (14 M, 17 F)	31.0 (19–72)	15.6 (13–18)
Mild dementia	Met DSM-III-R criteria for AD; MMSE score >21	16 (10 M, 6 F)	75.4 (54–88)	12.7 (8–18)
Honest-respondent groups combined	All of above	228 (112 M, 116 F)	52.8 (18–88)	14.6 (6–22)

NOTE: CT, computed tomography; CVA, cerebrovascular accident; LD, learning disability; AD, Alzheimer's disease; MRI, magnetic resonance imaging, M, male, F, female.
SOURCE: Adapted from Boone et al. (2002a).

performance produced such scores. Therefore, E-scores of 22 or greater are typically associated with invalid performance.

Boone et al. (2002b) also noted other indicators of invalid performance on the DCT: longer than seven-second mean grouped time, more than three errors, and a ratio of ungrouped to grouped time of less than 1.5. Sensitivities of these indicators are low, suggesting that these findings are relatively uncommon even in those with verified noncredible responding; however, specificities tend to be high, meaning that these signs are almost never present in honest responders.

Robles et al. (2015) suggest that the DCT (Boone et al., 2002a version) may be used in Spanish-speaking individuals with low education, though cutoff scores may need to be adjusted to maintain specificity (Table 15–10). Their sample comprised male monolingual Spanish speakers from Los Angeles and Mexico with low level of acculturation to the United States (age mean = 28.23, *SD* = 8.74, range = 18–49; education mean = 6.66, *SD* = 2.54, range = 0–10). Note that although the sample was divided into two educational groups, the impact of education on the DCT was not significant.

EVIDENCE FOR RELIABILITY

Boone et al. (2002a) did not provide data on reliability, arguing that credibility of responding is not a stable trait or skill. Our view is that test-retest reliability need not be demonstrated among those with incentives to malinger; however, it would be important to know that persons with legitimate deficits reliably produce valid scores.

In an original study by An et al. (2012), healthy undergraduate students participating in neuropsychological evaluation for extra course marks were given the DCT, TOMM, and VSVT over two sessions. In the first session, 45% failed the DCT and 65% failed the VSVT. In session two, 75% failed the DCT and 25% failed the VSVT. No one failed the TOMM. Performance in session one was highly predictive of performance in session two. However, in a replication study, Ross et al. (2016) reported much lower failure rates: 5% and 3% for sessions one and two, respectively. Unlike An et al. (2012), the authors of this study did not find temporal stability of invalid performance across the two sessions despite a shorter retest interval. The authors surmised that the differences in findings could be attributed to methodological factors such as the small sample size, ethnic differences, and non-native English-speaking status of many in the An et al. (2012) sample. More research in different samples is needed to clarify the temporal stability of DCT scores.

TABLE 15–10 Dot Counting Test (DCT) Cutoff Scores Associated with ≥90% Specificity in Monolingual Spanish-Speaking Males with Low Education and Low Level of Acculturation to the United States

	EDUCATION	
	0–6 YEARS (*N* = 56)	7–10 YEARS (*N* = 59)
Age	29.27 (*SD* = 8.86)	27.25 (*SD* = 8.59)
Education	4.59 (*SD* = 1.96)	8.63 (*SD* = 1.00)
E-score	≥16 (91%)	≥16 (90%)
Ungrouped time (in seconds)	≥9.0 (93%)	≥6.5 (90%)
Grouped time (in seconds)	≥4.9 (91%)	≥4.9 (90%)
Total errors	≥5 (92%)	≥5 (93%)
Ungrouped	≥4 (92%)	≥4 (91%)
Grouped	≥2 (94%)	≥2 (95%)

NOTE: Values in parenthesis represent specificity. Boone et al. (2002a) version used.
SOURCE: Adapted from Robles et al. (2015).

EVIDENCE FOR INTERNAL RELIABILITY

Not reported.

EVIDENCE FOR TEST-RETEST RELIABILITY, MEASURING CHANGE, AND PRACTICE EFFECTS

Not reported.

EVIDENCE FOR VALIDITY

WITHIN-TEST RELATIONSHIPS

Total errors correlate modestly with grouped time (r = .25) and with the ratio of ungrouped to grouped time (r = –.34). However, the amount of shared variance among scores does not exceed 12%, suggesting that speed and accuracy of dot-counting performance are separable constructs (Boone et al., 2002a). Of note, Binks et al. (1997) found that dot-counting accuracy appeared to be more important than the time scores in detecting noncredible performance.

CORRELATIONS WITH AND COMPARISONS TO OTHER PVTS

The DCT shows moderately high correlations with other measures assessing feigning of cognitive symptoms (e.g., b Test, r = .60; Rey Fifteen-Item, r = –.43 to –.56; WRMT, r = .41; Nelson et al., 2003; Sumanti et al., 2006; Portland Digit Recognition Test, r = –.41, Youngjohn et al., 1995), suggesting that the task provides somewhat overlapping information regarding performance validity compared to other measures but also contributes unique variance.

Of note, the association between the DCT E-score and Digit Span (age-corrected scaled score) is high (r = –.75; 56% shared variance), indicating that these two measures may provide somewhat redundant information (Nelson et al., 2003).

There is evidence that PVTs that employ the forced-choice recognition procedure are more sensitive than the DCT to invalid performance (Burton et al., 2012; Hiscock et al., 1994; Martin et al., 1996; Rose et al., 1998; Strauss et al., 2002; see also Vickery et al., 2001 for a meta-analytic review of various procedures). For example, the DCT does not appear useful in distinguishing forensic cases from clinical controls and those involved in capital murder cases compared to the TOMM and Rey Fifteen-Item (Burton et al., 2012). Similarly, Vilar-Lopez et al. (2008) found that the TOMM had better sensitivity than the DCT for identifying noncredible performance in Spanish examinees, some of whom were identified as malingering based on Slick et al. (1999) criteria. The authors noted that the DCT ratio score was both correlated with severity of symptom reporting ($r = -.36$) and had a high rate of misclassification of genuine impairment.

CORRELATIONS WITH AND COMPARISONS TO SVTS

Correlations are modest between the DCT and SVTs comprised of validity indicators on measures of psychopathology such as the Minnesota Multiphasic Personality Inventory (MMPI-2), Millon Clinical Multiaxial Inventory, Personality Assessment Inventory (PAI), and Structured Interview of Reported Symptoms (SIRS; Boone et al., 1995; Green et al., 2012; Sumanti et al., 2006; Youngjohn et al., 1995). In a stress claim workers' compensation sample ($N = 233$), 15% failed based on the DCT E-score; those who failed showed elevations on the somatic, anxiety, anxiety-related, depression, schizophrenia, and suicide scales on the PAI (Sumanti et al., 2006).

Overall, the DCT appears sensitive to exaggeration of neuropsychological deficits but not necessarily to self-reported psychopathology or other symptoms, as is the case for many PVTs. PVTs and SVTs tend to have some overlapping variance but may tap different dimensions of exaggeration.

CLINICAL STUDIES

CLASSIFICATION ACCURACY WITH REGARDS TO SLICK ET AL. (1999) AND OTHER MALINGERING CRITERIA

There exist few studies on the DCT's utility to predict malingering based on multidimensional malingering criteria such as the Slick et al. (1999) malingered neurocognitive dysfunction criteria or Bianchini et al. (2005) malingered pain-related disability criteria. Only one independent study utilizing a Spanish sample is available (Vilar-Lopez et al., 2008). As can be seen in Table 15–11, the DCT E-score yielded moderate sensitivity to Slick-defined malingering while maintaining specificity above 90% compared to the other DCT indices, although it is important to note that the cutoff score used in this study (≥7) was much lower than standard cutoffs. Nevertheless, the authors cautioned against the use of the DCT in Spanish populations in their study of malingering due to unacceptable classification errors; in this study, TOMM classification rates were superior.

Personal Injury Litigants. Like most PVTs, the efficacy of the test in detecting noncredible performance is dependent on the setting. For example, Boone et al. (2002a, 2002b) found that the task was able to discriminate a noncredible performance group of personal injury claimants from groups displaying credible performance. Using the DCT E-score, sensitivity was about 70% in this sample, and specificity was about 90% in a variety of clinical groups.

Mild Traumatic Brain Injury (TBI). Vilar-Lopez et al. (2008) in particular cautioned on using the DCT as a performance validity measure in Spanish population with mild TBI or postconcussive symptoms. Nevertheless, PVTs such as the DCT have utility for interpreting baseline and post-concussion performance of athletes. In one study, 11% of high-school football athletes undergoing baseline neuropsychological assessments failed the DCT (Hunt et al., 2007). Only about 2% failed the Rey Fifteen-Item Plus Recognition test. Performance on Trail Making Test

TABLE 15–11 Classification Accuracy of the Dot Counting Test (DCT) and Test of Memory Malingering (TOMM) in the Vilar-Lopez et al. (2008) Spanish Sample

	SENSITIVITY (%)		SPECIFICITY (%)	
	MALINGERING[a]	ANALOG MALINGERERS	NON-COMPENSATION SEEKING	COMPENSATION-SEEKING—VALID PERFORMANCE
N	10	54	30	14
DCT grouped time >7 seconds	30	35	100	92
DCT Errors >3	48	11	85	83
DCT Ratio >1.5	80	70	79	42
DCT E-score ≥7	40	48	100	92
TOMM Trial 2 <45	100	85	100	81

NOTE: PVT, Performance Validity Test; DCT grouped time, average time necessary to count the dots on the grouped cards; DCT errors, sum of the errors on the grouped and non-group cards; DCT ratio, mean time required to count the dots on the grouped cards divided by the mean time required to count the dots on the non-grouped cards; DCT E-score, mean time for non-grouped items + mean time for grouped items + number of errors.

[a] Based on Slick et al. (1999) malingering criteria.

SOURCE: Adapted from Vilar-Lopez et al. (2008).

(TMT-B), Symbol Digit Modalities Test (SDMT), Digit Span, Hopkins Verbal Learning Test (HVLT), and dominant Finger Tapping Test were significantly worse for those who failed the DCT than for those who passed the DCT. These findings suggest that inclusion of a PVT such as the DCT at concussion baseline testing is useful to validate test results.

Criminal Defendants. In a study of criminal defendants, Green et al. (2012) reported that the DCT E-score differentiated between a group of forensic psychiatry inpatients charged with felony offences and deemed incompetent to stand trial suspected of feigning by their treating psychiatrist from a genuine group (area under the curve [AUC] = .69). However, the DCT E-scores yielded a moderate sensitivity of 42%, with somewhat adequate specificity (86%). At a base rate of 21%, a PPV of 44%, an NPV of 85%, and an overall hit rate of 77% were obtained in this sample.

Boone et al. (2002a, 2002b) suggested that individuals in different settings may take different approaches to feigning. For example, prison inmates may slow their performance on both tasks, whereas civil litigants may slow grouped time to approximate ungrouped time and commit errors (Boone et al., 2002a, b). Additional studies are needed to confirm these findings.

Dementia. Some studies have shown DCT performance to be preserved in the context of actual memory impairment (e.g., Arnett & Franzen, 1997; Wernicke-Korsakoff syndrome, see Pachana et al., 1998), although cognitive status does affect performance, and the task should not be used with examinees who have extensive cognitive impairments (e.g., dementia, stroke) because their cognitive problems may well interfere with accurate assessment of performance validity (Back et al., 1996; Boone et al., 2002a; Dean et al., 2009; Hayes et al., 1997). As seen in Tables 15–12 and 15–13, the specificity of the DCT to noncredible performance decreases as MMSE scores decline, with an increasingly high false-positive rate as dementia severity increases, and high rates of false-positive errors are seen across dementia subtypes.

TABLE 15–12 Specificity of Dot Counting Test (DCT) E-Scores on Different Mini-Mental State Examination (MMSE) Bands and Probable Dementia Etiology

	SPECIFICITY (%)
Overall sample	50
MMSE <15 (*N* = 13)	8
MMSE 15–20 (*N* = 18)	44
MMSE 21–30 (*N* = 26)	77
Alzheimer's disease (*N* = 39)	54
Vascular dementia (*N* = 11)	27
Frontotemporal dementia (*N* = 4)	50

NOTE: Based on a sample of nonlitigating patients with dementia of mixed etiologies. *N* = 80; age mean = 63.5 years, *SD* = 15.1, range = 23–97; MMSE scores mean = 18.5, *SD* = 6.0, range = 1–29. DCT E-score >17 defines failure.

SOURCE: Dean et al. (2009).

TABLE 15–13 Cumulative Frequency of Total Scores on the Dot Counting Test (DCT) in Individuals with Low IQ (FSIQ <75)

TOTAL DOT COUNTING SCORE	N	%	CUMULATIVE %
5	1	1.4	1.4
10	1	1.4	2.9
11	2	2.8	5.7
12	1	1.4	7.1
13	1	1.4	8.6
14	1	1.4	10.0
15	4	5.6	15.7
16	4	5.6	21.4
17	1	1.4	22.9
18	2	2.8	25.7
19	1	1.4	27.1
21	3	4.2	31.4
22	2	2.8	34.3
23	3	4.2	38.6
24	6	8.5	47.1
25	2	2.8	50.0
26	3	4.2	54.3
27	6	8.5	62.9
28	1	1.4	64.3
29	3	4.2	68.6
30	4	5.6	74.3
32	2	2.8	77.1
33	1	1.4	78.6
34	3	4.2	82.9
36	2	2.8	85.7
37	3	4.2	90.0
38	2	2.8	92.9
40	1	1.4	94.3
46	2	2.8	97.1
49	1	1.4	98.6
50	1	1.4	100

SOURCE: Marshall and Happe (2007).

Low IQ. In some studies, individuals who have low intellectual functioning show a high rate of failure on the DCT when the recommended cutoff score is used (Marshall & Happe, 2007). Only about 21% pass the DCT, whereas more than 90% pass other embedded PVTs such as the California Verbal Learning Test (CVLT-II) Forced Choice Recognition, Logical Memory Rarely Missed Index, and Vocabulary-Digit Span Difference Score. Marshall and Happe (2007) provide data on a sample with low intellectual functioning who were not seeking compensation or in litigation (FSIQ <75, mean = 63, range = 51–74). As these individuals score very low on the DCT, the cutoff score must be adjusted to a very high value to achieve 90% specificity. Instead, the authors suggested that clinicians use Table 15–13 to evaluate whether the score obtained by their examinee is unusual in those with low intellectual functioning.

By contrast, Hurley and Deal (2006) reported that in their non-compensation-seeking sample of individuals with FSIQ of less than 79, the DCT yielded the least rate of misclassification relative to the TOMM, Rey Fifteen-Item, and SIRS: only one individual was misclassified by failing the

DCT, suggesting that the DCT may have promise as a PVT in those with low intellectual functioning.

Psychiatric Conditions. Psychiatric disturbance (e.g., depression, psychosis) appears to have little impact on test scores (Back et al., 1996; Boone et al., 2002a, 2002b; Green et al., 2012; Lee et al., 2000; Weiss & Rosenfeld, 2010) unless the individuals are seeking compensation (Sumanti et al., 2006).

Other Populations. In general, research utilizing undergraduate samples tends to be affected by a high rate of noncredible performance (An et al., 2012; DeRight & Jorgensen, 2015). However, inconsistent findings have been reported regarding the frequency of DCT failures in undergraduate research samples, ranging from 45% or higher to 5% or less (An et al., 2012; Ross et al., 2016). Regardless, these studies suggest that use of PVTs such as the DCT may be needed to clarify the validity of cognitive test results in research that uses undergraduate students.

COMMENT

The DCT appears to be a unique test that uses a paradigm other than the usual forced-choice memory format used by most PVTs. The Boone et al. version is the preferred version due to superior norms and classification accuracy data.

The test appears to be relatively unaffected by age or educational level and has been used in a variety of clinical groups, including brain injury, dementia, and low IQ, and in diverse cultural and linguistic groups. However, the evidence to date suggests that the DCT does not perform as well as other PVTs such as the TOMM in identifying noncredible performance.

To our knowledge, the Boone et al. (2002a) cutoff scores have not been extensively validated using multidimensional malingering criteria and the only study that utilized Slick-defined criteria for malingering produced disappointing findings, although the E-score showed decent classification accuracy. Additional research on its sensitivity and specificity to criteria-defined malingering is needed. Additional independent validation in groups where performance validity is a concern is also needed, including military samples, disability claimants, and other clinical groups known to have high base rates of invalid performance such as ADHD and chronic pain. Like most PVTs, the DCT is not impervious to cognitive impairment and should be used cautiously in those with dementia or low IQ.

Like most PVTs, the test appears to display moderate sensitivity and high specificity at recommended cutoffs. Positive findings imply invalid performance, but use of the task in isolation may result in an unacceptable number of false negatives, a problem not unique to this test. Therefore, the clinician is encouraged to supplement this task with other PVTs, particularly forced-choice procedures, in line with general recommendations on PVT usage.

The influence of ethnicity bears discussion. Although the lack of linguistic requirement of the DCT may suggest utility in non–English-speaking samples, the research to date has been mixed. Some studies suggest that monolingual Spanish-speakers perform in the valid range on the DCT with minor adjustment (Robles et al., 2015), while others have reported an unacceptably high rate of misclassification in non–English-speaking samples (Vilar-Lopez et al., 2008; Weiss & Rosenfeld, 2010; Weiss & Rosenfeld, 2016).

REFERENCES

An, K. Y., Zakzanis, K. K., & Joordens, S. (2012). Conducting research with non-clinical healthy undergraduates: Does effort play a role in neuropsychological test performance? *Archives of Clinical Neuropsychology, 27*(8), 849–857.

Arnett, P. A., & Franzen, M. D. (1997). Performance of substance abusers with memory deficits on measures of malingering. *Archives of Clinical Neuropsychology, 12,* 513–518.

Back, C., Boone, K. B., Edwards, C., Burgoyne, K., & Silver, B. (1996). The performance of schizophrenics on three cognitive tests of malingering, Rey 15-Item Memory test, Rey Dot Counting, and Hiscock Forced-Choice Method. *Assessment, 3,* 449–458.

Bianchini, K. J., Greve, K. W., & Glynn, G. (2005). On the diagnosis of malingered pain-related disability: Lessons from cognitive malingering research. *The Spine Journal, 5*(4), 404–417.

Binks, P. G., Gouvier, W. D., & Waters, W. F. (1997). Malingering detection with the Dot Counting Test. *Archives of Clinical Neuropsychology, 12,* 41–46.

Boone, K. B. (2013). *Clinical practice of forensic neuropsychology: An evidence-based approach.* New York: Guilford.

Boone, K. B., Lu, P., Back, C., King, C., Lee, A., Philpott, L., Shamieh, E., & Warner-Chacon, K. (2002b). Sensitivity and specificity of the Rey Dot Counting Test in patients with suspect effort and various clinical samples. *Archives of Clinical Neuropsychology, 17,* 625–642.

Boone, K., Lu, P., & Herzberg, D. S. (2002a). *The Dot Counting Test.* Los Angeles: Western Psychological Services.

Boone, K. B., Sadovnik, I., Ghaffarian, S., Lee, A., Freeman, D., & Berman, N. G. (1995). Rey 15-Item Memory and Dot Counting scores in a "stress" claim worker's compensation population: Relationship to personality (MCMI) scores. *Journal of Clinical Psychology, 5,* 457–463.

Burton, V., Vilar-López, R., & Puente, A. E. (2012). Measuring effort in neuropsychological evaluations of forensic cases of Spanish speakers. *Archives of Clinical Neuropsychology, 27*(3), 262–267.

Dean, A. C., Victor, T. L., Boone, K. B., Philpott, L. M., & Hess, R. A. (2009). Dementia and effort test performance. *The Clinical Neuropsychologist, 23*(1), 133–152.

DeRight, J., & Jorgensen, R. S. (2015). I just want my research credit: Frequency of suboptimal effort in a non-clinical healthy undergraduate sample. *The Clinical Neuropsychologist, 29,* 101–117.

Frederick, R. I. (2002). A review of Rey's strategies for detecting malingered neuropsychological impairment. *Journal of Forensic Neuropsychology, 2,* 1–25.

Green, D., Rosenfeld, B., Belfi, B., Rohlehr, L., & Pierson, A. (2012). Use of measures of cognitive effort and feigned psychiatric symptoms with pretrial forensic psychiatric patients. *International Journal of Forensic Mental Health, 11*(3), 181–190.

Hayes, J. S., Hale, D. B., & Gouvier, W. D. (1997). Do tests predict malingering in defendants with mental retardation? *The Journal of Psychology, 131,* 575–576.

Hiscock, C. K., Branham, J. D., & Hiscock, M. (1994). Detection of feigned cognitive impairment: The two-alternative forced-choice method compared with selected conventional tests. *Journal of Psychopathology and Behavioral Assessment, 16,* 95–110.

Hunt, T. N., Ferrara, M. S., Miller, L. S., & Macciocchi, S. (2007). The effect of effort on baseline neuropsychological test scores in high school football athletes. *Archives of Clinical Neuropsychology, 22*(5), 615–621.

Hurley, K. E., & Deal, W. P. (2006). Assessment instruments measuring malingering used with individuals who have mental retardation: Potential problems and issues. *Mental Retardation, 44*(2), 112–119.

Lee, A., Boone, K. B., Lesser, I., Wohl, M., Wilkins, S., & Parks, C. (2000). Performance of older depressed patients on two cognitive malingering tests: False positive rates for the Rey 15-Item Memorization and Dot Counting tests. *The Clinical Neuropsychologist, 14,* 303–308.

Lezak, M. D. (1983). *Neuropsychological assessment.* New York: Oxford University Press.

Lezak, M. D., Howieson, D. B., Bigler, E. D., & Tranel, D. (2012). *Neuropsychological assessment* (5th ed.). New York: Oxford University Press.

Lezak, M. D., Howieson, D. B., & Loring, D. W. (2004). *Neuropsychological assessment* (4th ed.). New York: Oxford University Press.

Marshall, P., & Happe, M. (2007). The performance of individuals with mental retardation on cognitive tests assessing effort and motivation. *The Clinical Neuropsychologist, 21*(5), 826–840.

Martin, R. C., Hayes, J. S., & Gouvier, W. D. (1996). Differential vulnerability between postconcussion self-report and objective malingering tests in identifying mild head injury. *Journal of Clinical and Experimental Neuropsychology, 18,* 265–275.

Nelson, N. W., Boone, K., Dueck, A., Wagener, L., Lu, P., & Grills, C. (2003). Relationships between eight measures of suspect effort. *The Clinical Neuropsychologist, 17,* 263–272.

Pachana, N. A., Boone, K. B., & Ganzell, S. (1998). False positive errors on selected tests of malingering. *American Journal of Forensic Psychology, 16,* 17–25.

Paul, D., Franzen, M. D., Cohen, S. H., & Fremouw, W. (1992). An investigation into the reliability and validity of two tests used in the detection of simulation. *International Journal of Clinical Neuropsychology, 14,* 1–9.

Rey, A. (1941). L' examen psychologique dans les cas d'encephalopathie traumatique. *Archives de Psychologie, 28,* 286–340.

Robles, L., López, E., Salazar, X., Boone, K. B., & Glaser, D. F. (2015). Specificity data for the b Test, Dot Counting Test, Rey-15 Item plus recognition, and Rey Word Recognition Test in monolingual Spanish-speakers. *Journal of Clinical and Experimental Neuropsychology, 37*(6), 614–621.

Rose, F. E., Hall, S., & Szalda-Petree, A. D. (1998). A comparison of four tests of malingering and the effects of coaching. *Archives of Clinical Neuropsychology, 13,* 349–363.

Ross, T. P., Poston, A. M., Rein, P. A., Salvatore, A. N., Wills, N. L., & York, T. M. (2016). Performance invalidity base rates among healthy undergraduate research participants. *Archives of Clinical Neuropsychology, 31*(1), 97–104.

Strauss, E., Slick, D. J., Levy-Bencheton, J., Hunter, M., MacDonald, S. W. S., & Hultsch, D. F. (2002). Intraindividual variability as an indicator of malingering in head injury. *Archives of Clinical Neuropsychology, 17,* 423–444.

Sumanti, M., Boone, K. B., Savodnik, I., & Gorsuch, R. (2006). Noncredible psychiatric and cognitive symptoms in a workers' compensation 'stress' claim sample. *The Clinical Neuropsychologist, 20*(4), 754–765.

Vickery, C. D., Berry, D. T. R., Inman, T. H., Harris, M. J., & Orey, S. A. (2001). Detection of inadequate effort on neuropsychological testing: A meta-analytic review of selected procedures. *Archives of Clinical Neuropsychology, 16,* 45–73.

Vilar-López, R., Gómez-Río, M., Santiago-Ramajo, S., Rodríguez-Fernández, A., Puente, A. E., & Pérez-García, M. (2008). Malingering detection in a Spanish population with a known-groups design. *Archives of Clinical Neuropsychology, 23*(4), 365–377.

Weiss, R. A., & Rosenfeld, B. (2016, August 15). Identifying feigning in trauma-exposed African immigrants. *Psychological Assessment.* Advance online publication. http://dx.doi.org/10.1037/pas0000381.

Weiss, R., & Rosenfeld, B. (2010). Cross-cultural validity in malingering assessment: The Dot Counting Test in a rural Indian sample. *International Journal of Forensic Mental Health, 9*(4), 300–307.

Youngjohn, J. R., Burrows, L., & Erdal, K. (1995). Brain damage or compensation neurosis? The controversial post-concussion syndrome. *The Clinical Neuropsychologist, 9,* 112–123.

MEDICAL SYMPTOM VALIDITY TEST (MSVT)

TEST NAME	**Medical Symptom Validity Test (MSVT)**
DOMAIN	Performance validity
AGE RANGE	In adults, has been used in a variety of age ranges
ADMINISTRATION TIME	5 minutes, and an additional 10-minute delay
SCORING FORMAT	Computerized
REFERENCE	Green, P. (2004a). *Medical Symptom Validity Test (MSVT)*. Edmonton, AB, Canada: Green's Publishing. www.wordmemorytest.com

DESCRIPTION

The Medical Symptom Validity Test (MSVT) is a computerized PVT involving verbal memory that is briefer and easier than the WMT, after which it is modeled (Green, 2004a; see the WMT review elsewhere in this chapter). Specifically, the MSVT has a shorter item list, a shorter interval between presentation and memory testing, and simpler foils. Surveys vary in the frequency of its usage but place it third for stand-alone PVT usage behind the TOMM and WMT in general neuropsychology practice (Martin, Schroeder, & Odland, 2015). It appears to be much less frequently used by neuropsychologists in forensic practice or in assessment of military veterans even though there is a significant body of literature in the latter group (Young, Roper, & Arentsen, 2016; LaDuke, Barr, Brodale, & Rabin, 2017).

The MSVT is comprised of two primary performance validity subtests (i.e., the Effort subtests) and two Memory subtests. Details on administration, items, and format are not provided to preserve test security. Please see original source for details.

Effort subtests are designed to be sensitive to feigning and exaggeration but relatively insensitive to veritable cognitive impairment including memory deficits. The three primary MSVT Effort scores include Immediate Recognition (IR), Delayed Recognition (DR), and Consistency (CNS), the latter calculated based on the consistency of responding between IR and DR. The Memory scores include the Paired Associates (PA) and Free Recall (FR) scores (Table 15–14).

The MSVT, along with other PVTs by Green (WMT, Non-Verbal MSVT [NV-MSVT]), have a unique feature in that they are designed to be able to differentiate between failure due to noncredible performance and failure due to severe cognitive compromise. This is done by examining the profile of scores generated and gradient of subtest difficulty according to a specific algorithm, the Genuine Memory Impairment Profile (GMIP). They also potentially allow screening of memory skills, although the effectiveness of the Memory subtests at measuring memory per se has not been as well studied in the MSVT as in other of Green's tests such as the WMT. There is also a "Stealth Version" of the test that is designed to help with detecting individuals who have been coached on the test, which is deliberately not discussed in detail in the manual to maintain test security on detection methods.

TABLE 15–14 Medical Symptom Validity Test (MSVT) Scores and Abbreviations

IR	Immediate Recognition
DR	Delayed Recognition
CNS	Consistency
PA	Paired Associates
FR	Free Recall
GMIP	Genuine Memory Impairment Profile

NOTE: The GMIP and related terms such as Dementia Profile and Severe Impairment Profile all denote the profile analysis method designed to differentiate test failure caused by severe cognitive impairment and test failure caused by noncredible performance. Some differences in definitions are addressed in the text. The preferred term is GMIP.

Importantly, the manual has a section instructing users how to describe MSVT results in their reports; this includes protecting the integrity of the test by not naming the test specifically as a PVT, not describing in detail the rationale for interpretation, and not including score graphs in the examinee's report, general recommendations that should apply to all PVTs.

ADMINISTRATION

Administration details, including set-up and installation instructions, are provided in the manual (Green, 2004a). The test is presented via computer, with instructions provided by the examiner. A reading level of Grade 3 or higher is recommended. Testing is quite brief, typically taking about five minutes, with an additional 10 minutes for the delay interval.

The manual indicates that it is advisable but not necessary to make sure the examinee is on task during the IR trial, but the examiner should leave the room when it is clear that the examinee has responded several times, whether responses are right or wrong. No feedback or assistance is then given, as normative data for IR and DR were all obtained with the examiner out of the room (Green, 2004a). The examiner then re-enters the room to administer the PA and FR subtests.

Some studies involving dementia patients have had the examiner remain in the room and control the mouse if the examinee was unfamiliar with computers (Howe, Anderson, Kaufman, Sachs, & Loring, 2007; Suesse et al., 2015). However, the general instruction that the examinee leave the room is recommended for all examinees. Although testing time is typically quite brief in most examinees, testing of severely cognitively impaired persons, such as institutionalized persons with advanced dementia, can be very challenging, taking 45 to 90 minutes in one study (Suesse et al., 2015).

Items can also be presented orally by the examiner, although this is not the preferred method. The oral version is described as less sensitive than the computerized version and not generally recommended unless the computerized version cannot be administered. In a sample of consecutive clinical patients described in the manual, agreement between the computerized MSVT and oral MSVT was 81%. With regard to the oral administration, Howe and Loring examined the performance of two German dementia samples from the manual who were administered the test orally and found similar performance levels to a US sample given the computerized version, indicating that sensory input modality does not affect results, at least not in dementia patients (Howe & Loring, 2009). Note that the examiner stayed in the room and assisted with mouse use in the computerized study, which may have also yielded better concordance with the oral version, which by necessity requires examiner presence throughout the test.

SCORING

A scoring report is generated by the computer program. Notation of the pass or fail status is provided based on whether any one of the examinee's three Effort scores fall below a specific cutoff (see manual for cutoff). Results are presented graphically (e.g., line chart or bar chart that displays percentage correct or line chart displaying *z* scores), and raw scores are presented in table format. Comparator groups can be selected for comparison to the examinee's scores (see "Normative Data"). Advanced interpretation is provided by the computerized Advanced Interpretation Program for the test (Green, 2011a). Compared to the standard program, the Advanced Interpretation Program updates the interpretation rules and provides new comparison groups; it also directs users to apply Criterion D of the Slick, Sherman, and Iverson malingering criteria (Slick, Sherman, & Iverson, 1999) to the determination of whether examinees meet the Genuine Memory Impairment Profile on the MSVT (P. Green, personal communication, May 2018).

Step-by-step guidelines for interpretation are also provided in the manual. As the manual describes, Effort scores would not be expected to be normally distributed. FR subtest scores are said to be normally distributed, however.

Genuine Memory Impairment Profile, Dementia Profile, and Severe Impairment Profile. The MSVT and other PVTs by Green have a unique feature in that they are designed to be able to differentiate between failure due to feigning/exaggeration and failure due to severe cognitive compromise. When interpreting MSVT results in people who score below Effort cutoffs, in order to rule out false positives (i.e., ensure that results of people with severe cognitive deficits are not erroneously identified as noncredible), the gradient of difficulty of the subtests is considered. Specific formulas have been derived to do this that will not be discussed here for security purposes, other than to say that the determination is based on the overall profile of scores across all subtests (Effort and Memory scores) according to specific algorithms (Manual).

Using the algorithm, scores that do not fit the expected profile of people with cognitive impairment are deemed invalid (i.e., due to noncredible responding), whereas scores that fit the pattern expected in cognitive impairment are considered a reliable reflection of neurological compromise rather than feigning or exaggeration. Based on this, the MSVT can therefore yield three kinds of results: (1) passing all Effort tests (credible responding), (2) failing Effort tests and not meeting criteria for cognitive impairment according to profile analysis (noncredible responding), and (3) failing Effort tests but meeting criteria for cognitive impairment based on profile analysis (credible responding with Effort score failure attributed to a known neurological condition; Reslan & Axelrod, 2017).

Unfortunately, it is challenging to get a good grasp of the MSVT profile analysis approach as both the manual and studies in the literature at times use different terms and different criteria to define the process. In the literature, the MSVT profile-based approach has been variously called the Dementia Profile, the Genuine Memory Impairment Profile (GMIP), and the Severe Impairment Profile (SIP), and not always using the same criteria. The manual refers to a Dementia Profile; its derivation and validation are not very clearly described: the Dementia Profile is determined based on four criteria in one section (Appendix B) but five criteria in a different section (Appendix F, included in manuals after April 2006). Similarly, studies have used three to five criteria to define the dementia/severe impairment profile. For example, the SIP has been defined by either three specific criteria ("SIP3") or five specific criteria ("SIP5"; Dunham & Denney, 2016). According to Dunham and

Denney (2016), the SIP3 is equivalent to the GMIP and is provided in the computerized Advanced Interpretation Program for the test and the SIP5 is equivalent to the Dementia Profile: that is, based on five criteria, not three. However, the manual does not make these distinctions. Some authors have defined the GMIP as referring to failure on the Memory subtests only, with passing on the Effort subtests, which would be discrepant with both the SIP3 and SIP5 (e.g., Chafetz & Biondolillo, 2013). See also "Clinical Studies: Dementia" and "Clinical Studies: Low IQ" in this review for more information on the use of profile analysis.

Given the variability in the literature and based on recommendation by the test author, the term "GMIP" should be used to refer to profile analysis criteria, and the method for doing so should follow that provided in the Advanced Interpretation Program, including application of Crierion D of the Slick et al. criteria (P. Green, personal communication, June 2018). Criterion D specifies that invalid performance cannot be fully accounted for by psychiatric, developmental, or neurological disorders that result in significantly diminished capacity to appreciate laws or mores against malingering or inability to conform behavior to such standards. Based on this rationale, by definition, any independently functioning examinee failing the Effort tests and yielding a GMIP profile on Memory tests would be ineligible for the GMIP (Armistead-Jehle & Denney, 2015) and would therefore be deemed as providing noncredible performance. See "Clinical Studies" and "Comment" for more discussion of this topic.

DEMOGRAPHIC EFFECTS

AGE

Although the manual reports that age does not meaningfully impact Effort scores, independent research suggests some impact of age in samples that include older age groups. In a sample of 100 German-speaking Swiss persons aged 18 to 60 (Giger & Merten, 2013), age was related to some Effort scores (IR and CNS), with lower performance with older age. Memory scores do appear to decrease with age, as would be expected for tests tapping memory (Giger & Merten, 2013).

GENDER

Less information is available on gender effects, but available evidence suggests no significant effect of gender on Effort scores (Giger & Merten, 2013). Gender effects on Memory scores have not been well studied.

EDUCATION AND IQ

Education does not affect performance on Effort scores (Armistead-Jehle, 2010; Giger & Merten, 2013; Bashem et al., 2014). Giger and Merten (2013) reported that verbal intelligence as measured by a vocabulary test was related to IR and CNS scores; however, no associations were reported in a study on TBI between MSVT Effort scores and predicted IQ (Bashem et al., 2014). Education effects on Memory scores have not been well studied, but there does appear to be an effect of education, with better-educated people having higher Memory scores (Table 15–15).

ETHNICITY, NATIONALITY, AND LINGUISTIC EFFECTS

There appear to be minimal cross-cultural and cross-linguistic effects on the test. Interestingly, participants appear to be able to pass the MSVT Effort tests well above cutoffs even when the test is administered in a language that they are not familiar with. This was demonstrated in a small study of Canadian children and adults who did not speak French but who passed the MSVT administered in French, indicating minimal linguistic effects in a very small sample (N = 8 to 12). However, lower scores were obtained on Memory subtests in this study, indicating some linguistic effects on these subtests, as would be expected.

There are a number of studies in different languages, particularly in German by Merten and colleagues (e.g., Giger & Merten, 2013; Gorny & Merten, 2006; Merten et al., 2005). As well, there are simulator data in the manual on non-English-speaking populations (e.g., French, Portuguese, German). In a US sample, Armistead-Jehle (2010) reported that ethnicity was not related to MSVT failure in a military sample with presumed mild TBI. Two dementia samples described in the manual who were administered the test orally in German had similar performance levels to a US sample who were given the computerized version,

TABLE 15–15 MSVT Age- and Education-Stratified Normative Data

LEVEL OF EDUCATION	AGE GROUP	IR	DR	CNS	PA	FR
Primary	18–40	99.3 (1.9)	97.9 (5.7)	98.6 (3.8)	78.6 (23.4)	65.0 (10.0)
	41–60	98.0 (3.5)	98.0 (4.8)	96.5 (5.3)	74.0 (24.1)	69.0 (13.5)
Secondary	18–40	99.8 (0.9)	99.6 (1.3)	99.5 (1.6)	93.6 (11.9)	82.3 (11.2)
	41–60	99.1 (1.9)	99.5 (2.0)	98.6 (3.2)	90.7 (12.8)	77.6 (14.2)
Tertiary	18–40	99.7 (1.3)	99.0 (2.8)	98.7 (3.0)	96.7 (8.2)	84.0 (12.6)
	41–60	99.6 (1.5)	99.6 (1.5)	99.1 (2.0)	97.3 (6.5)	81.8 (17.4)

NOTE: IR = Immediate Recognition; DR = Delayed Recognition; CNS = Consistency; PA = Paired Associates; FR = Free Recall.

SOURCE: Giger and Merten (2013).

indicating that language of administration does not appear to affect results (Howe & Loring, 2009).

NORMATIVE DATA

Interpretation of the MSVT is based on specific cutoffs but it is not clear from the manual what kind of sample the original cutoffs were derived from. According to the manual, even children with low intelligence have almost error-free scores on the Effort subtests.

Although Memory subtests can be affected by neurologic compromise, these subtests are also designed to be fairly easy, and high scores would be expected for most examinees. For example, the manual describes high scores (i.e., ≥88%) in a clinical sample of children 13 years of age, patients with moderate to severe brain injury, a clinical sample of adult patients who passed Effort subtests, and a sample of patients with severe brain injury (see manual for more details). Memory scores appear to vary more in independent research on the test depending on the sample but are affected in those with cognitive deficits (e.g., Carone, 2008).

HEALTHY CONTROLS

A variety of datasets are presented in the manual and scoring program (see Source). Although the Effort scores are designed to be interpreted according to specific cutoffs, normative data would be helpful for interpreting Memory scores. Giger and Merten (2013) present data on 100 German-speaking Swiss persons age 18 to 60, subdivided by age and education. Participants were volunteers, 49% female, and with an average age of 39.4 years (SD = 11.9). Participants were excluded if presenting with intellectual disability, brain injury, psychiatric treatment, or alcohol dependence, or if a psychologist or psychology student. The mean verbal intelligence score according to a vocabulary test was 104.2 (SD = 10.6). Data are broadly consistent with results provided in the manual, suggesting that most people perform well on Effort measures, with more variable and generally lower performance on Memory measures (Table 15–15).

GMIP AND PROFILE ANALYSIS

The manual makes reference to data provided by Brockhaus on the mean difference across MSVT subtests in 30 dementia patients, which appear to form the basis of the GMIP analysis criteria. However, the demographic and clinical characteristics of this sample are not clearly provided, nor whether additional groups were also used to derive or validate the criteria is (e.g., simulators, known malingerers). See "Scoring" and "Clinical Studies" for more information on profile analysis.

COMPARISON GROUPS

The manual and scoring program provide MSVT data for a number of comparison groups, including simulators, honest-responder volunteers, child groups, adult outpatient groups, patients with dementia, and patients with soft-tissue injuries involved in independent medical examination. The data are potentially quite useful, although not provided in a way that is easy to look up in the manual. The examiner selects the comparator group of most interest given the examinee characteristics. Guidelines for selecting appropriate comparator groups are discussed in the manual, and examples of interpretation are provided. The Advanced Interpretation Program facilitates this process.

EVIDENCE FOR RELIABILITY

No information on the reliability of Effort or Memory scores is available to our knowledge apart from a concussion baseline study indicating almost identical scores on repeat testing for IR, DR, CNS, and PA using an earlier version of the MSVT, with more variability noted for FR (Broglio, Ferrara, Macciocchi, Baumgartner, & Elliott, 2007).

EVIDENCE FOR VALIDITY

There are numerous studies by the test author that uniformly support the test's validity. The following review of validity evidence emphasizes independent studies on the test; this review will also focus mostly on nonsimulator studies as much as possible, as simulator studies tend to yield higher accuracy statistics than when PVTs are used in actual clinical samples.

WITHIN-TEST RELATIONSHIPS

MSVT Effort variables tend to be highly correlated (e.g., r = .61 to .81 in healthy people, Giger & Merten, 2013; r = .72 to .89 in mild TBI, Armistead-Jehle & Hansen, 2016; Spearman's rho =.55 to .91 in stimulators, Bashem et al., 2014). The association between Effort and Memory subtests has not been well studied in the literature, but also points to high intercorrelations (e.g., r = .50 to .77, Armistead-Jehle & Hansen, 2016).

FACTOR-ANALYTIC STUDIES

Factor analyses provide evidence that the MSVT Effort scores tap a dimension common with other PVTs that is relatively distinct from questionnaires that assess symptom report veracity (SVTs) and standard neuropsychological tests. However, results are more mixed regarding the MSVT Memory scores. For example, the MSVT Effort scores loaded on a PVT factor with other measures of response validity such as the TOMM and RDS in a confirmatory factor analysis in a veteran sample; cognitive measures and self-reported symptoms including SVTs from the MMPI-2 loaded on two other factors separate from the PVT factor (Van Dyke et al., 2013). In another study, the MSVT, NV-MSVT, and memory subtests from the Repeatable

Battery for the Assessment of Neuropsychological Status (RBANS) were subjected to a factor analysis in military service members with self-reported mild TBI (Armistead-Jehle & Hansen, 2016). This yielded a two-factor solution reflecting (1) a PVT factor with loadings from MSVT and NV-MSVT Effort scores but also with loadings from memory subtests such as PA, and (2) a memory factor with loadings from the RBANS memory subtests along with MSVT FR and NV-MSVT FR memory subtests. Notably, the authors concluded that PA measures performance validity independent of memory functioning; however, Effort and Memory subtests did not separate cleanly in this factor analysis, and the two factors themselves were fairly highly correlated, which may reflect either properties of the tests themselves or of the sample.

COMPARISONS TO OTHER PVTS

WMT AND NV-MSVT

More independent research on the associations between the MSVT and its counterparts, the WMT and NV-MSVT is needed. According to the manual, the MSVT is easier than the MSVT, but independent research on correlations and comparison of detection accuracy rates between the two tests is scarce, to our knowledge, although it is nevertheless assumed to be quite high given their common format and content. As noted, the MSVT is considered an easier test than the WMT and yields a lower failure rate.

Data from one research group indicate that the MSVT is more difficult (i.e., has a slightly higher failure rate) than its nonverbal counterpart, the NV-MSVT; MSVT Effort scores are nevertheless moderately to highly correlated with NV-MSVT Effort scores, indicating that the tests tap a common construct ($r = .77$; Armistead-Jehle & Hansen, 2011; Armistead-Jehle et al., 2016). Intercorrelations between MSVT Memory subtests and NV-MSVT Memory subtests are lower but still in the moderate to high range ($r = .31$ to $.59$; Armistead-Jehle & Hansen, 2016).

TOMM

Studies on the TOMM indicate that the MSVT and TOMM are fairly highly correlated; studies comparing detection rates are mixed, but compared to the TOMM, the MSVT does not appear to have the same issues with high false-positive rates that have been reported for the WMT (see review elsewhere in this chapter) and to have a more balanced sensitivity and specificity rate. For example, in a comparison of PVTs, TOMM sensitivity was slightly higher than that of the MSVT (50% and 45%, respectively), but the MSVT had higher specificity (94%; Bashem et al., 2014). Nearly equivalent discrimination ability between the MSVT and TOMM in social security disability claimants has also been found, including similar proportions of definite malingerers defined by below-chance performance (Chafetz et al., 2007; Chafetz, 2008). In one study, variables from the TOMM were highly accurate predictors of MSVT performance in a sample of veterans (Denning, 2014).

Some studies indicate higher sensitivity for the MSVT compared to the TOMM. For example, in one of the few studies using Slick et al. (1999) malingering criteria, 60% of social security disability claimants met probable malingered neurocognitive dysfunction criteria using the MSVT as part of the criteria, compared to 46% when the TOMM was used instead (Chafetz, 2008). In another study of active-duty and veteran soldiers, 32% failed the MSVT versus 23% failing the TOMM (Whitney et al., 2013). Similarly, in a mixed clinical veteran samples, MSVT failure rates exceeded those of the TOMM (e.g., 37% vs. 21%). However, if MSVT cut scores were adjusted downward to 70% instead of the recommended cutoff, failure rates were similar to those of the TOMM and of embedded indicators such as the CVLT Forced Choice. Reducing the MSVT cutoff to 70% was therefore found to best identify verified malingerers using the WMT while maintaining optimal specificity/false-positive rate (Axelrod & Schutte, 2011).

OTHER STAND-ALONE PVTS

The MSVT demonstrates moderate to large correlations with some but not all PVTs, indicating some degree of shared variance but also unique aspects to noncredible performance detection. Giger and Merten (2013) reported low correlations between the MSVT and other PVTs in healthy people such as the Amsterdam Short-Term Memory Test (ASTM); however, significant correlations were found for the Morel Emotional Numbing Test (MENT), a PVT for assessing feigned posttraumatic stress disorder (PTSD) ($r = -.21$ to $-.45$). One study showed high correlations with the ACS Word Choice (reviewed elsewhere in this chapter), but much lower ability to detect exaggeration for Word Choice compared to the MSVT (Bashem et al., 2014). The MSVT also correlates very highly with a scale developed specifically for detecting malingering in social security disability evaluations, the Symptom Validity Scale (SVS), especially for IR and DR scores compared to CNS ($r = -.79$, $-.80$, and $-.50$, respectively; Chafetz et al., 2007). Of note, Sollman and Berry (2011) concluded that the MSVT had the smallest effect size compared to other PVTs such as the VSVT, but this study was based on very few MSVT studies and involved simulators, not verified malingerers.

EMBEDDED PVTS

As would be the case for most PVTs, studies show lesser but still notable correlations between the MSVT and embedded PVTs compared to stand-alone PVTs. With regard to embedded validity indices, the MSVT has been reported to be highly related to the Rey Auditory Verbal Learning Test (RAVLT) Noncredible score but unrelated to RDS in a military sample (Whitney, Shepard, Williams, Davis, & Adams, 2009). On the whole, the MSVT identifies many more exaggerating examinees than do Digit Span-type embedded validity indicators (Whitney et al., 2013; see also Giger & Merten, 2013). MSVT failure correlates highly with failure on the RBANS Effort Index ($r = .56$) but the MSVT is superior to the RBANS in detecting noncredible performance (Armistead-Jehle & Hansen, 2011).

Some studies report equivalent failure rates for the MSVT and embedded PVTs such as CVLT-II Forced Choice (Bashem et al., 2014). Others report more failures with MSVT than CVLT-II Forced Choice, but adjusting the MSVT cut score downward to 70% instead of the recommended cutoff yields fairly similar failure rates (Axelrod & Schutte, 2011). In terms of concordance between measures, the MSVT and the CVLT-II Forced Choice have an overall agreement of 72%, but the MSVT identifies more exaggerators (Axelrod & Schutte, 2011).

MSVT failure is virtually uncorrelated with failure on validity indices from computerized neurocognitive test batteries such as ImPACT, Automated Neuropsychological Assessment Metrics (ANAM), and Axon in high school and college athletes undergoing baseline testing for concussion (Nelson, Pfaller, Rein, & McCrea, 2015). However, the MSVT has superior sensitivity to detection of coached and uncoached malingering compared to ImPACT validity indices in college athletes (Schatz & Glatts, 2013). Whether validity indices from these computerized batteries have been sufficiently validated as PVTs remains to be determined and may partially account for low intercorrelations with the MSVT, which has better validation evidence.

In low-failure groups such as research samples, the general trend of higher MSVT failure rates is still apparent, with a somewhat higher 9% MSVT failure rate compared to embedded indices whose failure rates range from 4% to 7%, including the CVLT-II Forced Choice, RDS, and Test of Variables of Attention (TOVA) Symptom Exaggeration Index (Clark et al., 2014).

CORRELATIONS TO SVTS AND OTHER STANDARDIZED QUESTIONNAIRES

Overall, as is the case for most PVTs, studies on concordance with SVTs indicate that the two kinds of measures tap somewhat separate dimensions of feigning that would be expected to overlap to different degrees depending on the sample studied (e.g., more overlap would be expected when examinees are motivated to exaggerate both cognitive and psychological problems and less overlap when examinees are motivated to exaggerate only cognitive deficits).

For example, the MSVT Effort subtests correlate moderately with MMPI-2 validity scales in military samples, including indices tapping cognitive exaggeration such as RBS, FBS, and Henry-Heilbronner Index (HHI), but also those tapping psychological exaggeration such as F, Fb, and Fp, with the latter group of indices showing slightly smaller correlations overall (Whitney et al., 2013; see the review of the MMPI-2 in Chapter 16 for more information on these MMPI-2 validity indices). Among MMPI-2 validity indices, HHI, an MMPI-2 validity index derived from Slick et al. (1999) malingering criteria, shows the largest effect sizes between those who fail and pass the MSVT, accounting for the most variance in MSVT scores (26%). Notably, similar-sized correlations are also found between the MSVT Memory scores and MMPI-2 validity scales.

With regard to the PAI, in veterans screening positive for TBI, PAI validity scales such as the Negative Impression (NIM), the Malingering Index, and the Rogers Discriminant Function do not differentiate between those who fail and pass the MSVT, suggesting little overlap between MSVT and PAI validity indices (Armistead-Jehle, 2010). Other psychological/clinical conditions in this sample also appear unrelated to MSVT failure (e.g., PTSD, substance use disorder). Notably, unlike the validity indices of the MMPI-2, PAI validity indices are designed to detect psychological and not cognitive overreporting, which may account for the lack of significant associations with MSVT.

In healthy people, correlations with the Structured Inventory of Malingered Symptomatology (SIMS), a scale for identifying feigning of psychological and cognitive deficits (see review in Chapter 16), are low for IR, but in the moderate range for DR and CNS ($r = -.35$ to $-.41$; Giger & Merten, 2013).

The MSVT is moderately correlated with the Memory Complaints Inventory, a self-report questionnaire by the same author (Green, 2004b), with lower scores associated with more memory complaints and with those failing the MSVT having significantly higher Memory Complaints Inventory scores (Armistead-Jehle, Grills, Bieu, & Kulas, 2016). Although more research on the association between the tests across samples is needed, as MSVT performance worsens, memory complaints increase.

CORRELATIONS WITH NEUROPSYCHOLOGICAL TESTS

Overall, there are relatively few studies on the association between the MSVT and standard measures of neuropsychological function; these generally indicate moderate to low associations depending on the test domain, as would be expected for a PVT. More studies of this kind would be useful in particular to clarify whether the Memory scores can function as bona fide memory measures.

In acute moderate to severe TBI, Effort scores are unrelated to standard memory measures, but Memory scores demonstrate moderate to high correlations with tests such as the WMS-IV Visual Reproduction and CVLT-II; correlations with memory tests are highest for FR compared to PA ($r = .49$ to $.60$, vs. $.33$ to $.34$; Macciocchi, Seel, Yi, & Small, 2017). Interestingly, IR, DR, and CNS also have modest correlations with attention tests such as the Symbol Digit Modalities Test and Letter-Number Sequencing in this population, possibly due to the fact that some of the patients in this particular study still had acute posttraumatic amnesia that may have affected both attention tests and MSVT performance, although relatively modestly.

Failure on the MSVT is associated with general suppression of test scores on other neuropsychological measures, as has also been demonstrated for tests such as the WMT. For example, results presented in the manual suggest that in a sample of adult outpatients, CVLT performance declined proportionally to performance on the MSVT, with the highest learning score found in those with the highest MSVT scores.

Similarly, failure on the MSVT is related to lower scores on cognitive test variables (e.g., RBANS scales), with effect sizes generally moderate in size according to Cohen's conventions (Armistead-Jehle et al., 2016). A composite of MSVT/NV-MSVT performance predicts performance on neuropsychological tests in active-duty military service members who sustained a concussion, along with age (Armistead-Jehle et al., 2016). Notably, MSVT Effort scores correlate moderately with RBANS subtests measuring memory to about the same degree as do MSVT Memory scores (Armistead-Jehle & Hansen, 2016). Last, failure on the MSVT and on one other PVT in research samples of veterans is associated with poor cognitive test performance (Clark et al., 2014).

CLINICAL STUDIES

CLASSIFICATION ACCURACY WITH REGARDS TO SLICK ET AL. (1999) AND OTHER MALINGERING CRITERIA

A high rate of failure on the MSVT has been noted in specific populations motivated to do poorly on neuropsychological tests (i.e., examinees seeking compensation) in contrast to low failure rates in normative groups (2% of cases; Giger & Merten, 2013), research samples (9%; Clark et al., 2014), and in patients motivated to do well such as preoperative deep-brain stimulation candidates hoping to be approved for surgery (10%; Suesse et al., 2015) and low-IQ parents seeking reunification with their children after child protective services involvement (0%; Chafetz & Biondolillo, 2012). Additionally, the MSVT has been used as a reference standard to evaluate performance of other PVTs and SVTs (e.g., Denning, 2014; Schutte et al., 2011; Whitney et al., 2013). However, there are few studies on the validation of MSVT cutoffs for predicting malingering as defined by established and widely used criteria, including the Slick et al. (1999) criteria for malingered neurocognitive dysfunction or the Bianchini et al. criteria for malingered pain-related disability (Bianchini et al., 2005). Nevertheless, one small study evaluating this question indicates that current cutoffs appear effective at detecting verified malingering. Specifically, of four patients failing the MSVT among 23 military veterans, all met Slick et al. malingering criteria, indicating 100% sensitivity and specificity for verified malingering using existing MSVT cutoffs (Whitney et al., 2009).

Below-chance performance on the MSVT, a stringent criterion considered equivalent to definite malingering (but which misses a substantial proportion of actual malingerers), has been reported in 12% of social services disability claimants, about the same rate as captured by the TOMM (Chafetz et al., 2007). Among compensation-seeking low-IQ examinees, 45% reach Slick et al. criteria when the MSVT is used as part of the criteria versus a 7% and 0% rate of Slick-criteria verified malingering in examinees motivated to do well, such as those seeking employment or reunification with their children after child protective services intervention (Chafetz et al., 2011).

In contrast, in another study involving a clinical sample with a low base rate of compensation seeking, only 28% of those failing the MSVT met Slick et al. (1999) criteria for presumed malingered neurocognitive dysfunction. The others failed for a variety of reasons unrelated to malingering, such as dementia or cognitive impairment, technical and visual problems, or otherwise unexplained failure (Suesse et al., 2015), suggesting that current cutoffs may need adjustment to capture verified malingerers without causing an undue number of false positives in some settings (i.e., settings with a low base rate of malingering). One study in a mixed veterans sample suggests that lowering the cutoff for failure to 70% instead of the recommended 85% yields failure rates similar to those of the TOMM and of embedded indicators such as the CVLT Forced Choice while maintaining an optimal specificity/false-positive rate (Axelrod & Schutte, 2011). However, this adjustment needs further validation in samples of verified malingerers.

Litigants and Disability Claimants. An effective PVT is expected to yield high failure rates in litigants and disability claimants, and this is the case for the MSVT, at least in social services disability evaluations where the test has been most often studied in independent research (e.g., Chafetz & Biondolillo, 2013; Chafetz, 2008; Chafetz et al., 2011). Compared to the WMT, there are comparatively few studies on the use of the MSVT in litigants and nonmilitary disability claimants.

Criminal Defendants. To our knowledge, there is no independent published research on the use of the MSVT in this group.

Military Samples. An effective PVT would be expected to yield high failure rates in military samples with secondary gain, and this is the case for the MSVT. MSVT failure rates in military samples vary depending on the type of military sample (Denning & Shura, 2017), with, in decreasing order, disability-related evaluations, clinical/research samples, and research-only samples, the latter not being characteristic of the vast majority of military settings where neuropsychologists conduct evaluations. For example, 58% of a sample of US veterans referred for neuropsychological assessment for mild TBI scored below MSVT cutoffs (Armistead-Jehle, 2010). In another study of active-duty and veteran military personnel, 32 to 34% failed the MSVT (Whitney, 2013; Whitney et al., 2013). Failure rates of 17% in a military poly-trauma sample (Whitney et al., 2009) and 15% in active-duty service members with high officer representation (Armistead-Jehle et al., 2016) have also been reported.

In a VA sample, not only was being "service connected" (deemed by Veterans Benefits as having one or more conditions caused/exacerbated by military service) more likely related to failure, but so was a depression diagnosis (Armistead-Jehle, 2010). Other clinical variables in this sample were not related to failure (e.g., PTSD, substance use disorder). Failure on the MSVT and on one other PVT in a research sample of veterans was associated with poor cognitive test performance and increased psychological symptom severity, as well as diagnoses of TBI, PTSD, and other Axis I diagnoses (Clark et al., 2014), demonstrating the link between PVT failure and clinical diagnoses as reflecting a common factor of over-reporting of symptomatology.

TBI. The manual presents data indicating that the mean MSVT score is lower in those with mild TBI compared to those with severe TBI (e.g., 77% vs. 93%), consistent with lower motivation or greater symptom exaggeration in patients with mild TBI. However, compared to other PVTs by the same author, notably the WMT, there are comparatively few independent studies on the use of the test in TBI, particularly in civilian TBI. Nevertheless, these studies demonstrate utility of the MSVT in mild to severe TBI.

Notably, adults from a concussion management program, most of whom had presumed mild TBI and were compensation-seeking, had much higher MSVT failure rates than did children with confirmed moderate to severe neurological dysfunction due to brain injury, stroke, or developmental disabilities (21% vs. 5%), a pattern that indicates exaggeration and that is not neurologically defensible (Carone, 2008). Of the adults failing the MSVT, about half also had a profile analysis suggestive of noncredible performance. Of note, adults who passed the MSVT had higher FR scores than children, demonstrating expected group differences for a score tapping memory processes; no differences were found for PA, however, even though this score also purportedly taps memory.

MSVT performance appears to be adversely affected by posttraumatic amnesia. In acute moderate to severe TBI, those with significant posttraumatic amnesia after TBI had high failure rates on IR, DR, and CNS (22%, 34%, and 44% failures, respectively; Macciocchi, Seel, Yi, & Small, 2017). All of these patients met criteria for the GMIP. Nevertheless, even acutely, the majority of moderate to severe TBI patients on average scored above cutoffs (e.g., Macciocchi et al., 2017). According to the authors, patients oriented to time, place, and injury status do not fail the MSVT despite severe deficits on neuropsychological testing and requiring care in an inpatient neurorehabilitation setting for activities of daily living. Nevertheless, in the early days post-injury, the test should only be administered after posttraumatic amnesia has resolved (Macciocchi et al., 2017); thus, moderate to severe TBI patients seen post-acutely after resolution of posttraumatic amnesia would not be expected to have failing scores on the test. Of note, memory scores were low in this study, particularly for FR, demonstrating some sensitivity of this score to acute memory impairment after TBI; less of an effect was found for PA.

With regard to expected failure rates for baseline concussion testing, high-school and college athletes undergoing baseline testing for concussion have a negligible failure rate on the MSVT, which is inconsistent with the notion that these athletes attempt to "sandbag" (intentionally underperform) baseline testing (2%; Nelson et al., 2015).

Psychiatric Conditions. To our knowledge, there are no independent studies of the test in psychiatric samples.

Chronic Pain. To our knowledge, there are no independent studies of the test in chronic pain.

Epilepsy and Psychogenic Nonepileptic Seizures. There are few studies of the test in this population. One study reported low rates of failure of the MSVT in people with psychogenic nonepileptic seizures (e.g., 5%; O'Brien et al., 2015).

ADHD and Learning Disabilities. To our knowledge, there are no independent studies of the test in people with ADHD or learning disabilities.

Dementia. In people with dementia or severe cognitive impairment, the MSVT is designed to improve accurate detection of noncredible performance by using an approach called "profile analysis," variously named in different publications as the GMIP, Dementia Profile, or SIP (i.e., SIP3 and SIP5; see "Scoring"; note that GMIP is the preferred term). The literature on dementia and MSVT is complex and at times contradictory. Although some studies show utility of the approach in reducing false positives in those with severe cognitive disorders, others provide mixed results.

The GMIP has been examined in two ways: (1) accuracy in detection of malingering and noncredible performance, and (2) accuracy in detection of dementia. These are two very different kinds of validation. Usually in PVT validation studies, sensitivity refers to the proportion of noncredible examinees correctly identified as noncredible, and specificity refers to the proportion of credible examinees correctly identified as honest respondants. In some MSVT studies (e.g., Howe & Loring, 2009), sensitivity has instead been defined as the proportion of examinees with dementia correctly identified as having dementia and specificity as the proportion of examinees without dementia correctly identified as not having dementia, which is a different usage of the test. This needs to be borne in mind when comparing classification accuracy statistics across different studies. As noted by McGuire and colleagues in their review of PVTs in dementia, studies that involve only those exerting credible effort (i.e., dementia patients) cannot possibly investigate the sensitivity of PVTs as there are no true positives in their sample (i.e., verified malingerers); they noted that the majority of MSVT studies on dementia are of this variety. Nevertheless, the MSVT and related tests such as the WMT and NV-MSVT were felt to be superior to other PVTs in the assessment of people with dementia, although data are preliminary given small samples sizes in the case of the MSVT in particular (McGuire, Crawford, & Evans, 2019).

To our knowledge, there is only one MSVT dementia study involving verified malingerers; it shows that the GMIP is effective at dementia detection in those failing the MSVT who actually have dementia, but less accurate at detecting malingerers. As well, patients may meet criteria for the GMIP for reasons other than having dementia (Suesse et al., 2015).

Studies involving simulated malingerers attempting to feign dementia also indicate that the GMIP can be faked. In one study, simulators were able to produce both the three-criteria and the five-criteria GMIP (the so-called SIP3 and SIP5). Although the SIP3 identified a memory impairment group residing in long-term care with high accuracy (94%), as did the SIP5 (96%), fewer than half of simulators feigning dementia were correctly identified by the SIP3 or SIP5 (Dunham & Denney, 2016). Nevertheless, a revised profile analysis using lower cut scores similar to those of Axelrod and Shutte (2011) combined with logistic regression weighting showed much higher sensitivity while retaining excellent specificity to detection of feigning (.84 and .96; Dunham & Denney, 2016). A flowchart outlining criteria is available directly from the authors (kathrynjdunham@hotmail.com or Denney@PsychologistSpringfield.com). Replication in clinical groups is needed before applying the Dunham and Denney profile analysis, but initial findings are promising.

Some authors have raised questions about the validity of the GMIP based on research showing that those meeting criteria do not differ from those not meeting criteria. For example, in a mixed clinical sample of veterans, 47% failed according to standard MSVT cutoffs; of these failures, about half met criteria for the GMIP, with the remaining not meeting GMIP criteria and therefore assumed to have provided noncredible responding (Axelrod & Schutte, 2010). However, the two groups performed fairly similarly on other cognitive tests and PVTs; those meeting criteria for the GMIP differed only in motor speed from those not meeting criteria, but not in terms of IQ or memory, which is at odds with the view that those meeting the GMIP criteria did so because of bona fide cognitive impairment (i.e., about a 50% fail rate). The two groups also had similar pass rates on other PVTs such as the TOMM and CVLT-II Forced Choice, raising questions about the accuracy of the GMIP to identify failure due to cognitive impairment versus exaggeration. Similarly, in a larger veteran sample without dementia, and looking at quantitative criteria only, of those who failed the MSVT, 81% met quantitative criteria for the GMIP, but differences between these patients and those who failed the MSVT were minimal in terms of number of failures on other stand-alone or embedded PVTs, cognitive test performance, or self-reported symptoms (Reslan & Axelrod, 2017). The authors concluded that the quantitative GMIP criteria are not efficient at differentiating between cognitive impairment and noncredible performance and that noncredible performance should always be assumed when there is no disabling neurological condition to explain MSVT Effort failure. They recommended additional study of the GMIP algorithm.

There does appear to be value in combining tests to better identify noncredible performance in the setting of suspected dementia. For example, although half of sophisticated dementia simulators (i.e., psychology students) are able to produce a GMIP yielding a 54% sensitivity to detecting simulators (Armistead-Jehle & Denney, 2015), combining the MSVT with the WMT significantly increases the detection of feigners to 84%; combining the MSVT and the NV-MSVT detects 100% of feigners, thereby correctly identifying the feigners who would have been missed by the MSVT used alone. Of the three tests, the NV-MSVT has the highest accuracy for detecting feigners using the GMIP, and the MSVT had the lowest accuracy. In a small study by the test author and colleagues ($N = 20$), similar results were reported: 100% of dementia patients in long-term care failed the MSVT Effort subtests and met criteria of the GMIP, but 40% of simulators were not detected as such by the GMIP approach. Using the MSVT in combination with the NV-MSVT reduced the percentage of incorrectly identified simulators to 20%, demonstrating the utility of using both tests together, with an impressive 80% sensitivity and 100% sensitivity (Singhal et al., 2009). Although replication in clinical groups with verified malingerers is needed, this study offers promising results that combining the MSVT with other similar PVTs eliminates some of the limitations of the GMIP on its own.

MSVT failure rates increase with dementia severity, but the majority of people with dementia will be correctly identified as such by the GMIP. For example, 83% of advanced dementia cases fail the test, with the majority meeting criteria for the GMIP (Howe et al., 2007). However, use of the GMIP significantly reduces invalid protocols in dementia patients from 42–43% to 3–6% (Howe et al., 2007; Howe & Loring, 2009).

In sum, studies show that in populations with few to no malingerers (i.e., no incentives to fail) and a high base rate of dementia, the GMIP can be used with confidence to predict dementia, with a PPV of 90% (Howe & Loring, 2009). However, a negative GMIP does not fully exclude dementia. Again, the MSVT is not a test designed a priori to detect dementia, so this is not surprising. However, when incentives to fail are present, studies show that the GMIP cannot necessarily be used with confidence to attribute MSVT test failure to cognitive deficits.

Low IQ. Independent studies support the use of the test in examinees with low intellectual ability, at least in IQs of 60 and above. Studies by the author indicate that IQs in the range of 46 to 70 in children and adults are not sufficient to explain failure on the MSVT (Green & Flaro, 2016; Green & Flaro, 2015). There is also a case study of a low-IQ child providing an almost perfect performance on the test (Carone, 2014).

With regard to Effort score failure rates, as already noted, independent studies indicate that low-IQ social services disability claimants seeking compensation for inability to work fail the MSVT at much higher rates than other low-IQ persons with motivation to do well on the test, such as applicants for a rehabilitation service who are seeking work and vocational training or parents seen by child protection services seeking reunification with their children (rates of 52%, 13%, and 0%, respectively; Chafetz et al., 2011). Well-motivated child protection examinees do not fail the MSVT, with a 100% pass rate in the IQ range of 60 to 75 (Chafetz & Biondolillo, 2013).

The utility of the GMIP (SIP) in differentiating between MSVT failure due to low IQ and failure due to noncredible performance is less clear. Chafetz and Biondolillo found that the GMIP is easily produced by low-IQ malingerers whose malingering status has been validated by established malingering criteria (i.e., incentive to do poorly and failure on two PVTs, one being the MSVT). Of confirmed malingerers among a social security disability sample, 28% produced a SIP5 profile (i.e., a GMIP comprised of five specific criteria) compared to only 6% of examinees with no evidence of malingering. Even more confirmed malingerers (50%) met SIP3 criteria (i.e., a GMIP comprised of three specific criteria). They concluded that a high proportion of low-IQ compensation-seeking social security disability claimants produce the GMIP, compared to few low-IQ well-motivated child protection claimants with no evidence of malingering. No examinees motivated to do well who had IQs between 60 and 75 produced the GMIP, although some examinees with IQs below 60 did so. The authors concluded that criterion malingerers produce an intolerably high rate of cognitive impairment profiles on the MSVT and that it is the appearance of impairment that is being feigned with the GMIP, not genuine cognitive impairment, at least when IQs are 60 and above.

Thus, studies by Chafetz and colleagues suggest that the GMIP works for IQs below 60, but that the GMIP cannot be trusted to identify impairment when there is compensation-seeking in low-IQ examinees. They note circularity in the GMIP: the method is used to identify true impairment but is only overturned if the examinee does not have true impairment. They concluded that when the GMIP occurs in examinees motivated to fail, it is more likely due to feigning than to actual impairment; when it occurs in well-motivated examinees with intellectual disability or dementia and without incentives to fail, the GMIP may assist in characterizing impairment (Chafetz & Biondolillo, 2013).

Resistance to Coaching. Explicit and detailed coaching improves performance on the MSVT (Gorny & Merten, 2006; Weinborn et al., 2012), especially when focused on test performance rather than symptom coaching. However, the test remains quite resistant to coaching, with only 20% of coached simulators managing to pass the MSVT; interestingly, recognizing the MSVT as a PVT does not necessarily lead to passing the test (Gorny & Merten, 2006). Classification accuracy remains very high in undergraduate simulators despite both symptom- and test-specific coaching, with an accuracy about equal to that of the TOMM and NV-MSVT (Weinborn et al., 2012).

NEUROANATOMICAL CORRELATES AND IMAGING STUDIES

No information is available.

COMMENT

There is considerable evidence for the validity of the MSVT, and it appears to be an impressive and effective verbal PVT overall. The test typically loads with other PVTs in factor analyses, correlates with most other validated PVTs, and tends to be at least or more sensitive and specific as most other PVTs. Failure rates are clearly higher in compensation-seeking groups compared to normative and well-motivated samples, as would be expected. As with most PVTs, use of the MSVT in dementia or other groups with severe cognitive impairment, such as low-IQ examinees, should be done cautiously (see "Limitations"), as there is mixed evidence of accuracy across studies. There is more evidence that FR taps memory than PA, which in some studies is associated more with PVT-type measures than memory per se. More research on the Memory subtests would be useful to support their use as memory tests, although FR in particular shows promise.

The MSVT follows in the footsteps of the WMT as a frequently cited and researched PVT, although its research literature is not as large or as extensive, nor has it been validated in as many different types of clinical samples. Similar in design to the WMT, the MSVT is simpler (e.g., shorter item list, shorter interval between presentation and memory testing, simpler foils) and is thus attractive to time-strapped clinicians who assess people who may struggle to tolerate longer, more complex tests. However, these advantages may be gained at the expense of lower sensitivity to malingering detection compared to the WMT, a test already known for its high sensitivity and higher false-positive rate compared to other PVTs (see the review of the WMT elsewhere in this chapter). On the other hand, the MSVT may for the same reasons be a welcome alternative to the WMT, which has been criticized for having too high a sensitivity at the expense of specificity (i.e., thereby identifying too many valid tests as invalid). In his review, Carone concluded that the MSVT should be used as a supplement rather than a substitute for the WMT unless there are significant time demands (Carone, 2009). We would propose that the MSVT stands in its own right as a valid alternative to the WMT and may in fact be the preferred test in some settings due to its lower risk of false positives; in certain groups with a strong body of research, it appears particularly useful (i.e., military samples and social security disability claimants).

Supplementing the MSVT with the NV-MSVT appears effective at increasing detection of noncredible performance and reducing false positives, and the combined use of these two brief PVTs, one verbal and one nonverbal, appears ideal. Combining all three tests has also been recommended (Armistead-Jehle & Denney, 2015), although the research appears to show that using two of the three tests is sufficient; the two-test approach is also supported by the test author (P. Green, personal communication, May 2018). Combining the MSVT with the TOMM, another nonverbal PVT with extensive usage in neuropsychology, requires study but seems a potentially useful combination given positive findings on combined use of the WMT and TOMM (see WMT review elsewhere in this chapter). Among stand-alone nonverbal PVTs, the TOMM does have considerably more validation evidence than the NV-MSVT as of this writing.

The balance of evidence suggests that demographic factors typically do not impact Effort scores, whereas age and education appear to affect Memory scores, as would be expected. In terms of normative data, the test offers a number of comparator groups, and Giger and Merten (2013) have presented normative data stratified by age and education, which may be of particular utility in interpreting Memory scores (see "Normative Data").

Although quite popular, the MSVT is not as commonly used as the WMT, and the literature reflects this—there are simply fewer studies on its use in several critical sample groups, most notably verified malingerers using accepted malingering criteria such as the Slick et al criteria, as well as in litigants, criminal defendants, psychiatric patients, ADHD, and chronic pain samples. Studies in some groups in particular, such as TBI, are fewer compared to the body of literature that exists for other PVTs such as the WMT and TOMM. However, this may change as the advantages of the MSVT become better known (i.e., acceptable false-positive rate/high specificity and considerably briefer administration time).

Like the WMT and NV-MSVT, the MSVT is unique in its design as it offers both Effort tests and Memory tests that progress along a gradient of difficulty; the resultant profile analysis may minimize false positives in people with cognitive impairment. However, one obvious and major limitation is that the GMIP can be faked—this may not be known by most users. Blind reliance on discounting malingering when the criteria for the GMIP are met is highly discouraged. When the GMIP occurs in examinees motivated to fail, the GMIP appears equally or more likely to be due to feigning than to actual impairment. However, when it occurs in well-motivated examinees with intellectual disability or dementia and without incentives to fail, the GMIP may assist in characterizing impairment (Chafetz & Biondolillo, 2013).

Users should recall the main tenet of the GMIP: that is, if the examinee is *not* dependent on others in daily life, then the criteria for the GMIP are not met, by definition. The test author states that the GMIP must be used in conjunction with Criteria D of the Slick et al. malingering criteria (Slick et al., 1999) to be effective at differentiating invalid performance from cognitive impairment. Criteria D specifies that behaviors meeting necessary criteria for malingering must not be fully accounted for by psychiatric, neurological, or developmental factors that result in significantly diminished capacity to appreciate laws or mores against malingering or inability to conform behavior to such standards, and are not the product of an informed, rational, and volitional effort aimed at least in part toward acquiring or achieving external incentives.

Some have criticized a somewhat circular reasoning within the GMIP and suggest the numerical algorithm should not depend on clinical criteria outside of the test results themselves. We see no problem with including Criterion D of the Slick criteria to aid in interpreting scores as this provides a bridge between purely actuarial approaches and purely clinical approaches to detecting malingering and exaggeration. However, more clarity, consistency, and validation of this approach are needed in the manual, scoring program, and related publications, including further validation of the cutoffs and algorithm using verified malingerers.

The use of different terminologies for profile analysis—GMIP, Dementia Profile, SIP (i.e., the SIP5 and SIP3)—defined by three to five criteria depending on the source can lead to confusion for users. Additionally, studies may or may not use a profile analysis correction, which complicates comparison of failure rates in the literature (Dunham & Denney, 2016). Again, "GMIP" is the recommended term and should be used when referring to profile analysis criteria.

From a practical perspective for users, the manual is not easily organized for rapid reference and is difficult to follow. Information on deriving the GMIP is also not clearly laid out in the manual, although this may have been updated in the computer program or in later editions. Information on the Stealth Version designed to detect coaching is lacking in the manual and in research studies and so remains unvalidated as of this writing. Analysis of scores is based in reference to comparator groups. Generally, these results are from various clinics, have small sample sizes in some cases, and quality control measures are not described, so their representativeness and generalizability when making important diagnostic clinical decisions in the individual examinee are not clear.

The administration instructions require that the examiner leave the room during the test; it is not clear that this procedure was followed in all MSVT research studies, particularly those involving dementia patients. Examinees with sensorimotor difficulties can be administered the oral version, although this is not a recommended practice.

As is the case for all PVTs, the MSVT offers information on the credibility of the examinee's test scores but does not speak to the cause of invalid scores. Use of multidimensional criteria to ascertain the basis for failure is necessary in this regard, including examining congruence between clinical characteristics, adaptive living skills, neuropsychological profile, and context of assessment (e.g., presence of incentive vs. no discernible incentive). Additional research providing data on reliability estimates for the Memory scores, in particular, and comparative performance in diverse groups would augment the literature on the test, although there is independent research on use of the test in other languages, most notably German.

REFERENCES

Armistead-Jehle, P. (2010). Symptom validity test performance in U.S. veterans referred for evaluation of mild TBI. *Applied Neuropsychology, 17*(1), 52–59. https://doi.org/10.1080/09084280903526182

Armistead-Jehle, P., Cooper, D. B., & Vanderploeg, R. D. (2016). The role of performance validity tests in the assessment of cognitive functioning after military concussion: A replication and extension. *Applied Neuropsychology: Adult, 23*(4), 264–273. https://doi.org/10.1080/23279095.2015.1055564

Armistead-Jehle, P., & Denney, R. L. (2015). The detection of feigned impairment using the WMT, MSVT, and NV-MSVT. *Applied Neuropsychology: Adult, 22*(2), 147–155. https://doi.org/10.1080/23279095.2014.880842

Armistead-Jehle, P., Grills, C. E., Bieu, R. K., & Kulas, J. F. (2016). Clinical utility of the Memory Complaints Inventory to detect invalid test performance. *The Clinical Neuropsychologist, 30*(4), 610–628. https://doi.org/10.1080/13854046.2016.1177597

Armistead-Jehle, P., & Hansen, C. L. (2011). Comparison of the Repeatable Battery for the Assessment of Neuropsychological Status Effort Index and stand-alone symptom validity tests in a military sample. *Archives of Clinical Neuropsychology, 26*(7), 592–601. https://doi.org/10.1093/arclin/acr049

Armistead-Jehle, P., & Hansen, C. L. (2016). Factor analysis of the MSVT, NV-MSVT, and RBANS Memory subtests. *Archives of Clinical Neuropsychology, 31*(5), 465–471. https://doi.org/10.1093/arclin/acw033

Axelrod, B. N., & Schutte, C. (2010). Analysis of the dementia profile on The Medical Symptom Validity Test. *The Clinical Neuropsychologist, 24*(5), 873–881. https://doi.org/10.1080/13854040903527295

Axelrod, B. N., & Schutte, C. (2011). Concurrent validity of three forced-choice measures of symptom validity. *Applied Neuropsychology, 18*(1), 27–33. https://doi.org/10.1080/09084282.2010.523369

Bashem, J. R., Rapport, L. J., Miller, J. B., Hanks, R. A., Axelrod, B. N., & Millis, S. R. (2014). Comparisons of five performance validity indices in bona fide and simulated traumatic brain injury. *The Clinical Neuropsychologist, 28*(5), 851–875. https://doi.org/10.1080/13854046.2014.927927

Bianchini, K. J., Greve, K. W., & Glynn, G. (2005). On the diagnosis of malingered pain-related disability: Lessons from cognitive malingering research. *The Spine Journal, 5*(4), 404–417. https://doi.org/10.1016/j.spinee.2004.11.016

Broglio, S. P., Ferrara, M. S., Macciocchi, S. N., Baumgartner, T. A., & Elliott, R. (2007). Test-retest reliability of computerized concussion assessment programs. *Journal of Athletic Training, 42*(4), 509–514.

Carone, D. A. (2008). Children with moderate/severe brain damage/dysfunction outperform adults with mild-to-no brain damage on the Medical Symptom Validity Test. *Brain Injury, 22*(12), 960–971. https://doi.org/10.1080/02699050802491297

Carone, D. A. (2009). Test review of the Medical Symptom Validity Test. *Applied Neuropsychology, 16*(4), 309–311. https://doi.org/10.1080/09084280903297883

Carone, D. A. (2014). Young child with severe brain volume loss easily passes the Word Memory Test and Medical Symptom Validity Test: Implications for mild TBI. *The Clinical Neuropsychologist, 28*(1), 146–162.

Chafetz, M. D. (2008). Malingering on the social security disability consultative exam: Predictors and base rates. *The Clinical Neuropsychologist, 22*(3), 529–546. https://doi.org/10.1080/13854040701346104

Chafetz, M. D., Abrahams, J. P., & Kohlmaier, J. (2007). Malingering on the social security disability consultative exam: A new rating scale. *Archives of Clinical Neuropsychology, 22*(1), 1–14. https://doi.org/10.1016/j.acn.2006.10.003

Chafetz, M. D., & Biondolillo, A. (2012). Validity issues in Atkins death cases. *The Clinical Neuropsychologist, 26*(8), 1358–1376. https://doi.org/10.1080/13854046.2012.730674

Chafetz, M. D., & Biondolillo, A. M. (2013). Feigning a severe impairment profile. *Archives of Clinical Neuropsychology, 28*(3), 205–212. https://doi.org/10.1093/arclin/act015

Chafetz, M. D., Prentkowski, E., & Rao, A. (2011). To work or not to work: Motivation (not low IQ) determines symptom validity test findings. *Archives of Clinical Neuropsychology, 26*(4), 306–313. https://doi.org/10.1093/arclin/acr030

Clark, A. L., Amick, M. M., Fortier, C., Milberg, W. P., & McGlinchey, R. E. (2014). Poor performance validity predicts clinical characteristics and cognitive test performance of OEF/OIF/OND veterans in a research setting. *The Clinical Neuropsychologist, 28*(5), 802–825. https://doi.org/10.1080/13854046.2014.904928

Denning, J. H. (2014). Combining the Test of Memory Malingering Trial 1 with behavioral responses improves the detection of effort test failure. *Applied Neuropsychology: Adult, 21*(4), 269–277. https://doi.org/10.1080/23279095.2013.811076

Denning, J. H., & Shura, R. D. (2017). Cost of malingering mild traumatic brain injury-related cognitive deficits during compensation and pension evaluations in the veterans benefits administration. *Applied Neuropsychology. Adult*, 1–16. https://doi.org/10.1080/23279095.2017.1350684

Dunham, K. J., & Denney, R. L. (2016). Development of the Poor Validity Profile Analysis for the Medical Symptom Validity Test. *Archives of Clinical Neuropsychology, 31*(8), 944–953. https://doi.org/10.1093/arclin/acw060

Giger, P., & Merten, T. (2013). Swiss population-based reference data for six symptom validity tests. *Clínica Y Salud, 24*(3), 153–159.

Gorny, I., & Merten, T. (2006). Symptom information—Warning—Coaching: How do they affect successful feigning in neuropsychological assessment? *Journal of Forensic Neuropsychology, 4*(4), 71–97. https://doi.org/10.1300/J151v04n04_05

Green, P. (2004a). *Medical Symptom Validity Test (MSVT)*. Edmonton, AB, Canada: Green's Publishing.

Green, P. (2004b). *Memory Complaints Inventory (MCI)*. Edmonton, AB, Canada: Green's Publishing.

Green, P. (2011a). *Advanced Interpretation (AI) program*. Edmonton, AB, Canada: Green's Publishing.

Green, P. (2011b). Comparison between the Test of Memory Malingering (TOMM) and the Nonverbal Medical Symptom

Validity Test (NV-MSVT) in adults with disability claims. *Applied Neuropsychology, 18*(1), 18–26.

Green, P., & Flaro, L. (2015). Results from three performance validity tests (pvts) in adults with intellectual deficits. *Applied Neuropsychology. Adult, 22*(4), 293–303. https://doi.org/10.1080/23279095.2014.925903

Howe, L. L. S., & Loring, D. W. (2009). Classification accuracy and predictive ability of the Medical Symptom Validity Test's Dementia Profile and General Memory Impairment Profile. *The Clinical Neuropsychologist, 23*(2), 329–342. https://doi.org/10.1080/13854040801945060

Howe, L. L. S., Anderson, A. M., Kaufman, D. A. S., Sachs, B. C., & Loring, D. W. (2007). Characterization of the Medical Symptom Validity Test in evaluation of clinically referred memory disorders clinic patients. *Archives of Clinical Neuropsychology, 22*(6), 753–761. https://doi.org/10.1016/j.acn.2007.06.003

LaDuke, C., Barr, W., Brodale, D. L., & Rabin, L. A. (2017). Toward generally accepted forensic assessment practices among clinical neuropsychologists: A survey of professional practice and common test use. *The Clinical Neuropsychologist, 1–20*. https://doi.org/10.1080/13854046.2017.1346711

Martin, P. K., Schroeder, R. W., & Odland, A. P. (2015). Neuropsychologists' validity testing beliefs and practices: A survey of North American professionals. *The Clinical Neuropsychologist, 29*(6), 741–776. https://doi.org/10.1080/13854046.2015.1087597

McGuire, C., Crawford, S., & Evans, J. J. (2019). Effort testing in dementia assessment: A systematic review. *Archives of Clinical Neuropsychology, 34*(1), 114–131. https://doi.org/10.1093/arclin/acy012

Merten, T., Green, P., Henry, M., Blaskewitz, N., & Brockhaus, R. (2005). Analog validation of German-language symptom validity tests and the influence of coaching. *Archives of Clinical Neuropsychology, 20*(6), 719–726. https://doi.org/10.1016/j.acn.2005.04.004

Nelson, L. D., Pfaller, A. Y., Rein, L. E., & McCrea, M. A. (2015). Rates and predictors of invalid baseline test performance in high school and collegiate athletes for three computerized neurocognitive tests (CNTs): ANAM, Axon, and ImPACT. *The American Journal of Sports Medicine, 43*(8), 2018–2026. https://doi.org/10.1177/0363546515587714

O'Brien, F. M., Fortune, G. M., Dicker, P., O'Hanlon, E., Cassidy, E., Delanty, N., . . . Murphy, K. C. (2015). Psychiatric and neuropsychological profiles of people with psychogenic nonepileptic seizures. *Epilepsy & Behavior, 43*, 39–45. https://doi.org/10.1016/j.yebeh.2014.11.012

Reslan, S., & Axelrod, B. N. (2017). Evaluating the Medical Symptom Validity Test (MSVT) in a sample of veterans between the ages of 18 to 64. *Applied Neuropsychology. Adult, 24*(2), 132–139. https://doi.org/10.1080/23279095.2015.1107565

Schatz, P., & Glatts, C. (2013). "Sandbagging" baseline test performance on ImPACT, without detection, is more difficult than it appears. *Archives of Clinical Neuropsychology, 28*(3), 236–244. https://doi.org/10.1093/arclin/act009

Schutte, C., Millis, S., Axelrod, B., & VanDyke, S. (2011). Derivation of a composite measure of embedded symptom validity indices. *The Clinical Neuropsychologist, 25*(3), 454–462. https://doi.org/10.1080/13854046.2010.550635

Singhal, A., Green, P., Ashaye, K., Shankar, K., & Gill, D. (2009). High specificity of the Medical Symptom Validity Test in patients with very severe memory impairment. *Archives of Clinical Neuropsychology: The Official Journal of the National Academy of Neuropsychologists, 24*(8), 721–728. https://doi.org/10.1093/arclin/acp074

Slick, D. J., Sherman, E. M., & Iverson, G. L. (1999). Diagnostic criteria for Malingered Neurocognitive Dysfunction: Proposed standards for clinical practice and research. *The Clinical Neuropsychologist, 13*(4), 545–561. https://doi.org/10.1076/1385-4046(199911)13:04;1-Y;FT545

Sollman, M. J., & Berry, D. T. R. (2011). Detection of inadequate effort on neuropsychological testing: A meta-analytic update and extension. *Archives of Clinical Neuropsychology, 26*(8), 774–789. https://doi.org/10.1093/arclin/acr066

Suesse, M., Wong, V. W. C., Stamper, L. L., Carpenter, K. N., & Scott, R. B. (2015). Evaluating the clinical utility of the Medical Symptom Validity Test (MSVT): A clinical series. *The Clinical Neuropsychologist, 29*(2), 214–231. https://doi.org/10.1080/13854046.2015.1022226

Van Dyke, S. A., Millis, S. R., Axelrod, B. N., & Hanks, R. A. (2013). Assessing effort: Differentiating performance and symptom validity. *The Clinical Neuropsychologist, 27*(8), 1234–1246. https://doi.org/10.1080/13854046.2013.835447

Weinborn, M., Woods, S. P., Nulsen, C., & Leighton, A. (2012). The effects of coaching on the Verbal and Nonverbal Medical Symptom Validity Tests. *The Clinical Neuropsychologist, 26*(5), 832–849. https://doi.org/10.1080/13854046.2012.686630

Whitney, K. A. (2013). Predicting test of memory malingering and medical symptom validity test failure within a Veterans Affairs Medical Center: Use of the Response Bias Scale and the Henry-Heilbronner Index. *Archives of Clinical Neuropsychology, 28*(3), 222–235. https://doi.org/10.1093/arclin/act012

Whitney, K. A., Shepard, P. H., & Davis, J. J. (2013). WAIS-IV Digit Span variables: Are they valuable for use in predicting TOMM and MSVT failure? *Applied Neuropsychology, 20*(2), 83–94. https://doi.org/10.1080/09084282.2012.670167

Whitney, K. A., Shepard, P. H., Williams, A. L., Davis, J. J., & Adams, K. M. (2009). The Medical Symptom Validity Test in the evaluation of Operation Iraqi Freedom/Operation Enduring Freedom soldiers: A preliminary study. *Archives of Clinical Neuropsychology, 24*(2), 145–152. https://doi.org/10.1093/arclin/acp020

Young, J. C., Roper, B. L., & Arentsen, T. J. (2016). Validity testing and neuropsychology practice in the VA healthcare system: Results from recent practitioner survey (.). *The Clinical Neuropsychologist, 30*(4), 497–514. https://doi.org/10.1080/13854046.2016.1159730

NON-VERBAL MEDICAL SYMPTOM VALIDITY TEST (NV-MSVT)

TEST NAME	**Non-Verbal Medical Symptom Validity Test (NV-MSVT)**
DOMAIN	Performance validity
AGE RANGE	In healthy adults, norms up to age 76; higher age ranges in clinical groups
ADMINISTRATION TIME	5 minutes, and an additional 10-minute delay
SCORING FORMAT	Computerized
REFERENCE	Green, P. (2008). *Green's Non-Verbal Medical Symptom Validity Test (NV-MSVT) for Windows user's manual.* Edmonton, AB, Canada: Green's Publishing. www.wordmemorytest.com

DESCRIPTION

The Non-Verbal Medical Symptom Validity Test (NV-MSVT) is a brief computerized PVT; it is the third published test in the suite of PVTs published by Paul Green, after the WMT and MSVT, both reviewed elsewhere in this chapter. According to the manual, the NV-MSVT was introduced due to a need for a nonverbal PVT that requires little administration time and has acceptable sensitivity to noncredible performance and few false positives when tested in persons with dementia. To this end, the emphasis is on profile analysis of scores as opposed to simple cutoffs. Similar in structure in a number of ways to the WMT and MSVT, the NV-MSVT differs in that images are used instead of words; target-foil differentiation is also expanded.

The NV-MSVT is comprised of four performance validity subtests (Effort subtests) and two memory subtests (Memory subtests). The test begins with List Presentation during which items are presented and named by the examinee, followed by the Effort subtests of Immediate Recognition (IR), Delayed Recognition (DR), Delayed Recognition Archetypes (DRA), and Delayed Recognition Variations (DRV). A consistency score is also derived based on agreement between IR and DR (CNS). The two Memory subtests are Paired Associates (PA) and Free Recall (FR; Table 15–16).

The NV-MSVT and the other PVTs by Green (WMT, MSVT) have a unique feature in that they are designed to be able to differentiate between failure due to noncredible performance and failure due to severe cognitive compromise. This is done by examining the profile of scores generated and the gradient of subtest difficulty according to a specific algorithm, the GMIP. The test also potentially allows screening of memory skills, although the effectiveness of the Memory subtests at measuring memory per se has not been as well studied in the NV-MSVT as in other of Green's tests such as the WMT.

According to the manual, naming is incorporated at various points to increase depth of processing to enhance the probability of recognition; most subtests involve visual identification of items, but FR assesses recall by having the examinee verbally recall previously presented items. The test includes so-called *archetypal images* that are deemed to be more easily and automatically recalled than other image types.

ADMINISTRATION

Administration details, including set-up and installation instructions, are provided in the manual (Green, 2008). The examinee must have adequate vision to identify items, but due to the visual nature of the task, no a priori reading level is required. The test is presented via computer, with instructions provided by the examiner. Testing is quite brief, typically taking about five minutes, with an additional 10 minutes for the delay interval. Testing of advanced dementia patients can be extremely lengthy and challenging (Singhal et al., 2009) and so is not recommended in most clinical settings. The examiner does not leave the room during testing, in contrast to other tests by Green reviewed in this volume.

TABLE 15–16 Non-Verbal Medical Symptom Validity Test (NV-MSVT) Scores and Abbreviations

IR	Immediate Recognition
DR	Delayed Recognition
DRA	Delayed Recognition Archetypes
DRV	Delayed Recognition Variations
CNS	Consistency
PA	Paired Associates
FR	Free Recall
GMIP	Genuine Memory Impairment Profile

NOTE: The GMIP and related terms such as Dementia Profile and Severe Impairment Profile all denote the profile analysis method designed to differentiate test failure caused by severe cognitive impairment and test failure caused by noncredible performance. The preferred term is GMIP.

SCORING

A report is generated by the scoring program. Failing occurs when the *mean* of either five or four specific Effort scores are below a specific cutoff. This differs from the WMT and MSVT, where failure is defined as having one out of three Effort scores below a specific cutoff. Memory subtest data (PA and FR) are also included. Results are presented graphically (e.g., line chart or bar chart that displays percentage correct or line chart displaying *z* scores), and raw scores are presented in table format. Comparator groups can be selected for comparison to the examinee's scores (see "Normative Data").

Notably, failing on Effort tests does not automatically indicate an invalid profile; rather, this is determined via profile analysis of multiple scores. Specific formulas have been derived to do this that will not be discussed here for security purposes, other than to say that the determination is based on the overall profile of scores across all subtests (Effort and Memory scores) according to specific algorithms. Although this is not clearly indicated in the manual, this process is the Genuine Memory Impairment Profile (GMIP) algorithm, variously termed the Dementia Profile and Severe Impairment Profile in various other sources. GMIP is, however, the preferred term (P. Green, personal communication, June 2018). Specifically, when an examinee fails the test, a second set of criteria are examined to determine whether the failure was due to noncredible performance or to severe cognitive impairment, that is, to a GMIP. This is done according to three more criteria that examine inconsistencies and variability across subtests (manual).

Advanced interpretation is provided by the computerized Advanced Interpretation Program for the test (Green, 2011). Compared to the standard program, the Advanced Interpretation Program updates the interpretation rules and provides new comparison groups; it also directs users to apply Criterion D of the Slick, Sherman, and Iverson malingering criteria (Slick et al., 1999) to the determination of whether examinees meet the GMIP (P. Green, personal communication, May 2018). According to the test author, Criterion D of the Slick criteria must be applied to correctly use the GMIP. Criterion D specifies that invalid performance cannot be fully accounted for by psychiatric, developmental, or neurological disorders that result in significantly diminished capacity to appreciate laws or mores against malingering or inability to conform behavior to such standards. Based on this rationale, by definition, any independently functioning examinee failing the Effort tests and yielding a GMIP profile on Memory tests would be ineligible for the GMIP and would therefore be deemed as providing noncredible performance. However, the manual does not specify this criterion, and so it is unclear if this important distinction is obvious to all users.

Using the GMIP algorithm, scores that do not fit the expected profile of people with cognitive impairment are deemed invalid (i.e., due to noncredible responding), whereas scores that fit the pattern expected in cognitive impairment are considered a reliable reflection of neurological compromise rather than feigning or exaggeration. Based on this, the NV-MSVT can therefore yield three kinds of results: (1) passing all Effort tests (credible responding), (2) failing Effort tests and not meeting criteria for cognitive impairment according to profile analysis (noncredible responding), and (3) failing Effort tests but meeting criteria for cognitive impairment based on profile analysis and therefore meeting criteria for the GMIP (credible responding with Effort score failure attributed to a known neurological condition; Reslan & Axelrod, 2017). Henry and colleagues provide a useful flowchart depicting the algorithm underlying the GMIP process which can be helpful in understanding how the criteria work (Henry et al., 2010).

The manual indicates that an isolated low DRA score, in the context of other Effort scores above cutoff, is not necessarily indicative of invalid performance but if this pattern is noted it should be interpreted cautiously. The manual states that the most common reason for a low DRA score is not ensuring that the examinee names all items on List Presentation and IR.

DEMOGRAPHIC EFFECTS

AGE

Age appears to be correlated with Effort scores in some but not all samples; FR is correlated with age, as expected for a score tapping memory. The manual presents mixed clinical data on children showing little change in Effort scores from age 7 to 18 years, with near-ceiling scores; the FR memory score, in contrast, does increase with age. In adult neurological patients, an independent study found age effects, with NV-MSVT performance decreasing with age; age was moderately correlated with Effort, but correlations were particularly high for FR ($r = -.54$; Henry et al., 2010).

GENDER

To our knowledge, there are no independent studies examining gender effects.

EDUCATION AND IQ

Research on the influence of education and IQ is mixed but does indicate associations with performance in some samples. For example, in a sample of adults seeking custody of their children, Effort scores were correlated with years of education (Spearman's rho = .31; manual). However, in a neurologic patient group, NV-MSVT scores were not correlated with education (Henry et al., 2010). To our knowledge, there are no independent studies on IQ in adults.

ETHNICITY, NATIONALITY, AND LINGUISTIC EFFECTS

The test has been used in a number of countries according to data presented in the manual. However, differential effects of culture and ethnicity across groups are not reported. Because this test is nonverbal and visually based, effects of language would be expected to be minimized compared to verbal PVTs, although even these appear to have minimal cross-cultural effects (see WMT and MSVT reviews elsewhere in this chapter). There is independent research supportive of its clinical usage in German patients (Henry et al., 2010).

NORMATIVE DATA

Interpretation of the NV-MSVT is based on specific cutoffs defining passing or failing the test. However, although the manual makes reference to numerous unpublished and published datasets and case studies, as noted by others (Henry et al., 2010), specific information on how cutoffs were derived and on which specific clinical groups they are based is not clearly laid out in the manual.

HEALTHY CONTROLS

In the manual, there is reference to a sample of 40 healthy volunteers with scores at or higher than 95% on Effort subtests and scores of 78% on FR. The sample is not clearly described in terms of recruitment and demographics, but, according to the author, normative data on healthy controls are not critical to the test because interpretation rests on cutoffs not norms. Nevertheless, data on healthy people are useful for determining the presence of age effects and for establishing the validity of the Memory subtests in particular.

Henry and colleagues provide data on healthy, community-dwelling adults given the German version of the test ranging in age from 50 to 76 (mean = 63 years, *SD* = 7.1). The sample was relatively well-educated (mean of 15.8 years, *SD* = 3.0) and screened for dementia using the MMSE, and for any neurological, psychiatric, or neurological disease. Note that the mouse was controlled by the examiner during test administration in this sample. These data demonstrate near perfect performance on Effort subtests in healthy people and provide a benchmark for interpretation of Memory scores (see Table 15–17).

TABLE 15–17 Non-Verbal Medical Symptom Validity Test (NV-MSVT) Means and Standard Deviations for Well-Educated Older Controls (*N* = 50)

SCORE	*M*	*SD*	RANGE
NV-MSVT IR	99.9	0.7	95–100
NV-MSVT DR	96.9	5.2	75–100
NV-MSVT CNS	96.8	5.2	75–100
NV-MSVT DRA	96.2	6.4	65–100
NV-MSVT DRV	96.2	5.3	80–100
NV-MSVT PA	99.6	2.0	90–100
NV-MSVT FR	81.0	13.8	40–100
Criterion A1	97.7	2.6	88–100

NOTE: Criterion A1 = Mean of IR, DR, CNS, DRV, and PA.

SOURCE: Adapted from Henry et al. (2010).

PROFILE ANALYSIS AND THE GMIP

Profile analysis is paramount to interpretation. The manual states that profile scores from dementia and simulator groups are the most informative to understand the quality of performance on the NV-MSVT. Performance is deemed adequate when the mean of specific scores is higher than a given value outlined in the manual. If this is not met, additional criteria are evaluated (i.e., Criterion B1 through B3, as defined in the manual). These criteria will not be detailed here, but essentially the results are first evaluated with respect to the cutoff scores of the Effort subtests, then Criteria B1 to B3 rely on the expected gradient of difficulty between subtests, with some subtests believed to yield distinctly higher rates of accuracy than others.

Using the criteria listed is reported to yield high specificity for avoiding false positives in people with dementia. Using this approach, the manual reports 70% sensitivity and 100% specificity in volunteer simulators, and no honestly responding person was incorrectly classified. In contrast to Effort scores, FR is "like any other memory test" (p. 24) and interpretation involves comparison to the appropriate comparator group selected in the reporting function. Of note, Effort scores show an extreme negative skew, whereas FR scores are more dispersed in an approximation of a normal distribution.

The manual contrasts the dementia profile that conforms to the expected gradient of difficulty on the NV-MSVT with what the author has termed a "Pinocchio Principle," named after the shape of the graph of results, an implausible profile involving PA because it does not conform to the expected gradient of difficulty on profile analysis. No independent research has validated this score pattern, to our knowledge.

COMPARISON GROUPS

Comparator groups provided by the test author in the manual or scoring program can be used to determine which group of patients a specific examinee most closely resembles. There are various comparator groups, including children with fetal alcohol disorder, volunteer simulators, patients with dementia, and so on. The comparator groups included in the computer program are from "independent investigators from around the world" who contributed scores ranging from an *N* of 1 (i.e., "one healthy adult making a good effort and one asked to simulate impairment," p. 65, manual) to multiple datasets from people with dementia. Of note, comparator groups are added as the program develops, with many consisting of unpublished datasets contributed by clinicians and researchers directly to the author.

EVIDENCE FOR RELIABILITY

No data on reliability are available to our knowledge.

EVIDENCE FOR VALIDITY

There are numerous datasets described in the manual and a smaller number of published studies by the test author that uniformly support the test's validity. The following review of validity evidence emphasizes independent studies on the test; this review will avoid simulator studies as much as possible (i.e., studies on people instructed to feign deficits on the test) as these tend to yield higher accuracy statistics than when PVTs are used in actual clinical samples, although some simulator data are provided here when other data are lacking.

WITHIN-TEST RELATIONSHIPS

In terms of score intercorrelations, the Effort scores and PA appear to have moderately to high associations with each other, but FR demonstrates lower correlations with the rest of the NV-MSVT scores (Armistead-Jehle & Hansen, 2016). This suggests that FR may measure a slightly distinct domain than the other NV-MSVT scores, most likely memory. Based on data provided in the manual, in general, NV-MSVT Effort variables correlate highly with WMT DR and MSVT DR (Green, 2008).

FACTOR-ANALYTIC STUDIES

One factor analysis provides evidence that the NV-MSVT Effort scores tap a dimension common to other PVTs that is relatively distinct from standard memory tests. The NV-MSVT, MSVT, and memory subtests from the RBANS were subjected to a factor analysis in military service members with self-reported mild TBI (Armistead-Jehle & Hansen, 2016). This yielded a two-factor solution reflecting (1) a PVT factor with loadings from NV-MSVT and MSVT Effort scores, but also with loadings from memory subtests such as PA and (2) a memory factor with loadings from the RBANS memory subtests along with NV-MSVT FR and MSVT FR memory subtests. Notably, the authors concluded that PA measures performance validity independent of memory functioning; however, Effort and Memory subtests did not separate cleanly in this factor analysis, and the two factors themselves were fairly highly correlated, which may reflect either properties of the tests themselves or of the sample.

COMPARISONS TO OTHER STAND-ALONE PVTS

There are relatively few independent studies on comparisons to other stand-alone PVTs. However, these studies indicate that the NV-MSVT fares quite well in comparison to the WMT and MSVT and does not necessarily have lower sensitivity than either test, as has been reported in the manual.

Specifically, based on data provided in the manual, and in general, NV-MSVT Effort variables correlate highly with WMT DR and MSVT DR (Green, 2008), consistent with all three tests tapping a common performance validity dimension. However, correlations for all Effort scores are not provided.

In terms of relative sensitivity of the three tests to noncredible performance, research presented by the test author indicates that the WMT is the most sensitive of the tests, followed by the MSVT and then the NV-MSVT (see manual for details). Independent studies indicate that, in some cases, the NV-MSVT is the more sensitive test. While NV-MSVT failure rate is reported at 15%, slightly lower than 20% in an active-duty military sample (Armistead-Jehle & Hansen, 2011), in simulators, the NV-MSVT was best at identifying feigning compared to the WMT and MSVT using the GMIP, although all three were effective. When the test was used in combination with either the WMT or MSVT, sensitivity was 100% (i.e., all feigners were correctly detected; Armistead-Jehle & Denney, 2015). Similarly, the NV-MSVT is associated with the highest sensitivity in identifying feigned impairment among the three tests in knowledgeable simulators (Armistead-Jehle & Denney, 2015).

Compared to the TOMM, data presented by the author indicate consistently higher sensitivity for the NV-MSVT (manual). Green (2011) also reported that in a group of consecutively evaluated outpatients referred for disability assessment, 26% of the mild TBI group failed the NV-MSVT compared to 10% failing the TOMM. A subset of individuals passed the TOMM and failed the NV-MSVT (11% of sample). This group showed a response pattern more indicative of feigning than severe cognitive impairment based on relative performance on items of varying difficulty and comparison to performance of people with dementia (Green, 2011).

In contrast, independent research studies show higher sensitivity for the NV-MSVT in some studies, while others show equivalent prediction accuracy. For example, although the tests agree in 84% of cases, twice as many non-head-injury disability claimants fail the NV-MSVT (21%) compared to the TOMM (9%); the NV-MSVT also has higher sensitivity to invalidity than the TOMM but equivalent specificity when the WMT and MSVT are used as reference standards for invalidity (Armistead-Jehle & Gervais, 2011). NV-MSVT failure rates of 15% have also been reported, slightly higher than the TOMM at 11% (Armistead-Jehle & Hansen, 2011). In ADHD, the NV-MSVT and TOMM show similar prediction accuracy for feigned and genuine ADHD, but both are superior to PVTs such as the b Test as well as SVTs designed to detect invalid ADHD symptoms or psychiatric malingering (Jasinski et al., 2011; Sollman et al., 2010; Williamson et al., 2014). In studies on the effects of coaching, both measures show similar detection rates for invalidity (Weinborn et al., 2012).

EMBEDDED PVTS

There are few independent studies on associations with embedded PVTs. These generally indicate lower associations than with stand-alone PVTs, as would be expected. For example, correlations between the NV-MSVT Effort scores and Reliable Digit Span (RDS) were variable in a group of older neurologic patients; correlations were minimal for IR and CNS, but moderate for DR ($r = .31$; Henry et al., 2010). As well, in an ADHD study, the NV-MSVT was superior to RDS in identifying those feigning ADHD (Williamson et al., 2014). Similarly, although NV-MSVT failure correlates highly with failure on the RBANS Effort Index ($r = .58$), the NV-MSVT is superior to the RBANS in detecting noncredible performance in a military sample (Armistead-Jehle & Hansen, 2011).

CORRELATIONS WITH NEUROPSYCHOLOGICAL TESTS

As is the case for other PVTs, failure is related to lower scores on other cognitive tests, and the test correlates with measures of neuropsychological functioning. NV-MSVT Memory scores in particular demonstrate strong correlations with other memory tests, but FR in particular demonstrates surprisingly high correlations with verbal memory tests despite its visual content.

For example, in a multiple regression with various demographic and clinical variables, a composite based on NV-MSVT/MSVT along with age predicted performance on neuropsychological tests in active-duty military service members who sustained a concussion (Armistead-Jehle et al., 2016a). Those who failed either the NV-MSVT or MSVT had lower scores on cognitive test variables (e.g., RBANS), with effect sizes generally moderate in size according to Cohen's conventions. Similarly, Effort scores are modestly to moderately correlated with RBANS memory scores in service members with a history of concussion; notably, the FR memory score correlates more highly with measures of verbal memory than of visual memory ($r = .43$ to RBANS List Learning, $r = .26$ with Figure Recall; Armistead-Jehle & Hansen, 2016). PA does not appear to demonstrate as strong or consistent a level of association to RBANS memory scores.

In neurologic patients, NV-MSVT Effort tests show modest to large correlations with the MMSE ($r = .47$ to $.65$), verbal memory (RAVLT), and language (Boston Naming Test [BNT]), with lesser but still significant correlations with some executive and working memory tasks (figural fluency, Digit Span, Corsi Block Tapping, Go/No Go tasks), but the tests are uncorrelated with reaction time tasks (Henry et al., 2010). Notably, there was no relation between passing or failing the NV-MSVT and MMSE performance. NV-MSVT Memory measures show strong correlations with memory measures, particularly between FR and RAVLT delayed recall ($r = .75$), providing support for the validity of the FR as a memory test. In contrast, PA had its largest correlations with the BNT, although it, too, demonstrated very high correlations with RAVLT memory scores (Henry et al., 2010).

CORRELATIONS WITH SVTS AND STANDARDIZED QUESTIONNAIRES

To our knowledge, there are no independent studies on concordance with well-known SVTs, such as invalidity scales from the MMPI-2 or PAI measuring psychological or cognitive symptom overreporting. However, the MSVT is modestly correlated with the Memory Complaints Inventory, a self-report questionnaire by the same author (Green, 2004), with lower scores associated with more memory complaints, and with those failing the NV-MSVT having significantly higher Memory Complaints Inventory scores (Armistead-Jehle et al., 2016b). Although more research on the association between the tests across samples is needed, as MSVT performance worsens, memory complaints increase.

In feigned ADHD, the NS-MSVT surpasses SVTs designed to detect invalid responding on ADHD questionnaires (e.g., Inconsistency Index from the Conners Adult ADHD Rating Scale; CAARS), as well as SVTs designed to detect psychiatric malingering, such as the Miller Forensic Assessment of Symptoms Test (M-FAST; Sollman et al., 2010).

With regard to measures of psychopathology, NV-MSVT scores are not related to depression (Beck Depression Inventory [BDI]) in healthy people (Henry et al., 2010). In a multiple regression with various demographic and clinical variables in active-duty military service members who sustained a concussion, those who failed either the NV-MSVT or MSVT had higher PAI somatic and depressive symptoms (Armistead-Jehle et al., 2016a).

CLINICAL STUDIES

To our knowledge, there exist no studies that validate the NV-MSVT cutoffs against established malingering criteria such as the Slick et al. (1999) criteria for malingered neurocognitive dysfunction or the Bianchini et al. criteria for malingered pain-related disability (Bianchini et al., 2005). Similarly, there do not appear to be as many independent studies involving TBI, criminal defendants, or people with low IQ as there are for other tests such as the WMT, TOMM, and MSVT, among others.

Litigants and Disability Claimants. Non-head-injury disability claimants have a 21% failure rate on the NV-MSVT (Armistead-Jehle & Gervais; 2011), with a very low rate of cases meeting GMIP criteria (4%). There are no studies on social security disability claimants to our knowledge as there are for the MSVT (see review elsewhere in this chapter).

Criminal Defendants. There are no independent studies on this clinical group to our knowledge. The manual presents data on examinees with end-stage renal disease who were in a prison system, but generalizability to most criminal/forensic settings is unknown.

Military Samples. There are a small number of studies in this clinical group from the same research group, compared to a more extensive literature for other PVTs such as the WMT and MSVT. Compared to these tests, NV-MSVT studies show a lower rate of failure in military samples; this may relate more to the number of studies available than to the sensitivity of the test. For example, in an active-duty military sample, NV-MSVT failure rate was 15%, lower than the MSVT at 20%, but higher than the TOMM at 11% (Armistead-Jehle & Hansen, 2011). In one study of active-duty service members with concussion with high officer representation, 11% failed the NV-MSVT compared to 15% failing the MSVT (Armistead-Jehle et al., 2016a). Many more participants met actuarial criteria for the GMIP on the MSVT than on the NV-MSVT; none met the clinical criteria of being dependent on others for everyday activities.

TBI. There are, to our knowledge, no independent studies on TBI using the NV-MSVT. Studies by the test author and datasets presented in the manual report higher failure rates in mild than moderate to severe TBI, consistent with the test's sensitivity to noncredible performance. For example, 26% of a mild TBI group failed the NV-MSVT, but no examinees with moderate to severe brain injury failed the test (Green, 2011).

Chronic Pain. There are no independent studies on this clinical group to our knowledge.

Dementia. There are few independent studies on the GMIP in dementia and none involving differentiating verified malingerers from people with dementia. As noted by McGuire and colleagues in their review of PVTs in dementia, studies that involve only those exerting credible effort (i.e., dementia patients) cannot possibly investigate the sensitivity of PVTs as there are no true positives in their sample (i.e., verified malingerers); they noted that the majority of MSVT studies on dementia are of this variety. Nevertheless, the NV-MSVT and related tests such as the WMT and MSVT were felt to be superior to other PVTs in the assessment of people with dementia, although data are preliminary given the small number of independent studies (McGuire et al., 2019). One study reported low specificity for the NV-MSVT but did not use the GMIP to correct for false positives (Rudman et al., 2011). Other datasets supportive of the test's usage in dementia are provided in the manual.

To our knowledge, there is only one independent study on the use of the GMIP in dementia patients. Henry, Merten, Wolf, and Harth (2010) reported that the NV-MSVT performed well in dementia patients, with very high specificity for dementia. They administered the NV-MSVT to neurologic patients, 32% of whom had a dementia diagnosis, and compared them to healthy participants. In all, 36% of dementia patients did not have a GMIP, and only one control was incorrectly classified as demented via the GMIP (2%). They noted than an impulsive response style in otherwise nondemented patients may contribute to false positives on the GMIP. In this study, DRA was the only subtest in which dementia patients scored the same as controls; dementia patients also scored much lower on PA than controls and even lower on FR, demonstrating sensitivity to memory impairment for these scores. Nevertheless, Henry and colleagues noted some limitations of the approach, including that the manual is unclear about how cases who meet criteria for the GMIP but have no evidence of dementia clinically are to be dealt with and the degree to which clinical information is to be considered to make decisions, noting that clear decision rules would be helpful (Henry et al., 2010). They concluded that the GMIP has high specificity for noncredible performance in neurological patients and healthy people (i.e., does not incorrectly identify them as feigning), but that the sensitivity of the NV-MSVT to noncredible performance (i.e., identification of persons putting forth noncredible performance) still needs to be demonstrated.

In a study by the author and colleagues, all severe dementia patients failed the test ($N = 10$), and all met criteria for the GMIP (Singhal et al., 2009). However, 40% of simulators were not detected by the GMIP approach. Using the NV-MSVT in combination with the MSVT reduced the percentage of incorrectly identified simulators to 20%, with an impressive 80% sensitivity and 100% specificity for feigning when both tests are used together (Singhal et al., 2009). Although replication in clinical groups with verified malingerers and larger samples is needed, this study offers promising results that combining the NV-MSVT with the MSVT eliminates some of the limitations of using the GMIP from either test alone.

Similarly, an independent simulation study supports the combined use of tests to differentiate noncredible performance from dementia using the GMIP, with better sensitivity for the NV-MSVT than for the WMT or MSVT. Very few sophisticated dementia simulators (i.e., psychology students) are able to produce a GMIP, yielding a 94% sensitivity to detecting simulators (Armistead-Jehle & Denney, 2015). Combining the NV-MSVT with the WMT or MSVT significantly increased the detection of feigners to 100%, thereby correctly identifying the feigners who would have been missed by the NV-MSVT used alone. Of the three tests, the NV-MSVT had the highest accuracy for detecting feigners using the GMIP, and the MSVT had the lowest accuracy.

It is possible that differences between how tests define the GMIP affect GMIP detection rates. In one study of active-duty service members with concussion with high officer representation (Armistead-Jehle et al., 2016a), much fewer participants met actuarial GMIP criteria for the NV-MSVT compared to the MSVT. Notably, the NV-MSVT requires a higher number of criteria to meet the GMIP requirements compared to the MSVT (see also Armistead-Jehle & Denney, 2015).

Low IQ. There are no independent studies on this clinical group to our knowledge. See manual for datasets and research presented by the test author supportive of its usage in this group. For example, the manual presents data on parents seeking custody of their children and notes that despite some having cognitive deficits, they performed extremely well on Effort subtests, with no failures noted. Comparatively speaking, the MSVT in particular has more studies on its use in low-IQ examinees.

ADHD. There is promising research on the NV-MSVT's capacity to detect feigned ADHD supporting its routine use in ADHD assessment, although none has included verified malingerers to date. Specifically, the test has been used in college students demonstrating generally large effect sizes in discriminating feigned versus genuine ADHD (Jasinski et al., 2011; Sollman et al., 2010; Williamson et al., 2014). Generally, the NV-MSVT yields low to moderate sensitivity and high specificity in these studies, similar to most other PVTs examined. Approximately 21% of college students seeking ADHD evaluations fail the NV-MSVT (Leppma et al., 2018).

Resistance to Coaching. Of note, explicit and detailed coaching can impact performance, although classification accuracy remains high according to one study examining this question (Weinborn et al., 2012). Specifically, the NV-MSVT had a specificity of 96% in college undergraduates subjected to various conditions of coaching. Overall, resistance to coaching was considered equivalent between the NV-MSVT, MSVT, and TOMM.

NEUROANATOMICAL CORRELATES AND IMAGING STUDIES

There are some supportive data presented by the author on this topic. In a study by the author, litigants and disability claimants who passed the NV-MSVT had a 47% rate of abnormalities on computed tomography (CT) or magnetic resonance imaging (MRI). In contrast, 0% failing the NV-MSVT had imaging abnormalities, the opposite pattern expected if failure were related to degree of neurological compromise (Green, 2011). The manual also described two cases of patients who had undergone nondominant temporal lobectomy also passing Effort tests despite poor performance on the FR (45% correct).

COMMENT

The NV-MSVT is similar in structure to Green's other PVTs (WMT, MSVT), but importantly, it is visual, nonverbal, and was developed to act as a PVT that requires little administration time and has acceptable sensitivity to invalidity yet few false positives when tested in persons with dementia. To this end, the emphasis is on profile analysis of scores as opposed to simple cutoffs, and this is emphasized more in the NV-MSVT than in the other tests by Green. In contrast to the WMT and MSVT, there is no base reading level required, and the test should thus be applicable to a broader range of examinees. The NV-MSVT includes both Effort tests and Memory tests that progress along a gradient of difficulty.

There is good evidence for the validity of the NV-MSVT as an effective PVT, although its independent research base is less than those of its counterparts, the WMT and MSVT. NV-MSVT subtests tend to be correlated with each other and tend to show high agreement with other PVTs. Research presented in the manual suggests WMT is the most sensitive, followed by the MSVT and then the NV-MSVT, which is in turn reported to be comparatively more sensitive than the TOMM. However, independent research is more mixed on this question, with some studies showing superiority for the NV-MSVT. Available evidence suggests that, overall, Memory scores tend to show stronger relationships with demographic factors than do Effort scores, with some mixed results regarding relationships between the NV-MSVT and education. Like other PVTs, failure on the NV-MSVT is generally related to lower scores on other tests; research suggests that NV-MSVT variables, regardless of whether they emphasize Effort or Memory, are correlated with cognitive tests. Compensation-seeking appears to affect performance, as would be expected for a PVT.

The test is designed to be used in conjunction with the WMT and MSVT (Green, 2008), but using two out of the three tests appears sufficient to detect most examinees with noncredible performance (P. Green, personal communication, June 2018); independent research suggests that one of the tests should be the NV-MSVT. Some have noted that if there is Effort score failure and no GMIP across the three PVTs, the data are exceedingly unlikely to be reflective of genuine responding (Armistead-Jehle & Denney, 2015).

Notably, the NV-MSVT requires that *mean* performance across subtests falls below a specific cutoff compared to failure on *one of three* subtests for the WMT and MSVT. It also includes a larger number of individual criteria to meet the GMIP requirements compared to the WMT and MSVT; these differences may affect detection rates, although more study is needed on this question.

The FR is designed to be used as a memory test (Green, 2008); PA appears to correlate more with Effort scores. Comparatively speaking, the research on FR as a memory test is quite positive, demonstrating high correlations with memory tests and age-related changes, as would be expected for a memory test. Of note, isolated low scores (e.g., DRA) can occur that are likely not indicative of invalid performance.

Practical aspects include a briefer and less demanding administration than tests such as the TOMM, which require the examiner to flip pages in a stimulus book, but downsides include not being able to pause the test or correct inadvertent examinee responses once the test administration begins (Wager & Howe, 2010).

The test has limitations that users should be aware of. There exist no studies that validate the NV-MSVT cutoffs against established malingering criteria such as the Slick et al. (1999) criteria for malingered neurocognitive dysfunction or the Bianchini et al. (2005) criteria for malingered pain-related disability. Similarly, as of this writing, there do not appear to be any independent studies involving TBI, criminal defendants, or people with low IQ as there are for other tests such as the WMT, TOMM, and MSVT, among others. Research on well-known SVTs (e.g., MMPI-2 validity scales) is also needed.

Despite its name, the NV-MSVT is actually not as nonverbal a task as other nonverbal PVTs, most notably the TOMM. Verbal demands include naming pictures and recalling stimuli verbally (Wager & Howe, 2010), and the test demonstrates high correlations with verbal memory tests in studies examining this question. It may therefore best be described as a combined verbal and nonverbal PVT, which in no way takes away from its validity as an effective PVT. In fact, adding a verbal element may make it a better PVT because, according to the author, verbal PVTs outperform nonverbal ones (Green, 2008). However, in people with severe verbal deficits, the TOMM may be more appropriate as it is a truly nonverbal PVT (excluding the fact that items on both tests can be covertly verbally encoded by the examinee if they choose to do so).

Like the WMT and MSVT, the NV-MSVT is unique in its design as it offers both Effort tests and Memory tests that progress along a gradient of difficulty; the resultant profile analysis may minimize false positives in people with cognitive impairment. However, one obvious and major limitation is that the GMIP can be faked—this may not be known by most users (see MSVT review elsewhere in this chapter). Blind reliance on discounting malingering when the actuarial criteria for the GMIP are met is discouraged. Although similar research on the NV-MSVT is lacking, independent studies on the MSVT indicate that when the GMIP occurs in examinees motivated to fail, the GMIP appears equally or more likely to be due to feigning than to actual impairment. However, when it occurs in well-motivated examinees with intellectual disability or dementia and without incentives to fail, the GMIP may assist in characterizing impairment (Chafetz & Biondolillo, 2013).

Users should recall the main tenet of the GMIP: that is, if the examinee is *not* dependent on others in daily life, then the criteria for the GMIP would not be met, by definition. The test author states that the GMIP must be used in conjunction with Criteria D of the Slick et al. malingering criteria (Slick et al., 1999) to be effective at differentiating invalid performance from cognitive impairment. Criteria D specifies that behaviors meeting necessary criteria for malingering must not be fully accounted for by psychiatric, neurological, or developmental factors that result in significantly diminished capacity to appreciate laws or mores against malingering or inability to conform behavior to such standards, and are not the product of an informed, rational, and volitional effort aimed at least in part toward acquiring or achieving external incentives.

Some have criticized a somewhat circular reasoning within the GMIP and suggest the numerical algorithm should not depend on clinical criteria outside of the test results themselves. We see no problem with including Criterion D of the Slick criteria to aid in interpreting scores as this provides a bridge between purely actuarial approaches and purely clinical approaches to detecting malingering and exaggeration. However, more clarity, consistency, and validation of this approach are needed in the manual, scoring program, and related publications, including further validation of the cutoffs and algorithm using verified malingerers. Criterion D of the Slick malingering criteria is not part of the GMIP algorithm described in the manual but is used in the Advanced Interpretation Program, making it difficult to compare results across studies that have used different criteria.

From a practical perspective for users, the manual is difficult to follow and not organized for rapid reference. Similarly, the manual emphases score patterns thought to reveal noncredible performance such as the "Pinocchio Principle," referring to a specific difference between two scores on the test indicative of feigning (Green, 2008). There is no validation on the Pinocchio Principle in independent studies, to our knowledge, and so reliance on profiles with more empirical support (Effort score failure, GMIP) makes sense until there is further research. Analysis of scores is based on reference to comparator groups. Generally, these results are from various clinics, have small sample sizes in some cases, and quality control measures are not described, so their representativeness and generalizability when making important diagnostic clinical decisions in the individual examinee are not clear.

Last, as is the case for all PVTs, the NV-MSVT offers information on the credibility of the examinee's test scores but does not speak to the cause of invalid scores. Use of multidimensional criteria to ascertain the basis for failure is necessary, including examining congruence between clinical characteristics, adaptive living skills, neuropsychological profile, and context of assessment (e.g., presence of incentive vs. no discernible incentive). Additional research providing data on reliability estimates for the Memory scores, in particular, and comparative performance in diverse ethnic, cultural, and linguistic groups would augment the literature on the test.

REFERENCES

Armistead-Jehle, P., Cooper, D. B., & Vanderploeg, R. D. (2016a). The role of performance validity tests in the assessment of cognitive functioning after military concussion: A replication and extension.

Applied Neuropsychology. Adult, 23(4), 264–273. https://doi.org/10.1080/23279095.2015.1055564

Armistead-Jehle, P., & Denney, R. L. (2015). The detection of feigned impairment using the WMT, MSVT, and NV-MSVT. *Applied Neuropsychology. Adult, 22*(2), 147–155. https://doi.org/10.1080/23279095.2014.880842

Armistead-Jehle, P., & Gervais, R. O. (2011). Sensitivity of the Test Of Memory Malingering and the Nonverbal Medical Symptom Validity Test: A replication study. *Applied Neuropsychology, 18*(4), 284–290. https://doi.org/10.1080/09084282.2011.595455

Armistead-Jehle, P., Grills, C. E., Bieu, R. K., & Kulas, J. F. (2016b). Clinical utility of the Memory Complaints Inventory to detect invalid test performance. *The Clinical Neuropsychologist, 30*(4), 610–628. https://doi.org/10.1080/13854046.2016.1177597

Armistead-Jehle, P., & Hansen, C. L. (2011). Comparison of the Repeatable Battery for the Assessment of Neuropsychological Status Effort Index and stand-alone symptom validity tests in a military sample. *Archives of Clinical Neuropsychology, 26*(7), 592–601. https://doi.org/10.1093/arclin/acr049

Armistead-Jehle, P., & Hansen, C. L. (2016). Factor analysis of the MSVT, NV-MSVT, and RBANS Memory subtests. *Archives of Clinical Neuropsychology, 31*(5), 465–471. https://doi.org/10.1093/arclin/acw033

Bianchini, K. J., Greve, K. W., & Glynn, G. (2005). On the diagnosis of malingered pain-related disability: lessons from cognitive malingering research. *The Spine Journal, 5*(4), 404–417. https://doi.org/10.1016/j.spinee.2004.11.016

Chafetz, M. D., & Biondolillo, A. M. (2013). Feigning a severe impairment profile. *Archives of Clinical Neuropsychology, 28*(3), 205–212. https://doi.org/10.1093/arclin/act015

Green, P. (2004). *Memory Complaints Inventory (MCI).* Edmonton, AB, Canada: Green's Publishing.

Green, P. (2008). *Green's Non-Verbal Medical Symptom Validity Test (NV-MSVT) user's manual for Microsoft Windows.* Edmonton, AB, Canada: Green's Publishing.

Green, P. (2011). Comparison between the Test of Memory Malingering (TOMM) and the Nonverbal Medical Symptom Validity Test (NV-MSVT) in adults with disability claims. *Applied Neuropsychology, 18*(1), 18–26. https://doi.org/10.1080/09084282.2010.523365

Henry, M., Merten, T., Wolf, S. A., & Harth, S. (2010). Nonverbal Medical Symptom Validity Test performance of elderly healthy adults and clinical neurology patients. *Journal of Clinical and Experimental Neuropsychology, 32*(1), 19–27. https://doi.org/10.1080/13803390902791653

Jasinski, L. J., Harp, J. P., Berry, D. T. R., Shandera-Ochsner, A. L., Mason, L. H., & Ranseen, J. D. (2011). Using symptom validity tests to detect malingered ADHD in college students. *The Clinical Neuropsychologist, 25*(8), 1415–1428. https://doi.org/10.1080/13854046.2011.630024

Leppma, M., Long, D., Smith, M., & Lassiter, C. (2018). Detecting symptom exaggeration in college students seeking ADHD treatment: Performance validity assessment using the NV-MSVT and IVA-Plus. *Applied Neuropsychology. Adult, 25*(3), 210–218. https://doi.org/10.1080/23279095.2016.1277723

McGuire, C., Crawford, S., & Evans, J. J. (2019). Effort testing in dementia assessment: A systematic review. *Archives of Clinical Neuropsychology, 34*(1), 114–131.. https://doi.org/10.1093/arclin/acy012

Reslan, S., & Axelrod, B. N. (2017). Evaluating the Medical Symptom Validity Test (MSVT) in a sample of veterans between the ages of 18 to 64. *Applied Neuropsychology. Adult, 24*(2), 132–139. https://doi.org/10.1080/23279095.2015.1107565

Rudman, N., Oyebode, J. R., Jones, C. A., & Bentham, P. (2011). An investigation into the validity of effort tests in a working age dementia population. *Aging & Mental Health, 15*(1), 47–57. https://doi.org/10.1080/13607863.2010.508770

Singhal, A., Green, P., Ashaye, K., Shankar, K., & Gill, D. (2009). High specificity of the Medical Symptom Validity Test in patients with very severe memory impairment. *Archives of Clinical Neuropsychology, 24*(8), 721–728. https://doi.org/10.1093/arclin/acp074

Slick, D. J., Sherman, E. M., & Iverson, G. L. (1999). Diagnostic criteria for malingered neurocognitive dysfunction: proposed standards for clinical practice and research. *The Clinical Neuropsychologist, 13*(4), 545–561. https://doi.org/10.1076/1385-4046(199911)13:04;1-Y;FT545

Sollman, M. J., Ranseen, J. D., & Berry, D. T. R. (2010). Detection of feigned ADHD in college students. *Psychological Assessment, 22*(2), 325–335. https://doi.org/10.1037/a0018857

Wager, J. G., & Howe, L. L. S. (2010). Nonverbal Medical Symptom Validity Test: Try faking now! *Applied Neuropsychology, 17*(4), 305–309. https://doi.org/10.1080/09084282.2010.525093

Weinborn, M., Woods, S. P., Nulsen, C., & Leighton, A. (2012). The effects of coaching on the verbal and nonverbal medical symptom validity tests. *The Clinical Neuropsychologist, 26*(5), 832–849. https://doi.org/10.1080/13854046.2012.686630

Williamson, K. D., Combs, H. L., Berry, D. T. R., Harp, J. P., Mason, L. H., & Edmundson, M. (2014). Discriminating among ADHD alone, ADHD with a comorbid psychological disorder, and feigned ADHD in a college sample. *The Clinical Neuropsychologist, 28*(7), 1182–1196. https://doi.org/10.1080/13854046.2014.956674

REY FIFTEEN-ITEM TEST (FIT)

TEST NAME	**Rey Fifteen-Item Test (FIT)**
DOMAIN	Performance validity
AGE RANGE	Adults
ADMINISTRATION TIME	5 minutes
SCORING FORMAT	Hand scored
REFERENCES	Boone, K. B., Salazar, X., Lu, P., Warner-Chacon, K., & Razani, J. (2002). The Rey 15-Item Recognition Trial: A technique to enhance sensitivity of the Rey 15-Item Memorization Test. *Journal of Clinical and Experimental Neuropsychology, 24*, 561–573. Griffin, G. A., Glassmire, D. M., Henderson, E. A., & McCann, C. (1997). Rey II: Redesigning the Rey Screening Test of malingering. *Journal of Clinical Psychology, 53*, 757–766. Paul, D. S., Franzen, M. D., Cohen, S. H., & Fremouw, W. (1992). An investigation into the reliability and validity of two tests used in the detection of dissimulation. *International Journal of Clinical Neuropsychology, 14*, 1–9. Rey, A. (1964). *L'examen clinique en psychologie*. Paris: Presses Universitaires de France.

DESCRIPTION AND ADMINISTRATION

The Rey Fifteen-Item Test (FIT) is also called the Fifteen-Item Memory Test or Rey's Memory Test. This test is used to assess exaggeration and feigning of memory complaints. It was originally developed by André Rey, who developed an interest in detecting malingering partly in response to accusations by insurance companies that most, if not all, claimants were probably only feigning impairment (Frederick, 2002). The FIT (Rey, 1964) is probably the best known of Rey's procedures (Frederick, 2002). Lezak (1983, Lezak et al., 2012) adapted the task. Although it has decreased in popularity, it is still one of the most commonly used performance validity measures (Dandachi-Fitzgerald et al., 2013; Martin et al., 2015; Sharland & Gfeller, 2007; Slick et al., 2004; Young et al., 2016). It consists of 15 items. Details on administration, items, and format are not provided to preserve test security. Please see original source or the third edition of this volume for details. In reality, because this is primarily a test of immediate memory and attention and because of item redundancy, the FIT is actually rather easy and examinees need recall only three or four ideas to recall most of the items. Individuals who are feigning memory problems are thought to misjudge the difficulty of the task and thus to perform more poorly than all but those examinees with severe intellectual impairment. In their discussion of the FIT, Lezak et al. (2004, 2012) suggested that anyone who is not significantly impaired can recall at least three of the five character sets or nine of the 15 items.

A number of authors have suggested various modifications of the FIT to increase the sensitivity of the test (see "Evidence for Validity"). For example, Paul, Franzen, Cohen, and Fremouw (1992) developed a 16-item version of the FIT. Griffin, Glassmire, Henderson, and McCann (1997) redesigned the figures, increasing the internal logic and pattern redundancy (FIT-II). Boone, Salazar, Lu, Warner-Chacon, and Razani (2002) included a recognition trial after the recall trial (Rey Fifteen-Item Recognition Trial; FIT+). The examinee is requested to recognize the 15 stimuli out of 15 targets and 15 foils.

SCORING

A number of scores can be computed. Typically, examiners record the total number of items recalled correctly, regardless of their spatial location. The range is 0 to 15. One can also record the number of correct rows in proper sequence; that is, the number of rows that are in the correct place in the 3 × 5 matrix and that contain all of the correct items arranged in the correct order. The range is 0 to 5. One can also sum the number of symbols correctly placed within a row. Analysis of type of error (e.g., rotations, distortions, perseverations) may also be of some use (e.g., Erdal, 2004; Greiffenstein et al., 1996; Griffen et al., 1996; also see "Evidence for Validity").

DEMOGRAPHIC EFFECTS

AGE

Modest associations have been reported between number correct and age. For example, Schretlen et al. (1991) found that, in adults, the number of items recalled was inversely related to age ($r = -.25$). Others have also reported that scores on the FIT decline with advancing age (e.g., Boone et al., 2002; Griffin et al., 1997; Philpott & Boone, 1994), although the amount of shared variance tends to be small (i.e., <10%).

GENDER

No difference between males and females was reported in one study (Constantinou & McCaffrey, 2003).

EDUCATION AND IQ

Level of education affects scores in adults, with scores increasing with higher levels of education (e.g., Back et al., 1996; Boone et al., 2002; Robles et al., 2015). Intellectual level is also related to performance on the test ($r = .38$ to .81; e.g., Griffin et al., 1997; Love et al., 2014; Schretlen et al., 1991). Therefore, the FIT may be inappropriate for individuals with less than average education/IQ (see Evidence for Validity for more discussion).

ETHNICITY, NATIONALITY, AND LINGUISTIC EFFECTS

The FIT appears robust to cultural/language factors, at least among male monolingual Spanish-speakers from Los Angeles and Mexico and may be suitable for this population (Robles et al., 2015; see "Normative Data" for more information).

NORMATIVE DATA

For the standard FIT, cutoff scores of 7 items correct or fewer (Lee et al., 1992), 8 items or fewer (Bernard & Fowler, 1990; Schretlen et al., 1991), 9 items or fewer (Greiffenstein et al., 1996; Lezak et al., 2004, 2012; Taylor et al., 2003), and 11 items (Hiscock et al., 1994) have been suggested to determine noncredible performance in adults (see "Evidence for Validity"). Adjusting the cutoff score higher tends to increase the FIT's sensitivity but at the expense of its specificity.

Although most researchers focus on the total number of items recalled, some have suggested more complex scoring schemes involving appraisals of item placement and accuracy of reproductions. For example, examiners can use a cutoff of fewer than two rows in the proper location (Arnett et al., 1995) or fewer than nine symbols accurately placed within rows (Greiffenstein et al., 1996).

The five rows that comprise the FIT differ in degree of difficulty. In nonlitigating brain-injured individuals, recall of the three rows follows a sequential order, with the most frequent qualitative error misordering of the fourth row (Morgan, 1991). In honest responders, perseverations/repetitions of correct stimuli and errors in the correct placement of rows appear to be relatively common; however, other types of errors are rare (e.g., dyslexic errors, such as letter reversals; gestalt errors, such as >3 items in a row, embellishments, or confabulatory errors; Griffin et al., 1996; Lee et al., 2000). It is important to bear in mind, however, that some of these errors (e.g., confabulations) may occur commonly in the context of low IQ or dementia (Hays et al., 2000). Additionally, the response mode (recalling the items vertically or horizontally) appears to have an impact on performance on the FIT (McGuire, 2006). In a TBI group, 17% reproduced the items vertically and obtained FIT scores that were lower than those who reproduced the items horizontally. About 57% of the latter group obtained more than 9 correct items whereas only one (9%) in the "vertical" group obtained scores of greater than 9. Similar findings were found in a non-neurological clinical group. McGuire (2006) suggested a number of strategies to minimize the impact of response mode, including spacing the test stimuli in a way that they would be naturally grouped in rows or including instruction for the clinician to gesture across the row as a cue to the respondent.

If the recognition trial is also given (FIT+), Boone et al (2002) suggest a combination cutoff score (Total FIT score + [Recognition score – false positives]) of less than 20 to indicate "failed" performance. Boone et al. (2002) suggested that sensitivity is increased by 50% relative to recall alone when the recognition trial is added (i.e., to >70%), with no appreciable loss in specificity (i.e., >90%). Note that patients with intellectual disability and dementia were excluded from the study, which probably enhanced specificity values. With a base rate of suspect performance of 28%, a combined score computed as recall correct plus recognition correct minus false-positive recognitions of 20 or less yielded a PPV of 78% and an NPV of 90%.

As the FIT is sensitive to intellectual disability such that a very low cutoff is needed to maximize specificity while maintaining sensitivity, use of a cutoff score may not be meaningful. Rather, clinicians may use Tables 15–18 and 15–19 to evaluate whether the score obtained by their examinee with intellectual disability is unusual. The sample is based on forensic inpatients without potential motivation to feign ($N = 21$, average FSIQ = 60.89, $SD = 6.8$, range = 45–73).

For male monolingual Spanish-speakers from Los Angeles and Mexico with low level of acculturation to the United States (age mean = 28.23, $SD = 8.74$, range = 18–49; education mean = 6.66, $SD = 2.54$, range = 0–10), FIT+ cutoff scores are adjusted for education because previous cutoffs for the FIT+ were inadequate for this sample (Robles et al., 2015). Table 15–20 presents the education-adjusted cutoff scores with a specificity of greater than 90%.

TABLE 15–18 Frequency of Number of Correct Items on the Rey Fifteen-Item Test (FIT) Recall

NUMBER OF ITEMS CORRECT	N	%	CUMULATIVE %
0	2	2.8	2.9
1	1	1.4	4.3
2	2	2.8	7.1
3	7	9.9	17.1
4	4	5.6	22.9
5	2	2.8	25.7
6	13	18.3	44.3
7	6	8.5	52.9
8	2	2.8	55.7
9	11	15.5	71.4
10	4	5.6	77.1
11	3	4.2	81.4
12	8	11.3	92.9
13	1	1.4	94.3
14	3	4.2	98.6
15	1	1.4	100

SOURCE: Marshall et al. (2007).

Morse et al. (2013) gave the FIT+ to noncredible litigants who failed two or more PVTs, credible litigants, patients with learning disability, and a mixed neuropsychology clinic sample not in litigation. In their sample, 29% of those in litigation met criteria for invalid performance. To maintain at least 90% specificity, a combination cutoff of less than 21 yielded a sensitivity of 70%. Sensitivity, specificity, PPV, and NPV data at various cutoff scores and base rates are presented in Tables 15–21 and 15–22. Almost 50% of noncredible litigants made at least one of four false-positive recognition errors, and only 11% of the other three groups combined made at least one error.

TABLE 15–19 Frequency of Total Scores on the Rey Fifteen-Item Test (FIT+)

TOTAL SCORE	N	%	CUMULATIVE %
0	2	2.8	2.9
1	1	1.4	4.3
2	3	4.2	8.6
3	1	1.4	10.0
4	3	4.2	14.3
5	5	7.0	21.4
6	2	2.8	24.3
7	5	7.0	31.4
8	4	5.6	37.1
9	3	4.2	41.4
10	5	7.0	48.6
11	2	2.8	51.4
12	6	8.5	60.0
13	2	2.8	62.9
14	3	4.2	67.1
15	1	1.4	68.6
16	1	1.4	70.0
17	2	2.8	72.9
18	3	4.2	77.1
19	4	5.6	82.9
20	4	5.6	88.6
22	1	1.4	90.0
23	2	2.8	92.9
24	2	2.8	95.7
25	1	1.4	97.1
27	1	1.4	98.6
30	1	1.4	100

SOURCE: Marshall et al. (2007).

TABLE 15–20 Rey Fifteen-Item Test (FIT+) Education-Adjusted Cutoff Scores for Male Monolingual Spanish Speakers

	EDUCATION			
	0–6 YEARS		7–10 YEARS	
	CUTOFF	SPECIFICITY (%)	CUTOFF	SPECIFICITY (%)
Combination Score	≤10	91	≤18	91
Total Recall	≤5	93	≤8	90
Recall Intrusions	≥3	93	≥1	93
Recognition Correct	≤4	93	≤8	93
Recognition False Positives	≥4	94	≥2	95

SOURCE: Adapted from Robles et al. (2015).

EVIDENCE FOR RELIABILITY

EVIDENCE FOR INTERNAL RELIABILITY

Not available.

EVIDENCE FOR TEST-RETEST RELIABILITY, MEASURING CHANGE, AND PRACTICE EFFECTS

Information regarding test-retest reliability is not available for the standard protocol. However, Paul et al. (1992) devised a 16-item version of the FIT (described earlier) and gave the task to community volunteers. On retesting after a two-week interval, community dwellers achieved a reliability coefficient of .48 due to the fact that healthy participants typically obtain perfect scores on both tests, which rose to .88 under simulation conditions.

EVIDENCE FOR INTERRATER RELIABILITY

Goldberg and Miller (1986) reported that independent raters showed 95% agreement for items correct and 97% agreement for rows correct scores, indicating high interrater agreement.

EVIDENCE FOR VALIDITY

RELATIONSHIPS WITH OTHER PVTS

The FIT shows modest to moderate correlations with other PVTs (r = .19 to .78; e.g., b Test, Dot Counting, TOMM, WRMT; McCaffrey et al., 2003; Nelson et al., 2003; Sumanti et al., 2006), with shared variances tending to be less than 50% (Nelson et al., 2003). Therefore, the FIT may provide some nonredundant information regarding performance validity compared to other PVTs.

TABLE 15–21 Sensitivity and Specificity of Rey Fifteen-Item Test (FIT+) Cutoff Scores for Noncredible Litigants, Credible Litigants, Patients with Learning Disability, and a Mixed Neuropsychology Clinic Sample Not in Litigation

	SENSITIVITY (%)		SPECIFICITY (%)		
CUTOFF SCORES	NONCREDIBLE LITIGANTS	CREDIBLE LITIGANTS	NONCREDIBLE LITIGANTS WHO FAILED ONE PVT	CLINICAL PATIENTS	LEARNING DISABILITY
Recall Correct					
<12	73	69	69	72	65
<11	65	77	74	85	73
<10	60	86	87	96	86
<9	48	94	96	100	99
Recognition Correct					
<13	79	67	71	74	69
<12	60	79	81	81	78
<11	52	85	91	91	89
<10	50	90	91	96	91
<9	47	92	95	100	95
Combination Score					
<26	76	65	67	70	69
<25	74	70	72	79	75
<24	74	79	79	85	79
<23	73	88	86	86	82
<22	71	91	92	93	86
<21	70	93	94	95	92
<20	66	93	85	98	93
<19	61	94	96	100	94

NOTE: Combination score, Recall Correct + (Recognition Correct – False Positives).
SOURCE: Morse et al. (2013).

Ideally, a test designed to detect invalid performance should be sensitive to faking but insensitive to genuine memory disturbance. However, the FIT appears to fall far short of this ideal. In general, honest responders achieve higher scores on the test than dissimulating responders, but the sensitivity of the FIT in identifying deception has been reported to be weak and lower than that of other tests in some studies (e.g., b Test, Digit Memory Test, TOMM, VSVT; Flaherty et al., 2015; Shum et al., 2004; Vallabhajosula & van Gorp, 2001; Vickery et al., 2001; Vilar-Lopez et al., 2008; Whitney et al., 2008), but comparable in other studies (e.g., TOMM, DCT; Burton et al., 2012; Marshall & Happe, 2007; Paradis et al., 2013). In Spanish patients with mild TBI or post-concussive syndrome divided based on compensation-seeking status and suspected exaggeration, the FIT did not perform as well as the VSVT and b Test (Vilar-Lopez et al., 2008).

TABLE 15–22 PPV and NPV for Rey Fifteen-Item Test (FIT+) Combination Score at Base Rates of 15%, 28%, and 40% Based on a Litigation and Disability Sample

	15% BASE RATE		29% BASE RATE		40% BASE RATE	
	PPV (%)	NPV (%)	PPV (%)	NPV (%)	PPV (%)	NPV (%)
<26	30	92	48	89	62	83
<25	36	64	54	89	68	83
<24	40	95	60	87	70	83
<23	46	95	65	87	75	84
<22	49	94	70	88	80	83
<21	57	94	73	88	84	84
<20	60	93	80	87	87	83
<19	64	92	84	87	88	83

NOTE: Combination score, Recall Correct + (Recognition Correct – False Positives), PPV, positive predictive value, NPV, negative predictive value.
SOURCE: Morse et al. (2013).

Some studies find that the FIT appears to be as effective as the TOMM in identifying invalid performance (Burton et al., 2012; Paradis et al., 2013) although performance may vary depending on the setting (Flaherty et al., 2015; Love et al., 2014; Whitney et al., 2008). For example, Spanish-speaking individuals from a private neuropsychology practice involved in capital murder cases performed similarly to individuals from a community clinic on the TOMM and FIT, with about 8% failing the FIT and 10% failing the TOMM (Burton et al., 2012). In a forensic group, 33% failed the FIT and 48% failed the TOMM (Burton et al., 2012). Similarly, 48% of defendants undergoing evaluation for competency to stand trial failed the FIT but 65% failed the TOMM (Paradis et al., 2013).

By contrast, Flaherty et al. (2015) reported that among veterans undergoing neuropsychological evaluation for mild TBI, about 77% obtained a perfect score on the FIT and less than 2% failed based on a standard cutoff of less than 9, while 27% failed the TOMM. Notably, only two out of 13 who failed both TOMM and Reliable Digit Span failed the FIT, suggesting that the FIT may not be sufficiently sensitive as a PVT in this setting. Whitney et al. (2008) also reported that veterans were more likely to fail the TOMM than the FIT-II (Griffith et al., 1997).

In their study, the FIT-II identified one-third to one-half of those identified by TOMM as exhibiting noncredible performance. The majority of those identified as exhibiting valid performance on the TOMM were identified by the FIT-II; however, the FIT-II qualitative methods yielded relatively high false-positive rates of 13 to 35% (Whitney et al., 2008). Likewise, the FIT yielded remarkably higher false-positive rates (24 to 38%) than the TOMM (<5%) among forensic inpatients with mild intellectual disability without potential motivation to feign symptoms (Love et el., 2014).

Compared to the DCT, the FIT/FIT+ is superior in identifying invalid performance among Spanish-speakers involved in capital murder cases or other forensic cases (e.g., personal injury, social security disability, or workers' compensation from a private neuropsychology practice; Burton et al., 2012) but not high-school football athletes undergoing concussion baseline assessments (Hunt et al., 2007). In addition, the FIT+ and the DCT are equivocal in identifying invalid performance in those with FSIQ of less than 75 who are not seeking compensation or in litigation (Marshall et al., 2007).

RELATIONSHIPS WITH SVTS

There appears to be little relationship between various MMPI-2 validity scales (e.g., F, F-K) and scores on the FIT (Greiffenstein et al., 1995; McCaffrey et al., 2003) or PAI validity indices (i.e., NIM, MAL, RDF; $r < .30$; Sumanti et al., 2006). The implication is that the FIT is measuring a different construct than the MMPI-2/PAI symptom validity scales.

RELATIONSHIPS WITH OTHER NEUROPSYCHOLOGICAL TESTS

As already noted, the test is also moderately to highly related to IQ (see "Demographic Effects"). A high correlation between MMSE and the FIT ($r = .74$) has been reported in pretrial homicide defendants (Myers et al., 2013). However, Myers et al. (2012) reported that the MMSE may be more useful than the FIT in identifying noncredible performance in these patients. Based on independent information, they found a 17% prevalence rate of noncredible performance in their sample. Using an MMSE cutoff of less than 24, 67% of noncredible responders were identified, with a false-positive rate of 7%, a PPV of 67%, and an NPV of 93%. By contrast, the FIT only identified 50% of noncredible responders and showed a false-positive rate of 14%, with a PPV of 43% and an NPV of 89%.

CLINICAL STUDIES

To our knowledge, no studies have been conducted to validate the FIT based on multidimensional malingering criteria such as the Slick et al. (1999) criteria for malingered neurocognitive dysfunction. Although not a study on classification accuracy, Cottingham et al. (2014) found that the reason for seeking evaluation may impact performance on the FIT+ even if the examinees met the criteria for Slick-defined malingering. They divided outpatients in university neuropsychology clinics and private practice settings who met Slick et al. (1999) criteria into groups based on litigation or disability-seeking status. Individuals seeking disability performed worse than those in litigation on the FIT+, with a sensitivity to malingering much higher (60%) than in those in litigation (36%). No differences in sensitivity rates among individuals seeking disability for mild or moderate-severe TBI were found; however, sensitivity rates were higher in individuals seeking disability for psychiatric reasons on the FIT+ than in those seeking disability for TBI. The authors surmised that the reason for seeking disability plays a role in the type of symptoms an individual may choose to feign.

While not strictly using Slick et al. (1999) defined malingering, Greiffenstein et al. (1994) tested a sample of 106 postconcussion patients with and without overt signs of invalid performance such as improbable poor performance on two or more neuropsychological measures and contradiction between collateral sources and symptom history on a battery of neuropsychological tests (e.g., RAVLT, WMS, WMS-R) and a number of PVTs, including the FIT. Probable malingering could not be differentiated from seriously brain-injured patients on free-recall measures from the Wechsler scales and the RAVLT. In contrast, probable malingers performed poorly on the performance validity measures, including the FIT, although the Portland Digit Recognition Test achieved a better hit rate.

In a study that used failures on two PVTs as the criterion for malingering in veterans undergoing neuropsychological evaluation for mild TBI ($N = 257$), the FIT yielded lower rates of failure relative to the TOMM (Trial 1 <41) and Digit Span (age-corrected scaled score <7) when the latter two measures were used as the criterion (Flaherty et al., 2015). About 77% obtained perfect scores on the FIT. Less than 2% failed based on a standard cutoff of less than 9. By contrast, about 16% failed Digit Span and 27% failed the TOMM. Among those who failed both PVTs, only two of the 13 failed the FIT. As such, the authors concluded that the FIT may not be useful as a PVT in this population.

Disability Claimants and Litigants. The FIT and DCT were minimally correlated to PAI validity indices in a sample of "stress claim" workers' compensation examinees ($N = 233$), suggesting that these tests assess different aspects of noncredible presentation (Sumanti et al., 2006). In this sample, the DCT E-score was failed by 15% and the FIT was failed by 8%, while 5% failed both, and between 9% and 29% failed the PAI validity scales. In sum, noncredible performance was not uncommon in this population of claimants, but the FIT demonstrated the lowest sensitivity of all these measures.

Criminal Defendants. Findings on the use of FIT in criminal forensic cases are inconsistent. In one study, the FIT identified 50% of pretrial homicide defendants who were noncredible responders and yielded a false-positive rate of 14% (Myers et al., 2013). Among pre-trial psychiatric patients hospitalized to restore their competency to stand trial, use of the FIT+ instead of the FIT improved the sensitivity to 64% in a noncredible group but decreased specificity to 75% in a genuine responder group (Stimmel et al., 2012). Paradis et al. (2013) reported that in defendants undergoing evaluation about their competency to stand trial, a higher number of those who failed the FIT had psychotic disorders than those who passed. Other psychiatric diagnoses such as affective disorders did not affect whether the individuals passed or failed the FIT.

Dementia. Patients with focal memory disturbance, as well as those with more extensive cognitive impairment, may perform poorly on the task. For example, Morgan (1991) examined 60 nonlitigating participants with mild to severe memory impairment and found that 12 of them failed the FIT when a criterion of three rows or nine items was used. Philpott and Boone (1994) gave the FIT to patients with Alzheimer's disease (AD) who varied with respect to level of cognitive impairment from mild to severe according to scores on the MMSE and to healthy adults, aged 46 to 80 years. They found that performance on the FIT varied with severity of dementia. Only two of the 49 patients with AD obtained a FIT score greater than 9. Even patients with mild cognitive decline exhibited a high rate of failure on this test. Dean et al. (2009) tested the utility of various performance validity indicators, including the FIT, in a sample of nonlitigating patients with dementia of mixed etiologies. Poor specificity was observed for FIT+ (i.e., 26% for recall cutoff of <9; 56% for FIT+ cutoff of <20). Specificity decreased from 33% to 0% as the MMSE score approached less than 15. Regardless of dementia etiology, specificity remained low (AD = 6%, vascular dementia = 27%, frontotemporal dementia = 25% for FIT; AD = 20%, vascular dementia = 7%, frontotemporal dementia = 33% for FIT+).

Low IQ. Marshall et al. (2007) reported that in their sample of individuals with FSIQ of less than 75 (mean = 63, range = 51–74) who were not seeking compensation or in litigation, only 17% passed the FIT+. By contrast, more than 90% passed the CVLT-II Forced Choice Recognition, Logical Memory Rarely Missed Index, and Vocabulary-Digit Span Difference Score. In forensic inpatients with mild intellectual disability without potential motivation to feign symptoms (average FSIQ = 60.89, *SD* = 6.8, range = 45–73), the FIT cutoff score must be decreased to less than 6 to maintain a specificity of at least 90% (Love et al., 2014). As such, the FIT should not be used in this population.

Psychiatric Conditions. Depression appears to have relatively little impact on test scores, at least when outpatients are evaluated. Lee et al. (2000) assessed a sample of older adult outpatients with major depression and found that about 5% failed the FIT using the cutoffs of less than 9 total items and less than 9 spatial score (number of items accurately placed within a row). By contrast, Guilmette et al. (1994) used a cutoff score of 7 items and found that 20% of depressed psychiatric inpatients would have been classified as possible invalid responders. Finally, Back et al. (1996) reported that in a sample of 30 patients with schizophrenia, 13% obtained a score of less than 9.

Learning Disability. Performance on the FIT (recall/recognition) does not appear to be contaminated by mild learning disorders. Boone et al. (2002) found that learning-disabled college students performed well on the tasks. However, it remains to be determined whether performance is contaminated by more severe learning disorders or in non-university students.

NEUROANATOMICAL CORRELATES AND IMAGING STUDIES

No imaging studies have been completed to our knowledge.

COMMENT

The FIT has fallen in popularity as a PVT among neuropsychologists in recent years even though it remains one of the top five stand-alone PVTs used by neuropsychologists (Dandachi-Fitzgerald et al., 2013; Martin et al., 2015; Sharland & Gfeller, 2007; Young et al., 2016). Low cost, ready availability, and ease of administration probably account for its popularity in the past, but its low accuracy likely contributed to its decline.

The FIT does not appear to compare well with other PVTs such as the TOMM among veterans, those with mild TBI, or those seeking compensation or in litigation. The available evidence suggests that the FIT may provide complementary information to that of other PVTs, partially because an individual may choose to feign different symptoms (e.g., memory vs. nonmemory). More importantly, it appears to be sensitive to genuine cognitive dysfunction including dementia, amnesia, and intellectual disability and is insufficiently sensitive to noncredible performance even in the absence of validation studies based on multidimensional malingering criteria (e.g., Flaherty et al., 2015; Sumanti et al., 2006; Vickery et al., 2001). One potential approach to improve sensitivity to feigning is to include the recognition trial in the administration (Boone et al., 2002). However, it should be noted that the FIT, even with the addition of the recognition trial, does not meet the Daubert standard for admissibility of scientific evidence based on its failure to achieve a criterion PPV of 80% or higher using a base rate of noncredible performance of 30% according to some authors (Vallabhajosula & van Gorp, 2001).

The FIT should not be used in isolation. If clinicians choose to use the FIT in combination with other measures, its greatest utility may be in detecting blatant strategies to feign cognitive dysfunction (Millis & Kler, 1995; Palmer et al., 1995). In such cases, the test should be given at the very beginning of the evaluation, before the patient is exposed to more difficult tests and subsequently understands the simplicity of the procedure (Iverson & Franzen, 1996). The use of the test in patients with severe brain dysfunction is not recommended. In fact, if poor scores occur on the FIT, clinicians should first consider the possibility of low IQ and/or severe neurological disturbance before drawing conclusions about the validity of scores (e.g., Dean et al., 2009; Love et al., 2014; Marshall et al., 2007). We recommend the use of other well-established standalone PVTs such as the TOMM, WMT, or MSVT in addition to or in place of the FIT.

REFERENCES

Arnett, P. A., Hemmeke, T. A., & Schwartz, L. (1995). Quantitative and qualitative performance on Rey's 15-Item Test in neurological patients and dissimulators. *The Clinical Neuropsychologist, 9,* 17–26.

Back, C., Boone, K. B., Parks, C., Burgoyne, K., & Silver, B. (1996). The performance of schizophrenics on three cognitive tests of malingering, Rey 15-Item Memory Test, Rey Dot Counting, and Hiscock forced-choice method. *Assessment, 3,* 449–457.

Bernard, L. C., & Fowler, W. (1990). Assessing the validity of memory complaints: Performance of brain-damaged and normal individuals on Rey's task to detect malingering. *Journal of Clinical Psychology, 46,* 432–436.

Boone, K. B., Salazar, X., Lu, P., Warner-Chacon, K., & Razani, J. (2002). The Rey 15-Item Recognition Trial: A technique to enhance sensitivity of the Rey 15-Item Memorization Test. *Journal of Clinical and Experimental Neuropsychology, 24,* 561–573.

Burton, V., Vilar-López, R., & Puente, A. E. (2012). Measuring effort in neuropsychological evaluations of forensic cases of Spanish speakers. *Archives of Clinical Neuropsychology, 27*(3), 262–267.

Constantinou, M., & McCaffrey, R. J. (2003). Using the TOMM for evaluating children's effort to perform optimally on neuropsychological measures. *Child Neuropsychology, 9,* 81–90.

Cottingham, M. E., Victor, T. L., Boone, K. B., Ziegler, E. A., & Zeller, M. (2014). Apparent effect of type of compensation seeking (disability versus litigation) on performance validity test scores may be due to other factors. *The Clinical Neuropsychologist, 28*(6), 1030–1047.

Dandachi-FitzGerald, B., Ponds, R. W. H. M., & Merten, T. (2013). Symptom validity and neuropsychological assessment: A survey of practices and beliefs of neuropsychologists in six European countries. *Archives of Clinical Neuropsychology, 28*(8), 771–783. https://doi.org/10.1093/arclin/act073

Dean, A. C., Victor, T. L., Boone, K. B., Philpott, L. M., & Hess, R. A. (2009). Dementia and effort test performance. *The Clinical Neuropsychologist, 23*(1), 133–152.

Erdal, K. (2004). The effects of motivation, coaching, and knowledge of neuropsychology on the simulated malingering of head injury. *Archives of Clinical Neuropsychology, 19,* 73–88.

Flaherty, J. M., Spencer, R. J., Drag, L. L., Pangilinan, P. H., & Bieliauskas, L. A. (2015). Limited usefulness of the Rey Fifteen-Item Test in detection of invalid performance in veterans suspected of mild traumatic brain injury. *Brain Injury, 29*(13-14), 1630–1634.

Frederick, R. I. (2002). A review of Rey's strategies for detecting malingered neuropsychological impairment. *Journal of Forensic Neuropsychology, 2,* 1–25.

Goldberg, J. O., & Miller, H. R. (1986). Performance of psychiatric inpatients and intellectually deficient individuals on a task that assesses the validity of memory complaints. *Journal of Clinical Psychology, 42,* 792–795.

Greiffenstein, M., Baker, W. J., & Gola, T. (1994). Validation of malingered amnesia measures with a large clinical sample. *Psychological Assessment, 6,* 218–224.

Greiffenstein, M. F., Baker, W. J., & Gola, T. (1996). Comparison of multiple scoring methods for Rey's malingered amnesia measures. *Archives of Clinical Neuropsychology, 11,* 283–293.

Greiffenstein, M. F., Gola, T., & Baker, W. J. (1995). MMPI-2 validity scales versus domain specific measures in detection of factitious traumatic brain injury. *The Clinical Neuropsychologist, 9,* 230–240.

Griffin, G. A., Glassmire, D. M., Henderson, E. A., & McCann, C. (1997). Rey II: Redesigning the Rey Screening Test of malingering. *Journal of Clinical Psychology, 53,* 757–766.

Griffin, G. A. E., Normington, J., & Glassmire, D. (1996). Qualitative dimensions in scoring the Rey Visual Memory Test of malingering. *Psychological Assessment, 8,* 383–387.

Guilmette, T. J., Hart, K. J., Giuliano, A. J., & Leininger, B. E. (1994). Detecting simulated memory impairment: Comparison of the Rey Fifteen-Item Test and the Hiscock Forced-Choice Procedure. *The Clinical Neuropsychologist, 8,* 283–294.

Hays, J. R., Emmons, J., & Stallings, G. (2000). Dementia and mental retardation on the Rey 15-Item Visual Memory Test. *Psychological Reports, 86,* 179–182.

Hiscock, C., Branham, J., & Hiscock, M. (1994). Detection of feigned cognitive impairment: The two-alternative forced-choice method compared with selected conventional tests. *Journal of Psychopathology and Behavioral Assessment, 16,* 95–109.

Hunt, T. N., Ferrara, M. S., Miller, L. S., & Macciocchi, S. (2007). The effect of effort on baseline neuropsychological test scores in high school football athletes. *Archives of Clinical Neuropsychology, 22*(5), 615–621.

Iverson, G. L., & Franzen, M. D. (1996). Using multiple object memory procedures to detect simulated malingering. *Journal of Clinical and Experimental Neuropsychology, 8,* 1–14.

Lee, A., Boone, K. B., Lesser, I., Wohl, M., Wilkins, S., & Parks, C. (2000). Performance of older depressed patients on two cognitive malingering tests: False positive rates for the Rey 15-Item Memorization and Dot Counting tests. *The Clinical Neuropsychologist, 14,* 303–308.

Lee, G. P., Loring, D. W., & Martin, R. C. (1992). Rey's 15-Item Visual Memory Test for the detection of malingering: Normative observations on patients with neurological disorders. *Psychological Assessment, 4,* 43–46.

Lezak, M. D. (1983). *Neuropsychological Assessment* (2nd ed.). New York: Oxford University Press.

Lezak, M. D., Howieson, D. B., Bigler, E. D., & Tranel, D. (2012). *Neuropsychological assessment* (5th ed.). New York: Oxford University Press.

Lezak, M. D., Howieson, D. B., & Loring, D. W. (2004). *Neuropsychological assessment* (4th ed.). New York: Oxford University Press.

Love, C. M., Glassmire, D. M., Zanolini, S. J., & Wolf, A. (2014). Specificity and false positive rates of the Test of Memory Malingering, Rey 15-Item Test, and Rey Word Recognition Test among forensic inpatients with intellectual disabilities. *Assessment, 21*(5), 618–627.

Marshall, P., & Happe, M. (2007). The performance of individuals with mental retardation on cognitive tests assessing effort and motivation. *The Clinical Neuropsychologist, 21*(5), 826–840.

Martin, P. K., Schroeder, R. W., & Odland, A. P. (2015). Neuropsychologists' validity testing beliefs and practices: A survey of North American professionals. *The Clinical Neuropsychologist, 29*(6), 741–776. https://doi.org/10.1080/13854046.2015.1087597

McCaffrey, R. J., O'Bryant, S. E., Ashendorf, L., & Fisher, J. M. (2003). Correlations among the TOMM, Rey-15, and MMPI-2 validity scales in a sample of TBI litigants. *Journal of Forensic Neuropsychology, 3,* 45–53.

McGuire, B. E. (2006). Response mode and performance on the Rey 15-Item test: A preliminary study. *Brain Injury, 20*(6), 647–651.

Millis, S. R., & Kler, S. (1995). Limitations of the Rey Fifteen-Item test in the detection of malingering. *The Clinical Neuropsychologist, 9,* 241–244.

Morgan, S. F. (1991). Effect of true memory impairment on a test of memory complaint validity. *Archives of Clinical Neuropsychology, 6,* 327–334.

Morse, C. L., Douglas-Newman, K., Mandel, S., & Swirsky-Sacchetti, T. (2013). Utility of the Rey-15 recognition trial to detect invalid performance in a forensic neuropsychological sample. *The Clinical Neuropsychologist, 27*(8), 1395–1407.

Myers, W. C., Hall, R. C. W., & Tolou-Shams, M. (2013). Prevalence and assessment of malingering in homicide defendants using the mini-mental state examination and the Rey 15-Item Memory Test. *Homicide Studies: An Interdisciplinary & International Journal, 17*(3), 314–328.

Nelson, N. W., Boone, K., Dueck, A., Wagener, L., Lu, P., & Grills, C. (2003). Relationships between eight measures of suspect effort. *The Clinical Neuropsychologist, 17,* 263–272.

Palmer, B. W., Boone, K. B., Allman, L., & Castro, D. B. (1995). Co-occurrence of brain lesions and cognitive deficit exaggeration. *The Clinical Neuropsychologist, 9,* 68–73.

Paradis, C. M., Solomon, L. Z., Owen, E., & Brooker, M. (2013). Detection of cognitive malingering or suboptimal effort in defendants undergoing competency to stand trial evaluations. *Journal of Forensic Psychology Practice, 13*(3), 245–265.

Paul, D. S., Franzen, M. D., Cohen, S. H., & Fremouw, W. (1992). An investigation into the reliability and validity of two tests used in the detection of dissimulation. *International Journal of Clinical Neuropsychology, 14,* 1–9.

Philpott, L. M., & Boone, K. B. (1994). *The effects of cognitive impairment and age on two malingering tests: An investigation of the Rey Memory Test and Rey Dot Counting Test in Alzheimer's patients and normal middle aged/older adults.* Paper presented to the International Neuropsychological Society, Cincinnati, Ohio.

Rey, A. (1964). *L'examen clinique en psychologie.* Paris: Presses Universitaires de France.

Robles, L., López, E., Salazar, X., Boone, K. B., & Glaser, D. F. (2015). Specificity data for the b Test, Dot Counting Test, Rey-15 Item plus recognition, and Rey Word Recognition Test in monolingual Spanish-speakers. *Journal of Clinical and Experimental Neuropsychology, 37*(6), 614–621.

Schretlen, D., Brandt, J., Krafft, L., & Van Gorp, W. (1991). Some caveats using the Rey 15-Item Memory Test to detect malingered amnesia. *Psychological Assessment, 3,* 667–672.

Sharland, M. J., & Gfeller, J. D. (2007). A survey of neuropsychologists' beliefs and practices with respect to the assessment of effort. *Archives of Clinical Neuropsychology, 22*(2), 213–223.

Shum, D. H. K., O'Gorman, J. G. O., & Alpar, A. (2004). Effects of incentive and preparation time on performance and classification accuracy on standard and memory-specific memory tests. *Archives of Clinical Neuropsychology, 19,* 817–823.

Slick, D. J., Sherman, E. M., & Iverson, G. L. (1999). Diagnostic criteria for malingered neurocognitive dysfunction: Proposed standards for clinical practice and research. *The Clinical Neuropsychologist, 13*(4), 545–561.

Slick, D. J., Tan, J. E., Strauss, E. H., & Hultsch, D. F. (2004). Detecting malingering: A survey of experts' practices. *Archives of Clinical Neuropsychology, 19,* 465–473.

Stimmel, M., Green, D., Belfi, B., & Klaver, J. (2012). Exploring the accuracy and utility of the Rey Fifteen-Item Test (RMT) with recognition trial in a forensic psychiatric population. *The International Journal of Forensic Mental Health, 11*(1), 51–58.

Sumanti, M., Boone, K. B., Savodnik, I., & Gorsuch, R. (2006). Noncredible psychiatric and cognitive symptoms in a workers' compensation 'stress' claim sample. *The Clinical Neuropsychologist, 20*(4), 754–765.

Taylor, L. A., Kreutzer, J. S., & West, D. D. (2003). Evaluation of malingering cut-off scores for the Rey 15-Item Test: A brain injury case study series. *Brain Injury, 17,* 295–308.

Vallabhajosula, B., & van Gorp, W. G. (2001). Post-Daubert admissibility of scientific evidence on malingering of cognitive deficits. *Journal of the American Academy of Psychiatry and the Law, 29,* 207–215.

Vickery, C. D., Berry, D. T. R., Inman, T. H., Harris, M. J., & Orey, S. A. (2001). Detection of inadequate effort on neuropsychological testing: A meta-analytic review of selected procedures. *Archives of Clinical Neuropsychology, 16,* 45–73.

Vilar-López, R., Gómez-Río, M., Caracuel-Romero, A., Llamas-Elvira, J., & Pérez-García, M. (2008). Use of specific malingering measures in a Spanish sample. *Journal of Clinical and Experimental Neuropsychology, 30*(6), 710–722.

Whitney, K. A., Hook, J. N., Steiner, A. R., Shepard, P. H., & Callaway, S. (2008). Is the Rey 15-item Memory Test II (Rey II) a valid symptoms validity test? Comparison with the TOMM. *Applied Neuropsychology, 15*(4), 287–292.

Young, J. C., Roper, B. L., & Arentsen, T. J. (2016). Validity testing and neuropsychology practice in the VA healthcare system: Results from recent practitioner survey. *The Clinical Neuropsychologist, 30*(4), 497–514. https://doi.org/10.1080/13854046.2016.1159730

TEST OF MEMORY MALINGERING (TOMM)

TEST NAME	**Test of Memory Malingering (TOMM)**
DOMAIN	Performance validity
AGE RANGE	In adults, to 90 years
ADMINISTRATION TIME	15 minutes, not including 15-minute delay interval
SCORING FORMAT	Hand scored
REFERENCE	Tombaugh, T. N. (1996). *Test of Memory Malingering (TOMM).* North Tonawanda, NY: Multi-Health Systems. www.mhs.com

DESCRIPTION

The Test of Memory Malingering (TOMM; Tombaugh, 1996) is a very popular test used to assess exaggeration and feigning of memory impairment. It is the PVT most commonly used by neuropsychologists in North America and Europe (Dandachi-FitzGerald et al., 2013; Martin et al., 2015; Sharland & Gfeller, 2007; Young et al., 2016). It involves recognition of pictorial stimuli, which were chosen because the literature suggests that recognition memory for pictures is remarkably robust in older adults and in various neurologically impaired populations.

The test involves two learning trials and a retention trial (i.e., Trial 1, Trial 2, and Retention). Further details on administration, items, and format are not provided to preserve test security. Please see original source for details.

ADMINISTRATION

See manual. Tombaugh (1996) suggested that the two learning trials are usually sufficient to assess invalid performance. However, use of the retention trial helps corroborate results (see "Within-Test Relationships" for further discussion of this issue).

Most clinicians use the original version, which involves direct administration by an examiner. However, there exists a computerized version that appears to give equivalent results to the standard booklet version, at least in undergraduate volunteers and a simulation paradigm (Rees et al., 1998; Vanderslice-Barr et al., 2011). However, differences may arise in the context of clinical evaluations, with the computerized version yielding a higher sensitivity to noncredible performance. The computerized version may also be preferred in order to avoid imprecise administration procedures (Tombaugh, 2002).

The BNT has similar test presentation format as the TOMM and is thought to influence TOMM performance if given before the TOMM. Ryan et al. (2010) disputed this concern by testing the performance of undergraduate volunteers on the TOMM and BNT. They found lower TOMM Trial 1 scores when the BNT was given first, but only one of 36 individuals scored less than 45 on TOMM Trial 1, and no one scored below this standard cutoff on Trial 2 or Retention. Administration of Wechsler Picture Completion before the TOMM also did not affect TOMM performance. These results suggest that test administration order has minimal effect TOMM performance.

SCORING

One point is given for each correct answer provided on the recognition and retention trials. Therefore, the maximum score on each trial is 50. The standard scoring procedures are by far the most commonly used for cutoffs in the literature. Recommended cutoffs across studies are shown in Table 15–23a and 15–23b.

In addition to the standard scoring, alternate indices have also been developed based on learning theories and consistency of responding. Davis and colleagues (2012) developed three Response Consistency indices (CNS) by comparing the consistency of responding on pairs of trials: TOMM-C1 = Trials 1 and 2; TOMM-C2 = Trial 1 and Retention; TOMM-C3 = Trial 2 and Retention. Pairs of responses are scored as consistent or inconsistent, and the inconsistent responses are summed and subtracted from 50 to yield a total CNS score. A score of 50 would reflect all items correct or all items wrong. Based on a study using undergraduate volunteer simulators, cutoff scores were TOMM-C1 less than 45, TOMM-C2 less than 45, and TOMM-C3 less than 48 to maintain the specificity higher than 90%. The sensitivity of the CNS indices was 38% to 42% for coached simulators and 47% to 51% for naïve simulators. Relative to the original CNS cutoff scores, the cut scores may be adjusted to TOMM-C1 less than 37, TOMM-C2 less than 37, and TOMM-C3 less than 46 to

TABLE 15–23A Test of Memory Malingering (TOMM) Cutoff Scores, Sensitivity, Specificity, PPV, and NPV Data for Various Populations for the Detection of Malingered Neurocognitive Dysfunction and Malingered Pain-Related Disability

						BASE RATE 20%		BASE RATE 30%		BASE RATE 40 TO 50%	
REFERENCE	POPULATION	CRITERION	CUTOFF	SENSITIVITY (%)	SPECIFICITY (%)	PPV (%)	NPV (%)	PPV (%)	NPV (%)	PPV (%)	NPV (%)
Buddin et al. (2014)	Forensic outpatients	Slick et al. (1999) criteria	Trial 2 < 45	44	97	–	–	–	–	–	–
			Retention < 45	48	97	–	–	–	–	–	–
			ACI ≥ 10	76	85	–	–	–	–	–	–
			IFFI ≥ 3	76	94	–	–	–	–	–	–
Green et al. (2012)	Forensic psychiatry inpatients charged with felony offences and deemed incompetent to stand trial	Slick et al. (1999) criteria	Trial 2 < 45	41	88	45	86	45	86	–	–
Greve et al. (2008)	TBI patients	Slick et al. (1999) criteria using psychometric indicators from the WAIS and MMPI	Trial 2 < 45	48	98	–	–	93	–	–	–
			Retention < 45	56	95	–	–	93	–	–	–
Greve et al. (2008)	Chronic pain patients	Slick et al. (1999) criteria using psychometric indicators from the WAIS and MMPI	Trial 2 < 45	40	98	–	–	92	–	–	–
			Retention < 45	35	98	–	–	90	–	–	–
Greve et al. (2009b)	Pain–related disability compared to TBI and dementia	Malingered pain–related disability	Trial 1 < 42	53	95	–	–	–	–	–	–
			Trial 2 and/or Retention < 45	38	100	–	–	–	–	–	–
Jones (2013)[a]	Active–duty military members assessed for mild head injuries, majority with incentive to feign	Larrabee et al. (2007) refinement of Slick et al. (1999) criteria	Trial 1 ≤ 44	91	93	76	98	85	96	90	94
			Trial 2 ≤ 48	95	100	10	99	100	98	10	97
			Retention ≤ 48	100	100	100	100	100	100	100	100
O'Bryant et al. (2007a)	Forensic referrals to a medical center outpatient neuropsychology clinic for mixed clinical conditions	Slick et al. (1999) criteria	Trial 1 ≤ 41	79	90	67	95	78	91	84	87
Smith et al. (2014)	Low-IQ patients	Slick et al. (1999) criteria	Trial 1 ≤ 38	58	91	–	–	–	–	–	–
			Trial 2 ≤ 48	73	100	–	–	–	–	–	–

NOTE: TBI, traumatic brain injury; ACI, Albany Consistency Index (Gunner et al., 2012); IFFI, Invalid Forgetting Frequency Index (Buddin et al., 2014); MMPI, Minnesota Multiphasic Personality Inventory; WAIS, Wechsler Adult Intelligence Scale; PPV, Positive Predictive Value; NPV, Negative Predictive Value.

[a] Users may refer to the article for additional data on cutoffs and positive and negative predictive values.

increase sensitivity up to 72% while maintaining specificity higher than 90% in a clinical sample of veterans.

The Albany Consistency Index (ACI; Gunner et al., 2012) is calculated by quantifying the consistency of responses across all TOMM trials (consistently incorrect, inconsistent, or consistently correct). Each item is coded 1 for correct or 0 for incorrect and then compared across all three trials to code for consistency of responses (Table 15–24). A cutoff of 10 or more inconsistent responses is indicative of noncredible performance.

TABLE 15-23B Test of Memory Malingering (TOMM) Cutoff Scores, Sensitivity, Specificity, PPV, and NPV for Various Populations Using Other Criteria Indicative of Malingering

						BASE RATE 20%		BASE RATE 30%		BASE RATE 40–50%	
REFERENCE	POPULATION	CRITERION	CUTOFF	SENSITIVITY (%)	SPECIFICITY (%)	PPV (%)	NPV (%)	PPV (%)	NPV (%)	PPV (%)	NPV (%)
Armistead & Gervais (2011)	Non–head–injury disability claimants	WMT	Trial 2 < 45	21	99	–	–	92	72	–	–
Bauer et al. (2007)	Mild head injury litigants	TOMM Trial 2 and/ or Retention < 45	Trial 1 < 39	90	>90	74	97	–	–	88	93
Fazio et al. (2015)	Criminal forensic setting	Failure on at least two other standalone PVTs (i.e., CARB, VIP, Rey FIT, VSVT, MSVT)	Trial 2 or Retention < 45	68	87	57	92	–	–	78	80
Fazio et al. (2015)	Criminal forensic setting	Failure on at least two other standalone PVTs (i.e., CARB, VIP, Rey FIT, VSVT, MSVT)	Trial 1 ≤ 39	68	89	61	92	73	87	–	–
Greve et al. (2009b)	Pain-related disability compared to TBI and dementia	PDRT, WMT, RDS, Digit Span, PSI, WMI, and CVLT Recognition hits	Trial 1 < 42	53	95	–	–	–	–	–	–
			Trial 2 and/or Retention < 45	38	100	–	–	–	–	–	–
Haber & Fichtenberg (2006)	Moderate–to–severe TBI patients and compensation–seeking mild TBI patients	RDS	Trial 2 < 45	76	100	–	–	–	–	–	–
Hilsabeck et al. (2011)	Mixed clinical sample of veterans without incentives	Trial 2 and/or Retention	Trial 1 < 39	87	96	–	–	–	–	–	–
Horner et al. (2006)	Mixed clinical sample of veterans	Trial 2	Trial 1 ≤ 35	96	92	–	–	–	–	–	–
			Trial 1 ≤ 27	48	100	–	–	–	–	–	–
		Retention	Trial 1 ≤ 35	100	87	–	–	–	–	–	–
			Trial 1 ≤ 27	67	100	–	–	–	–	–	–
Wisdom et al. (2012)	Patients with epilepsy on an epilepsy monitoring unit	Trial 2 and/or Retention	Trial 1 ≤ 39	77	93	73	94	–	–	88	86

NOTE: TBI, traumatic brain injury; CARB, Computerized Assessment of Response Bias; CVLT Recognition hits, California Verbal Learning Test Recognition Hits; MSVT, Medical Symptom Validity Test; PDRT, Portland Digit Recognition Test; PSI, Processing Speed Index; RDS, Reliable Digit Span; Rey FIT, Rey Fifteen-Item Test; WMI, Working Memory Index; WMT, Word Memory Test; VIP, Validity Indicator Profile; VSVT, Victoria Symptom Validity Test; PPV, Positive Predictive Value; NPV, Negative Predictive Value.

[a] Users may refer to the article for additional data on cutoffs and positive and negative predictive values.

The ACI has been found to be more sensitive than traditional TOMM cutoffs for identifying invalid performance defined as WMT failure. In a sample of medico-legal cases with mixed neurological conditions, the ACI yielded a sensitivity of 71%, a specificity of 100%, and a classification accuracy of 79%. Standard TOMM scoring yielded much lower rates, at 33% sensitivity, 96% specificity, and 65% classification accuracy.

TABLE 15-24 Consistency Coding for the Test of Memory Malingering (TOMM) Albany Consistency Index (ACI)

Consistently Incorrect	Incorrect on all three trials
Inconsistent	Incorrect on one trial OR two trials
Consistently Correct	Correct on all three trials

SOURCE: Adapted from Gunner et al. (2012).

As the ACI may falsely identify a pattern of consistent and valid learning across trials as invalid performance, Buddin et al. (2014) developed the Invalid Forgetting Frequency Index (IFFI) to identify patterns of "invalid forgetting" across trials while taking into account consistent, valid learning. IFFI is scored by coding every item as 0 (for incorrect response) or 1 (for correct response). Responses that are consistently correct or consistently incorrect across all three TOMM trials (labeled as Consistency pattern) are considered Valid Responding, as are the patterns showing Learning across trials (i.e., 001 or 011). The other patterns of responding are considered Invalid Responding. The sum of the valid response patterns is then subtracted from the ACI to form the IFFI. The cutoff for IFFI is 3 or more Inconsistent Response Patterns in order to achieve a specificity over 90% (Table 15–23a).

In addition to correct responses, the computerized version also allows examination of response latencies. Rees et al. (1998) found that response latencies are longer (on average by about 1–2 seconds) for simulators.

DEMOGRAPHIC EFFECTS

AGE

Some have reported that age has little impact on test scores (Tombaugh, 1996, 1997). Others have noted that TOMM performance decreases in a linear fashion with increasing age, accounting for up to 33% of variance (Rivera et al., 2015). Moderately strong relationships between age and Trial 2, and age and the Retention trial in older adults have also been reported (r = -.40 and -.50, respectively; Teicher & Wagner, 2004).

GENDER

Gender has no impact on test scores (Constantinou & McCaffrey, 2003; Donders, 2005; Paradis et al., 2013; Rivera et al., 2015).

EDUCATION AND IQ

Education has little relation to performance in adults with at least six years of education (Gervais et al., 2004; Green et al., 2012; Teichner & Wagner, 2004; Tombaugh, 1996). There are some suggestions that those with less than six years of education may perform worse on the TOMM than those with more education (Rivera et al., 2015; Strutt et al., 2012). Those diagnosed with mild intellectual disability or low IQ are able to pass the TOMM (Love et al., 2014; Simon, 2007; Smith et al., 2014), although moderate to severe cognitive deficit appears to have an impact (see "Evidence for Validity").

ETHNICITY, NATIONALITY, AND LINGUISTIC EFFECTS

No differences in TOMM performance between a Spanish sample and the original North-American sample were found by Vilar-Lopez et al. (2008). Spanish-speaking patients with TBI residing in the United States who were classified as valid performers according to Slick et al. (1999) malingering criteria also obtained scores well above standard cutoffs, suggesting that TOMM performance may not be impacted by language (Strutt et al., 2012).

NORMATIVE DATA

The test was developed on samples of community-dwelling individuals, ranging in age from 16 to 84 years, and on a sample of patients referred for neuropsychological evaluation (see Table 15–25). Tombaugh (1996, 1997) reported that performance on Trial 2 was very high for honest responders regardless of neurological dysfunction (except in the case of dementia). More than 95% of adults living in the community obtained a score of 49 or 50 on the second trial. Moreover, scores for different clinical samples showed that most nondemented individuals obtained a perfect score on Trial 2. In contrast, simulators tended to score below 45 on Trial 2 or on the Retention trial. Accordingly, Tombaugh (see Source) recommends that any score lower than 45 on Trial 2 or on Retention should raise concern about invalid performance. Others (Powell et al., 2004; Teichner & Wagner, 2004) have also reported that nondemented adults obtain high scores on the TOMM, with a cutoff point of 5 or more errors on Trial 2 or on the Retention trial both yielding a high rate of correct classification.

Tombaugh (see Source) recommends that, rather than using the score of 45 as a rigid cutoff, it should be viewed as a guideline, with the likelihood of invalid performance increasing as the score deviates further from the performance of specific clinical samples (see tables 3–5 and 3–7 in the Source as well as Table 15–23a and 15–23b in this chapter).

Clinicians may use published sensitivity and specificity data found in Table 15–23a and 15–23b to calculate the PPV and NPV corresponding to their clinical practice and base rate of feigning to assess the probability of false positives or false negatives associated with a given diagnostic decision using the following formulas as outlined by O'Bryant and Lucas (2006):

$$\text{PPV} = \frac{(\text{SN} \times \text{BR})}{(\text{SN} \times \text{BR}) + [(1 - \text{SP}) \times \text{RC}]}$$

$$\text{NPN} = \frac{(\text{SP} \times \text{RC})}{(\text{SP} \times \text{RC}) + [(1 - \text{SN}) \times \text{BR}]}$$

Where PPV is the positive predictive value, NPV is the negative predictive value, SN is sensitivity, SP is specificity, BR is base rate, and RC is remaining cases (or 1 BR).

TABLE 15–25 Characteristics of the Test of Memory Malingering (TOMM) Standardization Sample

CHARACTERISTIC	STANDARDIZATION SAMPLE	CLINICAL SAMPLE
Sample size	70 community-dwelling adults	135 inpatients and outpatients at the Boston VA diagnosed with a variety of disorders including amnesia, multiple sclerosis, Parkinson's disease, aphasia, dementia, head injury; 23 head-injured individuals involved in a study in Ottawa, Canada, were also included
Sample type	Community-dwelling individuals participating in studies of aging on memory; recruited at shopping centers, social organizations, work, psychology classes, word of mouth	138 consecutive patients referred for neuropsychological examination at the Boston VA (3 excluded because of severe dementia); 23 head-injured participants in a study for a PhD thesis
Age	17–73 years (*M* = 37.8, *SD* = 14.2)	19 –90 years (*M* = 56.2, *SD* = 18.8)
Geographical location	Ottawa, Canada	Boston, USA, and Ottawa, Canada
Education	7–20 years (*M* = 12.7, *SD* = 1.9)	4–21 years (*M* = 12.7, *SD* = 2.8)
Gender (Male/Female)	44 Men 26 Women	Not reported
Ethnicity	Not reported	Not reported
Screening	Any person with a self-reported history of neurological disease, psychiatric illness, head injury, or stroke was excluded	Not involved in litigation or compensation seeking

SOURCE: Adapted from Tombaugh (1996).

EVIDENCE FOR RELIABILITY

EVIDENCE FOR INTERNAL RELIABILITY

According to Tombaugh (personal communication, November, 1996), coefficient alphas (*n* = 40) were very high for each trial (Trial 1 = .94, Trial 2 = .95, Retention = .94).

EVIDENCE FOR TEST-RETEST RELIABILITY, MEASURING CHANGE, AND PRACTICE EFFECTS

No information is available.

EVIDENCE FOR VALIDITY

FACTOR-ANALYTIC STUDIES

Walters et al. (2009) examined the latent structure of the TOMM using taxometric analysis, a method to identify latent classes or single dimensions in a set of scores, to see if it measures a dimension or category of credible versus noncredible performance in a sample of compensation-seeking individuals (*N* = 527). Results suggested dimensional latent structure of feigning on the TOMM, suggesting that feigning on the TOMM falls along a continuum and the use of cutoff scores is arbitrary. As such, the context and referral question should be considered when choosing a cutoff score. Furthermore, given the dimensional nature, a dichotomous decision of valid versus invalid may not be appropriate but instead an indeterminate category should be created for marginal scores.

Supporting these findings, Mossman et al. (2018) submitted outpatient forensic cases without severe cognitive impairment such as dementia or intellectual disability to latent class modeling and based group membership (feigning vs. not feigning) on Bayesian inferences without using external criteria. They reported that about 66% had scores of greater than 45 on Trial 1, the score supportive of genuine responding based on statistical inferences, and 16% obtained scores of 42 to 45. About 8% had scores between 37 to 40, which may suggest feigning, and 11% had scores of 36 or less, which is almost certainly feigning according to their statistical inferences. On Trial 2, 6% obtained scores of 45 to 48, with scores of 47 and 48 indicative of feigning, and 10% had scores of less than 45, which is highly likely feigning. However, they found that scores of 49 and 50 on Trial 2 did not rule out feigning.

Factor analysis of the TOMM and Wechsler Adult Intelligence Scale (WAIS-R) in patients with mild TBI involved in litigation or seeking disability revealed TOMM loadings on the same factor as WAIS-R Arithmetic, Digit Span, and all Performance subtests (Digit Symbol, Picture Completion, Block Design, Picture Arrangement, and Object Assembly). Williams noted that these WAIS-R subtests are possibly most sensitive to feigning strategies, perhaps because it is easier to feign slowed responding or intentional wrong responses on these subtests than on the Verbal subtests (Williams, 2011).

When the TOMM is submitted to factor analysis along with psychiatric or cognitive test measures, the TOMM loads on a separate factor reflecting performance validity (Ruocco et al., 2008; Van Dyke et al., 2013). For example, when the TOMM was entered into a confirmatory factor analysis along with WAIS-IV FSIQ, CVLT-II, TMT-B, MSVT, WAIS-IV Reliable Digit Span, Post-traumatic Checklist-Military version (PCL-M), MMPI-2 F scale,

MMPI-2 Fake Bad Scale (FBS), MMPI-2 Response Bias Scale (RBS), and Postconcussive Symptom Questionnaire (PCSQ), a three-factor model appeared to be the strongest and most parsimonious, yielding cognitive performance, performance validity, and self-reported symptoms as separate factors. The TOMM loaded on the same factor as other performance validity indicators including the RDS and the MSVT, while the PCL-M, F scale, RBS, FBS, and PCSQ loaded on the same self-reported symptoms factor. As such, poor scores on SVTs may not necessarily be associated with poor cognitive performance, and PVTs should be examined separately from SVTs (van Dyke et al., 2013). In another study, RDS and TOMM loaded on one factor and the MCMI-III validity indices loaded on the other with different passing rates on these tests (Ruocco et al., 2008). Therefore, these studies suggest that both neuropsychological and psychiatric validity measures should be given as they measure different aspects relevant to detection of invalid results.

WITHIN-TEST RELATIONSHIPS

There is strong evidence that use of Trial 1 alone may be sufficient as a screening measure in a variety of settings as presented in Table 15–23a and 15–23b (Bauer et al., 2007; Fazio et al., 2017; Hilsabeck et al., 2011; Horner et al., 2006; O'Bryant et al., 2007a, 2008; Wisdom et al., 2012). O'Bryant et al. (2008) reported that in their sample of healthy community-dwelling older adults and mixed clinical cases, all who scored 45 or higher on Trial 1 obtained 45 or higher on Trial 2 and Retention. Using the TOMM Trial 1 also resulted in fairly similar results as the standard TOMM within a criminal forensic setting (Fazio et al., 2017). In mild head injury litigants, Trial 1 of less than 39 yielded high sensitivity and specificity (≥90%) against Trial 2 and/or Retention, and users may refer to the source article to adjust cutoff scores appropriate for their setting (Bauer et al., 2007). In a mixed clinical sample of veterans without incentives, no one obtained a Trial 1 score of 25 or lower. A Trial 1 score of 41 or greater yielded 100% specificity but a cutoff of 39 or greater improved the sensitivity to 87% while maintaining the specificity at 96% (Hilsabeck et al., 2011). Similarly, among epilepsy patients on an epilepsy monitoring unit, 99% of those who passed Trial 1 also passed Trial 2 and Retention, indicating that the likelihood of subsequent Trial 2 or Retention failure is very low (Wisdom et al., 2012). These cutoffs are suitable discontinuation scores for invalid performance, indicating that the test can be discontinued without additional administration of Trial 2 and Retention.

The manual indicates that the Retention trial is optional if the examinee passes Trial 2. However, Greve and Bianchini (2006) reported that about 3% of their 300 TBI and chronic pain patients involved in personal injury litigation or workers' compensation claims obtained less than 45 on the Retention trial despite passing Trial 2. As such, these authors recommend always administering the Retention trial because early termination may miss a minority of noncredible responders. On the other hand, Booksh et al. (2007) argued that the use of the Retention trial should remain optional because the manual also noted that 3% of cases scored below the cutoff on the Retention trial; however, these cognitively impaired patients reported in the manual were not involved in litigation. They noted that Trial 1 alone has been shown to yield acceptable PPV and NPV, and, in general, administration time affects a clinician's decision to use PVTs, and requiring the administration of Retention will not increase the frequency of PVT use. In their response, Greve and Bianchini (2007) clarified that the Retention trial should not be dropped if the TOMM is the only well-validated PVT administered.

RELATIONSHIPS WITH AND COMPARISONS TO OTHER PVTS

Tombaugh (1996, 2002) cautioned that interpretation of the TOMM involves many factors and that examinees may fail one type of PVT more than another because of the relevance of the test material to their presenting complaints.

In an early study, Tan et al (2002) used a simulation paradigm to compare the efficacy of the TOMM, the WMT, and the VSVT. Although all tasks differentiated groups, the TOMM proved least effective. Using suggested cutoffs from the test manuals, the TOMM misclassified 4% of the controls as suspect, whereas both the VSVT and the WMT correctly classified all controls into their group. All simulators were accurately identified by the WMT; 12% were not identified by the VSVT, and 20% were not identified by the TOMM.

Below-chance performance on the test is rare, as is the case for most PVTs, apart from some criminal defendant samples where this may occur more frequently (see Paradis et al., 2013). Greve et al. (2009a) examined the rates of below-chance performance on TOMM, Portland Digit Recognition Test (PDRT), and WMT in a large private practice forensic sample (N = 1,032) with alleged TBI, alleged toxic exposure, and chronic pain. The TOMM yielded slightly less below-chance performance (2%) than the WMT (3%) and PDRT (4%). The easy portion of both PDRT and WMT yielded smaller rates of below-chance performance than the hard portion whereas TOMM did not show any differences between trials.

The evidence comparing the TOMM and WMT is equivocal. In a criminal forensic setting, the TOMM (68%) yielded better sensitivity than the WMT (56%) but weaker specificity (87% and 95%, respectively) based on a criterion of failure on at least two standalone PVTs (Fazio et al., 2015). In a study by Greve et al. (2008), TBI and chronic pain patients were divided into malingering and honest responder groups based on Slick et al. (1999) malingering criteria. Although the WMT was more sensitive than the TOMM in identifying noncredible responders, it yielded a 20% higher false-positive rate in the TBI patients (Greve et al., 2008). Notably, Greiffenstein et al. (2008) argued that comparing three WMT indices to one TOMM index may inflate WMT sensitivity. They compared the performance of compensation-seeking individuals with mild neurological trauma on various combinations of TOMM and WMT. Using only TOMM Trial 2 compared against any of the three WMT subtests resulted in very low failure rates on the TOMM relative to the WMT, yielding a 72% agreement rate. When all three TOMM trials were used, the failure rates increased, yielding a 77% agreement rate. The WMT only showed a 5% advantage over the TOMM in this case. The authors concluded that the WMT is not necessarily superior to the TOMM. See also the WMT review elsewhere in this chapter for more discussion of the TOMM compared to the WMT.

Evidence exists that the TOMM is less affected by distraction or dual-task interference than the WMT (Batt et al., 2008; Eglit et al., 2017). When a distraction was introduced during task administration, 75% failed the WMT whereas only 33% failed the TOMM (Batt et al., 2008). Participants who had to perform an *n*-back task while learning the TOMM stimuli were still able to pass the TOMM based on familiarity-based recognition memory even though recollection-based recognition was affected on the TOMM. The latter study suggests that even when there was no conscious recollection of the stimuli, participants were still able to pass the TOMM using familiarity-based recognition memory, which generally explained more of the classification accuracy on the TOMM than WMT (Eglit et al., 2007).

The TOMM appears more efficient than the Rey Fifteen-Item Test at detecting invalid performance even though scores on the TOMM and on the Rey Fifteen-Item Test are highly correlated with one another (.78 to .89). The TOMM identifies more than twice as many litigants or veterans as noncredible responders than the Rey Fifteen-Item Test (McCaffrey et al., 2003; Whitney et al., 2008).

Studies on the TOMM and MSVT indicate that the two tests are fairly highly intercorrelated; studies comparing detection rates provide mixed results, with some but not all studies indicating higher MSVT sensitivity (see the MSVT review elsewhere in this chapter for more details). For example, the MSVT appears at least comparable or more sensitive than the TOMM (Axelrod & Schutte, 2011; Bashem et al., 2014). In a consecutively referred clinical sample in a VA medical center, failure rates were 21% and 37% on the TOMM Trial 2 and the MSVT easy subtest, respectively, with 77% classification agreement. In order to obtain passing rates comparable to the MSVT, the TOMM cutoff needed to be adjusted up, to less than 49 (Axelrod & Schutte, 2011).

The TOMM and NV-MSVT generally have between 84% and 90% agreement, but the NV-MSVT may be better than the TOMM in identifying invalid performance (Armistead-Jehle & Gervais, 2011; Green, 2011), although some studies show equivalent prediction accuracy (see the NV-MSVT review elsewhere in this chapter for more details). For example, in a study by the NV-MSVT author, among disability claimants with TBI, more than twice the examinees failed the NV-MSVT compared to the TOMM (Green, 2011). Similarly, Armistead-Jehle and Gervais (2011) reported that of their 345 non-head-injury disability claimants, 21% failed the NV-MSVT and 9% failed the TOMM, with more cases failing the NV-MSVT and passing the TOMM than vice versa. More importantly, using the WMT as external criterion for performance validity, NV-MSVT yielded higher sensitivity than TOMM while maintaining high specificity, suggesting that the NV-MSVT is superior to the TOMM as a performance validity measure. These findings will require replication with an external malingering criterion such as the Slick et al. (1999) criteria.

Compared to embedded performance validity indicators such as the Forced Choice trial of the CVLT-II, Moore and Donders (2004) examined TBI patients from a rehabilitation facility and found that the TOMM and the CVLT-II FC were equally sensitive to invalid test performance. There was strong but not perfect agreement between the two instruments. Axelrod and Schutte (2011) provided further support for the equivalence of the TOMM and CVLT-II FC in a consecutively referred clinical sample in a VA medical center. Failure rates were comparable between the TOMM and CVLT-II FC (21% and 23%, respectively), with 88% classification agreement between these two indicators.

The TOMM is more often perceived as a measure of performance validity than other tests (WMT, VSVT), at least when administered face-to-face by an examiner (Tan et al., 2002; but see Tombaugh, 1997). It is possible that people may be slightly more disinclined to feign nonverbal (picture recognition) as opposed to verbal (word recognition) memory deficits. Regardless, evidence to date recommends the use of multiple PVTs tapping various cognitive domains.

RELATIONSHIPS WITH AND COMPARISONS TO SVTS AND STANDARDIZED QUESTIONNAIRES

There is evidence that MMPI-2 validity scales that tap exaggeration of psychopathology measure a different construct than PVTs (see the review of MMPI-2 in Chapter 16). McCaffrey et al. (2003) found that MMPI-2 validity scales did not correlate with any trials on the TOMM, with the exception of the Fb scale, which was negatively correlated with TOMM Trial 1 ($r = -.34$).

Correlations between the TOMM and SIRS, a structured interview for malingering of psychopathology, are low to high ($r = -.14$ to $-.50$). Gottfried and Glassmire (2016) reported that the SIRS yielded slightly more invalid performance (57%) than the TOMM (51%) in their sample of forensic psychiatric inpatients assessed for competency to stand trial; however, 37% had invalid performance on both measures. Those feigning cognitive problems were 1.68 times more likely to feign psychiatric symptoms. Those feigning psychiatric symptoms were 1.86 times more likely to feign cognitive problems. As such, clinicians involved in such work are encouraged to assess for both cognitive deficit and psychiatric symptom exaggeration.

The relationship between TOMM scores and psychiatric symptoms may be minimal (Green et al., 2012; O'Bryant et al., 2007b). For example, O'Bryant and colleagues (2007b) found low correlations between TOMM Trial 1 and BDI-II or State-Trait Anxiety Inventory (STAI) (r = −.25 to −.37) and no correlation between TOMM Trial 2 or Retention and BDI-II or STAI scores.

However, TOMM performance may be related to somatization. Whiteside et al. (2010) examined the relationship between TOMM Trial 2 performance and PAI clinical scales in a sample of clinical and forensic referrals. TOMM Trial 2 and the Somatic Complaints scale (SOM) were modestly correlated (ρ = −.26), especially the Conversion subscale (SOM-C). Those who reported normal SOM scores obtained higher TOMM scores (Trial 2 M = 48.9, *SD* = 4.2) than those who reported extremely elevated SOM scores (Trial 2 M = 44.2, *SD* = 10.2).

RELATIONSHIPS WITH NEUROPSYCHOLOGICAL TESTS

Overall, the TOMM displays only modest correlations with standard neuropsychological tests. In mild and moderate TBI, correlations between Trial 2 and overall neuropsychological functioning are low to moderate while Retention is not correlated with neuropsychological functioning (Gfeller & Roskos, 2013). In general neurological samples, correlations with cognitive tests appear moderate, except for those involving Digit Span, which are low (Merten et al., 2007). TOMM performance appears only modestly related to measures of learning and memory, including free-recall measures of visual and verbal learning such as Visual Reproduction from the WMS-R, CVLT, and the Word List subtest from the Learning and Memory Battery (LAMB), with correlations ranging from .20 to .35 (Tombaugh, 1996).

CLINICAL STUDIES

As can be seen in Table 15–23a, multiple studies using Slick et al. (1999) malingering criteria and Bianchini et al. (2005) malingered pain-related disability criteria are generally consistent in showing that a TOMM Trial 2 cutoff of less than 45 yields acceptable sensitivity in a variety of settings while maintaining specificity at an acceptable 90% (i.e., <10% false-positive rate). Furthermore, in active-duty military members and among patients with low intelligence (FSIQ ≤75), a higher Trial 2 cutoff of 48 or lower yields high sensitivity with 100% specificity. In addition, combining the TOMM and WMT shows particular promise in detection of malingering, including both malingered neurocognitive dysfunction and malingered pain-related disability, with better sensitivities than either test used alone (see the WMT review elsewhere in this chapter for classification accuracy data and cutoffs).

In forensic outpatients who meet the Slick et al. (1999) malingering criteria, comparisons of the standard TOMM scores and derived TOMM scores such as IFFI and ACI reveal that the IFFI is as effective as the ACI and superior to TOMM Trial 2 or Retention used in isolation in identifying malingering cases while maintaining high specificity. Prediction accuracy is highest for IFFI followed by ACI and Retention, and last, by Trial 2 (80%, 78%, 78%, and 75%, respectively; Buddin et al., 2014).

Standard cutoffs yield low sensitivity for malingered pain-related disability in those with chronic pain (Greve et al., 2009b). Adjusting the cutoff of Trial 1 to less than 35, Trial 2 to less than 46, and Retention to less than 46 improves sensitivity to 50% while maintaining specificity at a high level (99%).

TBI. A number of studies have examined TOMM performance in TBI. For example, on average, patients with moderate to severe brain injury obtain Trial 2 scores of greater than 44 despite impairment on visual memory tests (Haber & Fichtenberg, 2006; Table 15–23a and 15–23b). Patients with TBI or postconcussion syndrome who are classified as valid performers using Slick et al. (1999) criteria or independent PVTs also perform well above standard cutoffs whereas the malingering cases perform at chance or significantly lower than the valid group (Strutt et al., 2012; Vilar-Lopez et al., 2008). TBI patients who perform noncredibly on the TOMM are not different from those who pass the TOMM on demographic, psychiatric, or substance abuse history or self-reported depression and anxiety (Locke et al., 2008). The only difference is in disability status, in which more of those who fail than pass the TOMM are on disability. It is notable that other objective variables such as severity of brain injury or employment status are not associated with TOMM performance, suggesting that the TOMM is insensitive to cognitive impairments associated with brain injury; other factors such as a "cry for help" or "diagnosis threat" in those who are on disability have been noted by some authors as possibly accounting for TOMM failure (Locke et al., 2008), although these factors are unlikely explanations of PVT failure in the overall literature.

Criminal Defendants. Within a criminal forensic setting, individuals suspected of feigning incompetence to stand trial (e.g., those facing murder charges or other felony offences) tend to produce low scores on the TOMM (Heinze & Purisch, 2001; Weinborn et al., 2003), with up to 26% scoring below chance (Paradis et al., 2013). Using the cutoffs described in the test manual, specificity tends to be high (90% or higher), although sensitivity is lower but still quite respectable in these settings (about 60% to 67%).

Dementia. Profound cognitive impairment appears to affect performance. Using a criterion cutoff score of 45 on Trial 2, Tombaugh's studies (Rees et al., 1998; Tombaugh, 1996, 1997) revealed specificity rates greater than 90% when considering cognitively impaired, aphasic, and non–compensation-seeking TBI patients. However, correct classification of demented patients was poor. About a quarter of nonlitigating patients diagnosed with moderate to severe dementia performed below the cutoff of 45 on Trial 2 (Merten et al., 2007; Walter et al., 2014). In contrast, patients with mild cognitive impairment (MCI) and healthy older adults perform almost perfectly on Trial 2 and on the Retention trial (Merten et al., 2007; Teicher & Wagner, 2004; Walter et al., 2014). As seen in Table 15–26, the specificity of TOMM decreases with decreasing MMSE performance in nonlitigating patients with dementia of mixed etiologies (Dean et al., 2009). Taken together, the TOMM may be used in those with MCI but is unsuitable as a performance validity measure in those with suspected moderate to severe dementia. Colby (2001) suggested that false-positive errors are reduced without a substantial decline in sensitivity when a cutoff of more than 14 errors on Trial 2 and Retention combined (or >13 errors if only Trial 2 is given) is used and dementia cannot be ruled out.

By contrast, there is a suggestion that even those with clinically obvious neurological symptoms are able to pass the TOMM, more so if they obtain an MMSE score of greater than 23 (Merten et al., 2007), yielding a greater than 83% passing rate. In contrast, the WMT yields a passing rate of 50 to 58%. As such, the authors suggested that the TOMM appears insensitive to clinically obvious neurological symptoms, though it may still be affected if the MMSE score is low.

Low IQ. Individuals diagnosed with mild intellectual disability are able to pass the TOMM with very low false-positive rates (<5%; Love et al., 2014; Simon, 2007). For example, Simon (2007) reported that 21 forensic inpatients with intellectual disability obtained passing scores (M = 48.7, *SD* = 1.9 on Trial 2 and M = 49.4, *SD* = 1.1 on Retention) with only one participant obtaining a score at the cutoff (Trial 2 = 45).

TABLE 15–26 Specificity of the Test of Memory Malingering (TOMM) in Dementia According to Mini-Mental State Examination (MMSE) Scores

SAMPLE	SPECIFICITY (%)
Overall Sample (*N* = 20)	45
MMSE <15 (*N* = 2)	0
MMSE 15–20 (*N* = 9)	33
MMSE 21–30 (*N* = 8)	63

NOTE: Based on TOMM Trial 2 <45. Note small *N*s.

SOURCE: Adapted from Dean et al. (2009).

With regard to feigning low IQ, the TOMM appears to yield low sensitivity when false positives are minimized for identifying feigned intellectual disability. Shandera et al. (2010) reported that using the standard Trial 2 cutoff score, the TOMM yielded a sensitivity of 40%, a specificity of 88%, and an overall hit rate of 64% to identify community volunteers instructed to feign intellectual disability. The cutoff score must be adjusted to less than 30 in order to maintain a specificity above 90%, though at the expense of sensitivity (24%). Although the TOMM shows low sensitivity for feigning of intellectual disability, it is the only measure that yields a low false-positive rate among 11 PVTs, including Letter Memory Test, Digit Memory Test (36-item short version), b Test, oral WMT, and WAIS-III derived indices (age-corrected Digit Span subtest scale score, Vocabulary-Digit Span, Mittenberg Discriminant Function, RDS; Shandera et al., 2010).

It is important to note that there are differences in the performance of credible individuals with low IQ and noncredible individuals. Using Slick et al. (1999) criteria, Smith et al. (2014) reported that a credible low-IQ group outperformed a malingering group on a large number of cognitive tests, including intelligence, attention, visuospatial skill, processing speed, verbal learning/recognition, and visual memory, but they performed worse on language, math skills, and executive skills. Weinborn et al. (2003) provided support for the use of a cutoff of more than 14 errors on Trial 2 and Retention combined (or >13 errors if only Trial 2 is given) among examinees with mild intellectual disability.

Chronic Pain. The experience of pain (e.g., low, high) within the assessment appears to be unrelated to test scores (Etherton et al., 2005; Gervais et al., 2004). In fact, in one study, patients with fibromyalgia with self-reported high level of depression (BDI-II in the moderate range on average), chronic pain (intense pain as measured by the Multidimensional Pain Inventory), and pain-related disability obtained almost perfect average TOMM Trial 2 and Retention trial scores. No one failed the TOMM, suggesting that the TOMM is not affected by these factors (Iverson et al., 2007). Even when patients with fibromyalgia fail the TOMM, their TOMM performance is not associated with self-report of pain, fatigue, or depression (Kalfon et al., 2016).

Psychiatric Conditions. Depression, including severe depression (Ashendorff et al., 2004; Paradis et al., 2013; Rees et al., 2001; Yanez et al., 2006) and anxiety (Ashendorff et al., 2004) do not adversely affect performance on the TOMM. One study suggested that cognitive impairment associated with psychosis generally does not impair TOMM performance to a level that would produce a false-positive finding (Duncan, 2005). Another study of 58 patients with schizophrenia or schizoaffective disorder found a

17 to 28% failure rate on the TOMM, with a range of invalid scores between 34 and 40 (Hunt et al., 2014). Colby's (2001) cutoffs may help to reduce the risk of false positives in cases of severe psychotic mental illness (Weinborn et al., 2003). However, those who fail the TOMM are more likely to report a higher number of neuropsychiatric symptoms (Gfeller & Roskos, 2013; Hilsabeck et al., 2011).

To detect feigned psychiatric illnesses, the TOMM appears adequate, at least in simulator studies. Weiss and Rosenfeld (2016) provided data suggesting that the TOMM may have high specificity to detect those feigning distress. They asked African immigrants in the United States with or without PTSD to feign distress-related symptoms. The TOMM misclassified 13% of the low PTSD group and none of the high PTSD group as feigning, but correctly classified 43% of the feigning group. In a sample of chronically mentally ill outpatients in a psychiatric hospital and community simulators instructed to feign mental illness, a TOMM Trial 2 score of 45 or less yielded a sensitivity of 62% and a specificity of 94%. At a base rate of 25%, PPV was 78% and NPV was 88% (Pivovarova et al., 2009).

Epilepsy and Psychogenic Nonepileptic Seizures. Patients with video-electroencephalogram (EEG) monitoring confirmed psychogenic nonepileptic seizures (PNES) are more likely than those with epilepsy or epilepsy and PNES to fail the TOMM, though the number of failures is generally fairly small (9 to 12%; Cragar et al., 2006; Wisdom et al., 2012). As such, the TOMM may help in differential diagnosis in this setting.

ADHD. Studies using verified clinical groups with feigned ADHD are scant, but studies using simulated feigned ADHD are promising. Use of standard TOMM cutoffs to detect feigned ADHD in undergraduate volunteers yields sensitivity rates in the 35% to 47% range (Jasinski et al., 2011; Sollman et al., 2010). In one undergraduate simulator study, sensitivity of TOMM Trial 2 and Retention to ADHD exaggeration was low (35% to 38%) despite 100% specificity (Jasinski et al., 2011). In another coached undergraduate simulator study, sensitivity to feigned ADHD was 47% and specificity was 97% for Trial 2 and Retention, whereas Trial 1 yielded a sensitivity of 87% but slightly lower specificity (83%; Sollman et al., 2010).

Resistance to Coaching. Evidence on the impact of coaching on the TOMM has been mixed. In one study, DenBoer and Hall (2007) found that coaching appeared to increase the chances of escaping detection on the TOMM. In another study (Jelicic et al., 2011), undergraduate simulators were coached on symptoms of brain injury or about PVTs but no differences in TOMM performance were found between the two feigning groups. A specificity of 100% was obtained, and sensitivity ranged from 80% to 87% for the feigning groups on Trial 2 and 80% to 97% on Retention, suggesting that the TOMM may be resistant to coaching. Last, Davis et al. (2012) found that coached undergraduate simulators performed better than naïve simulators on standard TOMM trials but no differences were seen between the simulators on the Davis et al. (2012) Response Consistency Indices (CNS), suggesting that the influence of coaching may be reduced when the CNS indices are used.

NEUROANATOMICAL CORRELATES AND IMAGING STUDIES

Studies do indicate some neuroanatomical correlates to TOMM performance. Among veterans with mild TBI without incentives to feign, those who failed the TOMM showed decreased brain metabolism in ventromedial prefrontal cortex, suggesting dysfunction in this brain region (Spadoni et al., 2015). Similarly, temporal lobe dysfunction might affect Retention performance, but not to a degree that TOMM performance falls below the cutoff for invalid performance (Hill et al., 2003).

COMMENT

The TOMM has become one of the most frequently used PVTs among neuropsychologists likely because of its simplicity and brevity, but also because of the impressive body of literature supporting its use as a PVT. In fact, use of Trial 1 alone has shown adequate utility as a screening measure in appropriate settings, and numerous studies have been conducted in various settings, with adjusted cutoff scores recommended for specific populations. The TOMM cutoffs have also been validated against Slick et al. (1999) malingering criteria in several studies and against malingered pain-related disability. Moreover, alternative indices such as the Albany Consistency Index (Gunner et al., 2012) and the Invalid Forgetting Frequency Index (Buddin et al., 2014) have been developed and appear to hold promise, although more studies are needed to clarify their use. It has also been suggested that the TOMM possesses sufficient validity to meet the Daubert criteria for admissibility of scientific evidence in the courtroom (Vallabhajosula & van Gorp, 2001; Tombaugh, 2002).

The TOMM appears to be more sensitive than the Rey Fifteen-Item Test and equivalent to the CVLT-II FC embedded indicator in identifying noncredible performance. Comparisons to the WMT, MSVT, and NV-MSVT are mixed, but suggest that these tests might be more appropriate in some circumstances. Combining the TOMM and WMT might be particularly promising as part of a PVT battery (see also WMT, MSVT, and NV-MSVT reviews elsewhere in this chapter). Specificity is high in many clinical, forensic, and compensation-seeking settings, resulting in few false positives other than in dementia or intellectual disability. Although those with MCI or mild intellectual disability can still pass the TOMM, the test is not recommended for use in moderate intellectual disability or moderate to severe dementia. It is also worth noting that below-chance scores are rare on the TOMM, and, as such, scores below recommended cutoffs are sufficient to suggest noncredible performance. Generally speaking, below-chance scores on PVTs identify few malingerers in the broader malingering literature.

Financial incentives, disability status, and premorbid psychiatric maladjustment raise the probability of invalid performance, but factors such as depression, anxiety, pain, and distraction do not necessarily negatively affect TOMM performance. Therefore, low scores should not be attributed to these conditions. However, it is worth noting that those who fail the TOMM are more likely to endorse psychiatric symptoms as is the case for many PVTs, particularly in settings involving malingering criminal defendants who tend to exaggerate both cognitive and psychiatric symptoms.

The task may be of value when assessing examinees from other cultures and therefore has a broader range of application than other PVTs that use word lists or other language-based content. Spanish samples and Spanish speakers living in the United States perform similarly to the original North-American sample, suggesting that TOMM performance may not be impacted by language (Vilar-Lopez et al., 2008; Strutt et al., 2012). Recall, too, that Tombaugh (1996) found that even patients with aphasic disturbances achieve high scores on the TOMM. However, there is some evidence that those with limited education may perform poorly on the TOMM. The impact of illiteracy on the TOMM is unknown at this time.

Studies suggest that the test is relatively insensitive to coaching. However, the test publisher has noted instances of individuals searching the Internet for information about feigned cognitive dysfunction in order to evade detection. Accordingly, as a precaution, the publisher recommends that the respondent not see the name of the test at any time during the administration, a recommended practice for all PVTs.

REFERENCES

Armistead-Jehle, P., & Gervais, R. O. (2011). Sensitivity of the Test of Memory Malingering and the Nonverbal Medical Symptom Validity Test: A replication study. *Applied Neuropsychology, 18*(4), 284–290.

Ashendorf, L., Constantinou, M., & McCaffrey, R. J. (2004). The effect of depression and anxiety on the TOMM in community-dwelling older adults. *Archives of Clinical Neuropsychology, 19,* 125–130.

Axelrod, B. N., & Schutte, C. (2011). Concurrent validity of three forced-choice measures of symptom validity. *Applied Neuropsychology, 18*(1), 27–33.

Bashem, J. R., Rapport, L. J., Miller, J. B., Hanks, R. A., Axelrod, B. N., & Millis, S. R. (2014). Comparisons of five performance validity indices in bona fide and simulated traumatic brain injury. *The Clinical Neuropsychologist, 28*(5), 851–875.

Batt, K., Shores, E. A., & Chekaluk, E. (2008). The effect of distraction on the Word Memory Test and Test of Memory Malingering performance in patients with a severe brain injury. *Journal of the International Neuropsychological Society, 14*(06), 1074.

Bauer, L., O'Bryant, S. E., Lynch, J. K., McCaffrey, R. J., & Fisher, J. M. (2007). Examining the Test of Memory Malingering Trial 1 and Word Memory Test Immediate Recognition as screening tools for insufficient effort. *Assessment, 14*(3), 215–222.

Booksh, R., Aubert, M., & Andrews, S. (2007). Should the retention trial of the Test of Memory Malingering be optional? A reply. *Archives of Clinical Neuropsychology, 22*(1), 87–89.

Buddin, W. H., Schroeder, R. W., Hargrave, D. D., Von Dran, E. J., Campbell, E. B., Brockman, C. J., . . . Baade, L. E. (2014). An examination of the frequency of invalid forgetting on the Test of Memory Malingering. *The Clinical Neuropsychologist, 28*(3), 525–542.

Colby, F. (2001). Using the binomial distribution to assess effort: Forced-choice testing in neuropsychological settings. *Neurorehabilitation, 16,* 253–265.

Constantinou, M., & McCaffrey, R. J. (2003). Using the TOMM for evaluating children's effort to perform optimally on neuropsychological measures. *Child Neuropsychology, 9,* 81–90.

Cragar, D. E., Berry, D. T. R., Fakhoury, T. A., Cibula, J. E., & Schmitt, F. A. (2006). Performance of patients with epilepsy or psychogenic non-epileptic seizures on four measures of effort. *The Clinical Neuropsychologist, 20*(3), 552–566.

Dandachi-FitzGerald, B., Ponds, R. W., & Merten, T. (2013). Symptom validity and neuropsychological assessment: A survey of practices and beliefs of neuropsychologists in six European countries. *Archives of Clinical Neuropsychology, 28*(8), 771–783.

Davis, J. J., Wall, J. R., & Whitney, K. A. (2012). Derivation and clinical validation of consistency indices on the Test of Memory Malingering. *Archives of Clinical Neuropsychology, 27*(7), 706–715.

Dean, A. C., Victor, T. L., Boone, K. B., Philpott, L. M., & Hess, R. A. (2009). Dementia and effort test performance. *The Clinical Neuropsychologist, 23*(1), 133–152.

DenBoer, J. W., & Hall, S. (2007). Neuropsychological test performance of successful brain injury simulators. *The Clinical Neuropsychologist, 21*(6), 943–955.

Donders, J. (2005). Performance on the Test of Memory Malingering in a mixed pediatric sample. *Child Neuropsychology, 11,* 221–227.

Duncan, A. (2005). The impact of cognitive and psychiatric impairment or psychotic disorders on the Test of Memory Malingering (TOMM). *Assessment, 12,* 123–129.

Eglit, G. M. L., Lynch, J. K., & McCaffrey, R. J. (2017). Not all performance validity tests are created equal: The role of recollection and familiarity in the Test of Memory Malingering and Word Memory Test. *Journal of Clinical and Experimental Neuropsychology, 39*(2), 173–189.

Etherton, J. L., Bianchini, K. J., Greve, K. W., & Ciota, M. A. (2005). Test of Memory Malingering performance is unaffected by laboratory-induced pain: Implications for clinical cue. *Archives of Clinical Neuropsychology, 20,* 375–384.

Fazio, R. L., Denning, J. H., & Denney, R. L. (2017). TOMM Trial 1 as a performance validity indicator in a criminal forensic sample. *The Clinical Neuropsychologist, 31*(1), 251–267.

Fazio, R. L., Sanders, J. F., & Denney, R. L. (2015). Comparison of performance of the Test of Memory Malingering and Word Memory Test in a criminal forensic sample. *Archives of Clinical Neuropsychology, 30*(4), 293–301.

Gervais, R. O., Rohling, M. L., Green, P., & Ford, W. (2004). A comparison of WMT, CARB, and TOMM failure rates in non-head injury disability claimants. *Archives of Clinical Neuropsychology, 19,* 475–487.

Gfeller, J. D., & Roskos, P. T. (2013). A Comparison of insufficient effort rates, neuropsychological functioning, and neuropsychiatric symptom reporting in military veterans and civilians with chronic traumatic brain injury: Military and civilian TBI. *Behavioral Sciences & the Law, 31*(6), 833–849.

Gottfried, E., & Glassmire, D. (2016). The relationship between psychiatric and cognitive symptom feigning among forensic inpatients adjudicated incompetent to stand trial. *Assessment, 23*(6), 672–682.

Green, D., Rosenfeld, B., Belfi, B., Rohlehr, L., & Pierson, A. (2012). Use of measures of cognitive effort and feigned psychiatric symptoms with pretrial forensic psychiatric patients. *International Journal of Forensic Mental Health, 11*(3), 181–190.

Green, P. (2011). Comparison between the Test of Memory Malingering (TOMM) and the Nonverbal Medical Symptom Validity Test (NV-MSVT) in adults with disability claims. *Applied Neuropsychology, 18*(1), 18–26.

Greiffenstein, M. F., Greve, K. W., Bianchini, K. J., & Baker, W. J. (2008). Test of Memory Malingering and Word Memory Test: A new comparison of failure concordance rates. *Archives of Clinical Neuropsychology, 23*(7–8), 801–807.

Greve, K., & Bianchini, K. (2006). Should the Retention trial of the Test of Memory Malingering be optional? *Archives of Clinical Neuropsychology, 21*(1), 117–119.

Greve, K., & Bianchini, K. (2007). Choosing to know less: A response to Booksh, Aubert, and Andrews. *Archives of Clinical Neuropsychology, 22*(2), 231–234.

Greve, K. W., Binder, L. M., & Bianchini, K. J. (2009a). Rates of below-chance performance in forced-choice symptom validity tests. *The Clinical Neuropsychologist, 23*(3), 534–544.

Greve, K., Etherton, J., Ord, J., Bianchini, K., & Curtis, K. (2009b). Detecting malingered pain-related disability: Classification accuracy of the Test of Memory Malingering. *The Clinical Neuropsychologist, 23*(7), 1250–1271.

Greve, K. W., Ord, J., Curtis, K. L., Bianchini, K. J., & Brennan, A. (2008). Detecting malingering in traumatic brain injury and chronic pain: A comparison of three forced-choice symptom validity tests. *The Clinical Neuropsychologist, 22*(5), 896–918.

Gunner, J. H., Miele, A. S., Lynch, J. K., & McCaffrey, R. J. (2012). The Albany Consistency Index for the Test of Memory Malingering. *Archives of Clinical Neuropsychology, 27*(1), 1–9.

Haber, A. H., & Fichtenberg, N. L. (2006). Replication of the Test of Memory Malingering (TOMM) in a traumatic brain injury and head trauma sample. *The Clinical Neuropsychologist, 20*(3), 524–532.

Heinze, M., & Purisch, A. D. (2001). Beneath the mask: Use of psychological tests to detect and subtype malingering in criminal defendants. *Journal of Forensic Psychology Practice, 1,* 23–52.

Hill, S. K., Ryan, L. M., Kennedy, C. H., & Malamut, B. L. (2003). The relationship between measures of declarative memory and the Test of Memory Malingering in patients with and without temporal lobe dysfunction. *Journal of Forensic Neuropsychology, 3,* 1–18.

Hilsabeck, R. C., Gordon, S. N., Hietpas-Wilson, T., & Zartman, A. L. (2011). Use of Trial 1 of the Test of Memory Malingering (TOMM) as a screening measure of effort: Suggested discontinuation rules. *The Clinical Neuropsychologist, 25*(7), 1228–1238.

Horner, M. D., Bedwell, J. S., & Duong, A. (2006). Abbreviated form of the Test of Memory Malingering. *International Journal of Neuroscience, 116*(10), 1181–1186.

Hunt, S., Root, J. C., & Bascetta, B. L. (2014). Effort testing in schizophrenia and schizoaffective disorder: Validity Indicator Profile and Test of Memory Malingering performance characteristics. *Archives of Clinical Neuropsychology, 29*(2), 164–172.

Iverson, G. L., Page, J. L., Koehler, B. E., Shojania, K., & Badii, M. (2007). Test of Memory Malingering (TOMM) scores are not affected by chronic pain or depression in patients with fibromyalgia. *The Clinical Neuropsychologist, 21*(3), 532–546.

Jasinski, L. J., Harp, J. P., Berry, D. T. R., Shandera-Ochsner, A. L., Mason, L. H., & Ranseen, J. D. (2011). Using symptom validity tests to detect malingered ADHD in college students. *The Clinical Neuropsychologist, 25*(8), 1415–1428.

Jelicic, M., Ceunen, E., Peters, M. J. V., & Merckelbach, H. (2011). Detecting coached feigning using the test of Memory Malingering (TOMM) and the Structured Inventory of Malingered Symptomatology (SIMS). *Journal of Clinical Psychology, 67*(9), 850–855.

Jones, A. (2013). Test of Memory Malingering: Cutoff scores for psychometrically defined malingering groups in a military sample. *The Clinical Neuropsychologist, 27*(6), 1043–1059.

Kalfon, T., Gal, G., Shorer, R., & Ablin, J. N. (2016). Cognitive functioning in fibromyalgia: The central role of effort. *Journal of Psychosomatic Research, 87,* 30–36.

Locke, D. E., Smigielski, J. S., Powell, M. R., & Stevens, S. R. (2008). Effort issues in post-acute outpatient acquired brain injury rehabilitation seekers. *NeuroRehabilitation, 23*(3), 273–281.

Love, C. M., Glassmire, D. M., Zanolini, S. J., & Wolf, A. (2014). Specificity and false positive rates of the Test of Memory Malingering, Rey 15-Item Test, and Rey Word Recognition Test among forensic inpatients with intellectual disabilities. *Assessment, 21*(5), 618–627.

McCaffrey, R. J., O'Bryant, S. E., Ashendorf, L., & Fisher, J. M. (2003). Correlations among the TOMM, Rey-15, and MMPI-2 validity scales in a sample of TBI litigants. *Journal of Forensic Neuropsychology, 3,* 45–53.

Martin, P. K., Schroeder, R. W., & Odland, A. P. (2015). Neuropsychologists' validity testing beliefs and practices: A survey of North American professionals. *The Clinical Neuropsychologist, 29*(6), 741–776. https://doi.org/10.1080/13854046.2015.1087597

Merten, T., Bossink, L., & Schmand, B. (2007). On the limits of effort testing: Symptom validity tests and severity of neurocognitive symptoms in nonlitigant patients. *Journal of Clinical and Experimental Neuropsychology, 29*(3), 308–318.

Moore, B. A., & Donders, J. (2004). Predictors of invalid neuropsychological test performance after traumatic brain injury. *Brain Injury, 18,* 975–984.

Mossman, D., Wygant, D. B., Gervais, R. O., & Hart, K. J. (2018). Trial 1 versus Trial 2 of the Test of Memory Malingering: Evaluating accuracy without a "gold standard." *Psychological Assessment, 30*(1), 74–85. https://doi.org/10.1037/pas0000449

O'Bryant, S. E., Engel, L. R., Kleiner, J. S., Vasterling, J. J., & Black, F. W. (2007a). Test of Memory Malingering (TOMM) Trial 1 as a screening measure for insufficient effort. *The Clinical Neuropsychologist, 21*(3), 511–521.

O'Bryant, S. E., Finlay, C. G., & O'Jile, J. R. (2007b). TOMM Performances and self-reported symptoms of depression and anxiety. *Journal of Psychopathology and Behavioral Assessment, 29*(2), 111–114.

O'Bryant, S. E., Gavett, B. E., McCaffrey, R. J., O'Jile, J. R., Huerkamp, J. K., Smitherman, T. A., & Humphreys, J. D. (2008). Clinical utility of Trial 1 of the Test of Memory Malingering (TOMM). *Applied Neuropsychology, 15*(2), 113–116.

O'Bryant, S. E., & Lucas, J. A. (2006). Estimating the predictive value of the Test of Memory Malingering: An illustrative example for clinicians. *The Clinical Neuropsychologist, 20*(3), 533–540.

Paradis, C. M., Solomon, L. Z., Owen, E., & Brooker, M. (2013). Detection of cognitive malingering or suboptimal effort in defendants undergoing competency to stand trial evaluations. *Journal of Forensic Psychology Practice, 13*(3), 245–265.

Pivovarova, E., Rosenfeld, B., Dole, T., Green, D., & Zapf, P. (2009). Are measures of cognitive effort and motivation useful in differentiating feigned from genuine psychiatric symptoms? *International Journal of Forensic Mental Health, 8*(4), 271–278.

Powell, M. R., Gfeller, J. D., Hendricks, B. L., & Sharland, M. (2004). Detecting symptom- and test-coached simulators with the Test of Memory Malingering. *Archives of Clinical Neuropsychology, 19,* 693–702.

Rees, L. M., Tombaugh, T. N., & Boulay, L. (2001). Depression and the Test of Memory Malingering. *Archives of Clinical Neuropsychology, 16,* 501–506.

Rees, L. M., Tombaugh, T. N., Gansler, D. A., & Moczynski, N. P. (1998). Five validation experiments of the Test of Memory Malingering (TOMM). *Psychological Assessment, 10,* 10–20.

Rivera, D., Perrin, P. B., Weiler, G., Ocampo-Barba, N., Aliaga, A., Rodríguez, W., . . . Arango-Lasprilla, J. C. (2015). Test of Memory Malingering (TOMM): Normative data for the Latin American Spanish speaking adult population. *NeuroRehabilitation, 37*(4), 719–735.

Ruocco, A. C., Swirsky-Sacchetti, T., Chute, D. L., Mandel, S., Platek, S. M., & Zillmer, E. A. (2008). Distinguishing between neuropsychological malingering and exaggerated psychiatric symptoms in a neuropsychological setting. *The Clinical Neuropsychologist, 22*(3), 547–564.

Ryan, J. J., Glass, L. A., Hinds, R. M., & Brown, C. N. (2010). Administration order effects on the Test of Memory Malingering. *Applied Neuropsychology, 17*(4), 246–250.

Shandera, A. L., Berry, D. T. R., Clark, J. A., Schipper, L. J., Graue, L. O., & Harp, J. P. (2010). Detection of malingered mental retardation. *Psychological Assessment, 22*(1), 50–56.

Sharland, M., & Gfeller, J. (2007). A survey of neuropsychologists' beliefs and practices with respect to the assessment of effort. *Archives of Clinical Neuropsychology, 22*(2), 213–223.

Simon, M. J. (2007). Performance of mentally retarded forensic patients on the test of memory malingering. *Journal of Clinical Psychology, 63*(4), 339–344. https://doi.org/10.1002/jclp.20351

Slick, D. J., Sherman, E. M., & Iverson, G. L. (1999). Diagnostic criteria for malingered neurocognitive dysfunction: Proposed standards for clinical practice and research. *The Clinical Neuropsychologist, 13*(4), 545–561.

Slick, D. J., Tan, J. E., Strauss, E. H., & Hultsch, D. F. (2004). Detecting malingering: A survey of experts' practices. *Archives of Clinical Neuropsychology, 19,* 465–473.

Smith, K., Boone, K., Victor, T., Miora, D., Cottingham, M., Ziegler, E., . . . Wright, M. (2014). Comparison of credible patients of very low intelligence and noncredible patients on neurocognitive performance validity indicators. *The Clinical Neuropsychologist, 28*(6), 1048–1070.

Sollman, M. J., Ranseen, J. D., & Berry, D. T. R. (2010). Detection of feigned ADHD in college students. *Psychological Assessment, 22*(2), 325–335.

Spadoni, A. D., Kosheleva, E., Buchsbaum, M. S., & Simmons, A. N. (2015). Neural correlates of malingering in mild traumatic brain injury: A positron emission tomography study. *Psychiatry Research: Neuroimaging, 233*(3), 367–372.

Strutt, A. M., Scott, B. M., Lozano, V. J., Tieu, P. G., & Peery, S. (2012). Assessing sub-optimal performance with the Test of Memory Malingering in Spanish speaking patients with TBI. *Brain Injury, 26*(6), 853–863.

Tan, J. E., Slick, D. J., Strauss, E., & Hultsch, D. F. (2002). How'd they do it? Malingering strategies on symptom validity tests. *The Clinical Neuropsychologist, 16,* 495–505.

Teicher, G., & Wagner, M. T. (2004). The Test of Memory Malingering (TOMM): Normative data from cognitively intact, cognitively impaired, and elderly patients with dementia. *Archives of Clinical Neuropsychology, 19,* 455–464.

Tombaugh, T. N. (1996). *Test of Memory Malingering (TOMM).* North Tonawanda, NY: Multi-Health Systems.

Tombaugh, T. N. (1997). The Test of Memory Malingering (TOMM): Normative data from cognitively intact and cognitively impaired individuals. *Psychological Assessment, 9,* 260–268.

Tombaugh, T. N. (2002). The Test of Memory Malingering (TOMM) in forensic neuropsychology. *Journal of Forensic Neuropsychology, 2,* 69–96.

Vallabhajosula, B., & van Gorp, W. G. (2001). Post-Daubert admissibility of scientific evidence on malingering of cognitive deficits. *Journal of the American Academy of Psychiatry and the Law, 29,* 207–215.

Vanderslice-Barr, J. L., Miele, A. S., Jardin, B., & McCaffrey, R. J. (2011). Comparison of computerized versus booklet versions of the TOMM™. *Applied Neuropsychology, 18*(1), 34–36.

Van Dyke, S. A., Millis, S. R., Axelrod, B. N., & Hanks, R. A. (2013). Assessing effort: Differentiating performance and symptom validity. *The Clinical Neuropsychologist, 27*(8), 1234–1246.

Vilar-Lopez, R., Gomezrio, M., Santiagoramajo, S., Rodriguezfernandez, A., Puente, A., & Perezgarcia, M. (2008). Malingering detection in a Spanish population with a known-groups design. *Archives of Clinical Neuropsychology, 23*(4), 365–377.

Walter, J., Morris, J., Swier-Vosnos, A., & Pliskin, N. (2014). Effects of severity of dementia on a symptom validity measure. *The Clinical Neuropsychologist, 28*(7), 1197–1208.

Walters, G. D., Berry, D. T. R., Rogers, R., Payne, J. W., & Granacher, R. P. (2009). Feigned neurocognitive deficit: Taxon or dimension? *Journal of Clinical and Experimental Neuropsychology, 31*(5), 584–593.

Weinborn, M., Orr, T., Woods, S. P., Canover, E., & Feix, J. (2003). A validation of the Test of Memory Malingering in a forensic psychiatric setting. *Journal of Clinical and Experimental Neuropsychology, 25,* 979–990.

Weiss, R. A., & Rosenfeld, B. (2017). Identifying feigning in trauma-exposed African immigrants. *Psychological Assessment, 29*(7), 881–889.

Whiteside, D., Clinton, C., Diamonti, C., Stroemel, J., White, C., Zimberoff, A., & Waters, D. (2010). Relationship between suboptimal cognitive effort and the clinical scales of the Personality Assessment Inventory. *The Clinical Neuropsychologist, 24*(2), 315–325.

Whitney, Kriscinda A., Hook, J. N., Steiner, A. R., Shepard, P. H., & Callaway, S. (2008). Is the Rey 15-Item Memory Test II (Rey II) a valid symptom validity test?: Comparison with the TOMM. *Applied Neuropsychology, 15*(4), 287–292.

Williams, J. M. (2011). The malingering factor. *Archives of Clinical Neuropsychology, 26*(3), 280–285.

Wisdom, N. M., Brown, W. L., Chen, D. K., & Collins, R. L. (2012). The use of all three Test of Memory Malingering trials in establishing the level of effort. *Archives of Clinical Neuropsychology, 27*(2), 208–212.

Yanez, Y., Fremouw, W., Tennant, J., Strunk, J., & Coker, K. (2006). Effects of severe depression on TOMM performance among disability-seeking outpatients. *Archives of Clinical Neuropsychology, 21*(2), 161–165.

Young, S., Jacobson, R., Einzig, S., Gray, K., & Gudjonsson, G. H. (2016). Can we recognise malingerers? The association between malingering, personality traits and clinical impression among complainants in civil compensation cases. *Personality and Individual Differences, 98,* 235–238.

VICTORIA SYMPTOM VALIDITY TEST (VSVT)

TEST NAME	**Victoria Symptom Validity Test (VSVT)**
DOMAIN	Performance validity
AGE RANGE	18+ years
ADMINISTRATION TIME	15 to 20 minutes
SCORING FORMAT	Computerized
REFERENCE	Slick, D., Hopp, G., Strauss, E., & Thompson, G. B. (1997). *Victoria Symptom Validity Test.* Odessa, FL: Psychological Assessment Resources. www.parinc.com

DESCRIPTION

The Victoria Symptom Validity Test (VSVT) is a PVT used to assess exaggeration and feigning of memory complaints. The VSVT is a modification of the original Hiscock and Hiscock (1989) two-alternative forced-choice recognition task. It measures digit recall, and item difficulty is manipulated, making items appear more difficult than they actually are. Details on administration, items, and format are not provided to preserve test security. Please see original source for details. The test is divided into Easy and Difficult items based on increases in retention interval. Response time is also recorded. Below-chance performance at $p < .05$ is labeled as invalid, and performance significantly above chance at $p < .05$ is labeled as valid. A third category, labeled "Questionable," consists of scores that fall within the remaining 90% confidence interval of chance performance. Because below-chance performance rarely captures most malingerers, newer cutoffs have been identified based on more recent research (see "Normative Data" and "Clinical Studies").

ADMINISTRATION

Test presentation is controlled by the computer program. The examiner should ensure that the examinee is properly oriented to the monitor and keyboard. The examiner may input responses for examinees who are unable to use both hands for the keyboard. Examinees should be familiar with reading Arabic numerals.

SCORING

Test scoring is provided by the computer program. The following summary information is provided.

1. The number of correct trials for each block and item difficulty level, along with the maximum number of correct items on Easy, Difficult, and Total trials.
2. *Z* scores derived from a binomial probability curve centered at chance-level performance (50% correct). A *z* score of 0 indicates exact chance-level performance, with half of the items passed. *Z* scores are translated directly to *p* values, indicating the likelihood of an examinee's obtaining a particular score by chance alone (i.e., responding randomly). High positive scores ($z > 1.65$) indicate better-than-chance performance, and low negative scores ($z < -1.65$) represent worse-than-chance performance
3. Bias, the tendency to use one hand more than the other. Scores can range from −1 (using only the left hand) to +1 (using only the right hand). High scores (< .6) raise the question of a perceptual defect (e.g., visual field), motoric defect, or some other unusual response set
4. Mean response latency and standard deviation of Easy and Difficult items in milliseconds

The main score for interpretation is the Difficult items correct score. Performance on the Easy items can be viewed as a baseline indicator of general adherence and attention to the task (Doss et al., 1999); that is, if an examinee obtains an almost perfect score on the Easy items, there seems to be less likelihood that a low score on the Difficult items can be attributed to an attention deficit.

Slick et al. (1996) noted that steep drops in scores across retention intervals were unusual in bona fide brain-injured individuals. Furthermore, it is rare for any non–compensation-seeking patient to obtain scores of 0 to 5 (where 8 is the highest possible score) on any of the six blocks of scores referred to in the VSVT printout (Grote et al., 2000).

With regard to response latency, Slick et al. (1996) suggested that average response times in excess of four seconds in patients who do not appear to be confused or disoriented may be indicative of noncredible responding. Based on an examination of non–compensation-seeking and compensation-seeking patients, Grote et al. (2000) suggested alternative criteria: three seconds for the Easy items and four seconds for the Difficult items.

SD scores for response latencies are provided on the scoring printout. Compensation-seeking patients tend to be more variable in their response latencies than non–compensation-seeking clients. Grote et al. (2000) recommended a cutoff for the standard deviation score of 1.9 seconds or less (but see Jones, 2013, in "Clinical Studies").

DEMOGRAPHIC EFFECTS

AGE

In adults, age has no effect (Grote et al., 2000; Keary et al., 2013; Slick et al., 1997; Strauss et al., 2002) or little effect on accuracy (Loring et al., 2005, 2007).

GENDER

Similarly, gender has no impact on test scores (Slick et al., 1997; Strauss et al., 2002).

EDUCATION

Years of education do not influence accuracy scores on the VSVT (Keary et al., 2013; Slick et al., 1997; Strauss et al., 2002).

ETHNICITY, NATIONALITY, AND LINGUISTIC EFFECTS

There are few cross-cultural studies. No differences in VSVT performance have been reported in a Spanish sample compared to North-American norms (Vilar-Lopez et al., 2007).

NORMATIVE DATA

The test does not employ normative data. Instead, interpretation relies on binomial probability theory (Slick et al., 1996, 1997). This approach provides an indicator of the validity of the respondent's performance relative to what would be predicted on the basis of chance alone (i.e., if a respondent had endorsed items in a completely random manner). The manual provides qualitative classifications of Valid, Questionable, and Invalid for Total, Easy, and Difficult scores based on above-chance, at chance, and below-chance performance. These are the guidelines used in the computer-generated report. However, these values have been shown to be too conservative, missing many examinees who exaggerate deficits on the test. Hence, values derived from actual patient groups are preferred. See "Clinical Studies" for details.

EVIDENCE FOR RELIABILITY

EVIDENCE FOR INTERNAL RELIABILITY

Slick et al. (1997) reported that alphas for the Easy, Difficult, and Total scores were high, at .82, .87, and .89, respectively.

EVIDENCE FOR TEST-RETEST RELIABILITY, MEASURING CHANGE, AND PRACTICE EFFECTS

The VSVT was administered twice to 31 healthy participants and 27 compensation-seeking patients (Slick et al., 1997). The median retest interval was 14 days for controls and 31 days for compensation-seeking patients (range = 1–550 days). Test-retest correlations for selected measures from the VSVT were low (.53 to .54 for latency measures) among the control sample, most likely a reflection of restriction of range. Among the compensation-seeking group, correlations were higher (.56 for Easy reaction time to .84 for Total items correct). All of the control participants obtained the same classification at retest (valid) as they did at first testing. Among the compensation-seeking patients, 86% obtained the same classification at retest. An et al. (2012) administered the VSVT and other PVTs over two sessions of about 80 days apart to a small sample of healthy, nonclinical undergraduate students who participated in neuropsychological evaluation for extra course marks. Test-retest reliability was in the moderate to high range (r = .66 to .77), suggesting that performance in session 1 is predictive of performance in session 2. Overall, these findings suggest that the VSVT exhibits adequate reliability and suggests that changes in classification across test-retest intervals likely reflect the VSVT's sensitivity to changes in performance credibility (Thompson, 2002).

There is evidence that noncredible responders, including those with considerable experience with regard to head injury, tend to be more inconsistent across serial testings. Using an analog design, Strauss et al. (1999, 2002) found that simulators fluctuated more than controls in terms of their accuracy on Difficult items and response latency. Successful feigning of the same level of performance across different test sessions appears to require higher levels of self-monitoring or more sophisticated knowledge of human behavior than most noncredible responders possess. Therefore, evaluation of response consistency across test occasions may increase the accuracy of detection. Clinicians should consider changes of 3 or more points up or down on the Difficult items as increasing the index of suspicion.

EVIDENCE FOR VALIDITY

FACTOR-ANALYTIC STUDIES

Latent structure of the VSVT was explored using taxometric analysis, a method to identify latent classes or single dimensions in a set of scores to see if it measures a dimension or category of adequate versus inadequate performance validity. Findings suggest a categorical measure of adequate versus inadequate performance validity in an outpatient clinical, nonlitigating sample (Frazier et al., 2007). By contrast, a sample of compensation-seeking individuals yielded a dimensional latent structure of feigning, suggesting that use of cutoff scores may not be appropriate in this population (Walters et al., 2009). These studies suggest that the context and referral question are important for the interpretation of the VSVT, as is the case for all PVTs.

Nelson et al. (2007) examined whether cognitive and psychological validity reflect distinct constructs using exploratory factor analysis of VSVT Total, TOMM Trial 2, and Letter Memory Test (LMT), along with MMPI-2 validity scales based on a sample of compensation-seeing individuals. A four-factor solution was obtained, representing the following: underreporting of psychological symptoms (MMPI-2 Lie, Defensiveness, and Superlative scales), overreporting of neurotic symptoms (MMPI-2 FBS, Response Bias Scale, and Malingered Depression scales), insufficient cognitive effort (VSVT, TOMM, LMT), and overreporting of psychotic/rarely endorsed symptoms (MMPI-2 Infrequency Psychopathology, Fb and Dissimulation scales).

INTERCORRELATIONS

Moderate correlations between VSVT accuracy and latency measures (r = –.37 to –.64) have been reported in a sample of neurology-based outpatient neuropsychology clinic patients, of which 16% were in litigation or seeking compensation (Haggerty et al., 2007). Similarly, moderate correlation was reported between Difficult and Easy items while response latencies for Difficult and Easy were highly correlated in a sample of patients with severe TBI in an acute neurorehabilitation inpatient program (S_{rho} = .52 and S_{rho} = .89, respectively; Macciochi et al., 2006). The authors suggest the use of only one indicator (Easy vs. Difficult response latency) to determine performance validity, not both, as they are correlated (Haggerty et al., 2007). Given these and other studies, particularly those on the sensitivity of the Difficult items to exaggeration of deficits, the Difficult items would be the recommended score for interpretation.

COMPARISONS WITH OTHER PVTS

Moderate to large correlations are observed between the VSVT and TOMM (r = .66) and VSVT and LMT (r = .78) in compensation-seeking individuals, suggesting that these tests likely measure similar constructs (Nelson et al., 2007; see also Tan et al., 2000). There is also evidence based on meta-analysis that the task shows superior classification accuracy compared with the WMT, TOMM, b Test, and the Rey Fifteen-Item Test (Sollman & Berry, 2011; Vickery et al., 2001). The VSVT Difficult items have also proved to be better predictors of instructional set than Dot Counting, Reliable Digit Span, or Vocabulary Minus Digit Span measures (Strauss et al., 1999, 2002), consistent with other research showing that forced-choice recognition tasks achieve the best hit rates in the detection of noncompliance (e.g., Greiffenstein et al., 1994; Rose et al., 1998). Among patients with schizophrenia without overt incentive to feign symptoms, the VSVT shows a 1% failure rate while the WMT yields a 15% failure rate, suggesting that the WMT may be overly sensitive in this group (Strauss et al., 2015).

CORRELATIONS WITH OTHER SVTs

Correlations between MMPI-2 validity scales and VSVT scores are in the small to medium range (Slick et al., 1996). Higher MMPI-2 Infrequency (F) scale scores are associated with lower VSVT Easy scores (r = –.29). Of note, Easy and Difficult item correlations with the FBS appear higher (.42 and .43, respectively), consistent with the notion that the FBS scale has greater utility than F-scale scores in the context of exaggerated neurotrauma claims. However, when participant classifications from the two tests are compared, a low rate of agreement is found between the MMPI-2 and the VSVT. This is not surprising as PVTs and SVTs tend to measure different aspects of exaggeration.

Similarly, in a study that examined the relationship between the VSVT and PAI validity scales (Inconsistency, Positive Impression [PIM], Negative Impression [NIM], and Infrequency scales) using a neuropsychological sample, only the PAI NIM was significantly but quite modestly correlated with all VSVT indicators (r = –.12 to .17), suggesting that these two tests measure different aspects of validity (Haggerty et al., 2007). As such, both cognitive and psychological validity measures should be administered when completing assessments in a compensation-seeking context (Haggerty et al., 2007; Nelson et al., 2007).

RELATIONSHIPS WITH OTHER NEUROPSYCHOLOGICAL TESTS AND SCALES

Evidence for divergent validity has been demonstrated by small to moderate correlations between the VSVT and scores on tests designed to measure dissimilar constructs. The VSVT is moderately to modestly correlated with WAIS-III indices and WMS-III indices in clinical, nonlitigating samples (r = .27 to .39; Frazier et al., 2007; Keary et al., 2013), with the largest correlation observed between VSVT Difficult items and WMS-III Working Memory Index, followed by WAIS-III FSIQ (r = .39 and .38, respectively; Keary et al., 2013). However, working memory appears to mediate the relationship between FSIQ and VSVT Difficult items. As such, Keary et al. (2013) recommended the use of other PVTs that have lower working memory demands, such as TOMM or WMT in epilepsy and other neurological populations where working memory deficits may be prominent (but see Grote et al., 2000; Loring et al., 2005; Macciochi et al., 2006). Response times to Easy and Difficult items show considerably less divergent validity, being moderately correlated (.32 to .53) with Digit Span and with measures with heavy processing-speed components (e.g., Stroop, Trails), suggesting caution in the interpretation of response times.

Moderate correlation has also been reported with the MATRICES Cognitive Consensus Battery (MCCB) in a sample of patients with schizophrenia (r = .39; Strauss et al., 2015) and with the Token Test in a sample of patients with severe TBI in an acute neurorehabilitation inpatient program (S_{rho} = .31; Macciochi et al., 2006). In another study, no memory test (e.g., RAVLT, Rey Figure) shared more than 5% of its variance with the VSVT (Slick et al., 1996). The VSVT was also not correlated to reading-based premorbid functioning (Wechsler Test of Adult Reading [WTAR]), the Brief Psychiatric Rating Scale, the Scale for the Assessment of Negative Symptoms, or the Level of Function Scale (Strauss et al., 2015). In sum, these studies indicate that the VSVT is largely unaffected by level of cognitive function except for working memory.

CLINICAL STUDIES

Jones (2013) provide cutoff scores for identifying Slick-defined malingering in a military sample, a majority of whom had mild TBI. Most individuals in the sample had potential incentive to feign symptoms. Cutoffs for detection of probable to definite malingering with at least 90% specificities are presented in Table 15–27, along with sensitivity, PPV, and NPV at various base rates. Easy items yielded the lowest sensitivities while the sensitivities for the Difficult and Total scores were high. Cutoffs of 22, 19, and 43 for Easy, Difficult, and Total scores, respectively, had 90% specificity (Table 15–27) and so appear to be recommended cutoffs for use in identifying exaggeration without unduly raising the false-positive rate. Cutoff scores of 19, 17, and 40 for Easy, Difficult, and Total scores, respectively, yielded PPVs of 100% at all base rates. To obtain at least a specificity of 90% using reaction time data, cutoffs of four seconds or more and five seconds or more for the Easy and Difficult items, respectively, could be used, but the sensitivities were low.

Compensation-Seeking Examinees. Compensation-seeking individuals obtain lower scores on this task (especially on the Difficult items) than do honest respondents and non–compensation-seeking examinees (Doss et al., 1999; Grote et al., 2000; Slick et al., 1994, 1996; Strauss et al., 1999, 2002; Suchy et al., 2012; Tan et al., 2002).

Slick et al. (1996) found that no healthy individual or non–compensation-seeking patient obtained a score of 15 or less on the Difficult items. Grote et al. (2000) found that 93% of 30 non–compensation-seeking patients with intractable epilepsy had VSVT Difficult scores of 21 or greater, compared with only 36% of 53 compensation-seeking patients. Loring et al. (2005) reported that 89% of 97 nonlitigating patients with intractable epilepsy obtained scores of at least 21/24 on the Difficult VSVT items. Based on these clinical data, we agree with Grote et al. (2000) that scores between 16 and 20 correct on the Easy or Difficult items should not be thought of as valid simply because they are above chance level, but instead as a level of performance that is rarely seen among non–compensation-seeking patients with documented brain injury.

Based on taxometric analysis in a clinical, nonlitigant sample, Frazier et al. (2007) found that the Total and Difficult indicator sets produced similar base rates (.14 and .13, respectively) while the Easy set produced a low base rate (.02), suggesting that Easy items are much less sensitive to noncredible performance. When the base rates of this study were compared to existing classification systems, standard VSVT cutoffs were found to be insensitive while the Difficult items cutoff of 21 or lower suggested by Grote et al. (2000) was found to produce false-positive errors.

Loring et al. (2007) examined performance on the VSVT in a heterogeneous clinical sample from an outpatient neuropsychology clinic comprising general referrals, referrals for TBI with no known external incentives, and compensation-seeking examinees. The compensation-seeking group was more likely to obtain invalid scores on VSVT Difficult (≤7/24; Table 15–28). When a cutoff of 17/24 or less was used, the compensation-seeking group had a 44% failure rate; with a cutoff of 20/24 or less, the failure rate was 60%, much higher for the compensation-seeking than the clinical groups.

Individuals who produce invalid protocols take about twice as long to respond as those who produce valid protocols. Although slowing of response (and inconsistency

TABLE 15–27 Victoria Symptom Validity Test (VSVT) Cutoffs, Sensitivity, Specificity, PPV, and NPV for Predicting Malingered Neurocognitive Dysfunction (MND) at Various Base Rates in a Military Sample

			BASE RATE 15% OR LESS		BASE RATE 30%		BASE RATE 40–50%	
CUTOFF	SENSITIVITY (%)	SPECIFICITY (%)	PPV (%)	NPV (%)	PPV (%)	NPV (%)	PPV (%)	NPV (%)
Easy ≤ 22	52	95	54	95	82	82	91	66
Difficult ≤ 19	91	93	59	99	85	96	93	91
Total ≤ 43	91	90	50	99	80	96	90	91
Easy minus Difficult ≥ 5	80	96	69	98	90	92	95	83

NOTE: Criterion = Probable to Definite MND; N = 234, majority had mild traumatic brain injury. Divided into "not malingering group," (passed all PVTs and SVTs; N = 122), "probable-to-definite malingerers" (failed one of the SVTs; N = 46), and "probable malingerers" (failed at least three PVTs or SVTs; N = 66) based on Larrabee et al. (2007) and Larrabee (2008) refinement of Slick et al. (1999) criteria. MND, Malingered Neurocognitive Dysfunction; PPV, positive predictive value; NPV, negative predictive value.

SOURCE: Adapted from Jones (2013).

TABLE 15–28 Victoria Symptom Validity Test (VSVT) Difficult Item Performance and Classification Rates for Various Neurological/Non-neurological Conditions

			VSVT DIFFICULT ITEM CUTOFF SCORE RANGES				
			≤7	8–15	16–24	≤17	≤20
	N	MEAN (*SD*)	PROPORTION OF GROUP (%)				
Dementia	50	20.3 (4.0)	0	12	88	22	38
Cerebrovascular	38	20.7 (3.9)	0	13	87	16	29
Multiple sclerosis	19	21.2 (3.7)	0	11	89	11	26
Mixed	27	21.2 (3.9)	0	7	93	11	26
Memory complaints	163	21.4 (3.8)	1	10	90	15	22
Clinical TBI	49	20.7 (4.1)	0	12	88	18	29
Compensation-seeking	25	16.5 (7.1)	20	20	60	44	60

NOTE: *N* = 297 non-TBI referrals, *N* = 49 TBI with no known external incentives referrals, and *N* = 25 compensation-seeking group. Dementia group includes Alzheimer's disease, Huntington's disease, HIV dementia, and frontotemporal dementia. Cerebrovascular group includes stroke, transient ischemic attacks, arteriovenous malformation, lupus, and vascular dementia. Mixed neurologic group includes neurocysticercosis, hypothalamic tumor, B12 deficiency, coronary artery bypass graft, astrocytoma, meningioma, meningitis, oligodendroglioma, colloid cyst, normal pressure hydrocephalus, Parkinson's disease, and Korsakoff's. The memory complaint group had memory complaints but was without neurologic cause on neurologic or neuropsychological evaluation. Compensation-seeking group includes referrals for independent medical examination and workers' compensation. TBI, traumatic brain injury.

SOURCE: Loring et al. (2007).

of response) tends to occur more commonly among those with suspect performance, the diagnostic utility of the accuracy score on the Difficult items appears to be greater (e.g., Grote et al., 2000; Strauss et al., 1999, 2002). Haggerty et al. (2007) found that an invalid group based on a standard VSVT cutoff showed longer response latency than a valid group, especially on Difficult items, in their neurology-based outpatient neuropsychology clinic patients. Table 15–29 presents the likelihood ratios of invalid responding for VSVT response latency. Response latency appears to be useful to detect invalid performance, although the authors indicated that longer response latency should only be used in high base-rate settings.

Dementia. Loring et al. (2007) examined performance on the VSVT in a heterogeneous clinical sample and found that when a cutoff of 17/24 or lower was used for Difficult items, failure rates were 22% in a dementia group; 38% failed when the cutoff was raised to 20 or less. These results indicate that the test is not appropriate for use with people who have severe cognitive dysfunction.

Contrary to these findings, others have concluded that severe cognitive impairment has minimal impact on the VSVT (Doss et al., 1999; Grote et al., 2000; Slick et al., 2003). For example, Slick et al. (2003) examined six nonlitigating patients with severe memory impairment whose scores on conventional memory tasks were generally below the first percentile (e.g., due to aneurysm of the anterior cerebral artery, Korsakoff's disease). Despite their obvious impairment, they obtained perfect scores on the Easy items (24/24) and near-perfect scores (≥22) on the Difficult items. Doss et al. (1999) noted that one of their patients with a diagnosis of probable dementia was able to obtain scores well above chance on the VSVT (Easy items, 23/24; Difficult items, 20/24) despite extremely low scores on traditional memory tasks. Patients with severe TBI in an acute neurorehabilitation inpatient program ($N = 71$) also

TABLE 15–29 Likelihood Ratios and Post-Test Probabilities of Invalid Responding for Victoria Symptom Validity Test (VSVT) Response Latencies Across Four Percentile Ranges

			POST-TEST PROBABILITIES				
			BASE RATE				
RESPONSE LATENCY	PERCENTILE	LIKELIHOOD RATIO*	5%	10%	15%	25%	50%
Easy items							
0–1833	1–50	0.20	.01	.02	.03	.06	.17
1834–2438	51–75	0.57	.03	.06	.09	.16	.36
2439–3292	75–90	2.83	.13	.24	.33	.49	.74
3293+	90+	4.50	.19	.33	.44	.60	.82
Difficult items							
0–2921	1–50	0.14	.01	.02	.02	.04	.12
2922–3745	51–75	0.27	.01	.03	.05	.08	.21
3746–5470	75–90	1.49	.07	.14	.21	.33	.60
5471+	90+	12.60	.40	.58	.69	.81	.93

NOTE: *N* = 300; age mean = 44.70, *SD* = 13.0, range = 18–78; 52% female; education mean = 13.8, *SD* = 2.5, range = 8–20; 16% in litigation or seeking compensation. *Likelihood ratio = likelihood ratio of invalid responding if response latency is within given percentile/score range.

SOURCE: Haggerty et al. (2007).

performed in the valid range on the VSVT, scoring between 23 and 24 on Easy, 21 and 23 on Difficult, and 44 and 47 on the Total score (Macciochi et al., 2006). These data demonstrate that valid scores can occur in patients with obvious, grossly impaired function, including severe attentional disturbance, impaired consciousness, severe visual perception deficits, and poor verbal fluency (Macciochi et al., 2006). Nevertheless, some of the mean performances in these studies are close to the cutoff for invalidity found in other studies (i.e., ≤22, ≤19 for Easy and Difficult; Jones, 2013), and so more independent studies of dementia patients and severely impaired patients are needed to determine at what level of impairment the test may not be as accurate.

Low IQ. There is a dearth of studies in low-IQ samples compared to most other PVTs. Loring et al. (2007) reported that no one with intellectual disability or FSIQ in the 50s obtained less-than-chance performance in their heterogeneous clinical sample; however, less-than-chance performance identifies few invalid protocols, and so more studies on the ability of the test to discriminate between deficits caused by low IQ and those related to feigning are needed.

Psychiatric Conditions. Depression has little impact on VSVT performance (Slick et al., 1996). However, poor performance on VSVT Difficult is associated with more physical anhedonia and global neuropsychological deficits in patients with schizophrenia (Strauss et al., 2015). More studies in psychiatric samples are needed.

Epilepsy. A number of studies reported that the majority of non–compensation-seeking, nonlitigating patients with intractable epilepsy have VSVT Difficult scores 21 or higher (Grote et al., 2000; Loring et al., 2005). However, in one study based on non–compensation-seeking, nonlitigating adults with medically refractory focal epilepsy being considered for surgery, 87% scored in the valid range, 8% in the questionable range, and 5% scored between 11 and 17 based on Difficult items at 21 or higher for valid performance, 18 to 20 for questionable, and less than 18 for invalid performance. The most common scores were 23 or 24 (65%). The group classification did not differ as a function of age of seizure onset or duration of epilepsy. Although no one obtained scores significantly below chance, failures on the VSVT in this population can occur even in the absence of overt external incentive, commensurate with the expected base rate of invalid performance in most nonlitigating clinical groups (i.e., 10%; Keary et al., 2013). To our knowledge, the VSVT has not been used in PNES.

ADHD and Reading Disorder. To our knowledge, there are no studies on ADHD or reading disorder using bona fide clinical groups. One study employed a simulation paradigm; Frazier et al. (2008) evaluated the utility of the VSVT and Validity Indicator Profile (VIP) in detecting noncredible performance in ADHD and reading disorder assessments using an undergraduate analog malingerer design study. Simulators in the ADHD group reported that the strategies they utilized included feigning problems in attending to information (90%) while the rest feigned slowed and inconsistent responding or difficulty organizing information. Strategies utilized by the reading disorder group included difficulty with reading accuracy or slowed reading. In this sample, a VSVT Difficult cutoff score of 19 was comparable to a cutoff of 21 in detecting simulation while minimizing false positives (0%). VSVT Easy, on the other hand, was less effective in detecting simulation of ADHD or reading disorder. The largest effect size was observed on VIP Nonverbal total score and VSVT Difficult items in the ADHD and reading disorder groups, although the latter group obtained poorer performance than the former. The VIP Nonverbal total score provided independent information over and above VSVT Difficult in the ADHD group while no scores added additional information over and above VSVT Difficult items in the reading disorder group, suggesting that VIP Nonverbal total may be better than VSVT Difficult in identifying dissimulation of ADHD symptoms while VSVT Difficult appears more suited for identifying dissimulation of reading disorder.

Other Conditions. Increased skin conductance but not heart rate was seen in undergraduate volunteers asked to exaggerate symptoms compared to those asked to try their best during the decision-making phase on the VSVT (Vilar-Lopez et al., 2011). Skin conductance normalized after responding, suggesting an emotional activation in the decision to respond incorrectly. Those asked to exaggerate committed more errors and had longer response times than those asked to try their best, who made very few errors. Accordingly, there is potential to use both PVTs and psychophysiological measures to identify exaggeration although more studies are needed.

The question of whether confronting individuals who failed a PVT affects their subsequent performance on the assessment was examined by Suchy et al. (2012). Patients with multiple sclerosis (MS) were given the VSVT, of which 11% failed the VSVT (Difficult ≤16). Half were confronted about their PVT failure and encouraged to try their best while the other half were not. They found that the invalid group reported more depressive symptoms than the valid group. On repeating the VSVT immediately after confrontation, overall improvements were seen. Difficult items showed greater improvement (19 of the 28 cases) than Easy items, although those who improved still performed lower than the valid group on the VSVT. The group that was not confronted performed worse than the valid and confronted group on the WMS-III, who performed similarly, thus suggesting that confrontation improves both VSVT and WMS-III performance. The authors suggested that confrontation may improve the chances of valid performance while allowing a discussion of the reason for noncredible responding during the feedback session in clinical settings. Whether confrontation should be applied in other settings is debatable.

Resistance to Coaching. Expertise with head injury (e.g., head-injured individuals, professionals working with head-injured individuals) does not affect the test's sensitivity (Strauss et al., 2002). In terms of face validity, the WMT fares best, with about one third of individuals perceiving it to be a legitimate measure of memory, followed by about one quarter who perceive the VSVT in this way (Tan et al., 2002).

NEUROANATOMICAL CORRELATIONS AND IMAGING STUDIES

None reported.

COMMENT

The VSVT is an interesting PVT in that it measures digit recall in an easily administered computer format. It has adequate reliability, is unaffected by age, gender, or education, and appears sensitive to changes in performance credibility. Computer administration allows for recording of response latency, which may provide additional information about the validity of test performance. The evidence to date suggests that the VSVT Difficult item cutoff of 19 or less has utility for identifying exaggeration or feigning of cognitive deficits. The presence of profound memory impairment affects VSVT performance minimally, although use of the VSVT in dementia, epilepsy, or other groups where working memory deficits are prominent is discouraged. It also has a left-right preference score that could alert clinicians to one of the few conditions that might cause spurious false-positive results on the VSVT (e.g., left neglect).

In initial studies, the test authors relied on binomial probability theory for VSVT interpretation. This resulted in quite conservative cutoff values for suspect performance (i.e., at or below chance). Later studies have suggested some empirically based cutoff scores for the VSVT that may serve to enhance its sensitivity. These demonstrate that scores at the bottom of the Valid range are more sensitive to invalid performance, particularly on the Difficult items.

Despite some advantages, the number of studies on the VSVT since publication in 1997 is relatively limited compared to other standalone PVTs such as the TOMM, WMT, and MSVT, among others. Specifically, more studies examining the sensitivity and specificity of the VSVT using an external criterion such as malingering criteria are needed, and there are only a few studies in compensation-seeking examinees, although these mostly appear quite favorable. There are no studies in criminal forensic settings, and more studies are needed in disability claimants and psychiatric samples, as well as in dementia and low-IQ examinees. There are, to our knowledge, no specific studies on malingered pain-related disability or somatoform disorders, where exaggeration is common, nor in clinical samples of ADHD or reading disability examinees, although simulation data appear promising. The test also does not have much data on how it performs cross-culturally except for one Spanish sample described here. As noted, the test requires some degree of working memory and so is not appropriate for all examinees, although this question deserves further study.

Last, the test's interpretation of scores rests on binomial probability theory based on whether the examinee's performance is above, at, or below chance; basing interpretation on this method will miss many feigning examinees and so reliance on cut scores derived from more recent studies is preferred compared to the qualitative classifications of Valid, Questionable, and Invalid provided by the test's computer scoring.

REFERENCES

An, K. Y., Zakzanis, K. K., & Joordens, S. (2012). Conducting research with non-clinical healthy undergraduates: Does effort play a role in neuropsychological test performance? *Archives of Clinical Neuropsychology, 27*(8), 849–857.

Doss, R. C., Chelune, G. J., & Naugle, R. I. (1999). Victoria Symptom Validity Test: Compensation-seeking vs. non-compensation-seeking patients in a general clinical setting. *Journal of Forensic Neuropsychology, 14*, 5–20.

Frazier, T. W., Frazier, A. R., Busch, R. M., Kerwood, M. A., & Demaree, H. A. (2008). Detection of simulated ADHD and reading disorder using symptom validity measures. *Archives of Clinical Neuropsychology, 23*(5), 501–509.

Frazier, T. W., Youngstrom, E. A., Naugle, R. I., Haggerty, K. A., & Busch, R. M. (2007). The latent structure of cognitive symptom exaggeration on the Victoria Symptom Validity Test. *Archives of Clinical Neuropsychology, 22*(2), 197–211.

Greiffenstein, M. F., Baker, W. J., & Gola, T. (1994). Validation of malingered amnesia measures with a large clinical sample. *Psychological Assessment, 6*, 218–224.

Grote, C. L., Kooker, E. K., Garron, D. C., Nyenhuis, D. L., Smith, C. A., & Mattingly, M. L. (2000). Performance of compensation seeking and non-compensation seeking samples on the Victoria Symptom Validity Test: Cross validation and extension of a standardization study. *Journal of Clinical and Experimental Neuropsychology, 22*, 709–719.

Guilmette, T. J., Hart, K. J., Giuliano, A. J., & Leininger, B. E. (1994). Detecting simulated memory impairment: Comparison of the Rey Fifteen-Item Test and the Hiscock Forced-Choice Procedure. *The Clinical Neuropsychologist, 8*, 283–294.

Haggerty, K. A., Frazier, T. W., Busch, R. M., & Naugle, R. I. (2007). Relationships among Victoria Symptom Validity Test indices and Personality Assessment Inventory validity scales in a large clinical sample. *The Clinical Neuropsychologist, 21*(6), 917–928.

Hiscock, M., & Hiscock, C. K. (1989). Refining the forced choice method for the detection of malingering. *Journal of Clinical and Experimental Neuropsychology, 11*, 967–974.

Jones, A. (2013). Victoria symptom validity test: Cutoff scores for psychometrically defined malingering groups in a military sample. *The Clinical Neuropsychologist, 27*(8), 1373–1394.

Keary, T. A., Frazier, T. W., Belzile, C. J., Chapin, J. S., Naugle, R. I., Najm, I. M., & Busch, R. M. (2013). Working memory and intelligence are associated with Victoria Symptom Validity Test Hard item performance in patients with intractable epilepsy. *Journal of the International Neuropsychological Society, 19*(3), 314–323.

Larrabee, G. J. (2008). Aggregation across multiple indicators improves the detection of malingering: Relationship to likelihood ratios. *The Clinical Neuropsychologist, 22*(4), 666–679. https://doi.org/10.1080/13854040701494987

Larrabee, G. J., Greiffenstein, M. F., Greve, K. W., & Bianchini, K. J. (2007). Refining diagnostic criteria for malingering. *Assessment of Malingered Neuropsychological Deficits*, 334–371.

Loring, D. W., Larrabee, G. J., Lee, G. P., & Meador, K. J. (2007). Victoria Symptom Validity Test performance in a heterogeneous clinical sample. *The Clinical Neuropsychologist, 21*(3), 522–531.

Loring, D. W., Lee, G. P., & Meador, K. J. (2005). Victoria Symptom Validity Test performance in non-litigating epilepsy surgery candidates. *Journal of Clinical and Experimental Neuropsychology, 27*, 610–617.

Macciocchi, S. N., Seel, R. T., Alderson, A., & Godsall, R. (2006). Victoria Symptom Validity Test performance in acute severe traumatic brain injury: Implications for test interpretation. *Archives of Clinical Neuropsychology, 21*(5), 395–404.

Nelson, N. W., Sweet, J. J., Berry, D. T. R., Bryant, F. B., & Granacher, R. P. (2007). Response validity in forensic neuropsychology: Exploratory factor-analytic evidence of distinct cognitive and psychological constructs. *Journal of the International Neuropsychological Society, 13*(3), 440–449.

Rose, F. E., Hall, S., & Szalda-Petree, A. D. (1998). A comparison of four tests of malingering and the effects of coaching. *Archives of Clinical Neuropsychology, 13*, 349–363.

Slick, D. (1996). *The Victoria Symptom Validity Test: A new clinical measure of response bias* (Unpublished doctoral dissertation). University of Victoria, British Columbia, Canada.

Slick, D., Hopp, G., Strauss, E., Hunter, M., & Pinch, D. (1994). Detecting dissimulation: Profiles of simulated malingerers, traumatic brain-injury patients, and normal controls on a revised version of Hiscock and Hiscock's forced choice memory test. *Journal of Clinical and Experimental Neuropsychology, 16*, 472–481.

Slick, D., Hopp, G., Strauss, E., & Thompson, G. B. (1997). *Victoria Symptom Validity Test.* Odessa, FL: Psychological Assessment Resources.

Slick, D. J., Sherman, E. M. S., & Iverson, G. L. (1999). Diagnostic criteria for malingered neurocognitive dysfunction: Proposed standard for clinical practice. *The Clinical Neuropsychologist, 13*, 545–561.

Slick, D. J., Tan, J. E., Strauss, E., Mateer, C. A., Harnadek, M., & Sherman, E. M. S. (2003). Victoria Symptom Validity Test scores of patients with profound impairment: Nonlitigant case studies. *The Clinical Neuropsychologist, 17*, 390–394.

Sollman, M. J., & Berry, D. T. R. (2011). Detection of inadequate effort on neuropsychological testing: A meta-analytic update and extension. *Archives of Clinical Neuropsychology, 26*(8), 774–789. https://doi.org/10.1093/arclin/acr066

Strauss, E., Hultsch, D. F., Hunter, M., Slick, D. J., Patry, B., & Levy-Bencheton, J. (1999). Using intraindividual variability to detect malingering in cognitive performance. *The Clinical Neuropsychologist, 14*, 420–432.

Strauss, E., Slick, D. J., Levy-Bencheton, J., Hunter, M., MacDonald, S. W. S., & Hultsch, D. F. (2002). Intraindividual variability as an indicator of malingering in head injury. *Archives of Clinical Neuropsychology, 17*, 423–444.

Strauss, G. P., Morra, L. F., Sullivan, S. K., & Gold, J. M. (2015). The role of low cognitive effort and negative symptoms in neuropsychological impairment in schizophrenia. *Neuropsychology, 29*(2), 282–291.

Suchy, Y., Chelune, G., Franchow, E. I., & Thorgusen, S. R. (2012). Confronting patients about insufficient effort: The impact on subsequent symptom validity and memory performance. *The Clinical Neuropsychologist, 26*(8), 1296–1311.

Tan, J. E., Slick, D. J., Strauss, E., & Hultsch, D. F. (2002). How'd they do it? Malingering strategies on symptom validity tests. *The Clinical Neuropsychologist, 16*, 495–505.

Thompson, G. B., III. (2002). The Victoria Symptom Validity Test: An enhanced test of symptom validity. *Journal of Forensic Neuropsychology, 2*, 43–67.

Vickery, C. D., Berry, D. T. R., Inman, T. H., Harris, M. J., & Orey, S. A. (2001). Detection of inadequate effort on neuropsychological testing: A meta-analytic review of selected procedures. *Archives of Clinical Neuropsychology, 16*, 45–73.

Vilar-López, R., Santiago-Ramajo, S., Gómez-Río, M., Verdejo-García, A., Llamas, J. M., & Pérez-García, M. (2007). Detection of malingering in a Spanish population using three specific malingering tests. *Archives of Clinical Neuropsychology, 22*(3), 379–388.

Vilar-López, R., Pérez-García, M., Sánchez-Barrera, M. B., Rodríguez-Fernández, A., & Gómez-Río, M. (2011). Symptom validity testing and its underlying psychophysiological response pattern: A preliminary study. *Archives of Clinical Neuropsychology, 26*(2), 133–143.

Walters, G. D., Berry, D. T. R., Rogers, R., Payne, J. W., & Granacher, R. P. J. (2009). Feigned neurocognitive deficit: Taxon or dimension? *Journal of Clinical and Experimental Neuropsychology, 31*(5), 584–593.

WORD CHOICE

TEST NAME	**Word Choice**
DOMAIN	Performance validity
AGE RANGE	16 to 69 years
ADMINISTRATION TIME	5 minutes
SCORING FORMAT	Computerized or hand scored
REFERENCE	Pearson. (2009a). *Advanced Clinical Solutions for WAIS-IV and WMS-IV: Clinical and Interpretive Manual.* San Antonio, TX: Pearson. Pearson. (2009b). *Advanced Clinical Solutions for WAIS-IV and WMS-IV: Technical Manual.* San Antonio, TX: Pearson. www.pearsonclinical.com

DESCRIPTION

Word Choice is a subtest of the Advanced Clinical Solutions for WAIS-IV and WMS-IV (ACS; Pearson, 2009a). The ACS consists of additional subtests and procedures for enhancing the clinical utility of the WAIS-IV and WMS-IV, with particular utility in diagnostic and forensic assessments (see also Holdnack et al., 2013). Word Choice is a forced-choice PVT, similar in format to the WRMT Words subtest. Details on administration, items, and format are not provided to preserve test security. Please see original source for details.

Although it can be used alone, Word Choice is designed to be combined with other performance indicators from the WAIS-IV and WMS-IV to determine invalid performance. Specifically, the combined number of raw scores below the cutoff for Word Choice, Logical Memory II Recognition, Verbal Paired Associates II Recognition, Visual Reproduction II Recognition, and Reliable Digit Span (RDS) can be evaluated in aggregate to provide a more powerful multi-test method to detect invalid responding. Combined PVTs provide more accurate prediction than individual tests for a given false positive/specificity rate (Larrabee, 2014). Furthermore, as noted in the manual, failure on a single PVT, including Word Choice, is insufficient for properly detecting invalid performance, as failing one PVTs occurs in honestly responding examinees.

ADMINISTRATION

See ACS manual for details. A stimulus book, Word Choice card, and record form are required.

SCORING

STANDARD SCORING APPROACH

Essentially, the total Word Choice score is interpreted by comparing the obtained score to overall base rates of scores in a clinical sample based on the notion that unusually low scores signal invalid performance. Invalid performance can be inferred in two ways: (1) by an unusually low Word Choice score compared to the clinical sample, unusual being defined by frequency of occurrence in the clinical sample, and (2) by a high number of unusually low scores across the five ACS PVTs compared to base rates in the clinical sample.

Unlike most other PVTs, the appropriate cutoff is selected by the user from set categories of 25% or less, 15% or less, 10% or less, 5% or less, and 2% or less, based on cumulative frequencies in the clinical sample. Percentages based on the number of ACS PVTs falling in these different categories are provided based on one, two, three, four, or five ACS scores below the designated cutoff.

Importantly, the manual indicates that users should employ the entire set of PVTs available in ACS rather than using a single PVT such as Word Choice in isolation and provides base rates across the five validity indicators at the different base-rate cutoffs. Scores can also be compared to base-rate information from healthy individuals provided according to education, ethnicity, and intellectual level, again according to the categories of 25% or less, 15% or less, 10% or less, 5% or less, and 2% or less.

To simplify interpretation and keep false positives to a rate of 10% or less, as is recommended in the field, we recommend using the 10% or less cutoff for determining invalidity and using a failure rate of two or more low scores out of five possible scores on the ACS PVTs to infer invalid performance. Other cut scores and base rates may be appropriate depending on the clinical scenario, but this combination of scores appears most straightforward and least liable to over- or underdetect invalid performance in most cases.

ADDITIONAL SCORING APPROACHES

One study by Erdodi and colleagues indicates that time to completion may augment clinical sensitivity; although

TABLE 15-30 Word Choice Critical-Item Index Scores

INDEX	ITEMS
CR-7	9, 11, 13, 17, 33, 39, 43
CR-5	9, 13, 17, 33, 39
CR-3	9, 33, 39

NOTE: Score based on number of errors on the specific set of critical items. Used by permission of the author.

more studies are needed, a total Word Choice completion time of about three minutes (i.e., ≥171 seconds) was associated with invalid performance, particularly when combined with the total score (Erdodi et al., 2017a).

Another study from the same authors suggests that scores from three sets of critical items may also improve prediction of noncredible performance. Specifically, three critical-item indexes comprised of combinations of 7, 5, and 3 items (i.e., termed CR-7, CR-5, and CR-3) improved classification accuracy over and above the total score (Erdodi et al., 2017b). To derive these indexes, errors are summed over the specific items. The items and cutoffs are shown in Table 15–30; see "Clinical Studies" for sensitivity and specificity.

DEMOGRAPHIC EFFECTS

AGE

Age effects were negligible in one study (Bashem et al., 2014). To our knowledge, there is no other information on age effects.

GENDER

To our knowledge, there is no information on gender effects.

EDUCATION AND IQ

Education effects are minimal in some clinical studies (Bashem et al., 2014; Miller et al., 2011). However, although data are not available for Word Choice itself, education effects are apparent in healthy individuals on the ACS PVTs, as shown in the manual and reproduced in Table 15–31. For example, one low ACS score is found in 27% of people with eight years of education or less, and in 17% of those with 9 to 11 years of education (i.e., a low score defined as at or below the 10th percentile in the clinical sample).

Similarly, although correlation to premorbid IQ appears negligible (Bashem et al., 2014), the manual indicates that 25% of individuals with mild intellectual disability obtain low scores on Word Choice (i.e., a low score defined as at or below the 10th percentile in the clinical sample). Similarly, when all five ACS PVTs are considered together, low-IQ individuals do not do well on ACS tests, with 19% of borderline and 38% of mild intellectual disability cases having one low score on the five ACS indices (Table 15–31).

TABLE 15-31 Percentages of Nonclinical Standardization Cases with One or More Scores Below the 10% Cutoff According to Education, Ethnicity, and IQ on Combined ACS Validity Indicators Including Word Choice

		ONE LOW SCORE	TWO LOW SCORES
Total Sample		7	1
Education	≤8 years	27	2
	9–11 years	17	4
	12 years	6	0
	13–15 years	5	1
	≥16 years	4	0
Ethnicity	White	4	1
	African American	12	1
	Hispanic	11	1
	Asian	7	0
IQ (WAIS-IV GAI)	69 or less	38	6
	70–84	19	2
	85–99	7	1
	100–114	4	0
	115 or higher	0	0

NOTE: Low score frequencies based on administration of all five ACS validity indicators including Word Choice, LM II Recognition, VPA II Recognition, VR II Recognition, and RDS. Low score defined as at or below the 10th percentile in the clinical sample. GAI, General Ability Index.

SOURCE: Adapted from Pearson (2009).

ETHNICITY, NATIONALITY, AND LINGUISTIC EFFECTS

The manual provides information on low scores based on administration of the five ACS indices, but not on Word Choice alone. These indicate the presence of ethnicity effects. Specifically, although rates were low for white examinees, 12% and 11% of African American and Hispanic examinees obtained one low score on ACS indices, defined as a score falling below the 10th percentile for the clinical group. However, having two low scores was found to be rare in both these groups. Notably, although we focus on the 10% cutoff here, some cutoffs were associated with unacceptably high false-positive rates in these groups, notably the 15% cutoff which is associated with low scores in 19% and 16% of African Americans and Hispanics, and the 25% cutoff, associated with a 33% and 36% rate for African Americans and Hispanics, respectively.

NORMATIVE DATA

Word Choice was validated on a sample of 352 clinical patients between the ages of 16 and 69 with a variety of neurological, psychiatric and developmental conditions from the WMS-IV clinical sample. The clinical sample included persons with moderate to severe TBI, temporal lobectomy, schizophrenia, major depressive disorder, mild intellectual disability, autistic disorder, Asperger's disorder, reading disorder, mathematics disorder, and ADHD. Demographics are not provided in the ACS manuals; these are described in the WMS-IV Technical Manual (Wechsler, 2009). For the Word Choice validation, the clinical sample purposefully excluded those with moderate intellectual disability and probable Alzheimer's disease due to the known high failure rate in these groups on PVTs.

Word Choice was also administered to healthy individuals from the WMS-IV standardization sample who were also administered the WAIS-IV; although specific *Ns* are not provided in either the Word Choice or ACS manual, this is presumably the sample of 1,250 individuals referenced in the WMS-IV manual. These data provide failure rates from a demographically representative sample of US cases according to education level, ethnicity, and IQ based on WAIS-IV GAI score (Pearson, 2009a, 2009b).

The test was also administered to 50 individuals instructed to feign impairment (i.e., Simulator Group). In addition, a group of 50 individuals were administered only the recognition portion of the test without having seen any of the test items and therefore provide performance data based on guessing alone (i.e., No Stimulus Group).

At a cutoff at or below the 10th percentile in the clinical sample, significant percentages of clinical examinees obtain one low score among the five ACS indices, including 19% of the overall sample, 30% of TBI, 17% of temporal lobectomy, 35% of schizophrenia, 63% of intellectual disability, and 27% of autistic disorder. When two low scores are required for invalidity, percentages across groups are much more acceptable (all <10%), with the exception of intellectual disability, where four low scores are required (Manual). However, the manual is very clear that single scores should not be interpreted as evidence of invalidity. Table 15–32 shows the percentages of clinical cases with one or more low scores (defined as below the clinical group 10% cutoff) on Word Choice and on all the ACS validity indicators combined.

TABLE 15–32 Percentages of Clinical Cases with One or More Low Scores (Defined as Below the Clinical Group 10% Cutoff) on Word Choice and Combined ACS Validity Indicators

	PERCENT WITH LOW SCORE ON WORD CHOICE	PERCENT WITH ANY ONE LOW ACS SCORE	PERCENT WITH ANY TWO LOW ACS SCORES
Total clinical sample	10[a]	19	5
Moderate-severe TBI	15	30	6
Temporal lobectomy	5	17	0
Schizophrenia	25–15	35	7
Major depression	10–5	12	2
Mild intellectual disability	25	63	31
Autistic disorder	10–5	27	9
Asperger's disorder	2	9	3
Reading disorder	10	7	0
Mathematics disorder	15–10	14	0
ADHD	10–5	9	3

NOTE: Low score frequencies based on administration of all five ACS validity indicators including Word Choice, LM II Recognition, VPA II Recognition, VR II Recognition, and RDS.

[a] Selected cumulative percentage cutoff of 10%.

SOURCE: Adapted with permission from Pearson (2009).

Of note, the theoretical, 90% confidence interval for random guessing on the test is 20 to 30, with the actual pure guessing group obtaining scores between 21 and 34 (Holdnack et al., 2013). A full 100% of the guessing group and 50% of simulators had scores below the 10 or less base rate cutoff for the overall clinical sample on Word Choice.

EVIDENCE FOR RELIABILITY

EVIDENCE FOR INTERNAL RELIABILITY

Not available.

EVIDENCE FOR TEST-RETEST RELIABILITY, MEASURING CHANGE, AND PRACTICE EFFECTS

Not available.

EVIDENCE FOR VALIDITY

FACTOR-ANALYTIC STUDIES

To our knowledge, this is unavailable.

CORRELATIONS WITH AND COMPARISONS TO OTHER PVTS AND SVTS

The test demonstrates modest to high correlations with other PVTs, particularly PVTs that also measure recognition memory. For example, in a TBI sample, Bashem and colleagues found large correlations with MSVT ($r > .50$), modest correlations with the TOMM and CVLT-II Forced Choice, but negligible correlations with RDS. As well, in identifying invalid performance, Word Choice had the lowest concordance with RDS but better concordance with other PVTs such as MSVT (Bashem et al., 2014), indicating that Word Choice and RDS may measure different aspects of invalid performance. Of note, Word Choice scores are uncorrelated to injury severity and time since injury after TBI (Bashem et al., 2014).

In a mixed sample comprised mostly of persons with TBI, Word Choice and WRMT Words were highly related ($r = .66$), but overall scores were lower on the WRMT. As well, more individuals obtained perfect scores on Word Choice (43% vs. 15%; Davis, 2014), raising the possibility that Word Choice is too easy in comparison. Others have also found that Word Choice is significantly easier than the WRMT, even though both tests are similar in format (Erdodi et al., 2014). This is attributed to the fact that the two tests have differences in word frequency, imageability, and concreteness of items, factors that affect recognition memory performance (Davis, 2014). Incidentally, although the WRMT is used as a PVT, it was originally designed to detect brain damage, whereas Word Choice was designed specifically to be insensitive to brain damage.

Davis (2014) found a concordance rate between Word Choice and other PVTs of 81% for WMT, 84% for RDS,

90% for CVLT Forced Choice, and 87% for indices from the RCFT, TMT, and WCST.

In a veteran sample, correlations with the WMT were large; this was the case both for WMT indices tapping primarily performance validity and those tapping memory performance (r = .67 to .78); in contrast, correlation to the TOMM was minimal and nonsignificant (r = .24; Bain & Soble, 2019).

Although Word Choice is felt to be resistant to coaching, the TOMM is the more sensitive measure; more simulators fail the TOMM despite coaching on how to pass it and are therefore correctly identified as feigning (i.e., 83% vs. 75%; Barhon et al., 2015).

To date, there are no studies involving well-known self-report SVTs, including the MMPI-2/MMPI-RF-2, PAI, or other SVTs that tap cognitive, somatic, or psychiatric overreporting.

CORRELATIONS WITH OTHER NEUROPSYCHOLOGICAL TESTS AND STANDARDIZED QUESTIONNAIRES

There are no studies to date on correlations with other neuropsychological tests and standardized questionnaires. However, the test appears fairly resistant to the effects of distraction, as shown in one study by equivalent group means when the standard administration was compared to administration during a distractor task (i.e., simultaneously adding orally presented numbers every three seconds while completing Word Choice; Barhon et al., 2015). However, the test is not completely impervious to distraction; when the cumulative percentages from this study are examined, it is apparent that distraction does have some effect on the test. For instance, 100% of the no-distraction group had scores of 48 or more, compared to only 52% of the distraction group (Barhon et al., 2015). However, this did not appear to meaningfully affect the false-positive rate as only 4% of the distraction group obtained scores below the cutoff for invalidity.

There is some evidence that Word Choice is more prone to the effects of genuine cognitive impairment than other PVTs such as the TOMM. In one study in veterans with a 40% WMT failure base rate, regression analyses showed that both Word Choice and TOMM contributed unique aspects to prediction of WMT failure. However, when individuals with cognitive impairment were examined, TOMM prediction efficacy remained, but Word Choice prediction efficacy declined, indicating that Word Choice performance was more reliant on intact cognition than was the TOMM. Specifically, among cognitively impaired veterans, although a TOMM score of 44/45 had excellent sensitivity and specificity (.83 and .94, respectively), the Word Choice cut score had to be increased to 47 to maintain an acceptable specificity, causing a significant decrease in its sensitivity (Bain & Soble, 2019).

There may be "equivocal zones" on the test—that is, scores that fall between the optimal cut score for identifying valid performance and the optimal cut score for identifying noncredible performance—indicative of neither valid nor invalid performance. On TOMM and Word Choice, these equivocal zones were different for cognitively unimpaired (i.e., TOMM score of 44, Word Choice score of 45 to 46) and cognitively impaired participants (i.e., TOMM score of 41, Word Choice score of 43 to 46; Bain & Soble, 2019).

CLINICAL STUDIES

Looking at multiple ACS PVTs together as described in the manual, failure on a single PVT (defined as a score falling at a ≤10% base rate in the clinical group) is common in several conditions, occurring in about a third or more of moderate to severe TBI, schizophrenia, and autistic disorder, and in two-thirds of persons with mild intellectual disability. Looking at failure on two PVTs defined as a score falling at a 10% or lower base rate, almost all the clinical groups had a low rate of failures, except for intellectual disability; as many as 30% of people with intellectual disabilities failed with this criterion. In contrast, all groups including intellectual disability had a low base rate of having three PVTs with scores falling at the ≤ 10% base rate (manual). Having more than four scores at or below the 10% base rate cutoff was rare in individuals with intellectual disability. More than two scores at or below the 2% base rate is unusual for all the clinical samples including mild intellectual disability—but this strict cutoff will not identify many exaggerators. For comparison, applying a 10% base rate cutoff from the clinical sample, in the nonclinical WMS-IV standardization sample, 7% had one score below the cutoff, but only 1% had two or more scores below the cutoff.

Of note, manual data indicate that reliance on one low ACS score to infer invalid performance is insufficient in several groups, including those with education below 12 years, non-white/non-Asian ethnicity, and IQ below 85 due to the risk of false positives. In contrast, using two low scores appears to be a useful criterion for detecting invalid performance, with a low risk of false positives regardless of education level, ethnicity, or IQ.

There are no studies on Word Choice's capacity to predict malingering based on multidimensional malingering criteria such as the Slick et al. (1999) malingered neurocognitive dysfunction criteria or Bianchini et al.'s malingered pain-related disability criteria (2005). However, a small number of studies have demonstrated the test's ability to predict PVT failure defined as failing two or more PVTs (Tables 15–33 and 15–34). Although not technically equivalent to multidimensional malingering criteria, failure on two or more PVTs is equated with an extremely high probability of malingering in most studies.

Erdodi and colleagues validated Word Choice against a composite PVT estimate comprised of 11 stand-alone and embedded PVTs from a variety of tests, including the FIT, CVLT-II, WMS-IV, WCST, and fluency tasks (Erdodi

TABLE 15–33 Word Choice Classification Accuracy at Cutoffs Yielding Minimum Acceptable Specificities (≥90%) for Prediction of Failure on Two or More PVTs

STUDY	GROUP	CRITERION	N	CUTOFF	SENSITIVITY (%)	SPECIFICITY (%)
Erdodi et al. (2017)	Mixed neuropsychological sample, mostly psychiatric and TBI	Failure on three or more PVTs	202	≤45	41	95
Davis (2014)	Mixed neuropsychological sample, mostly TBI	Failure on two or more PVTs	46	≤45	75	96
				≤43	38	96

NOTE: TBI, traumatic brain injury.

et al., 2017b); noncredible performance was defined as failure on three or more PVTs. A Word Choice cutoff of 45 or less was associated with .41 sensitivity and .95 specificity.

In a mixed sample of mainly TBI patients, a cutoff of 43 or less had a modest sensitivity of .38 at an excellent specificity of .96 in identifying examinees who failed two other PVTs (Davis, 2014), failure on two PVTs being extremely predictive of invalid performance. However, a slightly higher cutoff of 45 had even better prediction. Overall, based on this and on direct comparison to the WMT, Davis (2014) concluded that Word Choice appears useful as an adjunctive PVT, optimally to be used in combination with other PVTs based on the fact that its sensitivity was low compared to other freestanding PVTs, in the range reported for most embedded PVTs.

Similarly, using failure on two PVTs as the criterion for invalid performance in a moderate to severe TBI sample, Miller and colleagues found that, used in combination with the other ACS PVTs consisting of RDS and recognition trials from the WMS-IV Logical Memory, Verbal Paired Associates, and Visual Reproduction, Word Choice showed excellent diagnostic discrimination. Used alone, Word Choice also achieved excellent discrimination, with large effect sizes, but not as large as all five ACS indices combined (Miller et al., 2011). Cross-validation with subgroups from the WMS-IV standardization sample indicated strong support for the five-score model, with lesser results for the use of Word Choice alone (Holdnack et al., 2013).

TABLE 15–34 Word Choice Critical Item (CR) Cutoffs, Sensitivity, and Specificity for Prediction of PVT Failure (≥.90 Specificity)

	CUTOFF (NUMBER OF FAILED ITEMS)	SENSITIVITY (%)	SPECIFICITY (%)
CR-7	≥2	34	99
	≥3	25	99
CR-5	≥1	49	95
	≥2	27	100
	≥3	16	100
CR-3	≥1	40	95
	≥2	22	100
	=3	5	100

NOTE: PVT failure defined as three or more failures on an index comprised of 11 embedded and standalone PVTs. CR-7 = set of 7 critical items; CR-5 = set of 5 critical items; CR-3 = set of 3 critical items.

SOURCE: Adapted from Erdodi et al. (2017a).

There is some evidence that time to completion scores augment clinical prediction. In one study, time to completion of 171 seconds or more was associated with a .49 sensitivity and .93 specificity in detecting PVT failure in a mixed neurological/psychiatric sample, defined as failure on three or more scores on nine PVTs (i.e., FIT, embedded PVTs from the WAIS-IV, WMS-IV, WCST, CVLT-II, RFCT, Animals, and FAS; Erdodi et al., 2017a). Time to completion of 202 seconds or more was associated with a sensitivity of .50 and specificity of .92 using a PVT composite defined as failure on three or more of five PVTs (i.e., recognition memory paradigms from the CVLT-II, RCFT, and WMS-IV Logical Memory, Verbal Paired Associates, and Visual Reproduction). Combining the time-to-completion score with the total score significantly improved prediction; combining accuracy and time to completion (≥171 seconds) was associated with .54 sensitivity and .83 sensitivity for predicting failure on the nine-item PVT index and five-item PVT prediction, respectively, at specificities greater than .90. Using the time score in addition to the total score improved sensitivity by 6%, a non-negligible amount. The authors concluded that a completion time of about three minutes on Word Choice suggests noncredible performance.

The Word Choice critical items also appear of some utility in detection of noncredible performance using multiple PVT failures as the criterion. Failing two items on the CR-7 and one item on either the CR-5 or CR-3 all had adequate specificities at sensitivities greater than .95 at identifying noncredible performance (Table 15–30 and Table 15–34; Erdodi et al., 2017a).

Using group membership as the criterion for validation, a lesser criterion for establishing PVT validity than diagnostic criteria or failure on multiple PVTs, Bashem and colleagues reported that other PVTs markedly outperformed Word Choice in identifying correct group membership for individuals with moderate to severe TBI and simulators coached to feign memory problems. Specifically, the TOMM, MSVT, and CVLT-II Forced Choice were all superior to Word Choice, which had medium effect sizes, in differentiating individuals with TBI from simulators. Using cutoffs from the manual, they found a sensitivity of .41, but a specificity of only .84, which was much lower than those associated with the TOMM and MSVT, both of which had sensitivities of .45 to .50 at specificities greater than .90 (Bashem et al., 2014). Compared to other PVTs such as the TOMM and MSVT, Word Choice had poor classification accuracy, although it surpassed RDS, which had the lowest classification accuracy of all. In particular, Word Choice added little to prediction accuracy if two strong PVTs were already included, particularly when these PVTs were the TOMM and CVLT Forced Choice, but also if these were the TOMM and MSVT. Taking Word Choice as an example, the authors emphasized that in PVT administration, more is not always better, as adding more PVTs with limited prediction value can increase examinee fatigue and needlessly increase false-positive rates while doing little to improve diagnostic accuracy. Note that other researchers have reported excellent prediction at slightly higher cut scores (Table 15–33).

NEUROANATOMICAL CORRELATES AND IMAGING STUDIES

Studies are lacking as of this writing.

COMMENT

Word Choice is a promising choice among PVTs. It is derived from a large clinical sample, and it allows multivariate interpretation of results combining invalid scores using all five ACS validity indicators, a method that is more sophisticated than that provided by most PVTs which tend to rely on a single cutoff score and which have not all been validated for use in combination with other PVTs. In addition, these combined Word Choice/ACS validity indicators provide information on expected base rates by education, ethnicity, and intellectual level, information that is lacking for most PVTs (Nijdam-Jones & Rosenfeld, 2017). As well, Word Choice is still relatively new, and this may be an advantage over other measures such as the TOMM. Because it is not yet widely known in medicolegal settings or on the Internet, it may be less vulnerable to coaching by attorneys (Barhon et al., 2015). These are all clear advantages over other PVTs.

Of note, although the manual provides multiple cutoffs for determining invalidity, the use of the 10% cutoff will be the most useful metric as it minimizes false positives while not being overly restrictive in terms of sensitivity to invalid performance (i.e., specificity of .90 or false-positive rate of 10%). We recommend using the simple guideline of using two ACS PVT scores at the 10% cutoff as the criterion for invalid performance. Alternatively, three or more scores at the 15% clinical base rate may also be considered (Holdnack et al., 2013). Importantly, research is emerging demonstrating the sole use of Word Choice for identifying invalid performance, with excellent sensitivity and specificity using a 15% cutoff score (e.g., Table 15–33; Erdodi et al., 2017b; Davis, 2014). Alternatively, users may select the more extreme 2% cutoff (Holdnack et al., 2013), but this will result in significantly lower sensitivity to invalid performance.

To date, Word Choice cutoffs have not been validated using multidimensional malingering criteria such as those by Slick and colleagues for malingered neurocognitive disorder (Slick et al., 1999) or by Bianchini and colleagues for malingered pain-related disability (Bianchini et al., 2005), unlike some PVTs reviewed in this volume. Holdnack et al. (2013) do provide guidelines on how to use the ACS tests to detect malingering as per Slick et al. (1999) criteria. Although validated in independent research using multiple PVT failures as the criterion, Word Choice needs clinical research on its sensitivity and specificity to malingering defined by accepted and commonly used criteria. Additionally, no universally accepted cut score for the test has been established across clinical groups (Bain & Soble, 2019), but this will likely emerge as the test continues to be increasingly used in the field.

Because the user chooses the cutoff for invalidity, interpretation can be confusing for those not familiar with the concept of using cumulative percentages to identify suspect scores; there is no defined, one-size-fits-all cutoff for invalidity as is the case for most other PVTs. Essentially, the total Word Choice score is interpreted by comparing the obtained score to the overall base rate of the score in a clinical sample according to five possible specific base rates (i.e., ≤25%, ≤15%, ≤10%, ≤5%, and ≤2%). The user is instructed to decide a priori which of these cutoffs will be used to determine invalidity, and the number of unusually low scores defined by this cutoff is then examined across the five PVTs provided by the ACS to provide an overall base rate of low scores. Although this is a very logical, theoretically sound method, it is at times difficult for the average user to rapidly grasp how the test works. For some clinicians, this may be too many choices and too much complexity; as already noted, we recommend simply using the 10% or less cutoff and requiring failure on two ACS PVTs to infer invalid performance.

Detailed interpretive guidelines that would assist the user are provided in an additional Technical manual provided only in electronic format, separate from the Administration Manual provided in the test kit. Although this comprises a relatively minor, more logistical than clinical barrier to interpretation, it does reduce the likelihood that some users will take the time to fully understand how the test works. Of note, although a priori—not post hoc—selection of cutoffs for invalidity is recommended (Holdnack et al., 2013), the test's provision of all possible base rates at all cutoffs may raise the risk of post hoc cherry-picking of cutoffs according to conscious or unconscious examiner biases. On the other hand, the wealth of data available does provide rich detail for advanced users who may welcome the availability of multiple, different cutoffs for different clinical and research scenarios.

As noted by the test authors, using a single score such the Word Choice Total score to determine invalidity carries an unacceptably high risk of false positives, particularly in some ethnic and educational subgroups and in some clinical conditions. Others have also concluded that the test should not be used alone as an indicator of validity (Bashem et al., 2014; Davis, 2014), particularly due to its relatively low sensitivity (Erdodi et al., 2014). This guideline also applies to most PVTs reviewed in this volume.

With regard to influence of bona fide cognitive deficits on performance, the test authors recommend that for low-functioning examinees, the most restrictive cutoffs be used, with multiple failed indicators needed for invalidity. However, a more effective strategy to avoid false positives would be to avoid administering the test to examinees with major cognitive impairments such as dementia and moderate intellectual disability, as would be recommended for most PVTs. Word Choice is not robust against cognitive impairment, but this is also true of most PVTs; Word Choice may be more prone to effects of cognitive impairment than other PVTs such as the TOMM, at least in the one study that examined this question, but further comparative research is needed to confirm this.

Word Choice is very similar to already existing PVTs, most obviously the Words subtest of the WRMT, in its number of items, stimulus type, and response format, although Word Choice differs in difficulty level (easier) and sensitivity to invalid performance (lower).

Although there is some research on TBI, additional validation in other clinical groups where performance validity is a concern is needed, including military samples, criminal defendants, disability claimants, and clinical groups known to have high base rates of malingering (e.g., ADHD, chronic pain, somatoform disorders). More studies involving honestly responding clinical groups are also needed, including neurological and psychiatric patients. Similarly, the test is in need of studies on correlations with other neuropsychological tests and with SVTs such as the MMPI-2/MMPI-2-RF, in particular.

Last, as the authors note, Word Choice and other ACS indicators are only designed to detect invalid performance, not whether the examinee provided their best effort or best performance (Holdnack et al., 2013). The term "suboptimal effort" in the manual has been replaced by the terms "invalid performance" and "negative bias" in more recent work by the test authors to better describe what the tests actually measures (Holdnack et al., 2013).

REFERENCES

Bain, K. M., & Soble, J. R. (2019). Validation of the Advanced Clinical Solutions Word Choice Test (WCT) in a mixed clinical sample: Establishing classification accuracy, sensitivity/specificity, and cutoff scores. *Assessment, 26*(7), 1320–1328. 1073191117725172. https://doi.org/10.1177/1073191117725172

Barhon, L. I., Batchelor, J., Meares, S., Chekaluk, E., & Shores, E. A. (2015). A comparison of the degree of effort involved in the TOMM and the ACS Word Choice Test using a dual-task paradigm. *Applied Neuropsychology. Adult, 22*(2), 114–123. https://doi.org/10.1080/23279095.2013.863775

Bashem, J. R., Rapport, L. J., Miller, J. B., Hanks, R. A., Axelrod, B. N., & Millis, S. R. (2014). Comparisons of five performance validity indices in bona fide and simulated traumatic brain injury. *The Clinical Neuropsychologist, 28*(5), 851–875. https://doi.org/10.1080/13854046.2014.927927

Bianchini, K. J., Greve, K. W., & Glynn, G. (2005). On the diagnosis of malingered pain-related disability: Lessons from cognitive malingering research. *The Spine Journal, 5*(4), 404–417. https://doi.org/10.1016/j.spinee.2004.11.016

Davis, J. J. (2014). Further consideration of Advanced Clinical Solutions Word Choice: comparison to the Recognition Memory Test-words and classification accuracy in a clinical sample. *The Clinical Neuropsychologist, 28*(8), 1278–1294. https://doi.org/10.1080/13854046.2014.975844

Erdodi, L. A., Kirsch, N. L., Lajiness-O'Neill, R., Vingilis, E., & Medoff, B. (2014). Comparing the Recognition Memory Test and the Word Choice Test in a mixed clinical sample: Are they equivalent? *Psychological Injury and Law, 7*(3), 255–263.

Erdodi, L. A., Tyson, B. T., Abeare, C. A., Zuccato, B. G., Rai, J. K., Seke, K. R., . . . Roth, R. M. (2017b). Utility of critical items within the Recognition Memory Test and Word Choice Test. *Applied Neuropsychology. Adult,* 1–13. https://doi.org/10.1080/23279095.2017.1298600

Erdodi, L. A., Tyson, B. T., Shahein, A. G., Lichtenstein, J. D., Abeare, C. A., Pelletier, C. L., . . . Roth, R. M. (2017a). The power of timing: Adding a time-to-completion cutoff to the Word Choice Test and Recognition Memory Test improves classification accuracy. *Journal of Clinical and Experimental Neuropsychology, 39*(4), 369–383. https://doi.org/10.1080/13803395.2016.1230181

Holdnack, J. A., Millis, S., Larrabee, G. J., & Iverson, G. L. (2013). Assessing performance validity with the ACS. In J. A. Holdnack, L. W. Drozdick, L. G. Weiss, & G. L. Iverson (Eds.), *WAIS-IV, WMS-IV, and ACS: Advanced clinical interpretation* (pp. 331–365). New York: Elsevier.

Larrabee, G. J. (2014). False-positive rates associated with the use of multiple performance and symptom validity tests. *Archives of Clinical Neuropsychology, 29*(4), 364–373. https://doi.org/10.1093/arclin/acu019

Miller, J. B., Millis, S. R., Rapport, L. J., Bashem, J. R., Hanks, R. A., & Axelrod, B. N. (2011). Detection of insufficient effort using the Advanced Clinical Solutions for the Wechsler Memory Scale, Fourth Edition. *The Clinical Neuropsychologist, 25*(1), 160–172. https://doi.org/10.1080/13854046.2010.533197

Nijdam-Jones, A., & Rosenfeld, B. (2017). Cross-cultural feigning assessment: A systematic review of feigning instruments used with linguistically, ethnically, and culturally diverse samples. *Psychological Assessment, 29*(11), 1321–1336. https://doi.org/10.1037/pas0000438

Pearson. (2009a). *Advanced Clinical Solutions for WAIS-IV and WMS-IV: Clinical and interpretive manual.* San Antonio, TX: Pearson.

Pearson. (2009b). *Advanced Clinical Solutions for WAIS-IV and WMS-IV: Technical manual.* San Antonio, TX: Pearson.

Slick, D. J., Sherman, E. M., & Iverson, G. L. (1999). Diagnostic criteria for malingered neurocognitive dysfunction: proposed standards for clinical practice and research. *The Clinical Neuropsychologist, 13*(4), 545–561. https://doi.org/10.1076/1385-4046(199911)13:04;1-Y;FT545

Wechsler, D. (2009). *Technical and interpretive manual for the Wechsler Memory Scale* (4th ed.). San Antonio, TX: Pearson.

WORD MEMORY TEST (WMT)

TEST NAME	**Word Memory Test (WMT)**
DOMAIN	Performance validity
AGE RANGE	In healthy adults, norms up to age 80; higher age ranges in clinical groups
ADMINISTRATION TIME	20 minutes
SCORING FORMAT	Computerized
REFERENCE	Green, P. (2003). *Green's Word Memory Test for Microsoft Windows.* Edmonton, AB, Canada: Green's Publishing. www.wordmemorytest.com

DESCRIPTION

The Word Memory Test (WMT; Green, 2003) is a PVT designed to measure exaggeration and feigning of memory complaints. The WMT is widely used, second only to the TOMM in popularity. Like all PVTs, its usage among neuropsychologists has increased steadily over time; ranked as being used often by 16% of respondents in 2007 (Sharland & Gfeller, 2007), it is now used by 58% of North-American neuropsychologists and 48% of neuropsychologists in forensic practice (LaDuke et al., 2017), and it is the third-most often used PVT by neuropsychologists in the veterans' healthcare system after the TOMM and FIT (Young et al., 2016). It has had some penetrance in Europe as well, but PVT usage there remains comparatively lower overall (Dandachi-FitzGerald et al., 2013).

Details on administration, items, and format will not be provided to preserve test security. Please see original source for details. Briefly, the WMT provides two kinds of scores: (1) Effort scores (performance validity scores) and (2) Memory scores. Performance validity is assessed with the Immediate Recognition (IR) and Delayed Recognition (DR) subtests, and with the Consistency (CNS) score, defined as the consistency of responses across the two recognition trials (IR and DR), expressed as a percentage. Failure is defined according to specific cutoff values. The performance validity subtests are followed by memory subtests intended to be sensitive to verbal memory impairment. These include Multiple Choice (MC), Paired Associates (PA), Free Recall (FR), and Long Delayed Free Recall (LDFR) subtests. In all, three performance validity scores (IR, DR, CNS) and four memory scores (MC, PA, FR, LDFR) are generated by the test. These scores and their abbreviations are also presented in Table 15–35.

The WMT subtests have differing levels of subtest difficulty that produce a characteristic pattern of scores in honest responders; deviations from this pattern increase the index of suspicion for invalid performance. The Genuine Memory Impairment Profile (GMIP) is a three-part algorithm used to determine valid and invalid responding in those with cognitive deficits. Details of this process will not be provided here to protect test security but can be found in the manual.

Originally published in 2003, the manual was revised somewhat in 2005 to expand the number of comparison groups; the test structure remains the same. The test is available in a number of languages, including English, German, Dutch, Spanish, Turkish, Russian, Hebrew, Danish, Portuguese, and French (see manual and Merten et al., 2009, for more details on the German version).

Importantly, the manual has a section instructing users how to describe WMT results in their reports; this includes protecting the integrity of the test by not naming the test specifically as a PVT, not describing in detail the rationale for WMT interpretation, and not including score graphs in the examinee's report, which is a general recommendation that should apply to all PVTs.

ADMINISTRATION

See manual for details. The WMT is administered via computer. The test can be successfully completed by examinees with a Grade 3 reading level (Green & Flaro, 2003). When taking the WMT, examinees are given assistance with reading and understanding the task instructions as needed. If there is a question about reading ability, the examiner

TABLE 15–35 Word Memory Test (WMT) Scores and Abbreviations

Effort Scores	IR	Immediate Recognition
	DR	Delayed Recognition
	CNS	Consistency
Memory Scores	MC	Multiple Choice
	PA	Paired Associates
	FR	Free Recall
	LDFR	Long Delayed Free Recall
Profile Analysis	GMIP	Genuine Memory Impairment Profile

can ask the examinee to say each word aloud as it appears (Green, 2003). If there is an error, the examiner corrects the word immediately. If the examinee is expected to have difficulty on the computerized task (e.g., reading difficulty, visual difficulties), the test can be given orally, but this is not the recommended procedure (Green & Flaro, 2015).

The manual indicates that, for most adults, it is not necessary to stay in the room for the list presentation and that, in fact, once the person has responded several times on IR, whether right or wrong, the examiner is instructed to leave the room and then to re-enter the room to administer other nonverbal-memory tasks while awaiting the DR subtest, to occur 30 minutes later. The manual indicates that all normative data with adults were gathered by leaving the person unattended during the IR and DR subtests. The examiner is permitted to stay in the room if the examinee is very young or elderly, with interventions kept at a minimum. The remainder of the instructions are described in the manual.

One small study in adults with ADHD suggests that not having the examiner in the room may lead to higher failure rates compared to when the examiner is present, possibly due to an observer effect (Sullivan et al., 2007). Other studies have described administering the test with the examiner in the room and controlling the mouse in individuals with suspected MCI or dementia (Green et al., 2011), but standard administration has also been used with these patients too (Robinson et al., 2018).

SCORING

The computer program indicates whether the test is valid or invalid by indicating whether the results were a clear pass, clear fail, or a result in between, according to whether the examinee's scores on one out of the three Effort scores were below a specific cutoff (see manual for specific cutoff). The scoring printout shows the examinee's results graphically (e.g., percentage correct for each subtest, number of standard deviations above or below the mean compared to a reference group) and as a list of raw scores on all measures. Tables are provided so that scores can be compared with the mean scores obtained from each of a number of reference groups, including patients with moderate to severe brain injury, neurological patients, patients with normal verbal memory, patients with impaired verbal memory, and healthy controls.

The program flags low scores, alerting the examiner that if the examinee has severe cognitive impairment or dementia, interpretation using the GMIP process is recommended (details in manual). Notably, failing on Effort tests does not automatically indicate an invalid profile; rather, this is determined via profile analysis of multiple scores via the GMIP. Specific formulas have been derived to do this that will not be discussed here for security purposes other than to say that the determination is based on the overall profile of scores across all subtests (Effort and Memory scores) according to specific algorithms. Specifically, when an examinee fails the test, a second set of criteria are examined to determine whether the failure was due to noncredible performance or to severe cognitive impairment (i.e., to a GMIP; see manual).

Advanced interpretation is provided by the computerized Advanced Interpretation Program for the test. Compared to the standard program, the Advanced Interpretation Program updates the interpretation rules and provides new comparison groups; it also directs users to apply Criterion D of the Slick, Sherman, and Iverson malingering criteria (Slick et al., 1999) to the determination of whether examinees meet the GMIP (P. Green, personal communication, May 2018). According to the test author, Criterion D of the Slick criteria must be applied to correctly use the GMIP. Criterion D specifies that invalid performance cannot be fully accounted for by psychiatric, developmental, or neurological disorders that result in significantly diminished capacity to appreciate laws or mores against malingering or inability to conform behavior to such standards. Based on this rationale, by definition, any independently functioning examinee failing the Effort tests and yielding a GMIP profile on Memory tests would be ineligible for the GMIP and would therefore be deemed as providing noncredible performance. However, the manual does not specify this criterion, and so it is unclear if this important distinction is obvious to all users.

Using the GMIP algorithm, scores that do not fit the expected profile of people with cognitive impairment are deemed invalid (i.e., due to noncredible responding), whereas scores that fit the pattern expected in cognitive impairment are considered a reliable reflection of neurological compromise rather than feigning or exaggeration. Based on this, the WMT can therefore yield three kinds of results: (1) passing all Effort tests (credible responding), (2) failing Effort tests and not meeting criteria for cognitive impairment according to profile analysis (noncredible responding), and (3) failing Effort tests but meeting criteria for cognitive impairment based on profile analysis and therefore meeting criteria for the GMIP (credible responding with Effort score failure attributed to a known neurological condition; Reslan & Axelrod, 2017).

Of note, response time measurement may have promise in increasing the detection of feigning on the WMT (Nijdam-Jones & Rosenfeld, 2017), although more research on this scoring method is needed before it can be applied clinically.

DEMOGRAPHIC EFFECTS

AGE

According to the test author, Effort scores on the WMT appear largely invariant to demographic effects, including age (Green, 2003; Green et al., 2002; Green et al., 2011).

However, in healthy adults, Rienstra et al. (2009) found mild age effects on the Effort scores. Most studies note that age is associated with the Memory scores, as would be expected if they tap verbal memory (Green, 2003). Although the healthy sample in the manual has few individuals older than age 60, memory scores were noted to decrease with age in a healthy Dutch and Canadian combined sample with age extending to 80 years (*rs* = –.32 to –.38; Rienstra et al., 2009). Green, Montijo, and Brockhaus (2011) likewise reported that in patients with possible or probable dementia, age correlated with Memory scores to a moderate degree (*r* = –.26 to –.34), as it did in a possible MCI subsample (*r* = –.28 to –.33).

GENDER

Most studies indicate that gender does not impact performance (Green et al., 2002; Martins & Martins, 2010; Rienstra et al., 2009). One study in a large military sample found that all females passed the WMT but 27% of males failed it (McCormick et al., 2013), which may have more to do with the sample than with the WMT as other military studies have found no gender effects (Armistead-Jehle & Buican, 2012; Russo, 2012).

EDUCATION AND IQ

Although the author notes that education does not influence scores (Green, 2003; Green et al., 2002), other studies report otherwise. Rienstra et al. (2009) found education effects for both Effort and Memory scores up to the moderate range (*r* = .16 to .31) and that, overall, age and education explained about 20% of the variance on WMT memory scores. Education was also moderately related to FR in one study on neurological patients (Davis & Wall, 2014), which makes sense for a memory score.

Consistent with an education effect, Memory scores are significantly related to reading level (*r* = .40 to .61, Green & Flaro, 2003). According to the author, with regard to reading level, having a specific reading disability does not, in itself, affect WMT performance as long as the individual's reading level is above Grade 2 (Green & Flaro, 2003).

Findings regarding the Effort scores and IQ are mixed; although the author reports no association with IQ, most PVTs have significant correlations with IQ; evidence from a small ADHD study indicates significant correlations with DR and CNS (*r* = .38 to .45; Sullivan et al., 2007; see "Clinical Studies" for more discussion of IQ effects). Memory scores do increase with increasing verbal IQ, as would be expected (Green, 2003).

ETHNICITY, NATIONALITY, AND LINGUISTIC EFFECTS

The test is available in a number of languages and has been used cross-culturally in a number of simulations studies (see manual); there is also a study by the author on a Portuguese version in a clinical sample with memory impairment (Green et al., 2011). Independent studies also support its use in diverse groups. In direct comparison a similar pattern of performance of Dutch and Canadian samples has been described (Rienstra et al., 2009). In a US sample, no ethnicity effects were observed in a large military sample with more than 35% minority status (McCormick et al., 2013). In addition, the test has also been used in Spanish, Dutch, and German studies, among others (e.g., Brooks et al., 2012; Gorissen et al., 2005; Merten et al., 2009). One study found worse WMT performance in Spanish speakers with fibromyalgia compared to English speakers, with a failure rate of 56% versus 32%, respectively (Brooks et al., 2012); higher failures rates in some minority groups have been reported for other PVTs (see "Word Choice," for example).

NORMATIVE DATA

Interpretation of the WMT is based on specific cutoffs defining passing or failing the test. Cutoffs were initially set at the 2nd percentile relative to 157 patients with moderate to severe head injury or other neurological disorders, after excluding 10% of individuals in whom there was strong independent evidence of invalid performance (e.g., worse than chance scores on other tests; Green & Flaro, 2003). Cutoffs were subsequently increased (Green, 2003) based on data showing that healthy adult controls obtain perfect scores on the WMT (Iverson et al., 1999) and that nearly perfect scores are obtained in adults and children with neurological disease or intellectual disability. Accordingly, Green recommended that scores below specific cutoffs on the Effort subtests should raise concerns about invalid performance, with rare exceptions such as in people with dementia who need 24-hour care or in very young children with less than Grade 3 reading level, equivalent to the 5th percentile of people with severe brain injuries or neurological disease (manual). With regard to the Memory trials, Green (2003) indicates that, although MC and PA can be affected by actual neurological impairment, they are fairly easy to complete correctly even for those with severe brain injuries.

Although not designed to provide norm-referenced scores, the test manual includes a small sample of healthy people that can be used for comparison, in addition to comparison to numerous clinical samples. These were 40 healthy volunteers who responded to a general advertisement in a restaurant in Edmonton, Alberta (Green, 2003; Rienstra et al., 2009). Each received a free lunch for participating; the mean age was 36.7 (*SD* = 11.4) with a range of 16 to 68 years; mean education was 14.6 years (*SD* = 1.7) with a range from 10 to 16 years, and the sample was 55% female. No information is provided on ethnicity, but this is presumed to be a mainly Caucasian sample given its city of origin. The sample is also described as employed and as slightly brighter than average with a mean estimated IQ of 110 based on WAIS-R Vocabulary of 11.8 (*SD* = 3.9).

Norm-based data would be particularly useful for validating Memory scores. Rienstra et al. (2009) provide reference data for the WMT on 155 individuals comprised of 110 Dutch individuals combined with the original sample of 40 healthy Canadians described in the manual. The sample was stratified to represent gender, age, and education levels. Three age groups range from 20 to 40, 41 to 65, and 66 to 80, with an average age of 49.8 years (*SD* = 18.4). The Dutch sample had an average education level of 13.9 years (*SD* = 3.3) and was 53% female. Participants with psychiatric, neurologic, substance abuse, or developmental disorders were excluded, as were those who failed the WMT. Education was defined according to three levels corresponding to primary education (*M* = 9.5, *SD* = .90), average junior vocational training (*M* = 13.5, *SD* = .90), and senior vocational or academic education (*M* = 17.7, *SD* = 1.5). Note that the Dutch sample was tested in their homes by an examiner; whether the examiner followed the standard procedure (i.e., leaving the room during test administration) is not specified.

These data are provided in Table 15–36 according to age and education. Regression equations to calculate standard scores for FR and LDFR corrected for age and education are provided in Figure 15–1. Overall, visual inspection suggests a gradient of performance consistent with data from the manual, with Effort scores highest and the more challenging Memory tests comparatively lower. Importantly, some concerns have been raised about the adequacy of these norms with regard to producing appropriate age-corrected memory scores. Using these norms, 40% of individuals with normal memory based on CVLT-II produced WMT Memory age-corrected scores in the impaired range (Davis & Wall, 2014).

WMT data on a Portuguese version for a small sample of 27 mostly highly-educated, healthy adults with a mean age of 32 years (*SD* = 2.8) are shown in Table 15–37. Normative data from other countries and languages would be of benefit for validating the Memory scores.

In addition to these data, the test provides comparison data to 1,250 patients in the author's practice and 1,244 in a colleague's practice, also in Edmonton, Canada (Green, 2003), in addition to multiple other datasets of various patients and conditions which presumably continue to accrue over time as the test is used in more samples. Accordingly, comparisons to appropriate clinical groups can be done by selecting appropriate comparison groups from the wide variety available through the scoring program and by referring to the test manual. Scores are also provided by age and verbal IQ in the manual.

Of note, some have noted that clinical cases used as comparison data are not equivalent to normative data collected from individuals who have been screened for neurologic, medical, and psychiatric conditions (Davis, 2014); comprehensive norms have therefore been recommended for the test, particularly for the memory scores, which are subject to age and education effects (Soble et al., 2016).

EVIDENCE FOR RELIABILITY

EVIDENCE FOR INTERNAL RELIABILITY

To our knowledge, this is not available for the English-language version, but a Portuguese translation had very high internal consistency (alpha = .95; Martins & Martins, 2010).

EVIDENCE FOR TEST-RETEST RELIABILITY

In a study of 20 healthy individuals tested at various sites and with various test-retest intervals ranging from one day to one week, the mean score of all three WMT Effort trials had extremely high reliability (r = .97); MC and PA test-retest reliability was also extremely high (r = .99), as was FR reliability (r = .92; Manual).

EVIDENCE FOR VALIDITY

WITHIN-TEST CORRELATIONS

WMT scores correlate strongly with one another. Green (2003) reported that in 1,207 consecutive outpatients, correlations were very high between IR and DR (r = .88),

TABLE 15–36 Means and Standard Deviations (*SDs*) for Word Memory Test (WMT) Subtests by Age and Education (*N* = 155)

LEVEL OF EDUCATION	AGE	IR	DR	CNS	MC	PA	FR	LDFR
Low	20 to 40	98.4 (2.2)	98.4 (2.3)	97.2 (3.6)	91.3 (6.4)	88.3 (9.4)	65.3 (9.4)	62.8 (22.5)
	41 to 65	97.1 (4.1)	98.6 (3.2)	96.7 (4.2)	88.5 (11.6)	82.0 (17.2)	65.6 (17.7)	60.0 (15.9)
	66 to 80	97.5 (2.2)	97.2 (2.5)	95.0 (3.5)	80.0 (12.3)	78.3 (12.1)	50.9 (8.5)	53.1 (9.7)
Average	20 to 40	98.3 (2.7)	98.4 (2.9)	98.2 (3.2)	94.8 (7.3)	92.5 (10.5)	65.5 (16.4)	67.3 (16.9)
	41 to 65	98.0 (2.9)	97.8 (2.8)	95.5 (4.4)	89.1 (8.3)	87.1 (10.4)	56.8 (12.5)	59.5 (16.1)
	66 to 80	96.3 (4.2)	98.0 (2.9)	95.3 (4.7)	87.3 (13.6)	85.0 (14.4)	57.6 (15.9)	57.7 (15.2)
High	20 to 40	99.7 (.82)	99.3 (1.3)	98.8 (1.9)	97.6 (3.5)	97.2 (3.3)	78.4 (12.2)	81.6 (11.8)
	41 to 65	98.8 (2.1)	99.2 (1.4)	99.7 (.85)	96.6 (5.5)	94.8 (6.2)	68.2 (11.2)	71.5 (9.0)
	66 to 80	96.6 (4.4)	96.1 (4.7)	95.8 (5.1)	82.5 (16.7)	81.3 (20.1)	54.5 (13.9)	55.3 (18.5)

SOURCE: Rienstra et al. (2009).

(1) Standard scores FR subset

$$\text{Expected FR score} = 59.4 - 0.31 \times \text{age} + 1.4 \times \text{education}$$

$$\text{T-score FR} = 50 + 10 \times \frac{\text{observed FR} - \text{expected FR}}{\text{SEE}}$$

$$\text{T-score FR} = 50 + 10 \times \frac{\text{observed FR} - (59.4 - 0.31 \times \text{age} + 1.4 \times \text{education})}{13.7}$$

(2) Standard scores LDFR

$$\text{Expected LDFR score} = 51.2 - 0.37 \times \text{age} + 1.76 \times \text{education} + 4.78 \times \text{gender}$$

$$\text{T-score LDFR} = 50 + 10 \times \frac{\text{observed LDFR} - \text{expected LDFR}}{\text{SEE}}$$

$$\text{T-score FR} = 50 + 10 \times \frac{\text{observed LDFR} - (51.2 - 0.37 \times \text{age} + 1.76 \times \text{education} + 4.78 \times \text{gender})}{14.9}$$

N.B. Education = years of full-time formal education.

Figure 15–1 *Regression formulas to calculate age- and education-corrected standard scores for the WMT.*
SOURCE: Reproduced with permission from Rienstra et al. (2009).

MC and PA (*r* = .90), and FR and LDFR (*r* = .86). IR, DR, and CNS also correlate highly in other samples such as mild TBI (*r* = .74 to .92; Heyanka et al., 2015).

FACTOR-ANALYTIC STUDIES

There are few factor-analytic studies on the WMT. In one study, WMT Effort variables loaded separately from CVLT-II memory variables, forming a PVT factor with the TOMM; CVLT-II Forced Choice, an embedded PVT, loaded with other CVLT-II variables but not with the WMT or TOMM (Heyanka et al., 2015). To our knowledge, there are no factor-analytic studies of the WMT Memory subtests with other memory tests.

TABLE 15–37 Word Memory Test (WMT) Means and Standard Deviations (*SDs*) for a Primarily University-Educated Portuguese Sample

	MEAN	*SD*
IR	97.3	4.3
DR	99.1	3.4
CNS	97.1	5.0
MC	90.5	14.0
PA	85.3	21.8
FR	72.3	16.8

NOTE: *N* = 29. Demographic characteristics as follows: male:female ratio = 1:2.2, education = less than 6 years (10%), 7–11 years (7%), 12 years (7%), University (72%), Master's degree (3%).

SOURCE: Adapted from Martins & Martins (2010).

CORRELATIONS WITH OTHER PVTs

Overall, WMT Effort scores are highly related to those of other stand-alone PVTs. This includes moderate to high correlations with the TOMM in a variety of samples (e.g., >.68, Green, 2007; Green et al., 1997; .64 to .75, Heyanka et al., 2015; Merten et al., 2007) and high correlations with the CARB, ASTM, and 21-Item Test.

Correlations with embedded PVTs are less strong than those for standalone PVTs, but still substantial in most cases. With regard to embedded PVTs, Effort scores on the WMT are moderately correlated with CVLT-II Forced Choice scores (*r* = .47 to .55, Heyanka et al., 2015). Similarly, WMT IR and DR are highly correlated with List Recognition, a component of the RBANS Effort Index, an embedded PVT (*r* = .66). Smaller correlations are found with RBANS Digit Span, also a component of the Effort Index (*r* = .21 to .23; Young et al., 2012). Modest to moderate correlations are found with Reliable Digit Span (*r* = .24 to .28, Merten et al., 2007, 2009).

In ADHD, WMT CNS correlates moderately with multiple other PVTs, with correlations ranging from .34 to .36 with Dot Counting and Reliable Digit Span, but not with CVLT Forced Choice (Marshall et al., 2010). In a college simulation sample, standalone PVTs such as the FIT as well as other tests used as PVTs such as Finger Tapping and Digit Span were correlated with WMT Effort scores, but also subtantially with WMT Memory scores (*r* = .35 to .66 and *r* = .21 to .63, respectively, Demakis et al., 2015).

SENSITIVITY VERSUS OTHER PVTS

There is a large body of independent literature demonstrating that the WMT is more sensitive to invalid performance than other PVTs. Although this literature is quite compelling, some have noted that there may be methodological issues at play and that the test's high sensitivity may come at the cost of too many false positives.

In addition to studies by the test author, independent studies show superior WMT sensitivity across clinical groups, including studies in litigants and disability claimants, military samples, TBI, ADHD, and PTSD, among others. For example, the WMT yielded more below-chance scores than the TOMM in a private practice sample of 1,032 examinees with mild TBI, toxic exposure, and chronic pain (Greve et al., 2009). In a mixed litigation and disability sample, WMT failure rate was 45%, equivalent to the VSVT but higher than the TOMM at 18% (Miele et al., 2012). In active-duty military personnel, the WMT detected many more instances of noncredible performance compared to the ACS (38% vs. only 6%; Armistead-Jehle & Buican, 2013). In a study in criminal defendants, the WMT had better predictive accuracy for malingering than the VIP (Fazio & Denney, 2018). In malingered ADHD, the WMT had better prediction accuracy than stand-alone PVTs such as the b Test and Dot Counting, as well as embedded PVTs from the Conners CPT, RDS, and CVLT-II Forced Choice, with 64% sensitivity at a specificity 90% or greater (Marshall et al., 2010). In alleged PTSD, the WMT identified many more people than did the RDS (51% vs. 23%, Merten et al., 2009). Last, Mossman, Wygant, and Gervais (2012) reported that Bayesian estimates using Monte Carlo methods suggested the WMT had the best classification accuracy when compared to the CARB and TOMM (WMT = .93, CARB = .77, and TOMM = .77). If false-positive rates were held constant at .02, true-positive rates remained highest for the WMT (WMT = 65%, CARB = 35%, and TOMM = 49%).

Importantly, Greiffenstein and colleagues concluded that there are methodological issues in comparative research on WMT sensitivity because of asymmetrical concordance analyses—for example, defining WMT failure as failure on one out of three Effort scores while defining TOMM failure otherwise (e.g., one out of one score), therefore biasing sensitivity estimates in favor of the WMT. Specifically, they compared failure rates using equivalent criteria on the WMT and TOMM (i.e., failure on any one of three scores). Using the same failure criteria, the WMT and TOMM yielded similar failure rates in a sample of 473 compensation-seeking persons with remote neurologic trauma (Greiffenstein et al., 2008). Similarly, there are differences in how other PVTs define failure, which may affect equivalence; for example, ACS failure may be defined as two or more failures on a possible five tests using a 10% base rate level, while WMT failure rests on failure on one of three possible scores (see the review of Word Choice elsewhere in this chapter).

With regard to false positives, a meta-analysis indicated that the WMT, like other PVTs, is associated with large effect sizes and excellent sensitivity to feigning (.75; Sollman & Berry, 2011) but has lower specificity than other PVTs such as the TOMM (.69 vs. .94), with a mean false-positive rate of about 30% compared to less than 10% for other PVTs.

CORRELATIONS WITH AND COMPARISONS TO SVTS AND OTHER QUESTIONNAIRES

The WMT appears to have modest to high associations with SVTs that measure exaggeration of psychopathology depending on whether psychopathology is part of the exaggeration profile of the particular examinee group. In feigned ADHD, the WMT clearly outperforms SVTs in the identification of malingerers.

In veterans, correlations between the WMT and MMPI-2 validity indices are modest, ranging from .20 for RBS and F, and .16 for FBS, even though the RBS in particular was developed based on prediction of failure on one of three PVTs, one of which was the WMT. Notably, the WMT was not correlated with the HHI (Young et al., 2011), an MMPI-2 SVT based on Slick malingering criteria (see the reviews of MMPI-2 and MMPI-2-RF in Chapter 16).

With regard to psychopathology, an association has been reported between failure on the WMT and over-reporting of symptoms (Gervais et al., 2001), which may underlie purported relationships between depression and WMT failure. Accordingly, patients who fail the WMT appear more likely to produce elevated complaints of subjective distress, as indexed by the MMPI-2 (Williamson et al., 2003). In alleged PTSD, the WMT is fairly highly correlated with two well-known SVTs designed to detect exaggeration of psychopathology, the SIMS and the MENT ($r = -.49$ and $-.66$, respectively). Both the WMT and the SIMS have equivalent fail rates of 51% in this population, with MENT fail rates slightly lower at 40% (Merten et al., 2009). In alleged PTSD, lower WMT scores are correlated with higher psychological symptoms as measured by the SCL-90-R ($r = -.54$; Merten et al., 2009). In a study on college simulators, WMT scores were modestly related to a measure of psychopathy (Demakis et al., 2015).

There are few studies on the relationship between the WMT and pain scales, but in fibromyalgia, WMT IR, DR, and CNS scores are moderately related to MCMI-III Debasement, a validity scale measuring exaggeration of symptoms ($r = -.42$ to $.43$; Brooks et al., 2012). In this population, WMT is also related to Somatoform, Depression, Dysthymia, and Anxiety scales.

In ADHD, the WMT outperforms other SVTs but does have some common variance with SVTs. In malingered ADHD, the WMT detects more malingerers than questionnaire-based exaggeration scales for ADHD (i.e., the Clinical Assessment of Attention Deficit Disorder—Adult Infrequency scale; Marshall et al., 2010). In adults seen for suspected ADHD, WMT failure is associated with elevations on a validity index from the Conners Adult ADHD Rating Scale (CAARS; Cook et al., 2016), and those who fail the WMT report higher ADHD symptoms as measured by the CAARS, indicating that ADHD evaluations should always include a PVT such as the WMT to rule out exaggeration (Sullivan et al., 2007). In ADHD, WMT failure is not related to MMPI-2-RF or PAI scales designed to detect exaggeration (FBS and NIM, respectively; Cook et al., 2016; Sullivan et al., 2007), consistent with the view that most existing SVTs have poor sensitivity for detecting feigned ADHD.

CORRELATIONS WITH OTHER NEUROPSYCHOLOGICAL TESTS

PVTs should be as insensitive as possible to actual cognitive impairment. Studies from the author demonstrate that WMT Effort trials are very easy even for adults with significant neurological impairment (e.g., moderate to severe head injury, MS, tumor, ADHD, conduct disorder; Green & Flaro, 2003; Green et al., 1999, 2001, 2002; Williamson et al., 2003). A mixed clinical sample described in the manual also performed well on Effort subtests despite poor scores on the CVLT. Data presented essentially suggest a ceiling or near-ceiling effect on scores sensitive to performance validity in both patients and controls.

Generally speaking, it is well established that PVT failure is related to performance on other tests. Accordingly, the more poorly examinees perform on the WMT, the lower their CVLT LDFR scores (manual). Similarly, examinees who fail the WMT have been shown to have lower performance on neuropsychological tests (Armistead-Jehle & Buican, 2012; see review by Armistead-Jehle & Green, 2016; Lange et al., 2012; Strauss et al., 2015; Suhr et al., 2011), including the TMT, WRMT, Category Test, and Finger Tapping Test (manual; note that some of these tests are also used as PVTs). For example, in a sample of service members, examinees who failed the WMT performed worse than those who passed, with small effect sizes for visual and verbal reasoning, but large effect sizes for attention, motor skills, processing speed, and memory (Armistead-Jehle & Buican, 2012). Low scores on the WMT therefore are associated with a general suppression of test scores, in particular learning and memory tests (Gervais et al., 2001, 2004; Green & Flaro, 2003; Green et al., 2001, 2002), but other domains are also affected (e.g., smell identification, Green et al., 2003; mood, Rohling et al., 2002; see Green, 2007, for a review). Therefore, failure on the WMT validity components suggests invalid results on other tests as well (Green et al., 2002). Fox (2011) reported that in patients who failed either the WMT or the Computerized Test of Attention and Memory, there was no correlation between performance on neuropsychological tests and brain damage. In those patients who passed PVTs, the relationship with brain damage and neuropsychological test performance was retained, however. Thus, as reported in other research as well, performance validity can exert a more prominent effect on performance than pathology.

With regard to mental status, the WMT correlates fairly highly with the MMSE in neurological patients, but only modest correlations are found with other neuropsychological tests such as the TMT, Digit Span, Block Design, and reaction time (Merten et al., 2007). With regard to memory, independent studies do show that Effort scores on the WMT are correlated moderately to highly with the CVLT-II (Total Words and Long-Delay Free Recall, $r = .43$ to .57, Heyanka et al., 2015), contrary to data presented in the manual.

The use of the WMT as a memory test has been studied less than its use as a PVT. Studies by the author and colleagues show that the WMT memory measures (MC, PA, FR, LDFR) show moderately strong correlations with independent verbal memory measures such as the CVLT and CVLT-II (Armistead-Jehle et al., 2015).

However, other studies show that the WMT Memory scores may not have expected relationships to criterion variables compared to other standard memory tests. Donders and Strong (2013) examined the utility of WMT Memory scores in a TBI sample that passed the WMT. They found that, unlike the CVLT-II, which showed expected associations with coma duration and differences between brain injury severity groups, the WMT Memory subtests were not related to brain injury severity variables. Furthermore, WMT Memory variables did not correlate distinctly or uniquely with any CVLT-II variables tapping common constructs such as multiple-choice performance. WMT Memory scores also had poor sensitivity in identifying patients with memory impairments on the CVLT-II. Although WMT Memory variables and CVLT-II variables were moderately correlated (range $r = .36$ to .53), use of the WMT MC, PA, FR, and LDFR as measures of memory in TBI was not supported.

Similarly, Davis (2016) found no significant correlations between length of posttraumatic amnesia and WMT memory scores in a TBI sample, but found moderate to high correlations with FR when only non-medicolegal cases were considered; TBI severity groups differed on FR, but not on MC or PA. Notably, the FR did not contribute to prediction over and above that of the CVLT-II Total score to predict TBI severity. In a study of individuals with mixed neurological diagnoses, all the WMT memory variables were highly correlated with CVLT-II memory scores ($r = .65$ to .76), with FR in particularly very highly correlated with CVLT-II Total ($r = .81$). However, using norm-referenced scores based on the Rienstra et al. norms (Table 15–36), many more individuals scored in the impaired range on WMT memory scores than on CVLT-II scores, with 50% of individuals having at least one impaired score on the WMT versus 17% for the CVLT-II. In total, 44% of those with nonimpaired profiles on the CVLT-II performed in the impaired range on the WMT, raising serious concerns about these norms for the WMT (Davis & Wall, 2014).

CLINICAL STUDIES

The WMT has been used in almost every population where feigning and exaggeration of cognitive problems are a concern, including litigants, disability claimants, and criminal defendants, as well as a wide variety of clinical conditions associated with elevated rates of malingering and exaggeration such as mild brain injury, military samples, ADHD, learning disability, pain disorders, PTSD, and nonepileptic seizures. It has also been well studied in conditions associated with cognitive impairment where PVT failure might indicate false positives rather than malingering, including MCI, dementia, and intellectual disability, and some severe psychiatric conditions such as schizophrenia. Notably, despite the many studies by the test author and his colleagues, as well as the numerous independent studies supportive of the use of the test across different populations, there are only a handful of studies on the test's ability to predict verified malingering based on established malingering criteria.

Failure rates follow expected PVT failure rates based on sample characteristics. Failure rates are approximately 45–60% in medical-legal TBI referrals (Flaro et al., 2007; Miele et al., 2012), 49–68% in veterans (McCormick et al., 2013; Armistead-Jehle & Buican, 2012; Young et al., 2011), 22–48% in adults referred for ADHD (Cook et al., 2016; Suhr et al., 2011; Sullivan et al., 2007), 51% in patients reporting PTSD seen for independent evaluation (Merten et al., 2009), 51% in people with PNES (Drane et al., 2006), 46% in complex regional pain syndrome type 1 (Greiffenstein et al., 2013), 32% in people with fibromyalgia (Brooks et al., 2012), and 15% in learning disability (Sullivan et al., 2007). In samples seeking disability benefits for pain, WMT failure rates are also high (e.g., more than 40%; Gervais et al., 2004). Most studies find relatively low base rates of failure in college undergraduates (<1–3%, depending on the variable; Ross et al., 2016).

In comparison, people who are highly motivated to perform well on neuropsychological evaluations, such as parents seeking custody of their children, have a pass rate as high as 98% (Flaro et al., 2007).

Of note, the method for determining failure on the WMT can vary across studies; although the majority follow the manual's definition of failure (i.e., one of three Effort scores below the cutoff), some studies have used a more stringent failure rate of more than one subtest failure (e.g., Suhr et al., 2011).

The gold standard for PVTs is to be able to accurately detect verified malingerers; that is, examinees who meet multidimensional malingering criteria such as Malingered Neurocognitive Dysfunction criteria (MND; Slick et al., 1999) or Malingered Pain-Related Disability criteria (MPRD; Bianchini et al., 2005). In addition, malingering can be defined as failing two or more PVTs; although not equivalent to multidimensional malingering criteria, failure on two or more PVTs is equated with an extremely high probability of malingering in most studies.

Although the WMT has been used as a reference standard for malingering in numerous studies to validate other PVTs, there are surprisingly few studies that show the test's accuracy in predicting malingering itself. To our knowledge, there are only four studies on the calibration of the WMT with regard to malingering criteria: one involving TBI litigants and pain patients (Greve et al., 2008), two on an overlapping sample of criminal defendants (Fazio et al., 2015, Fazio & Denney, 2018), and one in ADHD (Marshall et al., 2010). As noted by Fazio et al. (2015), these kinds of studies are critical in establishing Daubert admissibility requirements, in addition to being necessary to calibrate cutoffs to detect bona fide malingering. These studies indicate that the WMT is prone to a high rate of false positives in TBI and criminal defendants unless adjusted cutoffs or the GMIP are used, or unless the test is used in conjunction with another PVT such as the TOMM. Standard cutoffs appear to work well in chronic pain and ADHD, and the GMIP works well in criminal defendants. These studies are reviewed in the following sections, with data presented in Tables 15–38 and 15–39 for cutoffs with acceptable false-positive rates.

Litigants and Disability Claimants. Research on litigants and disability claimants is described in detail in the manual, as well as in research by authors who contributed data (e.g., Gervais et al., 2001; Gervais, 2004; see also Armistead-Jehle et al., 2015). Surprisingly, despite the multiple large-*N* studies involving litigants and disability claimants, to our knowledge, none has used multidimensional criteria (i.e., verified malingers) to validate WMT cutoffs. Although this isn't technically specified, a portion of the Greve et al. (2008) TBI sample was presumably litigants or disability claimants as all the verified malingerers had external incentives to perform poorly.

Criminal Defendants. In the criminal setting, where there tend to be a number of low-IQ examinees, the standard WMT Effort cutoffs appear to have very high sensitivity but inadequate specificity to malingering as defined by failure on two independent PVTs (.95 to 1.00, and .67 to 68, respectively; Fazio et al., 2015; Fazio & Denney, 2018). In contrast to the WMT's false-positive rate that was as high as 33%, the TOMM had a false-positive rate of 13%. However, when the GMIP approach was used on

TABLE 15–38 Word Memory Test (WMT) Classification Accuracy for Cutoffs with Acceptable Specificities (≥90%) for Prediction of Malingered Neurocognitive Dysfunction (MND), Malingered Pain-Related Disability (MPRD), or Other Malingering Criteria at Different Base Rates

							BASE RATE 15% OR LESS		BASE RATE 30%		BASE RATE 40–50%	
STUDY	GROUP	CRITERION	N	CUTOFF	SENSITIVITY (%)	SPECIFICITY (%)	PPV (%)	NPV (%)	PPV (%)	NPV (%)	PPV (%)	NPV (%)
Greve et al. (2008)	TBI	Slick et al. (1999) Malingered Neurocognitive Dysfunction criteria	70	IR ≤ 75.0 DR ≤ 77.5 CNS ≤ 72.5	59 63 63	88 88 93	– – –	– – –	73 74 83	– – –	– – –	– – –
Greve et al. (2008)	Chronic pain	Bianchini et al. (2005) Malingered Pain-Related Disability criteria	100	IR ≤ 87.5 DR ≤ 87.5 CNS ≤ 87.5	60 57 55	90 88 88	– – –	– – –	76 72 71	– – –	– – –	– – –
Fazio et al. (2015)	Criminal defendants	MND defined as failure on two PVTs	79	GMIP	56	95	54	95	82	83	91	68
Fazio & Denney (2018)	Criminal defendants	MND defined as failure on two PVTs	60	GMIP	72	96	66	97	88	89	95	78
Marshall et al. (2010)	ADHD	Noncredible ADHD based on Slick et al. (1999) probable MND	53	WMT	64	91	54	93	74	85	–	–

NOTE: GMIP, Genuine Memory Impairment Profile; MND, Malingered Neurocognitive Dysfunction; PVT, Performance Validity Test.

WMT scores, the false-positive rate dropped to 5% or less while retaining adequate sensitivity of .56 to .72 (specificity of .95 to .96; Table 15–38). Another approach to reduce false positives while increasing detection of malingering was to combine the test with the TOMM. Specifically, in comparison to the TOMM, the WMT has better positive predictive power, but the TOMM has better negative predictive power. In other words, the WMT is more prone to false positives and the TOMM to false negatives. Therefore, combining the WMT GMIP and the TOMM yields better prediction of malingering in criminal defendants than either used alone (i.e., .68 sensitivity and .92 specificity; see Table 15–39).

Similar findings were reported for another PVT, the Validity Indicator Profile (VIP; Table 15–39). In a sample of malingering and nonmalingering criminal defendants, the standard WMT Effort cutoffs exhibited an excessive false-positive rate (33%), but with perfect sensitivity (1.00). However, when the GMIP was used, both sensitivity and specificity were excellent (.72 and .96, respectively). Adding the Validity Indicator Profile did not meaningfully increase sensitivity when both tests were used together, but did yield perfect specificity (i.e., no false positives; Fazio & Denney, 2018).

TBI. Only one study to our knowledge has calibrated the WMT against established malingering criteria in TBI. Greve, Ord, Curtis, Bianchini, and Brennan (2008) found that when using the standard Effort cutoffs, the WMT had good sensitivity to verified malingering in TBI but had a high false-positive rate of 20% or more, with CNS in particular misclassifying 30% of nonmalingering TBI patients as malingering. In comparison, the TOMM produced acceptable false-positive rates at its published cutoffs. Greve et al. (2008) concluded that although the WMT detected 50% more TBI malingerers, it did so with a 15 times higher false-positive rate compared to the TOMM when using the publisher's cutoffs. Reducing the WMT IR cutoff to 75.0 or less, the DR cutoff to 77.5 or less, and the CNS cutoff to 72.5 or less substantially improved prediction by reducing false positives (Table 15–38). Combining the WMT with the TOMM also increased the accurate detection of malingerers without increasing false positives, with good sensitivity and specificity (Table 15–39). Some have questioned whether the WMT is an appropriate test for people with brain injury, concluding that the test is more difficult for people with severe TBI than the TOMM, leading to an unacceptable rate of false positives, which means that the test may not meet Daubert standards (Batt et al., 2008). See others for more debate on this question, as well as the manual for research on TBI by the author and colleagues (e.g., Bowden et al., 2006; Rohling & Demakis, 2010).

TABLE 15–39 Combined Word Memory Test (WMT) and Test of Memory Malingering/Validity Indicator Profile (TOMM/VIP) Classification Accuracy for Cutoffs with Acceptable Specificities (≥90%) for Prediction of Malingering Based on Slick et al. (1999) or Bianchini et al. (2005) Malingering Criteria

							BASE RATE 15% OR LESS		BASE RATE 30%		BASE RATE 40–50%	
STUDY	GROUP	MALINGERING CRITERION	N	FAILURE CRITERIA	SENSITIVITY (%)	SPECIFICITY (%)	PPV (%)	NPV (%)	PPV (%)	NPV (%)	PPV (%)	NPV (%)
Greve et al. (2008)	TBI	Malingered Neurocognitive Dysfunction (MND)	70	WMT + TOMM	67	91	–	–	80	–	–	–
Greve et al. (2008)	Chronic Pain	Malingered Pain-Related Disability	100	WMT + TOMM	53	93	–	–	80	–	–	–
Fazio et al. (2015)	Criminal defendants	MND defined as failure on two PVTs	79	WMT GMIP + TOMM	68	92	100	95	100	82	100	66
Fazio & Denney (2018)	Criminal defendants	MND defined as failure on two PVTs	60	WMT GMIP + VIP	39	100	100	94	100	79	100	62

NOTE: GMIP, Genuine Memory Impairment Profile; MND, Malingered Neurocognitive Dysfunction; PVT, Performance Validity Test; VIP, Validity Indicator Profile.

As already noted, the WMT Memory scores may be less sensitive to TBI severity than the CVLT-II and may not be suitable as measures of memory for clinical decision making in this group (Davis, 2016).

Military Samples. To our knowledge, there are no WMT studies to date on verified malingering using established malingering criteria in military samples. Failure rates in military samples vary significantly, with estimates ranging from 19% to 55% (McCormick et al., 2013) based on a variety of military samples including active-duty outpatients referred to TBI clinics or general neuropsychology services, or assessed as part of Medical Evaluation Board disability assessments (Armistead-Jehle & Buican, 2012; Jones et al., 2012; Lange et al., 2012). WMT failure rates in active-duty samples with a history of concussion are much higher in disability versus clinical contexts (Grills & Armistead-Jehle, 2016). Military personnel with PTSD have higher rates of WMT failure than those without (34% vs. 19%), as do those with depression (McCormick et al., 2013).

Pain Disorders. Using established malingering criteria, in a pain sample, the standard WMT Effort cutoffs had excellent accuracy for detecting verified malingering based on Bianchini's criteria for Malingered Pain-Related Disability, with sensitivities greater than .50 and specificities greater than .95. False positives were not elevated in these pain patients, supporting the use of the existing cutoffs as appropriate for detecting malingering in pain conditions (Greve et al., 2008; see Table 15–39).

Studies on examinees with pain disorders indicate that it is the presence of external incentives that determines WMT performance, not the presence of pain. Gervais and colleagues found that in fibromyalgia, base rates of WMT failure were elevated in disability claimants but not in those with no external incentives (30% vs. 4%), including a zero fail rate in rheumatoid arthritis, a painful medical condition without external incentives. Furthermore, fibromyalgia patients seeking disability had higher failure rates than those already on disability (44% vs. 23% Gervais et al., 2001). Consistent with the view that it is not pain per se that affects WMT scores but rather the presence of external incentives, pain at the time of the assessment does not affect test performance (Gervais et al., 2004; see also manual).

Using the same definition of failure—that is, any two scores failed—WMT had higher sensitivity than TOMM (46% vs. 33%) in complex regional pain syndrome, a condition in which three-quarters of patients meet criteria for probable MPRD (Greiffenstein et al., 2013).

ADHD. With regard to predicting malingering of ADHD based on multidimensional criteria, the WMT shows good accuracy for detecting feigned ADHD based on criteria similar to the Slick et al. (1999) MND criteria, with .64 specificity and .90 sensitivity, better than prediction accuracy for the Conners CPT, b Test, Dot Counting, Reliable Digit Span, and CVLT-II Forced Choice, and better than a questionnaire-based exaggeration scale for ADHD (i.e., the Clinical Assessment of Attention Deficit—Adult Infrequency scale; Marshall et al., 2010). However, the authors caution that relying only on the WMT alone to determine feigning leads to a high false-positive rate and that the determination of exaggeration in ADHD needs to be based on failure on two PVTs, consistent with general recommendations for PVT use in other conditions.

In adults referred for possible ADHD, failure rates vary between 32% and 48%, compared to only 15% in adults referred for possible learning disability (Sullivan et al., 2007). Suhr et al. (2011) reported a 33% failure rate using one WMT subtest failed and 22% with a more stringent criteria of two subtests failed.

In ADHD, those who fail the WMT have a 77% rate of impaired performance on the Conners CPT, compared to 44% for those with bona fide ADHD (Suhr et al., 2011), demonstrating that continuous performance tasks are vulnerable to noncredible performance and that PVTs should be used in the evaluation of people with ADHD.

Epilepsy and PNES. In temporal lobe epilepsy, there are a significant number of false positives on WMT Effort subtests, but the GMIP shows utility in ruling out false positives attributable to severe memory problems. However, in differentiating between left and right temporal epilepsy, there are smaller effect sizes compared to the RAVLT.

In one study, the WMT did not improve classification of left and right temporal lobectomy patients over and above the RAVLT, even though there were differences in FR scores between the two groups in the expected direction (Soble et al., 2016). However, it was superior to the WMS-IV Logical Memory subtest and functioned as a bona fide memory tests in this clinical group, with the odds of having right temporal epilepsy increasing 8% with each 1-point increase in WMT FR percent correct score. The authors noted that FR was more accurate when age was taken into account; the provision of comprehensive age-adjusted norms would likely increase the clinical utility of the FR in comparison to existing verbal memory tests as its age-based healthy norms are quite limited at present.

In another study, 19% of people with epilepsy failed the WMT, compared to 51% of people with PNES (Drane et al., 2006). However, once those deemed false positives were removed from the epilepsy group ($N = 4$), the rate in epilepsy fell to 8%.

Dementia. Studies in MCI and dementia indicate that the test is failed at a higher than expected rate in these conditions and at a higher rate than other PVTs such as the TOMM. For example, Merten, Bossink, and Schmand (2007) reported that 90% of patients with AD failed the WMT, compared to 30% failing TOMM Trial 2 (Robinson et al., 2018). In severe Parkinson's disease patients undergoing deep brain stimulation, 37% had scores in the caution range, and 10% failed the test despite high motivation to do well (Rossetti et al., 2017).

However, use of the WMT GMIP may yield good sensitivity and specificity to detecting invalid responding without an unduly raised false-positive rate. For example, in a Portuguese sample, 67% of patients with MCI failed the test based on Effort scores (Martins & Martins, 2010), but using the GMIP criteria instead yielded acceptable classification accuracy statistics. Green et al. (2011) reported that when the WMT was interpreted via profile analysis based on relative performance of easy vs. difficult subtests, the specificity of WMT was 98% or greater. However, Robinson et al. (2018) found that the GMIP did not function effectively in an older mixed dementia sample of veterans with possible secondary gain. Using the standard cut scores, 83% of dementia patients and 60% of MCI patients failed the WMT. While almost all of those failing met criteria for the GMIP, using corroboration from chart review to detect malingerers, GMIP sensitivity was less than 13% even though specificity was very high at 97%, indicating that attaining an acceptable false-positive rate came at the cost of poor detection of malingerers. They concluded that the practical utility of the GMIP in veterans with external incentives was questionable.

In memory clinics, the rate of patients with suspected memory problems who fail the WMT using the GMIP is overall quite low (7%), albeit somewhat higher in younger patients (13%). Of note, in MCI patients with credible performance on the WMT, there are high correlations between left hippocampal volumes and memory tests, whereas the association disappears in those who fail the WMT, supporting the use of the test in memory clinics to identify the minority of patients who present with conditions mimicking bona fide memory deficits (Rienstra et al., 2013a).

There is also evidence that the GMIP is a useful predictor of dementia and provides information relevant to the clinical diagnosis of dementia. The GMIP has excellent sensitivity and specificity with regard to CDR ratings of dementia at baseline and at two-year follow-up (Rienstra et al., 2013b), and patients with the GMIP profile have poorer neuropsychological scores than those who pass the WMT, including on the MMSE, RAVLT, fluency tasks, Stroop, Clock Drawing, and Block Design, with memory tests showing the largest effect sizes. At two years, 66% of the GMIP group had declined on the CDR versus only 17% in the group who passed the WMT, and those who declined had lower neuropsychological test scores and a higher rate of dementia and MCI diagnoses at follow-up. Two of 12 cases identified as having noncredible performance on the WMT were shown to have degenerative diseases.

Psychiatric Conditions. Failure rates are somewhat elevated in psychiatric conditions, as is the case for most PVTs, particularly when disability claims are involved, but also in clinical patients. For example, nonmilitary disability claimants with PTSD are reported to have a failure rate of 20% (Demakis et al., 2008). In schizophrenia, results are mixed. In one study, about 15% failed the test, all of whom passed the VSVT based on published cutoffs, with failure thought to relate to negative symptoms such as avolition and anhedonia (Strauss et al., 2015). In comparison, Gorissen et al. (2005) found that 72% of patients with schizophrenia and no external incentives failed the oral version of the WMT. Notably, as many as 25% of psychiatric controls also failed the test, most of whom had an anxiety disorder. This may have been due to a higher rate of cognitive impairment and worse symptomatology in this study as patients had been referred for cognitive evaluations. Nevertheless, this raises the possibility that fewer false positives may have been obtained if the GMIP had been used. In this study, WMT scores were significantly related to negative symptoms and general psychopathology.

Low IQ. According to the author, persons of low intelligence typically perform above cutoffs on the WMT (Green & Flaro, 2015, 2016). A small number of cases studies of patients with developmental delay, extremely poor adaptive function and significant brain pathology also indicate that these patients can pass the test (Carone, 2014).

However, there have been mixed results in independent studies. Shandera and colleagues found good sensitivity but an excessive false-positive rate in a simulation design involving individuals with intellectual deficits who received the oral version of the WMT (sensitivity: .68 to .80 for IR, DR, and CNS, but with specificity of .25 to .42). In this study, the TOMM fared much better, with specificities of .88 and higher (Shandera et al., 2010).

Green and Flaro (2015) comment that prior studies on adults with intellectual disability may have included people not trying their best, as many were collecting disability payments and therefore may have had an incentive to perform poorly. They therefore tested a group of adults with intellectual disability who were seeking custody of their children and who therefore would have incentive to do well on cognitive testing ($N = 14$ given the WMT). High- and low-IQ parents seeking custody failed the WMT at rates of 5% and 14%, a nonsignificant difference. Despite these small *N*s and the need for replication, the authors present a compelling rationale for determining the presence of incentives to perform poorly in samples of people with intellectual disability, as larger studies of people with and without motivation to fail certainly support the view of intrinsic external incentives fueling some claims of intellectual disability (Shandera et al., 2010).

Distraction and Medication Effects. Some studies show that the WMT has higher cognitive demands than the TOMM and that it is more prone to interference from distraction, which explains its higher rate of failures in clinical groups with cognitive impairments (Batt et al., 2008; Eglit et al., 2017). For example, Batt et al. (2008) found that 75% of severe head injury examinees failed the WMT under a distraction condition, compared to 33% failing the TOMM. However, one study showed that when the GMIP approach is used, failure rates are closer to that of the TOMM even in the presence of distraction caused by dual-task interference (Eglit et al., 2017).

In a randomized, double-blind, placebo-controlled crossover study, Loring et al. (2011) reported that 21% of healthy volunteers failed the WMT while on lorazepam versus 4% on placebo, with effects on IR, CNS, and some delayed memory scores (excepting DR). The authors hypothesized this may be due to transient impairments of alertness affecting WMT performance. The authors stated that "under certain circumstances, medications can impact [PVT] results with poor [PVT] scores unrelated to apparent intentional attempts at response distortion" (p. 809). The implication is that the WMT is not immune to the effects of cognitive impairment, be it temporary (drug effects, seizure effects) or permanent (dementia, low IQ). With relevance to epilepsy, they also noted that seizure in the 24 hours prior to testing may also be a confounding factor in WMT interpretation and may contribute to WMT failure (Loring et al., 2011).

Resistance to Coaching. In terms of face validity compared to other PVTs, the WMT fares best, with about one-third of participants perceiving it to be a legitimate measure of memory, followed by about one-quarter for the VSVT and 10% for the TOMM (Tan et al., 2002). Coaching of individuals on how to avoid detection improves performance, although such individuals still perform worse than controls (Dunn et al., 2003). Of note, a 2006 study found that, compared to the TOMM and VSVT, the WMT had the least information available online, suggesting better test security (Bauer & McCaffrey, 2006).

NEUROANATOMICAL CORRELATES AND IMAGING STUDIES

To date, the WMT is unique among PVTs in that it has a considerable number of studies showing its neuroanatomic underpinnings. Neuroimaging research suggests that WMT performance relies on a widespread network of circuits associated with cognitive effort and that the test is performed differently after TBI.

In a small case study involving three nonlitigating amnesic patients with focal bilateral hippocampal atrophy, amnesic individuals scored above cutoffs on WMT Effort scores but had poor performance on WMT Memory subtests (Goodrich-Hunsaker & Hopkins, 2009). Other case studies include patients with removal of the left anterior hippocampus and parahippocampal gyrus with associated impaired FR memory performance who nevertheless passed the Effort scores (Carone et al., 2014).

Allen, Wu, and Bigler (2011) reported on an unusual case whereby functional MRI (fMRI) data from the WMT were collected one year previous and one year subsequent to a mild TBI. In this person, response times were slower post-injury but accuracy was not compromised. However, broader areas of recruitment were noted on fMRI, interpreted as indicative of increased cognitive demand subsequent to mild brain injury. In another study, clear differences were noted in TBI patients compared to controls, suggesting that the brain processes the WMT differently post-injury; interestingly, invalid performance on the WMT in simulators was associated with a generalized pattern of activation (Wu et al., 2010). Similarly, Larsen, Allen, Bigler, Goodrich-Hunsaker, and Hopkins (2010) had 10 healthy participants complete the WMT under valid and simulated invalid performance conditions. Trials with valid performance were associated with activation in dorsolateral prefrontal cortex, superior parietal lobe, anterior cingulate, lingual cortices (bilateral), and anterior insula/frontal operculum. Invalid performance conditions showed similar activation patterns, but with activation more broadly represented.

Some research also suggests that WMT Memory scores depend on hippocampal integrity. In credible older adults with suspected MCI, hippocampal volume was moderately correlated with WMT Effort performance, but more highly correlated with WMT Memory scores (r = .34 to .46, vs. r = .50 to .56; Rienstra et al., 2013a). Correlations between the memory measures and hippocampal volume were found only in suspected MCI patients who passed PVTs (TOMM or WMT; r = .49) and were nonsignificant in those who scored below cutoffs.

COMMENT

The WMT is one of the most commonly used, frequently cited, and well researched of the PVTs and has served as a reference standard in many studies that have evaluated other PVTs. Unique in its design and ingenious in its paradigm, it offers both PVTs and memory tests that progress along a gradient of difficulty. Most notably, it includes an algorithm for use in examinees with severe cognitive deficits such as low IQ or dementia (the GMIP), which appears to generally eliminate the false-positive problem that plagues most PVTs when used in these groups.

The test is easy, and high performance levels are expected in the majority of credible examinees. The manual and scoring program include a multitude of comparator groups (e.g., moderate to severe brain injury, neurology patients) to which the results can be compared for reference purposes. WMT scores are generally associated with excellent internal and test-retest reliability.

Research largely supports the WMT's validity. Overall, the WMT correlates well with many other PVTs and is one of the most sensitive of the PVTs, although some studies have indicated that this may be accomplished at the cost of more false positives. Although many persons with cognitive impairment perform within established cutoffs, there is evidence that false positives can occur in patients with severe cognitive impairment. In these patients, use of simple cutoffs is ill advised, and the use of the GMIP is indicated. For this reason, it is important to administer all the WMT subtests, not just the Effort subtests.

Memory scores on the WMT have been less studied. At present, these appear to have some promise in tapping verbal memory, but they do not perform as well as standard memory tests in clinical groups such as TBI and general neuropsychology referrals. This may in part be due to the lack of large-scale norms that could correct for age effects which affect memory scores on the test.

The WMT has been used in a wide variety of clinical groups. Although it has considerable research evidence to support its use in screening for exaggeration and feigning in clinical conditions associated with cognitive deficits, including litigants, disability claimants, criminal defendants, TBI, chronic pain, and other conditions, it also has considerable utility in conditions associated with psychopathology, such as depression and PTSD. In the criminal setting, where many examinees have low IQs, the WMT GMIP proves particularly effective for ruling in malingering without unduly increasing false positives (Fazio et al., 2015). In ADHD, the WMT appears to be much more effective at detecting malingerers than questionnaire-based invalidity scales. The use of the GMIP shows promise in tracking progression of dementia but needs further study for this usage. Last, the test has some compelling neuroimaging research findings.

Importantly, the manual has a section instructing users how to describe WMT results in their reports; this includes protecting the integrity of the test by not naming the test specifically as a PVT, not describing in detail the rationale for WMT interpretation, and not including score graphs in the examinee's report, which is a general recommendation that should apply to all PVTs.

Some have concluded that the test has unacceptably high false-positive rates in the identification of malingering (Fazio & Denney, 2018; Greve et al., 2008) and that the previously assumed high sensitivity compared to other PVTs is simply an artifact of its methods for defining failure as it requires failure on only one of its three possible Effort scores. Independent research using multidimensional malingering criteria suggests that the cutoff scores from the manual may be too high in some groups such as TBI, identifying too many people with scores below the cutoff and therefore increasing false positives. Lower cutoffs of 72.5 to 77.5 have been suggested instead as more appropriate. Nevertheless, standard cutoffs appear appropriate for use identifying malingering in pain patients, and false-positive rates in other groups can be ameliorated by the use of the GMIP or by using an additional PVT such as the TOMM. The test would benefit from more validation research using multidimensional malingering criteria such as Slick et al. and Bianchini et al. criteria for MND and MPRD to better calibrate and validate cutoffs across different groups. The WMT GMIP has also not been as well studied in independent research as it has for the MSVT, where questions have been raised about effectiveness in dementia and low-IQ examinees.

Users should recall the main tenet of the GMIP: that is, if the examinee is *not* dependent on others in daily life, the examinee would not meet criteria for the GMIP, by definition. The test author states that the GMIP must be used in conjunction with Criteria D of the Slick et al. malingering criteria (Slick et al., 1999) to be effective at differentiating invalid performance from cognitive impairment. Criteria D specifies that behaviors meeting necessary criteria for malingering must not be fully accounted for by psychiatric, neurological, or developmental factors that result in significantly diminished capacity to appreciate laws or mores against malingering or inability to conform behavior to such standards and are not the product of an informed, rational, and volitional effort aimed at least in part toward acquiring or achieving external incentives.

Some have criticized a somewhat circular reasoning within the GMIP and suggest the numerical algorithm should not depend on clinical criteria outside of the test results themselves. We see no problem with including Criterion D of the Slick criteria to aid in interpreting scores, as this provides a bridge between purely actuarial approaches and purely clinical approaches to detecting malingering and exaggeration. However, more clarity, consistency, and validation of this approach are needed in the manual, scoring program, and related publications, including further validation of the cutoffs and algorithm using verified malingerers. Criterion D of the Slick malingering criteria is not part of the GMIP algorithm described in the manual but is used in the Advanced Interpretation Program, making it difficult to compare results across studies that have used different criteria.

There are small to moderate effects of age and education, with more pronounced effects on memory scores. Most studies have focused on the Effort scores and not on Memory scores. Memory subtests are in need of comprehensive, stratified norms for clinical diagnostic making, with the norms presented in the manual insufficient for use as memory test norms. The original sample of healthy people described in the manual is small and has a limited age range, with few individuals older than age 60. Similarly, although the Dutch/Canadian sample from Rienstra et al. (2009) is an improvement over the norms in the manual, it may have some limitations for application to North-American populations based on some evidence that the norms overidentify memory impairment (Davis & Wall, 2014). Independent research on the WMT Memory measures indicates that these are not appropriate for clinical evaluation of memory functioning, at least in TBI, where this has been studied. More study on this question is needed. Of note, few studies have included the LDFR score.

The standard instructions require that the examiner leave the room during the test; it is not clear that this procedure was followed in all WMT research studies. Examinees with sensorimotor difficulties can be administered the oral version, although this is not a recommended practice. From a practical perspective, the manual contains a lot of information on normative and clinical samples but is not well organized for rapid reference.

Although it has an impressive number of translations and has been used in other languages and other countries, the test could use more studies focused explicitly on the influence of ethnicity, as would most PVTs (Nijdam-Jones & Rosenfeld, 2017), as well as validation in North-American Spanish-speaking and Asian populations.

Last, like all PVTs, the WMT is a test that offers information regarding the validity of scores produced by examinees but does not inform as to the cause of invalid performance when noncredible performance is detected. Failure does not equate malingering, and clinical judgment must be brought to bear using the framework of multidimensional malingering criteria to ascertain the basis for failure, including examining congruence between clinical characteristics, adaptive living skills, and neuropsychological profile. The clinical characteristics of an examinee who fails the test therefore needs to be carefully evaluated before making conclusions about causality or intent, as is the case whenever an examinee fails a PVT.

REFERENCES

Allen, M. D., Wu, T. C., & Bigler, E. D. (2011). Traumatic brain injury alters Word Memory Test performance by slowing response time and increasing cortical activation: An fMRI study of a symptom validity test. *Psychological Injury and Law*, *4*(2), 140–146. https://doi.org/10.1007/s12207-011-9105-4

Armistead-Jehle, P., & Buican, B. (2012). Evaluation context and symptom validity test performances in a U.S. military sample. *Archives of Clinical Neuropsychology*, *27*(8), 828–839. https://doi.org/10.1093/arclin/acs086

Armistead-Jehle, P., & Buican, B. (2013). Comparison of select Advanced Clinical Solutions embedded performance validity measures to the Word Memory Test in the detection of suboptimal performance validity. *Archives of Clinical Neuropsychology*, *28*(3), 297–301. https://doi.org/10.1093/arclin/act017

Armistead-Jehle, P., & Green, P. (2016). Model for the effects of invalid styles of response. *Applied Neuropsychology: Adult*, *23*(6), 449–458. https://doi.org/10.1080/23279095.2016.1178646

Armistead-Jehle, P., Green, P., Gervais, R. O., & Hungerford, L. D. (2015). An examination of the Word Memory Test as a measure of memory. *Applied Neuropsychology. Adult*, *22*(6), 415–426. https://doi.org/10.1080/23279095.2014.953678

Batt, K., Shores, E. A., & Chekaluk, E. (2008). The effect of distraction on the Word Memory Test and Test of Memory Malingering performance in patients with a severe brain injury. *Journal of the International Neuropsychological Society: JINS*, *14*(6), 1074–1080. https://doi.org/10.1017/S135561770808137X

Bauer, L., & McCaffrey, R. (2006). Coverage of the Test of Memory Malingering, Victoria Symptom Validity Test, and Word Memory Test on the Internet: Is test security threatened? *Archives of Clinical Neuropsychology*, *21*(1), 121–126. https://doi.org/10.1016/j.acn.2005.06.010

Bianchini, K. J., Greve, K. W., & Glynn, G. (2005). On the diagnosis of malingered pain-related disability: Lessons from cognitive malingering research. *The Spine Journal*, *5*(4), 404–417. https://doi.org/10.1016/j.spinee.2004.11.016

Bowden, S. C., Shores, E. A., & Mathias, J. L. (2006). Does effort suppress cognition after traumatic brain injury? A re-examination of the evidence for the Word Memory Test. *The Clinical Neuropsychologist*, *20*(4), 858–872. https://doi.org/10.1080/13854040500246935

Brooks, L., Johnson-Greene, D., Lattie, E., & Ference, T. (2012). The Relationship between performances on neuropsychological symptom validity testing and the MCMI-III in patients with fibromyalgia. *The Clinical Neuropsychologist*, *26*(5), 816–831. https://doi.org/10.1080/13854046.2012.662999

Carone, D. A. (2014). Young child with severe brain volume loss easily passes the word memory test and medical symptom validity test: implications for mild TBI. *The Clinical Neuropsychologist*, *28*(1), 146–162. https://doi.org/10.1080/13854046.2013.861019

Carone, D. A., Green, P., & Drane, D. L. (2014). Word Memory Test profiles in two cases with surgical removal of the left anterior hippocampus and parahippocampal gyrus. *Applied Neuropsychology: Adult*, *21*(2), 155–160. https://doi.org/10.1080/09084282.2012.755533

Cook, C. M., Bolinger, E., & Suhr, J. (2016). Further validation of the Conners Adult Attention Deficit/Hyperactivity Rating Scale

Infrequency Index (CII) for detection of noncredible report of attention deficit/hyperactivity disorder symptoms. *Archives of Clinical Neuropsychology, 31*(4), 358–364. https://doi.org/10.1093/arclin/acw015

Dandachi-FitzGerald, B., Ponds, R. W. H. M., & Merten, T. (2013). Symptom validity and neuropsychological assessment: A survey of practices and beliefs of neuropsychologists in six European countries. *Archives of Clinical Neuropsychology, 28*(8), 771–783. https://doi.org/10.1093/arclin/act073

Davis, J. J. (2014). Further consideration of Advanced Clinical Solutions Word Choice: Comparison to the Recognition Memory Test-words and classification accuracy in a clinical sample. *The Clinical Neuropsychologist, 28*(8), 1278–1294. https://doi.org/10.1080/13854046.2014.975844

Davis, J. J. (2016). Reconsidering the Word Memory Test as a memory measure in traumatic brain injury. *Archives of Clinical Neuropsychology.* https://doi.org/10.1093/arclin/acw058

Davis, J. J., & Wall, J. R. (2014). Examining verbal memory on the Word Memory Test and California Verbal Learning Test-Second Edition. *Archives of Clinical Neuropsychology, 29*(8), 747–753. https://doi.org/10.1093/arclin/acu030

Demakis, G. J., Gervais, R. O., & Rohling, M. L. (2008). The effect of failure on cognitive and psychological symptom validity tests in litigants with symptoms of post-traumatic stress disorder. *The Clinical Neuropsychologist, 22*(5), 879–895. https://doi.org/10.1080/13854040701564482

Demakis, G., Rimland, C., Reeve, C., & Ward, J. (2015). Intelligence and psychopathy do not influence malingering. *Applied Neuropsychology: Adult, 22*(4), 262–270. https://doi.org/10.1080/23279095.2014.920842

Donders, J., & Strong, C.-A. H. (2013). Does Green's Word Memory Test really measure memory? *Journal of Clinical and Experimental Neuropsychology, 35*(8), 827–834. https://doi.org/10.1080/13803395.2013.824557

Drane, D. L., Williamson, D. J., Stroup, E. S., Holmes, M. D., Jung, M., Koerner, E., . . . Miller, J. W. (2006). Cognitive impairment is not equal in patients with epileptic and psychogenic nonepileptic seizures. *Epilepsia, 47*(11), 1879–1886. https://doi.org/10.1111/j.1528-1167.2006.00611.x

Dunn, T. D., Shear, P. K., Howe, S., & Ris, M. D. (2003). Detecting neuropsychological malingering: Effects of coaching information. *Archives of Clinical Neuropsychology, 18,* 121–134.

Eglit, G. M. L., Lynch, J. K., & McCaffrey, R. J. (2017). Not all performance validity tests are created equal: The role of recollection and familiarity in the Test of Memory Malingering and Word Memory Test. Journal of Clinical and *Experimental Neuropsychology, 39*(2), 173–189. https://doi.org/10.1080/13803395.2016.1210573

Fazio, R. L., & Denney, R. L. (2018). Comparison of performance of the VIP and WMT in a criminal forensic sample. *Archives of Clinical Neuropsychology, 33*(8), 1069–1079. https://doi.org/10.1093/arclin/acy001

Fazio, R. L., Sanders, J. F., & Denney, R. L. (2015). Comparison of performance of the Test of Memory Malingering and Word Memory Test in a criminal forensic sample. *Archives of Clinical Neuropsychology, 30*(4), 293–301. https://doi.org/10.1093/arclin/acv024

Flaro, L., Green, P., & Robertson, E. (2007). Word Memory Test failure 23 times higher in mild brain injury than in parents seeking custody: The power of external incentives. *Brain Injury, 21*(4), 373–383. https://doi.org/10.1080/02699050701311133

Fox, D. D. (2011). Symptom validity test failure indicates invalidity of neuropsychological tests. *The Clinical Neuropsychologist, 25*(3), 488–495. https://doi.org/10.1080/13854046.2011.554443

Gervais, R. (2004). A comparison of WMT, CARB, and TOMM failure rates in non-head injury disability claimants. *Archives of Clinical Neuropsychology, 19*(4), 475–487. https://doi.org/10.1016/j.acn.2003.05.001

Gervais, R. O., Rohling, M. L., Green, P., & Ford, W. (2004). A comparison of WMT, CARB, and TOMM failure rates in non-head injury disability claimants. *Archives of Clinical Neuropsychology, 19,* 475–487.

Gervais, R. O., Russell, A. S., Green, P., Allen, L. M., Ferrari, R., & Pieschl, S. D. (2001). Performance validity testing in fibromyalgia patients with disability incentives. *Journal of Rheumatology, 28,* 1892–1899.

Goodrich-Hunsaker, N. J., & Hopkins, R. O. (2009). Word memory test performance in amnesic patients with hippocampal damage. *Neuropsychology, 23*(4), 529–534. https://doi.org/10.1037/a0015444

Gorissen, M., Sanz, J. C., & Schmand, B. (2005). Effort and cognition in schizophrenia patients. *Schizophrenia Research, 78*(2–3), 199–208. https://doi.org/10.1016/j.schres.2005.02.016

Green, P. (2003). *Green's Word Memory Test for Microsoft Windows.* Edmonton, AB, Canada: Green's Publishing.

Green, P. (2007). The pervasive influence of performance validity on neuropsychological tests. *Physical Medicine and Rehabilitation Clinics of North America, 18*(1), 43–68.

Green, P., Allen, L. M., & Astner, K. (1997). *The Word Memory Test: A user's guide to the oral and computer-administered forms, US Version 1.1.* Durham, NC: CogniSyst.

Green, P., & Flaro, L. (2003). Word Memory Test performance in children. *Child Neuropsychology, 9,* 189–207.

Green, P., & Flaro, L. (2015). Results from three performance validity tests (PVTs) in adults with intellectual deficits. *Applied Neuropsychology. Adult, 22*(4), 293–303. https://doi.org/10.1080/23279095.2014.925903

Green, P., & Flaro, L. (2016). Results from three performance validity tests in children with intellectual disability. *Applied Neuropsychology. Child, 5*(1), 25–34. https://doi.org/10.1080/21622965.2014.935378

Green, P., Iverson, G., & Allen, L. (1999). Detecting malingering in head injury litigation with the Word Memory Test. *Brain Injury, 13,* 813–819.

Green, P., Lees-Haley, P., & Allen, L. (2002). The Word Memory Test and the validity of neuropsychological test scores. *Forensic Neuropsychology, 2,* 97–124.

Green, P., Montijo, J., & Brockhaus, R. (2011). High specificity of the Word Memory Test and Medical Symptom Validity Test in groups with severe verbal memory impairment. *Applied Neuropsychology, 18*(2), 86–94. https://doi.org/10.1080/09084282.2010.523389

Green, P., Rohling, M. L., Iverson, G. L., & Gervais, R. O. (2003). Relationships between olfactory discrimination and head injury severity. *Brain Injury, 17,* 479–496.

Green, P., Rohling, M. L., Lees-Haley, P. R., & Allen, L. M. (2001). Performance validity has a greater effect on test scores than severe brain injury in compensation claimants. *Brain Injury, 15,* 1045–1060.

Greiffenstein, M., Gervais, R., Baker, W. J., Artiola, L., & Smith, H. (2013). Symptom validity testing in medically unexplained pain: A chronic regional pain syndrome type 1 case series. *The Clinical Neuropsychologist, 27*(1), 138–147. https://doi.org/10.1080/13854046.2012.722686

Greiffenstein, M. F., Greve, K. W., Bianchini, K. J., & Baker, W. J. (2008). Test of Memory Malingering and Word Memory Test: A new comparison of failure concordance rates. *Archives of Clinical Neuropsychology, 23*(7–8), 801–807. https://doi.org/10.1016/j.acn.2008.07.005

Greve, K. W., Binder, L. M., & Bianchini, K. J. (2009). Rates of below-chance performance in forced-choice symptom validity tests. *The Clinical Neuropsychologist, 23*(3), 534–544. https://doi.org/10.1080/13854040802232690

Greve, K. W., Ord, J., Curtis, K. L., Bianchini, K. J., & Brennan, A. (2008). Detecting malingering in traumatic brain injury and chronic pain: A comparison of three forced-choice symptom validity tests. *The Clinical Neuropsychologist, 22*(5), 896–918. https://doi.org/10.1080/13854040701565208

Grills, C. E., & Armistead-Jehle, P. (2016). Performance validity test and neuropsychological assessment battery screening module performances in an active-duty sample with a history of concussion. *Applied Neuropsychology. Adult, 23*(4), 295–301. https://doi.org/10.1080/23279095.2015.1079713

Heyanka, D. J., Thaler, N. S., Linck, J. F., Pastorek, N. J., Miller, B., Romesser, J., & Sim, A. H. (2015). A factor-analytic approach to the validation of the Word Memory Test and Test of Memory Malingering as measures of performance validity and not memory. *Archives of Clinical Neuropsychology, 30*(5), 369–376. https://doi.org/10.1093/arclin/acv025

Iverson, G., Green, P., & Gervais, R. (1999). Using the Word Memory Test to detect biased responding in head injury litigation. *Journal of Cognitive Rehabilitation, 17*, 4–8.

Jones, A., Ingram, M. V., & Ben-Porath, Y. S. (2012). Scores on the MMPI-2-RF Scales as a function of increasing levels of failure on cognitive symptom validity tests in a military sample. *The Clinical Neuropsychologist, 26*(5), 790–815. https://doi.org/10.1080/13854046.2012.693202

LaDuke, C., Barr, W., Brodale, D. L., & Rabin, L. A. (2017). Toward generally accepted forensic assessment practices among clinical neuropsychologists: A survey of professional practice and common test use. *The Clinical Neuropsychologist*, 1–20. https://doi.org/10.1080/13854046.2017.1346711

Lange, R. T., Pancholi, S., Bhagwat, A., Anderson-Barnes, V., & French, L. M. (2012). Influence of poor performance validity on neuropsychological test performance in U.S. military personnel following mild traumatic brain injury. *Journal of Clinical and Experimental Neuropsychology, 34*(5), 453–466. https://doi.org/10.1080/13803395.2011.648175

Larsen, J. D., Allen, M. D., Bigler, E. D., Goodrich-Hunsaker, N. J., & Hopkins, R. O. (2010). Different patterns of cerebral activation in genuine and malingered cognitive performance validity during performance on the Word Memory Test. *Brain Injury, 24*(2), 89–99. https://doi.org/10.3109/02699050903508218

Loring, D. W., Marino, S. E., Drane, D. L., Parfitt, D., Finney, G. R., & Meador, K. J. (2011). Lorazepam effects on Word Memory Test Performance: A randomized, double-blind, placebo-controlled, crossover trial. *The Clinical Neuropsychologist, 25*(5), 799–811. https://doi.org/10.1080/13854046.2011.583279

Marshall, P., Schroeder, R., O'Brien, J., Fischer, R., Ries, A., Blesi, B., & Barker, J. (2010). Effectiveness of symptom validity measures in identifying cognitive and behavioral symptom exaggeration in adult Attention Deficit Hyperactivity Disorder. *The Clinical Neuropsychologist, 24*(7), 1204–1237. https://doi.org/10.1080/13854046.2010.514290

Martins, M., & Martins, I. P. (2010). Memory malingering: evaluating WMT criteria. *Applied Neuropsychology, 17*(3), 177–182. https://doi.org/10.1080/09084281003715709

McCormick, C. L., Yoash-Gantz, R. E., McDonald, S. D., Campbell, T. C., & Tupler, L. A. (2013). Performance on the Green Word Memory Test following Operation Enduring Freedom/Operation Iraqi Freedom-era military service: Test failure is related to evaluation context. *Archives of Clinical Neuropsychology, 28*(8), 808–823. https://doi.org/10.1093/arclin/act050

Merten, T., Bossink, L., & Schmand, B. (2007). On the limits of performance validity testing: Symptom validity tests and severity of neurocognitive symptoms in nonlitigant patients. *Journal of Clinical and Experimental Neuropsychology, 29*(3), 308–318. https://doi.org/10.1080/13803390600693607

Merten, T., Thies, E., Schneider, K., & Stevens, A. (2009). Symptom validity testing in claimants with alleged posttraumatic stress disorder: Comparing the Morel Emotional Numbing Test, the Structured Inventory of Malingered Symptomatology, and the Word Memory Test. *Psychological Injury and Law, 2*(3–4), 284–293. https://doi.org/10.1007/s12207-009-9057-0

Miele, A. S., Gunner, J. H., Lynch, J. K., & McCaffrey, R. J. (2012). Are embedded validity indices equivalent to free-standing symptom validity tests? *Archives of Clinical Neuropsychology, 27*(1), 10–22. https://doi.org/10.1093/arclin/acr084

Mossman, D., Wygant, D. B., & Gervais, R. O. (2012). Estimating the accuracy of neurocognitive performance validity measures in the absence of a "gold standard." *Psychological Assessment, 24*(4), 815–822. https://doi.org/10.1037/a0028195

Nijdam-Jones, A., & Rosenfeld, B. (2017). Cross-cultural feigning assessment: A systematic review of feigning instruments used with linguistically, ethnically, and culturally diverse samples. *Psychological Assessment, 29*(11), 1321–1336. https://doi.org/10.1037/pas0000438

Reslan, S., & Axelrod, B. N. (2017). Evaluating the Medical Symptom Validity Test (MSVT) in a sample of veterans between the ages of 18 to 64. *Applied Neuropsychology. Adult, 24*(2), 132–139. https://doi.org/10.1080/23279095.2015.1107565

Rienstra, A., Groot, P. F. C., Spaan, P. E. J., Majoie, C. B. L. M., Nederveen, A. J., Walstra, G. J. M., . . . Schmand, B. (2013a). Symptom validity testing in memory clinics: Hippocampal-memory associations and relevance for diagnosing mild cognitive impairment. *Journal of Clinical and Experimental Neuropsychology, 35*(1), 59–70. https://doi.org/10.1080/13803395.2012.751361

Rienstra, A., Klein Twennaar, M., & Schmand, B. (2013b). Neuropsychological characterization of patients with the WMT Dementia Profile. *Archives of Clinical Neuropsychology, 28*(5), 463–475. https://doi.org/10.1093/arclin/act026

Rienstra, A., Spaan, P. E. J., & Schmand, B. (2009). Reference data for the Word Memory Test. *Archives of Clinical Neuropsychology, 24*(3), 255–262. https://doi.org/10.1093/arclin/acp035

Robinson, J. S., Collins, R. L., Miller, B. I., Pacheco, V. H., & Wisdom, N. M. (2018). The Severe Impairment Profile: A conceptual shift. *Archives of Clinical Neuropsychology, 33*(2), 238–246. https://doi.org/10.1093/arclin/acx069

Rohling, M. L., & Demakis, G. J. (2010). Bowden, Shores, & Mathias (2006): Failure to replicate or just failure to notice: Does effort still account for more variance in neuropsychological test scores than TBI severity? *The Clinical Neuropsychologist, 24*(1), 119–136. https://doi.org/10.1080/13854040903307243

Rohling, M. L., Green, P., Allen, L. M., & Iverson, G. L. (2002). Depressive symptoms and neurocognitive test scores in patients passing symptom validity tests. *Archives of Clinical Neuropsychology, 17*, 205–222.

Ross, T. P., Poston, A. M., Rein, P. A., Salvatore, A. N., Wills, N. L., & York, T. M. (2016). Performance invalidity base rates among healthy undergraduate research participants. *Archives of Clinical Neuropsychology, 31*(1), 97–104. https://doi.org/10.1093/arclin/acv062

Rossetti, M. A., Collins, R. L., & York, M. K. (2017). Performance validity in deep brain stimulation candidates. *Archives of Clinical Neuropsychology*, 1–7. https://doi.org/10.1093/arclin/acx081

Russo, A. C. (2012). Symptom validity test performance and consistency of self-reported memory functioning of Operation Enduring Freedom/Operation Iraqi Freedom Veterans with positive Veteran Health Administration comprehensive traumatic brain injury evaluations. *Archives of Clinical Neuropsychology, 27*(8), 840–848. https://doi.org/10.1093/arclin/acs090

Shandera, A. L., Berry, D. T. R., Clark, J. A., Schipper, L. J., Graue, L. O., & Harp, J. P. (2010). Detection of malingered mental retardation. *Psychological Assessment, 22*(1), 50–56. https://doi.org/10.1037/a0016585

Sharland, M. J., & Gfeller, J. D. (2007). A survey of neuropsychologists' beliefs and practices with respect to the assessment of effort. *Archives of Clinical Neuropsychology, 22*(2), 213–223. https://doi.org/10.1016/j.acn.2006.12.004

Slick, D. J., Sherman, E. M., & Iverson, G. L. (1999). Diagnostic criteria for malingered neurocognitive dysfunction: Proposed standards for clinical practice and research. *The Clinical Neuropsychologist, 13*(4), 545–561. https://doi.org/10.1076/1385-4046(199911)13:04;1-Y;FT545

Soble, J. R., Osborn, K. E., Mattingly, M. L., Vale, F. L., Benbadis, S. R., Rodgers-Neame, N. T., & Schoenberg, M. R. (2016). Utility of Green's Word Memory Test Free Recall subtest as a measure of verbal memory: Initial evidence from a temporal lobe epilepsy clinical sample. *Archives of Clinical Neuropsychology, 31*(1), 79–87. https://doi.org/10.1093/arclin/acv084

Sollman, M. J., & Berry, D. T. R. (2011). Detection of inadequate performance validity on neuropsychological testing: A meta-analytic update and extension. *Archives of Clinical Neuropsychology, 26*(8), 774–789. https://doi.org/10.1093/arclin/acr066

Strauss, G. P., Morra, L. F., Sullivan, S. K., & Gold, J. M. (2015). The role of low cognitive performance validity and negative symptoms in neuropsychological impairment in schizophrenia. *Neuropsychology, 29*(2), 282–291. https://doi.org/10.1037/neu0000113

Suhr, J. A., Sullivan, B. K., & Rodriguez, J. L. (2011). The relationship of noncredible performance to Continuous Performance Test scores in adults referred for Attention-Deficit/Hyperactivity Disorder evaluation. *Archives of Clinical Neuropsychology, 26*(1), 1–7. https://doi.org/10.1093/arclin/acq094

Sullivan, B. K., May, K., & Galbally, L. (2007). Symptom exaggeration by college adults in Attention-Deficit Hyperactivity Disorder and learning disorder assessments. *Applied Neuropsychology, 14*(3), 189–207. https://doi.org/10.1080/09084280701509083

Tan, J. E., Slick, D. J., Strauss, E., & Hultsch, D. F. (2002). How'd they do it? Malingering strategies on symptom validity tests. *The Clinical Neuropsychologist, 16,* 495–505.

Williamson, D. J. G., Green, P., Allen, L., & Rohling, M. L. (2003). Evaluating performance validity with the Word Memory Test and Category Test—or not: Inconsistencies in a compensation-seeking sample. *Journal of Forensic Neuropsychology, 3,* 19–44.

Wu, T. C., Allen, M. D., Goodrich-Hunsaker, N. J., Hopkins, R. O., & Bigler, E. D. (2010). Functional neuroimaging of symptom validity testing in traumatic brain injury. *Psychological Injury and Law, 3*(1), 50–62. https://doi.org/10.1007/s12207-010-9067

Young, J. C., Baughman, B. C., & Roper, B. L. (2012). Validation of the Repeatable Battery for the assessment of neuropsychological status—performance validity index in a veteran sample. *The Clinical Neuropsychologist, 26*(4), 688–699. https://doi.org/10.1080/13854046.2012.679624

Young, J. C., Kearns, L. A., & Roper, B. L. (2011). Validation of the MMPI-2 Response Bias Scale and Henry–Heilbronner Index in a U.S. veteran population. *Archives of Clinical Neuropsychology, 26*(3), 194–204. https://doi.org/10.1093/arclin/acr015

Young, J. C., Roper, B. L., & Arentsen, T. J. (2016). Validity testing and neuropsychology practice in the VA healthcare system: Results from recent practitioner survey. *The Clinical Neuropsychologist, 30*(4), 497–514. https://doi.org/10.1080/13854046.2016.1159730

16 | SYMPTOM VALIDITY

MINNESOTA MULTIPHASIC PERSONALITY INVENTORY-2 (MMPI-2)

TEST NAME	**Minnesota Multiphasic Personality Inventory-2 (MMPI-2)**
DOMAIN	Symptom validity (see other sources for the use of the test in assessing psychopathology)
AGE RANGE	18 to 90 years
ADMINISTRATION TIME	1 to 2 hours
SCORING FORMAT	Computerized, mail-in, or hand scored
REFERENCES	Butcher, J. N., Graham, J. R., Ben Porath, Y. S., Tellegen, A., Dahlstrom, W. G., & Kaemmer, B. (2001). *MMPI-2, Minnesota Multiphasic Personality Inventory–2: Manual for administration, scoring, and administration* (revised ed.). Minneapolis: University of Minnesota Press. Ben-Porath, Y. S., Graham, J. R., & Tellegen, A. (2009). *The MMPI-2 Symptom Validity (FBS) scale: Development, research findings, and interpretive recommendations*. Minneapolis: University of Minnesota Press. www.pearsonclinical.com

DESCRIPTION

The Minnesota Multiphasic Personality Inventory-2 (MMPI-2; Butcher et al., 2001) is a self-report questionnaire that ranks as one of the most popular psychological assessment measures among neuropsychologists (Rabin et al., 2016). Details on general interpretation are available in the original source and in numerous publications and will not be covered here in order to provide an exclusive focus on the MMPI-2 as a symptom validity tool. Specifically, this review will focus primarily on the use of the MMPI-2 validity scales in detecting feigning in contexts relevant to neuropsychologists, such as feigning of cognitive and physical deficits in evaluations for personal injury, disability, and criminal-forensic matters. For an overview of the MMPI-2's utility in the detection of feigned psychopathology, please see other comprehensive sources (e.g., Butcher et al., 2015; Greene, 2008; Nichols, 2011).

Among measures used by neuropsychologists to assess symptom validity, the MMPI-2 is the second-most frequently used scale with symptom validity tests (SVTs), employed by almost 30% of neuropsychologists who use SVTs (Martin et al., 2015). Previously the most commonly used scale (Sharland & Gfeller, 2007), it now trails one step behind the MMPI-2-RF, also reviewed in this chapter. However, the number of studies on the MMPI-2 validity scales still largely outstrips those of the MMPI-2-RF.

The MMPI really pioneered an approach to detecting test validity that we now expect to find in most well-designed, comprehensive standardized psychological questionnaires, namely, the inclusion of three broad types of scales: (1) scales to measure item completion and item consistency, (2) scales to measure underreporting of symptoms, and (3) scales to measure overreporting of symptoms.

Here, we focus on core MMPI-2 validity scales to detect overreporting of cognitive and somatic symptoms, both developed by neuropsychologists: the Symptom Validity Scale (FBS; formerly known as the Fake Bad Scale but still retaining its FBS acronym) and the Response Bias Scale (RBS). In addition, we review two lesser-known scales, the Henry-Heilbronner Index (HHI) and the Cognitive Complaints Scale (CCS).

The MMPI-2 test publisher provides English, Spanish, Hmong, and French-Canadian versions (www.pearsonclinical.com). Several other translations exist in more than 20 other languages as of this writing, available through the University of Minnesota Press (https://www.upress.umn.edu/test-division/translations-permissions/available-translations), including three versions in Spanish for use in Mexico/Central America, Spain/South America/Central America, and the United States, respectively.

MMPI-2 CLINICAL SCALES AND RESTRUCTURED CLINICAL SCALES

The MMPI itself was published in 1940, with a revision and restandardization produced in 1989 to improve the adequacy of the normative base and item content (Butcher et al., 1989). The Restructured Clinical (RC) scales were published later (Tellegen et al., 2003); these were based on the original items but designed to improve interpretation and more closely parallel modern models of psychopathology (see also the review of MMPI-2-RF elsewhere in this chapter). The test was again revised extensively in 2008 to create the MMPI-2-RF (Ben-Porath & Tellegen, 2008), but the original MMPI-2 continues to generate a significant amount of research and continues to be used by a large number of clinicians.

The ten main MMPI-2 Clinical scales are often simply known by their number (e.g., "Scale 8"). These include Hypochondriasis (Hs), Depression (D), Hysteria (Hy), Psychopathic Deviate (Pd), Masculinity-Femininity (Mf), Paranoia (Pa), Psychasthenia (Pt), Schizophrenia (Sc), Hypomania (Ma), and Social Introversion (Si). These are listed in Table 16–1 for reference purposes as they will not be discussed in detail here. The RC scales are listed in Table 16–2.

The test also includes Content and Supplementary scales; the ten Content Scales include Anxiety, Fears, Obsessiveness, Depression, Health Concerns, Bizarre Mentation, Anger, Cynicism, Antisocial Practices, Type A, Low Self-Esteem, Social Discomfort, Family Problems, Work Interference, and Negative Treatment Indicators. See the manual for more information on the Content and Supplementary scales.

MMPI-2 VALIDITY SCALES

Validity scales measuring item completion and item consistency are shown in Table 16–3. Scales that tap underreporting (i.e., L scale, K scale) tend to be elevated in groups attempting to minimize problems (e.g., personnel evaluations, custody evaluations) but not in most neuropsychological contexts. These are shown in Table 16–4 but will not be reviewed in detail here. Table 16–5 shows the main MMPI-2 scales for assessing overreporting of psychopathology, known as the F-Family of scales. Last, the cognitive and somatic overreporting scales are shown in Table 16–6; these are critical scales for neuropsychological assessment in particular.

TABLE 16–1 MMPI-2 Clinical Scales

SCALE	NAME	DESCRIPTION
1	Hypochondriasis (HS)	Tendency to deny good health and report a variety of physical symptoms
2	Depression (D)	Symptoms of depression including depressed mood, low self-esteem, and feelings of inadequacy
3	Hysteria (HY)	Somatic complaints and a tendency to deny psychological or social problems
4	Psychopathic Deviate (PD)	Antisocial behavior, alienation, rebellion, disrupted family relations, impulsiveness, legal/work/substance abuse problems
5	Masculinity-Femininity (MF)	Patterns of interest and attitudes that tend to follow gender stereotypes
6	Paranoia (PA)	Ideas of being misunderstood, persecuted, treated unfairly
7	Psychasthenia (PT)	Tendency to be anxious, worry, obsess, ruminate
8	Schizophrenia (SC)	Disturbed thinking, mood, and behavior
9	Hypomania (MA)	High activity/energy level, excitability, sociability, impulsivity, optimism, grandiosity
10	Social Introversion (SI)	Introversion, withdrawal

HOW TO ASSESS SYMPTOM VALIDITY USING THE MMPI-2

To properly assess validity, MMPI-2 interpretation should follow a sequential process starting first with assessing form completion (Cannot Say), then consistency using Variable Response Inconsistency (VRIN) and True Response Inconsistency (TRIN), and then moving on

TABLE 16–2 MMPI-2 Restructured Clinical (RC) Scales

SCALE	ABBREVIATION	SCALE NAME
RCd	DEM	Demoralization
RC1	SOM	Somatic Complaints
RC2	LPE	Low Positive Emotions
RC3	CYN	Cynicism
RC4	ASB	Antisocial Behavior
RC6	PER	Ideas of Persecution
RC7	DNE	Dysfunctional Negative Emotions
RC8	ABX	Aberrant Experiences
RC9	HPM	Hypomanic Activation

TABLE 16–3 Core MMPI-2 Validity Scales Measuring Item Completion and Consistency

COMPLETENESS AND CONSISTENCY SCALES		
CNS	Cannot Say	Reflects the number of unanswered items; may reflect defensiveness if above 30; scores above 35 invalidate the profile
VRIN	Variable Response Inconsistency	Based on 49 unique items generating 67 item pairs with similar or opposite content, scored based on whether item pairs are discrepant or not; high T scores indicate that items may have been answered indiscriminately, and that the profile is not valid; scores at 90 or above indicate an invalid profile; high scores may also indicate a nay-saying bias indicative of trying to fake good
TRIN	True Response Inconsistency	Based on 20 items with opposite content; high scores indicate a tendency to indiscriminately answer "True" to items; very low scores indicate a tendency to indiscriminately answer "False" to items; scores at or above 90 indicate an invalid profile

SOURCE: Adapted from information presented in Butcher (1998) and Greene (2008).

to assessing accuracy (underreporting and overreporting scales; Greene, 2008; see Figure 16–1). Not following this process raises the risk of false positives; that is, erroneously identifying inconsistent responding due to inattention, incapacity, or uncooperativeness as purposeful symptom exaggeration. This is because elevations on inconsistency scales can elevate overreporting scales in the absence of symptom distortion.

CANNOT SAY SCALE

The Cannot Say scale is sometimes seen as merely a clerical scale alerting the clinician to whether sufficient items

TABLE 16–4 Core MMPI-2 Validity Scales Measuring Underreporting

UNDERREPORTING SCALES		
L	Lie	Consists of items reflective of socially desirable traits that are unlikely to be true in the majority of people, and that reflect an unsophisticated or virtuous test-taking attitude; scores of 65 and above indicate that the examinee is presenting themselves in an overly positive light
K	Correction Scale	Consists of items reflective of the willingness to disclose personal information; designed to reduce false negatives on the L scale; scores of 65 and above indicate uncooperativeness, unwillingness, lack of insight, or reluctance to disclose personal information; intelligence and educational level need to be taken into account in interpreting the scale

SOURCE: Adapted from information presented in Butcher (1998) and Greene (2008).

TABLE 16–5 Core MMPI-2 Validity Scales Measuring Overreporting of Psychopathology

F-FAMILY OF SCALES		
F	Infrequency	Consists of a variety of items reflective of psychopathology with low endorsement (< 10%) in the original normative group; endorsement of F items suggest exaggeration, inaccurate self-appraisal, confusion, or faking of mental illness; sensitive to rare psychotic or other rarely endorsed psychological symptoms; scores at or above 90 indicate an invalid profile; all F items appear in the first 370 items of the MMPI-2
Fb	Back F	Designed to detect deviant responding on the last half of the MMPI-2 not covered by F, and also include items with low endorsement (<10%) in the normative sample; interpretation depends on the F score (i.e., some examinees may change their approach to items mid-way through the test, and provide a normal F but abnormal Fb); sensitive to rare psychotic or other rarely endorsed psychological symptoms
Fp	Infrequency—Psychopathology	Consists of items with low endorsement in psychiatric inpatients and in the normative sample, designed to be less prone to elevations in bona fide severe psychiatric conditions and more sensitive to exaggeration of psychopathology; scores at or above 90 indicate an invalid profile

SOURCE: Adapted from information presented in Butcher (1998) and Greene (2008).

TABLE 16–6 MMPI-2 Validity Scales for Measuring Overreporting of Cognitive and Somatic Symptoms

Core Validity Scales		
FBS	Symptom Validity Scale[a]	Designed specifically for personal injury cases to detect noncredible symptom presentation; sensitive to exaggeration of somatic and nonpsychotic symptoms
RBS	Response Bias Scale	Designed to detect cognitive malingering; items specifically selected on basis of ability to predict PVT failure in non-TBI disability claimants
Additional Validity Scales		
HHI	Henry-Heilbronner Index	Designed to detect somatic malingering; items were selected based on their ability to identify Slick et al. (1999) defined malingering in a sample with high prevalence of traumatic brain injury
CCS	Cognitive Complaints Scale	Designed to detect feigned cognitive symptoms in mild traumatic brain injury, the scale consists of items reflecting cognitive complaints only, with cut scores derived from mild traumatic brain injury samples and validated against failure on two or more PVTs; high scores suggest exaggeration of cognitive symptoms

NOTE: PVT, performance validity test; TBI, traumatic brain injury.

[a]Formerly known as the Fake Bad Scale.

SOURCE: Adapted from information presented in Butcher (1998), Greene (2008), and Nelson et al. (2006).

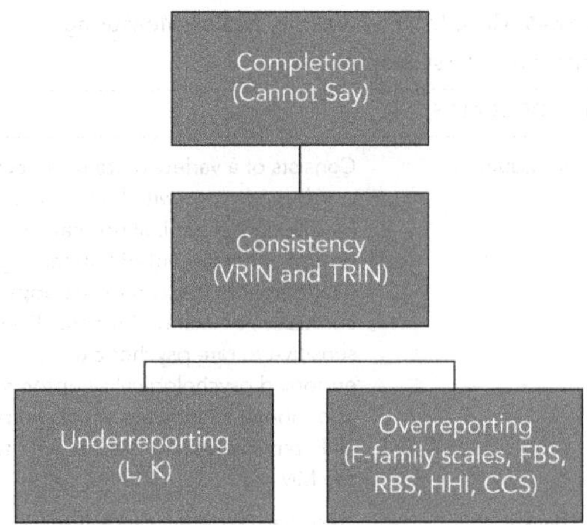

Figure 16–1 Steps for Assessing Validity on the Minnesota Multiphasic Personality Inventory-2 (MMPI-2).
SOURCE: Adapted from Greene (2008).

have been completed to allow scoring, but it is more than that. Because so few normative and clinical examinees omit items, a high number of omitted items can indicate defensiveness, paranoia, or frank refusal to cooperate with the assessment process. Although some conclude that malingerers tend not to omit items because one must endorse items in order to malinger successfully, some groups such as criminal defendants suspected of malingering make a high number of item omissions, supporting the view that deliberately skipping items may be a strategy to appear too impaired to complete the test (Greene, 2008). Scores of 30 or more indicate possible defensiveness, and scores of 35 or more invalidate the protocol.

VRIN AND TRIN

Once it is determined that sufficient items have been completed, interpretation of validity moves to determining the reliability of reporting, assessed via the consistency scales of VRIN and TRIN. Response consistency must be assessed before moving on to assessing validity scales indicative of over- or underreporting to guard against misidentification of inconsistent responding as malingering (Greene, 2008). VRIN is unaffected by pathology, with no differences between normative and clinical groups; poor consistency may be due to inadequate reading skills, low education or IQ, confusion due to psychiatric illness, active substance abuse, cognitive deficits, or noncompliance (Greene, 2008). Different cut scores have been recommended for VRIN; Greene (2008) proposed general guidelines for interpretation, reproduced in Table 16–7.

TABLE 16–7 General Guidelines for Interpreting VRIN

RAW SCORE	INTERPRETATION
≤7	High probability of consistent responding
8–15	Unclear whether items were completed consistently or not; check other MMPI-2 validity indices
≥16	High probability of inconsistent responding

SOURCE: Adapted from Greene (2008).

TRIN is similar to VRIN, except that items within item pairs are opposite in content rather than similar. This allows detection of all-True or all-False item responding, which will not be detected by VRIN. There is comparatively less research on TRIN, although one study shows that very low raw TRIN scores may indicate "faking good" due to a nay-saying bias and denial of problems (Hartmann & Hartmann, 2014).

F-FAMILY OF SCALES: OVERREPORTING OF PSYCHOPATHOLOGY

The MMPI-2 includes several psychopathology overreporting scales available either as part of the automatic scoring package or proposed in the literature; depending on the scale, the majority of these minimally tap cognitive or physical symptoms. These include the Infrequency scale (F), the Back F scale (Fb), the Infrequency-Psychopathology scale (Fp), the Infrequency minus K Correction (F – K), and the original and revised Gough's Dissimulation Index (Ds2 and Dsr2, respectively), as well as more recently derived scales for detecting feigned psychopathology such as the Malingered Depression (MD) scale, Malingered Mood Disorder Scale (MMDS), and Psychosocial Distress Scale (PDS). The Meyers Index assesses exaggeration of psychological symptoms by weighing seven MMPI-2 validity scales including the FBS. The reader is encouraged to consult other sources for more information on these scales (e.g., Aguerrevere et al., 2008; Boone, 2013; Greene, 2008; Heilbronner & Henry, 2013; Henry et al., 2008; Sweet et al., 2006).

Although the F-family of scales (F, Fb, Fp) have proved useful in distinguishing persons feigning various types of psychiatric disorders from true patients and healthy controls, their use in forensic neuropsychological settings has produced unsatisfactory results. This is because persons feigning neuropsychological conditions such as brain injury tend to endorse high rates of cognitive and somatic rather than psychiatric symptoms, causing the F scales to be minimally sensitive in these settings (Boone, 2013). F-family scales may be most appropriate to assess for exaggeration of psychotic symptoms—an uncommon scenario in personal injury or disability evaluations, but not infrequent in criminal defendants attempting to avoid criminal responsibility. Like all overreporting scales, F scales can be elevated due to random responding (Greene, 2008), and this needs to be ruled out before inferring exaggeration of psychopathology.

SYMPTOM VALIDITY SCALE (FBS)

The FBS is the best-known of the core MMPI-2 validity scales most relevant to neuropsychological assessment.

Developed by Lees-Haley et al. (1991), previously known as the Fake Bad Scale, and now renamed the Symptom Validity Scale, it is a 43-item scale comprised of items endorsed infrequently by personal injury claimants with bona fide symptoms (Greene, 2008). According to critics, the FBS was renamed because the original name was found prejudicial in a judicial opinion in which its admissibility was denied (Nichols & Gass, 2015). It was originally derived to detect malingering in personal injury cases who were claiming emotional distress but not symptoms related to brain injury or neuropsychological problems (Heilbronner & Henry, 2013). However, it has come to be used by neuropsychologists to detect malingered neurocognitive dysfunction as well. Items cover both social desirability and symptom exaggeration, with most FBS items taken from Clinical Scales 1 and 3 (i.e., Hypochondriasis and Hysteria) and RC1 (Somatic Complaints). Consequently, FBS is thought to measure exaggeration of somatic symptoms more than exaggeration of psychiatric symptoms (Nelson et al., 2006). In addition, FBS is thought to be uniquely related to cognitive feigning (Slick et al., 1996; Greiffenstein et al., 2002) as it correlates more highly with Slick-defined malingering (i.e., Slick et al., 1999) and performance validity tests (PVTs) than do F scales, although some studies show that other scales such as RBS and HHI are equally or more suited in this regard, most obviously because their items were derived specifically to predict PVT failure or Slick et al. malingering criteria, respectively. However, FBS contains few cognitive items. The FBS is one of the core MMPI-2 validity scales automatically calculated by the scoring program.

RESPONSE BIAS SCALE (RBS)

Like the FBS, the RBS is a core validity scale on the MMPI-2. The RBS consists of 28 items selected for their ability to predict feigned cognitive symptoms (Gervais et al., 2007). The scale was derived in a sample of non–brain-injured disability claimants using failure on one PVT out of three as the criterion for group membership (i.e., failure on either the Test of Memory Malingering [TOMM], Word Memory Test [WMT], or Computerized Assessment of Response Bias [CARB]). Items are varied, with items from Clinical scales 7 and 8 (Psychasthenia and Schizophrenia) and RC1 (Somatic Complaints). It has few cognitive items, but relatively more than does FBS. The scale therefore taps somatic concerns, dysphoria, anxiety, cognitive problems, and delusions of control (Nichols, 2011). Items have a significant degree of overlap with those of FBS, which, in addition to tapping a similar construct may account for their high intercorrelations in most studies (see "Evidence for Validity"). Like the FBS, RBS is one of the core MMPI-2 validity scales automatically calculated by the scoring program.

HENRY-HEILBRONNER INDEX (HHI)

The HHI (Henry et al., 2006) is not as well-known as the FBS and RBS and is currently not part of the core MMPI-2 validity indexes automatically provided by the scoring program but can be obtained by contacting the author (ghenry0249@aol.com). It is reported to measure exaggeration, overreporting, and malingering of physical symptoms (i.e., "somatic malingering"). It consists of 15 items derived from the FBS and Shaw and Matthew's Pseudoneurologic Scale, the latter originally developed to differentiate psychiatric from neurological patients (for details, see Henry et al., 2006). Unlike other scales, item selection was based on item correlations with malingering group membership defined by Slick et al. (1999) malingering criteria in a sample with a high prevalence of brain injuries. Of the 15 items on the HHI, 11 can be found on the FBS.

COGNITIVE COMPLAINTS SCALE (CCS)

The CCS is a 13-item scale developed by Henry, Heilbronner, and colleagues (Henry et al., 2014), developers of the HHI. It is also not currently part of the core MMPI-2 validity indexes automatically provided by the scoring program but can be obtained by contacting the author (ghenry0249@aol.com). The CCS was developed to serve as a better indicator of feigned cognitive problems given that existing MMPI-2 validity scales had few items specifically tapping cognitive symptoms. According to the authors, only two of 43 FBS items, nine of 28 RBS items, and two of 15 HHI items tap cognitive problems. The derivation of an index with more items tapping cognition was therefore thought to increase predictive validity with regard to PVT failure (Henry et al., 2014). Items were initially selected based on rational analysis, followed by nonparametric item response theory scaling in order to identify items that discriminated between examinees who passed and failed two or more PVTs. According to the authors, one distinct advantage of the scale is that it shares very few items with the FBS and HHI (two items) and RBS (four items), nor are items found on the traditional F-family set of scales.

ADMINISTRATION

Details regarding MMPI-2 administration procedures can be found in the original source. Computer administration and computer scoring are highly recommended to reduce errors in transcription and scoring, and to reduce administration time. For most examinees, the item-by-item computer administration confers an advantage over booklet and response sheet administration due to the lower demands on attention and visual scanning required to track items and transcribe answers to an answer sheet.

Of note, although breaks are permitted, allowing the examinee to complete the MMPI-2 at home is not recommended because norms were generated under carefully controlled conditions, factors affecting validity cannot be controlled, and responses may be influenced by others, or possibly even completed by someone other than the examinee. A Grade 8 reading ability is necessary, although Nichols (2011) reports that a Grade 9 reading level is required for some items.

SCORING

Generally speaking, hand-scoring is possible with the use of various scoring keys but is highly discouraged given the potential for errors and the amount of time required. Entering data from booklet administration into the scoring program also introduces potential for errors, so careful review or double-scoring is required to ensure accurate scores. Computer administration eliminates both these problems and is therefore highly recommended.

The FBS and RBS are automatically calculated as part of the standard MMPI-2 scoring program. At present, the HHI and CCS are not part of the standard MMPI-2 scoring software but item lists and scoring criteria can be obtained directly from the author (ghenry0249@aol.com).

Scores for the FBS and RBS are provided as raw scores and T scores on the MMPI-2 scoring program, along with interpretations. However, it is highly recommended that cutoff scores appropriate for the examinee and the setting be consulted for interpretation rather than relying exclusively on the MMPI-2 scoring program and interpretive software (see "Clinical Studies"). HHI and CCS scores can be interpreted by using suggested cutoff values (see "Clinical Studies").

Importantly, when interpreting MMPI-2 clinical and content scales, T scores of 65 or greater are usually considered clinically significant; this is not necessarily the case for validity indices. Very high T scores may be required on some validity scales to reach the invalid range (e.g., T > 90 and T > 100; see "Clinical Studies").

DEMOGRAPHIC EFFECTS

AGE

There is scant information on age and MMPI-2 validity scales, although age is unrelated to CCS scores in the original validation sample (Henry et al., 2014).

GENDER

Gender differences have been reported for FBS. Women tend to score about two points higher than men (Greiffenstein et al., 2007), and there are larger effect sizes for women (Nelson et al., 2010) that are present across samples with various ethnicities (Dean et al., 2008). Separate cutoffs are therefore usually provided for men and women. However, in a large personal injury sample, Lee and colleagues found no evidence of clinically meaningful gender bias in prediction of PVT test failure for men and women using the publisher's recommended FBS cutoff scores (Lee et al., 2012). The influence of gender on other MMPI-2 validity scales such as RBS, HHI, and CCS has not been well studied, although one meta-analytic study shows no gender effects for RBS (Ingram & Ternes, 2016).

EDUCATION AND IQ

Education effects have not been extensively studied but appear minimal. Education accounted for less than 3% of shared variance in FBS scores in a sample with mixed ethnicities (Dean et al., 2008). No effects of education are found for RBS (Ingram & Ternes, 2016). The CCS is reported to be unrelated to education (Henry et al., 2014).

ETHNICITY, NATIONALITY, AND LINGUISTIC EFFECTS

In one study involving Caucasian, Hispanic, and African Americans, no significant differences in FBS scores were reported (Dean et al., 2008). There is surprisingly little information on ethnicity for other scales such as the RBS, and validity indicator information is lacking on translated versions of the MMPI-2 (Nijdam-Jones & Rosenfeld, 2017).

NORMATIVE DATA

MMPI-2 STANDARDIZATION SAMPLE

General MMPI-2 norms were developed from a sample of 2,600 community-dwelling individuals recruited by ads, directories, and mailing lists (Butcher et al., 2001). In comparison to the 1990 US Census data, there was some underrepresentation of Hispanics and Asian Americans, as well as of the extremes of the age distribution. In contrast, each validity scale reviewed here was developed based on samples of examinees not included in the original MMPI-2 standardization sample. These are described next. Note that recommended cutoffs may be derived from these original validation samples or from later cross-validation samples, depending on the scale (see "Clinical Studies").

FBS VALIDATION SAMPLE

The FBS sample consisted of 45 personal injury cases from the private practice of the FBS first author, 25 of whom were identified as malingerers (Lees-Haley et al., 1991). FBS items were selected based on their ability to distinguish between malingerers and nonmalingerers; exact criteria for determination of malingering were not clearly provided, nor were details regarding injuries or referral sources (Butcher et al., 2008). Because of this, some of its more vocal critics have concluded that the FBS is at best a scale that differentiates personal injury litigants from nonlitigants, not malingerers from nonmalingerers (Butcher et al., 2008). However, there is a large body of research supporting its validity as a tool effective at detecting malingering (see "Clinical Studies").

RBS VALIDATION SAMPLE

The RBS was developed based on 1,212 non–brain-injured disability claimants from the private practice of the RBS's first author with relatively equal representation of men and women and an average education of 12 years; ethnicity was not reported. They were classified as either valid or invalid based on failure on one of three PVTs (i.e., either the TOMM, WMT, or CARB). The scale was then validated on a separate sample of more than 300 disability claimants with mixed diagnoses such as anxiety, depression, pain, and traumatic brain injury (TBI) passing or failing the WMT or Medical Symptom Validity Test (MSVT), some of whom were from the same private practice that also provided patients for the original study (Gervais et al., 2007). Since then, the RBS has been validated in civil litigants, disability and criminal samples, and in veteran samples, among others (Nelson et al., 2007; Whitney et al., 2008; Wygant et al., 2010).

HHI VALIDATION SAMPLE

The HHI scale was developed using data from 119 adults, 45 of whom were seen for personal injury or disability evaluations and determined to be malingering based on Slick et al. (1999) probable and definite malingering criteria. Although precise numbers can only be estimated from the study, it appears that more than 50% of this malingering group had diagnoses of brain injury. In addition, 74 nonlitigating brain-injured patients, mostly mild brain injury, served as the nonmalingering group. Education was reported for some subgroups, with an average education of about 14 years in the malingering group; no information on ethnicity is provided.

CCS VALIDATION SAMPLE

The CCS was developed based on 100 adults with mild TBI who were either litigants or disability claimants, and classified as either passing or failing PVTs based on failure on two or more of the TOMM, WMT, and Victoria Symptom Validity Test (VSVT). In addition, a mild brain injury, no-incentive control group was included for comparison. Gender distribution was approximately equal, and the sample had an average education between 12 and 14 years and was generally Caucasian (>90%; Henry et al., 2014).

EVIDENCE FOR RELIABILITY

EVIDENCE FOR INTERNAL RELIABILITY

There is information on internal reliability for some but not all MMPI-2 validity scales reviewed here. FBS internal reliability is low to marginal in the normative sample (alpha = .55 to .60, Ben-Porath et al., 2009), with higher reliabilities in personal injury samples (i.e., .86 for men, .85 for women; Butcher et al., 2003) that exceed those for both F and Fb (Lees-Haley & Fox, 2004). HHI internal reliability is also reported as high (alpha = .88; Henry et al., 2006).

EVIDENCE FOR TEST-RETEST RELIABILITY, MEASURING CHANGE, AND PRACTICE EFFECTS

Although some experts in the field advocate that test-retest reliability is not necessary for PVTs and SVTs, our stance is that it is important to demonstrate reliability in honest responders, including both healthy samples and in individuals with medical, neurological, and psychiatric conditions of interest. The FBS monograph reports an adequate one-week test-retest reliability of .72 for a subsample of the normative sample (N = 193), a value similar to that of the F-family scales. No information on any effects of repeat administration on test means were reported. To our knowledge, there exists no other information on the reliability of MMPI-2 validity indices.

EVIDENCE FOR VALIDITY

FACTOR-ANALYTIC STUDIES

Overall, factor-analytic studies of the MMPI-2 show that FBS, RBS, and HHI tap a somatic and cognitive overreporting factor, a dimension separate from the psychopathologic overreporting inherent to the F-family of scales, but also separate from that measured by PVTs. For example, in a military sample, FBS, HHI, and RBS loaded together on a factor tapping cognitive and somatic overreporting that was separate from the F-family scales, which loaded together on a second factor comprised of F, Fb, and Fp and deemed to reflect overreporting of psychopathology (Jones & Ingram, 2011). With regard to PVTs, a four-factor model emerged when Nelson and colleagues examined MMPI-2 validity indices along with PVTs, with MMPI-2 scales loading on three factors characterized as underreporting of psychological symptoms, overreporting of neurotic symptoms, and overreporting of psychotic symptoms, with PVTs such as the VSVT and TOMM clustering together on a separate factor (Nelson et al., 2007). Specifically, FBS and RBS loaded together on a single overreporting factor, while F-scales and other overreporting scales loaded on a separate factor. Although the study points to the separate dimensions tapped by SVTs and PVTs, the authors acknowledge that MMPI-2 item overlap may have contributed to the factor solution as well.

Another confirmatory factor analysis in a veteran sample yielded three distinct factors; the first factor comprised of standard cognitive tests, the second of PVTs (Reliable Digit Span, TOMM, MSVT), and a third factor reflecting both self-reported symptoms and symptom validity measures from the MMPI-2 (F, FBS, RBS) along with posttraumatic stress disorder (PTSD) and postconcussive scales (Van Dyke et al., 2013).

A factor analysis of the FBS in a veteran sample yielded three factors deemed tiredness/distractibility, claimed virtue of self/others, and stomach/head discomfort, the latter discriminating between veterans who passed and failed PVTs. However, structural discordance related to the claimed virtue factor, behaviors commonly denied by healthy individuals, was thought to introduce systematic error variance in this sample, which the authors felt indicated content ambiguity for the FBS (Gass & Odland, 2014).

Although methodological details are not provided, principal components analysis of the HHI by its authors indicates one dominant factor comprised mostly of items reflecting physical symptoms, consistent with the interpretation of the scale as measuring "somatic malingering" (Henry et al., 2006). To our knowledge, factor-analytic studies have not yet been conducted on the CCS.

MMPI-2 VALIDITY SCALE INTERCORRELATIONS AND COMPARISONS

Correlations between FBS, RBS, and HHI range from modest to high, with most studies showing a fair degree of association depending on the sample. FBS, RBS, and HHI validity scales tend to be moderately to highly intercorrelated; not surprisingly, the degree of correlation between scales often relates to the degree of item overlap. Specifically, there is a high degree of shared items between FBS and HHI, and between FBS and RBS, so significant intercorrelations are not surprising. In a veteran sample, FBS, RBS, and HHI correlations ranged from .73 to 80, with particular high correlations between FBS and HHI (r = .86) and RBS and HHI (r = .80). High correlations between FBS and RBS are also reported in simulators (Sullivan & Elliott, 2012). Given the high correlations and item overlap between FBS and HHI, one author has called the HHI "FBS lite" (Dionysus et al., 2011).

In TBI litigants, Dionysus and colleagues found that FBS and HHI were most highly correlated, followed by RBS and HHI, and finally, FBS and RBS (r = .73, .65, and .51, respectively; Dionysus et al., 2011). Despite the high correlations between scales, in this group, RBS and FBS significantly increased prediction of malingering compared to the HHI, and HHI did not contribute to further incremental validity over RBS and FBS. Similar findings are reported by others in litigants with TBI and clinical patients, with very high correlations between FBS and HHI, but also between RBS and HHI (r = .79, r = .73; Tsushima et al., 2011). In contrast, other studies show that the highest association are between RBS and HHI and find that these two scales generally perform better than FBS (Jones & Ingram, 2011).

In some studies, RBS correlates with overreporting of psychopathology (F-scales) in criminal samples but not disability samples, consistent with the notion that criminal defendants tend to exaggerate both cognitive and psychiatric symptoms whereas disability samples exaggerate cognitive and somatic symptoms (Wygant et al., 2010; see also Sullivan et al., 2013; Sullivan & Elliott, 2012). Correlational studies for the CCS are lacking as of this writing.

CORRELATIONS WITH AND COMPARISONS TO OTHER PVTS AND SVTS

Most studies show moderate correlations between PVTs and the MMPI-2 FBS, RBS, and HHI validity scales, with lower correlations between PVTs and F-family scales in most but not all studies. Importantly, despite the fact that RBS was specifically derived and validated using PVT failure as its criterion for invalidity, RBS is not necessarily more highly correlated with PVT performance than other scales such as FBS and HHI, scales whose items were selected based on malingering and not PVT failure. Most researchers agree that the moderate correlations between PVTs and MMPI-2 validity indicators such as FBS, RBS, and HHI support the general view that PVTs and SVTs such as those from the MMPI-2 tap different aspects of malingering and exaggeration and are complementary and necessary aspects of comprehensive neuropsychological assessment.

In terms of specific PVTs, the FBS correlates fairly well with the VSVT, the Portland Digit Recognition Test, the Rey Fifteen-Item Test (FIT), and Reliable Digit Span (Slick et al., 1996; Greiffenstein et al., 2002; Larrabee, 2003b). In one study, compared to embedded PVTs derived from the Benton Visual Form Discrimination, Finger Tapping, Reliable Digit Span, and Wisconsin Card Sorting Test (WCST), the FBS was the single most sensitive measure for discriminating definite malingerers from those with moderate-severe TBI (Larrabee, 2005).

The RBS also correlates moderately with PVTs such as the MSVT, TOMM, and CARB in studies by the RBS authors (rs = −.32 to −.44; Gervais et al., 2008), although one might expect higher correlations given how the scale was constructed (i.e., performance on these exact PVTs served as the criterion for selecting items). Similar-sized correlations have been reported between the RBS and TOMM, and between the HHI and the TOMM in veterans (r = −.31 to −.43, Whitney et al., 2008), with only marginally higher correlations for the RBS versus the HHI. Whitney et al. (2008) found marginally higher effect sizes for RBS than HHI in predicting failure on the TOMM in their mixed veterans sample, but both had very large effect sizes compared to F-family scales and were superior to the FBS. Similarly, compared to the FBS and F scales, the RBS was best at predicting PVT performance in civil litigants (Smart et al., 2008). The RBS appears effective in classifying individuals as having passed or failed a PVT using optimal classification tree analysis; in comparison, the FBS is not a significant predictor (Smart et al., 2008). The authors noted that variable classifications and moderate effect strengths indicated that correspondence among MMPI-2 scales and PVTs is inconsistent and that PVTs should never be omitted in favor of MMPI-2 validity scales in a forensic context.

In contrast, in a veteran sample, Young and colleagues found only modest correlations between MMPI-2 validity indexes and the WMT, with correlations in the range of .15 to .20 for FBS, RBS and HHI, as well as for F-family scales (Young et al., 2011). Furthermore, they found no incremental validity in using RBS to predict WMT performance beyond that already provided by F-type scales and FBS. Wygant and colleagues found that the RBS and FBS were relatively equivalent at discriminating between disability claimants passing a PVT (WMT or TOMM), and RBS and Fp were relatively equivalent at discriminating between criminal defendants passing a PVT (Wygant et al., 2010). As well, although RBS added incremental validity in the disability sample over other MMPI-2 validity scales, it did not in improve prediction in criminal defendants.

Studies on the association between the CCS and PVTs are lacking as of this writing.

CORRELATIONS WITH OTHER NEUROPSYCHOLOGICAL TESTS AND QUESTIONNAIRES

The RBS is highly correlated with subjective memory complaints in non-head-injured disability claimants as measured by the Memory Complaints Inventory (MCI; Green, 2004), whereas the FBS and the F-family scales show only moderate to high correlations with this scale (Gervais et al., 2008). However, the RBS does not appear to correlate with objective memory testing as measured by the California Verbal Learning Test (CVLT) once those failing PVTs are excluded (Gervais et al., 2008), thus providing further evidence that RBS taps exaggeration and not cognitive functioning per se. Overall, there is not an extensive literature on the associations between FBS, RBS, HHI, and CCS and other neuropsychological tests and standardized questionnaires.

The RBS has been used in combination with PVTs and the MCI (Green, 2004) to identify malingering as defined by the Slick et al. (1999) criteria. Guidelines to do so are reproduced in Table 16–8, based on non-traumatic-brain-injury litigants (Gervais et al., 2008). They are designed to help users differentiate between overexaggeration of memory complaints related to psychiatric/somatoform disorders and volitional exaggeration related to malingering. Further validation is needed before generalizing to other kinds of clinical populations, but these guidelines show promise in the use of combined tools to maximize accurate interpretation in clinical settings.

TABLE 16–8 Interpretive Guidelines for the Response Bias Scale (RBS) in Combination with PVT and Memory Complaints Inventory (MCI) Results

RBS T SCORE	INTERPRETATION
<50	Minimal memory or other cognitive symptoms reported; consider denial or "fake good" attitude if cognitive testing reveals deficits. PVT failure unlikely. If PVT failed, consider passive factors such as disengagement or disinterest rather than active negative response bias.
50–64	Minor memory or cognitive symptoms may be reported, consistent with cognitive test results. If F, Fb, and Fp T scores <80, consider emotional factors contributing to memory complaints. PVT failure unlikely. If PVT failed, consider passive factors such as lack of engagement in testing. If F, Fb, and Fp T scores >80, symptom exaggeration is possible. Rule out possible MND as per Slick et al. (1999) criteria.
65–79	Increasing memory complaints; if F, Fb, and Fp T scores <80, complaints are probably related to emotional factors. If F, Fb, and Fp T scores >80 or PVT failed, consider volitional symptom exaggeration; rule out possible MND.
80–99	Exaggerated memory complaints are likely; this T-score range is associated with MCI scores 1.5 SD above moderate to severe brain injury; probability of PVT failure as high as 67%. If F, Fb, and Fp T scores <80, memory complaints may be related to emotional factors. If F, Fb, or Fp T scores >80, exaggerated psychopathology is possible. If PVT failed, exaggerated memory complaints are probable; rule out probable MND.
100+	Memory complaints are exaggerated; this T-score range is associated with MCI scores 2 SDs above moderate to severe brain injury; probability of PVT failure is 77–100%. If F, Fb, or Fp T scores >100, malingered psychopathology is probable. If PVT failed, exaggeration of memory complaints is confirmed. If PVT passed, rule out coaching. Rule out probable or definite MND.

NOTE: PVT, performance validity test; F, Infrequency; Fb, Infrequency Back; Fp, Infrequency Psychopathology; MND, malingered neurocognitive dysfunction as per Slick et al. (1999) criteria; MCI, Memory Complaints Inventory.

SOURCE: Gervais et al. (2008), used with permission.

CLINICAL STUDIES

Overall, the clinical literature on FBS, RBS, HHI, and CCS generally includes known-groups studies primarily consisting of compensation-seeking individuals (litigation, disability, and military), with fewer studies on criminal defendants. In terms of clinical populations with higher than average base rates of malingering, the majority of studies have involved TBI, with comparatively few studies on psychiatric patients. Most importantly, all of the MMPI-2 validity indices have been evaluated in terms of their ability to predict malingering based on Slick et al. (1999) criteria. Other studies have also validated cutoffs based on prediction of PVT failure, which is a lesser criterion of validity but which still contributes to incremental validity.

Incidentally, not much is known about the use of MMPI-2 SVTs in specific populations at high risk of false positives on PVTs, namely low-IQ examinees and dementia patients, as the MMPI-2 is virtually never used in these groups. Studies on resistance to coaching appear to be lacking, as are neuroanatomical correlations and imaging studies, which exist for a small number of PVTs (e.g., WMT).

FBS DIAGNOSTIC ACCURACY WITH REGARDS TO SLICK ET AL. (1999) OR OTHER MALINGERING CRITERIA

Overall, over the years, evidence supportive of higher cutoffs has begun to accumulate, particularly from more recent studies based on the use of malingering criteria and recommended specificity rates to reduce false-positive risk (i.e., ≥90% specificity). Earlier studies including the initial validation study suggested cutoffs such as 20, 21, and 24 (e.g., Greiffenstein et al., 2002; Larrabee, 2003b, 2003c; Lees-Haley, 1992; Lees-Haley et al., 1991). For example, Greiffenstein, Fox, and Lees-Haley (2007) examined a large sample combined from a variety of conditions (N = 1,052) and determined that a cutoff of 22 or higher had a specificity of .90, a cutoff of 25 or higher had a specificity of .95, and a cutoff of 28 or higher had a specificity of .99; that is, false-positive rates of 10%, 5%, and 1%, respectively. Based on these data, a cutoff of 23 for men and 26 for women (T score of 80) was deemed to suggest possible exaggeration according to the test publisher (Ben-Porath et al., 2009).

A statement from the MMPI-2 University of Minnesota Press indicates that raw scores above 22 (i.e., cutoff ≥23) should raise concerns about the validity of symptoms and that raw scores above 28 (i.e., cutoff of ≥29) should raise very significant concerns about validity. The latter is associated with a very low false-positive rate of erroneously identifying results of those reporting genuine health problems as invalid (Ben-Porath & Tellegen, 2017).

Studies using Slick et al. (1999) criteria for probable or definite malingered neurocognitive dysfunction are remarkably consistent in showing that when specificity is held at .90 (i.e., at an acceptable false-positive rate of <10%) an FBS cutoff of at least 25 or more is required, although a substantial proportion of malingerers are missed by this cutoff. Recommended cutoffs and classification accuracy statistics are shown in Table 16–9 for studies using the Slick et al. criteria. These and other studies tend toward the consensus view that FBS scores of 30 or more are highly indicative of malingering and are extremely unlikely to result in false positives (Greve et al., 2006; Meyers et al., 2002; Larrabee, 2003a, 2003b). In TBI, the FBS also correlates with the number of separate criteria met for malingered neurocognitive dysfunction, with higher FBS scores related to a higher probability of meeting malingering criteria (Greve et al., 2006). Of note, in our review, we could not find a criminal sample that employed Slick et al. criteria for the determination of malingering, so these cutoffs apply to litigants, disability claimants, military samples, and to TBI. To our knowledge, there are no studies on prediction of malingered pain-related disability based on Bianchini et al. malingering criteria (2005).

As is always the case for PVTs and SVTs, any increase in the cutoff score to decrease false positives will result in a decrease in sensitivity to detection of malingering. However, FBS sensitivities remain relatively acceptable even with maintaining the .90 standard for specificity, which is not always the case for other MMPI-2 validity indices reviewed here (e.g., RBS). In the studies reviewed here, sensitivity ranged from .37 to .64, and PPV ranged from .83 to .92 at a 40 to 50% base rate, all of which demonstrates considerable support for the use of the scale (Table 16–9).

Of note, none of these studies suggest different cutoffs for men and women; however, gender was typically not examined separately in these studies, and one study involved primarily males (i.e., military sample from Jones, 2016).

Greve and colleagues provide cumulative frequencies across different clinical conditions to compare individual examinees' raw scores to various clinical groups including TBI, cerebrovascular disease, memory disorder, and psychiatric conditions; these are shown in Table 16–10 (Greve et al., 2006).

TABLE 16–9 Symptom Validity Scale (FBS) Classification Accuracy for Cutoffs with Acceptable Specificities (≥90%) for Prediction of Malingered Neurocognitive Dysfunction (MND)

STUDY	GROUP	MND CRITERION	N	RAW SCORE CUTOFF	SENSITIVITY (%)	SPECIFICITY (%)
Henry et al. (2006)	Personal injury/disability and non-litigants (>50% TBI)	Probable or Definite MND	119	≥24	64	92
Larrabee (2003b)	Mild TBI litigants and moderate to severe TBI litigant/nonlitigants	Definite MND	55	≥25	62	93
Dionysus et al. (2011)	TBI litigants	Probable MND	79	≥25	60	90
Jones (2016)	Mild TBI active duty military	Probable or Definite MND	300	≥25	37	92
Greve et al. (2006)	TBI, with and without incentives	Probable or Definite MND	259	≥28	46	96
Peck et al. (2013)	TBI litigants	Probable MND	45	≥28	39	93

NOTE: MND, malingered neurocognitive dysfunction; TBI, traumatic brain injury.

Cutoff scores and T scores that were not provided in original sources were estimated/extrapolated from the MMPI-2 Technical Manual, and so may not map exactly onto values provided in original sources.

TABLE 16–10 Symptom Validity Scale (FBS) Raw Score Cumulative Percentages for Malingering and Nonmalingering Patients with Various Neurological Conditions

	MALINGERING	NONMALINGERING						
	TBI (*N* = 96)	MILD TBI (*N* = 51)	MODERATE-SEVERE TBI (*N* = 46)	CVA (*N* = 51)	MEMORY DISORDER (*N* = 20)	PSYCHIATRIC (*N* = 22)	TOTAL NON-TBI (*N* = 132)	
FBS								*FBS*
39	0							*39*
38	1							*38*
37	1							*37*
36	2							*36*
35	5							*35*
34	10							*34*
33	14		0					*33*
32	18		2					*32*
31	22		2					*31*
30	27		2					*30*
29	33		2					*29*
28	41	4	2	0			*0*	*28*
27	46	14	4	2			*1*	*27*
26	50	24	7	4		0	*2*	*26*
25	52	33	9	6		5	*4*	*25*
24	59	43	9	12		5	*6*	*24*
23	62	47	15	12		5	*8*	*23*
22	65	49	17	12		9	*9*	*22*
21	68	53	22	12		27	*14*	*21*
20	71	57	24	16	0	36	*19*	*20*
15	85	78	52	55	40	77	*52*	*15*
5	100	100	100	100	100	100	*100*	*5*

NOTE: Total Non-TBI: All non-TBI diagnoses, including cerebrovascular accident (CVA), memory disorder, psychiatric, encephalopathy, infection, seizure, multiple sclerosis, substance abuse, academic problems, lupus, and no diagnosis. TBI, traumatic brain injury.

SOURCE: Adapted from Greve et al. (2006).

OTHER CLINICAL STUDIES ON THE FBS

In their large meta-analysis of FBS research, Nelson et al. (2010) found large effect sizes for the FBS compared to medium effect sizes for F-family scales, particularly in TBI (Nelson et al., 2010).

In one study on concussion, an elevated FBS was the most prevalent finding in individuals with late postconcussive syndrome and PTSD, more frequent than MMPI-2 F and PVTs including the TOMM, Reliable Digit Span, finger tapping, and grip strength; dually diagnosed individuals had higher failure rates than those with postconcussive syndrome only (Greiffenstein & Baker, 2008). Importantly, the authors noted that in these cases, the differential diagnosis should include somatization, factitious disorder, and personality disorders in addition to malingering, supporting the view that an elevated FBS is not synonymous with malingering.

FBS requires more study in its ability to detect exaggeration of chronic pain, although initial results are promising (Nelson et al., 2010). With regard to differentiating between intentional exaggeration (i.e., malingering) versus unintentional exaggeration (i.e., somatization and conversion disorders), Peck and colleagues found that individuals with psychogenic nonepileptic seizures, a form of unintentional symptom exaggeration due to psychopathology, obtained FBS scores between those of nonmalingering and malingering TBI patients. They concluded that the MMPI-2 could serve as a useful measure for differentiating between somatic symptom disorders and malingering, something that PVTs are less able to do according to these authors (Peck et al., 2013).

The FBS does not appear to be associated with medical or sleep variables in medical inpatients undergoing sleep studies, indicating minimal influence on scores from medical impairment (Greiffenstein, 2010). Scores are also not influenced by whether they were obtained during plaintiff versus defense forensic examination (Greiffenstein et al., 2010).

RBS: DIAGNOSTIC ACCURACY WITH REGARDS TO SLICK ET AL. (1999) OR OTHER MALINGERING CRITERIA

The RBS has been used in several studies, with most supporting the utility of the scale to detect exaggeration of cognitive and somatic symptoms. Although the initial validation study by Gervais and colleagues (Gervais et al., 2007) used failure on a PVT as the gold-standard criterion for establishing cutoffs rather than malingering as defined by multidimensional malingering criteria, several studies are indeed supportive of RBS in predicting malingered neurocognitive dysfunction. Although some researchers conclude that prior RBS studies may have used methods that fall short of recommended guidelines for malingering research, including reliance on weak classification methods and group statistics (Sullivan et al., 2013), the RBS has not been criticized with the same vehemence and tenacity as has the FBS, even though both scales appear to function quite similarly in neuropsychological studies of detection of exaggeration and malingering.

Table 16–11 shows RBS classification accuracy statistics to predict Slick et al. (1999) and Bianchini et al. (2005) malingering criteria for cutoffs associated with acceptable specificities (i.e., cutoffs that keep the false-positive rate at ≤10%). With one exception, these indicate that cutoffs closer to a T score of 90 and over (i.e., 88 to 114, depending on the sample) are optimal. Generally speaking, cutoffs closer to 95 were needed in these studies for identifying verified malingering. This contrasts with the cutoffs suggested by the publisher, which include 80 to 99 for possible overreporting and more than 100 for likely overreporting. Note that some studies are based on the MMPI-2-RF, which uses the same RBS scale. Overall, sensitivities range from .13 to .73 for a minimum specificity of .90, with PPVs of .50 to .89 at base rates of 40 to 50% in these studies (Table 16–11). At an average PPV of .72, this is lower than the FBS, but both measures appear to be effective at malingering detection.

Nguyen et al. (2015) found that to maintain 90% specificity and ensure an acceptable rate of false positives, much higher RBS cutoffs had to be employed than are provided in the manual (i.e., T scores of ≥101 to 114, depending on the group; see Table 16–11 for raw score equivalents). Similarly, Schroeder et al. (2012) found that an RBS cutoff of 16 or higher (T score of >92) provided a 43% sensitivity rate with a specificity of greater than 90% in TBI litigants, but that a higher cutoff was required in psychiatric patients (i.e., T score >105). Different cutoffs are likely needed in different settings. For example, higher cutoffs are reported in veteran and criminal settings using PVTs as validation; however, these cutoffs have not yet been validated using malingering criteria per se (e.g., criminal defendants, ≥20; Wygant et al., 2010; veterans, ≥17; Whitney et al., 2008; Young et al., 2011).

Of note, the mid-range cutoffs presented here are close to those suggested in the original RBS validation study, which suggested a raw score cutoff of 17 or greater or T score higher than 100 (Gervais et al., 2007). Of note, one study with a recommended cutoff of 17 or greater involved disability claimants that were from the same private practice as those of the original RBS validation study (Tarescavage et al., 2013). Lower cutoffs may be optimal in military samples, as shown by the optimal cutoff of 15 or greater in the Jones study (2016). Higher cutoffs are recommended in psychiatric patients, equivalent to 20 or more raw score points or 114 or more T-score points.

Schroeder and colleagues (2012) provide RBS T-score cumulative frequencies for groups defined by Slick-criteria

TABLE 16–11 Response Bias Scale (RBS) Classification Accuracy for Cutoffs with Acceptable Specificities (≥90%) for Prediction of Malingered Neurocognitive Dysfunction (MND) or Malingered Pain-Related Disability (MPRD)

STUDY	GROUP	CRITERION	N	RAW SCORE CUTOFF	T SCORE CUTOFF	SENSITIVITY (%)	SPECIFICITY (%)
Bianchini et al. (2017)	Chronic pain patients	Probable or Definite MPRD	501	≥12	≥80	73	≥ 90
Dionysus et al. (2011)	TBI litigants	Probable MND	79	≥14	≥88	54	93
Sullivan et al. (2013)	Mixed incentive (43% TBI)	Possible, Probable or Definite MND	83	≥14	≥88	27	90
Jones (2016)	Mild TBI active duty military	Probable or Definite MND	300	≥15	≥92	52	93
Schroeder et al. (2012)	TBI litigants	Probable or Definite MND	48	≥16	>92	43	92
Peck et al. (2013)	TBI litigants	Probable MND	45	≥16	≥96	50	92
Tarescavage et al. (2013)	Disability claimants	Probable or Definite MND	863	≥17	>100	34	92
Nguyen et al. (2015)	Disability/Civil forensic—medical symptoms	Defined as passed or failed Slick criteria	49	≥17	≥100	16	93
Nguyen et al. (2015)	Disability/Civil forensic—neurological symptoms	Defined as passed or failed Slick criteria	74	≥18	≥105	13	90
Wygant et al. (2011)	Disability claimants (pain and TBI)	Probable or Definite MND/MPRD	251	≥19	>105	34	93
Nguyen et al. (2015)	Disability/Civil forensic—psychiatric symptoms	Defined as passed or failed Slick criteria	66	≥20	≥114	18	94

NOTE: RBS given as part of the MMPI-2-RF or MMPI-2.

MND, malingered neurocognitive dyfunction; MPRD, malingered pain-related disability; TBI, traumatic brain injury.

Cutoff scores and T scores that were not provided in original sources were estimated/extrapolated from the MMPI-2 Technical Manual and so may not map exactly onto values provided in original sources.

TABLE 16–12 Response Bias Scale (RBS) T Score Cumulative Frequencies for Malingering, Traumatic Brain Injury, Epilepsy, Neurological, and Psychiatric Patients

RBS T SCORE	TBI FAIL SLICK CRITERIA	TBI PASS SLICK CRITERIA	EPILEPSY	MIXED NEUROLOGICAL	MIXED PSYCHIATRIC
29	100%	100%	100%	100%	100%
33	100	100	100	100	100
38	100	100	98	100	100
42	100	100	98	100	100
46	100	92	92	100	100
50	100	92	88	100	100
54	100	81	78	90	93
59	100	77	70	76	79
63	100	69	56	57	79
67	100	62	42	52	64
71	100	50	24	48	64
76	95	42	22	43	57
80	86	31	14	33	43
84	81	23	8	14	43
88	67	19	4	5	43
92	57	12	2	5	36
97	43	8	2	0	29
101	38	4	2	0	21
105	33	4	2	0	14
109	14	0	2	0	0
114	10	0	0	0	0
118	5	0	0	0	0
120	5	0	0	0	0

NOTE: TBI, traumatic brain injury; TBI Fail Slick Criteria, TBI failing Slick criteria group; TBI Pass Slick Criteria, TBI passing Slick criteria group; Epilepsy, Epileptic Seizure group; Mixed Neurological, Mixed neurological group; Mixed Psychiatric, Mixed psychiatric group.

Data collected as part of the MMPI-2-RF, which uses identical items to the MMPI-2.

SOURCE: From Schroeder et al. (2012). Used with permission.

malingering as well as for neurological and psychiatric patients. These are reproduced in Table 16–12 and can be useful for clinicians to compare to scores of individual examinees. Most importantly, these frequencies show that a significant number of neurological patients have RBS T scores greater than 80, and an even higher percentage of psychiatric patients have scores greater than 90, scores that are typically flagged by the MMPI-2 scoring program as indicative of possible overreporting.

OTHER CLINICAL STUDIES ON THE RBS

Generally speaking, studies using failure on PVTs as the criterion for invalidity indicate higher cut scores for an acceptable balance of sensitivity and specificity. A cut score of 17 or greater provided a sensitivity of .25 and specificity of .95 in the original study at predicting PVT failure (Gervais et al., 2007). Since then, raw scores of about 15 to 17, equivalent to T scores between 90 and 100 have also been recommended based on PVT failure as criterion (Wygant et al., 2010). Specifically, a cut score of 20 was needed in a veteran sample to reach an adequate specificity of greater than .90 (Young et al., 2011). Using a single PVT (TOMM) as the criterion for malingering, a cut score of 17 or greater provided a sensitivity and specificity of .50 and .92 in a veterans sample; the higher cutoff of 19 or greater reached an impressive .96 specificity, but with sensitivity unacceptably low (Whitney et al., 2008). Similarly, in a sample of criminal defendants, a cutoff of 17 or greater demonstrated an acceptable sensitivity of .59 and specificity of .89 (Wygant et al., 2010). Lower specificity has been reported in other studies (Young et al., 2011) compared to the original validation study of Gervais et al. (2007).

The ability of different MMPI-2 validity indices to predict litigation status (personal injury and disability) versus nonlitigation status was explored in a study by Tsushima et al. (2011), who found the RBS superior to other indices including the FBS and HHI in identifying examinees involved in litigation or disability evaluations.

As was found with the FBS, Peck and colleagues found that individuals with psychogenic nonepileptic seizures, a form of unintentional symptom exaggeration due to psychopathology, obtained scores between those of nonmalingering and malingering brain injury patients on the RBS, demonstrating utility of the RBS to help differentiate between somatic disorders and malingering (Peck et al., 2013).

HHI: DIAGNOSTIC ACCURACY WITH REGARDS TO SLICK ET AL. (1999) AND OTHER MALINGERING CRITERIA

Unlike the other MMPI-2 validity scales, the HHI was developed using malingering defined by Slick et al. (1999) criteria in its item selection. According to its authors, the HHI is superior to the FBS in identifying malingerers

(Henry et al., 2006); at a specificity of .89 and using the recommended cutoff of 8 or greater, the HHI classified 86% of examinees compared to 81% for FBS. Although this is a marginally better rate, it does require cross-validation. In brain injury litigants, Dionysus et al. (2011) found that a higher HHI cutoff (≥12) was predictive of malingering according to Slick et al. (1999) criteria; the recommended cutoff of 8 or greater produced unacceptably high false positives. The same cutoff was found to be acceptable in a military sample to accurately detect Slick-defined malingering without raising the false-positive rate to unacceptable levels (Jones, 2016). HHI classification accuracy statistics and cutoffs are shown in Table 16–13. Although the recommended cutoff from its authors is not included because it fails to reach the criterion of .90 specificity, a cutoff of 9 or greater is shown in the table with its related statistics, which are all fairly respectable, and although based on fewer studies, show marginally higher sensitivity and PPV compared to FBS and RBS (Tables 16–9 and 16–11). To our knowledge, there are no validation studies on predicting malingered pain-related disability.

OTHER CLINICAL STUDIES ON THE HHI

In terms of using PVTs as the gold standard for noncredible reporting, Young et al. (2011) found that the HHI had strong sensitivity for prediction of PVT failure in veterans at the usual cutoff of 8 or greater but had unacceptably low specificity. They opined that the difficulties in finding an acceptable cutoff in some groups may relate to the fact that the scale has fewer items than other MMPI-2 validity scales, precluding a range of alternate cutoffs for use in different settings. With only 15 items in the scale, a score of 14 or greater had only a .85 specificity, leaving very little room to attain the recommended specificity of .90.

Of note, the HHI may have some utility in detecting noncredible Attention-Deficit/Hyperactivity Disorder (ADHD) symptom reporting. Although Fp had better classification accuracy overall, HHI classification accuracy was respectable, and, using a cutoff of 9 or greater, it had better sensitivity and specificity than either the FBS or the RBS at their own recommended cutoffs (≥23 and ≥17, respectively) for detecting simulated ADHD symptoms (Young & Gross, 2011). This finding needs further validation in confirmed ADHD malingering groups but shows promise for the HHI as a measure to use in adult ADHD, a condition associated with elevated rates of noncredible symptom reporting.

CCS: DIAGNOSTIC ACCURACY WITH REGARDS TO SLICK ET AL. (1999) AND OTHER MALINGERING CRITERIA AND CLINICAL STUDIES

The CCS has not yet been validated with regard to Slick et al. malingering criteria; however, it uses a validation criterion that some equate with noncredible performance (i.e., failure on two PVTs). In the validation study, using a CCS cut score of 12 or higher yielded a sensitivity of .30 and a specificity of .94 to failure on two PVTs. According to the authors, litigation status more than doubles the CCS score; in addition, more than 50% of examinees in the failed PVT group reached the cutoff versus only 4% of the nonlitigating mild brain injury examinees. No studies on prediction of somatic malingering exist to our knowledge.

Studies are needed to compare the CCS scale to other MMPI-2 validity scales. However, the scale is of interest given its validation in mild brain injury and the use of two or more PVTs as the derivation criterion, which is a more optimal and validated approach than validity indexes that used failure on one PVT only as the criterion (i.e., RBS). Its sole focus on cognitive items rather than mixed item content is also potentially useful for fulfilling criteria C5 of the Slick et al. (1999) malingering criteria; that is, the requirement for evidence of exaggeration of neurocognitive dysfunction from self-report (Henry et al., 2014). However, the scale may be hampered by too few items and an apparent ceiling effect given an optimal cutoff of 12 and a total of 13 items only (G. Larrabee, personal communication, March 2018).

COMMENT

The exaggeration of cognitive, somatic, and psychiatric symptoms are each distinctive aspects of noncredible symptom reporting (e.g., Greiffenstein et al., 1995, 2002;

TABLE 16–13 Henry-Heilbronner Index (HHI) Classification Accuracy at Cutoffs Yielding Minimum Acceptable Specificities (≥90%) for Prediction of Malingered Neurocognitive Dysfunction (MND)

STUDY	GROUP	CRITERION	N	CUTOFF	SENSITIVITY (%)	SPECIFICITY (%)
Henry et al. (2006)	Personal injury, disability and non-litigants (> 50% TBI)	Probable MND	119	≥9	73	95
Dionysus et al. (2011)	TBI litigants	Probable MND	79	≥12	41	93
Jones (2016)	Mild TBI active duty military	Probable or Definite MND	300	≥12	42	94

NOTE: TBI, traumatic brain injury; MND, malingered neurocognitive dysfunction.

McCaffrey et al., 2003; Slick et al., 1996; Temple et al., 2003; see also Larrabee, 2003d). Some individuals may feign one type (e.g., cognitive disturbance) but not another (e.g., psychiatric disorder); others may show a different pattern (e.g., somatic and cognitive exaggeration only). In almost all settings where neuropsychologists conduct evaluations, there is a need to screen for exaggeration in all three of these domains. The MMPI-2 has the potential to tap all these dimensions of exaggeration in one scale and remains the most well researched scale in neuropsychology with regard to malingering identification.

Of all the MMPI-2 validity scales reviewed here, the most useful and most validated are the FBS and RBS, followed by the HHI. All three tap the dimension of somatic overreporting, while F-family scales tap overreporting of psychopathology. They also tap cognitive malingering as shown by associations with PVTs and malingered neurocognitive dysfunction, although all three scales contain few cognitive items. CCS, a new scale, contains only cognitive items, but needs more validation research.

Nevertheless, there are several vocal critics of the FBS in particular, most notably Butcher, Nichols, and colleagues (e.g., Arbisi & Butcher, 2004; Butcher et al., 2015; Butcher et al., 2008; Nichols, 2011). Specifically, the scale has been criticized for lack of clarity, a variable yardstick for recommended cutoffs, and unacceptable specificities in some groups (Butcher et al., 2008). In addition, the FBS has been criticized for containing a high number of items on physical symptoms and as therefore being prone to false-positive errors in groups with physical problems, including implying intentional faking in those with somatoform disorders and in those with bona fide physical conditions experiencing psychological distress (Butcher et al., 2008). In particular, Butcher and colleagues caution against using the FBS on the grounds that it is biased against women, people with disabilities, those exposed to trauma, and those "faking good." Some have criticized the FBS for including problematic items related more to involvement in litigation than to overreporting (i.e., the so-called "litigation response syndrome," a collection of symptoms identified in an early publication of one of the FBS authors) and conclude that the FBS measures credible symptoms related to the experience of being in litigation rather than exaggeration of symptoms and that the use of the scale in civil litigation carries a high risk of being discredited (Nichols & Gass, 2015).

Butcher and colleagues also note three *Frye* challenges in Florida (i.e., on its admissibility based on scientific soundness and acceptability in the professional community); all three resulted in exclusion (Butcher et al., 2008). Nichols also notes a number of examples of courts ruling against testimony involving the FBS under *Frye* and *Daubert* standards between 2006 and 2015 (Nichols, 2017). Butcher and colleagues advise that expert testimony based on this scale should be excluded from consideration in court, that it has the potential for misuse in clinical evaluations, and that clinicians should avoid using the scale entirely (see also Nichols, 2011).

These criticisms have resulted in numerous rebuttals over the years (e.g., Arbisi, 2017; Greve & Bianchini, 2004; Lees-Haley & Fox, 2004; Larrabee et al., 2017b). For example, Larrabee and colleagues (Larrabee et al., 2017a) provide convincing evidence of the FBS's validity as a measure of symptom exaggeration, including its common acceptance by the professional community as the most widely used SVT among neuropsychologists and cite the literature on significant associations between FBS and PVTs, noting that neither litigants who pass PVTs nor nonlitigating medical patients with physical, emotional, and cognitive symptoms produce elevated FBS scores. They conclude that the FBS measures noncredible symptom reporting and not litigation stress and that the literature supports the admissibility of the FBS under both *Frye* and *Daubert* criteria. The FBS does indeed have a large number of validity studies and continues to show equivalent and in some cases superior ability to differentiate between groups compared to other MMPI-2 validity scales (Nelson et al., 2010). Arguments invoking gender bias do not appear convincing given large-scale medico-legal samples showing no gender biases when the publisher's cutoffs are employed (Lee et al., 2012). Our own view is that the literature—particularly the multiple studies showing utility relating to detection of malingering according to established criteria reviewed here—is supportive of its use in neuropsychological medicolegal evaluation, as long as the appropriate cutoffs are used. Misuse seems more related to using an inappropriately low cut score rather than reflective of any fundamental flaw with the scale. Overall, we agree with Arbisi that it is time to move on from criticizing the FBS to accepting it as one of the best available validity indicators for identifying overreporting of symptoms (Arbisi, 2017).

Of note, the criteria used to develop the main MMPI-2 validity scales reviewed here differ: namely, FBS and HHI were specifically created to identify malingering, whereas RBS (and CCS) were created based on the ability to predict PVT failure. In terms of the quality of the definition of malingering used as the criterion in these validation studies, HHI is the only validity index to use the multidimensional Slick et al. malingering criteria in its item validation, whereas FBS validation was based on a definition of malingering determined by its author and never fully technically elucidated. Nevertheless, the FBS has been validated in a number of subsequent studies using the Slick et al. criteria, albeit with higher cutoff values than suggested in the original validation study. In comparison, HHI was developed on recognized malingering criteria, but needs additional validity literature.

RBS, in comparison, was derived based on its ability to predict PVT failure and not malingering per se, defined by failure on a single PVT rather than on established malingering criteria. Failure on a single PVT as an indicator of invalid performance has subsequently been found to increase false-positive risk; failure on one PVT has indeed been used to define *nonmalingering* in some studies (e.g., Peck et al., 2013). Most guidelines indicate that failure on two PVTs is required to correctly infer invalid performance. Technically speaking, one might also therefore wonder why one would include the RBS in an evaluation if actual PVTs are also being administered. Furthermore, when examinees fail the RBS but pass actual PVTs, it is unclear how this should be interpreted clinically. Nevertheless, if appropriate cut scores are employed, an elevated RBS is a reliable predictor of exaggeration of overreporting of *symptoms* (as opposed to exaggeration of cognitive *performance deficits* as measured by PVTs). Furthermore, the RBS has been repeatedly validated as an effective predictor of Slick-defined malingering at a cutoff of 14 or higher and, as such, appears equally effective as the FBS, although its sensitivity to detect malingering is marginally lower than that of FBS at the same specificity criterion of .90 (see Tables 16–9 and 16–11). As Greve and colleagues have so cogently pointed out, at a given acceptable specificity (false-positive rate) for a specific cutoff, the index with the best sensitivity and best positive predictive value (PPV) is always preferred, particularly given the legal standard of "more likely than not" which is satisfied if a positive predictive value of .51 or greater is obtained at a base rate that matches that of the setting in which the examinee was seen (Greve et al., 2006). At a 40 to 50% base rate of malingering, FBS marginally outstrips RBS in terms of sensitivity and PPV.

Although some might be tempted, using RBS as a proxy PVT measure instead of an actual PVT is discouraged given the only partial overlap between these measures. Although the RBS has been deemed by some as possibly serving as a proxy for PVTs in cases where PVTs were not administered, Wygant et al. (2010) note that symptom exaggeration as detected by the RBS may not be accompanied by PVT failure in individual examinees. Wygant et al. suggest that the RBS could be used as a screening measure in some settings where PVTs are not routinely administered, followed by administration of PVTs if the RBS is flagged. We would offer that prediction of PVT failure is rarely the point of administering the MMPI-2 as part of a neuropsychological evaluation and that the RBS should simply be used as an index reflective of the validity of symptom self-report, whether or not PVTs are administered.

Technically speaking, CCS is a promising scale that is at least a theoretical improvement over RBS as it was validated using failure on two PVTs instead of one PVT and is of interest because of its singular focus on cognitive symptoms. The CCS needs more study but has interesting potential.

Importantly, individual MMPI-2 scales should not be used in isolation to diagnose malingering. In addition, significant elevations do not necessarily confirm malingering or intentional exaggeration for other reasons; rather, they indicate that the symptom report is exaggerated and does not accurately reflect the person's actual status, although the more extreme the score, the more likely that it does indicate intentional exaggeration and malingering (Greve et al., 2006). Generally speaking, as with all SVTs, elevated validity scales on the MMPI-2 can occur in the presence of bona fide cognitive impairment, physical conditions, or psychopathology; in these cases, the MMPI-2 can only inform on the accuracy of the examinee's self-description, not conclusively rule in or rule out the presence of genuine problems (Greene, 2008).

Researchers appropriately raise concerns about the utility of MMPI-2 scales such as the RBS and HHI across all settings (Young et al., 2011), and highlight that sample-specific factors may affect the appropriateness of cutoffs. In addition, studies indicate that FBS, RBS, and HHI are not technically independent SVTs, as most scales are at least moderately intercorrelated and have item overlap. FBS and HHI in particular have significant item overlap and, as such, may not fulfill guidelines that recommend use of multiple independent SVTs in the detection of noncredible symptom reporting.

There are no studies, to our knowledge, on MMPI-2 validity indices from translated versions of the MMPI-2. Similarly, there is scant research on the MMPI-2 validity scales from countries other than the United States, Canada, and Australia. There is a general paucity of research on ethnicity, although a small number of studies are favorable.

It is necessary to note that the length of the MMPI-2 is a significant barrier to widespread usage in non-forensic settings, with many clinicians avoiding its routine use in clinical evaluations. Readers are encouraged to nevertheless consider using the scale because the sophistication of its validity indexes and its massive research base is far in excess of those of briefer tools. An obvious alternative to the MMPI-2 is the MMPI-2-RF, which has almost all of the advantages of the MMPI-2 without the length. On the other hand, as noted in the MMPI-2-RF review later in this chapter, both scales are nevertheless cumbersome to use due to their complexity but also because their interpretation is not as intuitive as that of briefer scales or of more comprehensive scales based directly on models of psychopathology found in the Diagnostic and Statistical Manual of Mental Disorders (DSM) such as the Personality Assessment Inventory (PAI).

Although there are a number of studies involving personal injury litigants and disability cases, the field is in need of more MMPI-2 studies on other high malingering base rates groups such as ADHD, although there is promising preliminary research on the utility of the HHI. Generally speaking, persons with somatic symptom disorders obtain scores between those of valid responders and malingerers on the FBS and most other MMPI-2 validity indexes reviewed here, but more research on somatic symptom disorder and malingered pain-related disability is also needed.

In addition, there are scant neuropsychological studies validating FBS, RBS, and HHI cutoffs on psychiatric patients, a group that tends to require higher cutoffs on SVTs (e.g., see the Structured Inventory of Malingered Symptomatology [SIMS] reviewed elsewhere in this chapter) due to the risk of false positives. Similarly, all the MMPI-2 SVTs reviewed here would benefit from more studies on their ability to predict malingering in criminal defendants using established malingering criteria.

Lastly, although as of this writing there is scant research on the validity scales of the new Minnesota Multiphasic Personality Inventory-3 (MMPI-3; Ben-Porath & Tellegen, 2020), the RBS is unchanged and the FBS is based on the MMPI-2-RF and so past research should be applicable to these scales.

REFERENCES

Aguerrevere, L. E., Greve, K. W., Bianchini, K. J., & Meyers, J. E. (2008). Detecting malingering in traumatic brain injury and chronic pain with an abbreviated version of the Meyers Index for the MMPI-2. *Archives of Clinical Neuropsychology, 23*(7–8), 831–838. https://doi.org/10.1016/j.acn.2008.06.008

Arbisi, P. A. (2017). Form vs function, fighting the last war: A reflection on the exchange between Larrabee, Bianchini, Boone, and Rohling (2017) and Nichols (2017) over Nichols and Gass (2015). The Fake Bad Scale (FBS): malingering or ligation response syndrome—Which is it? *The Clinical Neuropsychologist,* 1–6. https://doi.org/10.1080/13854046.2017.1365933

Arbisi, P. A., & Butcher, J. N. (2004). Failure of the FBS to predict malingering of somatic symptoms: Response to critiques by Greve and Binachini and Less Haley and Fox. *Archives of Clinical Neuropsychology, 19,* 341–345.

Ben-Porath, Y. S., Graham, J. R., & Tellegen, A. (2009). *The MMPI-2 Symptom Validity (FBS) scale: Development, research findings, and interpretive recommendations.* Minneapolis: University of Minnesota Press.

Ben-Porath Y. S., & Tellegen, A. (2008). *Minnesota Multiphasic Personality Inventory-2 Restructured Form (MMPI-2-RF): Manual for administration, scoring, and interpretation.* Minneapolis: University of Minnesota Press.

Ben-Porath, Y., & Tellegen, A. (2017). *MMPI-2 Symptom Validity Scale (FBS).* University of Minnesota Press. Retrieved from https://www.upress.umn.edu/test-division/mtdda/mmpi-2-symptom-validity-scale-fbs.

Ben-Porath, Y. S., & Tellegen, A. (2020). *Minnesota Multiphasic Personality Inventory – 3 (MMPI-3).* Bloomington, MN: NCS Pearson.

Bianchini, K. J., Aguerrevere, L. E., Curtis, K. L., Roebuck-Spencer, T. M., Frey, F. C., Greve, K. W., & Calamia, M. (2017). Classification accuracy of the Minnesota Multiphasic Personality Inventory-2 (MMPI-2)-Restructured Form validity scales in detecting malingered pain-related disability. *Psychological Assessment.* https://doi.org/10.1037/pas0000532

Bianchini, K. J., Greve, K. W., & Glynn, G. (2005). On the diagnosis of malingered pain-related disability: Lessons from cognitive malingering research. *Spine Journal, 5*(4), 404–417. https://doi.org/10.1016/j.spinee.2004.11.016

Boone, K. B. (2013). *Clinical practice of forensic neuropsychology: An evidence-based approach.* New York: Guilford Press.

Butcher, J. N. (1998). *MMPI-2 User's guide for the Minnesota Report: Reports for forensic settings.* Minneapolis: University of Minnesota Press.

Butcher, J. N., Arbisi, P. A., Atlis, M. M., & McNulty, J. L. (2003). The construct validity of Lees-Haley Fake Bad Scale: Does this scale measure somatic malingering and feigned emotional distress? *Archives of Clinical Neuropsychology, 18,* 473–485.

Butcher, J. N., Dahlstrom, W. G., Graham, J. R., Tellegen, A. M., & Kaemmer, B. (1989). *MMPI-2, Minnesota Multiphasic Personality Inventory–2: Manual for administration and scoring.* Minneapolis: University of Minnesota Press.

Butcher, J. N., Gass, C. S., Cumella, E., Kally, Z., & Williams, C. L. (2008). Potential for bias in MMPI-2 assessments using the Fake Bad Scale (FBS). *Psychological Injury and Law, 1*(3), 191–209.

Butcher, J. N., Graham, J. R., Ben Porath, Y. S., Tellegen, A., Dahlstrom, W. G., & Kaemmer, B. (2001). *MMPI-2, Minnesota Multiphasic Personality Inventory-2: Manual for administration, scoring, and administration* (revised ed.). Minneapolis: University of Minnesota Press.

Butcher, J. N., Hass, G. A., Greene, R. L., Nelson, L. D., & Association, A. P. (2015). *Using the MMPI-2 in forensic assessment.* Washington, DC: American Psychological Association.

Dean, A. C., Boone, K. B., Kim, M. S., Curiel, A. R., Martin, D. J., Victor, T. L., . . . Lang, Y. K. (2008). Examination of the impact of ethnicity on the Minnesota Multiphasic Personality Inventory-2 (MMPI-2) Fake Bad Scale. *The Clinical Neuropsychologist, 22*(6), 1054–1060. https://doi.org/10.1080/13854040701750891

Dionysus, K. E., Denney, R. L., & Halfaker, D. A. (2011). Detecting negative response bias with the Fake Bad Scale, Response Bias Scale, and Henry–Heilbronner Index of the Minnesota Multiphasic Personality Inventory-2. *Archives of Clinical Neuropsychology, 26*(2), 81–88. https://doi.org/10.1093/arclin/acq096

Gass, C. S., & Odland, A. P. (2014). MMPI-2 Symptom Validity (FBS) Scale: Psychometric characteristics and limitations in a Veterans Affairs neuropsychological setting. *Applied Neuropsychology. Adult, 21*(1), 1–8. https://doi.org/10.1080/09084282.2012.715608

Gervais, R. O., Ben-Porath, Y. S., Wygant, D. B., & Green, P. (2007). Development and validation of a Response Bias Scale (RBS) for the MMPI-2. *Assessment, 14*(2), 196–208. https://doi.org/10.1177/1073191106295861

Gervais, R. O., Ben-Porath, Y. S., Wygant, D. B., & Green, P. (2008). Differential sensitivity of the Response Bias Scale (RBS) and MMPI-2 validity scales to memory complaints. *The Clinical Neuropsychologist, 22*(6), 1061–1079. https://doi.org/10.1080/13854040701756930

Green, P. (2004). *Memory Complaints Inventory.* Edmonton, Canada: Green's Publishing.

Greene, R. L. (2008). Malingering and defensiveness on the MMPI-2. In R. Rogers (Ed.), *Clinical assessment of malingering and deception* (3rd ed., pp. 159–181). New York: Guilford.

Greiffenstein, M. F. (2010). The MMPI-2 Symptom Validity Scale (FBS) not influenced by medical impairment: a large sleep center investigation. *Assessment, 17*(2), 269–277. https://doi.org/10.1177/1073191109358823

Greiffenstein, M. F., & Baker, W. J. (2008). Validity testing in dually diagnosed post-traumatic stress disorder and mild closed head injury. *The Clinical Neuropsychologist, 22*(3), 565–582. https://doi.org/10.1080/13854040701377810

Greiffenstein, M. F., Baker, W. J., Gola, T., Donders, J., & Miller, L. (2002). The Fake Bad Scale in atypical and severe closed head injury litigants. *Journal of Clinical Psychology, 58,* 1591–1600.

Greiffenstein, M. F., Baker, W. J., Tsushima, W. T., Boone, K., & Fox, D. D. (2010). MMPI-2 validity scores in defense- versus plaintiff-selected examinations: A repeated measures study of examiner effects. *The Clinical Neuropsychologist, 24*(2), 305–314. https://doi.org/10.1080/13854040903456222

Greiffenstein, M. F., Fox, D., & Lees-Haley, P. R. (2007). The MMPI-2 Fake Bad Scale in detection of noncredible brain injury claims. In K. B. Boone (Ed.), *Assessment of feigned cognitive impairment: A neuropsychological perspective* (pp. 210–235). New York: Guilford Press.

Greiffenstein, M. F., Gola, T., & Baker, W. J. (1995). MMPI-2 validity scales versus domain specific measures of detection of factitious traumatic brain injury. *The Clinical Neuropsychologist, 9,* 230–240.

Greve, K. W., & Bianchini, K. J. (2004). Response to Butcher et al.: The construct validity of the Lees-Haley Fake-Bad Scale. *Archives of Clinical Neuropsychology, 19,* 337–339.

Greve, K. W., Bianchini, K. J., Love, J. M., Brennan, A., & Heinly, M. T. (2006). Sensitivity and specificity of MMPI-2 validity scales and indicators to malingered neurocognitive dysfunction in traumatic brain injury. *The Clinical Neuropsychologist, 20*(3), 491–512. https://doi.org/10.1080/13854040590967144

Hartmann, E., & Hartmann, T. (2014). The impact of exposure to Internet-based information about the Rorschach and the MMPI-2 on psychiatric outpatients' ability to simulate mentally healthy test performance. *Journal of Personality Assessment, 96*(4), 432–444. https://doi.org/10.1080/00223891.2014.882342

Heilbronner, R. L., & Henry, G. K. (2013). Psychological assessment of symptom magnification in mild traumatic brain injury cases. In D. A. Carone and S. S. Bush (eds.), *Mild traumatic brain injury: Symptom validity assessment and malingering* (pp. 183–202). New York: Springer Publishing.

Henry, G. K., Heilbronner, R. L., Mittenberg, W., & Enders, C. (2006). The Henry-Heilbronner Index: A 15-item empirically derived MMPI-2 subscale for identifying probable malingering in personal injury litigants and disability claimants. *The Clinical Neuropsychologist, 20*(4), 786–797. https://doi.org/10.1080/13854040500287749

Henry, G. K., Heilbronner, R. L., Mittenberg, W., Enders, C., & Roberts, D. M. (2008). Empirical derivation of a new MMPI-2 scale for identifying probable malingering in personal injury litigants and disability claimants: The 15-item Malingered Mood Disorder Scale (MMDS). *The Clinical Neuropsychologist, 22*(1), 158–168. https://doi.org/10.1080/13825580601025916

Henry, G. K., Heilbronner, R. L., Mittenberg, W., Hellemann, G., & Myers, A. (2014). Development of the MMPI-2 cognitive complaints scale as an embedded measure of symptom validity. *Brain Injury, 28*(3), 357–363. https://doi.org/10.3109/02699052.2013.865272

Ingram, P. B., & Ternes, M. S. (2016). The detection of content-based invalid responding: A meta-analysis of the MMPI-2-Restructured Form's (MMPI-2-RF) overreporting validity scales. *The Clinical Neuropsychologist, 30*(4), 473–496. https://doi.org/10.1080/13854046.2016.1187769

Jones, A. (2016). Cutoff scores for MMPI-2 and MMPI-2-RF Cognitive-Somatic validity scales for psychometrically defined malingering groups in a military sample. *Archives of Clinical Neuropsychology.* https://doi.org/10.1093/arclin/acw035

Jones, A., & Ingram, M. V. (2011). A comparison of selected MMPI-2 and MMPI-2-RF validity scales in assessing effort on cognitive tests in a military sample. *The Clinical Neuropsychologist, 25*(7), 1207–1227. https://doi.org/10.1080/13854046.2011.600726

Larrabee, G. J. (2003a). Exaggerated MMPI-2 symptom report in personal injury litigants with malingered neurocognitive deficit. *Archives of Clinical Neuropsychology, 18,* 673–686.

Larrabee, G. J. (2003b). Detection of symptom exaggeration with the MMPI-2 in litigants with malingered neurocognitive deficit. *The Clinical Neuropsychologist, 17,* 54–68.

Larrabee, G. J. (2003c). Detection of malingering using atypical performance patterns on standard neuropsychological tests. *The Clinical Neuropsychologist, 17,* 410–425.

Larrabee, G. J. (2003d). Exaggerated pain report in litigants with malingered neurocognitive dysfunction. *The Clinical Neuropsychologist, 17,* 395–410.

Larrabee, G. J. (2005). Assessment of malingering. In G. J. Larrabee (Ed.), *Forensic neuropsychology: A scientific approach.* New York: Oxford University Press.

Larrabee, G. J., Bianchini, K. J., Boone, K. B., & Rohling, M. L. (2017a). The MMPI-2/MMPI-2-RF Symptom Validity Scale (FBS/FBS-r) is not a measure of "litigation response syndrome": commentary on Nichols and Gass (2015). *The Clinical Neuropsychologist,* 1–9. https://doi.org/10.1080/13854046.2017.1364423

Larrabee, G. J., Bianchini, K. J., Boone, K. B., & Rohling, M. L. (2017b). The validity of the MMPI-2/MMPI-2-RF Symptom Validity Scale (FBS/FBS-r) is established: Reply to Nichols (2017). *The Clinical Neuropsychologist, 31*(8), 1401–1405. https://doi.org/10.1080/13854046.2017.1363293

Lee, T. T. C., Graham, J. R., Sellbom, M., & Gervais, R. O. (2012). Examining the potential for gender bias in the prediction of symptom validity test failure by MMPI-2 symptom validity scale scores. *Psychological Assessment, 24*(3), 618–627. https://doi.org/10.1037/a0026458

Lees-Haley, P. R. (1992). Efficacy of the MMPI-2 validity scales and MCMI-II modifier scales for detection of spurious PTSD claims: F, F-K, Fake-Bad scale, ego strength, subtle-obvious subscales, Dis, and Deb. *Journal of Clinical Psychology, 48,* 681–689.

Lees-Haley, P. R., English, L. T., & Glenn, W. G. (1991). A Fake-Bad-Scale for personal injury claimants. *Psychological Reports, 68,* 203–210.

Lees-Haley, P. R., & Fox, D. D. (2004). Commentary on Butcher, Arbisi, Atlis, & McNulty (2003) on the Fake Bad Scale. *Archives of Clinical Neuropsychology, 19,* 333–336.

Martin, P. K., Schroeder, R. W., & Odland, A. P. (2015). Neuropsychologists' validity testing beliefs and practices: A survey of North American professionals. *The Clinical Neuropsychologist, 29*(6), 741–776. https://doi.org/10.1080/13854046.2015.1087597

McCaffrey, R. J., O'Bryant, S. E., Ashendorf, L., & Fisher, J. M. (2003). Correlations among the TOMM, Rey-15, and MMPI-2 validity scales in a sample of TBI litigants. *Journal of Forensic Neuropsychology, 3,* 45–53.

Meyers, J. E., Millis, S. R., & Volkert, K. (2002). A validity index for the MMPI-2. *Archives of Clinical Neuropsychology, 17,* 157–169.

Nelson, N. W., Hoelzle, J. B., Sweet, J. J., Arbisi, P. A., & Demakis, G. J. (2010). Updated meta-analysis of the MMPI-2 symptom validity scale (FBS): Verified utility in forensic practice. *The Clinical Neuropsychologist, 24*(4), 701–724. https://doi.org/10.1080/13854040903482863

Nelson, N. W., Sweet, J. J., Berry, D. T. R., Bryant, F. B., & Granacher, R. P. (2007). Response validity in forensic neuropsychology: exploratory factor analytic evidence of distinct cognitive and psychological constructs. *Journal of the International Neuropsychological Society, 13*(3), 440–449. https://doi.org/10.1017/S1355617707070373

Nelson, N. W., Sweet, J. J., & Demakis, G. J. (2006). Meta-analysis of the MMPI-2 fake bad scale: utility in forensic practice. *The Clinical Neuropsychologist, 20*(1), 39–58. https://doi.org/10.1080/13854040500459322

Nguyen, C. T., Green, D., & Barr, W. B. (2015). Evaluation of the MMPI-2-RF for detecting overreported symptoms in a civil forensic and disability setting. *The Clinical Neuropsychologist, 29*(2), 255–271. https://doi.org/10.1080/13854046.2015.1033020

Nichols, D. S. (2011). *Essentials of MMPI-2 assessment.* New York: John Wiley & Sons.

Nichols, D. S. (2017). Fake Bad Scale: The case of the missing construct, a response to Larrabee, Bianchini, Boone, and Rohling (2017). *The Clinical Neuropsychologist,* 1–5. https://doi.org/10.1080/13854046.2017.1365934

Nichols, P. D., & Gass, C. S. (2015). The Fake Bad Scale: Malingering or litigation response syndrome—which is it? *Archives of Assessment Psychology, 5*(1), 5–10.

Nijdam-Jones, A., & Rosenfeld, B. (2017). Cross-cultural feigning assessment: A systematic review of feigning instruments used with linguistically, ethnically, and culturally diverse samples. *Psychological Assessment, 29*(11), 1321–1336. https://doi.org/10.1037/pas0000438

Peck, C. P., Schroeder, R. W., Heinrichs, R. J., Vondran, E. J., Brockman, C. J., Webster, B. K., & Baade, L. E. (2013). Differences in MMPI-2 FBS and RBS scores in brain injury, probable malingering, and conversion disorder groups: a preliminary study. *The Clinical Neuropsychologist, 27*(4), 693–707. https://doi.org/10.1080/13854046.2013.779032

Rabin, L. A., Paolillo, E., & Barr, W. B (2016). Stability in test-usage practices of clinical neuropsychologists in the United States and Canada over a 10-year period: A follow-up survey of INS and NAN members. *Archives of Clinical Neuropsychology, 31,* 206–230.

Schroeder, R. W., Baade, L. E., Peck, C. P., VonDran, E. J., Brockman, C. J., Webster, B. K., & Heinrichs, R. J. (2012). Validation of MMPI-2-RF validity scales in criterion group neuropsychological samples. *The Clinical Neuropsychologist, 26*(1), 129–146. https://doi.org/10.1080/13854046.2011.639314

Sharland, M. J., & Gfeller, J. D. (2007). A survey of neuropsychologists' beliefs and practices with respect to the assessment of effort. *Archives of Clinical Neuropsychology, 22,* 213–223.

Slick, D. J., Hopp, G., Strauss, E., & Spellacy, F. J. (1996). Victoria Symptom Validity Test: Efficiency for detecting feigned memory impairment and relationship to neuropsychological tests and MMPI-2 validity scales. *Journal of Clinical and Experimental Neuropsychology, 18,* 911–922.

Slick, D. J., Sherman, E. M.S., & Iverson, G. (1999). Diagnostic criteria for malingered neurocognitive dysfunction: Proposed standards for clinical practice and research. *The Clinical Neuropsychologist, 13,* 545–561.

Smart, C. M., Nelson, N. W., Sweet, J. J., Bryant, F. B., Berry, D. T. R., Granacher, R. P., & Heilbronner, R. L. (2008). Use of MMPI-2 to predict cognitive effort: A hierarchically optimal classification tree analysis. *Journal of the International Neuropsychological Society, 14*(5), 842–852. https://doi.org/10.1017/S1355617708081034

Sullivan, K. A., & Elliott, C. (2012). An investigation of the validity of the MMPI-2 response bias scale using an analog simulation design. *The Clinical Neuropsychologist, 26*(1), 160–176. https://doi.org/10.1080/13854046.2011.647084

Sullivan, K. A., Elliott, C. D., Lange, R. T., & Anderson, D. S. (2013). A known-groups evaluation of the response bias scale in a neuropsychological setting. *Applied Neuropsychology, Adult, 20*(1), 20–32. https://doi.org/10.1080/09084282.2012.670149

Sweet, J. J., Malina, A., & Ecklund-Johnson, E. (2006). Application of the new MMPI-2 Malingered Depression scale to individuals undergoing neuropsychological evaluation: Relative lack of relationship to secondary gain and failure on validity indices. *The Clinical Neuropsychologist, 20*(3), 541–551. https://doi.org/10.1080/13854040590967135

Tarescavage, A. M., Wygant, D. B., Gervais, R. O., & Ben-Porath, Y. S. (2013). Association between the MMPI-2 restructured form (MMPI-2-RF) and malingered neurocognitive dysfunction among non-head injury disability claimants. *The Clinical Neuropsychologist, 27*(2), 313–335. https://doi.org/10.1080/13854046.2012.744099

Tellegen, A., Ben-Porath, Y. S., McNulty, J. L., Arbisi, P. A., Graham, J. R., & Kaemmer, B. (2003). *The MMPI–2 restructured clinical scales: Development, validation, and interpretation.* Minneapolis: University of Minnesota Press.

Temple, R. O., McBride, A. M., Horner, M. D., & Taylor, R. M. (2003). Personality characteristics of patients showing suboptimal effort. *The Clinical Neuropsychologist, 17,* 402–409.

Tsushima, W. T., Geling, O., & Fabrigas, J. (2011). Comparison of MMPI-2 validity scale scores of personal injury litigants and disability claimants. *The Clinical Neuropsychologist, 25*(8), 1403–1414. https://doi.org/10.1080/13854046.2011.613854

Van Dyke, S. A., Millis, S. R., Axelrod, B. N., & Hanks, R. A. (2013). Assessing effort: Differentiating performance and symptom validity. *The Clinical Neuropsychologist, 27*(8), 1234–1246. https://doi.org/10.1080/13854046.2013.835447

Whitney, K. A., Davis, J. J., Shepard, P. H., & Herman, S. M. (2008). Utility of the Response Bias Scale (RBS) and other MMPI-2 validity scales in predicting TOMM performance. *Archives of Clinical Neuropsychology, 23*(7), 777–786. https://doi.org/10.1016/j.acn.2008.09.001

Wygant, D. B., Sellbom, M., Gervais, R. O., Ben-Porath, Y. S., Stafford, K. P., Freeman, D. B., & Heilbronner, R. L. (2010). Further validation of the MMPI-2 and MMPI-2-RF Response Bias Scale: findings from disability and criminal forensic settings. *Psychological Assessment, 22*(4), 745–756. https://doi.org/10.1037/a0020042

Young, J. C., & Gross, A. M. (2011). Detection of response bias and noncredible performance in adult attention-deficit/hyperactivity disorder. *Archives of Clinical Neuropsychology, 26*(3), 165–175. https://doi.org/10.1093/arclin/acr013

Young, J. C., Kearns, L. A., & Roper, B. L. (2011). Validation of the MMPI-2 Response Bias Scale and Henry-Heilbronner index in a US veteran population. *Archives of Clinical Neuropsychology, 26*(3), 194–204. https://doi.org/10.1093/arclin/acr015

MINNESOTA MULTIPHASIC PERSONALITY INVENTORY-2 RESTRUCTURED FORM (MMPI-2-RF)

TEST NAME	**Minnesota Multiphasic Personality Inventory-2 Restructured Form (MMPI-2-RF)**
DOMAIN	Symptom validity (see other sources for using the test to assess psychopathology or personality)
AGE RANGE	18 to 85 years
ADMINISTRATION TIME	25 to 35 minutes for computer administration, 35–50 minutes for booklet administration
SCORING FORMAT	Computerized, mail-in, or hand scored
REFERENCES	Ben-Porath Y. S., Tellegen A. (2011a). *Minnesota Multiphasic Personality Inventory-2 Restructured Form (MMPI-2-RF): Manual for administration, scoring, and interpretation.* Minneapolis: University of Minnesota Press. Ben-Porath Y. S., Tellegen A. (2011b). *Minnesota Multiphasic Personality Inventory-2 Restructured Form (MMPI-2-RF): Technical manual.* Minneapolis: University of Minnesota Press. www.pearsonclinical.com

DESCRIPTION

The Minnesota Multiphasic Personality Inventory-2 Restructured Form (MMPI-2-RF; Ben-Porath & Tellegen, 2011) is a briefer, revised version of the MMPI-2, also reviewed in this chapter. The MMPI-2-RF and MMPI-2 are both self-report questionnaires that rank as the most popular psychological assessment measures among neuropsychologists (Rabin et al., 2016) and are used by 78% of forensic neuropsychologists in particular (LaDuke et al., 2017). In terms of its specific usage as a scale with an SVT, the MMPI-2-RF is the most frequently used scale, employed by more than 35% of neuropsychologists who use SVTs, with the MMPI-2 a close second at 30% (Martin et al., 2015).

Details on general interpretation are available in the original source and in numerous publications and will not be covered here in order to provide an exclusive focus on the MMPI-2-RF as a symptom validity tool, with only a brief review of clinical scales that measure cognitive and neurological symptoms because these are potentially useful as SVTs and are new to the test. Specifically, this review focuses primarily on the use of the MMPI-2-RF in detecting exaggeration in contexts relevant to neuropsychologists, such as feigning of cognitive and somatic symptoms in personal injury, disability, and criminal-forensic settings. For an overview of the MMPI-2-RF's utility in the detection of feigned psychopathology specifically, please see other comprehensive sources (e.g., Greene, 2010; Nichols, 2011).

The test publisher provides English, Spanish, and French-Canadian versions, with online administration and scoring (www.pearsonclinical.com). As of this writing, other translations are available in Croatian, Dutch-Flemish, French, Italian, Korean, Spanish for Mexico and Central America, Spanish for Spain, South America and Central America, and Spanish for the United States (https://www.upress.umn.edu/test-division/translations-permissions/available-translations). As of this writing, there appear to be more translations for the MMPI-2 than for the MMPI-2-RF.

CLINICAL CONTENT OF THE MMPI-2-RF

The MMPI was originally published in 1940, then revised and renormed in 1989 to create the MMPI-2. The MMPI-2 introduced new Content Scales but kept the Clinical Scales from the original MMPI derived through empirical keying. Specifically, MMPI-2 Clinical Scales were constructed based on items that differentiated between specific clinical groups and normative samples, regardless of item content. This differs from scales constructed from items based on theoretical models that are then validated on clinical groups in a second step. Because of known problems with the Clinical Scales, such as very high intercorrelations and heterogeneous, atheoretical content resulting from empirical keying, in 2003, the MMPI-2 Restructured Clinical (RC) scales were added to the MMPI-2, while still retaining the older Clinical Scales (Tellegen & Ben-Porath, 2011). These new RC scales were based on original MMPI-2 items but were designed to reduce shared items between scales and minimize scale intercorrelations; this would help improve

TABLE 16–14 MMPI-2-RF Higher-Order (H-O) Scales

ABBREVIATION	SCALE NAME
EID	Emotional/Internalizing Dysfunction
THD	Thought Dysfunction
BXD	Behavioral/Externalizing Dysfunction

interpretation and more closely parallel modern models of psychopathology (Nichols, 2011). In 2008, the MMPI-2-RF was published with the RC scales as its core, completely eliminating the older Clinical Scales in favor of 50 new and revised scales based on a dramatically reduced number of items (see Ben-Porath & Tellegen, 2008, for details on item number, content, and administration). The standardization sample is the same as in the MMPI-2 but norms are not divided by gender and are based on a smaller normative set comprised of equal numbers of men and women, reportedly adopted because of civil rights legislation prohibiting the use of gendered norms in personnel screening (Ben-Porath & Tellegen, 2008).

The MMPI-2-RF is comprised of three overarching Higher-Order scales measuring three broad dimensions: Emotional/Internalizing Dysfunction, Thought Dysfunction, and Behavioural/Externalizing Dysfunction (Table 16–14). The nine main clinical scales are the RC scales; these measure more specific aspects of psychopathology (Table 16–15), in addition to the Demoralization Scale (RCd) which is different from the other RC scales in that it measures a general factor associated with a sense of nonspecific psychological distress, suffering, the sense of "patienthood," and general emotional problems. This general factor arose in the original MMPI-2 because the original Clinical Scales were based on differences between "normals" and clinical patients, resulting in a high representation of this "patienthood" factor in all the Clinical Scales and contributing to high, nonspecific scale intercorrelations and reduced discriminative ability between scales (Tellegen & Ben-Porath, 2011). In the MMPI-2-RF, this general factor was then extracted from the other RC scales to increase discriminative ability of the RC scales. RC scales of specific relevance to neuropsychologists include RC1 (Somatic Complaints), RC2 (Low Positive Emotions), and RC7 (Dysfunctional Negative Emotions), measuring aspects of somatization, depression, and anxiety.

TABLE 16–15 MMPI-2-RF Restructured Clinical (RC) Scales

SCALE	ABBREVIATION	SCALE NAME
RCd	DEM	Demoralization
RC1	SOM	Somatic Complaints
RC2	LPE	Low Positive Emotions
RC3	CYN	Cynicism
RC4	ASB	Antisocial Behavior
RC6	PER	Ideas of Persecution
RC7	DNE	Dysfunctional Negative Emotions
RC8	ABX	Aberrant Experiences
RC9	HPM	Hypomanic Activation

TABLE 16–16 MMPI-2-RF Specific Problems (SP) Scales with Relevance to Physical Symptoms and Cognitive Symptoms

ABBREVIATION	SCALE	DESCRIPTION	NUMBER OF ITEMS
MLS	Malaise	Nonspecific, generalized sense of poor health and physical debilitation, sense of physical incapacity	8
HPC	Head Pain Complaints	Head and neck pain	8
NUC	Neurological Complaints	Dizziness, numbness, weakness, involuntary movement	10
COG	Cognitive Complaints	Memory problems, intellectual limitations, concentration problems, confusion	10

SOURCE: Adapted from information presented in Ben-Porath and Tellegen (2011).

In addition, the MMPI-2-RF has 23 Specific Problems scales, which provide a more fine-grained analysis than the RC scales; five of these have particular relevance to neuropsychology as they tap somatic, neurological, and cognitive symptoms (Table 16–16). Of these, the Cognitive Complaints scale in particular is of interest; it covers items pertaining to memory, concentration, forgetfulness, reading comprehension, and poor stress tolerance (Gervais et al., 2009). Also of interest are the Head Pain Complaints and Neurological Complaints scales.

Interestingly, there have been comparatively few studies on the effect of malingering on MMPI-2-RF RC and Specific Problem scales. However, in disability claimants with pain or TBI meeting criteria for probable or definite malingering, Wygant and colleagues found significantly elevated scores on all of the RC scales with the exception of RC4 and RC9 (antisocial and hypomanic symptoms) and on all the Specific Problems scales measuring somatic and cognitive symptoms, including Malaise, Head Pain Complaints, Neurological Complaints, and Cognitive Complaints. Those with possible malingering had scores of intermediate severity on the same scales, halfway between probable/definite malingering and nonmalingering groups (Wygant et al., 2011).

The MMPI-2-RF also has five scales designed to measure personality based on a five-factor model of personality (i.e., the PSY-5 scales) which will not be discussed in detail here.

MMPI-2-RF VALIDITY SCALES

The MMPI-2-RF has nine validity scales that cover both non–content-based invalid responding (i.e., failure to respond to items or responding in a fixed or random manner regardless of item content) and content-based invalid responding (i.e., portraying oneself as functioning better or worse than indicated by objective assessment, but responding in a content-specific manner; Forbey et al., 2013). The validity scales include a variety of SVTs: shortened versions of original MMPI-2 validity scales, new scales designed exclusively for the MMPI-2-RF, and original MMPI-2 validity scales. Comparisons of the MMPI-2-RF to the MMPI-2 therefore depend on which scale is being examined. Here, we focus mostly on scales that have been developed to detect overreporting, exaggeration, or feigning of cognitive and somatic symptoms.

Non–content-based invalid responding scales measure item completion and consistency; these reflect the extent to which the examinee cooperated with the testing process, measuring both the percent of items completed and the consistency of responses to similar items (i.e., Cannot Say; Variable Response Inconsistency, VRIN-r; True Response Inconsistency, TRIN-r). Of note, some inconsistency scales have been associated with a greater risk of PVT failure, suggesting that some scales—TRIN in particular—may reflect an uncooperative test-taking attitude in addition to inconsistency (Gervais et al., 2017). Content-based invalid responding scales either tap underreporting (i.e., L-r scale, K-r scales, known as Uncommon Virtues and Adjustment Validity, respectively), or overreporting. Underreporting scales tend to be elevated in groups attempting to minimize problems (e.g., personnel evaluations, custody evaluations), but not in most neuropsychological contexts. See the review of the MMPI-2 earlier in this chapter for further information on completion, consistency, and underreporting scales.

Although the F-family of scales (F-r, Fb-r, Fp-r) has proved useful in distinguishing between persons feigning various types of psychiatric disorders from true patients and healthy controls, their use in civil forensic neuropsychological settings has produced unsatisfactory results. This is because persons feigning neuropsychological conditions such as brain injury tend to endorse high rates of cognitive and somatic rather than psychiatric symptoms, causing the F scales to be minimally sensitive in most of these settings (Boone, 2013). For a brief overview of validity scales measuring overreporting of psychopathology (i.e., F, Fb, Fp), see the review of the MMPI-2 earlier in this chapter.

The main MMPI-2-RF overreporting validity scales included with the test are as follows: Symptom Validity Scale-Restructured (FBS-r), Response Bias Scale (RBS), and Infrequent Somatic Responses (Fs). The Henry-Heilbronner Index Restructured (HHI-r) can also be derived. Each of these will be discussed in turn. The MMPI-2-RF also contains a number of somatic scales such as Head Pain Complaints, Neurological Complaints, and Cognitive Complaints; these may also have potential to tap overreporting of symptoms although are less studied than the MMPI-2-RF SVTs.

SYMPTOM VALIDITY SCALE-RESTRUCTURED (FBS-R)

The Symptom Validity Scale-Restructured (FBS-r) contains 30 of the original 43 items from the MMPI-2 Fake Bad Scale developed by Lees-Haley et al. (1991), now renamed the Symptom Validity Scale (FBS). FBS-r is thought to measure exaggeration of somatic and cognitive symptoms more than exaggeration of psychiatric symptoms. However, the vast majority of items tap somatic overreporting and aspects of psychological distress, with only a few items directly related to cognition. See the earlier MMPI-2 review for more information on how the scale was developed and on its original validation sample. The FBS-r is one of the core MMPI-2-RF validity scales automatically calculated by the scoring program.

RESPONSE BIAS SCALE (RBS)

The RBS is the same scale that appears in the MMPI-2 and is included in its entirety in the MMPI-2-RF. Briefly, it includes 28 items selected for their ability to predict feigned cognitive symptoms using failure on a PVT as the criterion for item selection (Gervais et al., 2007). Like the FBS, the majority of items tap somatic overreporting and aspects of psychological distress, with only a few items directly related to cognition. See the earlier MMPI-2 review for more information on how the scale was developed and on its original validation sample. The RBS is one of the core MMPI-2-RF validity scales automatically calculated by the scoring program.

INFREQUENT SOMATIC RESPONSES (FS)

The Infrequent Somatic Responses scale (Fs) is new to the MMPI-2-RF and not available in the MMPI-2. This is a potentially interesting scale; somatic overreporting is a common feature of exaggeration in many neuropsychological populations such as mild TBI, pain disorders, nonepileptic seizures, and some potentially compensable medical conditions with unclear etiology, such as fibromyalgia and chronic fatigue syndrome (see Boone, 2017, for a review of somatic symptom disorders). Fs consists of 16 items designed to detect overreporting of physical complaints; items were derived based on low endorsement (<25%) in a large sample of examinees with medical conditions as well as chronic pain (*N* >55,000). The Fs is one of the core MMPI-2-RF validity scales automatically calculated by the scoring program.

HENRY-HEILBRONNER INDEX (HHI-R)

The HHI-r (Henry et al., 2013) measures exaggeration, overreporting, and malingering of physical symptoms (i.e., "somatic malingering"). It consists of 11 items from the original MMPI-2 HHI (Henry et al., 2006). It has few items that tap cognition. Unlike other scales, item selection was based on item correlations with group membership defined by Slick et al. (1999) malingering criteria in a sample with a high prevalence of brain injuries. Specific items are listed in the original source (Henry et al., 2013). See the earlier MMPI-2 review for more information on how the scale was developed and on its original validation sample.

The HHI-r is not automatically provided in the MMPI-2-RF scoring program and must be derived by hand.

STEPS TO ASSESSING SYMPTOM VALIDITY USING THE MMPI-2-RF

Properly assessing validity means following a sequential process starting first with assessing content nonresponsiveness; that is, assessing form completion (Cannot Say), followed by response consistency (VRIN-r and TRIN-r). Next, one assesses content-responsiveness; that is, scales that detect overreporting (i.e., F-family of scales including Fs, as well as FBS-r, RBS, HHI-r) and underreporting (i.e., L-r and K-r). Because overreporting scales are elevated by random or fixed responding (e.g., random responding, or answering all "True"), not following this sequential interpretation process raises the risk of false positives (i.e., erroneously identifying inconsistent responding due to inattention, incapacity, or uncooperativeness as purposeful symptom exaggeration). Interestingly, some scales are much more susceptible to the influence of non-content-based invalid responding (i.e., F-family scales, Fs, RBS, L-r) than others (FBS-r, K-r; Burchett et al., 2016). See also the earlier MMPI-2 review for more information.

Importantly, overreporting scales such as FBS-r, RBS, and Fs do not inform on the intentionality of the examinee. Overreporting scales can be elevated due to intentional overreporting (i.e., cognitive or somatic malingering) or unintentional overreporting (i.e., psychiatric somatic conditions). However, the degree of overreporting (mild vs. severe), in most cases, can provide useful information for inferring intentionality based on the likelihood of a given score elevation in malingering versus bona fide clinical groups (see "Clinical Studies"). In other words, the more extreme the elevation, the greater the likelihood of malingering.

ADMINISTRATION

Details regarding MMPI-2-RF administration can be found in the manual. Computer administration and computer scoring are highly recommended to reduce errors in transcription and scoring. Anecdotally, we find that examinees are less overwhelmed by computer administration compared to booklet/answer sheet administration as only one item is presented at a time. We have therefore had better completion rates with computer administration than booklet administration in examinees with cognitive or psychiatric issues.

According to the authors, administration time ranges from 25 to 35 minutes for examinees with intact cognition using the computer version, to 35 to 50 minutes for examinees completing the test by hand using the booklet and answer sheet. One study found slightly longer administration times on a tablet compared to laptop administration (Menton et al., 2017).

A Grade 5 to 7 reading ability is recommended, although Nicholls (2011) reports that a Grade 9 reading level is required for some items. This is slightly lower than required for the MMPI-2.

Although breaks are permitted during administration, allowing the examinee to complete the test at home is not advised because norms were generated under carefully controlled conditions, factors that can affect validity cannot be controlled, and responses may be influenced by others at home (and indeed someone else may have completed the instrument; Butcher & Pope, 1992).

SCORING

Generally speaking, hand-scoring is possible with the use of various scoring keys but is highly discouraged given potential for errors and the amount of time required. However, given the number of items, entering hand-completed scores from an answer sheet into the scoring program can also result in scoring errors, so careful review or double scoring is required to ensure accurate scores. Computer administration eliminates both these problems.

The FBS-r, RBS, and Fs are automatically calculated as part of the standard MMPI-2-RF scoring program. At present, the HHI-r is not part of the standard scoring software, but scoring criteria can be obtained directly from the author (ghenry0249@aol.com).

Scores for the FBS-r, RBS, and Fs are provided as raw scores and T scores by the MMPI-2-RF scoring program, along with suggested interpretations. However, it is highly recommended that cutoff scores appropriate for the examinee and the setting be consulted for interpretation rather than relying exclusively on the MMPI-2 interpretive software (see "Clinical Studies"). HHI-r scores should also be interpreted by using recommended cutoff values (see "Clinical Studies").

When interpreting MMPI-2-RF RC and other clinical scales, T scores of 65 or greater are usually considered high; this is not necessarily the case for validity indices. Very high T scores may be required on some scales to demonstrate invalidity, in the range of T greater than 90 and T greater than 100 (see Table 16–17 and "Clinical Studies").

AGE

There is scant information on age and MMPI-2-RF validity scales. Age was found to be a significant moderator for FBS-r but not for RBS or Fs in one meta-analytic study (Ingram & Ternes, 2016).

GENDER

Ingram and Ternes reported no gender effects in their meta-analysis of MMPI-2-RF validity scales including FBS-r, RBS, and Fs (Ingram & Ternes, 2016). Similarly, Schroeder et al. (2012) found no differential gender effects on optimal cutoffs for FBS-r.

TABLE 16–17 Overview and Interpretive Guidelines for MMPI-2-RF Validity Scales for Measuring Overreporting in Neuropsychological Assessment

Core Validity Scales		
FBS-r	Symptom Validity Scale—Restructured[a]	Designed specifically for personal injury cases to detect noncredible symptom presentation; sensitive to exaggeration of somatic and nonpsychotic symptoms; T scores of 80–99 raise concerns about possible overreporting or could reflect credible symptoms in individuals with substantial medical conditions; scores of 100 or higher indicate that overreporting of cognitive and somatic symptoms has likely occurred, affecting the interpretability of the Somatic Complaints (RC1) scale and COG scale
RBS	Response Bias Scale	Designed to detect cognitive malingering; items specifically selected on basis of ability to predict PVT failure in non-TBI disability claimants; T scores of 80–99 raise concerns about possible overreporting or could reflect credible symptoms in individuals with substantial emotional conditions; scores of 100 or higher indicate that overreporting of memory symptoms has likely occurred; scores on the COG scale may be invalid
Fs	Infrequent Somatic Responses	Designed to detect overreporting of physical complaints; items based on low endorsement (<25%) in a large sample of examinees with medical conditions including chronic pain; T scores of 80–99 raise concerns about possible overreporting or could reflect credible symptoms in individuals with substantial medical conditions; scores of 100 or higher indicate that overreporting of somatic symptoms has likely occurred, affecting the interpretability of the Somatic Complaints (RC1) scale and its related Specific Problems scales (i.e., MLS, GIC, HPC, NUC, and COG)
Additional Validity Scales		
HHI-r	Henry-Heilbronner Index—Restructured	Designed to detect somatic malingering, items were selected based on their ability to identify Slick et al. (1999) defined malingering in a sample with high prevalence of TBI

[a]Formerly known as the Fake Bad Scale (FBS).

NOTE: MLS, Malaise; GIC, Gastrointestinal Complaints; HPC, Head Pain Complaints; NUC, Neurological Complaints; COG, Cognitive Complaints.

SOURCE: Adapted from information presented in Ben-Porath and Tellegen (2011).

EDUCATION AND IQ

Education effects have not been well studied, although education effects were not found for FBS-r, RBS, or Fs in a meta-analysis of MMPI-2-RF validity scales (Ingram & Ternes, 2016). Correlations with IQ are minimal (see "Evidence for Validity").

ETHNICITY, NATIONALITY, AND LINGUISTIC EFFECTS

There is little information on ethnicity and MMPI-2-RF validity scales (Nijdam-Jones & Rosenfeld, 2017), including on its translated versions.

NORMATIVE DATA

The original MMPI-2 norms on which the MMPI-2-RF depends were developed from a sample of 2,600 community-dwelling individuals recruited by ads, directories, and mailing lists according to the 1990 Census (Butcher et al., 2001). From this sample, 2,276 individuals were retained in the MMPI-2-RF, divided equally according to gender and cross-validated with a contemporary validation sample.

However, the cutoffs for each of the validity scales reviewed here were originally developed based on samples that were not part of the original MMPI-2 or MMPI-2-RF standardization sample. Details on these samples are provided in the review of MMPI-2, elsewhere in this chapter. As already noted, the Fs validation sample was based on a sample of more than 55,000 medical and chronic pain patients. Note that recommended cutoffs for validity scales may be derived from these original validation samples or from later cross-validation samples, depending on the scale (see "Clinical Studies").

EVIDENCE FOR RELIABILITY

EVIDENCE FOR INTERNAL RELIABILITY

The manual presents internal reliabilities for several samples, including normative, outpatient mental health, and inpatient psychiatric samples. Alphas for validity scales are fairly low overall in the normative sample (alpha = .39 to .56 for FBS-r, RBS, and Fs, respectively), but low to adequate in clinical samples (alpha = .60 to .76). The same pattern occurs for the somatic Specific Problems scale internal reliabilities (e.g., Head Pain Complaints, Neurological Complaints, Cognitive Complaints), which are low in the normative sample (alpha = .52 to .69), but quite respectable in clinical samples (alpha = .71 to .84; Technical Manual). Other studies show that FBS-r has acceptable internal consistency in non-forensic samples (alpha = .75) and that the Cognitive Complaints scale has an internal consistency of .82 in disability claimants (Gervais et al., 2009). Of note, equivalent reliabilities have been reported for the tablet and laptop versions of the MMPI-2-RF (Menton et al., 2017).

EVIDENCE FOR TEST-RETEST RELIABILITY, MEASURING CHANGE, AND PRACTICE EFFECTS

One-week test-retest reliabilities are presented for a subset of the normative sample in the Technical Manual ($N = 193$). Although FBS-r and RBS reliabilities are adequate ($r = .72$ and .71, respectively), Fs reliability is low ($r = .51$). Of note, among F-scales, the Fs is an exception, as the other F scales have adequate to high reliabilities (i.e., F-r, Fp-r, $r = .82$ and .71). Normative sample reliabilities for the somatic Specific Problems scales such as Head Pain Complaints and Cognitive Complaints are also quite respectable (i.e., $r = .74$

to .82), with the exception of Neurological Complaints, which is low (r = .54). Equivalent test-retest reliabilities have been reported for tablet and laptop versions of the MMPI-2-RF (Menton et al., 2017). The manual makes no mention of practice effects, or rather, effects of prior exposure, which in some questionnaires can yield lower scores on retest.

EVIDENCE FOR VALIDITY

MMPI-2-RF VERSUS MMPI-2

MMPI-RF-2 and MMPI-2 versions of FBS-r/FBS have very high intercorrelations, as would be expected given overlapping content (manual; note: RBS is the same in both tests). Similarly, correlations between HHI-r and HHI in a military sample were extremely high (r = .97; Jones, 2016). Nevertheless, studies find that the MMPI-2-RF overreporting scales outperform those of the MMPI-2 in the prediction of malingering of cognitive, somatic, and psychological symptoms, even though the MMPI-2-RF contains fewer items (Chmielewski et al., 2017; Gervais et al., 2010). In epilepsy, the scales are relatively similar in their ability to identify people with nonepileptic seizures (Locke et al., 2010).

FACTOR-ANALYTIC STUDIES

Gass and Odland (2012) conducted a factor analysis of FBS-r and reported that it had two higher order dimensions (i.e., Somatic Complaints and Optimism/Virtue) but that it had a discordant factor structure in that some items from the first factor were negatively correlated with items from the second factor. Seven first-order factors were found to underlie the FBS-r, consisting of distractible/overwhelmed, stomach pain, headache, anthropic optimism, escape wish, virtue, and neck pain. Factor-analytic studies of other MMPI-2-RF SVT scales or combining MMPI-2-RF SVT and clinical scales are lacking to our knowledge.

MMPI-2-RF VALIDITY SCALE INTERCORRELATIONS AND COMPARISONS

Overall, correlations between FBS-r, RBS, and Fs range from modest to high, with most studies showing a fair degree of association depending on the sample. Not surprisingly, the degree of correlation between scales, at least in the case of FBS-r and RBS, may relate to the degree of item overlap because both have items from RC1. Fs was specifically designed not to contain items from that scale. In the normative sample, correlations between FBS-r, RBS, and Fs are in the moderate range (r = .30 to .47; Technical Manual). Intercorrelations in clinical samples described in the manual tend to be high, in the .60 to .70 range.

In a study involving criminal defendants deemed incompetent to stand trial, all the validity scales were highly intercorrelated, with the highest correlations found between FBS-r and RBS, followed by RBS and Fs; however, correlations between FBS-r and Fs were also quite large (rs = .81, .75, and .66, respectively; Grossi et al., 2017). Similar correlations are reported in other criminal and disability samples between FBS-r, RBS, and Fs (r = .63 to .77; Wygant et al., 2010). Intercorrelations between scales are also fairly high in epilepsy and nonepileptic seizure samples (r = .53 to .57; Wershba et al., 2015). In some cases, RBS correlates more highly with overreporting of psychopathology (F scales) in criminal samples than in disability samples, consistent with the notion that criminal defendants tend to exaggerate both cognitive and psychiatric symptoms whereas disability samples exaggerate mainly cognitive and somatic symptoms (Grossi et al., 2017).

Overall, correlational studies indicate that the scales are moderately to highly correlated and are not therefore independent in terms of shared variance as one would expect for measures tapping a similar dimension of overreporting and which in some cases share some items.

CORRELATIONS WITH AND COMPARISONS TO OTHER PVTS

As is the case for the original MMPI-2, most studies show moderate correlations between MMPI-2-RF validity scales and PVTs, with lower correlations between PVTs and F-family scales in most but not all studies. Despite the fact that RBS was specifically derived using PVT failure as its criterion for invalidity, both RBS and FBS-r are predictive of PVT performance, although RBS tends to be more consistently so. Evidence for Fs is more mixed. Of note, studies on correlates of HHI-r are lacking (but see corresponding section in the MMPI-2 review for some validation evidence for the original HHI).

For example, neither FBS-r nor Fs is related to injury severity in brain injury litigants, but both instead predict PVT performance (Youngjohn et al., 2011). Perhaps not surprisingly, MMPI-2-RF clinical scales that tap somatic and cognitive complaints such as the Head Pain Complaints scale are even better predictors of PVT failure in this group, with nonspecific physical symptoms (Malaise scale) the best predictor of all, suggesting that the somatic scales may also be effective at detecting overreporting and, in some cases, be stronger predictors than the validity scales themselves.

In one study in non–head-injury disability claimants, RBS demonstrated the highest correlations with PVTs compared to FBS-r and Fs, with modest to moderate correlations with PVTs such as the WMT, MSVT, Non-Verbal Medical Symptom Validity Test (NV-MSVT), TOMM, CARB, Reliable Digit Span, and CVLT recognition indices (Tarescavage et al., 2013). Fs demonstrated the weakest correlation with PVTs, even weaker than validity indices designed for detection of feigned psychopathology such as the F-r and Fp-r.

In military service members with mild TBI who underwent a medical board evaluation, a disability evaluation process for determining fitness for duty that typically has a high PVT and SVT failure rate, more than 57% exceeded cutoffs for invalid results on the MMPI-2-RF, with the same percentage failing the WMT. However, correlations between the two tests were nonsignificant, indicating that different individuals failed these tests. The highest percentage of individuals had elevations on RBS and F scales (Armistead-Jehle et al., 2017). These results suggest that, in some settings, even though examinees may fail SVTs or PVTs, failure on both SVTs and PVTs may be a relatively infrequent event, even when the base rate of exaggeration is high.

In criminal defendants who are incompetent to stand trial, the largest correlations between MMPI-2-RF indices and PVTs were for RBS, followed by Fs and FBS-r (*rs* = –.55, –.47, and –.39, respectively; Grossi et al., 2017). The RBS also had the largest effect sizes in predicting TOMM failure compared to the other MMPI-2-RF validity indices, but this was comparable to F-r. RBS scores were not correlated with an exaggeration index that taps feigned cognitive dysfunction from the SIRS, often considered the gold standard test for exaggeration of psychopathology. However, both contributed to predicting TOMM failure, again demonstrating that malingering criminal defendants typically exhibit a combination of feigned cognitive and psychiatric symptoms.

Somewhat surprisingly, RBS was not predictive of PVT failure in adults with ADHD referred to a university psychology clinic (Cook et al., 2016), which the authors interpreted as supporting the need for ADHD-specific measures of noncredible presentation.

CORRELATIONS WITH AND COMPARISONS TO OTHER SVTS AND COMPREHENSIVE QUESTIONNAIRES

Correlations with PAI overreporting validity scales indicate that the PAI's Negative Impression Management scale (NIM) has the highest correlations with MMPI-2-RF validity scales, followed by the PAI Malingering scale (MAL); the PAI's Rogers Discriminant Function scale (RDF) has only low to modest associations with MMPI-2-RF validity scales (Crighton et al., 2017). Among the scales, RBS is most correlated with NIM (*r* = .62), followed by FBS-r (*r* = .41). These correlations are particularly impressive because the PAI validity scales are not geared toward detection of somatic and cognitive feigning, as are FBS-r and RBS, but rather target feigned psychopathology.

In disability claimants, FBS-r and Fs demonstrate moderate correlations with an SVT designed to detect exaggeration of psychopathology, the Miller Forensic Assessment of Symptoms Test (M-FAST; *rs* = .41 to .47; Chmielewski et al., 2017). Both FBS-r and Fs T scores of greater than 100 had excellent specificity in predicting malingering of psychopathology on the M-FAST but with low sensitivity (i.e., specificity of greater than .90, but with .20 to .30 sensitivity, respectively).

One question that arises in evaluations is whether other questionnaires that don't include validity indicators can be interpreted when MMPI-2-RF validity scales are elevated. One study on college students, prisoners, and psychiatric patients indicates that when MMPI-2-RF validity scales are elevated, examinees also overreport on other questionnaires in a similar fashion, even when these tests do not include validity scales themselves and even when these collateral measures are administered up to 10 days after the MMPI-2-RF (Forbey et al., 2013; see also Crighton et al., 2017).

CORRELATIONS WITH OTHER MMPI-2-RF SCALES

Not many studies have examined how the validity scales relate to other MMPI-2-RF scales, and correlations between validity scales and other scales are lacking in the manual. In nonforensic referrals, the biggest predictor of FBS-r is MMPI-2-RF Anxiety, accounting for 45% of the variance in FBS-r scores (Gass & Odland, 2012). With regard to correlations with subjective memory concerns, in disability claimants, RBS demonstrates the highest correlations with memory complaints as measured by the MMPI-2-RF Cognitive Complaints scale (*r* = .80), but correlations involving FBS-r and Fs are also quite large (*r* = .60 to .61; Gervais et al., 2009). One study found that Cognitive Complaints was not correlated with memory performance in Korsakoff's syndrome patients and patients with alcohol-related cognitive impairment (Walvoort et al., 2016). These patients showed no elevations on Cognitive Complaints despite severe memory problems. The authors concluded that this could have been due to the fact that alcohol impairs meta-memory and self-awareness, but further study is needed.

CORRELATIONS WITH OTHER NEUROPSYCHOLOGICAL TESTS AND QUESTIONNAIRES

With regard to correlations with other neuropsychological tests, FBS-r is unrelated to cognitive performance, including verbal ability, perceptual reasoning, working memory, processing speed, learning, memory, and executive functioning as tapped by well-known neuropsychological tests such as the Wechsler Adult Intelligence Scale (WAIS-III/IV), Wechsler Memory Scale (WMS-III/IV), and Delis-Kaplan Executive Function System (D-KEFS; Martin et al., 2015). Although RBS is correlated with most of these cognitive domains, the relationship disappears when PVT failure is accounted for. These findings demonstrate that genuine cognitive deficits do not affect either FBS-r or RBS scores in individuals referred for neuropsychological assessment. Similarly, Gervais and colleagues reported no associations of FBS-r, RBS, or Fs with CVLT scores when controlling for PVT performance (Gervais et al., 2010).

RBS correlations with subjective memory concerns as measured by the Memory Complaints Inventory (MCI; Green, 2004) are quite large ($r = .61$), and larger than those for FBS-r and Fs, paralleling the higher RBS correlations with the MMPI-2-RF Cognitive Complaints scale (Gervais et al., 2009, 2010). Similarly, FBS-r, RBS, and Fs are all highly related to self-reported memory complaints in active service members with a history of concussion, again with the highest correlations obtained with RBS (*rs* = .55 to .68; Armistead-Jehle et al., 2016).

Gervais and colleagues suggest that when both RBS and Cognitive Complaints are elevated, memory complaints are likely to be exaggerated. They also provide interpretive guidelines incorporating the MMPI-2-RF, the MCI, and PVTs based on data from disability claimants (Gervais et al., 2010). These guidelines are designed to help users differentiate between emotionally related overexaggeration of memory complaints (related to psychiatric/somatoform disorders) from volitional exaggeration (due to malingering). Further validation is needed before generalizing to other kinds of clinical populations, but these guidelines show promise in the use of combined tools to maximize accurate interpretation in clinical settings (see Table 16–18 for interpretation guidelines).

With regard to associations with measures of psychopathology, FBS-r and Fs are not related to ratings of psychotic symptoms in first-episode psychosis patients, but RBS demonstrates very modest associations ($r = .21$ to .24, Purdon et al., 2011).

With regard to somatic exaggeration, FBS-r and Fs have been used in conjunction with pain questionnaires such as the Modified Somatic Perception Questionnaire and Pain Disability Index and found to be related to Waddell signs (i.e., nonorganic signs of somatic amplification) in pain patients (Wygant et al., 2017).

CLINICAL STUDIES

Validation against accepted multidimensional malingering criteria is critical for determining the validity and utility of SVTs and particularly for validating cutoffs that will be used in clinical practice. The MMPI-2-RF validity indices have been evaluated in terms of their ability to predict malingering based on Slick et al. (1999) criteria for malingered neurocognitive dysfunction, as well as on prediction of malingered pain-related disability as per Bianchini and colleagues (Bianchini et al., 2005). Other studies have also validated cutoffs based on prediction of PVT failure, which is a lesser criterion of validity because PVT failure is not synonymous with malingering as defined by multifactorial criteria, but which still contributes to incremental validity.

COMPARATIVE EFFICACY OF FBS-R, RBS, FS, AND HHI-R AT DETECTING MALINGERING

Studies directly comparing FBS-r, RBS, and Fs in populations relevant to neuropsychologists, generally speaking, indicate that FBS-r and RBS are more effective than Fs at detecting feigning in neuropsychological contexts, although there is some mixed evidence that Fs may have unique potential in helping differentiate between somatic malingering and genuine somatic conditions. There are at present too few studies on the HHI-r to comment on its utility.

Nguyen and colleagues found that FBS-r and RBS scores were higher in disability claimants who failed the Slick et al. malingering criteria (i.e., including failure on

TABLE 16–18 Interpretive Guidelines for the RBS in Combination with PVTs and the Memory Complaints Inventory (MCI)

T < 50 (Raw 0–4)	Minimal memory or other cognitive symptoms reported. Consider denial or "fake good" attitude, if cognitive testing reveals deficits. SVT failure is unlikely. If SVT(s) failed, consider passive factors such as disengagement or disinterest rather than active negative response bias.
T = 50–64 (Raw 5–8)	Minor memory or cognitive symptoms may be reported, consistent with cognitive test results. If F-r < 79 T, Fp-r < 70 T, Fs and FBS-r < 80 T, consider emotional factors contributing to memory complaints. SVT failure is unlikely. If SVT(s) failed, consider passive factors such as lack of engagement in testing. If F-r ≥ 79, Fp-r > 70, Fs or FBS-r > 80 T, rule out possible MND (Slick et al., 1999).
T = 65–79 (Raw 9–11)	Increasing memory complaints. If F-r < 79 T, Fp-r < 70 T, Fs, and FBS-r < 80 T, complaints are probably related to emotional factors. If F-r ≥ 79, Fp-r > 70, Fs or FBS-r > 80 T, or SVT(s) failed, consider volitional symptom exaggeration. Rule out possible or probable MND.
T = 80–99 (Raw 12–16)	Exaggerated memory complaints are likely. *T* scores are associated with mean MCI score 1.5 SD above moderate to severe brain injury. Probability of SVT failure as high as 67%. If F-r < 79 T, Fp-r < 70 T, Fs and FBS-r < 80 T, memory complaints may be related to emotional factors. If F-r ≥ 79, Fp-r > 70, Fs or FBS-r > 80 T, exaggerated psychopathology and somatic/cognitive symptoms are possible. If SVT(s) failed, exaggerated memory complaints are probable. Rule out probable MND.
T = 100+ (Raw 17+)	Memory complaints are exaggerated, *T* scores are associated with mean MCI score 2 SD above moderate to severe brain injury. Probability of SVT failure is 77–100%. If F-r, Fp-r, Fs, or FBS-r > 100, malingered psychopathology is probable. If SVT(s) failed, exaggeration of memory complaints is confirmed. If SVT(s) passed, rule out coaching. Rule out probable or definite MND.

SOURCE: Used with permission from Gervais et al. (2010).

two PVTs) compared to those who passed and that this was the case for both those with neurological symptoms and those with psychiatric symptoms, but not those with medical symptoms such as chronic fatigue syndrome (Nguyen et al., 2015). Effect sizes for FBS-r were quite large in psychiatric disability claimants and medium in size in neurological disability claimants, with relatively similar results for RBS. However, Nguyen et al. (2015) found that Fs did not differentiate between those who failed and passed Slick et al. criteria among disability claimants with neurological symptoms.

Similarly, compared to RBS and Fs, Schroeder and colleagues found that FBS-r had the highest sensitivity in identifying brain injury litigants failing Slick et al. criteria, even though all three measures had good specificity for their respective optimal cutoffs (i.e., specificity >.90 at T-score cutoffs of >92, >83, and >89, respectively; Schroeder et al., 2012). Furthermore, the same cutoff could be applied to a psychiatric group without raising the rate of false positives, a situation not applicable to RBS, which required a higher cutoff in psychiatric patients.

Other studies show that FBS-r also differentiates well between noncredible somatic simulators and genuine medical patients, with large effect sizes, but it is not as effective as Fs in differentiating between somatic malingering and genuine somatoform conditions (Sellbom et al., 2012). Of note, RBS did not contribute significantly to prediction in this study.

In a chronic regional pain syndrome sample with a high rate of malingered pain-related disability, with nearly half the sample failing at least two PVTs, FBS-r was the most frequently failed SVT, with 50% of the sample having a score of 80 or greater and 22% with a score of 90 or greater; RBS showed the next-highest failure rate, followed by Fs (Greiffenstein et al., 2013). FBS-r also showed the largest effect sizes in differentiating patients with nonepileptic seizures from those with epilepsy, along with RC1, Malaise, and Neurological Complaints (Locke et al., 2010). A cut score of 83 had optimal specificity (.91) but low sensitivity for identifying nonepileptic seizures (.23) at a base rate of greater than 50%.

FBS-r is the least elevated of the validity scales in patients with first-episode psychosis, demonstrating a relative lack of susceptibility to spurious elevations in severe psychiatric disease (Purdon et al., 2011). Cumulative frequency counts for FBS-r in first-episode psychosis are shown in Table 16–19 for reference purposes. At an FBS-r cutoff recommended by the manual of greater than 100, 0% of the sample was identified as feigning, compared to 6% for RBS and 5% for Fs. All of these are acceptable rates, indicating that none of the scales will erroneously overidentify psychiatric patients as overreporting. However, as shown in the table, using the MMPI-2-RF publisher's recommendation that T scores of 80 to 99 identifies "possible" overreporting, only 10% of psychiatric patients would be misdiagnosed based on FBS-r, compared to 26% and 25% of patients based on RBS and Fs.

TABLE 16–19 FBS-r, RBS, and Fs Cumulative Percentages in Severe Psychiatric Conditions

≥	FBS-R	*RBS*	*FS*	≥
120	0	1	2	*120*
110	0	3	3	*110*
100	0	6	5	*100*
90	1	11	18	*90*
80	10	26	25	*80*
70	20	41	42	*70*
60	48	57	55	*60*
50	73	83	85	*50*
40	94	98	100	*40*
30	100	100	100	*30*

Sample consisting of 130 patients seen for first-episode psychosis, with most having schizophrenia-spectrum disorders.

SOURCE: Adapted from Purdon et al. (2011).

Other studies show that FBS-r demonstrates large effect sizes in differentiating honest from nonhonest responders and is minimally influenced by contextual factors such as diagnosis and respondent group (Ingram & Ternes, 2016). Similarly, regarding concerns that FBS-r is susceptible to genuine somatic and cognitive symptoms, Arbisi and colleagues found that elevations on FBS-r in soldiers with mild TBI were no larger than in those without mild brain injury or PTSD, suggesting that elevations on FBS-r cannot be attributed solely to neurological conditions (Arbisi et al., 2011).

However, other studies show better efficacy for the RBS. For example, compared to FBS-r, RBS had larger effect sizes in differentiating disability claimants according to Slick et al. malingering criteria (Tarescavage et al., 2013). However, combining MMPI-2-RF validity scales significantly improved sensitivity and specificity over use of single validity indicators, with potential utility for clinical practice (Table 16–20). Use of three validity indicators was associated with excellent specificity and a PPV of .82, and use of four indicators with an even higher PPV of .85.

Notably, the largest study on malingered pain-related disability to date also showed that RBS was superior to FBS-r and Fs at detecting malingering (Bianchini et al., 2017). Cumulative percentages of malingering and nonmalingering chronic pain patients at different MMPI-2-RF cutoffs are shown in Table 16–21.

In military service members with mild TBI who underwent a medical board evaluation, the highest percentage of individuals had elevations on RBS, along with one of the F scales (Armistead-Jehle et al., 2017). Comparison of MMPI-2-RF validity indicators in another military sample showed that RBS performed best overall at predicting malingering based on Slick et al. criteria compared to FBS-r, and Fs, followed closely by HHI-r (Jones, 2016). Of note, this is the only study, to our knowledge, comparing the HHI-r to other MMPI-2-RF validity indicators.

TABLE 16–20 Classification Accuracy for Combined MMPI-2-RF Validity Scales in Disability Claimants for Prediction of Malingered Neurocognitive Dysfunction (MND) at Different Base Rates

NUMBER OF ELEVATED VALIDITY SCALES	SENSITIVITY (%)	SPECIFICITY (%)	BASE RATE = 15% OR LESS		BASE RATE = 30%		BASE RATE = 40–50%	
			PPV (%)	NPV (%)	PPV (%)	NPV (%)	PPV (%)	NPV (%)
1	50	81	23	94	53	79	72	62
2	42	89	30	93	62	78	79	61
3	27	94	33	92	66	75	82	56
4	11	98	38	91	70	72	85	52
5	0	100	*n/a*	*n/a*	*n/a*	*n/a*	*n/a*	*n/a*

Based on T-score cutoffs of F-r ≥100, FP-r ≥70, Fs ≥90, FBS-r ≥90, and RBS ≥90.

NOTE: PPV, positive predictive value; NPV, negative predictive value.

SOURCE: Adapted from Tarescavage et al. (2013).

RBS demonstrates large effect sizes in differentiating honest from nonhonest responders and, like FBS-r, is minimally influenced by contextual factors such as diagnosis and respondent group (Ingram & Ternes, 2016). Peck and colleagues found that individuals with psychogenic nonepileptic seizures, a form of somatic symptom exaggeration due to psychopathology, obtained scores between those of nonmalingering and malingering brain-injury patients on the RBS, demonstrating utility of the RBS to help differentiate between somatic disorders and malingering (Peck et al., 2013). See the MMPI-2 review in this chapter for other clinical studies involving the RBS, including diagnostic accuracy in studies using PVTs as the criterion.

There appear to be differences in validity scores across different types of samples. For example, in criminal defendants, RBS does not add incremental predictive validity over the standard F scales to identifying individuals who fail PVTs. However, in disability samples, RBS adds incremental predictive validity, but likely not meaningfully more than the FBS-r (Wygant et al., 2010). Furthermore, RBS cutoffs need to be higher in criminal samples to maintain an optimal balance of sensitivity and specificity for identifying PVT failure (i.e., >100 to 120).

Study results on Fs are mixed. In one of the few studies to include actual somatoform patients, Fs (along with Fp-r) was associated with the best differentiation between somatoform, somatic malingering, and medical patients, even though somatoform patients scored higher on FBS-r and RBS (Sellbom et al., 2012). Somatoform patients also scored higher on malaise and cognitive complaints scales (MAL and COG), whereas somatic malingerers scored high on gastrointestinal complaints (GIC). Other studies show lower detection rates. Fs had the smallest effect size in identifying Slick-defined malingering in a military sample even though effect sizes were still substantial (i.e., >1.0; Jones, 2016), similar to large effect sizes in differentiating between honest and dishonest responders in a meta-analysis of MMPI-2-RF validity scales (Ingram & Ternes, 2016). In epilepsy, Fs is elevated in patients with nonepileptic seizures, but FBS-r is still a better predictor of group membership (Locke et al., 2010). In the largest study on malingered pain-related disability, Fs was

TABLE 16–21 Cumulative Percentages for MMPI-2-RF FBS-r, RBS, and Fs T Scores for Chronic Pain Patients with and without Malingered Pain-Related Disability (MPRD)

T SCORE ≥	FBS-R		RBS		FS		T SCORE ≥
	NON-MPRD	MPRD	NON-MPRD	MPRD	NON-MPRD	MPRD	
120		0		7		3	120
115		1		10		8	115
110		1		14		8	110
105		7		22		15	105
100		11		30	0	15	100
95		26		40	9	22	95
90	0	36		50	9	33	90
85	7	52	0	60	9	33	85
80	16	71	10	73	13	47	80
75	24	78	19	78	13	47	75
70	40	86	29	85	16	65	70
65	47	89	35	86	24	77	65
60	67	94	52	91	24	77	60
55	69	96	52	93	40	88	55
50	91	100	87	98	76	97	50

NOTE: Non-MPRD, *N* = 45; MPRD, *N* = 214.

SOURCE: Adapted from Bianchini et al. (2017).

much weaker at detecting malingering compared to FBS-r and RBS, with RBS having the best classification accuracy overall (Bianchini et al., 2017). This is despite the fact that Fs was deliberately created to identify somatic overreporting.

Fs taps rarely-endorsed symptoms in genuine medical patients, but it also appears to have utility in criminal forensic settings where examinees may be more likely to endorse these atypical symptoms (Nguyen et al., 2015; Sellbom et al., 2010; Wygant et al., 2010). However, FBS-r still has larger effect sizes in identifying malingering criminal defendants in some studies, but not as large as those of the traditional F scales such as F-r and Fp-r (Sellbom et al., 2010). This study also shows how criminal defendants tend to malinger symptoms across psychopathological, cognitive, and somatic domains, whereas disability claimants are more restricted to cognitive and somatic symptoms.

FBS-R CUTOFFS AND CLASSIFICATION ACCURACY FOR PREDICTING MALINGERING

Optimal cutoffs and classification accuracy statistics are shown in Table 16–22 for studies using the Slick et al. or Bianchini et al. malingering criteria. Studies using Slick et al. (1999) malingered neurocognitive dysfunction are fairly consistent in showing that when specificity is held at .90 (i.e., <10% false-positive rate), FBS-r cutoffs of ≥ 20 to 24 or higher, equivalent to T scores of ≥ 90 to 100 or higher, are required to maintain an acceptable false-positive rate for identifying malingering, with generally acceptable sensitivities—although sensitivities are not optimal in some groups, indicating that many malingerers are missed by the scale. Lower cutoffs are reported in military samples, with ranges between 80 and 86, while higher cutoffs of 25 or more raw score points or 105 T-score points are reported in disability claimants with primarily psychiatric symptoms. The one study on Bianchini et al. (2005) malingered pain-related disability indicates that lower cutoffs are sufficient in chronic pain patients (i.e., T ≥85) to identify malingerers while not erroneously overidentifying honest responders.

The studies reviewed here (Table 16–22) suggest caution in adopting the publisher's recommendation that scores between 80 and 99 may reflect possible noncredible reporting; instead, with few exceptions, malingering was consistently identified across studies at T-score values of about 90 and higher, excepting examinees with primarily psychiatric symptoms where even higher cutoffs are required. The manual uses a cutoff of greater than 100 for likely malingering.

As is always the case for PVTs and SVTs, any increase in the cutoff score to decrease false positives will result in a decrease in sensitivity to detection of malingering—the proverbial price to pay for avoiding false positives. FBS-r sensitivities vary significantly across samples when the .90 standard for specificity is maintained. In the studies

TABLE 16–22 FBS-r Classification Accuracy for Cutoffs with Acceptable Specificities (≥90%) for Prediction of Malingered Neurocognitive Dysfunction (MND) or Malingered Pain-Related Disability (MPRD)

STUDY	GROUP	CRITERION	*N*	RAW SCORE CUTOFF	T SCORE CUTOFF	SENSITIVITY (%)	SPECIFICITY (%)
Jones (2016)	Military, mild TBI	Probable or Definite MND	300	≥17	≥80	43	92
Bianchini et al. (2017)	Chronic pain patients	Probable or Definite MPRD	501	≥18	≥85	52	≥90
Schroeder et al. (2012)	TBI litigants	Probable or Definite MND	48	≥20	≥90	48	96
Nguyen et al. (2015)	Disability/civil forensic—neurological symptoms[a]	Defined as passed or failed Slick criteria[b]	74	≥22	≥96	30	90
Nguyen et al. (2015)	Disability/civil forensic—medical symptoms[c]	Defined as passed or failed Slick criteria[b]	49	≥22	≥96	11	90
Tarescavage et al. (2013)	Disability claimants	Probable or Definite MND	863	≥24	>100	10	97
Wygant et al. (2011)	Disability claimants, pain and TBI	Probable or Definite MND/MPRD	251	≥24	>100	14	95
Nguyen et al. (2015)	Disability/civil forensic—psychiatric symptoms[d]	Defined as passed or failed Slick criteria[b]	66	≥25	≥105	18	91

NOTE: TBI, traumatic brain injury.

Cutoff scores and T scores that were not provided in original sources were estimated/extrapolated from the MMPI-2-RF Technical Manual and so may not map exactly onto values provided in original sources.

[a]Patients with alleged neurological conditions such as traumatic brain injury, CVAs, dementia or other neurological conditions.

[b]Defined as passing or failing two PVTs.

[c]Patients reporting diverse medical problems including medically unexplained symptoms and chronic pain.

[d]Patients reporting primarily psychiatric conditions such as depression and anxiety.

TABLE 16–23 Cumulative Percentages for MMPI-2-RF FBS-r, RBS, and Fs T Scores for Disability Claimants with and without Malingered Neurocognitive Dysfunction (MND)

	FBS-R		RBS		FS		
T SCORE ≥	NOT MND	MND	NOT MND	MND	NOT MND	MND	T SCORE ≥
120	—	—	—	1.3	2.3	4.2	120
115	—	—	0.2	2.1	5.3	6.3	115
110	—	0.4	0.5	2.9	5.3	6.3	110
105	0.9	2.9	3.4	10.8	7.8	9.6	105
100	3.0	4.2	7.8	13.3	7.8	9.6	100
95	8.0	11.7	12.2	20.4	12.4	15.0	95
90	13.3	19.2	16.3	24.6	17.9	25.0	90
85	24.8	33.8	20.4	31.3	17.9	25.0	85
80	39.4	48.3	31.4	44.6	25.9	35.4	80
75	46.1	54.6	40.1	52.5	25.9	35.4	75
70	59.2	68.8	46.8	60.0	37.2	49.6	70
65	65.4	75.4	54.6	68.3	50.5	63.3	65
60	80.3	87.1	64.9	74.2	50.5	63.3	60
55	84.6	90.0	72.0	81.3	68.1	75.4	55
50	94.5	95.8	89.0	94.2	84.4	89.2	50
45	97.2	97.9	94.0	97.9	84.4	89.2	45
40	98.2	99.2	97.7	99.6	100	100	40
35	100	100	99.5	99.6	100	100	35
30	100	100	100	100	100	100	30

NOTE: Not MND, *N* = 436; MND = 187.

SOURCE: Adapted from Tarescavage et al. (2013).

reviewed here, sensitivity ranged from .10 to .48, and PPV ranged from .40 to .90 at a 40 to 50% base rate (Table 16–22). In some of these studies, sensitivities were inadequate for clinical use, and PPV was only acceptable at high base rates of malingering. Of note, the original FBS in the MMPI-2 appears to yield slightly better classification accuracy statistics (see the review of the MMPI-2 presented earlier in this chapter).

Notably, when examinees were divided according to presenting problem based on neurological, somatic, or psychiatric symptoms, Nguyen et al. (2015) found that to maintain an acceptable 90% specificity rate and minimize false positives, different FBS-r cutoffs had to be employed than are provided in the MMPI-2-RF manual (i.e., T scores of ≥96 to 105, depending on the group; see Table 16–22 for raw score equivalents). With regard to prediction of malingered psychopathology, FBS-r T scores greater than 100 have excellent specificity but marginal sensitivity (Chmielewski et al., 2017).

Cumulative percentages for FBS-r, RBS, and Fs are provided for disability claimants with and without malingered neurocognitive dysfunction in Table 16–23 from the Tarescavage et al. study (2013; Table 16–23).

RBS CUTOFFS AND CLASSIFICATION ACCURACY FOR PREDICTING MALINGERING

Table 16–24 shows RBS classification accuracy statistics to predict Slick et al. (1999) and Bianchini et al. (2005) malingering criteria for cutoffs associated with acceptable specificities (i.e., cutoffs that keep the false positive rate at ≤10%). With one exception, these indicate that cutoffs closer to a T score of 90 and higher (i.e., 88 to 114, depending on the sample) are optimal. Generally speaking, cutoffs closer to 95 were needed in these studies for identifying verified malingering. This contrasts with the cutoffs suggested by the publisher, which include 80 to 99 for possible overreporting and greater than 100 for likely noncredible reporting. Note that some studies are based on the MMPI-2, which uses the same RBS scale. Overall, sensitivities range from .13 to .73 for a minimum specificity of .90, with PPVs of .50 to .89 at base rates of 40 to 50% in these studies (Table 16–24). As with the FBS-r, in some of these studies, sensitivities were inadequate for clinical use, and PPV was only acceptable at high base rates of malingering.

Nguyen et al. (2015) found that to maintain 90% specificity and ensure an acceptable rate of false positives, much higher RBS cutoffs had to be employed than are provided in the manual (i.e., T scores of ≥101 to 114, depending on the group; see Table 16–24 for raw score equivalents). Similarly, Schroeder et al. (2012) found that an RBS cutoff of over 16 (T score of >92) provided a 43% sensitivity rate with a specificity of greater than 90% in TBI litigants but that a higher cutoff was required in psychiatric patients (i.e., T score >105). Different cutoffs are likely needed in different settings. For example, higher cutoffs are reported in veteran and criminal settings using PVTs as validation; however, these cutoffs have not yet been validated using malingering criteria per se (e.g., criminal defendants, ≥20; Wygant et al., 2010; veterans, ≥17; Whitney et al., 2008; Young et al., 2011).

Of note, the mid range cutoffs presented here are close to those suggested in the original RBS validation study,

TABLE 16–24 Response Bias Scale (RBS) Classification Accuracy for Cutoffs with Acceptable Specificities (≥90%) for Prediction of Malingered Neurocognitive Dysfunction (MND) or Malingered Pain-Related Disability (MPRD)

STUDY	GROUP	CRITERION	N	RAW SCORE CUTOFF	T SCORE CUTOFF	SENSITIVITY (%)	SPECIFICITY (%)
Bianchini et al. (2017)	Chronic pain patients	Probable or Definite MPRD	501	≥12	≥80	73	≥90
Dionysus et al. (2011)	TBI litigants	Probable MND	79	≥14	≥88	54	93
Sullivan et al. (2013)	Mixed incentive (43% TBI)	Possible, Probable or Definite MND	83	≥14	≥88	27	90
Jones (2016)	Mild TBI active duty military	Probable or Definite MND	300	≥15	≥92	52	93
Schroeder et al. (2012)	TBI litigants	Probable or Definite MND	48	≥16	>92	43	92
Peck et al. (2013)	TBI litigants	Probable MND	45	≥16	≥96	50	92
Tarescavage et al. (2013)	Disability claimants	Probable or Definite MND	863	≥17	>100	34	92
Nguyen et al. (2015)	Disability/civil forensic—medical symptoms	Defined as passed or failed Slick criteria	49	≥17	≥101	16	93
Nguyen et al. (2015)	Disability/civil forensic—neurological symptoms	Defined as passed or failed Slick criteria	74	≥18	≥105	13	90
Wygant et al. (2011)	Disability claimants (pain and TBI)	Probable or Definite MND/MPRD	251	≥19	>105	34	93
Nguyen et al. (2015)	Disability/civil forensic—psychiatric symptoms	Defined as passed or failed Slick criteria	66	≥20	≥114	18	94

NOTE: RBS given as part of the MMPI-2-RF or MMPI-2.

TBI, traumatic brain injury.

Cutoff scores and T scores that were not provided in original sources were estimated/extrapolated from the MMPI-2-RF Technical Manual and so may not map exactly onto values provided in original sources.

which suggested a raw score cutoff of 17 or higher or T of greater than 100 (Gervais et al., 2007). Of note, one study with a recommended cutoff of 17 or higher involved disability claimants who were from the same private practice as those of the original RBS validation study (Tarescavage et al., 2013). Lower cutoffs may be optimal in military samples, as shown by the optimal cutoff of 15 or higher in the Jones study (2016). Higher cutoffs are recommended in psychiatric patients, equivalent to 20 or more raw score points or 114 or more T-score points.

Schroeder and colleagues (2012) provide RBS T-score cumulative frequencies for groups defined by Slick-criteria malingering as well as for neurological and psychiatric patients. These can be found in the MMPI-2 review earlier in this chapter. Most importantly, these frequencies show that a significant number of neurological patients have RBS T scores greater than 80, and an even higher percentage of psychiatric patients have scores of greater than 90, scores that are typically flagged by the scoring program as indicative of possible overreporting of noncredible symptoms.

FS CUTOFFS AND CLASSIFICATION ACCURACY FOR PREDICTING MALINGERING

Findings on the ability of the Fs to predict Slick-defined or Bianchini-defined malingering are mixed. All studies required a raw score of 6 or more, equivalent to a T score of 84 or above to maintain an adequate false-positive rate. Higher rates are needed in psychiatric samples to accomplish this, in the range of more than 115 T-score points. Table 16–25 shows Fs values for acceptable specificities (>.90) across studies using verified malingering as the validation criterion. Based on these and other studies reviewed earlier, sole reliance on the Fs to detect malingering is not recommended. For example, the Fs scale failed to differentiate between disability claimants with and without malingering presenting with neurological or medical complaints (Nguyen et al., 2015).

HHI-R CUTOFFS AND CLASSIFICATION ACCURACY FOR PREDICTING MALINGERING

Unlike the other MMPI-2-RF validity scales, the HHI-r was developed using malingering criteria as defined by Slick et al. (1999) in its item selection. The scale shows excellent sensitivity at recommended specificity values in the validation study (Table 16–26). For example, a score of 7 or higher had a specificity over .90 and sensitivity of .69, and a score of 10 or higher was associated with a 100% positive predictive power for malingered neurocognitive dysfunction (i.e., with no false-positive errors). However, in a military sample, Jones (2016) found that a score of 9 or higher was required for adequate specificity and reported much lower sensitivity than in the validation study (Table 16–26). However, PPV

TABLE 16–25 Fs Classification Accuracy for Cutoffs with Acceptable Specificities (≥90%) for Prediction of Malingered Neurocognitive Dysfunction (MND) or Malingered Pain-Related Disability (MPRD)

STUDY	GROUP	CRITERION	N	RAW SCORE CUTOFF	T SCORE CUTOFF	SENSITIVITY (%)	SPECIFICITY (%)
Schroeder et al. (2012)	TBI litigants	Probable or Definite MND	48	≥6	≥84	43	96
Bianchini et al. (2017)	Chronic pain patients	Probable or Definite MPRD	501	≥6	≥85	33	≥90
Jones (2016)	Mild TBI active duty military	Probable or Definite MND	300	≥6	≥91	32	94
Nguyen et al. (2015)	Disability/civil forensic—medical symptoms	Defined as passed or failed Slick criteria	49	≥6	≥91	16	83
Nguyen et al. (2015)	Disability/civil forensic—neurological symptoms	Defined as passed or failed Slick criteria	74	≥7	≥99	20	90
Wygant et al. (2011)	Disability claimants (pain and TBI)	Probable or Definite MND/MPRD	251	≥7	≥95	38	96
Tarescavage et al. (2013)	Disability claimants	Probable or Definite MND	863	≥7	>100	20	92
Nguyen et al. (2015)	Disability/civil forensic—psychiatric symptoms	Defined as passed or failed Slick criteria	66	≥9	≥115	36	94

NOTE: TBI, traumatic brain injury.

Cutoff scores and T scores that were not provided in original sources were estimated/extrapolated from the MMPI-2-RF Technical Manual and so may not map exactly onto values provided in original sources.

values are fairly impressive, with an average of .86 at a 40 to 50% base rate of malingering.

USE IN DEMENTIA AND LOW-IQ GROUPS

Not much is known about the use of the MMPI-2-RF SVTs in specific populations at high risk of false positives when PVTs are used to detect exaggeration—namely, in low-IQ examinees and dementia patients—because the MMPI-2-RF is virtually never used in these groups. One notable exception is the study by Carone and Ben-Porath, who document that a 65-year-old woman with severe dementia was able to produce an accurate MMPI-2-RF (Carone & Ben-Porath, 2014).

NEUROANATOMICAL CORRELATES AND IMAGING STUDIES

To our knowledge, there are no neuroanatomical correlates or imaging studies on MMPI-2-RF validity scales; these exist only for a small number of PVTs (e.g., WMT).

COMMENT

The exaggeration of cognitive, somatic, and psychiatric symptoms comprises distinct aspects of malingering. In almost all settings where neuropsychologists conduct evaluations, there is a need to screen for exaggeration in all three of these domains. Like the MMPI-2, the MMPI-2-RF SVTs tap these dimensions of exaggeration. The MMPI-2 and MMPI-2-RF also contain, by an extremely large margin, the most well-researched SVTs in neuropsychology. Although the MMPI-2 may have a larger base of studies overall given its longer life span, the MMPI-2-RF is quickly catching up, with an increasingly large pool of scientific publications on its use since its publication in 2008. Importantly, some studies find that the MMPI-2-RF validity scales outperform those of the MMPI-2 in the prediction of malingering of cognitive, somatic, and psychological symptoms even though the MMPI-2-RF contains fewer items.

As a general recommendation for all SVTs, individual MMPI-2-RF scales should not be used in isolation to

TABLE 16–26 HHI-r Classification Accuracy at Cutoffs Yielding Minimum Acceptable Specificities (≥90%) for Prediction of Malingered Neurocognitive Dysfunction (MND) at Different Base Rates

							BASE RATE 20% OR LESS		BASE RATE 30%		BASE RATE 40–50%	
STUDY	GROUP	CRITERION	N	CUTOFF	SENSITIVITY (%)	SPECIFICITY (%)	PPV (%)	NPV (%)	PPV (%)	NPV (%)	PPV (%)	NPV (%)
Henry et al. (2013)	Personal injury, disability and non-litigants (> 50% TBI)	Probable MND	119	≥7	69	93	72	92	81	87	87	82
Jones (2016)	Mild TBI active duty military	Probable or Definite MND	300	≥9	38	93	38	93	70	78	85	60

NOTE: TBI, traumatic brain injury; PPV, positive predictive value; NPV, negative predictive value.

SOURCE: Adapted from Henry et al. (2013) and Jones (2016).

diagnose malingering. In addition, significant elevations do not necessarily confirm malingering (i.e., intentional exaggeration); rather, they indicate that the symptom report is exaggerated and does not accurately reflect the person's actual status—although the more extreme the score, the more likely it reflects intentional exaggeration (Greve et al., 2006). Generally speaking, as with all SVTs, elevated validity scales on the MMPI-2-RF can co-occur with bona fide cognitive impairment, physical conditions, or psychopathology; in these cases, SVTs can only inform on the accuracy of the examinee's self-description (exaggeration or no exaggeration), not conclusively rule in or rule out the presence of other genuine problems (Greene, 2008).

Of the MMPI-2-RF validity scales reviewed here, the most useful and most validated appear to be the FBS-r and the RBS, although HHI-r demonstrates impressive PPVs in two studies to date. Both FBS-r and RBS appear to tap the dimension of somatic and cognitive overreporting, complementing F-family scales that tap overreporting of psychopathology. Nevertheless, it should be noted that both FBS-r and RBS contain very few items actually tapping cognition, even though the scales do predict malingering according to Slick et al. criteria. As such, they are best considered mixed SVTs that tap primarily somatic overreporting along with psychological distress and, to some degree, cognitive overreporting—a relatively distinct dimension of malingering compared to the psychiatric malingering tapped by F-family SVTs. In head-to-head comparison, FBS-r appears to have particular utility in brain injury litigants, somatic malingerers, nonepileptic seizures, and chronic pain and may be less susceptible to spurious elevations due to psychiatric conditions. In comparison, RBS is best at predicting PVT failure, may have specific utility in military samples, and may be especially sensitive to malingered pain-related disability.

As Greve and colleagues have pointed out, at a given acceptable specificity (false-positive rate) for a specific cutoff, the index with the best sensitivity and best PPV will be preferable, particularly given the legal standard of "more likely than not" that is satisfied if a PPV of .51 or greater is obtained at a base rate that matches that of the setting in which the examinee was seen (Greve et al., 2006). At a 40 to 50% base rate of malingering, RBS appears to marginally outstrip FBS-r in terms of sensitivity and PPV. Overall, Fs is more limited in comparison and does not actually appear to be better at detecting somatic malingering than the RBS and FBS-r in most studies, even though it was expressly developed for this purpose. However, combining multiple MMPI-2-RF validity scales appears to significantly improve sensitivity and specificity over use of single validity indicators, with potential utility for clinical practice (Table 16–20).

Notably, although the FBS has been vehemently criticized over the years (see the review of the MMPI-2 earlier in this chapter), there does not appear to be the same degree of resistance to acceptance of FBS-r in the MMPI-2-RF literature (but see Nichols, 2011). The research reviewed here demonstrates that it is a well-validated tool for the purposes for which it was designed, although sensitivity is not optimal in some studies on malingering (i.e., the scale will miss malingering examinees). This applies to the RBS as well. Despite the fact that RBS was specifically derived to detect PVT failure, both RBS and FBS-r are predictive of PVT performance, although RBS tends to be more consistently so.

Technically speaking, the criteria used to develop the main MMPI-2-RF validity scales reviewed here differ—namely, FBS-r and HHI-r were specifically created to identify malingering, RBS was created to predict PVT failure, and Fs was designed to detect somatic exaggeration. In terms of the quality of the definition of malingering used as the criterion in these validation studies, HHI-r is the only validity index to use the Slick et al. malingering criteria in its validation study, whereas FBS-r validation was based on a definition of malingering determined by its author and never clearly elucidated according to some critics (see the review of the MMPI-2). Nevertheless, the FBS-r has been validated in a number of studies using the Slick et al. criteria, whereas HHI-r needs additional validation before being accepted into routine clinical practice. RBS, in comparison, was derived based on ability to predict PVT failure and not malingering per se, defined by failure on a single PVT rather than on established malingering criteria. Failure on a single PVT as an indicator of invalid performance has subsequently been found to increase false-positive risk; failure on one PVT has indeed been used to define *nonmalingering* in some studies (e.g., Peck et al., 2013). Nevertheless, the RBS predicts the likelihood of malingering as defined by multidimensional criteria and appears equally or more effective as FBS-r in predicting the likelihood of malingering (see the MMPI-2 review for more discussion of validation via PVTs vs. malingering diagnostic criteria for the RBS).

Sample-specific factors may affect the appropriateness of cutoffs. In addition, FBS-r, RBS, and Fs are not technically independent SVTs as they may share items, are all at least moderately intercorrelated, and may therefore not technically fulfill guidelines that recommend use of multiple independent SVTs in the detection of noncredible symptom reporting. However, many PVTs show at least moderate intercorrelations, with an average correlation of about .30 (Berthelson et al., 2013), so some degree of construct overlap is expected for all SVTs, particularly those taken from the same instrument. Notably, the use of combined MMPI-2-RF validity indicators significantly increases sensitivity and PPV to malingering over the use of single scales.

Overall, the clinical literature on FBS-r, RBS, Fs, and HHI-r generally includes known-groups studies primarily consisting of compensation-seeking individuals (litigation, disability, and military), with fewer studies on criminal defendants. In terms of clinical populations with higher than average base rates of malingering, the majority of studies have involved disability and TBI, with comparatively few studies on psychiatric patients. Studies show that different cutoffs are likely needed in different settings, and cutoffs needed for veteran and criminal settings have not yet been validated using malingering criteria per se. Higher scores are required to ensure adequate specificity in those with psychiatric symptoms. The field is in need of more studies on other high-malingering base rates groups such as ADHD; more research on somatic symptom disorder and psychiatric patients is also needed. All the scales reviewed here would benefit from more studies on their ability to predict malingering in criminal defendants using established malingering criteria.

The inclusion of internal and test-retest reliability data in the MMPI-2-RF manual is an asset, as this meets standards for tools designed for clinical use; this is not the case for a number of PVTs and SVTs in common usage. Only Fs has questionable test-retest reliability based on these data. Lack of association between FBS-r and RBS and cognitive tests provides strong evidence for their validity as SVTs and supports their use in neuropsychological assessment of persons with cognitive impairment. Some research indicates that the MMPI-2-RF validity scales can serve as proxies for validity scales on other questionnaires that don't include their own validity indicators because examinees overreport on other questionnaires in a similar fashion.

Practically speaking, although briefer than the MMPI-2, the length of the MMPI-2-RF is still a significant barrier to widespread use in nonforensic settings. Readers are nevertheless encouraged to consider using the scale in routine clinical evaluations as the sophistication of its validity indexes and its massive research base is far in excess of those of briefer tools for assessing psychopathology or cognitive self-report. On the other hand, both the MMPI-2 and MMPI-2-RF are extremely complex measures; require considerable time, effort, and training by the clinician to be used effectively; and are somewhat cumbersome to interpret when used as screening measures or diagnostic tools in clinical settings. They are also quite expensive compared to other scales and do not have the intuitive theoretical simplicity of scales derived a priori on current models of psychopathology such as DSM; this leads many clinicians to prefer briefer clinical scales or comprehensive measures, such as the PAI, which are more straightforward for making clinical diagnoses.

Research on other SVTs and PVTs demonstrate that classification accuracy varies when using these tools in culturally diverse populations (Nijdam-Jones & Rosenfeld, 2017). Despite its impressive publication base and high clinical usage among neuropsychologists, the MMPI-2-RF is still lacking in studies on culturally diverse populations, and this is a major limitation. Clinicians need to be aware that cutoffs derived from samples that differ linguistically, ethnically, or culturally from the individual examinee may lead to diagnostic errors.

Lastly, although as of this writing there is scant research on the validity scales of the new MMPI-3 (Ben-Porath & Tellegen, 2020), the MMPI-3 FBS and RBS are unchanged from the MMPI-2-RF and so past research should be applicable to these scales. There is also a high degree of item overlap between MMPI-2-RF and MMPI-3 with approximately 80% of the same items retained in the MMPI-3 F, Fp, and Fs.

REFERENCES

Arbisi, P. A., Polusny, M. A., Erbes, C. R., Thuras, P., & Reddy, M. K. (2011). The Minnesota Multiphasic Personality Inventory-2 Restructured Form in National Guard soldiers screening positive for posttraumatic stress disorder and mild traumatic brain injury. *Psychological Assessment, 23*(1), 203–214. https://doi.org/10.1037/a0021339

Armistead-Jehle, P., Cole, W. R., & Stegman, R. L. (2017). Performance and symptom validity testing as a function of medical board evaluation in US military service members with a history of mild traumatic brain injury. *Archives of Clinical Neuropsychology*, 1–5. https://doi.org/10.1093/arclin/acx031

Armistead-Jehle, P., Grills, C. E., Bieu, R. K., & Kulas, J. F. (2016). Clinical utility of the Memory Complaints Inventory to detect invalid test performance. *The Clinical Neuropsychologist, 30*(4), 610–628. https://doi.org/10.1080/13854046.2016.1177597

Ben-Porath, Y. S., & Tellegen, A. (2008, 2011). *MMPI-2-RF (Minnesota Multiphasic Personality Inventory-2 Restructured Form): Manual for administration, scoring, and interpretation*. Minneapolis: University of Minnesota Press.

Ben-Porath, Y. S., & Tellegen, A. (2011). *MMPI-2-RF (Minnesota Multiphasic Personality Inventory-2 Restructured Form): User's guide for reports* (2nd ed.). Minneapolis: University of Minnesota Press.

Ben-Porath, Y. S., & Tellegen, A. (2020). Minnesota Multiphasic Personality Inventory – 3 (MMPI-3). Bloomington, MN: NCS Pearson.

Berthelson, L., Mulchan, S. S., Odland, A. P., Miller, L. J., & Mittenberg, W. (2013). False positive diagnosis of malingering due to the use of multiple effort tests. *Brain Injury, 27*(7–8), 909–916. https://doi.org/10.3109/02699052.2013.793400

Bianchini, K. J., Aguerrevere, L. E., Curtis, K. L., Roebuck-Spencer, T. M., Frey, F. C., Greve, K. W., & Calamia, M. (2017). Classification accuracy of the Minnesota Multiphasic Personality Inventory-2 (MMPI-2)-Restructured Form validity scales in detecting malingered pain-related disability. *Psychological Assessment.* https://doi.org/10.1037/pas0000532

Bianchini, K. J., Greve, K. W., & Glynn, G. (2005). On the diagnosis of malingered pain-related disability: Lessons from cognitive malingering research. *Spine Journal, 5*(4), 404–417. https://doi.org/10.1016/j.spinee.2004.11.016

Boone, K. B. (2013). *Clinical practice of forensic neuropsychology: An evidence-based approach.* New York: Guilford Press.

Boone, K. B. (2017). *Neuropsychological evaluation of somatoform and other functional somatic conditions.* New York: Routledge.

Burchett, D., Dragon, W. R., Smith Holbert, A. M., Tarescavage, A. M., Mattson, C. A., Handel, R. W., & Ben-Porath, Y. S. (2016). "False feigners": Examining the impact of non-content-based invalid responding on the Minnesota Multiphasic Personality Inventory-2 Restructured Form content-based invalid responding indicators. *Psychological Assessment, 28*(5), 458–470. https://doi.org/10.1037/pas0000205

Butcher, J. N. (1998). *MMPI-2 user's guide for the Minnesota Report: Reports for forensic settings.* Minneapolis: University of Minnesota Press.

Butcher, J. N., Graham, J. R., Ben Porath, Y. S., Tellegen, A., Dahlstrom, W. G., & Kaemmer, B. (2001). *Manual for administration, scoring, and administration* (revised ed.). Minneapolis: University of Minnesota Press.

Butcher, J. N., Hass, G. A., Greene, R. L., Nelson, L. D., & Association, A. P. (2015). *Using the MMPI-2 in forensic assessment.* Washington, DC: American Psychological Association.

Butcher, J. N., & Pope, K. S. (1992). The research base, psychometric properties, and clinical uses of the MMPI-2 and MMPI-A. *Canadian Psychology, 33,* 61–78.

Carone, D. A., & Ben-Porath, Y. S. (2014). Dementia does not preclude very reliable responding on the MMPI-2 RF: A case report. *The Clinical Neuropsychologist, 28*(6), 1019–1029. https://doi.org/10.1080/13854046.2014.930182

Chmielewski, M., Zhu, J., Burchett, D., Bury, A. S., & Bagby, R. M. (2017). The comparative capacity of the Minnesota Multiphasic Personality Inventory-2 (MMPI-2) and MMPI-2 Restructured Form (MMPI-2-RF) validity scales to detect suspected malingering in a disability claimant sample. *Psychological Assessment, 29*(2), 199–208. https://doi.org/10.1037/pas0000328

Cook, C. M., Bolinger, E., & Suhr, J. (2016). Further validation of the Conner's Adult Attention Deficit/Hyperactivity Rating Scale Infrequency Index (CII) for detection of noncredible report of attention deficit/hyperactivity disorder symptoms. *Archives of Clinical Neuropsychology, 31*(4), 358–364. https://doi.org/10.1093/arclin/acw015

Crighton, A. H., Tarescavage, A. M., Gervais, R. O., & Ben-Porath, Y. S. (2017). The generalizability of overreporting across self-report measures: An investigation with the Minnesota Multiphasic Personality Inventory-2-Restructured Form and the Personality Assessment Inventory in a civil disability sample. *Assessment, 24*(5), 555–574. https://doi.org/10.1177/1073191115621791

Forbey, J. D., Lee, T. T. C., Ben-Porath, Y. S., Arbisi, P. A., & Gartland, D. (2013). Associations between MMPI-2-RF validity scale scores and extra-test measures of personality and psychopathology. *Assessment, 20*(4), 448–461. https://doi.org/10.1177/1073191113478154

Gass, C., & Odland, A. (2012). Minnesota Multiphasic Personality Inventory–2 Revised Form Symptom Validity Scale–Revised (MMPI–2–RF FBS–r; also known as Fake Bad Scale): Psychometric characteristics in a nonlitigation neuropsychological setting. *Journal of Clinical and Experimental Neuropsychology, 34*, 561–70. https://doi.org/10.1080/13803395.2012.666228

Gervais, R. O., Ben-Porath, Y. S., & Wygant, D. B. (2009). Empirical correlates and interpretation of the MMPI-2-RF Cognitive Complaints (COG) scale. *The Clinical Neuropsychologist, 23*(6), 996–1015. https://doi.org/10.1080/13854040902748249

Gervais, R. O., Ben-Porath, Y. S., Wygant, D. B., & Green, P. (2007). Development and Validation of a Response Bias Scale (RBS) for the MMPI-2. *Assessment, 14*(2), 196–208. https://doi.org/10.1177/1073191106295861

Gervais, R. O., Ben-Porath, Y. S., Wygant, D. B., & Sellbom, M. (2010). Incremental validity of the MMPI-2-RF overreporting scales and RBS in assessing the veracity of memory complaints. *Archives of Clinical Neuropsychology, 25*(4), 274–284. https://doi.org/10.1093/arclin/acq018

Gervais, R. O., Tarescavage, A. M., Greiffenstein, M. F., Wygant, D. B., Deslauriers, C., & Arends, P. (2017). Inconsistent responding on the MMPI-2-RF and uncooperative attitude: Evidence from cognitive performance validity measures. *Psychological Assessment*. https://doi.org/10.1037/pas0000506

Green, P. (2004). *Memory Complaints Inventory*. Edmonton, Canada: Green's Publishing.

Greene, R. L. (2008). Malingering and defensiveness on the MMPI-2. In R. Rogers (Ed.), *Clinical assessment of malingering and deception* (3rd ed.; pp. 159–181). New York: Guilford.

Greene, R. L. (2010). *The MMPI-2/MMPI-2-RF: An interpretive manual* (3rd ed.). New York: Allyn & Bacon.

Greiffenstein, M., Gervais, R., Baker, W. J., Artiola, L., & Smith, H. (2013). Symptom validity testing in medically unexplained pain: A chronic regional pain syndrome type 1 case series. *The Clinical Neuropsychologist, 27*(1), 138–147. https://doi.org/10.1080/13854046.2012.722686

Greve, K. W., Bianchini, K. J., Love, J. M., Brennan, A., & Heinly, M. T. (2006). Sensitivity and specificity of MMPI-2 validity scales and indicators to malingered neurocognitive dysfunction in traumatic brain injury. *The Clinical Neuropsychologist, 20*(3), 491–512. https://doi.org/10.1080/13854040590967144

Grossi, L. M., Green, D., Einzig, S., & Belfi, B. (2017). Evaluation of the Response Bias Scale and Improbable Failure Scale in assessing feigned cognitive impairment. *Psychological Assessment, 29*(5), 531–541. https://doi.org/10.1037/pas0000364

Henry, G. K., Heilbronner, R. L., Algina, J., & Kaya, Y. (2013). Derivation of the MMPI-2-RF Henry-Heilbronner Index-r (HHI-r) scale. *The Clinical Neuropsychologist, 27*(3), 509–515. https://doi.org/10.1080/13854046.2012.739644

Henry, G. K., Heilbronner, R. L., Mittenberg, W., & Enders, C. (2006). The Henry-Heilbronner Index: A 15-item empirically derived MMPI-2 subscale for identifying probable malingering in personal injury litigants and disability claimants. *The Clinical Neuropsychologist, 20*(4), 786–797. https://doi.org/10.1080/13854040500287749

Ingram, P. B., & Ternes, M. S. (2016). The detection of content-based invalid responding: A meta-analysis of the MMPI-2-Restructured Form's (MMPI-2-RF) overreporting validity scales. *The Clinical Neuropsychologist, 30*(4), 473–496. https://doi.org/10.1080/13854046.2016.1187769

Jones, A. (2016). Cutoff scores for MMPI-2 and MMPI-2-RF Cognitive-Somatic validity scales for psychometrically defined malingering groups in a military sample. *Archives of Clinical Neuropsychology*. https://doi.org/10.1093/arclin/acw035

LaDuke, C., Barr, W., Brodale, D. L., & Rabin, L. A. (2017). Toward generally accepted forensic assessment practices among clinical neuropsychologists: A survey of professional practice and common test use. *The Clinical Neuropsychologist*, 1–20. https://doi.org/10.1080/13854046.2017.1346711

Lees-Haley, P. R., English, L. T., & Glenn, W. G. (1991). A Fake-Bad-Scale for personal injury claimants. *Psychological Reports, 68*, 203–210.

Locke, D. E. C., Kirlin, K. A., Thomas, M. L., Osborne, D., Hurst, D. F., Drazkowski, J. F., . . . Noe, K. H. (2010). The Minnesota Multiphasic Personality Inventory-2-Restructured Form in the epilepsy monitoring unit. *Epilepsy & Behavior, 17*(2), 252–258. https://doi.org/10.1016/j.yebeh.2009.12.004

Martin, P. K., Schroeder, R. W., Heinrichs, R. J., & Baade, L. E. (2015). Does true neurocognitive dysfunction contribute to Minnesota Multiphasic Personality Inventory-2nd Edition-Restructured Form Cognitive Validity Scale scores? *Archives of Clinical Neuropsychology, 30*(5), 377–386. https://doi.org/10.1093/arclin/acv032

Martin, P. K., Schroeder, R. W., & Odland, A. P. (2015). Neuropsychologists' validity testing beliefs and practices: A survey of North American professionals. *The Clinical Neuropsychologist, 29*(6), 741–776. https://doi.org/10.1080/13854046.2015.1087597

Menton, W. H., Crighton, A. H., Tarescavage, A. M., Marek, R. J., Hicks, A. D., & Ben-Porath, Y. S. (2017). Equivalence of laptop and tablet administrations of the Minnesota Multiphasic Personality Inventory-2 Restructured Form. *Assessment*. https://doi.org/10.1177/1073191117714558

Nguyen, C. T., Green, D., & Barr, W. B. (2015). Evaluation of the MMPI-2-RF for detecting overreported symptoms in a civil forensic and disability setting. *The Clinical Neuropsychologist, 29*(2), 255–271. https://doi.org/10.1080/13854046.2015.1033020

Nichols, D. S. (2011). *Essentials of MMPI-2 assessment*. New York: John Wiley & Sons.

Nijdam-Jones, A., & Rosenfeld, B. (2017). Cross-cultural feigning assessment: A systematic review of feigning instruments used with linguistically, ethnically, and culturally diverse samples. *Psychological Assessment, 29*(11), 1321–1336. https://doi.org/10.1037/pas0000438

Peck, C. P., Schroeder, R. W., Heinrichs, R. J., Vondran, E. J., Brockman, C. J., Webster, B. K., & Baade, L. E. (2013). Differences in MMPI-2 FBS and RBS scores in brain injury, probable malingering, and conversion disorder groups: a preliminary study. *The Clinical Neuropsychologist, 27*(4), 693–707. https://doi.org/10.1080/13854046.2013.779032

Purdon, S. E., Purser, S. M., & Goddard, K. M. (2011). MMPI-2 Restructured Form overreporting scales in first-episode psychosis.

The Clinical Neuropsychologist, 25(5), 829–842. https://doi.org/10.1080/13854046.2011.585141

Rabin, L. A., Paolillo, E., & Barr, W. B. (2016). Stability in test-usage practices of clinical neuropsychologists in the United States and Canada over a 10-year period: A follow-up survey of INS and NAN members. *Archives of Clinical Neuropsychology, 31*(3), 206–230. https://doi.org/10.1093/arclin/acw007

Schroeder, R. W., Baade, L. E., Peck, C. P., VonDran, E. J., Brockman, C. J., Webster, B. K., & Heinrichs, R. J. (2012). Validation of MMPI-2-RF validity scales in criterion group neuropsychological samples. *The Clinical Neuropsychologist, 26*(1), 129–146. https://doi.org/10.1080/13854046.2011.639314

Sellbom, M., Toomey, J. A., Wygant, D. B., Kucharski, L. T., & Duncan, S. (2010). Utility of the MMPI-2-RF (Restructured Form) validity scales in detecting malingering in a criminal forensic setting: a known-groups design. *Psychological Assessment, 22*(1), 22–31. https://doi.org/10.1037/a0018222

Sellbom, M., Wygant, D., & Bagby, M. (2012). Utility of the MMPI-2-RF in detecting noncredible somatic complaints. *Psychiatry Research, 197*(3), 295–301. https://doi.org/10.1016/j.psychres.2011.12.043

Slick, D. J., Sherman, E. M. S., & Iverson, G. (1999). Diagnostic criteria for malingered neurocognitive dysfunction: Proposed standards for clinical practice and research. *The Clinical Neuropsychologist, 13*, 545–561.

Sullivan, K. A., Elliott, C. D., Lange, R. T., & Anderson, D. S. (2013). A known-groups evaluation of the response bias scale in a neuropsychological setting. *Applied Neuropsychology. Adult, 20*(1), 20–32. https://doi.org/10.1080/09084282.2012.670149

Tarescavage, A. M., Wygant, D. B., Gervais, R. O., & Ben-Porath, Y. S. (2013). Association between the MMPI-2 restructured form (MMPI-2-RF) and malingered neurocognitive dysfunction among non-head injury disability claimants. *The Clinical Neuropsychologist, 27*(2), 313–335. https://doi.org/10.1080/13854046.2012.744099

Tellegen, A., & Ben-Porath, Y. S. (2008, 2011). *MMPI-2-RF (Minnesota Multiphasic Personality Inventory-2 Restructured Form): Technical manual.* Minneapolis: University of Minnesota Press.

Walvoort, S. J. W., van der Heijden, P. T., Wester, A. J., Kessels, R. P. C., & Egger, J. I. M. (2016). Self-awareness of cognitive dysfunction: Self-reported complaints and cognitive performance in patients with alcohol-induced mild or major neurocognitive disorder. *Psychiatry Research, 245*, 291–296. https://doi.org/10.1016/j.psychres.2016.08.007

Wershba, R. E., Locke, D. E. C., & Lanyon, R. I. (2015). Analysis of Minnesota Multiphasic Personality Inventory-2-Restructured Form response bias indicators as suppressors or moderators in a medical setting. *Psychological Assessment, 27*(2), 733–737. https://doi.org/10.1037/a0038802

Whitney, K. A., Davis, J. J., Shepard, P. H., & Herman, S. M. (2008). Utility of the Response Bias Scale (RBS) and other MMPI-2 validity scales in predicting TOMM performance. *Archives of Clinical Neuropsychology, 23*(7), 777–786. https://doi.org/10.1016/j.acn.2008.09.001

Wygant, D., Anderson, J., Sellbom, M., Rapier, J., M. Allgeier, L., & Granacher, R. (2011). Association of the MMPI2 Restructured Form (MMPI2RF) Validity Scales with structured malingering criteria. *Psychological Injury and Law, 4*, 13–23. https://doi.org/10.1007/s12207-011-9098-z

Wygant, D. B., Arbisi, P. A., Bianchini, K. J., & Umlauf, R. L. (2017). Waddell non-organic signs: New evidence suggests somatic amplification among outpatient chronic pain patients. *Spine Journal, 17*(4), 505–510. https://doi.org/10.1016/j.spinee.2016.10.018

Wygant, D. B., Sellbom, M., Gervais, R. O., Ben-Porath, Y. S., Stafford, K. P., Freeman, D. B., & Heilbronner, R. L. (2010). Further validation of the MMPI-2 and MMPI-2-RF Response Bias Scale: Findings from disability and criminal forensic settings. *Psychological Assessment, 22*(4), 745–756. https://doi.org/10.1037/a0020042

Young, J. C., Kearns, L. A., & Roper, B. L. (2011). Validation of the MMPI-2 Response Bias Scale and Henry–Heilbronner Index in a US veteran population. *Archives of Clinical Neuropsychology, 26*(3), 194–204. https://doi.org/10.1093/arclin/acr015

Youngjohn, J. R., Wershba, R., Stevenson, M., Sturgeon, J., & Thomas, M. L. (2011). Independent validation of the MMPI-2-RF Somatic/Cognitive and Validity scales in TBI litigants tested for effort. *The Clinical Neuropsychologist, 25*(3), 463–476. https://doi.org/10.1080/13854046.2011.554444

PERSONALITY ASSESSMENT INVENTORY (PAI)

TEST NAME	**Personality Assessment Inventory (PAI)**
DOMAIN	Symptom validity (see other sources for information on assessing psychopathology and personality with the PAI)
AGE RANGE	18 to 89
ADMINISTRATION TIME	40 to 60 minutes
SCORING FORMAT	Computerized or hand scored
REFERENCE	Morey, L.C. (2007). *Personality Assessment Inventory.* Lutz, FL: Psychological Assessment Resources. www.parinc.com

DESCRIPTION

The Personality Assessment Inventory (PAI; Morey, 2007) is a well-known standardized self-report questionnaire for assessing psychopathology and personality. It is used routinely by about 35% of neuropsychologists, including general and forensic neuropsychologists (LaDuke et al., 2017; Rabin et al., 2016). In terms of its specific usage as an SVT, the PAI is used by almost 30% of neuropsychologists who use SVTs and is the third-most-often used scale with SVTs behind the MMPI-2 and MMPI-2-RF, also reviewed in this chapter (Martin et al., 2015). The PAI is shorter than the MMPI-2 and similar in length to the MMPI-2-RF.

This review focuses primarily on the use of the PAI as a symptom validity tool to detect exaggeration and malingering in contexts relevant to neuropsychologists, such as overreporting of cognitive and somatic symptoms in evaluation of personal injury, disability, and criminal behavior. For an overview of the PAI's utility in the detection of feigned psychopathology specifically, please see other comprehensive sources (Morey, 2003; Blais et al., 2010).

CLINICAL CONTENT OF THE PAI

In contrast to the MMPI-2 whose clinical scales were initially empirically derived to distinguish between clinical groups, PAI clinical scales were developed a priori on theoretical grounds to measure discrete clinical constructs (Morey, 2007). The 11 clinical scales cover major categories of pathology corresponding to DSM nosology, including neurotic-spectrum disorders (i.e., Somatic Complaints, Anxiety, Anxiety-Related Disorders, Depression), psychotic-spectrum disorders (i.e., Mania, Paranoia, Schizophrenia), and behavior disorder or impulse control problems (i.e., Borderline, Antisocial, Alcohol Problems, Drug Problems). The PAI also contains five treatment scales that measure constructs relevant to treatment and two interpersonal scales (see Table 16–27).

To ensure adequate depth of coverage, the scales were designed to include items that address the multidimensionality and full range of severity of the construct. As a consequence, most of the clinical scales are divided into subscales, each of which taps an important component of the superordinate construct. For example, the Depression scale is comprised of three subscales covering affective, cognitive, and physiological components of depression (Table 16–27).

The Somatic Complaints (SOM) scale is of particular potential utility for neuropsychologists in identifying overreporting of somatic symptoms in neuropsychological populations. It was designed to measure symptoms related to somatoform disorders and comprises three subscales. The Conversion subscale measures dramatic symptoms commonly found in conversion disorders; the Somatization subscale covers more routine physical complaints diagnostic through their frequency rather than for their content, and the Health Concerns subscale taps preoccupation with health and physical functioning. Each has eight items.

The PAI is available in US Spanish and European Spanish through the publisher; there are also other translations in circulation, including French, Danish, Korean, and Hebrew translations.

SHORT FORMS

The PAI Short Form is comprised of the first 160 items of the full-length PAI; it can be derived in cases of incomplete administration, other unusual clinical circumstances, or in some research or screening situations; validity studies are scant. There is also a 22-item Personality Assessment Screener (PAS, Morey, 1997), intended as a very brief screen covering 10 different clinical problems based on items from the PAI with maximum sensitivity, including negative affect, acting out, health problems, psychosis,

TABLE 16–27 Overview of Personality Assessment Inventory (PAI) Clinical Scales and Subscales

	SCALE	SUBSCALES
Clinical Scales	Somatic Complaints (SOM)	Conversion Somatization Health Concerns
	Anxiety (ANX)	Cognitive Affective Physiological
	Anxiety-Related Disorders (ARD)	Obsessive-Compulsive Phobias Traumatic Stress
	Depression (DEP)	Cognitive Affective Physiological
	Mania (MAN)	Activity Level Grandiosity Irritability
	Paranoia (PAR)	Hypervigilance Persecution Resentment
	Schizophrenia (SCZ)	Psychotic Experiences Social Detachment Thought Disorder
	Borderline Features (BOR)	Affective Instability Identity Problems Negative Relationships Self-Harm
	Antisocial Features (ANT)	Antisocial Behaviors Egocentricity Stimulus Seeking
	Alcohol Problems (ALC) Drug Problems (DRG)	
Treatment Consideration Scales	Aggression (AGG)	Aggressive Attitude Verbal Aggression Physical Aggression
	Suicidal Ideation (SUI) Stress (STR) Nonsupport (NON) Treatment Rejection (RXR)	
Interpersonal Scales	Dominance (DOM) Warmth (WRM)	

SOURCE: Adapted from Morey (2007). Reproduced by special permission of the Publisher, Psychological Assessment Resources, Inc. (PAR), 16204 North Florida Avenue, Lutz, Florida 33549, from the Personality Assessment Inventory by Leslie C. Morey, PhD, Copyright 1991, 2007 by PAR. Further reproduction is prohibited without permission of PAR.

social withdrawal, hostility, suicidal ideation, alienation, alcohol problems, and anger problems. The PAS does not have any validity scales. Due to limited research on either scale in neuropsychological populations, the full PAI is recommended for most evaluation contexts.

PAI VALIDITY SCALES

The PAI contains four main validity scales; additional supplementary validity scales will not be reviewed here. Relevant validity scales are shown in Tables 16–28 and 16–29. Like other major scales such as the MMPI-2-RF, the PAI provides an assessment of two main facets of invalid responding: non–content-based invalid responding (i.e., failure to respond to items, or responding to items in a fixed or random manner, regardless of content), and content-based invalid responding (i.e., choosing items that portray oneself as functioning better or worse than indicated by objective assessment; Forbey et al., 2013). The latter type of invalid responding taps the dimension of overreporting of symptoms and is usually the focus when malingering or symptom amplification is a possibility—although malingerers may also choose items randomly or erratically in order to appear impaired.

Among non–content-based invalid responding scales, the PAI Inconsistency scale (ICN) reflects the extent to which the examinee cooperated with the testing process as reflected by consistency of responses to items of similar content.

Infrequency (INF) also measures consistency of responding across the item set, using neutral items placed throughout the scale designed to detect general inattention to item content. Note that the PAI Infrequency (INF) scale is not an "infrequency" scale akin to infrequency scales of the MMPI-2/MMPI-2-RF, which were all designed specifically to detect overreporting of symptoms; that is, endorsement of clinically infrequent symptoms (i.e., F, Fp, Fs). Instead, PAI INF items contain no relevant clinical content per se but are simply included throughout the scale to test whether the examinee is attending to items; the items are designed to detect random responding, not exaggeration (Table 16–28).

The PAI's content-based invalid responding scales tap two dimensions: underreporting and overreporting of symptoms. Generally speaking, underreporting scales tend to be elevated in groups attempting to minimize problems (e.g., personnel evaluations, custody evaluations), but not in most groups seen by neuropsychologists. The PAI's Positive Impression Management (PIM) scale measures this dimension of invalidity (Table 16–28) along with other underreporting scales detailed in the manual.

Here, we focus mostly on PAI scales that measure symptom overreporting, that is, Negative Impression Management (NIM), the Malingering Index (MAL), and the Rogers Discriminant Function (RDF). Each is described in more detail in Table 16–29. Importantly, the PAI does not include any scales specifically developed to identify cognitive or somatic overreporting, including overreporting of neurological symptoms, dimensions of exaggeration that are critical in neuropsychological evaluation and that are well covered by the MMPI-2 and MMPI-2-RF (see reviews earlier in this chapter).

NEGATIVE IMPRESSION MANAGEMENT (NIM)

NIM is comprised of items capturing bizarre or unlikely symptoms infrequently endorsed by normative and clinical samples, although these may be endorsed in severe mental disorders. The author is clear that an elevated NIM does not equate malingering; rather, the test is deemed invalid due to a response style consisting of extreme distortion of the self-report. NIM was derived based on a college sample instructed to malinger severe mental illness. As noted in the manual, groups instructed to feign obtain much higher

TABLE 16–28 Personality Assessment Inventory (PAI) Validity Scales Measuring Consistency and Underreporting of Symptoms

	DESCRIPTION	NUMBER OF ITEMS
Inconsistency (ICN)	Measures how consistently items with similar content were completed; consists of pairs of items with similar content; T scores from 64 to 72 indicate some inconsistency in responding; scores of 73 and over suggest that the respondent did not attend consistently to items, and the protocol is deemed invalid (note: random protocols yield scores of 73)	10 item pairs
Infrequency (INF)	Items with very high or low endorsement rates in the normative and clinical samples; items are neutral in content and designed to be responded to in a consistent way regardless of clinical status; high scores may reflect random responding due to confusion, reading difficulties, scoring errors, or possibly an idiosyncratic response style; T scores between 60 and 74 indicate some degree of unusual responding; scores of 75 and over suggest that the examinee did not completely attend to items (note: random protocols yield scores of 86).	8
Positive Impression (PIM)	Suggests an enhanced positive impression, with the presentation of very favorable self-presentation and the denial of minor faults; items are rarely endorsed in normative and clinical samples; elevations tend to be quite rare in clinical samples and are therefore interpretively significant if found; moderate elevations from 57 to 67 indicate some positive impression management, either covert or overt defensive styles, with scores of 68 and higher indicative of questionable validity.	9

SOURCE: Adapted from Morey (2007). Reproduced by special permission of the Publisher, Psychological Assessment Resources, Inc. (PAR), 16204 North Florida Avenue, Lutz, Florida 33549, from the Personality Assessment Inventory by Leslie C. Morey, PhD, Copyright 1991, 2007 by PAR. Further reproduction is prohibited without permission of PAR.

NIM scores than those of actual clinical patients. NIM is thus more useful for identifying feigning of severe pathology versus milder forms, with more effectiveness at detection of feigned psychosis compared to feigned PTSD, anxiety, or depression (manual). Among approaches used by SVTs, NIM is based on the rare symptoms detection strategy (Sellbom & Bagby, 2008).

MALINGERING INDEX (MAL)

The MAL score is based on what the author describes as eight "configural features of the PAI profile" that tend to be found more frequently among those simulating mental disorders. These scale cut points were derived based on performance of a college sample instructed to malinger severe psychiatric illness; the statistical methods through which this was done are not clearly explained in the manual. MAL is calculated according to specific criteria shown in Table 16–30, with one point awarded per criterion for a maximum of eight points. Among approaches used by SVTs, MAL is based on detection of unlikely patterns of psychopathology based on symptom combinations (Sellbom & Bagby, 2008).

Importantly, NIM is a component of MAL. Similarly, both MAL and RDF include depression, treatment rejection, paranoia, and antisocial clinical scales as part of their scoring criteria (see Tables 16–29 and 16–30).

ROGERS DISCRIMINANT FUNCTION (RDF)

To calculate the RDF, T scores for certain PAI scales are multiplied by a specific coefficient listed in the manual and summed with a constant. Notably, weights for approximately half of the scales are negative, and thus values for these scales are subtracted from the sum to provide the final RDF score. The scale was developed based on a discriminant function that differentiated simulators from psychiatric patients. The manual cautions reliance on the RDF in

TABLE 16–29 Overview of Personality Assessment Inventory (PAI) Validity Scales Measuring Overreporting of Symptoms

	DESCRIPTION	NUMBER OF ITEMS
Negative Impression Management (NIM)	Suggests an exaggerated unfavorable impression; items comprised of bizarre or unlikely symptoms infrequently endorsed by normative and clinical samples, although these are more frequently endorsed in clinical samples such that scores will be elevated in severe mental disorders; elevated scales do not equate malingering; rather, these show that the test is invalid due to extreme distortion of the self-report; T scores between 73 and 83 suggest some exaggeration of complaints and symptoms; scores between 84 and 91 may indicate "a cry for help" or an extremely negative evaluation of oneself and one's life; high scores of 92 and up are strongly suggestive of careless responding, extremely negative self-presentation, or malingering; scores greater than 110 often indicate deliberate negative distortion (note: random protocols yield scores of 96)	9
Malingering Index (MAL)	Consists of 8 "configural features of the PAI profile" that tend to be found more frequently among those simulating mental disorders; scores of 84 or higher raise the possibility of malingering of mental disorder; scores of 111 or greater are highly unusual (see manual for more details on this scale)	
Rogers Discriminant Function (RDF)	Developed to distinguish between profiles of bona fide patients and those simulating psychiatric disorders, involving weighted combinations of 20 PAI scores identified by a discriminant function; scores of 59 or greater suggest malingering of mental disorders	

SOURCE: Adapted from Morey (2007). Reproduced by special permission of the Publisher, Psychological Assessment Resources, Inc. (PAR), 16204 North Florida Avenue, Lutz, Florida 33549, from the Personality Assessment Inventory by Leslie C. Morey, PhD, Copyright 1991, 2007 by PAR. Further reproduction is prohibited without permission of PAR.

forensic and correctional settings due to inconsistent results in prior studies. Like MAL, RDF is based on detection of unlikely patterns of psychopathology based on symptom combinations (Sellbom & Bagby, 2008). See Table 16–31 for RDF components.

ADMINISTRATION

Details regarding administration procedures can be found in the manual. According to the authors, administration time ranges from 40 to 50 minutes for examinees with intact cognition, to 90 minutes for examinees with attention or psychomotor problems. A Grade 4 reading ability is recommended. The test can be administered via computer.

Like all standardized questionnaires, allowing the examinee to complete the test at home is not advised because norms were generated under carefully controlled conditions, factors affecting validity cannot be observed, and responses may be influenced by or completed by others.

SCORING

Although hand-scoring is available, computer scoring is highly recommended to reduce errors in transcription and scoring.

DEMOGRAPHIC EFFECTS

Most of the information available on demographic effects is on NIM; demographic effects on MAL and RDF, to our knowledge, are lacking.

AGE

Age has minimal impact on NIM scores, accounting for less than 2% of variance. Visual inspection of standardization means suggests that younger examinees score slightly higher than older age groups, with about a three to four T-score point difference (manual). Age is not considered in the derivation of T scores.

TABLE 16–30 Personality Assessment Inventory (PAI) MAL Score Components

MAL SCORE COMPONENTS
NIM
INF minus ICN
NIM minus INF
Depression and Treatment Rejection
Mania (Irritability) minus Mania (Grandiosity)
Paranoia (Persecution) minus Paranoia (Hypervigilance)
Paranoia (Persecution) minus Paranoia (Resentment)
Antisocial Features (Egocentricity) minus Antisocial Features (Antisocial Behaviors)

NOTE: NIM, Negative Impression Management; INF, Infrequency; ICN, Inconsistency; components are awarded one point each if present and summed.

SOURCE: Adapted from Morey (2007). Reproduced by special permission of the Publisher, Psychological Assessment Resources, Inc. (PAR), 16204 North Florida Avenue, Lutz, Florida 33549, from the Personality Assessment Inventory by Leslie C. Morey, PhD, Copyright 1991, 2007 by PAR. Further reproduction is prohibited without permission of PAR.

GENDER

Gender also has a negligible effect on NIM scores, accounting for less than 1% of variance in scores and appearing to exert less than one T-score point on visual inspection of means (manual). Gender effects were not found in workers' compensation cases scoring above or below PAI validity cutoffs in one study (Sumanti et al., 2006). No other information on gender effects appears available.

EDUCATION AND IQ

About 5% of variance in NIM scores is attributable to education effects. Visual inspection of means in the manual indicates higher NIM scores with lower education, with about an eight-point T-score difference between groups defined by four to 11 years of education versus 16 years or more years of education (manual). Education effects were not found for workers' compensation cases who scored above or below PAI validity cutoffs in one study (Sumanti et al., 2006). See "Correlations with Neuropsychological Tests" for a discussion of IQ effects.

ETHNICITY, NATIONALITY, AND LINGUISTIC EFFECTS

Ethnicity accounts for less than 3% of variance in NIM scores, with four to five T-score differences on visual inspection of means, indicating slightly higher NIM scores in African American and other ethnicities versus Caucasians; it is unclear if these reflect meaningful differences (manual). One study suggests that NIM performed similarly in English and Spanish versions of the PAI at identifying simulators (Fernandez et al., 2008). No other information on demographic effects appears available.

NORMATIVE DATA

Norms were developed from a US 1995 Census-matched sample of 1,000 community-dwelling individuals stratified according to age, gender, and ethnicity (Table 16–32). Data were also gathered from a sample of 1,050 college students and a sample of 1,265 clinical subjects, the latter drawn from a wide variety of clinical facilities, including outpatient psychiatric settings, inpatient psychiatric settings, medical settings, substance abuse programs, and correctional settings, with, in descending order of prevalence, individuals with diagnoses of affective disorders, alcohol-related disorders, adjustment disorders, personality disorders, drug-related disorders, anxiety disorders, schizophrenia, so-called organic disorders, and somatization disorders (manual).

The NIM scale validation study used a sample of 44 college students enrolled in a class on abnormal psychology and instructed to feign psychiatric disorder. The MAL scale was also developed based on the same simulation sample as the NIM scale; detailed statistical information on how the index was derived is not provided in the manual, except that it is composed of "eight configural features" of the PAI profile observed more frequently in the simulators than in actual clinical patients.

TABLE 16–31 Personality Assessment Inventory (PAI) RDF Score Components

RDF SCORE COMPONENTS
ICN
INF
Stress
Treatment Rejection
Somatic Complaints (Conversion)
Somatic Complaints (Health Concerns)
Anxiety (Affective)
Anxiety (Physiological)
Anxiety-Related Disorders (Obsessive-Compulsive)
Anxiety-Related Disorders (Phobias)
Anxiety-Related Disorders (Traumatic Stress)
Depression (Cognitive)
Paranoia (Hypervigilance)
Paranoia (Resentment)
Schizophrenia (Psychotic Experiences)
Schizophrenia (Thought Disorder)
Borderline (Identity Problems)
Borderline (Negative Relationships)
Borderline (Self-Harm)
Antisocial Features (Egocentricity)

NOTE: INF, Infrequency; ICN, Inconsistency; T scores on each scale are multiplied by a specific value listed in the manual and summed with a constant to provide the RDF raw score; notably, weights for approximately half of the scales are negative, and thus values for these scales are subtracted from the sum to provide the final RDF score.

SOURCE: Adapted from Morey (2007). Reproduced by special permission of the Publisher, Psychological Assessment Resources, Inc. (PAR), 16204 North Florida Avenue, Lutz, Florida 33549, from the Personality Assessment Inventory by Leslie C. Morey, PhD, Copyright 1991, 2007 by PAR. Further reproduction is prohibited without permission of PAR.

TABLE 16–32 Characteristics of the Personality Assessment Inventory (PAI) Standardization Sample

Sample size	1,000 adults selected from an initial sample of 1,462 adults residing in the United States
Age	18 to 89
Geographic location	12 states in the United States representing both rural and urban areas
Sample type	Individuals drawn from directories and special appeals to community groups
Education	Mean = 13.7
Gender	48% Men 52% Women
Ethnicity	Ethnic composition for Caucasian, African American and Other categories comparable to 1995 US Census
Screening	No more than 33 items could be left blank

Age groupings of 18 to 29, 30 to 49, 50 to 59, and 60 and older.

SOURCE: Adapted from Morey (2007). Reproduced by special permission of the Publisher, Psychological Assessment Resources, Inc. (PAR), 16204 North Florida Avenue, Lutz, Florida 33549, from the Personality Assessment Inventory by Leslie C. Morey, PhD, Copyright 1991, 2007 by PAR. Further reproduction is prohibited without permission of PAR.

The RDF was also developed based on a simulation sample described in an older publication (Rogers et al., 1996) but not in the manual. The simulation sample consisted of 246 simulators (undergraduates and doctoral students) who were compared to genuine clinical patients with schizophrenia, depression, and generalized anxiety. A discriminant function was derived to differentiate the two groups based on weighted combinations of 20 scores. Although the original sample had modest to moderate predictive power, cross-validation to a second sample had lower specificity according to the manual (i.e., 80% sensitivity, 81% specificity). Detailed statistical information on the discriminant function derivation is not provided in the manual.

EVIDENCE FOR RELIABILITY

EVIDENCE FOR INTERNAL RELIABILITY

NIM has adequate internal reliability in normative and clinical samples, above .70, with similar reliabilities according to ethnicity (Caucasian vs. African American; manual); reliabilities for the college sample are somewhat low (alpha = .63). No information is provided on MAL or RDF reliabilities in the manual. High PAI reliabilities have been reported in pain patients (Karlin et al., 2005) and in mixed neuropsychological samples (Busse et al., 2014).

EVIDENCE FOR TEST-RETEST RELIABILITY, MEASURING CHANGE, AND PRACTICE EFFECTS

Test-retest reliabilities are adequate for NIM in a combined community and college sample ($N = 155$) with an approximate retest interval of 26 days ($r = .75$), with a mean T-score difference of 3.0; that is, lower scores at retest (manual). The manual also presents mean test-retest correlations for NIM across three studies, which are also adequate overall ($r = .74$). No information is provided on MAL or RDF test-retest reliabilities.

EVIDENCE FOR VALIDITY

FACTOR-ANALYTIC STUDIES

In a four-factor solution in the clinical sample, NIM appears to load on a general psychological distress factor along with PAI clinical scales measuring clinical syndromes and subjective distress, including anxiety, depression, schizophrenia, borderline traits, somatic symptoms, and paranoia (i.e., ANX, DEP, ARD, SCZ, BOR, SOM, and PAR, respectively), as described in the manual. See manual for a listing of other factor-analytic studies, some of which identified a separate validity factor. In an independent study, a three-factor solution was found in a mixed neuropsychological sample, with TOMM scores on the first factor, NIM and PIM scores on the second factor, and INF scores on the third factor (Whiteside et al., 2009).

PAI SCALE INTERCORRELATIONS

Across studies, NIM and MAL tend to be highly correlated. NIM is a component of MAL, so this is expected. RDF typically shows lower correlations with NIM and MAL. For example, NIM and MAL tend to be highly correlated in mixed neuropsychological samples ($r = .71$); both have lower correlations with RDF (Gaasedelen et al., 2017). A similar pattern is reported in veterans between NIM and MAL ($r = .69$), with again, lower correlations between NIM and RDF ($r = .21$; Braxton et al., 2007). In inmates, NIM and MAL are reported to be very highly correlated ($r = .80$), but NIM and RDF have more modest correlations ($r = .41$; Edens et al., 2007). Similar results are reported in workers' compensation cases (Sumanti et al., 2006).

With regard to correlations with PAI clinical scales, NIM correlates highly with several clinical scales in the standardization sample and in the clinical sample. Its highest correlations in the standardization and PAI clinical sample are to the Schizophrenia scale ($r = .69, .76$, respectively), along with very high correlations with Somatic Complaints, Anxiety, Anxiety-Related Disorders, Paranoia, Borderline Features, and Suicidal Ideation (i.e., all *rs* >.52 to .68; manual).

No information is provided on correlations with clinical scales for MAL and RDF in the manual. However, both scales are comprised of clinical scales, so high associations would be expected. In one study in prisoners, NIM and MAL both demonstrated substantial correlations with PAI clinical scales that measure psychopathology ($r = .47$ to .84); in contrast, RDF was not correlated with PAI clinical scales in this group (Edens et al., 2007).

CORRELATIONS AND COMPARISONS TO PVTS

Overall, PAI overreporting validity scales show modest to low associations with PVTs, including the MSVT, NV-MSVT, VSVT, TOMM, Dot Counting Test, and FIT. As well, PAI overreporting scales are not always clearly elevated in those who fail PVTs. Of PAI indices, NIM tends to be the most correlated with PVTs, and RDF the least. For example, in mixed neuropsychological samples, correlations between NIM and VSVT scores are reported as modest (Haggerty et al., 2007), and correlations between NIM and TOMM are in the medium range ($r = .33$ to .38), indicating some degree of shared variance (Whiteside et al., 2009). In workers' compensation cases, correlations between NIM and PVTs such as Dot Counting and FIT are modest to moderate (absolute value *rs* = .26 and .30, respectively); correlations for MAL are slightly lower, and correlations involving RDF approach zero (Sumanti et al., 2006). In examinees with ADHD or learning disability, including suspected malingerers, there is a clear lack of association between PAI validity scales and WMT scores (Sullivan et al., 2007).

In veterans with mild TBI, no differences in NIM scores were found for those who passed or failed the MSVT; results were similar for MAL and RDF (Armistead-Jehle, 2010). However, those failing the MSVT had an average T score nearing 80, suggesting an element of exaggeration; MAL and RDF were not elevated in these examinees. In a military concussion sample, the failure rate for NIM was 8% using a T-score cutoff of 72 as the criterion, significantly lower than the PVT failure rate, at 17%. However, those who failed either the MSVT or NV-MSVT had significantly higher NIM, Somatic Complaints, and Depression scores (Armistead-Jehle et al., 2016).

Other research indicates that Somatic Complaints, and Conversion in particular, are related to TOMM performance, with modest correlations in mixed neuropsychological samples ($r = -.25$; $r = -.29$, respectively; see also Sumanti et al., 2006). However, this relationship is attenuated when NIM is accounted for, as it is likely the stronger predictor. Overall, elevations on NIM, Somatic Complaints, and particularly Conversion may have promise as indicators of increased risk of invalid performance on cognitive tests (Whiteside et al., 2010), although no studies have provided cross-validation and combined cutoffs for these scales.

CORRELATIONS AND COMPARISONS TO OTHER SVTS

PAI scales, particularly NIM, demonstrate high associations with several other SVTs, including validity scales from the MMPI-2, MMPI-2-RF, as well as with the SIMS. It also correlates highly with the SIRS, a scale often considered the gold standard for identification of malingering of psychopathology. However, the PAI may be less sensitive overall to malingering in neuropsychological populations compared to some of these SVTs, especially those from the MMPI-2-RF. This likely relates to the fact that, unlike the MMPI-2-RF, the PAI lacks scales specifically geared toward detection of cognitive and somatic malingering.

For example, with regard to the MMPI-2, the PAI identified fewer invalid protocols in a veterans sample (Braxton et al., 2007), a finding reported by other studies, and this despite lower cutoffs for PAI validity scales. In contrast, positive distortion detection was equivalent for the two scales. This suggests that the PAI may be less effective at detecting overreporting compared to the MMPI-2. In this study, correlations between NIM and MMPI-2 validity scales were large, including correlations with F and Fp ($r = .77$, $r = .55$, respectively; Braxton et al., 2007). On the original MMPI, NIM is most correlated with F ($r = .54$), with only modest correlations with other validity scales (manual).

With regard to the MMPI-2-RF, in disability claimants, NIM is highly correlated with MMPI-2-RF validity scales tapping cognitive, somatic, and psychiatric overreporting, including RBS and F-r ($r = .62$ and .72, respectively), with substantial correlations with Fp-r and Fs ($r = .54$) and lower but still moderate correlations with FBS-r (r = .41). A similar pattern is found for MAL, but with more modest correlations overall (r = .25 to .49). In comparison, correlations between RDF and MMPI-2-RF indices are minimal (r = .13 to .25; Crighton et al., 2017). The authors concluded that, overall, individuals overreporting psychiatric, cognitive, and somatic complaints appeared to perform similarly on the PAI and MMPI-2-RF, but there were smaller effect sizes found on the PAI for somatic-cognitive overreporting likely due to the absence of these specialized scales on the PAI.

Among PAI invalidity scales, in civil disability claimants, NIM scores demonstrated the largest effect sizes in identifying exaggerators based on MMPI-2-RF validity scales, with average T scores of over 80 in psychiatric overreporters and of over 72 in somatic-cognitive overreporters (Crighton et al., 2017); MAL had slightly lower effects sizes, and differences for RDF were negligible. For psychiatric overreporting, 30% had NIM scores above a T-score cutoff of 92, with 27% and 41% with elevations on MAL and RDF. For somatic and cognitive overreporting, 19% had NIM T-score elevations higher than 92, with 20% and 28% having elevations on MAL and RDF, respectively.

NIM correlations with the SIRS and SIMS, two commonly used scales to determine exaggeration of symptoms, are very high in inmates (r = .75, r = .84, respectively; Edens et al., 2007). In comparison, MAL and RDF correlations with SIRS and SIMS are much lower, although still notable (r = .40 to .57), with RDF the least correlated with other SVTs. NIM and SIRS are also highly correlated in criminal defendants (r = .76); correlations for MAL are lower but still substantial (r = .58), and correlations for RDF are negligible (Kucharski et al., 2007).

CORRELATIONS WITH NEUROPSYCHOLOGICAL TESTS

Although research has focused almost exclusively on NIM, PAI validity indices appear to have minimal association with cognitive test performance. For example, NIM was unrelated to neuropsychological test performance in a military concussion sample, as measured by the TMT, word fluency, and RBANS. Compared to PVTs such as MSVT and NV-MSVT that accounted for about 15% of variance, NIM accounted for only .04% of variance in test performance (Armistead-Jehle et al., 2016). Similarly, other PAI clinical scales such as Somatic Complaints, Anxiety, and Depression accounted for only negligible amounts of variance in neuropsychological performance. No information was presented on MAL and RDF.

Some researchers suggest that PAI validity scales may be influenced by cognitive or attention deficits and, in fact, that elevations on these validity scales may indicate the presence of cognitive deficits. However, methodological limitations of these studies preclude these conclusions, most evidently the lack of PVTs to exclude exaggeration as a factor in both cognitive deficits and PAI validity scale elevations. Specifically, some studies report that PAI validity scales are associated with performance on IQ, motor, visual-spatial, and, in particular, attention tests (Aikman & Souheaver, 2008). Others have found that in psychiatric outpatients, those who have invalid PAI profiles have, on average, low average to borderline IQ and that when IQ is controlled for, attention problems as measured by the Trail Making Test (TMT-A), Digit Span, and Digit Symbol predict PAI invalidity (Sinclair et al., 2015). Furthermore, the same authors found that cognitive impairments as measured by the WMS-IV Brief Cognitive Status Examination predicted PAI profile invalidity (Sinclair et al., 2015). Last, incarcerated examinees with significant mental illness who had invalid PAI profiles had lower WAIS-IV scores, particularly on the Working Memory Index, with WAIS-IV subtests explaining 20% of the variance in PAI invalidity (Matlasz et al., 2017). These findings require replication with a cognitive battery that includes PVTs to differentiate between genuine cognitive impairment and exaggeration.

CORRELATIONS WITH OTHER QUESTIONNAIRES

PAI validity index scores would be expected to correlate with other questionnaires tapping psychological distress. This is because NIM has substantial correlations with PAI clinical scales in the standardization sample and, in the case of MAL and RDF, because these scales include clinical scales as part of their composite scores.

For example, NIM is moderately related to depression and anxiety in both clinical and college student samples as measured by a variety of scales including Beck scales (r = .40 to .53), as well as suicide probability scales (r >.40, manual). NIM is also highly correlated with neuroticism and inversely correlated with agreeableness as measured by the NEO-PI personality scale, with lesser associations with extraversion, openness, and consciousness (manual). Correlations with clinician ratings of psychiatric symptoms are on the whole modest, with some higher correlations found for suspiciousness (manual). Information on associations to psychopathology scales is not provided for MAL and RDF in the manual.

In active service members with a history of concussion, NIM is highly correlated with subjective memory concerns as measured by the Memory Complaints Inventory (MCI; Green, 2004), with quite a large correlation (r = .62). Those with scores above the NIM cutoff had higher MCI scores. In comparison, MAL correlations are modest (r = .34), and RDF is completely uncorrelated with memory complaints, suggesting limited validity for the RDF scale in this sample.

CLINICAL STUDIES

Although there have been a number of studies involving simulators, we focus our review here almost exclusively on known-groups studies as these represent a more stringent and relevant criterion for determining validity. This is because simulation designs are known to inflate sensitivity estimates compared to when tests are used in real clinical groups. Of note, PAI validity indicators have yielded mixed results even in simulation designs aimed at detecting overreporting of psychopathology, a goal for which they were designed (see Sellbom & Bagby, 2008). In all, most studies provide some evidence on the utility of NIM and, to some degree, of MAL, but limited evidence for the RDF in neuropsychological groups.

There are no studies on the PAI's capacity to predict malingering based on multidimensional malingering criteria such as the Slick malingered neurocognitive dysfunction criteria or Bianchini's malingered pain-related disability criteria (Slick et al., 1999; Bianchini et al., 2005). However, two studies have demonstrated the test's ability to predict PVT failure defined as failing two or more PVTs. Although not technically equivalent to multidimensional malingering criteria, failure on two or more PVTs has been used as a proxy for malingering in studies examining this question. Of note, using failure on two or more PVTs as the criterion for malingering in these studies allows examination cognitive malingering prediction but not prediction of other kinds of malingering (e.g., somatic, psychiatric). Overall, there is some evidence for the utility of NIM in identifying malingering, but with less than optimal sensitivity. There is limited evidence supportive of the effectiveness of MAL and particularly of RDF at detecting malingering in neuropsychological settings.

For instance, in a study involving a mixed neuropsychological sample, a NIM T-score cutoff of 79 had a specificity of greater than .90 for malingering defined as failure on two PVTs, but at a very low sensitivity of only .16; MAL and RDF yielded similar classification accuracy statistics indicative of limited sensitivity to malingering. Raising the T-score cutoff to 86 marginally increased specificity while yielding even lower sensitivity (Gaasedelen et al., 2017). The authors concluded that there was limited evidence to support the use of RDF in detecting exaggerated cognitive dysfunction. Furthermore, they concluded that even when NIM and MAL are within the valid range, clinicians cannot be confident of having ruled out cognitive malingering.

Similarly, in another study, NIM had limited utility in identifying suspected malingerers from controls and clinical patients in a psychoeducational evaluation sample. Specifically, failure on two embedded PVTs from the WAIS-III was used as evidence of invalid performance in college students completing psychoeducational evaluations for ADHD, learning disorder, or other problem. NIM had extremely low sensitivity at the recommended T-score cutoff of 73 (.16 sensitivity to suspected invalid performance, at .83 to .95 specificity, depending on the comparison group). MAL did not fare much better, but RDF showed slightly higher sensitivity, at .26, but at the price of unacceptably low specificities (Musso et al., 2016).

In another study involving prisoners where probable malingering was identified by clinical judgment of an intake psychiatrist, a NIM T-score of 77 or higher had good sensitivity and specificity (.58 and .97) in differentiating malingerers from controls, but very poor specificity in differentiating malingerers from genuinely disordered patients (specificity of .50). MAL and RDF had slightly better specificities, but not at a level that would be feasible for clinical practice as there was an unacceptable false positive rate for both scales in clinical patients (i.e., specificity of .73; Edens et al., 2007).

Criminal Defendants. In criminal defendants, there is some supportive evidence for the use of NIM when the SIRS, a well-validated semi-structured interview, is used as the criterion for malingering. For example, one study found that NIM but not MAL or RDF successfully differentiated between malingerers and nonmalingerers with acceptable sensitivity and specificity (Kucharski et al., 2007). At a T score of 92, NIM sensitivity was .71 and specificity was .89. Another study involving criminal defendants found that NIM outperformed MAL, but RDF failed to demonstrate better than chance prediction. However, at a T score of 92 or higher, NIM scores had good sensitivity to SIRS-defined malingering (.78) but less than optimal specificity (.84). The authors concluded that RDF should not be used in criminal forensic settings (Boccaccini et al., 2006).

TBI. Studies in TBI indicate that patients tend to have elevations on PAI clinical scales, but that these are more frequent in those who fail PVTs. Furthermore, although NIM does not seem to be elevated by genuine symptoms of brain injury, it is not a strong predictor of exaggeration in this group, possibly due to lack of adequate coverage of somatic and cognitive overreporting (Keiski et al., 2015).

For example, several studies involving TBI indicate that when individuals with invalid profiles are excluded, the most common PAI elevations are on the Somatic Complaints, Depression, and Schizophrenia scales, but not on NIM, indicating that NIM is not elevated by genuine brain dysfunction (Demakis et al., 2007; Kennedy et al., 2015; Till et al., 2009). Similarly, compensating-seeking individuals with mild TBI have higher NIM scores than non–compensation-seeking patients, along with elevations on PAI scales measuring somatic concerns, anxiety, and depression (Whiteside et al., 2012). However, NIM is only mildly elevated in compensation-seeking patients, with a mean T score of 63, well below the recommended cutoffs for overreporting and with only medium effect size in differentiating the groups. Mild TBI patients failing PVTs and SVTs have higher PAI clinical scale scores than those who pass (Lange et al., 2012); fully 70% of patients with invalid performance have at least five PAI clinical scale elevations.

In those who pass PVTs/SVTs, only 32% of mild and 17% of severe TBI patients have five or more PAI clinical scale elevations.

Pain Disorders. There is a need for more research on pain, including malingering of pain and response patterns in somatoform disorders. In one study involving chronic pain patients, mean scores on NIM, MAL, and RDF were all clearly below cutoffs for overreporting (T scores of 49 to 58), but all the Somatic Complaints subscales were elevated, above 70, particularly Somatization. College students instructed to feign pain obtained higher NIM and Somatic Complaints scores than the genuine pain patients, but NIM itself provided only modest incremental prediction over chance in identifying the simulators; similar results were reported for MAL and RDF (Hopwood et al., 2010). There are no studies to date on actual malingering pain patients, but there are studies supporting the use of the test in chronic pain patients (Karlin et al., 2005).

ADHD. The PAI appears to have limited efficacy in detecting malingering of ADHD-type symptoms. Specifically, in examinees with ADHD or learning disability, including suspected feigners, very few patients obtain elevated scores on any of the PAI validity indices, and none elevates NIM in particular, even though a substantial proportion has invalid WMT scores (Sullivan et al., 2007). Other studies have reported a lack of sensitivity of the NIM scale to exaggerated or malingered ADHD, with one study reporting good results with the RDF, albeit with ADHD simulators rather than verified ADHD malingerers (Smith, Cox, Mowle, & Edens, 2017). In a college sample seen for psychoeducational assessments and with external incentives (i.e., seeking ADHD medication or academic accommodations), NIM was higher in the nonincentive group, contrary to hypothesis, but with the RDF showing higher means in the incentive group (Pella et al., 2012). However, the proportion of examinees scoring beyond the NIM, RDF, and MAL cut scores was similar between incentive and no-incentive groups.

Attempts to derive new PAI scales that could identify individuals with ADHD have not yet produced satisfactory classification rates (Watson & Liljequist, 2015), although one set of new PAI validity measures appears promising based on good sensitivity and specificity using ADHD simulators and genuine ADHD (Aita et al., 2017).

Nonepileptic Seizures. The PAI has also been used to identify patients with nonepileptic seizures, a form of somatic symptom disorder, with some success using the Somatic Complaints scale, particularly its conversion subscale (Locke et al., 2011). Interestingly, these efforts have not typically included the overreporting validity scales such as NIM, MAL and RDF; this may be because these are not typically elevated in this population (e.g., Purdom et al., 2012).

COMMENT

As a comprehensive clinical tool, the PAI has several strengths. It includes a number of clinical scales that would be of particular use in certain settings, including substance abuse, aggression potential, suicide potential, and treatment resistance. It also has personality disorder scales, which are particularly useful in personality assessment and in assessing people in counseling or therapy settings. It is an inherently appealing and easy-to-use clinical tool when clinical diagnoses are needed because its clinical scales fit DSM nosology. However, as a tool for identifying overreporting, exaggeration, and invalid symptom reporting in high-stakes neuropsychological settings where malingering occurs, it requires more study. Although its validity scales have been evaluated in a variety of populations of interest to neuropsychologists, including veterans, military samples, disability claimants, and criminal defendants, compared to the MMPI-2 and MMPI-2-RF, its clinical research base is much more shallow in terms of validation as a tool suitable for detection of malingering and exaggeration.

One distinct advantage of the PAI is that it has well-described and comprehensive information on internal and test-retest reliability for its validity scales, including information on clinical and demographic variables such as ethnicity and educational level. Good reliability is an important characteristic of tests for malingering (Smith, 2008). However, reliability data are provided for NIM, but not MAL or RDF. The influence of demographic effects on the latter two are generally unknown, a distinct weakness when the test is to be used in diverse populations.

Of note, PAI items are scored according to a Likert scale rather than a dichotomous scale, as is the MMPI-2-RF. According to the author, PAI items may therefore capture more variability in the construct being measured and better assess reliability with fewer items as items capture aspects of both frequency and intensity (Morey, 2007). While this may be an asset in clinical evaluation, is not clear that this has translated into better detection of invalid responding.

The biggest weakness by far of the PAI validity indices is that they are simply not as effective as other SVTs at detecting malingering in neuropsychological populations. This is likely due to the fact that none of the scales were designed to identify the type of malingering most commonly found in these populations, namely, combined cognitive, somatic, and psychiatric overreporting. In addition, it is not altogether clear that the PAI overreporting indices are as effective as other SVTs in detecting malingering of psychiatric symptoms, most notably compared to the MMPI-2 and MMPI-2-RF validity scales. For example, although not reviewed here, research suggests that MMPI-2 validity scales outperform those of the PAI in identifying feigned psychopathology in neuropsychological groups, including feigned PTSD (Lange et al., 2010). In her review of the test, Boone found that PAI cutoffs derived from correctional settings had some value, although MAL in particular had very low sensitivity; she concluded that these cutoffs are probably not suitable for civil litigation settings, as these claimants typically do not malinger the severe psychopathology seen in correctional settings (Boone, 2012).

The test may be better at identifying who is not malingering versus who is (Kucharski et al., 2007; Sellbom & Bagby, 2008), but even this is not always clear, as specificity is less than optimal in several studies of the PAI. Some research indicates that the Somatic Complaints clinical scale may be more effective in identifying cognitive feigning than any of the actual PAI validity scales. The test would greatly benefit from derivation of new indices sensitive to neuropsychological malingering and from more research on neuropsychological groups. In the past, the MMPI-2 lagged behind the PAI in terms of known-groups studies, but this is clearly no longer the case (see the reviews of MMPI-2 and MMPI-2-RF elsewhere in this chapter). High-stakes assessment where malingering is a concern certainly requires using the most validated instruments available.

Most notably, compared to other SVTs that have been intensely and repeatedly scrutinized by experts in the field (see the MMPI-2-RF review earlier in this chapter and the FBS scale in particular), there is surprisingly little research on the PAI's MAL and RDF. These validity indices have simply not been examined with the same careful (or vehement) attention as have other SVTs in the field of neuropsychology. In particular, independent validation of components of the MAL index is needed, as is independent validation and replication of the discriminant function underlying the RDF.

From a technical and psychometric perspective, the PAI overreporting scales also fall short in terms of their development compared to other SVTs reviewed here. Specifically, NIM was not specifically created as a malingering index and has never been clearly validated as such. MAL and RDF were both developed based on simulators, not verified clinical malingerers, a method that will overestimate sensitivity to malingering. This has been borne out by research to date, which has produced disappointing sensitivities overall in clinical groups. In comparison, the MMPI-2 and MMPI-2-RF have scales and validation samples more geared toward neuropsychological malingering, including validation samples composed of verified clinical malingerers based on accepted multidimensional malingering criteria such as Slick et al. (1999) criteria and cutoffs validated with established malingering criteria and PVT failure.

The overlapping content of some of the PAI validity indices is also problematic. Guidelines for neuropsychologists recommend using more than one and ideally multiple independent SVTs to detect invalid responding. Using NIM and MAL as independent validity indicators will not work as NIM is a component of MAL, and the two scales are as a result highly correlated with each other. Similarly, MAL and RDF both include depression, treatment rejection, paranoia, and antisocial clinical scales as part of their criteria and therefore also have overlapping content. Of course, overlapping SVT content is not a problem specific to the PAI; most notably, shared items occur for the FBS and RBS scales of the MMPI-2/MMPI-2-RF. Generally speaking, combining multiple SVTs increases detection accuracy. There is, to our knowledge, no research using combined PAI indices, which could potentially increase effectiveness.

In the past, the PAI had advantages compared to the original MMPI: it had a lower reading level, shorter length, non-overlapping scales, and clinical scales more closely aligned with accepted frameworks for classifying psychopathology, such as the DSM. However, with the release of the MMPI-2 and MMPI-2-RF, these advantages are less clear. Both the MMPI-2 and MMPI-RF-2 now also have theoretically driven and non-overlapping clinical scales, and the PAI and MMPI-2-RF are roughly equivalent in terms of length. The reading-level advantage remains (i.e., Grade 4 for the PAI, vs. Grades 5 to 9 for the MMPI-2/MMPI-2-RF), in addition to the ease of use and intuitive nature of the PAI's clinical scales, which is no small point. Of note, PAI validity indicators have an extremely limited number of items compared to validity indicators from the MMPI-2 and MMPI-2-RF, many of which are long enough to comprise their own standalone scales. This may be one reason for the lower effectiveness of PAI validity scales compared to the MMPI-2-RF. For example, on the MMPI-2 and MMPI-2-RF, FBS and FBS-r have 43 and 30 items, respectively; RBS has 28 items, and HHI and HHI-r have 15 and 11 items, respectively. In comparison, the PAI's NIM has only 9 items, similar to the MMPI-2-RF Fs, which has 8 items, and which is one of the weaker MMPI-2-RF validity scales. The PAI MAL and RDF, although comprised of more elements than NIM, have not fared as well in validation research.

From a purely practical standpoint, fully understanding the PAI validity scales is not an easy undertaking; relevant information appears to be presented in at least five different sections of the 385-page manual. Ensuring clarity for users, in our opinion, is an important part of test validity. This too, unfortunately, is not a problem specific to the PAI: the MMPI-2 and MMPI-2-RF SVTs are even more complex, with relevant user information spread across several manuals and publications.

Overall, of the three PAI scales, NIM would be the preferred scale based on research on neuropsychological and non-neuropsychological samples. MAL is somewhat in between, and RDF is the least predictive of malingering and exaggeration. Nevertheless, a determination of invalid responding should not be based solely on a high NIM score, particularly since the majority of malingerers will be missed by the scale. Therefore, high-stakes assessment of neuropsychological populations requires using additional or alternate SVTs. Nevertheless, the PAI's positive features may make it an appealing choice for clinical settings with low base rates of malingering and where compensation seeking and secondary gain are not at stake. Notably, the PAI appears to be especially insensitive to exaggeration in ADHD, which may relate to the fact that the PAI lacks cognitive overreporting scales or that few SVTs including the PAI are geared towards detection of ADHD symptoms. PVTs fare much better in this regard (e.g., WMT, TOMM, NV-MSVT).

REFERENCES

Aikman, G. G., & Souheaver, G. T. (2008). Use of the Personality Assessment Inventory (PAI) in neuropsychological testing of psychiatric outpatients. *Applied Neuropsychology, 15*(3), 176–183. https://doi.org/10.1080/09084280802324283

Aita, S. L., Sofko, C. A., Hill, B. D., Musso, M. W., & Boettcher, A. C. (2017). Utility of the Personality Assessment Inventory in detecting feigned Attention-Deficit/Hyperactivity Disorder (ADHD): The Feigned Adult ADHD index. *Archives of Clinical Neuropsychology*, 1–13. https://doi.org/10.1093/arclin/acx113

Armistead-Jehle, P. (2010). Symptom validity test performance in US veterans referred for evaluation of mild TBI. *Applied Neuropsychology, 17*(1), 52–59. https://doi.org/10.1080/09084280903526182

Armistead-Jehle, P., Cooper, D. B., & Vanderploeg, R. D. (2016). The role of performance validity tests in the assessment of cognitive functioning after military concussion: A replication and extension. *Applied Neuropsychology. Adult, 23*(4), 264–273. https://doi.org/10.1080/23279095.2015.1055564

Bianchini, K. J., Greve, K. W., & Glynn, G. (2005). On the diagnosis of malingered pain-related disability: Lessons from cognitive malingering research. *Spine Journal, 5*(4), 404–417. https://doi.org/10.1016/j.spinee.2004.11.016

Blais, M. A., Baity, M. R., & Hopwood, C. J. (2010). *Clinical applications of the Personality Assessment Inventory*. New York : Routledge. Retrieved from https://trove.nla.gov.au/version/35626929

Boccaccini, M. T., Murrie, D. C., & Duncan, S. A. (2006). Screening for malingering in a criminal-forensic sample with the Personality Assessment Inventory. *Psychological Assessment, 18*(4), 415–423. https://doi.org/10.1037/1040-3590.18.4.415

Boone, K. B. (2012). *Clinical practice of forensic neuropsychology: An evidence-based approach*. New York: Guilford.

Braxton, L. E., Calhoun, P. S., Williams, J. E., & Boggs, C. D. (2007). Validity rates of the Personality Assessment Inventory and the Minnesota Multiphasic Personality Inventory-2 in a VA Medical Center setting. *Journal of Personality Assessment, 88*(1), 5–15. https://doi.org/10.1080/00223890709336829

Busse, M., Whiteside, D., Waters, D., Hellings, J., & Ji, P. (2014). Exploring the reliability and component structure of the Personality Assessment Inventory in a neuropsychological sample. *The Clinical Neuropsychologist, 28*(2), 237–251. https://doi.org/10.1080/13854046.2013.876100

Crighton, A. H., Tarescavage, A. M., Gervais, R. O., & Ben-Porath, Y. S. (2017). The generalizability of overreporting across self-report measures: An investigation with the Minnesota Multiphasic Personality Inventory-2-Restructured Form and the Personality Assessment Inventory in a civil disability sample. *Assessment, 24*(5), 555–574. https://doi.org/10.1177/1073191115621791

Demakis, G. J., Hammond, F., Knotts, A., Cooper, D. B., Clement, P., Kennedy, J., & Sawyer, T. (2007). The Personality Assessment Inventory in individuals with traumatic brain injury. *Archives of Clinical Neuropsychology, 22*(1), 123–130. https://doi.org/10.1016/j.acn.2006.09.004

Edens, J. F., Poythress, N. G., & Watkins-Clay, M. M. (2007). Detection of malingering in psychiatric unit and general population prison inmates: A comparison of the PAI, SIMS, and SIRS. *Journal of Personality Assessment, 88*(1), 33–42. https://doi.org/10.1080/00223890709336832

Fernandez, K., Boccaccini, M. T., & Noland, R. M. (2008). Detecting over- and underreporting of psychopathology with the Spanish-language Personality Assessment Inventory: Findings from a simulation study with bilingual speakers. *Psychological Assessment, 20*(2), 189–194. https://doi.org/10.1037/1040-3590.20.2.189

Forbey, J. D., Lee, T. T. C., Ben-Porath, Y. S., Arbisi, P. A., & Gartland, D. (2013). Associations between MMPI-2-RF validity scale scores and extra-test measures of personality and psychopathology. *Assessment, 20*(4), 448–461. https://doi.org/10.1177/1073191113478154

Gaasedelen, O. J., Whiteside, D. M., & Basso, M. (2017). Exploring the sensitivity of the Personality Assessment Inventory symptom validity tests in detecting response bias in a mixed neuropsychological outpatient sample. *The Clinical Neuropsychologist, 31*(5), 844–856. https://doi.org/10.1080/13854046.2017.1312700

Green, P. (2004). *Memory Complaints Inventory (MCI)*. Edmonton, AB: Green's Publishing.

Haggerty, K. A., Frazier, T. W., Busch, R. M., & Naugle, R. I. (2007). Relationships among Victoria Symptom Validity test indices and Personality Assessment Inventory validity scales in a large clinical sample. *The Clinical Neuropsychologist, 21*(6), 917–928. https://doi.org/10.1080/13854040600899724

Hopwood, C. J., Orlando, M. J., & Clark, T. S. (2010). The detection of malingered pain-related disability with the Personality Assessment Inventory. *Rehabilitation Psychology, 55*(3), 307–310. https://doi.org/10.1037/a0020516

Karlin, B. E., Creech, S. K., Grimes, J. S., Clark, T. S., Meagher, M. W., & Morey, L. C. (2005). The Personality Assessment Inventory with chronic pain patients: Psychometric properties and clinical utility. Journal of Clinical Psychology, 61(12), 1571–1585. https://doi.org/10.1002/jclp.20209

Keiski, M. A., Shore, D. L., Hamilton, J. M., & Malec, J. F. (2015). Simulation of traumatic brain injury symptoms on the Personality Assessment Inventory: An analogue study. *Assessment, 22*(2), 233–247. https://doi.org/10.1177/1073191114539380

Kennedy, J. E., Cooper, D. B., Reid, M. W., Tate, D. F., & Lange, R. T. (2015). Profile analyses of the Personality Assessment Inventory following military-related traumatic brain injury. *Archives of Clinical Neuropsychology, 30*(3), 236–247. https://doi.org/10.1093/arclin/acv014

Kucharski, L. T., Toomey, J. P., Fila, K., & Duncan, S. (2007). Detection of malingering of psychiatric disorder with the Personality Assessment Inventory: An investigation of criminal defendants. *Journal of Personality Assessment, 88*(1), 25–32. https://doi.org/10.1080/00223890709336831

LaDuke, C., Barr, W., Brodale, D. L., & Rabin, L. A. (2017). Toward generally accepted forensic assessment practices among clinical neuropsychologists: A survey of professional practice and common test use. *The Clinical Neuropsychologist*, 1–20. https://doi.org/10.1080/13854046.2017.1346711

Lange, R. T., Pancholi, S., Bhagwat, A., Anderson-Barnes, V., & French, L. M. (2012). Influence of poor effort on neuropsychological test performance in US military personnel following mild traumatic brain injury. *Journal of Clinical and Experimental Neuropsychology, 34*(5), 453–466. https://doi.org/10.1080/13803395.2011.648175

Lange, R. T., Sullivan, K. A., & Scott, C. (2010). Comparison of MMPI-2 and PAI validity indicators to detect feigned depression and PTSD symptom reporting. *Psychiatry Research, 176*(2–3), 229–235. https://doi.org/10.1016/j.psychres.2009.03.004

Locke, D. E. C., Kirlin, K. A., Wershba, R., Osborne, D., Drazkowski, J. F., Sirven, J. I., & Noe, K. H. (2011). Randomized comparison of the Personality Assessment Inventory and the Minnesota Multiphasic Personality Inventory-2 in the epilepsy monitoring unit. *Epilepsy & Behavior: E&B*, 21(4), 397–401. https://doi.org/10.1016/j.yebeh.2011.05.023

Martin, P. K., Schroeder, R. W., & Odland, A. P. (2015). Neuropsychologists' validity testing beliefs and practices: A survey of North American professionals. *The Clinical Neuropsychologist, 29*(6), 741–776. https://doi.org/10.1080/13854046.2015.1087597

Matlasz, T. M., Brylski, J. L., Leidenfrost, C. M., Scalco, M., Sinclair, S. J., Schoelerman, R. M., . . . Antonius, D. (2017). Cognitive status and profile validity on the Personality Assessment Inventory (PAI) in offenders with serious mental illness. *International Journal of Law and Psychiatry, 50,* 38–44. https://doi.org/10.1016/j.ijlp.2016.10.003

Morey, L. C. (2003). *Essentials of PAI assessment.* Hoboken, NJ: Wiley.

Morey, L. C. (2007). *Personality Assessment Inventory.* Lutz, FL: Psychological Assessment Resources.

Morey, L. C. (1997). *Personality Assessment Screener.* Lutz, FL: Psychological Assessment Resources.

Musso, M. W., Hill, B. D., Barker, A. A., Pella, R. D., & Gouvier, W. D. (2016). Utility of the Personality Assessment Inventory for detecting malingered ADHD in college students. *Journal of Attention Disorders, 20*(9), 763–774. https://doi.org/10.1177/1087054714548031

Pella, R. D., Hill, B. D., Shelton, J. T., Elliott, E., & Gouvier, W. D. (2012). Evaluation of embedded malingering indices in a non-litigating clinical sample using control, clinical, and derived groups. *Archives of Clinical Neuropsychology, 27*(1), 45–57. https://doi.org/10.1093/arclin/acr090

Purdom, C. L., Kirlin, K. A., Hoerth, M. T., Noe, K. H., Drazkowski, J. F., Sirven, J. I., & Locke, D. E. C. (2012). The influence of Impression Management Scales on the Personality Assessment Inventory in the epilepsy monitoring unit. *Epilepsy & Behavior: E&B, 25*(4), 534–538. https://doi.org/10.1016/j.yebeh.2012.10.005

Rabin, L. A., Paolillo, E., & Barr, W. B. (2016). Stability in test-usage practices of clinical neuropsychologists in the United States and Canada over a 10-year period: A follow-up survey of INS and NAN members. *Archives of Clinical Neuropsychology, 31*(3), 206–230. https://doi.org/10.1093/arclin/acw007

Rogers, R., Sewell, K. W., Morey, L. C., & Ustad, K. L. (1996). Detection of feigned mental disorders on the Personality Assessment Inventory: a discriminant analysis. *Journal of Personality Assessment, 67*(3), 629–640. https://doi.org/10.1207/s15327752jpa6703_15

Sellbom, M., & Bagby, R. M. (2008). Response styles on multiscale inventories. In R. Rogers (Ed.), *Clinical assessment of malingering and deception* (3rd ed., pp. 182–206). New York: Guilford.

Sinclair, S. J., Walsh-Messinger, J., Siefert, C. J., Antonius, D., Baity, M. R., Haggerty, G., . . . Blais, M. A. (2015). Neuropsychological functioning and profile validity on the Personality Assessment Inventory (PAI): An investigation in multiple psychiatric settings. *Bulletin of the Menninger Clinic, 79*(4), 305–334. https://doi.org/10.1521/bumc.2015.79.4.305

Slick, D. J., Sherman, E. M., & Iverson, G. L. (1999). Diagnostic criteria for malingered neurocognitive dysfunction: Proposed standards for clinical practice and research. *The Clinical Neuropsychologist, 13*(4), 545–561. https://doi.org/10.1076/1385-4046(199911)13:04;1-Y;FT545

Smith, G. P. (2008). Brief screening measures for the detection of feigned psychopathology. In R. Rogers (Ed.), *Clinical assessment of malingering and deception* (3rd ed., pp. 323–342). New York: Guilford.

Smith, S. T., Cox, J., Mowle, E. N., & Edens, J. F. (2017). Intentional inattention: Detecting feigned attention-deficit/hyperactivity disorder on the Personality Assessment Inventory. *Psychological Assessment, 29*(12), 1447–1457. https://doi.org/10.1037/pas0000435

Sullivan, B. K., May, K., & Galbally, L. (2007). Symptom exaggeration by college adults in attention-deficit hyperactivity disorder and learning disorder assessments. *Applied Neuropsychology, 14*(3), 189–207. https://doi.org/10.1080/09084280701509083

Sumanti, M., Boone, K. B., Savodnik, I., & Gorsuch, R. (2006). Noncredible psychiatric and cognitive symptoms in a workers' compensation "stress" claim sample. *The Clinical Neuropsychologist, 20*(4), 754–765. https://doi.org/10.1080/13854040500428467

Till, C., Christensen, B. K., & Green, R. E. (2009). Use of the Personality Assessment Inventory (PAI) in individuals with traumatic brain injury. *Brain Injury, 23*(7), 655–665. https://doi.org/10.1080/02699050902970794

Watson, J., & Liljequist, L. (2015). Using the Personality Assessment Inventory to identify ADHD-like symptoms. *Journal of Attention Disorders.* https://doi.org/10.1177/1087054714567133

Whiteside, D., Clinton, C., Diamonti, C., Stroemel, J., White, C., Zimberoff, A., & Waters, D. (2010). Relationship between suboptimal cognitive effort and the clinical scales of the Personality Assessment Inventory. *The Clinical Neuropsychologist, 24*(2), 315–325. https://doi.org/10.1080/13854040903482822

Whiteside, D. M., Dunbar-Mayer, P., & Waters, D. P. (2009). Relationship between TOMM performance and PAI validity scales in a mixed clinical sample. *The Clinical Neuropsychologist, 23*(3), 523–533. https://doi.org/10.1080/13854040802389169

Whiteside, D. M., Galbreath, J., Brown, M., & Turnbull, J. (2012). Differential response patterns on the Personality Assessment Inventory (PAI) in compensation-seeking and non-compensation-seeking mild traumatic brain injury patients. *Journal of Clinical and Experimental Neuropsychology, 34*(2), 172–182. https://doi.org/10.1080/13803395.2011.630648

STRUCTURED INVENTORY OF MALINGERED SYMPTOMATOLOGY (SIMS)

TEST NAME	**Structured Inventory of Malingered Symptomatology (SIMS)**
DOMAIN	Symptom validity
AGE RANGE	18+ years
ADMINISTRATION TIME	10 minutes
SCORING FORMAT	Online scoring available, but can be hand scored
REFERENCE	Widows, M. R., & Smith, G. P. (2005). Structured Inventory of Malingered Symptomatology (SIMS). Lutz, FL: Psychological Assessment Resources, Inc. www.parinc.ca

DESCRIPTION

The Structured Inventory of Malingered Symptomatology (SIMS; Widows & Smith, 2005) is a self-report SVT designed to detect malingering. It is aimed at the detection of malingered psychiatric disorders but also malingered cognitive and neurological disorders. Specifically, three of five subscales cover amnestic symptoms, neurological symptoms, and intellectual deficits, of particular relevance to neuropsychologists. The test can therefore be used to assess the validity of neurocognitive symptoms, ideally in conjunction with individually administered PVTs, although the test is designed to stand on its own. Because of the range of items covering cognitive, neurological, and psychiatric symptoms, the SIMS is designed to be suitable for a variety of types of evaluations, including those conducted in medico-legal, disability, criminal, correctional, and clinical settings.

The SIMS contains five 15-item scales: Amnestic Disorders, Low Intelligence, Neurologic Impairment, Affective Disorders, and Psychosis (Table 16–33). These scales contain items reflecting unusual, bizarre, or illogical symptoms that would not usually be present in genuine psychiatric conditions, that represent an unsophisticated knowledge of clinical conditions, or that would not be endorsed by the vast majority of examinees. It also includes some items reflecting symptoms of genuine disorders, but which would be of low frequency or atypical (i.e., Affective Disorders scale).

According to the test authors, the SIMS was designed for screening, not diagnosis. As such, a determination of malingering should not be based exclusively on SIMS results. Instead, positive identification by the SIMS should raise strong suspicion of malingering that can then be further evaluated based on a more comprehensive evaluation with multiple sources of data to confirm the classification. The SIMS can, however, provide information on the specific nature of overreporting (i.e., cognitive, psychiatric, or neurological) through analysis of scale score elevations.

The test is available in other languages. Several publications have employed the Dutch version (e.g., Merckelbach & Smith, 2003). The SIMS is also available in Spanish (www.par.inc) and in German (Cima et al., 2003).

ADMINISTRATION

Administration instructions are printed on the record form and further detailed in the manual; the scale can also be administered online via computer. A fifth-grade reading level is required. The manual notes that examinees with significant cognitive incapacity or with gross psychosis, agitation, or incoherence should not be administered the SIMS.

SCORING

The scale contains both negative and positive items, the latter reverse scored. Scoring is very straightforward and typically takes about 10 minutes, less if scored via computer.

The manual recommends a Total score cutoff of 14 to identify examinees reporting an unusually high number of

TABLE 16–33 Structured Inventory of Malingered Symptomatology (SIMS) Total and Subscale Descriptions

SCALE	DESCRIPTION
Amnestic Disorders	Memory symptoms incompatible with bona fide memory disorders
Neurologic Impairment	Illogical or atypical neurological symptoms
Low Intelligence	Logic questions correctly answered by the vast majority of examinees
Affective Disorders	Atypical depression or anxiety symptoms
Psychosis	Bizarre or unusual symptoms not usually found in bona fide psychosis
Total Score	Overall estimate of the likelihood of feigning of psychiatric or cognitive symptoms

SOURCE: Adapted from Widows and Smith (2005). Reproduced by special permission of the Publisher, Psychological Assessment Resources, Inc. (PAR), 16204 North Florida Avenue, Lutz, Florida 33549, from the Structured Inventory of Malingered Symptomatology by Glenn P. Smith, PhD, Copyright 1993, 1997, 2005 by PAR. Further reproduction is prohibited without permission of PAR.

symptoms that would be atypical in patients with genuine psychiatric or cognitive disorders. This cutoff was derived from analog malingerer data (i.e., people simulating malingering), not from actual clinical malingerers. The authors acknowledge that although other sources recommend higher cutoffs, a cut score of 14 increases the probability that all potential malingerers are identified; these can then be further assessed or referred for more extensive evaluation. The recommended cutoff thereby reduces false negatives. However, what this means, of course, is that more genuinely responding examinees will be identified as malingerers by the test (i.e., thereby increasing false positives). The approach of maximizing false negatives over false positives is consistent with the use of the test as a screener. However, higher minimum cutoffs seem more appropriate, given the literature, and because of the high personal costs for examinees to be erroneously identified as not providing credible responses. For example, cutoffs with better specificity (i.e., a lower false-positive rate) include >19 and >24 in groups with severe psychiatric or neurological comorbidity (see the section "Clinical Studies" for further discussion).

Van Impelen, Merckelbach, Jelicic, and Merten (2014) provide what are essentially metanorms on the SIMS. Their large, comprehensive meta-analysis of the SIMS includes more than 30 studies, 3,000 participants, and 4,000 SIMS protocols, covering nonclinical samples, honestly responding patient groups, claimants, and criminal defendants. These data indicate that a Total score cutoff of greater than 14 is too low for most clinical purposes and that a score greater than 16 or 20 seems more diagnostically accurate to identify noncredible responding across a variety of clinical settings. Van Impelen et al. (2014) note that a high score does not necessarily indicate malingering per se; it simply points to an invalid profile. They note that it is important to rule out other explanations that may also explain high scores (i.e., frustration, defiance, fatigue, incomprehension).

Subscale cutoffs are detailed in the manual, which notes that these demonstrate utility for identifying specific types of exaggeration. Subscale cutoffs have been less extensively validated than the Total cutoff. However, van Impelen et al. (2014), in their comprehensive meta-analysis, conclude that the Amnestic Disorders, Neurological Impairment, and Affective Disorders subscales show high sensitivity in their respective clinical subgroups, but that the Low Intelligence subscale seems relatively insensitive to noncredible intellectual deficits.

Rogers, Robinson, and Gillard (2014) developed alternative scales for the SIMS based on rare symptoms (RS) and symptom combinations (SC), both of which were developed with empirical means by examinations of base rates of symptom endorsement and item correlations in inpatients with genuine disorders asked to feign greater disabilities (see Table 16–34 for derivation, and Table 16–35 for diagnostic accuracy statistics at different base rates). The SC scale demonstrates large effect size (Cohen's $d = 2.0$) and appears most effective at ruling out examinees with a high likelihood of genuine disorders compared to standard SIMS subscales. Although these data are compelling, more research on these new scores is needed.

TABLE 16–34 Items for Additional Detection-Based Scales for the Structured Inventory of Malingered Symptomatology (SIMS)

SCALE	ITEMS
Rare Symptoms (RS)	3, 8, 14, 21, 28, 34, 40, 42, 56, 58, 63, 67, 69, 73, 75
Symptom Combinations (SC)	4–74, 5–60, 20–24, 25–61, 25–64, 27–61, 35–60, 47–59, 47–74, 48–65, 52–66, 56–67, 56–75

SOURCE: Adapted from Rogers et al. (2014).

NORMATIVE DATA

SIMS cutoffs were derived in an analog simulation study at four universities and community colleges (476 undergraduate volunteers, 71% female, 90% Caucasian, mean age = 24.4). The sample was divided into an initial validation sample and a cross-validation sample, each of which was divided into either an honest responder group or one of six experimental conditions spanning simulated psychosis, amnesia, depression, low intelligence, neurological impairment, and "faking bad." Cutoff scores were developed for each scale to optimally detect the most analog malingerers while minimizing misidentification of honest responders. From these and related analyses, the Total score was identified as the best score, with an efficiency rating of 95%.

Van Impelen et al. (2014) provide meta-data on weighted means and confidence intervals for a variety of groups, including nonclinical controls, honest patients, honest claimants, and honest defendants, as well as scores for noncredible claimants and clinical defendants, who obtain the highest means by far than any other group on the SIMS (Table 16–36). These means can be used as a benchmark when evaluating examinee scores on the SIMS. They also clearly demonstrate the incremental increase in SIMS scores as one moves from groups with low probability of exaggeration (e.g., controls, honest patients) to those with high probability (feigning claimants, criminal defendants). However, these means also demonstrate that adhering to the published cutoff of >14 would be inadequate, as the raw score distribution of honestly responding examinees overlaps and in some cases exceeds this cutoff (Table 16–37). Overall, the SIMS does tap genuine symptomatology, and so higher cutoffs are needed in clinical groups for the test to be effective without erroneously capturing honest responders.

TABLE 16–35 Effectiveness of Rare Symptoms (RS) and Symptom Combination (SC) Scales at Ruling in Suspected Feigning on the Structured Inventory of Malingered Symptomatology (SIMS)

				BASE RATE = 15%		BASE RATE = 25%	
SCALE	CUTOFF	SENSITIVITY (%)	SPECIFICITY (%)	PPV (%)	NPV (%)	PPV (%)	NPV (%)
Rare Symptoms (RS)	RS > 6	42	98	79	91	88	84
Symptom Combinations (SC)	SC > 6	67	98	85	94	92	90

SOURCE: Adapted from Rogers et al. (2014).

DEMOGRAPHIC EFFECTS

AGE

Although not extensively studied, age does not appear to majorly affect scores. For example, age was uncorrelated to SIMS scores in a Dutch study of psychiatric examinees (Dandachi-FitzGerald et al., 2011).

GENDER

Van Impelen et al. (2014) report no gender effects in their comprehensive meta-analysis.

EDUCATION AND IQ

Education is inversely correlated with SIMS scores in clinical samples. IQ effects are modest in nonclinical controls (van Impelen et al., 2014), but clinical samples with lower IQ are more likely to fail the test (Dandachi-FitzGerald et al., 2011). Possible reasons for this may include more blatant exaggeration in low-IQ individuals, difficulty understanding SIMS items in low-IQ persons, or a higher likelihood of detection of the true purpose of the SIMS in high-IQ individuals (Dandachi-FitzGerald et al., 2011).

ETHNICITY, NATIONALITY, AND LINGUISTIC EFFECTS

Compared to some PVTs and SVTs, the SIMS has been used in a fair degree of research involving ethnically diverse groups. For example, van Impelen et al. (2014) note that nonclinical Dutch examinees obtain lower SIMS scores than English, Spanish, and German examinees (Table 16–36). The test has also been used in a Dutch study of asylum seekers from the Middle East, Russia, and Africa, where there are high incentives for showing elevated psychiatric symptoms in order to stay in the host country for medical reasons (van der Heide & Merckelbach, 2016). In this study, high scores were more associated with incentives than with low Dutch language proficiency. The SIMS has also been used effectively in forensic samples with high representation of African Americans (e.g., Vitacco et al., 2007).

EVIDENCE FOR RELIABILITY

EVIDENCE FOR INTERNAL RELIABILITY

Internal reliabilities are high, ranging from .82 for the Psychosis scale to .88 for the Total score (manual). Additional studies show excellent reliabilities for the Total score in criminal defendants and asylum seekers of diverse ethnic backgrounds (.91 to .96; van der Heide & Merckelbach, 2016; Vitacco et al., 2007); subscale reliabilities tend to be somewhat lower but generally acceptable. Of note, lower Total internal reliability has been reported in a study of undergraduate honest responders (.72) but with subscale scores much below acceptable standards, ranging from .24 to .59 (Merckelbach & Smith, 2003).

EVIDENCE FOR TEST-RETEST RELIABILITY, MEASURING CHANGE, AND PRACTICE EFFECTS

Test-retest reliability based on a small number of honest undergraduate responders re-evaluated after three weeks indicates adequate stability over time for the Total score and no changes in Total score means ($r = .72$; manual). As well, three-week test-retest reliability was extremely high in a small group of undergraduates tested with the German version (Cima et al., 2003). High test-retest correlations have also been reported in mixed-ethnicity asylum seekers tested over several weeks, albeit with a very small sample ($N = 9, r = .91$; van der Heide & Merckelbach, 2016).

EVIDENCE FOR VALIDITY

CONTENT-RELATED VALIDITY

SIMS items were selected based on a review of the literature and of existing SVTs to find items to distinguish between five types of malingering, namely, malingering of psychosis, low intelligence, affective disturbance, neurological impairment, and amnesia. Scale items were selected based on expert agreement and interrater reliability (manual).

FACTOR-ANALYTIC STUDIES

A factor analysis of the initial development sample data ($N = 238$) yielded a four-factor solution supportive of four of the five SIMS scales except for the Neurologic Impairment scale, which instead loaded primarily with the Psychosis scale. Nevertheless, the Neurologic Impairment scale was retained due to good expert agreement ratings on the scale (manual).

TABLE 16–36 Weighted Structured Inventory of Malingered Symptomatology (SIMS) Means, Standard Deviations (SDs), and 95% Confidence Intervals for Various Diagnostic Groups Based on Over 4,000 SIMS Protocols

SCALE	*N*	WEIGHTED MEAN SIMS RAW SCORE	WEIGHTED SD	95% CONFIDENCE INTERVAL OF WEIGHTED MEAN
Nonclinical controls (Dutch)	688	4.7	3.4	3.5–5.9
Nonclinical controls (English, German, Spanish)	648	7.6	4.1	5.9–9.2
Honest criminal defendants	141	13.2	8.4	10.9–15.5
Honest claimants	563	13.5	6.3	11.9–15.1
Honest patients	742	16.1	8.8	13.4–18.9
Feigning claimants	238	23.7	8.7	20.4–27.0
Feigning criminal defendants	102	38.2	14.6	33.6–42.8

NOTE: For honestly-responding groups, honesty was assumed but not always confirmed by validity testing.

SOURCE: Adapted from van Impelen et al. (2014) based on an overall *N* of 4,810 SIMS protocols; see original reference for further details.

CORRELATIONS AND COMPARISONS TO OTHER SVTS AND PVTS

With regard to other SVTs, correlations with the SIRS, a gold standard criterion measure for feigned mental disorders, are high in veterans with PTSD and in prisoners in mental health units (r = .54 to .81; Edens et al., 2007; Freeman et al., 2008). There is a significant degree of shared variance between the two instruments (e.g., 29 to 66%; reviewed in van Impelen et al., 2014).

Correlations with the PAI validity scales such as the Rogers Discriminant Function (RDF), Malingering Index (MAL), and Negative Impression Management (NIM) are moderate to very high in prison inmates (r = .45, .68, and .84, respectively, Edens et al., 2007). This is despite their differing item content, with the PAI not geared toward detecting cognitive malingering. Nevertheless, the SIMS was superior in the detection of simulators and suspected malingerers within this population (.90 and .85 sensitivity versus .76 and .58 sensitivity for the PAI, respectively). However, neither measure reached optimal specificity among patients with genuine disorders (.40 and .50, respectively), a level inadequate for clinical use due to excessive false-positive errors.

With regard to PVTs, the SIMS is as sensitive as the TOMM at detecting coached feigning of cognitive problems (.87 and .86 sensitivity, respectively; Jelicic et al., 2011). However, it was more sensitive than the WMT in detecting feigned whiplash (Merten et al., 2008, as cited in van Impelen et al., 2014).

In compensation claimants, correlations with the WMT are moderate (rs = –.44 to –.49), but with more shared variance between SIMS and WMT (19 to 24%) than between SIMS and other PVTs, as summarized by van Impelen et al. (2014).

The SIMS demonstrated modest correlations with the Amsterdam Short-Term Memory (ASTM), a forced-choice PVT, in a clinical sample referred for neuropsychological assessment in which a third had a diagnosis of ADHD (r = –.22; Dandachi-FitzGerald et al., 2011). SIMS failure rate was 21%, a detection rate equivalent to that of the ASTM (Dandachi-FitzGerald et al., 2011).

CORRELATIONS WITH OTHER NEUROPSYCHOLOGICAL TESTS

Failing the SIMS appears to be more related to elevated psychiatric symptoms on scales such as the SCL-90 than with performance on neuropsychological tests, including the Rey Auditory Verbal Learning Test (RAVLT), Stroop, and concept-shifting tasks, in contrast to forced-choice PVT failure which is more associated with memory performance (Dandachi-FitzGerald et al., 2011). Overall, there are comparatively few studies of the relationship between the SIMS and neuropsychological performance.

TABLE 16–37 Diagnostic Accuracy for Structured Inventory of Malingered Symptomatology (SIMS) Cutoff of >16 for Different Groups, with Base Rates Based on 31 Studies (*N* >3,000)

					BASE RATE = 10%		BASE RATE = 30%		BASE RATE = 50%	
SCALE	*N*	CUTOFF	SENSITIVITY (%)	SPECIFICITY (%)	PPV (%)	NPV (%)	PPV (%)	NPV (%)	PPV (%)	NPV (%)
Nonclinical adults	1,487	>16	92	99	91	99	98	97	99	93
Honest patients	377	>16	–	59	20	99	49	95	69	88
Claimants	730	>16	91	70	25	99	57	95	75	89
Criminal defendants	108	>16	100	67	25	100	56	100	75	100

NOTE: Based on an overall *N* of 3,652; honest patients' honesty assumed but not confirmed by validity testing. See original reference for values for cutoff of >14. PPV, positive predictive value; NPV, negative predictive value.

SOURCE: Adapted from van Impelen et al. (2014).

CORRELATIONS WITH OTHER SCALES AND QUESTIONNAIRES

Correlations between the SIMS and measures of depression and anxiety are moderate to high (r = .39 to .71), indicating that the SIMS is sensitive to psychopathology as measured by scales such as the SCL-90 and PAI (Dandachi-FitzGerald et al., 2011; Edens et al., 2007; Merckelbach & Smith, 2003). SIMS scores are also related to higher levels of childhood trauma (r = –.41; Geraerts et al., 2006).

CLINICAL STUDIES

Overall, there is an impressive body of literature supporting the clinical validity of the SIMS in a variety of clinical populations and settings, including validation of SIMS cutoffs for the detection of malingering. For example, Van Impelen and colleagues (van Impelen et al., 2014) reviewed 10 studies of known groups (i.e., compensation claimants, criminal defendants, prisoners) and concluded that the SIMS was fairly effective at discriminating between noncredible and honestly responding groups, with large effect sizes (Cohen's d = 1.0–3.0). However, although the sensitivity of recommended cutoffs was adequate (.75 to 1.00 for cutoffs of >14 or >16), specificities varied widely (.37 to .93), and were at times alarmingly low. Notably, the criterion measure in the majority of studies was the SIRS (Table 16–37).

Using the Slick, Sherman, and Iverson (1999) criteria for malingered neurocognitive dysfunction and the Bianchini, Greve, and Glynn (2005) criteria for malingered pain-related disability to identify verified malingerers, Wisdom, Callahan, and Shaw (2010) reported large effect sizes for the SIMS using a variety of SIMS cutoffs in patients referred for assessment of brain injury or trauma for personal injury or disability reasons (Table 16–38). Only a very high cutoff (>24) provided optimal specificity, thereby ensuring no false positives, but at a cost of reduced sensitivity. A cutoff of >21 had a specificity of .73 (i.e., incorrectly identifying almost a quarter of honest examinees as noncredible); the standard cutoff of >14 had a specificity of only .64, causing even more nonmalingerers to be falsely identified as noncredible. A cutoff of >24 identified all genuinely responding examinees as credible while maintaining good sensitivity to verified malingerers (sensitivity and specificity of .55 and 1.00, respectively). Notably, this study had a very high base rate of malingering (67%), making it unlikely that similar effectiveness would be obtained in settings with lower malingering base rates. Vossler-Thies et al. (2013, as cited in van Impelen et al., 2014) also reported large effect sizes for detection of malingering as defined by the Slick et al. (1999) criteria using a SIMS cutoff of >16 in a sample of claimants, but accuracy statistics were not reported.

TABLE 16–38 Cutoffs, Diagnostic Accuracy, and Effect Sizes of the Structured Inventory of Malingered Symptomatology (SIMS) at Detecting Malingering Based on Established Malingering Criteria by Slick et al. (1999) and Bianchini et al. (2005)

CUTOFF	SENSITIVITY (%)	SPECIFICITY (%)
>14	96	64
>21	68	73
>24	55	100

NOTE: Personal injury and disability sample with base rate of malingering of 67%. Malingering defined based on Slick et al. (1999) and Bianchini et al. (2005).

SOURCE: Adapted from Wisdom et al. (2010).

In their detailed meta-analysis (Table 16–37), van Impelen et al. (2014) concluded that the SIMS is able to differentiate between experimental feigners and honest responders, with effect sizes between 0.5 and 4.7 depending on the type of group. Specifically, nonclinical controls had much lower scores than honestly responding patient groups. This means that SIMS scores increase in the presence of genuine symptoms. Although they concluded that a cutoff of >16 is acceptable in nonclinical controls (i.e., specificity of .88 to 1.00), in honest patients with genuine symptomatology, this is largely unacceptable due to high false-positive errors (i.e., specificity of .23 to .83). Sensitivity values are, however, more consistent and more optimal across studies (.87 to 1.00; Table 16–37).

Litigants and Disability Claimants. SIMS scores are higher in litigants than in nonlitigating examinees, and scores above the cutoff occur more frequently in litigating examinees with psychogenic symptoms or crime-related amnesia, demonstrating the SIMS's sensitivity to differential prevalence of malingering in different groups (van Impelen et al., 2014). More research in litigants and in disability claimants is needed.

Criminal Defendants. Although not extensively studied in criminal and correctional settings, research indicates that the standard cutoff from the manual is too low, identifying too many genuinely responding examinees in criminal forensic settings as noncredible. For example, in criminal defendants undergoing mandatory competency to stand trial evaluations for violent crimes and using the SIRS to define malingering, although sensitivity was perfect using the recommended cutoff of >14 (i.e., all malingerers correctly identified), this came at a cost of unacceptably high false-positive rate; 35% of nonmalingering examinees were erroneously identified as noncredible (Vitacco et al., 2007). SIMS subscales were similarly inadequate in terms of their specificity using the cutoffs provided in the manual. In comparison, the Miller Forensic Assessment of Symptoms Test (M-FAST), a scale for identifying overreporting of psychopathology, was much more effective in this group.

Similar results were reported in prison inmates from a mental health unit. Specifically, the SIMS was able to detect suspected malingerers identified as such by psychiatrists

(.85 sensitivity) but at the cost of severely inadequate specificity (.40), thereby causing an unacceptable number of false-positive errors (i.e., too many nonmalingering examinees scoring above the cutoff of >14; Edens et al., 2007). The scale did well when used in nonclinical, general population examinees, but this is not a group in which it would typically be used. Alternatively, the authors noted that its high sensitivity might be useful for screening in all potential malingerers, who could then be subjected to a second, more rigorous and comprehensive set of assessment procedures to assess malingering, consistent with the purpose of the test. In most clinical settings where neuropsychologists operate, this would be a burdensome and atypical way to use the test.

TBI. There is little research on the use of the SIMS in this group. One study on postconcussive disorders and PTSD found that the Amnestic Disorders subscale was the best at differentiating between these two feigning groups (Parks et al., 2016).

Psychiatric Patients. Van Impelen compiled the data on psychiatric studies and found that the diagnostic accuracy of the SIMS may be suboptimal in schizophrenia (van Impelen et al., 2014). SIMS scores are elevated in patients with sexual pathologies and antisocial personality traits in forensic patients (Cima et al., 2003).

Low IQ. The SIMS includes a subscale specifically designed to detected malingered intellectual deficit, but, to our knowledge, the test has not been used much in genuinely responding and malingering low-IQ groups. However, there is some evidence that the SIMS has lower specificity in low-IQ individuals than in other clinical groups (Graue et al., 2007); that is, it identifies too many genuinely responding low-IQ examinees as being noncredible.

ADHD. There are very few studies of the test in this group, likely because people with ADHD tend not to exaggerate psychiatric or neurological symptoms; as well, as of this writing, SVTs have not been as effective in the detection of malingered ADHD as have PVTs. Nevertheless, the SIMS failure rate was 21% in a clinical sample referred for neuropsychological assessment where the most common diagnosis was ADHD, a detection rate equivalent to that of the ASTM, a forced-choice PVT (Dandachi-FitzGerald et al., 2011), demonstrating the potential usefulness of the scale in this group.

Chronic Pain and Somatic Conditions. More research in this group is needed. A SIMS failure rate of 23% has been reported in patients with medically unexplained neurological symptoms (van Beilen et al., 2009), but with nonpsychogenic neurological patients showing higher failure rates than healthy controls.

Psychogenic Nonepileptic Seizures. Although there exist few studies, the scale appears to have utility in this clinical group. In one study, patients with epilepsy from a Veterans' Affairs medical center had a mean score of 14, compared to a mean score of 22 for patients with psychogenic nonepileptic events (Benge et al., 2012). In this sample, the Neurologic Impairment and Affective Disorders subscales were best at predicting individuals with psychogenic nonepileptic seizures. To attain a specificity of .90 or higher (i.e., an optimal level recommended to minimize false positives), a Total score of 23 or above was required, yielding a sensitivity of .39. Scores of 6 or more on the Neurological scale and 8 or more on the Affective scale also had optimal specificity of .90 or above, with sensitivities of .40 and .26, respectively. To maintain acceptable prediction without increasing false positives, cutoffs were much higher than those in the manual, which may have been in part related to the nature of the sample (military, exposed to trauma, psychiatric comorbidity). Overall, high SIMS scores increased confidence in identifying nonepileptic seizures in patients with high comorbidity (Benge et al., 2012), albeit at higher cutoffs than those in the manual, consistent with other studies in different clinical groups.

Resistance to Coaching. The SIMS appears generally resistant to coaching about cognitive disorders, including examinees provided with information about brain injury and instructed not to overexaggerate symptoms, retaining high sensitivity to feigning (90%), a level superior to PVTs such as the ASTM (Jelicic et al., 2011). Compared to the TOMM, the SIMS appears equally resistant to coaching (Jelicic et al., 2011).

In a study on feigned whiplash, SIMS sensitivity dropped after forewarning participants, but WMT sensitivity was unaffected by forewarning. Although both measures were identified as such by the majority of participants, more participants identified the SIMS as an SVT than identified the WMT as a PVT (69% vs. 56%, Merten et al., 2008, as cited in van Impelen et al., 2014). However, another study on PTSD found much lower rates of examinees correctly identifying the SIMS and WMT as SVTs/PVTs (i.e., 28% vs. 16%; Merten et al., 2010, as cited in van Impelen et al., 2014).

NEUROANATOMICAL CORRELATES AND IMAGING STUDIES

Not available.

COMMENT

The SIMS is intended to serve as a screening SVT to assist in identifying malingering, including malingering of neurocognitive and neurological symptoms. It is one of the few stand-alone questionnaire-based SVTs with relevance to neuropsychology, as it covers overreporting of psychiatric, cognitive, and neurological symptoms. Most other SVTs are embedded as part of much more lengthy, comprehensive multidimensional questionnaires (e.g., MMPI-2, MMPI-2-RF, PAI), and so the SIMS has appeal as a way to rapidly screen for validity of symptom reporting. Unlike many other similar measures, the SIMS has demonstrated utility in linguistically and culturally diverse groups. The test also demonstrates solid reliability data, including test-retest information, the latter often lacking in published PVTs. Studies have also demonstrated its resistance to coaching.

Thanks to the meta-data presented by van Impelen et al. (2014), there is an incredibly large dataset consisting of more than 30 studies and 3,000 examinees and based on more than 4,000 SIMS protocols. This meta-analysis provides a useful benchmark with which to compare examinee scores and shows unequivocally that the test is sensitive to differential prevalence of malingering among clinical groups (e.g., lowest scores in honest responders, highest scores in criminal defendants). Most importantly, it has been validated against established malingering criteria, where a cutoff of >24 has acceptable specificity (i.e., does not have an excessively high false-positive rate).

From an administration standpoint, the SIMS is relatively brief, easy to score, and does not require sophisticated training to administer. It also has a well-written manual organized for easy reference. It may be particularly useful when long inventories (e.g., MMPI-2-RF, PAI) are not possible due to time constraints or examinee limitations. On the other hand, the SIMS appears better at ruling out feigning than at ruling it in (van Impelen et al., 2014), but this is the case for all SVTs and PVTs when cutoffs with acceptable specificities are used.

In terms of limitations, SIMS studies cover a number of nonclinical, clinical, and feigning groups but nevertheless do not have as much validation evidence relevant to neuropsychological evaluation compared to other longer scales, such as the MMPI-2 and MMPI-2-RF, which have extensive validation in neuropsychological groups. More research on litigants, disability claimants, brain injury patients, ADHD, and pain disorders is needed. However, the SIMS has an extensive literature on exaggeration of psychopathology and a number of studies in criminal forensic settings.

The manual's published cut score of >14 is too low for clinical evaluation of malingering. Scores above this cutoff may indicate psychological distress and overestimate exaggeration in genuinely responding patients. Use of higher cutoffs such as >24 means some genuine feigners will be missed and that only blatant exaggerators may be detected (van Impelen et al., 2014), which may be an acceptable trade-off. Caution is recommended in settings with low base rates of malingering, where most SVTs/PVTs also fare poorly due to modest PPVs.

There is fairly strong evidence for the utility of the Total score, less so for subscales, even though subscale data would have particular utility in differentiating between neurocognitive and psychiatric overreporting. The Amnestic and Neurological Disorders subscales seem to have fair sensitivity in clinical groups, but the Low Intelligence subscale seems more problematic in terms of detecting feigned intellectual deficits.

Users should be aware that the SIMS does not include an inconsistency scale designed to detect random or other noncompliant response styles—for example, responding all "True" or all "False"—a feature of most SVTs. The test could also use more studies on relationships to other well-known SVTs and standard neuropsychological measures.

As some have noted, its name is misleading because there is no such thing as a "malingering test"; some have also recommended that the test should not include symptoms reflective of genuine psychopathology as this raises the risk of false positives in honest patients (van Impelen et al., 2014). Last, as is the case for all SVTs and PVTs, identification of exaggerated or feigned symptoms on the SIMS does not preclude the presence of genuine cognitive deficits or psychiatric disorder (Widows & Smith, 2005). As noted in the manual, high scores do not necessarily confirm malingering; they simply point to an invalid profile, with other explanations needing to be examined as well (i.e., frustration, defiance, fatigue, incomprehension), although as scores increase, so does the probability of malingering.

REFERENCES

Benge, J. F., Wisdom, N. M., Collins, R. L., Franks, R., Lemaire, A., & Chen, D. K. (2012). Diagnostic utility of the Structured Inventory of Malingered Symptomatology for identifying psychogenic non-epileptic events. *Epilepsy & Behavior, 24*(4), 439–444. https://doi.org/10.1016/j.yebeh.2012.05.007

Bianchini, K. J., Greve, K. W., & Glynn, G. (2005). On the diagnosis of malingered pain-related disability: Lessons from cognitive malingering research. *Spine Journal, 5*(4), 404–417. https://doi.org/10.1016/j.spinee.2004.11.016

Cima, M., Hollnack, S., Kremer, K., Knauer, E., Schellbach-Matties, R., Klein, B., & Merckelbach, H. (2003). [The German version of the Structured Inventory of Malingered Symptomatology: SIMS]. *Der Nervenarzt, 74*(11), 977–986. https://doi.org/10.1007/s00115-002-1438-5

Dandachi-FitzGerald, B., Ponds, R. W. H. M., Peters, M. J. V., & Merckelbach, H. (2011). Cognitive underperformance and symptom overreporting in a mixed psychiatric sample. *The Clinical Neuropsychologist, 25*(5), 812–828. https://doi.org/10.1080/13854046.2011.583280

Edens, J. F., Poythress, N. G., & Watkins-Clay, M. M. (2007). Detection of malingering in psychiatric unit and general population prison inmates: a comparison of the PAI, SIMS, and SIRS. *Journal of Personality Assessment, 88*(1), 33–42. https://doi.org/10.1080/00223890709336832

Freeman, T., Powell, M., & Kimbrell, T. (2008). Measuring symptom exaggeration in veterans with chronic posttraumatic stress disorder. *Psychiatry Research, 158*(3), 374–380. https://doi.org/10.1016/j.psychres.2007.04.002

Geraerts, E., Jelicic, M., & Merckelbach, H. (2006). Symptom overreporting and recovered memories of childhood sexual abuse. *Law and Human Behavior, 30*(5), 621–630. https://doi.org/10.1007/s10979-006-9043-y

Graue, L. O., Berry, D. T. R., Clark, J. A., Sollman, M. J., Cardi, M., Hopkins, J., & Werline, D. (2007). Identification of feigned mental retardation using the new generation of malingering detection instruments: Preliminary findings. *The Clinical Neuropsychologist, 21*(6), 929–942. https://doi.org/10.1080/13854040600932137

Jelicic, M., Ceunen, E., Peters, M. J. V., & Merckelbach, H. (2011). Detecting coached feigning using the Test of Memory Malingering (TOMM) and the Structured Inventory of Malingered Symptomatology (SIMS). *Journal of Clinical Psychology, 67*(9), 850–855. https://doi.org/10.1002/jclp.20805

Merckelbach, H., & Smith, G. P. (2003). Diagnostic accuracy of the Structured Inventory of Malingered Symptomatology (SIMS) in detecting instructed malingering. *Archives of Clinical Neuropsychology, 18*(2), 145–152.

Parks, A. C., Gfeller, J., Emmert, N., & Lammert, H. (2016). Detecting feigned postconcussional and posttraumatic stress symptoms with the Structured Inventory of Malingered Symptomatology (SIMS). *Applied Neuropsychology. Adult,* 1–10. https://doi.org/10.1080/23279095.2016.1189426

Rogers, R., Robinson, E. V., & Gillard, N. D. (2014). The SIMS Screen for feigned mental disorders: The development of detection-based scales. *Behavioral Sciences & the Law, 32*(4), 455–466. https://doi.org/10.1002/bsl.2131

Slick, D. J., Sherman, E. M., & Iverson, G. L. (1999). Diagnostic criteria for malingered neurocognitive dysfunction: Proposed standards for clinical practice and research. *The Clinical Neuropsychologist, 13*(4), 545–561. https://doi.org/10.1076/1385-4046(199911)13:04;1-Y;FT545

van Beilen, M., Griffioen, B. T., Gross, A., & Leenders, K. L. (2009). Psychological assessment of malingering in psychogenic neurological disorders and non-psychogenic neurological disorders: Relationship to psychopathology levels. *European Journal of Neurology, 16*(10), 1118–1123. https://doi.org/10.1111/j.1468-1331.2009.02655.x

van der Heide, D., & Merckelbach, H. (2016). Validity of symptom reports of asylum seekers in a psychiatric hospital: A descriptive study. *International Journal of Law and Psychiatry, 49*(Pt A), 40–46. https://doi.org/10.1016/j.ijlp.2016.05.007

van Impelen, A., Merckelbach, H., Jelicic, M., & Merten, T. (2014). The Structured Inventory of Malingered Symptomatology (SIMS): A systematic review and meta-analysis. *The Clinical Neuropsychologist, 28*(8), 1336–1365. https://doi.org/10.1080/13854046.2014.984763

Vitacco, M. J., Rogers, R., Gabel, J., & Munizza, J. (2007). An evaluation of malingering screens with competency to stand trial patients: A known-groups comparison. *Law and Human Behavior, 31*(3), 249–260. https://doi.org/10.1007/s10979-006-9062-8

Widows, M. R., & Smith, G. P. (2005). *Structured Inventory of Malingered Symptomatology (SIMS).* Lutz, FL: Psychological Assessment Resources, Inc.

Wisdom, N. M., Callahan, J. L., & Shaw, T. G. (2010). Diagnostic utility of the structured inventory of malingered symptomatology to detect malingering in a forensic sample. *Archives of Clinical Neuropsychology, 25*(2), 118–125. https://doi.org/10.1093/arclin/acp110

CREDITS

TABLE 2–7

Urbina, S. (2014). *Essentials of psychological testing* (2nd ed.). Hoboken, NJ: Wiley. Reproduced with permission from John Wiley & Sons.

TABLE 3–2

Resnick, P. J., West, S. G., & Wooley, C. N. (2018). The malingering of posttraumatic disorders. In R. Rogers & S. D. Bender (Eds.), *Clinical assessment of malingering and deception* (4th ed., pp. 188–211). New York: Guilford Press. Used with permission.

TABLE 3–4

Sherman, E. M. S., Slick, D. J., & Iverson, G. I. (2020). Multidimensional malingering criteria for neuropsychological assessment: A twenty-year update of the Malingered Neurocognitive Dysfunction criteria. *Archives of Clinical Neuropsychology*. Reprinted by permission of Oxford University Press.

TABLE 4–16

Martin, P. K., Hunter, B. P., Rach, A. M., Heinrichs, R. J., & Schroeder, R. W. (2017). Excessive decline from premorbid functioning: detecting performance invalidity with the WAIS-IV and demographic predictions. *The Clinical Neuropsychologist*, 31(5), 829–843. https://doi.org/10.1080/13854046.2017.128426. Reproduced with permission from Taylor & Francis.

TABLE 5–13

Saklofske, D. H., Zhu, J., Miller, J. L., Weiss, L. G., Babcock, S. E., Cayton, T. G., . . . Coalson, D. L. (2012). The Cognitive Proficiency Index for the Canadian edition of the Wechsler Adult Intelligence Scale–Fourth Edition. *Canadian Journal of Behavioural Science / Revue Canadienne Des Sciences Du Comportement*, 44(2), 117–123. Reproduced with permission from the American Psychological Association.

TABLE 5–14

Saklofske, D. H., Zhu, J., Miller, J. L., Weiss, L. G., Babcock, S. E., Cayton, T. G., . . . Coalson, D. L. (2012). The Cognitive Proficiency Index for the Canadian edition of the Wechsler Adult Intelligence Scale–Fourth Edition. *Canadian Journal of Behavioural Science / Revue Canadienne Des Sciences Du Comportement*, 44(2), 117–123. https://doi.org/10.1037/a0026734

TABLE 6–2

Reproduced with permission from CNS Vital Signs.

TABLE 6–3

Reproduced with permission from CNS Vital Signs.

TABLE 6–5

Source: Reprinted from Iverson, G. L., Brooks, B. L., Langenecker, S. A., & Young, A. H. (2011). Identifying a cognitive impairment subgroup in adults with mood disorders. *Journal of Affective Disorders*, 132(3), 360–367. https://doi.org/10.1016/j.jad.2011.03.001, with permission from Elsevier.

TABLE 6–22

Reproduced with permission from Cambridge University Press.

TABLE 7–4

Reproduced with permission from John Wiley & Sons, Inc.

TABLE 8–20

Sandford, J. A., & Sandford, S. E. (2016). IVA-2™: Integrated Visual and Auditory Continuous Performance Test. Richmond, VA: Brain Train, Inc. Used with permission.

TABLE 8–39

Gonzalez, R., Miller, S. W., Carey, C. L., Woods, S. P., Rippeth, J. D., Schweinsburg, B. C., . . . Heaton, R. K. (2006). Association Between Dyads and Correct Responses on the Paced Auditory Serial Addition Task (PASAT). *Assessment*, 13(4), 381–384. http://doi.org/10.1177/1073191106286567

TABLE 8–59

Gonzalez, H., Whitfield, K., West, B., Williams, D., Lichtenberg, P., & Jackson, J. (2007). Modified-Symbol Digit Modalities Test for African Americans, Caribbean Black Americans, and non-Latino Whites: Nationally representative normative data from the National Survey of American Life. *Archives of Clinical Neuropsychology*, 22(5), 605–613. http://doi.org/10.1016/j.acn.2007.04.002

TABLE 8–63

Pena-Casanova, J., Quinones-Ubeda, S., Quintana-Aparicio, M., Aguilar, M., Badenes, D., Molinuevo, J. L., . . . for the NEURONORMA Study Team. (2009). Spanish Multicenter Normative Studies (NEURONORMA Project): Norms for Verbal Span, Visuospatial Span, Letter and Number Sequencing, Trail Making Test, and Symbol Digit Modalities Test. *Archives of Clinical Neuropsychology*, 24(4), 321–341. http://doi.org/10.1093/arclin/acp038

TABLE 8–66

Vogel, A., Stokholm, J., & Jørgensen, K. (2013). Performances on Symbol Digit Modalities Test, Color Trails Test, and modified Stroop test in a healthy, elderly Danish sample. *Aging, Neuropsychology, and Cognition*, 20(3), 370–382. http://doi.org/10.1080/13825585.2012.725126

FIGURE 8–6

Leark, R., Greenberg, L. M., Kindschi, C., Dupuy, T. R., & Hughes, S. (2017). T.O.V.A: Test of Variables of Attention: Professional Manual. Los Alamitos, CA: The T.O.V.A. Company.

TABLE 9–31

Sugawara, N., Yasui- Furukori, N., Umeda, T., Sato, Y., Kaneda, A., Tsuchimine, S., ... Kaneko, S. (2010). Clock drawing performance in a community-dwelling population: Normative data for Japanese subjects. *Aging & Mental Health*, 14(5), 587–592. https://doi.org/10.1080/13607860903586086. Reproduced with permission from Taylor & Francis.

TABLE 9–32

Sugawara, N., Yasui-Furukori, N., Umeda, T., Sato, Y., Kaneda, A., Tsuchimine, S., ... Kaneko, S. (2010). Clock drawing performance in a community-dwelling population: Normative data for Japanese subjects. *Aging & Mental Health*, 14(5), 587–592. https://doi.org/10.1080/13607860903586086. Reproduced with permission from Taylor & Francis.

TABLE 9–33

Sugawara, N., Yasui-Furukori, N., Umeda, T., Sato, Y., Kaneda, A., Tsuchimine, S., ... Kaneko, S. (2010). Clock drawing performance in a community-dwelling population: Normative data for Japanese subjects. *Aging & Mental Health*, 14(5), 587–592. https://doi.org/10.1080/13607860903586086. Reproduced with permission from Taylor & Francis.

TABLE 9–34

Sugawara, N., Yasui-Furukori, N., Umeda, T., Sato, Y., Kaneda, A., Tsuchimine, S., ... Kaneko, S. (2010). Clock drawing performance in a community-dwelling population: Normative data for Japanese subjects. *Aging & Mental Health*, 14(5), 587–592. https://doi.org/10.1080/13607860903586086. Reproduced with permission from Taylor & Francis.

TABLE 9–85

Van Den Berg, E., Nys, G. M. S., Brands, A. M. A., Ruis, C., Van Zandvoort, M. J. E., & Kessels, R. P. C. (2009). The Brixton Spatial Anticipation Test as a test for executive function: Validity in patient groups and norms for older adults. *Journal of the International Neuropsychological Society*, 15(5), 695. Reproduced with permission from Cambridge University Press.

TABLES 9–88 and 9–89

Izaks, G. J., Joosten, H., Koerts, J., Gansevoort, R. T., & Slaets, J. P. (2011). Reference data for the Ruff Figural Fluency Test stratified by age and educational level. *PloS One*, 6(2), e17045. http://doi.org/10.1371/journal.pone.0017045

TABLE 9–92

Woods, D. L., Wyma, J. M., Herron, T. J., & Yund, E. W. (2016). A computerized test of design fluency. *PloS One*, 11(5), e0153952

TABLE 9–167

Dikmen, S. S., Heaton, R. K., Grant, I., & Temkin, N. R. (1999). Test-retest reliability and practice effects of expanded Halstead-Reitan neuropsychological test battery. *Journal of the International Neuropsychological Society*, 5, 346–356. Reproduced with permission from Cambridge University Press.

FIGURE 9–7

Kingery, L. R., Schretlen, D. J., Sateri, S., Langley, L. K., Marano, N. C., & Meyer, S. M. (2006). Interrater and test–retest reliability of a fixed condition Design Fluency Test. *The Clinical Neuropsychologist*, 20(4), 729– 740. http://doi.org/10.1080/13854040500350992. Reproduced with permission from Taylor & Francis.

FIGURE 9–16

Crawford, J. R., Moore, J. W., & Cameron, I. M. (1992). Verbal fluency: A NART-based equation for estimation of premorbid performance. *British Journal of Clinical Psychology*, 31, 327–329. Reproduced with permission from John Wiley & Sons.

TABLE 10–5

© 2004 The Author(s). This is an Open Access article distributed under the terms of the Creative Commons Attribution 4.0 license (unless stated otherwise) which permits unrestricted use, distribution, and reproduction in any medium, provided the original work is properly cited.

TABLE 10–6

© 2004 The Author(s). This is an Open Access article distributed under the terms of the Creative Commons Attribution 4.0 license (unless stated otherwise) which permits unrestricted use, distribution, and reproduction in any medium, provided the original work is properly cited.

TABLE 10–8

Reproduced by special permission of the Publisher, Psychological Assessment Resources, Inc. (PAR), 16204 North Florida Avenue, Lutz, Florida 33549.

TABLE 10–12

Schretlen et al. (2010). Reproduced by special permission of the Publisher, Psychological Assessment Resources, Inc. (PAR), 16204 North Florida Avenue, Lutz, Florida 33549, from *The Calibrated Neuropsychological Normative System*, by David J. Schretlen, PhD, ABPP, S. Marc Testa, PhD and Godfrey D. Pearlson, MD, Copyright 2010 by PAR. Further reproduction is prohibited without permission from PAR.

TABLE 10–16

© Goretti et al.; licensee BioMed Central Ltd. This is an Open Access article distributed under the terms of the Creative Commons Attribution License (http://creativecommons.org/licenses/by/4.0), which permits unrestricted use, distribution, and reproduction in any medium, provided the original work is properly credited. The Creative Commons Public Domain Dedication waiver (http://creativecommons.org/publicdomain/zero/1.0/) applies to the data made available in this article, unless otherwise stated.

TABLE 10–51

Miotto, E. C., Campanholo, K. R., Rodrigues, M. M., Serrao, V. T., de Lucia, M. C. S., & Scaff, M. (2012). Hopkins Verbal Learning Test-Revised and Brief Visuospatial Memory Test-Revised: Preliminary normative data for the Brazilian population. *Arquivos De Neuro-Psiquiatria*, 70(12), 962–965. Reproduced with permission from the Brazilian Psychiatric Association.

TABLE 10–87

Reproduced with permission from John Wiley & Sons, Inc.

TABLE 10–88

Tremblay, M., Potvin, O., Callahan, B. L., Belleville, S., Gagnon, J. F., Caza, N., ... Macoir, J. (2015). Normative data for the Rey–Osterrieth and the Taylor Complex Figure tests in Quebec-French people. *Archives of Clinical Neuropsychology*, 30(1), 78–87. Reproduced with permission from Oxford University Press.

TABLE 10–89

Tremblay, M., Potvin, O., Callahan, B. L., Belleville, S., Gagnon, J. F., Caza, N., ... Macoir, J. (2015). Normative data for the Rey–Osterrieth and the Taylor Complex Figure tests in Quebec-French people. *Archives of Clinical Neuropsychology*, 30(1), 78–87. Reproduced with permission from Oxford University Press.

TABLE 10–95

Blaskewitz, N., Merten, T., & Brockhaus, R. (2009). Detection of suboptimal effort with the Rey Complex Figure Test and Recognition trial. *Applied Neuropsychology*, 16(1), 54–61. Reproduced with permission from Taylor & Francis.

FIGURE 10–2

Geffen, G. M., Butterworth, P., & Geffen, L. B. (1994). Test-retest reliability of a new form of the Auditory Verbal Learning Test (AVLT). *Archives of Clinical Neuropsychology*, 9, 303–316. Reproduced with permission from Oxford University Press.

FIGURE 10–6

Ferman, T. J., Lucas, J. A., Ivnik, R. J., Smith, G. E., Willis, F. B., Petersen, R. C., & Graff-Radford, N. R. (2005). Mayo's Older African American Normative Studies: Auditory-Verbal Learning Test norms for African American elders. *The Clinical Neuropsychologist*, 19, 214–228. Reproduced with permission from Taylor & Francis.

TABLE 11–3

Pineda, D. A., Rosselli, M., Ardila, A., Mejia, S. E., Romero, M. G., & Perez, C. (2000). The Boston Diagnostic Aphasia Examination-Spanish version: The influence of demographic variables. *Journal of the International Neuropsychological Society*, 6, 802–814. Reproduced with permission from Cambridge University Press.

TABLE 11–7

Miotto, E. C., Sato, J., Lucia, M. C. S., Camargo, C. H. P., & Scaff, M. (2010). Development of an adapted version of the Boston Naming Test for Portuguese speakers. *Revista Brasileira de Psiquiatria*, 32(3), 279–282. Reproduced with permission from the Brazilian Psychiatric Association.

TABLE 11–21

Miotto, E. C., Sato, J., Lucia, M. C. S., Camargo, C. H. P., & Scaff, M. (2010). Development of an adapted version of the Boston Naming Test for Portuguese speakers. *Revista Brasileira de Psiquiatria*, 32(3), 279–282. Reproduced with permission from the Brazilian Psychiatric Association.

TABLE 11–36

Silvestre, G., Iglesias, R. M., & Silvestre, E. (2018). Boston Naming Test norms for the Dominican population. *Aphasiology*, 32(3), 340–365. https://doi.org/10.1080/02687038.2017.1338662. Reproduced with permission from Taylor & Francis.

TABLE 11–37

Silvestre, G., Iglesias, R. M., & Silvestre, E. (2018). Boston Naming Test norms for the Dominican population. *Aphasiology*, 32(3), 340–365. https://doi.org/10.1080/02687038.2017.1338662. Reproduced with permission from Taylor & Francis.

TABLE 12–12

Whiteside, D., Wald, D., & Busse, M. (2011). Classification accuracy of multiple visual spatial measures in the detection of suspect effort. *The Clinical Neuropsychologist*, 25(2), 287–301. Reproduced with permission from Taylor & Francis.

TABLE 13–5

Reproduced courtesy of Sensonics International, Haddon Heights, NJ, USA. Copyright © 2013, Sensonics International.

FIGURE 14–2

Matthews, C. G., & Klove, K. (1964). *Instruction manual for the Adult Neuropsychology Test Battery.* Madison, WI.: University of Wisconsin Medical School.

TABLE 15–15

Copyright © 2013 Colegio Oficial de la Psicología de Madrid. Published by Elsevier España S.L.

TABLE 15–18

Marshall, P., Schroeder, R., O'Brien, J., Fischer, R., Ries, A., Blesi, B., & Barker, J. (2010). Effectiveness of symptom validity measures in identifying cognitive and behavioral symptom exaggeration in adult Attention Deficit Hyperactivity Disorder. *The Clinical Neuropsychologist*, 24(7), 1204–1237. Reproduced with permission from Taylor & Francis.

TABLE 15–21

Morse, C. L., Douglas-Newman, K., Mandel, S., & Swirsky-Sacchetti, T. (2013). Utility of the Rey-15 recognition trial to detect invalid performance in a forensic neuropsychological sample. *The Clinical Neuropsychologist*, 27(8), 1395–1407. Reproduced with permission from Taylor & Francis.

TABLE 15–22

Morse, C. L., Douglas-Newman, K., Mandel, S., & Swirsky-Sacchetti, T. (2013). Utility of the Rey-15 recognition trial to detect invalid performance in a forensic neuropsychological sample. *The Clinical Neuropsychologist*, 27(8), 1395–1407. Reproduced with permission from Taylor & Francis.

TABLE 15–31

Adapted with permission from Pearson. (2009a). *Advanced Clinical Solutions for WAIS-IV and WMS-IV: Clinical and interpretive manual.* San Antonio, TX: Pearson.

TABLE 15–36

Rienstra, A., Spaan, P. E. J., & Schmand, B. (2009). Reference data for the Word Memory Test. *Archives of Clinical Neuropsychology*, 24(3), 255–262. https://doi.org/10.1093/arclin/acp035. Reproduced with permission from Oxford University Press.

FIGURE 15–1

Rienstra, A., Spaan, P. E. J., & Schmand, B. (2009). Reference data for the Word Memory Test. *Archives of Clinical Neuropsychology*, 24(3), 255–262. https://doi.org/10.1093/arclin/acp035. Reproduced with permission from Oxford University Press.

TABLE 16–7

Greene, R. L. (2008). Malingering and defensiveness on the MMPI-2. In R. Rogers (Ed.), *Clinical assessment of malingering and deception* (3rd ed.; pp. 159–181). New York: Guilford. Reproduced with permission from the publisher.

TABLE 16–8

Gervais, R. O., Ben-Porath, Y. S., Wygant, D. B., & Green, P. (2008). Differential sensitivity of the Response Bias Scale (RBS) and MMPI-2 validity scales to memory complaints. *The Clinical Neuropsychologist*, 22(6), 1061–1079. https://doi.org/10.1080/13854040701756930. Reproduced with permission from Taylor & Francis.

TABLE 16–12

Schroeder, R. W., Baade, L. E., Peck, C. P., VonDran, E. J., Brockman, C. J., Webster, B. K., & Heinrichs, R. J. (2012). Validation of MMPI-2-RF validity scales in criterion group neuropsychological samples. *The Clinical Neuropsychologist*, 26(1), 129–146. https://doi.org/10.1080/13854046.2011.639314. Reproduced with permission from Taylor & Francis.

TABLE 16–18

Gervais, R. O., Ben-Porath, Y. S., Wygant, D. B., & Sellbom, M. (2010). Incremental validity of the MMPI-2-RF overreporting scales and RBS in assessing the veracity of memory complaints. *Archives of Clinical Neuropsychology*, 25(4), 274–284. https://doi.org/10.1093/arclin/acq018. Reproduced with permission from Oxford University Press.

TABLE 16–38

Wisdom, N. M., Callahan, J. L., & Shaw, T. G. (2010). Diagnostic utility of the structured inventory of malingered symptomatology to detect malingering in a forensic sample. *Archives of Clinical Neuropsychology*, 25(2), 118–125. https://doi.org/10.1093/arclin/acp110. Reproduced with permission from Oxford University Press.

FIGURE 16–1

Greene, R. L. (2008). Malingering and defensiveness on the MMPI-2. In R. Rogers (Ed.), *Clinical assessment of malingering and deception* (3rd ed.; pp. 159–181). New York: Guilford. Reproduced with permission from the publisher.

LIST OF ACRONYMS

2 & 7 Test	Ruff 2 & 7 Selective Attention Test
3MS	Modified Mini-Mental State Examination
7MS	7 Minute Screen
ACE-III	Addenbrooke's Cognitive Examination-III
ACI	Albany Consistency Index
ACS	Advanced Clinical Solutions
AD	Alzheimer's disease
ADAS-Cog	Alzheimer's Disease Assessment Scale-Cognitive
ADHD	attention-deficit/hyperactivity disorder
Adjusting-PSAT	Adjusting-Paced Serial Addition Test
ADLs	activities of daily living
AIDS	acquired immunodeficiency syndrome
ALS	amyotrophic lateral sclerosis
aMCI	amnestic mild cognitive impairment
AN	anorexia nervosa
APM	Advanced Progressive Matrices
ASD	autism spectrum disorder
ASTM	Amsterdam Short-Term Memory Test
BADS	Behavioural Assessment of the Dysexecutive Syndrome
BDAE	Boston Diagnostic Aphasia Examination
BDI—II	Beck Depression Inventory—Second Edition
BDNF	brain-derived neurotrophic factor
BICAMS	Brief International Cognitive Assessment for MS
BNT	Boston Naming Test
BNT-2	Boston Naming Test, Second Edition
BRIEF-A	Behavior Rating Inventory of Executive Function-Adult Version
BTA	Brief Test of Attention
BVMT-R	Brief Visuospatial Memory Test—Revised
BVRT-5	Benton Visual Retention Test Fifth Edition
CANTAB	Cambridge Neuropsychological Test Automated Battery
CARB	Computerized Assessment of Response Bias
CAT	Category Test
CATA	Conners Continuous Auditory Test of Attention
CBD	corticobasal degeneration
CBS	Cognitive Bias Scale
CBS	corticobasal syndrome
CCS	Cognitive Complaints Scale
CDR	Clinical Dementia Rating
CDT	Clock Drawing Test
CEFI	Comprehensive Executive Function Inventory
CELF-4	Clinical Evaluation of Language Fundamentals—Fourth Edition
CERAD	Consortium for the Establishment of a Registry for Alzheimer's Disease
CET	Cognitive Estimation Test
CHC	Cattell–Horn–Carroll
CIND	cognitive impairment-no dementia
CIS	clinically isolated syndrome
CMS	Children's Memory Scale
CNS	Cannot Say scale
CNS	central nervous system
CNS	Response Consistency Index
CNS VS	CNS Vital Signs
CNT	Computerized Neurocognitive Test
COG	Cognitive Complaints Scale
COI	condition of interest
COWA	Controlled Oral Word Association Test
CPM	Colored Progressive Matrices
CPT 3	Conners Continuous Performance Test 3rd Edition
CPT II	Conners Continuous Performance Test II
CSF	cerebrospinal fluid
CV	coefficient of variation
CVA	cerebrovascular accident
CVLT	California Verbal Learning Test
CVLT-II	California Verbal Learning Test—Second Edition
CVMT	Continuous Visual Memory Test
D-KEFS	Delis–Kaplan Executive Function System
DAI	diffuse axonal injury
DART	Danish Adult Reading Test
DCT	Dot Counting Test
DEX	Dysexecutive Questionnaire
DLB	Dementia with Lewy bodies
DRS	Dementia Rating Scale
DRS-2	Dementia Rating Scale—2
EBMT	East Boston Memory Test
ECT	electroconvulsive therapy
EDPF	Excessive Decline from Premorbid Functioning

EEG	electroencephalogram
EI	Emotional Intelligence
EXAMINER	Executive Abilities: Measures and Instruments for Neurobehavioral Evaluation and Research
F	Infrequency scale
FAR	Feifer Assessment of Reading
Fb	Back F scale
FBS	Symptom Validity Scale (formerly Fake Bad Scale)
FBS-r	Symptom Validity Scale—Restructured (formerly Fake Bad Scale)
FCSRT	Free and Cued Selective Reminding Test
FHS	Framingham Heart Study
FIT	Rey Fifteen-Item Test
FloPS	Frontal Lobe Personality Scale
Fp	Infrequency—Psychopathology scale
Fp-r	Infrequent Psychopathology Responses—Restructured scale
F-r	Infrequent Responses—Restructured scale
FrSBe	Frontal Systems Behavior Scale
FRT	Benton Facial Recognition Test
Fs	Infrequent Somatic Responses scale
FSIQ	Full-Scale Intelligence Quotient
FTD	frontotemporal dementia
FTT	Finger Tapping Test
G theory	Generalizability theory
GABA	gamma-aminobutyric acid
GDS	Geriatric Depression Scale
GMIP	Genuine Memory Impairment Profile
GPCOG	General Practitioner Assessment of Cognition
GPT	Grooved Pegboard Test
HAND	HIV-associated neurocognitive disorder
HBT	Hayling and Brixton Tests
HD	Huntington's disease
HHI	Henry-Heilbronner Index
HHI-r	Henry-Heilbronner Index—Restructured
HIV	human immunodeficiency virus
HRNES	Halstead Russell Neuropsychological Evaluation System
HVLT-R	Hopkins Verbal Learning Test—Revised
HVOT	Hooper Visual Organization Test
IADLs	instrumental activities of daily living
ICC	intraclass correlation coefficient
IFFI	Invalid Forgetting Frequency Index
ILS	Independent Living Scale
ImPACT	Immediate Post-Concussion Assessment and Cognitive Testing
IQ	intelligence quotient
IQCODE	Informant Questionnaire on Cognitive Decline in the Elderly
IRBD	Idiopathic REM Sleep Behavior Disorder
IRT	item response theory
IVA-2	Integrated Visual and Auditory Continuous Performance Test, Second Edition
JLO	Judgment of Line Orientation
K	Adjustment Validity scale
K-BIT	Kaufman Brief Intelligence Test
KBIT-2	Kaufman Brief Intelligence Test, Second Edition
KBNA	Kaplan Baycrest Neurocognitive Assessment
K-r	Adjustment Validity—Restructured scale
KR20 coefficient	Kuder–Richardson reliability coefficient
L	Uncommon Virtues scale
LHO	left hemibody onset
L-r	Uncommon Virtues—Restructured scale
LR-	negative likelihood ratio
LR+	positive likelihood ratio
MAE	Multilingual Aphasia Examination
MAL	Malingering Index
MCCB	Measurement and Treatment Research to Improve Cognition in Schizophrenia (MATRICS) Cognitive Consensus Battery
MCI	Memory Complaints Inventory
MCI	mild cognitive impairment
MDMA	3,4-methylenedioxymethamphetamine
MDS	multidimensional scaling
MENT	Morel Emotional Numbing Test
MFQ	Memory Functioning Questionnaire
MMA	mixed martial arts
MMPI-2	Minnesota Multiphasic Personality Inventory—2
MMPI-2-RF	Minnesota Multiphasic Personality Inventory—2 Restructured Form
MMPI-3	Minnesota Multiphasic Personality Inventory—3
MMSE	Mini-Mental State Examination
MMSE-2	Mini-Mental State Examination, 2nd Edition
MMSE-2:BV	Mini-Mental State Examination, 2nd Edition, Brief Version
MMSE-2:EV	Mini-Mental State Examination, 2nd Edition, Expanded Version
MNCD	mild neurocognitive disorder
MND	malingered neurocognitive dysfunction
MOAANS	Mayo's Older African Americans Normative Studies
MOANS	Mayo's Older Americans Normative Studies
MoCA	Montreal Cognitive Assessment
MPRD	Malingered Pain-Related Disability
MS	multiple sclerosis
MSA	multiple system atrophy
MSFC	Multiple Sclerosis Functional Composite
MSVT	Medical Symptom Validity Test
MWCST	Modified Wisconsin Card Sorting Test
NAART	North American Adult Reading Test

NAB	Neuropsychological Assessment Battery
NART	National Adult Reading Test
NEO PI-R	NEO Personality Inventory—Revised
NEURONORMA project	Spanish Multicenter Normative Studies
NFT	neurofibrillary tangles
NIM	Negative Impression Management scale
NINCDS-ARDA	National Institute of Neurological Disorders and Stroke–Alzheimer's Disease and Related Disorders Association
NPV	negative predictive value
NV-MSVT	Non-Verbal Medical Symptom Validity Test
OCD	obsessive-compulsive disorder
OKLAHOMA	Oklahoma Longitudinal Assessment of Health Outcomes in Mature Adults
OMC	Orientation-Memory-Concentration test
OPIE-IV	Oklahoma Premorbid Intelligence Estimate-IV
PAF	pure autonomic failure
PAI	Personality Assessment Inventory
PASAT	Paced Auditory Serial Addition Test
PCA	posterior cortical atrophy
PCS	postconcussive syndrome
PD	Parkinson's disease
PD-MCI	Parkinson's Disease—Mild Cognitive Impairment
PDD	Parkinson's disease dementia
PDRT	Portland Digit Recognition Test
PIM	Positive Impression Management scale
PNES	psychogenic nonepileptic seizure
PPV	positive predictive value
PPVT-R	Peabody Picture Vocabulary Test, Revised
PASAT	Paced Auditory Serial Addition Test
PSP	progressive supranuclear palsy
PTSD	posttraumatic stress disorder
PVSAT	Paced Visual Serial Addition Test
PVT	Performance validity test
RAVLT	Rey Auditory Verbal Learning Test
RBANS	Repeatable Battery for the Assessment of Neuropsychological Status
RBMT-3	Rivermead Behavioural Memory Test—Third Edition
RBS	Response Bias Scale
RCFT	Rey–Osterrieth Complex Figure Test
RCI	Reliable Change Index
RDF	Rogers Discriminant Function
RDS	Reliable Digit Span
REM	rapid-eye movement
RFFT	Ruff Figural Fluency Test
RHO	right hemibody onset
RIAS-2	Reynolds Intellectual Assessment Scales, Second Edition
RIST-2	Reynolds Intellectual Screening Test, Second Edition
RMT	Warrington Recognition Memory Test
RNBI	Ruff Neurobehavioral Inventory
ROC	receiver operating characteristic
RUDAS	Rowland Universal Dementia Assessment Scale
SB5	Stanford-Binet Intelligence Scales-Fifth Edition
SDMT	Symbol Digit Modalities Test
SE_D	standard error of the difference
SE_E	standard error of estimation
SEM	standard error of measurement
SE_P	standard error of prediction
SE_Y	standard error for individual predicted scores
SIMS	Structured Inventory of Malingered Symptomatology
SIP	Severe Impairment Profile
SIRS	Structured Interview of Reported Symptoms
SLAS	Singapore Longitudinal Ageing Studies
SLE	Systemic Lupus Erythematosus
SMMSE	Severe Mini-Mental State Examination
SMT	Sniff Magnitude Test
SOM	Somatic Complaints scale
SRB	standardized regression-based change scores
SRT	Selective Reminding Test
STMS	Short Test of Mental Status
STW	Spot-the-Word Test
SVS	Symptom Validity Scale
SVT	Symptom Validity Test
TBI	traumatic brain injury
TEA	Test of Everyday Attention
TIA	transient ischemic attack
TICS	Telephone Interview for Cognitive Status
TLE	temporal lobe epilepsy
TMS	transcranial magnetic stimulation
TMT	Trail Making Test
TOMM	Test of Memory Malingering
TONI-4	Test of Nonverbal Intelligence, Fourth Edition
TOPF	Test of Premorbid Functioning
T.O.V.A.	Test of Variables of Attention
TPT	Tactual Performance Test
TRIN	True Response Inconsistency scale
TRIN-r	True Response Inconsistency—Restructured scale

TT	Token Test
UPSIT	University of Pennsylvania Smell Identification Test
VaD	Vascular dementia
VMI	Beery Buktenika Developmental Test of Visual Motor Integration
VRIN	Variable Response Inconsistency scale
VRIN-r	Variable Response Inconsistency—Restructured scale
VST	Victoria Stroop Test
VSVT	Victoria Symptom Validity Test
WAB	Western Aphasia Battery
WAIS	Wechsler Adult Intelligence Scale
WAIS-III	Wechsler Adult Intelligence Scale-III
WAIS-IV	Wechsler Adult Intelligence Scale—Fourth Edition
WAIS-R	Wechsler Adult Intelligence Scale—Revised
WASI	Wechsler Abbreviated Scale of Intelligence
WASI-II	Wechsler Abbreviated Scale of Intelligence, Second Edition
WAT	Word Accentuation Test
WCST	Wisconsin Card Sorting Test
WCST-64	Wisconsin Card Sorting Test 64-Card Version
WIAT-II	Wechsler Individual Achievement Test—Second Edition
WIAT-III	Wechsler Individual Achievement Test—Third Edition
WISC-III	Wechsler Intelligence Scale for Children—Third Edition
WISC-IV	Wechsler Intelligence Scale for Children—Fourth Edition
WJ III ACH	Woodcock-Johnson III Tests of Achievement
WJ IV Cog	Woodcock-Johnson IV Tests of Cognitive Abilities
WMH	white matter hyperintensity
WMS-III	Wechsler Memory Scale—Third Edition
WMS-IV	Wechsler Memory Scale—Fourth Edition
WMS-R	Wechsler Memory Scale—Revised
WMT	Word Memory Test
WRAT-3	Wide Range Achievement Test 3
WRAT-4	Wide Range Achievement Test 4
WRAT-R	Wide Range Achievement Test—Revised
WRMT	Warrington Recognition Memory Test
WTAR	Wechsler Test of Adult Reading

TEST INDEX

Tables or figures are indicated by an italic *t* or *f* following the page number.

SUBJECT INDEX

Tables or figures are indicated by an italic *t* or *f* following the page number.